The 5-Minute Pediatric Consult

Fourth Edition

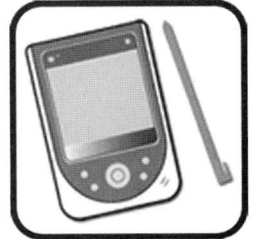
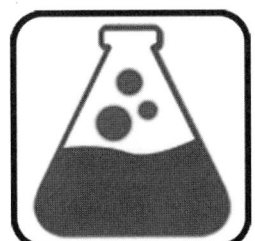
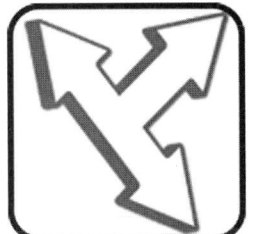
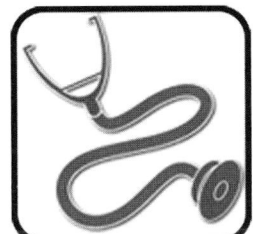
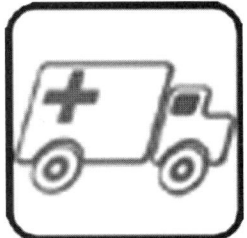
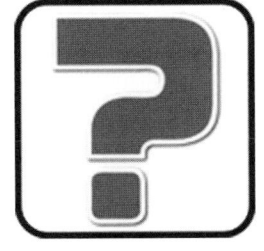

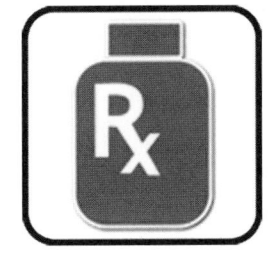

The 5-Minute Pediatric Consult

Fourth Edition

EDITOR

M. WILLIAM SCHWARTZ, M.D.

EMERITUS PROFESSOR OF PEDIATRICS

UNIVERSITY OF PENNSYLVANIA SCHOOL OF MEDICINE

AND SENIOR PHYSICIAN AT

CHILDREN'S HOSPITAL OF PHILADELPHIA

PHILADELPHIA, PENNSYLVANIA

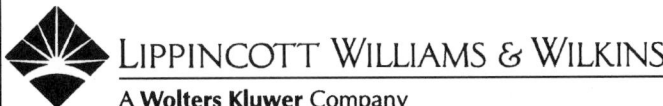

LIPPINCOTT WILLIAMS & WILKINS
A **Wolters Kluwer** Company
Philadelphia · Baltimore · New York · London
Buenos Aires · Hong Kong · Sydney · Tokyo

Acquisitions Editor: Anne Sydor
Developmental Editors: Joyce Murphy and Stacey Sebring
Project Manager: Bridgett Dougherty
Senior Manufacturing Manager: Ben Rivera
Marketing Manager: Kathleen Neely
Design Coordinator: Terry Mallon
Compositor: TechBooks
Printer: Edwards Brothers

First edition, 1997
Second edition, 2000
Third edition, 2003

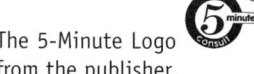

The 5-Minute Logo is a registered trademark of Lippincott Williams & Wilkins. This mark may not be used without written permission from the publisher.

Printed in the USA

Library of Congress Cataloging-in-Publication Data

The 5-minute pediatric consult / editor, M. William Schwartz.—4th ed.
  p.;cm.
  Includes bibliographical references and index.
  ISBN 0-7817-5452-6 (hardcover: alk. paper)
  1. Pediatrics—Handbooks, manuals, etc.   I. Schwartz, M. William, 1935–
 II. Title: Five-minute pediatric consult.
  [DNLM: 1. Pediatrics—Handbooks. WS 39 Z99 2005]
 RJ48 .A15 2005
 618.92—dc22   2005008673

Care has been taken to confirm the accuracy of the information presented and to describe generally accepted practices. However, the authors, editors, and publisher are not responsible for errors or omissions or for any consequences from application of the information in this book and make no warranty, expressed or implied, with respect to the currency, completeness, or accuracy of the contents of the publication. Application of this information in a particular situation remains the professional responsibility of the practitioner.

The authors, editors, and publisher have exerted every effort to ensure that drug selection and dosage set forth in this text are in accordance with current recommendations and practice at the time of publication. However, in view of ongoing research, changes in government regulations, and the constant flow of information relating to drug therapy and drug reactions, the reader is urged to check the package insert for each drug for any change in indications and dosage and for added warnings and precautions. This is particularly important when the recommended agent is a new or infrequently employed drug.

Some drugs and medical devices presented in this publication have Food and Drug Administration (FDA) clearance for limited use in restricted research settings. It is the responsibility of the health care provider to ascertain the FDA status of each drug or device planned for use in their clinical practice.

10 9 8 7 6 5 4 3 2 1

TO

Susan and my girls and boys, my treasures

MWS

Robert, Rosemary and my Parents

LB

Dana, Nishan, Tavid, and Aram

PB

Drs. Ed Baik Chung, and OkHyung Kang, Dennis, Marissa and Emma Lee

EC

Marisa Weiss, Elias, Henry, and Isabel

DF

Elyse, Nathaniel, and Rebecca

AM

Brandie, Mitchell, Caroline, Chloe, my parents, and GG

CS

Sarah, Meghan, and Lauren

RT

and special accolades to Cheryl Kosmowski, our managing editor, and Joyce Murphy at Lippincott and Doug English at TechBooks who capably and calmly made sure that we did our job so they could produce this volume.

Preface

Early in the history of this book, an editor informed me that the second edition offered an opportunity to correct the mistakes of the first; the third edition was the polished product. She did not describe the features of the fourth edition as that seemed too far in the future and the chances of moving into a fourth edition seemed to be a remote idea. The fourth edition is a chance to add new authors with fresh ideas to the team. Even though I did not think it was possible, there are new topics such as SARS and knee pain to mention a few. A new edition is a chance to update the bibliography and remove a few split infinitives. Making sure that the information is current and accurate remains the biggest challenge.

Most satisfying is observing the continued use of the text in offices, emergency departments and resident lounges. A Spanish language version should be available when this edition is published and other translations are in progress. As expected, the number of PDA versions rises each year as the information is current and the format of the 5 Minute texts lends itself to the rapid retrieval of information. We look forward to electronic versions that can be updated as new facts are published.

Once again, the final version of this edition was sent to Lippincott, Williams & Wilkins several months before the deadline—a tribute to the associate editors, managing editors, and authors for their hard work and cooperation. Each one, in individual styles, managed to make the assignments and receive the chapters in good spirit without raising voices or making threats. My thanks to the team of Lou Bell, Peter Bingham, Esther Chung, David Friedman, Andy Mulberg, and the new member, Ronn Tanel. Charlie Schwartz took care of lists and tables in his usual capable manner. Cheryl Kosmowski made sure all the work was done, lost files were found, and the project was complete. Her skills, pleasant personality, and dedication served as the infrastructure of this and previous editions. She is our special treasure.

Special thanks to the staff of Lippincott, Williams & Wilkins of Wolters Kluwer Health for their help and support. Although he is no longer with the company, Tim Hiscock arranged for the beginning of the revision. He was a special friend and colleague whom we miss but wish him well in his new position. Ann Sydor took over the book as we completed the manuscripts. Joyce Murphy, as she has done in the past three editions, took the chapters and put them into correct formats and sizes to enable the production people to finish the job. We appreciate their professionalism and interest.

As we move on, it is reassuring that the additions of the last edition on smallpox and anthrax proved to be chapters of interest but not ones that were consulted because of actual cases. We hope the next edition will include new treatments that eradicate infections and cures for oncologic diseases without adding information about new threats to our health and peace.

Contributing Authors

Unless otherwise indicated, faculty appointments are at the University of Pennsylvania School of Medicine, and hospital appointments are at Children's Hospital of Philadelphia, Pennsylvania.

AKINYEMI AJAYI, M.D., D.A.B.S.M.
University of Ilorin, Nigeria MBBS
Director, Pediatric Pulmonary Medicine, Florida
    Hospital, Orlando
Medical Director, The Children's Sleep Laboratory-Orlando
Medical Director, Orlando Pediatric Pulmonary and Sleep
    Associate, Pennsylvania

EVALINE A. ALESSANDRINI, M.D., M.S.C.E.
Assistant Professor, Department of Pediatrics
Emergency Medicine and Epidemiology
Attending Physician
Division of Emergency Medicine

JULIAN L. ALLEN, M.D.
Professor of Pediatrics
Chief, Division of Pulmonary Medicine and Cystic
    Fibrosis Center
Robert Gerard Morse Chair in Pulmonary Medicine

CRAIG A. ALTER, M.D.
Division of Endocrinology
Clinical Associate Professor of Pediatrics

TIMOTHY ANDREWS, M.D.
Fellow, Allergy & Immunology

LEE R. ATKINSON-McEVOY, M.D.
Attending Physician
Division of General Academic Pediatrics
Children's Memorial Hospital
Chicago, Illinois

J. CHRISTOPHER AUSTIN, M.D.
Assistant Professor of Urology
University of Iowa Carver College of Medicine
Pediatric Urologist
Children's Hospital of Iowa

MARK L. BAGARAZZI, M.D.
Director, Worldwide Regulatory Affairs
Vaccine/Biologics, Merck Research Laboratories
West Point, Pennsylvania

ROBERT BALDASSANO, M.D.
Associate Professor of Pediatrics
University of Pennsylvania
Attending Physician
Division of Gastroenterology and Nutrition

QASIM BASHIR, M.D.
Chief Resident Neurology
University of Vermont
Fletcher Allen Health Care

LEE A. SAVIO BEERS, M.D.
Children's National Medical Center
Division of General; Community Pediatrics
Assistant Professor of Pediatrics
The George Washington University Medical Center

NATHANIEL S. BEERS, M.D., M.P.A.
Continuity Clinic Director
Medical Director, Developmental Behavioral
    Evaluation Center
Children's National Medical Center
Assistant Professor of Pediatrics
The George Washington University
School of Medicine and Health Sciences

LOUIS M. BELL, M.D.
The Patrick S. Pasquariello Professor of Pediatrics
Department of Pediatrics
Chief, Division of General Pediatrics

SUZANNE BENO, M.D.
Fellow in Pediatric Emergency Medicine

A.G. CHRISTINA BERGQVIST, M.D.
Assistant Professor of Neurology and Pediatrics
Division of Neurology

AMANDA BERRY BSN, MSN, CPNP
Pediatric Nurse Practitioner
DOVE Center, Division of Urology

ANITA BHANDARI, M.D.
Attending Pulmonologist

SUMIT BHARGAVA, M.B.B.S., M.D.
Section of Respiratory Medicine
Assistant Professor of Pediatrics
Department of Pediatrics
Yale University School of Medicine
Pediatric Pulmonologist
Kansas City, Kansas

GIL BINENBAUM, M.D.
Division of Ophthalmology

PETER M. BINGHAM, M.D.
Clinical Associate Professor of Neurology & Pediatrics
Fletcher Allen Health Care
University of Vermont

GEOFFREY L. BIRD, M.D. F.A.A.P.
Staff Cardiac Intensivist, Cardiac ICU
Assistant Professor of Anesthesia, Department of
    Anesthesiology and Critical Care Medicine
Assistant Professor of Pediatrics, Department
    of Pediatrics

JULIE A. BOOM, M.D.
Assistant Professor of Pediatrics
Baylor College of Medicine
Director, Immunization Project
Texas Children's Hospital

JAMES T. BOYD, M.D.
Assistant Professor
Department of Neurology
University of Vermont
Fletcher Allen Health Care
Burlington, Vermont

AMY R. BROOKS-KAYAL, M.D.
Assistant Professor of Neurology and Pediatrics
Attending Neurologist

KURT A. BROWN, M.D.
Associate Director, Clinical Research
AstraZeneca LP
Wilmington, Delaware

VALERIE I. BROWN, M.D., Ph.D.
Assistant Professor of Pediatrics
Attending Physician
Blood and Bone Marrow Transplant Program
Division of Oncology

ANN B. BRUNER, M.D.
Clinic Physician
Student Health and Wellness Center
Johns Hopkins University
Baltimore, Maryland

LEAH W. BURKE, M.D., M.A.T.
Associate Professor of Pediatrics and Medicine
University of Vermont College of Medicine
Attending Physician, Fletcher Allen Health Care

DAVID M. BUSH, M.D., Ph.D.
Major, V.S.A.F., M.C.
Staff Pediatric Cardiologist

San Antonio Military Pediatric Center
Assistant Clinical Professor, Pediatrics
University of Texas Health Science Center
Uniformed Services University of Health Sciences

EVAN BUXBAUM, M.D. M.P.H.
Department of Pediatrics
Vermont Children's Hospital
Burlington, Vermont

KRISTEN W. CALCAGNI, M.D.
Fellow, Department of Pediatrics
Section of Endocrinology
Yale University School of Medicine
New Haven, Connecticut

JAMES M. CALLAHAN, M.D., F.A.A.P., F.A.C.E.P
Associate Professor of Emergency Medicine
and Pediatrics
Director, Pediatric Emergency Medicine Fellowship
SUNY Upstate Medical University
Attending Physician, Pediatric Emergency Department
University Hospital, Syracuse, New York

CARLA CAMPBELL, M.D., M.S.
Clinical Associate Professor of Pediatrics
Department of Pediatrics
Medical Director
Lead Evaluation Clinic

DOUGLAS CANNING, M.D.
Professor of Surgery
Director, Division of Urology

WILLIAM B. CAREY M.D.
Division of General Pediatrics
Clinical Professor of Pediatrics

CHRISTINE A. CARMAN-DILLON, M.D.
Division of Plastic Surgery

MICHAEL C. CARR, M.D., Ph.D.
Assistant Professor of Urology
Attending Surgeon, Pediatric Urology

AARON E. CARROLL, M.D., M.S.
Assistant Professor of Pediatrics
Children's Health Services Research
Department of Pediatrics
Indiana University School of Medicine
Indianapolis, Indiana

RUBEN W. CERRI, M.D.
Gastroenterology and Nutrition Fellow
Alfred I duPont Hospital for Children
Wilmington, Delaware

ELIZABETH CANDELL CHALOM, M.D.
Director, Pediatric Rheumatology
St. Barnabas Medical Center
Livingston, New Jersey
Clinical Assistant Professor of Pediatrics
University of Medicine and Dentistry of New Jersey

CINDY W. CHRISTIAN, M.D.
Associate Professor of Pediatrics
Chair, Child Abuse and Neglect Prevention

THOMAS H. CHUN, M.D.
Assistant Professor
Department of Pediatrics
Department Psychiatry and Human Behavior
Brown University
Providence, Rhode Island

ESTHER K. CHUNG, M.D., M.P.H.
Assistant Professor of Pediatrics
Thomas Jefferson College of Medicine
Philadelphia, Pennsylvania
Active Staff, Department of Pediatrics
A.I. duPont Hospital for Children
Wilmington, Delaware

RUSSELL G. CLAYTON SR., D.O.
Division of Pulmonary Disease

MICHELE CLEMENT, M.D.
Department of Urology

SUSAN E. COFFIN, M.D., M.P.H.
Medical Director, Infection Prevention and Control
Division of Infectious Diseases
Department of Pediatrics

MERYL S. COHEN, M.D.
Assistant Professor of Pediatrics
Interim Director, Echocardiography Laboratory

MITCHELL I. COHEN, M.D.
Arizona Pediatric Cardiology Consultant
Section Chief, Pediatric Cardiology
Phoenix Children's Hospital
Clinical Associate of Pediatrics
University of Arizona School of Medicine

MATTHEW J. COX, M.D.
Co-director, REACH Program
Children's Medical Center Pediatric Medicine
Dallas, Texas

LUCY S. CRAIN, M.D.
Department of Pediatrics
University of California
San Francisco, California

PETER B. CRINO, M.D.
Department of Neurology
Hospital of the University of Pennsylvania

RANDY Q. CRON, M.D., Ph.D.
Assistant Professor of Pediatrics
Department of Pediatrics
Division of Rheumatology

MONICA H. DARBY, B.Sc.
Staff Pharmacist
Department of Pharmacy Services

RICHARD S. DAVIDSON, M.D.
Associate Professor
Division of Orthopedics

SUZANNE DAWID, M.D., Ph.D.
Fellow, Infectious Disease

RALPH J DEBERARDINIS, M.D. Ph.D.
Fellow, Medical Genetics

MARK DITMAR, M.D.
Clinical Assistant Professor of Pediatrics
Jefferson Medical College
Director, Pediatric Hospitalist Program
AtlantiCare Regional Medical Center
Pomona, New Jersey

DENNIS J. DLUGOS, M.D.
Assistant Professor of Neurology & Pediatrics

AARON DONOGHUE, M.D.
Instructor
Fellow, Divisions of Critical Care and Emergency Medicine

JOHN P. DORMANS, M.D.
Chief of Orthopaedic Surgery
Professor of Orthopaedic Surgery

HENRY R. DROTT, Ph.D.
Director of Clinical Chemistry Lab

NANCY A. DRUCKER, M.D.
Associate Professor, Pediatrics
University of Vermont
Fletcher Allen Health Care

DENNIS R. DURBIN, M.D., M.S.C.E
Associate Professor of Pediatrics and Epidemiology
University of Pennsylvania
Attending Physician
Division of Emergency Medicine

GARY A. EMMETT, M.D., F.A.A.P.
Clinical Associate Professor of Pediatrics
Thomas Jefferson University
Director of General Pediatrics
Thomas Jefferson University Hospital
Director of Jefferson duPont Children Health Center

DON E. ESLIN, M.D.
Attending Physician
Division of Hematology/Oncology
Nemours Children's Clinic and Arnold Palmur Hospital
Orlando, Florida

STEPHEN J. FALCHEK, M.D.
Instructor in Pediatrics and Neurology
Thomas Jefferson University
Director, Epilepsy Program
AI duPont
Hospital for Children

JOEL A. FEIN, M.D., M.P.H.
Associate Professor of Pediatrics and Emergency Medicine
Attending Physician
Emergency Department

MICHAEL A. FERGUSON, M.D.
Chief Resident, Pediatrics
Clinical Instructor of Pediatrics
The University of Vermont College of Medicine
Vermont Children's Hospital at Fletcher Allen Health Care

RICHARD S. FINKEL, M.D.
Associate Clinical Professor, Pediatrics and Neurology
Director, Neuromuscular Program

MICHAEL J. FISHER, M.D.
Assistant Professor of Pediatrics
Attending Physician, Division of Oncology/Neuro-Oncology

JONATHAN T. FLEENOR, M.D., F.A.A.P., F.A.C.C.
Uniformed Services University, Bethesda, MD
Assistant Professor: Uniformed Services University,
  Bethesda, MD
Pediatric Cardiologist: Naval Medical Center San Diego

JOHN M. FLYNN, M.D.
Attending Surgeon
Division of Orthopedic Surgeon
Associate Professor of Orthopaedics

MATTHEW ISAAC FOGG, M.D.
Fellow, Division of Allergy and Immunology

BRIAN J. FORBES M.D., Ph.D.
Attending Surgeon, Division of Ophthalmology
Assistant Professor of Ophthalmology

DAVID F. FRIEDMAN, M.D.
Clinical Assistant Professor of Pediatrics

THEODORE J. GANLEY, M.D.
Orthopaedic Director of Sports Medicine
Assistant Professor of Orthopaedic Surgery

LYNETTE A. GILLIS, M.D.
Assistant Professor
Department of Pediatrics
Division of Pediatric Gastroenterology, Hepatology
and Nutrition
  and Division of Medical Genetics
Vanderbilt University Medical Center
Nashville, Tennessee

JILL P. GINSBERG, M.D.
Assistant Professor of Pediatrics
Division of Oncology

KENNETH R. GINSBERG, M.D.
Associate Professor of Pediatrics
Division of Adolescent Medicine

KELLY C. GOLDSMITH, M.D.
Division of Hematology/Oncology

SCOTT M. GOLDSTEIN, M.D.
Clinical Assistant Professor of Ophthalmology
Tri county Eye Physicians and Surgeons
Southampton, Pennsylvania

JOHN M. GOOD, M.D., F.A.A.P.
General Pediatrics
Lovelace Sandia Health Systems
Clinical Faculty
University of New Mexico

VANI GOPALAREDDY M.B.B.S.
Fellow, Pediatric Gastroenterology
AI Dupont Children's Hospital
Wilmington, Delaware

MARC H. GORELICK, M.D., M.S.C.E.
Associate Professor of Pediatrics
and Epidemiology
Medical College of Wisconsin; Medical Director
Emergency Department
Children's Hospital of Wisconsin
Milwaukee, Wisconsin

JANE M. GOULD, M.D.
Research Associate Department of Microbiology
Attending Staff Physician

WILLIAM R. GRAESSLE, M.D.
Assistant Professor
Director, Pediatric Medical Education
Department of Pediatrics
UMDNJ-Robertwood Johnson Medical School
Camden Cooper Hospital
Camden, New Jersey

ROSE C. GRAHAM-MAAR, M.D.
Clinical Instructor of Pediatrics
Fellow, Division of Gastroenterology & Nutrition

ERNEST M. GRAHAM, M.D.
Assistant Professor, Department of Gyn-OB
Div. of Maternal-Fetal Medicine
Johns Hopkins University School of Medicine

ANDRES J. GRECO, M.D.
Pediatric Nephrology Fellow
Division of Nephrology

JEANNE GREENBLATT, M.D.
Clinical Assistant Professor
University of Vermont
Department of Psychiatry
Burlington, Vermont

ADDA GRIMBERG, M.D.
Assistant Professor of Pediatrics
Division of Endocrinology and Diabetes

BLAZE ROBERT GUSIC, M.D.
Clinical Assistant Professor of Pediatrics
Attending Physician

J. NINA HAM, M.D.
Fellow
Division of Endocrinology and Diabetes

OLGA T. HARDY, M.D.
Fellow
Division of Endocrinology and Diabetes

CHERYL L. HAUSMAN, M.D.
Medical Director
Primary Care Center at University Center

EUGENE R. HERSHORIN, M.D.
Associate Professor of Clinical Pediatrics
Medical Director—Behavioral Pediatrics Clinic
Associate Director—Masters of Pediatrics
Director—Masters of Developmental
and Behavioral Pediatrics
University of Miami School of Medicine

Y. LILY HIGGINS, M.S., M.D.
Instructor of Pediatrics
Thomas Jefferson University Hospital
Dupont Hospital for Children

IVOR BRADEN HORN, M.D., M.P.H.
Assistant Professor of Pediatrics
The George Washington University School
  of Medicine and Health Sciences
Children's National Medical Center

MALAKA B. JACKSON, M.D.
Fellow
Division of Endocrinology and Diabetes

ZEV JACOBSON, M.D.
Assistant Professor of Pediatrics
Division of Cardiology

CYNTHIA R. JACOBSTEIN, M.D.
Clinical Assistant Professor
Department of Pediatrics
Division of Emergency Medicine

DOUGLAS A. JACOBSTEIN, M.D.
Fellow
Division of Gastroenterology and Nutrition

HELEN ANITA JOHN-KELLY, M.D.
Assistant Professor of Pediatrics
Columbia University, College of Physicians and Surgeons
Director, Pediatric Gastroenterology
New York Hospital, Queens

CHRISTOPHER JUSTINICH, M.D., F.R.C.P.(C)
Head
Pediatric Gastroenterology
Queen's University

JONATHAN KALTMAN, M.D.
Fellow, Pediatric Cardiology

ROBERT K. KAMEI, M.D.
Clinical Professor of Pediatrics
University of California, San Francisco

PETER B. KANG, M.D.
Instructor in Neurology, Harvard Medical School
Assistant in Neurology, Children's Hospital Boston
Associate, Howard Hughes Medical Institute

TAMMY I. KANG, M.D.
Assistant Professor
Division of Hematology

WILLIAM J. KATOWITZ, M.D.
Division of Ophthalmology

LORRAINE KATZ, M.D.
Assistant Professor
Division of Endocrinology

ANDREA KELLY, M.D.
Assistant Professor of Pediatrics
Endocrinology/Diabetes

KARA M. KELLY, M.D.
Associate Professor of Clinical Pediatrics
Division of Pediatric Oncology
Columbia University College of Physicians & Surgeons
Morgan Stanley Children's Hospital of New York-Presbyterian

THOMAS L. KENNEDY III, M.D.
Professor of Clinical Pediatrics
Department of Pediatrics
The Yale University School of Medicine
New Haven, Connecticut
Chairman, Department of Pediatrics
Bridgeport Hospital
Bridgeport, Connecticut

HANS B. KERSTEN, M.D.
Assistant Professor of Pediatrics
Drexel University College of Medicine
St. Christopher's Hospital for Children

FEMIDA KHERANI, M.D.
Division of Pediatric Ophthalmology

JASON Y. KIM, M.D.
Fellow, Pediatric Infectious Diseases
University of Michigan Medical Center
C.S. Mott Children's Hospital
Attending Physician
Division of Pediatric Infectious Diseases

TERRY KIND, M.D., M.P.H.
Assistant Professor of Pediatrics
Children's National Medical Center
The George Washington School of Medicine and Health Sciences

RICHARD E. KIRSCHNER, M.D., F.A.C.S., F.A.A.P.
Associate Professor of Surgery
Associate Professor

THOMAS F. KOLON, M.D.
Assistant Professor of Pediatric Urology
Assistant Professor of Urology

WENDY J. KOWALSKI, M.D.
Attending Physician
Division of Neonatology
Lehigh Valley Hospital
Allentown, Pennsylvania

RICHARD M. KRAVITZ, M.D.
Assistant Professor of Pediatrics
Director, Pediatric Sleep Lab
Division of Pediatric Pulmonary Diseases
Duke University Medical Center

JANET L. KWIATKOWSKI, M.D.
Assistant Professor of Pediatrics
Attending Hematologist

THOMAS LAHIRI, M.D., F.A.A.P.
Assistant Professor of Pediatrics
University of Vermont College of Medicine
Director, Pediatric Pulmonology
Vermont Children's Hospital

JANE LAVELLE, M.D.
Associate Professor of Pediatrics
Associate Director of Emergency Medicine

KAREN LECOMTE, M.D.
Instructor in Neurology
University of Vermont/Fletcher Allen Health Care
Burlington, Vermont

P. NELSON LE, M.D.
Heart Failure and Transplant Fellow
Division of Cardiology

DIVA D. DE LEÓN, M.D.
Assistant Professor of Pediatrics
Attending Physician
Division of Endocrinology and Diabetes

MARY B. LEONARD, M.D., M.S.C.E.
Assistant Professor of Pediatrics and Epidemiology

LEONARD J. LEVINE, M.D.
Fellow, Adolescent Medicine
Instructor in Pediatrics

JANET M. LI-TEMPEST, M.D.
Pediatrician, Gallup Indian Medical Center
Gallup, New Mexico

CHRIS A. LIACOURAS, M.D.
Professor of Pediatrics
Division of Gastroenterology

DANIEL J. LICHT, M.D.
Assistant Professor of Neurology and Pediatrics

KAREN LIQUORNIK, M.D.
Division of Gastroenterology

GRANT T. LIU, M.D.
Professor of Neurology and Ophthalmology
Neuro-ophthalmogist
Division of Ophthalmology

KATHLEEN GRAHAM LOMAX, M.D.
Associate Director
Medical Affairs
Gastroenterology, Eisai Inc.
Teaneck, New Jersey

KATHLEEN LOOMES, M.D.
Division of Gastroenterology

JEFFREY P. LOUIE, M.D.
Instructor
Department of Emergency Medicine
Children's Hospital and Clinics
St. Paul, Minnesota
Adjunct Clinical Instructor
University of Minnesota School of Medicine
Mineapolis, Minnesota

GORDANA LOVREKOVIC M.D.
Assistant Professor, Department of Pediatrics
Section of Pediatric Pulmonology
Medical College of Georgia
Augusta, Georgia

DAVID W. LOW, M.D.
Plastic Surgery

SAMUEL D. MALDONADO, M.D., M.P.H.
Senior Director
Global Regulatory Affairs
Johnson and Johnson

PETAR MAMULA, M.D.
Assistant Professor of Pediatrics
Division of Gastroenterology

YANG MAO-DRAAYER, M.D., Ph.D.
University of Vermont
College of Medicine
Fletcher Allen Hospital

BRADLEY S. MARINO, M.D., M.P.P.
Assistant Professor of Anesthesia & Pediatrics
Department of Anesthesiology, Critical
Care Medicine, & Pediatrics
Divisions of Critical Care Medicine & Cardiology

JONATHAN E. MARKOWITZ, M.D., M.S.C.E.
Attending Physician and Director, Inpatient Gastroenterology
Division of GI & Nutrition
Assistant Professor of Pediatrics

ERIC D. MARSH, M.D., Ph.D.
Clinical Neurophysiology Fellow
Division of Neurology

MARIA R. MASCARENHAS, M.B.B.S
Associate Professor of Pediatrics
Section Chief Division of Gastroenterology & Nutrition
Attending Gastroenterologist

PAUL S. MATZ, M.D.
Assistant Professor of Pediatrics
Drexel University College of Medicine
St. Christopher's Hospital for Children
Division of Ambulatory Pediatrics

OSCAR H. MAYER, M.D.
Clinical Associate in Pediatrics
Division of Pulmonary Medicine
Department of Pediatrics

STEPHEN J. McGEADY, M.D.
Associate Professor of Pediatrics
Thomas Jefferson University

ERIN E. McGINTEE, M.D.
Fellow, Allergy and Immunology

MARGARET M. McNAMARA, M.D., F.A.A.P.
Assistant Clinical Professor
University of California San Francisco

D. ELIZABETH McNEIL, M.D.
Division of Neurology

DEVENDRA I. MEHTA, M.B.B.S., M.Sc., M.R.C.P.
Assistant Professor of Pediatrics, Thomas
Jefferson University
Director of the Pediatric GI and Nutrition Fellowship
Alfred I. DuPont Hospital for Children
Pediatric Gastroenterologist, Nemours Children's
Clinic—Wilmington

JONDAVID MENTEER, M.D.
Assistant Professor of Pediatrics
Keck School of Medicine at U.S.C.
Attending Physician, Division of Cardiology
Children's Hospital of Los Angeles

KEVIN E.C. MEYERS, M.B., B.Ch.
Assistant Professor of Pediatrics, Pediatric Nephrologist

MONTE D. MILLS, M.D.
Director, Division of Ophthalmology
Assistant Professor

JANE E. MINTURN, M.D., Ph.D.
Instructor
Department of Pediatrics
Division of Oncology

NAHUSH A. MOKADAM, M.D.

CYNTHIA J. MOLLEN, M.D., M.S.C.E.
Assistant Professor
Department of Pediatrics
Attending Physician
Division of Emergency Medicine

THOMAS J. MOLLEN, M.D.
Clinical Associate and Attending Physician
Division of Neonatology

LINDA V. MUIR, M.D.
Sacred Heart Medical Center
Spokane, Washington

ANDREW E. MULBERG, M.D.
Adjunct Associate Professor of Pediatrics
Director, Global Drug Development
Johnson & Johnson Pharmaceutical Research &
Development, LLC

LAURA T. MULREANY, M.D.
Major, Medical Corps., US Army
Chief, Pediatric Pulmonology
Director, Cystic Fibrosis Center
Department of Pediatrics
Tripler Army Medical Center, Honolulu, Hawaii
Assistant Clinical Professor of Pediatrics
Uniformed Services University of the Health Sciences,
Bethesda, MD
Assistant Clinical Professor of Pediatrics
John A. Burns School of Medicine
University of Hawaii at Manoa, Honolulu, Hawaii

MICHAEL P. MULREANY, M.D.
Lieutenant Colonel, Medical Corps, US Army
Chief, Pediatric Cardiology
Tripler Army Medical Center, Honolulu, Hawaii
Assistant Clinical Professor, Pediatrics
John A. Burns School of Medicine—University of Hawaii,
Honolulu, Hawaii

FRANCES M. NADEL, M.D., M.S.C.E.
Assistant Professor of Clinical Pediatrics
Department of Pediatrics
Attending Physician
Division of Emergency Medicine

KEITH NAGEL, M.D.
Assistant Professor of Pediatrics
University of Vermont
Burlington, Vermont

SETH L. NESS M.D., Ph.D.
Clinical Fellow
CNS Therapeutic Area
Johnson & Johnson Pharmaceutical Research &
Development L.L.C.

JASON NEWLAND, M.D.
Division of Infections Diseases

MICHAEL E. NORMAN, M.D.
(Retired) Department of Pediatrics
North Carolina Medical Center
Charlotte, North Carolina

CYNTHIA F. NORRIS, M.D.
Clinical Associate in Pediatrics
Attending Physician, Medical Director
Hematology Acute Care Unit

KEVIN C. OSTERHOUDT, M.D., M.S.C.E.
Assistant Professor of Pediatrics
Attending Physician
Division of Emergency Medicine
Associate Medical Director
The Poison Control Center
Philadelphia, Pennsylvania

HOWARD B. PANITCH M.D.
Associate Professor of Pediatrics
Director of Clinical Programs
Division of Pulmonary Medicine

RITA PANOSCHA, M.D.
Assistant Professor of Pediatrics at
  OHSU (Oregon Health Sciences University)
Child Development and Rehabilitation Center

SUSAN L. PERLMAN, M.D.
Clinical Professor of Neurology
David Geffen School of Medicine at UCLA
Director, Neurogenetics Clinic/Ataxia Center

ELENA PEREZ, M.D.
Immunologic and Infectious Diseases

FRANK PESSLER, M.D., Ph.D.
Division of Rheumatology

NADJA G. PETER, M.D.
Clinical Associate
Craig-Dalsimer Division of Adolescent Medicine
Hospital of the University of Pennsylvania

SHANNON CONNOR PHILLIPS, M.D.
Director, Pediatric Hospitalist Program
The Children's Hospital at the Cleveland Clinic
Assistant Professor of Pediatrics
Cleveland Clinic Lerner College of Medicine of
  Case Western Reserve University

VICTOR M. PIÑEIRO-CARRERO, M.D., F.A.A.P.
Division Chief
Gastroenterology and Nutrition
Nemours Children's Clinic

JONATHAN R. PLETCHER, M.D.
University of Pennsylvania
Medical Director
Adolescent Care Center

CHARLES A. POHL, M.D.
Clinical Associate Professor of Pediatrics
Associate Dean for Student Affairs and Career
  Counseling
Jefferson Medical College of Thomas
Jefferson University

BRENDA E. PORTER, M.D.
Division of Neurology

JILL C. POSNER, M.D., M.S.C.E.
Assistant Professor of Pediatrics
Attending Physician, Emergency Department

GRAHAM E. QUINN, M.D., M.S.C.E.
Professor of Ophthalmology
Attending Physician, Ophthalmology

LESLIE RAFFINI, M.D.
Assistant Profesor
Division of Hematology

ADAM J. RATNER, M.D., M.P.H.
Division of Infectious Diseases

DANIEL H. REIRDEN, M.D.
Fellow, Craig-Dalsimer Division of Adolescent Medicine
Instructor

SUSAN R. RHEINGOLD, M.D.
Assistant Professor
Attending Physician

DAVID L. ROBINOWITZ, M.D.
Clinical Fellow
Pediatric Pulmonary Medicine
University of California, San Francisco

J. FERNANDO DEL ROSARIO, M.D.
Assistant Professor of Pediatrics
Thomas Jefferson University of Medical College/A.I. duPont
  Hospital for Children

HOWARD M. ROSENBERG, D.D.S., M.ED.
Associate Professor
Department of Pediatric Dentistry
School of Dental Medicine; University of Pennsylvania

ALISHA J. ROVNER, B.A.
Doctoral Candidate, Human Nutrition
Center for Human Nutrition
Johns Hopkins Bloomberg School of Public Health

MARIANNE RUBY, M.D.
Clinical Instructor in Gynecology
Thomas Jefferson University

RICHARD M. RUTSTEIN, M.D.
Medical Director, Special Immunology Service
Associate Professor of Pediatrics

MATTHEW J. RYAN, M.D.
Clinical Instructor of Pediatrics
Fellow, Division of Gastroenterology & Nutrition

SULAGNA C. SAITTA, M.D.
Division of Genetics

ANN E. SALERNO, M.D.
Fellow in Pediatric Nephrology

DENISE A. SALERNO, M.D., F.A.A.P.
Associate Professor of Pediatrics
Pediatric Clerkship Director
Temple University Children's Medical Center
Temple University School of Medicine

ZUHAIR SAYANY, D.M.D.
B.A. (Psych) 1987, University of Pennsylvania
D.M.D 1990, University of Pennsylvania School of Dental Medicine
Diplomate, American Board of Pediatric Dentistry
Clinical Affiliate Children's Hospital of Philadelphia
Attending Staff, (1995–2002)
Assistant Professor University of Pennsylvania S.D.M. (until 2002)
Currently in Private Practice of Pediatric Dentistry in Cherry Hill,
  New Jersey

THOMAS F. SCANLIN, M.D.
Director, Cystic Fibrosis Center
Professor of Pediatric

VERED YEHEZKELY SCHILDKRAUT, M.D.
Division of Pediatric Gastroenterology and Nutrition
Meyer Children's Hospital, Rambam Medical Center
Haifa, Israel

EUGENE SCHNEIDER, M.D.
Assistant Director
CNS—Clinical Development & Medical Affairs
Forest Research Institute

SETH L. SCHULMAN, M.D.
Adjunct Associate Professor of Pediatrics
Associate Director, Clinical Research & Development
Wyeth Research

AMY H. SCHULTZ, M.D.
Assistant Cardiologist
Division of Cardiology
Instructor, Department of Pediatrics

CAROLYN SCHWARTZ, M.D.
Private practice–Morehill Pediatrics
Phoenixville, Pennsylvania

CHARLES SCHWARTZ, M.D., F.A.A.P.
Assistant Clinical Professor of Pediatrics at the University
  of Pennsylvania
School of Medicine
General Pediatrician–PennCare for Kids
Phoenixville, Pennsylvania

MITCHELL ROBERT SCHWARTZ, M.D.
Private Practice-Philadelphia, Pennsylvania

M. WILLIAM SCHWARTZ, M.D.
Emeritus Professor of Pediatrics
Senior Physician

SEPEHR SEKHAVAT, M.D.
Fellow, Cardiology
Clinical Instructor, Department of Pediatrics

STEVEN M. SELBST
Professor of Pediatrics
Jefferson Medical College/ Thomas Jefferson University
Philadelphia, Pennsylvania
Vice Chair for Education
Department of Pediatrics
Jefferson Medical College/A.I. duPont Hospital for Children
Wilmington, Delaware

EDISIO SEMEAO, M.D.
Assistant Clinical Professor
Department of Pediatrics

STEPHEN E. SHAFFER, M.D.
Clinical Assistant Professor
Department of Pediatrics, Jefferson Medical
College of Thomas Jefferson University, Philadelphia, Pennsylvania
Chief, Division of Gastroenterology, duPont
Hospital for Children
Wilmington, Delaware

SAMIR S. SHAH, M.D.
Assistant Professor of Pediatrics, Department of Pediatrics
Division of General Pediatrics and Infectious Diseases

RAANAN SHAMIR, M.D.
Associate Professor, Bruce Rappaport School of Medicine
Technion-Institute of Technology
Director, Division of Pediatric Gastroenterology and Nutrition
Meyer Children's Hospital, Rambam Medical Center
Haifa, Israel

KATHY N. SHAW, M.D., M.S.C.E.
Professor of Pediatrics at the Children's Hospital of Philadelphia
Chief, Division of Emergency Medicine

DAVID D. SHERRY, M.D.
Director, Clinical Rheumatology
Professor of Pediatrics

ASEEM R. SHUKLA, M.D.
Assistant Professor of Surgery
Mayo Clinic College of Medicine
Nemours Children's Clinic
Jacksonville, Florida

LAURA N. SINAI, M.D., M.S.C.E.
General Pediatrics, Charlotte, North Carolina

V. BEN SIVARAJAN M.D., F.R.C.P.C, F.A.A.P
Fellow, Division of Cardiology
Clinical Instructor

KIM SMITH-WHITLEY, M.D.
Assistant Professor
Division of Hematology

SABRINA E. SMITH, M.D., Ph.D.
Instructor
Department of Neurology

HOWARD M. SNYDER III, M.D.
Professor of Surgery in Urology
Associate Director Pediatric Urology
Senior Surgeon

RAMAN SREEDHARAN, M.D., D.C.H., M.R.C.P.C.H.
Fellow in Pediatric Gastroenterology
AI duPont Hospital for Children

KATHLEEN E. SULLIVAN, M.D., Ph.D.
Associate Professor of Pediatrics

JULIE W. STERN, M.D.
Clinical Assistant Professor
Divisions of Hematology & Oncology
(MD Northwestern University Medical School)

JOHN I. TAKAYAMA, M.D., M.P.H.
Director, Department of Interdisciplinary Medicine
National Center for Child Health and Development, Japan

RONN E. TANEL, M.D.
Assistant Professor
Department of Pediatrics

Attending Cordiologist
Division of Cordiology

DANNA TAUBER, M.D., M.P.H.
Drexel University College of Medicine
Assistant Professor
St Christopher's Hospital for Children
Attending Physician
Division of Pulmonary Medicine
St. Christopher's Hospital for Children

GREGORZ TELEGA, M.D.
Division of Gastroenterology
Children's Hospital of Wisconsin Milwaukee, Wisconsin

BRUCE TEMPEST, M.D.
Medical Director (ret.) USPHS
Consultant, Gallup Indian Medical Center
Indian Health Service, USPHS

MEENA THAYU, M.D.
Fellow GI and Nutrition
Department of Pediatrics

OLAFUR THORARENSEN, M.D.
Division of Neurology

PAUL S. THORNTON M.B., B.Ch., M.R.C.P.I.
Medical Director of Diabetes and Endocrinology
Cook Children's Medical Center, Forth Worth, Texas

NICHOLAS TSAROUHAS, M.D.
Associate Professor of Clinical Pediatrics
Department of Pediatrics
Medical Director
Emergency Transport Services
Attending Physician
Division of Emergency Medicine

JOHN TUNG, M.B.B.S., B.Sc., M.R.C.P.
Attending Pediatric Gastroenterologist
AI duPont Children's Hospital
Wilmington, Delaware

PAUL P. WANG, M.D.
Associate Director
Pfizer Global Research & Development
Groton, Connecticut

DROR WASSERMAN, M.D.
Tel Aviv Medical Center
Maccabi Healthcare Organization, Israel

BARBARA WATSON M.B., CH.B., D.C.H., M.R.C.P.
(LONDON, U.K.)
Associate Professor of Pediatrics Jefferson
Medical College
Affiliate of Albert Einstein Medical Center

STUART A. WEINZIMER, M.D.
Assistant Professor, Department of Pediatrics, Section
of Endocrinology
Yale University School of Medicine
Attending Physician, Yale-New Haven Medical Center,
New Haven, Connecticut

PETER C. WILMONT, D.O.
Fellow, Pediatric Gastroenterology
AI duPont Hospital for Children
Wilmington, Delaware

GEORGE A. WOODWARD, M.D., M.B.A.
Professor of Pediatrics
University of Washington School of Medicine
Seattle, Washington
Chief, Division of Emergency Medicine
Director, Emergency Services
Children's Hospital and Regional Medical Center
Seattle, Washington

PAIGE L. WRIGHT, M.D.
Attending Physician
Children's Hospital at Regional Medical Center
Assistant Professor Department of Pediatrics
University of Washington School of Medicine
Academic Faculty, Emergency Services Department
Children's Hospital and Regional Medical Center
Seattle, Washington

HSI-YANG WU, M.D.
Assistant Professor of Urology
University of Pittsburgh
Attending Physician, Department of Urology
Children's Hospital of Pittsburgh

ALBERT C. YAN, M.D.
Director, Pediatric Dermatology
Assistant Professor, Pediatrics and Dermatology

THEOKLIS ZAOUTIS, M.D.
Assistant Professor
Department of Pediatrics
Attending Physician
Division of Infectious Diseases

STEPHEN A. ZDERIC, M.D.
Attending Urologist
Associate Professor of Urology in Surgery

KAREN PAUL ZIMMER, M.D., M.P.H.
Fellow, General Academic Pediatric Fellowship
at Johns Hopkins University School of Medicine

RAEZELLE ZINMAN, M.D.
Clinical Professor of Pediatrics
Division of Pulmonary Medicine

KATHLEEN MARY WHOLEY ZSOLWAY, D.O.
Clinical Assistant Professor of Pediatrics
Attending Physician, Medical Director
General Pediatrics Faculty Practice

Contents

SECTION III: SYNDROMES GLOSSARY / 915

SECTION IV: CARDIOLOGY LABORATORY / 921

Ilana Zeltser

SECTION V: SURGICAL GLOSSARY / 929

Aaron E. Carroll, Nahush A. Mokadam

SECTION VI: LABORATORY VALUES / 933

Henry R. Drott

SECTION VII: TABLES / 937

Charles Schwartz

DEVELOPMENT

GROWTH CHART

IMMUNIZATION

SECTION VIII: MEDICATIONS / 985

Monica Darby

SECTION I
Chief Complaints

Abdominal Mass

 Database

DEFINITION

Either an unusually enlarged abdominal or retroperitoneal organ (i.e., hepatomegaly, splenomegaly, or enlarged kidney) or a defined fullness in the abdominal cavity not directly associated with an abdominal organ.

 Differential Diagnosis

STOMACH

- Gastroparesis
- Duplication
- Foreign body/bezoar
- Gastric torsion
- Gastric tumor (lymphoma, sarcoma)

SPLEEN

- Infiltrative disease (Gaucher, Niemann-Pick)
- Langerhans cell histiocytosis
- Leukemia
- Hematologic (hemolytic disease, sickle cell disease, hereditary spherocytosis/elliptocytosis)

INTESTINE

- Feces (constipation)
- Meconium ileus
- Duplication
- Volvulus
- Intussusception
- Intestinal atresia or stenosis
- Inflammatory bowel disease complications (abscess, phlegmon)
- Appendiceal or Meckel diverticulum abscess
- Toxic megacolon
- Mesenteric/omental cyst
- Mesenteric fibromatosis
- Lymphoma, Adenocarcinoma
- Carcinoid
- Foreign body
- Duodenal hematoma (trauma)

PANCREAS

- Pseudocyst (trauma)
- Pancreatoblastoma

LIVER

- Endocrinologic (glycogen storage disease)
- Infectious (hepatitis A, B, C)
- Congenital hepatic fibrosis
- Tumor (hepatic adenoma, hepatoblastoma, hepatocellular carcinoma)
- Vascular (hamartoma, hemangioma, hemangioendothelioma)
- Cystic disease (Caroli disease)
- Focal nodular hyperplasia

BLADDER

- Posterior urethral valves
- Neurogenic bladder

OVARY

- Cysts (dermoid, follicular)
- Torsion
- Germ cell tumor

KIDNEY

- Hydronephrosis/ureteropelvic obstruction[1]
- Polycystic/multicystic kidney disease[1]
- Wilms tumor
- Renal vein thrombosis
- Mesoblastic nephromas

PERITONEAL

- Ascites
- Teratoma

UTERUS

- Pregnancy
- Hematocolpos
- Hydrometrocolpos

ADRENAL

- Adrenal hemorrhage
- Adrenal abscess
- Neuroblastoma
- Pheochromocytoma

GALLBLADDER

- Choledochal cyst
- Hydrops
- Obstruction (stone, stricture, trauma)

ABDOMINAL WALL

- Umbilical/inguinal/ventral hernia
- Omphalocele/gastroschisis
- Trauma (rectus hematoma)
- Tumor (fibroma, lipoma, rhabdomyosarcoma)

OTHER

- Lymphangioma
- Fetus-in-fetu

Approach to the Patient

GENERAL GOALS

Abdominal masses in children are often found by an unsuspecting parent during bathing or by a physician during a routine physical examination. Most masses have no specific signs or symptoms. In children, abdominal masses require immediate attention. When evaluating a pediatric abdominal mass, an organized approach is paramount in determining its etiology.

Phase 1: Determine the location of the abdominal mass and its association with intraabdominal organs.

Phase 2: Perform diagnostic tests; the abdominal x-ray and ultrasound are the most efficient way to start the evaluation.

Phase 3: Treatment (see Laboratory Aids)

[1]Most common in newborns

 Data Gathering

HISTORY

Question: Weight loss?
Significance: Tumor, inflammatory bowel disease

Question: Fever?
Significance: Abscess, malignancy

Question: Jaundice?
Significance: Liver/biliary disease

Question: Hematuria or dysuria?
Significance: Renal disease

Question: Vomiting?
Significance: Intestinal obstruction

Question: Frequency and quality of bowel movements?
Significance: Constipation, intussusception, compression of bowel by mass

Question: Bleeding or bruising?
Significance: Coagulopathy

Question: History of abdominal trauma?
Significance: Pancreatic pseudocyst

Question: Sexual activity?
Significance: Pregnancy

Question: What is the age of the patient?
Significance: The age of the patient is often a helpful clue in investigating the cause of the abdominal mass. In neonates, the most common origin of abdominal masses is the genitourinary system (cystic kidney disease, hydronephrosis). In infants and preschool-aged children, the most common malignant tumors are Wilms tumor and neuroblastoma. In adolescent-aged girls, ovarian disorders, hematocolpos, and pregnancy are more common causes of abdominal masses.

Physical Examination

Finding: General appearance
Significance: Ill-appearing or cachexia point toward infection or malignancy

Finding: Location of abdominal mass
Significance: Helps to narrow differential diagnosis

Left lower quadrant—Constipation, ovarian process, ectopic pregnancy

Left upper quadrant—Anomaly of the kidney or spleen (mass)

Right lower quadrant—abscess (inflammatory bowel disease), intestinal phlegmon, appendicitis, intussusception, ovarian process, ectopic pregnancy

Right upper quadrant—involves liver, gallbladder, biliary tree, or intestine

Epigastric—Abnormality of the stomach (bezoar, torsion), pancreas (pseudocyst), or enlarged liver

Suprapubic—Pregnancy, hydrometrocolpos, hematocolpos, posterior urethral valves

Flank—Renal disease (cystic kidney, hydronephrosis, Wilms tumor)

Finding: Characteristics of abdominal mass
Significance: Mobility, tenderness, firmness, smoothness, and/or irregularity of the surface of the mass can provide clues to its significance

Finding: Hard and immobile mass
Significance: Tumor

Finding: Extension of mass across midline or into pelvis
Significance: Tumor, hepatomegaly, splenomegaly

Finding: Percussion of mass
Significance: Dullness indicates a solid mass; tympany indicates a hollow viscus

Finding: Shifting dullness, fluid wave
Significance: Ascites

Finding: Skin examination
Significance: Bruising and petechiae may occur with coagulopathy related to liver disease and malignant infiltration of bone marrow; café au lait spots are associated with neurofibromas

Finding: Lymphadenopathy or lymphadenitis
Significance: More systemic process, either malignant or infectious

The abdomen of a normal infant and child should be completely soft and nontender. As a child ages, an increase in abdominal wall musculature may give greater resistance on examination, but the normal abdomen should continue to be soft to deep palpation. Palpation of an abdominal mass is abnormal and should be further evaluated.

 ## Laboratory Aids

Test: CBC
Significance: Anemia or hemolysis

Test: Chemistry panel
Significance:

- Renal disease (BUN, creatinine)
- Liver disease (ALT, AST, alkaline phosphatase, albumin)
- Gallbladder disease (bilirubin, GGT)
- Pancreatic disease (amylase/lipase)
- Intestinal disease (hypoalbuminemia)

Test: Uric acid, lactate dehydrogenase
Significance: Elevated in the setting of rapid cell turnover of solid tumors

Test: Plain abdominal x-ray studies
Significance: Rule out intestinal obstruction, identify calcifications, stool pattern

Test: Abdominal ultrasound
Significance: Can usually identify the origin of the mass and differentiate between solid and cystic tissue; disadvantages are operator variability and a limited exam when bowel gas obscures underlying abdominal tissues

Test: Computed tomography (CT) scan
Significance: Can provide more detail when there is overlying gas or bone; if malignancy is suspected should do chest, abdomen, and pelvis CT

Test: Magnetic resonance imaging
Significance: Vascular lesions of liver, major vessels, and tumors

Test: Radioisotope HIDA scan
Significance: Liver, gallbladder

Test: Intravenous urography or voiding cystourethrography
Significance: Wilms tumor, cystic kidney disease, posterior urethral valves

Test: Upper gastrointestinal (GI), barium enema
Significance: May be of benefit when the mass involves the intestine

Test: Endoscopy
Significance: Can be of benefit when the mass involves the intestine

Test: Laparoscopy
Significance: Can be useful for direct intraperitoneal visualization and biopsy of abdominal masses

Emergency Care

- Patients who present with an abdominal mass and signs and/or symptoms of intestinal obstruction (intussusception, volvulus, gastric torsion, bezoar, foreign body)
- Toxic megacolon
- Ovarian torsion
- Ectopic pregnancy
- Biliary obstruction (stone, hydrops)
- Fever

- Pancreatitis (pseudocyst) requires immediate hospitalization.

Initial diagnostic studies should include plain abdominal x-ray studies, an abdominal ultrasound, and a surgical consultation. The remaining causes of abdominal masses require urgent care and timely evaluation.

Issues for Referral

Except for the diagnosis of constipation, the presence of an abdominal mass requires immediate attention and diagnostic studies should be performed expeditiously at a facility capable of diagnosing pediatric disorders.

Clinical Pearls

- In neonates, a palpable liver edge can be normal; the total liver span is most important
- In infants, a full bladder is often mistaken for an abdominal mass.
- In infants, most abdominal masses are of renal origin and nonmalignant.
- Severe constipation in older children and adolescents can present as a large, hard mass extending from the pubis past the umbilicus.
- Gastric distension should be considered in all children who present with a tympanitic epigastric mass.

BIBLIOGRAPHY

Golden CB, Feusner JH. Malignant abdominal masses in children: quick guide to evaluation and diagnosis. *Pediatr Clin North Am* 2002;49(6):1369–1392.

Liacouras CA. Abdominal Masses. In: Altschuler SM and Liacouras CA, eds. *Clinical Pediatric Gastroenterology.* Philadelphia: Churchill Livingstone, 1998:1–3.

Mahaffey SM, Rychman RC, Martin LW. Clinical aspects of abdominal masses in children. *Semin Roentgenol* 1988;23:161–174.

Merten DF, Kirks DR. Diagnostic imaging of pediatric abdominal masses. *Pediatr Clin North Am* 1985;32:1397–1426.

Schwartz MW. Abdominal masses. In: Schwartz MW, Curry TA, Charney ED, et al, eds. *Principle and Practice of Clinical Pediatrics.* Chicago: Yearbook, 1987:139–144.

Squires RH. Abdominal masses. In: Walker WA, Durie PR, Hamilton JR, et al, eds. *Pediatric Gastrointestinal Disease: Pathophysiology, Diagnosis, Management,* 3rd Ed. Philadelphia: BC Decker, 2000:150–163.

Swischuk LE, Hayden CK Jr. Abdominal masses in children. *Pediatr Clin North Am* 1985;32: 1281–1298.

Authors: Rose C. Graham-Maar and Chris A. Liacouras

Abdominal Pain

 Database

DEFINITION

Abdominal pain is a frequent complaint in the pediatric age group. Pain may be acute or chronic, focal, or nonspecific. A child's complaint of abdominal pain can originate from gastrointestinal (GI) and non-GI causes but also commonly can be the manifestation of referred pain from extraabdominal sites.

 Differential Diagnosis

CONGENITAL/ANATOMIC

- Incarcerated hernia
- Intestinal adhesions
- Intussusception
- Malrotation with volvulus
- Ovarian torsion
- Testicular torsion
- Uteropelvic junction obstruction

INFECTIOUS

- Cystitis and urinary tract infections
- Fitz-Hugh-Curtis syndrome
- Gastroenteritis (bacterial, viral, or parasitic)
- Helicobacter pylori gastritis
- Mononucleosis with splenic enlargement/rupture
- Otitis media
- Pharyngitis
- Pelvic inflammatory disease
- Peritonitis
- Pneumonia
- Psoas abscess
- Sepsis
- Tuboovarian abscess
- Varicella

TOXIC, ENVIRONMENTAL DRUGS

- Anticholinergic drugs
- Caustic ingestions
- Intestinal foreign body
- Heavy metal (i.e., lead) ingestion
- Mushroom poisoning
- Sympathomimetic drugs

TRAUMA

- Child abuse
- Duodenal hematoma
- Perforated viscus
- Splenic hematoma/rupture

TUMOR

- Any tumor, benign or malignant, leading to viscous obstruction
- Leukemia
- Lymphoma
- Nephroblastoma
- Wilms tumor

GENETIC/METABOLIC

- Diabetic ketoacidosis

ALLERGIC/INFLAMMATORY

- Appendicitis
- Cholecystitis
- Eosinophilic gastroenteritis
- Hemolytic-uremic syndrome
- Henloch-Schonlein purpura
- Hepatitis
- Inflammatory bowel disease
- Mesenteric adenitis
- Necrotizing enterocolitis
- Pancreatitis
- Peptic ulcer or gastritis
- Esophagitis or duodenitis

FUNCTIONAL

- Depression
- Functional abdominal pain
- Malingering
- Munchausen syndrome (+/- by proxy)

MISCELLANEOUS

- Abdominal migraine
- Cholelithiasis
- Colic
- Constipation
- Dysmenorrhea
- Ectopic pregnancy
- Endometriosis
- Ileus
- Intestinal pseudoobstruction
- Irritable bowel syndrome
- Lactose intolerance
- Mittelschmerz
- Nephrolithiasis
- Ovarian cyst
- Pregnancy
- Porphyria
- Sickle-cell disease
- Typhlitis

Approach to the Patient

GENERAL GOALS

One must decide if abdominal pain complaints require emergent, urgent, or nonimmediate intervention.

Phase 1: Careful and complete history and physical examination to narrow this extensive DDx.

Phase 2: Directed laboratory evaluations should be made to support more likely portions of the DDx. If a narrowed differential is difficult to formulate, every effort should be made to assure that the patient is clinically stable. A limited blood and/or radiographic evaluation screening with:

- CBC
- ESR

Comprehensive metabolic panel (i.e., Na +, K +, Cl −, CO2, BUN, Creatinine, glucose, total protein, albumin, ALT, Uric acid, LDH) Abdominal x-ray for significant abnormalities could be made to ensure there are no significant abnormalities above one's clinical suspicion.

Phase 3: Institute appropriate therapy related to diagnosis.

Data Gathering

HISTORY

Question: Location of pain?
Significance: Pain etiology. See Table 2.

Question: Duration of pain?
Significance: Acute versus chronic illness

Question: Onset and progression of symptoms?
Significance: Evolution of painful process

Question: Frank hematochezia?
Significance: Colonic bleeding or massive upper GI bleeding

Question: Abdominal distension?
Significance: Distension of an abdominal viscus by air, stool, or fluid

Question: Radiation of pain?
Significance: Certain entities characteristically have radiation of pain (i.e., pancreatitis to the back, appendicitis to the right lower quadrant)

Question: Pain relieved by bowel movements?
Significance: Etiology may be related to colonic distension (by air or stool) or inflammation (colitis)

Question: Bowel movement pattern, decrease in frequency or change in caliber?
Significance: Constipation

Question: Relationship to emesis
Significance: Usually upper intestinal tract disorders

 ## Physical Examination

Finding: Location of pain
Significance: See Table 2.

Finding: Reexamination by the same healthcare provider for changing characteristics
Significance: Evolution of abdominal process

Finding: Rebound tenderness
Significance: Peritonitis and the potential need for surgical intervention

Finding: Rectal examination
Significance: Peritoneal irritation, further localization of pain, masses, presence and consistency of stool, and/or occult heme

 ## Laboratory Aids

Test: CBC with differential
Significance: Total white count is nonspecific and may be a poor indicator of intestinal inflammation

Test: ESR
Significance: Nonspecific indicator of systemic inflammation

Test: Urinalysis
Significance: General screen for urinary tract abnormalities

Test: Two position abdominal x-ray
Significance: Possible clue to ileus, intussusception, intestinal obstruction, retained feces or gas

 ## Emergency Care

Every effort should be made to ensure that the patient is clinically stable. Frequent evaluation of vital signs and physical examination are a means of assessing evolving pain and ensuring that the patient is well enough for potential discharge.

Issues for Referral

Persistent abdominal pain without clear etiology or chronic gastrointestinal diseases should be referred to a pediatric gastroenterologist.

Clinical Pearls

- The farther the complaint of pain is away from the periumbilical region, the more likely the pain etiology represents organic disease.
- True nighttime waking with pain is more often correlated with organic disease than functional pain.

BIBLIOGRAPHY

Alfven G. One hundred cases of recurrent abdominal pain in children: diagnostic procedures and criteria for a psychosomatic diagnosis. [erratum appears in *Acta Paediatr* 2003;May;92(5):641]. *Acta Paediatrica* 2003;92(1):43–49.

Ball TM, Weydert JA. Methodological challenges to treatment trials for recurrent abdominal pain in children. *Arch Pediatr Adolesc Med* 2003;157(11):1121–1127.

Crushell E, et al. Importance of parental conceptual model of illness in severe recurrent abdominal pain. *Pediatrics* 2003;112(6 Pt 1):1368–1372.

Hyams JS. Functional gastrointestinal disorders. *Curr Opin Pediatr* 1999:Oct; 11(5):375–378.

Apley J. Psychosomatic aspects of gastrointestinal problems in children. *Clinics in Gastroenterology* 1977;6:311–320.

Zeiter DK, Hyams JS. Recurrent abdominal pain in children. *Pediatr Clin North Am* 2002;Feb;49(1):53–71.

Author: Kurt A. Brown, M.D.

Abnormal Bleeding

 ## Database

DEFINITION

Abnormal bleeding may present as: (1) frequent or significant mucocutaneous bleeding (epistaxis, bruising, gum bleeding or menorrhagia); (2) bleeding in unusual sites such as muscles, joints or internal organs; or (3) excessive postsurgical bleeding.

 ## Differential Diagnosis

Abnormal bleeding can be the result of an acquired or congenital disorder of platelets, the endothelial cell wall or coagulation factors. Platelet disorders may be quantitative or qualitative, disorders of the endothelial cell are often inflammatory, and disorders of co-agulation factors may be singular or multiple.

THROMBOCYTOPENIA: DEFECTIVE PRODUCTION

Congenital/Genetic

- Thrombocytopenia with absent radii (TAR) syndrome
- Amegakaryocytic thrombocytopenia
- Fanconi anemia
- Metabolic disorders
- Wiskott-Aldrich syndrome
- Bernard-Soulier syndrome
- Other rare familial syndromes (e.g., May-Hegglin anomaly)

Acquired

- Aplastic anemia
- Drug-associated marrow suppression
- Virus-associated marrow suppression (e.g., HIV)
- Chemotherapy
- Radiation injury
- Nutritional deficiencies (e.g., vitamin B_{12} and folate)

Marrow Infiltration

- Neoplasia (e.g., leukemia, neuroblastoma)
- Histiocytosis
- Osteopetrosis
- Myelofibrosis
- Hemophagocytic syndromes
- Storage diseases

THROMBOCYTOPENIA: INCREASED DESTRUCTION

- Idiopathic thrombocytopenic purpura (ITP)
- Neonatal alloimmune thrombocytopenia
- Maternal autoimmune thrombocytopenia
- Drug-induced (heparin, sulfonamides, digoxin, chloroquine)
- Sepsis/DIC
- Infection: viral, bacterial, fungal, rickettsial
- Microangiopathic process (e.g., TTP/HUS)
- Kasabach-Merritt syndrome
- Hypersplenism

PLATELET FUNCTION DISORDERS

- Storage pool disorders (e.g., dense granule deficiency, Hermansky-Pudlak syndrome)
- Platelet receptor abnormalities (e.g., Glanzmann thrombasthenia, ADP receptor defect)
- Drugs (e.g., aspirin, NSAIDs, guaifenesin, antihistamines, phenothiazines, anticonvulsants)
- Uremia
- Paraproteinemia

COAGULATION DISORDERS

Prolongation of aPTT

- Deficiency of factor VIII, IX, XI, or XII*
- Acquired inhibitor or lupus anticoagulant*
- von Willebrand disease (vWD) (PTT may be normal)

Prolongation of PT

- Mild vitamin K deficiency
- Liver disease, mild to moderate
- Deficiency of factor VII
- Factor VII inhibitor

Prolongation of PT and aPTT

- Liver disease, severe
- DIC
- Severe vitamin K deficiency
- Hemorrhagic disease of the newborn
- Deficiency of factors II, V, or X or fibrinogen
- Dysfibrinogenemia
- Hypoprothrombinemia associated with a lupus anticoagulant

Normal Screening Laboratory Tests

- vWD
- Factor XIII deficiency
- $\alpha 2$ antiplasmin deficiency
- Plasminogen activator inhibitor-I deficiency

VESSEL WALL DISORDERS

Congenital

- Hereditary hemorrhagic telangiectasia
- Ehlers-Danlos syndrome
- Osteogenesis imperfecta
- Marfan syndrome

Acquired

- Vasculitis (SLE, HSP, etc.)
- Scurvy

Approach to the Patient

- **Phase 1:** Includes a thorough history and physical examination as well as standard screening laboratory tests: PT/aPTT and platelet count. A familial history is an important component of this phase.

- **Phase 2:** If a bleeding disorder is suspected but the initial screening tests are negative, then testing for vWD, factor XIII deficiency, and dysfibrinogenemia is warranted. A bleeding time should be performed at this phase if a platelet dysfunction is suspected.

*Factor XII deficiency and lupus anticoagulant not associated with abnormal bleeding.

- **Phase 3:** Any abnormal screening tests need further evaluation with additional testing to define the specific disorder (e.g., factor assays, platelet aggregations).

 ## Data Gathering

HISTORY

By taking into account the patient's age, sex, clinical presentation, past medical history, and family history, the most likely cause of bleeding can usually be determined.

Question: Age of patient?
Significance: Serious congenital bleeding disorders usually present in the first year of life

Question: Sex of patient?
Significance: Hemophilia is X-linked

Question: Family history of bleeding?
Significance: Should suggest an inherited bleeding disorder

Question: Bleeding in unusual places without significant trauma (intracranial, joints, etc.)?
Significance: Significant factor deficiency-hemophilia

Question: Several surgeries in the past without bleeding?
Significance: An inherited bleeding disorder is unlikely

Question: Poorly controlled epistaxis?
Significance: Localized trauma (nose-picking) can cause epistaxis, unilateral epistaxis

Question: Sepsis?
Significance: DIC

Question: Mucocutaneous bleeding (gum bleeding, bruises, epistaxis, menorrhagia)?
Significance: Platelet disorder, vWD

Question: Petechiae?
Significance: Platelet disorders, vWD

Question: Recent medications?
Significance: Aspirin and other drugs affect platelet function

Question: Presence of renal or liver disease?
Significance: Azotemia contributes to bleeding. Liver disease reduces clotting factors.

Question: Severe malnutrition?
Significance: Scurvy, vitamin K deficiency, decreased hepatic synthesis of coagulation factors

Question: Sudden onset of petechiae?
Significance: ITP

 ## Physical Examination

Finding: Petechiae in skin and mucous membranes
Significance: Disorder of platelet number or function, vWD

Finding: Small bruises in unusual places?
Significance: Possible platelet disorder, vWD

Finding: Large bruises or palpable bruises?
Significance: Coagulation deficiencies, severe platelet disorders, or vWD

Finding: Delayed wound healing?
Significance: Factor XIII deficiency and dysfibrinogenemia

Finding: Purpura localized to lower body (buttocks, legs, ankles)?
Significance: Henoch-Schönlein purpura (HSP)

 ## Laboratory Aids

Phase 1: Initial Laboratory Screening

- Platelet count
- PT and aPTT

Phase 3: Discriminating Laboratory Studies for Abnormal Phase 1 Tests

When thrombocytopenia is present:

- Inspection of blood smear (screening for bone marrow diseases)
- Mean platelet volume (elevated in destructive causes, low in Wiskott-Aldrich)
- Bone marrow aspiration (rarely necessary)

When DIC is suspected (infection, liver disease, massive trauma, PT/aPTT prolonged):

- Fibrinogen
- D-dimer or fibrin split products
- Peripheral smear inspection for RBC fragments

Prolonged aPTT

- Inhibitor screen (50:50 mixing study of patient's and normal plasma)
- If aPTT fully corrects:

—Specific factor assays in the following order: VIII, IX, XI, XII
—If partial or no correction after mixing study:
—Inhibitor is present
—Confirmatory test for the presence of a lupus anticoagulant with a platelet neutralizing procedure

Prolonged PT

- Specific factor levels (II, VII, X)
- Inhibitor screen should also be considered for prolonged PT

Prolonged PT and aPTT

- Test for DIC, liver disease, and fibrinogen disorders, as described previously
- Vitamin K deficiency, moderate to severe
- Factor assays: V, X, II (prothrombin) and fibrinogen

Phase 2: Screening tests normal, bleeding disorder suspected

- Qualitative platelet defect suspected

—Bleeding time (not suggested for young children)

—Platelet aggregation and ATP release studies with ristocetin, collagen, thrombin, arachidonic acid and ADP

- vWD suspected

—Factor VIII:C
—von Willebrand factor (vWF; VIIIR:Ag)
—Ristocetin cofactor or von Willebrand factor activity
—vWF multimeric analysis- once diagnosis of vWD has been established

- Thrombin time or fibrinogen assay to screen for hypo- or dysfibrinogenemia

—Factor XIII deficiency suspected
—Factor XIII assay (urea clot lysis study)

PITFALLS OF TESTING

Bleeding Time

- Prolonged when platelets below 100,000/mm3
- Affected by medications such as aspirin, NSAIDs, antihistamines
- Does not correlate well with bleeding risk
- Accurate result depends on proper technique

PT and aPTT

- Normal ranges age dependent
- Polycythemia (Hct. 65%) or too little blood collected may result in a spuriously high result
- Heparin contamination in samples from arterial or venous catheter
- vWD Studies
- Normal ranges depend on patient's ABO blood group type
- Values fluctuate over time and may periodically be normal in affected individuals
- May require repeated testing to make diagnosis

 ## Emergency Care

- Pressure, elevation, and ice are generally helpful for most bleeding disorders when active bleeding is present.
- More definitive care is dictated by the nature of the underlying hemostatic defect. Platelet transfusions are useful in disorders of thrombocytopenia due to decreased production and for intrinsic qualitative platelet disorders but not for immune platelet disorders. Frozen plasma should only be used in severe cases when the exact diagnosis is not readily available but a defect in coagulation is suspected.
- Head injuries in patients with thrombocytopenia or hemophilia require immediate medical attention.

Common Questions and Answers

Q: What are the proper preoperative screening tests for bleeding disorders prior to elective surgery such as tonsillectomy?

A: A thorough personal history, familial history, and physical examination are by far the most important screening tests. A bleeding time is not recommended. A CBC and PT/aPTT are often requested by the surgeon, but normal results do not ensure that a bleeding complication will not occur. Overall the sensitivity and specificity of these screening tests is poor.

Q: Bruising is a normal part of childhood. How does one know when bruising is "too much"?
A: Small bruises seen only on the arms and legs of an active child probably reflect trauma rather than a bleeding disorder.

Issues for Referral

Indications

- If the history and physical examination suggest the presence of a bleeding disorder, or if the screening tests are abnormal, the patient should be referred to a pediatric hematologist.
- If von Willebrand disease is suspected, referral to a pediatric hematologist is usually necessary to determine the exact type and for testing that will assess the patient's response to ddAVP therapy.
- Patients with hemophilia should have regular visits to a hemophilia treatment center for follow-up and coordination of care.

Clinical Pearls

Children with bleeding disorders are more likely to have large bruises (greater than 5 cm), hematomas (palpable bruises), and bruises on more than one body part.
The aPTT may be extremely prolonged in patients with deficiencies of the contact factors (pre-Kallikrein, HMWK, factor XII). These deficiencies do not result in bleeding. Bleeding from a single site, such as menorrhagia or epistaxis alone, is more likely to be a result of local causes.

BIBLIOGRAPHY

Buchanan GR. Bleeding signs in children with idiopathic thrombocytopenic purpura. [Review. Tutorial] *J Pediatr Hematol/Oncol* 2003;25(Suppl 1):S42–S46.

Hayward CP. Inherited platelet disorders. *Curr Opin Hematol* 2003;10(5):362–368.

Koreth R, et al. Measurement of bleeding severity: a critical review. *Transfusion* 2004;44(4):605–617.

Laposata M, et al. *The Clinical Hemostasis Handbook.* Chicago: Year Book, 1989.

Manno CS. Difficult pediatric diagnoses—bruising and bleeding. *Pediatr Clin North Am* 1991;38:637–655.

Pramanik AK. Bleeding disorders in neonates. *Pediatr Rev* 1992;13(5):163–173.

Schafer AI. Thrombocytosis. *N Eng J Med* 2004;350(12):1211–1219.

Author: Leslie Raffini

Allergic Child

 Database

DEFINITION

The allergic child has the tendency toward IgE-mediated reactions in response to pollens, molds, environmental allergens, drugs, insect stings or foods. These reactions may manifest as any of the following: eczema, allergic rhinitis, asthma, angioedema, hives, or anaphylaxis.

 Differential Diagnosis

EYES

- Physical and chemical irritants
- Viral or bacterial infection

NOSE

- Recurrent upper respiratory tract infections
- Rhinitis medicamentosum—reaction to nasal sprays
- Drugs that cause nasal congestion

—Oral contraceptives
—Reserpine
—Guanethidine
—Propranolol
—Thioridazine
—Tricyclic antidepressants
—Aspirin

- Airway irritants

—Smoke
—Environmental pollution
—Cold air

- Kartagener syndrome—sinusitis, bronchiectasis, immobile cilia
- Cystic fibrosis
- Sinusitis

LUNGS

- Airway irritants

—Smoke
—Environmental pollution
—Cold air

- Gastroesophageal reflux
- Foreign body aspiration
- Anatomic defect in airway
- Cystic fibrosis
- Kartagener syndrome
- Immune deficiency

SKIN

- Viral exanthems
- Autoimmune disorders
- Physical and chemical irritants

 Data Gathering

HISTORY

The history may reveal seasonal or year round symptoms.
Specific questions are best asked systematically in a review of systems format.

Ears

- Otitis
- Myringotomy tubes
- Hearing loss

Nasal

- Frequent URIs
- Sinusitis
- Polyps
- Epistaxis
- Snoring
- Sneezing
- Rhinitis
- Deviated septum
- Obstruction
- Itch
- Mouth breathing
- Nasal discharge

Throat

- Sore throat
- Throat clearing
- Postnasal drip
- Palate itch
- Tonsillitis
- Tonsillectomy
- Croup

Chest

- Day cough
- Night cough
- Sputum production
- Pain
- Wheeze
- Shortness of breath
- Cyanosis

Eyes

- Itching
- Tearing
- Discharge
- Swelling
- Redness
- Rubbing

Gastrointestinal

- Anorexia
- Nausea
- Vomiting
- Diarrhea
- Constipation
- Gas
- Belching
- Abdominal pain
- Fatty or foul-smelling stools

Skin

- Eczema
- Hives
- Angioedema
- Contact dermatitis
- Seborrheic dermatitis
- Skin infections
- Pruritus

Genitourinary

- Dysuria
- Burning
- Polyuria
- Hematuria
- Enuresis

Headache

- Location
- Character
- Frequency
- Duration
- Nausea
- Vomiting
- Scotomata

Other important questions include:

Question: Does your child have food or drug allergies?

Significance: This question should be asked at every office visit. Be sure to ask what type of reaction the child had (many types of intolerances are called allergies by parents). Generally, allergies are IgE-mediated reactions resulting in wheezing, allergic rhinitis, hives, angioedema, eczema, or anaphylaxis. Intolerances generally include a nonspecific rash, diarrhea, gas, headache, or hyperactivity.

Question: Has your child ever been stung by a bee, and, if so, what was the reaction?
Significance: Systemic reactions are an indication for referral to an allergist for venom desensitization. Venom desensitization can be potentially lifesaving. Ask parents if they know the type of bee involved with the reaction. (Honeybees are the only bees that leave their stinger at the sting site.)

Question: Does anyone in your family have hayfever (allergic rhinitis), asthma, or eczema?
Significance: Familial history of atopy increases the likelihood of atopy in other family members.

Questions to ask regarding the environment:

Question: Do you have a basement?
Significance: Damp basements are a source of mold spores.

Question: Are there any damp areas in your home?
Significance: Damp areas serve to propagate mold growth in the home.

Question: Do you have forced air or radiator heat?
Significance: Forced air heat tends to blow allergen-laden dust around the home.

Question: How do you cool your home?
Significance: Opening outside windows lets the pollens from outside into the house.

Question: Do you have a humidifier?
Significance: Molds can grow in the water, and increased ambient humidity will raise the dust mite population in the home.

Question: Are there any smokers in the home?
Significance: Cigarette smoke is an airway irritant and can exacerbate respiratory difficulties.

Question: Are there any pets in the home, at school, or in day care?
Significance: Animal dander is a common aeroallergen. Pets should be excluded from the bedroom if a child has allergic stigmata (a pet that sleeps on the patient's bed is a common problem). If a child has severe allergies or asthma related to pet exposure, the animal should be removed from the home.

Question: Are there many stuffed animals or books in the bedroom?
Significance: Dust mites love these dust collectors, and they should be removed from the bedroom. Environmental control efforts should be focused on the bedroom as children typically spend more than one third of their time sleeping. Patients can have significant allergen exposure during sleep.

Question: Does the bedroom have carpeting?
Significance: Hardwood or tile floors are best to keep the dust mite population under control.

Question: How often do you wash the bedding, what type of pillow do you have, and is the mattress encased in plastic?
Significance: To keep the dust mite population under control the bedding should be washed in hot water at least once every 2 weeks (hot water kills dust mites), the pillow should be fiber filled, and the mattress should be encased in plastic.

Question: Where does the patient spend most of his time?
Significance: Allergenic exposure where most of the patient's time is spent is most important.

Question: Does the patient attend day care?
Significance: Day care is a major source of upper respiratory tract infections, which can mimic allergies and exacerbate reactive airway disease.

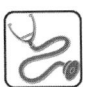 ## Physical Examination

A complete physical examination is essential to rule out systemic disease that can mimic allergies (i.e., clubbing, anatomic obstruction, heart murmur, etc.)

Finding: Ocular allergic signs
Significance: Allergic shiners are due to passive congestion in the nose, which impedes the venous return to the vessels under the eyes.

• Cobblestoning of the conjunctiva is associated with allergic conjunctivitis.
• Dennie-Morgan line, infraorbital folds associated with suborbital edema secondary to atopy.
• Clear stringy discharge is the characteristic eye discharge seen in allergic conjunctivitis.

Finding: Nasal allergic signs
Significance: Pale edematous nasal mucosa is characteristic of allergic rhinitis.

• Nasal crease across the bridge of nose is secondary to repeated upward rubbing of the nose.
• Clear nasal discharge with or without occlusion is characteristic of allergic rhinitis.

Finding: Ears allergic signs
Significance: Fluid in the middle ear, or retracted tympanic membranes may be associated with eustachian tube dysfunction seen with allergic inflammation.

Finding: Throat allergic signs
Significance: Cobblestoning of posterior pharynx secondary to submucosal lymphoid hyperplasia can be seen in allergic patients.

Finding: Lungs allergic signs
Significance: Wheezes, rhonchi, decreased air entry, and chronic obstruction can be secondary to allergic responses.

Finding: Skin allergic signs

Significance: Eczema, hives, angioedema, and dermatographism are all characteristic of allergic skin.

 ## Laboratory Aids

Test: Immediate hypersensitivity
Significance: Skin prick tests to suspected allergens based on history.

• These are the study of choice because of their low cost, high sensitivity, rapid results, and documented excellent correlation with clinical sensitivity especially to pollens and animal dander.
• Intradermal skin tests are reserved for patients who have a negative prick test and a suspicious history. These studies are more sensitive than prick tests but less specific, and pose a greater risk of systemic reactions.
• RAST tests (radioallergosorbent tests) measures free serum IgE to a specific antigen to which a particular patient may be sensitized. In children, these tests are primarily reserved for patients at risk for a severe systemic reaction from skin testing (i.e., Latex allergic patients), or in patients in whom skin testing is not feasible (i.e., patients with extensive skin disease). These tests are less sensitive than skin prick and intradermal tests. These tests are starting to be used more frequently in the diagnosis of food allergy although skin testing is still preferred.
• Serum IgE levels have a low sensitivity and, generally, are of little help.
• Presence of blood eosinophilia. Eosinophils in the blood or respiratory secretions may be indicative of an allergic diathesis.

Test: Baseline laboratory
Significance: Baseline pulmonary function studies should be obtained on asthmatic children, or in children with an allergic history to evaluate for obstructive disease.

Emergency Care

ANAPHYLAXIS

• Subcutaneous epinephrine 1:1,000
• Diphenhydramine
• Ranitidine
• Methylprednisolone
• Volume expander to correct hypotension

ACUTE ASTHMA

• Oxygen
• Inhaled β-agonist
• Subcutaneous epinephrine 1:1,000
• Steroids
• Magnesium or Terbutaline if life-threatening episode

 ## Common Questions and Answers

Q: Do children outgrow allergies?
A: In general, environmental allergies that cause rhinitis and asthma persist into

adulthood. However, most children outgrow food allergies to milk, egg, soy, wheat, and other foods. Children may rarely outgrow peanut, tree nut, or shellfish allergy.

Q: Can allergic children acquire more allergies?
A: Allergic children have the biologic potential to become sensitized to many environmental allergens. The goal should be to limit exposure to these antigens to prevent sensitization.

Q: If a parent is allergic to a specific allergen, can the child inherit this allergy?
A: Children inherit the tendency to be allergic, but they do not inherit specific allergies.

Q: What treatments are available?
A: Specific environmental control (as determined by skin testing), antihistamines, topical steroids, and immunotherapy.

Issues for Referral

• A patient failing medical management of upper respiratory or ocular allergies with routine antihistamine/decongestant medications. The allergist can help identify triggers contributing to the allergic symptomatology.
• Poorly controlled asthma not responding to intermittent inhaled β-agonists or an asthmatic who is symptomatic between exacerbations, or one that has an atypical pattern of exacerbations.
• Asthmatics with frequent hospitalizations or steroid-dependent asthmatics should also be referred.
• Patients who are absent from school frequently due to allergic or asthmatic symptoms.
• Patients with limited activities due to allergies or asthma.
• Strong seasonal history to respiratory complaints
• Systemic reaction to bee sting
• Difficult to manage eczema (atopic dermatitis)
• Recurrent croup
• Food allergy
• History of anaphylaxis
• Egg allergic patient who require influenza vaccine
• Drug allergy
• Latex allergy

BIBLIOGRAPHY

Fireman P. Diagnosis of allergic disorders. *Pediatr Rev* 1995;16(5):178–183.

Hopkin JM. Asthma and allergy-disorders of civilization? *Q J Med* 1998;91(3):169–170.

Middleton E, Reed CE, Adkinson NF, et al. *Allergic Principles and Practice.* 4th Ed. Philadelphia: Mosby, 1993.

Sites DP, Terr AI, Parslow TG. *Basic and Clinical Immunology.* 8th Ed. Englewood Cliffs, NJ: Prentice Hall, 1994.

Authors: Mathew Fogg
Christopher A. Smith 3rd edition

Alopecia (Hair loss)

 Database

DEFINITION

Alopecia is the absence of hair where it normally grows. Alopecia can be categorized as either acquired or congenital. Acquired and congenital causes of alopecia have diffuse and localized forms. Previous classifications of hair loss have included scarring and nonscarring forms. However, scarring may be difficult to appreciate, and some causes of hair loss have scarring at one time but not at another. For diagnostic purposes, it is more useful to classify hair loss as congenital versus acquired and further as circumscribed (localized) versus diffuse. This classification should be used when considering the various etiologies in the differential diagnosis.

 Differential Diagnosis

INFECTIOUS

- Tinea capitis
- Varicella
- Syphilis

CONGENITAL

- Aplasia cutis congenita
- Incontinentia pigmenti
- Oculomandibulofacial syndrome (sparse hair, hypoplastic teeth, cataracts, short stature)
- Goltz syndrome (alopecia, focal dermal hypoplasia, strabismus, nail dystrophy)
- Triangular alopecia of the frontal scalp
- Focal dermal hypoplasia
- Hair shaft defects (trichodystrophies)
- Ectodermal dysplasias
- Nevi
- Progeria

NUTRITIONAL

- Zinc deficiency
- Marasmus
- Kwashiorkor
- Hypervitaminosis A
- Celiac disease

ENDOCRINOLOGIC

- Androgenetic alopecia
- Hypothyroidism
- Hyperthyroidism
- Hypoparathyroidism
- Hypopituitarism
- Diabetes mellitus

RHEUMATOLOGIC

- Systemic lupus erythematosus
- Scleroderma

TRAUMA

- Traction alopecia
- Trichotillomania
- Scalp electrode scar from in utero monitoring

TOXIN

- Radiation
- Medications (e.g., anticoagulants, antimetabolites)
- Heavy metals (e.g., arsenic, lead)

MISCELLANEOUS

- Alopecia areata (autoimmune)
- Telogen effluvium
- Darier disease (keratotic crused papules, keratosis follicularis)
- Lichen planus
- Burn

Approach to the Patient

GENERAL GOALS

Phase 1: Attempt to classify the alopecia in order to aid in diagnosis and subsequent treatment plan. In taking the history, assess whether the loss is acquired or congenital.

Phase 2: In performing the physical examination, assess if the hair loss is localized or diffuse.
Recognize whether the alopecia is treatable or likely to be self-limited.
Consider most likely diagnoses first (tinea capitis, traumatic alopecia, alopecia areata)

Phase 3: Identify whether there are associated abnormalities that may be part of a syndrome.
Determine if there is an endocrine abnormality or a toxin/medication effect that should be addressed. Refer or consult with a specialist when necessary.

Hints for Screening Problem

- Consider the most likely diagnoses first.
- Specific questions can include whether they have seen an increased amount of hair in the brush or in the shower/tub drain, whether their hair appears or feels thinner, whether they have noted patches of hair loss or broken hairs.

 Data Gathering

HISTORY

Question: Is the hair loss congenital or acquired?
Significance: Most cases of alopecia are acquired and, of these, tinea capitis is most common, followed by traumatic alopecia and alopecia areata.

Question: Was there a recent stressful event?
Significance: Telogen effluvium is suggested when alopecia is preceded by a psychologically or physically stressful event 6–16 weeks prior to the onset of hair loss. Growing hairs convert rapidly to resting hairs. Spontaneous regrowth is expected unless the stressful event recurs.

Question: Does the child suck his/her thumb?
Significance: Trichotillomania is frequently associated with a finger sucking habit.

Question: Is anyone else currently (or recently) affected?
Significance: Tinea capitis can be spread by close contact with other infected individuals.

Question: Has a family member had patches of alopecia that resolved?
Significance: There is a family history in 10%–42% of cases of alopecia areata.

Question: Have there been any exposures to medication, chemicals, or heavy metals?
Significance: Exposures associated with alopecia include antimetabolites, anticoagulants, antithyroid medications, lead and arsenic.

 Physical Examination

Finding: Is the hair loss localized or diffuse?
Significance: Most cases of alopecia are localized and, of these, tinea capitis is the most common.

Finding: Are there any associated systemic signs or any nonscalp findings?
Significance: May signify a genetic syndrome or endocrine abnormality.

Finding: Scalp appears normal
Significance: In alopecia areata, the scalp appears normal. In tinea capitis, scalp is often scaly and may be erythematous.

Finding: Areas of hair loss with broken hair stubs amidst scaly and/or erythematous scalp
Significance: Referred to as "black-dot" alopecia.

Finding: Bizarre configuration and irregular outline of hair loss. Hairs of varying lengths.
Significance: Distinguishes traction/traumatic alopecia from alopecia areata.

Finding: S[...]ts
Significanc[...]
associated [...]
black dot [...]is.

Finding: F[...]
decreased [...]
Significanc[...]
androgene[...]

Finding: [...]h
small nod[...]
increased [...]
Significan[...]
hair) is a [...]
Other hai[...]
fragility i[...]
trichorrhe[...]s
kinky hai[...]y.

Finding: [...]ic
changes and fine stippling
Significance: Nail defects are seen in
10%-20% of cases of alopecia areata. The fine
stippling has been described as a "hammered
brass" appearance. Nail defects accompanying
localized alopecia along with syndactyly,
strabismus, and dermal hypoplasia may be
found in Goltz syndrome. In ectodermal
dysplasias, the nails, hair, teeth, or glands
may be affected.

Finding: Occipital or cervical
lymphadenopathy
Significance: Found with infectious causes of
alopecia, such as tinea capitis.

Finding: Pubic hair and eyebrow hair loss
Significance: Found in a form of alopecia
areata called alopecia universalis, where
nearly all body hair is lost (alopecia totalis
involves the loss of all scalp hair). Body hair
loss such as pubic hair or eyebrow hair may
also occur in trichotillomania.

Laboratory Aids

Test: Potassium hydroxide exam (KOH)
Significance: Can use this test when assessing
for tinea capitis as a cause of alopecia.
Hyphae and spores within hair shaft indicate
tinea capitis, usually caused by *Trichophyton
tonsurans*. With Microsporum, spores surround
the hair shaft.

Test: Fungal culture
Significance: Recommended for use when
assessing for tinea capitis as a cause of
alopecia. Definitive results may take up to
several weeks, may treat pending results.
Using a cotton tipped applicator, culturette,
toothbrush or direct plating on Sabouraud
dextrose agar, culture will be positive for
Trichophyton tonsurans in >90% of cases in
North America. Less common are *Microsporum
canis*, *Microsporum audouinii*, *Trichophyton
mentagrophytes*, and *Trichophyton
schoenleinii*.

Test: Dermatophyte Testing Medium (DTM)
Significance: Can use this test when assessing
for tinea capitis as a cause of alopecia,
although definitive results may take from days
to weeks. If dermatophyte colonies grow on
the media, the phenol red indicator in the
agar will turn from yellow to red.

Test: Wood light (lamp) examination
Significance: When the fluorescent light of a
Wood lamp shines upon scalp infections with
tinea capitis caused by *Microsporum canis*,
Microsporum audouinii, or *Trichophyton
schoenleinii*, the scalp will fluoresce green.
However, *Trichophyton tonsurans* does not
fluoresce.

Test: Thyroid testing, glucose levels
Significance: With diffuse alopecia, consider
endocrine tests if other relevant symptoms
occur

Test: Scalp biopsy
Significance: Can help to distinguish alopecia
areata and trichotillomania. In alopecia
areata, hair follicles become small but
continue to produce fine hairs; there is
mitotic activity in the matrix and often
inflammation is present. In contrast, in
trichotillomania, follicles are not small, yet
they are usually in a transitional (catagen)
phase and no longer produce normal hair
shafts. There is keratinous debris, fibrosis,
and clumps of dark melanin pigment present.
Significant inflammation is absent.

Test: Hair pluck
Significance: Used to determine the ratio of
telogen (resting) to anagen (growing) hairs.
More than 25% telogen hairs are indicative of
telogen effluvium. Approximately 50 hairs are
plucked (can be with one short firm tug using
a hemostat 1 cm from scalp) and examined
under a low power lens.

Emergency Care

• Alopecia itself does not require emergency
care.
• If alopecia signifies a toxic exposure or an
endocrine abnormality, the underlying
condition may require prompt diagnosis and
treatment.
• Infectious causes of alopecia (such as with
tinea capitis) should be treated promptly.

Common Questions and Answers

Q: When can children with tinea capitis return
to school?
A: Once treatment with a systemic antifungal
has begun, the child may return to school. A
topical shampoo, such as selenium sulfide or
ketoconazole shampoo is recommended to
decrease fungal shedding and risk of spread
to others.

Q: Will the hair grow back?
A: For the 3 most common causes of alopecia
(accounting for 90% of cases) in children
(tinea capitis, alopecia areata, and traction
alopecia) hair will regrow.

Q: Where can parents and patients gain
additional information and psychologic
support?
A: There is a National Alopecia Areata
Foundation (http://www.naaf.org) and a
National Foundation for Ectodermal Dysplasia
(http://www.nfed.org). More information is
available by searching "alopecia" at The
National Library of Medicine's health
information site http://medlineplus.gov.

Issues for Referral

• Consider referral to Dermatology with any
case of alopecia that is not acquired and
localized.
• When alopecia has an endocrine or genetic
cause, consider referral to the appropriate
subspecialist. Treatment may require a
multidisciplinary approach.

Clinical Pearls

• Topical antifungals alone are not adequate
to treat tinea capitis.
• Other than reassurance and waiting, there
is no proven therapy for alopecia areata
(although topical or intralesional steroids may
be tried).
• Patients often deny trichotillomania, and
direct confrontation is rarely helpful.
• Many normal healthy newborns lose their
hair in the first few months of life. Telogen
effluvium accounts for this loss. It may be
exacerbated by friction from bed sheets,
especially in atopic infants.
• Normally, 50 to 100 hairs are shed and
simultaneously replaced every day, on
average.

ICD-9-CM 704.00

BIBLIOGRAPHY

American Academy of Pediatrics. Tinea Capitis.
In: Pickering LK, ed. Red Book: 2003 *Report of
the Committee on Infectious Diseases*. 26th
Ed. Elk Grove Village, IL: American Academy
of Pediatrics, 2003:617–618.

Hantash BM, Schwartz RA. Traction alopecia
in children. *Cutis* 2003;71:18–20.

McMichael AJ. Hair and scalp disorders in
ethnic populations. *Dermatol Clin*
2003;21:629–644.

Price VH. Androgenetic alopecia in
adolescents. *Cutis* 2003;71:115–121.

Vasiloudes P, et al. Bald spots: remember the
"big three." *Contemp Pediatr* 1997;14:76–91.

Whiting DA. Chronic telogen effluvium.
Dermatol Clin 1996;14:723–31.

Author: Terry Kind

Back Pain

Database

DEFINITION

• Back pain refers to any condition in which a patient has complaints of discomfort of the thoracic, lumbar, or sacral spine.
• Back pain can result from a variety of causes, involving the bony or muscular structures of the back, intervertebral discs, spinal cord, or peripheral nerves.
• Inheritance patterns for some of the congenital (e.g., scoliosis, Scheuermann kyphosis) and inflammatory/rheumatologic causes of back pain have been described.
• There is a 30%–50% lifetime incidence of back pain in adolescents. Eight percent of adolescents report recurrent or chronic back pain. Discitis and osteomyelitis are most commonly seen in children less than 10 years of age. Spondylolysis, spondylolisthesis, Scheuermann kyphosis, herniated disc, tumors, and apophyseal ring fractures are usually seen in children over 10 years.

COMPLICATIONS

Depending on the underlying etiology, complications of missed diagnosis or improper management can include paralysis or other permanent neuromuscular injury, and neoplastic/paraneoplastic or infectious syndromes.

PROGNOSIS

• Prognosis is dependent on the underlying cause of back pain. The majority, if properly diagnosed and treated, do well, without significant sequelae.
• It is not possible to predict when spondylolysis will worsen or progress to spondylolisthesis, or the future course of Scheuermann kyphosis.

Differential Diagnosis

CONGENITAL

• Tethered cord
• Syringomyelia (may also be traumatic)

INFLAMMATORY

• Ankylosing spondylitis
• Enteropathic arthritis
• Intervertebral disc calcification

INFECTIOUS

• Tuberculosis
• Discitis
• Epidural abscess

TRAUMA

• "Musculotendinous" strain
• Spondylolysis (stress fracture of posterior vertebral elements, thought to be a repetitive stress injury)
• Spondylolisthesis (anterior displacement or "slip" of the vertebral body, associated with bilateral spondylolysis)
• Herniated disc
• Apophyseal ring fracture (fracture separating the vertebral body and cartilaginous ring apophysis)
• Epidural hematoma (traumatic or due to bleeding diathesis)

NEOPLASTIC

Bony

• Osteoid osteoma, osteoblastoma
• Osteosarcoma
• Ewing sarcoma
• Aneurysmal bone cyst

Metastatic/Other

• Leukemia, lymphoma
• Eosinophilic granuloma
• Glioma
• Neuroblastoma
• Rhabdomyosarcoma

DEVELOPMENTAL

• Scheuermann kyphosis (excessive kyphosis/"hunchback" due to abnormal ossification causing "wedging" of the vertebral bodies)
• Painful scoliosis

REFERRED

• Pyelonephritis
• Pancreatitis

PSYCHOGENIC

Data Gathering

Warning signs of potentially serious causes of back pain in children include:

• Young age (less than 4 years old)
• Chronic interference with normal activity (e.g., school, sports, play)
• Duration of pain longer than 4 weeks
• Associated fever, weight loss, or other systemic symptoms
• Postural shift of trunk
• Any neurologic abnormality
• Limitation of spinal motion (e.g., bending forward, straight leg raise)
• Painful or left thoracic scoliosis

HISTORY

Question: Onset, duration, and frequency of pain?
Significance: Fleeting or short duration of pain is rarely serious.

Question: Interference with activity?
Significance: Often a marker of severe disease.

Question: Physical activity and trauma history?
Significance: Spondylolysis and spondylolisthesis are more commonly seen in children who repeatedly twist, bend, or hyperextend their spine (e.g., participate in gymnastics, diving, tennis, contact sports, weightlifting, etc.). Heavy lifting may contribute to Scheuermann kyphosis. Trauma causes one third of herniated disc injuries.

Question: Use of backpack?
Significance: Carrying a backpack with >15% of one's body weight may cause back pain.

Question: Pain aggravated by activity and/or relieved by rest?
Significance: Overuse conditions, spondylolysis, or spondylolisthesis is likely.

Question: Radiation of pain?
Significance: Pain that shoots down the legs is suggestive of a herniated disc, spondylolisthesis, epidural abscess, or osteoid osteoma.

Question: Motor, sensory, or bowel/bladder symptoms?
Significance: Consider syringomyelia or spinal cord abnormalities (e.g., congenital, tumors, or herniated disc).

Question: Growth history?
Significance: Adolescents during growth spurts are more prone to musculotendinous strain.

Question: Previous history of scoliosis?
Significance: Idiopathic scoliosis is rarely painful or functionally limiting.

SPECIAL QUESTIONS

Pain that awakens the child from sleep and/or relief with NSAIDs. Osteoid osteoma and osteoblastoma often present with nighttime back pain and/or recurrent back pain relieved by NSAIDs.
Pain aggravated by prone position is suggestive of an epidural abscess.

Physical Examination

Finding: Inspect for any occult abnormalities
Significance: Sacral dimples, hair tufts, vascular anomalies, café-au-lait spots, or discrepancies in limb length. If the head is not midline, consider syringomyelia, tumor, spondylolisthesis, or herniated disc. Shortened waistline and flattening or "heart shaped" buttocks are often seen in spondylolisthesis.

Finding: With the child's feet together and knees and hips straight, observe the child from the back and side, both standing and through full range of motion of the spine.
Significance: This evaluates the patient for scoliosis, kyphosis, and range of motion. Lumbar lordosis should "reverse" when the child bends over; if it does not, significant pathology should be suspected.
During forward flexion: if thoracic kyphosis is accentuated, suspect Scheuermann kyphosis; if stiffness is observed, consider inflammatory, infectious, or neoplastic causes. Stiffness during extension is typical of discitis.

Finding: Palpate for any point or focal tenderness
Significance: Fractures often manifest with point tenderness.

Finding: Assess neurologic function
Significance: In young children, this may be evaluated by observing gait, heel- and toe-walking, and rising from a squat. Complete examination of the lower body, including examination of sensation and rectal tone, should be performed. Any abnormal neurologic findings should be thoroughly investigated.

Finding: Abnormal gait
Significance: Consider spondylolisthesis (short stride or "pelvic waddle") or herniated disc.

Finding: Hamstring tightness and/or decreased hip flexion
Significance: May be seen in spondylolisthesis and discitis.

Finding: With the patient supine, examine the abdomen and have the patient perform a straight leg raise
Significance: Limitation in leg raise or radiating pain is suggestive of neurologic abnormality. Lack of abdominal reflexes may suggest syringomyelia.

SPECIFIC TESTS

• Standing hyperextension (bending backward) often reproduces the lower lumbar pain of spondylolysis.
• A bony "ledge"/step-off on palpation of the lumbar spine or an anterior bony mass on rectal examination is sometimes appreciated with spondylolisthesis.
• Asymmetry of lower extremity muscle circumference may be a sign of nerve impingement due to a herniated disc.

 ## Laboratory Aids

Test: Plain radiographs (AP and lateral, and if warranted, oblique and flexion/extension views) of the spine are indicated if any worrisome signs or symptoms are present.
Significance: Spondylolysis has the appearance of a "collar" (lucent line) on the "Scottie dog's" neck.

Test: Bone or SPECT scan
Significance: More sensitive for occult or subtle lesions, and should be obtained if a serious etiology is clinically suspected.

Test: MRI
Significance: The preferred examination for suspected neurologic or disc injury.

Test: Blood tests (e.g., sed rate, HLA-B27, ANA, rheumatoid factor, blood culture)
Significance: Indicated only if infectious or rheumatologic etiologies are considered.

Test: Bacterial cultures (needle aspiration or open biopsy)
Significance: Positive in only 25%–50% of discitis patients. Routine biopsy, therefore, is not recommended in cases of suspected discitis. Staphylococcal species are the most frequently recovered organism.

 ## Therapy

• If no warning signs are present, conservative management with rest, activity modification, ice or heat (whichever is appropriate), acetaminophen or ibuprofen, muscle relaxants, physical therapy, and close follow-up is reasonable. A back brace may also be helpful in spondylolisthesis and Scheuermann kyphosis.
• Conservative medical treatment is indicated for spondylolysis and spondylolisthesis of less than 50% slip. Surgical treatment is warranted for slip greater than 50% or persistent back pain.
• Antistaphylococcal medications are indicated in cases of discitis. The choice between oral or intravenous medications depends on the severity of the patient's symptoms.
• There is limited evidence in adults that lumbar supports are effective in treating low back pain.

 ## Follow-Up

• Patients managed conservatively should be reevaluated within 2 weeks.
• All patients should be instructed to follow-up immediately for any worsening symptoms.

PREVENTION

• When the child has recuperated, back muscle strengthening and hamstring stretching exercises may be helpful.
• If the child uses a backpack, the maximum load should be 10%-15% of their body weight.
• When participating in sports, appropriate protective equipment should be used and proper technique should be emphasized.
• In athletes, training more than 15 hours per week has been associated with increased risk of injury.
• In adult studies, lumbar supports do not appear to be effective at preventing low back pain.

PITFALLS

• Missed diagnosis of a serious cause of back pain.
• Plain films are often normal, even in cases with serious causes.

 ## Common Questions and Answers

Q: Which children should have activity restrictions?
A: "High-risk" children (e.g., those with spinal or bony abnormalities, or familial histories of spondylolysis) should avoid hyperextension and contact sports.

Q: When can/should the child resume normal activities?
A: "Low-risk" children, with a normal neurologic exam, can resume activity or sports when they are pain free.

BIBLIOGRAPHY

Gerbino PG, Micheli LJ. Back injuries in the young athlete. *Clin Sports Med* 1995;14(3):571–590.

Ginsburg GM, Bassett GS. Back pain in children and adolescents: evaluation and differential diagnosis. *J Am Acad Orthop Surg* 1997;5(2):67–78.

Jellema P, van Tulder MW, van Poppel MNM, et al. Lumbar supports for prevention and treatment of low back pain. *Spine* 2001;26(4):377–386.

Mackenzie WG, et al. Backpacks in children. *Clin Orthop Rel Res* 2003;409:78–84.

Mason DE. Back pain in children. *Pediatr Ann* 1999;28(12):727–738.

Payne WK, Ogilvie JW. Back pain in children and adolescents. *Pediatr Clin North Am* 1996;43(4):899–917.

Trainor TJ, Wiesel SW. Epidemiology of back pain in the athlete. *Clin Sports Med* 2002;21(1):93–103.

Author: Thomas H. Chun

Behavioral or Psychiatric Problems

Database

DEFINITION

Behavioral, developmental, or psychosocial problems that require medical or psychiatric treatment, or that cause the child significant impairment. Epidemiologic research indicates that between 14% and 20% of American children have moderate to severe psychiatric disorders. Unfortunately, research also shows that 30% of children with mental retardation and other developmental disabilities, and 50%–80% of children with other mental health problems are not recognized by their primary care providers.

Differential Diagnosis

ORGANIC CAUSES

- CNS infections or parainfectious syndromes
- Substance abuse, toxic ingestions, medication adverse effects
- Intracranial trauma or other injury
- CNS tumors
- Endocrine disorders

—Thyroid or adrenal dysfunction

- Metabolic disorders

—Abnormal glucose
—Sodium
—Potassium
—Calcium

- Migraines
- Seizure disorders
- Hematologic disorders

—Porphyria
—Severe anemia

- Hypoxia
- Other cardiopulmonary disturbances

Among psychobehavioral disorders, many disorders have similar symptoms.

- Attention deficit/hyperactivity disorder (ADHD) may be difficult to distinguish from mood (depression or bipolar disorder), anxiety (including school phobia), posttraumatic stress, and tic disorders, substance abuse, hearing or vision impairment, and learning disabilities.
- Social withdrawal may be a sign of depression, neglect, pervasive developmental disorder (PDD), sensory impairment (e.g., deafness), or learning disability.
- Psychotic symptoms are seen not only in psychotic disorders, but also in mood disorders (depression, bipolar disorder), borderline personality disorder, and substance abuse.
- Aggressive or violent behavior is not a diagnosis unto itself, but can represent a final common pathway of depression, psychosis, delirium, substance abuse, ADHD (uncommon), physical or sexual abuse, or family dysfunction.

Approach to the Patient

GENERAL GOALS

Phase 1: Assess the patient for safety (i.e., suicidality, homicidality, and adequate support and supervision at home).

Phase 2: Rule out organic causes.

Phase 3: As organic causes are being investigated, establish psychiatric/psychologic causes as a possible diagnosis.

Phase 4: Work with the family to accept possibility of psychiatric/psychologic diagnosis and if necessary, facilitate referral to mental health services.

HINTS FOR SCREENING PROBLEMS

- Parents and children often are reluctant to discuss psychosocial issues. Standard developmental checklists in pediatric encounter forms often are inadequate for this purpose. Asking "Do you have any concerns about your child's behavior or emotional well-being?" has been suggested as a way to increase the likelihood of identifying such problems.
- There is strong evidence for a genetic risk of bipolar disorder (manic-depression), schizophrenia, and depression. There is growing evidence that other conditions, e.g., anxiety, ADHD, PDD, and tic disorders, may be genetically transmissible. Twin studies (monozygotic versus dizygotic) suggest that personality disorders have a significant genetic component.
- Many disorders, e.g., ADHD (between 3:1 to 9:1), depression (1:2), etc., have distinct male/female preponderance.
- Suicide is epidemic. Eight percent of high school students attempt suicide, 25% of which require medical attention. Fifty percent of attempters seek medical care in the month preceding their attempt, 25% in the preceding week.
- Conservative estimates of the prevalence of depression in children and adolescents range from 5%–10%.
- Eating disorders, while relatively uncommon (0.5%–1% prevalence), have a 5%–15% mortality rate.

Data Gathering

HISTORY

- A psychobehavioral assessment should include a history of the presenting complaint, a past medical, developmental, and behavioral/psychiatric history, and a complete familial history and review of systems.
- The "SHADSSS" mnemonic is a useful inventory of psychosocial functioning. It is structured such that the least threatening topics are asked first, the most intimate last. All of these areas of psychosocial functioning should be assessed in all patients.

—School (in school? grades? relationships with peers and teachers?)
—Home (living situation? relationship with parents? siblings?)
—Activities (how do patients spend their free time?)
—Depression
—Substance abuse (including alcohol and tobacco)
—Sexuality (including abuse, STDs, and pregnancy)
—Safety (suicidality, homicidality, plans for revenge or violence)

Children do not exist in a vacuum. All families should receive a family assessment. Families/support systems are crucial for the ultimate success of any treatment plan. At a minimum, a family assessment should include a discussion of:

- Constitution of household, custody/visitation arrangements
- Who supervises the child or provides child care
- Stressors on the family (emotional, financial, interpersonal, violence within the family, involvement with law enforcement or social services, etc.)
- Strategies used by the family in coping with conflicts, problems, stressors, etc.

Physical Examination

A thorough physical examination should be performed on all patients. The goal is to detect any abnormalities suggestive of an organic cause for the patient's symptoms (see Differential Diagnosis).

Behavioral or Psychiatric Problems

 ## Laboratory Aids

There is no set of "routine" laboratory tests that should be ordered to rule out an organic etiology of the behavioral or psychiatric symptoms. Tests should be performed on the basis of clinical suspicion.

SPECIFIC RESOURCES

• The use of screening questionnaires (see Bibliography), parent monitoring forms/diaries, and direct observation of parent–child interactions can be used, depending on the practitioner's experience, familiarity, and confidence with these modalities, as well as the practice setting. Screening for maternal depression may also be important in detecting psychosocial dysfunction.
• The Pediatric Symptom Checklist (PSC) is a well-validated 35-item, easily scored, parent-report screen of emotional and behavioral problems. It can be completed in 5 minutes and is easily administered in an office waiting area. The Child Behavior Checklist (CBCL) provides more in-depth assessment, but is more difficult to administer and score. A multitude of other screening tools have been developed, which are of varying utility to the pediatric practitioner.
• Conners Rating Scales alone are not sufficient to diagnose ADHD. It is a clinical diagnosis, based on pervasive inattention, hyperactivity, or impulsivity across different settings.
• Published in 1996 by the American Academy of Pediatrics, the *Diagnostic and Statistical Manual for Primary Care* (DSM-PC), child and adolescent version, is the result of collaborative efforts by pediatricians (primary care, and behavioral and developmental specialists), and child psychiatrists, psychologists, and neurologists. It provides a concise, user-friendly guide for diagnosing mental disorders in children and adolescents.

Clinical Pearls

• Children on psychotropic medications should be monitored for adverse effects.
• Stimulants: frequent assessment of growth, heart rate, and blood pressure every 3 to 6 months. Those on pemoline (Cylert) should have LFTs checked every 6 to 12 months.
• Tricyclic antidepressants: baseline ECG (before starting medication), and ECGs 1 month after starting medications and every 6 months thereafter.
• Antipsychotics: reassessment at 2, 4, and 12 weeks after starting medication, and every 3 to 6 months thereafter for adverse effects (dystonia, anticholinergic symptoms, movement disorders).
• "Atypical" antipsychotics: frequently cause significant weight gain and may cause impaired glucose tolerance and prolong QTc. Patients' weight should be closely monitored, as well as any signs of diabetes mellitus. An ECG should be obtained before and after starting zisprasidone.

PITFALLS

• Not asking about behavioral or psychiatric problems. Parents are often reluctant to talk about such problems, thinking such problems are stigmatizing.
• Missed psychiatric diagnosis, especially suicidality, homicidality, or plans for revenge or violence.
• Confusing the degree of medical severity of a suicide attempt with the degree of suicide intent, i.e., "(S)he isn't significantly injured, so (s)he isn't seriously suicidal." Children and adolescents often misjudge the lethality of their suicide methods. All attempts must be taken seriously.
• Deciding on a diagnosis and/or treatment without a complete evaluation. Many psychiatric disorders can present in similar fashion (see Differential Diagnosis). The success of any treatment plan, as well as avoidance of erroneously "labeling" a child (with an incorrect diagnosis), depends on an accurate diagnosis, based on a thorough biopsychosocial evaluation.
• Many patients with primary psychiatric disorders will present with vague physical complaints. All patients with such complaints should be screened for psychiatric problems.
• Delay in diagnosis or referral for treatment, e.g., prognosis for learning disabilities and hearing impairment, is associated with timely intervention.

 ## Common Questions and Answers

Q: When should a child be referred to a specialist?
A: Whenever there is uncertainty about diagnosis or management, or when the treatment needs of the patient exceed the practitioner's capacity to provide them.

Q: How do you get children and families to talk about their problems?
A: There is no "trick." Being a patient, empathetic, nonjudgmental listener is the best strategy.

Q: What constitutes a psychiatric emergency?
A: Any situation where the safety or functioning of the child, family, or another person is endangered.

BIBLIOGRAPHY

Achenbach TM, Ruffle TM. The child behavior checklist and related forms for assessing behavioral/emotional problems and competencies. *Pediatr Rev* 2000;21(8): 265–271.

American Academy of Child and Adolescent Psychiatry: Practice parameter for the assessment and treatment of children and adolescents with suicidal behavior. *J Am Acad Child Adol Psychiatry* 2001;40(Suppl):24S–51S.

American Academy of Pediatrics, ADHD subcommittee. Clinical practice guideline: diagnosis and evaluation of the child with ADHD. *Pediatrics* 2000;105(5):1158–1170.

Cantwell DP. Attention deficit disorder: a review of the past 10 years. *J Am Acad Child Adolesc Psychiatry* 1996;35(8):978–987.

Casidy LJ, Jellinek MS. Approaches to recognition and management of childhood psychiatric disorders in pediatric primary care. *Pediatr Clin North Am* 1998;45(5):1037–1052.

Clark LR, Ginsburg KR. How to talk to your teenage patients. *Contemp Adolesc Gynecol* 1995;Winter:23–27.

Glascoe FP. Early detection of developmental and behavioral problems. *Pediatr Rev* 2000;21(8):272–279.

Green WH. *Child and Adolescent Clinical Psychopharmacology*. 3rd Ed., Philadelphia: Lippincott Williams & Wilkins, 2001.

Roberts RE, et al. Prevalence of psychopathology among children and adolescents. *Am J Psych* 1998;155(6): 715–725.

Stancin T, Palermo TM. A review of behavioral screening practices in pediatric settings: do they pass the test? *J Dev Behav Pediatr* 1997;18(3):183–194.

Wolralch ML. Diagnostic and statistical manual for primary care (DSM-PC) child and adolescent version: design, intent, and hopes for the future. *J Dev Behav Pediatr* 1997;18(3):171–182.

Author: Thomas H. Chun

Bruising

 Database

DEFINITION

Bruises are the result of extravasation of blood into the skin. Conventional usage often groups petechiae and bruises (or ecchymoses) together as purpura and defines them as follows:

- Petechiae: flat, red, or reddish purple, 1 to 3 mm, nonblanching
- Ecchymoses: larger than petechiae, due to local extravasation, nonpulsatile, sometimes palpable, color depends on age of lesion

 Differential Diagnosis

CONGENITAL/ANATOMIC

- Coagulation factor abnormality: hemophilia, von Willebrand disease
- Platelet defect: Bernard-Soulier syndrome, Glanzmann thrombasthenia, and storage pool defects
- Congenital alloimmune or isoimmune thrombocytopenia
- Neonatal extramedullary hematopoiesis
- Hereditary hemorrhagic telangiectasia

INFECTIOUS

- Meningococcemia
- Viral infections (coxsackieviruses, echoviruses)
- Rocky Mountain spotted fever (RMSF)
- Syphilis
- Pertussis—secondary to severe cough
- Septic or fat emboli
- DIC—acquired factor deficiency

TOXIC, ENVIRONMENTAL, DRUGS

- Warfarin—acquired factor deficiency
- Corticosteroids—striae caused by increased capillary fragility
- Aspirin and ibuprofen—cause a qualitative platelet abnormality
- Sulfonamides
- Bismuth
- Chloramphenicol

TRAUMA

- Normal activity
- Child abuse
- Valsalva, crying, forceful coughing
- Cupping or coin rubbing
- Tight garments

TUMOR (QUANTITATIVE PLATELET ABNORMALITY)

- Bone marrow replacement–leukemia, myelofibrosis

GENETIC/METABOLIC

- Uremia
- Vitamin C deficiency
- Vitamin K deficiency—due to antibiotics, biliary atresia, malabsorption (acquired factor deficiency)

ALLERGIC/INFLAMMATORY/VASCULITIC

- Henoch-Schönlein purpura (HSP)
- Bone marrow failure—aplastic anemia (including Fanconi, PNH)
- Increased destruction—idiopathic thrombocytopenic purpura, Evan syndrome, lupus
- Nephrotic syndrome
- Collagen vascular disease
- Ehlers-Danlos syndrome
- Snake bite (copperhead)

MISCELLANEOUS (DISORDERS THAT SIMULATE BRUISES)

- Ataxia telangiectasia
- Cherry angiomata
- Kaposi sarcoma

Approach to the Patient

GENERAL GOAL

To determine if the etiology of the bruising is due to thrombocytopenia, a coagulation disorder, or an extrinsic factor (such as trauma, infection, etc.).

Phase 1: Determine if the history of bruising and/or petechiae is acute or chronic in onset and if there is known trauma versus spontaneous lesions (see table, Most Common Causes of Bruising).

The acute onset of diffuse subcutaneous bleeding with bruises of different ages may indicate severe thrombocytopenia. Generally, children will not bruise or develop petechiae spontaneously until the platelet count is under 20,000/mm^2. ITP, leukemia, aplastic anemia, etc., can cause this bleeding. A hematologist should be consulted, because of the risk of potentially life-threatening bleeding.

Chronic history of recurrent bleeding, such as mucosal, deep muscle or joint bleeding, may indicate an inherited coagulation defect such as von Willebrand disease or hemophilia. The familial history may be positive, although von Willebrand disease often goes undiagnosed into adulthood if there has been no challenge such as surgery.

Phase 2: Perform screening tests for bleeding disorders to categorize the abnormality.

- Platelet count to assess level of thrombocytopenia
- PT/PTT: Prolongation of either one or both of these may aid in the diagnosis of von Willebrand disease, coagulation factor deficiencies, liver disease, and vitamin K deficiency.
- Bleeding time: Prolongation may indicate the presence of a platelet aggregation disorder or von Willebrand disease.

 Data Gathering

HISTORY

Question: At what age was the bruising first noticed?
Significance: Significant bruising in the neonatal period may indicate neonatal thrombocytopenia, congenital infections, and sepsis with DIC. Hemophilia more typically presents with bleeding in the neonatal period, such as with circumcision. Other inherited coagulation disorders, such as von Willebrand disease, may not be diagnosed until a child is older, as these tend to be mild in nature and may be uncovered with preoperative testing or postoperative bleeding complications. ITP may occur at any age.

Question: What is the pattern or distribution of the bruises?
Significance: The pattern of bruising, especially in a younger child, may indicate normal toddler activity, child abuse, or religious practices such as coining (common among Southeast Asians) in which warm or hot coins are rubbed on the skin to help in the healing process.

Question: What medications is the child taking?
Significance: Use of aspirin, ibuprofen, cough syrups with guaifenesin, and some antihistamines cause platelet dysfunction by inhibiting cyclooxygenase and, therefore, interfering with the release of platelet granules. Use of these drugs may also unmask an otherwise mild inherited bleeding disorder.

Question: Are there any signs or symptoms of systemic illness or infection?
Significance: Infections such as meningococcemia or viruses and collagen vascular diseases may present with ecchymosis or petechiae.

Question: Is there any familial history of a bleeding diathesis, easy bruisability, or heavy menstrual bleeding?
Significance: A positive familial history of inherited disorders of coagulation factors or platelet aggregation may aid in directing the workup. A negative familial history does not rule out any of these disorders, however.

Physical Examination

Question: Does the child appear well or systemically ill?
Significance: A well appearance is often found in those with ITP, though there is often a history of an antecedent viral illness. An ill appearance should raise concerns about malignancy, infection (especially meningococcemia), or other acquired coagulation factor deficiencies such as those seen with liver failure.

Question: What is the distribution of the bruises?
Significance: Bruising in unusual locations such as the back, genitalia, or thorax should raise suspicions of child abuse, especially if the lesions are in different stages of healing (see table, How to Estimate the Age of Bruises) or suggest the pattern of a hand, belt, etc. Purpura confined mostly to the legs are typical of HSP. Most toddlers will have multiple ecchymoses in the pretibial regions that occur with normal activity. Petechiae entirely above the nipple line is consistent with Valsalva maneuver, severe cough, and viral infections.

Question: Is the bleeding confined to the skin surface or are deeper tissues such as muscles and joints involved?
Significance: Hemophilia generally causes deeper bleeding, although bruising is common in the infant and younger child.

Question: Are the mucous membranes involved?
Significance: Severe thrombocytopenia, streptococcal pharyngitis, varicella, measles, and other viral infections can cause this finding. Von Willebrand disease can also present with gingival bleeding.

Question: Is there hepatosplenomegaly or lymphadenopathy?
Significance: Involvement of the reticuloendothelial system can be found with malignancies such as leukemia or with viral or bacterial infections.

Question: Are there other congenital abnormalities?
Significance: Syndromes such as Fanconi anemia and thrombocytopenia absent radii (TAR) may present with upper extremity limb malformations and bruising.

Most Common Causes of Bruising

Trauma (either accidental or intentional)
Infectious (viral etiology more common than bacterial)
Thrombocytopenia
Henoch-Schönlein purpura
Inherited coagulation defects (hemophilia, von Willebrand disease)

 ## Laboratory Aids

Test: CBC
Significance: Platelet count is the most important, however, abnormalities of WBC or Hgb may aid in the diagnosis of bone marrow infiltration or failure.

Test: PT
Significance: Elevation may indicate warfarin ingestion or factor VII deficiency or vitamin K deficiency.

Test: aPTT
Significance: Prolongation is seen with hemophilia and may be seen in von Willebrand disease.

Test: Both PT and PTT
Significance: Both are prolonged in DIC, liver failure, and vitamin K deficiency.

Test: Bleeding time
Significance: Lengthened in platelet aggregation disorders and with drug effects.

Test: Fibrinogen
Significance: Decreased in liver failure, DIC

Test: Urinalysis
Significance: Hematuria and/or proteinuria may indicate HSP, nephrotic syndrome, or other vasculitis.

 ## Emergency Care

Factors that make this an emergency include:

• Severe thrombocytopenia below 10,000–20,000/mm^3 carries a higher risk of spontaneous internal bleeding including intracranial bleeding.
• Bleeding or bruising accompanied by evidence of leukemia or other malignancy.
• Evidence of sepsis (DIC) or meningococcemia.

 ## Common Questions and Answers

Q: Is hemophilia always diagnosed in the newborn period?
A: No. A familial history may provide clues, but a significant number of patients represent a spontaneous mutation. Additionally, not all boys with hemophilia will bleed with circumcision and the diagnosis may not be made until the infants become more active.

Q: What is a common cause of bruising among girls?
A: Girls may first come to attention at menarche and be diagnosed at that time with von Willebrand disease. Rarely, girls whose fathers have hemophilia may be unfavorably "lyonized" and, therefore, have decreased factor levels consistent with mild hemophilia.

Issues for Referral

• ITP should be referred to a hematologist especially if the child is older, because there is a higher risk of chronic ITP or an underlying disorder such as lupus.
• Prolonged PT/PTT/BT often requires referral to work up an inherited or acquired coagulation defect.
• Any concern about a malignancy, liver failure, or child abuse.

Clinical Pearls

• The amount of bruising may or may not correlate with the amount of internal bleeding that has occurred. Hemophiliacs can significantly drop their hemoglobin during a thigh or psoas bleed without having much in the way of ecchymosis.
• A child presenting with ITP may have bruises and petechiae from head to toe without changing the hemoglobin much at all.

BIBLIOGRAPHY

Berntorp E. Progress in haemophilic care: ethical issues. *Haemophilia* 2002;8(3): 435–438.

Buchanan GR. Bleeding signs in children with idiopathic thrombocytopenic purpura. *J Pediatr Hematol/Oncol* 2003;25(Suppl 1): S42–S46.

Horton TM, et al. Case series of thrombotic thrombocytopenic purpura in children and adolescents. *J Pediatr Hematol/Oncol* 2003;25(4):336–339.

Manno CS. Difficult pediatric diagnoses: bleeding and bruising. *Pediatr Clin North Am* 1991;38(3):637–655.

Wight J, Paisley S. The epidemiology of inhibitors in haemophilia A: a systematic review. *Haemophilia* 2003;9(4):418–435.

Author: Julie W. Stern

Chest Pain

 Database

DEFINITION

Chest pain is a common pain syndrome in childhood (see table, Most Common Causes of Pediatric Chest Pain).

 Differential Diagnosis

MUSCULOSKELETAL DISORDERS

- Chest wall strain
- Costochondritis
- Direct chest trauma
- Slipping rib syndrome

CARDIAC PATHOLOGY

- Arrhythmia (supraventricular tachycardia, premature ventricular contractions)
- Coronary-artery anomalies
- Coronary-artery aneurysms (Kawasaki disease)
- Infections (myocarditis, pericarditis)
- Myocardial infarction/ischemia
- Structural abnormalities

—Aortic stenosis
—Hypertrophic cardiomyopathy
—Pulmonic stenosis
—Mitral valve prolapse
—Severe coarctation of the aorta

GASTROINTESTINAL DISORDERS

- Caustic ingestions
- Esophageal foreign bodies
- Esophagitis (sometimes tetracycline, "pill," induced)

PSYCHOGENIC CAUSES

- Anxiety
- Hyperventilation

RESPIRATORY DISORDERS

- Asthma
- Cough (prolonged)
- Pleural effusion

Most Common Causes of Pediatric Chest Pain

Idiopathic
Musculoskeletal
   Chest wall strain
   Costochondritis
   Direct trauma
Respiratory conditions
   Asthma, cough, pneumonia
Gastrointestinal problems
   Esophagitis, esophageal foreign body
Psychogenic—stress related
Cardiac pathology

- Pneumonia
- Pneumothorax—spontaneous, trauma-related, drug-related (cocaine)
- Pneumomediastinum
- Pulmonary embolism

MISCELLANEOUS

- Breast mass
- Cigarette smoke
- Pleurodynia
- Precordial catch syndrome
- Shingles
- Sickle cell crises
- Thoracic tumor

Approach to the Patient

GENERAL GOAL

Identify the rare child with a serious etiology for chest pain (see table, Important Physical Findings on General Examination of Child with Chest Pain).

Phase 1: Is the patient in acute distress? If so, begin emergency management and proceed rapidly to find the cause of pain.

Phase 2: For the majority of stable children with chest pain, determine whether laboratory tests are needed to help identify the etiology.

Phase 3: Treat specific conditions as appropriate. Begin analgesics, reassure the family and arrange for follow-up care.

HINTS FOR SCREENING PROBLEM

Take a thorough history and perform a careful physical examination. Examine the chest last—do not focus only on this area. Use laboratory tests sparingly, only to confirm clinical suspicions.

 Data Gathering

HISTORY

Question: How severe, how often is the pain?
Significance: Constant, frequent severe pain is more likely to be distressing, interruptive of daily activity. Serious etiology is not well correlated with frequency, severity of pain.

Question: What is the type of pain? Its location?
Significance: Burning pain is associated with esophagitis. Sharp, stabbing pain relieved by sitting up or leaning forward is typical of pericarditis. Young children do not describe or localize chest pain well.

Question: When was the onset of pain?
Significance: Acute pain (<48 hours) is more likely to have an organic etiology. Chronic pain (>6 months) is more likely to be psychogenic, idiopathic. In an older child with sudden onset of pain consider an arrhythmia, pneumothorax, or musculoskeletal injury. In a young child with sudden onset of pain consider a foreign body (coin) in the esophagus, or injury.

Question: Is the pain induced by exercise?
Significance: Exercise-induced chest pain may be related to serious cardiac disease or asthma.

Question: Recent trauma or muscle overuse?
Significance: Musculoskeletal (chest wall) pain

Question: Eaten spicy foods? Taken tetracycline or other pills?
Significance: Esophagitis. Teens often take pills with little water and then lie down. The undissolved pill may lodge in the esophagus and cause pain.

Question: Recent use of cocaine?
Significance: Hypertension, tachycardia, myocardial ischemia, or pneumothorax

Question: Use of oral contraceptives or recent leg trauma?
Significance: Pulmonary embolism. This is very rare in the pediatric age group.

Question: Recent significant stress (e.g., move, death of loved one, serious illness)?
Significance: Psychogenic pain. We know children have headaches and abdominal pain related to stress. Chest pain may also relate to unusual stress.

Question: Associated complaints?
Significance: Fever may imply pneumonia, myocarditis, pericarditis. Syncope, palpitations may imply cardiac arrhythmias or severe anemia. Joint pain, rash may relate chest pain to collagen vascular disease. Pain that resolves with parental attention may indicate an emotional etiology.

Question: Positive familial history?
Significance: Hypertrophic cardiomyopathy is often familial. Those with this disorder may have familial history positive for sudden death. When there is a positive familial history of heart disease or chest pain, the parents may be unusually concerned about the symptom in a child. The child often has a nonorganic etiology.

Question: Past medical history?
Significance: Previous Kawasaki disease, long-standing insulin-dependent diabetes mellitus, and sickle cell disease may have serious cardiac or pulmonary complications leading to chest pain. Marfan syndrome has increased risk for aortic dissection, pneumothorax. Asthma has increased risk for pneumonia, pneumothorax. Collagen vascular disease has increased risk for pleural effusion, pericarditis. Most underlying structural cardiac lesions rarely produce chest pain.

Physical Examination

Finding: Child is in significant distress
Significance: Requires emergency care; stabilization. Consider pneumothorax, arrhythmia.

Finding: Child appears chronically ill
Significance: Chest pain may be found in serious illness such as malignancy (Hodgkin lymphoma), or systemic lupus erythematosis.

Finding: Fever
Significance: Consider pneumonia, myocarditis, pericarditis.

Finding: Skin bruising present
Significance: Chest pain may be related to unrecognized trauma.

Finding: Abdominal pathology
Significance: Pain may be referred to the chest.

Finding: Arthritis present
Significance: Collagen vascular disease may manifest as pleural effusion, chest pain.

Finding: Unusually anxious child
Significance: Underlying stress may lead to pain.

Finding: Breast enlargement, asymmetry, tenderness
Significance: Physiologic breast changes in young teens may be painful. Consider pregnancy in teenage girls.

Finding: Rales, decreased breath sounds, wheezing
Significance: May suggest pneumonia, asthma with overuse of chest wall muscles.

Finding: Subcutaneous emphysema palpable on chest or neck
Significance: Pneumothorax, pneumomediastinum

Finding: Heart murmur, rub, arrhythmia
Significance: Congenital heart disease, cardiac infection such as myocarditis, pericarditis, supraventricular tachycardia, ventricular tachycardia

Finding: Tenderness of chest wall, costochondral junctions
Significance: Musculoskeletal pain

 ## Laboratory Aids

Test: Electrocardiogram
Significance: Obtain if history suggests cardiac pathology. For example:

- Acute onset of pain
- Pain on exertion
- Pain associated with syncope, dizziness, palpitations
- History of congenital heart disease
- Serious associated medical problems (Kawasaki disease, diabetes mellitus)
- Use of cocaine

Obtain also if physical examination is abnormal. For example:

- Respiratory distress
- Cardiac abnormality
- Fever
- Significant trauma

Test: Chest radiograph
Significance: Same as for electrocardiogram. Also, obtain if history suggests cardiac or pulmonary pathology, tumor, Marfan syndrome, or foreign body (coin ingestion). Also, obtain if physical examination suggests decreased breath sounds, or palpation of subcutaneous air.

Test: Holter monitor
Significance: Arrange for this study if cardiac arrhythmia is suspected. Electrocardiogram may fail to detect intermittent arrhythmia.

Test: Exercise stress test, pulmonary function tests
Significance: Obtain if pain is induced by exertion.

Test: Drug screen
Significance: Obtain if cocaine use is suspected.

 ## Emergency Care

Factors that make this an emergency include:

- Pneumothorax: may present with severe sudden chest pain, respiratory distress, cyanosis, hypotension.
- Cardiac arrhythmia: ventricular tachycardia or supraventricular tachycardia in an older child may progress to heart failure or a lethal rhythm.
- Cocaine intoxication: may present with pneumothorax, cardiac arrhythmia, hypertension.
- Direct chest trauma: may lead to cardiac contusion, and arrhythmia.
- Caustic ingestions or esophageal foreign bodies require prompt attention.

 ## Common Questions and Answers

Q: How common is chest pain in children?
A: Chest pain is a common pain syndrome reported in 6 of 1,000 children who present to an urban emergency department. The complaint is less common than abdominal pain or headache. Although children of all ages may complain of chest pain, the mean age is approximately 12 years.

Q: Is follow-up important?
A: Yes. Serious pathology is unlikely to be found if not diagnosed initially. However, watch for signs of exercise-induced asthma or for emotional problems that were not obvious initially. Ensure that the child returns to normal activity when appropriate.

Q: What is the prognosis for most children with chest pain?
A: Most children with chest pain have an excellent prognosis. About 40% of children with chest pain will have continued symptoms for 6 to 24 months.

Issues for Referral

- Acute distress
- Significant trauma
- History of heart disease or related serious medical problem
- Pain with exercise, syncope, palpitations, dizziness
- Serious emotional disturbance
- Esophageal foreign body, caustic ingestion
- Pneumothorax, pleural effusion

Clinical Pearls

- Chest pain in children is rarely related to cardiac pathology.
- Not all children with chest pain have a benign etiology.
- Pain associated with exertion, syncope, dizziness is concerning for heart disease.
- If the child is febrile, consider pneumonia, or viral myocarditis.
- Treat specific etiology when found.
- Over-the-counter analgesics (acetaminophen, ibuprofen) suffice for most pain.
- Antacids may be diagnostic and therapeutic for esophagitis pain.
- Rest, heat, relaxation techniques may be useful.
- Avoid expensive, invasive laboratory studies with chronic pain and normal physical examination, benign history.

BIBLIOGRAPHY

Gumbiner CH. Precordial catch syndrome. *South Med J* 2003;96:38–41.

Lam JC, Tobias JD. Follow-up survey of children and adolescents with chest pain. *South Med J* 2001;94:921–924.

Owens TR. Chest pain in the adolescent. *Adol Med: State of the Art Rev* 2001;12:95–104.

Selbst SM, Ruddy RM, Clark BJ, et al. Pediatric chest pain; a prospective study. *Pediatrics* 1988;82:319–323.

Selbst SM. Chest pain in children; consultation with the specialist. *Pediatr Rev* 1997;18:169–173.

Washington RL. Sudden deaths in adolescent athletes caused by cardiac conditions. *Pediatr Ann* 2003;32:751–756.

Author: Steven M. Selbst

Coma

 ## Database

DEFINITION

Coma is defined as a state in which the patient is unresponsive with eyes closed, usually lasting less than 24 hours. Coma is a medical emergency, and immediate attention/intervention is required for abnormalities in breathing, circulation, glucose, or electrolytes. Coma should be differentiated from the following:

- Lethargy: a patient who is incoherent but arousable and has a tendency to sleep.
- Stupor: a state of somnolence, the patient is only responsive transiently to pain.
- Delirium: a confused, agitated patient with fragmented attention, concentration, and memory.
- Vegetative state: chronic state with clear sleep/wake cycles and no signs of cognition.
- Locked-in: must be distinguished from coma; cognitive functions are intact, though the patient may appear unconscious.

CAUSES OF COMA

- Trauma: bleeds (epi/subdural, intracerebral), cerebral swelling, diffuse axonal injury
- Intoxication (seizure or psychotropic medications, street drugs)
- Hypoxia/ischemia
- Infection: meningitis, encephalitis, toxic shock, subdural empyema, systemic shock
- Metabolic disorders: Hypoglycemia (salicylate or ethanol intoxication, hyperinsulinemia), Diabetic ketoacidosis (rarely neurologic deterioration on initiation of insulin therapy), Reye syndrome; electrolyte abnormalities (Na, K, Ca, Mg), hepatic/uremic encephalopathy, inborn errors of metabolism, hormonal abnormalities (thyroid, adrenal, pituitary), hypothermia/hyperthermia
- Tumor
- Seizure: nonconvulsive status, spike and wave stupor
- Vascular: hemorrhage from arteriovenous malformation (AVM), aneurysm, coagulopathy, infarction, cerebral venous thrombosis, hypertensive encephalopathy
- Hydrocephalus: ventriculoperitoneal (VP) shunt obstruction, mass/bleed obstructing ventricular outflow

PATHOPHYSIOLOGY

Dysfunction of the reticular-activating system in the brainstem or bilateral cerebral dysfunction.

COMPLICATIONS OF ACUTE COMA

- Respiratory failure
- Deep venous thrombosis
- Pneumonia (aspiration and infectious)

 ## Differential Diagnosis

DISORDERS MIMICKING COMA

- Psychogenic coma: patient may resist passive eye opening, regards self in mirror, and avoids passive arm fall over face
- Locked-in state: complete paralysis with normal cerebral function. May occur in severe neuromuscular disorders (acute polyneuropathy) or in ventral pontine lesions (hemorrhage, demyelination)

 ## Data Gathering

HISTORY

- Head trauma
- Ingestion/Drugs/Toxins (in home, given by acquaintances)
- Fever (and other symptoms of infection or preceding viral illness)
- Headache (nausea, vomiting, and other signs of increasing pressure or meningitis)
- Seizures
- Diabetes
- Preexisting neurologic disease including previous episodes of coma

 ## Physical Examination

- Vital signs: look for bradycardia, hypertension, and abnormal respiratory pattern (Cushing triad for cerebral herniation)
- Look for signs of head trauma: raccoon eyes, Battle sign (ecchymosis at mastoid equals basilar skull fracture), retinal hemorrhages, bulging fontanelle
- Signs of meningitis: nuchal rigidity, Kernig and Brudinski signs (fallible)
- Neurologic: verbal or motor response to voice, touch, pain; eye opening/fixation; pupil symmetry/reactivity; spontaneous movements/posturing; worsening of these signs may indicate increased intracranial pressure (ICP)
- Reflexes: specific to rostral brainstem function (pupillary light reflex, corneal reflex, jaw jerk) and to caudal brainstem function (oculocephalic reflex [eye deviation with passive head rotation], gag, spontaneous respirations)

 ## Laboratory Aids

Initial blood studies obtained with placement of an IV line include:

- Glucose, electrolytes, BUN/creatinine, calcium, CBC
- Arterial blood gas
- Toxicology screen
- Ammonia, liver transaminases
- Radiology—first, noncontrast head CT scan to look for hemorrhage, may be followed by contrasted images or MRI to look for infection/mass lesions
- Cervical spine series (CT or lateral and AP x-ray studies)—indicated if evidence of trauma by history or on examination. Spine must be stabilized until injury is ruled out
- Lumbar puncture, to rule out infection, bleeding; defer until after CT if focal examination or signs of increased ICP. If question of "traumatic tap," spin out red cells promptly and examine fluid for xanthochromia
- EEG—helpful to rule out nonconvulsive status epilepticus

Emergency Care

- First priority is stabilization of respiratory and hemodynamic status (A,B,Cs).
- Endotracheal intubation—often required for airway protection and adequate oxygenation.
- Large-bore IV lines should be placed and isotonic fluids administered as needed to replace intravascular volume and maintain adequate blood pressure.
- If finger-stick glucose determination is low, give 2 to 4 mL of 25% dextrose (D25) per kilogram intravenously (D10 if young infant).
- If ingestion is suspected, administer naloxone (0.01 mg/kg IV).
- When there is evidence of increased ICP:

—Hyperventilate to decrease blood CO_2 to 25 to 30 torr and give mannitol (0.5–1 g/kg IV). Can also give Dexamethasone, 1 to 2 mg/kg IV
—Fluids given should be isotonic and the volume limited to maintain adequate perfusion.
—Elevate head to 30 degrees above horizontal to maximize cerebral venous drainage.
—Hospitalization is in the intensive care unit for close monitoring for changes in respiratory status or signs of increased ICP.
—IV antibiotics should be given if infection is suspected.

 ## Therapy

As per underlying etiology of the coma

Follow-Up

PROGNOSIS

Prognosis depends on underlying etiology. Complete recovery frequently seen after toxic-metabolic coma. In contrast, patients with coma resulting from severe head trauma or hypoxic injury often have significant neurologic sequelae and require long-term physical, occupational, and cognitive therapies.

PITFALLS

- Be aware of psychogenic coma and locked in states (see above)
- Loss of protective airway reflexes signals impending respiratory failure.

 ## Common Questions and Answers

Q: What is the role of EEG in the diagnosis of coma?
A: EEG is useful in diagnosis of psychogenic coma (should be normal) and in coma from nonconvulsive status epilepticus (shows electrographic seizures), and in possible herpes encephalitis (temporal or frontal sharp activity).

Q: Should anticonvulsants be given to comatose victims of trauma?
A: While no clear evidence exists that anticonvulsants improve outcome or reduce incidence of posttraumatic seizures, they are often given for posttraumatic intracranial hypertension, bleeding, and/or edema as seizures are known to raise ICP.

Issues for Referral

Neurosurgical intervention may be required in cases of head trauma, hemorrhage, mass lesion, or hydrocephalus. Neurology consultation is usually indicated.

Clinical Pearls

Trauma and near-drowning are the leading causes of coma in children, and boys are more often victims of trauma/near-drowning than girls.

BIBLIOGRAPHY

Jacinto SJ, Gieron-Korthals M, Ferreira, JA. Predicting outcome in hypoxic-ischemic brain injury. *Pediatr Clin North Am* 2001;48(3): 647–660.

Tasker RC. Neurolocal critical care. *Curr Opin Pediatr* 2000;12(3):222–226.

Trubel HK, et al. Outcome of Coma in Children. *Curr Opin Pediatr* 2003;15: 283–287.

Authors: Amy R. Brooks-Kayal and Eric Marsh

Cough

Database

DEFINITION

Cough is a symptom of a variety of underlying conditions, which results from a complex reflex phenomenon initiated by cough receptors and mediated in the brainstem's cough center. These receptors are located throughout the large- to medium-sized airways (but not the lower airways), pharynx, paranasal sinuses, external auditory canal, and stomach, and are triggered by thermal, chemical, mechanical, or inflammatory stimuli. The resultant high-velocity expiration, which removes airway secretions, is generally reflexive, but may sometimes be voluntarily initiated or suppressed.

Differential Diagnosis

Infection and reactive airway disease are the most common causes of cough in all age groups and should always be considered.

CAUSES OF ACUTE COUGH

- Infection
- Reactive airway disease (RAD)
- Sinusitis
- Irritative
- Allergic
- Foreign body

CAUSES OF CHRONIC COUGH

- Infection
- Asthma or asthmatic bronchitis
- Sinusitis
- Irritative/postinfectious
- Allergic
- Foreign body (FB)
- Gastroesophageal reflux (GER)
- Habitual or psychogenic
- Anatomic abnormalities

—Tracheoesophageal fistula
—Tracheobronchomalacia
—Laryngeal cleft
—Polyps
—Adductor vocal cord paralysis
—Pulmonary sequestration
—Bronchogenic cyst
—Cystic hygroma
—Vascular ring
—Tumor

- Cystic fibrosis (CF)
- Ciliary dyskinesia syndromes
- Immunodeficiency states

—Human immunodeficiency virus (HIV)
—Immunoglobulin deficiencies (IgA, IgG)
—Phagocytic defects
—Complement deficiency

- Pulmonary hemosiderosis
- Angiotensin-converting enzyme inhibitors
- External auditory canal irritation

Approach to the Patient

GENERAL GOAL

The presenting symptom of cough is a familiar one to most physicians and accounts for nearly 7% of chief complaints to pediatricians. Cough is an easily identifiable symptom that frequently provokes parental concern and can be troublesome to the physician. The possible etiologies of cough are diverse, and may range from a minor illness to a life-threatening condition. Therefore, a stepwise approach is required in an effort to prevent a costly and lengthy investigation. In particular, a thorough history and physical examination are of paramount importance in the evaluation.

Phase 1: Complete history and physical examination to determine time course and severity of cough and to ascertain whether it represents a significant problem of respiratory function or a serious underlying disease.

Phase 2: Initiate focused workup and treatment plan depending on differential diagnosis (see previous section).

Phase 3: Refer to pediatric pulmonologist if concerned about significant pathology or if cough persists for prolonged period (see following section).

Data Gathering

HISTORY

Question: Is the cough acute or chronic?
Significance: Generally considered to be chronic if present longer than 3 to 4 weeks. Although there is significant overlap, differential diagnosis varies depending on the time course.

Question: How is this problem different in children as compared with adults?
Significance: Differential diagnosis varies considerably based on the patient's age.

Question: Is there a recent history of upper respiratory infection (URI)?
Significance: Consider serial URIs (children have average of 6 to 8 per year with each often lasting up to 2 to 3 weeks), postinfectious/ irritative, or sinusitis (which complicates up to 5% of URIs).

Question: What are the associated symptoms?
Significance:

- Fever, nasal discharge suggests infection.
- Fever with chills or night sweats suggests tuberculosis (TB); may also have weight loss with TB.
- Sputum production indicates bronchiectasis or other lower airway pathology.
- With rhinorrhea, halitosis, headache or facial edema, consider sinusitis.
- With respiratory distress, suspect RAD.

Question: What is the quality of the cough?
Significance:

- Productive cough suggests lower airway infection, CF/bronchiectasis.
- Dry cough suggests RAD, fungal infection.
- Barking cough is usually associated with croup.
- Honking or brassy cough is typical in habitual or psychogenic cough.

Question: What is the pattern of the cough?
Significance:

- Chronic nighttime cough suggests RAD.
- With nighttime/early morning cough, consider sinusitis.
- Seasonal cough suggests allergy.

Question: Are there any known triggers of cough (e.g., smoke, cold air, dust, URI)?
Significance: Consider irritant, allergic, or reactive airway disease.

Question: Is there any personal or familial history of atopy?
Significance: Consider RAD.

Question: Is there a history of recurrent infections?
Significance: Consider immunodeficiency, CF. Also consider pulmonary sequestration if patient has recurrent pneumonias in the same location.

Question: Is there any relation of cough to feedings?
Significance: Consider aspiration, GER, tracheoesophageal fistula in infants.

Question: Is there a history of a choking episode?
Significance: Consider retained foreign body, although there may not be a history of a choking episode in this case, and cough may be episodic as FB moves along respiratory tract.

Question: Is there failure to thrive?
Significance: Rule out tuberculosis, CF, immunodeficiency.

Physical Examination

Finding: Patient's general appearance
Significance:

- Evidence of failure to thrive—consider tuberculosis, CF, immunodeficiency.
- Cyanosis or pallor—rule out hypoxemia.
- Signs of respiratory distress such as tachypnea, accessory muscle use—most likely RAD or infection.

Finding: Barrel chest
Significance: Suggests air-trapping due to chronic disease.

Finding: Clubbing
Significance: May be seen with bronchiectasis.

Finding: Nasal polyps
Significance: May be associated with allergic conditions or CF.

Finding: Tracheal deviation
Significance: Suggests mediastinal mass or FB aspiration.

Finding: Signs of atopic disease
Significance: Eczema, allergic shiners, transverse nasal crease, rhinitis, mucosal cobblestoning, injected conjunctivae suggest allergy, RAD.

Finding: Rhinorrhea/purulent posterior pharyngeal drainage, sniffling, halitosis, periorbital edema, sinus tenderness
Significance: Sinusitis

Finding: Wheezing
Significance: Polyphonic inspiratory or expiratory wheezes suggest RAD, while monophonic or fixed wheezes should make one consider FB or mass/congenital lesion.

 ## Laboratory Aids

Laboratory investigation should reflect a rational, stepwise approach based on likely etiologies after a thorough history and physical examination.

Test: Chest radiograph
Significance:

• Infiltrates may suggest pneumonia, bronchiolitis, pneumonitis, TB, CF, bronchiectasis, FB.
• Volume loss may be seen with FB aspiration; sometimes need to obtain lateral decubitus views in young children who cannot cooperate with inspiratory/expiratory views.
• Hyperinflation suggests RAD or CF.
• Mediastinal nodes may indicate infection (especially TB, fungus) or malignancy.

Test: Wright peak flow (WPF) rate; complete pulmonary function tests
Significance:

• Easy to perform WPF in the primary care office with the proper flow meter.
• Helpful to get prebronchodilator and postbronchodilator rates if RAD suspected.
• Standardized tables available with values based on height and race.
• Pulmonary function tests may be indicated for diagnosis of RAD (e.g., cough variant type) and for assessment of severity or treatment of asthmatics.

Test: Mantoux test-purified protein derivative (PPD)
Significance: Rule out tuberculosis.

Test: Microbiology workup as indicated; e.g., Polymerase Chain Reaction (PCR) for Pertussis, Direct Fluorescent Antibody (DFA) for viral panel, culture for Chlamydia
Significance: Aids in precise diagnosis and treatment as needed

Test: Paranasal sinus computed tomographic scan
Significance: Should be used judiciously to evaluate sinus disease

Test: Complete blood count
Significance: Eosinophilia suggests atopic disease or, rarely, parasitic infection; anemia should prompt one to consider chronic disease or, rarely, pulmonary hemosiderosis.

Test: Sputum sample must contain alveolar macrophages.
Significance:

• Eosinophils suggest asthmatic process or hypersensitivity reaction of lung.
• Polymorphonuclear cells suggest infection.
• Predominance of macrophages suggests postinfectious hyperresponsive cough receptors.
• Hemosiderin staining suggests pulmonary hemosiderosis.
• Lipid-laden macrophages suggest recurrent aspiration.
• Routine or special cultures based on likely pathogens.

Test: Serum IgE
Significance: Significant elevation indicates allergy or, rarely, parasites.

Test: Sweat chloride test
Significance: Cystic fibrosis. Need to be sure that laboratory has experience with this test.

Test: Immune workup
Significance: HIV; immunoglobulins

Test: Barium swallow or pH probe
Significance: Reflux

Test: Bronchoscopy
Significance: To remove FB or obtain tissue samples.

 ## Emergency Care

• Cough should be considered an emergency if there are associated signs or symptoms of respiratory distress.
• Routine emergency airway assessment (i.e., ABCs) should be undertaken on presentation and appropriate supportive measures started in cases in which there is concern.
• Refer for additional treatment as outlined previously.

Common Questions and Answers

Q: Is whooping cough still a problem despite routine childhood immunization?
A: Yes. Pertussis often goes unrecognized as a cause of acute and chronic cough, particularly in infants who have not completed their immunization series and in adolescents (and adults) in whom immunity from vaccination will have waned.

Q: Is it possible for children to have asthma if they have never wheezed?
A: Yes, there is cough-variant reactive airway disease. However, it is important to demonstrate a clear response to bronchodilators in such children in order to avoid overdiagnosis of asthma.

Issues for Referral

The vast majority of cases of cough, even when chronic, can be diagnosed and managed by the primary care physician. Factors that may prompt you to make a referral include:

• The cough is unresponsive to treatment.
• The cause is likely to be an anatomic malformation or FB aspiration.
• There appears to be involvement of other organ systems (e.g., failure to thrive, GER, congestive heart failure, immunodeficiency, unusual infection).
• Hemoptysis.

Clinical Pearls

• The goal is to treat the underlying cause of the cough, not the symptom.
• To avoid overuse of antibiotics, parents should be informed that viral URIs can cause cough that commonly lasts 2 to 3 weeks.
• Educate parents about the beneficial function of cough to remove irritants and about the potential harm of suppressing a productive cough or cough secondary to RAD.
• Specific pharmacologic interventions:

—RAD: bronchodilators ± inhaled antiinflammatory agents, oral or inhaled steroids, removal of irritants
—Infection: appropriate antibiotics
—Over-the-counter cough medicines are widely prescribed and overused. Cough suppressants have not been shown to be efficacious in children under 5 years, and have been associated with significant toxicity in this age group.

• Self-hypnosis is a safe, effective treatment for children with habitual cough.

BIBLIOGRAPHY

Anbar RD, Hall HR. Childhood habit cough treated with self-hypnosis. *J Pediatr* 2004;144(2):213–217.

Committee on Drugs. Use of codeine and DM-containing cough remedies in children. *Pediatrics* 1997;99(6):918–920.

de Jongste JC, Shields MD. Cough: Chronic cough in children. *Thorax* 2003;58(11): 998–1003.

Taylor JA, Novack AH, Almquist JR, et al. Efficacy of cough suppressants in children. *J Pediatr* 1993;122(5):799–802.

Todokoro M, et al. Childhood cough variant asthma and it relationship to classic asthma. *Ann Allergy Asthma Immunol* 2003;90(6): 652–659.

Author: Margaret McNamara

Crying

 ## Database

DEFINITION

Crying is usually a normal physiologic response to distress, discomfort, or unfulfilled needs. Crying is felt to be potentially pathologic if it is interpreted by caregivers as differing in quality and duration without apparent explanation and/or persists without consolability beyond a reasonable time (generally 1 to 2 hours).

 ## Differential Diagnosis

CONGENITAL/ANATOMIC

- Intussusception
- Gastroesophageal reflux/esophagitis
- Volvulus
- Gaseous destention (2° to improper feeding or burping)
- Incarcerated hernia
- Peritonitis (acute abdomen)
- Testicular/ovarian torsion
- Constipation
- Anal fissure
- Meatal ulceration
- Glaucoma
- Urinary retention (secondary to posterior urethral valves)
- Cardiac—anomalous coronary artery, hypoxia

INFECTIOUS

- Otitis media/externa
- Urinary tract infection/pyelonephritis
- Stomatitis/gingivitis
- Meningitis/encephalitis
- Discitis
- Gastroenteritis
- Arthritis, septic
- Osteomyelitis
- Perianal cellulitis
- Balanitis
- Dermatitis (especially pruritic as in scabies or painful as in staphylococcal scalded skin syndrome)

TOXIC, ENVIRONMENTAL, DRUGS

- Neonatal drug withdrawal
- Prenatal/perinatal cocaine exposure
- Immunization reactions (especially DTP)
- Cow milk intolerance
- Isolated fructose intolerance
- Drug reactions (especially antihistamines, pseudoephedrine, phenylpropanolamine), including maternal medications in breast milk
- Vitamin A toxicity
- Carbon monoxide exposure
- Emotional/physical neglect

TRAUMA

- Corneal abrasion
- Foreign body (hypopharynx, eye, ear, nose)
- Skull fracture/subdural hematoma
- Intracranial hemorrhage
- Retinal hemorrhage
- Other fractures (especially extremities)
- Hair tourniquet syndrome (encircling finger, toe, penis, clitoris)
- Open diaper pin
- Bite (human, animal, insect)

GENETIC/METABOLIC

- Sickle cell crisis
- Phenylketonuria
- Hypothyroidism
- Electrolyte abnormalities (especially sodium)
- Hypoglycemia
- Hypocalcemia
- Inborn error of metabolism

ALLERGIC/INFLAMMATORY

- Cow milk allergy
- Celiac disease (gluten enteropathy)

FUNCTIONAL

- Parental expectations/responses

MISCELLANEOUS

- Overstimulation
- Persistent night awakening
- Night terrors
- Congestive heart failure
- Caffey disease (infantile cortical hyperostosis)
- Dysrhythmia (especially supraventricular tachycardia)
- Autism
- Teething
- Headache/migraine
- Temperament
- Colic
- Discomfort (cold, heat, itching, hunger)

Approach to the Patient

GENERAL GOAL

Decide if the crying represents a normal physiologic response, a protracted multifactorial physiologic/developmental response (colic), or a potentially pathologic problem.

Phase 1: How urgent is the need for evaluation? A classic and difficult triage issue. One must identify the periodicity of the problem, associated symptoms, impression of wellness, and parental anxiety/reliability.

Phase 2: When in doubt, particularly if "colic" seems unlikely, see the patient as soon as possible.

 ## Data Gathering

HISTORY

Question: Onset after 1 month of age or persistent in infants older than 4 months?
Significance: Colic less likely as a cause.

Question: First episode?
Significance: Recurrent episodes, particularly with a diurnal pattern, are more likely due to colic.

Question: Fever?
Significance: Potential need for evaluation of meningitis, other infections.

Question: Do attempts at consolation make the crying worse?
Significance: Paradoxically increased crying (especially with lifting, rocking) can be seen in meningitis, peritonitis, long-bone fractures, arthritis.

Question: Stridor?
Significance: Implies possible upper airway obstruction (mechanical, functional).

Question: Expiratory grunting?
Significance: Higher likelihood of significant pathologic cause of crying (especially cardiac, respiratory, and/or infectious disease).

Question: Cold symptoms and/or day-care attendance?
Significance: Increased likelihood of otitis media.

Question: Vomiting?
Significance: Higher likelihood of pathologic gastrointestinal cause (e.g., obstruction, G-E reflux with possible esophagitis), particularly in infant <3 months, or CNS disease.

Question: What is the pattern of feeding?
Significance: Over/underfeeding, excessive air swallowing, inadequate burping, improper formula preparation may contribute to excessive crying.

Question: Recent fall or trauma?
Significance: Possible fracture, increased intracranial pressure, abuse.

Physical Examination

Finding: Tympanic membrane with loss of landmarks, poor mobility; swollen canal
Significance: Otitis media, otitis externa, foreign body

Finding: Tenderness on palpation of extremities, clavicle or scalp; painful or decreased range of motion of joints
Significance: Suggests fracture, subluxation, osteomyelitis, septic arthritis

Finding: Conjunctival redness, eye tearing, scratches near the eye
Significance: Suggests corneal abrasion (fluorescein testing of eye warranted) or foreign body in eye (eversion of lid recommended).

Finding: Impacted or bloody stool on rectal exam, abdominal mass
Significance: Constipation or intussusception

Finding: Geographic scars, frenulum tears, retinal hemorrhages, suspicious bruises, burns, decreased weight/height ratio
Significance: Neglect/abuse (physical, emotional)

Finding: Bulging or full fontanel (especially in upright, quiet infant)
Significance: Possible increased intracranial pressure (ICP) (meningitis, subdural hematoma, vitamin A toxicity)

Finding: Edema of individual toes, fingers, or penis
Significance: Hair tourniquet syndrome

Finding: Tender swelling in inguinal or scrotal area
Significance: Incarcerated hernia, testicular torsion

Finding: Heart rate >200 with minimal variability
Significance: Possible supraventricular tachycardia

Laboratory Aids

Test: Stool for occult blood
Significance: Possible intussusception, anal fissure

Test: Fluorescein testing of eye
Significance: Corneal abrasion (may occur without significant conjunctival redness)

Test: Urinalysis/urine culture
Significance: Urinary tract infection

Test: Urine toxicology screen
Significance: Drug withdrawal (neonatal), ingestions, passive exposures (e.g., cocaine)

Test: Pulse oximetry
Significance: Hypoxia (from cardiac causes) may cause increased irritability

Test: Electrolyte panel/blood glucose
Significance: Endocrine or metabolic disturbance, especially if abnormal sodium, hypoglycemia, significant acidosis or elevated anion gap

Emergency Care

Factors that make this an emergency include:

- Suspicion of meningitis: stiff neck, bulging fontanel, fever (especially infants <2 to 3 months)
- Suspicion of intestinal obstruction: vomiting (especially bilious or projectile), mass on abdominal palpation, and/or bloody stools
- Suspicion of incarcerated hernia or testicular/ovarian torsion
- Evidence of cardiac compromise (congestive heart failure [CHF], supraventricular tachycardia [SVT]): tachycardia, poor perfusion (capillary refill >3 seconds, poor distal pulses), rales
- Evidence of acute dehydration: weight loss, decreased urine output, orthostatic changes, poor perfusion
- Evidence of child abuse or neglect

Common Questions and Answers

Q: What is the most likely cause of inconsolable crying in the first few months of life?
A: Without question, infantile colic. A practitioner needs to be familiar with the clinical pattern of infantile colic, so that deviations from this most common pediatric syndrome are readily recognized.

Q: Is teething a common cause of excessive crying?
A: Grandparents everywhere insist that it is (as well as a common cause of fever, diarrhea, rashes, etc.). Objective data do not support a strong association. Be careful in ascribing symptoms and signs to teething. Trust the grandparents, but verify.

Issues for Referral

Factors that may help alert you to make a referral include: ill versus well-appearing. Although observation alone is less reliable in infants <3 months, judgment of an infant to be ill-appearing (e.g., pallor, grunting, poor arousability, poor response to social overtures) warrants more urgent and extensive evaluation. Weight loss or abnormal development implies a much higher likelihood of an organic cause of repetitive bouts of crying.

Clinical Pearls

- Quality of cry: Objective acoustic analyses of cries may become a common future modality to distinguish pathologic from physiologic crying. However, subjective interpretation can be helpful.

—High-pitched (shrill, piercing) crying in short bursts: associated with CNS pathology, especially with increased intracranial pressure
—High-pitched crying in longer bursts: seen in small for gestational age (SGA) infants, neonatal drug withdrawal
—Hoarse crying: seen in hypothyroidism, laryngeal diseases, hypocalcemic tetany
—Weak crying: may be seen in neuromuscular disorders, such as Hoffman-Werdnig syndrome, infant botulism, and/or the very ill infant
—Cat-like cry: as noted on every pediatric board exam for the last 35 years, a mewing cry can be associated with cri du chat syndrome (5p syndrome or absence of short arm of chromosome 5)

- Neonatal drug withdrawal has other characteristic findings in addition to excessive crying.

—Wakefulness
—Irritability
—Tremulousness, temperature variation, tachypnea
—Hyperactivity, high-pitched persistent cry, hyperacusis, hyperreflexia, hypertonia
—Diarrhea, diaphoresis, disorganized suck
—Rub marks, respiratory distress, rhinorrhea
—Apnea, autonomic dysfunction
—Weight loss or failure to gain weight
—Alkalosis (respiratory)
—Lacrimation

BIBLIOGRAPHY

Barr RG, Hopkins B, Green JA, eds. *Crying as a Sign, a Symptom, and a Signal*. London: Cambridge University Press, 2000.

Committee on Drugs. Neonatal drug withdrawal. *Pediatrics* 1998;101(6)72: 1079–1088.

Corwin MJ, Lester BM, Golub HL. The infant cry: what can it tell us? *Curr Probl Pediatr* 1996;26(9):325–334.

Poole SR. The infant with acute, unexplained, excessive crying. *Pediatrics* 1991;88(3): 450–455.

Trocinski DR, Pearigen PD. The crying infant. *Emerg Clin North Am* 1998;16(4):895–910.

Author: Mark F. Ditmar

Diarrhea

 Database

DEFINITION

Diarrhea should be considered whenever there is an increase in frequency, volume, or liquidity of patient's stool as compared with their normal bowel movement pattern. While an adult excretes 100 to 200 g of stool each day, a child typically passes 10 g/kg in each 24 hours. Diarrhea also can be characterized by duration. Chronic diarrhea is generally defined as the persistence of loose or more frequent stools for more than 2 weeks. Tenesmus, perianal discomfort, and incontinence may also occur. Diarrhea is caused whenever there is an alteration in the normal intestinal fluid-electrolyte balance. Malabsorption, maldigestion, cellular electrolyte pump dysfunction, and intestinal colonization or invasion by microorganisms can cause diarrhea.

 Differential Diagnosis

ACUTE DIARRHEA

- Dietary causes

—Sorbitol, fructose
—Intolerance to specific foods (beans, fruit, peppers, etc.)

- Infectious causes

—Bacterial (*Salmonella, Shigella, Campylobacter, Yersinia, Plesiomonas, Aeromonas, Escherichia coli*)
—Viral (rotavirus, Norwalk agent, adenovirus)

- Medication

—Antibiotics
—Laxatives: Magnesium-containing

CHRONIC DIARRHEA

- Allergic/autoimmune

—Milk/soy protein allergy
—Eosinophilic enteritis
—Henoch-Schönlein purpura
—AIDS
—IgA deficiency
—Combined immunodeficiency
—Vasculitis
—Autoimmune enteropathy

- Anatomic abnormalities

—Short intestine
—Malrotation

- Bile salt malabsorption
- Celiac disease
- Congenital causes

—Cystic fibrosis
—Villous atrophy
—Holovisceral myopathy

DISACCHARIDASE DEFICIENCY

- Hirschsprung enterocolitis
- Encopresis
- Endocrine disorders

—Hyperthyroidism
—Diabetes
—Congenital adrenal hyperplasia

- Infectious causes

—Bacterial
—Viral
—Parasites (*Giardia, Entamoeba, Cryptosporidium*)
—*Clostridium difficile*
—Bacterial overgrowth

- Inflammatory bowel disease

—Ulcerative colitis
—Crohn disease

- Intestinal lymphangiectasia: primary and secondary
- Irritable bowel syndrome
- Lactose intolerance (primary, secondary, congenital)
- Medication
- Necrotizing enterocolitis
- Pancreatic dysfunction

—Shwachman syndrome
—Chronic pancreatitis

- Postinfectious diarrhea
- Pseudo-obstruction
- Secretory tumors (VIPoma, somatostatinoma, gastrinoma)

—Hemolytic uremic syndrome

Approach to the Patient

GENERAL GOAL

Determine the type of diarrhea (osmotic versus secretory).

Phase 1: Secretory Diarrhea: Absorption of intestinal fluid and electrolytes is accomplished through multiple cellular pumps transporting sodium, glucose, and amino acids. Factors that interrupt these pumps (cholera toxin, prostaglandin E, VIP, secretin) can cause a severe active isotonic secretory state manifested by profuse diarrhea, dehydration, and acidosis.

Phase 2: Osmotic Diarrhea: In general, the solute composition of intestinal fluid is similar to plasma. Osmotic diarrhea occurs when poorly absorbed or nonabsorbable solute is present in the intestinal lumen. This can occur with the ingestion of nonabsorbable sugars or cathartics, with carbohydrate malabsorption secondary to mucosal damage, with maldigestion secondary to pancreatic or hepatic dysfunction, with rapid transit of intestinal fluid, or with a rare congenital transport defect.

 Data Gathering

HISTORY

Question: Has the diarrhea lasted less than 2 weeks?
Significance: A distinction should be made between acute and chronic diarrhea. The cause of acute diarrhea is almost always related to an infection, a medication, or the addition of a new food.

Question: Travel history?
Significance: Questions should be asked regarding travel to areas where drinking water is contaminated (e.g., Mexico—*Entamoeba*) or the ingestion of infected meat (*E. coli*) or fresh water (well water) infected with *Giardia*.

Question: Is the patient an adolescent who is concerned about his or her weight?
Significance: Laxative abuse causing an osmotic diarrhea is common among adolescents who have an eating disorder.

Question: Does the patient have other systemic symptoms?
Significance: Systemic symptoms such as fever, gastrointestinal bleeding, rash, or vomiting should be ascertained. Specific infections and inflammatory bowel disease have associated systemic symptoms.

Question: Hematochezia?
Significance: The occurrence of acute, bloody stools and fever generally indicates a bacterial infection or amebiasis; however, these same symptoms coupled with thrombocytopenia, anemia, and azotemia, or with a purpuric rash can indicate hemolytic uremic syndrome or Henoch-Schönlein purpura (HSP), respectively. Chronic bloody diarrhea, abdominal pain, and weight loss are characteristic of inflammatory bowel disease.

Question: What is the age of the child?
Significance: The age of the child is important because a number of diseases present between birth and 3 months of life including congenital villus/transport abnormalities, cystic fibrosis, or milk/soy allergy. In a previously well infant who had a recent viral illness with subsequent protracted diarrhea, the diagnosis of postviral enteritis should be suspected. This disorder is characterized by severe mucosal injury resulting in disaccharidase deficiency and prolonged malabsorption. Chronic nonspecific diarrhea should be considered in otherwise normal preschool-aged children who have 2 to 10 watery stools/day without other symptoms and/or etiology. Lactose intolerance commonly occurs in many older children and adults, with over a 95% occurrence rate in some ethnic groups.

Question: Chronic diarrhea with weight loss?
Significance: Inflammatory or immunologic disorders such as ulcerative colitis, Crohn disease, and celiac disease must be considered.

Question: Water supply?
Significance: Patients may acquire *Giardia* infection from well water or water from some rural areas.

Physical Examination

Finding: What are the child's growth parameters?
Significance: Previous measurements are necessary to make an accurate evaluation. Findings of a chronically malnourished child with years of unsuspected weight loss or poor growth velocity would indicate a divergent differential diagnosis from that of a healthy-appearing child with normal growth.

Finding: Does the child have arthritis?
Significance: Arthritis and diarrhea can occur in diseases such as inflammatory bowel disease, celiac disease, HSP, and specific bacterial infections.

Finding: Is there nailbed clubbing?
Significance: Cystic fibrosis.

Finding: Is there a right lower quadrant mass?
Significance: A right lower quadrant mass could suggest an abscess (Crohn disease, appendiceal abscess).

Laboratory Aids

Test: Stool culture
Significance: Stool examination not only for blood/mucus/inflammatory cells and microorganisms is important in determining the etiology of the diarrhea. Stool cultures for parasites (*Giardia, Entamoeba*), bacterial pathogens (*Salmonella, Campylobacter, Shigella, Yersinia, Aeromonas, Plesiomonas*), and *C. difficile* toxin should be obtained in all children with unexplained diarrhea.

Test: Stool Gram stain
Significance: Useful in determining the presence of polymorphonuclear leukocytes suggesting a colitis.

Test: Stool pH
Significance: Useful in identifying carbohydrate malabsorption; normal stool pH is 5 to 6.

Test: Hemoccult
Significance: Documents blood.

Test: 72-hour quantitative fecal fat evaluation
Significance: A sensitive test for steatorrhea. Patients need to be placed on a high-fat diet (3 g/kg) for 3 days. During this time, all stools are collected and frozen, and on completion the amount of ingested fat is compared to excreted fat. When malabsorption is present, disorders of pancreatic function (cystic fibrosis, Shwachman syndrome) or severe intestinal disease should be suspected.

Test: Lactose breath test
Significance: A noninvasive test that measures hydrogen levels in expired air and is based on the principle that hydrogen gas is produced by colonic bacterial fermentation of malabsorbed carbohydrates. When abnormal in older healthy-appearing children, primary lactose deficiency is suggested. However, in young children, secondary lactase deficiency should be considered and small-bowel disease should be suspected.

Test: D-xylose test
Significance: Based on the principle that D-xylose absorption occurs independently of bile salts, pancreatic secretions, and intestinal disaccharidases. A specific dose of D-xylose (0.5 gm/kg, maximum 25 g) is given orally after an 8 hour fast and the serum level of D-xylose is determined after 1 hour. Typically, disorders that alter or disrupt the intestinal mucosa produce abnormal results.

Test: Endoscopy and colonoscopy
Significance: Direct visualization of the intestinal mucosa but intestinal culture, disaccharidase, pancreatic enzyme evaluation and intestinal biopsy can be performed.

Management

• Rehydration is the cornerstone of treatment.

—Oral rehydration therapy with glucose concentrations of 74–111 mmol/L is recommended.
—Breast feeding should continue during episodes of gastroenteritis, as its promotes mucosal healing and recovery
—It has been traditionally believed that bowel rest was beneficial for formula fed infants. Many studies have shown that return feeding after 4–6 hours also promotes faster recovery
—Intravenous rehydration is indicated for patients who are severely dehydrated and unable to tolerate oral feedings

• Antibiotics

—*V. cholerae, Shigella,* and *Giardia lamblia* require antimicrobial therapy
—Prolonged courses of enteropathogenic *E. coli., Yersinia* in sickle cell patients, and *Salmonella* species infections in the very young febrile infant or when associated with bacteremia also require antimicrobial therapy

• Micronutrients

—Zinc supplementation during episodes of acute diarrhea has been shown to decrease severity and duration as well as preventing future episodes in malnourished children.

• Probiotics

—*Lactobacillus rhamnosus* GG has been shown to shorten the duration of illness as well as viral shedding in patients with rotavirus diarrhea and decrease the duration of antibiotic-associated diarrhea.

Emergency Care

Diarrhea can lead to dehydration. Any child suspected of clinical dehydration should be closely observed. If oral rehydration is ineffective, intravenous therapy is indicated. In addition, rarely acute right lower abdominal pain with diarrhea may indicate appendicitis. Culture-negative gastrointestinal bleeding associated with severe abdominal pain and diarrhea should always be treated urgently.

Issues for Referral

Because the occurrence of diarrhea in children is quite common, the decision to pursue an evaluation rests with the primary care physician. Children who present with growth failure, noninfectious heme-positive diarrhea, or unexplained chronic diarrhea should be considered for referral to a pediatric gastroenterologist.

BIBLIOGRAPHY

Ali SA, Hill DR. Giardia intestinalis. *Curr Opin Infect Dis* 2003;16(5):453–460.

Baldas sano RN, Liarcouras, CA. Chronic diarrhea: A practical approach for the pediatrician. *Pediatr Clin North Am* 1991;38: 667–685.

Fontaine O. Oral rehydration therapy: a critical component in integrated management of childhood illness. *J Pediatr Gastroenterol Nutr* 2000;30(5):490.

Gore JI, Surawicz C. Severe acute diarrhea. *Gastroenterol Clin North Am* 2003;32(4): 1249–1267.

Ryan ET, et al. Illness after international travel. *N Engl J Med* 2002;347(7):505–516.

Thielman NM, Guerrant RL. Clinical practice. Acute infectious diarrhea. *N Engl J Med* 2004;350(1):38–47.

Waters V, Ford-Jones EL, Petric M, et al. Etiology of community-acquired pediatric viral diarrhea: a prospective longitudinal study in hospitals, emergency departments, pediatric practices and child care centers during the winter rotavirus outbreak, 1997 to 1998. Rotavirus Epidemiology Study for Immunization Study Group. *Pediatr Infect Dis J* 2000;19(9):843–848.

Author: Meena Thayu, M.D.

Dyspnea

Database

DEFINITION

Shortness of breath. A subjective feeling of having difficulty breathing.

Differential Diagnosis

CONGENITAL

- Subglottic stenosis
- Vocal cord paralysis
- Macroglossia
- Pierre Robin sequence
- Laryngeal atresia
- Pulmonary sequestration
- Pulmonary hypoplasia

INFECTIOUS

- Lower airway

—Bronchiolitis
—Pertussis
—Pneumonia
—Tuberculosis

- Upper Airway

—Croup
—Epiglottitis
—Tracheitis
—Peritonsillar abscess

TOXIC, ENVIRONMENTAL, DRUGS

- Aspiration

—Fluid
—Foreign body
—Carbon monoxide poisoning
—Methemoglobinemia

- Smoke inhalation

TUMORS/CYSTS

- Head/neck

—Dermoid cysts
—Brachial cleft cysts
—Lingual thyroid
—Hemangioma
—Teratoma
—Papilloma
—Brainstem tumor

- Thoracic

—Teratoma
—Cystic hygroma
—Bronchogenic cyst
—Pericardial cyst
—Neurogenic tumor
—Lymphoma
—Leukemia

- Abdominal mass

—Hepatic mass
—Hepatoblastoma
—Neuroblastoma

- Allergy

—Anaphylaxis

- Pulmonary

—Asthma
—Atelectasis
—Pneumothorax
—Pleural effusion
—Hemorrhage
—Embolism

- Cardiac

—Pulmonary edema

- Renal

—Renal failure causing fluid overload
—Metabolic acidosis

- Hematology

—Anemia
—Sickle cell crisis/acute chest syndrome

- Muscle weakness

—Duchenne muscular dystrophy
—Spinal muscle atrophy

- Miscellaneous

—High altitude
—Exercise
—Psychogenic hyperventilation
—Anxiety/panic disorders

Approach to the Patient

The general goal is to identify the organ system responsible for the dyspnea and to determine whether the process is acute or chronic.

Phase 1: Determine if the cause is respiratory or cardiac in nature. If it is one of these two is the patient clinically stable and can the patient protect his or her airway? It is important to identify those who will need intensive/emergency care and those who can be worked up in the office.

Phase 2: Inquire about the duration of symptoms the circumstances around the onset of the dyspnea. History and physical exam should focus on respiratory and cardiology. If these two have been ruled out, other etiologies must be evaluated.

Phase 3: Appropriate use of laboratory tests and imagings.

Data Gathering

HISTORY

Question: Onset of dyspnea? What was the patient doing at the time of onset (if acute)?
Significance: In a small child, acute onset may be related to aspiration of a foreign body or liquid. If the patient was unsupervised, foreign body is a high probability. If the dyspnea occurred over days, other respiratory, cardiac or renal should be suspected.

Question: Any fever, cough, chest pain, runny nose?
Significance: This would suggest an infectious etiology. The chest pain could be related to a pneumothorax which can occur spontaneously in some individuals

Question: Any one at home sick or have respiratory problems/Illness?
Significance: Leading toward infection. However in some cases of congenital heart disease a respiratory virus like RSV can make a otherwise stable patient into a critically ill child.

Question: Is there history of wheezing or asthma?
Significance: Children who have a history of wheezing are like to reexacerbate their lung disease.

Question: Has the child ever been hospitalized or had respiratory problem in the past?
Significance: Children who have been hospitalized for respiratory problem are likely to have subsequent difficulty with other respiratory problems.

Question: Any history of cardiac problems or ever been diagnosed with a murmur?
Significance: In the absence of an infectious type or wheezing type of history, a murmur can help the examiner focus on the cardiac exam.

Physical Examination

LUNG EXAMINATION

Finding: Crackles or rhonchi auscultate
Significance: Lower lung disease such as pneumonia or bronchiolitis. Fluid overload can cause bilateral crackles

Finding: Wheezing auscultated
Significance: Wheezing is usually heard on expiration. Suggest obstructive lung disease like asthma or reactive airways disease or anaphylaxis

Finding: Distant or absent breath sounds
Significance: Foreign body aspiration blocking air movement. Pneumothorax should also be suspected.

Finding: Barking cough
Significance: Croup, which is usually caused by parainfluenza virus.

Finding: Symptoms worse in supine position
Significance: Could be secondary to pulmonary edema or compression by a mediastinal mass.

Finding: Egophony auscultate
Significance: Pleural effusion should be suspected.

HEART EXAMINATION

Finding: Loud murmur or gallop auscultated
Significance: Cardiac disease in which pulmonary edema can be etiology of the dyspnea.

Finding: Cyanosis
Significance: Poor oxygen perfusion

Finding: Low blood pressure and poor skin perfusion
Significance: the patient can be in shock. Quick identification of the type of shock is needed to correct the underlying problem.

Finding: Clubbing of the digits
Significance: Suggests chronic disease like cystic fibrosis or cardiac disease

Finding: Drooling, with mouth open in an ill-appearing child
Significance: Suggests epiglotitis and need for careful evaluation (see epiglotitis)

Finding: Abdominal mass palpated
Significance: Could be causing compression of lungs

Finding: Ascites or edema
Significance: Fluid overload either from renal or cardiac etiology

 Laboratory Aids

CHEST RADIOGRAPH

Significance: Look for appearance of the lung fields for the different types of pneumonia. Evaluate the heart size and the pulmonary vascularity for fluid overload. Hyperinflation suggests an obstructive pulmonary disease like asthma. A hyperinflated (usually right lobe) darkened lobe is suspicious of a foreign body that is present. Seeing a shift in the heart and seeing a lung edge are common in pneumothorax or effusion. Fluid in the costophrenic angle suggests an effusion.

PULSE OXIMETRY

Significance: A rapid assessment of oxygen perfusion.

ARTERIAL BLOOD GAS

Significance: A more detailed assessment of oxygenation and acidosis. A blood gas will also delineate metabolic versus respiratory acidosis and also can show if compensation has occurred.

COMPLETE BLOOD COUNT WITH DIFFERENTIAL

Significance: First an elevated white blood count with a left shift differential can be a sign of infection. If the patient has pallor, the hemoglobin can be evaluated to see if the patient is anemic. A CBC also can be helpful in patients in which leukemia or other oncologic diseases are suspected.

MANTOUX (PPD)

Significance: With a history of family members with tuberculosis or immigrants from a country where TB is prevalent, a PPD should be placed with anergy panel.

Issues for Referral

Factors that may help alert you to make a referral or an emergency:

• Any patient that has unstable vital signs, inability to oxygenate, and will need critical care services.
• Any patient with a suspected foreign body aspiration will need a surgical consult that is able to provide bronchcosopy.
• If asthma is suspected, use criteria as noted in asthma (see Asthma).
• Any patient with epiglotitis will need an Otolaryngologist to evaluate the patient under general anesthesia (see Epiglotitis).

• Anaphylaxis is a medical emergency and mandates immediate action. Epinephrine, Benadryl, and possibly steroids are the drugs of choice for treatment.
• Any patient that has a pneumothorax may require surgical aspiration or chest tube placement (see Pneumothorax).
• Any patient in whom an oncologic process is suspected should be referred to a tertiary care center with a critical care unit with a pediatric oncologist is recommended (see Leukemia).

Clinical Pearls

• A child who presents with dyspnea, anxiety, or panic disorder should only be considered after the more serious etiologies have been ruled out.
• If hyperventilation is suspected, a brown paper bag can be useful to break the cycle of hypocarbia.

 Questions and Answers

Q: Is dyspnea, in most cases, pulmonary in nature?

A: Yes, it is in most cases. However if infectious, foreign body, and asthma etiologies are ruled out, nonrespiratory causes must be investigated.

BIBLIOGRAPHY

Diagnosis and treatment. *Pediatrics in Review* 1987;9(6):191–196.

Denny FW. Acute respiratory infections in children: etiology and epidemiology. *Pediatrics in Review* 1987;9(5):135–146.

Dibs SD, Baker MD. Anaphylaxis in children: a 5-year experience. *Pediatrics* 1997;99(1):E7.

Holroyd HJ. Foreign body aspiration: potential cause of coughing and wheezing. *Pediatrics in Review* 1988;10(2):59–63.

McIntosh K. Respiratory syncytial virus infections in infants and children: diagnosis and treatment. *Pediatr Rev* 1987;9(6): 191–196.

Schidlow DV, Callahan CW. Pneumonia. *Pediatrics in Review* 1996;17(9):300–309.

Segel GB. Anemia. *Pediatrics in Review* 1988;10(3):77–88
Author: Charles Schwartz

Dysuria

 Database

DEFINITION

Painful urination

 Differential Diagnosis

CONGENITAL/ANATOMIC

- Meatal stenosis
- Urethral stricture
- Posterior urethral diverticula
- Urethral stones
- Urethral valves
- Ureterocele
- Ectopic ureter
- Vesicovaginal fistula

INFECTIOUS

- Viral infection
- Gonorrhea
- Chlamydia
- Herpes simplex
- Tuberculosis
- Cystitis
- Candida
- Urethritis
- Pinworms
- Prostatitis

TOXIC, ENVIRONMENTAL, DRUGS

- Bubble-bath urethritis
- Cytoxan

TRAUMA

- Diaper dermatitis
- Foreign body
- Bicycle injury
- Masturbation
- Sexual abuse
- Irritation—sand, tight pants

TUMOR

- Sarcoma botryoides

GENETIC/METABOLIC

- Cystinuria

ALLERGIC INFLAMMATORY

- Food allergy
- Stevens-Johnson syndrome
- Contact dermatitis such as poison ivy

FUNCTIONAL

- Attention mechanism

MISCELLANEOUS

- Appendicitis

Approach to the Patient

GENERAL GOALS

Determine the cause and begin treatment.

Phase 1: Rule out common causes such as trauma, infection, chemical irritant, constipation, and masturbation. Consider attention-getting behavior.

Phase 2: Continue investigation—look for congenital problems that cause infection, strictures. Metabolic disease and allergies.

Phase 3: Begin treatment.

HINTS FOR SCREENING PROBLEMS

Ask about medications and food allergens. Ask about special situations such as sand in bathing suit to cause irritation.

 Data Gathering

HISTORY

Question: Do the symptoms occur at any special time of day?
Significance: May indicate an attention mechanism if occurs before school.

Question: What kinds of medicine do you take?
Significance: Some medications such as cytoxin will cause irritation of the urethra.

Question: Have there been any new foods or known food allergens?
Significance: Milk and citrus fruits can cause dysuria in certain patients. Best determined if symptoms regress on elimination of possible offending food.

Question: Do you use bubble bath?
Significance: Bubble bath is fun but depletes the protective lipids in the urethra

Question: Any signs of bleeding?
Significance: Can indicate trauma, infection, or congenital anomalies. Calcium excretion can cause dysuria as well as hematuria.

Question: Fever?
Significance: Common sign of urinary tract infection.

Question: Frequency?
Significance: Both frequency and dysuria are common findings in urinary tract infections.

Question: Past history of urologic operations?
Significance: Antireflux surgery may have a side effect of dysuria.

Question: What have you taken for the discomfort?
Significance: Although cranberry juice is used for many urinary problems, the volume needed is usually more than what can be easily ingested.

Question: Quality and strength of the urinary stream?
Significance: Patients with posterior urethral valves have small, frequent voidings with low pressure because of the obstruction in the posterior urethra.

Question: Sexual activity?
Significance: Urethritis from gonorrhea or Chlamydia

Physical Examination

Finding: Any signs of redness or ecchymoses?
Significance: May indicate trauma from masturbation or abuse

Finding: Any bleeding?
Significance: Seen in trauma, tumors, and infection

Finding: Any change in behavior?
Significance: This symptom may be an attention-seeking device

Finding: Abnormal swelling?
Significance: May occur in trauma or rare tumors

Finding: Abnormal urethra?
Significance: Prolapsed urethra or diverticula

Finding: Grape-like structures in vagina?
Significance: Sarcoma botryoides

Finding: Abdominal pain?
Significance: Intraabdominal abscess or low-lying inflamed appendix can cause dysuria

 ## Laboratory Aids

Test: Urinalysis
Significance: Most urinary tract infections will have white cells in the urine.

Test: Urine culture
Significance: Check for infection.

Test: Ultrasound
Significance: Not routinely requested unless a congenital anomaly is suspected.

Test: Metabolic screens
Significance: If sediment shows crystals; if familial history of metabolic disease.

Test: Urinary screen for gonorrhea and Chlamydia
Significance: DNA amplification by PCR or ligase chain reaction on freshly voided urine has 95% sensitivity and 100% specificity.

 ## Common Questions and Answers

Q: How does bubble bath cause dysuria?
A: The bubble bath depletes lipids that protect the urethra, causing the tissue to swell and become inflamed.

Q: Can allergies cause dysuria?
A: It is difficult to directly prove allergies as a cause of dysuria. However, in some cases, elimination of certain foods such as spices, citrus fruits, or known skin allergens have improved symptoms.

Q: How do children get infected with gonococcus?
A: This is a red flag of sexual abuse, which must be investigated.

Q: Which viruses cause dysuria?
A: Adenovirus has been identified.

Issues for Referral

- Evidence of congenital anomaly
- Increasing severity of symptoms
- Failure to respond to symptomatic or specific treatment

Clinical Pearls

- Sometimes difficult to differentiate dysuria from frequency, which may cause an uncomfortable feeling or pressure that is described by the child as "pain."
- Discharge with dysuria suggests gonococcal or Chlamydia infection.
- Low-lying inflamed appendix may cause bladder irritation and dysuria.
- Urethral prolapse may present as hematuria or frequency.

BIBLIOGRAPHY

Anonymous. 1998 Guidelines for treatment of sexually transmitted diseases. Centers for Disease Control and Prevention. *MMWR* 1998; 47(RR-1):1–111.

Claudius H. Dysuria in adolescents. *Western Journal of Medicine* 2000;172(3):201–205.

Hellerstein S, Linebarger JS. Voiding dysfunction in pediatric patients. *Clin Pediatr (Phila)* 2003;42(1):43–49.

Lee HJ, Pyo JW, Choi EH et al. Isolation of adenovirus type from the urine of children with acute hemorrhagic cystitis. *Pediatr Infect Dis J* 1996;15(7):633–634.

Rushton HG. Urinary tract infections in children. Epidemiology, evaluation, and management. *Pediatr Clin North Am* 1997; 44(5):1133–1169.

Authors: Caroline Schwartz and William Schwartz

Earache

Database

DEFINITION

- Primary otalgia refers to pain originating from the ear structures.
- Secondary otalgia is the sensation of ear pain as a result of referred pain from other areas of the head and neck. Secondary pain is referred through cranial and cervical nerves that share distributions with the ear.

Differential Diagnosis

PRIMARY OTALGIA

Infectious

- Acute otitis media
- Otitis externa
- Varicella virus
- Herpes simplex virus
- Cellulitis
- Furunculosis (localized abscess of cartilaginous portion of ear canal (outer third))
- Mastoiditis
- Myringitis (inflammation and blisters on the tympanic membrane)
- Perichondritis (inflammation of auricle without ear lobe involvement)

Trauma

- Foreign body
- Lacerations, abrasions
- Blunt trauma
- Barotrauma (injury to middle ear arising from abrupt changes in pressure (airplanes, scuba diving))
- Thermal injury to auricle
- Caustic burns from hearing aid batteries

Tumor

Rare in pediatric patients, but may involve any of the ear structures including skin, bone, vascular, and neural components

- Rhabdomyosarcoma
- Lymphoma
- Pheochromocytoma

Allergic/Inflammatory

- Otitis media with effusion
- Eczema
- Psoriasis
- Allergic reaction to topical antibiotic and cerumenolytic agents.

Functional

- Eustachian tube dysfunction

Miscellaneous

- Impacted cerumen

—Eosinophilic granuloma
—Wegener granulomatosis

- Aural neuralgia (brief sharp pain localized deep in ear without radiation; unknown etiology)

SECONDARY OTALGIA

Infectious

- Dental abscess

—Gingivitis

- Stomatitis due to herpes simplex or coxsackie viruses
- Tonsillitis
- Peritonsillar abscess
- Retropharyngeal abscess
- Mumps
- Sinusitis
- Cervical adenitis
- Laryngitis
- Sialadenitis
- Ramsay Hunt syndrome (viral neuritis of facial nerve due to herpes zoster)

Trauma

- Dental trauma
- Penetrating injuries to the oropharynx
- Lacerations
- Posttonsillectomy/adenoidectomy
- Burn (caustic, thermal or electrical)
- Injuries to the neck and C-spine, including fractures and muscle tension

Tumor

- Oropharyngeal/laryngeal tumors
- Intracranial tumors (rarely will present with ear pain)

Allergic/Inflammatory

- Allergic rhinitis
- Cervical spine arthritis

Miscellaneous

- Aphthous ulcers (canker sores)
- Foreign body lodged in piriform sinus or esophagus
- Esophagitis
- Temporomandibular joint (TMJ) disease
- Migraine
- Thyroid inflammation
- Psychogenic (rarely)
- "Pillow otalgia" (otalgia due to sleep position)

Approach to the Patient

General Goals

The primary determination is whether or not the child needs acute/emergent treatment for life-threatening disease. Ear pain may arise from disease involving almost any part of the head and neck; therefore, history taking and physical examination should be directed toward assessing symptoms from the entire region, not just the ear. Preceding symptoms and a history of events leading up to the onset of pain are of particular importance, as there are classic historic features to many of the diseases of the ear (e.g., URI symptoms with otitis media, wrestling history with auricle disease, swimming history with otitis externa).

Phase 1: Each encounter should begin with a careful history and physical examination. If the examination of the ear does not reveal the cause of pain, thoroughly examine the entire head and neck region.

Phase 2: An abnormal audiogram or tympanogram may help to determine if ear pathology is present when physical examination is normal.

Phase 3: Referral to an otorhinolaryngologist and/or dentist is indicated in cases of ear pain without identifiable cause.

Data Gathering

HISTORY

Question: Duration of symptoms?
Significance: Acute onset suggests recent trauma or infection. Acute otitis media is the most common cause of acute onset pediatric otalgia.

Question: Severity of pain?
Significance: Severe pain is usually otogenic.

Question: Precipitating factors?
Significance: Pain increased with auricle movement is seen with otitis externa, furunculosis, perichondritis, and cellulitis. Pain increased with jaw movement suggests TMJ disease or furunculosis.

Question: Associated symptoms?
Significance: Symptoms that point to primary otalgia include aural discharge, deafness, tinnitus, and vertigo.

Question: Hoarseness?
Significance: Suggestive of oropharyngeal or laryngeal pathology including infections, foreign body, and GER.

Question: Choking/coughing?
Significance: Consider foreign body, mass, or GER.

Question: Location of additional pain or symptoms?
Significance: If referred pain, will likely have symptoms at primary site as well.

Question: Fever?
Significance: Suggestive of infectious etiology.

Question: Trauma and barotrauma?
Significance: Ask about recent ear cleaning, falls, accidents, air travel, diving.

Question: History of recurrent otitis media?
Significance: Consider otitis media with effusion, cholesteatoma.

Physical Examination

Finding: Intense pain elicited by traction on pinna
Significance: Suggestive of otitis externa or furunculosis.

Finding: Areas of trauma
Significance: There may be an isolated abrasion or laceration; however, inspect carefully for hemotympanum, associated injuries, and evidence of a basilar skull fracture.

Finding: Foreign bodies
Significance: May be isolated, or associated with otitis externa; there are several case reports of foreign bodies found behind the tympanic membrane.

Finding: Bulging, red, immobile tympanic membrane
Significance: Consistent with acute otitis media.

Finding: Retracted, immobile tympanic membrane
Significance: Suggests otitis media with effusion and eustachian tube dysfunction.

Finding: Redness, swelling, or tenderness of auricle
Significance: With lobe involvement may be seen with cellulitis; without lobe involvement may be seen with perichondritis.

Finding: Normal ear examination
Significance: Suggests secondary otalgia. Be sure to examine head and neck carefully (see subsequent findings).

Finding: Dental caries
Significance: Multiple dental caries should raise the suspicion of a possible dental abscess.

Finding: Vesicles on the auricle or in the ear canal
Significance: Chickenpox and herpes zoster may involve the auricle and ear canal.

Finding: Tonsillar asymmetry or uvular deviation from midline
Significance: May represent peritonsillar cellulitis/abscess or mass.

Finding: Assess facial-nerve and other cranial nerve function.
Significance: Bell palsy may be a complication of acute otitis media. Other cranial nerve dysfunction suggests possible intracranial lesion.

Finding: Ear protrudes anteriorly or laterally placed auricle
Significance: This is present in mastoiditis, a complication of supurative otitis media.

Laboratory Aids

The history and physical examination are usually sufficient to make the diagnosis.

Test: Audiometry
Significance: Assess for hearing loss suggestive of primary otalgia.

Test: Tympanometry
Significance: Useful in assessment of otitis media with effusion, eustachian-tube dysfunction, and tympanostomy tube obstruction.

Test: Culture of aural discharge
Significance: Indicated when otitis externa or otitis media with perforation of the tympanic membrane does not resolve as expected with routine antibiotic usage.

Test: Computed tomography (CT) scan(s)
Significance: Important if symptoms suggest retropharyngeal mass/abscess (neck), to rule out sinusitis in complicated cases (sinus study), or to further evaluate for mastoiditis (mastoid).

Test: Magnetic resonance imaging (MRI) or CT scan of head
Significance: Rarely needed unless intracranial lesion is suspected.

Test: Blood tests
Significance: Not routinely useful.

Emergency Care

Disorders with potential to cause airway compromise (e.g., mass lesions, foreign bodies, abscess, penetrating injuries, posttonsillectomy complications):

- Establish "ABCs" as indicated.
- Consult otorhinolaryngologist (ORL).
- Hospitalize.

Trauma resulting in hearing loss, significant bleeding, or fractures:

- Establish "ABCs" as indicated.
- Promptly consult ORL.
- Do not attempt to remove debris from ear if suspected basilar skull fracture (can introduce bacteria).
- Hospitalize as indicated.

Infectious etiologies that cause toxic-appearing or "septic" child:

- Establish "ABCs" as indicated.
- Hospitalize and administer intravenous antibiotics.

Issues for Referral

Factors that may alert you to make a referral to ORL when otalgia is primary in origin include:

- Pain with unexplained hearing loss, vertigo, tinnitus
- Unexplained or persistent otorrhea
- Suspected neoplasm
- History suggestive of severe barotrauma
- Acute otitis media with complications

- Foreign bodies that cannot be removed easily from the ear
- Potential for auricle destruction (e.g., perichondritis can lead to permanent deformation, cauliflower ear)
- Ear pain without an identifiable source

Therapy

- Therapy is directed at the identified underlying cause.
- Pain medication such as topical benzocaine for acute otitis media, and acetaminophen or ibuprofen is always important, as many of the infectious etiologies are exquisitely painful.

Follow-Up

Varies depending on the underlying diagnosis.

Common Questions and Answers

Question: Which nerves are involved in referred pain to the ear?
Answer: Sensory innervation of the ear arises from branches of the fifth (trigeminal), seventh (facial), ninth (glossopharyngeal), and tenth (vagus) cranial nerves as well as the second and third cervical nerves.

Question: What is the most common source of referred ear pain?
Answer: Dental disease.

Question: What are the most common organisms in otitis externa?
Answer: Pseudomonas aeruginosa, Staphylococcus aureus, Staphylococcus epidermidis, streptococci, *Enterobacter aerogenes, Proteus mirabilis, Klebsiella pneumoniae, Candida, Aspergillus.*

Question: What are the most common organisms in acute otitis media?
Answer: Streptococcus pneumoniae, Haemophilus influenzae, Moraxella catarrhalis, and viral agents.

BIBLIOGRAPHY

Janvrin S. Middle ear pain and trauma during air travel. *Clinical Evidence* 2002;(7):466–468.

LeLiever WC. Nonotologic otalgia. *JAMA* 1990;264:2302.

Leung AK, Fong JH, Leong AG. Otalgia in children. *J Natl Med Assoc* 2000;92:254–260.

Licameli GR. Diagnosis and management of otalgia in the pediatric patient. *Pediatr Ann* 1999;28(6):364–368.

Yellon R. The spectrum of reflux-associated otolaryngologic problems in infants and children. *Am J Med* 1997;103:125S–129S.

Zenian J. Pillow otalgia. *Arch Otolaryngo Head Neck Surg* 2001;127:1288.

Author: Laura N. Sinai

Edema

Database

DEFINITION

Edema is the presence of an abnormal amount of fluid in the extracellular spaces of the body. Edema is usually secondary to low albumin, obstruction of venous or lymphatic channels, or trauma.

CAUSES

- Excessive losses

—Renal loss of protein
—Gastrointestinal

- Inadequate production

—Liver disease
—Malnutrition

- Local trauma
- Increased hydrostatic pressure

—Congestive heart failure
—Pericardial effusion
—Venous obstruction
—Lymphatic obstruction

Differential Diagnosis

LOCALIZED

- Trauma—pressure or sun damage
- Infection
- Allergy
- Lymphatic obstruction (less common)
- Bee stings or insect bites

GENERALIZED

Congenital

- Lymphatic obstruction of legs or thoracic duct
- Infection
- Hepatitis and liver failure
- Pericarditis

Toxic, Environmental, Drugs

- Sodium poisoning
- Toxic effect on liver and/or heart (chemotherapy)
- Cirrhosis

Tumor

- Obstruction of venous return from enlarged abdominal lymph nodes
- Genetic/metabolic
- Sickle cell renal failure

Allergic Inflammatory

- Protein-losing enteropathy

Miscellaneous

- Nephrotic syndrome
- Renal failure
- Congestive heart failure
- Pericarditis
- Gastrointestinal protein loss
- Postpericardiotomy or congenital heart surgery
- Endocrine—sodium retention, hypothyroidism
- Hepatobiliary diseases

Approach to the Patient

GENERAL GOALS

Determine the cause of swelling. Is it localized, are there any losses of protein, or is there underproduction of protein? Determine the serum protein/albumin, which would make you consider increased losses or decreased production.

Phase 1: Is the swelling localized as seen in trauma, lymphatic, or venous obstruction?

Phase 2: Are there urinary or gastrointestinal losses? This will be associated with decreased serum albumin. Most likely the source of the loss is renal disease and less frequently gastrointestinal losses.

Phase 3: Search for other causes of edema such as insect bites, pericardial effusion, metabolic disease.

Data Gathering

HISTORY

Question: Is the edema localized or generalized?
Significance: See Differential Diagnosis section.

Question: Is the patient asymptomatic or in some distress specifically due to the edema?
Significance: Determines treatment urgency.

Question: Is there evidence of cardiac, renal, or gastrointestinal disease?
Significance: These are the major causes of edema.

Question: Has waist size become larger? Are shoes difficult to put on?
Significance: Evidence of edema in body.

Question: What is the salt intake in diet?
Significance: In some patients, excess salt contributes to edema.

Question: Is there shortness of breath?
Significance: There may be ascites, which compresses the diaphragm, or causes pleural effusions.

Question: Is there chronic diarrhea?
Significance: Seen in protein-losing enteropathy or lymphatic obstruction.

Question: Have any urinalyses been performed in the past?
Significance: May help date the onset of the problem.

Question: History of allergies?
Significance: Allergies will commonly cause swelling around the eyes or face.

Physical Examination

Finding: Dependent edema
Significance: Lumbosacral area pretibial pressure to detect edema scrotum/labia

Finding: Percussion of chest
Significance: Pleural effusion

Finding: Shifting dullness
Significance: Early signs of ascites

Finding: Soft ear cartilage
Significance: Common finding in nephrotic syndrome

Finding: Pitting edema
Significance: Pitting edema is seen in cases of protein loss and obstruction of venous/lymphatic flow, whereas nonpitting edema is seen in salt poisoning.

Laboratory Aids

DISCRIMINATING LABORATORY TESTS

Test: Dipstick urinalysis
Significance: If there is generalized edema with heavy proteinuria and hypoalbuminemia, the presumptive diagnosis is always nephrotic syndrome until proven otherwise.

Test: Serum albumin
Significance: If there is generalized edema with no proteinuria but hypoalbuminemia, consider cardiac, gastrointestinal, or hepatobiliary disease and direct additional studies to evaluate these three organ systems specifically. If there is either localized edema or generalized edema but a normal urinalysis and a normal serum albumin, consider other unusual causes for edema such as mechanical or lymphatic obstruction, certain endocrine disorders, or the effects of drugs or toxins.

Test: Stool albumin
Significance: Seen in protein-losing enteropathy.

Issues for Referral

Referral to a specialist for edema is indicated for the following reasons:

- Nephrotic edema with impaired glomerular function—pediatric nephrologist
- Protein-losing enteropathy or hepatobiliary disease—pediatric gastroenterologist
- Congestive heart failure secondary to occult cardiac disease-pediatric cardiologist
- Endocrine-mediated edema—pediatric endocrinologist
- Lymphatic or other mechanical obstructions—vascular surgeon or pediatric surgeon, if readily available

Emergency Care

Any child or adolescent with an edema-forming state that compromises either cardiorespiratory function or the vascular integrity of a peripheral organ or limb should be referred immediately to an appropriate specialist for emergency care.

Clinical Pearls

- If edema is massive, the patient may awaken with swollen eyelids. Place blocks under the head of the bed to keep head elevated.
- If there is scrotal edema, jockey shorts will help support scrotum and protect the skin from breaking down.

Common Questions and Answers

Q: At what level of serum albumin will edema occur?
A: Edema is generally associated with serum albumin below 2.5 g/dL.

Q: Why does pericardial effusion cause edema?
A: The pericardial effusion is associated with decreased lymphatic flow and increased venous pressure.

Q: Is there a certain group of allergens that will cause edema?
A: No special allergens are associated with edema. The usual causes include such foods as peanuts and drugs such as penicillin.

BIBLIOGRAPHY

Dudin A, Othman A. Acute periorbital swelling: evaluation of management protocol. *Pediatr Emerg Care* 1996;12(1):16–20.

Holliay MA, Segar WE. Reducing errors in fluid therapy management. *Pediatrics* 2003;111(2):424–425.

Jacobs ML, Rychik J, Byrum CJ, et al. Protein-losing enteropathy after Fontan operation: resolution after baffle fenestration. *Ann Thorac Surg* 1996;61(1):206–208.

Kelsch RC, Sedman AB. Nephrotic syndrome. *Pediatr Rev* 1993;14:30–38.

Molina JF, Brown RF, Gedalia A, et al. Protein losing enteropathy as the initial manifestation of childhood systemic lupus erythematosus. *J Rheumatol* 1996;23(7):1269–1271.

Moritz ML, Ayus JC. Prevention of hospital acquired hyponatremia: A case for using isotonic saline. *Pediatrics* 2003;111(2):227–230.

Rosen FS. Urticaria, angioedema, anaphylaxis. *Pediatr Rev* 1992;13:387–390.

Vande Walle JG, Donckerwolcke RA. Pathogenesis of edema formation in the nephrotic syndrome. *Pediatr Nephrol* 2001;16(3):283–293.

Author: Michael E. Norman

Failure to Thrive

Database

DEFINITION

- Failure to thrive (FTT) is a term used to describe infants and children who fail to meet standards for appropriate growth. FTT is more a sign or symptom of an underlying problem than a final diagnosis or disease state. FTT can occur due to inadequate intake, inadequate absorption, excess metabolic demand or defective utilization.
- The Gomez formula is the ratio of the child's current weight for age divided by the expected weight for age (50th percentile) and can be used to assess the degree of malnutrition: if the ratio is 75% to 90% the FTT is considered mild; moderate, if the ratio is 60% to 74%; and severe, if the ratio is less than 60%.

Differential Diagnosis

CONGENITAL/ANATOMIC

- Congenital syndromes
- Chromosomal abnormalities (e.g., Down syndrome)
- Congenital heart disease
- Hirschsprung disease
- Pyloric stenosis
- Malrotation
- Vascular slings

INFECTIOUS

- Urinary tract infection
- Chronic sinusitis
- Human immunodeficiency virus (HIV)
- Hepatitis
- Tuberculosis
- Parasitic infection

TOXINS, ENVIRONMENTAL, DRUGS

- Inadequate caloric intake due to emotional deprivation
- Maternal depression
- Poor feeding techniques
- Poor child–caregiver interactions
- Improper formula preparation
- Lack of proper environment for mealtimes
- Parental drug/alcohol abuse
- Child abuse/neglect
- Lead/mercury poisoning
- Hypervitaminosis
- Fetal exposure to alcohol/anticonvulsants

GENETIC/METABOLIC

- Malabsorption (lactase deficiency, celiac disease)
- Cystic fibrosis
- Diabetes mellitus
- Thyroid disease
- Pituitary disease
- Adrenal disease
- Rickets
- Parathyroid disease
- Galactosemia
- Aminoaciduria
- Organic acidurias
- Storage diseases
- Hypercalcemia

ALLERGIC/INFLAMMATORY

- Food allergies
- Inflammatory bowel disease
- Chronic lung disease, including aspiration

FUNCTIONAL

- Gastroesophageal reflux (GER)
- Chronic constipation

NEUROLOGIC

- Cerebral palsy
- Oral-motor dysfunction
- Structural abnormalities
- Degenerative diseases
- Diencephalic syndrome

RENAL

- Chronic renal insufficiency
- Renal tubular acidosis

HEMATOLOGIC

- Sickle cell disease
- Thalassemia
- Iron-deficiency anemia

ORTHOPAEDIC

- Osteogenesis imperfecta
- Chondrodystrophies

MISCELLANEOUS

- Upper airway obstruction, including adenoidal hypertrophy
- Acquired heart disease
- Dental abnormalities (caries, infection)

Approach to the Patient

GENERAL GOALS

Determine whether the patient has growth failure by measuring the child's weight, height, and head circumference accurately, plotting them on standard growth curves, and comparing them to previous growth points.

Phase 1: Is the malnutrition acute or chronic, symmetric or asymmetric? With acute malnutrition, weight is the first parameter to be affected, leading to wasting. After weeks to months of malnutrition, stunted linear growth occurs. Finally, with long-standing and/or severe malnutrition, head circumference is affected. Symmetric FTT suggests long-standing malnutrition, chromosomal abnormalities, congenital infection, or teratogenic exposures as etiologies.

When growth failure is recognized, the prenatal, developmental, and nutritional history must be complete. Search for indicators of diminished intake, excessive losses, and medical diseases. The physical examination should be thorough. The laboratory evaluation is guided by the results of the history and physical examination. Although some laboratory tests can be useful in the evaluation of FTT, random screening in search of a medical diagnosis is usually unrevealing, and is not recommended.

Phase 2: If the history and physical examination suggest a medical disease as a cause of the growth failure, appropriate diagnostic evaluation should be done. In the majority of cases, the cause of growth failure is environmental or psychosocial. Medical diseases are identified in fewer than 50% of children hospitalized for growth failure and even less frequently in children evaluated in the outpatient setting.

Phase 3: If organic disease is excluded, begin education and psychosocial interventions to improve nutrition.

HINTS FOR SCREENING PROBLEM

Always plot growth on the same standardized growth chart so that the child's percentiles are known and can be compared to percentiles at previous ages.

Data Gathering

HISTORY

Question: What is the child's typical daily diet?
Significance: Because FTT is commonly an environmental problem, and represents undernutrition, the child's feeding history may yield clues to the problem. For example, some toddlers who have not yet been weaned from the bottle may have excess fluid but poor caloric intake. Others may be drinking excess water, juice, or tea. Have the parent describe in detail what the child eats and drinks each day, the daytime schedule, how formula is prepared. Determine who is responsible for meal preparation, when and where the child eats, and what problems the parent identifies related to mealtime.

Question: Does the child have a medical problem that explains the FTT?
Significance: Ask about symptoms that would lead you to believe the child has a medical illness, including vomiting, diarrhea, abdominal distension, exercise intolerance, developmental problems, etc.

Question: Are there indications of parental stress, drug abuse, or other family factors that may be contributing to the child's growth failure?
Significance: Children do not live in isolation, and growth failure may be a manifestation of family dysfunction.

Physical Examination

Start with a complete physical examination. Observe the interaction between the parent and the child, especially during a feeding.

Finding: Changing growth patterns on a plotted growth chart.
Significance: In practice, FTT is identified when a child's weight falls below the 5th percentile for age, when the weight falls more than two major percentile groups, or when the weight for height is below 80% of the median.

Finding: Look for wasted, thin extremities, with loose skin hanging from the buttocks; temporal wasting; thin, sparse hair or alopecia.
Significance: Signs of malnutrition

Finding: Cheilosis, or cracking and irritation at the corners of the mouth.
Significance: Riboflavin and other vitamin B complex deficiencies

Finding: Edema
Significance: Protein deficiency

Finding: Oropharyngeal abnormalities (dental caries, tonsillar hypertrophy, submucosal clefts, etc.).
Significance: These factors may interfere with eating.

Finding: Neurologic abnormalities
Significance: Cerebral palsy and other neurologic abnormalities may result in oral-motor dysfunction, swallowing incoordination, and difficulty eating.

Finding: Dysmorphic features
Significance: Suggestive of a genetic disorder, which may be associated with poor growth

Finding: Bruises, burns, patterned cutaneous injuries
Significance: Such injuries should raise the suspicion for child physical abuse.

Laboratory Aids

The majority of children with FTT have no laboratory abnormalities. Avoid extensive, random laboratory evaluation.

Test: A complete blood count (CBC)
Significance: Rule out iron-deficiency anemia, neutropenia, leukemia

Test: Lead level
Significance: Rule out lead poisoning, which may be associated with impaired appetite

Test: Urinalysis and urine culture
Significance: Screens for urinary tract infection and renal tubular acidosis

Test: Purified protein derivative (PPD) test (contains 5 tuberculin units of PPD)
Significance: To rule out tuberculosis

Test: Comprehensive metabolic (or chemistry) panel
Significance: Assess for underlying metabolic problems and renal insufficiency. These tests are indicated to help prevent the refeeding syndrome. The refeeding syndrome includes potentially dangerous disorders in serum phosphorus, calcium, potassium, and other minerals and electrolytes at the time of reintroduction of nutrition, in severely malnourished children.

Emergency Care

SEVERE MALNUTRITION

• Children meeting criteria for severe malnutrition are at risk for refeeding syndrome, and should be hospitalized.
• Early hospitalization of the severely malnourished child focuses on slowly introducing nutrition while avoiding potentially life-threatening changes in serum electrolytes. In the most severe cases, life support, and hyperalimentation are needed. Hospitalization provides a controlled environment in which to assess the causes of growth failure, and to determine the child's caloric needs for catch-up growth.
• Therapy aimed at improving and sustaining the child's nutrition needs to continue well after the child has been discharged from the hospital and requires frequent weight checks, careful monitoring, and family support. Clinicians with access to dieticians should seek their expertise.

Common Questions and Answers

Q: How can you differentiate between FTT and alternative diagnoses related to growth?
A: Recognize that 3% of the population will naturally fall below the 3rd percentile using the most recent growth charts from the Centers for Disease Control and Prevention (CDC). These children usually are proportional (normal weight for height). Growth velocity and height for weight determinations may be helpful in identifying children with malnutrition.

Q: How quickly will a child respond to nutritional therapy?
A: Initiation of catch-up growth depends on the severity of the malnutrition. Initially, weight gains of 2 to 3 times the normal growth rate for age may be observed. Weight gain will precede improvements in height. Months of refeeding are required to restore the patient's weight for height, stature, and head circumference.

Issues for Referral

• Indications of child abuse or neglect: in every state, laws require that physicians report suspected child abuse and neglect to child welfare agencies for investigation.
• Multidisciplinary team referral: for children with moderate FTT, those who do not improve after therapy has been initiated, or families with psychosocial problems, nutritionists, nurses, social workers, feeding specialists, and psychologists can contribute to the continual assessment and care of the child and family.

Clinical Pearls

• Remember that medical and psychosocial causes of malnutrition often coexist and should be considered.
• Remember to ask about how much juice the infant or toddler drinks. This is a very common cause of FTT.
• In cases of moderate-severe FTT, it may be necessary to increase the caloric density of the child's foods, as many malnourished children cannot increase the volume of food ingested to meet the requirement for catch-up growth. A diet with approximately 30%–35% more energy and nearly twice the amount of protein is needed for catch-up growth.
• Provide a multivitamin.
• Continued, close follow-up of the malnourished child is essential to prevent recurrent growth failure and to monitor the child's development, which can be adversely affected in moderate and severe growth failure.

BIBLIOGRAPHY

Chatoor I. Feeding disorders in infants and toddlers: diagnosis and treatment. *Child & Adolesc Psych Clin North Am* 2002;11(2): 163–183.

Gahagan S, Holmes R. A stepwise approach to evaluation of undernutrition and failure to thrive. *Pediatr Clin North Am* 1998;45: 169–187.

Wright C. Identification and management of failure to thrive: a community perspective. *Arch Dis Child* 2000;82:5–9.

Zenel JA. Failure to thrive: a general pediatrician's perspective. *J Pediatr Rev* 1997;18(11):371–378.

Authors: Cindy W. Christian and Matthew J. Cox

Fever and Petechiae

 Database

DEFINITION

Petechiae are defined as small hemorrhages into the superficial layers of the skin. Petechiae are less than 3 mm in size, and manifest as a reddish-purple, macular, nonblanching skin rash. Purpura are larger skin hemorrhages and are purple in color. Purpura are often macular, like petechiae, but may be raised or tender.

CAUSES

Petechiae, when accompanied by fever, most often has an infectious etiology. Multiple organisms are associated with fever and petechiae. Less commonly, fever and petechiae may be caused by other entities such as acute leukemia, idiopathic thrombocytopenic purpura (ITP), and bacterial endocarditis.

- Bacterial

—*Neisseria meningitidis*
—*Streptococcus pneumoniae*
—*Hemophilus influenzae* type b
—*Staphylococcus aureus*
—*Streptococcus pyogenes*
—*Escherichia coli*

- Viral

—Enterovirus
—Adenovirus
—Influenza
—Parainfluenza
—Epstein-Barr virus
—Rubella
—Respiratory syncytial virus
—Hepatitis viruses
—Rickettsial
—*Rickettsia rickettsii*
—Ehrlichiosis

PATHOPHYSIOLOGY

Petechiae may result from several different mechanisms.

- Disruption of vascular integrity—due to infections, vasculitis, or trauma
- Platelet deficiency or dysfunction—typically thrombocytopenia due to sepsis, disseminated intravascular coagulation (DIC), ITP, or leukemia
- Factor deficiencies (more likely to manifest as ecchymoses and deep bleeding)

EPIDEMIOLOGY

- Although there is no strong epidemiologic data, the presentation of fever and petechiae is rare compared to the presentation of fever alone.
- A great majority of patients (between 70% and 80%) presenting with fever and petechiae have defined or presumed viral infections. These are most often caused by enterovirus or adenovirus.
- Several prospective studies have documented that between 2% and 15% of children presenting with fever and petechiae will have an invasive bacterial disease, most commonly *Neisseria meningitides*.
- Infants and toddlers are at greatest risk of having an invasive bacterial infection with fever and petechiae.
- Teenagers and young adults are most commonly affected by outbreaks of meningococcemia, presenting with fever and petechiae.
- Streptococcal pharyngitis may cause fever and petechiae in the well-appearing child.
- Other etiologies, such as acute leukemia, ITP, and Henoch-Schonlein Purpura (HSP) are responsible for between 5% and 10% of cases of fever and petechiae.

COMPLICATIONS

- Complications of fever and petechiae are related to the underlying etiology.
- Most common complications of invasive bacterial disease causing fever and petechiae include sepsis and meningitis.
- Morbidity from *Neisseria meningitides* includes neurologic deficits, limb loss, and skin sloughing necessitating skin grafts. Mortality is estimated to be between 7% and 20%.

PROGNOSIS

- Prognosis is dependent upon the underlying etiology.
- As most cases of fever and petechiae are due to viral infections, particularly enteroviruses and adenoviruses, the prognosis is excellent.
- Studies demonstrate that the mortality rate of meningococcemia is between 7% and 20%.

 Differential Diagnosis

- Viral infections (see causes above)
- Invasive bacterial infections, most commonly *Neisseria meningitidis* and less often *Staphylococcus aureus*, *Escherichia coli*, *Streptococcus pneumoniae*, and *Hemophilus influenzae* type b. *Streptococcus pneumoniae* and *Hemophilus influenzae* type b are less common because of widespread childhood immunization.
- Streptococcal pharyngitis due to *Streptococcus pyogenes*
- Rickettsial infections—diagnosis aided by season, history of tick bite accompanied by fever, petechiae, headache, and myalgias
- Stress petechiae in the distribution of the superior vena cava (SVC) after significant coughing or vomiting
- Coining or other traumatic etiologies
- Acute leukemias—diagnosis aided by clinical findings of pallor, adenopathy and hepatosplenomegaly, and laboratory findings.
- Idiopathic thrombocytopenic purpura—diagnosis aided by findings of mucous membrane bleeding and isolated thrombocytopenia on laboratory testing.
- Henoch Schonlein purpura—diagnosis aided by clinical findings consistent with HSP, including palpable purpura on the buttocks and lower extremities, usually in the absence of fever.
- Endocarditis—aided by a history of congenital heart disease, cardiac surgery or rheumatic fever.

 Data Gathering

HISTORY

Important historical factors to obtain include:

- Age of the child
- Any underlying immunodeficiency
- Immunizations received
- Exposure to infectious contacts, particularly *Neisseria meningitidis*
- Duration and height of fever
- Duration and progression of rash
- Excessive coughing or vomiting
- Pallor or other bleeding
- Level of activity, excess fatigue
- Travel or history of tick bites
- History of trauma in location of rash

Physical Examination

Important physical examination components on which to concentrate:

- Vital signs, particularly noting tachycardia or hypotension
- Mental status
- Meningismus/nuchal rigidity
- Character of rash—petechiae or purpura, body distribution, number of lesions, progression during examination

Important physical examination findings suggesting specific diagnoses:

- Pallor, adenopathy, organomegaly (suggesting leukemia, EBV infection)
- Mucous membrane bleeding (suggesting thrombocytopenia such as occurs in ITP)
- Myalgias, centripetal rash distribution (suggesting Rocky Mountain spotted fever)

 ## Laboratory Aids

- All children with fever and petechiae require laboratory testing. At a minimum, children should receive a complete blood count with differential and a blood culture.
- Children older than 12 to 18 months of age with fever and petechiae should have a throat culture performed.
- Children who are ill-appearing may warrant coagulation studies, including a prothrombin (PT) time, partial thromboplastin (PTT) time, and disseminated intravascular coagulation (DIC) screen.
- Emerging literature suggests that C-reactive protein may assist in identifying those children with fever and petechiae at greatest risk for invasive bacterial disease.
- Viral testing, including cultures, serology, and antibody immunofluorescence are not routinely required and may be ordered at the discretion of the managing practitioner based upon exposures, need for specific therapeutic interventions, admission to the hospital, and severity of illness.

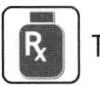 ## Therapy

SPECIFIC

- The management of children who are ill-appearing, have meningismus or purpura consists of a full sepsis evaluation, admission to the hospital with parenteral antibiotics, and fluids and vasoactive infusions to maintain normal hemodynamics.
- Prudent antibiotic choices would be those effective against meningococcal and streptococcal disease, including third generation cephalosporins such as cefotaxime or ceftriaxone.
- Doxycycline should be administered if rickettsial disease is considered.

- Vancomycin should be administered to children with suspected pneumococcal meningitis.
- Since sporadic as opposed to epidemic cases of meningococcemia appear to occur in children in the first 2 years of life, and these children have less competent immune systems in fighting encapsulated organisms, full sepsis evaluations and admission for all children in this young age group is recommended.
- The well-appearing child with fever and petechiae and a positive streptococcal antigen test may be treated as an outpatient with antistreptococcal antibiotics.
- Nontoxic-appearing children greater than 2 years of age with fever and petechiae should have a CBC with differential, blood culture and PT, PTT drawn.
- Although no one factor is 100% sensitive in identifying children with IBD, a constellation of factors is useful in identifying children with fever and petechiae in whom IBD is unlikely. Multiple studies have demonstrated well-appearing children with a normal white blood cell count (WBC between 5,000 and 15,000), a normal absolute neutrophil count (ANC between 1,500 and 9,000), an absolute band count <500 and petechiae limited to above the nipple line are exceedingly unlikely to have an invasive bacterial infection. A recent European study demonstrated that no children with a C-reactive protein level less than 6 had IBD.
- After a several hour period of observation, children who remain well-appearing, are not tachycardic, whose petechiae have not progressed, and whose laboratory studies are normal may be considered for management as outpatients.
- Empiric antibiotic use should be decided on a case-by-case basis. There are no studies investigating the efficacy of antibiotic therapy in the outpatient management of patients with fever and petechiae. However, this author recommends the use of parenteral ceftriaxone as *Neisseria meningitides*, the most likely bacterial pathogen in this circumstance, has such a high morbidity and mortality.

PREVENTION

Vaccine Recommendations

- All children should complete the *Streptococcus pneumoniae* and *Hemophilus influenzae* type b immunization series that begins at 2 months of age.
- Routine childhood immunization with meningococcal vaccine is not recommended. Immunization is recommended for children older than 2 years of age and older who are high-risk, defined as asplenic, and those with terminal complement deficiencies.
- Practitioners should consider immunizing college students who will be living in a dormitory for the first time, given that their risk of invasive disease is higher.

Chemoprophylaxis is recommended for close contacts of patients with meningococcal disease. Ideally, treatment with rifampin, ceftriaxone, or ciprofloxacin should begin within 24 hours.

 ## Follow-Up

- Children managed as outpatients must be told to return immediately for progression of rash or worsening illness, be followed up in 12 to 18 hours, and their cultures should be monitored closely.
- Most children with viral etiologies have little progression of their petechiae, and are clinically better within several days with the resolution of fever.

PITFALL

Unsuspected invasive bacterial disease is the most common pitfall with fever and petechiae. A thorough history and physical exam, accompanied by laboratory testing and a period of close observation may minimize missed serious diagnoses.

 ## Common Questions and Answers

Q: What is the most common etiology of fever and petechiae in children?
A: Viruses are the most common overall cause of fever and petechiae in children. The most common invasive bacterial disease causing fever and petechiae in children in the 21st century is *Neisseria meningitidis*.

Q: Is there ever a role for outpatient management of children with fever and petechiae?
A: Practitioners may consider outpatient management in well-appearing children >2 years of age with a normal white blood cell count (WBC between 5,000 and 15,000), a normal absolute neutrophil count (ANC between 1,500 and 9,000), an absolute band count <500 and petechiae limited to above the nipple line after a period of observation in which they have normal vital signs and no progression of petechiae.

BIBLIOGRAPHY

Mandl KD, Stack AM, Fleisher GR. Incidence of bacteremia in infants and children with fever and petechiae. *J Pediatr* 1997;131:398–404.

Neilsen HE, et al. Diagnostic assessment of haemorrhagic rash and fever. *Arch Dis Child* 2001;85:160–165.

Wells LC, et al. The child with a nonblanching rash: How likely is meningoccal disease? *Arch Dis Child* 2001;85:218–222.

Author: Evaline A. Alessandrini

Fever of Unknown Origin

 Database

DEFINITION

Fever of unknown origin (FUO) implies: (1) A febrile illness (38.3°C on multiple occasions); (2) present for >14 days; and (3) no apparent source despite careful history taking, physical examination, and preliminary laboratory studies.

 Differential Diagnosis

CAUSES

FUO is more often an unusual presentation of a common disease than a common presentation of an unusual disease. In recent studies, 40% to 60% of children have resolution of fever without identification of a specific cause. This may be a result of earlier diagnosis of cases previously presenting as FUO using new technologies such as MRI and detection of genomic material of pathogens by polymerase chain reaction. Possible etiologies include:

Common Infectious Causes

—Respiratory infections (otitis media, sinusitis, pneumonia, pharyngitis)
—Systemic viral syndrome
—Urinary tract infection
—Bone or joint infection
—Enteric infection (*Salmonella, Yersinia enterocolitica, Yersinia pseudotuberculosis, Campylobacter jejuni*)

Less Common Infectious Causes

—Tuberculosis (TB)
—Cat-scratch disease
—Infectious mononucleosis (Epstein-Barr virus, EBV; cytomegalovirus, CMV)
—Lyme disease
—Rickettsial disease (Rocky Mountain spotted fever, ehrlichiosis)
—Malaria
—Central nervous system infection (bacterial or viral meningoencephalitis, intracranial abscess)
—Dental or periodontal abscess
—Subacute bacterial endocarditis (SBE)
—HIV infection
—Acute rheumatic fever

Other Infectious Causes

—Q fever
—Brucellosis
—Toxoplasmosis
—Syphilis
—Parvovirus B19
—Endemic fungi (histoplasmosis, blastomycosis, cocciciodiomycosis)
—Psittacosis
—Chronic meningococcemia

Possible Noninfectious Causes

—Collagen vascular disease (juvenile rheumatoid arthritis, JRA; systemic lupus erythematosus, dermatomyositis, sarcoidosis, vasculitis syndrome)
—Malignancy
—Kawasaki syndrome
—Inflammatory bowel disease (IBD)
—Drug fever
—Hyperthyroidism
—Factitious fever or Munchausen syndrome by proxy
—Centrally mediated fever
—Periodic fever syndrome

Approach to the Patient

GENERAL GOALS

Find the cause of the fever and begin treatment of the underlying illness.

Phase 1: Attempt to diagnose more common causes of fever. Observe the pattern of fever. Determine whether constitutional symptoms (e.g., growth failure, developmental arrest) suggest a serious underlying disease.

Phase 2: Begin invasive studies to seek rarer forms of fever such as lymphoma, brucellosis, SBE.

Phase 3: Reexamine patient and repeat tests to reconsider etiologies such as JRA, sarcoidosis, factitious fever.

 Data Gathering

HISTORY

Question: What have the temperatures been and how were they measured (tympanic, oral, axillary, rectal)?
Significance: As many a 50% of children referred for evaluation of FUO have multiple unrelated infections, parental misinterpretation of normal temperature variation, or complete absence of fever at time of evaluation. Parents are sometimes told to add a 1–2°F "correction" onto a temperature measured in the axilla to better approximate the core temperature. Such practices may further cloud the evaluation of the febrile child.

Question: Exposure to animals, including rodents, and household contacts with occupational exposure to animals?
Significance: Cat-scratch disease, brucellosis, tularemia, leptospirosis, and lymphocytic choriomeningitis virus (exposure to house mice)

Question: Travel history, including past residence?
Significance: Malaria, endemic fungi (e.g., coccidioidomycosis, blastomycosis), tuberculosis

Question: Ingestion of raw meat, fish, or unpasteurized milk?
Significance: Trichinosis, brucellosis

Question: Pica or dirt ingestion?
Significance: Toxocara canis or *Toxoplasma gondii*

Question: Change in behavior or activity?
Significance: Brain tumor, TB, EBV, Rocky Mountain spotted fever

Question: Pattern of fever?
Significance: May correlate with underlying etiology. A fever diary kept by the parent or caretaker may provide more objective documentation of the fever pattern than simple recall.

Question: Medications (including over-the-counter medications and eye drops)?
Significance: Drug fever, atropine-induced fever, methylphenidate, and antibiotics (especially penicillin, cephalosporins, and sulfonamides)

Question: Well-water ingestion?
Significance: Giardiasis

Physical Examination

Finding: Impaired weight gain or linear growth
Significance: Collagen vascular disease, malignancy, IBD

Finding: Toxic appearance
Significance: Kawasaki syndrome

Finding: Conjunctivitis
Significance: Kawasaki, adenovirus, measles

Finding: Ophthalmologic examination
Significance: Brain tumor, TB, systemic lupus erythematosus, Kawasaki (uveitis)

Finding: Sinus tenderness, nasal discharge, or halitosis
Significance: Sinusitis

Finding: Pharyngitis
Significance: Kawasaki syndrome, EBV, SBE

Finding: Tachypnea
Significance: SBE, pneumonia

Finding: Rales
Significance: Histoplasmosis, sarcoidosis, coccidioidomycosis

Finding: Cardiac murmur, gallop, or friction rub
Significance: SBE, acute rheumatic fever, pericarditis

Finding: Hepatosplenomegaly
Significance: Hepatitis, EBV, CMV

Finding: Rectal abnormalities
Significance: Pelvic abscess, IBD

Finding: Arthritis
Significance: JRA, IBD

Finding: Bony tenderness
Significance: JRA, leukemia, osteomyelitis

 ## Laboratory Aids

The laboratory evaluation for a child with FUO should be directed toward the most likely diagnostic possibilities. Consider the following initial studies:

Test: CBC with differential and careful examination of WBC morphology
Significance: Kawasaki, cyclic neutropenia, malignancy, ehrlichiosis, babesiosis

Test: Blood cultures
Significance: Endocarditis, salmonellosis, other bloodstream infections

Test: Urinalysis and urine culture
Significance: UTI, Kawasaki (sterile pyuria)

Test: ESR, C-reactive protein, or procalcitonin
Significance: Collagen-vascular disease, IBD, occult infection

Test: Tuberculin skin test (by PPD)
Significance: TB

Additional studies to be considered include:

Test: Chest x-ray or sinus CT
Significance: TB, endemic fungi, sinusitis

Test: Stool bacterial culture and examination for ova and parasites
Significance: Salmonella, Giardia

Test: Bone marrow examination and culture
Significance: Salmonella, histoplasmosis, malignancy

Test: Chest and/or abdominal CT scan
Significance: TB, liver abscess, hepatosplenic cat-scratch disease

Test: Gallium or bone scan
Significance: Osteomyelitis

Test: Specific antibody testing
Significance: Depending on clinical suspicion, consider: CMV IgM or viral detection in blood, streptococcal enzyme titers (ASO, anti-DNase B), and antibodies for EBV, cat-scratch, Lyme disease, HIV, hepatitis A, B, or C, Rocky Mountain spotted fever, ehrlichiosis, toxoplasmosis, brucellosis, Q fever, leptospirosis, tularemia, dengue fever.

• Other studies to consider: lumbar puncture, stool testing for *Clostridium difficile* toxins A and B, evaluation for immune deficiency, rapid viral antigen testing of nasopharyngeal aspirates.

 ## Common Questions and Answers

Q: How do you explain factitious fever?
A: The patient may twirl the thermometer under the tongue. If left unattended, the child may place the thermometer under hot water or shake it to elevate temperature reading. Take the temperature of the patient's freshly voided urine specimen measured concurrently with the oral temperature to dispel suspicion of factitious fever.

Q: Do all of the above tests need to be performed?
A: A "shotgun" approach to testing is rarely useful in making the diagnosis. Initial studies should include a CBC, liver function tests, blood culture, urinalysis, urine culture, stool culture, and stool ova and parasite testing. Repeated history and physical exam combined with the results of previous testing should guide the subsequent evaluation.

BIBLIOGRAPHY

Brook I. Unexplained fever in young children: how to manage severe bacterial infection. *BMJ* 2003;327(7423):1094–1097.

Calello DP, Shah SS. The child with fever of unknown origin. *Pediatr Case Rev* 2002;2:226–239.

Jacobs RF, Schutze GE. Bartonella henselae as a cause of prolonged fever and fever of unknown origin in children. *Clin Infect Dis* 1998;26:80–84.

McCarthy PL. Fever without apparent source on clinical examination. *Curr Opin Pediatr* 2003;15(1):112–120.

McCarthy PL, Baron MA, et al. Fever without apparent source on clinical examination, lower respiratory infections in children, other infectious diseases, and acute gastroenteritis and diarrhea of infancy and early childhood. *Curr Opin Pediatr* 1997;9(1):105–126.

McClung HJ. Prolonged fever of unknown origin in children. *Am J Dis Child* 1972;124:544–550.

Miller LC, Sisson BA, Tucker LB, et al. Prolonged fevers of unknown origins in children, patterns of presentation and outcome. *J Pediatr* 1996;129:419–423.

Shah SS. Fever. In: Shah SS, Ludwig S, eds. *Pediatric Complaints and Diagnostic Dilemmas: A Case-Based Approach*. Philadelphia: Lippincott Williams & Wilkins, 2004:291–317.

Steele RW, et al. Usefulness of scanning procedures for diagnosis of fever of unknown origin in children. *J Pediatr* 1991;119:526–530.

Author: Samir S. Shah

Hematuria

Database

DEFINITION

Hematuria is defined as >5 red blood cells per high-power field using a standard urinalysis technique on a centrifuged sample. This correlates with a urine dipstick reaction of 1+ or greater.

Differential Diagnosis

CAUSES

- Hematuria may originate at any site along the urinary tract.
- Factitious causes—urine appears bloody, but no red blood cells are present.

FACTIOUS CAUSES—ENDOGENOUS PIGMENTS

- Myoglobin
- Hemoglobin
- Bile pigments
- Urate crystals ("pink diaper" syndrome)
- Beets, blackberries

FACTIOUS CAUSES—EXOGENOUS PIGMENTS

- Food and beverage dyes
- Drugs that cause urinary discoloration

—Phenazopyridine (Pyridium)
—Deferoxamine
—Rifampin
—Sulfa
—Others

- *Serratia marcescens*

GLOMERULAR CAUSES

Common

- Strenuous exercise
- Acute postinfectious glomerulonephritides
- IGA nephropathy
- Thin basement membrane disease (benign familial hematuria)

Uncommon

- Membranoproliferative glomerulonephritis
- Nephritis of systemic disease (Henoch-Schönlein or systemic lupus)
- Alport syndrome, hereditary nephritis

NONGLOMERULAR (INTERSTIAL) RENAL CAUSES

Common

- Pyelonephritis
- Hypercalciuria/nephrolithiasis/ nephrocalcinosis
- Renal trauma (contusion)
- Hemoglobinopathies (sickle cell [SC] disease, SC trait, SC disease)
- Ureteropelvic junction obstruction

Uncommon

- Drug-induced interstitial nephritis (penicillins, cephalosporins, NSAIDs, phenytoin)
- Cystic disease (simple cyst, polycystic kidney disease)
- Neoplasm—Wilms tumor
- Coagulopathy
- Renal venous thrombosis, renal arterial thrombosis

URINARY TRACT CAUSES

Common

- Bladder catheterization, foley catheter
- Cystitis (bacterial, viral, occasionally chemical)
- Meatal stenosis
- Urethritis
- "Terminal hematuria" syndrome (trigonitis)
- Perineal trauma or irritation

Uncommon

- Bladder tumor
- Polyp
- Urethral or bladder trauma
- Foreign body in bladder or urethra

External Causes of "Hematuria"

- Menstrual contamination
- Diaper rash

Approach to the Patient

GENERAL GOALS

Phase 1: Determine if the pigment in urine is from blood or other source. Are red blood cells present?

Phase 2: Determine the source of bleeding, i.e., kidney, bladder, urethra.

Phase 3: Select those who will require referral versus those who simply require follow-up.

Data Gathering

HISTORY

Question: Prior episodes of any gross hematuria, or abnormal urinalyses?
Significance: Chronic versus acute process

Question: Medications and diet?
Significance: Food or drug pigment, drug nephrotoxicity

Question: Antecedent infection or concurrent infection? Streptococcal pharyngitis or impetigo?
Significance: Antecedent suggests postinfectious glomerulonephritis (GN). Concurrent URI or gastroenteritis suggests IgA nephropathy.

Question: Any precipitating factors (trauma, exercise)?
Significance: Renal contusion, exercise hematuria, or myoglobinuria

Question: Voiding symptoms, dysuria, urgency, frequency?
Significance: Suggests bacterial or viral (adenovirus) hemorrhagic cystitis

Question: Renal colic or other pain?
Significance: Suggests stones

Question: Fever, rash, arthritis?
Significance: Signs or symptoms of systemic illness, immune mediated process

Question: Bleeding from any other source (e.g., gums, gastrointestinal)?
Significance: Suggests coagulopathy.

Question: Symptomless "terminal" hematuria
Significance: trigonitis

Question: Hematuria in family members?
Significance: Familial benign hematuria or Alport syndrome

Question: Premature deafness in family members?
Significance: Suggests Alport syndrome

Question: Sickle cell disease in family members?
Significance: Suggests sickle nephropathy, papillary necrosis or hemoglobinuria

Question: Kidney failure or identified kidney disease/nephritis in family members?
Significance: Suggests hereditary nephritis, cystic disease

Clinical Aids in Distinguishing the Origin of Hematuria

TEST FOR	GLOMERULAR OR RENAL	EXTRARENAL
Urine color	Brown, "tea" or "cola" colored, cloudy, red	Red, pink
Clots	Usually absent	Frequently present
RBC casts	Frequently present	Never present
Red-cell morphology	Dysmorphic or distorted	Normal RBC shape
Urine stream	Constantly bloody	More bloody at initiation (suggesting distal urethral origin) or termination (suggesting trigonitis)

Physical Examination

Finding: HEENT examination—periorbital edema
Significance: Glomerulonephritis, renal failure, volume overload

Finding: Back examination—flank tenderness
Significance: pyelonephritis, renal calculi, large cysts

Finding: Genital examination—blood at urethral meatus
Significance: Urethral trauma

Finding: Perineal examination—skin breakdown, irritation
Significance: External source of bleeding or infection

Finding: Extremities—pretibial edema, arthritis
Significance: Glomerulonephritis, volume overload, systemic illness

Finding: Skin and mucosal examination—petechial, vasculitic rash, ulcerations
Significance: Systemic illness (lupus, HSP)

Laboratory Aids

Test: Repeat urinalysis to confirm persistent microscopic hematuria. Patient should be told not to exercise prior to the urine collection.
Significance: Two of three positive specimens over 2 to 3 weeks should be documented in an otherwise well child before diagnostic evaluation of microscopic hematuria

Test: Gross and microscopic analyses of fresh urine specimen
Significance: Absence of red blood cells suggests factitious hematuria. Red blood cell casts—diagnostic for glomerulonephritis. White blood cells—suggests cystitis. White blood cell casts—suggests pyelonephritis.

Test: Screening of the family members for occult hematuria
Significance: Familial benign hematuria or Alport syndrome

Test: Screening for hypercalciuria (random urine calcium:creatinine ratio >0.2 in children >6 years old; >0.6 in children 6 to 12 months old; >0.8 under 6 months of age)—if elevated, 24-hour urine calcium collection >4 mg/kg per day.
Significance: Hypercalciuria

Test: Urine culture—bacterial, viral
Significance: Cystitis, *Serratia marcescens*, Adenovirus

Test: Serum electrolytes, BUN and creatinine
Significance: Impaired renal function suggests inflammation, infection, or obstruction

Test: Evaluation for glomerulonephritis
Significance: Hematuria in combination with proteinuria, edema, hypertension, or impaired renal function.

Test: Streptococcal serology (ASOT, streptozyme)
Significance: Acute postinfectious glomerulonephritis

Test: Complement studies (C3, C4)
Significance: Hypocomplementemic glomerulonephritis—immune complex mediated (lupus nephritis, postinfectious GN, membranoproliferative GN)

Test: Antinuclear antibody titer (ANA)
Significance: Vasculitis (lupus)

Test: Quantitation of proteinuria and serum albumin concentration
Significance: 3 to 4 + proteinuria, urine protein/creatinine ratio >2, hypoalbuminemia suggests glomerular disease/nephrosis

Test: CBC with platelets, coagulation times
Significance: May suggest hemolysis, clotting disorder, systemic illness

Test: Hemoglobin electrophoresis should be considered in Black patients.
Significance: Sickle cell disease or sickle trait may cause hematuria

IMAGING STUDIES

Every child with gross hematuria should have imaging of the kidneys and urinary tract. It may or may not be indicated in children with microscopic hematuria.

Renal ultrasound

Abdominal CT

Helical CT without contrast
Significance: Study of choice for the visualization of stones

ADDITIONAL INVESTIGATIONS

Test: Audiometry for all boys with familial hematuria or family history of premature hearing impairment
Significance: Hereditary (Alport) nephritis

Follow-Up

The well child with asymptomatic isolated hematuria and a negative workup should be reassessed annually with a complete physical examination and a urinalysis. If hematuria is persistent, periodic assessment of renal function, blood pressure, and evaluation for proteinuria should also be performed.

PROGNOSIS

- Majority of children with asymptomatic isolated microscopic hematuria detected on a well-child examination will not be found to have serious underlying pathology and will simply require longitudinal follow-up.
- Children with asymptomatic microscopic or gross hematuria combined with proteinuria have a high likelihood of glomerular disease.
- Benign familial hematuria is a diagnosis of exclusion and has an excellent prognosis. However, children should be examined yearly for the development of hypertension, proteinuria.

PITFALLS

- Positive test for blood on urine dipstick may be myoglobin or hemoglobin. If the urinary sediment does not show red cells, investigate for problems such as rhabdomyolysis (elevated CPK) or hemolysis.

BIBLIOGRAPHY

Ahn JH, Morey AF, McAninch JW. Workup and management of traumatic hematuria. *Emerg Med Clin North Am* 1998;16(1):145–164.

Cohen RA, Brown RS. Clinical practice: microscopic hematuria. *N Engl J Med* 2003;348(23):2330–2338.

Feld LG, Meyers KE, Kaplan BS, et al. Limited evaluation of microscopic hematuria in pediatrics. *Pediatrics* 1998;102(4):E42.

Meglic A, Cavic M, Hren-Vencelj H, et al. Chlamydial infection of the urinary tract in children and adolescents with hematuria. *Pediatr Nephrol* 2000;15(1–2):132–133.

Patel HP, Bissler JJ. Hematuria in Children. *Pediatr Clin North Am* 2001;48(6):1519–1537.

Piqueras AI, White RH, Raafat F, et al. Renal biopsy diagnosis in children presenting with haematuria. *Pediatr Nephrol* 1998;12(5):386–391.

Author: Ann Salerno

Hemolysis

Database

DEFINITION

The premature destruction of red blood cells (RBCs) either intravascularly or extravascularly leading to a shortened red cell survival time.

Differential Diagnosis

See table, Common Mechanisms of Hemolysis.

CONGENITAL/ANATOMIC

- ABO and Rh incompatibility between infant and mother
- Cardiac lesions with turbulent flow, left-sided more common than right-sided
- Prosthetic heart valve (especially aortic)
- Kasabach-Merritt syndrome
- Hypersplenism

INFECTIOUS

- Congenital infections with syphilis, rubella, cytomegalovirus (CMV), and toxoplasmosis
- Malaria
- Bartonellosis
- *Clostridium perfringens* (via a toxin)
- *Mycoplasma pneumoniae*
- HIV
- Hemolytic uremic syndrome (HUS)

TOXIC, ENVIRONMENTAL, DRUGS

- Immune-complex "innocent bystander" mechanism

—Quinidine
—Acetaminophen
—Amoxicillin
—Cephalosporins
—Isoniazid
—Rifampin

- Immune-complex drug-adsorption mechanism

—Penicillin
—Cephalosporins
—Erythromycin
—Tetracycline
—Isoniazid

- Drug-induced autoimmune hemolytic anemia

—α-Methyldopa

Common Mechanisms of Hemolysis

ACQUIRED DISORDERS	HEREDITARY DISORDERS
Infectious	Hemoglobinopathies
Drug-induced	Red blood cell (RBC) membrane defects
Immune mediated	RBC enzyme defects
Microangiopathic	

- Toxic drug-induced hemolysis
—Ribavirin (generally mild and not clinically significant)

- Snake and spider venoms
- Extensive burns

TRAUMA (MECHANICAL HEMOLYSIS)

- Cardiac hemolysis
- Abnormal microcirculation

—Thrombotic thrombocytopenic purpura (TTP)
—Disseminated intravascular coagulopathy (DIC)
—Malignant hypertension
—Eclampsia
—Hemangiomas
—Renal graft rejection

- "March" hemoglobinuria (a result of prolonged physical activity)

TUMOR

- Lymphomas
- Thymoma
- Lymphoproliferative disorders

GENETIC/METABOLIC

- RBC membrane defects

—Hereditary spherocytosis (HS)
—Hereditary elliptocytosis (HE)
—Pyropoikilocytosis
—Paroxysmal nocturnal hemoglobinuria

- Enzyme defects

—Pyruvate kinase deficiency (PK)
—Glucose-6-phosphate dehydrogenase deficiency (G-6-PD)

- Thalassemias (β-thalassemia major is the most severe)
- Hemoglobinopathies

—Sickle cell anemia (Hgb SS and SC variants)
—Unstable hemoglobins

ALLERGIC/INFLAMMATORY/IMMUNE

- Autoimmune hemolytic anemia (AIHA)

—Warm antibody mediated
—Cold antibody mediated
—Hemolytic transfusion reaction

Approach to the Patient

GENERAL GOALS

Establish existence of hemolysis versus other causes of anemia such as blood loss, hypoproduction, and so on.

Phase 1: Determine acuity and severity of the hemolysis. If the process has been acute in onset, there will be evidence of unstable vital signs and possibly heart failure. Parents may give a history of a rapid deterioration of the child's physical and/or mental state. Patients with a chronic hemolytic anemia that has progressed slowly over time may have a "critically low" hemoglobin level, yet may be

well compensated with fairly normal vital signs (except for tachycardia). A complete blood count (CBC) with a corrected reticulocyte count will help determine if there is an appropriate bone marrow response to the level of anemia, and, therefore, whether the process is acute or chronic in onset.

Phase 2: Determine the cause of the hemolysis. Treatment approaches will vary depending on the underlying etiology.

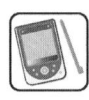

Data Gathering

HISTORY

Question: Is the patient pale, fatigued, or jaundiced? Is there a history of tea-colored urine?
Significance: The presence of hemoglobinuria is a sign of intravascular hemolysis, while pallor, fatigue, and jaundice may occur with either intravascular or extravascular hemolysis.

Question: Is there a history of anemia, splenectomy, or early cholecystectomy in multiple family members?
Significance: While hereditary membrane defects and enzyme deficiencies are autosomal-dominant and X-linked disorders, respectively, a negative familial history does not always rule out these diagnoses. In some cases, the diagnosis of HS has not been identified, yet multiple members of a family have had their gallbladders removed at an early age, which may indicate the presence of this defect. Thalassemia (especially β-thalassemia) and sickle cell anemia may present in early childhood with chronic hemolysis with or without a familial history.

Question: Is there a history of travel?
Significance: Malaria is endemic to Africa, India, and parts of Central America.

Question: What drugs is the patient taking? What is the diet history? Specifically ask about exposure to fava beans, mothballs, and antibiotics.
Significance: Drugs can themselves cause hemolysis or can induce hemolysis if there is an underlying disorder such as G-6-PD deficiency.

Question: How old was the child at the first signs and symptoms of hemolysis (pallor or jaundice)?
Significance: Hereditary causes of hemolysis are most often chronic or recurrent, although the diagnosis may be delayed until the child is older if the process is mild. Acute, acquired hemolytic disorders may also recur (such as AIHA, Evan syndrome, lupus, etc.).

Physical Examination

Question: What is the general appearance of the child? Is there any vital sign instability?
Significance: Acute processes such as autoimmune hemolytic anemia (both warm and cold antibody mediated) may present with a child in extremis. Tachycardia is a common finding in nearly all cases of acute hemolysis. Blood pressure instability is a late finding. More chronic processes such as HS, G-6-PD, and PK deficiencies, thalassemia, intermedia, or sickle cell disease may be picked up on routine physical or laboratory examination. These children often appear well (except for jaundice) but may become more anemic with an acute illness.

Question: Is there an underlying systemic illness?
Significance: Hemolysis that is a secondary problem (i.e., caused by infection, tumors, etc.) may be found incidentally during evaluation of the primary process.

Question: Is there any hepatosplenomegaly or lymphadenopathy?
Significance: Splenomegaly, often impressive, as well as hepatomegaly are common findings in extravascular hemolysis. Hepatomegaly may be more pronounced if the child is in heart failure as a consequence of acute, severe anemia. Remember that splenomegaly may be either the cause of, or more frequently, a result of a hemolytic process. If significant lymphadenopathy is present, look for any underlying etiology like lymphoproliferative disorders or other tumors.

Question: What is the skin exam?
Significance: Pallor is nearly a universal finding in acute hemolysis and in exacerbations of chronic hemolysis. Jaundice is more common in intravascular hemolysis. The presence of ecchymoses or petechiae suggest DIC or thrombocytopenia.

 ## Laboratory Aids

Test: CBC with differential and reticulocyte count
Significance: The level of anemia and the reticulocyte count must be interpreted together. Chronic hemolysis as a consequence of HS, for example, may have a nearly normal hemoglobin but usually has an increased reticulocyte count. With a rapid fall in Hgb, as in acute autoimmune hemolytic anemia, the reticulocyte count may be low at the start, rise in response to anemia, and fall during recovery. Thrombocytopenia should raise suspicions about TTP or HUS.

Test: Peripheral blood smear
Significance: Fragmented RBCs, schistocytes, and helmet cells are seen in DIC, TTP, HUS, and cardiac valve hemolysis. Other findings on the smear that may be helpful in the diagnosis are spherocytes (HS and warm AIHA), target cells (hemoglobin C and thalassemias), and acanthocytes (anorexia nervosa).

Test: Bilirubin
Significance: Total and unconjugated bilirubins are elevated in most cases.

Test: Urinalysis
Significance: Hemoglobinuria is present in intravascular hemolysis. This is established by a urine dipstick positive for heme with no intact red cells microscopically. Myoglobinuria can also give this picture.

Test: Coombs test
Significance: Direct Coombs test (direct antiglobulin test or DAT) detects antibodies or complement fragments present on the patient's RBCs, while the indirect antiglobulin test detects antibodies in the patient's serum that can bind normal RBCs. The DAT provides direct evidence of immune-mediated hemolysis. Warm antibody AIHA is caused by an IgG antibody that coats RBCs, which are subsequently removed by the spleen. Cold antibody AIHA is caused by an IgM antibody that binds RBCs, fixes complement, and can cause both extravascular as well as intravascular hemolysis.

Test: Haptoglobin, hemopexin, and lactate dehydrogenase (LDH)
Significance: In intravascular hemolysis, haptoglobin levels may be undetectable, hemopexin is reduced and LDH is significantly increased. In extravascular hemolysis, haptoglobin is decreased (but detectable) and LDH may be increased, but not to the level seen in intravascular hemolysis.

Test: Bone marrow aspiration
Significance: Rarely indicated, but if performed, erythroid hyperplasia should be present.

Emergency Care

Factors that constitute an emergency include:

- Hemoglobin under 5 g/dL, especially with signs of cardiovascular compromise, requires immediate attention. Attempts to stabilize cardiovascular compromise with volume should be undertaken with care, as hemodilution may occur. Transfusion may be difficult in autoimmune hemolysis because of potential problems with cross matching.
- Renal failure may accompany severe hemolysis in TTP or HUS.
- Hemolysis in the neonatal period secondary to ABO or Rh incompatibility may require exchange transfusion either for anemia or for hyperbilirubinemia.

 ## Common Questions and Answers

Q: When are blood transfusions indicated in patients with active hemolysis?
A: Patients with severe, acute hemolysis that is causing cardiovascular compromise may require a transfusion if the process cannot be stopped with standard therapy (steroids for warm AIHA, plasmapheresis for TTP, etc.). Transfusions must be given slowly if the hemolytic process has been chronic and the patient's blood volume is expanded.

Q: Can hemolysis always be identified on a peripheral blood smear?
A: No. Schistocytes, fragments, spherocytes, targets, or other morphology may provide clues to specific diagnoses but are not always present. The presence of a hemolytic process is inferred from a fall in hemoglobin, rise in the reticulocyte count, and elevation of the bilirubin and LDH levels.

Issues for Referral

- Most patients with severe, acute hemolysis, either primary or as a consequence of an underlying chronic hemolytic disorder, will need to be evaluated by a hematologist.
- Suspected RBC membrane and enzyme defects, as well as hemoglobinopathies, should be referred at least for initial evaluation. Ongoing involvement of a hematologist will depend on the ultimate diagnosis.
- Hereditary RBC membrane defects may be mild and may be diagnosed at an older age. Although these disorders are autosomal dominant, 20% of these patients represent new spontaneous mutations and have no affected family members.
- Blood for diagnostic RBC enzyme studies must be drawn prior to transfusion.

BIBLIOGRAPHY

Lo L, Singer ST. Thalassemia: current approach to an old disease. *Pediatr Clin North Am* 2002;49(6):1165–1191, v.

Old JM. Screening and genetic diagnosis of haemoglobin disorders. *Blood Rev* 2003;17(1):43–53.

Shah S, Vega R. Hereditary spherocytosis. *Pediatr Rev* 2004;25(5):168–172.

Tabbara IA. Hemolytic anemias. Diagnosis and management. *Med Clin North Am* 1992;76(3):649–668.

Author: Julie W. Stern

Hepatomegaly

Database

DEFINITION

Liver enlargement beyond age-adjusted normal values. Can be a common component of many diverse disease processes seen in infants and children.

Differential Diagnosis

CONGENITAL/ANATOMIC

- Alagille syndrome
- Biliary atresia
- Choledochal cyst
- Congenital hepatic fibrosis
- Obstruction of the common bile duct as a result of stones, strictures, or tumors

INFECTIONS

- Viral infections

—Hepatitis types A–E
—Cytomegalovirus (CMV)
—Epstein-Barr virus (EBV)
—Coxsackievirus

- Congenital infections

—Toxoplasmosis
—Rubella
—CMV
—Herpes
—Human immunodeficiency virus (HIV)

- Parasitic infections

—Amebiasis
—Flukes
—Schistosomiasis
—Malaria

- Fungal disease

—Candidiasis
—Histoplasmosis

- Sexually transmitted disease

—Gonococcal perihepatitis
—Syphilis
—HIV

- Zoonotic diseases

—Brucellosis

- Leptospirosis
- Hepatic abscess
- *Bartonella henselae*
- *Pasteurella multocida*
- Tuberculosis
- Septicemia

TOXIC, METABOLIC, DRUGS

- Drug-induced hepatitis

—Acetaminophen
—Alcohol
—Corticosteroids
—Erythromycin
—Hypervitaminosis A
—Iron
—Isoniazid
—Nitrofurantoin
—Oral contraceptives
—Phenobarbital
—Valproate

TRAUMA

- Hemorrhage
- Subcapsular hematoma
- Traumatic cyst

TUMOR

- Benign tumors
- Hemangioma
- Hemangioendothelioma
- Mesenchymal hamartoma
- Focal nodular hyperplasia
- Adenoma

—Malignant tumors
—Hepatoblastoma
—Hepatocellular carcinoma

Metastatic tumors
Histiocytic disease

GENETIC/METABOLIC

- α_1-Antitrypsin deficiency
- Amyloidosis
- Beckwith-Wiedemann syndrome
- Chédiak-Higashi syndrome
- Crigler-Najjar syndrome
- Cystic fibrosis
- Diabetes mellitus
- Galactosemia
- GM_1 gangliosidoses
- Glycogen storage diseases
- Hematochromatosis
- Hereditary fructose intolerance
- Homocystinuria
- Lipidoses
- Mucopolysaccharidoses
- Urea cycle defects
- Wilson disease
- Zellweger syndrome

ALLERGIC/INFLAMMATORY

- Chronic active hepatitis
- Sclerosing cholangitis
- Sarcoidosis
- Systemic inflammatory disease

—Juvenile rheumatoid arthritis
—Systemic lupus erythematosus
—Inflammatory bowel disease

MISCELLANEOUS

- Congestive heart failure
- Extramedullary hematopoiesis
- Pulmonary hyperinflation
- Restrictive pericarditis
- Veno-occlusive disease
- Malnutrition
- Reye syndrome
- Total parenteral nutrition

Approach to the Patient

- All patients with hepatomegaly should have a laboratory evaluation including complete blood count with differential, comprehensive metabolic panel (including liver function tests, total protein and albumin, total and direct bilirubin, basic electrolytes, and glucose), a prothrombin time, and a partial prothrombin time.
- A detailed history and physical examination will direct the practitioner to any additional laboratory testing or appropriate radiologic evaluation.

Data Gathering

HISTORY

Question: Any prenatal history suggesting possible TORCH infection or HIV infection?
Significance: TORCH infections and HIV may cause hepatomegaly, although the liver involvement with HIV is usually secondary to disseminated opportunistic infections or neoplastic processes, rather than from the primary infection itself.

Question: Any history of blood product transfusions?
Significance: Hepatitis C is the most common cause of transfusion-associated hepatitis and the diagnosis should be considered in any child who had received transfusions prior to 1990.

Question: Any history of sexual activity or intravenous drug use?
Significance: Consider not only hepatitis B and HIV, but also gonococcal perihepatitis (Fitz-Hugh–Curtis syndrome), and syphilis.

Question: Any foreign travel?
Significance: Increased risk for parasitic infections or liver abscess.

Question: Any shellfish ingestion?
Significance: Contaminated shellfish has been the source of several large outbreaks of hepatitis A.

Question: What medications is the patient taking?
Significance: Many pharmaceuticals have hepatotoxic side effects. Remember to ask about nonprescription and recreational drug use, as vitamin A, alcohol, and certain mushroom species (*Amanita phalloides*) can be hepatotoxic.

Question: Any other chronic illnesses present?
Significance: Patients with heart disease may have liver enlargement as a result of congestive heart failure. Patients with cystic fibrosis can have focal biliary cirrhosis. Patients with diabetes mellitus often have hepatomegaly secondary to increased glycogen secretion. Severely anemic patients have hepatomegaly because of extramedullary hematopoiesis.

Question: Has the patient received total parenteral nutrition (TPN)?
Significance: Cholestasis, bile duct proliferation, fatty infiltration, and early cirrhosis are all well-described complications of TPN.

Question: Any itching?
Significance: Pruritus can be a subtle sign of cholestasis.

Physical Examination

Finding: Where is the liver edge?
Significance: In children younger than 2 years of age, the liver edge can extend from 1 to 3 cm below the right costal margin in the midclavicular line. In older children, the liver edge rarely extends beyond 2 cm. Verify all suspected cases of hepatomegaly by checking the liver span.

Finding: What are signs of chronic liver disease?
Significance: The liver is usually firm and enlarged, though actually may decrease in size eventually with advanced disease. Splenomegaly, caput medusae, spider angiomas, esophageal varices, and hemorrhoids suggest portal hypertension. Ascites may develop as a result of elevated hydrostatic pressures and decreased oncotic pressures secondary to hypoalbuminemia. Also look for signs of occult bleeding or bruising as a result of impaired vitamin K production.

Finding: Is splenomegaly present?
Significance: Splenic enlargement in the context of chronic liver disease implies portal hypertension. Splenomegaly in the context of other signs of viral illness like adenopathy, fever, malaise, and pharyngitis suggests acute viral hepatitis. Splenomegaly in the absence of these signs suggests storage disease or hematologic malignancy.

Finding: Are there conditions present that may be mimicking hepatomegaly?
Significance: Pulmonary hyperinflation, subdiaphragmatic abscesses, retroperitoneal mass lesions, or rib cage anomalies may all downwardly displace a normal-sized liver mimicking hepatomegaly.

Laboratory Aids

Test: Complete blood count with differential (CBC); aminotransferase and alanine aminotransferase (AST and ALT).
Significance: Elevations reflect the amount of damage to hepatocytes.
Elevations >1,000 indicate severe damage.

Test: Prothrombin time and partial prothrombin time (PT and PTT)
Significance: Good indicators of the liver's synthetic function. Elevations can occur with an acute injury or illness. Combined with albumin level, this test can be a sensitive indicator of chronic liver disease as well.

Test: γ-Glutamyltransferase (GGT) and alkaline phosphatase
Significance: Elevations of GGT out of proportion to elevations in AST and ALT can indicate an obstructive or infiltrative abnormality. If an elevated GGT is associated with elevations in bilirubin, cholesterol, and alkaline phosphatase, an obstructive process is more likely.

Test: Ammonia level
Significance: Rising ammonia levels with a prolongation of the PT and PTT suggests liver failure.

Test: Hepatitis profile
Significance: Should be obtained in all patients with appropriate prodromal illness.

Test: Mono spot
Significance: While this is a nonspecific heterophile antibody test for EBV infection, it can be predictive in association with an elevation of the atypical lymphocyte count. There is a high false-negative rate as well in children less than 4 years of age. EBV titer is the only confirmatory test.

Test: A-fetoprotein (AFP) and carcinoembryonic antigen (CEA)
Significance: Tumor markers for hepatoblastoma and hepatocellular carcinoma, respectively.

Test: TORCH titers
Significance: Consider in newborns with hepatomegaly.

Test: Serum immunoglobulins, antinuclear antibody (ANA), smooth muscle antibody (SMA), antimicrosomal antibody, etc.
Significance: Additional autoimmune evaluation is indicated for those patients with chronic active hepatitis.

Test: Abdominal ultrasound
Significance: Should be performed on all patients with acholic stools, asymmetric liver enlargement, or abdominal mass.

Test: Serum ceruloplasmin level and urinary excretion of copper
Significance: Decreased ceruloplasmin levels and increased urinary excretion of copper characterize Wilson disease, especially after the administration of oral D-penicillamine. Consider the diagnosis for patients with unexplained liver disease.

Emergency Care

Indications for immediate hospitalization include:

- Persistent anorexia and vomiting
- Mental status changes
- Worsening jaundice
- Relapse of symptoms after initial improvement

- Known exposure to a liver toxin
- Rising PT
- Rising ammonia level
- Bilirubin >20 mg/dL
- AST >2,000
- Development of new ascites
- Hypoglycemia
- Leukocytosis and thrombocytopenia

Common Questions and Answers

Q: Why does cholestasis cause pruritus?
A: This probably reflects an abnormal accumulation of bile acids in the skin.

Q: When following patients with chronic liver disease, are there any differences in their nutritional needs?
A: Patients may have impaired fat absorption, and therefore may have deficiencies of fat soluble vitamins A, D, E, and K, which may become evident as anemia, neuropathy, rickets, pathologic fractures, visual disturbances, or skin changes. Also consider supplementing the diet with medium-chain triglycerides, which are more easily absorbed. There may also be higher than normal requirements of trace minerals as well.

Q: What is the etiology of TPN cholestasis?
A: Certain amino acids present in TPN have been shown to increase the serum levels of bile acids, which may in turn affect peristalsis in the gallbladder. Fasting may also decrease the normal hormonal stimulation of bile secretion.

Clinical Pearls

- Until age 2, girls have a slightly larger liver span than boys.
- A Reidel lobe is a normal variant in which the right lobe of the liver appears elongated as a result of its adhesion to the mesocolon.
- The majority of cases of hepatic failure in children are as a result of acute viral hepatitis. Toxic exposure accounts for 25% of cases, with the most common drug being acetaminophen.
- Administration of vitamin K in an attempt to correct PT can be a valuable assessment of the liver's synthetic function.
- Fetor hepaticus is a sweetish odor that can be detected on the breath and urine of patients with liver failure.
- Asterixis or liver flap is rare in children.

BIBLIOGRAPHY

Roy C, Silverman A, Alagille D. *Pediatric Clinical Gastroenterology*. St. Louis: Mosby, 1995.

Author: John M. Good

Hypogammaglobulinemia

 Database

DEFINITION

Hypogammaglobulinemia is a humoral immunodeficiency signified by low or absent immunoglobulin levels, as compared with age-matched controls, and defective specific antibody production.

 Differential Diagnosis

- Selective IgA deficiency
- For details, refer to the topics Immune Deficiency, Common Variable Immunodeficiency (CVID), and Immune A Deficiency.
- X-linked agammaglobulinemia (XLA) (Bruton agammaglobulinemia)

—Intrinsic defect in B-cell maturation as a result of mutations in the gene on the X chromosome encoding a B-cell–associated tyrosine kinase. The protein is involved in cytoplasmic signal transduction.
—All immunoglobulin isotypes are significantly decreased or absent.
—Significant reduction or absence of B cells
—Bacterial infections with pyogenic encapsulated organisms as a result of *Staphylococcus aureus, Streptococcus Pneumoniae, Haemophilus influenzae,* and *Pseudomonas* species
—Recurrent respiratory tract infections including otitis, sinusitis, bronchitis, and pneumonia
—Associated complications include arthritis of the large joints, chronic meningoencephalitis as a result of echoviruses, chronic diarrhea as a result of *Giardia lamblia,* neutropenia, autoimmune hemolytic anemia, dermatomyositis, and an increased incidence of lymphoreticular malignancies.
—Patients are also susceptible to viral infections, particularly enteroviruses. Live viral vaccines are contraindicated in these patients because some patients have vaccine-associated poliomyelitis.

- Hyper-IgM syndrome

X-LINKED HYPER IGM (XHIM)

—Defect is caused by mutations in the gene encoding the CD40 ligand surface molecule on T cells. This leads to defective T-cell signaling for B-cell immunoglobulin class switching.
—Normal to elevated IgM levels with low to absent IgG, IgA, and IgE
—Recurrent upper respiratory tract infections, otitis, pneumonia, sinusitis
—Associated complications include autoimmune hemolytic anemia/thrombocytopenia/neutropenia, opportunistic infections with *Pneumocystis carinii,* and lymphoproliferative disease.

CD40 MUTATION

—Type I integral membrane glycoprotein encoded by gene chromosome 20 defect results in defective B-cell class switching
—Autosomal recessive form of hyper IgM clinically similar to XHIM
—Activation-dependant cytidine deaminase (AID) mutation
—AID is an RNA-editing enzyme encoded by a gene on chromosome 12p13 expressed in germinal center B cells. Deficiency of AID causes impaired terminal differentiation of B cells and failure of isotype switching
—Extreme elevation of IgM with low to absent IgG, IgA, and IgE
—Lymphoid hyperplasia unlike XHIM in which there is minimal lymphoid tissue
—Older at age of onset no susceptibility to *Pneumocystis carinii*

- Transient hypogammaglobulinemia of infancy

—It is difficult to differentiate this from the normal physiologic nadir of IgG that occurs between 3 and 6 months of age as a result of the loss of maternally derived immunoglobulin.
—This nadir is normally short lived.
—Affected infants have abnormally prolonged delay in the onset of their own immunoglobulin production to compensate for this nadir.
—The cause is unknown.
—Self-limited, most infants recover by 18 to 36 months.
—Clinical course is typically benign. Therapy with intravenous immunoglobulin (IVIG) should be considered only in infants with severe recurrent infections.
—This syndrome is frequently seen in infants with a familial history of SCID or other immunodeficiencies.

- Selective IgG subclass deficiency (the four subclasses of IgG, in decreasing order of serum levels: IgG1, IgG2, IgG3, and IgG4)

—Total serum IgG levels can be normal even when one subclass is low or absent.
—Deficiency of IgG3 is most common in adults while deficiency of IgG2 is seen more frequently in children.
—IgG2 deficiency has been associated with an inability to respond to polysaccharide antigens.
—The clinical significance of IgG subclass deficiency has not been fully defined. Many patients have been described as having an increased frequency of upper and lower respiratory tract infections while others are asymptomatic.
—There is no consensus on standard therapy for these patients in regard to replacement IVIG.

- Kappa-chain deficiency

—Absence of the kappa subtype of light chains in immunoglobulin molecules
—Described in two families
—Associated with variable defects in specific antibody formation

- Immunodeficiency with thymoma

—Seen in adults, typically between 40 and 70 years old
—Associated with significantly decreased to absent IgG, IgA, and IgM

- Secondary causes of hypogammaglobulinemia

—Viruses: Epstein-Barr virus (EBV), cytomegalovirus (CMV), congenital rubella
—The mechanism by which antibody responses and immunoglobulin production are altered in infected patients is not clearly defined.
—Infectious mononucleosis has been associated with defective specific antibody responses to neoantigens and impaired in vitro B-cell function in normal individuals. These defects are transient and resolve within 6 to 8 weeks after the onset of the disease. A disastrous response to EBV infection is seen in X-linked lymphoproliferative syndrome. These patients develop fatal infectious mononucleosis, marrow aplasia, B-cell lymphoma, and agammaglobulinemia.
—HIV, CMV, and rubella infections have been associated with abnormal specific antibody responses.

DRUGS

- Immunosuppressive/chemotherapeutic agents, phenytoin
- The associated defects in immune function and antibody production usually resolve after the therapy is discontinued.

OTHER

- Protein-losing enteropathy
- Intestinal lymphangiectasia
- Nephrotic syndrome
- The hypogammaglobulinemia is a result of direct loss through the gastrointestinal (GI) tract or kidneys.
- Lymphoreticular malignancies have been associated with various immune defects and decreased immunoglobulin production.

 Data Gathering

HISTORY

A detailed history for recurrent infection is key to evaluating suspected humoral immunodeficiency.

- Patients with humoral immunodeficiencies usually present with recurrent infections as a result of encapsulated bacteria, such as *H. influenzae* type B and *S. pneumoniae.*
- It is important to rule out hypogammaglobulinemia in patients with recurrent infections because replacement therapy with intravenous IgG is readily available.

Question: At what age did the recurrent infections start?
Significance: Patients with hypogammaglobulinemia usually present after 3 to 6 months of age. Late onset of infections may be more consistent with CVID.

Question: What type of infections have been diagnosed?
Significance: Hypogammaglobulinemia typically results in bacterial infections with encapsulated organisms.

Question: Have there been recurrent severe infections such as meningitis, sepsis, and osteomyelitis?
Significance: Some of the congenital immunodeficiency syndromes are signified by specific infections such as chronic meningoencephalitis with echoviruses, vaccine-associated poliomyelitis, and *P. carinii* pneumonia.

Question: Is there a familial history of immunodeficiencies?
Significance: Previously affected males suggests an X-linked inheritance pattern.

Question: Early infant deaths?
Significance: Early infant deaths as a result of overwhelming infection may indicate a previously undiagnosed congenital immunodeficiency.

Question: Any other associated signs or symptoms?
Significance: Many of the congenital immunodeficiencies have associated arthritis, autoimmune disease, chronic lung disease, and GI manifestations.

Physical Examination

In general, patients should be examined for signs of acute and chronic infections.

Finding: Growth parameters
Significance: Children with significant, recurrent infections and GI disease related to immunodeficiency may present with failure to thrive.

Finding: Signs of chronic otitis media or conjunctival recurrent disease
Significance: Patients with XLA frequently have signs of chronic conjunctivitis.

Finding: Gingivitis and stomatitis
Significance: May occur with the neutropenia-associated hypogammaglobulinemia syndromes.

Finding: Lymphoid tissue
Significance: Absence of tonsillar tissue and palpable lymph nodes is suggestive of X-linked agammaglobulinemia.

Finding: Lymphadenopathy and tonsillar hypertrophy
Significance: Can be seen in hyper-IgM syndrome and CVID. Persistently enlarged nodes should be investigated.

Finding: Wheezes, rales
Significance: Acute pneumonia or chronic lung disease

Finding: Hepatosplenomegaly or masses
Significance: May be seen in hyper-IgM syndrome and CVID. Abdominal masses should be investigated promptly to rule out malignancy.

Finding: Arthritis, clubbing
Significance: Arthritis can be seen in patients with XLA and CVID. Clubbing can be seen in the presence of chronic lung disease/bronchiectasis.

Laboratory Aids

Test: Complete blood count with differential
Significance: Autoimmune hemolytic anemia, neutropenia, and thrombocytopenia can be seen in XLA, hyper-IgM, and CVID.

Test: Quantitative immunoglobulin levels
Significance: Each isotype should be measured (IgG, IgA, IgM, IgE). A normal or elevated IgM level in face of low to absent IgG, IgA, is characteristic of hyper-IgM syndrome.

Test: Serial testing of immunoglobulins
Significance: Should be done in infants suspected of transient hypogammaglobulinemia to document subsequent normalization of immunoglobulin levels.

Test: Qualitative antibody levels
Significance: Isohemagglutinins are primarily IgM antibodies to the main blood groups. They should be present in normal patients. However, they will be absent in patients with AB blood type. In addition, their presence is inconstant in children under 1 year of age.

Test: Antibody titers to tetanus, diphtheria, *S. pneumoniae*, and *H. influenzae* type B measured postvaccination.
Significance: The ability to mount a protective antibody response to childhood vaccinations may indicate a less severe clinical course in hypogammaglobulinemia.

Test: B-cell enumeration
Significance: Numbers of peripheral B-cell will be decreased to absent in XLA and rare in CVID. They are usually normal in other hypogammaglobulinemia syndromes.

Test: Total lymphocyte count (derived from the CBC with differential)
Significance: Lymphocyte enumeration is done using monoclonal antibodies to cell-specific CD surface markers measured by flow cytometry.

Test: Chest and sinus radiography and CT scans
Significance: May be helpful in evaluating for acute and chronic disease. Bronchiectasis can be a long-term sequela of chronic pulmonary infection.

- Prompt and appropriate antibiotic therapy is an important part of routine treatment.
- There may be a role for prophylactic antibiotics in patients with persistent recurrent infections.
- Replacement therapy with IVIG is the primary therapeutic modality for XLA, hyper-IgM syndrome, and CVID. Usual initiating doses are 200 to 400 mg/kg every 3 to 4 weeks. Nadir IgG levels should be greater than 300 mg/dL.

- Patients receiving IVIG therapy should not receive routine vaccinations; they are passively immunized with the therapy.
- Therapy is usually lifelong in patients with documented humoral immunodeficiency.

Common Questions and Answers

Q: When should I make a referral?
A: Refer any patient suspected of having a primary humoral immunodeficiency to a specialist in allergy and immunology. These are patients with chronic disease who require prolonged follow-up and good communication between the referring physician and specialist.

BIBLIOGRAPHY

Conley ME, Rohrer J. Minegishi Y: X-linked agammaglobulinemia. *Clinical Reviews in Allergy and Immunology* 2000;19(2):183–204.

Ferrari S, Giliani S, Insalaco A, et al. Mutations of CD40 gene cause an autosomal recessive form of immunodeficiency with hyper IgM. *Proc Natl Acad Sci* 2001;98:12614–12619.

Huston DP, Kavanaugh AF, Rohane PW, et al. Immunoglobulin deficiency syndromes and therapy. *J Allergy Clin Immunol* 1991;87:1–17.

Minegishi Y, Lavoie A, Cunningham-Rundles C, et al. Mutations in activation-induced cytidine deaminase in patients with hyper IgM syndrome. *Clin Immunol* 2000;97:203–210.

Ochs HD, Smith CI. X-linked agammaglobinemia: a clinical and molecular analysis. *Medicine* 1996;75(6):287–299.

Ochs HD, Winkelstein JA. Disorders of the B-cell system. In: Stiehm ER, ed. *Immunologic Disorders in Infants and Children.* 4th Ed. Philadelphia: WB Saunders, 1996:296–338.

Rosen FS, Cooper MD, Wedgwood RJP. The primary immunodeficiencies. *N Engl J Med* 1995;333:431–440.

Schaffer FM, Ballow M. Immunodeficiency: the office work-up. *J Respir Dis* 1995;16:523–541.

Skull S, Kemp A. Treatment of hypogammaglobulinaemia with intravenous immunoglobulin, 1973–1993. *Arch Dis Child* 1996;74(6):527–530.

Woroniecka M, Ballow M. Office evaluation of children with recurrent infection. *Pediatr Clin North Am* 2000;47(6):1211–1224.

Author: Timothy Andrews

Immune Deficiency—Primary

 Database

DEFINITION

- Immunodeficiencies represent a defect in host defense.
- Can be either congenital or acquired.
- Certain immunodeficiencies lead to specific types of infections, although others are associated with a more global predisposition to infection.

PATHOPHYSIOLOGY

- B-cell dysfunction: leads to antibody deficiency; poor opsonization of bacteria, loss of immunologic memory. The hallmark of B-cell disorders is recurrent infections with organisms typical for that age group.
- T-cell dysfunction: loss of cytolytic activity against viruses, loss of cytokines required for regulation of the immune response. Patients are vulnerable to viral infections, chronic indolent infections such as fungi, and opportunistic infections. May have autoimmune disease as a result of impaired regulation.
- Complement deficiency: complement serves as a major opsonin to tag pathogens for removal. Complement deficiencies are associated with systemic lupus erythematosus, infections with encapsulated organisms, or infections with neisserial species.
- Neutrophil disorders: either a result of qualitative or quantitative dysfunction; impaired phagocytosis of bacteria.

GENETICS

The immunodeficiencies are generally autosomal recessive although there are several important exceptions.

- X-linked (properdin deficiency, X-linked agammaglobulinemia, X-linked hyper-IgM, X-linked severe combined immunodeficiency, X-linked chronic granulomatous disease, X-linked lymphoproliferative syndrome).
- Hyper-IgE syndrome—typically autosomal dominant.
- IgA deficiency and common variable immunodeficiency are polygenic.

EPIDEMIOLOGY

- Most common immunodeficiency is IgA deficiency with an estimated prevalence of 1:500 people.
- 1:3,000 for chromosome 22q11.2 deletion syndrome (DiGeorge syndrome)
- 1:200,000 for chronic granulomatous disease.

COMPLICATIONS

- Bronchiectasis
- Deafness
- Autoimmune disease
- Lymphoreticular malignancies occur in patients with T-cell disorders.

- Live viral vaccines administered to patients with T-cell dysfunction can result in unchecked viremia.
- Oral polio vaccine administered to patients with agammaglobulinemia can cause meningoencephalitis.

PROGNOSIS

- Most antibody deficiencies have an excellent prognosis. Transient or developmental deficiencies of IgG or IgG subclasses typically resolve by 2 years of age.
- Antibody deficiencies such as X-linked agammaglobulinemia or common variable immunodeficiency have a good prognosis with IVIG treatment.
- The treatment of neutrophil disorders remains problematic and most children with chronic granulomatous disease will not have a full life expectancy.
- Patients with T-cell disorders for whom bone marrow transplantation is not performed can do well if the defect is mild and if they do not suffer from autoimmune disease, malignancy, or recurrent infections.

 Differential Diagnosis

- Chronic inflammation of mucous membranes such as that as a result of reflux or allergies can lead to recurrent infections.
- Ciliary Obstruction
- Secondary immunodeficiency.

—Immunocompromise as a result of chemotherapy and immunosuppressive drugs

- Malnutrition, intercurrent viral infections such as EBV and CMV, toxin exposure, and medications such as Dilantin and gold.

—Inborn errors of metabolism.
—Chromosomal syndromes.

- HIV infection.

BRIEF DESCRIPTIONS OF CONGENITAL OR PRIMARY IMMUNODEFICIENCIES

Defects in Antibody Production

- X-linked agammaglobulinemia. Onset of symptoms after 6 months; sinopulmonary infections with typical bacterial pathogens. Markedly decreased immunoglobulins and B cells are characteristic.
- Hyper-IgM syndrome. Usually presents with recurrent bacterial infections; *Pneumocystis carinii* is seen in some infants; intermittent neutropenia is common. Decreased IgG, IgE, IgA with normal or increased IgM.
- Common variable immunodeficiency. Usually presents with recurrent bacterial infections; most commonly arises in the second or third decade of life (but is seen in all ages). Immunoglobulin levels and function gradually decline; often an associated mild T-cell defect.
- IgG subclass deficiency. IgG2 subclass deficiency is seen as a transient developmental delay in the acquisition of humoral immunity. May also precede the

---

development of common variable immunodeficiency and can rarely be seen as an isolated defect.

- IgA deficiency. The most common congenital immunodeficiency (1:500); most are asymptomatic. Symptoms can be seen at any age; typically sinopulmonary infections; increased risk of allergy, autoimmune disease, and anaphylaxis from blood products.
- Transient hypogammaglobulinemia of infancy. A developmental delay of immunoglobulin production; function is intact; typically resolves between 9 and 15 months.

T-Cell Defects

- Severe combined immunodeficiency. Most common presentation is a respiratory virus that fails to clear or chronic diarrhea. Failure to thrive, thrush, and *Pneumocystis carinii* pneumonia are also common; see Section 2.
- Chromosome 22q11.2 deletion syndrome (DiGeorge syndrome/velocardiofacial syndrome). See DiGeorge Syndrome.
- Chronic mucocutaneous candidiasis. There are multiple forms of this disorder. One form is also called autoimmune polyendocrino-pathy—candidiasis—ectodermal dystrophy (APECED) and has a very strong association with polyendocrinopathies and ectodermal dysplasia. The other types are more likely to have an associated T-cell defect. Infants have extensive or recurrent Candida; predisposition to other infections is modest.

Neutrophil Defects

- Autoimmune neutropenia of infancy. Most common neutrophil defect of childhood; usually detected at about 6 to 12 months of age; often resolves by 2 years of age.
- Congenital neutropenia. Infections may be skin infections or sinopulmonary; patients have either absent or markedly low neutrophil counts, which are consistent.
- Leukocyte adhesion deficiency. Approximately 10% have delayed separation of the umbilical cord; most common presentations are recurrent skin ulcers and periodontitis.
- Chronic granulomatous disease. Recurrent skin abscesses common, deep hepatic abscesses, and pulmonary abscesses are also seen. Typical organisms are *Staphylococcus aureus* and Pseudomonas; Aspergillus and Candida are also seen; age of onset is usually 1 to 3 years.

Immunodeficiency Syndromes

- Ataxia telangiectasia. Progressive cerebellar ataxia beginning at about 12 months; ocular telangiectasias beginning at about 5 to 15 years; recurrent sinopulmonary infections; α-fetoprotein is elevated, IgA and IgG2 are diminished.
- Wiskott-Aldrich syndrome. Clinical triad of eczema, thrombocytopenia, and recurrent infections. IgM low; IgG normal or slightly low; IgA and IgE elevated; platelets range from 20K to 90K and are small.

- Hyper-IgE syndrome. Recurrent infections of the skin, lungs, middle ears, and sinuses; *S. aureus* is a major cause of infection and pulmonary infections typically heal with pneumatoceles.
- X-linked lymphoproliferative syndrome. Four main types of presentation: acute EBV infection with hemophagocytosis, lymphoma, hypogammaglobulinemia, and aplastic anemia. Family history is key to diagnosis.
- Chédiak-Higashi syndrome. Pigmentary dilution, progressive neuropathy, and frequent infections; associated with a hemophagocytic process. Neutrophil counts are low and neutrophils have giant inclusions.

Miscellaneous

- Complement deficiency. Deficiencies of C5 to C9 are associated with Neisseria infections; deficiencies of C1, C2, C4 are associated with lupus and recurrent bacterial infections. C3 deficiency is associated with glomerulonephritis and severe recurrent infections.
- Familial hemophagocytic lymphohistiocytosis. A defect in natural killer cell function; presents with fever, pancytopenia and hepatosplenomegaly; usually before 5 years of age.

SECONDARY IMMUNODEFICIENCIES

- HIV infection
- Malignancy
- Viral suppression
- Nephrotic syndrome
- Malnutrition
- Medications
- Splenectomy

Approach to the Patient

GENERAL GOALS

- Immunologic laboratory evaluations are performed according to the suspected type of immunodeficiency. A patient with recurrent sinopulmonary infections with typical organisms could have a defect in antibody production. Therefore, laboratory evaluations should focus on the quantity and function of antibodies.
- Patients with chronic viral infections or opportunistic infections might have a T-cell defect. These patients would benefit from an evaluation of T-cell production and function.
- Neutrophil disorders typically present with skin abscesses or ulcers or deep infections with Staphylococcus or Pseudomonas. Patients with these problems would benefit from an evaluation of neutrophil numbers and function.
- In certain patients it may be difficult to differentiate between viral processes and bacterial processes. In these cases, a CBC and differential, IgG, IgA, IgM levels, and diphtheria and tetanus titers are a useful screen to evaluate for the most common immunodeficiencies.

 ## Data Gathering

HISTORY

- Family history (possible maternally inherited disorders)
- Number and duration of infections (to determine whether the problem is one of clearance, or frequency)
- Types of infections (infections of skin are frequently as a result of neutrophil problems, whereas recurrent infections of a single site imply an anatomic problem). Opportunistic infections are associated with both neutrophil defects and T-cell defects.
- HIV risk factors.

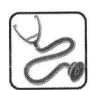 ## Physical Examination

- The physical examination should be directed at defining organ damage as a result of infection, the presence of any current infections, the presence of any syndromic features, the presence of signs of autoimmune disease, and the characterization of accessible lymphoid organs. Examination of lymph nodes, tonsils, liver, and spleen will reveal hypoplasia or expansion.

 ## Laboratory Aids

TESTS

- CBC
- Quantitative immunoglobulins
- Antibody responses to immunizations (must be certain that the child has been immunized)
- T-cell enumeration
- T-cell function measured as proliferation in response to maximal stimuli (PHA, PWM, ConA) or physiologic stimuli (recall antigens)
- Neutrophil respiratory burst assay (nitroblue tetrazolium, dichlorofluorescein, rhodamine)
- CH50: total hemolytic complement
- HIV ELISA and Western blot: If positive in children under 15 months of age, HIV infection should be confirmed with HIV PCR.

 ## Emergency Care

Suspected severe combined immunodeficiency requires isolation, CMV negative/irradiated blood products, and a prompt evaluation.

 ## Therapy

Bone Marrow Transplantation

- Severe combined immunodeficiency (SCID)
- Wiskott-Aldrich syndrome
- X-linked lymphoproliferative syndrome

- Chédiak-Higashi syndrome
- Familial hemophagocytic lymphohistiocytosis

Thymus Transplantation

Severe chromosome 22q11.2 deletion syndrome (DiGeorge syndrome)

Intravenous Immunoglobulin Replacement

- X-linked agammaglobulinemia
- Hyper-IgM
- Common variable immunodeficiency
- IgG subclass deficiency (infrequently)

Prophylactic Antibiotics/Antifungals

- IgG subclass deficiency
- Chronic mucocutaneous candidiasis
- Ataxia telangiectasia
- Hyper-IgE syndrome
- Chronic granulomatous disease

 ## Common Questions and Answers

Q: I have many patients with recurrent episodes of green rhinorrhea. Do these episodes all need to be treated with antibiotics and should the child have an immunologic evaluation?
A: Many viral infections cause green rhinorrhea and thus do not require antibiotics. Children with no other infections may be safely observed.

Q: Does a child with thrush require evaluation?
A: A child with severe thrush in the absence of risk factors should have an evaluation for T-cell dysfunction, HIV, and the possibility of chronic mucocutaneous candidiasis of childhood. Moderate thrush or recurrent simple thrush does not require evaluation unless it is occurring in an older child.

Q: A newborn in my practice still has his umbilical cord attached at 6 weeks. Is that abnormal and does it require an evaluation for leukocyte adhesion deficiency?
A: A completely healthy appearing cord at 6 weeks does not require any evaluation.

Clinical Pearls

- Boys with X-linked agammaglobulinemia and X-linked hyper-IgM do not have tonsils and adenoids
- Children and adults with hyper-IgE syndrome develop abscesses that are not painful.

BIBLIOGRAPHY

Conley ME, Notarangelo L, Etzioni A. Diagnostic criteria for primary immunodeficiencies. *Clin Immunol* 1999;93:190–197.

Noroski L, Shearer WT. Screening for primary immunodeficiencies in the clinical immunology laboratory. *Clin Immunol Immunopathol* 1998;86:237–245.

Author: Kathleen E. Sullivan

Jaundice

Database

- Jaundice is derived from the French word *jaune,* which means "yellow."
- Jaundice—a yellow or green/yellow hue to the skin, sclera, and mucous membranes that can be appreciated at serum levels greater 2 mg/dL. Intensity of color is directly related to the serum bilirubin level.
- Unconjugated bilirubin: 80% is a result of hemoglobin turnover and 20% is from degradation of hepatic and renal heme proteins. It is a hydrophobic compound that must be carried to the liver by albumin for processing.
- Conjugated bilirubin: conjugated to glucuronic acid in the liver, a water-soluble derivative that helps lipid emulsification and absorption.
- Conjugated hyperbilirubinemia (direct hyperbilirubinemia) is defined as a direct-reacting fraction of serum bilirubin greater then 2 mg/dL or greater then 20% of the total bilirubin.
- The most common causes of pathologic jaundice:

—Newborn period: biliary atresia, idiopathic neonatal hepatitis, α_1-antitrypsin deficiency and infection.
—Older child: autoimmune hepatitis, viral hepatitis, Wilson disease, biliary obstruction

Differential Diagnosis

UNCONJUGATED HYPERBILIRUBINEMIA
Congenital/Anatomical

- Placental dysfunction/insufficiency resulting in polycythemia (e.g., infants of diabetic mothers)
- Upper GI tract obstruction (e.g., pyloric stenosis, duodenal web, or atresia)
- Congenital hypothyroidism

Infectious

- Sepsis

Trauma/Delivery Complications

- Cephalohematoma/bruising
- Delayed cord clamping, twin-twin transfusion, maternal-fetal transfusion leading to polycythemia.
- Intrauterine hypoxia (secondary to cocaine abuse, high altitude) resulting in polycythemia
- Induction of labor with oxytocin
- Prematurity

Genetic/Metabolic

- Inherited red cell enzyme, membrane defects (e.g., spherocytosis, G-6-PD deficiency, phosphokinase deficiency, elliptocytosis)

- Red cell abnormalities (sickle cell anemia, thalassemia)
- Defect in hepatic bilirubin conjugation (e.g. Crigler-Najar types I and II, Gilbert's)
- Inborn errors of metabolism

Allergic/Inflammatory/Immunologic

- Isoimmunization (ABO, Rh, Kell, other incompatibility)

Functional

- Physiological jaundice-peaks during the day
- Breast feeding-associated jaundice
- Swallowed maternal blood
- Increased bilirubin load as a result of infant bleeding from a clotting disorder
- Familial benign unconjugated hyperbilirubinemia in mother and neonate (Lucey-Driscoll syndrome)

Conjugated Hyperbilirubinemia
Congenital

- Extrahepatic biliary atresia
- Choledochal cysts and other abnormalities of the choledochopancreatic ductal junction
- Spontaneous perforation of the bile duct
- Bile or mucous plug or biliary sludge
- Gallstones
- Cystic dilation of the intrahepatic bile ducts
- Congenital hepatic fibrosis/polycystic kidney and liver disease

Infectious Etiologies

- Bacterial

—Gram-negative sepsis
—Urinary tract infection/pyelonephritis

- Viral

—Cytomegalovirus (CMV)
—Echovirus
—Herpes simplex virus
—Rubella
—Epstein-Bar virus
—HIV
—Hepatitis A, B, C, D, E

- Toxoplasmosis
- *Pneumocystis carinii*
- *Entamoeba histolytica*
- *Mycobacterium tuberculosis*
- *M. avium-intracellulare*
- Syphilis

Toxic/Environmental/Drugs

- Postnecrotizing entercolitis (NEC)
- Postshock or postasphyxia (ischemic injury to liver)
- Drugs: acetaminophen, valproate, chlorpromazine, Amanita toxin
- Hyperalimentation (TPN)

Tumor

- Neuroblastoma, hepatic, biliary, pancreatic, duodenal, peritoneal
- Porta hepatis nodes

Genetic/Metabolic

- Arteriohepatic dysplasia (Alagille syndrome)
- Progressive familial intrahepatic cholestasis (PFIC) (including Byler disease and MDR3 deficiency)
- Benign recurrent intrahepatic cholestasis (BRIC)
- Defects in bile acid metabolism
- Defects in amino acid metabolism
- Defects in lipid metabolism

—Wolman disease
—Niemann-Pick disease
—Gaucher disease

- Defects in carbohydrate metabolism

—Galactosemia
—Hereditary fructose intolerance
—Glycogenosis type IV
—Zellweger syndrome

- Defects in mitochondrial DNA and respiratory chain defects
- α_1 antitrypsin deficiency
- Cystic fibrosis
- Multiple acyl coenzyme A dehydrogenase deficiency
- Wilson disease (older children)
- Inherited noncholestatic conjugated jaundice syndromes (e.g., Dubin-Johnson and Rotor syndrome)
- Familial benign recurrent cholestasis
- Hereditary cholestasis with lymphedema (Aegenaes syndrome)

Allergic/Inflammatory/Immunologic

- Sclerosing cholangitis
- Idiopathic neonatal hepatitis
- Neonatal iron storage disease
- Idiopathic hypopituitarism
- Chronic active hepatitis

Approach to the Patient

- **Step 1:** Determine if the patient labs show an elevated conjugated or unconjugated hyperbilirubinemia.
- **Step 2:** If unconjugated hyperbilirubinemia

—obtain CBC and indices
—reticulocyte count
—Coombs test.

- If Coombs positive, then diagnosis is isoimmune.
- If Coombs negative, then consider polycythemia, extravascular bleed, or RBC structural or enzyme defects.
- **Step 3:** If conjugated hyperbilirubinemia

—ALT, AST, GGTP (γ-glutamyltranspeptidase)
—PT/PTT/INR
—Ultrasound of the liver/pancreas/gallbladder and biliary tree
—Rule out those causes of direct hyperbilirubinemia that may adversely affect the outcome if diagnosis is delayed
  —biliary atresia
  —tyrosinemia
  —galactosemia
  —inborn error bile acid synthesis
  —hereditary fructose intolerance
  —neonatal iron storage disease.

Data Gathering

HISTORY

Question: Does the patient have unexplained itching?
Significance: Cholestatic liver disease (conjugated hyperbilirubinemia)

Question: Does the patient have a history of poor school performance, change in mental status, handwriting?
Significance: Wilson disease

Question: Is there a history of other family members having prolonged jaundice or hepatic failure in infancy?
Significance: A sibling with prolonged neonatal jaundice, death, or significant illness may suggest an underlying inborn error of metabolism, such as tyrosinemia, galactosemia, etc.

Question: Is there a history of intravenous drug abuse or exposure to blood or blood products, especially prior to 1992?
Significance: The patient may have transfusion-associated hepatitis, e.g., hepatitis C.

Physical Examination

Finding: Scratch marks
Significance: Pruritis secondary to cholestasis

Finding: Spider angiomata, palmer erythema
Significance: Chronic liver disease

Finding: Petechiae, purpura, microcephaly
Significance: Thrombocytopenia, secondary to congenital TORCH infection

Finding: Heart murmur
Significance: Alagille syndrome (peripheral pulmonic stenosis)

Finding: Ascites
Significance: Hypoalbuminemia, generally caused by only four major causes: nephrotic syndrome, protein-losing enteropathy, malnutrition, liver failure.

Finding: Urine for bile acid analysis
Significance: Inborn error of bile acid metabolism

Finding: Acholic stool
Significance: Severe cholestasis; in the newborn, highly suggestive of biliary atresia; in the older child, may also suggest biliary obstruction secondary to gallstones, mass

Laboratory Aids

Test: Total with fractionalization into unconjugated, conjugated bilirubin, and delta fractions
Significance: Direct versus indirect hyperbilirubinemia

If unconjugated hyperbilirubinemia, investigation is initiated with:

Test: CBC with indices, reticulocyte count, and peripheral blood smear for red blood cell morphology
Significance: Polycythemia in neonate, hemolysis or other red cell evidence of increased destruction

Test: Coombs test
Significance: Isoimmune and autoimmune hemolytic anemia

Test: PT/PTT/INR, platelet count
Significance: Coagulopathy associated with hemorrhage that causes an increased bilirubin load

Test: Sepsis evaluation (blood, urine, and spinal fluid)
Significance: Sepsis can impair conjugation and excretion of bilirubin, result in poor feeding with bile sludging and subsequent formation of gallstones.

Test: Free T3, T4, and TSH
Significance: Congenital hypothyroidism

Test: Serum aminotransferases (AST, ALT)
Significance: Ongoing liver inflammation/destruction

Test: Alkaline phosphatase/GGTP
Significance: Biliary tree obstruction/cholestasis.

Test: Serum albumin, PT, PTT fibrinogen, cholesterol
Significance: Liver synthetic function.

Test: Stool color
Significance: Acholic (white) stools suggest biliary atresia as a result of the lack of bile salts in the stool.

Test: Urine dipstick for glucose and reducing substances
Significance: Positive reducing substances seen in galactosemia and hereditary fructose intolerance.

Test: α_1-antitrypsin serum levels and Pi genotype.
Significance: Serum α_1-antitrypsin levels will be low in inherited protease inhibitor deficiency. Caution that high or normal levels can be falsely elevated as a result of the fact that α_1-antitrypsin is an acute phase reactant.

Test: Ultrasound
Significance: A noninvasive method to examine the overall liver appearance, size, and density. Allows for examination of the biliary tree and gallbladder to rule out choledochal cysts, sludge/stones, and ductal dilatation indicating possible obstruction.

Test: Hepatobiliary scintigraphy (HIDA scan)
Significance: Biliary secretion into the duodenum and exclusion of biliary atresia or extrahepatic biliary obstruction

Test: Percutaneous liver biopsies
Significance: Liver pathology: hepatocyte and other cell histology, fibrosis and pathological features

Common Questions and Answers

Q: Are there any characteristic findings in neonatal jaundice that are specifically concerning?
A: These findings are concerning until proven otherwise:

- Development of jaundice before 36 hours
- Persistent jaundice beyond 10 days
- Serum bilirubin concentration greater then 12
- Elevation of direct bilirubin greater then 2 mg/dL or 20% of total bilirubin at any time

Q: Are there any ethnic/social factors associated with higher bilirubin levels?
A: Factors that have been associated with high serum bilirubin levels are low birth weight, certain ethnic groups (Asian, Native American, Greek), delayed meconium passage after birth, breast-feeding. Factors that been associated with lower serum levels in neonates include maternal smoking, black race, and certain drugs, such as Phenobarbital.

WHEN TO REFER?

- Lack of excretion on HIDA scan suggestive of obstruction
- Presence of choledochal cyst or dilated biliary ducts seen on US
- Abnormal metabolic screen
- Evidence of decompensated liver disease

—PT >20s
—Albumin <3.0 g/dL
—Ascites
—Encephalopathy
—Bilirubin >20mg/dL
—AST/ALT >300 (impending fulminant liver failure)

Clinical Pearls

- Treat Crigler-Najar Type II syndrome promptly with phototherapy and phenobarbital to prevent kernicterus
- Older children with Wilson disease may present with profound hemolysis and may have predominantly unconjugated hyperbilirubinemia with severe parenchymal liver disease and fulminant liver failure.

BIBLIOGRAPHY

Davenport M, Betalli P, D'Antiga L, et al. The spectrum of surgical jaundice in infancy. *J Pediatr Surg* 2003;38(10):1471–1479.

Kanegawa K, Ak asaka Y, Kitamura E, et al. Sonographic diagnosis of biliary atresia in pediatric patients using the "triangular cord" sign versus length and contraction. *Am J Roentgenol* 2003;181(5):1387–1390.

Takaya J, Munoyuki M, Tokuhara D, et al. Congenital dilation of the bile duct: changes in diagnostic tools over the past 19 years. *Pediatr Int* 2003;45(4):383–387.

Authors: Peter C. Wilmot and J. Fernando del Rosario

Learning Problems

Database

DEFINITION

Learning disorders, or learning disabilities, are defined in the *Diagnostic and Statistical Manual of Mental Disorders,* 4th edition (DSM-IV) as academic achievement that is substantially below the level expected for age, schooling, and general intellectual ability, and that cannot be accounted for by psychosocial factors. A learning disability may affect reading, writing, spelling, or math, and any given child may have more than one learning disability. Learning disabilities have neurobiological and genetic roots. Reading disorder, which is also known as dyslexia and is the most frequently diagnosed type of learning disorder, is characterized by impairments in phonological processing.

EPIDEMIOLOGY

Learning disorders have an estimated incidence of 10% or more in school-aged children. Learning disorders typically are not evident until academic demands are placed on the affected children. Psychiatric comorbidity is frequent, either as a complication of learning problems or as an etiologic factor in their development.

Differential Diagnosis

Children's school problems may result from a specific learning disorder, or may be the secondary effect of some other medical or psychosocial problem.

- Attention deficit/hyperactivity disorder (ADHD) may present as a learning problem, especially when the inattentive and distractible symptoms of the diagnosis are greater than the hyperactive symptoms. ADHD may be difficult to distinguish from a learning disorder, and the two also may be found comorbidly. Careful psychoeducational assessment may be needed to clarify these diagnoses.
- Sensory impairments: Hearing or vision impairments may cause learning problems. School screening results should be confirmed in children with learning problems.
- Neurologic: Absence seizures and other nonconvulsive epileptic disorders are much less common than ADHD but may mimic its symptoms. Narcolepsy also is associated with learning problems. Neurodegenerative disorders such as Niemann-Pick disease, adrenoleukodystrophy, ceroid lipofuscinosis, and subacute sclerosing panencephalitis may rarely present as school-age learning problems.
- Mental retardation: In some cases, borderline and mild mental retardation are not recognized until school entrance.

- Genetics: Some genetic syndromes may show subtle dysmorphology that is not noted until learning problems arise. Examples are sex chromosome aneuploidies, fragile X syndrome in both boys and girls, neurofibromatosis, tuberous sclerosis, and velocardiofacial/DiGeorge syndrome.
- Nutritional, toxicologic, infections: Lead intoxication, chronic malnutrition, iron-deficiency, hypothyroidism, and HIV infection may have insidious effects on cognitive function.
- Iatrogenic interventions: Medical therapies may compromise learning abilities; for example, treatment with antiepileptic drugs and other medications that affect cognition.
- Psychosocial: Issues related to family stress, peer relationships, illness, or adolescence may present as academic difficulty. Conversely, behavior problems at home or at school always should prompt evaluation of school functioning.
- Psychiatric comorbidity occurs commonly. Adjustment disorders, mood disorders, oppositional defiant disorder, conduct disorder, tic disorders, substance abuse, and other behavior problems may precede or follow the presentation of learning problems. Less commonly, psychotic disorders, personality disorders, and obsessive-compulsive disorder may underlie learning problems.
- Speculative etiologies: Food allergies, "developmental optometric" disorders, and exposure to food preservatives or sugar are widely discussed but are essentially unproven causes of learning problems.

Approach to the Patient

GENERAL GOAL

Determine whether the learning problems result from a primary medical or psychosocial condition. If no such condition is identified, then the patient may have a specific learning disability. The pediatrician also is in a good position to identify social and environmental factors that may be associated with learning problems, and can coordinate the appropriate medical, psychiatric, and/or psychoeducational evaluation, with consultation as indicated. Early identification of learning problems and appropriate intervention help to prevent the cascade of negative consequences triggered by poor academic achievement.

Phase 1a: Identify and address medical factors that may affect learning (e.g., sensory impairments, lead intoxication, absence seizures, iatrogenic interventions). Consider subtle genetic syndromes (e.g., fragile X syndrome in girls) that may cause learning problems without causing other major medical abnormalities.

Phase 1b: Screen for psychiatric conditions, and for social and environmental factors that may be associated with learning problems. Psychosocial stresses may exacerbate learning difficulties, or be a primary etiologic factor. If indicated, refer to appropriate consultants.

Phase 2: For patients with learning problems that are suspected to be primary (i.e., specific learning disabilities), a complete psychoeducational evaluation is indicated. If ADHD is present, treatment may be directed by the primary care physician or by a subspecialist.

Data Gathering

HISTORY

Question: When and how does the child fail in his or her daily academic pursuits?
Significance: For specific learning disabilities, problems may occur in only one class. For attention deficit, problems may be broad-based and may emerge as children move into more formal didactic settings. With borderline mental retardation or other chronic problems, there may be a long history of developmental concerns.

Question: Recent or new decline in school performance?
Significance: Consider new pathophysiologic processes, such as psychosocial issues, new vision or hearing impairment, side effect from new medication, or neurodegenerative disorder (rare).

Question: Reaction to the learning problem (mood, anxiety)?
Significance: Poor school performance commonly leads to depression, poor self-esteem, and possible behavior problems.

Question: Past medical history? Medications? Review of systems? Psychosocial stresses?
Significance: Identify factors that may affect learning. Early language delays are common among children with learning disorders.

Question: Family history?
Significance: May be positive for learning or attention problems that are similar to the child's.

Physical Examination

Finding: Subtle dysmorphology
Significance: May suggest the presence of a genetic syndrome or a pattern of malformation resulting from teratogenic fetal exposures (e.g., alcohol, phenytoin, etc.).

Finding: Abnormal neurological examination
Significance: Any focal signs demand additional evaluation. Soft signs (neuromaturational signs) are often present in children with learning problems, but are nonspecific.

Finding: Abnormal audiology or vision screening
Significance: May be direct cause of learning problem.

Laboratory Aids

Behavioral screening should be performed, but no laboratory studies are routinely indicated. The history and physical examination may provide specific indications for further testing.

Test: Standardized behavior questionnaires
Significance: Diagnosis of attention deficit disorder is critically dependent on input from teachers and parents. Psychiatric complications, such as depression, should also be considered.

Test: Lead level, thyroid functions, karyotype, HIV testing, hearing and vision testing, EEG, neuroimaging
Significance: Each of these can be considered if the history or physical exam provides specific indications.

Test: Psychoeducational evaluation
Significance: A comprehensive psychoeducational evaluation serves as the cornerstone of diagnosis and educational intervention. This testing must be performed individually, and should include general intelligence and academic achievement testing. Federal law requires schools to provide comprehensive evaluations on written request by the parents to the school principal. (Specific information for each state can be obtained from the National Dissemination Center for Children with Disabilities (800-695-0285; www.nichcy.org). Many centers outside the school system (e.g., hospital-based centers) also conduct evaluations of children with learning problems.

Test: Neuropsychological evaluation
Significance: For children who do not respond to first-line educational interventions, more extensive neuropsychological testing may elucidate specific cognitive strengths and weaknesses that may be helpful in developing an effective educational plan.

Issues for Referral

Referrals to medical and psychological professionals may be helpful for both diagnostic and therapeutic purposes. When a specific medical etiology is suspected, the choice of subspecialist for referral will be clear. When no specific etiology is apparent, consider referral to a clinician experienced with learning disabilities. This consultant may assist in comprehensive diagnostic formulation, pharmacologic treatment when indicated, developmental follow-up, and advocacy.

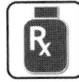

Therapy

- For children with learning disorders, specialized educational approaches and tutoring are the centerpieces of treatment. This is often provided through Resource Room assistance or alternative classroom placement. In addition, the child may benefit from classroom accommodations such as preferential seating, extra time for test-taking, use of electronic word processors, and provision of written rather than verbal instructions. For children with ADHD, behavioral therapy and pharmacologic therapy may also be required to optimize their potential for learning.
- Treatment is most effective when it employs a team approach, inclusive of parents, teachers, and other therapists.
- Grade retention, which only provides a repeat of the same educational approaches that have already failed the child, will not be helpful.

Follow-Up

Children with learning disabilities require continued monitoring of academic progress. Even when the initial learning problems are resolved, later difficulties may arise in writing, note-taking, composition, organization, and with more abstract academic topics.

Clinical Pearls

- Comorbidity and symptomatic overlap are common among ADHD, specific learning disabilities, and other psychiatric disorders. Students who have a learning disability or are depressed may show symptoms of inattention. Academic or attention difficulties may lead to spiraling psychological problems, from depression or damaged self-esteem to conduct disorder and school dropout.
- Normal attention and activity in the physician's office do not rule out ADHD. Many children with ADHD show significant difficulties with inattention and distractibility, but little hyperactivity. Even children with severe ADHD may appear attentive in the intimidating and artificial milieu of the doctor's office, or when engaged in highly motivating and highly reinforcing computer games.

BIBLIOGRAPHY

Buttross S. Attention deficit-hyperactivity disorder and its deceivers. *Curr Probl Pediatr* 2000;30(2):37–50.

Eden GF, Moats L. The role of neuroscience in the remediation of students with dyslexia. *Nature Neurosci* 2002;5(Suppl):1080–1084.

Grigorenko EL. Developmental dyslexia: an update on genes, brains, and environments. *J child Psychol Psychiat Allied Discipl* 2001;42(1):91–125.

Hechtman L. Assessment and diagnosis of attention-deficit/hyperactivity disorder. *Child Adolesc Psychiatr Clin North Am* 2000;9(3):481–498.

Levy SE. Pediatric evaluation of the child with developmental delay. *Child Adolesc Psychiatr Clin North Am* 1996;5(4):809–826.

Mannuzza S, Klein RG. Long-term prognosis in attention-deficit/hyperactivity disorder. *Child Adolesc Psychiatr Clin North Am* 2000; 9(3):711–726.

Mazzocco MM. Advances in research on the fragile X syndrome. *Mental Ret Devel Disabil Res Rev* 2000;6(2):96–106.

O'Brien G. Adult outcome of childhood learning disability. *Devel Med Child Neurol* 2001;43(9):634–638.

Reiff MI. Adolescent school failure: failure to thrive in adolescence. *Pediatr Rev* 1998; 19(6):199–207.

Author: Paul P. Wang

Leukocytosis

 Database

DEFINITION

An increase in white blood cell count above normal for age. The most frequent cause is an increase in the total neutrophil count but leukocytosis may result from an increase in any type of white blood cell, such as lymphocytosis, monocytosis, eosinophilia, or basophilia (see tables, causes of Neutrophilia, Causes of Lymphocytosis, Causes of Eosinophilia, and Causes of Monocytosis).

 Differential Diagnosis

INFECTIOUS

- Bacterial

—Streptococcus (especially pneumoniae)
—*Staphylococcus aureus*
—Haemophilus
—Neisseria
—Brucella
—Bartonella (cat-scratch disease)
—*Clostridium difficile*
—Pertussis

- Viral

—Infectious mononucleosis
—Cytomegalovirus (CMV)
—Rubella
—Mumps
—Hepatitis

- Fungal

—Aspergillus

- Parasitic

—Toxocara
—Toxoplasma
—Trichinella
—Tapeworms
—Strongyloides
—Coccidioidomycosis

- Tuberculosis
- Syphilis
- Acute infectious lymphocytosis

—Benign viral mediated lymphocytosis (often >25,000/mm^3)

- Kawasaki disease

Causes of Neutrophilia

Bacterial infections
Inflammatory states
Acute hemorrhage
Stress
Drugs
    Corticosteroids, Epinephrine
Metabolic disorders
    Uremia, Acidosis
Myeloproliferative disorders
    Myelofibrosis, Polycythemia vera, CML
Sickle cell disease

CONGENITAL/ANATOMIC

- Down syndrome
- Sickle cell disease
- Fanconi anemia
- Thrombocytopenia with absent radii
- Leukocyte adhesion factor deficiency

DRUGS

- Corticosteroids
- B-agonists
- Epinephrine
- Lithium
- Granulocyte colony-stimulating factor (G-CSF)
- Granulocyte-macrophage colony-stimulating factor (GM-CSF)

TRAUMA

- Acute hemorrhage
- Severe burns
- Splenectomy

TUMOR

- Leukemia
- Lymphoma
- Myeloproliferative disorders

GENETIC/METABOLIC

- Hyperthyroidism
- Acidosis

INFLAMMATORY

- Juvenile rheumatoid arthritis (JRA)
- Rheumatoid arthritis (RA)
- Inflammatory bowel disease (IBD)
- Chronic granulomatous disease (CGD)
- Pulmonary eosinophilic syndromes

—Transient infiltrates associated with a peripheral eosinophilia

ALLERGIC

- Asthma
- Seasonal or drug allergies
- Eczema
- Psoriasis

HEMATOLOGIC

- Severe hemolysis

Causes of Lymphocytosis

Viral infections: CMV, EBV, Pertussis, Hepatitis, Toxoplasmosis
Acute infectious lymphocytosis
Chronic Infections: Tuberculosis, Brucellosis Syphilis
Malignancy: Acute lymphocytic leukemia, Lymphoma
Relative Lymphocytosis: Addison disease, Thyrotoxicosis, Splenic sequestration

STRESS

- Anxiety
- Overexertion/exercise
- Seizures
- Anesthesia

ARTIFACTUAL

- Nucleated RBCs
- Clumped platelets on a mechanical differential

Approach to the Patient

Phase 1: Is the WBC count dangerously elevated?

- WBC of 100,000/mm^3 can increase blood viscosity, causing stroke or infarct of end organs. Patients with WBC counts this high almost always have a malignant bone marrow process (leukemia, myeloproliferative disorder).

Phase 2: Which white blood cell line is elevated?

- An elevated neutrophil count is more likely with bacterial infections and a lymphocytosis is usually associated with viral infections. Eosinophilia is often indicative of an allergic disorder.
- Pitfall: Many laboratories provide only machine-generated differentials. If there are any abnormalities, a manual differential must be obtained. It may be necessary to review the smear with a hematologist or pathologist.

Phase 3: The degree of elevation can be indicative of the diagnosis.

- Most elevations of WBC count are in the 10,000 to 20,000/mm^3 range. A WBC count in the 30,000/mm^3 range is more consistent with pertussis, pneumococcal infection, or acute infectious lymphocytosis. Higher counts are worrisome for malignant processes or leukemoid reactions.

Causes of Eosinophilia

Allergic disorders: Asthma, Urticaria, Drug hypersensitivity
Skin disorders: Eczema, Psoriasis, Pemphigus
Parasitic infections
Fungal infections
Immunologic disorders: RA, SLE, Eosinophilia-myalgia syndrome
Malignancies: non-Hodgkin lymphoma, Hodgkin disease
Myeloproliferative Disorders: CML, PV, Myelofibrosis
Hypereosinophilic syndromes
Hereditary eosinophilia
Hematologic disorders: Fanconi anemia, Thrombocytopenia with absent radii
Congenital neutropenias
Inflammatory disorders: GI, Sarcoidosis, Polyarteritis nodosa

Data Gathering

HISTORY

Question: Is there any evidence for infection, such as fever, rash, or swelling?
Significance: Infection is the most common etiology for leukocytosis. Fever can also be a symptom of inflammatory diseases such as JRA or CGD.

Question: Does the patient have any other medical problems?
Significance: Patients with sickle cell disease have an elevated WBC count probably secondary to chronic inflammation or marrow expansion. Children with Down syndrome can have a benign leukemoid reaction, especially in the first few months of life, that resolves spontaneously.

Question: Is the patient on any medications?
Significance: Corticosteroids will increase the neutrophil precursors. Epinephrine can cause a transitory increase in neutrophil count.

Question: Is there a familial history of any inflammatory diseases?
Significance: For example, collagen vascular disease such as RA, thyroid, Crohn disease.

Question: Has the patient lost weight, been fatigued, had night sweats, or been pale?
Significance: Malignancy must be ruled out.

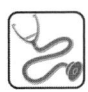
Physical Examination

Finding: Lymphadenopathy or hepatosplenomegaly?
Significance: Points toward a possible viral etiology but is also of concern for malignancy

Finding: Are joints tender or swollen?
Significance: JRA, septic arthritis, SLE

Finding: Mongoloid features?
Significance: Down syndrome

Causes of Monocytosis

Infection
  Tuberculosis
  Malaria
  Brucellosis
  Bacterial endocarditis
Inflammatory disease
  Collagen vascular disease
  Sarcoid
  RA
  Crohn, ulcerative colitis
  SLE
Malignancy
  Hodgkin disease
  Acute myelocytic leukemia
  Myelodysplastic syndromes

Laboratory Aids

Test: WBC count including differential.
Significance: If neutrophilia is present, think of bacterial infections. Pneumonia, urinary tract infections, and soft tissue infections are the most likely to cause a leukocytosis. One may also see Döhle bodies, toxic granulations, or vacuolization in WBCs in bacteremia. A recovering or stressed marrow may have an increase in monocytes or eosinophils. Look for leukemic blasts.

Test: Hemoglobin/platelet count
Significance: If either is low, consider a marrow infiltrative process or a marrow that is hyperstimulated to compensate for a low hemoglobin or platelet count.

Test: Chemistry panel
Significance: Evaluate LFTs for possible viral etiology. Uric acid and LDH are elevated in leukemia and lymphoma.

Test: Cultures
Significance: Blood, urine, stool, throat, etc.

Test: Monospot, heterophil Ab, EBV titers
Significance: Screen for infectious mononucleosis. Monospot can be falsely negative in younger children.

Test: Leukocyte alkaline phosphatase
Significance: Elevated in infection but not in leukemia. Helps to differentiate CML from a leukemoid reaction.

Test: ANA
Significance: Screen for rheumatologic etiology.

Test: Bone marrow biopsy and aspirate
Significance: Necessary if any other blood cell line is abnormally low or if the WBCs appear dysmorphic. Need to rule out malignancy, myelodysplasia, or other marrow processes. Send cytogenetics when possible.

Test: Chest radiograph
Significance: Pneumonia, tuberculosis

Issues for Referral

- WBC counts greater than 50,000/mm³
- Associated thrombocytopenia or anemia
- Any indication of malignancy
- Any indication of a rheumatologic etiology
- Inability to find an etiology with a persistent leukocytosis

Emergency Care

- If the leukocytosis is >100,000/mm³ and the patient has symptoms of end-organ failure, emergent leukapheresis should be considered. If the patient's condition is hemodynamically stable, avoid red cell transfusions, which will increase the blood viscosity. If the platelet count is <20,000/mm³ transfuse platelets to prevent hemorrhagic infarcts.

Clinical Pearls

Beware of any differential that has a high percentage of monocytes or atypical lymphocytes whether machine generated or manual. Leukemic blasts are similar appearing to these cell types under the microscope.

Common Questions and Answers

Q: What does "left-shifted" mean?
A: There are increased numbers of early granulocyte precursors (metamyelocytes, myelocytes, bands) seen in the peripheral smear with a bandemia and neutrophilia. Often seen with bacterial infections or marrow recovery from a suppressing drug/virus.

Q: Infectious mononucleosis (IM) and acute lymphocytic leukemia (ALL) have many similar signs and symptoms. How can I differentiate them?
A: Both can present with fever, malaise, headache, prominent lymphadenopathy, organomegaly, and suppressed hemoglobin and platelet counts. IM tends to be associated with a sore throat and children with ALL are more likely to complain of bony pain. The easiest way to differentiate the two is a careful exam of the peripheral smear. A heterophil AB or monospot can be sent and, if positive, help with the diagnosis of IM.

Q: What are the signs and symptoms of acute infectious lymphocytosis (AIL)?
A: AIL is probably caused by several viruses from which the child can be totally asymptomatic except for a significant lymphocytosis (40,000 to 80,000/mm³). On review of the peripheral smear there is a prevalence of small, mature lymphocytes. There can also be an eosinophilia. As a rule there is no anemia or thrombocytopenia. The lymphocytosis resolves spontaneously.

BIBLIOGRAPHY

Abramson N, Melton B. Leukocytosis: basics of clinical assessment. *Am Fam Physician* 2000;62(9):2053–2060.

Hoffbrand AV, Pettit JE, eds. *Color Atlas of Clinical Hematology.* 3rd Ed. St. Louis: Mosby-Wolfe, 2000.

Peterson L, Hrisinko MA. Benign lymphocytosis and reactive neutrophilia. *Clin Lab Med* 1993;13(4):863–877.

Author: Susan R. Rheingold

Lower GI Bleeding

 ## Database

DEFINITION

Lower gastrointestinal (GI) bleeding refers to bleeding from the lower GI tract, distal to the Ligament of Treitz. It can be hematochezia (passage of bright red or dark blood per rectum) or melena (passage of dark, black, or tarry stools).

 ## Differential Diagnosis

- The majority of patients with lower GI bleeding have a fissure or infection.
- Mucosal lesions are more likely to be associated with antecedent occult bleeding.
- In most patients the bleeding stops spontaneously.

REASONS FOR LOWER GI BLEEDING AT DIFFERENT AGES

Neonatal Period

- Anal fissure
- Necrotizing enterocolitis
- Enteric infections
- Allergic colitis
- Lymphonodular hyperplasia (LNH)
- Upper GI source
- Duplication cyst
- Enterocolitis with Hirschsprung disease
- Meckel diverticulum
- Vascular malformations
- Shock with ischemic bowel
- Hemorrhagic disease of the newborn
- Stress ulcers

Infancy

- Anal fissure
- Enteric infections
- Allergic colitis
- Intussusception
- Meckel diverticulum
- LNH
- Upper GI source
- Duplication cyst
- Enterocolitis with Hirschsprung disease
- Vascular malformation
- Shock with ischemic bowel
- Gangrenous bowel

Preschool Age

- Anal fissure
- Enteric infections
- Polyps
- Parasites
- Meckel diverticulum
- Intussusception
- LNH
- Inflammatory bowel disease (IBD)
- Enterocolitis with Hirschsprung disease
- Hemolytic uremic syndrome
- Shock with ischemic bowel
- Gangrenous bowel

- Vascular malformation
- Child abuse
- Perianal streptococcal cellulitis

School Age

- Anal fissure
- Enteric infections
- IBD
- Intussusception
- Meckel diverticulum
- Polyps
- Henoch Schönlein purpura (HSP)
- Hemolytic uremic syndrome (HUS)
- Parasites
- Child abuse
- Vascular malformations
- Perianal streptococcal cellulitis

Adolescent

- Anal fissure
- Enteric infections
- IBD
- HUS
- Intussusception
- Midgut volvulus
- Vascular malformations
- LNH
- Parasites
- Hemorrhoids

Approach to the Patient

GENERAL GOALS

Determine location of bleeding, the cause, and begin stabilization and treatment

Phase 1: Determine if there is blood or other cause of red or black stools.

Phase 2: Assess patient to determine etiology; follow history, physical, and laboratory.

Phase 3: Stabilize patient, decide if emergency treatment is needed or if referral is appropriate. (See Emergency Care.)

HINTS FOR SCREENING PROBLEM

- The rate of bleeding will determine the clinical presentation.
- The more rapid the rate, the larger the volume of lower GI bleeding, and greater the drop in hemoglobin and change in pulse and blood pressure.
- Any significant blood loss will lead to pallor, tachycardia, orthostasis, poor capillary refill, CNS changes (restlessness, confusion), and hypotension.
- Hypotension may not be seen even in the face of significant blood loss, because vasoconstriction will occur to maintain blood pressure until decompensation.
- Initial hemoglobin values may be unreliable since a delay in hemodilution may falsely result in near-normal values.
- In newborn, determine if this is swallowed maternal blood.

 ## Data Gathering

HISTORY

Question: Is this really blood?
Significance: Get a history and check if any recently ingested foods resemble blood, e.g., red dye, beets, Jell-O, Kool-Aid.

Question: Color of blood?
Significance: If bright red, then site of bleeding is probably in left colon, rectosigmoid, or anal canal; if darker red, then from right colon; if melena or tarry, then bleeding is proximal to ileocecal valve.

Question: Location of blood in relation to the stool?
Significance: In colitis the blood will be mixed with the stool, with a fissure it will be in streaks on the outer aspect of the stool.

Question: Consistency of the stool?
Significance: If diarrhea, more likely to be colitis; if hard, then more likely to be a fissure.

Question: Painful stools?
Significance: Suggest anal fissure or local proctitis.

Question: Painless rectal bleeding?
Significance: Associated with polyps and Meckel diverticulum.

Question: Abdominal pain?
Significance: Can be seen with colitis, IBD, or surgical abdomen.

Question: Any underlying known GI disease, previous GI surgery?
Significance: Past history of colitis, Hirschsprung disease, necrotizing enterocolitis.

Question: Any history of jaundice, hepatitis, liver disease, neonatal history?
Significance: Suggestive of portal vein thrombosis (sepsis, shock, exchange transfusion, omphalitis, IV catheters), portal hypertension, and variceal bleeding.

Question: Any familial history of bleeding diathesis?
Significance: von Willebrand disease, hemophilia

Question: Any medications that can cause bleeding—heparin, warfarin?

Question: Any associated symptoms?
Significance:

- Mouth ulcers
- Weight loss
- Joint pains as in IBD
- Petechiae
- Renal insufficiency
- History of ingestion of uncooked meat as in HUS
- Purpuric rash as in HSP
- Severe abdominal pain and vomiting as in a surgical abdomen

Physical Examination

Finding: Skin
Significance:

- Petechiae
- Ecchymosis
- Purpura
- Hemangiomas
- Evidence of chronic liver disease

—Spider angiomata
—Palmar erythema

- Jaundice

Finding: HEENT: freckles on buccal mucosa
Significance: Peutz-Jeghers syndrome

Finding: Mouth ulcers
Significance: Crohn disease

Finding: Abdomen: hepatosplenomegaly, ascites
Significance: Portal hypertension

Finding: Isolated splenomegaly
Significance: Cavernous transformation of the portal vein

Finding: Rectal examination: evidence of any perianal disease
Significance: Source of bleeding

- IBD, bright red blood in the perianal area or on the examining glove
- Polyps bright red blood in stool

 Laboratory Aids

Test: CBC
Significance: Iron-deficiency anemia. If there is leukopenia, anemia, and thrombocytopenia think chronic liver disease and portal hypertension. If there is anemia with normal RBC indices, then there is truly an acute cause for bleeding. If RBC indices indicate iron-deficiency anemia, think of varices or a mucosal lesion, i.e., chronic blood loss. If thrombocytopenia, think Hemolytic uremic syndrome (HUS).

Test: Coagulation profile
Significance: If PT and PTT are abnormal, then think of liver disease or disseminated intravascular coagulation (DIC) with sepsis. If DIC screen is negative, think liver disease.

Test: Renal function tests (BUN, creatinine, urine analysis)
Significance: Abnormal in HUS, HSP

Test: Liver function tests
Significance: Abnormal in chronic liver disease

Test: Stool tests
Significance: Stool culture (Salmonella, Shigella, Campylobacter, Yersinia, Aeromonas, *Escherichia coli*), stool for *Clostridium difficile* toxin A and B, three stool samples for ova and parasites (amoeba). Stool smears for white blood cells (not always positive in colitis) and eosinophils (not always positive in allergic colitis).

Test: Abdominal x-ray
Significance: Helpful in surgical abdomen (dilated bowel, air-fluid levels, perforation), constipation (presence of excessive stool), or colitis (edematous bowel, thumb-printing) and toxic megacolon.

Test: Lower and upper endoscopy
Significance: Full colonoscopy to the terminal ileum helpful in diagnosing IBD. Upper endoscopy diagnostic in massive upper GI bleeds presenting with hematochezia. Enteroscopy involves the passage of a special endoscope further in the small bowel allowing for the identification of rare lesions in the proximal 60 to 120 cm of the jejunum.

Test: Barium tests
Significance: Barium enema is diagnostic and therapeutic in intussusception. Contraindicated in moderate and severe colitis. Air contrast barium enema is helpful in diagnosing mucosal lesions (polyps). Upper GI series with small bowel follow through is helpful in evaluating anatomy and Crohn's disease and its complications (fistula, sometimes ulcer may be identified). Enteroclysis or small bowel enema provides good mucosal detail.

Test: Meckel scan
Significance: Diagnostic for Meckel diverticulum that secrete acid. There may be false negatives if the Meckel diverticulum has different tissue expression.

Test: Bleeding scan
Significance: Useful in the patient in whom endoscopy was not diagnostic. Technetium sulfur colloids versus tagged RBC scan. The former detects rapid bleeding but can miss small bleeds, especially if patient is not bleeding during the scan. The latter can detect small bleeds, especially if intermittent.

Test: Angiography
Significance: Useful in detecting vascular causes for GI bleeding. Can also be therapeutic.

Test: Video capsule endoscopy
Significance: Useful in detecting distal small bowel hemorrhage. Not appropriate for younger children.

 Emergency Care

- If patient critical, stabilize the patient with intravenous fluids and blood products.
- Order laboratory tests: CBC, PT/PTT, DIC screen, liver function tests, blood type, and crossmatch.
- Insert an NG tube and lavage with saline if it is unclear whether the patient is having hematochezia as a result of massive bleeding from the upper GI tract.
- Monitor patient's vital signs and hemoglobin as necessary.
- Make appropriate diagnosis and institute appropriate therapy, i.e., abdominal x-ray, colonoscopy, bleeding scans.

PITFALLS

- Make sure red substance in stool is really blood and not food coloring.
- Initial hemoglobin if normal may be misleading.

Common Questions and Answers

Q: What is the most common cause of lower GI bleeding?
A: Throughout all age groups fissures are the leading cause followed by infections. However, in infancy, the most common cause is a fissure, in toddlers and young children—polyps, and in older children—IBD.
Q: What common foods cause stools to be red? black?
A: Red: Raspberries, cranberries, artificial coloring in cereal. Black: Bismuth, licorice.

Issues for Referral

The following patients should be referred to a specialist:

- Any patient with significant acute lower GI bleeding after initial stabilization.
- Patients with less acute bleeding for whom an easily identifiable cause has not been found (e.g., fissures, infection, intussusception, Meckel diverticulum); patients with chronic or recurrent lower GI bleeding.

Clinical Pearls

- Anal fissure: Treat the underlying constipation (mineral oil, lactulose, high-fiber diet). Local therapy consists of sitz baths, local emollient cremes, and steroid suppositories.
- Polyp: Colonoscopy and polypectomy.
- Intussusception: Barium enema is both diagnostic and permits hydrostatic reduction.
- Parasites. Antiparasitic drugs.
- Surgery: In cases of massive or persistent bleeding with no identifiable site, exploratory laparotomy with intraoperative endoscopic evaluation of the entire bowel to identify mucosal lesions eluding diagnosis by conventional means may be required.

BIBLIOGRAPHY

Chaibou M, Tucci M, Dugas MA, et al. Clinically significant upper gastrointestinal bleeding acquired in a pediatric intensive care unit. *Pediatrics* 1998;102(4 Pt 1):933–938.

Lawrence WW, Wright JL. Causes of rectal bleeding in children. *Pediatr Rev* 2001;22(11):394–395.

Leung AK, Wong AL. Lower gastrointestinal bleeding in children. *Pediatr Emerg Care* 2002;18(4):319–323.

Squires RH. Gastrointestinal bleeding. *Pediatr Rev* 1999;20(3):95–101.

Authors: Maria R. Mascarenhas and Meena Thayu

Mediastinal Mass

 ## Database

DEFINITION

Any mass in the anterior, posterior, or middle mediastinum. The anterior mediastinum includes the thymus and other structures anterior to the pericardium. The middle mediastinum is a vascular space that contains the pericardium, heart, great vessels, ascending aorta, and the aortic arch. The posterior mediastinum contains the tracheobronchial tree, esophagus, descending aorta, and neural structures.

 ## Differential Diagnosis

CONGENITAL/ANATOMIC

- Thoracic meningocele
- Large normal thymus in neonate
- Bronchogenic cyst
- Pericardial cyst
- Aortic aneurysm

INFECTIOUS

May cause mediastinal adenopathy and/or pulmonary nodules.

- Tuberculosis
- Histoplasmosis
- Aspergillosis
- Coccidioidomycosis
- Blastomycosis

TOXIC, ENVIRONMENTAL, DRUGS

- Foreign body in the trachea or esophagus

TUMOR

- Benign

—Thymoma
—Teratoma/dermoid cyst
—Lymphangioma/cystic hygroma
—Hemangioma
—Pheochromocytoma
—Ganglioneuroma
—Neurofibroma

- Malignant

—Hodgkin lymphoma
—Non-Hodgkin lymphoma
—Leukemia
—Neuroblastoma
—Rhabdomyosarcoma
—Ganglioneuroblastoma
—Neurofibrosarcoma
—Ewing sarcoma
—Malignant germ cell tumor

ALLERGIC, INFLAMMATORY

- Sarcoid

Approach to the Patient

GENERAL GOAL

Promptly establish diagnosis and begin treatment as indicated. Leukemia and lymphoma may progress rapidly and become life-threatening. If you suspect a malignancy, the child should be immediately referred to an oncologist.

Phase 1: Identify and treat life-threatening complications promptly.

- Superior vena cava (SVC) syndrome—mass compression of the SVC resulting in decreased blood flow to the heart.
- Tracheal compression
- Spinal cord compression
- Pleural and/or pericardial effusion
- Tumor lysis syndrome—metabolic triad of hyperkalemia, hyperuricemia, and hyperphosphatemia

Phase 2:

- If mass appears solid, attempt to obtain a tissue diagnosis via biopsy or excision of mass
- If mass appears cystic, surgical intervention may or may not be indicated
- If patient exhibits signs of infection (fever, cough, etc.), obtain appropriate cultures, place PPD and anergy panel and begin broad-spectrum antibiotics

COMPLICATIONS

- Superior vena cava (SVC) syndrome: mass compressing the SVC resulting in decreased blood flow to the heart. Signs and symptoms include edema and cyanosis of the face, neck, and upper extremities, plethora, distended neck veins, cough, dyspnea, orthopnea, headache, anxiety, and confusion. Symptoms are exacerbated when child is recumbent.
- Tracheal compression: mass compression of the trachea resulting in respiratory compromise. Signs and symptoms include stridor, cough, dyspnea, orthopnea.
- Spinal cord compression: neurologic symptoms vary depending on the level of the lesion.
- Pleural and pericardial effusions: resulting in respiratory distress or cardiac tamponade.
- Infection: may be the primary mass (tuberculosis) or a complication of the mass (infected cyst, infected nodes).
- Horner syndrome: ptosis, miosis, and anhydrosis resulting from compression of the cervical sympathetic nerve trunk.
- Esophageal narrowing or erosion: may result in feeding difficulty or bleeding.

 ## Data Gathering

HISTORY

Question: Symptoms of respiratory distress: stridor cough, dyspnea, orthopnea, wheezing?
Significance: May indicate tracheal compression.

Question: Headache, syncope, dyspnea, orthopnea, anxiety, facial swelling, eye edema?
Significance: Seen in SVC syndrome.

Question: Systemic symptoms: fever, weight loss, night sweats, fatigue?
Significance: Associated with infection and malignancies.

 ## Physical Examination

Finding: Decreased breath sounds, wheezing, stridor
Significance: Mass may be impinging on trachea or bronchi.

Finding: Edema and cyanosis of face, neck, and upper extremities
Significance: Seen in SVC syndrome.

Finding: Venous distension (jugular and superficial chest veins)
Significance: Seen in SVC syndrome.

Finding: Conjunctival edema, retinal vessel engorgement
Significance: Seen in SVC syndrome.

Finding: Lymphadenopathy and/or hepatosplenomegaly
Significance: Suggests lymphoma/leukemia.

Finding: Generalized bruises, petechiae, mucosal bleeding
Significance: Suggests thrombocytopenia, which can be seen in leukemia.

Finding: Horner syndrome
Significance: Can be seen in neuroblastoma. Typically a posterior mediastinal mass.

Mediastinal Mass

 Laboratory Aids

Test: Chest radiograph (lateral film required)
Significance: Establish size and location of mass.

Test: CBC with differential
Significance: Anemia, thrombocytopenia, or leukocytosis frequently noted in leukemia or lymphoma syndromes.

Test: LDH, uric acid, electrolytes, BUN, Creatinine
Significance: Frequently abnormal in leukemia or lymphoma syndromes.

Test: Pulse oximetry
Significance: Helpful to assess tissue oxygenation.

Test: Computed tomography (CT) of the chest (if patient can tolerate recumbency)
Significance: Define size, location, and consistency of mass.

Test: Diagnostic

- Lymph node aspiration/biopsy
- Bone marrow aspiration/biopsy
- PPD skin test for tuberculosis

Test: Diagnostic and therapeutic: pleurocentesis or pericardiocentesis, biopsy, or excision of mass
Significance: Establish tissue diagnosis and relieve symptoms.

PROCEDURE

- Avoid supine position in suspected SVC syndrome.

Clinical Pearls

Do not treat a patient who has no history of asthma with steroids without a chest radiograph to confirm that there is no mediastinal mass.

General Therapy

Therapy will be based on the diagnosis and may include:

- Chemotherapy and/or radiation therapy for malignant tumors
- Surgical excision alone for benign tumors.
- Antibiotics for infectious processes

 Emergency Care

If symptoms are progressing rapidly or there is evidence of SVC syndrome, tracheal compression, or spinal cord compression, steroids or radiation may be required.

PITFALLS

Circulatory collapse or respiratory failure can occur in children with SVC syndrome and/or tracheal compression. Avoid:

- General anesthesia: try to make the diagnosis with local or no anesthesia.
- Sedation: may cause irreversible respiratory depression.
- Supine position: keep head elevated to increase venous return.
- Placing intravenous line in the upper extremities as a result of poor venous return: try to use lower extremities.
- Long delays in establishing diagnosis: leukemia and lymphomas grow quickly and can rapidly impinge on vital structures.

Common Questions and Answers

Q: What should be done if the child is asymptomatic and mediastinal mass is an incidental finding on CXR?
A:

- Careful history and physical with specific attention to pulmonary, cardiac, and hematologic systems
- Vital signs to include temperature and pulse OX
- CBC, differential, ESR, tumor lysis labs
- PPD, anergy panel
- CT of chest
- Referral to oncologist, surgeon, or infectious disease specialist, pending above results

Q: When should an oncologist be consulted?
A: With any of the following:

- Rapidly enlarging mass
- Signs and symptoms of tracheal compression, SVC syndrome, or spinal cord compression
- Hepatosplenomegaly, lymphadenopathy, bruises, or petechiae on physical examination
- Anemia, thrombocytopenia, or leukocytosis suggesting bone marrow involvement
- Malignant histology is demonstrated with biopsy
- When help is needed in establishing the diagnosis

BIBLIOGRAPHY

Bower RJ, Kiesewetter WB. Mediastinal masses in infants and children. *Arch Surg* 1977; 112:1003–1009.

Buckley JA, et al. CT evaluation of mediastinal masses in children: spectrum of disease with pathologic correlation. *Clin Rev Diagn Imaging* 1998;39(5):365–392.

Hudson MM, Donaldson SS. Hodgkin's disease. *Pediatr Clin North Am* 1997;44:891–906.

Kelly KM, Lange B. Oncologic emergencies. *Pediatr Clin North Am* 1997;44:809–829.

Maity A, Goldweins JW, Lange BW, et al. Mediastinal masses in children with Hodgkin's disease. *Cancer* 1992;69(11):2755–2760.

Ricketts RR. Clinical management of anterior mediastinal tumors in children. *Semin Pediatr Surg* 2001;10:161–168.

Robie DK, Gursoy MH, Pokorny WJ. Mediastinal tumors—airway obstruction and management. *Semin Pediatr Surg* 1994;3:259–266.

Saenz NC, Schnitzer JJ, Eraklis AE, et al. Posterior mediastinal masses. *J Pediatr Surg* 1993;28:172–176.

Shad A, Magrath I. Non-Hodgkin's lymphoma. *Pediatr Clin North Am* 1997;44:863–890.

Shamberger RC, Holzman RS, Griscom NJ, et al. Prospective evaluation by computed tomography and pulmonary function tests of children with mediastinal masses. *Surgery* 1995;118(3):468–473.

Authors: Don E. Eslin
Leslie Raffini, 3rd edition

Microcytic Anemia

 Database

DEFINITION

Microcytic anemia is a term used to describe a low hemoglobin level and reduced red cell size.

- The mean corpuscular volume (MCV), which measures red cell size, varies with age. Thus, adult normal values cannot be applied to young children. Newborns have larger red cells with a mean MCV of 108 fL, and a lower limit of normal of 98 fL. The MCV then gradually declines. At 2 weeks of age, the lower limit of normal is 86 fL, and by 2 months, it is 77 fL. From age 6 months to 2 years, the lower limit of normal is 70 fL, from 2 to 5 years it increases to 75 fL, from 6 to 12 years, it is 77 fL, and from 13 to 18 years, it is 78 fL.
- A quick estimate of the lower limit of normal for MCV for children over a year old can be made with the following formula:

—Lower limit of normal MCV = 70 + age (years)

PATHOPHYSIOLOGY

The hemoglobin molecule is made up of heme and globin components. Disorders of the production of either of these components may result in a microcytic anemia. Heme production requires iron, and therefore it is affected by iron deficiency or inadequate iron utilization as is seen in the anemia of chronic inflammation. Inadequate production of the porphyrin component of the heme molecule can also impair heme synthesis and such disorders are known as sideroblastic anemias. Sideroblastic anemias can be inherited or acquired. Disorders of globin chain synthesis include the thalassemias and hemoglobin E disease. See Thalassemia chapter.

EPIDEMIOLOGY

- Iron deficiency anemia occurs with a prevalence of 1% to 5% in the United States. Young children and adolescent females are at greatest risk.
- β-thalassemia mutations are common in Mediterranean countries, Southeast Asia, China, Africa, and India.
- Hemoglobin E mutations are common in certain Southeast Asian countries, particularly Cambodia, Laos, and Thailand.
- α-thalassemia mutations occur in the Chinese subcontinent, Malaysia, Indochina, and Africa

 Differential Diagnosis

METABOLIC

- Iron deficiency (most common)

ENVIRONMENTAL

- Chronic lead poisoning

CONGENITAL

- Thalassemia syndromes
- Hemoglobin E trait (single gene affected) or disease (2 genes affected)
- Selected congenital hemolytic anemias with unstable hemoglobin

INFLAMMATORY

- Recent or chronic inflammation or infection. Anemia of chronic inflammation (also known as anemia of chronic disease) may cause a microcytic anemia or normocytic anemia.

—Common causes of anemia of chronic inflammation include chronic infection, rheumatoid arthritis, systemic lupus erythematosus, inflammatory bowel disease (may also be a component of iron deficiency), and malignancy

MISCELLANEOUS

- Sideroblastic anemia (rare in children)

Approach to the Patient

Review of the child's history, red cell indices, and peripheral blood smear should guide further laboratory evaluation. General guidelines for evaluating a patient with microcytic anemia include:

- Initially identify severe anemia that requires inpatient observation and possible blood transfusion.
- Consider chronic lead intoxication early. If history is suspicious (e.g., peeling paint, pica, etc.), draw lead level to make diagnosis.
- Iron deficiency is the most common cause of microcytic anemia. Screen by history as described below. If history is suspicious, consider therapeutic iron trial prior to additional workup.
- If suspicious of a thalassemia syndrome, send hemoglobin electrophoresis, with hemoglobin A2 quantification. Complete blood counts and hemoglobin electrophoresis from parents may also be helpful.

 Data Gathering

HISTORY

Question: What is the child's age?
Significance: Microcytic anemia in children age 9 months to 3 years and in adolescence is most commonly as a result of iron deficiency. Term infants are born with adequate iron stores for 6 months and therefore should not have nutritional iron deficiency causing anemia. β-thalassemia major often presents in first year of life as fetal hemoglobin production declines.

Question: What does the child's diet include?

- Evaluate dietary iron intake as appropriate for age. Iron in breast milk is more bioavailable (50% vs. 10%) than iron in formula.

—Infants who are exclusively breast-fed after 6 months are at an increased risk for iron deficiency if they do not receive supplements.
—Infant formulas and cereals should be iron-fortified. In preschool children and adolescents assess intake of high iron-containing foods including red meats, fish, poultry, beans, and peanut butter.

- Introduction of whole cow's milk before the age of 1 year provides little dietary iron and can cause occult intestinal bleeding leading to iron loss.

—High intake of milk also causes a decreased appetite for other foods with a higher iron content.
—Cow's milk intake of greater than 24 ounces daily is a risk factor for iron deficiency.

- History of pica suggests iron deficiency and/or lead intoxication.

Question: Is there any history of blood loss?
Significance: Blood loss decreases iron stores. Ask about loss from stool, urine, chronic nosebleeds, and menorrhagia.

Question: Was the child born prematurely or was there a history of blood loss at birth?
Significance: Premature infants have lower total body iron stores and an increased growth rate that leads to increased iron requirements. Significant blood loss at birth can deplete iron stores.

Question: What is the child's ethnic background? Is there any familial history of anemia?
Significance: α-thalassemia is most common among children of African or Asian descent. β-thalassemia is most common in children of Mediterranean, Asian, or African descent. Hemoglobin E occurs most commonly in children of Southeast Asian descent.

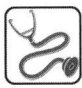 ## Physical Examination

Finding: Child's general appearance
Significance: Most children with mild to moderate microcytic anemia are well appearing with a normal physical examination.

Finding: Irritability or pallor
Significance: Anemia is likely more severe than usual. Irritability is a common finding with iron deficiency.

Finding: Cardiovascular examination
Significance: Check for instability including tachycardia, hypotension, and presence of a gallop. Flow murmurs are common with chronic anemia.

Finding: Abnormal sclerae
Significance: Blue sclera is associated with iron deficiency (very rare). Icterus is seen with severe thalassemia syndromes and hemolytic anemias.

Finding: Mouth lesions
Significance: Glossitis and stomatitis are signs of iron deficiency.

Finding: Splenic enlargement
Significance: Splenic enlargement may be seen with thalassemia syndromes depending on the severity. The spleen is a site of extramedullary hematopoiesis and clears abnormal red cells.

 ## Laboratory Aids

PATIENT

Test: Complete blood count (CBC)
Significance: Low hemoglobin level and low MCV for age

Test: Red cell distribution width (RDW)
Significance: Measures the variation in red cell size. It is elevated in iron deficiency and normal in thalassemia trait, infection, and lead poisoning.

Test: Peripheral blood smear
Significance: Microcytosis and hypochromia. Marked poikilocytosis and anisocytosis with iron deficiency and thalassemia syndromes. Basophilic stippling with lead poisoning. Target cells are found with heterozygous or homozygous hemoglobin E.

Test: Ferritin
Significance: Serum ferritin reflects tissue iron stores. It is reduced in iron deficiency. Ferritin is an acute phase reactant and is increased with infection, inflammation, and liver disease. It is normal or increased in thalassemia.

Test: Serum iron
Significance: Reduced in iron deficiency. Normal in thalassemia (unless chronically transfused which leads to increased iron levels). Normal or reduced in infection or inflammatory states.

Test: Transferrin saturation
Significance: Transferrin saturation measures the iron available for hemoglobin synthesis. Low in iron deficiency and chronic infection. Normal in thalassemia.

Test: Lead level
Significance: Increased in lead intoxication.

Test: Hemoglobin electrophoresis with quantification
Significance: Increased hemoglobin A_2 in β-thalassemia trait, and normal in α-thalassemia trait and other microcytic anemias. Iron deficiency anemia may cause a reduction in hemoglobin A_2 production. If microcytosis persists after iron is replenished, hemoglobin electrophoresis should be repeated.

Test: Soluble transferrin receptor
Significance: Indicator of increased tissue iron demand. It is increased in iron deficiency anemia and also in thalassemia syndromes, but not with the anemia of chronic inflammation.

Test: Bone marrow aspirate
Significance: Bone marrow aspirate is rarely needed to establish diagnosis. Iron stores can be assessed by hemosiderin staining. In sideroblastic anemias, greater than 10% of the nucleated red cell precursors are ringed sideroblasts.

FAMILY STUDIES

- **Test:** CBC
- **Test:** Peripheral blood smear
- **Test:** Hemoglobin electrophoresis

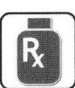 ## Therapy

- Consider therapeutic trial of iron supplementation if history is suspicious.
- May require initial inpatient observation in cases of severe anemia.
- Red cell transfusion only if evidence of cardiovascular compromise (rarely indicated).
- Removal of environmental exposure and possible chelation for lead poisoning to prevent central nervous system toxicity.
- No treatment is needed for α or β-thalassemia trait and Hemoglobin E trait or disease. Iron therapy is not indicated. If concomitant iron deficiency is suspected, iron studies should be sent and treatment commenced if iron deficiency is documented.

 ## Follow-Up

In iron deficiency, the reticulocyte count begins to increase in 3 to 4 days and the hemoglobin concentration should rise by at least 1 g/dL in 2 to 4 weeks following iron supplementation. Children with thalassemia trait have a persistent mild, microcytic anemia that is not clinically significant, but require genetic counseling as they become older. Children with other thalassemia syndromes (β-thalassemia major, hemoglobin H disease) should be referred to a hematologist.

PITFALLS

Lead poisoning and iron deficiency can occur concurrently because iron deficiency causes increased lead absorption. If history is concerning for increased lead exposure in cases of documented iron deficiency, send lead levels.

 ## Common Questions and Answers

Q: What is a therapeutic iron trial and when is it indicated?
A: A therapeutic iron trial is a trial of oral iron therapy without additional laboratory testing in a patient with a microcytic anemia and a history of dietary deficiency or known history of blood loss. An increase in the hemoglobin concentration of 1 g/dL or greater after 2 to 4 weeks of therapy confirms the diagnosis of iron deficiency. If the hemoglobin level does not increase, additional laboratory testing is necessary and other diagnoses should be considered.

Q: How does infection affect the diagnosis of anemia?
A: Common childhood infections can be associated with a mild microcytic anemia. Acute infection also affects some of the laboratory tests used to diagnose the cause of microcytic anemia. With infection there is a shift of iron from serum to storage sites. Serum iron is reduced and ferritin increases. It is, therefore, preferable to evaluate a microcytic anemia 3 to 4 weeks after an infection resolves.

BIBLIOGRAPHY

Grantham-McGregor S, Ani C. A review of studies on the effect of iron deficiency on cognitive development in children. *J Nutr* 2001;131(2S-2):649S–666S; discussion 666S–668S.

Hoffbrand AV, Herbert V. Nutritional anemias. *Semin Hematol* 1999;36(4 Suppl 7):13–23.

Pappas DE. Iron deficiency anemia. *Pediatr Rev* 1998;19:321–322.

Wharton BA. Iron deficiency in children: detection and prevention. *Br J Hematol* 1999;106:270–280.

Authors: Janet L. Kwiatkowski, MD
Suzanne Shuslerman, 3rd edition

Pallor

Database

DEFINITION

Pallor is defined as paleness of the skin and may be a reflection of anemia or poor peripheral perfusion. Anemia is age-dependent.

Differential Diagnosis

CONGENITAL

- Hemoglobinopathies

—Sickle cell syndromes
—Thalassemia syndromes
—Other unstable hemoglobins

- Erythrocyte membrane defects

—Hereditary spherocytosis
—Elliptocytosis
—Stomatocytosis
—Pyropoikilocytosis
—Infantile pyknocytosis

- Erythrocyte enzyme defects

—Glucose-6-phosphate dehydrogenase (G-6-PD) deficiency
—Pyruvate kinase deficiency

- Diamond-Blackfan anemia

—Congenital pure red-cell aplasia (rare)

- Fanconi anemia

—Constellation of varied cytopenias
—Multiple congenital anomalies
—Abnormal bone marrow chromosomal fragility

INFECTIOUS

- Septic shock
- Infection-related bone marrow suppression

—Parvovirus B19 infection

- Infection-related hemolytic anemias

—Epstein-Barr virus
—Influenza
—Coxsackievirus
—Varicella
—Cytomegalovirus
—*Escherichia coli*
—Pneumococcus
—Streptococcus
—*Salmonella typhi*
—Mycoplasma

NUTRITIONAL/TOXIC/DRUGS

- Iron-deficiency anemia

—Common cause of anemia in children, especially under the age of 3 years and in female adolescents

- Plumbism

—Anemia usually as a result of coexisting iron deficiency. Very high lead levels associated with altered heme synthesis

- Vitamin B12 and/or folate deficiency
  —Results in a megaloblastic anemia

- Medication-induced bone marrow suppression

—Chemotherapy
—Antibiotics, especially trimethoprim-sulfamethoxazole

- Drug-related hemolytic anemia

—Antibiotics
—Antiepileptics
—Azathioprine
—Isoniazid
—Nonsteroidal anti-inflammatory drugs

TRAUMA

- Acute blood loss

TUMOR

- Leukemia with bone marrow infiltration
- Metastatic tumors with bone marrow infiltration

GENETIC/METABOLIC

- Metabolic derangements

—Severe electrolyte disturbance
—pH disturbance
—Inborn errors

- Schwachmann-Diamond syndrome

—Marrow hypoplasia with associated pancreatic insufficiency and associated failure to thrive

OTHER

- Transient erythroblastopenia of childhood

—Acquired pure red blood cell aplasia

- Aplastic anemia

—Bone marrow failure syndrome with at least 2 of the 3 blood cell lines eventually affected

- Systemic diseases

—Anemia of chronic disease
—Chronic renal disease
—Uremia

- Hypothyroidism
- Sideroblastic anemia

—Defective iron utilization within the developing erythrocytes

- Autoimmune and isoimmune hemolytic anemias
- Microangiopathic hemolytic anemias

—Thrombotic thrombocytopenic purpura (TTP)
—Hemolytic uremic syndrome (HUS)
—Disseminated intravascular coagulation (DIC)

- Mechanical destruction

—Vascular malformation
—Abnormal or prosthetic cardiac valves

Approach to the Patient

Determine first that the child appears pale, not simply fair-skinned. Second, decide if there is a medical emergency associated with circulatory failure. If not, the goal is to investigate the etiology and then intervene appropriately.

Phase 1: Assess for signs of shock—if present, initiate emergency procedures as required to stablize the patient, such as airway, breathing, and circulating.

Phase 2: If patient is stable, perform history, physical examination, and CBC with reticulocyte count to establish time of onset of pallor, associated symptoms, and level of anemia.

Phase 3: Specific diagnostic workup based on findings in phase 2.

Data Gathering

HISTORY

Question: Onset? Acute versus chronic
Significance: Helps with differential diagnosis

Question: Associated symptoms? Weight loss, fever, night sweats, Cough, and/or bone pain?
Significance: Suggests an underlying systemic illness, such as leukemia, infection or rheumatologic disorder

Question: Jaundice, scleral icterus, dark urine?
Significance: Suggests hemolysis

Question: Age between 6 months and 3 years, or adolescent females?
Significance: Peak age ranges for iron deficiency

Question: Age less than 6 months?
Significance: May represent a congenital anemia or isoimmunization

Question: Male?
Significance: Some red-cell enzyme X-linked defects, such as G-6-PD and phosphoglycerate kinase deficiencies are sex linked.

Question: African-American?
Significance: Hemoglobins S and C, α-and β-thalassemia trait, G-6-PD deficiency

Question: Southeast Asian?
Significance: Hemoglobin E and α-thalassemia

Question: Mediterranean descent?
Significance: β-Thalassemia and G-6-PD deficiency

Question: Premature infant?
Significance: Increased risk of both iron and vitamin E deficiency. Exaggerated hyperbilirubinemia can be the presenting symptom of isoimmune hemolytic or other congenital hemolytic anemia.

Question: Pica?
Significance: Often associated with both plumbism and iron deficiency

Question: Medications?
Significance: Can cause bone marrow suppression and/or hemolysis.

Question: Mild intake?
Significance: Cow's milk before age 12 months and high milk intake are associated with iron deficiency.

Question: Recent trauma and/or surgery?
Significance: Blood loss can result in iron deficiency.

Question: Recent infection?
Significance: Can be associated with hemolysis or bone marrow suppression.

Question: Familial history?
Significance: Some of the congenital hemolytic anemias are autosomal dominant. Familial history of splenectomy and/or early cholecystectomy can be a clue for a previously undiagnosed hemolytic anemia.

 ## Physical Examination

Finding: Rapid respiratory rate, decreased blood pressure, weak pulses, slow capillary refill
Significance: Indications of uncompensated anemia and/or shock

Finding: Frontal bossing and prominence of the malar and maxillary bones
Significance: Extramedullary erythropoiesis

Finding: Enlarged spleen
Significance: Hemolytic anemias, malignancy, infection

Finding: Glossitis
Significance: Vitamin B12 deficiency

Finding: Scleral interus or jaundice
Significance: May indicate hemolysis

Finding: Systolic flow murmur
Significance: Anemia

Finding: Bruits
Significance: May indicate vascular malformations

Finding: Petechiae and bruising
Significance: May indicate an associated thrombocytopenia, coagulopathy, or vasculitis

Finding: Dysmorphic features
Significance: Both Diamond-Blackfan and Fanconi's anemia are associated with other congenital defects, including thumb abnormalities, short stature, congenital heart disease.

 ## Laboratory Aids

Test: Complete blood count (CBC) with red cell indices.
Significance: Establishes the diagnosis of anemia, distinguishes by size—normocytic, macrocytic, microcytic

Test: Reticulocyte count
Significance: Distinguishes between decreased production and increased destruction of red cells

Test: Coombs test and antibody screen
Significance: Identifies immune-mediated red-cell destruction

Test: Peripheral blood smear
Significance: Specific morphologic findings can be diagnostic

Test: Iron studies: iron-binding capacity, serum Fe, ferritin, transferrin
Significance: Diagnosis of iron deficiency anemia or anemia of chronic disease

Test: Hgb electrophoresis with quantification
Significance: Establish diagnosis of hemoglobinopathy

Test: Lead studies: serum lead, free erythrocyte protoporphyrin
Significance: Diagnosis of plumbism

Test: Stool guaiac
Significance: Looks for occult blood loss

Test: Osmotic fragility
Significance: Diagnosis of red cell membrane defects (spherocytosis)

Test: Quantitative red-cell enzyme assays
Significance: Diagnosis of inherited RBC enzyme deficiencies

Test: Serum folate, RBC folate, and serum vitamin B12 levels
Significance: Diagnosis of deficiency of these vitamins

Test: Bone marrow aspiration and biopsy
Significance: Diagnosis of malignancy or bone marrow failure syndrome

Issues for Referral

- Severe or unexplained anemia
- Anemias other than dietary iron deficiency or thalassemia trait
- Recurrent iron deficiency—may suggest ongoing bleeding or iron malabsorption.
- All bone marrow failure or infiltrative processes

 ## Emergency Care

- Severe anemia of unclear etiology with hemodynamic instability: transfuse with packed red blood cells cautiously. In an antoimmune hemolytic process, the child is at risk for a transfusion reaction. Obtain blood for diagnostic studies before transfusion if possible.
- If there is circulatory failure without anemia, treatment requires intensive monitoring and access to critical care in an emergency room or ICU. Fluid resuscitation and/or inotropic pressor support as needed.
- Acute blood loss: treat circulatory failure as described. Transfuse with packed red blood cells, platelets, and fresh frozen plasma as needed.
- Malignancies: Emergency care should be directed toward treatment of circulatory failure and possible associated infection, and then to rapid diagnosis and treatment of the malignancy. Consultation with an oncologist should be sought as soon as possible.

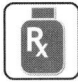 ## Therapy

Iron deficiency anemia—treat with 4 to 6 mg/kg elemental iron divided 2 to 3 times daily. This is absorbed best with acidic drinks, including orange juice; dairy products decrease absorption. The reticulocyte should improve 72 hours after starting iron therapy, the hemoglobin may take a week to rise. Iron should be continued for at least 3 months to replenish iron stores.

Clinical Pearls

- Parents often fail to notice pallor of gradual onset. Grandparents or others who see child less often may be the first to suspect pallor.

BIBLIOGRAPHY

Glader BE. Hemolytic anemia in children. *Clin Lab Med* 1999;19(1):87–111.

Graham EA. The changing face of anemia in infancy. *Pediatr Rev* 1995;15:175–183.

Monzon CM, Beaver D, Dillon TD. Evaluation of erythrocyte disorders with mean corpuscular volume (MCV) and red cell distribution width (RDW). *Clin Pediatr* 1987;26:632–638.

Segal G, Hirsh M, Feig S. Managing anemia in pediatric office practice: part 1. *Pediatr Rev* 2002;23:75–84.

Sills RH. Indications for bone marrow examination. *Pediatr Rev* 1995;16:226–228.

Authors: Leslie Raffini
Debra L. Friedman, 3rd edition

Proteinuria

Database

DEFINITION

Protein may be found in the urine of healthy children. The term proteinuria is used to indicate urinary protein excretion beyond the upper limit of normal, which is 100 mg/m^2 per day or 4 mg/m^2 per hour in children and 150 mg per day in adults.

Proteinuria greater than 40 mg/m^2 per hour is considered as nephrotic range and usually is associated with other features of the nephrotic syndrome.

PATHOPHYSIOLOGY

Approximately 50% of the normally excreted protein consists of Tamm-Horsfall protein, a glycoprotein secreted by the ascending loop of Henle. Small quantities of plasma proteins filtered by the glomeruli, mainly albumin (up to 30% of the total urinary protein), but also immunoglobulin, transferrin, and β_2-microglobulin, comprise the rest. Proteinuria may be the result of an increased permeability of the glomeruli to the passage of serum proteins (glomerular proteinuria) or decreased reabsorption of low molecular weight proteins, such us $\beta_2\beta$-microglobulin, by the renal tubules (tubular proteinuria).

CLASSIFICATION

• Transient proteinuria is most often associated with fever in excess of 38.3°C, cold stress, dehydration, and exercise. Transient proteinuria is not considered to be associated with underlying renal disease and by definition is absent on subsequent urine examinations.

• Orthostatic proteinuria is defined as elevated protein excretion when the subject is upright, but normal protein excretion during recumbency. It most commonly occurs in school-age children and rarely exceeds 1 g/m^2 per day. These children need follow-up by the primary physicians to monitor the first morning urine for protein.

If present they require evaluation by a nephrologist (see Questions and Answers).

• Persistent or fixed proteinuria is defined as urinary dipstick ≥1+ in the first morning urine specimen on multiple occasions for a period >3 months. Fixed proteinuria requires prompt confirmation and referral to nephrology because it may be a result of glomerular, or less frequently, to tubular disorders.

Glomerular Proteinuria: The amount of proteinuria may range from <1 to >30 g per day. It is usually found in the context of edema, hypertension, abnormal glomerular filtration rate, and hematuria. The major marker is albumin.

Tubular Proteinuria: rarely exceeds 1 g per day and it is not associated with edema. It may be associated with other defects of proximal tubular function (glucosuria, phosphaturia, and aminoaciduria) and tubular interstitial processes. The major marker is $\beta_2\beta$-microglobulin.

Differential Diagnosis

IDIOPATHIC NEPHROTIC SYNDROME

• Minimal change nephritic syndrome (MCNS)
• Mesangial proliferation
• Focal and segmental glomerulosclerosis (FSGS)
• Membranous nephropathy

NEPHROTIC SYNDROME FROM GENETIC CAUSES

• Finnish-type congenital nephrotic syndrome
• Familial FSGS (AR or AD)
• Diffuse mesangial sclerosis
• Denys-Drash syndrome

ACQUIRED GLOMERULAR DISEASE

• Idiopathic glomerulonephritis (membranoproliferative GN)
• Lupus nephritis
• IgA nephropathy
• Systemic vasculitides
• Subacute bacterial endocarditis
• Diabetes mellitus
• Hypertension
• Hemolytic uremic syndrome
• Hyperfiltration secondary to nephron loss (with or without sclerosis)

GENETIC DISORDERS

• Nail-patella syndrome
• Alport syndrome
• Fabry disease
• Glycogen storage disease
• Cystic fibrosis
• Hurler syndrome (MPS type-1)
• α_1-antitrypsine
• Mitochondrial disorders (usually tubular proteinuria)
• Gaucher disease
• Dent disease (X-linked nephrolithiasis)
• Cystinosis
• Wilson disease

ONCOLOGIC/HEMATOLOGIC

• Sickle cell disease
• Renal vein thrombosis
• Leukemia
• Lymphoma

INFECTIOUS

• Poststreptococcal GN
• HIV nephropathy
• Hepatitis B and C
• Malaria
• Syphilis (can present as congenital nephrotic syndrome)
• Pyelonephritis

DRUGS/TOXINS

• Bee sting
• Food allergens
• Antibiotic-induced interstitial nephritis
• Penicillamine
• Gold salts
• NSAIDs
• Heavy metals (mercury, lead)

MISCELLANEOUS

• Tubular interstitial nephritis
• Acute tubular necrosis
• Reflux nephropathy
• Hypothyroidism
• Congestive heart failure

Data Gathering

HISTORY

• General symptoms related, such as fatigue, general malaise, reduced appetite
• Weight changes
• Facial swelling (in the mornings) and lower limb swelling (in the afternoon)
• Symptoms related to rheumatological conditions (skin rash, joint pain or stiffness, abdominal pain, mood changes)
• Changes in the aspect of the urine (foamy) or color (red, tea-color)
• Cough, shortness of breath
• Limb pain (leukemia, Fabry disease)
• Allergic diseases
• Recent illnesses (pharyngitis and upper respiratory infections) or frequent episodes of fever (lymphoma, malignancies)
• Heavy or vigorous exercise
• Medications and herbal/folk medicines
• Illicit drugs use and risk factors for STD in adolescents and adults (HIV, syphilis)
• UTI in the past (reflux nephropathy)
• Polydipsia/polyuria/dysfunctional voiding
• Visual acuity (retinitis pigmentosa)
• Hearing loss
• Prenatal ultrasound and neonatal history (use of umbilical lines)
• Family history of renal, rheumatological diseases, hearing loss, mental retardation, miscarriages

Physical Examination

Special attention has to be taken to the following systems/organs:

GENERAL

- Hypertension
- Growth and development
- Dysmorphic features

HEENT

- Periorbital edema
- Malar rash
- Cataracts

LYMPHADENOPATHY

CHEST

- Pericardial/pleural effusions
- Heart murmurs

ABDOMEN

- Ascites
- Abdominal bruits
- Hepatosplenomegaly
- Abdominal mass
- Costovertebral or suprapubic tenderness

GENITALIA

- Scrotal edema or scrotal pain
- Ambiguous genitalia

SKIN

- Purpuric or petechial rash
- Angiokeratomas
- Pallor

EXTREMITIES

- Pitting-dependent edema
- Arthralgias/arthritis
- Dystrophic nails
- Dystrophic limbs (elbow, patella)

 ## Laboratory Aids

DIPSTICK TESTING

- A semiquantitative routine screening test for proteinuria is performed in the office
- It is reported as negative, trace (10–20 mg/dL), 1+ (>30 mg/dL), 2+ (>100 mg/dL), 3+ (>300 mg/dL), and 4+ (>1,000 mg/dL).
- A negative or trace result in a concentrated urine specimen (specific gravity >1,020) is normal.
- It primarily detects albuminuria.
- False-positive results can occur with alkaline (pH >8.0) or concentrated urine (specific gravity >1,025). False-negative results can be a result of dilute urine.
- Should be always done in the first morning urine

24-HOUR COLLECTION OF URINE FOR PROTEIN AND CREATININE

- It is indicated for quantification of proteinuria and to confirm the diagnosis.
- Normal range is <100 mg/m^2 per day or <4 mg/m^2 per hour.
- The amount of creatinine is useful to determine that the specimen is truly a 24-hour collection, which is usually 15–20 mg/kg ideal body weight in females and 20–25 mg/kg ideal body weight in males.
- The 24-hour collection can be split into standing and recumbent collection for assessment of orthostatic proteinuria.

SPOT RATIO FOR PROTEIN/CREATININE RATIO (ON FIRST MORNING URINE)

- It has a high correlation with timed collection.
- Normal values are <0.2 mg protein/mg creatinine in children >2 years old and <0.5 mg protein/mg creatinine in children 6–24 months old.
- It is the simplest method to quantitate proteinuria.

MICROALBUMINURIA/ ALBUMIN–CREATININE INDEX

- It is used to assess risk of progressive glomerulopathy in patients with diabetes mellitus with disease duration of more than 5 years.
- Normal value is <30 mg urine albumin/g creatinine on first morning urine.
- With positive results a test should be repeated in 3–6 months to substantiate diagnosis and treatment.
- Additional tests depend on the presence of nephrotic syndrome, red blood cell casts, and/or hematuria in urinalysis and/or hypertension: comprehensive metabolic panel, serum albumin, serum cholesterol, complement levels (C3 and C4), streptozyme, or ASO titers.
- If evidence or suspicion for SLE, dsDNA antibodies are also needed. Antinuclear antibodies (ANA) have a very low specificity and should not be done.

 ## Common Questions and Answers

Q. When to refer to nephrology?
A. Patients with one of the following: fixed proteinuria, associated hypertension, associated hematuria, clinical evidence of nephrotic syndrome, evidence of systemic diseases associated with proteinuria, low complement levels, and patients with significant family history for severe renal disease and that have developed similar symptoms.

Q. When are imaging studies indicated?

- In patients with associated hypertension, abnormal renal function, patients with hematuria, patients with history of nephrolithiasis.
- The best initial study is kidney and bladder ultrasound. Some conditions can be associated with nephrocalcinosis.

Q. Which are usual indications for renal biopsy in a patient referred from a primary care physician with asymptomatic proteinuria?
A. Fixed proteinuria <1 g per day and one of the following: hematuria, decreased GFR, persistent hypocomplementemia, and/or hypertension. Proteinuria >1 g per day.

BIBLIOGRAPHY

Bergstein JM. A practical approach to proteinuria. *Pediatr Nephrol* 1999;13:697–700.

Dalton RN, Haycock GB. Laboratory investigation. In: Barrat TM, Avner ED, Harmon WE, eds. *Pediatric Nephrology*. 4th Ed. Baltimore: Williams & Wilkins 1999:343–364.

Eddy AA, Symons JM. Nephrotic syndrome in childhood. *Lancet* 2003;362:629–639.

Hogg RJ, Portman RJ, Milliner D, et al. Evaluation and management of proteinuria and nephrotic syndrome in children: recommendations from a pediatric nephrology panel established at the National Kidney Foundation Conference on Proteinuria, Albuminuria, Risk, Assessment, Detection, and Elimination (PARADE). *Pediatrics* 2000;105(6):1242–1249.

Author: Andres Greco

Pruritus

Database

DEFINITION

Itching, an unpleasant cutaneous sensation that provokes the desire to rub or scratch the skin to obtain relief.

Differential Diagnosis

CONGENITAL/ANATOMICAL

- Cholestasis secondary to biliary obstruction (e.g., Alagille syndrome)

INFECTIONS

- Pinworms (*Enterobius vermicularis*)
- Swimmer's itch (as a result of fresh water mammalian or avian schistosomes)
- Seabather eruption (affects swimmers and divers in marine waters off Florida, in the Gulf of Mexico, and the Caribbean Sea attributed to various organisms but recently to the larvae of the schyphomedusa [jellyfish], *Linuche unguiculata*).
- Herpes viruses: primary varicella infection or zoster; herpes simplex
- *Borrelia burgdorferi*: erythema chronicum migrans lesion of Lyme disease
- *Streptococcus pyogenes*: sandpaper rash of scarlet fever
- *Tinea corporis*
- *Toxocara canis*

TOXIC

- Contact dermatitis

—Allergens
—Plants (Rhus dermatitis—poison ivy/oak)
—Cosmetics—Dyes—Medications
—Irritants—Soaps—Detergents
—Excrement—Wool—Fiberglass

ENVIRONMENTAL

- Papular urticaria: bites of fleas, mosquitoes, etc.
- Pediculosis (lice)
- Mites: scabies (*Sarcoptes scabei*), chiggers (*Enterobicula alfreddugesi*), etc.
- Subcutaneous foreign body
- Phytophotodermatitis occurs when skin is exposed to sunlight after contact with an offending plant

DRUGS

- Systemic use of medications: aspirin, barbiturates, chloroquine, erythromycin, gold, griseofulvin, iodine contrast dyes, isoniazid, opiates, phenothiazines, vitamin A

ALLERGIC, INFLAMMATORY

- Atopic dermatitis (eczema)
- Psoriasis
- Seborrheic dermatitis

MISCELLANEOUS

- Burns
- Nonspecific urticaria
- Pityriasis rosea
- Asteatotic eczema–"winter itch"
- Xerosis (dry skin)—from excess bathing with or without strong detergents or low humidity, idiopathic

Approach to the Patient

GENERAL GOALS

Determine severity and if pruritus is isolated or as a result of an underlying systemic illness primarily by assessing the presence or absence of associated signs and symptoms, especially rash.

Phase 1: Assess the severity of illness. Pruritus will rarely be an element of a medical emergency except in cases of anaphylaxis or erythema multiforme-major.

Phase 2: A thorough review of potential precipitating events and the duration of symptoms will help determine if the itch is isolated or if there are any associated signs or symptoms. Pruritus with or without rash may be a manifestation of systemic illness.

Phase 3: A thorough history and examination should narrow the differential diagnosis considerably, enabling the clinician to determine the underlying cause of the complaint in the majority of cases. Laboratory tests may be indicated in cases in which the diagnosis is unclear.

HINTS FOR SCREENING PROBLEM

- Is a new or recurrent problem.

—If it is new, one should ask if there is anything new in the child's life that may be associated with the onset of pruritus (with or without rash). This is often the most revealing question as one may find that the child recently came in contact with a new item, which is known to be a contact irritant (see table, Potential Contact Irritants).

Data Gathering

HISTORY

Question: How severe is the pruritus? On a scale of 1 to 10? Compared to a mosquito bite? Is it severe enough to interfere with the daily routine of the child (e.g., wakes the child from sleep)?
Significance: Waking from sleep may point to a more severe form resulting from systemic disease.

Question: Has anything new or different been introduced to the child, especially anything that comes in contact with his/her skin?
Significance: See table, Potential Contact Irritants.

Question: How often and with what products is the child bathed?
Significance: Different soaps or detergents contain additives that may be allergenic. Changes in soaps may be important as stated previously. Some soaps cause excessive dryness or contain heavy fragrances. Children who are bathed frequently with anything more than water may develop dry and irritated (pruritic) skin.

Question: Has the child been hiking or camping in a wooded area?
Significance: May be from rhus dermatitis, from poison ivy.

Question: Are there any underlying illness(es) or associated symptoms?
Significance: For example, pruritus associated with night sweats and fever may point to hematopoietic malignancy. There is a long list of illnesses that are associated with pruritus (see table, Causes of Pruritus in Children).

Question: Does anyone who has frequent contact with the child also complaining of itching?
Significance: This may identify a common source of a contact irritant. For example, one will often see multiple family members affected by scabies or lice.

Question: Has this ever happened before?
Significance: Atopic dermatitis will present as chronic or recurrent pruritic skin lesions.

Potential Contact Irritants

Shoes	Clothing	Diapers	Cosmetics
Dyes (for hair, etc.)	Detergents	Excrement	Plants (e.g., cacti)
Jewelry (nickel)	Systemic medications	Topical medications	Foods
Wool	Fiberglass	Animals	Capsaicin in hot peppers*

*Acts as an irritant when first applied but actually decreases pruritus if applied repeatedly over weeks.

Physical Examination

Finding: If rash is present, what is the appearance?
Significance:

• Lesions appear in crops with varicella zoster, scabies, insect bites
• Lesions are in groups of 3 or 4 with a central punctum in scabies
• Papular lesions occur with insect bites, chiggers, pediculosis, contact dermatitis, pityriasis rosea, urticaria (wheal), and atopic dermatitis
• Lichenification (plaque and scale formation) occur with psoriasis, xerosis, tinea, atopic dermatitis
• Serpiginous lesions occur with cutaneous larva migrans and myiasis (or maggots)
• Vesicular lesions occur with varicella (generalized), scabies, poison ivy (linear), and atopic dermatitis
• Dry skin (xerosis) occurs with atopic dermatitis
• Christmas tree pattern occurs with pityriasis rosea

Finding: What is the location of the itch and/or rash?
Significance:

• Generalized distribution occurs with varicella
• Anus: consider pinworms
• Back: consider pityriasis rosea
• Axillae and/or genital/diaper area: consider seborrheic dermatitis and scabies
• Dorsal foot: consider shoe dermatitis from rubber or tanning agents

• Exposed surfaces: consider swimmer's itch and poison ivy
• Finger, ear lobe, wrist, or necklace distribution: consider irritant contact dermatitis (e.g., nickel)
• Nipples: scabies (burrows)
• Interdigital areas and ulnar borders: consider tinea pedis, scabies (burrows)
• Palms and/or soles: consider biliary cirrhosis
• Plantar foot: consider cutaneous larva migrans
• Scalp: consider pediculosis (nits found cemented to hair shaft) and tinea capitis

Finding: Abnormal affect or mood?
Significance: If after an exhaustive search there appears to be no physiological basis for the itch, one must consider whether the complaint is psychosomatic or as a result of neurotic excoriation.

Finding: Enlargement of liver, spleen or lymph nodes
Significance: Pruritus may be the initial manifestation of lymphoma.

Laboratory Aids

Test: Complete blood count including differential.
Significance: Presence of eosinophilia suggests atopy or parasitic infections.

Test: Wood lamp examination, KOH preparation.
Significance: Screen for tinea infections.

Test: Skin scraping in oil under cover slip.
Significance: Verify presence of mites in scabies.

Test: Perianal adhesive tape slide (preferably early morning).
Significance: Verify pinworm.

Test: Serum for hepatic and renal function.
Significance: Screen for underlying disease.

Test: Urine β-HCG
Significance: Investigate presence of cholestasis associated with pregnancy.

Test: Skin biopsy
Significance: Usually not of value since histologic changes are as a result of scratching

Clinical Pearls

• Pruritus that is worse at night is seen with scabies or pinworm.
• If the child was recently swimming in fresh water, one should consider swimmer's itch, caused by fresh water mammalian or avian schistosomes.

Common Questions and Answers

Q: Are some antihistamines better than others for pruritus?
A: Possibly, there is conflicting evidence, but several studies have shown that older systemic antihistamines that cause more somnolence are actually more effective at alleviating pruritus than newer, longer-acting antihistamines (e.g., astemizole, loratadine, terfenadine, cetirizine).

Q: Do topical antihistamines alleviate pruritus?
A: Not usually, except for pruritus seen with insect bites and urticaria. Use of topical antihistamines for pruritus or rash that is widespread should be discouraged, because toxicity may occur as a result of systemic absorption.

Q: Does scratching make the pruritus better or worse?
A: Worse, scratching leads to the release of the mediators of inflammation including histamine that in turn, leads to more pruritus thus creating a vicious cycle.

Q: Are there any useful adjuncts to reduce pruritus?
A: Yes, keeping skin moist with moisturizers and avoiding dry environments. Avoid overwashing especially with hot water and/or alkaline soaps.

BIBLIOGRAPHY

Charlesworth EN, Beltrani VS. Pruritic dermatoses: overview of etiology and therapy. *Am J Med* 2002;113(Suppl 9A):25S–33S.

Millikan LE. Pruritus: unapproved treatments or indications. *Clin Dermatol* 2000; 18:149–152.

Wahlgren CF. Itch and atopic dermatitis: an overview. *J Dermatol* 1999;26:770–779.

Author: Mark L. Bagarazzi

Causes of Pruritus in Children

MOST COMMON	LESS COMMON	RARE
Atopic dermatitis (eczema)	Anaphylaxis	Collagen—vascular disorders
Contact dermatitis	Cholestasis: Drug-induced	Congenital ectodermal disorders
Allergens: plants ("poison ivy"), cosmetics, dyes, medications	(e.g., total parenteral nutrition, estrogens, phenothiazine, allopurinol),	Systemic infections: HIV/AIDS, Parvovirus B19, Giardiasis, Ascariasis
Irritants: soaps, detergents and other chemicals, excrement, wool, fiberglass	Extrahepatic biliary obstruction, biliary cirrhosis	Endocrinological disorders: Carcinoid syndrome, Diabetes mellitus,
Cutaneous infections: Varicella-zoster virus (chicken pox), Tinea infections, pinworm	Cutaneous infections: Cutaneous larva migrans— "creeping eruption", Hookworm, Cercariasis Trichinosis	Hyper/hypothyroidism, Hypoparathyroidism Neurologic syndromes: cerebral abscess or tumor,
Papular urticaria—bites of fleas, mosquitoes, etc.	Myiasis (maggots)	multiple sclerosis
Pediculosis (lice)	Neurotic excoriation	Erythropoeitic protoporphyria
Mites—scabies (*Sarcoptes scabei*), chiggers (*Enterobicula alfreddugesi*), etc.	Chronic renal failure—with or without "uremic frost"	Psychosomatic disorders Hematopoietic neoplasms
Seborrheic dermatitis	Hematopoietic neoplasms: Hodgkin disease,	Polycythemia vera Mastocytosis
Xerosis (dry skin)— Excess bathing Low humidity	Lymphoma, leukemia Iron-deficiency anemia	

Short Stature

Database

DEFINITION

Short stature is defined as height below the 3rd percentile, but many pediatricians use the 5th percentile as the cutoff.

• Growth failure refers to downward crossing of the height percentile over the normal curves and eventually leads to short stature. With evidence of growth failure, diagnostic evaluation is required, even if short stature is not yet present.

• Failure to thrive refers to infants and children who fail to gain weight and often lose weight. They may or may not be short and are underweight for height.

Differential Diagnosis

EXTREMES OF NORMAL GROWTH

• Familial short stature

—Short parent(s)
—Normal height velocity
—Normal age of onset of puberty
—Normal bone age
—Short stature throughout childhood
—Final adult height close to the midparental height and around the 3rd or 5th percentile

• Constitutional short stature/delay of growth

—Height percentile below the target range defined by parental heights
—Delayed bone age
—Reduced height velocity (especially in late childhood—below 25th percentile)
—Associated with delay of puberty
—Positive family history, usually boys
—Final adult height in the normal range and commensurate with target height

• Idiopathic short stature

—Used to categorize patients otherwise normal, who cannot be diagnosed with a variant of normal growth or any of the causes of short stature. May not always turn out to be a true normal variant.
—This is a diagnosis of exclusion and groups patients whose calculated predicted height is more than 2 SD below the midparental height, whose height is below the 5th percentile, with or without delay of skeletal maturation, and without identifiable diagnosis after appropriate evaluation.

PRIMARY SHORT STATURE

• Usually the consequence of an abnormality of the skeletal system. Bone age often not delayed or only delayed mildly.

• Skeletal defect can be primary or secondary to a metabolic abnormality. These may lead to disproportionate short stature and/or significant dysmorphism. Occasionally, the skeletal abnormalities are subtle and do not lead to disproportionate short stature.

• Skeletal dysplasia

—Osteochondrodysplasia
—Genetic transmission—many cases represent new mutation
—Defects in growth of tubular bones and/or axial skeleton
—Typical radiologic findings on skeletal survey x-ray
—More common forms include: achondroplasia, hypochondroplasia

• Short stature as a result of congenital error of metabolism

—Diffuse skeletal involvement
—Mostly autosomal recessive inheritance
—Dysmorphic features
—Typical biochemical abnormalities
—More common type: mucopolysaccharidosis

• Chromosomal abnormalities

—Autosomes or sex chromosomes
—Usually associated with other somatic abnormalities or mental retardation
—Clinical findings may be subtle (mosaicism)
—More common forms: Trisomy 21, −18, −13, and Turner syndrome

• Intrauterine growth retardation (IUGR)

—Often with poor postnatal growth
—Cause for IUGR may come from mother, fetus, or placenta
—Primordial dwarfism: as a result of intrinsic fetal defect leading to both prenatal and postnatal growth failure (may be associated with specific genetic anomaly)
—IUGR is seen in congenital infection, fetal exposure to toxin, placental abnormalities, maternal disease, Russell-Silver syndrome and other congenital anomalies.

SECONDARY SHORT STATURE

• Malnutrition

—Especially under 2 years of age (most common in first 6 months of life)
—Caloric—malnutrition and/or protein—malnutrition
—Vitamin and mineral deficiencies (vitamin D, iron, zinc deficiency)

• Chronic illness

—Many chronic diseases present first with poor growth
—Cardiovascular: VSD, PDA, TOF, TGV, AS, PS, aortic coarctation, AV canal
—Pulmonary: asthma, CF, BPD
—GI/liver: inflammatory bowel disease (IBD), celiac disease, malabsorption, short bowel syndrome, chronic gastroenteritis, CF
—Renal: NS, CGN, RTA, CRF, nephrogenic DI, uropathy, congenital anomalies

—Metabolic: poorly controlled diabetes mellitus, storage disorders
—Chronic infections (HIV) and immune deficiencies
—Hematopoietic: anemia, leukemia, SCD

• Drugs

—Corticosteroids
—Sex steroids
—Methylphenidate, dextroamphetamine

• Psychosocial growth retardation
• Endocrine short stature

—Among secondary short stature, endocrine causes are least frequent

Approach to the Patient

GENERAL GOAL

Determine if the patient has short stature and/or growth failure. Determine if height alone is affected, or if growth problem includes weight and head circumference.

Phase 1: Determine if patient's profile fits normal variant of growth.

Phase 2: Determine if patient's profile fits with pathologic short stature.

Phase 3: Screening evaluation, referral to pediatric endocrinologist or observation.

Data Gathering

HISTORY

Question: Is the child short for his/her parents?
Significance: Midparental height is calculated to estimate the expected target height. To calculate midparental height for a boy, add his father's height to his mother's height plus 13 cm, and divide by 2. To calculate midparental height for a girl, add her mother's height to her father's height minus 13 cm, and divide by 2. If the child's height percentile is out of keeping with the calculated target height, this is likely significant.

Question: What is the child's growth (or height) velocity?
Significance: Height velocity for a specific interval can be annualized and plotted on a height velocity curve. This becomes an important criterion in a patient's growth and is different from height at any point in time, which, for a major part, is a representation of the influence of things past.

Question: What is the weight-to-height ratio?
Significance: Usually increased in hypothyroidism, Cushing syndrome, pseudohypoparathyroidism, and growth hormone deficiency. Normal or decreased in emotional deprivation, anorexia, chronic renal failure, renal tubular acidosis, IBD, malabsorption, malnutrition, lung and heart disease.

Question: Were there any complications during pregnancy, labor, and delivery?
Significance: Clues from the pregnancy can provide information about possible maternal disorders, intrauterine drug exposure, or placental abnormalities that lead to IUGR. Birth trauma can be associated with hypopituitarism.

Question: Familial history. What are the heights of the parents and grandparents? What are the heights of the siblings? Was puberty on time in both parents? Any history of endocrine disorder or chronic illness affecting a major organ system?
Significance: Calculate midparental height. If short stature is running in the family, this could point toward familial or genetic short stature, isolated growth hormone deficiency, or skeletal dysplasia. Delayed pubertal maturation in the parents is important for a diagnosis of constitutional growth delay. Disorders such as diabetes mellitus and insipidus, thyroiditis, hypophosphatemic rickets, arthritis, and IBD can affect different family members.

Question: What is the social situation?
Significance: Emotional stresses affect growth and development, either directly (abnormal growth hormone production), or indirectly (inadequate nutrition).

Question: What are current eating habits and how is the past dietary history? Any evidence of underutilization of calories ingested?
Significance: Estimate approximate total daily caloric intake. Detect deficiencies in certain nutrients, or the existence of abnormal eating habits (malabsorption, rickets, anorexia, inadequate parenting).

Question: Any chronic illness? Any hospitalization, surgery, or trauma to the head?
Significance: Chronic disorders can present with growth failure first, without specific symptoms (rheumatoid arthritis, celiac disease), and a previous hospitalization or surgery could be a clue for an underlying pathology (jaundice and hepatitis—chronic liver disease, asthma exacerbation and high-dose corticosteroids, head trauma and pituitary insufficiency).

The history should be completed by obtaining a detailed review of systems, with specific questions inquiring about the occurrence of headache, vomiting, visual disturbance (brain tumor), anorexia, diarrhea, or constipation (bowel disease, hypothyroidism), polyuria and polydypsia (diabetes mellitus, diabetes insipidus, and renal problems), and medication as well as activity pattern, sleep hygiene, and general development.

 Physical Examination

Finding: Abnormal upper/lower segment ratio
Significance: Primary short stature

Finding: Low weight/height ratio
Significance: Points toward malnutrition

Finding: Edema
Significance: Chronic renal failure

Finding: Frontal bossing, flat nasal bridge, and truncal fat deposition
Significance: Growth hormone deficiency

Finding: Abdominal distension and gluteal wasting
Significance: Malabsorption and celiac disease

Finding: Webbed neck, increased carrying angle, shield chest
Significance: Turner syndrome

Finding: Smooth tongue
Significance: Iron deficiency

Finding: Round face, ear lobe abnormality, and mental retardation
Significance: Pseudohypoparathyroidism

Finding: Temporal thinning of the hair, sparse hair, dry hair
Significance: Hypothyroidism, growth hormone deficiency, hypopituitarism

Finding: Delayed pubertal maturation
Significance: Turner syndrome, constitutional delay, hypopituitarism, hypothyroidism, IBD, chronic renal disease

Finding: Leg bowing, rachitic rosary, widening of wrists
Significance: Rickets, malabsorption

 Laboratory Aids

If no specific cause found, screening tests are indicated.

Test: Complete blood count and differential
Significance: Anemia, infection, leukemia

Test: Sedimentation rate
Significance: Infection, inflammation

Test: Electrolyte panel, glucose
Significance: Renal disorders, diabetes mellitus, and insipidus

Test: Metabolic panel
Significance: Malnutrition, liver problem, bone disorder, pseudohypoparathyroidism

Test: Urinalysis
Significance: Urinary tract infection, diabetes, renal disorder, metabolic problem

Test: Thyroxine and thyroid-stimulating hormone
Significance: Hypothyroidism, hypopituitarism

Test: X-ray study of the left hand and wrist
Significance: Bone age determination

Test: Karyotype
Significance: Turner syndrome in short girls, chromosomal disorders

Test: IGF-I and IGFBP-3 concentrations
Significance: Shows little fluctuation over 24 hours, but interpretation of values needs to take age-related norms into account. IGF-I and IGFBP-3 are low in GH-deficiency, but can also be low as a result of hypothyroidism, chronic illness, or poor nutrition. Normal IGF-I and IGFBP-3 concentrations make growth hormone deficiency less likely.

Issues for Referral

- Flat growth curve, delayed bone age, abnormal thyroid test, poorly controlled diabetes, physical findings consistent with growth hormone deficiency, hypothyroidism, rickets
- Protein-losing enteropathy, malabsorption, hepatic disorder
- Chronic lung disease, abnormal sweat chloride test
- Congenital heart disease, occult cardiac disease
- Elevated creatinine, low serum bicarbonate, abnormal urinalysis

Growth failure is usually a relatively slow or subacute process and, therefore, does not require emergency workup. It is of basic importance, however, to pay special attention to correct measurements of height, weight, and head circumference, and to evaluate the abnormally growing child adequately.

BIBLIOGRAPHY

Bryant J, Cave C, Milne R. Recombinant growth hormone for idiopathic short stature in children and adolescents. *Cochrane Database Syst Rev* 2003;(4):CD004440.

Lee PA, Kendig JW, Kerrigan JR. Persistent short stature, other potential outcomes, and the effect of growth hormone treatment in children who are born small for gestational age. *Pediatrics* 2003;112(1 Pt 1):150–162.

Wheeler PG, Bresnahan K, Shephard BA, Lau J, Balk EM. Short stature and functional impairment: a systematic review. *ARCH Pediatr Adolesc Med* 2004;158(3):236–243.

Authors: Mitchell R.M. Schwartz
Philippe F. Backeljauw, 3rd edition

Sore Throat

Database

DEFINITION

Sore throat or pain with swallowing is a common presenting complaint in the pediatric population. The majority of cases have an infectious etiology, with viral causes being the most common.

Differential Diagnosis

INFECTIOUS

• Pharyngitis/Tonsillitis

—Respiratory and other viruses: adenovirus/influenza/ parainfluenza; Epstein-Barr virus (EBV); Cytomegalovirus; Human immunodeficiency virus
—Bacterial: Group A β-hemolytic streptococcus (*Streptococcus pyogenes*); groups C and G streptococci; diphtheria; *Neisseria gonorrhoeae;* anaerobic bacteria; tularemia; Chlamydia; Mycoplasma; *Arcanobacterium haemolyticum*
—Stomatitis: Herpes simplex virus, coxsackievirus
—Peritonsillar cellulitis/abscess
—Retropharyngeal abscess
—Epiglottitis/supraglottitis

ENVIRONMENTAL

• Irritative pharyngitis: exposure to smoke or dry air

TRAUMA

• Foreign body: either retained or causing laceration to posterior pharynx
• Burns: hot liquids/foods
• Voice overuse

TUMOR

• Rare in pediatric population

ALLERGIC/INFLAMMATORY

• Allergens causing chronic postnasal drip that leads to irritant pharyngitis

MISCELLANEOUS

• Kawasaki disease
• Psychogenic pain
• Referred pain

Approach to the Patient

GENERAL GOAL

The majority of cases of sore throat have an infectious cause, with most (~70% to 80%) of these having a viral etiology. Once the life-threatening and/or noninfectious causes have been excluded, the goal is to determine if the pharyngitis is caused by group A β-hemolytic streptococci (GABS), which should be treated with antibiotics, or one of the many other infectious etiologies.

Phase 1: Use history and physical exam to separate infectious from noninfectious causes. If etiology seems infectious, consider throat culture for group A streptococci infection.

Data Gathering

HISTORY

Question: Sore throat in association with fever, headache, and/or abdominal pain?
Significance: Common association of symptoms present in group A streptococci pharyngitis.

Question: Sore throat in association with fever, upper respiratory infection symptoms (cough, rhinorrhea, conjunctivitis)?
Significance: More suggestive of viral pharyngitis.

Question: Presence of drooling, voice changes?
Significance: Possibility of more severe infectious etiology, including retropharyngeal or peritonsillar abscess, epiglottitis.

Question: Foreign body exposure?
Significance: Retained foreign body (e.g., fishbone) or laceration/irritation from foreign body.

Question: Irritant exposure (e.g., dry air from heating or cooling system)?
Significance: Pharyngeal mucosal drying.

Question: Immunization status and travel history?
Significance: Possibility of diphtheria in the nonimmunized or incompletely immunized patient, especially if recent travel to countries of the former Soviet Union.

Question: Sexual activity (including oral sex and possibility of abuse)?
Significance: Gonococcal pharyngitis.

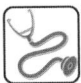

Physical Examination

Finding: Pharyngeal erythema with or without exudate
Significance: Suggestive of infectious etiology, though does not reliably differentiate viral from bacterial causes

Finding: Tender cervical adenopathy
Significance: Suggestive of infectious etiology; anterior cervical nodes described in classic GABS infection; posterior cervical nodes $\pm$ hepatosplenomegaly suggest possibility of EBV.

Finding: Stridor/drooling
Significance: Raises concern for etiologies that may cause airway obstruction

Finding: Asymmetric enlargement of tonsillar pillar with deviation of uvula away from enlarged side
Significance: Peritonsillar abscess

Finding: Mild erythema with cobblestoning of posterior pharyngeal mucosa
Significance: Suggests allergic or irritant etiology

Finding: Vesicular or ulcerative lesions in oropharynx
Significance: Suggestive of viral etiologies including herpes simplex (lesions commonly in anterior oropharynx) or coxsackievirus (lesions commonly in posterior oropharynx)

Laboratory Aids

Test: Throat swab for strep antigen test with subsequent culture if antigen test is negative.
Significance: Useful for definitive diagnosis of group A streptococci infection. A negative antigen test should be followed by throat culture to improve sensitivity.

Test: Lateral neck x-ray
Significance: Enlarged epiglottis suggests epiglottitis; widened prevertebral soft tissue space suggestive of retropharyngeal abscess.

Test: Complete blood count and Monospot if indicated
Significance: Atypical lymphocytosis/presence of heterophil antibodies suggestive of EBV infection. EBV titers (if indicated) should be sent in those less than 4 years of age because of low sensitivity ($\sim$50%) of Monospot in this age group.

Emergency Care

Factors that make sore throat an emergency include:

- Airway compromise

  —Epiglottitis
  —Retropharyngeal abscess
  —Peritonsillar abscess
  —Significant tonsillar hypertrophy
  —Diphtheria

The patient may present with toxic appearance, fever, drooling, voice change, and sitting in the sniffing position (to optimize airway). Make nothing by mouth (NPO), supplemental oxygen; consider airway adjuncts (e.g., NP airway), intravenous access to facilitate airway management (if patient able to tolerate). Consider anesthesia consult for endotracheal intubation in most controlled setting.

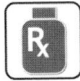

Therapy

- Penicillin is the drug of choice for treatment of GABS pharyngitis. Oral and intramuscular regimens are available. Macrolide antibiotics (e.g., erythromycin), clindamycin, or some first-generation cephalosporins (provided no allergy) may be used for those with penicillin allergy.
- The treatment of viral pharyngitis is largely supportive care, including fluids and pain control.

Common Questions and Answers

Q: What is the incidence of group A streptococci disease as the cause of pharyngitis?
A: Group A streptococci is the most common bacterial etiology of infectious pharyngitis. The incidence of this disease is approximately 15% to 30% of all cases of infectious pharyngitis.

Q: When must antibiotic therapy begin in group A streptococci pharyngitis in order to prevent rheumatic fever?
A: Antibiotics should be started within 9 days from the onset of symptoms in order to prevent this nonsuppurative complication of group A streptococci pharyngitis.

Issues for Referral

- Signs/symptoms of airway compromise—general toxicity, stridor, drooling. Patient may need emergent airway protection/stabilization.
- Fluctuant peritonsillar abscess—drainage may be done by otolaryngologist.
- Presence of foreign body—may need removal by otolaryngologist or x-ray to look for air in retropharyngeal soft tissue

Clinical Pearls

The clinical appearance of GABS pharyngitis may be indistinguishable from pharyngitis of viral etiologies. The therapy for these illnesses is different: antibiotics for group A streptococci versus symptomatic care for viral pharyngitis. The practitioner should perform diagnostic testing with rapid strep antigen and/or culture when GABS pharyngitis is considered. In general, it is not recommended to treat pending the culture results; rather, wait until the GABS pharyngitis is confirmed with a positive antigen or culture before starting antibiotics.

BIBLIOGRAPHY

Attia MW, Bennett JE. Pediatric pharyngitis. *Pediatric Case Reviews* 2003;3(4):203–210.

Bisno AL. Acute pharyngitis. *N Engl J Med* 2001;344(3):205–211.

Bisno AL. Acute pharyngitis: etiology and diagnosis. *Pediatrics* 1996;97(6 Pt 2): 949–954.

Fleisher GR. Sore throat. In: Fleisher GR, Ludwig S, eds. *Textbook of Pediatric Emergency Medicine.* Philadelphia: Lippincott Williams & Wilkins, 2000:581–585.

Gerber MA, Tanz RR. New approaches to the treatment of group A streptococcal pharyngitis. *Curr Opin Pediatr* 2001;13(1):51–55.

Schwartz B, et al. Pharyngitis-principles of judicious use of antimicrobial agents. *Pediatrics* 1998;101(1 Pt 2):171–174.

Shulman ST. Acute streptococcal pharyngitis in pediatric medicine: Current issues in diagnosis and management. *Pediatr Drugs* 2003;5(Suppl 1):13–23.

Author: Cynthia R. Jacobstein

Speech Delay

 Database

DEFINITION

• Speech delay is delay in the development of speech, the verbal expression of language.
• Language, the symbolic system used to communicate, is made up of receptive and expressive language.

—Receptive language is the ability of the person to process the language they are hearing or seeing.
—Expressive language is the ability to produce language to express oneself through speech, sign, or another means of communication.

Types of expressive language delays (these differ from speech disorders in that the speech sounds are intact and well formed):

• Verbal dyspraxia: little verbal output with very poor phonology
• Speech programming deficit disorder: sounds as if something is said, but there are little to no actual words

Mixed receptive and expressive delays:

• Verbal auditory agnosia: difficulty in understanding language as a result of the inability to hear parts of words, which leads to severe expressive delays.
• Phonologic/syntactic deficit disorder: language understood is better than the language spoken. Speech has poor organization of individual words and phrases.

EPIDEMIOLOGY

• Approximately 20% of 2-year-olds have delayed speech.
• At 5 years old, 19% have speech and language disorders (6.4% speech, 8% language, 4.6% both)
• 85% of children with language delays are boys.
• Articulation problems occur in 5% of school-age children and 10% of preschool-age children

GENETICS

• Higher prevalence of speech and language delays in first-degree relatives of affected persons with up to 30% of affected children having a first-degree relative with a speech or language delay.
• Twin concordance rates are 70% to 90% in monozygotic twins and 30% to 60% in dizygotic twins.

 Differential Diagnosis

INFECTION

• HIV encephalopathy

ENVIRONMENTAL

• Lack of stimulation
• Lead poisoning

CONGENITAL

• Hearing impairment
• Fragile X syndrome
• Down syndrome
• Muscular dystrophy
• Fetal alcohol syndrome/effects

NUTRITIONAL

• Malnutrition
• Iron deficiency

TUMORS

• Tuberous sclerosis
• Neurofibromatosis

DEVELOPMENTAL

• Constitutional language delay
• Mental retardation
• Autistic spectrum disorders
• Dysarthria
• Stuttering
• Apraxia
• Acquired hearing loss

 Data Gathering

HISTORY

• Focus on the concerns of the parents
• Birth history including prenatal care and exposures

Question: Ask about details of the developmental history.
Significance: Will allow one to determine if this is an isolated speech delay or global delay.

Question: Ask about trouble with chewing or excessive drooling for age.
Significance: Signs of oromotor dysfunction can be important in thinking about cause of delays and treatment.

Question: Ask about hearing and frequency of ear infections.
Significance: Children with undetected hearing loss are at higher risk for speech and language delays.

Question: Ask about the social abilities of the child.
Significance: Will help differentiate speech delays from autistic spectrum disorders.

Question: Ask about family history of speech/language delays, mental retardation and hearing loss.
Significance: Family history will encourage further exploration for less common causes of speech delay.

 Physical Examination

• Complete evaluation to assess the child's nutritional and physical health.
• Particular attention to assess for any dysmorphic features, or hearing or neurologic abnormalities.

Finding: Excessive drooling
Significance: Poor oromotor control suggestive of hypotonicity of the muscles that are required for adequate speech development.

Finding: Dysmorphic features.
Significance: Syndromes such as Down syndrome, Williams syndrome, fetal alcohol syndrome, fragile X syndrome, Angelman syndrome.

Finding: Abnormal tympanic membranes.
Significance: Chronic ear infections or congenital abnormalities of the TM can lead to hearing impairment, which can cause speech delays.

Finding: Skin lesions.
Significance: Café-au-lait patches and fibroma suggestive of neurofibromatosis, Shagreen patches suggestive of tuberous sclerosis.

Laboratory Aids

- Hearing evaluations—should be done in all children with speech delays; best if done by audiology. However, oto-acoustic emissions are being used by some providers to rule out hearing loss. Pure-tone audiometry has a significant false-negative rate, and should not be used to rule out hearing loss in children with speech delay.
- Developmental testing—if clinical suspicion of delays in other developmental domains.
- Screening tools for language delays

—Denver Developmental Screening Tool Revision II—commonly used but not as sensitive for language delays as other tools.
—Early Language Milestone Scale (2nd edition) (ELMS) sensitive for language screening.
—Clinical Linguistic and Auditory Milestone Scale (CLAMS) sensitive for language screening.

General guidelines for language milestones to help determine if a delay exists

—Four to 6 months	Babbling
—Eight to 9 months	Mama/Dada
—One year	Single word other than Mama/Dada; points to indicate wants
—Eighteen months	5 to 10 words
—Two years	2-word sentences, >50 words
—Three years	Stories, prepositions, naming objects
—Four years	Speech 100% understandable

- Formal speech and language evaluation—to determine the type of disorder and to recommend the best intervention for the child
- Genetic counseling and additional laboratory testing—should be considered based on history and physical findings.

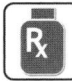 ## Therapy

- Children with hearing loss should be referred to an otolaryngologist (Ear, Nose, and Throat [ENT] specialist)
- Speech and language therapy—should be considered for all children with speech delays.
- Sign language—can be a mechanism to decrease a child's frustration as he or she is improving his or her verbal communication. This will not delay the onset of verbal language, but should help decrease frustration for the child.
- Augmentative communication devices (picture boards) may be helpful for children unable to sign.

 ## Follow-Up

- Children with isolated developmental language disorders will often improve and become normal with time. However, 20% to 60% of these children will have difficulties in the ability to learn to read and write later.
- Children with constitutional language delay will normalize and should have no academic delays.

PITFALLS

- Inadequate evaluation of hearing.
- Missing delays in other areas of development.
- Delays in referral to speech and language evaluations.
- Inadequate history and physical—missed seizure disorder, missed organic disease causing speech delays, missed genetic syndrome

 ## Common Questions and Answers

Q: Why should I send the child for hearing testing when he or she appears to hear normally in the office?
A: Children are very adept at using visual cues to figure out what is being asked of them. In addition, people often use gestures to indicate instructions to children, or use visual demonstrations. The level of receptive language delay and hearing loss is very difficult to predict without formal assessments.

Q: At what age should I refer a child for formal speech and language evaluation?
A: Children certainly develop at different rates, and some normal children will not have completed certain speech tasks by the expected age. However, any child who continues to lag at a follow-up visit should be evaluated more formally. In addition, a child who is having any behavioral problems, such as tantrums or aggressive behavior, should be evaluated by a developmental specialist. Finally, children with language concerns and delayed social skills should also be evaluated for autism.

BIBLIOGRAPHY

Coplan J. Normal speech and language development: an overview. *Pediatr Rev* 1995;16:91–100.

Guitar B and Belin-Frost G. Stuttering. In: Parker S and Zuckerman B (eds). *Behavioral and Developmental Pediatrics: A Handbook for Primary Care*. Boston, MA: Little, Brown and Company, 1995:294–296.

Kelly DP and Sally JI. Disorders of speech and language. In: Levine MD, Carey WB, Crocker AC eds. *Developmental-behavioral pediatrics*. 3rd Ed. Philadelphia: WB Saunders Company, 1999:621–631.

Law J, Garrett Z, Nye C. Speech and language therapy interventions for children with primary speech and language delay or disorder. *Cochrane Database Syst Rev* 2000;3:CD004110; 2000;21:147–158.

McCauley R. Articulation disorders. In: Parker S, Zuckerman B, eds. *Behavioral and Developmental Pediatrics: A Handbook for Primary Care*. Boston: Little, Brown and Company, 1995:70–72.

Plomin R. Genetic factors contributing to learning and language delays and disabilities. *Child Adolesc Psychiatr Clinic NA* 2001;10(2):259–77.

Simms MD, Schum RL. Preschool children who have atypical patterns of development. *Pediatr. Rev.* 2000;21:147–158.

Author: Nathaniel S. Beers

Speech Problems

 Database

DEFINITION

- Speech problems may occur in children with difficulties in speech, language or both.
- Speech problems can be broken down into the following categories:

Articulation Problems

- Articulation disorder: substituting sounds ("w" for "r"), leaving sounds out, or adding sounds to words.
- Apraxia: impairment of voluntary control of the muscles necessary to generate speech sounds.
- Dysarthria: inability to produce the sounds of speech but not as a result of inability to control the muscles.
- Phonologic disorder: phonologic errors inappropriate for age as a result of inaccurate production of a specific sound.

Voice Problems

- Hoarseness.
- Resonance: problems in resonance result in hypo- or hypernasal quality to sound production.
- Fluency problems like stuttering

EPIDEMIOLOGY

- At 5 years old, 19% have speech and language disorders. (6.4% speech, 8% language, and 4.6% both speech and language.)
- Articulation problems occur in 5% of school-aged children and 10% of preschool-aged children.

 Differential Diagnosis

INFECTIOUS

- Chronic/recurrent otitis media

ENVIRONMENTAL

- Lack of stimulation
- Lead poisoning

CONGENITAL

- Hearing impairment
- Fragile X syndrome
- Down syndrome
- Fetal alcohol syndrome/effects
- Cleft lip/palate

NUTRITIONAL

- Malnutrition
- Iron deficiency

TUMORS

- Tuberous sclerosis
- Neurofibromatosis

DEVELOPMENTAL

- Mental retardation
- Autistic spectrum disorders
- Dysarthria
- Apraxia

NEUROMUSCULAR

- Muscular dystrophy
- Acquired hearing loss
- Intracranial hearing loss
- Cerebral palsy
- Hydrocephalus

Approach to Patient

- Determine if there is an underlying cause for the delays (hearing impairment, oromotor tone).
- Determine if there are delays in other areas of development.
- Determine if the speech problems are new, or if there is a regression in skills.
- Refer to the appropriate provider for additional evaluations as needed.

 Data Gathering

The parent spends the most time with the child and is more likely to hear errors in speech than anyone else. Some parents may not be as aware of what is appropriate at various ages and may be overly or under concerned. Misarticulations or stuttering can be appropriate at some ages, but should resolve by a certain age.

Question: How much of the child's speech is intelligible?
Significance: The rule of four applies here. The amount of speech that should be understandable by a visiting family member is the child's age in years divided by 4. So a 2-year-old should have speech that is at least one-half understandable.

Question: Does you child have a problem with eating or drooling?
Significance: Problems beyond what is normal for age could suggest problems with apraxia or dysarthria.

Question: Does your child have trouble hearing?
Significance: Chronic hearing loss can lead to trouble in sound production. If the child is having distortions in sounds, she/he may have trouble in production.

Question: Does your child stutter? If so, is your child bothered by the stutter?
Significance: One of the major indicators for referral for stuttering is when a child is starting to have emotional reaction to either the stuttering or the teasing by others because of the stuttering.

Question: Did your child ever have skills that he or she lost?
Significance: Regressions can be seen in undetected chronic diseases (such as HIV, acquired hearing loss) but also in Landau Kleffner syndrome.

Past medical history, including birth history, is important.

Physical Examination

The goal of the physical exam in a child with speech problems is to rule out anatomic abnormalities or syndromes that may explain why a child is having difficulties with speech.

Finding: Hyper- or hyponasal speech.
Significance: hyponasal speech could suggest an obstruction of the upper airway, such as adenoid hypertrophy, although hypernasal suggests velopharyngeal insufficiency, such as cleft palate.

Finding: Dysmorphic features.
Significance: Signs of syndromes such as fetal alcohol syndrome, Williams syndrome, Down syndrome, Angelman syndrome.

Finding: Abnormal tympanic membrane (TM)
Significance: Signs of chronic ear infections or congenital abnormalities of TMs may lead to hearing impairments.

Finding: Pooling of food in mouth or excessive drooling.
Significance: Signs of poor oromotor control which can be helpful in assessing a child for apraxia and dysarthria.

Finding: Poor social skills
Significance: Speech problems and social communication problems are suggestive of autistic spectrum disorders.

Finding: Skin abnormalities
Significance: Findings consistent with neurofibromatosis or tuberous sclerosis. Also look for scars from tracheostomy.

- Watching a child eat or drink can be valuable in starting to think about why a child is having speech problems.
- A thorough neurologic exam and developmental screening will help determine the need for additional testing.

Laboratory Aids

Test: Hearing evaluation.
Significance: Hearing impairment can alter speech development.

- Pure tone audiometry: high false-negative rate, only useful in older children and those capable of cooperating.
- Otoacoustic emissions: useful for children of all ages as a screening tool for hearing impairment.
- Bilateral audio-evoked response testing: gold standard for hearing evaluations.

Test: Speech and language evaluation.
Significance: Comprehensive assessment of receptive and expressive language and extent of articulation difficulties.

Test: Modified barium swallow.
Significance: This is a good tool to assess children with excessive drooling or pocketing of food in their mouth. It will help in assessing for oromotor dysfunction.

Test: Genetic testing
Significance: Useful in children with physical or historical features suggestive of genetic syndromes.

Test: Electroencephalogram (EEG)
Significance: May help rule-out seizure disorder or Landau Kleffner syndrome. Used when the history or physical indicate need.

Therapy

Speech and language therapy should have the following goals:

- Progression in the normal developmental order
- Fixing errors in child's speech
- Encourage understanding of patterns and meanings of language
- Encourage flexibility in language
- Fine tuning of skills

SPEECH AND LANGUAGE PATHOLOGISTS

- All children with significant speech problems should be referred to speech and language pathologists.
- Stuttering should be referred when it is distressing to the child, or if the child is experiencing excessive repetitions (greater than 5 per 100 words), physical struggle with words (grimacing), trouble getting the word started, or behaviors to avoid speaking or saying particular words

1. Otolaryngologists: All children with hearing loss; and children with speech problems and history of chronic ear infections.
2. Developmental pediatrician: Children with speech problems and delays in other developmental areas including social skills. Also children with behavioral problems related to their delays (selective mutism, tantrums, aggressive behaviors).
3. Neurologist: Children with signs or symptoms of a seizure disorder, children with hypotonia or hypertonia, or children with regressions.
4. Geneticist: Children with dysmorphic features of unclear etiology; or for genetic counseling for parents if etiology clear.
5. Occupational therapist: Children with poor oromotor tone can benefit from therapy. This is sometimes done by speech pathologists.

Follow-Up

Children with speech problems should be followed on the regular well-child periodicity schedule.

Common Questions and Answers

Q: How do I assess a bilingual child?
A: Bilingual children should be assessed by the same criteria as any other child. The only difference is both languages should be taken into consideration when determining the extent of the vocabulary or syntax used.

Q: Are children with speech problems more likely to be mentally retarded?
A: All Children with mental retardation have speech delays. Children with isolated speech delays are not mentally retarded.

Q: How can parents help a child with speech problems?
A: Using multiple means of communication can be very valuable. Parents can use pictures of their child's favorite things or activities to help the child communicate and reduce his/her frustration level. Additionally, saying the word when the child points at objects can reinforce the use of language for requests.

BIBLIOGRAPHY

Coplan J. Normal speech and language development: An overview. *Pediatr Rev* 1995;16(3):91–100.

Guitar B, Belin-Frost G. Stuttering. In: Parker S, Zuckerman B, eds. *Behavioral and developmental pediatrics: a handbook for primary care.* Boston, Little, Brown and Company, 1995:294–296.

Kelly DP, Sally JI. Disorders of speech and language. In: Levine MD, Carey WB, Crocker AC, eds. *Developmental-behavioral pediatrics,* 3rd ed. Philadelphia, WB Saunders Company, 1999;621–631.

McCauley R. Articulation disorders. In: Parker S, uckerman B, eds. *Behavioral and developmental pediatrics: a handbook for primary care.* Boston, Little, Brown and Company, 1995:70–72.

Simms MD, Schum RL. Preschool children who have atypical patterns of development. *Pediatr Rev* 2000;21(5):147–158.

Toppelberg CO, Shapiro T. Language disorders: a 10-year research upate review. *J Amer Acad Child Adolesc Psychiatry* 2000;39:143–152.

Author: Nathaniel S. Beers

Splenomegaly

 Database

DEFINITION

A palpable spleen is found in most premature infants and in 30% of term infants. A spleen tip is still palpable in 10% of infants at 1 year of age and in 1% of children 10 years of age. Normal spleens are no larger than 6 cm at 3 months, 7 cm at 12 months, 9.5 cm at 6 years, 11.5 cm at 12 years, and no greater than 13 cm for adolescents. The clinical significance of splenomegaly found on radiologic study, but not palpable on physical exam requires other laboratory or clinical data to establish its importance. Normal spleens are soft, at the midclavicular line, and often palpable only on deep inspiration. Dullness on percussion beyond the 11th intercostal space suggests splenomegaly. A spleen edge palpated more than 2 cm below the costal margin is always an abnormal finding. Splenic tenderness is abnormal.

Physiology

ROLE OF THE SPLEEN

The spleen is a hematopoietic organ with two main parts: (a) white pulp contains the lymphoid tissue and (b) the red pulp is the red cell mass. The splenic sinusoids are lined with macrophages that destroy mutant or abnormal red cells. The spleen also serves as a reservoir for platelets. A normal size spleen can hold one-third of the circulating platelets although an enlarged spleen can hold up to 90% of the circulating platelet mass.

 Differential Diagnosis

INFECTION

BACTERIAL

- Bacteremia
- Pneumonia
- Sepsis
- Subacute bacterial endocarditis
- Salmonella
- Tuberculosis
- Brucellosis
- Staphylococcal shunt infections
- Tularemia
- Syphilis
- Leptospirosis

VIRAL

- Epstein-Barr virus (mononucleosis)
- Cytomegalovirus
- HIV
- Rubella
- Herpes
- Hepatitis A, B

RICKETTSIAL/PROTOZOAN

- Rocky Mountain spotted fever
- Malaria
- Toxoplasmosis
- Trypanosomiasis
- Babesiosis
- Schistosomiasis
- Visceral larval migrans
- Kala-azar

FUNGAL

- Histoplasmosis
- Coccidioidomycosis

BLOOD DISEASE: HEMOLYTIC DISEASES

- Hereditary spherocytosis
- Sickle cell disease in early childhood or during splenic sequestration crisis
- Thalassemia major autoimmune hemolytic anemia
- Hemoglobin C disease
- Pyruvate kinase deficiency
- Glucose-6-phosphate dehydrogenase deficiency
- Isoimmunization disorders
- Infantile pyknocytosis
- Iron-deficiency anemia (rare)
- Thrombocytopenic purpura

VASCULAR CONGESTIVE DISORDERS

- Cavernous transformation of the portal vein
- Congential hepatic fibrosis
- Splenic vein thrombosis

CIRRHOSIS SECONDARY TO

- Hepatitis
- Biliary atresia
- Wilson disease
- Cystic fibrosis
- α_1-Antitrypsin deficiency
- Tyrosinemia
- Hereditary fructose intolerance
- Hemosiderosis
- Thrombosis of the hepatic vein
- Budd-Chiari syndrome
- Congestive heart failure
- Constrictive pericarditis
- Galactosemia
- Congenital portal vein stenosis or atresia
- Splenic artery aneurysm
- Splenic hematoma
- Splenic hemangioma

METABOLIC DISEASES

- Gangliosidoses
- Mucolipidoses
- Metachromatic leukodystrophy
- Wolman disease
- Gaucher disease
- Niemann-Pick disease
- Amyloidosis
- Hyperlipoproteinemia
- Familial hemophagocytic reticulosis
- Porphyria
- Lysinuric protein intolerance
- Dibasic aminoaciduria
- Cystinosis

NEOPLASTIC DISEASES

- Leukemia
- Lymphoma
- Lymphosarcoma
- Neuroblastoma
- Histiocytosis X

MISCELLANEOUS

- Serum sickness
- Connective-tissue disorders
- Juvenile rheumatoid arthritis
- Systemic lupus erythematosus
- Sarcoidosis
- Beckwith-Wiedemann syndrome
- Infant of a diabetic mother
- Splenic hamartoma
- Cysts: congenital and posttraumatic
- Hyperparathyroidism
- Gingival fibromatosis and digital anomalies

NONSPLENIC LEFT QUADRANT ABDOMINAL MASSES

- Large kidney
- Retroperitoneal tumor
- Adrenal neoplasm
- Ovarian cyst
- Pancreatic cyst
- Mesenteric cyst

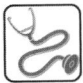

Physical Examination

Question: Is there swelling with slight pallor over the gum in which the tooth will erupt?
Significance: This is a normal finding.

Question: Is there bluish discoloration overlying the gum in which a tooth is expected?
Significance: This represents a hematoma, known as an "eruption cyst," which is a normal finding.

Question: Is the child irritable?
Significance: Irritability on physical examination suggests a more serious illness other than teething. In addition to the infectious etiologies noted, the child should be evaluated for hair tourniquet syndrome and/or corneal abrasion.

Question: Are there oral ulcers?
Significance: Viral enanthems, such as herpes or Coxsackie, should be considered.

Question: Is cervical lymphadenopathy present?
Significance: Oral, dental, or pharyngeal infections should be considered.

Question: Are there signs of dehydration, such as dry mucous membranes, absent tears, sunken fontanel, or tenting of the skin?
Significance: Infectious etiologies that result in poor oral intake or diarrhea should be considered.

Question: Is there oral erythema, and abrasions with excessive drooling?
Significance: The possibility of caustic ingestion should be explored.

Laboratory Aids

No laboratory tests are indicated in the otherwise healthy child with teething.

Common Questions and Answers

Q: What are some common remedies for relieving the pain caused by teething?
A: Children with teething should find temporary relief from biting or chewing on hard or cold items, such as refrigerated plastic teething rings, a cold wet washcloth, or teething biscuits. Gum massage with a clean finger may also provide relief.
Over-the-counter products containing benzocaine should be used with caution. Acetaminophen (15 mg/kg by mouth every 4 hours) or ibuprofen (10 mg/kg by mouth every 6 hours) may be used for pain relief as needed, but should not be given round-the-clock so as to mask fever. Remedies that have been used in the past and are no longer recommended include: alcoholic liquors, paregoric, 2% lidocaine solution, lancing the gums, and rubbing the gums with a thimble until the tooth breaks through the gum.

Q: What is the difference between natal teeth and neonatal teeth?
A: Natal teeth are present at birth, whereas neonatal teeth erupt during the first month of life. The incidence of natal teeth is 1:2,000 to 1:6,000 live births and usually involves the lower central incisor. Natal teeth can be associated with various conditions including Pierre Robin sequence, and cleft lip and/or palate. There is often a familial history of natal or neonatal teeth. Ninety-five percent of natal teeth are normal primary incisors that may have formed superficially and erupted early. Only 5% of natal teeth are supernumerary (extra) teeth. Therefore, if a natal tooth is removed, a primary tooth will not erupt in its place in most cases. Because primary teeth act as space holders for the secondary teeth, early loss of a primary tooth may result in significant crowding of the secondary teeth.

Q: Does primary tooth eruption in preterm infants occur at the same time as in full-term infants?
A: In healthy preterm infants who had relative uneventful neonatal courses, the first primary tooth erupts at the usual chronological age. In premature infants requiring prolonged oral intubation and/or who experience inadequate nutrition as a result of the severity of neonatal disease may have delays in tooth eruption. The initial eruption sequence remains the same (lower central incisors first).

Issues for Referral

• Children who have delayed eruption of their first primary tooth beyond 12 months require additional investigation for the following: adontia, osteodystrophies, hypothyroidism, hypopituitarism, rickets, Down syndrome, and Gardner syndrome. Most of these conditions require referral to a specialist for management.
• Children with premature eruption may have a familial cause; however, referral for evaluation of hyperpituitarism should be considered.
• Referral to a dentist should be considered for children with significant variation in eruption caused by dental infections, additional teeth in the path of eruption, insufficient space in the dental arch, and/or ectopic placement of teeth.
• Natal teeth that are stable and do not interfere with breast-feeding may remain. Loose natal teeth may need to be removed to prevent choking and aspiration. Natal teeth can interfere with breast-feeding and cause ulceration, which is another indication for removal.

BIBLIOGRAPHY

Jaber L, Cohen IJ, Mor A. Fever associated with teething. *Arch Dis Child* 1992;67: 233–234.

Kates GA, Needleman HL, Holmes LB. Natal and neonatal teeth: a clinical study. *J Am Dent Assoc* 1984;109:441–443.

Macknin ML, Piedmonte M, Jacobs J, et al. Symptoms associated with infant teething: a prospective study. *Pediatrics* 2000;105: 747–752.

Mofenson HC, Caraccio TR, Miller H, et al. Lidocaine toxicity from topical mucosal application. *Clin Pediatr* 1983;22:190–192.

Paynter AS, Alexander FW. Salicylate intoxication caused by teething ointment. *Lancet* 1979;2:1132.

Psoter WJ, Morse DE, Pendrys DG, Zhang H, Mayne ST. Median ages of eruption of the primary teeth in white and Hispanic children from Arizona. *Pediatr Dent* 2003;25:257–261.

Townes PL, Geertsma MA, White MR. Benzocaine induced methemoglobinemia. *Am J Dis Child* 1977;13:697–698.

Viscardi RM, Romberg E, Abrams RG. Delayed primary tooth eruption in premature infants: relationship to neonatal factors. *Pediatr Dent* 1994;16:23–28.

Wake M, Hesketh K, Lucas J. Teething and tooth eruption in infants: a cohort study. *Pediatrics* 2000;106:1374–1379.

Author: Julie A. Boom

Thrombosis

Database

DEFINITION

Pathologic arterial or venous intravascular occlusion by thrombus, which interferes with normal blood flow.
The following are common thrombotic events:

- Deep venous thrombosis (DVT): involves large systemic veins outside the CNS.
- Cerebral sinovenous thrombosis: involves the intracranial venous sinuses often with extension into the cerebral veins.
- Ischemic stroke: CNS arterial occlusion or insufficiency with infarction of brain tissue.
- Intracardiac thrombosis: mural, valvular, or foreign body associated.
- Femoral artery thrombosis: associated with vessel catheterization.
- Renal vein thrombosis: in the neonatal period; may be unilateral or bilateral.
- Myocardial infarction: Kawasaki disease or with severe familial hypercholesterolemia.
- Budd-Chiari syndrome: thrombosis of the hepatic vein.
- Portal vein thrombosis.

EPIDEMIOLOGY

- The incidence of venous thrombosis in children is estimated at 0.7 per 100,000 per year. It is likely that the actual incidence is higher.
- Two-thirds of children with thromboembolic disease have a predisposing underlying condition, the most common being an indwelling catheter.

COMPLICATIONS

- In deep venous thrombosis, pulmonary embolism is the most significant acute complication. Recurrent thrombosis and postphlebitic syndrome are common chronic complications.
- In arterial thromboembolic disease, the ischemic injury to the involved organ determines the acute and long-term complications.

Differential Diagnosis

PRIMARY PROTHROMBOTIC STATES

Inherited

- Factor V Leiden gene mutation
- Prothrombin 20210 gene mutation
- Protein C deficiency
- Protein S deficiency
- Antithrombin deficiency
- Homocystinemia (mild to moderate) from minor defects in enzymes such as methylenetetrahydrofolate reductase (MTHFR) or severe in homocystinuri
- Elevated lipoprotein (a) plasminogen deficiency
- Dysfibrinogenemia
- Heparin cofactor II deficiency

Acquired

- Antiphospholipid antibody syndrome

RISK FACTORS FOR THROMBOSIS

Neonatal

- Prematurity
- Maternal diabetes
- Umbilical catheters
- Sepsis
- Polycythemia
- Perinatal asphyxia

Malignancy/Bone Marrow Disorders

- Leukemia (hyperleukocytosis, APML)
- Myeloproliferative disorders
- Paroxysmal nocturnal hemoglobinuria

Medications

- L-Asparaginase
- Oral contraceptives
- Heparin (heparin-induced thrombocytopenia)
- Steroids

Anatomic

- Indwelling catheters
- Congenital heart disease
- Prosthetic heart valves
- Intracardiac baffles
- Tumor compression
- IVC atresia
- Thoracic outlet obstruction (Paget-Schroetter syndrome)

Disorders Associated with Thrombosis

- Nephrotic syndrome
- Inflammatory disorders (e.g., IBD, SLE)
- Liver disease
- Sickle cell disease
- Diabetes mellitus

Miscellaneous Risk Factors

- Infection
- Trauma
- Surgery
- Obesity
- Prolonged immobilization or paralysis
- Dehydration

Risk Factors/Conditions Specific for Arterial Disease

- Kawasaki disease
- Takayasu arteritis
- Hyperlipidemia

Data Gathering

HISTORY

Question: Current (or recent) central venous or arterial catheter?
Significance: Most significant risk factor for thrombosis

Question: Any of the risk factors (see list)?

Question: Is there a family history of thrombosis?
Thromboembolic disease is commonly overlooked.

Question: Personal history of thrombosis?
Significance: Patients with a history of thrombosis are an increased risk of recurrence.

Question: Neonatal seizure?
Significance: Common and often sole presenting sign for cerebral sinovenous thrombosis.

Question: Chest pain or shortness of breath?
Significance: Suggestive of pulmonary embolism

Physical Examination

Finding: Unilateral swelling/edema of a limb
Significance: Extremity DVT

Finding: Bilateral lower extremity edema of a limb
Significance: IVC thrombosis

Finding: Plethoric, swollen head and neck
Significance: Superior vena cava syndrome

Finding: Pale extremity with decreased perfusion/pulses
Significance: Arterial thrombosis

Finding: Abdominal mass and/or in neonate
Significance: Renal vein thrombosis

Finding: Tachypnea, shallow respirations
Significance: Pulmonary embolism

Finding: Unexplained hepatosplenomegaly
Significance: Hepatic or portal vein thrombosis

Finding: Superficial dilated cutaneous veins distal to the site of venous occlusion
Significance: Postphlebitic syndrome

Finding: Chronic discoloration (darkening) of the skin, ulcerations, pain, intermittent swelling
Significance: Postphlebitic syndrome

Laboratory Aids

General evaluation of the hemostatic system:

- PT/PTT/fibrinogen
- CBC with platelet count
- D-dimer

The following tests are used to investigate for a prothrombotic state:

Phase 1:

- Factor V Leiden mutation analysis by PCR
- Prothrombin 20210A allele by PCR
- Lupus anticoagulant screen (dRVVT, PTT)
- Anticardiolipin antibodies (IgG, IgM)
- Protein C activity
- Protein S, free and total
- Antithrombin activity
- Fasting homocysteine
- Lipoprotein (a)

Phase 2: For patients whose phase 1 studies are normal, but there is a strong family history

- Factor VIII activity
- Plasminogen
- Thrombin time or dysfibrinogenemia screen
- Activated protein C resistance clotting assay
- Heparin cofactor II
- Plasminogen activator inhibitor type 1

IMAGING

Contrast angiography—is the gold standard but invasive and sometimes technically difficult to perform in small children.

- Ultrasound—is the most commonly employed imaging study as a result of the noninvasiveness, absence of radiation, and ability to be performed at the bedside.
- In the diagnosis of upper extremity related DVT, often a combination of ultrasound and venography are necessary.

—Compression ultrasound of the upper central veins may be impeded by the distal end of the clavicle.
—Venography has a poor sensitivity for diagnosing thrombosis of the internal jugular veins.
—The recommended approach for diagnosis of an upper extremity thrombosis is to start with ultrasound and proceed to venography if the ultrasound is normal and there is a high clinical suspicion.

- Echocardiography may be useful in evaluating atrial thrombi, which may result from central venous catheters.
- Pulmonary angiography, ventilation-perfusion scans (V/Q), spiral CT are the imaging studies use for the diagnosis of pulmonary embolism, though none of these have been studied in children. V/Q scan or spiral CT (depending on the expertise at the institution) are the most common tests used for the diagnosis of PE in children. In patients with a PE, it is important to look for a source of thrombosis in the upper and lower extremities.
- Other diagnostic imaging options include CT and MR venography, which are noninvasive, although the sensitivity and specificity of these studies is not known. They may be particularly helpful in evaluating proximal thrombosis.
- For the diagnosis of cerebral sinovenous thrombosis, the most sensitive imaging study is brain MRI with venography (MRV).

PITFALLS

- Normal ranges for coagulation tests are age dependent: diagnosing an inherited deficiency in any of the anticoagulant proteins can be difficult in the neonatal period. Repeat testing at 6 to 12 months of age is necessary.
- Consumption can occur during acute thrombosis; therefore, low levels of the anticoagulant proteins must be repeated.
- Warfarin will decrease the levels of protein C and protein S.

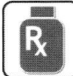

Therapy

- Therapy for acute thrombosis and long-term management is individualized.
- Consult someone with expertise in pediatric anticoagulant therapy.

DRUGS

- Unfractionated Heparin (uFH): Given as a bolus followed by an infusion, adjusted to maintain the aPTT 1.5 to 2.5 times baseline. Younger children require higher doses of heparin to achieve a therapeutic level.
- Low molecular weight heparin (LMWH): More predictable dose response. Given subcutaneously twice a day. Equivalent in efficacy to uFH in the acute management of uncomplicated DVT.
- Thrombolytics: Urokinase or recombinant tissue plasminogen activator. May be given systemically or locally. High risk of bleeding.
- Warfarin: An oral anticoagulant given as a loading dose to a patient already receiving heparin, adjusted to maintain the INR at 2.0 to 3.0 for treatment of DVT. Used for outpatient management.
- Aspirin: Beneficial in stroke, and other arterial events

Approach to the Patient

Phase 1: Perform complete history and examination; establish diagnosis using appropriate radiologic study

Phase 2: Laboratory studies (CBC, PT/PTT, D-dimer, antithrombin) and begin anticoagulation therapy with unfractionated heparin or LMWH. Patients with life- or limb-threatening thrombosis may require thrombolysis.

Phase 3: Complete work up for hyper-coagulable state; outpatient anticoagulation; follow thrombosis radiologically.

Follow-Up

- Growth of involved limbs, especially following an arterial event.
- Compression stocking may decrease risk of postphlebitic syndrome
- Medical risk factors such as oral contraception, use of catheters or prolonged immobilization should be controlled.

PITFALLS

Central venous catheter related thrombosis may be subtle despite extensive damage to the venous system. Recurrent line infection, line occlusion, and prominent venous collateral on the chest suggest UE DVT. The long-term consequences of this are not known.

Coumadin can cause purpura fulminans if started in an unheparinized patient.

Common Questions and Answers

Q: If an inherited prothrombotic condition is identified, should family members be tested?
A: If they have other risk factors for thrombosis such as malignancy, major surgery, oral contraceptives, obesity, and so on.

Q: When is it appropriate to use LMWH rather than unfractionated heparin?
A: There are several potential advantages to LMWH. The pharmacokinetics are much more predictable and frequent monitoring is not necessary. It is administered subcutaneously, not intravenous. The risk of bleeding may be slightly lower.

Q: When is it appropriate to use thrombolytic therapy?
A: Studies do not clearly demonstrate a role for thrombolytic therapy in DVT. However, if a thrombus extends on heparin therapy, a pulmonary embolus is suspected, or if the disturbance in blood flow causes ischemia, thrombolytic therapy can be used. Intracranial bleeding is a contraindication. For arterial thrombotic events, thrombolytic therapy is often the treatment of choice because of the rapid resolution of the clot and restoration of blood flow.

Q: What precautions should be taken for invasive procedures and for athletics when a patient is on anticoagulant therapy?
A: Lumbar punctures, arterial punctures, and surgical procedures should be avoided. If they are necessary, then the child should have the anticoagulant partially or fully reversed prior to the procedure. The child should not participate in contact sports such as football, karate, and boxing. For baseball, a helmet should be worn at all times.

Issues for Referral

- Pediatric hematologists should be consulted to assist in evaluating for primary hypercoagulable states and assisting in the management of anticoagulant therapy
- Radiologists should be consulted for choosing the best imaging study for diagnosis and follow-up.

BIBLIOGRAPHY

Andrew M, Monagle PT, Brooker L. *Thromboembolic Complications During Infancy and Childhood.* Hamilton, Ont: BC Decker, 2000.

Kearon C. Natural history of venous thromboembolism. *Circulation* 2003;107(23 Suppl 1):I22–I30.

van Ommen CH, Peters M. Venous thromboembolic disease in childhood. *Semin Thromb Hemost* 2003;29(4):391–404.

Authors: Leslie Raffini
J. Nathan Hagstrom, 3rd edition

Upper GI Bleeding

 Database

DEFINITION

Vomiting of blood whether bright red or dark constitutes upper gastrointestinal (GI) bleeding or hematemesis. This usually represents bleeding from the GI tract proximal to the ligament of Treitz. One has to differentiate upper GI (UGI) bleeding from hemoptysis (coughing up of blood), nose bleeds, and bleeding from the mouth and pharynx. Sometimes UGI bleeding can present with melena or the passage of tarry stools.

 Differential Diagnosis

- Ninety-five percent of the causes of UGI bleeding are as a result of mucosal abnormalities or esophageal varices.
- Mucosal lesions are more likely to be associated with antecedent occult bleeding.
- In about 80% to 95% of patients the bleeding stops spontaneously.
- Age of the patient is important.

NEONATAL PERIOD

- Swallowed maternal blood
- Hemorrhagic disease of the newborn
- Esophagitis/gastritis
- Stress ulcer
- Foreign body irritation
- Vascular malformation

INFANCY

- Esophagitis/gastritis
- Stress ulcer
- Mallory-Weiss tear
- Pyloric stenosis
- Vascular malformation
- Duplication cysts

PRESCHOOL AGE

- Esophageal varices
- Esophagitis/gastritis/ulcer
- Foreign body/bezoar
- Mallory-Weiss tear
- Vascular malformation

SCHOOL AGE

- Esophageal varices
- Esophagitis/gastritis/ulcer
- Mallory-Weiss tear
- Inflammatory bowel disease

Approach to the Patient

GENERAL GOALS

Determine the cause of the bleeding and begin treatment.

Phase 1: Determine if the vomitus truly contains blood, as red food coloring, fruit flavored drinks and juices, vegetables, and medicines may appear like blood. A pH buffered Gastroccult test identifies blood in the vomitus or gastric aspirate.

Phase 2: Assess severity of bleeding. Is there a change in vital signs, hematocrit, blood pressures, capillary filling, pulse?

Phase 3: Determine the site of bleeding and begin treatment. Examine airway for bleeding—epistaxis may contaminate vomitus to appear as UGI bleeding. Usually will require imaging or endoscopy.

HINTS FOR SCREENING PROBLEM

- Bright red blood signifies active bleeding.
- Darker blood or "coffee grounds" usually means that the blood has had some time to be denatured by gastric acid.
- The rate of bleeding will determine the clinical presentation. The more rapid the rate, the larger the volume of UGI bleeding and the greater the drop in hemoglobin and change in pulse and blood pressure. Slower bleeding usually presents with anemia and heme-positive stools.
- Any significant blood loss will lead to pallor, tachycardia, orthostasis, poor capillary refill, CNS changes (restlessness, confusion), and hypotension. Hypotension may not be seen even in the face of significant blood loss because vasoconstriction will occur to maintain blood pressure until decompensation.
- Initial hemoglobin values may be unreliable because a delay in hemodilution may falsely result in near normal values.
- Absence of blood in the emesis or in nasogastric lavage fluid does not rule out the UGI tract as the site of bleeding, because a competent pylorus may mask bleeding from a duodenal site. In fact, in some cases of massive UGI bleeding, the patient may not vomit blood but may pass large, black, tarry, or sticky stools, called melena.

 Data Gathering

HISTORY

Question: Amount of blood, i.e., drops versus 1 teaspoon versus 1 tablespoon? Any clots?
Significance: Indicates severity of bleeding.

Question: Vomitus contains blood?
Significance: Indicates bleeding from UGI tract or swallowed blood.

Question: Any recently ingested foods resemble blood, e.g., red food dye, beets, Jell-O, Kool-Aid, antibiotic syrups, food fibers?
Significance: Vomitus may not have blood.

Question: Can one determine the source of bleeding?
Significance: Hematemesis from the esophagus, stomach, or duodenum versus hemoptysis versus swallowed blood from the nose, mouth, or pharynx.

Question: Was the blood coughed or vomited?
Significance: Indicative of hemoptysis.

Question: Was it from the nose—swallowed and then vomited?
Significance: Not bleeding from the UGI tract.

Question: Was there prolonged vomiting preceding the bleeding?
Significance: Prolonged retching prior to hematemesis suggests a Mallory-Weiss tear.

Question: History of recent stress (burns, head trauma, surgery)?
Significance: Suggests an ulcer or gastritis.

Question: History of toxic ingestion?
Significance: May result in an ulcerated esophagus, which can bleed.

Question: Ingestion of certain medications?
Significance: Aspirin, steroids can lead to gastritis and ulcers. Ingestion of drugs (nonsteroidal antiinflammatory drugs) and alcohol can lead to gastritis.

Question: Abdominal pain and vomiting blood?
Significance: Suggests esophagitis, gastritis, and peptic ulcers

Question: Is there breast-feeding?
Significance: Cracked nipples in the mother can lead to the infant swallowing maternal blood and then having hematemesis.

Question: Is there history of gastroesophageal reflux?
Significance: Suggests esophagitis.

Question: Is there past history of GI disease?
Significance: Gastroesophageal reflux, peptic ulcer disease, or previous GI surgery may suggest that the current symptoms may be as a result of recurrence of disease.

Question: Is there history of jaundice, hepatitis, or liver disease?
Significance: Suggests portal hypertension and variceal bleeding.

Question: Was there any neonatal history of umbilical vein catheterization or infection?
Significance: Portal vein thrombosis (sepsis, shock, exchange transfusion, omphalitis, IV catheters) suggests portal hypertension and bleeding varices as a result of cavernous transformation of the portal vein.

Question: Familial history of bleeding?
Significance: Familial history of bleeding diathesis, e.g., von Willebrand disease, hemophilia.

 Physical Examination

Finding: Are there any skin petechiae, ecchymosis, hemangiomas?
Significance: Evidence of chronic liver disease (spider angiomata, palmar erythema, jaundice). Look for evidence of chronic liver disease and bleeding diathesis.

Finding: HEENT: Nasopharyngeal source of bleeding
Significance: Swallowed blood

Finding: Freckles on buccal mucosa
Significance: Osler-Weber-Rendu syndrome; Peutz-Jeghers syndrome

Finding: Oral thrush
Significance: Candida esophagitis

Finding: Oral mucosal lesions
Significance: Corrosive ingestions

Finding: Abdomen

- Hepatosplenomegaly
- Ascites

Significance: Portal hypertension

Finding: Isolated splenomegaly
Significance: Cavernous transformation of the portal vein; portal hypertension

Finding: Rectal examination
Significance: Heme-positive stool may or may not be present. If positive, confirms the presence of UGI bleeding.

 ## Laboratory Aids

Test: Gastroccult
Significance: If possible check the red substance for blood. In neonates, may need to check for fetal hemoglobin with the Apt test.

Test: CBC
Significance: If there is leukopenia, anemia, and thrombocytopenia, think chronic liver disease and portal hypertension. If there is anemia with normal RBC indices, then there is truly an acute cause for bleeding. If RBC indices indicate iron-deficiency anemia, think of varices or a mucosal lesion, i.e., chronic blood loss.

Test: Coagulation profile
Significance: If PT/PTT are abnormal, then think of liver disease or disseminated intravascular coagulation (DIC) with sepsis. If DIC screen is negative, think liver disease. Make sure, however, that blood sample was not contaminated with heparin.

Test: Bleeding time
Significance: Abnormal in patients with previous history (or family history) of bleeding disorders.

Test: Liver function tests
Significance: Abnormal in chronic liver disease

Test: Upper endoscopy
Significance: Useful, as diagnosis can be made in 75% to 90% of patients.

Test: Barium tests
Significance: Not as useful as esophagogastroduodenoscopy (EGD) but can identify a large ulcer. Air-contrast UGI better than regular UGI test.

Test: Bleeding scan
Significance: Useful in the patient with significant bleeding in whom endoscopy was not diagnostic. Can get two types of scans: technetium sulfur colloid or tagged RBC scan. The former detects very rapid bleeding but can miss small bleeds, especially if patient is not bleeding during the scan. The latter can detect small bleeds, especially if intermittent.

Test: Angiography
Significance: Useful in detecting vascular causes for UGI bleeding. Can also be therapeutic, i.e., injection of coils into a vascular malformation to occlude it. Invasiveness and need for specialized training are limitations.

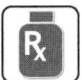 ## Therapy

Initial management of the emergency depends on diagnosis and clinical condition of the patient.

- Stabilize the patient with intravenous fluids and blood products if necessary.
- Order laboratory tests: CBC, PT/PTT, DIC screen, liver function tests, blood type, and crossmatch.
- Insert an nasogastric tube and lavage with saline to determine site as well as rate of ongoing bleeding. No need for cold saline.
- Monitor patient's vital signs and hemoglobin as necessary.
- Make appropriate diagnosis and institute appropriate therapy, i.e., EGD, bleeding scans.

DISEASE-SPECIFIC THERAPY

- Peptic ulcer disease

—Proton pump inhibitors
—H2 blockers
—Sucralfate
—Prokinetic agents

- Esophageal varices

—Vasopressin or somatostatin infusion
—Sclerotherapy or banding
—Sengstaken-Blakemore tube
—Portosystemic shunts

If bleeding stops quickly, then workup is less emergent.

 ## Follow-Up

- Monitor hemoglobin in the hospital until stable
- Once patient is discharged, monitor hemoglobin weekly as well as Hemoccult cards until stable.
- More specific follow-up depends on the underlying condition.

PREVENTION

- Avoid drugs that are likely to cause bleeding or gastritis especially in a susceptible patient.
- In patients with chronic GI conditions, optimize therapy and monitoring.
- Correct coagulopathy
- Prophylactic sclerotherapy or banding for patients with known variceal bleeds

PITFALLS

- Make sure the vomited material is really blood.
- A negative nasogastric aspirate for blood does not indicate the absence of UGI bleeding.
- Initial hemoglobin may not be accurate and serial hemoglobins should be obtained.

 ## Common Questions and Answers

Q: When do you refer a patient?
A: Any bleed—immediate referral if bleed is large, the patient is hemodynamically unstable, and bleeding will not stop. Patient with evidence of chronic iron deficiency anemia and heme-positive stools.

Q: What makes UGI bleeding an emergency?
A: Any persistent bleed with change in vital signs. Significant drop in hemoglobin.

BIBLIOGRAPHY

Ament M. Diagnosis and management of upper gastrointestinal bleeding in the pediatric patient. *Pediatr Rev* 1990;12:107–116.

Faubion WA, Perrault J. Gastrointestinal bleeding. In: Walker WA, Durie PR, Hamilton JR, et al., eds. *Pediatric Gastrointestinal Disease.* Philadelphia: BC Decker, 2000:164–178.

Fox VL. Gastrointestinal bleeding in infancy and childhood. *Gastroenterol Clin North Am* 2000;29(1):37–66.

Hassal E. Sclerotherapy for extrahepatic nonvariceal upper GI bleeding. *Med Clin North Am* 1993;77:973–992.

Sherman PM. Peptic ulcer disease in children—diagnosis, treatment and the implication of Helicobater pylor. *Gastroenterol Clin North Am* 1994;23(4):707–725.

Vinton NE. Gastrointestinal bleeding in infancy and childhood. *Gastroenterol Clin North Am* 1994;23(1):93–122.

Squires RH. Gastrointestinal bleeding. *Pediatr Rev* 1999;20(3):95–101.

Authors: Maria R. Mascarenhas and Meena Thayu

Vomiting

Database

DEFINITION

The expulsion of gastric contents through the mouth in varying degrees. Regurgitation is defined as small, effortless mouthfuls of food or stomach contents. Vomiting is usually associated with large, forceful amounts of stomach contents.

Differential Diagnosis

DISORDERS OF GASTROINTESTINAL TRACT

- Anatomic

—Esophageal: stricture, web, ring, atresia
—Stomach: pyloric stenosis, web, duplication
—Intestine: duodenal atresia, malrotation, duplication
—Colon: Hirschsprung disease, imperforate anus

- Motility

—Achalasia
—Gastroesophageal reflux
—Intestinal pseudo-obstruction

- Foreign body/bezoar
- Obstruction

—Intussusception
—Volvulus
—Incarcerated hernia

- Cholecystitis or cholelithiasis
- Eosinophilic enteritis
- Appendicitis
- Necrotizing enterocolitis
- Peritonitis
- Celiac disease
- Peptic ulcer
- Trauma

—Duodenal hematoma
—Pancreatitis (pseudocyst)

NEUROLOGIC

- Intracranial mass lesions

—Tumor
—Cyst
—Subdural hematoma

- Cerebral edema
- Hydrocephalus
- Pseudotumor cerebri
- Migraine (head, abdominal)
- Seizures

RENAL

- Obstructive uropathy

—Ureteropelvic junction obstruction
—Hydronephrosis
—Nephrolithiasis

- Renal insufficiency
- Glomerulonephritis
- Renal tubular acidosis

METABOLIC

- Inborn errors of metabolism

—Galactosemia
—Fructose intolerance
—Hereditary fructose intolerance
—Amino acid or organic acid metabolism
—Urea cycle defects
—Fatty acid oxidation disorders
—Lactic acidosis

INFECTION

- Sepsis
- Meningitis
- Urinary tract infection
- Parasites
- Giardia
- Ascaris
- Helicobacter pylori
- Otitis media
- Viral/bacterial

—Gastroenteritis
—Viral hepatitis (A, B, C)
—Bordetella pertussis

ENDOCRINE

- Diabetes

—Diabetic ketoacidosis (DKA)
—Gastroparesis

- Adrenal insufficiency

RESPIRATORY

- Pneumonia
- Sinusitis
- Laryngitis

IMMUNOLOGIC

- Milk/soy protein allergy
- Cryptosporidium (AIDS)
- Graft-versus-host disease
- Chronic granulomatous disease

OTHER

- Pregnancy
- Rumination
- Bulimia
- Psychogenic
- Cyclic emesis syndrome
- Overfeeding
- Medications

—Drugs
—Vitamin toxicity

- Vascular (superior mesenteric artery syndrome)

Approach to the Patient

Vomiting is a prominent feature of many disorders of infancy and childhood and is often the only presenting symptom of many diseases. Vomiting can occur as a defense mechanism to expel ingested toxins, as an abnormality of the vomiting center related to increased intracranial pressure, as a result of intestinal obstruction or anatomic/mucosal abnormalities, or as the result of a generalized metabolic disease. A full history should include medication and drug use, trauma, and, in adolescents, questions regarding feeding disorders (bulimia) and intercourse (pregnancy).

Data Gathering

HISTORY

Question: Fever?
Significance: Infectious causes of vomiting are common.

Question: Abdominal pain and frequent, forceful, or bilious emesis?
Significance: Often associated with anatomic or obstructive intestinal disorder

Question: Age of patient?
Significance: Pyloric stenosis and inborn errors of metabolism almost always present in infancy with vomiting, dehydration, and biochemical abnormalities.

Question: Mental retardation, pica, and patchy baldness?
Significance: Foreign body or hair ingestion and the development of a gastric bezoar

Question: Nausea and epigastric pain related to meals?
Significance: Often indicates gastritis, gastric emptying delay, or gallbladder disease

Question: Alleviated by meals?
Significance: Gastroesophageal reflux and gastric ulcer disease

Question: Alternating vomiting and lethargy?
Significance: Intussusception

Question: Chronic headaches, fatigue, weakness, weight loss, and early morning vomiting?
Significance: Neurologic causes of vomiting secondary to increased intracranial pressure

Question: Right- or left-sided abdominal pain?
Significance: Renal disease, inflammatory bowel disease

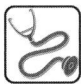 Physical Examination

A careful and complete physical examination can often provide excellent clues as to the cause of vomiting in children.

Finding: Visible bowel loops
Significance: Obstruction

Finding: Palpation for a mass effect and tenderness, and auscultation for evidence of absent bowel sounds or borborygmi (rumbling bowel sounds)
Significance: Intestinal obstruction

Finding: Rectal examination
Significance: Testing the stool for occult blood

Finding: Discoloration of skin and sclera
Significance: Jaundice (liver/gallbladder or metabolic disease)

Finding: Orange tint of sclera or skin
Significance: Hypervitaminosis A

Finding: Unusual odor
Significance: Metabolic disease

Finding: Chronic vomiting
Significance: Evidence of neurologic dysfunction, including nystagmus, head tilt, papilledema, abnormal reflexes, and weakness

Finding: Tense anterior fontanelle
Significance: May indicate meningitis, hydrocephalus, or vitamin A toxicity

Finding: Enlarged parotid glands and hypersalivation
Significance: Bulimia and other feeding disorders

Finding: Pelvic examination
Significance: Pregnancy, pelvic inflammatory disease, or ovarian disease

Laboratory Aids

Test: CBC
Significance: Anemia and iron deficiency can occur with intestinal duplication and obstruction, gastritis/esophagitis, and ulcer disease.

Test: Blood chemistry
Significance: Electrolyte abnormalities are found in pyloric stenosis, metabolic abnormalities, although an elevated ALT, total bilirubin, and GGT can indicate liver, gallbladder, or metabolic disease.

Test: Urinalysis
Significance: Pyelonephritis

Test: Amylase
Significance: Pancreatitis

Test: BUN/creatinine
Significance: If elevated—renal disease

Test: Urine culture
Significance: UTI

Test: Plain abdominal x-ray study
Significance: Obstruction

Test: Abdominal ultrasound
Significance: Liver, gallbladder, renal, pancreatic, ovarian, or uterine disease. In infants, abdominal ultrasound is the test of choice for pyloric stenosis. Useful when considering abdominal abscess and appendicitis.

Test: Contrast radiography
Significance: Intestinal anatomic abnormalities (malrotation, intussusception, volvulus)

Test: Computed tomography
Significance: Not generally indicated for evaluation of vomiting, although it is an effective tool when more anatomic abdominal detail is required (abscess, tumor).

Test: Endoscopy
Significance: Esophageal, gastric, and duodenal inflammation (esophagitis, gastritis, ulcer disease, celiac disease, eosinophilic enteritis) as well as for obtaining cultures for unusual infections (duodenal Giardia, Helicobacter pylori/cytomegalovirus gastritis).

Issues for Referral

- Chronic vomiting (2 to 3 weeks)
- Weight loss
- Severe abdominal pain or irritability
- Gastrointestinal bleeding
- Evidence of intestinal obstruction
- Serum electrolyte abnormalities
- Abnormal neurologic examination
- Dehydration
- Signs of an acute abdomen
- Lethargy

Emergency Care

Evidence of hematemesis, intestinal obstruction (bilious vomiting), dehydration, neurologic dysfunction, or an acute abdomen should be treated as a medical emergency, and hospitalization should be considered.

BIBLIOGRAPHY

Silverman A, Roy CC, eds. *Pediatric Clinical Gastroenterology*. 3rd Ed. St. Louis: Mosby, 1983.

Sondheimer J. Vomiting and regurgitation. In: Walker WA, Durie PR, Hamilton Jr, et al., eds. *Pediatric Gastrointestinal Disease*. St. Louis: Mosby, 1996;19.

Authors: Matthew J. Ryan
Chris A. Liacouras, 3rd edition

Weight Loss

Database

DEFINITION

Weight loss is a documented decrease in weight from a previous measurement. Outside of the newborn period (weight loss in the first 2 weeks is common), acute illnesses resulting in fluid loss, and obese adolescents voluntarily on a designed weight reduction program, weight loss is an unusual and worrisome symptom, regardless of the percentage decline.

Differential Diagnosis

CONGENITAL/ANATOMIC

- Congenital heart disease
- Pyloric stenosis
- Gastrointestinal malformation (duodenal atresia, annular pancreas, volvulus)
- Short bowel syndrome
- Lymphangiectasia
- Superior mesenteric artery syndrome
- Gastroesophageal reflux
- Immunodeficiency disorders
- Hirschsprung disease

INFECTIOUS

- Urinary tract infection
- Tuberculosis
- Stomatitis
- Osteomyelitis
- Human immunodeficiency virus
- Hepatitis
- Parasitic disease
- Abscess, intraabdominal
- Gastroenteritis
- Pericarditis
- Histoplasmosis
- Acute severe febrile illness (pyelonephritis, pneumonia, septic arthritis)

TOXIC, ENVIRONMENTAL, DRUGS

- Lead poisoning
- Mercury poisoning
- Vitamin A poisoning
- Chronic methylphenidate, dextroamphetamine, or valproic acid use
- Substance abuse, especially amphetamines and crack cocaine

TRAUMA

- Chronic subdural hematomas

TUMOR

- Diencephalic syndrome
- Leukemia
- Lymphoma
- Pheochromocytoma
- Other neoplasms

GENETIC/METABOLIC

- Diabetes mellitus
- Diabetes insipidus
- Hyperthyroidism
- Cystic fibrosis
- Schwachman syndrome
- Addison disease
- Hypercalcemia
- Congenital adrenal hyperplasia
- Lactose intolerance
- Renal tubular acidosis
- Chronic renal failure
- Hypopituitarism
- Inborn errors of metabolism
- Storage diseases
- Muscular dystrophy
- Lipodystrophy

ALLERGIC/INFLAMMATORY

- Inflammatory bowel disease
- Juvenile rheumatoid arthritis
- Systemic lupus erythematosus
- Sarcoidosis
- Pancreatitis
- Hepatitis
- Celiac disease (gluten enteropathy)

FUNCTIONAL/MISCELLANEOUS

- Malnutrition
- Child abuse
- Postoperative
- Dieting
- Rumination syndrome
- Depression/affective disorders
- Anorexia nervosa

—Inability to eat (new orthodontic appliances, loss of teeth, chronic mouth ulcerations)

- Chronic congestive heart failure
- Chronic pulmonary disease
- Chronic renal disease
- Iron deficiency
- Zinc deficiency
- Cerebral palsy
- Postinfectious malabsorption
- Factitious (e.g., scale error)

Approach to the Patient

GENERAL GOAL

Determine the acuity or chronicity and severity of weight loss, and the need for hospitalization.

Phase 1: Attempt to narrow the diagnostic possibilities by history and examination, particularly by assessing if the loss might be attributable to diminished intake, diminished absorption, or increased requirements.

Data Gathering

HISTORY

Question: Is the weight loss real?
Significance: Scale error, different scales, different technique (e.g., clothed versus unclothed)

Question: What is the child's diet?
Significance: A prospective 3-day dietary record can be very useful for demonstrating insufficient caloric intake

Question: Less than 2 weeks of age?
Significance: Physiologic weight loss, underfeeding, inappropriate feeding, inborn errors of metabolism, congenital heart disease, gastroesophageal reflux

Question: Less than 4 months?
Significance: Malnutrition, improper formula preparation, cystic fibrosis, gastroesophageal reflux, pyloric stenosis, congenital heart disease, congenital adrenal hyperplasia, inborn errors of metabolism

Question: 4 months to 8 years?
Significance: Chronic infection, cystic fibrosis, malabsorption, neglect/abuse, renal disease, liver disease, diabetes mellitus

Question: Older than 8 years?
Significance: Eating disorder, chronic infection, neoplasm, renal disease, liver disease, substance abuse, diabetes mellitus, inflammatory bowel disease, collagen vascular disease

Question: Cramping, bloating or abnormally greasy, voluminous stools?
Significance: Possible malabsorption

Question: Vomiting, especially projectile?
Significance: Suggestive of intestinal obstruction, G-E reflux, inborn errors of metabolism

Question: Polyuria, polydipsia, and polyphagia?
Significance: Possible diabetes mellitus

Question: Headaches, especially early morning?
Significance: Possible increased intracranial pressure, CNS malignancy

Question: Maternal history of multiple miscarriages, neonatal deaths, or consanguinity?
Significance: Possible inborn error of metabolism

Question: History of severe infections, persistent candidal infections?
Significance: Immunodeficiency, congenital or acquired

Question: Fear of fatness, preoccupation with food, distorted body image, and/or amenorrhea?
Significance: Possible eating disorder

Question: Delayed puberty?
Significance: Suggests chronic severe weight loss, pituitary abnormalities, anorexia nervosa

Question: Foreign travel?
Significance: Possible chronic infection (e.g., tuberculosis, parasitic disease)

Question: Tiring during feeding or difficulty feeding as a result of cough and dyspnea?
Significance: Suggests coronary heart failure in newborn/infant, hypothyroidism

Question: Increased appetite with weight loss?
Significance: Suggests hyperthyroidism, cystic fibrosis, pheochromocytoma

Question: Altered mental status, seizures, unusual body/fluid odors
Significance: Inborn error of metabolism

Question: Chronic sadness or irritability; insomnia or hypersomnia
Significance: Depression/affective disorder

 ## Physical Examination

Finding: Clubbing
Significance: Suggests chronic cardiac, pulmonary, or intestinal disease

Finding: Significant abdominal distension
Significance: Suggests celiac disease

Finding: Hypothermia, bradycardia
Significance: Suggests anorexia nervosa, hypothyroidism

Finding: Tachycardia, resting
Significance: Hyperthyroidism, pheochromocytoma, anemia, acute weight loss

Finding: Orthostatic changes
Significance: Significant weight loss, possibly acute

Finding: Hypotension, resting
Significance: Addison disease, anorexia nervosa, significant acute dehydration

Finding: Swollen joint
Significance: Juvenile rheumatoid arthritis, inflammatory bowel disease (IBD)

Finding: Muscle weakness
Significance: Connective tissue disorder, electrolyte abnormality, muscular dystrophy

Finding: Enlarged liver and/or spleen
Significance: Suggests malignancy, chronic infection, storage disease, inborn error of metabolism

 ## Laboratory Aids

Test: Complete blood count
Significance:

• Evidence of

—Anemia—macrocytic associated with folate/B12 deficiency, microcytic with iron deficiency or chronic infection
—Polycythemia—suggestive of chronic pulmonary or cardiac disease

—Neutropenia—suggestive of hematologic malignancy, Schwachman syndrome, immunodeficiency
—Lymphopenia—suggestive of immunodeficiency
—Eosinophilia—suggestive of parasitic disease
—Leukocytosis—suggestive of infection
—Thrombocytosis—suggestive of chronic infection, malignancy
—Lymphoblasts—suggestive of leukemia

Test: ESR
Significance: May be elevated in IBD, chronic infections, rheumatoid diseases

Test: Serum electrolytes
Significance: Abnormalities in dehydration, adrenal insufficiency (low Na, high K), renal disease, anorexia nervosa

Test: BUN, creatinine
Significance: Abnormal in renal disease, dehydration

Test: Stool for occult blood and pH
Significance: Occult blood suggests IBD

Test: Urinalysis
Significance: Hematuria and/or proteinuria suggest renal disease; glycosuria suggests diabetes mellitus; very low specific gravity suggests diabetes insipidus, chronic renal failure, hypercalcemia; pyuria suggests UTI; pH >6 suggests RTA (type I)

Test: Urine culture

Test: Serum protein levels
Significance: Very low levels imply impaired liver function, severe chronic weight loss or protein malabsorption

Test: Tuberculosis skin test

Test: Liver function tests
Significance: Evaluation for hepatitis, chronic liver disease

Depending on age and clinical findings, other tests to consider include thyroid function tests, sweat test, tests for malabsorption (e.g., lactose breath test, stool fat, stool for trypsin), tests for metabolic disease (e.g., plasma ammonia, lactate, serum/urine amino acids, urine organic acids), imaging studies (e.g., CT, MRI, bone scan), immunologic studies.

 ## Emergency Care

• Significant dehydration: abnormal vital signs with orthostasis, decreased urine output, decreased skin turgor, delayed capillary refill (>3 seconds). Mandates cardiovascular support (intravenous hydration) and a more urgent diagnosis (e.g., inborn error of metabolism, obstructive GI disease, congenital adrenal hyperplasia, diabetic ketoacidosis).
• Abnormal mental status, significant lethargy: May be seen in severe dehydration, hypoadrenalism, hypoxic states, toxic ingestions, renal or respiratory failure, increased intracranial pressure, severe electrolyte abnormalities.

• Increasing vomiting in the setting of known weight loss in infants: high risk for dehydration, hypoglycemia, and electrolyte abnormalities. Need to evaluate for treatable conditions (e.g., obstructive GI disease, inborn errors of metabolism, congenital adrenal hyperplasia, congenital heart disease) in which a delay is life-threatening.
• Severe malnutrition (weight loss >20% of ideal body weight): high risk for metabolic derangements, including dysrhythmias secondary to electrolyte abnormalities. Aggressive evaluation is warranted.

Common Questions and Answers

Q: How common is weight loss in the first 2 weeks of life?
A: Formula-fed babies may lose up to 7% of birth weight and breast-fed newborns up to 10% before regaining their birth weight by 2 weeks of age.

Issues for Referral

Weight loss is a diagnostic exigency—a cause must be found or the loss self-resolved. If a diagnosis is not uncovered in the setting of continued weight loss, referral to a pediatric diagnostic center is indicated.

Clinical Pearls

• Be certain that the weight loss is real. In some studies, up to 25% of weight loss is artifactual as a result of measurement errors (e.g., excessive movement of scale, dressed versus undressed patient).
• Newborns with weight loss, especially at the 2-week visit, may manifest passivity and paradoxical lack of interest in breast-feeding, although the reason for their problem is malnourishment as a result of inadequate intake (often from improper positioning or too infrequent feedings). They may not act "hungry." Observation of the feeding technique (by a practitioner with expertise or a lactation consultant) is vital.

BIBLIOGRAPHY

Kleinman RE, ed. *Pediatric Nutrition Handbook.* 5th ed. Elk Grove Village, IL: American Academy of Pediatrics, 2004.

Schechter M. Weight loss/failure to thrive. *Pediatr Rev* 2000;21:238–239.

Author: Mark F. Ditmar

Wheezing

Database

DEFINITION

• Wheezing is a continuous sound that is caused by turbulent airflow through an obstructed airway.

—Often described as musical in nature and with a variable pitch.
—Wheezing—expiratory sound; stridor as an inspiratory sound.
—Wheezing occurs from an obstruction in the intrathoracic airway, although stridor by itself is caused by an obstruction in the extrathoracic airway.
—If heard in both inspiration and expiration, there is a fixed obstruction or separate lesions in both the intrathoracic and extrathoracic airways.

Differential Diagnosis

EXTRATHORACIC

Nasal/Nasopharynx

• Acute—Nasal turbinate edema or secretions, foreign body
• Chronic—Adenoidal enlargement, nasal polyps, choanal stenosis, midface hypoplasia

Oropharynx

• Acute—Peritonsillar abscess, retropharyngeal abscess, palatine tonsillitis
• Chronic—Adenotonsillar hypertrophy, macroglossia, micrognathia

Hypopharynx

• Acute—Acute nasal, nasopharyngeal, or oropharyngeal obstruction
• Chronic—Hypopharyngeal hypotonia, glossoptosis, obesity, neoplasia

Larynx

• Acute—Laryngospasm, laryngotracheobronchitis (croup), epiglottitis, foreign body (large and irregular)
• Chronic—Laryngomalacia, papillomatosis, hemangioma, granuloma, congenital cyst or web, laryngocele

Glottis

• Acute—Vocal cord paralysis or paresis, vocal cord inflammation or polyp, psychogenic wheezing
• Chronic—Paradoxical vocal cord motion (vocal cord dysfunction), psychogenic wheezing, brainstem compression, injury to the vagus, glossopharyngeal or recurrent laryngeal nerves, papillomatosis

Subglottis/Extrathoracic Trachea

• Acute—Laryngotracheobronchitis (croup), bacterial rachitic, recent endotracheal extubation
• Chronic—Subglottic stenosis (congenital or after prolonged intubation), papillomatosis

INTRATHORACIC

Trachea (Extrinsic Compression)

• Acute—Uncommon
• Chronic—

—Vascular—(vascular ring/sling, pulmonary artery compression);
—Cardiac—(left main bronchus compression, recurrent laryngeal nerve compression "cardiovocal syndrome");
—Anterior mediastinum—lymphoma, thymoma, teratoma;
—Middle mediastinum—lymphoma, lymphadenopathy (tuberculosis, mycotic infection, sarcoidosis);
—Posterior mediastinum—Neurogenic tumors, esophageal duplication cyst, bronchogenic cyst

Trachea (Intramural Lesions)

• Acute—Uncommon
• Chronic—Tracheomalacia

—Congenital—Cartilagenous defect (Campbell-Williams syndrome), muscular defect (Mounier-Kuhn syndrome), s/p tracheoesopageal hernia repair, external compression/distortion, complete tracheal rings;
—Acquired—Chronic inflammation (recurrent infection, gastroesophageal reflux, recurrent aspiration), prolonged positive pressure ventilation, external compression

Trachea (Intralumenal Lesions)

• Acute—Foreign body (irregularly shaped and elongated), bacterial tracheitis (with chronic tracheostomy tube usage)
• Chronic—Tracheal granulomas, hemangioma, papillomatosis, tracheal web
• Bronchi/bronchioles
• Acute—Viral bronchiolitis, bronchopneumonia, foreign body (small, smooth shape), granuloma, neoplasia
• Chronic—Asthma, bronchopulmonary dysplasia, bronchomalacia, carcinoid, adenoma

Approach to the Patient

GENERAL GOALS

Phase 1: Determine the severity of the patient's general status and degree of respiratory distress and triage accordingly.

Phase 2: Construct a differential diagnosis.

Phase 3: Initiate appropriate therapies.

Data Gathering

HISTORY

Question: What is/has been the pattern of the wheezing?
Significance: A rapid onset suggests a foreign body or a postexposure exacerbation of asthma, a slow onset suggests an infection.

• Periods of recurrent wheezing suggests asthma.
• Nocturnal and early morning wheezing or coughing consistent with gastroesophageal reflux, sinusitis, and sensitivity to common household allergens.
• Wheezing in association with or soon after a meal can be seen in swallowing dysfunction and gastroesophageal reflux. Wheezing that worsens with crying is suggestive of tracheomalacia and/or bronchomalacia or a fixed intralumenal or extralumenal obstruction.

Question: Timing to exertion?
Significance: Exercise-induced asthma

Question: Multiple exacerbations with recurrent or chronic symptoms?
Significance: Recurrent cycles of exacerbations, with clearing in between, suggests a process such as asthma, cystic fibrosis, and bronchopulmonary dysplasia, although chronic or persistent wheezing is more common with fixed anatomic abnormalities.

Question: What are the triggers?
Significance: Common triggers include smoke, dust, animal dander, change in humidity or temperature, change in seasons (pollens, grasses, molds), exercise, infections, and inflammation of any sort.

Question: Is there a family history?
Significance: A positive family history of wheezing, asthma, allergic rhinitis, or atopy suggests a diagnosis of asthma.

Question: Did an episode of choking precede the onset of wheezing?
Significance: Foreign body aspiration.

Physical Examination

• Observe: assess the patient's degree of respiratory difficulty.

—Tachypnea
—Accessory muscle usage—use of intercostal and sternocleidomastoid muscles and abdominal musculature, and indicates increased expiratory effort to overcome airway obstruction.
—Subcostal retractions
—Nasal flaring—with increasing respiratory difficulty the nares will be dilated to decrease the resistance to air flow.

• Auscultate: Assess airflow, adventitious sounds, and the inspiratory to expiratory ratio.

—Aeration—decreased aeration is much worse prognostically than wheezing since it is directly related to the amount of aeration and ventilation. With decreased aeration wheezing may not be audible.
—Ratio of inspiration to exhalation—with increased intrathoracic airways obstruction the time needed to exhale will become greater because of a greater decrease in airway caliber during exhalation.

OTHER FINDINGS

• Presence of nasal crease, the "allergic salute" (e.g., rubbing the nose with the palm of the hand), atopic dermatitis, boggy nasal turbinates, clear postnasal drainage, allergic shiners, or Dennie lines.

Significance: Suggestive of allergic rhinitis, or atopic disease including asthma.

DIAGNOSTIC AIDS

• Bronchodilator responsiveness.

Significance: A postbronchodilator improvement in wheezing indicates a reversible process such as asthma. Worsening can be seen in disorders of airway wall rigidity such as bronchomalacia or tracheomalacia. No change can be seen in situations with foreign bodies, fixed airway obstruction, as a result of significant inflammation (e.g., status asthmaticus), or as a result of airway remodeling.

• Pulmonary function testing (spirometry)

Significance: Spirometry remains the standard and most helpful measure of pulmonary function, and normative data have been described in children more than 3 years of age.

• Pulse oximetry measurement of oxygen saturation (SpO_2).

Significance: Pulse oximetry is an insensitive measure of mild to moderate respiratory difficulty during wheezing, but oxyhemoglobin saturation below 92% may be seen in severe compromise.

• Arterial blood gas (ABG)

Significance: ABGs provide a direct measure of oxygenation (PaO_2) and ventilation ($PaCO_2$) and also can help to determine severity. A normal or high normal $PaCO_2$ in a tachypneic patient, where it should be low, may be a sign of impending respiratory failure.

• Chest radiography (anterioposterior and lateral)

Significance: It should be strongly considered in all patients with new-onset wheezing or an asymmetric lung exam. It can show findings suggestive of airway obstruction (hyperinflation, hyperlucency, flattening of the diaphragms). Asymmetry in aeration on right- and left-lateral decubitus films suggests foreign body on the side having the greatest air trapping.

• Microbiologic studies.

Significance: Positive bacterial culture of sputum is helpful in directing or focusing antibiotic therapy. Positive respiratory virus screen or culture (often within 12 hours) can prevent needless antibiotic therapy, may be helpful in prognosticating future disease.

• Tuberculosis skin test—Mantoux purified protein derivative (PPD)

Significance: Tuberculosis

• Complete blood count including eosinophil count, quantitative immunoglobulins, IgE, complement, HIV testing, allergy skin testing

Emergency Care

Factors that may indicate a respiratory emergency:

• Signs of mild to moderate respiratory difficulty—tachypnea, intercostal and suprasternal retractions, nasal flaring, head bobbing and exaggerated shoulder movement during breathing, abdominal breathing and subcostal retractions, relative difficulty speaking in complete sentences, significant wheezing, prolonged exhalation, and low $PaCO_2$ in the face of tachypnea.
• Signs of impending respiratory failure—cyanosis, fatigue, inability to speak in greater than 1- to 2-word phrases, altered mental status (i.e., confusion, agitation), decreased respiratory drive, inadequate ventilation (poor air flow), no audible wheezing, high normal or rising $PaCO_2$ in the face of tachypnea or respiratory distress.
• Determine which patients require assisted ventilation (i.e., bag-mask ventilation, noninvasive [nasal] ventilation, or endotracheal intubation).
• Lack of response to aggressive albuterol therapy, without a history of asthma or recurrent wheeze, or biphasic adventitious sounds should immediately raise the suspicion of a fixed lesion.

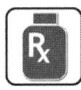

Therapy

• A trial of bronchodilator therapy (e.g., albuterol) may be both therapeutic and diagnostic of the reversible airway obstruction characteristic of asthma.
• For acute asthma exacerbation—corticosteroids PO or IV.
• In the acute setting ipratropium bromide may be helpful in reducing airway secretions and reducing airway obstruction, but of little value out of the acute setting.
• Antibiotics should be used in patients with suspected pneumonia.

Common Questions and Answers

Q: What percent of recurrent wheezing resolves by school age?
A: roughly 40% of children with one or more episodes of wheezing by 3 years clear by 6 years of age.

Q: Should chest radiographs be routinely obtained in children experiencing their first episodes of wheezing?
A: For a child with new-onset asymmetric wheezing a chest radiograph should be obtained. For a child with symmetric wheezing chest radiography will not likely be helpful and should be ordered judiciously.

Clinical Pearls

• "All that wheezes is not asthma": While most episodes of wheezing will represent viral infections or asthma, clinicians need to be mindful of alternative diagnoses. This is especially true in patients with first-time, persistent, or atypical episodes of wheezing.

The 3 "R's" of asthma:

—Recurrence: symptoms that occur multiple times with full resolution in between.
—Reactivity: symptoms that can be triggered during exposures (temperature extremes, smoke, dust, humid or dry air, aromas, etc.).
—Reversibility: symptoms that resolve with albuterol therapy.

BIBLIOGRAPHY

Bel EH. Clinical phenotypes of asthma. *Curr Opin Pulm Med* 2004;10(1):44–50.

Covar RA, Spahn JD. Treating the wheezing infant. *Pediatr Clin North Am* 2003;50(3): 631–54.

Expert Panel Report 2. Guidelines for the diagnosis and management of asthma: National Heart, Lung, and Blood Institute. National Asthma Education Program Expert Panel report NIH Publication No. 97-4051, April 1997.

Author: Hank Mayer

SECTION II
Specific Diseases

Abdominal Migraine (Epilepsy)

 Database

DEFINITION

Recurrent attacks of periumbilical pain, with nausea, vomiting, headache, pallor, perspiration, slowing of pulse rate.

PATHOLOGY

• Although nonspecific EEG changes are seen more commonly among these children, very few go on to develop signs of epilepsy. Children with abdominal migraine are more likely than controls to develop migraine headaches later in life; 10% of children who have migraine headaches are found in retrospect to have suffered from unexplained abdominal pain prior to the onset of headache. Adult migraine headache sufferers experience abdominal pain more frequently than tension headache sufferers.
• May involve neuronal activity originating in the hypothalamus with involvement of the cortex and autonomic nervous system. Serotonin is implicated, and blockade of serotonin receptors may prevent abdominal migraine.
• May involve some as yet ill-defined local intestinal vasomotor factor.

EPIDEMIOLOGY

• Mostly occurs in children between the ages of 3 and 10, peaking at about age 9
• More common in girls
• May affect as many as 1%–2% of children at some point in their lives
• Declining frequency toward adulthood

GENETICS

• Parents of affected children often have history of migraine headaches

 Differential Diagnosis

INFECTION

• *Giardia*
• Environmental: lead intoxication
• Tumors
• Metabolic: porphyria, lactose intolerance, female carriers of (X-linked) ornithine transcarbamoylase (OTC) gene mutation
• Psychosocial: functional abdominal pain/irritable bowel syndrome
• Surgical: appendicitis, intussusception, biliary colic
• Inflammation: inflammatory bowel disease, peptic ulcer disease, mesenteric adenitis
• Gastrointestinal: irritable bowel, gastroesophageal reflux, wandering spleen, cyclical vomiting, recurrent abdominal pain.
• Anatomic: Meckel diverticulum, ureteropelvic junction (UPJ) obstruction
• Miscellaneous: constipation, abdominal epilepsy—but has a shorter duration of pain (minutes), altered consciousness during event, abrupt onset, abnormal discharges in EEG in 80%

 Data Gathering

HISTORY

• Pain usually lasts less than 6 hours.
• Pain can be located anywhere in abdomen, but more often in upper quadrants.
• No abdominal pain in between attacks
• Repetition of identical abdominal crises, anywhere from one per week to several times a year
• Migraine in the history of patient or relatives
• Occasionally, presence of other migrainous syndromes such as nausea, vomiting, perspiration, body temperature changes, focal paresthesias, radiation of pain to a limb, general malaise
• Impaired consciousness—some degree of lethargy may occur

 Physical Examination

The physical examination is unremarkable, with a benign abdomen.

SPECIAL QUESTIONS

Ask about a family history of migraine headache or unexplained bouts of abdominal pain as children.

 Laboratory Aids

Test: Normal CBC, differential, sedimentation rate, urinalysis
Significance: R/O infection, i.e., urinary tract infection

Test: Stool heme test, and stool for cultures
Significance: Inflammatory bowel disease, GI causes of pain

Test: Lactose breath test
Significance: Lactose intolerance

Test: Lead test, porphyria workup (depending on situation)
Significance: Porphyria

Test: Urine organic acids, ammonia level
Significance: Underlying metabolic disorders may cause episodic vomiting.

Test: EEG
Significance: May help differentiate between abdominal migraine and abdominal epilepsy.

Test: Visual evoked response (VER) to red and white flash light
Significance: Has been shown to be helpful in diagnosing abdominal migraine, as children with clinically diagnosed abdominal migraine may display a specific fast-wave activity response compared to normal controls, or children with migraine headaches alone.

Test: Obstruction series
Significance: Intermittent or partial bowel obstruction

Test: Upper GI
Significance: To rule out anatomic abnormalities

Test: Ultrasound
Significance: To rule out tumor, chronic appendicitis, etc.

Test: Renal ultrasound
Significance: To rule out UPJ obstruction

Test: Barium enema
Significance: During painful crisis to rule out intussusception

Therapy

DRUGS

- Ergotamine, used for treatment of migraine headaches
- Serotonin receptor antagonists
- If EEG or other data point to possible epilepsy, empiric treatment with anticonvulsants may be considered and weighed against possible side effects of these agents.

PITFALLS

- Because it is usually a diagnosis of exclusion, many patients go through a large workup to rule out other causes of pain, sometimes including laparotomy.
- The medications must be given on a daily basis, as they are used in a prophylactic fashion. For the majority of patients, risks of side effects and complications from the use of these medications may outweigh the relief of pain, especially in children who are experiencing infrequent episodes.
- Even if a patient meets most criteria for abdominal migraine, various studies as outlined above should be done to ensure that a more serious disorder does not exist. Thus, abdominal migraine is a diagnosis of exclusion.

 Follow-Up

Most children outgrow abdominal migraines by early adolescence. However, a substantial percentage of them may then develop more typical migraine headaches.

 Common Questions and Answers

Q: Does this mean my child will develop migraine headaches?
A: There is an association between abdominal migraines in childhood and migraine headaches in later life. There is no good way to predict for sure whether your child will be a sufferer.

Q: I have two other younger children. What chance do they have of developing abdominal migraines?
A: Although there is a genetic tendency—i.e., abdominal migraines do tend to run in families—there is no known mendelian inheritance pattern. This is as opposed to a disease that is known to be recessive or dominant, such as cystic fibrosis, for which a probability can be given.

Q: What can I do to help my child during bouts of pain?
A: The parent should allow the child to do whatever makes him or her comfortable. This may mean rest, positioning, quiet, etc. Acetaminophen and other pain relievers may help to a certain degree. Whether the patient should be excused from school depends on various factors, such as the frequency, severity, and duration of the pain, as well as the age, maturity, and coping skills of the child.

ICD-9-CM 346.2

BIBLIOGRAPHY

Barlow CF. The periodic syndrome—cyclic vomiting and abdominal migraine. *Clin Dev Med* 1984;91:83–84.

Catto-Smith AG, Ranuh R. Abdominal migraine and cyclical vomiting. *Seminars in Pediatric Surgery* 2003;12(4):254–258.

Li BU, Balint JP. Cyclic vomiting syndrome: evolution in our understanding of a brain-gut disorder. *Advances in Pediatrics* 2000;47: 117–160.

Mortimer MJ, Kay J, Janon A, et al. Clinical epidemiology of childhood migraine in an urban general pediatric practice. *Dev Med Child Neurol* 1993;35:243–248.

Russell G, et al. Abdominal migraine: evidence for existence and treatment options. *Paediatric Drugs* 2002;4(1):1–8.

Symon DY. Abdominal migraine: a childhood syndrome defined. *Cephalalgia* 1986;6: 223–228.

Weydert JA, et al. Systematic review of treatments for recurrent abdominal pain. *Pediatrics* 2003;111(1):e1–e11.

Author: Karen Liquornik

Acetaminophen Poisoning

 Database

DEFINITION

• Acetaminophen poisoning may occur after acute or chronic overdose.
• A serum acetaminophen level above the treatment line of the Rumack-Matthew acetaminophen poisoning nomogram (p. XXX) after acute overdose should be considered possibly hepatotoxic.

PATHOPHYSIOLOGY

• The majority of absorbed acetaminophen is metabolized through formation of hepatic glucuronide and sulfate conjugates.
• Some acetaminophen is metabolized by the cytochrome P450 mixed-function oxidase system leading to the formation of the toxic N-acetyl-p-benzoquinoneimine (NAPQI).
• NAPQI is quickly detoxified by glutathione under usual circumstances.
• After overdose, glucuronidation enzyme pathways become saturated:

—Drug elimination half-life becomes prolonged
—Proportionately more NAPQI is produced
—Glutathione supply cannot meet detoxification demand
—Hepatotoxicity or renal toxicity may ensue

EPIDEMIOLOGY

• Analgesics are the most common drugs implicated in poisoning exposures among children less than 6 years of age.
• Acetaminophen preparations comprise approximately 47% of all analgesic poisoning exposures reported to poison control centers.
• Acetaminophen may be sold under many brand names, and is often an ingredient in combination pain-reliever preparations.
• Serious hepatotoxicity after single-acute overdose by young children is rare compared to adolescents.
• Most toddlers with acetaminophen hepatotoxicity suffered repeated, supratherapeutic dosing.

COMPLICATIONS

• 0–24 hours postingestion:

—Most patients will appear asymptomatic
—Anorexia, nausea, vomiting, diaphoresis may be present.
  • 24–72 hours postingestion:
—Right upper quadrant tenderness may occur
—Serum aminotransferases rise
—Liver function declines
—Renal function may decline
—May see secondary effects of hepatorenal failure
  • >72 hours–2 weeks postingestion:
—Fulminant liver failure occurs or liver failure resolves.

PROGNOSIS

• Among previously healthy children, hepatotoxicity is rare with single doses below 150 mg/kg.
• After single, acute acetaminophen overdose, likelihood of hepatotoxicity may be determined by using the Rumack-Matthew nomogram (p. XXX).
• N-acetylcysteine therapy prevents hepatic failure in greater than 99% of acetaminophen-poisoned patients if administered within 8 hours of overdose.
• Repetitive dosing of >75 mg/kg per day should be evaluated cautiously, especially in the presence of:

—Febrile illness
—Vomiting or malnourishment
—Anticonvulsant or isoniazid therapy

ASSOCIATED DISEASES

• Acetaminophen is often marketed in combination with other pharmaceuticals, which may complicate drug overdose situation.
• Adolescents frequently overdose on more than one drug preparation.

 Differential Diagnosis

• Infectious hepatitis
• Other drug-induced hepatitis

 Data Gathering

HISTORY

Question: Medical history of pain or fever?
Significance: Acetaminophen ingestion should be explored in any patient being treated for pain or fever.

Question: Amount of acetaminophen ingested?
Significance: A single, acute ingestion of less than 150 mg/kg (up to 7.5 g in adolescents) is unlikely to cause significant toxicity among otherwise healthy individuals.

Question: Timing of ingestion?
Significance: Allows application of the Rumack-Matthew nomogram.

Question: Sustained-release preparation?
Significance: Acetaminophen is now available in sustained release form.

Question: Medication list?
Significance: Use of isoniazid, or other CYP2E1 hepatic enzyme inducers may increase risk for toxicity.

 Physical Examination

Finding: Right upper quadrant tenderness
Significance: May suggest acetaminophen-induced hepatitis.

 Laboratory Aids

TESTS

Test: Serum acetaminophen level
Significance: Allows application of the Rumack-Matthew nomogram after acute overdose.

Test: Hepatic transaminases
Significance: Aspartate aminotransferase is the most sensitive of the widely available measures to assess acetaminophen hepatotoxicity. Begins to rise 12–36 hours after significant overdose.

Test: Liver and kidney function tests
Significance: As the AST rises it is important to follow liver and kidney function with tests such as serum glucose, prothrombin (PT) and partial thromboplastin (PTT) times, serum creatinine, plasma pH, and serum albumin.

Test: Salicylate level
Significance: May be a coingestant in the setting of analgesic drug overdose.

PITFALLS

• The Rumack-Matthew nomogram only applies to single, acute acetaminophen overdose scenarios.
• The PT/PTT may be slightly elevated due to direct effect of elevated blood acetaminophen concentrations or n-acetylcysteine therapy, without signifying liver injury.
• The decline of an elevated serum AST may indicate either liver recovery or profound liver failure and must be interpreted in context.

Therapy

SINGLE ACUTE OVERDOSE

- Activated charcoal, 1 g/kg (max ~ 75 g), may be administered if acetaminophen is judged to be present in the stomach or proximal intestine (usually within 2 hours of ingestion).
- N-acetylcysteine should be administered if a serum acetaminophen level obtained greater than 4 hours after overdose falls above the treatment line of the Rumack-Matthew nomogram.
- Patients presenting to medical care more than 7 hours postoverdose should be given a loading dose of n-acetylcysteine while waiting for the serum acetaminophen level.
- The oral n-acetylcysteine dose is 140 mg/kg loading dose, followed by 70 mg/kg maintenance doses every 4 hours for 17 additional doses (see Common Questions and Answers).
- In the presence of clinical liver injury, n-acetylcysteine therapy should be continued until liver recovery occurs.

REPEATED SUPRATHERAPEUTIC INGESTION

- Consider n-acetylcysteine therapy if:

—Ingestion of greater than 75 mg/kg or 7.5 g per day for consecutive days
—Patient is symptomatic
—AST is elevated
—Acetaminophen level is higher than would be expected given dosing and AST is normal.

- Consider the asymptomatic patient to be at minimal risk if AST is normal and serum acetaminophen is undetectable.

 ## Follow-Up

- Liver transplant should be considered for patients with:

—pH <7.30 after resuscitation, or
—PT >1.8 X control, plus
—Serum creatinine >3.3 mg/dL, plus
—Encephalopathy.

- Drug administration education should be offered to victims of chronic overdose.
- Home safety education should be provided after pediatric exploratory ingestions.
- Mental health services should be provided to victims of intentional overdose.

PITFALLS

- N-acetylcysteine therapy is less efficacious when administered greater than 8 hours after overdose, but should still be offered.
- Acetaminophen poisoning and n-acetylcysteine therapy are emetogenic.

—Chill and cover the n-acetylcysteine.
—Consider antiemetic therapy with drugs such as metoclopramide and/or ondansetron.
—N-acetylcysteine may be given slowly via nasogastric or nasoduodenal tube.

 ## Common Questions and Answers

Q: What is "short course" n-acetylcysteine (NAC) therapy?
A: The toxic NAPQI metabolite has a short biologic half-life. Some suggest that those patients with a nondetectable serum acetaminophen level paired with a normal AST 24 hours after ingestion do not need any further antidotal therapy.

Q: Can NAC be given intravenously?
A: This has been the standard-of-care in parts of Canada and Europe for years. In 2004, the United States Food and Drug Administration approved an intravenous form of NAC for use in adults. The oral form of NAC has been used orally, "off-label," in the United States with good success—guidance may be obtained from your regional poison control center (1–800–222–1222). The major complication of intravenous NAC therapy is the infrequent occurrence of an anaphylactoid-type systemic response.

BIBLIOGRAPHY

American Academy of Pediatrics. Committee on Drugs. Acetaminophen toxicity in children. *Pediatrics* 2001;108:1020–1024.

Bizovi KE, Smilkstein MJ. Acetaminophen. In: Goldfrank LR, Flomenbaum NE, Lewin NA, et al., eds. *Goldfrank's Toxicologic Emergencies*, 7th Ed. New York: McGraw-Hill, 2002: 480–501.

Kozer E, Koren G. Management of paracetamol overdose: current controversies. *Drug Safety* 2001;24:503–512.

Author: Kevin C. Osterhoudt

Acne

Database

DEFINITION

• Acne is a common disorder of the pilosebaceous units (pilosebaceous follicles and sebaceous glands) characterized by comedones and inflammation.
• Diagnosis includes:
—Acne vulgaris–common onset adolescence to early 20s; cosmetic or "pomade" acne
—Neonatal acne—common in first month of life, usually mild and only on face, caused by activation of neonatal sebaceous glands or follicles by maternal hormones
—Infantile acne—now considered different from neonatal acne. Acne is much less common in older infants, although occasionally preceded by persistent or progressive neonatal acne. Sebaceous glands or follicles are activated by a surge of intrinsic adrenal hormones to produce acne in the infant. Severe, persistent acne in infants associated with accelerated linear growth may be associated with an endocrinopathy and justifies referral for further endocrinologic evaluation.
—Acne conglobata—numerous deep, coalescing inflammatory nodules, cysts, often with sinus tracks on face and trunk, most common type of intense inflammatory acne.
—Pyoderma faciale—numerous large pustules and nodular furuncles
—Acne fulminans—rare, associated with fever, arthralgias, leukocytosis, and inflammatory bone lesions

Manifestations of acne range from mild to severe:
• Mild: comedones, occasional papules, may include focal inflammation
• Moderate: inflammatory lesions, comedones, papules, and pustules
• Severe: generalized and inflammatory nodulocystic acne

PATHOPHYSIOLOGY

Primary Cause

• Excessive sebum production by active sebaceous gland activity caused by androgen production (initially by adrenal glands or prepubertal adrenarche, then by the gonads or pubertal adrenarche). Sebum, dead skin cells and bacteria plug hair follicle, creating acne lesion or "pimple."

Other Contributing Causes

• *Propionibacterium acnes* (common skin anaerobe)—proliferates in excess sebum and follicular cell mixture
• Linoleic acid deficiency—increases surface epithelial desquamation
• Hormonal factors associated with
—Emotional stress:
—Menstruation is a topic of current research, as narrowing of sebaceous duct orifices during the midcycle has been observed. This contributes to sebaceous duct obstruction and blockage of sebum flow, and can result in comedone formation. In the presence of *P. acnes*

colonization, this further contribution to "flare ups" of premenstrual acne is well documented.
—Polycystic ovary disease is associated with pathologically elevated levels of dehydroepiandrosterone sulfate (DHEAS). Elevated androgens are implicated in increased sebum production, contributing to acne formation. Abnormally high levels of circulating androgens levels are found in females with severe acne or signs of virilization, and may also be elevated in females with milder acne and no overt evidence of virilization. Other females with mild acne and normal androgen levels may have increased end-organ responsiveness to androgen stimulation
• Comedogenic (pore clogging) cosmetics, creams, cocoa butter, pomades (especially those not designated "noncomedogenic") can physically obstruct pilosebaceous units (hair follicles and sebaceous glands, which are most numerous on the face, back, and upper chest
• Certain drugs cause acne. These include corticosteroids, adrenocorticotropic hormone (ACTH), androgens, iodides, phenytoin, bromides, isoniazid, lithium, halothane, rifampin, and others. Corticosteroids (systemic and topical) appear to sensitize the follicular epithelium to sebum comedogenesis. Steroid acne begins as red papules, succeeded by closed comedones, and later by open comedones. All 3 stages of lesions may be evident in chronic steroid acne.
• Environmental factors—prolonged work over fat cookers has been implicated in comedogenesis, as have mechanical trauma due to occlusive or tight clothing and behavioral habits (rubbing, stroking, squeezing the skin). Very humid environments and heavy sweating can cause keratin hydration and lead to swelling and obstruction of sebaceous ducts.

COMPLICATIONS

• Loss of self-esteem
• Embarrassment
• Overt behavioral and psychiatric pathology, including depression
• Potential keloid formation
• Permanent scarring, associated with nodulocystic acne
• Secondary infection, especially prevalent with concomitant eczema, folliculitis, poor hygiene, and skin picking
• SAPHO syndrome—recently reported, uncommon syndrome of synovitis, acne, pustulosis, hyperostosis, and osteomyelitis, associated with acne fulminans, acne conglobata, pustular psoriasis, and other severe skin conditions

PROGNOSIS

• Mild acne papules ("zits" or "pimples") may resolve in 5 to 7 days.
• Major improvement usually noted 2–4 weeks with effective treatment.
• Improves/resolves in >90% of individuals with proper care/treatment
• Severe scarring, keloid formation in fewer than 10% of patients with cystic acne, may justify steroid injection, dermabrasion or carbon dioxide laser ablation, and/or plastic surgery.

Differential Diagnosis

• Steroid folliculitis
• Periorofacial dermatitis
• Rosacea

Data Gathering

HISTORY

Question: Age of onset?
Significance: Average age of onset is 11 years (or Tanner stage II) in both sexes.

Question: Current skin care?
Significance: Comedogenic cosmetics, moisturizers, sunscreens, soaps, and abrasive cleansers may worsen acne.

Question: Noted provocative factors?
Significance: Provocative factors include stress, menstrual cycle, occupational exposures, head or facial gear (including ball caps, 'do rags, helmets), allergies, contact irritants.

Question: Past or current use of over-the-counter (OTC) or prescriptive medications for acne?

Question: Any other medications or drugs, prescriptive and nonprescriptive?
Significance: Steroids, phenytoin, other medications with androgenic side effects, may contribute.

Question: Any evidence for androgenic/hormonal disorder (amenorrhea, hirsutism, obesity)?

Question: Extent of concern with appearance?

Physical Examination

• Determine types, location, numbers and types of acne lesions present.
• Classify with respect to severity level, including scarring, hypopigmentation or hyperpigmentation.
• Document or use skin map to record details in the patient's record.
• Note any signs of hirsutism, striae, obesity.

Laboratory Aids

Laboratory or serologic tests are not routinely necessary or recommended for adolescents and young adults with acne.

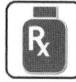

Therapy

Patient education: Dispel common myths about acne:
• Acne is not caused by dirt, lack of scrubbing the skin, too much chocolate, diet, too much or too little sex or masturbation.

• Medically indicated, prescribed antibiotics do not permanently impair the immune system (including long-term tetracyclines). However, resistant strains of *P. acnes* may be attributable to long-term treatment with oral or topical antibiotics. Changing or suspending use of antibiotic is recommended if decreased response to a previously effective antibiotic therapy is observed. Resumption of original antibiotic therapy after a few weeks suspension or changing to an alternate antibiotic, if needed, should be considered.

• Accutane (isotretinoin) is not warranted for every teenager with acne, and can have major side effects.

MILD ACNE (COMEDONES, PAPULES, FOCAL INFLAMMATION)

• General skin care: wash gently with nonabrasive, noncomedogenic soap 1–2 times per day. Harsh scrubbing may increase inflammation. Occasional/once daily astringent or alcohol pads may help remove excess oil or makeup without necessity of repeated washing. Use noncomedogenic cosmetics, if any.

• Add benzoyl peroxide (BP) gel 0.025% (bactericidal) or wash (5%) or tretinoin (Retin-A) 0.025–0.05% cream (topical retinoid) at bedtime, at least 20 minutes after washing.

Moderate acne (comedones, papules, pustules, local inflammation)

• General skin care
• BP 5% gel in the morning and 0.025% tretinoin (Retin-A) gel at bedtime
• Add topical antibiotics (BP combination with topical clindamycin) 1–2 times per day if any inflammation present.

Severe acne (comedones, pustules, plus nodular and cystic lesions)

• General skin care
• BP with clindamycin gel 1–2 times per day
• Tretinoin (Retin-A) 0.025–0.05% cream or 0.025% gel at bedtime
• Systemic antibiotics (e.g., tetracycline 500–1,000 mg b.i.d. or minocycline HCl, doxycycline, or erythromycin of recommended equivalent dose)

TOPICAL MEDICATIONS primarily work either as bactericidals and/or drying agents for the skin. (As noted, cytokine research shows that topical retinoids may block the cytokine pathway toward inflammation.)

• Benzoyl peroxide (bactericidal)—is drying and also synergistic with retinoids
• Clindamycin and erythromycin topicals—equally effective, although less bacterial resistance to clindamycin.
• Tretinoin (topical retinoid, vitamin A derivative)—photosensitizer, increases sunburn risk, drying. Gel formulation more drying and potent than cream or lotion formulation
• Adapalene gel 0.1% (Differin), a synthetic derivative of naphthoic acid with retinoid-like activity. Has comedolytic and antiinflammatory effects and reportedly better efficacy than Retin-A gel 0.025%. Less irritating than more familiar retinoids.

• Tazoretene (Tazorac) 0.05%, 0.1% gel newer retinoid-like compound
• Azeleic acid (Azelex) 20% cream, a dicarboxylic acid, FDA (Food and Drug Administration) as a topical treatment for acne, has antikeratinizing and antimicrobial properties and fewer side effects than other topicals; use b.i.d. instead of benzoyl peroxide and tretinoin, if scars or pustules are hyperpigmented, or if BP and retinoids are too irritating.

SURGICAL TREATMENT OPTIONS are generally reserved for dermatology specialists or plastic surgeons.

SYSTEMIC MEDICATIONS

ANTIMICROBIALS prevent and/or decrease colonization by *P. acnes* to eliminate inflammation in acne.

• Tetracycline—Dose: 250–500 mg q.d.–b.i.d. for age >8 years of age
• Minocycline for >8 years of age. Dose: 50–100 mg q.d.–b.i.d.
• Doxycycline—for >8 years of age. Dose: 50–100 mg q.d.–b.i.d.
• Erythromycin—Dose: 250–500 mg q.d.–b.i.d.; common GI upset, drug interactions with tegretol, digoxin, theophylline, terfenadine, others.

HORMONE PREPARATIONS work primarily by decreasing or modulating cyclic androgen level effects on acne provocation.

• Oral Contraceptives (OCPs): Low androgen-progestin component OCPs, such as Ortho Tri-Cyclen, approved by FDA for treatment of moderate acne in >15-year-old females. Prescriptive use and dose schedule recommended in consultation with gynecologist or adolescent medicine specialist.
• Spironolactone—oral, an effective androgen blocker at 50–200 mg per day dose. Common side effects—breast tenderness, menstrual irregularities, and hyperkalemia.

ORAL RETINOID

• Isotretinoin (Accutane): is reserved for treatment of severe, recalcitrant nodular acne, unresponsive to conventional therapy (including systemic antibiotics). Prescriptive recommendation of accutane should be restricted to dermatologists and/or to health care providers who have received intensive training and certification in its use. A single course of 15 to 20 weeks of accutane therapy effectively results in complete, prolonged remission in most patients with severe acne that has been unresponsive to conventional treatment. Recurrent acne develops within 3 years of initial isotretinoin treatment in the vast majority of patients. If indicated, a second course can be initiated no sooner than 8 weeks after completion of the 1st course of therapy. Successful isotretinoin treatment of acne reportedly results in normalization of linoleic acid levels in epidermal lipids. Isotretinoin is known to have numerous side effects, including hyperlipidemia, hearing impairment, hepatotoxicity, inflammatory bowel disease, vision impairment, arthralgias,

osteoporosis, acute pancreatitis, pseudotumor cerebri, depression, psychosis, and behavioral disorders. Of greatest concern is the extremely high risk for severe and potentially fatal birth defects in fetuses exposed to accutane in utero. Accutane must not be used by pregnant females. Less commonly, isotretinoin has been implicated in the causation of disseminated interstitial skeletal hyperostosis.

Follow-Up

• Patients with moderate acne requiring antibiotic treatment should initially be seen in 2 to 4 weeks, then at least every 3 to 4 months.
• Patients with keloids or scarring acne should be referred for dermatologic consultation.
• Encourage good daily skin care, and washing face and involved skin with a mild noncomedogenic soap (Cetaphil, Neutrogena) 1 to 2 times per day.
• Discourage harsh scrubbing of skin or frequent application of alcohol or astringents.
• Avoid comedogenic cosmetics, moisturizers, sun lotions, cocoa butter, oily hair and skin products.
• Avoid wearing hair on face, sweat bands, hats, or caps with forehead contact.
• Avoid picking or squeezing lesions, which may result in scarring.

Common Questions and Answers

Q: What's the best medication to use for mild acne?
A: Benzoyl peroxide gel and/or tretinoin (Retin-A) used nightly or on alternate nights, if skin is especially dry.

Q: Does chocolate cause acne?
A: No, diet is not thought to affect acne. Prolonged food preparation over hot grease can be comedogenic, as can topical application of cocoa butter and other comedogenic topical cosmetic products.

BIBLIOGRAPHY

Fagundes DS, et al. New therapy update—a unique combination formulation in the treatment of inflammatory acne. *Cutis* 2003;72:16–19.

Krowchuk DP, Lucky AW. Managing adolescent acne. *Adolesc Med* 2001;12:355–374.

Brown SK, Shalita AR. Acne vulgaris. *Lancet* 1998;351:1871–1876.

National Institute of Arthritis and Musculoskeletal and Skin Diseases. Questions and answers about acne. 2001, NIH publ. # 01-4998, 1–10.

Strasburger VC. Acne: what every pediatrician should know about treatment. *Pediatr Clin North Am* 1997;44:1505–1523.

Author: Lucy S. Crain

Acquired Hypothyroidism

 ## Database

DEFINITION

Hypothyroidism that occurs after the neonatal period.

PATHOPHYSIOLOGY

- There are myriad causes (see Differential Diagnosis).
- Decreased synthesis or release of thyroid hormone can result from thyroid gland dysfunction (primary hypothyroidism) or from pituitary/hypothalamic dysfunction leading to understimulation of the thyroid gland (secondary and tertiary hypothyroidism).

GENETICS

- A genetic predisposition exists in patients with chronic lymphocytic thyroiditis (CLT), the most common cause of acquired thyroiditis in nonendemic areas; 30% to 40% of patients have a family history of thyroid disease, and up to 50% of their first-degree relatives have thyroid antibodies.
- Associations of CLT with certain human leukocyte antigen (HLA) haplotypes are weak and not consistently reproducible.
- Autoimmune thyroid disease may be part of Schmidt syndrome (type II polyglandular autoimmune disease), which also involves Addison disease and type 1 diabetes mellitus. This incompletely penetrant autosomal-dominant disorder demonstrates stronger HLA linkage.
- Genetic syndromes associated with higher incidence of autoimmune thyroiditis:

—Down syndrome
—Turner syndrome (especially those with isochromosome Xq)

EPIDEMIOLOGY

- May develop at any age.
- CLT prevalence correlates with iodine intake, such that countries as the United States and Japan with the highest dietary iodine also have the highest CLT prevalence. Experiments with T cells from CLT patients and with NOD-H_2(h4) mice, a model for autoimmune thyroiditis, suggest that iodine increases the autoantigenicity of thyroglobulin.
- Autoimmune thyroid disorders occur more frequently in children and adolescents with type 1 diabetes mellitus.

COMPLICATIONS

- The most significant complication during childhood is impaired linear growth.
- Puberty can also be affected.
- Myxedema coma may occur.
- Encephalopathy of varied clinical presentation has been associated with high titers of thyroid antibodies, especially antimicrosomal, and responds well to corticosteroid treatment.

 ## Differential Diagnosis

IMMUNOLOGIC

- Chronic lymphocytic thyroiditis (often referred to as Hashimoto thyroiditis)
- Autoimmune polyendocrine syndrome (Schmidt syndrome)

INFECTIOUS

- Postviral subacute thyroiditis
- Associated with congenital infections

—Rubella
—Toxoplasmosis

ENVIRONMENTAL

- Goitrogen ingestion

—Iodides
—Expectorants
—Thioureas

IATROGENIC

- Following surgical thyroidectomy for thyroid cancer, hyperthyroidism, or extensive neck tumors.
- Following radioiodine ablative therapy for hyperthyroidism or thyroid cancer.
- Following irradiation to the head or neck for cancer treatment.
- Medications: lithium, amiodarone, iodine contrast dyes, tiratricol (an over-the-counter fat loss supplement).

METABOLIC

- Cystinosis
- Histiocytosis X

CONGENITAL

- Late-onset congenital-large ectopic gland

GENETIC SYNDROMES

- Down syndrome
- Turner syndrome

SECONDARY OR TERTIARY HYPOTHYROIDISM

- Hypothalamic or pituitary disease

CONSUMPTIVE HYPOTHYROIDISM

- Due to increased type 3 iodothyronine deiodinase activity in hemangiomas.

 ## Data Gathering

HISTORY

Question: Growth pattern?
Significance: Linear growth failure can be the first sign of thyroid dysfunction.

Question: Declining school performance?
Significance: Sensitive marker for lethargy and reduced focusing.

SYMPTOMS

Question: Any symptoms of hypothyroidism and their duration?
Significance: Early primary hypothyroidism can be asymptomatic. The presence of hypothyroid-related symptoms indicates progression from compensated to uncompensated hypothyroidism.

Question: Notice any thyroid gland enlargement? Its duration? Tenderness?
Significance: Goiter may be the presenting sign of acquired hypothyroidism. Tenderness suggests an infectious process.

Question: Any past medical history factors associated with hypothyroidism (e.g., genetic syndromes, radiation exposure, medications, history of diabetes)?
Significance: Any of these factors should raise the concern for possible acquired hypothyroidism.

Question: Family history of thyroid disease (hyper or hypo) or other autoimmune endocrinopathies
Significance: Family history of thyroid disease or other autoimmune endocrinopathies increases the risk of developing autoimmune thyroid disease.

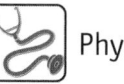 ## Physical Examination

Finding: Bradycardia
Significance: Thyroid hormone has cardiac effects.

Finding: Short stature (or fall-off on growth curve), and increased upper/lower segment ratio
Significance: Euthyroidism is required to maintain normal growth.

Finding: Goiter: note consistency, symmetry, nodularity, signs of inflammation
Significance: Goiter characteristics may give a clue regarding the cause of the hypothyroidism and provide a clinical marker to follow during therapy.

Finding: Myxedema (water retention)
Significance: Myxedema is not limited to the subcutaneous tissue. It may also lead to cardiac failure, pleural effusions, and coma.

Finding: Muscle hypertrophy, yet muscle weakness most obvious in arms, legs, and tongue.
Significance: Hypothyroidism causes disordered muscle function.

Finding: Delayed relaxation phase of deep tendon reflexes
Significance: Due to slowed muscle contraction, not a change in the transmission rate of the nervous impulse.

Finding: Pale, cool, dry, carotenemic skin
Significance: Due to decreased cell turnover.

Finding: Increase in lanugo hair
Significance: Can be seen in children with hypothyroidism and reversed with treatment.

SPECIAL QUESTIONS

Sexual development is an important factor because hypothyroidism can be associated with delayed puberty (due to low thyroid hormone level) as well as precocious puberty and galactorrhea (due to elevated TSH).

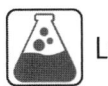 Laboratory Aids

TESTS

Test: T4 (low) and TSH (elevated)
Significance: Elevated TSH with normal T4 represents a state of compensated primary hypothyroidism.

Test: Free T4
Significance: The most sensitive marker for secondary/tertiary hypothyroidism (in which case, TSH elevation is lost and total T4 may still be in the low end of the normal range).

Test: Antithyroglobulin and antimicrosomal (antiperoxidase) antibodies
Significance: Markers for CLT.

IMAGING

Test: Head MRI
Significance: Suspected secondary/tertiary hypothyroidism; pituitary or hypothalamic lesion

The following conditions may test false-positive for acquired hypothyroidism:

Test: Thyroid-binding globulin deficiency
Significance: Low total T4, but normal free T4 and TSH

Test: Peripheral resistance to thyroid hormone
Significance: Normal/high total T4

Test: "Euthyroid sick" syndrome
Significance: Low T4 and T3; normal/low TSH; increased shunting to reverse T3

The following tests may be affected in acquired hypothyroidism:

Test: Serum creatinine
Significance: Elevated due to reduced glomerular filtration rate from the hypodynamic state of hypothyroidism

Test: Low density lipoprotein (LDL) cholesterol level
Significance: Elevated due to decreased LDL receptor expression

Test: Creatine kinase
Significance: Increased; hypothyroidism is a rare cause of rhabdomyolysis

 Therapy

l-THYROXINE (SYNTHETIC THYROID HORMONE) REPLACEMENT

- Indicated for the treatment of overt or compensated hypothyroidism.
- 2 to 5 μg/kg/d po, once daily
- Monitor T4 and TSH and titrate dose to maintain normalized TFTs.
- Duration of therapy

—Lifetime
—30% of children with CLT will undergo spontaneous remission, and reassessment of need for treatment can be done after growth is completed.

 Follow-Up

CHANGES IN TFTS

- Whenever starting medication or adjusting dose, check T4 and TSH 4 to 6 weeks later, to assess adequacy of the new dose.

WHEN TO EXPECT IMPROVEMENT

- Treated patients often resume growth at a rate greater than normal (catch-up growth).
- Other signs and symptoms resolve at a variable rate.
- Goiters in CLT may not completely regress with treatment (enlargement due to persistent inflammation does not correct, though TSH-mediated hypertrophy will).

SIGNS TO WATCH FOR TO INDICATE PROBLEMS

- Monitor response to treatment by measuring T4 and TSH levels to ensure compliance.

PROGNOSIS

- If patients are compliant, prognosis is excellent.
- In children in whom treatment has been delayed, catch-up growth may not fully normalize height to predicted values.

 Common Questions and Answers

Q: What happens if my child forgets a dose?
A: Give the dose as soon as you remember. If it is the next day, give two doses.

Q: How long will my child have to take these pills?
A: Probably for life.

Q: Are there any side effects from the medication?
A: No. The medication contains only the hormone that your child's thyroid gland is not making. The hormone is made synthetically, so there is also no infectious risk.

Q: If my child takes twice the dose, will his or her growth catch up faster?

A: Your child may grow a little faster but will also have adverse effects from having too much thyroid hormone.

Q: Does the medication have to be taken at any particular time of day?
A: No, but consistently choosing the same time of day helps to remember taking it. Do not take simultaneously with soy products or raloxifene (an antiestrogen medication) because they can cause malabsorption of levothyroxine.

Q: What if my child needs surgery?
A: Treatment of hypothyroidism such that the patient is euthyroid (normal thyroid status) prior to surgery is preferable whenever possible (only exception is ischemic heart disease requiring surgery). "Euthyroid sick" syndrome, which is common in very ill patients, should not be treated.

ICD-9-CM 244.9

BIBLIOGRAPHY

Ai J, et al. Autoimmune thyroid diseases: etiology, pathogenesis, and dermatologic manifestations. *J Amer Acad Dermatol* 2003;48:641–659.

Barbesino G, Chiovato L. The genetics of Hashimoto's disease. *Endocrinol Metab Clin North Am* 2000;29:357–374.

Betterle C, Volpato M, Greggio AN, et al. Type 2 polyglandular autoimmune disease (Schmidt syndrome). *J Pediatr Endocrinol Metab* 1996;(9 Suppl 1):113–123.

Hunter I, Greene SA, MacDonald TM, et al. Prevalence and aetiology of hypothyroidism in the young. *Arch Dis Child* 2000;83:207–210.

Pearce EN, et al. Thyroiditis. [erratum appears in *N Engl J Med.* 2003;349:620]. *New Engl J Med* 2003;348:2646–2655.

Ranke MB. Catch-up growth: new lessons for the clinician. *J Pediatr Endocrinol Metab* 2002;15(Suppl 5):1257–1266.

Roldan MB, Alonso M, Barrio R. Thyroid autoimmunity in children and adolescents with Type 1 diabetes mellitus. *Diabetes Nutr Metab Clin Exp* 1999;12:27–31.

Schmiegelow M, et al. A population-based study of thyroid function after radiotherapy and chemotherapy for a childhood brain tumor. *J Clin Endocrinol Metab* 2003;88:136–140.

Stathatos N, et al. Perioperative management of patients with hypothyroidism. *Endocrinol Metab Clin N Amer* 2003;32:503–518.

Surks MI, et al. Subclinical thyroid disease: scientific review and guidelines for diagnosis and management. *JAMA* 2004;291:228–238.

Vasconcellos E, Pina-Garza JE, Fakhoury T, et al. Pediatric manifestations of Hashimoto's encephalopathy. *Pediatr Neurol* 1999;20(5): 394–398.

Weber G, et al. Thyroid function and puberty. *J Pediatr Endocrinol Metab* 2003;16 (Suppl 2):253–257.

Authors: Adda Grimberg

Acute Lymphoblastic Leukemia

 ## Database

DEFINITION

Acute lymphoblastic leukemia (ALL) is a malignant disorder of lymphoblasts occurring as a result of indefinite clonal proliferation of a single lymphoblast that has undergone malignant transformation. This lymphoblastic clonal proliferation leads to overgrowth and the crowding out of normal bone marrow precursors, invasion of nonhematopoietic tissues, and suppression of differentiation of normal cells causing ineffective hematopoiesis.

CAUSES

• Unknown

Following factors have been associated:

• Genetic predisposition

—Identical twins
—Trisomy 21 (Down syndrome)
—Ataxia telangectasia
—Bloom syndrome
—Wiscott-Aldrich syndrome
—Congenital hypogammaglobulinemia

• Immunodeficiencies

—Prolonged immunosuppressive therapy is related to lymphoid malignancies
—Exposure to ionizing radiation (not diagnostic x-rays)
—Chemical exposure

EPIDEMIOLOGY

• Acute leukemia is the most common cancer of childhood
• Incidence of ALL is 1/1700 in children under the age of 15 years
• 75% to 80% of acute leukemia in childhood is ALL
• Peak incidence occurs between 2 and 5 years of age
• More common in whites and boys
• Other risk factors include in utero x-ray exposure and therapeutic postnatal radiation

COMPLICATIONS

Due to disease:

• Hyperleukocytosis (WBC >400,000): can lead to stroke
• Mediastinal mass (usually T-cell lineage): can lead to cardiorespiratory arrest
• Tumor lysis syndrome: can lead to renal failure, cardiac arrhythmias
• Coagulopathy: can lead to stroke and hemorrhage
• Severe anemia: can lead to CHF
• Hypercalcemia: can lead to renal failure, cardiorespiratory arrest
• Febrile neutropenia can lead to infections, shock, sepsis

Due to therapy:

• Cranial radiation (XRT)

—Brain tumors: Leukoencephalopathy and deterioration of intellectual functions/learning deficits
—Growth retardation: Decreased bone density

• Vincristine (VCR)
—Syndrome of inappropriate antidiuretic hormone—Footdrop (reversible)
—Hair loss

• L-asparaginase
—Pancreatitis
—Coagulopathy leading to cerebral infarcts or thrombosis

• Adriamycin/Doxorubicin/Daunorubicin
—Cardiac toxicity

• Cyclophosphamide
—Hemorrhagic cystitis
—Sterility

• Methotrexate (MTX)
—Hepatotoxicity

PROGNOSIS

• Remission induction in all risk categories with presently available therapy is 95%.
• Long-term survival overall approaches 80%
• Long-term survival in standard risk group is about 85% (>5 years after completion of therapy) and slightly higher for girls than for boys.
• Long-term survival in high-risk group is about 60% to 65%.

GENETICS

Increased risk of leukemia with:

• Trisomy 21 (up to 15% risk), Fanconi anemia, Bloom syndrome, Ataxia telangiectasia, Klinefelter syndrome, Schwachmann Diamond syndrome, Neurofibromatosis
• Congenital immunodeficiencies, e.g., Wiscott-Aldrich Syndrome
• 25% risk of ALL in monozygotic twin if one twin develops ALL before 5 years of age
• 2- to 4-fold higher risk in siblings than in general population

 ## Differential Diagnosis

NONMALIGNANT CONDITIONS

• Juvenile rheumatoid arthritis
• Infectious mononucleosis
• Acute infectious lymphocytosis
• Idiopathic thrombocytopenic purpura
• Pertussis and parapertussis
• Aplastic anemia

MALIGNANT CONDITIONS

• Neuroblastoma with bone marrow involvement
• Lymphoma with bone marrow involvement
• Rhabdomyosarcoma
• Retinoblastoma
• Acute myeloid leukemia

 ## Data Gathering

HISTORY

Question: Bleeding (cutaneous and mucosal); easy bruising; petichiae?
Significance: Low platelet count, coagulopathy

Question: Bone pains; arthralgia, limp?
Significance: Infiltrative disease of marrow

Question: Fatigue and pallor?
Significance: Anemia

Question: Stridor, orthopnea, shortness of breath, any respiratory distress?
Significance: Mediastinal mass, pleural effusion

Question: Oliguria, anuria?
Significance: Renal failure most likely from tumor lysis syndrome

Question: Ocular pain; blurred vision; photophobia?
Significance: Leukemia infiltration of orbit, optic nerve, retina, iris, cornea, or conjunctiva

Question: Headache, vomiting, seizures?
Significance: Leukemia infiltration of CNS

Physical Examination

Finding: Pallor
Significance: Anemia

Finding: Lymphadenopathy (generalized)
Significance: Infiltration with leukemia

Finding: Hepatosplenomegaly
Significance: Infiltration with leukemia

Finding: Sternal tenderness/bone tenderness
Significance: Bone marrow infiltration

Finding: Petechiae and purpura, subconjunctival and retinal hemorrhages
Significance: Thrombocytopenia

Finding: Hypopyon (layering of leukemia cells in anterior chamber of eye)
Significance: Leukemic infiltrate into eye

Finding: Painless testicular enlargement in boys
Significance: Testicular infiltration

Finding: Papilledema in CNS leukemia
Significance: Meningeal infiltration

Finding: Swelling of the face, orthopnea
Significance: Superior venacaval syndrome in presence of mediastinal mass

Finding: Subcutaneous nodules (leukemia cutis)
Significance: Leukemic infiltration of skin

Finding: Extremity weakness; numbness or tingling
Significance: Spinal cord compression

Laboratory Aids

Test: CBC
Significance: Increased white blood count
>10,000/mm³ in 50% of cases
>50,000/mm³ in 20% of cases

Neutropenia (<500/mm³) common
Hb <10 g/dL in 80% of cases
Thrombocytopenia (<100,000/mm³) in 75% of cases
Peripheral smear may show characteristic leukemic lymphoblasts

Test: Bone marrow aspirate
Significance: >25% leukemic lymphoblasts is diagnostic

Test: Immunophenotyping and cytogenetic studies on bone marrow aspirate
Significance: Diagnostic and prognostic

Test: Biochemical abnormalities
Significance: Tumor lysis syndrome
—Hyperuricemia, hyperphosphatemia, hypocalcemia, hyperkalemia, increased uric acid
—Slight abnormality of liver function tests due to leukemic infiltrate

Test: Chest x-ray
Significance: 5% to 10% cases have mediastinal mass

Test: CSF examination with lymphoblasts
Significance: CNS leukemia (5% at diagnosis)

PROGNOSTIC FACTORS

• Patients with any of the following criteria are at high risk for relapse and thus require more intensive therapy.

—Age <1 year or >10 years of age
—WBC count >50,000/mm³
—Translocations-t (9;22), t (4;11), t (1;19)
—Hypodiploidy (<46 chromosomes or DI <1.16 by karyotype)

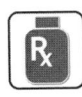 Emergency Care

• Hyperleukocytosis
• Spinal cord compression
• Mediastinal mass

 Therapy

• Stratified according to risk groups
• Risk assessment based on clinical features (age and initial WBC at time of diagnosis), biologic characteristics of lymphoblasts and bone marrow response to initial therapy.

—Low risk: triple trisomies 4,10,17 or t(12;21) (TEL/AML1) and age 1 to 10 years old; WBC <50,000 at diagnosis
—Standard risk: age 1 to 10 years old; WBC <50,000 at diagnosis; karyotype does not have t(9;22), t(4;11) regardless of age or WBC

—High risk: age 1 to 10 years old with WBC ≥50,000; age <1 or >10 years old regardless of WBC or karyotype;
—Very high risk: karyotype t(9;22), t(4;11) regardless of age or WBC; extreme hypodiploidy (<45 chromosomes or DI <0.81); failed induction therapy

• High-risk group refers to the high risk for failure of remission induction with standard therapy, and so this group of patients receives more intensive therapy
• Overall, there are four phases of therapy

—Induction
—Consolidation
—Delayed intensification
—Maintenance

• Induction: To achieve remission (<5% blasts in bone marrow)

—Vincristine
—Glucocorticoid steroids (Prednisone or dexamethasone)
—L-asparaginase
—Doxorubicin or daunorubicin
—Intrathecal methotrexate

• Consolidation and CNS prophylaxis: To prevent CNS disease

—Intrathecal MTX along with oral 6-mercaptopurine (6MP) and MTX
—Intrathecal MTX along with cranial radiation (1800 cGy), oral 6MP and MTX for slow early responders (>25% lymphblasts in bone marrow on d28 of induction)

• Delayed Intensification (one or two): To further decrease leukemic burden

—VCR
—Glucocorticoid steroids (Prednisone or dexamethasone)
—L-asparaginase
—Doxorubicin
—Cyclophosphamide
—Cytosine arabinoside (ARA-C)
—6 thioguanine (6TG)
—Intrathecal MTX

• Maintenance

—Treat for 2.5 years for girls and 3 years for boys
—Daily oral 6MP
—Weekly MTX and monthly pulses of VCR and glucocorticoid steroids
—Intrathecal MTX every 3 months

• CNS leukemia at diagnosis

—Cranial radiation (2,400 cGy)
—Triple intrathecal (MTX, ARA-C, Hydrocortisone), in addition to therapy above.

 Follow-Up

CBC every month for first year and then every 3 months for second year, then every 6 months for 5 years. Liver and renal function tests every 3 to 6 months. Cardiac evaluation yearly. Endocrine evaluation in children close to puberty.

• RELAPSE—reappearance of leukemia cells at any site in the body

—Responsiveness of recurrent ALL to therapy depends on duration of first remission (prognosis for early bone marrow relapse and for late bone marrow relapse is 10%–20% and 30%–40%, respectively)
—Most relapses occur during treatment or within the first 2 years after completion of therapy, but some initial relapses can occur >10 years after diagnosis
—Most common sites of relapse are bone marrow, CNS, testis

• Bone marrow relapse

—May present with anemia, leukocytosis, leukopenia, thrombocytopenia, hepatosplenomegaly, bone pain, fever, or sudden decrease in tolerance to chemotherapy
—Bone marrow relapse with or without extramedullary involvement usually points to poor clinical outcome

• Extramedullary relapse (CNS, testis)

—Patients who initially present with high WBC, t(9;22) karyotype, or CNS leukemia have a increased risk of CNS relapse

Common Questions and Answers

Q: Can the child on treatment for ALL go to school?
A: Yes.

Q: Will the hair fall out and child be sick for all 3 years on chemotherapy?
A: The hair usually falls out within a few weeks of initiating therapy and remains with alopecia for first 6 to 8 months and grows back once maintenance therapy begins. Most children feel well during the maintenance chemotherapy.

Q: Does the child need to be isolated from other children?
A: The child should be isolated from any child who has varicella or is obviously sick due to any other infection.

ICD-9-CM 204.0

BIBLIOGRAPHY

Pui CH, et al. Acute lymphoblastic leukemia. *N Engl J Med* 2004;350:1535–1548.

Pui CH. Acute lymphoblastic leukemia in children. *Curr Opin Oncol* 2000;12:3–12.

Rubnitz JE, Pui CH. Recent advances in the treatment and understanding of childhood acute lymphoblastic leukaemia. *Cancer Treatment Reviews* 2003;29:31–44.

Author: Valerie I. Brown

Acute Myeloid Leukemia

 Database

DEFINITION

Acute myeloid leukemia (AML) is a block in differentiation and an unregulated proliferation of myeloid progenitor cells.

PATHOPHYSIOLOGY

- Principal defect is a block in the differentiation of primitive myeloid precursor cells.
- Two predominant mechanisms have been identified:

—Defect at the level of transcriptional activation.
—Defects in the signaling pathway of hematopoietic growth factors. In particular the proto-oncogene Ras is mutated in up to one-third of patients with AML.

ETIOLOGY

- Exact cause unknown.
- Acquired risk factors

—Exposure to benzene
—Exposure to ionizing radiation
—Therapy induced from chemotherapy for a prior malignancy
—Alkylating agents such as cyclophosphamide, nitrogen mustard, chlorambucil, melphalan. Typically presents several years after therapy.
—Epipodophyllotoxins such as VP16, VM26. Typically occurs within 2 years after therapy and are characterized by rearrangements involving 11q23.

- Certain congenital syndromes carry an increased risk of AML

—Fanconi anemia
—Bloom syndrome
—Neurofibromatosis type I
—Down syndrome
—Severe congenital anemia, i.e., Kostmann disease treated with granulocyte colony-stimulating factor
—Diamond Blackfan anemia
—Paroxysmal nocturnal hemoglobinemia
—Li-Fraumeni syndrome

PATHOLOGY

- Bone marrow aspirate must contain >30% myeloblasts.
- Classified according to the French-American-British Classification (FAB)

—Divides AML into 7 subtypes—M1–M7

- Immunophenotyping

—Blasts positive for myeloid associated surface antigens (CD11b, CD13, CD14, CD15, CD33, or CD36) in 90% of cases
—Lymphoid markers, both T and B cell may be present in 30%–60% of pediatric patients
—CD41 and CD42 (megakaryocytic)

- Morphology

—Large blasts with low nuclear/cytoplasmic ratio
—Multiple nucleoli and cytoplasmic granules

- Cytochemistry

—Blasts are positive for myeloperoxidase and Sudan black and usually negative for periodic acid-Schiff (PAS) and terminal deoxynucleotide transferase (TdT)

CYTOGENETICS

- Only 20% to 30% of pediatric blasts have a normal karyotype vs. 40% to 50% in adults
- 60% of abnormal karyotypes fall into known subgroups
- Translocations or duplications of the MLL gene at 11q23 are found in many cases of therapy-induced AML as well as in infants
- Techniques such as fluorescence in situ hybridization, Southern blotting, and reverse transcriptase—polymerase chain reactions are becoming necessary diagnostic tools for AML

EPIDEMIOLOGY

- Seventh most common pediatric malignancy
- 500 children/year in the U.S.
- Incidence peaks at 2 years and again at 16 years
- Leukemia in first 4 weeks of life is usually AML
- Ratio of AML to ALL throughout childhood is 1:4
- Boys and girls equally affected

COMPLICATIONS AT DIAGNOSIS

- Bleeding—usually secondary to thrombocytopenia
- Disseminated intravascular coagulation (DIC) occurs in some types of AML, including APML (M3).

—Should be aggressively treated with fresh frozen plasma and platelet transfusions.

- Infection

—40% of patients are febrile at diagnosis.
—Empiric antibiotic therapy must be started after blood cultures are obtained.

- Leukostasis

—Intravascular clumping of blasts causing hypoxia, infarction, and hemorrhage.
—Usually with white blood count (WBC) >200,000/mm^3.
—Brain and lung are commonly affected organs.
—Leukophoresis or exchange transfusion may be indicated with patients who are symptomatic with extremely high blast counts.

- Tumor lysis syndrome

—Refers to the metabolic consequences from the release of cellular contents of dying leukemic cells.
—Hyperuricemia can lead to renal failure.
—Hyperkalemia, hyperphosphatemia, and secondary hypocalcemia can be life threatening.
—Patients should be hydrated with fluid containing bicarbonate and given allopurinol.

PROGNOSIS

- 85% achieve remission with intensive chemotherapy.
- About 30% to 40% achieve long-term survival (more than 5 years after diagnosis).

 Differential Diagnosis

- Myeloid blast crisis of chronic myeloid leukemia (Philadelphia chromosome positive)
- Acute lymphoblastic leukemia
- Leukemoid reaction
- Exaggerated leukocytosis

Data Gathering

HISTORY

• Children with AML can present with very few symptoms or with life-threatening sepsis or hemorrhage. Common symptoms include

—Fever: 30%–40%
—Pallor: 25%
—Weight loss/anorexia: 22%
—Fatigue: 19%
—Bleeding, i.e., cutaneous, mucosal, menorrhagia: 33%
—Bone or joint pain: 18%

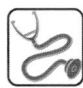
Physical Examination

• Signs of anemia

—Pallor, fatigue, headache, dyspnea, systolic flow murmur
—Signs of thrombocytopenia
—Petechiae, bruising, epistaxis, gingival bleeding

• Signs of infection

—Fever
—Lingering bacterial infections of lung, sinuses, gingiva, perirectal area, skin

• Other exam findings

—Hepatomegaly
—Splenomegaly
—Lymphadenopathy
—Gingival hyperplasia
—Papilledema, cranial nerve palsies (rare)
—Colorless or slightly purple subcutaneous nodules—"blueberry muffin" lesions of leukemia cutis (more commonly seen in neonates)

Laboratory Findings

• CBC

—Anemia, thrombocytopenia, elevated or low total WBC count

• Peripheral smear

—Myeloblasts may be seen

• Bone marrow aspirate

—>30% myeloblasts is diagnostic
—Confirm with immunophenotyping and cytochemistry

• PT/PTT fibrin spit products

—Can be elevated with some cases especially with acute promyelocytic leukemia (M3)
—Can have severe, life-threatening DIC

• Electrolytes—abnormalities associated with tumor lysis syndrome

—Hyperkalemia
—Hypocalcemia
—Hyperphosphatemia
—Hyperuricemia

• CSF for cell count and cytology

—>5 WBC/mm^3 is suggestive of CNS disease.
—5%–15% of cases have CNS involvement at diagnosis.

PROGNOSTIC FACTORS

Factors associated with low remission induction rate:

• WBC count >100,000/mm^3
• Monosomy 7
• Secondary AML or prior myelodysplastic syndrome
• FLT 3 mutation

Emergency Care

• Children with suspected AML should have immediate evaluation with physical exam, history, and laboratory data including CBC, PT/PTT, electrolytes, calcium, phosphorus, uric acid, creatinine.

Therapy

INDUCTION

• Most effective drugs for remission induction in AML are anthracyclines, e.g., doxorubicin, daunomycin, mitoxantrone, and cytarabine
• 6-thioguanine (6TG), VP-16, and dexamethasone are added in some regimens
• Remission rate is approximately 70%–85%
• High rate of remission induction with all trans-retinoic acid in acute promyelocytic leukemia
• Consolidation therapy usually with ARA-C and L-asparaginase
• Intrathecal ARA-C for CNS prophylaxis
• Maintenance with VP16, ARA-C, 6TG, daunomycin, dexamethasone
• Duration of therapy is usually 6–9 months
• Allogeneic bone marrow transplant may be the best treatment for AML in first remission

SUPPORTIVE CARE

• Hydration, alkalization, and allopurinol during induction
• Blood product support

—Avoid products from family members due to the possibility of allogeneic bone marrow transplant

• Broad-spectrum antibiotics and antifungal therapy for fever and neutropenia
• Prophylactic trimethoprim/sulfamethoxazole for *Pneumocystis*
• Nystatin/fluconazole for fungal prophylaxis
• Heparin may be needed for treatment of DIC.

Follow-Up

Blood counts monthly for first year, then every 3 months for the second year and then every 6 months. Liver and kidney function tests are done every 3 months. Cardiac function should be checked every 6 to 12 months. Endocrine function should be tested in pubertal children.

Common Questions and Answers

Q: Is an indwelling line required for therapy?
A: Always.

Q: Are repeated hospitalizations likely?
A: Repeated hospitalizations are needed for chemotherapy and infectious complications.

Q: Can the child go to school?
A: May be able to go intermittently during therapy.

ICD-9-CM 205.0

BIBLIOGRAPHY

Ebb DH, Weinstein HJ. Diagnosis and treatment of childhood AML. *Pediatr Clin North Am* 1997;44(4):847–862.

Golub TR, Weinstein HJ, Grier HE. Acute myelogenous leukemia. In: Pizzo PA, Poplack DG, eds. *Principles and Practices of Pediatric Oncology*. 3rd Ed. Philadelphia: Lippincott-Raven, 1997.

Hurwitz CA, Mounce KG, Grier HE. Treatment of patients with AML: review of clinical trials of past decade. *J Pediatr Hematol Oncol* 1995;17(3):185–197.

Kersey JH. Fifty years of studies of biology and therapy of childhood leukemia. *Blood* 1997;90(11):4243–4251.

Kottaridis PD, et al. Prognostic implication of the presence of LFT3 mutations in patients with acute myeloid leukemia. *Leuk Lymphoma* 2003;44(6):905–13.

Langmuir P, Aplenc R, Lange B. Acute myeloid leukemia in children. *Best Pract Res Clin Haematol* 2001;14(1):77–93.

A pediatric approach to the WHO classification of myelodysplastic and myeloproliferative disease. *Leukemia* 2003;17(2):277–82.

Author: Tammy Kang

Adenovirus Infection

Database

DEFINITION

Adenoviruses are ubiquitous nonenveloped double-stranded DNA viruses. There are 49 human serotypes.

PATHOPHYSIOLOGY

Adenoviruses may cause a lytic infection or a chronic/ latent infection. They also are capable of inducing oncogenic transformation of cells, although the clinical significance of this observation remains unclear.

EPIDEMIOLOGY

• Primary infection usually occurs early in life (by age 10 years) and is most often characterized by upper respiratory symptoms.
• Military trainees are especially susceptible to infection, probably due to crowded living conditions.
• Respiratory and enteric infections may occur at any time of year. Epidemics of respiratory disease occur in winter and spring.
• Transmission of respiratory disease occurs via contact with infected secretions. Transmission of enteric adenoviruses is via the fecal-oral route.
• Outbreaks of pharyngoconjunctival fever have been associated with inadequately chlorinated swimming pools.
• Has been identified as the most common infectious cause of myocarditis in children and adults.

COMPLICATIONS

• Bronchiolitis obliterans (rare), corneal opacities with visual disturbance (usually resolves spontaneously), congestive heart failure, dilated cardiomyopathy

PROGNOSIS

Most syndromes are self-limited.

ASSOCIATED ILLNESSES

• Respiratory infection responsible for 10% of all pediatric respiratory illnesses; may cause upper respiratory symptoms, pertussis-like syndrome; pneumonitis; lower respiratory tract disease associated with adenovirus types 4 and 7.
• Pharyngoconjunctival fever: Low-grade fever associated with conjunctivitis, pharyngitis, rhinitis, and cervical adenitis; 15% of patients may have meningismus; increased incidence in summer months; common-source outbreaks most often associated with type 3.
• Epidemic keratoconjunctivitis: Bilateral conjunctivitis with preauricular adenopathy; may persist for up to 4 weeks; corneal opacities may persist for several months; associated with types 8,19, and 37.
• Myocarditis: Preceeding viral illness; present with cardiovascular collapse, congestive heart failure, respiratory distress, or ventricular tachycardia. Prognosis is poor: high mortality, a large number require transplant, and a portion develop dilated cardiomyopathy.
• Hemorrhagic cystitis may cause microscopic or gross hematuria; if present, gross hematuria persists on average for 3 days; often associated with dysuria and urinary frequency; more common in males than females; associated with types 11 and 21.
• Infantile diarrhea: watery diarrhea associated with fever; symptoms may persist for 1 to 2 weeks; associated with types 40 and 41.
• Central nervous system (CNS) infection epidemics (associated with outbreaks of respiratory disease) and sporadic cases of encephalitis and meningitis have been observed; often associated with pneumonia.
• Miscellaneous adenoviruses have been associated with intussusception (isolated in up to 40% of cases), fatal congenital infection, disseminated disease in immunocompromised patients.

Differential Diagnosis

• Respiratory infection

—Influenza
—Parainfluenza
—RSV
—Human metapneumovirus
—Pertussis
—Mycoplasma pneumonia
—Bacterial pneumonia

• Pharyngoconjunctival fever

—Group A streptococcus
—Epstein-Barr virus
—Parainfluenza
—Enterovirus
—Measles

• Epidemic keratoconjunctivitis

—Herpes simplex
—Chlamydia
—Enterovirus

• Myocarditis

—Enteroviruses
—Parvovirus
—Herpes simplex
—Epstein-Barr virus
—Influenza
—Bacterial myocarditis

• Hemorrhagic cystitis

—Glomerulonephritis
—Vasculitis
—Renal tuberculosis

• Infantile diarrhea

—Rotavirus
—Norwalk agent
—Astrovirus
—Salmonella
—Shigella
—Campylobacter

• CNS infection

—Enterovirus
—Herpes simplex virus
—Mycoplasma
—Bacterial meningitis

Data Gathering

HISTORY

Question: Fever?
Significance: Nonspecific

Question: Rhinitis?
Significance: URI

Question: Laryngitis, sore throat?
Significance: URI

Question: Nonproductive or croupy cough?
Significance: Respiratory infection

Question: Headache, myalgias?
Significance: CNS infection

Question: Hematuria (gross or microscopic), dysuria, urinary frequency?
Significance: Hemorrhagic cystitis

Question: Watery diarrhea?
Significance: Enteric adenovirus

 ## Physical Examination

Finding: Head and neck—conjunctivitis, rhinitis, exudative pharyngitis, meningismus
Significance: Typical findings of adenovirus

Finding: Pulmonary tachypnea, wheezing, rales
Significance: Pneumonia

Finding: Tachycardia, tachypnea, gallop rhythm, hepatomegaly
Significance: Myocarditis

Finding: Abdominal tenderness, distension
Significance: Gastroenteritis

 ## Laboratory Aids

Test: CBC
Significance: Leukocytosis or leukopenia, often with left shift in the differential count

Test: Erythrocyte sedimentation rate
Significance: Often elevated

Test: Chest radiograph
Significance: Bilateral patchy interstitial infiltrates (lower lobes) or enlarged heart

Test: Echocardiogram
Significance: Poor ejection fraction, cardiomegaly

Test: Electrocardiogram
Significance: Low-voltage QRS, low amplitude or inverted T-waves, small or absent q wave in V5 and V6

Test: Viral isolation
Significance: From nasopharyngeal secretions, urine, conjuctivae, or stool

Test: Viral identification
Significance: Observe viral antigen in infected cells by immunofluorescence, amplify genome by PCR; highest yield from nasopharyngeal swab or stool.

Test: Serology
Significance: Diagnosis may be made by a documented 4-fold rise in serum antibody.

Precautions that Should Be Used for Hospital Patient

SYMPTOMS	TYPE OF PRECAUTIONS
Respiratory disease	Contact and droplet
Gastrointestinal	Contact
Conjunctivitis	Contact

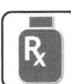 ## Therapy

Cidofovir has been shown to have some benefit in immunocompromised patients with disseminated disease. However, a high risk of developing a dose-limiting nephrotoxicity exists.

PREVENTION

Oral vaccines have been used by the military.

ICD-9-CM 079.0

Diarrhea secondary to adenoviral infection 008.62
Conjunctivitis-pharyngoconjuctival fever 007.2
Conjunctivitis 077.3
Myocarditis 422

BIBLIOGRAPHY

Baum SG. Adenovirus. In: Mandell GL, Douglas RG, Bennett JE, eds. *Principles and Practice of Infectious Diseases.* 4th Ed. New York Churchill. Livingstone 2001:1382–1387.

Bowles NE, et al. Detection of viruses in myocardial tissues by polymerase chain reaction. Evidence of adenovirus as a common cause of myocarditis in children and adults. *J Am Coll Cardiol* 2003;42(3):466–472.

Friedman RA, et al. Myocarditis. In: Feigin RD, Cherry JD, Demmler GJ, Kaplan SL, eds. *Textbook of Pediatric Infectious Diseases.* 4th Ed. Philadelphia: WB Saunders 2004: 390–413.

Krajden M, Brown M, Petrasek A, et al. Clinical features of adenovirus enteritis: a review of 127 cases. *Pediatr Infect Dis J* 1990;9: 636–641.

Leruez-Ville M, et al. Real-time blood plasma polymerase chain reaction for management of disseminated adenovirus infection. *Clin Infect Dis* 2004;38:45–52.

Wirsing von Konig CH, Rott H, Bogaerts H, et al. A serologic study of organisms possibly associated with pertussis-like coughing. *Pediatr Infect Dis J* 1998;17(7):645–649.

Authors: Jason Newland and Susan E. Coffin

Alcohol (Ethanol) Intoxication

 Database

DEFINITION

- Acute ingestion (accidental or intended) of alcohol, resulting in loss of inhibition, often associated with unruly/violent behavior, impaired judgment and/or coordination, diminished alertness/responsiveness, and sedation or coma.
- Accidental ingestion is more common in toddlers and younger children; frequency of intentional alcohol use increases with age.

ETIOLOGY

- Alcoholic beverages (water and ethanol) produced from fermentation/distillation of sugar from grapes (wine), grains/corn (beer/whiskey), potatoes (vodka) or sugar cane (rum). After distillation, alcohol is mixed into solution to make specific beverages; products marketed according to alcohol content or "proof" which is twice the percent. Alcohol content ranges from 3%–6% (6–12 proof) in beer to 40%–75% (80–150 proof) in vodka/rum/whiskey.
- Alcohol often consumed concurrently with other substances (licit and illicit) presenting mixed clinical picture of intoxication.

PATHOPHYSIOLOGY

- Effects of alcohol ingestion related to dose, time in which alcohol was consumed and then absorbed, and the patient's prior history of alcohol exposure.
- Alcohol absorption, decreased by presence of food in stomach and increased if liquid is carbonated, occurs rapidly and to a large extent in the small intestine.
- Minimal quantities of alcohol excreted in urine, sweat, and breath.
- Over 90% of alcohol oxidized in liver following zero-order kinetics primarily by alcohol dehydrogenase (ADH) and then acetaldyhyde dehydrogenase (ALDH); rate of metabolism is fixed (not related to dose or time) and is proportional to body weight. Ethnic/racial and gender variability exist as to quantity and efficacy of ADH.
- Ethanol is metabolized by ADH to acetaldehyde, then to acetate, and finally to either ketones, fatty acids, or acetone; ketosis and infrequently metabolic acidosis can occur.
- Respiratory acidosis can occur secondary to carbon dioxide retention from respiratory depression due to ethanol intoxication.
- Hypoglycemia occurs during acute ethanol intoxication due to impaired gluconeogenesis resulting from changes in the NADH/NAD+ ratio associated with ethanol metabolism.
- Alcohol impacts central nervous system (CNS) primarily through the γ-aminobutyric acid (GABA) and glutamate neurotransmitter systems.

EPIDEMIOLOGY

- Alcohol second only to caffeine in prevalence and incidence of use among substances of use/abuse.
- Over 75% of high school students have had >1 drink in their lifetime; 30% had their first drink before age 13.
- Nearly 50% of high school students report current alcohol use, and 30% report heavy drinking in the past 30 days (>5 drinks).
- Almost 1/3 of high school students have ridden in a car with a driver who has been drinking alcohol.
- In 2002, 41% of all traffic fatalities were alcohol-related motor vehicle crashes.

COMPLICATIONS

- Diuresis and dehydration
- Vasodilation and hypotension
- Vomiting, aspiration, potential respiratory arrest
- Hypoglycemia
- Metabolic acidosis
- Impaired mental status
- Engagement in risk-taking behaviors while intoxicated (i.e., other drug use, unprotected intercourse)
- CNS depression
- Gastritis
- Gastrointestinal bleeding
- Acute pancreatitis
- Motor vehicle accidents associated with driving while intoxicated
- Alcoholism
- Alcohol withdrawal following a period of intoxication in chronic users; symptoms include tachycardia, elevated blood pressure, irritability, nausea, vomiting, and tremor

 Differential Diagnosis

ENVIRONMENTAL

- Other ingestions (overdose of sedatives or illicit drugs, such as benzodiazepines, marijuana, narcotics, LSD, and PCP)
- Toxic exposures (ethylene glycol, methanol, carbon monoxide)
- Head trauma

INFECTION

- Meningitis
- Encephalitis
- Sepsis

TUMOR

- Brain tumor

METABOLIC

- Hypoglycemia
- Ketoacidosis
- Hyperammonemia
- Electrolyte imbalances (hyponatremia, hypernatremia)

MISCELLANEOUS

- Increased intracranial pressure from hydrocephalus, mass, other
- Stroke

 Data Gathering

HISTORY

Question: Any past medical history?
Significance: Baseline health will affect patient's response to alcohol; diabetics, for example, may have worse hypoglycemia.

Question: Were any other drugs ingested, and if so, what and how much?
Significance: Clinical effects of and treatment for other ingestions can vary depending on substance. Polysubstance ingestion may occur.

Question: Any past psychiatric history?
Significance: Evaluate for possible suicidal ideation.

Question: What are the details regarding the alcohol consumed? What type, how much, and over what time period?
Significance: May help predict clinical course. For example, the blood alcohol concentration (BAC) may continue rising if ingestion occurred recently.

 Physical Examination

Finding: Bruises, lacerations, fractures
Significance: May suggest trauma and raise concern about CNS injury.

Finding: Neurologic exam, including mental status
Significance: To assess degree of intoxication and consciousness, including patient's ability to protect his/her airway and/or risk for aspiration. Intoxication clinically presents with signs ranging from lack of coordination, slurred speech, and confusion (BAC of 20–200 mg/dL) to ataxia, nausea/vomiting (BAC 200–300 mg/dL) to amnesia, seizures, or coma (BAC >300 mg/dL).

Finding: Tachycardia, hypotension
Significance: May indicate dehydration

Finding: Fever
Significance: May suggest infection

Laboratory Aids

Test: Blood alcohol concentration (BAC)
Significance: BAC generally correlates with clinical picture; (see Physical Examination). In children, signs of intoxication may be present at levels of 50 mg/dL. Serum levels of 600–800 mg/dL can be fatal.

Test: Blood and/or urine toxicology screen
Significance: Concurrent ingestions are common.

Test: Acetaminophen level
Significance: Usually not part of the general serum toxicology screen. Consider if polysubstance ingestion suspected and/or if patient with suicidal ideation.

Test: Serum electrolytes
Significance: Alcohol is a diuretic; the associated nausea and vomiting seen with intoxication may result in severe dehydration. Ketosis and infrequently metabolic acidosis can occur.

Test: Serum glucose
Significance: Ethanol inhibits gluconeogenesis and can be associated with hypoglycemia.

Test: Blood gas
Significance: Can see both respiratory and metabolic acidosis.

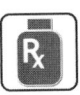 Therapy

- Assess airway, breathing and circulation (ABCs).
- Protect airway—the patient may require intubation and mechanical ventilation.
- Mainstay is supportive therapy, as no specific ethanol antidote exists.
- Appropriate trauma management as needed.
- Intravenous fluids for dehydration and hypotension.
- Intravenous dextrose for hypoglycemia.
- Because alcohol is absorbed rapidly, gastric lavage is only indicated if the patient is seen immediately after ingestion (within minutes).

 Follow-Up

- Refer to substance abuse specialist (addiction medicine, psychiatrist, or certified addictions counselor) for detailed evaluation and treatment.
- Refer for psychiatric evaluation if depression, anxiety, suicidal ideation, or any other mental health condition is suspected.
- Assess for other risk-taking behaviors, including: other substance use, sexual activity, use of motor vehicles while intoxicated, weapon carrying, and delinquency; and their sequelae, including pregnancy, sexually transmitted infections, and violence.

PREVENTION

- Promote family discussions about alcohol use and abuse.
- Provide safety recommendations to prevent accidental ingestions.

PITFALLS

- Most urine toxicology screens do not test for alcohol.
- Alcohol-drug interactions are common because acute intoxication reduces hepatic clearance for other drugs thereby increasing their serum concentrations.

 Common Questions and Answers

Q: How quickly does a person metabolize alcohol?
A: The liver metabolizes approximately 10 g of ethanol per hour, which corresponds to a decline in BAC of 18–20 mg/dL per hour.

Q: What is the legal level of BAC that defines driving under the influence of alcohol?
A: This varies by state, but generally is between 80–100 mg/dL.

Q: Why do some individuals, particularly of Asian descent, turn red or develop signs of pruritus after ingesting alcohol?
A: Flushing, pruritus, and nausea are due to high levels of acetaldehyde. Variations in the metabolic activity of dehydrogenase enzymes are associated with factors such as gender, history of alcohol use, and genetics. Decreased ALDH activity, which is more common in Native Americans and Asians, can result in increased levels of acetaldehyde.

ICD-9 CODE 980.0

BIBLIOGRAPHY

Centers for Disease Control and Prevention. National drunk and drugged driving prevention month—December 2003. *MMWR Morb Mortal Wkly Rep* 2003;52:1185–1186.

Clark DB, et al. Alcohol use disorders in adolescents. *Pediatr Drugs* 2002;4:493–502.

Coupey SM. Specific Drugs. In: Schydlower M, ed. *Substance Abuse: A Guide for Health Professionals.* 2nd Ed. Elk Grove Village, IL: American Academy of Pediatrics; 2002: 208–215.

Foxcroft DR, et al. Longer-term primary prevention for alcohol misuse in young people: a systematic review. *Addiction* 2003;98(4):397–411.

Yost DA. Acute care for alcohol intoxication. *Postgrad Med* 2002;112(6):14–26.

Author: Ann B. Bruner

Alpha-1 Antitrypsin Deficiency

 Database

DEFINITION

• Lethal hereditary disorder of Caucasian persons of European ancestry characterized by a reduced serum level of Alpha-1 antitrypsin (α-1-AT), a glycoprotein that is synthesized in large amounts by the liver, accounting for approximately 80% of circulating levels and in small amounts by circulating neutrophils and macrophages. Lung emphysema and chronic liver disease are phenotypes.

CAUSES

• Lowered levels of circulating α-1-AT. α-1-AT is a small 52 kDa glycoprotein that serves as an antiprotease and as the inhibitor of trypsin, pancreatic elastase, and macrophage proteases, such as neutrophil elastase, cathepsin G and proteinase 3. The result is unregulated protease activity with end organ damage in the liver and the lungs.

EPIDEMIOLOGY

• The incidence of PiZZ genotype is highest in the Caucasian population within North America, Australia and Europe.
• There has been an estimated 70,000 to 100,000 individuals affected in the North America. As many as 25 million people in the United States are carriers of a deficiency allele.
• More recent studies have shown a greater worldwide racial and ethnic distribution than previously felt. Individuals who are homozygotes or heterozygotes for the two most common defective alleles (PiS and PiZ), as well as individuals with carrier phenotypes, have been found in various populations of African blacks, Arabs and Jews in the Middle East, and Central, Far East and Southeast Asians.
• Felt to be significantly under-recognized.
• Most common metabolic cause of emphysema in adults and liver disease in children.

GENETICS

• Alpha$_1$-AT disease state is associated with a defective protease inhibitor that is a result of two codominantly inherited recessive alleles encoded on the long arm of chromosome 14. (14q32.19).
• The result of the mutation causes the protein to form intermolecular linkages in the glycoprotein that results in the accumulation of polymers within the endoplasmic reticulum of hepatocytes forming inclusion bodies that are not secreted.
• The normal functioning genotype of protease inhibitor (Pi) is PiMM. There are over 75 different codominant alleles, with only a few that results in defective protease inhibitors.
• Patients with PiZZ alleles have the most significant findings with serum levels of α-1-AT at levels 80%–90% lower than normal.
• Other intermediate genotypes: PiMS, PiMZ, PiSS and PiSZ, have not been definitively associated with hepatic disease. The Null gene is one that produces no detectable levels of α-1.
• The Null-Null phenotype is associated with the greatest risk for emphysema, yet this phenotype has not been associated with liver disease.

COMPLICATIONS

• Cirrhosis and early onset lower-lobe emphysema are common in the PiZZ phenotype.
• 12%–15% PiZZ phenotypes will develop liver disease.
• The course of liver disease is highly variable in affected individuals. Jaundice, acholic stools, and hepatomegaly are present during the first week of life, but the jaundice usually clears by the 4th month. Complete resolution of symptoms, chronic liver disease, or the development of cirrhosis may follow. Older children may present with manifestations of chronic liver disease or cirrhosis, with evidence of portal hypertension.
• Major dermatologic manifestation: Panniculitis, an inflammation of the fat just beneath the skin, causing the skin to harden and form lumps, patches, or lesions. It is likely that the damage is initiated by the destructive action of unrestrained neutrophils.

 Differential Diagnosis

Alpha-1-AT deficiency in infancy and childhood has diverse presentations. Patients in infancy most typically present with prolonged jaundice, hepatosplenomegaly with or without ascites and cirrhosis. Differential diagnoses include idiopathic neonatal hepatitis, cholestasis and cirrhosis. (see Chapter, Jaundice and Cirrhosis for a complete listing)

 Data Gathering

HISTORY

Question: How do neonates and young children present?
Significance: Highly variable presentation. Jaundice, hepatomegaly, and even acholic stools can present during the first weeks of life. The jaundice usually clears by age 2–4 months. Normal liver function, continued liver disease, or progression to cirrhosis may follow, depending on the clinical course.

Question: What is the usual adolescent/adults presentation?
Significance: Adolescents: hepatomegaly, jaundice and other signs of chronic liver disease, depends on the degree of liver involvement. Those with advanced liver disease may present with ascites and cirrhosis, as in adults.

 Physical Examination

Evidence of jaundice, hepatosplenomegaly and other stigmata of chronic liver disease is observed.

Laboratory Aids

- Serum levels of α-1-AT levels and genotype analysis of the Pi phenotype
- Definitive diagnosis is made by liver biopsy.
- Quantitative serum α-1-AT levels:

—PiMM: α-1-AT levels: 20 to 53 mmol/L.
—PiZZ: 2.5 to 7 mmol/L or less
—Pi null/null phenotype: no measurable levels of α-1-AT.
—False positives occur due to the fact that the protein acts as an acute-phase reactant.
—In retrospective studies, low levels of α-1-AT levels had a positive predictive value of 94% and a negative predictive value of 100%.

- Confirmation is made with examination of the phenotype by performing serum protein electrophoresis to determine the allele type.
- Definitive diagnosis with liver biopsy: eosinophilic cytoplasmic granules that stain intensely with periodic acid-Schiff (PAS) stain in periportal hepatocytes.

IMAGING TECHNIQUES

Ultrasound with Doppler study for evaluation of portal hypertension and/or for pretransplantation evaluation has been extremely useful.

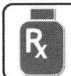 ## Therapy

DRUGS

- There is no specific definitive treatment for the disease. Specific symptoms are treated and palliative treatment is given. Prevention of potential complications is important.
- The avoidance of cigarette smoking and hepatotoxins.
- Ursodeoxycholic acid, a choleretic agent, is used at a dose of 20 to 30 mg/kg per day to manage the cholestasis and pruritus associated with liver disease.
- Augmentation therapy—Pooled human plasma derived α-1-AT has been used to restore circulating levels of the protease inhibitor to levels above the protective threshold. Studies have shown that this results in the decrease in the rate of decline in FEV1 and decreased mortality rate during the period of study.
- Future therapeutics: gene replacement therapy

DURATION

- Patients will require lifelong management of the symptoms of the disease. Treatment will need to be optimized based on the clinical findings and the needs of the patient.

SURGICAL

- Surgical treatment at this time consists of orthotopic liver transplantation for patients with end stage liver disease. Reoccurrence of the disease does not occur following transplantation.

 ## Follow-Up

PROGNOSIS

- One-fourth of the children will need a future liver transplant, as a result of worsening liver function and evidence of cirrhosis and portal hypertension.
- One-fourth will stabilize and liver function will normalize.
- One-fourth will slowly develop chronic liver disease and cirrhosis.
- One-fourth will have less severe impairment and live into adulthood.

 ## Common Questions and Answers

Q: Do all patients with PiZZ disease get liver involvement?
A: For those with the PiZZ phenotype, the risks of developing liver disease vary depending on the age of the patient, and prevention of further liver injury from other causes. Around 10% of newborns with the ZZ genotype have liver disease that leads to fatal childhood cirrhosis. The risk is slightly higher in adults. Overall, approximately 12%–15% of all ZZ genotypes develop liver disease.

Q: What is the usual medical course of this disease?
A: The disease course is variable. Approximately one-fourth of the children will need a liver transplant at some point, as a result of worsening liver function. One-fourth of the patients will have a stable course without any significant liver damage. One fourth will have a course of slow progression of liver disease and cirrhosis. The last fourth will have less severe liver impairment and live into adulthood.

BIBLIOGRAPHY

Coakley RJ. Alpha-1-antitrypsin deficiency: biological answers to clinical questions. *Am J Med Sci* 2001;321(1):33–41.

de Serres, Frederick J. Worldwide racial and ethnic distribution of alpha1 antitrypsin deficiency. *Chest* 2002;122(5):1818–1829.

Steiner SJ. Serum levels of alpha-1 antitrypsin predict phenotype expression of the alpha1-antitrypsin gene. *Dig Dis Sci* 2003;28(9):1793–1796.

Stoller JK. Augmentation therapy with alpha-1 antitrypsin: Patterns of use and adverse effects. *Chest* 2003;123(5):1425–1434.

Authors: Peter C. Wilmot and J. Fernando del Rosario

Altitude Illness

 Database

DEFINITION

- Acute mountain sickness (AMS): Failure to adapt to the hypoxic demands of altitude. Includes a group of clinical signs and symptoms seen in travelers to altitudes greater than 2,500 m.
- Mild mountain sickness: Headache in morning and on exertion, anorexia, nausea, dizziness, vomiting, shortness of breath on exertion, insomnia, irritability, periodic breathing (Cheyne-Stokes respiration), poor performance
- Moderate mountain sickness: Severe headache, lassitude (weariness, indifference, antisocial), weakness, anorexia, nausea, ataxia, decreased urine output, diminished judgment and coordination. Capable of activities with difficulty
- Severe mountain sickness: Insidious or acute onset, usually 2 to 4 days after ascent. Can progress to a life-threatening condition within hours. Can include pulmonary and cerebral edema
- High-altitude cerebral edema (HACE): Develops over 1–3 days after ascent, usually preceded by AMS. Headache, vomiting, lassitude, irritability, drowsiness, ataxia, slurred speech, cranial nerve paralysis, hyporeflexia hypereflexia or hyperreflexia, hemiparesis, hemiplegia, mental status changes (confusion, irrationality, depression, disorientation, amnesia, hallucinations, severe nightmares), decreased urine output, seizures, papilledema, coma, death.
- High-altitude pulmonary edema (HAPE): Often develops over several days and may be associated with or exacerbated by concurrent viral illness. Thought to be related to pulmonary hypertension (and resultant noninflammatory fluid leak) at altitude. Initially with dyspnea on exertion, then at rest, decreased exercise capability, dry cough, fatigue, tachypnea, low-grade temperature <38.5°C). Develop pink frothy sputum, cyanosis, wheezing, rales, tachycardia, low-grade fever, orthopnea.
- Other altitude related issues: High-altitude syncope, amnesia, edema (facial and extremity), retinopathy (hemorrhages), pharyngitis and bronchitis, flatus, immune suppression, thrombosis, coagulation abnormalities (thrombolic events), platelet changes, chronic mountain illness (Monge disease, polycythemia), weight loss.

PROGNOSIS AND COMPLICATIONS

- Excellent if recognized quickly, ascent stopped, and/or descent and therapy initiated
- Can be poor if symptoms go unrecognized or noted without appropriate descent and therapy
- Symptoms either insidious or acute onset, usually 2 to 4 days after ascent
  —Can become life-threatening within hours

ASSOCIATED ILLNESSES

- Ophthalmologic
  —Retinal vessel engorgement
  —Retinal hemorrhages: Usually resolves in 7 to 10 days without symptoms. 100% of people at 6,500 m (21,450 ft)
  —Macular hemorrhages: More severe, associated with visual changes.
  —Ultraviolet keratitis.

 Differential Diagnosis

ENVIRONMENTAL FACTORS

- Alcohol toxicity
- Hangover
- Drug effects
- Hypothermia
- Carbon monoxide poisoning

MEDICAL/METABOLIC

- Dehydration
- Viral illness

PSYCHOSOCIAL

- Exhaustion, sleep deprivation
- Personality traits (irritability)
- Insomnia

 Data Gathering

HISTORY

Question: Previous altitude illness?
Significance: Suggests symptoms in future with ascent to similar altitude.

Question: Location (altitude) where symptoms occurred, how did the patient arrive at that altitude, and what was the rate of ascent?
Significance: Rapid ascent minimizes time for natural acclimatization and increases risk of developing altitude illness.

Question: Exertion level?
Significance: Increased exertion on ascent may increase speed of symptom development.

Question: Medication, drug, or alcohol use, predisposing medical illness (asthma, restrictive lung disease)?
Significance: Underlying medical conditions, such as sickle cell disease, hypertension, sleep apnea, obstructive lung disease, cerebrovascular disease or concurrent infections, may predispose one to development of altitude illness. Medication use or presumed medical illness may mask or mimic signs and symptoms of altitude illness.

Question: Symptom complex (variable)?
Significance: Do symptoms fit with another illness or with classic (or progressive) altitude illness?

Question: Morning headache, progressive with ascent?
Significance: Suggests HACE.

Question: Insomnia, difficulty falling asleep, frequent waking?
Significance: Suggests hypoxia and development of altitude illness.

Question: Periodic breathing (hyperapnea to apnea)?
Significance: Suggests moderate to more advanced altitude illness.

Question: Gastrointestinal: anorexia, nausea, vomiting, abdominal cramps, flatus?
Significance: Potentially related to ascent.

Question: Pulmonary: dry cough, shortness of breath, sore throat, dyspnea on exertion and at rest, decreased exercise capability?
Significance: Potential progression to high altitude pulmonary edema (HAPE).

Question: Neurologic: lassitude, weariness, indifference, fatigue, irritability, dizziness, ataxia, weakness?
Significance: Progression to high altitude cerebral edema (HACE).

Question: Decreased urine output edema, fluid retention?
Significance: Indicative of fluid shifts, fluid losses, inadequate replacement, or dehydration.

 Physical Examination

Finding: Normal in early AMS
Significance: Physical examinations are nondescript early in development. Abnormalities usually occur after 12 to 24 hours at altitude (range, 2 to 96 hours).

 Laboratory Aids

Test: Chest x-ray study (CXR)
Significance: Vasocongestion, patchy or diffuse infiltrates; often worse than physical examination would suggest.

Test: ECG
Significance: Rule out myocardial etiology of symptoms or consequence of ascent.

Test: Toxicologic screen
Significance: Rule out medication effect for presenting symptoms.

Test: Electrolytes
Significance: Assess hydration status, fluid shifts, glucose.

Test: Arterial blood gas
Significance: Assess oxygenation, ventilation, and acid–base status.

Test: Carbon monoxide level
Significance: Ensure carbon monoxide poisoning not a factor in presentation.

Test: CBC
Significance: Assess oxygen carrying capacity of blood. Look for anemia, polycythemia, and platelet abnormalities.

Test: Ventilation and perfusion scan
Significance: Structural pulmonary assessment.

Test: Brain CT
Significance: Assess for structural abnormalities and cerebral edema.

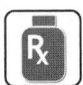

Therapy

GENERAL

- Suspect AMS
- Stop ascent
- Partial or full descent, Gamow portable hyperbaric chamber may be used as a stop gap until descent can be arranged
- Oxygen if available
- Fluids
- Consider acetazolamide to hasten acclimatization
- Avoid alcohol, codeine, sedative-hypnotics

—Red wine reported to perhaps have beneficial effect with regards to HAPE

- Avoid respiratory depressants

SPECIFIC

Mild AMS: Treatment may not be needed. Symptomatic headache relief with ibuprofen, acetaminophen, aspirin, prochlorperazine (Compazine). Temporal artery massage. Halt descent until symptoms improve.

- Moderate to severe AMS

—Descent
—Oxygen (relieves hypoxia, reduces pulmonary hypertension)
—Furosemide (be careful of volume depletion)
—Acetazolamide
—Consider dexamethasone (if allergic to sulfa or cannot take acetazolamide)
—Vasodilators (nifedipine, morphine)

- HACE: Descend immediately. Oxygen, furosemide, dexamethasone. Consider intubation and hyperventilation.
- HAPE

—Descend immediately
—Oxygen
—Furosemide
—Acetazolamide
—Vasodilators (nifedipine, morphine) and bronchodilators may be useful
—Consider antibiotics
—Positive-pressure breathing
—Pursed-lip breathing, mask, intubation
—Knee-chest position with abdominal squeeze
—Portable hyperbaric chamber
—Symptoms may recur when positive pressure removed.

MEDICATIONS

- Acetazolamide (Diamox, a carbonic anhydrase inhibitor)

—Diuretic which induces mild metabolic acidosis with concomitant reflex hyperventilation
—Hastens natural respiratory changes that occur during acclimatization

—Can help prevent AMS. Effectiveness in treating established AMS not clear.
—General guidelines for use
—Use in conjunction with (not in place of) gradual ascent, with passive transport to 3,000 m (9,850 ft) and rapid active transport
—Prophylaxis if previous history of AMS, history of periodic breathing, insomnia
—Treatment of early AMS
—May be useful if sulfa allergy is present
—Dosage: 5 to 10 mg/kg per day divided b.i.d. (125–500 mg b.i.d. or t.i.d. in adults), 24 hours prior to ascent and 1 to 2 days at altitude
—Side effects: mild diureses, paresthesias, nausea, drowsiness, taste changes, anorexia, blurred vision

- Dexamethasone (Decadron): Helpful for AMS treatment and early cerebral edema.
- Oxygen: Helpful at low flow at night (for headache, insomnia, cyanosis). Increases Pao_2.
- Nifedipine: Dosage: 20 mg sustained release q8–12 hours may be useful for treatment and prevention of HAPE, 24 hours prior to ascent and for 2 to 3 days at altitude.
- Diet: Increase fluid and calorie consumption with altitude and exertion. Increased carbohydrate diet. Avoid alcohol, tobacco, sedatives, recreational drugs.

Follow-Up

- Expect improvement with mild mountain sickness in 1 to 2 days.
- Moderate mountain sickness clears with descent and acclimation.
- Severe mountain sickness clears with descent and therapy.

PROGNOSIS

Good if recognized and treated appropriately. Poor if not recognized or treated appropriately

PREVENTION

- Avoid rapid ascent: Do not go too high too fast. Do not fly or drive to heights >3,000 m (>10,000 ft).
- Gradual acclimatization: Limit ascents to 300 m (1,000 ft) per day above 3,000 m (10,000 ft). Allow at least 24 hours for each 1,000 m (3,300 ft) gained. Exercise is not a substitute for acclimatization (or protection against AMS).
- Be aware and respectful of symptoms (even if minor): Assume symptoms secondary to AMS unless proven otherwise. Go no higher until symptoms resolve. Descend if worsening.
- Climb high, sleep low.
- Avoid alcohol, codeine, and sedative-hypnotics that are respiratory depressants.
- Exercise within individual capacity; avoid heavy exercise after passive ascent for at least 24 hours.
- Further investigation required regarding potential effectiveness of ginkgo biloba, garlic sildenafil, and theophylline in altitude illness prevention and/or therapy (no compelling clinical correlates to date)

Common Questions and Answers

Q: Can one develop AMS at moderate altitudes, such as during a ski vacation?
A: Yes, although the altitudes encountered rarely lead to the development of severe symptoms in this population.

Q: Will physical conditioning prior to ascent decrease the risk of developing altitude illness?
A: No, in fact better conditioning may inadvertently increase the risk of developing altitude illness as one may achieve higher altitudes more quickly.

Q: Are children more likely to develop HAPE than adults?
A: Children from low altitudes have no greater risk of developing HAPE than adults, however children who reside at high altitude are more likely than adults to develop reentry HAPE.

Q: Should everyone in whom a headache develops when at a higher than usual altitude be treated (pretreated) with acetazolamide?
A: No. One must weigh other options and severity of illness prior to decision to treat or provide prophylaxis for AMS.

Q: Should athletes avoid altitude in their training regimens?
A: No. In fact, living at altitude, but training at a lower altitude has been shown to improve performance, reportedly by an increase in erythropoietin.

BIBLIOGRAPHY

Bartsch P, et al. Update: High altitude pulmonary edema. *Adv in Experim Med & Biol* 2001;502:89–106.

Basnyat B, Murdoch DR. High-altitude illness. *Lancet* 2003;361(9373):1967–74.

Carpenter TC, Niermeyer S, Durmowicz AG. Altitude-related illness in children. *Curr Probl Pediatr* 1998;28(6):177–198.

Dumont L, Mardirosoff C, Tramer MR. Efficacy and harm of pharmacological prevention of acute mountain sickness: quantitative systematic review. *Br Med J* 2000;321(7256):267–272.

Kinsey CM, Roach R. Role of cerebral blood volume in acute mountain sickness. *Adv in Experim Med & Biol* 2003;543:151–159.

Kleinsasser A, Loeckinger A. Are sildenafil and theophylline effective in the prevention of high-altitude pulmonary edema? *Med Hypoth* 2002;59(2):223–225.

Sartori C, et al. Salmeterol for the prevention of high-altitude pulmonary edema. *N Engl J Med* 2002;346(21):1631–1636.

Woodward GA. Altitude Illness. *Clinical Pediatric Emergency Medicine: Environmental Emergencies* 2001;(3):168–178.

Authors: Paige L. Wright and George A. Woodward

Amblyopia

Database

DEFINITION

- Amblyopia is poor vision, usually just in one eye, resulting from poor visual input during early childhood (the critical period for visual development).
- Although the cause of amblyopia (refractive blur, strabismus, cataract) may be correctable, vision is not restored immediately due to poor neurovisual development.
- Early detection and treatment is essential, amblyopia can only be effectively treated in early childhood.

PATHOPHYSIOLOGY

- Equal, focused visual input from each eye is necessary for the visual system to develop normally. Any condition that prevents a clear, fusible (capable of being integrated into a single binocular image in the brain) image during the first 8–10 years of life may cause amblyopia.
- In general, the earlier the abnormal input, the greater the likelihood and severity of amblyopia. In an infant, amblyopia can result from as little as 1 week of abnormal visual input. Asymmetrical input between the two eyes (unilateral cataract, anisometropia, etc.) is more likely to cause amblyopia than symmetrically poor images, due to competitive influences between the two eyes. As a result, amblyopia is almost always unilateral.
- Bilateral amblyopia may result from severe, symmetrical bilateral image degradation such as bilateral cataract, bilateral high ametropia (high refractive error), etc.
- Visual acuity in amblyopic eyes varies from minimal impairment (20/25) to legal blindness (<20/200). Other significant impairments in amblyopic eyes may include reduced contrast sensitivity, reduced or absent binocularity and depth perception, and impaired or distorted spatial perception. Peripheral visual fields are preserved, and vision is never completely lost (no light perception) from amblyopia alone.

CLASSIFICATION

Amblyopia is generally classified by cause, with three primary types:

- Anisometropic amblyopia—resulting from asymmetrical refractive error and resultant unilateral blurring. This is the most common cause of amblyopia.
- Strabismic amblyopia—resulting from misalignment of the eyes, and subsequent lack of an image that can be "fused" or integrated into a single image in the brain. This is most likely with early onset, constant strabismus. Up to 60% of patients with strabismus will also have amblyopia.
- Deprivation amblyopia—resulting from optical imperfection (cataract, ptosis, corneal opacity, prolonged patching or bandage) which prevents the formation of a clear image in one or both eyes. Deprivation, especially if it begins early in life, is associated with the most severe amblyopia.

EPIDEMIOLOGY

- Large population based studies suggest that 2%–5% of the adult population has amblyopia.
- Amblyopia is the most common cause of unilateral vision loss in children and young adults.
- Despite screening programs and widely available treatment, amblyopia remains a significant cause of vision loss in developed countries.

Differential Diagnosis

Amblyopia is diagnosed by exclusion: residual vision loss after correction or elimination of all other optical and anatomic factors is defined as amblyopia. Conditions that cause vision loss without easily recognized pathology might be mistaken for amblyopia. In children, the differential diagnosis of vision loss in normal-appearing eyes includes:

- Uncorrected refractive error (hyperopia, myopia, astigmatism)
- Optic nerve hypoplasia
- Optic atrophy
- Compressive, toxic, or hereditary optic neuropathies
- Retinopathies, including Leber congenital amaurosis, Stargardt disease, retinitis pigmentosa, and others
- Central visual impairment (cortical blindness)
- Glaucoma
- Factitious or functional causes (hysterical blindness)

Data Gathering

HISTORY

- Age of onset of vision loss
- History of eye trauma, injury or surgery
- History of refractive error or glasses
- History of ptosis or ocular occlusion
- Family history of strabismus, anisometropia, or amblyopia

Physical Examination

Visual acuity is the single most significant sign in detection of amblyopia. Vision must be tested with each eye separately, with reliable occlusion (adhesive patch, opaque card, or plastic occluder). Since most amblyopia is monocular, testing vision with both eyes open is inadequate as a screening tool.

- In older children (>4 years) capable of reliable testing, monocular recognition visual acuity is tested by reading standard charts. Interocular difference of >1 line on the chart, or vision in either eye <20/40 that is not corrected with glasses should be investigated with full ophthalmologic examination. Charts may use illiterate symbols (pictures, numbers, E's) or letters.
- Younger children or children not capable of recognition visual acuity testing with charts can be tested by fixation preference, by induced tropia test (using vertical prism to induce diplopia and observing fixation preference).
- Binocularity tests such as Titmus stereopsis (3-D fly) will detect suppression, which is frequently associated with amblyopia.
- Other tests for amblyopic factors, while not directly measuring reduced vision, are useful for screening purposes, including
—Cover test, Hirschberg corneal light reflex test, and Bruchner tests for strabismus (see Strabismus chapter)
—Photoscreening, which uses the characteristics of the red reflex to detect amblyogenic factors such as optical aberrations and strabismus
—Inspection of the red reflex for cataract, optical opacities, and high refractive errors

Because the outcome of amblyopia depends entirely on early detection and treatment within the first few years of life, all children should be screened by monocular recognition visual acuity as early as possible (at the 3 or 4-year well child visit) and testing should be repeated annually until 8 years of age. Children with interocular difference of more than 1 line, or acuity in one or both eyes less than 20/40 should be referred for complete ophthalmologic evaluation and treatment. Children who are not capable of accurate visual acuity testing by 4 years should also be referred for complete evaluation.

Laboratory Aids

TESTS

Electrophysiologic testing using visual evoked cortical potential (VEP) is capable of detecting amblyopia. As typically performed, using very bright diffuse flashes, however, VEP is not sensitive enough to accurately detect amblyopia. Special VEP techniques using patterns (SVEP), however, show promise as a useful technique to measure resolution visual acuity in very young and nonverbal children. Psychophysical tests such as Teller preferential visual acuity testing have been used clinically to detect amblyopia and quantify visual acuity in young children, but are less useful for population-based screening because of the time and skill required to administer the tests.

Imaging studies of the optic nerves and posterior visual pathways may be useful in selected cases to exclude other causes of vision loss.

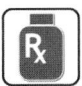

Therapy

Treatment for children with unilateral amblyopia consists of treating the underling cause of vision loss (strabismus, anisometropia, optical opacity, etc.) and forced preferential use of the amblyopic eye. The classic and most common treatment is occlusion with an adhesive patch worn over the opposite eye for several hours per day. The amount of time of occlusion necessary to reverse amblyopia depends on variables including the severity of amblyopia, cause of amblyopia, age, and other associated ocular conditions. Typically patches are worn from hours to full time, from a few weeks to months. Infants and very young children will require closer observation to prevent reversing the amblyopia to the previously preferred eye (occlusion amblyopia) from excessive patching.

Optical penalization of the opposite eye using topical cycloplegic eyedrops, such as atropine 1%, are another frequent therapy for amblyopia. Recent studies suggest that atropine penalization may be as effective as patching to treat mild or moderate amblyopia. Other treatments include:

• Occlusion of the opposite eye with opaque or translucent lens in glasses or opaque contact lens
• Optical penalization of the opposite eye with intentional overcorrection of refractive error (usually +3.00 diopters or more overcorrection)

Treatment should be attempted in amblyopic children within the "sensitive period" of birth to 8 years of age. Improvement of vision with treatment of older children has been reported, but is much less likely. Treatment is usually continued until visual acuity is equal to the opposite eye, or no further improvement is seen over several examinations with treatment.

The primary risk of treatment is overcorrection, with iatrogenic amblyopia in the occluded opposite eye.

In strabismic amblyopia, initiation of treatment for amblyopia need not wait for correction of the strabismus. In fact, the stability of the surgical strabismus correction is improved if amblyopia therapy is initiated prior to surgery. Treatment is usually continued until visual acuity in both eyes is equal, or until vision in the amblyopic eye shows no further improvement after several examinations over a period of time.

For bilateral amblyopia, correction of the underlying cause is the only treatment available.

Follow-Up

In general, the younger the patient, the more intensive the patching therapy, and the milder the amblyopia, the more frequent vision testing is necessary to ensure that vision in the opposite, occluded eye is not harmed. For full-time patching, testing is generally done at intervals of about 1 week per year of age, i.e., 2 weeks for a 2-year-old, etc.

• Children are clever at finding ways to avoid the temporary vision impairment from patching, and will peek or remove patches frequently. Parental encouragement and rewards, persistence, and close supervision are necessary for success. Older patients benefit from an explanation of the rational and potential long-term benefits of amblyopia therapy.
• In younger children, amblyopia may recur after successful treatment. Children should be retested frequently, and retreated if vision drops after finishing successful initial treatment. Testing should continue at least annually until the child is at least 8 years old.

PITFALLS

• Early vision testing is the most important tool for detection of amblyopia. Using age-appropriate charts (symbols, numbers, and letters) and well-trained testers will improve sensitivity and specificity of vision screening. Routine vision screening as a part of the annual well child examination beginning at age 4, as well as school screening programs, can detect amblyopia and potentially amblyopia-inducing factors in otherwise asymptotic children early enough for successful treatment.
• Vision testing in young children is difficult and sometimes unreliable. Children must be tested with each eye separately. Repeating the tests and adjunctive tests including the Titmus test (3-D fly), cover testing, photoscreening, and Bruchner red reflex test will increase the sensitivity of screening.
• Prompt referral of failures and children suspected of poor vision for complete ophthalmic examination is essential for successful amblyopia screening programs.
• Once treated, amblyopia may recur and vision should be retested regularly.
• Patients with strabismus, even if previously treated with glasses or surgery must be followed for amblyopia. Amblyopia is found in 40%–60% of patients with strabismus, and is not reversed by strabismus surgery.

Common Questions and Answers

Q. How long will patching be necessary?
A. It is not possible to predict exactly how long treatment will be necessary to restore vision. In general, the younger the patient, the milder the impairment, and the more intensive the patching, the more quickly vision is restored. In general, patching is usually continued for 1–4 months in most cases of anisometropic or strabismic amblyopia. Normalization of vision or lack of further improvement are usually treatment end-points.

Q. Will vision be normal after treatment?
A. The degree of recovery with amblyopia therapy depends on the density of the amblyopia, the cause, and the age at which treatment is initiated. In almost all children under 6–8 years of age, some visual improvement can be expected with amblyopia treatment, although not all patients will improve to 20/20 vision.

Q. Will patching eliminate the need for glasses?
A. No, patching does not influence the outcome of refractive errors (power of glasses, see chapter, Refractive Error). Glasses may still be needed after patching is completed.

Q. Will patching for amblyopia improve the strabismus?
A. No, in most cases patching for amblyopia will not eliminate strabismus or the need for strabismus surgery. However, in most cases it is best to begin amblyopia treatment before surgery to improve the surgical outcome.

Q. Is "vision therapy" without patching an effective treatment for strabismus?
A. Although eye exercises, pleioptics, and other vision therapies have been used to treat amblyopia, none is as effective as patching or other occlusive therapy. Current vision therapy techniques have not been proven to improve amblyopia.

Q. My child refuses to wear a patch. Are there alternatives to patching?
A. Yes, optical penalization with glasses, atropine cycloplegic penalization, and even contact lens occlusion can be effective. However, patching is the most reliable and effective treatment. Parental support, encouragement, and reward is essential for treatment compliance.

BIBLIOGRAPHY

Holmes JM, et al. Impact of patching and atropine treatment on the child and the family in the amblyopia treatment study. *Arch Ophthalmol* 2003;121:1625–1632.

The Pediatric Eye Disease Investigator Group. The course of moderate amblyopia treated with patching in children: experience of the amblyopia treatment study. *Am J Ophthalmol* 2003;136:620–629.

The Pediatric Eye Disease Investigator Group. A comparison of atropine and patching treatments for moderate amblyopia by patient age, cause of amblyopia, depth of amblyopia and other factors. *Ophthalmol* 2003;110: 1632–1637.

Repka MX, et al. A randomized trial fo patching regimens for treatment of moderate amblyopia in children. *Arch Ophthalmol* 2003;121:603–611.

Sengpien F, Blakemore C. The neural basis of supression and amblyopia in strabismus. *Eye* 1996;10:250–258.

Author: Monte D. Mills

Amebiasis

 Database

DEFINITION

- Clinical syndromes associated with *Entamoeba histolytica* infection.
- Most common clinical manifestation is intestinal amebiasis.
- Intestinal disease may be asymptomatic or have mild symptoms such as abdominal discomfort, flatulence, constipation, and occasionally diarrhea.
- Nondysenteric colitis is characterized by intermittent diarrhea and abdominal pain.
- Acute amebic colitis (dysenteric) is associated with grossly bloody stools with mucus, abdominal pain, and tenesmus.

CAUSES

- *Entamoeba histolytica* is nonflagellated protozoan parasite.
- Other species of the Entamoeba family are nonpathogenic including the morphologically identical *E. dispar*.

PATHOPHYSIOLOGY

- Fecal-oral transmission
- *E. histolytica* is excreted as cysts or trophozoites in the stool of infected patients.
- Ingested cysts are unaffected by gastric acid and produce trophozoites that colonize and invade the colon. The parasite has the ability to lyse human cells including colonic epithelium and immune effector cells such as neutrophils, macrophages, and lymphocytes. The host immune response contributes significantly to the destruction of host tissues.
- Amebas disseminate directly from the intestine to the liver in up to 10% of patients. Dissemination from the liver to the lung, heart, brain, and spleen has been described.
- The incubation period is typically 1–3 weeks but can range from a few days to months or years.

EPIDEMIOLOGY

- Spreads person to person via fecal-oral transmission.
- Less common modes of transmission include food and water. Sexual transmission can occur among homosexual males.
- Worldwide distribution involving an estimated to 10% or more of the world's population. Most common in tropical areas with infection rates as high as 20%–50%. The highest morbidity and mortality is seen in developing countries in Central America, South America, Africa, and Asia.
- Amebiasis accounts for 40–50 million cases of colitis worldwide and leads to 40,000–110,000 deaths annually.
- The estimated prevalence in the United States is 4%.
- The very young, the elderly, and patients with underlying immunosuppression or malnutrition are at highest risk for severe disease.

COMPLICATIONS

- Amebic liver abscess—second most common presentation of amebiasis, often not associated with amebic dysentery
- Ameboma—abdominal mass representing granulation tissue in the colon
- Extraintestinal manifestations of amebiasis are presumed to be a result of direct extension from liver abscesses. These include:
- Pericarditis
- Pleuropulmonary abscess or empyema
- Bronchohepatic fistula
- Genitourinary tract abscess
- Cerebral abscess
- Cutaneous amebiasis

 Differential Diagnosis

INFECTION

- *Salmonella*
- *Shigella*
- *Campylobacter*
- *Yersinia*
- *Clostridium difficile*
- *Escherichia coli* (enteroinvasive and enterohemorrhagic)
- Pyogenic abscess
- Echinococcal cyst

INFLAMMATORY BOWEL DISEASE

- Crohn disease
- Ulcerative colitis

MISCELLANEOUS

- Ischemic colitis
- Diverticulitis
- Arteriovenous malformations
- Hepatoma

 Data Gathering

The diagnosis is often missed in children because the disease is not included in the differential. Patients in whom the diagnosis should be considered include:

- Immigrants from or travelers to endemic areas
- Children with bloody stools or mucus in stools
- Children with hepatic abscess
- The febrile child with right upper quadrant pain and tenderness, abdominal pain, or discomfort
- The child with hepatomegaly, typically without jaundice.

Laboratory Aids

The diagnosis of amebiasis depends on the recognition of typical symptoms and:

ROUTINE LABORATORY TESTS

- Complete blood count typically reveals a leukocytosis.
- Transaminases are often not elevated.
- Occult blood is detected in stool.

MICROSCOPIC DIAGNOSIS

Identification of trophozoites or cysts in the stool.

- Serial stool samples, usually three, are recommended.
- Samples obtained within 1–2 hours of passage should be examined by wet mount and fixed in formalin and polyvinyl alcohol.
- Serial stool samples are necessary since cysts may be shed intermittently. Three serial stool samples will detect up to 70% of patients with amebic colitis and 50% of patients with hepatic abscess.
- Stool samples should not be contaminated by urine, water, barium, enema substances, laxatives, or antibiotics since these substances may destroy or interfere with identification of the trophozoites.

SEROLOGY

- Serum antiamebic antibodies are considered an adjunct to diagnosis. Approximately 85% of patients with amebic dysentery and 99% of patients with liver amebiasis will have positive serology.

RADIOGRAPHIC STUDIES

- Ultrasound, CT, or MRI of the liver.
- Chest radiographs in patients with hepatic amebiasis may reveal elevation of the right hemidiaphragm.

BIOPSY STUDIES

- Amebae are difficult to visualize in abscess aspirates and substantial risk is associated with CT or ultrasound-guided procedures including bleeding, peritonitis secondary to spillage of amebae or rupture of echinococcal cysts.
- Colonic or rectal mucosa visualized by colonoscopy reveals ulcerations and amebae can often be found around these lesions.

 ## Therapy

SPECIFIC

- The goal of treatment is the elimination of tissue-invading trophozoites and intestinal cysts.
- The choice of treatment regimens depends on the clinical presentation. Agents that are active against *E. histolytica* are divided into two categories: drugs with activity against intraluminal amebae and drugs with activity against extraintestinal and invasive amebiasis.

—Asymptomatic intestinal amebiasis—intraluminal agents
—Iodoquinol is the drug of choice. The recommended dosage is 30–40 mg/kg per day (max. 1,950 mg) given orally in three divided doses for 20 days.
—Alternative agents include diloxanide furoate (Furamide) at doses of 20 mg/kg per day (max. 1,500 mg/day) given orally in three divided doses OR paromomycin, 25–35 mg/kg per day given orally in three divided doses for 7 days.
—Acute amebic colitis or extraintestinal amebiasis
—Metronidazole (a tissue active agent) 35–50 mg/kg per day given orally in three divided doses for 10 days (max. 2,250 mg/day) PLUS a course of treatment with an intraluminal active agent (as above). Approximately one third of patients treated with metronidazole alone will relapse.

- Patients with large liver abscesses or who have failed medical therapy should be considered candidates for surgical or percutaneous drainage.

PREVENTION

- Treatment of drinking water
- Hand washing
- Appropriate disposal of human fecal waste
- Use of condoms

INFECTION CONTROL MEASURES

- Standard precautions are recommended for the hospitalized patient.

 ## Follow-Up

- Clinical improvement is expected within 72 hours of initiation of therapy
- Follow-up stool examination is always necessary to insure eradication of intestinal amebae
- For amebic abscesses, drainage should be considered if response to medical therapy has not occurred in 4 to 5 days

PITFALLS

Misdiagnosis is a common problem with amebiasis. Since it is not common in the United States, amebiasis may initially be misdiagnosed as bacterial dysentery.

BIBLIOGRAPHY

Haque R, et al. Amebiasis. *N Engl J Med* 2003;348(16):1565–1573.

Hotez PJ, Strickland AD. Amebiasis. In: Feigin RD, Cherry JD, eds. *Textbook of Pediatric Infectious Diseases*. 4th Ed. Vol 2. Philadelphia: WB Saunders 1998;208: 2389–2397.

Purdy JE, Petri WA Jr. Entamoeba histolytica (amebiasis). In: Long SS, Pickering LK, Pober CG, eds. *Principles and Practice of Pediatric Infectious Diseases*. New York: Churchill Livingstone, 1997;275:1380–1386.

Ravdin JI. Entamoeba histolytica (amebiasis). In: Mandell GL, Bennett JE, Dolin R, eds. *Principles and Practice of Infectious Diseases*. 5th Ed. Vol 2. Philadelphia: Churchill Livingstone 2000:2798–2810.

Stauffer W, Ravdin JI. Entamoeba histolytica: an update. *Current Opinion in Infectious Diseases*. 2003;16(5):479–485.

Authors: Jason Kim
Theoklis Zaoutis, 3rd edition

Anaerobic Infections

Database

DEFINITION

Anaerobes are organisms capable of growing in a reduced oxygen environment, either exclusively (obligate anaerobes) or in addition to growing in air (facultative anaerobes). They are components of the normal bacterial flora but can cause invasive disease in some circumstances.

PATHOPHYSIOLOGY

- Usually caused by endogenous organisms.
- Generally occurs when there is a break in a mucocutaneous barrier.
- Infections are often polymicrobial and include aerobic organisms.
- Increased risk associated with impaired host immunity or presence of devitalized tissue (due to surgery, trauma, and vascular insufficiency).
- Numerous virulence factors including exotoxins (e.g., *Clostridium* spp.), antiphagocytic capsule (e.g., *Bacteroides* spp.), endotoxin (e.g., *Fusobacterium* spp).
- Infections may be characterized by suppuration, abscess formation, tissue destruction, or systemic disease.

EPIDEMIOLOGY

- Less frequent in children than in adults, in whom anaerobes may account for up to 10% of bacteremic episodes.
- Some sites of infection (e.g., anaerobic infection in chronic otitis media) are common in children.

COMPLICATIONS

- Vary with nature of infection.

PROGNOSIS

- Determined by speed with which infection is appropriately treated with antibiotics and/or drainage.
- High rates of mortality associated with clinically apparent anaerobic bacteremia. Specific prognosis depends on the bacterial species involved and the status of the patient's immune system.
- Soft tissue infections caused by *Clostridium* spp. may cause up to 20% mortality despite aggressive therapy.

ASSOCIATED ILLNESSES

- Central nervous system (CNS) infections

—Brain abscess
—Subdural empyema
—Epidural abscess

- Head and neck infections

—Sinusitis (generally polymicrobial)
—Chronic otitis media
—Ludwig angina (infection of the submandibular space)
—Cervical adenitis
—Peritonsillar abscess
—Dental abscess
—Gingivitis
—Actinomycosis of jaw
—Lemiere syndrome (septic thrombophlebitis of the internal jugular vein due to Fusobacterium, often resulting in pulmonary abscess formation)

- Pleuropulmonary infections

—Aspiration of oral and/or gastrointestinal fluids
—Pneumonia, abscess formation
—Secondary to aspirated foreign bodies
—Actinomycosis

- Peritonitis/peritoneal abscess

—Appendiceal abscess
—Perforated viscus
—Postoperative complication
—Trauma related
—Actinomycosis

- Cholangitis

—Ascending infection may occur following biliary tract surgery (e.g., Kasai procedure)
—Infection is often polymicrobial.

- Bacteremia

—Often associated with focal primary site of involvement (GI disease, abscess)

- Soft tissue infection

—Paronychia
—Crepitant cellulitis
—Necrotizing fasciitis
—Gas gangrene (*Clostridium* spp.)

- Infected bite wounds

—Anaerobes isolated from 50% of human or animal bites.

- Likely pathogens not recovered from aerobic cultures.
- Failure of empiric antibiotic coverage that is not active against anaerobes.

Data Gathering

HISTORY

Question: Impaired mental status?
Significance: Increased risk of aspiration.

Question: History of thumb-sucking?
Significance: Anaerobes frequently isolated from paronychia.

Question: Recent surgery or trauma?
Significance: Poor drainage or devitalized tissue associated with anaerobic infection.

Question: Underlying immunodeficiency or chronic illness?
Significance: Impaired phagocytic function.

Question: Discharge with foul odor?
Significance: Characteristic of anaerobic infection.

Question: Lateral neck pain in association with respiratory distress?
Significance: Lemiere disease causes septic thrombophlebitis of the internal jugular vein and lung abscess.

Physical Examination

Finding: Location of infection
Significance: Increased incidence of anaerobic infections in the oropharyngeal, abdominal, and female genital tract.

Finding: Poor dentition
Significance: Increased colonization of oropharynx with anaerobic organisms.

Finding: Gas in tissue, crepitus
Significance: Infection with gas-forming organism

Finding: "Dishwater" pus
Significance: Characteristic of anaerobic infections

Laboratory Aids

Test: Gram stain
Significance: Small, pleomorphic gram-negative bacilli (*Bacteroides* spp.); large gram-positive organisms with "box-car" morphology (*Clostridium* spp.).

Test: Anaerobic cultures
Significance: Should be performed on tissue or aspirated fluid obtained in a sterile fashion from the infected site. Avoid sending a swab for culture. Specimens need to be transported promptly to the microbiology laboratory.

Test: X-ray studies
Significance: Air-fluid level, cavity formation, gas in tissue.

Test: Special imaging studies
Significance: CT and/or MRI scans often important to define anatomic location and extent of disease.

 ## Therapy

EMPIRIC DRUG THERAPY

- CNS infections
—Vancomycin + cefotaxime + metronidazole
- Head and neck infections
—Ampicillin-sulbactam or amoxicillin-clavulanate or clindamycin
- Pleuropulmonary infections
—Ampicillin-sulbactam or amoxicillin-clavulanate or clindamycin
- Peritonitis/peritoneal abscess
—Gentamicin + either ampicillin/sulbactam or cefoxitin
- Cholangitis
—Ampicillin/sulbactam + gentamicin
- Bacteremia
—Isolate-dependent
- Soft tissue infection
—Site dependent
- Infected bite wounds
—Amoxicillin/clavulinic acid

ADJUNCTIVE THERAPY

- Surgery
—Effective drainage of abscesses and debridement of devitalized tissue essential.
- Hyperbaric oxygen
—Especially for extensive Clostridial infections.

ICD-9-CM 041.84

BIBLIOGRAPHY

Bliss SJ, Flanders SA, Saint S. A pain in the neck. *N Engl J Med* 2004;350:1037–1042.

Brook I. Anaerobic infections in children. *Microbes and Infection* 2002;4:1271–1280.

Brook I. Clinical review: bacteremia caused by anaerobic bacteria in children. *Critical Care* 2002;6:205–211.

Correa AG. Clostridial intoxication and infection. In: Feigin RD, Cherry JD, Demmler GJ, Kaplan SL, eds. *Textbook of Pediatric Infectious Diseases*. 5th Ed. Philadelphia: WB Saunders 2004:1751–1758.

Author: Adam J. Ratner

Anaphylaxis

Database

DEFINITION

Anaphylaxis is an explosive antigen specific IgE-mediated response resulting in the release of potent biologically active mediators from mast cells and other inflammatory cells. However, non-IgE-mediated direct mast cell degranulation can result in a similar response. Patients may develop any combination of the following symptoms: cutaneous (urticaria/angioedema), respiratory (bronchospasm/laryngeal edema), cardiovascular (hypotension, arrhythmias, myocardial ischemia), and gastrointestinal (nausea, vomiting, pain, and diarrhea).

PATHOPHYSIOLOGY

Inducing agents stimulate mast cells to release inflammatory mediators either via an antigen-specific or antigen-nonspecific manner. These mediators may then act either locally or systemically. Mediator release results in the table Pathophysiology of Anaphylaxis.

EPIDEMIOLOGY

- Incidence 0.4 cases per million individuals annually
- Increased hospital incidence of 0.6 cases per 1,000 patients
- 400 to 800 deaths annually in the United States

COMPLICATIONS

- Pulmonary edema, pulmonary hemorrhage, and pneumothorax
- Laryngeal edema with or without airway obstruction
- Myocardial ischemia and infarction
- Death may result from asphyxiation from upper airway obstruction or profound shock or both.

PROGNOSIS

Excellent provided the trigger can be avoided.

Differential Diagnosis

GENETIC/METABOLIC

- Hereditary angioedema
- Systemic mastocytosis
- Pheochromocytoma
- Carcinoid

ALLERGIC/IMMUNOLOGIC

- Idiopathic
- Foods

—Insect stings
—Drugs
—Latex

- Nonimmunologic mast-cell degranulation
- Exercise-induced (may occur only after ingestion of a specific food)
- Serum sickness

MISCELLANEOUS

- Vasovagal collapse

COMMON CAUSES

- IgE-mediated

—Antibiotics (penicillin and others)
—Foreign protein agents (insect venom, latex antigens, fire ant venom, blood products and others)
—Therapeutic agents (allergen extracts, vaccines, and others)
—Foods (peanuts, nuts, shellfish, and others)

- Non-IgE-mediated "Anaphylactoid" reactions (activates histamine release from mast cells without protein binding to IgE)

—Radiocontrast media
—Opiates
—Dextran
—Vancomycin
—Polymyxin B
—Quaternary ammonium muscle relaxants (i.e., methyl scopolamine bromide, homatropine methylbromide, methantheline bromide, and ProBanthine bromide)

Approach to the Patient

GENERAL GOAL

Rapidly decide whether the symptoms the patient is experiencing are consistent with anaphylaxis (profuse rhinorrhea, urticaria, wheezing, throat tightness, tachycardia, and hypotension).

Phase 1: Initiate therapy for anaphylaxis. This generally includes: epinephrine 1:1000 administered subcutaneously, H1 antihistamines, H2 antihistamines, and rapid volume expansion if necessary.

Phase 2: Attempt to identify the agent that induced the anaphylactic reaction.

Data Gathering

HISTORY

Question: How long does it take for a patient to react to an offending allergen?
Significance: Anaphylactic reactions usually begin within seconds to minutes after contact with offending antigen. This can help the physician identify the responsible antigen.

Question: Can a patient have an anaphylactic reaction on their first exposure to an allergen?
Significance: A patient must have had a previous exposure to the offending allergen for sensitization to occur. Therefore, anaphylactic reactions should not occur on first exposure. Remember, however that infants can be sensitized through breast milk: therefore a baby may react upon "first" exposure to a food.

Question: What does the patient sense during an anaphylactic reaction?
Significance: Patients commonly describe an impending doom. This may be the first sign of an impending anaphylactic reaction.

Question: What organ systems are affected in an anaphylactic reaction?
Significance: The target organs may include: the heart, the lungs, the skin, the gastrointestinal tract, and the upper respiratory tract. Any or all of these target organs may be affected.

Question: What is the mechanism of fatal anaphylaxis?
Significance: Death may occur from upper airway obstruction and/or shock. When treating a patient with anaphylaxis upper airway obstruction, and hypotension should be taken very seriously.

Question: Has the patient had anaphylaxis in the past?
Significance: The patient likely knows the responsible allergen. Efforts should be directed toward allergen avoidance.

Pathophysiology of Anaphylaxis

PATHOLOGIC PROCESS	SIGN OR SYMPTOM	PUTATIVE MEDIATOR RESPONSIBLE
Vascular permeability	Urticaria, angioedema, laryngeal edema, abdominal swelling, cramps	Histamine (H1) leukotrienes, prostaglandins
Vasodilation	Flushing, headache	Histamine (H1 and H2), leukotrienes, prostaglandins
Smooth-muscle contraction	Wheezing, gastrointestinal cramps, diarrhea	Histamine (H1), leukotrienes, prostaglandins
Congestion	Rhinorrhea, bronchorrhea	Histamine (H2), prostaglandins, leukotrienes

Source: From Atkinson et al., with permission.

Question: Does the patient have autoinjectable epinephrine?
Significance: Most deaths from anaphylaxis are associated with delayed administration of epinephrine. Most patients with a history of anaphylaxis are candidates for autoinjectable epinephrine.

Question: Did the patient experience an insect sting, or is the patient allergic to any foods?
Significance: Insect or fire ant venom allergy can result in anaphylaxis. It is important to identify the insect if possible (remember honey bees leave their stinger at the sting site). Immunotherapy is indicated and effective for anaphylaxis in venom-allergic patients. Any food can cause anaphylaxis, but cow's milk, egg, soy, peanut, wheat, tree nut and shellfish are the most common.

Question: Does the patient have asthma or heart disease?
Significance: Asthma and cardiovascular disease are risk factors for death during anaphylaxis.

Question: Does the patient take any medications?
Significance: Beta-blockers make treatment of anaphylaxis more difficult. Alternative medications (glucagon) should be sought in patients with a history of anaphylaxis.

 ## Physical Examination

Finding: Angioedema
Significance: May be noted anywhere during a systemic allergic reaction, but it is much more significant if it involves the lips, tongue, mouth, or larynx (can result in airway obstruction).

Finding: Urticaria
Significance: Cutaneous manifestation of a systemic allergic reaction.

Finding: Profuse rhinorrhea
Significance: May signal upper respiratory tract involvement in a systemic allergic reaction.

Finding: Wheezing
Significance: Signals lower respiratory tract involvement in a systemic allergic reaction.

Finding: Tachycardia and hypotension
Significance: Signals cardiovascular involvement in a systemic allergic reaction. Tachycardia usually represents a compensatory mechanism in order to maintain the patient's blood pressure from fluid extravasation.

 ## Laboratory Aids

The treatment of anaphylaxis should never be withheld while awaiting laboratory confirmation.

Test: Plasma histamine
Significance: Plasma histamine is elevated during anaphylaxis but difficult to measure because of extremely short half life. Only useful in research setting.

Test: Serum tryptase
Significance: Serum tryptase is elevated during anaphylaxis. β-tryptase is elevated for several hours after the onset of anaphylaxis. This is the preferred test if available.

Test: Complete blood count
Significance: Hemoconcentration (as judged by an increased hematocrit or hemoglobin) is common as fluid exits the intravascular space during an anaphylactic reaction.

Test: Chest x-ray
Significance: The bronchospasm associated with anaphylaxis may result in air trapping and hyperinflated lung fields on chest x-ray.

Test: ECG
Significance: Anaphylaxis may show rhythm abnormalities, ischemic changes, or infarction on an ECG.

Test: Cardiac enzymes
Significance: Myocardial ischemia during anaphylaxis may result in a myocardial infarction, and elevated cardiac enzymes.

REFERRAL

Factors that may help alert you to make a referral include:

- History of idiopathic anaphylaxis. The allergist can help by testing to likely triggers.
- History of anaphylaxis to insect stings or fire ants. Anaphylaxis to insects or fire ants is an indication for venom desensitization.
- History of food anaphylaxis. The allergist can assist with an appropriate avoidance diet and support resources.
- History of latex anaphylaxis. The allergist can assist with strict latex avoidance precautions, and latex testing if the history is unclear.

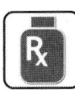 ## Therapy

- Subcutaneous epinephrine 1:1000 concentration. Early administration of epinephrine is essential.
- Maintain airway. Laryngeal edema can be managed with racemic epinephrine from a meter dose inhaler or nebulizer.
- A tourniquet may be applied (above the injection or sting site) to decrease venous blood return from the site of antigen entry.
- Supplement with oxygen, place in recumbent position and elevate legs. Patients during anaphylaxis have increased oxygen consumption.
- Diphenhydramine IV. H1 blockade is very important in the control of an anaphylactic reaction.
- Ranitidine IV. H1 blockade may be helpful in refractory anaphylaxis.
- Maintain blood pressure with volume expanders or pressors. Hypotension is a serious manifestation of anaphylaxis.
- Aminophylline may be added for wheezing.
- Hydrocortisone or another systemic steroid should be started. These are most helpful to prevent a late-phase reaction, and they are of little help during an immediate anaphylactic reaction.

 ## Follow-Up

- All patients who have had anaphylaxis should be discharged with epinephrine in an autoinjecting apparatus.
- Patients with a known trigger should be counseled on strict avoidance.
- All patients should follow up with an allergist.
- Patients not admitted to the hospital should be observed for several hours because late "biphasic" reactions can begin as late as 24 hours after the initial anaphylaxis. These patients are at risk for a second episode of anaphylaxis. Therefore, patients with anaphylaxis should be treated with steroids during the acute treatment, and they should be given a short course of oral corticosteroids to finish at home. In addition, these patients must be discharged with autoinjectable epinephrine (this will provide temporary relief so the patient will have time to seek medical assistance). Patients must know to seek immediate medical help if symptoms return.

 ## Common Questions and Answers

Q: When should the autoinjectable epinephrine be used?
A: It is intended for severe allergic reactions as manifested by any of the following: bronchospasm, angioedema of the lips or tongue, or hypotension (dizziness). The patient must seek immediate medical help if the autoinjectable epinephrine is required.

Q: Do patients outgrow this condition?
A: No. Subsequent reactions tend to have a more rapid onset, and tend to be more severe. Children may outgrow food-induced anaphylaxis.

Q: Who should be referred to an allergist?
A: All patients who have experienced anaphylaxis would benefit from consultation with an allergist. Patients with anaphylaxis from insect stings, fire ants and certain antibiotics can be desensitized. In addition, the allergist can be helpful in identifying obscure triggers of anaphylaxis.

BIBLIOGRAPHY

Bochner BS, Lichtenstein LM. Anaphylaxis. *N Engl J Med* 1991;324:1785–1790.

Cahaly RJ, Slater JE. Latex hypersensitivity in children. *Curr Opin Pediatr* 1995;7(6): 671–675.

Authors: Mathew Fogg
Christopher A. Smith, 3rd edition

Anemia of Chronic Disease

 Database

DEFINITION

Anemia that accompanies a variety of systemic diseases with the common features of chronicity and inflammation

PATHOPHYSIOLOGY

• Associated with collagen vascular disease, inflammatory bowel disease, malignancy, severe tissue injury, renal failure, and infections.

• Three common pathophysiologic factors

—Shortened red-cell survival—not seen in the anemia of all chronic disorders. The mechanism has not yet been defined.
—Impaired bone marrow erythropoietic response to the anemia with a blunted increase in red-cell production. Decreased marrow response to erythropoietin.
—Impaired iron utilization. Poor iron release from the reticuloendothelial system. This leads to a fall in plasma iron levels, a decrease in marrow sideroblasts, and a rise in red cell protoporphyrin concentration.

• Impaired erythroid progenitor response.
• Iron absorption may be normal or decreased.
• Cytokines such as interleukin-1 and interleukin-6 can activate ferritin synthesis. The ferritin can lead to sequestration of iron, which eventually is converted into hemosiderin.

EPIDEMIOLOGY

May be associated with chronic infections, collagen vascular disorders, other chronic inflammatory diseases, and cancer.

COMPLICATIONS

If severe, patients may be transfusion dependent and thus be at risk for complications associated with packed red blood cell transfusions.

 Differential Diagnosis

• Often confused with iron-deficiency anemia.
• In both iron deficiency and anemia of chronic disease

—Decreased plasma iron
—Decreased transferrin saturation
—Decreased marrow sideroblasts
—Elevated free erythrocyte protoporphyrin (FEP)
—Decreased reticulocyte count

• In anemia of chronic disease

—Mild to moderate anemia
—Mild anisocytosis
—Usually normochromic normocytic but can be hypochromic with microcytosis
—Decreased plasma iron
—Decreased iron-binding capacity
—Normal or slightly low transferrin saturation
—Decreased marrow sideroblasts
—Normal or elevated reticuloendothelial iron
—Elevated free erythrocyte protoporphyrin
—Normal or elevated ferritin

• In iron deficiency

—Decreased plasma iron
—Increased iron-binding capacity
—Decreased transferrin saturation
—Decreased marrow sideroblasts
—Decreased reticuloendothelial iron
—Increased free erythrocyte protoporphyrin
—Decreased serum ferritin

 Data Gathering

HISTORY

• Underlying disease process exists. Disease entities often associated with anemia of chronic disease include infections, both acute and chronic; inflammatory disease; collagen vascular diseases; malignancies, and renal failure.
• The anemia develops over the first month of the disease process and then remains fairly stable over time.

 Physical Examination

Various abnormal physical findings may be present depending on the underlying chronic disease process.
May have mild pallor but will not have signs of circulatory collapse.

Laboratory Aids

- Complete blood count with indices: normocytic, normochromic (can be microcytic, hypochromic) anemia with hematocrit rarely less than 20%
- Reticulocyte count: Usually in the normal range, but low for the level of anemia.
- Iron studies: Low plasma iron, with low total iron-binding capacity, low transferrin saturation by iron, normal or high ferritin, elevated FEP.
- Hemosiderin in bone marrow macrophages is increased if bone marrow aspiration is done and the aspirate is viewed with iron stains. This is generally not indicated.
- Albumin and transferrin: Both low.
- Acute-phase reactants like C-reactive protein may be elevated.

PITFALLS

If only the serum iron is obtained without the remainder of iron studies, the child may be inappropriately diagnosed with iron deficiency.

Anemia of chronic disease often coexists with other causes of anemia, including: occult blood loss, hemolysis, dietary iron deficiency, and drug-related marrow suppression.

 ## Therapy

DRUGS

Iron: There is no role for iron therapy unless there is coexisting iron-deficiency anemia.
Recombinant human erythropoietin: Effective, but indications for use are still not universally accepted. Often utilized in chronic renal failure. Has been used in inflammatory bowel diseases with good results. Should be used for more severe and symptomatic anemia where the underlying disease is likely to be prolonged and difficult to treat. May be used in childhood cancer to decrease the exposure to blood products.

OTHER THERAPIES

Treatment should be directed at the underlying disease process.
Transfusion of packed red blood cells is sometimes indicated intermittently in severe anemia with hemodynamic compromise.

 ## Follow-Up

Treatment of underlying disease process may promote slow resolution of associated anemia. Hematocrit increases about 6–8 weeks after start of recombinant human erythropoietin therapy. Continues to rise over 6 months.

 ## Common Question and Answer

Q: Does anemia that is associated with a chronic disease require further evaluation?
A: If the anemia fits within the general guidelines of diagnosis as outlined above, there is no need to pursue further investigation, except in specific cases. If there is an associated malignancy where marrow metastasis is possible, a bone marrow aspirate and biopsy should be done. In conditions with malabsorption, nutritional deficiencies and blood loss should be ruled out.

ICD-9-CM 281.9

BIBLIOGRAPHY

Andrews NB, Bridges KC. Disorders of iron metabolism and sideroblastic anemia. In: Nathan DG, Oski FA, eds. *Hematology of Infancy and Childhood*. 5th Ed. Philadelphia: WB Saunders 1998:450–451.

Goodnough LT, et al. Erythropoietin, iron, and erythropoiesis. *Blood* 2000;96(3):823–833.

Means RT. Erythropoietin in the treatment of anemia in chronic infectious, inflammatory, and malignant disease. *Curr Opin Hematol* 1995;2:210–213.

Means RT. Clinical application of recombinant erythropoietin in the anemia of chronic disease. *Hematol Oncol Clin North Am* 1994;8:933–944.

Stockman JA III, Ezekowitz AB. Hematologic manifestations of systemic diseases. In: Nathan DG, Oski FA, eds. *Hematology of Infancy and Childhood*. 5th Ed. Philadelphia: WB Saunders 1998:1841–1879.

Weiss G. Pathogenesis and treatment of anemia of chronic disease. *Blood Rev* 2002;16(2):87–96.

Author: Tammy I. Kang

Angioedema

 Database

DEFINITION

Hereditary angioedema is an autosomal-dominant disorder in which mutations in the C1-INH (C1 esterase inhibitor) gene results in a deficiency or an inactive form of plasma C1-INH. This permits unregulated activation of the complement and plasma kinin-forming pathways leading to angioedema.

COMMON CAUSES

Classic Hereditary Form

• Defect in one of the two genes coding for C1-INH on chromosome 11.

Acquired Forms

• In one form, normal amount and functionally normal C1-INH is secreted into the plasma, but it is bound to circulating antibodies that inactivate it (associated with benign and malignant monoclonal B-cell lymphoproliferative disorders).
• In the other form, an autoantibody not associated with lymphoproliferative disorders binds to C1-INH resulting in increased degradation of C1-INH.

PATHOPHYSIOLOGY

• Deficiency of C1-INH leads to unopposed activation of the first complement component, resulting in the formation of bradykinin, which produces angioedema.
• Angioedema may occur in the upper airway, gastrointestinal tract, and extremities.
• Life-threatening upper airway obstruction may develop.

GENETICS

• Autosomal dominant
• Mutations may be in either of two genes for C1-INH located on chromosome 11.
• Acquired forms lack a genetic predisposition (there is no mutation in the C1-INH gene).

COMPLICATIONS

• Life-threatening upper airway obstruction.
• Severe abdominal pain often mistaken for a surgical abdomen.

PROGNOSIS

Good with prophylactic and recombinant C1-INH therapies. Recombinant C1-INH is not available in the United States despite its proven clinical efficacy for treatment of acute attacks.

 Differential Diagnosis

TOXIC, ENVIRONMENTAL, DRUGS

Patients on angiotensin-converting enzyme (ACE) inhibitors

ALLERGIC INFLAMMATORY

• IgE-mediated allergic reactions

—Drug allergy
—Food allergy
—Contact allergy

• Transfusion reaction

TUMOR

Associated with neoplasms via unknown mechanism

GENETIC/METABOLIC

• Urticaria pigmentosa/mastocytosis
• Familial cold urticaria
• C3b inactivator deficiency
• Amyloidosis with deafness and urticaria
• Hereditary vibratory angioedema

PHYSICAL

• Physical urticarias

—Cold urticaria
—Cholinergic urticaria
—Pressure urticaria (angioedema)
—Vibratory angioedema
—Solar urticaria
—Aquagenic urticaria

• Exercise-induced anaphylaxis

RHEUMATOLOGIC

Collagen vascular disease

PSYCHOLOGICAL

• Panic attacks
• Globus hystericus
• Vocal cord dysfunction

MISCELLANEOUS

Idiopathic angioedema

 Data Gathering

HISTORY

Question: At what age did the recurrent episodes of subcutaneous and submucosal edema begin?
Significance: Recurrent episodes of angioedema usually begin at puberty.

Question: How are the episodes of angioedema characterized?
Significance: Angioedema episodes are characterized by edema of the upper airway, extremities, or bowels (can cause severe abdominal pain).

Question: Are the angioedema episodes associated with hives?
Significance: Episodes of angioedema are not associated with hives. However, patients may have an erythema marginatum rash which is nonpruritic.

Question: How long do the episodes of angioedema last?
Significance: The duration of an angioedema episode usually last 1 to 4 days.

Question: What triggers the angioedema episode?
Significance: Episodes of angioedema can be triggered by emotional stress, physical trauma such as surgery or dental procedures. Episodes can also be triggered by infection, menstruation, pregnancy, and estrogen-containing oral contraceptives.

Question: Do other family members have similar episodes of angioedema?
Significance: Angioedema can be inherited in an autosomal-dominant fashion. There may be other affected family members.

Question: Do the episodes of angioedema respond to epinephrine, antihistamines, or corticosteroids?
Significance: Angioedema related to C1 esterase inhibitor responds poorly to epinephrine, antihistamines, and corticosteroids.

Angioedema

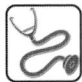 ## Physical Examination

Aside from angioedema, the physical examination is normal. Erythema marginatum may also be present.

 ## Laboratory Aids

GENERAL GOALS

Decide if the patient's symptoms are consistent with hereditary angioedema (recurrent angioedema after minor trauma, family history, onset at puberty, lack of hives, and poor response to epinephrine).

- Measure C1 esterase inhibitor level and function
- If C1 esterase inhibitor level is normal, and an acquired deficiency is suspected, order a functional assay of C1 esterase inhibitor. Samples for complement assays must be placed on ice immediately, otherwise the results may be falsely low.

Test: Direct measurement of C1-INH level and function (study of choice to identify the hereditary form of C1-INH deficiency). *Significance:* This is an antigenic assay. Affected patients may have a minimal quantity of C1-INH detected, and heterozygotes (carriers) have approximately one-half normal levels detected. Some patients may have normal levels of protein with reduced function.

Test: C1q
Significance: In acquired C1-INH deficiency levels of C1q will be reduced, while the C1q will be normal in the hereditary form.

Test: CH50
Significance: The CH50 is a general screen of the complement system, and if abnormal can indicate a deficiency of any of the complement components.

REFERRAL

Factors that may help alert you to make a referral include:

- Any patient diagnosed with angioedema. An allergist can help evaluate these patients for possible androgen prophylaxis therapy. In addition, they can assist in the creation of an emergency plan for management of acute attacks.
- Patients with difficult-to-control angioedema without an identified trigger. An allergist/immunologist can assist with the appropriate evaluation.

 ## Therapy

PROPHYLAXIS

- Anabolic steroids (Danazol or Stanozolol) cause increased production of C1-INH resulting in near-normal C2 and C4 levels (decreased degradation by activated C1), and a significantly decreased episode frequency. This therapy is indicated in patients with frequent or life-threatening episodes.
- Plasmin inhibitors (ϵ-aminocaproic acid or tranexamic acid) do not correct C2 and C4 levels, but are clinically effective.
- Recombinant C1-INH concentrate available outside the U.S. and is highly effective.

—Prior to dental and surgical procedures, doses of androgen should be increased for 1 to 2 weeks. In addition, some experts recommend treatment with fresh frozen plasma shortly before and immediately after surgery as this product contains C1-INH.

ACUTE ATTACKS

- Recombinant C1-INH concentrate (outside of U.S.)

—Increase dose of androgen at first symptoms of an attack
—Immediately seek medical care, airway should be protected if any compromise imminent

- Intermittent administration of subcutaneous epinephrine (this type of angioedema is usually poorly responsive, but in an emergent situation this may be considered).

MEDICAL MANAGEMENT

Treatment of the underlying condition often results in resolution of the angioedema.

 ## Follow-Up

- Patients should be seen at least annually.
- Follow-up should include:

—Review of triggers
—Prospective genetic counseling
—Reinforcement of the need for prophylaxis
—Review of attacks during the previous year
—Creation of an emergency plan for the administration of recombinant C1 esterase inhibitor during severe attacks

- Regular follow-up with an endocrinologist is indicated for patients requiring androgen steroid therapy

 ## Common Questions and Answers

Q: What is a good screening test for angioedema?
A: The CH50 is a good screening test. Patients with angioedema have a low CH50. Remember that the specimen must be placed on ice immediately. Failure to ice the specimen will result in a falsely low CH50.

Q: What are the side effects of the prophylactic androgen therapy?
A: The side effects include: masculinization, menstrual irregularities, enhanced epiphyseal growth plate closure, water retention, hypertension, cholestatic hepatitis, hepatic carcinoma, decreased spermatogenesis, and gynecomastia.

BIBLIOGRAPHY

Frigas E, Nzeako UC. Angioedema. Pathogenesis, differential diagnosis, and treatment. *Clin Rev in Allerg & Immunol* 2002;23(2):217–231.

Gratten C, Powell S, Humphreys F. Management and diagnostic guidelines for urticaria and angio-edema. *Br J Dermatol* 2001;144(4):708–714.

Kaplan AP. Clinical practice. Chronic urticaria and angioedema. *N Engl J Med* 2002;346(3):175–179.

Kozel MM, et al. Laboratory tests and identified diagnoses in patients with physical and chronic urticaria and angioedema: A systematic review. *J Am Acad Dermatol* 2003;48(3):409–416.

Authors: Mathew Fogg
Christopher A. Smith, 3rd edition

Ankylosing Spondylitis

 ## Database

DEFINITION

Ankylosing spondylitis is an inflammatory arthritis that tends to be asymmetric peripherally and to involve the insertion of tendons, ligaments, as well as the sacroiliac joints and spine.

CAUSES

- Idiopathic

PATHOLOGY

- Inflammatory synovitis of joints and calcification of the anterior and posterior longitudinal ligaments of the spine

EPIDEMIOLOGY

- Typically affects adolescent males
- About 1 per 1,000 white boys
- Much less common in blacks

GENETICS

- HLA-B27 associated

COMPLICATIONS

- Acute anterior uveitis
- Aortic insufficiency

 ## Differential Diagnosis

INFECTION

- Reiter syndrome caused by enteric pathogens or Chlamydia
- Whipple disease
- Intestinal-bypass-associated arthritis
- Discitis
- Pott disease

TUMORS

- Osteoid osteoma

TRAUMA

- Traumatic injury causing low back pain/spasm
- Herniated disc

METABOLIC

- Ochronosis

CONGENITAL

- Kyphosis

IMMUNOLOGIC

- Inflammatory bowel disease-associated arthropathy
- Pauciarticular juvenile rheumatoid arthritis

PSYCHOLOGICAL

- Feigning low back pain/stiffness

MISCELLANEOUS

- Psoriasis-associated arthritis
- SEA (seronegative enthesopathy and arthropathy) syndrome

 ## Data Gathering

HISTORY

Question: Ankylosing spondylitis
Significance: Signified by back pain of insidious onset that has been present for at least 3 months. There is usually a family history of a male relative with disease and inactivity stiffness resulting in gelling of peripheral joints and back.

 ## Physical Examination

Finding: Sacroiliac tenderness
Significance: Indicates site of inflammation

Finding: Pain on direct palpation at insertion of Achilles tendon and plantar fascia at calcaneal insertion
Significance: Indicates site of inflammation

Finding: Schober test of lumbar spine flexibility
Significance: Mark 15-cm span at mid-low back at level of iliac crest while patient is standing. Have patient flex back as far as possible. Remeasure span. Abnormal if less than 5 cm increase in span.

 ## Laboratory Aids

Test: CBC, ESR, HLA-B27, rheumatoid factor (RF), and antinuclear antibody (ANA) tests should be done.
Significance: Note that ESR is occasionally not elevated. RF and ANA are typically negative.

Test: Imaging
Significance: Sacroiliac views should be obtained to demonstrate evidence of pseudo-widening and/or sclerosis.

Test: False positives
Significance: HLA-B27 occurs in 8% of whites and 6% of blacks.

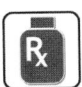 ## Therapy

DRUGS

- NSAIDs: naproxen, indomethacin, meclofenamate
- Disease-modifying drugs: sulfasalazine, methotrexate, and tumor necrosis factor inhibitors.

PHYSICAL THERAPY

Physical therapy is an essential component of treatment. Must encourage range-of-motion exercises and avoid prolonged neck flexion.

DURATION OF THERAPY

- May be lifelong

DIET

- Food intake should be good with NSAIDs
- Ensure folate intake with methotrexate

 ## Follow-Up

WHEN TO EXPECT IMPROVEMENT

Over weeks to several months should see some improvement in stiffness, synovitis, and range of motion.

SIGNS TO WATCH FOR TO INDICATE PROBLEMS

- Worsening stiffness
- Acute or chronic eye pain
- Chest pain or shortness of breath

PROGNOSIS

- Poor if disease remains active for 10 years or more

PITFALLS

Overdiagnosis in HLA-B27-positive individuals in whom other causes for joint swelling should be considered.

 ## Common Questions and Answers

Q: Should HLA-B27 be checked routinely in boys with back pain?
A: Detection of HLA-B27 alone should not precipitate an extensive workup because it is so common in the normal healthy population. However, the risk for developing a spondyloarthropathy is 16 times greater than in the HLA-B27-negative individual.

Q: Can affected individuals play contact sports?
A: This is probably not a good idea because as the spine fuses, the risk for fracture of the spine (especially the C-spine) increases. However, children with milder forms of disease, such as SEA syndrome should not be discouraged.

ICD-9-CM 720.0

BIBLIOGRAPHY

Bukulmez H, Colbert RA. Juvenile spondyloarthropathies and related arthritis. *Curr Opin Rheumatol* 2002;14:531–535.

Burgos-Vargas R. The juvenile-onset spondyloarthritides. *Rheum Dis Clin North Am* 2002;28:531–560.

Burgos-Vargas R, et al. The place of juvenile onset spondyloarthropathies in the Durban 1997 ILAR classification criteria of juvenile idiopathic arthritis. International League of Associations for Rheumatology. *J Rheumatol* 2002;29:869–874.

Homeff G, Burgos-Vargas R. TNF-alpha antagonists for the treatment of juvenile-onset spondyloarthritides. *Clin Exp Rheumatol* 2002;20(Suppl 28):S137–S142.

Sherry DD, Sapp LR. Enthesalgia in childhood: site-specific tenderness in healthy subjects and in patients with seronegative enthesopathic arthropathy. *J Rheumatol* 2003;30:1335–1340.

Tse SM, Laxer RM. Juvenile spondyloarthropathy. *Curr Opin Rheumatol* 2003;15:374–379.

Author: Randy Q. Cron

Anomalous Coronary Artery

 Database

DEFINITION

In this disorder, most commonly the left (rarely the right) coronary artery arises from the pulmonary trunk rather than the aorta.

CAUSES

- Abnormal septation of the conotruncus into aorta and pulmonary artery.
- Persistence of the pulmonary buds and involution of the aortic buds that will eventually form the coronary arteries.
- As yet unspecified genetic predisposition.

PATHOPHYSIOLOGY

- Collateral flow runoff tends to "steal" blood from the myocardial blood vessels into the pulmonary artery, resulting in myocardial ischemia.
- The diastolic blood pressure in the pulmonary artery is typically much lower than the main driving force for myocardial perfusion in patients with normal anatomy, namely diastolic aortic pressure.
- The fact that the left ventricle may be perfused with desaturated blood plays a less important role than the overall perfusion-related imbalance between myocardial oxygen demand and supply.

EPIDEMIOLOGY

- Rare anomaly
- The majority of patients with this anomaly present in infancy at around the age of 2 months.
- Of note, the literature includes many single case reports of newly diagnosed patients presenting as old as during the fourth to seventh decade.

 Differential Diagnosis

- Cardiomyopathy
- Mitral-valve incompetence
- Left ventricular failure from other causes
- Colic
- Bronchiolitis

 Data Gathering

HISTORY

- Paroxysms of poor feeding, pallor, and sweating
- Irritability (crying), especially after meals
- May have intractable congestive heart failure
- Sometimes asymptomatic
- Occasionally may be symptomatic in infancy and then gradually improve (with adequate coronary collateralization)
- Older children and adults may have dyspnea, syncope, or angina pectoris on effort
- Sudden death

 Physical Examination

- Signs of congestive heart failure, including cachexia, tachycardia, tachypnea, lethargy, diaphoresis, etc.
- Loud P_2 component of S_2
- Gallop rhythm
- Murmur: mitral incompetence or a continuous murmur reminiscent of a coronary arteriovenous fistula
- Diagnosis should be entertained in any infant presenting with cardiomegaly or perplexing cardiorespiratory symptoms.

 Laboratory Aids

Test: Chest x-ray study
Significance: Cardiomegaly, pulmonary edema

Test: Nuclear imaging
Significance: Thallium myocardial perfusion imaging shows reduced uptake in ischemic regions.

Test: Electrocardiography
Significance: Anterolateral infarct pattern in an infant (Q in I, aVL, V4-V6), abnormal R wave progression in precordial leads

Test: Echocardiogram
Significance: Attachment of coronary artery to pulmonary artery by two-dimensional imaging. Doppler interrogation shows flow passing from coronary artery to great artery rather than vice versa.

- Large right coronary artery
- Functional impairment, wall-motion abnormalities, and dilation of the left ventricle
- Echogenic papillary muscles
- Mitral regurgitation

Test: Cardiac catheterization
Significance: Angiographic and hemodynamic parameters can correlate with degree of cardiovascular dysfunction.

- Low cardiac output
- High filling pressures
- Pulmonary hypertension
- Aortic root angiography shows passage of contrast medium from normally connected right coronary artery to the left coronary arterial system to pulmonary artery

Test: Pulmonary artery angiogram
Significance: Shows reflux of contrast medium into the left coronary artery, and/or a "negative wash-in" of unopacified blood flowing from left coronary to pulmonary artery.

 Emergency Care

Attention to basic life support measures (airway, breathing, and circulation) and prompt referral to a pediatric cardiac center. An excess of procedures, interventions, and manipulation are poorly tolerated by this group of patients. Even with the full support of a tertiary center's experienced team, these measures are fraught with peril.

Therapy

The first priority is to safely institute supportive care measures while expeditiously planning for surgical intervention. Medical therapy alone has a very limited role in the current era.

SURGERY

- Direct reimplantation of the left coronary artery into the aorta using a button of pulmonary arterial tissue and/or an extension tube graft of anterior and posterior pulmonary arterial wall tissue sewn into a narrow cylinder to avoid tension, distortion, and stenosis.
- Creation of an aortopulmonary window and tunnel that directs blood from aorta to the left coronary ostium (Takeuchi procedure).
- Ligation of the origin of the left coronary artery (to prevent flow runoff into the pulmonary artery or "steal") is less frequently used, even in very ill infants.
- Ligation of origin of left coronary artery and reconstitution of flow with saphenous or internal mammary graft is less frequently used in the current era.

PROGNOSIS

- Untreated, 65% to 85% of those who present in infancy will die before the age of 1 year, usually after 2 months of age (when pulmonary vascular resistance falls).
- Few of those who present early improve spontaneously.
- Late results after surgery are excellent in many centers. Hospital mortality in larger selected series of these frequently moribund patients is at or below 5%, with very little subsequent attrition.
- Mitral regurgitation usually improves after surgery establishes a patent dual-coronary system, but this may take 6 to 12 months to be fully realized. Follow-up evaluation is warranted as mitral regurgitation may progress in spite of surgery and valve repair may be required later.

Common Questions and Answers

Q: How do you differentiate the crying from colic?
A: This is not easy, but clinical assessment should manifest the signs of congestive heart failure, shock, and low cardiac output that are decidedly atypical for the usual patient with colic. If the patient is still feeding, the crying in patients with this lesion classically occurs after meals when blood is shunted to the liver and intestines. This is not a highly sensitive finding, and concern should lead to further objective evaluation.

Q: How does one proceed with the evaluation?
A: In addition to history and physical examination findings, results of chest radiography, an ECG, and echocardiography may show the typical features discussed above.

ICD-9-CM 746.85

BIBLIOGRAPHY

Ando M, et al. Creation of a dual-coronary system for anomalous origin of the left coronary artery from the pulmonary artery utilizing the trapdoor flap method. *Eur J Cardiothorac Surg* 2002;Oct;22(4):576–581.

Azakie A, et al. Anatomic repair of anomalous left coronary artery from the pulmonary artery by aortic reimplantation: early survival, patterns of ventricular recovery and late outcome. *Ann Thorac Surg* 2003;75(5): 1535–1541.

Davis JA, Cecchin F, Jones TK, et al. Major coronary artery anomalies in a pediatric population: incidence and clinical importance. *J Am Coll Cardiol* 2001;37(2):593–597.

Dodge-Khatami A, et al. Anomalous origin of the left coronary artery from the pulmonary artery: collective review of surgical therapy. *Ann Thorac Surg* 2002;74(3):946–955.

Emmanouilides GC, Riemenschneider TA, Allen HD, et al, eds. *Moss and Adams' Heart Disease in Infants, Children and Adolescents Including the Fetus and Young Adult.* 5th Ed. Baltimore: Williams & Wilkins 1995:776–780.

Frommelt MA, et al. Detection of septal coronary collaterals by color flow Doppler mapping is a marker for anomalous origin of a coronary artery from the pulmonary artery. *J Am Soc Echocardiogr* 2002;15(3): 259–263.

Fyler C. *Nadas' Pediatric Cardiology.* Philadelphia: Henley & Belfus/St. Louis: Mosby 1992;51:715–718.

Michielon G, et al. Anomalous coronary artery origin from the pulmonary artery: correlation between surgical timing and left ventricular function recovery. *Ann Thorac Surg* 2003;76(2):581–588.

Pelliccia A. Congenital coronary artery anomalies in young patients: new perspectives for timely identification. *J Am Coll Cardiol* 2001;37(2):598–600.

Author: Geoffrey Bird

Anorexia Nervosa

 Database

DEFINITION

Anorexia nervosa (AN) is a potentially life-threatening, psychopathologic disorder of eating, involving profound weight loss and abnormal body image. Associated impact on nutritional status and multisystem involvement of the individual's health can be significant and potentially life-threatening. Diagnostic criteria:

- Weight loss or failure to attain expected weight gain leading to body weight less than 85% of normal weight for height (using Body Mass Index [BMI], growth charts with age appropriate norms)
- Disordered perception of personal body weight or shape, undue influence of body image on self-assessment, and/or denial of seriousness and abnormality of current low body weight
- Intense, abnormal fear of becoming fat or of weight gain, although significantly underweight for height
- In females, the absence of at least 3 consecutive menstrual periods (i.e., amenorrhea)
- DSM-IV specifies two types of AN:
—Restricting type: Absence of regular binge eating or purging (i.e., misuse of laxatives, enemas, or diuretics or self-induced vomiting) during the current episode of anorexia nervosa
—Binge eating/purging type: presence of regular purging or binge eating behaviors during the current episode of AN
- Additionally, eating disorder not otherwise specified (EDNOS), describes patients who present with emotional concerns similar to those with AN or bulimia, and are considered preanorexic, at risk, or subthreshold anorexia.

Spectrum of Severity

Mild: Weight proportionate (at or >90%) for height

- More exaggerated concern about body image and thinness than among normal adolescent and young adult populations in the United States
- Mild distortion of body image (self-perception as overweight)
- No symptoms or signs of excess weight loss are noted.
- Daily diet contains 1,000 calories or more
- No purging
- Exercise moderate, not excessive

Moderate: Increasing distortion of body image (escalating self-perception of being overweight)

- Weight <90% of average weight for height
- Symptoms and signs of weight loss
- Constant dieting
- Abnormal concern with weight (either avoiding being weighed or weighing him/herself frequently, sometimes several times daily)
- Excessive exercise (may approach obsessive exercise patterns)
- Diet contains <1,000 calories per day
- Withdrawal from family and friends
- Denial of weight loss, thinness, or the exist-ence of any problem with weight loss or thinness

Severe: Pathologic and dramatic distortion of body image plus ongoing weight loss

- Weight only 85% (or less) of height
- Ongoing determination to lose additional weight
- Signs and symptoms of malnutrition (may include bradycardia and/or hypotension)
- Denial regarding thinness
- Pathologic or unhealthy means of weight loss (consuming <1,000 calories/day, purging, enemas, laxatives, anorexic drugs)
- Markedly excessive exercise

Profound: Body weight 75% or less than expected for height, as well as continuing rapid weight loss

- Increasingly distorted perception of body image and denial of thinness
- Electrolyte imbalances
- Associated cardiac abnormalities (e.g., arrhythmias, prolonged QT interval, bradycardia)
- Hypotension, with potential cardiovascular collapse

EPIDEMIOLOGY

- Generally, more common in adolescents and young adults
- Much more prevalent in industrialized societies
- Bimodal distribution of early onset: 85%–95% female and later adult >40 year old onset: 24% male
- Age of presentation: 9 to 25 years; most common of onset: 14 and 18 years, occasional onset after age 40.
- U.S. average of 145 deaths annually attributable to AN

COMPLICATIONS

- Cardiac failure, dysrhythmia, hypotension, syncope
- Cardiac ventricular enlargement, cardio-ascular collapse, shock, and potential death
- Esophagitis, hematemesis (including Mallory-Weiss tear)
- Constipation, decreased intestinal, rectal prolapse
- Delayed gastric emptying
- Gastric dilatation and even rupture
- Pancreatitis
- Renal calculi
- Delayed onset of puberty, amenorrhea, infertility
- Convulsive seizures
- Peripheral neuropathies
- Severe bone loss, potential persistent osteopenia, and related growth arrest, fracture risk
- Depression, anxiety, obsessive-compulsive disorder, potential suicide risk (may be comorbid or coexistent diagnoses)
- Euthyroid sick syndrome
- Malnutrition and/or acute and chronic malnutrition states
- Anemia, leukopenia, thrombocytopenia

PROGNOSIS

- Mortality rate of AN is 0.56% per year (12 times the mortality rate among young females in general population)
- Most common causes of death: cardiac dysfunction or suicide

- 50% fully recover; 30% have partial recovery, including recurrences; 20% may have no substantial improvement in symptoms

 Differential Diagnosis

TUMORS

- Malignancy, including CNS malignancy

GASTROINTESTINAL

- Inflammatory bowel disease
- Gastroesophageal reflux disease

METABOLIC

- Diabetes mellitus
- Addison disease
- Estrogen deficiency

PSYCHIATRIC/EMOTIONAL

- Anxiety, depression, obsessive-compulsive disorder, suicidal ideation, psychosis
- Substance abuse
- Effects of domestic violence, physical/emotional/sexual abuse

 Data Gathering

HISTORY

- Weight changes (duration, extent, exact or estimated weight loss, including clothing sizes, past history)
- Diet patterns
- Menstruation history
- Exercise (type, frequency, duration, competitive, casual)
- Energy level
- Sleep (changes in patterns, duration, restfulness)
- Emesis, other purging, including laxatives, diuretics, enemas
- Anorexic drugs, caffeine, other stimulants
- Illicit drugs, alcohol, tobacco, addiction history and/or tendencies
- Other concomitant illnesses or family history of illnesses, including thyroid disorders, malignancies, diabetes mellitus, inflammatory bowel disease, psychiatric disorders

QUESTIONS TO ASK PATIENT

Question: How do you feel about your body size, i.e., too thin, too heavy, or just right for your height? How much would you like to weigh?

Question: When did you last weigh yourself? How often do you weigh yourself?

Question: What foods do you avoid? What foods make you feel anxious/guilty to eat? *Significance:* Fatty or high calorie foods may be specifically avoided by those with AN. Other questions to include:

- When did you last eat something? Drink something? What? How much?
- How did you feel after you last ate (or drank) something?
- Do you feel sick (nauseated, bloated, etc.) after you eat (and how often)?
- When did you last vomit after eating (was it spontaneous or provoked)?

Physical Examination

Finding: Flat affect, despondent
Significance: Depression, potential suicidal risk, poor self-image

Finding: Bradycardia, hypothermia, orthostasis, and/or hypotension
Significance: Volume depletion, dehydration, for cardiovascular collapse and shock

Finding: Dry skin, lanugo hair, carotinemic skin coloration
Significance: Chronic malnutrition and vitamin deficiency

Finding: Peripheral edema, acrocyanosis, diminished capillary refill
Significance: Increased severity of malnutrition and possible cardiovascular, electrolyte, and/or renal pathology

Finding: Bladder distension
Significance: Water loading to falsely increase weight for exam

Finding: Scars on knuckles, eroded dental enamel, parotid enlargement
Significance: Suggestive of self-induced vomiting, bulimia

Finding: Scars, old cuts, evidence of self-inflicted burns
Significance: Risk-taking behaviors

Laboratory Aids

No laboratory test is diagnostic for eating disorders, which are often a diagnosis of exclusion. Laboratory aids are necessary to assess medical complications of AN, as well as to rule out other differential diagnoses.

- Complete blood count (CBC)—screening for anemia, leukopenia, thrombocytopenia (all common in AN).
- Erythrocyte sedimentation rate.
- Serum electrolytes, Critical deficiencies of calcium and magnesium may present with neurologic changes, increased reflex tone, and compromised cardiac function.
- Electrocardiogram—if significant bradycardia (heart rate <50) is present or dysrhythmias due to electrolyte imbalance and/or cardiac conduction disorders are suspected.
- Thyroid function studies (TSH, T3, T4)—in initial diagnostic confirmation and to rule out hyperthyroidism or euthyroid sick syndrome with normal T3 and low normal TSH. Also indicated as part of work up for secondary amenorrhea.
- FSH/LH, and pregnancy test—especially in purging types of AN or bulimia to rule out cause of emesis, or if adrenal or ovarian malignancy is suspected. Also important in work up of secondary amenorrhea, along with estradiol, prolactin, and thyroid function tests
- Bone densitometry—if fractures and AN diagnosis, or if patient amenorrheic for >6 months.

Therapy

Inpatient hospitalization indicated for:

- Very low weight (75% or less of expected body weight)
- Excessive and rapid weight loss
- Acute electrolyte imbalance
- Cardiac disturbance
- Determination of need for parenteral or enteral rehydration and nutrition
- High suicide risk or psychosis
- Symptoms not responding to outpatient treatment
- Note: Specialized eating disorder centers are not readily available in all locations

Outpatient treatment management indicated for:

- Majority of mild and moderate eating disorders

Intervention may include any of the following:
- Patient and parent education
- Collaboration with experienced and knowledgeable treatment team (including primary care physician, dietitian/nutritionist, psychotherapist, or psychiatric social worker)
- Stabilize nutritional status and medical concerns
- Rehabilitation plan leading to gradual weight gain of 0.5 to 2.0 lbs/week with goal of achieving 90% of normal body weight over time
- Individual and family therapy
- Assessment of suicide risk and extent of any concomitant psychiatric pathology
- Appropriate limitations on exercise, as indicated
- Diet with adequate protein and fat, plus calcium (1,000–1,500 mg/day) and multivitamin supplementation (including vitamin D 400 IU/day)
- Psychiatric consultation and treatment for concomitant psychiatric illness
- Consider fluoxetine, desipramine, or imipramine for stabilization of recovery (with psychiatric/psychopharmacologic consultation), when weight at or <85% appropriate for height. (Note: Obtain baseline ECG to rule out prolonged QT interval before considering tricyclic antidepressants.)

Follow-Up

- Must be coordinated with patient, parents, primary health care providers and psychiatric consultant for moderate and severe AN.
- Should involve at least one key contact at school and/or work: teacher, coach, counselor.
- At least weekly follow-up appointments for 2 months or longer are warranted for patients with moderate or severe AN until weight gain and full activities are resumed.
- Resumption of weight gain should occur gradually over weeks.
- Resumption of academic and extracurricular activities, sports participation, and exercise must be monitored in view of general health, nutritional status.

SIGNS TO WATCH FOR TO INDICATE PROBLEMS

- Failure to regain weight or weight loss
- Noncompliance with scheduled follow-up appointments
- Unexcused or unwarranted school or work absenteeism
- Deterioration in academic performance, impaired cognitive abilities, distractibility
- Sleep disturbance, excessive fatigue
- Behavioral problems, acting out, risk-taking behaviors
- Depression, other symptoms or signs of psychopathology
- Electrolyte abnormalities, or other signs of recurrent AN or bulimia

PITFALLS

- Excessive rapid refeeding (may produce gastric bloating, edema, or congestive heart failure)
- Potential electrolyte imbalances during refeeding
- Premature hospital discharge
- Failure to detect comorbid psychiatric illness and/or addiction

Common Questions and Answers

Q: When can the patient resume regular school attendance?
A: As soon as possible, or when weight is at >85% of ideal body weight.

Q: When can the patient resume sports participation?
A: Exercise restrictions apply until there is no evidence of cardiac or electrolyte abnormalities.

Q: When can the patient safely be discharged from close monitoring and frequent follow-up medical care?
A: Individually determined, with consideration given to severity of the eating disorder, duration of symptoms, and compliance with treatment plan, as well as consistency of weight gain. At least annual physical examinations with detailed nutritional assessment are advised for the lifetime of individuals with significant eating disorders.

ICD-9-CM 307.1

BIBLIOGRAPHY

American Academy of Pediatrics, Committee on Adolescence. Identifying and treating eating disorders. *Pediatrics* 2003;111: 204–211.

Fisher M. The course and outcome of eating disorders in adults and in adolescents: a review. *Adolescent Medicine State of the Art Reviews* 2003;14(1):149–158.

Treasure J, Schmidt U. Anorexia nervosa. [Update in *Clin Evid* 2002;(8):903–913; PMID: 12603919], and *Clinical Evid* 2002;(7):824–833.

Author: Lucy S. Crain

Anthrax

Database

DEFINITION

Bacillus anthracis is a spore-forming, gram-positive rod that can cause acute infection (anthrax) in humans and animals.

PATHOPHYSIOLOGY

• After inhalation, wound inoculation, or ingestion, *B. anthracis* spores infect macrophages, germinate, and proliferate. Proliferation occurs at the site of infection and in regional lymph nodes. Replicating bacteria release toxins leading to edema, hemorrhage, and necrosis.
• The incubation period of anthrax depends on the route of transmission.

—Inhalational anthrax: Infection requires inhalation of >8,000 spores. Incubation period is 2 to 60 days.
—Cutaneous anthrax: Spores enter a cut or abrasion in the skin. Incubation period is 1 to 12 days.
—Gastrointestinal anthrax: Spores are ingested in undercooked, infected meat. Incubation period is 1 to 7 days. Infection occurs in the upper (oral-pharyngeal lesions) or lower (intestinal lesions) GI tract.

• Hematogenous spread of the bacteria causes infection at other sites including the CNS, liver, spleen, and kidney.

ASSOCIATED DISEASES

• If anthrax is intentionally released, physicians must be alert for diseases caused by other potential biologic warfare agents. These include plague, tularemia, Q fever, smallpox, and botulism.

EPIDEMIOLOGY

• Anthrax is primarily zoonotic. Most naturally acquired anthrax infections are cutaneous (95%). Inhalational (5%) and GI (<1%) forms are particularly rare.

—Prior to October of 2001, only 18 cases of inhalational anthrax were reported in the United States during the 20th century.
—No human-to-human spread of inhalational anthrax has been reported.
—Rare cases of human-to-human transmission of cutaneous anthrax has been reported after direct contact with infected skin lesions.

• Anthrax has been used as an agent of bioterrorism.

COMPLICATIONS

• Antibiotic therapy of cutaneous anthrax limits the likelihood of developing systemic symptoms but does not change the course of the eschar formation.
• Systemic dissemination of inhalational, cutaneous, or GI anthrax may lead to sepsis, meningitis, and death.

PROGNOSIS

• Inhalational anthrax

—Case fatality rates were previously estimated to be >85% once symptoms develop. However, early use of appropriate antibiotic therapy appears to improve survival.
—Survival rate is higher if symptoms develop >30 days after exposure.

• Cutaneous anthrax

—Case-fatality rate is 20% without antibiotic treatment and <1% with antibiotic treatment.

• GI anthrax

—Case-fatality rate is 25% to 60%.

Differential Diagnosis

• The prodromal illness of inhalational anthrax may resemble a lower respiratory tract infection although URI symptoms are characteristically absent.
• Patients with inhalational anthrax may have a widened mediastinum on CXR which may resemble an aortic aneurysm or bacterial mediastinitis.
• Necrotic skin lesions may resemble plague, tularemia, ecthyma gangrenosum, and brown recluse spider bite.
• Gastrointestinal anthrax may be confused with other infectious causes of enteritis (*Shigella, Salmonella, Yersinia, Campylobacter,* enterohemorrhagic *Escherichia coli, C. difficile* colitis), intussusception, Meckel diverticulum, and inflammatory bowel disease.

Data Gathering

HISTORY

• Inhalational anthrax

—Clinical presentation is a two-stage illness.
—Initial symptoms are nonspecific and last 1 to 3 days. They include low-grade fever, dry cough, headache, vomiting, chills, weakness, abdominal pain, and substernal discomfort. This stage is followed by a brief period of apparent recovery.
—Second-stage symptoms develop abruptly and include fever, hemoptysis, dyspnea, chest pain, and profuse diaphoresis. Death may occur within 1 to 2 days.

• Cutaneous anthrax

—Lesions develop on affected areas soon after exposure.
—Systemic symptoms of fever, malaise, and headache may occur.

• GI anthrax

—Oral-pharyngeal form causes sore throat, dysphagia, and fever.
—Intestinal form also causes nausea, vomiting, anorexia, severe abdominal pain, and bloody diarrhea.

Physical Examination

• Inhalational anthrax
• Tachypnea, hypoxia, cyanosis
• Stridor, rales, signs of pleural effusion
• Hemoptysis, hematemesis, melena
• Cutaneous anthrax
• Initial painless, pruritic macule or papule enlarges into a 1- to 3-cm round ulcer by the 2nd day
• 1- to 3-mm vesicles with clear or serosanguinous fluid surround the ulcer
• A painless, depressed, black eschar follows, often with extensive local edema
• Over 1 to 2 weeks, the eschar dries, loosens, and falls off, occasionally with scarring.
• Painful, regional lymphadenopathy may occur.
• GI anthrax
• Oral or esophageal ulcers, cervical lymphadenopathy
• Cecal or terminal ileal ulcers
• Massive ascites
• Acute abdomen
• Disseminated anthrax (potential complication of any of the above forms of anthrax)

—Sepsis syndrome: tachycardia, hypotension, septic shock
—Meningitis: meningismus, delirium, obtundation

Laboratory Aids

Test: Chest X-ray (or chest CT scan)
Significance: Inhalational anthrax causes a hemorrhagic mediastinitis. CXR shows a widened mediastinum and pleural effusions. No infiltrates are present.

Test: Gram stain smear and culture from vesicular fluid
Significance: Diagnose cutaneous anthrax. Gram stain reveals large, gram-positive, boxcar-shaped bacilli. Capsule is visible on polychrome methylene blue stain. *B. anthracis* grows readily on blood agar.

Test: Anthraxin skin test
Significance: Measures anthrax cell-mediated immunity. It is positive in 80% of patients within 72 hours of infection and >95% of cases within 3 weeks. The test was positive in 72% of patients >16 years after recovery.

Test: Serologic enzyme-linked immunosorbent assay (ELISA)
Significance: Measures antibodies to the lethal and edema toxins of *B. anthracis*. Positive if a single acute-phase titer is >1:32 or if there is a fourfold or greater rise between acute and convalescent titers collected 4 weeks apart.

Test: PCR, immunohistochemical staining

Test: Nasopharyngeal swab or induced respiratory secretion culture
Significance: Used for epidemiologic investigation. The sensitivity, specificity, and predictive value of nasal swab testing are unknown; therefore this test should not be used to guide the use of postexposure prophylactic antibiotics.

Test: Blood culture
Significance: Patient with cutaneous anthrax may have bacteremia with *B. anthracis* even without significant signs of systemic disease.

Test: Complete blood count

Test: Serum electrolytes, glucose, and calcium
Significance: Hypokalemia, acidosis, hypoglycemia, and hypocalcemia occurred during experimental anthrax infection in animals.

 ## Emergency Care

• When a person has had direct physical contact with a substance alleged to be anthrax, the following measures should be implemented:

—Wash exposed skin and articles of clothing with soap and water.
—Administer postexposure prophylaxis until the substance is proved not to be anthrax.
—Contact the public health department or the Centers for Disease Control and Prevention.

 ## Therapy

• Postexposure prophylaxis

—Ciprofloxacin 15 mg/kg (up to 500 mg) OR doxycycline 2 mg/kg (up to 100 mg) po b.i.d. for 60 days.
—In children, use ciprofloxacin for initial prophylaxis. Switch to amoxicillin or penicillin if susceptibility testing permits.

• Treatment

—For all forms of anthrax, begin with IV therapy and switch to oral therapy when clinically appropriate. Treat for 60 days (IV and po combined).
—Inhalational or GI anthrax: Ciprofloxacin 15 mg/kg (up to 400 mg) or doxycycline 2 mg/kg (up to 100 mg) IV every 12 h PLUS clindamycin or rifampin.
—Cutaneous anthrax: Ciprofloxacin or doxycycline IV.
—In children, begin therapy with ciprofloxacin (plus clindamycin or rifampin for inhalational/GI anthrax) and convert to penicillin G IV if susceptibility testing permits and when clinical improvement is documented.

 ## Follow-Up

INFECTION CONTROL

• Immediately notify the hospital epidemiologist, infection control department, or local health department of suspected cases.
• No data suggest that patient-to-patient transmission of inhalational anthrax occurs. Standard barrier isolation precautions are recommended for all hospitalized patients with all forms of anthrax infection. High-efficiency particulate air filter masks or other measures for airborne precautions are not indicated.
• There is no need to immunize or provide prophylaxis to patient contacts unless they, like the patient, were exposed to the aerosol.
• If anthrax is used as a bioweapon, spores may be detected on environmental surfaces. Inhalational anthrax is unlikely to be caused by secondary aerosolization of these spores.

PREVENTION

• Antibiotics are effective against germinating *B. anthracis* but not against the spores. Therefore, if prophylactic antibiotics are stopped prematurely, remaining spores can cause disease when they germinate. This phenomenon of delayed onset disease does not occur with cutaneous or GI exposures.
• In situations where the threat of transmission of *B. anthracis* spores is deemed credible, decontamination of skin and potential fomites (e.g., clothing) may be considered to reduce the risk for cutaneous and GI forms of the disease.

• AVA (anthrax vaccine adsorbed) is the only licensed human anthrax vaccine in the United States. Primary vaccination consists of subcutaneous injections at 0, 2, and 4 weeks, and three booster vaccinations at 6, 12, and 18 months. Annual booster injections are required to maintain immunity. Most common adverse event is injection-site discomfort (e.g., edema, pain, local hypersensitivity).

PITFALLS

• Failure to remember that the pulmonary disease caused by anthrax is a hemorrhagic mediastinitis with pleural effusions and NOT a bronchopneumonia.

 ## Common Questions and Answers

Q: Does the government have a plan in place if there were mass exposure to anthrax?
A: Yes. Under emergency plans, the federal government would ship appropriate antibiotics from its stockpile to wherever they are needed.

Q: Should individuals ask their physicians to write a prescription for ciprofloxacin (or other antibiotics) so they have prophylaxis available?
A: No. Ciprofloxacin and other antibiotics should not be prescribed unless there is a clearly indicated need. Additionally, indiscriminate prescribing and widespread use of ciprofloxacin could hasten the development of drug-resistant organisms.

Q: Can a person get screened or tested for anthrax?
A: No screening test is available to determine whether anthrax exposure has occurred. The only way exposure can be determined is through a public health investigation.

ICD-9-CM

Anthrax 022.9;

Cutaneous 022.0;

Pulmonary 022.1

BIBLIOGRAPHY

CDC. Use of anthrax vaccine in the United States: recommendations of the Advisory Committee on Immunization Practices (ACIP). *MMWR* 2000;49(RR-15):1–20.

CDC. Update: investigation of bioterrorism-related anthrax and interim guidelines for exposure management and antimicrobial therapy. *MMWR* 2001;50:909–919.

Sellman BR, Mourez M, Collier RJ. Dominant-negative mutants of a toxin subunit: an approach to therapy of anthrax. *Science* 2001;292:695–697.

Weber DJ, Rutala WA. Risks and prevention of nosocomial transmission of rare zoonotic diseases. *Clin Infect Dis* 2001;32:446–456.

Author: Samir S. Shah

Aplastic Anemia

 Database

DEFINITION

Aplastic anemia is a heterogeneous disorder within the bone marrow failure syndromes. It is characterized by a marked decrease or absence of blood precursors in the bone marrow and peripheral pancytopenia. The disorder exists in both acquired and congenital forms.

CAUSES

Acquired

- Idiopathic (70% of cases)
- Drugs (idiosyncratic)—e.g., chloramphenicol, nonsteroidal anti-inflammatory drugs, antiepiletics, quinacrine, cimetidine
- Hepatitis (often non-A, non-B, and non-C)
- HIV, EBV, HHV-6, CMV
- Chemicals/toxins such as insecticides (DDT, parathion); benzene, carbon tetrachloride
- Radiation
- Malnutrition—Kwashiorkor, marasmus, anorexia nervosa
- Paroxysmal nocturnal hemoglobinuria (PNH)
- Pregnancy
- Autoimmune mechanisms
- Preleukemia, myelodysplastic syndrome (MDS)

Congenital

- Fanconi anemia
- Dyskeratosis congenita
- Shwachman-Diamond syndrome
- Reticular dysgenesis
- Amegakaryocytic thrombocytopenia
- Familial

PATHOLOGY/PATHOPHYSIOLOGY

- Marked reduction in number of hematopoietic stem cells (CD34+)
- Autoimmune-mediated destruction of hematopoietic stem cell
- Aberrant cytokine production by host T-lymphocytes suppressing hematopoietic cell proliferation and triggering apoptosis of CD34 progenitor cells
- Stromal (supporting) cells within the bone marrow microenvironment are usually normal
- Genetic predisposition

GENETICS

- Most cases are sporadic
- Moderately correlated with specific histocompatibility antigen frequency (HLA-DR2 antigen is twice as frequent in aplastic anemia patients as in the unaffected population)
- Familial aplastic anemia is associated with congenital syndromes, with heterogeneous hematologic manifestations, and usually recognizable congenital physical anomalies. This diagnosis should always be considered even without a positive family history or obvious syndromic features. Testing for Fanconi anemia is considered mandatory in all new AA patients.

EPIDEMIOLOGY

- Annual incidence of 2 to 3 new cases per 1 million in the United States and Europe
- Incidence in Asia is about threefold higher than in West, likely related to environmental/infectious exposures.
- Two major age peaks: 15 to 25 years and over 60 years
- Males and females equally affected.

COMPLICATIONS

- Infection: overwhelming bacterial sepsis and fungal (Aspergillus) infections are most frequent cause of death.
- Hemorrhage: intracranial, especially if refractory to platelet transfusions
- Iron overload secondary to long-term red blood cell transfusions, with subsequent organ dysfunction if untreated.

PROGNOSIS

- In patients with severe aplastic anemia, 80% to 90% mortality at 2 years if untreated.
- Bone marrow transplant from HLA-identical sibling donor

—77% overall survival in children
—80% to 90% survival for the young, uninfected, and minimally transfused patient

- Bone marrow transplant from HLA-identical unrelated donor

—30% to 55% survival (due to older population, frequent graft rejection, more severe graft versus host disease, infection from delayed engraftment with prolonged neutropenia)

- Immunosuppressive therapy

—75% response rate (initial treatment)
—90% 5-year survival among responders

- Factors associated with poor outcome:

—Bleeding at presentation
—Severe pancytopenia (ANC $<200/mm^3$, platelet $<20,000/mm^3$)
—Prolonged pancytopenia (>1 month)
—Active infection at diagnosis

 Differential Diagnosis

- Acute leukemia
- Myelodysplastic syndrome
- Paroxysmal nocturnal hemoglobinuria
- Folate or B_{12} deficiency (macrocytic anemia)
- Acute drug reaction with bone marrow suppression
- Acute infection (viral) with bone marrow suppression, e.g., HIV-1, CMV, parvovirus B19, EBV
- Marrow infiltration by malignant tumors, e.g., non-Hodgkin lymphoma, neuroblastoma
- Hemophagocytic lymphohistiocytosis (i.e., familial erythrophagocytic lymphohistiocytosis)

 Data Gathering

HISTORY

Evidence of Bone Marrow Failure

- Pallor, lethargy, easy fatigue, weakness, and loss of appetite are signs of anemia. These may not be noticed by patient/parent due to slow onset of anemia (with compensation).
- Petechiae, easy and excessive bruising, prolonged epistaxis, gingival bleeding, hematuria and bloody stools are signs/symptoms of thrombocytopenia.
- Infections that do not respond to antibiotics, oral ulcers, and gingival hyperplasia may be signs of neutropenia.

EVIDENCE OF CAUSE

- Drug or toxin exposure (although usually not identified)
- History of hepatitis, jaundice, or other viral infections

 Physical Examination

- Cachexia suggests another etiology such as malignancy
- Excessive bruising, petechiae, and pallor as signs of severe thrombocytopenia and anemia. Skin hyperpigmentation or hypopigmentation may be seen with Fanconi anemia
- Oral mucosal ulcerations and bleeding, thrush, palatal petechiae, and gingival hypertrophy as signs of neutropenia, and thrombocytopenia
- Tachycardia and systolic ejection murmur from anemia
- Lymphadenopathy and hepatosplenomegaly suggest acute leukemia/malignant process, and are not associated with aplastic anemia.
- Perianal ulcerations/infection from neutropenia
- Skeletal anomalies, dysmorphic features may be signs of Fanconi anemia

Laboratory Aids

TO CONFIRM THE DIAGNOSIS

Test: CBC with differential and reticulocyte count

• Severe aplastic anemia (at least 2 of the following):

—Granulocyte count <500/mm3
—Platelet count <20,000/mm3
—Reticulocyte count (corrected for hematocrit) <1%

• Mild or moderate aplastic anemia (hypoplastic anemia)

—Less severe cytopenias

Test: Bone marrow aspirate and biopsy
Significance:

• Severe aplastic anemia

—Hypocellular with fatty infiltration
—Less than 25% cellularity on biopsy

• Mild or moderate aplastic anemia

—Normal or increased cellularity

Supplemental Laboratory Studies

• LFTs, hepatitis A, B, and C antibody panel
• Viral serologies: EBV, parvovirus B19 (IgG and IgM), VZV, CMV, HIV, HHV-6

TO EXCLUDE OTHER CAUSES

• Bone marrow aspirate for chromosomal analysis to rule out myelodysplastic syndromes, acute leukemia
• Diepoxybutane chromosome breakage study (on peripheral blood) to test for Fanconi anemia
• Flow cytometry to exclude paroxysmal nocturnal hemoglobinuria
• Red cell folate and vitamin B12 levels to detect deficiency causing pancytopenia with macrocytosis

Emergency Care

• Broad-spectrum antibiotics for febrile neutropenic patients. Consider antifungal therapy for patients with prolonged fevers.
• Platelet transfusions for bleeding. Maintain platelet count >10,000/mm^3 in nonbleeding adolescent/adult patients (single donor units, irradiated, leukocyte depleted)
• Red cell transfusions in severely anemic patients should be given slowly to prevent congestive heart failure (unless anemia is acute and due to blood loss rather than lack of production). Use irradiated, leukocyte-depleted, CMV safe red cell product from unrelated donors.

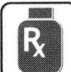 ## Therapy

• Bone marrow transplantation

—Treatment of choice for patients <40 years with severe aplastic anemia and HLA-identical sibling.
—Transplant early, minimize supportive transfusions.
—Alternative donor BMT should be used only for patients who have failed immunosuppressive therapy (>1 course of immunosuppressive treatment reduces success with BMT).
—Peripheral blood stem cell and umbilical cord blood regimens currently being tested.

• Immunosuppressive therapy

—Antithymocyte globulin (ATG), cyclosporine, methylprednisolone, and growth factors (G-CSF or GM-CSF)
—High-dose cyclophosphamide without BMT. This treatment was associated with a greater number of early deaths from infection than treatment with ATG/cyclosporine A.

• Androgens

—Used for the treatment of Fanconi anemia
—Effective in moderate and mild aplastic anemia, particularly if anemia is the most significant cytopenia

• Supportive therapy

—Transfusion support: family donors should not be used (to avoid alloimmunization), use CMV safe, irradiated, leuko-reduced product; minimize number of transfusions.
—Infectious disease support: pan culture and institute broad-spectrum parenteral antibiotics for fever/neutropenia; antifungal therapy for persistent fevers. The addition of G-CSF may lead to more rapid rise in neutrophil counts, although there are some reports of increased clonal transformation with its use. Maintain good hand washing and oral hygiene. Avoid raw fish, fruits, and vegetables. Avoid rectal temperatures. Long-term prophylactic antibiotics are not recommended.

 ## Follow-Up

TIME TO RECOVERY

Response to medical therapy is not immediate, but most responses to medical therapy, with some degree of blood count recovery, occur within 3 months of treatment. Hematologic recovery may be incomplete and some patients may remain cyclosporine dependent.

SIGNS OF RECOVERY

Signs of recovery include normalization of mean corpuscular volume (MCV), increasing reticulocyte, neutrophil and monocyte count. Full platelet recovery may take months.

RELAPSE

• Risk of relapse is 30% to 40% at 5 years; many respond to salvage therapy.
• Salvage therapy: second course of immunosuppressive therapy (50% salvage); matched-unrelated donor BMT (30 to 55% overall survival).

OTHER

• 8% to 15% risk of MDS and/or myeloid leukemia at 10 years. May be lower in children
• 15% risk of PNH at 5 years. May be lower in children

 ## Common Questions and Answers

Q: Can family members donate blood for a child with aplastic anemia?
A: This is not recommended, as transfusion with blood products from parents or siblings increases the risk of graft rejection of bone marrow in the setting of a related-donor bone marrow transplant.

Q: What activities should a child with aplastic anemia avoid?
A: Patients with low red blood cell counts should avoid excessive exercise or high-altitude exposure. Patients with low white blood cell counts are more susceptible to bacterial infections. Patients should avoid dental work, as this may introduce bacteria into the bloodstream through the mouth. Patients with low platelet counts should avoid contact sports, including football, hockey, lacrosse, skiing, etc.

Q: How does one learn more about experimental therapies for the treatment of aplastic anemia?
A: Inquiries to the National Institutes of Health (NIH) in Bethesda, Maryland, or to the hematology division of the nearest medical school or NIH-designated cancer center should result in information about the availability of experimental therapies.

ICD-9-CM 284.9

BIBLIOGRAPHY

Alter BP. Bone marrow failure syndromes in children. *Pediatr Clin N Am* 2002;49:973–988.

Ball SE. The modern management of severe aplastic anaemia. *Br J Haematol* 2000;110: 41–53.

Frickhofen N, Rosenfeld SJ. Immuno-suppressive treatment of aplastic anemia with antithymocyte globulin and cyclosporine. *Semin Hematol* 2000;37:56–68.

Horowitz MM. Current status of allogeneic bone marrow transplantation in acquired aplastic anemia. *Semin Hematol* 2000;37:30–42.

Young NS. Acquired aplastic anemia. *JAMA* 1999;281:271–278.

Authors: Janet L. Kwiatkowski, MD
Jane Mintirn, 3rd edition

Appendicitis

 ## Database

DEFINITION

Acute inflammation of the appendix

CAUSES

• Obstruction of appendiceal lumen by fecalith, calculi, or hyperplastic lymphoid tissue

PATHOLOGY

• Acute obstruction raises intraluminal pressure, leading to ischemia.
• Bacteria invade the appendiceal wall at sites of ulceration producing inflammation.
• Necrosis of appendiceal wall results in perforation with fecal contamination of the peritoneum.

EPIDEMIOLOGY

• The most common acute surgical emergency in childhood.
• Usually occurs in children greater than 2 years of age and rarely considered in children less than 3 years of age
• Peak incidence in teens and young adults aged 15 to 25.
• Affects 1 in 500 people each year worldwide.

 ## Differential Diagnosis

INFECTION

• Gastroenteritis (e.g., Yersinia, Campylobacter)
• Constipation
• Right lower lobe pneumonia
• Mesenteric adenitis
• Typhlitis
• Urinary tract infection
• Pelvic inflammatory disease, tuboovarian abscess, or ectopic pregnancy
• Parasitic infection: *Trichuris trichiura*, *Ascaris lumbricoides*

INFLAMMATORY

• Inflammatory bowel disease exacerbation
• Anaphylactic purpura
• Hemolytic uremic anemia
• Cholecystitis
• Pancreatitis
• Diverticulitis

GENETIC/METABOLIC

• Diabetes
• Sickle and sickle cell disease
• Renal stones
• Hypernatremia
• Crohn disease

MISCELLANEOUS

• Function abdominal pain
• Fecalith
• Torsion of testes or ovaries
• Ovarian cyst
• Endometriosis
• Small bowel obstruction
• Rupture of rectus abdominis

 ## Data Gathering

HISTORY

Question: Is there constipation and inability to pass gas?
Significance: These are considered traditional cardinal signs for irritation associated with peritoneal or abdominal mesentery.

Question: Is there nausea or vomiting?
Significance: Many surgeons feel that vomiting is the cardinal symptom associated with appendicitis.

Question: Is there fever?
Significance: Low-grade fever is common in appendicitis; higher fever can be an abscess or other infectious disease.

Question: Does the pain move or is there point tenderness associated in the right lower quadrant (RLQ)?
Significance: Typically, there is poorly localized, cramp-like midabdominal pain that migrates to the RLQ.

Question: Other classic features?

• Rectal tenderness
• Nausea, anorexia
• Patient prefers to lie still
• Rarely secretory diarrhea; more common in infants <2 years
• Change in bowel habits, especially diarrhea
• Guarding, i.e., voluntary contraction of the abdominal muscle

Significance: Appendicitis may be presenting with unusual features.

 ## Physical Examination

Finding: Focal peritoneal signs
Significance: Peritoneal irritation

Finding: Pain at McBurney point
Significance: Peritoneal irritation

Finding: Psoas sign
Significance: Peritoneal irritation

Finding: Abdominal rebound tenderness
Significance: Peritoneal irritation

Finding: Focal tenderness on rectal examination
Significance: Appendicitis or abscess

Finding: Following perforation, abdomen becomes rigid and tender with absent bowel sounds; patients often febrile, tachypneic, and tachycardic
Significance: Peritonitis

SPECIAL QUESTION

Question: Was the car ride painful, e.g., going over bumps?
Significance: Another way to elicit peritoneal irritation.

SPECIAL EXAMINATION TRICKS

• Palpation with stethoscope
• Jiggling bed should produce RLQ pain.
• Pain may be elicited by asking patient to cough or hop on right foot (psoas sign).

Laboratory Aids

TESTS

Test: CBC
Significance: Elevated white blood cell (WBC) count with left shift

IMAGING

Test: Abdominal x-ray
Significance:

- Often normal
- 8% to 10% show calcified fecalith
- Cecal-wall thickening
- Air-fluid levels suggesting small bowel obstruction
- Indistinct psoas margins
- Pneumoperitoneum (rare)

Test: Barium enema—not routine
Significance: May show evidence of RLQ mass or partial or complete nonfilling of appendix.

Test: Ultrasound
Significance: Edema, inflammation, and/or abscess formation

Test: CT abdomen
Significance: Gaining popularity for diagnostic problems.

Therapy

- IV fluids to correct hypovolemia, electrolyte abnormalities
- Exploratory laparotomy
- Emergency appendectomy; laparoscopic technique has been utilized and potentially associated with earlier return to activities of daily living
- Broad-spectrum antibiotics should be used if perforation is suspected.
- Nasogastric tube and pain medications may provide comfort preoperatively.
- Abscess may require external drainage.

Follow-Up

- Recovery rapid
- Prognosis excellent without perforation, good with perforation (mortality, 1%)

PITFALLS

- Position of appendix may vary, i.e., location of pain may vary
- Retroiliac appendix, poorly localized pain
- Retrocecal appendix, right upper quadrant (RUQ) pain
- Appendix in gutter, flank pain
- Pelvic appendix, pain on rectal examination, or diarrhea caused by direct irritation of sigmoid colon
- Appendicitis progresses rapidly in children; perforation often occurs due to delayed diagnosis
- Pain may resolve briefly following perforation.

DIETARY GUIDELINES

Postoperative

- Patient diet should consist of clear liquids, i.e., broth, juices, and herbal teas.
- Introduce foods high in beta-carotene.

Significance: beta-carotene soothes injured mucous membrane and heals tissue.

- Avoid gas-producing foods, e.g., nuts, legumes, broccoli.
- Introduce nutritional supplements or foods high in vitamin B-complex for strength, vitamin C for tissue repair, vitamin E for antioxidant, and zinc to aid healing tissue.

Common Questions and Answers

Q: Why is perforation more commonly observed in children with appendicitis?
A: There is more rapid progression of symptoms that may not follow the classic pattern of RLQ pain. Young children may not be capable of describing their pain. The mesentery in children is thin walled and less effective at walling off an infection.

Q: Is appendicitis genetically inherited?
A: Appendicitis does show a tendency to occur in families.

Q: How long is the typical postoperative recovery period?
A: Traditional recovery period rule of thumb is 6 weeks.

ICD-9-CM 541

BIBLIOGRAPHY

Alloo J, et al. Appendicitis in children less than 3 years of age: 1 28-year review. *Pediatr Surg Int* 2004;19(12):777–779.

Andersen BR, Kallehave FL, Anderson HK. Antibiotics versus placebo for prevention of postoperative infection after appendicectomy (Cochrane Review). *Cochrane Database Syst Rev* 2001:2.

Brender JD, Marcuse EK, Koepsell T, et al. Childhood appendicitis: factors associated with perforation. *Pediatrics* 1985;76:301–306.

Dorfman S, et al. The role of parasites in acute appendicitis of pediatric patients. *Invest Clin* 2003;44(4):337–340.

Kokoska ER, Minkes RK, Silen ML, et al. Effect of pediatric surgical practice on the treatment of children with appendicitis. *Pediatrics* 2001;107(6):1298–1301.

Lawrence J. Computed tomography in diagnosing suspected appendicitis. *Pediatrics* 2001;107(5):1231.

Lintula H, et al. The costs and effects of laparoscopic appendectomy in children. *Arch Pediatr Adolesc Med* 2004;158(1):11–12.

Author: Andrew E. Mulberg, M.D.

Arthritis—Juvenile Rheumatoid

Database

DEFINITION

• Juvenile rheumatoid arthritis (JRA) is chronic synovial inflammation of unknown etiology in at least one joint, for at least 6 weeks. Age of onset must be less than 16 years old. It can be subdivided into three major types.
• Pauciarticular JRA is JRA affecting less than five joints.

—Type I usually affects young girls. Peak age of onset is 1 to 6 years; 80% are antinuclear antibody (ANA)-positive.
—Type II (spondyloarthropathies) generally affects boys, many of whom are human leukocyte antigen (HLA)-B27 positive, in late childhood or adolescence.

• Polyarticular JRA affects five or more joints and can occur at any age, but peak ages of onset are 1 to 4 and 7 to 10 years.

—Rheumatoid factor positive (RF+) polyarticular JRA is like adult onset RA that occurs in a child. It is often quite aggressive.
—Rheumatoid factor negative (RF-) polyarticular JRA is usually less aggressive and easier to control.

• Systemic-onset JRA is characterized by high, spiking quotidian or diquotidian fevers and an evanescent pink/salmon-colored macular rash. Affected children may also have lymphadenopathy, hepatosplenomegaly, pericarditis, or pleuritis. The arthritis may not appear until weeks to months after the onset of the systemic symptoms. Systemic-onset JRA can occur at any age.

CAUSES

The etiology of JRA is unknown, but genetic predisposition, autoimmunity, and/or infection may play a role.

PATHOLOGY

• Chronic synovial inflammation

EPIDEMIOLOGY

• JRA affects approximately 70,000–100,000 children in the United States. The incidence varies from 3 to 23 per 100,000 per year.
• Girls are affected twice as often as boys, but pauciarticular type II usually affects boys more frequently (male/female ratio, 10:1).
• Approximately 50% to 60% of children with JRA have the pauciarticular type.
• 30% to 40% have the polyarticular type.
• 10% have systemic-onset JRA.

GENETICS

JRA is rare in siblings, but there have been many studies demonstrating increased frequencies of various HLA markers in JRA. Each marker may be associated with a different subtype of JRA. For example, HLA-DR4 seems to be associated with rheumatoid factor-positive (RF+) polyarticular JRA, HLA-DR1 is associated with pauciarticular disease without uveitis, and HLA-DR5 is associated with pauciarticular JRA with uveitis. HLA-B27 is associated with the spondyloarthropathies and HLA-A2 is associated with early onset pauciarticular JRA.

COMPLICATIONS

• Joint degeneration with loss of articular cartilage
• Soft tissue contractures
• Leg-length discrepancies
• Micrognathia
• Cervical spine dislocations
• Rheumatoid nodules
• Growth retardation
• Uveitis: pauciarticular JRA, especially with a positive ANA, is associated with a chronic uveitis, which can lead to loss of vision if not detected early with routine slit-lamp eye examinations.
• Pericarditis and pleuritis, as well as severe anemia, may develop in patients with systemic-onset JRA.
• Macrophage activation syndrome, or hemophagocytic syndrome, is a rare, but potentially lethal complication of systemic onset JRA, resulting from an overproduction of inflammatory cytokines. It may present as an acute febrile illness with pancytopenia and hepatosplenomegaly. Diagnosis is made by bone marrow aspiration. Treatment is often with high-dose steroids and cyclosporin.

Differential Diagnosis

• Monoarticular JRA

—Septic joint
—Toxic synovitis
—Trauma
—Hemarthrosis
—Villonodular synovitis

• Monoarticular or pauciarticular JRA

—Lyme disease
—Acute rheumatic fever or poststreptococcal arthritis
—Malignancies
—Sarcoidosis
—Inflammatory bowel disease

• Polyarticular JRA

—Viral or postviral illness (especially parvovirus)
—Lyme disease
—Lupus

• Systemic-onset JRA

—Infection
—Oncologic process (leukemia, lymphoma)
—Inflammatory bowel disease
—Lupus

Data Gathering

HISTORY

• Morning stiffness that improves after a warm shower/bath or with stretching and mild exercise is common in JRA. Many young children do not complain of pain, but walk with a limp or refuse to walk down the stairs in the morning.
• Joints often become sore/painful again in the late afternoon or evening.
• Patients with JRA generally do not complain of severe pain, but rather they avoid using joints that are particularly affected. If a child has severe pain in a joint, especially pain that seems out of proportion to the physical findings, diagnoses other than JRA should be entertained.
• In systemic JRA the fever curve is important to document. Between fever spikes the child is often completely afebrile. The rash is evanescent and the patients often have a history of fatigue, malaise, and weight loss.

Physical Examination

- Arthritis must be present in at least one joint in pauciarticular or polyarticular JRA. There may be restricted range of motion in the affected joints and soft tissue contractures as well.
- Enthesitis and sacroiliac tenderness are often seen in spondyloarthropathies.
- In systemic JRA the rash, if present, is almost pathognomonic for this disease.
- Lymphadenopathy and hepatosplenomegaly may be seen in systemic JRA.
- A careful cardiac and pulmonary examination must be done to look for pericarditis and pleuritis.

Laboratory Aids

- No laboratory finding is diagnostic for JRA.
- Many patients with JRA, especially the polyarticular and systemic types, have elevated sedimentation rates and anemia.
- Patients with systemic JRA often have a leukocytosis (predominantly neutrophils), a thrombocytosis, and an elevated ferritin level.
- ANA is a useful test in classifying patients with JRA and determining the risk of uveitis. It is positive in:

—80% of pauciarticular type I
—40% to 60% polyarticular
—15% normal population

- RF will be positive in 15% to 20% of patients with polyarticular arthritis and usually indicates a more aggressive form of arthritis.

IMAGING

- Radiography is often normal early in JRA.
- Later, if arthritis persists, bone demineralization, loss of articular cartilage, erosions, and joint fusion may be seen.

Therapy

DRUGS

- Nonsteroidal antiinflammatory drugs (NSAIDs)

—First-line therapy for JRA
—If there is no response to the initial NSAID after 4 to 6 weeks of an adequate dose, a different one should be tried. Patients will often respond differently to the various nonsteroidal drugs.
—If patients experience GI upset or excessive bruising, COX-2 inhibitors may be used.

- If NSAIDs are ineffective in controlling the disease, a second-line agent should be added, such as methotrexate, or sulfasalazine.
- Methotrexate: If the arthritis does not respond to NSAIDS, methotrexate is often

started. Laboratory values must be monitored closely in these patients, looking for bone marrow suppression or elevation of transaminase levels.
- Biologic agents are often added when patients don't respond adequately to methotrexate or cannot tolerate its side effects.

—Antitumor necrosis factor therapy is frequently used.

1. Etanercept is a receptor for TNF that is given subcutaneously once or twice a week
2. Infliximab is a chimeric antibody to TNF that is given intravenously every 4 to 8 weeks.
3. Adalimumab is a fully humanized antibody to TNF given subcutaneously every other week.

—Anti-IL-1 and anti-IL-6 therapy is currently being studied in children with JRA.

- Glucocorticoids

—In systemic JRA with high fevers, systemic glucocorticoids are often necessary, either as oral (daily or every other day) doses or as intravenous pulses, every 2 to 8 weeks. Steroids are also used for patients with polyarticular JRA whose arthritis is unresponsive to other medications. Because of the many side effects of systemic steroids, patients should be weaned off steroids as soon as possible.
—Intraarticular steroids are often used in patients with only one or two active joints.

- Medications such as cyclophosphamide or thalidomide are sometimes necessary to control severe systemic onset JRA.

PHYSICAL AND OCCUPATIONAL THERAPY

Physical and occupational therapy are important in the management of JRA. The goal is to maintain range of motion, muscle strength, and function.

DIET

Patients with systemic or polyarticular JRA, especially those on steroids, should maintain adequate calcium and vitamin D intake to minimize osteoporosis. Patients on methotrexate should take folate supplements daily, except on the days that the methotrexate is given.

WHEN TO EXPECT IMPROVEMENT

- Responses to treatments for JRA vary tremendously.

—Some patients may respond to NSAIDs within a week or two.
—Others take 4 to 6 weeks to improve and some may not respond at all.
—Steroids usually start to relieve symptoms within a few days.
—Methotrexate usually takes 4 to 8 weeks until a benefit is seen.
—Anti-TNF therapy can start decreasing symptoms in as little as 1 to 2 weeks, or it may take up to 3 months.

—Other second-line agents can take up to 16 weeks until the maximum benefit is seen.

- The waxing and waning nature of JRA itself adds to the variability of patient responses to treatments.

PROGNOSIS

- Varies considerably
- Children with pauciarticular JRA usually do well and often go into remission within a few years of starting treatment. They may have flares, however, even up to 10 years after being symptom-free and off all medications.
- Patients with polyarticular JRA who are RF+ often develop a severe arthritis that may persist into adulthood.
- RF—polyarticular patients generally do better and many outgrow their disease.
- 50% of patients with systemic-onset JRA will develop severe chronic polyarticular arthritis.

PITFALLS

Overdiagnosis: Arthritis must be present for at least 6 weeks before a patient can be diagnosed with JRA. Many viral illnesses can give joint pain and swelling that mimics JRA, but resolves within 4 to 6 weeks.

Common Questions and Answers

Q: Will the patient outgrow JRA?
A: Prognosis depends of the type of JRA. In some studies, up to 50% of patients with JRA still had active disease 10 years after diagnosis. Only 15%, however, had any loss of function.

Q: Will siblings of patients with JRA develop the disease?
A: Rarely, but it can occur.

ICD-9-CM 714.30

BIBLIOGRAPHY

Patel H, Goldstein D. Pediatric uveitis. *Pediatr Clin North Am* 2003;50(1):125–136.

Ravelli A. Macrophage activation syndrome. *Curr Opin in Rheumatol* 2002;14(5):548–552.

Schneider R, Passo MH. Juvenile rheumatoid arthritis. *Rheum Dis Clin North Am.* 2002;28(3):503–530.

Singsen BH. Epidemiology of rheumatic diseases of childhood. *Rheum Dis Clin North Am* 1990;16:581–599.

Towner SR, Michet CJ Jr, O'Fallon WM, et al. The epidemiology of juvenile arthritis in Rochester, Minnesota. *Arthritis Rheum* 1983;26:1208.

Tse SM, Laxer RM. Juvenile spondyloarthropathy. *Curr Opin in Rheumatol* 2003;15(4): 374–379.

Author: Elizabeth Candell Chalom

Ascaris Lumbricoides

 Database

DEFINITION

Ascaris lumbricoides is a large roundworm, 15 to 40 cm in length, which infects humans via eggs found in soil. Animals are not affected. Approximately one-fourth of the world's population is infested with this worm.

PATHOPHYSIOLOGY

- The life cycle begins when eggs are ingested from soil contaminated with human feces.
- Subsequently, the larvae are liberated in the small intestine.
- The rhabdoid larvae invade the venous system and travel to the portal circulation, inferior vena cava, and finally, pulmonary capillaries.
- They penetrate the alveoli, and are subsequently expelled by coughing across the epiglottis and swallowed. During the migration of the parasite through the pulmonary vessels, an eosinophilic response is evoked.
- The larvae become adult worms in the small intestine.
- The cycle takes 2 months.
- In the intestinal stage, mechanical obstruction from the mass of worms in the gut may be observed in children.

EPIDEMIOLOGY

- One female worm produces 200,000 eggs per day.
- Fertilized eggs must incubate in the soil for 2 to 3 weeks.
- The eggs are viable for up to 6 years in temperate climates; they survive freezing but not direct sunlight.
- All ages may be affected; however, children are more frequent hosts due to oral behavior.
- Ascariasis is more common where sanitation is poor and population dense.

COMPLICATIONS

- Bronchopneumonia may be seen during the migrational stage, producing fever, cough, dyspnea, wheeze, eosinophilia, and pulmonary infiltrates.
- Heavy infestations may cause abdominal pain, malabsorption, and growth failure.
- Children may experience obstruction (ileocecal), malabsorption, or intussusception.
- Perforation of a viscus, or migration into the appendix, biliary, or pancreatic ducts may rarely occur.

PROGNOSIS

- Once intestinal infection is detected and treated, the prognosis is excellent. If obstructive or respiratory complications have occurred, the prognosis is less favorable.
- The case fatality rate in the United States is 3%.

 Differential Diagnosis

- Ascariasis should be considered in the differential diagnosis when a patient presents with pneumonia and peripheral eosinophilia.
- The diagnosis of *Ascaris* infection should be considered whenever intestinal obstruction is seen in an endemic area.
- This infection may be associated with other parasites acquired from contaminated soil.

 Data Gathering

HISTORY

Question: Do patients infected with *Ascaris* always have symptoms?
Significance: The majority of patients with moderate infections are asymptomatic.

Question: Do patients actually see worms in their stool?
Significance: History or passage of large worms in the stool or vomitus is suggestive.

Question: What are pulmonary symptoms?
Significance: During the pulmonary stage, cough, dyspnea, fever, and pulmonary infiltrates in the presence of eosinophilia suggest the diagnosis.

Question: Are there symptoms of obstruction?
Significance: Rarely, the infection presents as intestinal obstruction, with an incidence of approximately 2 children per 1,000 infected.

Physical Examination

Chest: May have rales or wheezing if *Ascaris* is in the lungs.
Abdomen: Auscultate and palpate for signs of obstruction.

 ## Laboratory Aids

Test: Microscopic examination of stool specimens
Significance:

- Will demonstrate the characteristic eggs.
- During the pulmonary phase, eosinophils and larvae may be seen. However, stool may be negative during this early phase.
- No serologic tests are necessary, and are poorly specific to the diagnosis.

Test: Chest x-ray, if cough is present

Test: Abdominal plain film if abdominal signs or symptoms

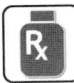 ## Therapy

- Either albendazole 400 mg as a single dose or mebendazole 100 mg twice daily for 3 days is currently considered to be first line therapy for symptomatic infection.
- A single dose of pyrantel pamoate (11 mg/kg; maximum, 1 g) is also effective.
- None of the above regimens are approved for children less than 2 years old; however, limited studies in this age group suggest that the medications are safe.
- Piperazine citrate (75 mg/kg/d for 2 days; maximum, 3.5 g) is suggested in cases of obstruction due to large worm bezoars to aid passage. It should not be administered with pyrantel pamoate.

PREVENTION

Infection Control

- With appropriate disposal of human excrement and with hand washing, this infection could be eliminated.
- In communities with high *Ascaris* carriage, biannual administration of pyrantel pamoate or mebendazole is effective.

 ## Follow-Up

Treatment as specified above is highly effective. Reexamination of stool specimens 3 weeks after therapy to determine that the eggs are eliminated can be considered but is not essential. Reinfection is problematic in endemic areas.

 ## Common Questions and Answers

Q: Where do children get this infection?
A: Commonly from playing in dirt contaminated with *Ascaris* eggs.

ICD-9-CM 127.0

BIBLIOGRAPHY

American Academy of Pediatrics. *Ascaris Lumbricoides* infections. In: Pickering LK, eds. *2003 Red book: Report of the Committee on Infectious Diseases.* 26th Ed. Elk Grove Village, IL: American Academy of Pediatrics, 2003:206–208.

O'Lorcain P, Holland CV. The public health importance of *Ascaris lumbricoides*. *Parasitology* 2000;121(Suppl):S51–S71.

Authors: Suzanne Dawid
Louis M. Bell, 3rd edition

Ascites

 Database

DEFINITION

Ascites is defined as effusion and pathologic accumulation of fluid in the abdominal cavity. Peritoneal fluid formation is a dynamic process of production and absorption. See table Analysis of Ascitic Fluid.

PATHOPHYSIOLOGY

The development of ascitic fluid may be sudden or insidious, associated with nonhepatic etiologies, or secondary to acute reduction in hepatocellular function in a marginally compensated liver.
Intraabdominal factors which result in a net flow of fluid and protein out of the mesenteric capillary bed are:

- Decreased plasma colloid osmotic pressure
- Increased capillary pressure
- Increased ascitic colloid osmotic fluid pressure
- Decreased ascitic fluid hydrostatic pressure

Accumulation of fluid occurs with:

- Inflammatory conditions, e.g., mesenteric adenitis, tuberculosis, pancreatitis, secondary to inflammation of visceral and/or parietal peritoneum
- Obstruction of portal vein flow and/or lymphatic flow by mass, tumor, or external pressure; tumors of abdominal viscera, retroperitoneum, thorax, or mediastinum (often characterized by chylous ascites)
- Primary (congenital) abnormalities of the lymphatics (Milroy disease), congenital neonatal ascites, secondary to GI tract trauma (ureteral rupture), hematologic diseases (hydrops secondary to hemolysis), congestive heart disease; and lysosomal storage diseases including sialidosis (neuraminidase deficiency), Salla disease, GM1 gangliosidosis, Gaucher disease, and Niemann-Pick type C
- Decreased plasma oncotic pressure secondary to hypoalbuminemia (increased losses: renal, gastrointestinal tract; decreased production: hepatic failure)
- Rupture of intraabdominal viscus or peritoneal/mesenteric cyst

ANALYSIS OF ASCITIC FLUID

- The initial evaluation of a patient with ascites should include a directed history, and focused physical examination. Paracentesis should be considered for all patients with ascites. It is usually not indicated in the initial diagnostic evaluation of ascites in the child with known liver disease. The other causes of ascites that occur more often in adults with liver disease, such as malignant or tuberculous ascites, are very rare in children. It is, however, important to know the usual composition of ascitic fluid in patients with liver disease without secondary complications.
- The serum ascites albumin gradient (SAAG) = serum albumin—ascitic albumin, is useful in determining the cause of ascites and subsequently guiding the management.
If greater or equal to 1.1 g/dl, it is a high gradient and represents portal hypertension. If lower than 1.1g/dl, it represents a normal gradient and excludes portal hypertension.

COMPLICATIONS

Infection

Ascitic fluid infection can be classified into three categories based on ascitic culture results, PMN count, and presence or absence of a surgical source of infection.
An abdominal paracentesis must be performed and ascitic fluid must be analyzed before a confident diagnosis of ascitic fluid infection can be made. The blood culture bottle should be injected with peritoneal fluid at the bedside in order to increase the culture's yield.

- Spontaneous ascitic fluid infection: infection of the peritoneal fluid of patients with ascites in the absence of secondary causes, such as bowel perforation or intraabdominal abscess.

Subtypes:

Spontaneous bacterial peritonitis, (SBP), (65%) and
Monomicrobial nonneutrocytic bacterascites (MNB)
Culture negative neutrocytic ascites (CNNA)

- Secondary bacterial peritonitis: there is an identified intraabdominal surgically treatable primary source of infection (e.g., perforated gut, perinephric abscess) that usually requires emergency surgical intervention.
- Polymicrobial bacterascites: This diagnosis should be suspected when the paracentesis is

traumatic or unusually difficult because of ileus, or when stool or air is aspirated into the paracentesis syringe (diagnostic of gut perforation by the paracentesis needle.) Antibiotic therapy should be started if there is a high index of suspicion and:

PMNs <250/mm³ no treatment
PMNs >250 <500 mm³ IV antibiotics if clinical suspicion high; or, wait and retap
PMNs >500 mm³ IV antibiotics (e.g., cefotaxime + ampicillin)
PMNs >500 mm³ Rule out secondary peritonitis

—An indication of therapeutic response is a decrease in the neutrophil count in the ascitic fluid by 50% from that detected on presentation. It is appropriate to treat according to sensitivies when cultures are available. The length of therapy depends on clinical response but should be a minimum of 10 days.

Other Complications

- Respiratory distress from decreased lung volume and diaphragmatic limitation
- Hepatic hydrothorax, large symptomatic pleural effusion that occurs in a cirrhotic patient in the absence of primary cardiopulmonary disease.
- Abdominal wall hernias with rupture
- Tense ascites with leakage (especially after paracentesis).

Conservative management consists of appropriate initial therapy for most of these except hernia rupture, which requires surgical reduction

PROGNOSIS

Depends on the etiology. If from nephrotic syndrome, will regress as proteinuria clears. If from liver failure, will depend on recovery of liver function. Cirrhosis complicated by ascites is associated with significant morbidity and mortality, related in part to the severe underlying liver disease and in part to the ascites per se. Once ascites appears, the expected mortality rate is approximately 50% in just 2 years. With liver transplantation, survival is improved dramatically.

 Differential Diagnosis

- Enlarged liver or spleen
- Mesenteric cyst: does not have shifting dullness when position is changed
- Intestinal obstruction

 Data Gathering

HISTORY

- The etiology for acute decompensation in hepatocellular function, i.e., massive bleeding, sepsis, superimposed infections, should be investigated.
- Use of umbilical catheters in newborn period
- Evidence of chronic liver disease
- Respiratory distress

Analysis of Ascitic Fluid

	COLOR	TRIGLYCERIDES	TOTAL FAT	WHITE BLOOD CELL COUNT
Cirrhotic	Straw	<250 mg/dL		WBC/mL (more than 75 leukocytes [PMNs] suggests inflammation)
Chylous	Yellow-white Creamy	400 mg/dL	Two times that of plasma	
Traumatic	Blood, bile, air, or intestinal contents			

- Exposure to hepatotoxins
- Mental retardation suggesting metabolic disease

 ## Physical Examination

- Vital signs
- Abdominal cavity circumference
- Weight
- Auscultation of the pericardium
- Neurologic examination to evaluate for encephalopathy
- Skin changes suggestive of chronic liver disease
- Special attention should be directed toward identification of a distended abdomen, fullness in the flanks, inverted umbilicus, and development of hernias, scrotal edema, rectal prolapse, and a prominent anterior wall.
- Techniques to detect free intraabdominal fluid include presence of a fluid wave, shifting dullness, and puddle sign (percuss abdomen with patient flexed at hip to detect dullness that may accurately detect fluid over 1 L).
- Other physical examination signs include splenomegaly and prominent abdominal veins (portal hypertension), cor pulmonale (congestive heart failure), pericardial friction rub (pericarditis), diffuse abdominal pain (peritonitis or visceral perforation), abdominal pain radiating to the back (pancreatitis), and lymphedema (lymphatic obstruction/trauma to the thoracic duct).

 ## Laboratory Aids

LABORATORY TESTS

- Complete white blood cell count
- Electrolytes
- Liver-function tests: transaminases, PT/PTT
- Total protein, albumin
- Amylase and lipase (to exclude pancreatitis)
- Creatinine and blood urea nitrogen
- Blood cultures
- Urine for specific gravity
- Viral serologies, including hepatitis B and C viruses, coxsackievirus, enteroviruses

IMAGING

- Abdominal radiography
- Ultrasound of the abdomen to differentiate between free and loculated fluid collection and the presence of intraabdominal masses
- Abdominal computed axial tomography

ABDOMINAL PARACENTESIS

Abdominal paracentesis is a safe procedure in the evaluation of etiologies of ascites. The two complications are perforation of the bowel and hemorrhage. With sterile conditions, a narrow-bore angiocatheter, usually 23-gauge, is inserted through the linea alba 2 cm below the umbilicus, using the Z-technique. Paracentesis is done for: Routine studies, including white blood cell count, culture, LDH, total protein, albumin,

glucose, Gram stain, amylase, cholesterol with triglycerides, and cytology.
Calculate serum-ascites albumin gradient (SAAG): SAAG 1.1 g/dL: portal hypertension very likely SAAG <1.1 g/dL: suspect other causes. These tests require approximately 10 to 20 mL of fluid.

- When glucose in the ascitic fluid is below 30 mg/dL, tuberculous peritonitis must be excluded.
- When ascitic amylase is greater than the normal serum amylase, pancreatitis is suggested.

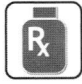 ## Therapy

The management of the ascites should be directed toward the underlying etiology. In a patient with cirrhosis, accumulation of ascites should be avoided by preventing complications such as esophageal hemorrhage, spontaneous bacterial peritonitis, hepatorenal syndrome, inferior vena cava obstruction, and renal and cardiac circulatory disturbances.

- Sodium intake should be restricted to 1 to 2 mEq/kg/day (low-salt diet).
- Water should be restricted to 50% to 75% of maintenance requirements in patients with significant water excess or profound hyponatremia.
- Diuretics may be used to promote negative sodium and water balance. Spironolactone (2–3 mg/kg/day). Furosemide could be added if no response to Spirolonactone. When diuretics are used, urine output and serum electrolytes should be closely monitored to prevent prerenal azotemia and decrease effective blood flow to the kidneys.

Refractory ascites: Diuretic-refractory ascites derives from a lack of response to dietary sodium restriction and maximal diuretic therapy. Treatment options are:

- Therapeutic abdominal paracentesis (large volume paracentesis) should be used only in resistant cases and for tense ascites, because ascitic fluid tends to reaccumulate. Paracentesis of volumes greater than 1 L should be accompanied by the IV infusion of salt-poor albumin during the procedure.
- LeVeen shunt (peritoneal-venous shunting) connects the peritoneal cavity with the superior vena cava near its entrance into the right atrium. The shunt is rarely used as a therapeutic option because of the high frequency of infection, obstruction, and other complications.
- Transjugular intrahepatic portosystemic shunting (TIPS) consists of a metallic stent that bridges the branches of the portal and hepatic veins. May be valuable in cases where portal hypertension is felt to be the underlying etiology of ascitic accumulation. Variceal hemorrhage remains the main indication for TIPS.
- Orthotopic liver transplantation (OLT) is the only curative therapy for refractory ascites from liver disease and the only definitive

treatment that has been shown to improve survival.

 ## Follow-Up

Weight and effects of diuretics should be assessed closely with attention to preservation of renal function. Urine and serum electrolytes should be monitored. Abdominal girth should be measured frequently. In cases of infection or peritonitis, a repeat paracentesis should be performed approximately 48 hours after the initiation of antibiotics for culture and white blood cell count.

PITFALLS

- With congenital ascites, evaluate for lysosomal storage diseases.
- When performing paracentesis, make certain that the fluid is ascitic and not intraluminal.
- Ultrasonography may be helpful to determine the location of this fluid.
- With new onset of ascites, make certain to evaluate for abdominal neoplasia.
- With marginally compensated liver disease, attempt to identify the source of the patient's acute decompensation.

 ## Common Questions and Answers

Q: What are primary considerations regarding neonatal ascites?
A: Exclude lysosomal storage and/or other metabolic diseases.

Q: What is the best test to discriminate the type of ascites?
A: Analysis of the peritoneal fluid collected by abdominal paracentesis is required for this purpose.

ICD-9-CM 789.5

BIBLIOGRAPHY

Sabri M, et al. Pathophysiology and management of pediatric ascites. *Curr Gastroenterol Rep* 2003;5(3):240–246.

Sabri M, et al. Pathophysiology and management of pediatric ascites. *Curr Gastroenterol Rep* 2003;5(3):240–246.

Wong F. The pathophysiologic basis for the treatment of cirrhotic ascites. *Clin Liver Dis* 2001;5(3):819–832.

Wongcharatrawee S, Garcia-Tsao G. Clinical management of ascites and its complications. *Clin Liver Dis* 2001;5:833–850.

Yu AS, Hu KQ. Management of ascites. *Clin Liver Dis* 2001;5(2):541–568.

Zervos EE. Management of medically refractory ascites. *Am J Surg* 2001;181(3):256–264.

Authors: Ruben W. Cerri
Stephen E. Shaffer
Dror Wasseeman, 3rd edition

Aspergillosis

Database

DEFINITION

The term aspergillosis is applied to the wide variety of illnesses that are caused by the fungi in the genus *Aspergillus*. Most human disease is caused by *Aspergillus fumigatus*; *Aspergillus flavus, Aspergillus niger*, other *Aspergillus* species may occasionally cause disease.

PATHOPHYSIOLOGY

• The most common portal of entry for *Aspergillus* is the respiratory tract; however damaged skin or operative wounds, the cornea, and the ear can also serve as sites of entry.
—The development of disease depends on the interaction between the organism (virulence) and the host, specifically host defense mechanisms.
—*Aspergillus* produces toxic metabolites such as elastase, cytotoxins, endotoxins, phospholipases, and various inhibitors of immune function.
—*Aspergillus* is an unusual pathogen in immunocompetent patients. The first line of defense in the lungs is the marcrophages. Neutrophils are also a key part of the host defense against *Aspergillus*.

• Conditions that alter the normal immunologic mechanisms predispose to invasive aspergillosis; leukemia (neutropenia), corticosteroids (decreased neutrophil mobilization and macrophage killing), chronic granulomatous disease (decreased oxidative mediated killing).

ASSOCIATED ILLNESSES

• Allergic bronchopulmonary aspergillosis (ABPA) is characterized by periodic episodes of wheezing, low-grade fever, eosinophilia on peripheral smear, transient infiltrates on chest x-ray film, and a cough productive of brown mucus plugs. ABPA is thought to represent a hypersensitivity response to *Aspergillus* colonization of the lungs. It occurs most commonly in patients with chronic respiratory disease (e.g., in children with cystic fibrosis).
• Otomycosis is a localized, noninvasive infection of the external ear seen in healthy hosts. It occurs more commonly in warm, wet climates.
• Sinusitis occurs in both healthy and immunocompromised patients. Healthy patients can present with signs and symptoms of chronic sinusitis or a mass (aspergilloma) in the maxillary or ethmoid sinuses. Immunocompromised patients present with invasive disease characterized by bony destruction, extension to contiguous sites such as the orbit or CNS.

—Noninvasive pulmonary aspergillosis (aspergillomas) are pulmonary fungus balls that grow in bronchogenic cysts or other lung cavities. They are the most frequent form of pulmonary aspergillosis.

• Invasive pulmonary aspergillosis occurs in the immunocompromised host, most commonly in patients with hematologic malignancy, solid organ transplantation, HIV infection or other patients receiving long-term immunosuppressive therapy. Invasion of blood vessels by *Aspergillus* leads to infarction, necrosis, and hematogenous dissemination.

EPIDEMIOLOGY

• *Aspergillus* species are saprophytic molds that are ubiquitous and worldwide, growing in soil, grain, dung, bird droppings, and decaying plant matter.
• Spores are resistant to desiccation, lightweight, and easily dispersed in air currents.
• Main route of transmission is via inhalation of airborne spores; person-to-person spread does not occur.
• Other than those with otomycosis or allergic bronchopulmonary disease, most patients infected with *Aspergillus* are immunocompromised in some way.
• Nosocomial outbreaks have occurred when ventilation or heating systems become contaminated, or when large numbers of spores become airborne during building construction or renovation.
• The incubation period has not been defined.

COMPLICATIONS

• Disseminated infection: defined as infection of two or more organs, can involve any of the previously discussed sites, as well as the CNS, heart, bones, or skin. Invasiveness depends on the immune state of the host, as well as the period of time and number of spores in the exposure.
• Patients with underlying diseases that predispose them to pulmonary cavitations, blebs, or cysts (such as asthma, chronic bronchitis, TB, sarcoid, histoplasmosis, and bronchiectasis) may develop an aspergilloma (fungus ball) after seeding their pulmonary secretions with *Aspergillus*. When the mass is large enough to be demonstrated on chest x-ray study, serum levels of IgG antibody to *Aspergillus* are characteristically high. Patients may present with hemoptysis, exacerbation of their underlying disease, or rarely, invasion or dissemination.

PROGNOSIS

• Good in noninvasive disease, such as simple otomycosis or paranasal sinusitis
• Immunosuppressed or severely neutropenic patients can have rapid extension or dissemination of disease; prognosis is often very poor. Early recognition and aggressive treatment and debridement are necessary.

Differential Diagnosis

• Other bacterial and fungal infections in immunocompromised hosts
• Allergic pneumonitis (other causes)
—Chronic bacterial sinusitis
• Neoplasm

Data Gathering

HISTORY

Question: Is there a history of the chronic otitis externa?
Significance: Associated with otomycosis

Question: Is there history of sinusitis that does not clear?
Significance: Indolent or noninvasive paranasal sinusitis presents with signs and symptoms of chronic sinusitis that are unresponsive to antibiotic therapy.

Question: Does an asthmatic patient cough up large, dark mucus plugs?
Significance: Allergic bronchopulmonary aspergillosis should be considered in the asthmatic patient with a history of expectorating dark mucus plugs, or a history of fleeting pulmonary infiltrates on chest x-ray (due to bronchial plugging).

Question: Is the patient immunocompromised?
Significance: Immunocompromised patients, especially those with prolonged neutropenia, are at highest risk for invasive aspergillosis. Patients with neutropenia, who are febrile for 1 week despite broad-spectrum antibiotics, are at increased risk of invasive fungal infection.

Physical Examination

• Otomycosis is characterized by a mass of black spores (*A. niger*) that start close to the eardrum and eventually fill the external canal, pain on tragal movement, and occasionally a purulent discharge. It is only rarely an invasive disease.
• Invasive sinus aspergillosis may present with severe pain, proptosis, monocular blindness, and bony destruction on x-ray films, with evidence of direct extension to the anterior fossa or orbit, or with widespread dissemination.
• Invasive pulmonary aspergillosis may be indistinguishable from other causes of pneumonia on physical examination. Findings may include fever, tachypnea, rales, hypoxemia, and hemoptysis (secondary to the angioinvasive potential of the organism).

 ## Laboratory Aids

• Isolation of *Aspergillus* species by culture is required for definitive diagnosis.
• *Aspergillus* can be recovered from samples of blood, CSF, sputum, urine, BAL sample, or tissue biopsy. Types of specimens collected are guided by history and physical examination.
• *Aspergillus* species recovered from cultures of the respiratory tract (e.g., sputum and nasal cultures) are usually a result of colonization in the immunocompetent host but may indicate of invasive disease in the immunocompromised host. The positive predictive value may be as high as 80% to 90% in patients with leukemia or bone marrow transplants.
• Microscopic examination of specially stained tissue samples, or of 10% potassium hydroxide wet preparation samples, which are positive for branching, septate hyphae are suggestive of *Aspergillus* or other fungal invaders.
• Elevated serum IgE eosinophilia, serum antibody for *Aspergillus* and an immediate-type skin test response to *Aspergillus* antigen are often present in patients with allergic aspergillosis and are helpful in establishing the diagnosis.
• Radiographic studies may include characteristic findings such as wedge-shaped pleural-based densities or cavities on plain radiographs. Findings on CT scans include the "halo sign" (an area of low attenuation surrounding a nodular lung lesion) initially (caused by edema or bleeding surrounding an ischemic area) and later the "crescent sign" (an air crescent near the periphery of a lung nodule, caused by contraction of infarcted tissue).
• Recent developments in early diagnosis include the use of: high-resolution chest CT, new rapid stain techniques and monoclonal antibodies for BAL samples, and serum ELISA for *Aspergillus galactomannan*.

 ## Therapy

• Allergic bronchopulmonary aspergillosis is frequently managed with oral or inhaled corticosteroids. In patients with corticosteroid-dependent allergic bronchopulmonary aspergillosis, the addition of itraconazole has been shown to be an effective adjunctive agent.
• If paranasal sinusitis is noninvasive, surgical drainage or debridement usually results in clearance of the infection.
• Otomycosis (most commonly secondary to *A. niger*) is often found in association with a bacterial external otitis. Debridement of the external canal and treatment of underlying bacterial external otitis usually produces a good therapeutic response.
• The newer azole antifungal agent voriconazole is considered primary therapy for invasive aspergillosis.
• Amphotericin B and the lipid-based amphotericin preparations remain appropriate second-line therapeutic options for patients who do not tolerate voriconazole or are not responding to therapy. For patients in whom amphotericin is being considered, the lipid-based formulations may be preferred as initial therapy in those with marginal renal function or in those receiving other nephrotoxic drugs.
• Itraconazole has been shown to be efficacious in the treatment of invasive aspergillosis. The oral form of itraconazole may be considered as an alternative to amphotericin for prolonged treatment once disease progression has been halted with IV amphotericin therapy.
• Surgical excision, in addition to amphotericin B, is sometimes required for localized debridement in invasive disease.

 ## Follow-Up

The course of illness is variable, depending on host immune function and location and invasiveness of disease.

PITFALLS

• Any immunocompromised patient with persistent fevers or signs of invasive infection not improving on treatment with broad-spectrum antibiotics must be evaluated for fungal infection and the empiric use of antifungal medications considered.
• The rare finding of diffuse nodular pneumonia in children may be indicative of an underlying diagnosis of chronic granulomatous disease and aspergillosis.

PREVENTION

Infection Control

• Hospitalized, immunosuppressed patients are at risk for invasive aspergillosis.
• Environmental measures to control airborne spread of conidiospores in hospitals during construction are indicated.
• Laminar-flow rooms with appropriate filters will significantly decrease contact with airborne conidiospores.

 ## Common Questions and Answers

Q: What are rare complications of aspergillosis?
A: Endocarditis, osteomyelitis, and cutaneous disease.

Q: Does person-to-person spread occur?
A: No. The principal route of transmission is inhalation of airborne spores.

ICD-9-CM 117.3

BIBLIOGRAPHY

American Academy of Pediatrics Aspergillosis. In: Pickering L, eds. *2003 Red Book: Report of the Committee on Infectious Diseases.* 25th Ed. Elk Grove Village, IL: American Academy of Pediatrics, 2003:208–210.

Blum MD, Wiederman BL. Aspergillus. In: Feigen RD, Cherry JD, eds. *Textbook of Pediatric Infectious Diseases.* 5th Ed. Philadelphia: WB Saunders, 2004:2550–2560.

Denning DW. Invasive Aspergillosis. *Clin Infect Dis* 1998;26:781–805.

Marr KA, et al. Aspergillosis. Pathogenesis, clinical manifestations, and therapy. *Infectious Dis Clin North Am* 2002;16(4):875–894.

Patterson TF. Combination antifungal therapy. *Pediatr Infect Dis J* 2003;22(6):555–556.

Steinbach WJ, Stevens DA. Review of newer antifungal and immunomodulatory strategies for invasive aspergillosis. *Clin Infect Dis* 2003;37(Suppl 3):S157–S224.

Stevens DA, Kan VL, Judson MA, et al. Practice guidelines for diseases caused by Aspergillus. *Clin Infect Dis* 2000;30:696–709.

Stevens DA, et al. Allergic Bronchopulmonary Aspergillosis in Cystic Fibrosis-State of the Art: Cystic Fibrosis Foundation Consensus Conference. *Clin Infect Dis* 2003;37(Suppl 3):S225–S264.

Author: Theoklis Zaoutis

Asplenia/Hyposplenia

 Database

DEFINITION

Hyposplenia and asplenia are defined by the functional capacity of the spleen to filter blood and perform immunogenic functions.

CAUSES

Hyposplenia/asplenia occurs secondary to: (1) surgical splenectomy, (2) congenital asplenia or (3) in association with certain diseases or illnesses. A complete listing of causes is given below (see Differential Diagnosis).

PATHOLOGY

• Most patients with hyposplenism have no problems handling antigens. However, if the spleen is minimally functional, problems develop. The major consequence is an inability to handle infections.
• The spleen is a major component of reticuloendothelial system; it is important both for antibody synthesis and removal of opsonized organisms. The encapsulated microbes such as pneumococcus, meningococcus and *Haemophilus* are usually handled by this mechanism.
• Under the age of 4 years where few alternate routes of bacterial clearance exist, significant pathology can result for the patient with impaired splenic function.
• Asplenia syndrome should be viewed separately as its morbidity is distinctly unfavorable. Asplenia syndrome is characterized by complex congenital heart defects, asplenia, and abdominal heterotaxy.

—The common associated anomalies include: atrioventricular canal defects, conotruncal anomalies, anomalous systemic pulmonary venous connections, and abnormalities of visceroatrial situs.
—The embryologic basis is thought to be a disturbance in embryogenesis in the fifth week of development that results in bilateral right-sidedness with abnormal pulmonary lobation in 80% of patients and abdominal heterotaxy in 72%. The mouse model and family history are suggestive of an autosomal-recessive inheritance pattern. A review of 519 autopsy cases calculated survival to be 2.6 months with death typically resulting from cardiorespiratory failure or infection.

 Differential Diagnosis

Diminished splenic function is found in:

• Normal infants
• Congenital asplenia
• Asplenia syndrome
• Old age
• Sequestration rises (sickle hemoglobinopathies, essential thrombocytosis, malaria, thrombosis of the splenic vessels)
• Autoimmune disorders (glomerulonephritis, SLE, rheumatoid arthritis, GVHD, sarcoid, Sjogren syndrome, Grave disease)
• Gastrointestinal disorders (celiac disease—30% to 50% are hyposplenic, Crohn disease, ulcerative colitis, dermatitis herpetiformis)
• Space-occupying lesions (tumors, amyloid, cysts)
• Splenic irradiation
• Postsplenectomy
• Bone marrow transplant

 Data Gathering

HISTORY

The history taking should be directed toward the differential diagnosis given above. However, in the apparently healthy child with no identified risk factors who presents with an overwhelming infection with an encapsulated organism, the hematologic smear should be examined.

 Physical Examination

On physical exam the spleen may be normal, large, or atretic. Therefore, the size of the spleen cannot be used as an index of splenic function. The size is most closely linked to the underlying etiology. Complete splenic replacement by cysts, neoplasm, or amyloid is an example of hyposplenic splenomegaly. Similarly, sequestration crises such as that associated with sickle cell and malaria clog the spleen with cellular debris, which results in increased spleen size and decreased function.

Asplenia/Hyposplenia

 Laboratory Aids

- The reduction or absence of splenic function can be determined by specific hematologic changes.
- Nonspecific changes include a modest increase in WBC and platelet count.
- The spleen normally removes intracellular debris such as Howell-Jolly bodies (nuclear remnants), Heinz bodies (denatured hemoglobin) and Pappenheimer bodies (iron granules). Findings of target cells, Howell-Jolly, Heinz, Pappenheimer bodies and pitted erythrocytes are indicative of hyposplenism or asplenia.
- Pits or pox on the red cell surface are the most sensitive indicator of hyposplenism. These are submembranous vacuoles that can be seen only in wet preparations of red cells fixed in 1% gluteraldehyde and viewed using direct interference-contrast microscopy.
- 51Cr-labeled heat damaged red cells can be used as a measure of the capacity of the spleen to clear particulate matter from the bloodstream.
- Size of the spleen can be determined by either ultrasound or CT scan.

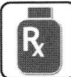 Therapy

- Immunization with a pneumococcal conjugate and/or polysaccharide vaccine should be carried out in all patients with hyposplenism. In those patients who will be undergoing splenectomy, the vaccine should be given prior to the operation.
- Reimmunization is recommended for children who received the pneumococcal conjugate and/or polysaccharide vaccine before 24 months of age.
- Children should also receive HiB vaccine.
- Quadrivalent meningococcal polysaccharide vaccine should be given to all asplenic patients 2 years of age and older.
- Antimicrobial prophylaxis should be strongly considered in all asplenic children less than 5 years of age and for at least 1 year after splenectomy. Oral penicillin is being replaced by amoxicillin-clavulanic acid, trimethoprim-sulfamethoxazole and cefuroxime due to increasing penicillin resistance.

PITFALLS

Under the age of 4 years, splenectomy is contraindicated because of the risk of developing bacterial infection.

 Common Questions and Answers

Q: What should I do if my child has a fever?
A: In hyposplenic patients, especially those under the age of 4 years, all fevers should be taken seriously. If the child is not on prophylactic penicillin, he/she should be treated for all symptomatic infections.

Q: Are there any special times I need to worry about infections?
A: In these patients dental work, especially tooth extraction, should always be covered with antibiotics.

ICD-9-CM 459.0

BIBLIOGRAPHY

Brigden ML. Detection, education and management of the asplenic or hyposplenic patient. *American Family Physician* 2001;63(3):499–506.

Phoon CK, Neill CA. Asplenia syndrome: insight into embryology through an analysis of cardiac and extracardiac anomalies. *Am J Cardiol* 1994;73:581–587.

Phoon CK, Neill CA. Asplenia syndrome—risk factors for early unfavorable outcome. *Am J Cardiol* 1994;73:1235–1237.

Red Book: 2003 Report of the Committee on Infectious Diseases. 26th Ed. Elk Grove Village, IL: American Academy of Pediatrics; 2003:80–81.

Suchy F. *Liver Disease in Children.* Philadelphia: Mosby, 1994.

Sumaraju V, et al. Infectious complications in asplenic hosts. *Infectious Disease Clinics of North America,* June 2001;15(2):551–565

Authors: Matthew Ryan
Barbara Haber, 3rd edition

Asthma

 Database

DEFINITION

- Characterized by three components:

—Reversible airway obstruction
—Airway inflammation
—Airway hyperresponsiveness to a variety of stimuli

DIAGNOSIS—THE THREE R'S

- Recurrence—symptoms are recurrent
- Reactivity—symptoms brought on by specific occurrence or exposure (trigger)
- Responsive—symptoms diminish in response to bronchodilator or antiinflammatory agent

PATHOPHYSIOLOGY AND CAUSES

- Immune and inflammatory responses in the airways triggered by an array of environmental antigens, irritants, or infectious organisms
- Atopy and asthma are related

—Eosinophilia and the ability to make excess IgE in response to antigen is associated with increased airway reactivity.
—Asthma is more common in children who have allergic rhinitis and eczema.

- Viral infections, particularly respiratory syncytial virus (RSV), during infancy may play a role in the development of asthma or may modify the severity of asthma.
- Exposure to cigarette smoke and other airway irritants influences the development and severity of asthma.
- Airway stimulated and primary inflammatory mediators released.
- Airway is invaded by inflammatory cells (mast cells, basophils, eosinophils, macrophages, neutrophils, B and T lymphocytes).
- Inflammatory cells respond to and produce various mediators (cytokines, leukotrienes, lymphokines), augmenting the inflammatory response.
- Airway epithelium is inflamed and becomes disrupted, and basal membrane is thickened.
- Airway smooth muscle is hyperresponsive, and bronchoconstriction ensues.
- Airway smooth muscle hypertrophy and airway epithelial hyperplasia are characteristic chronic changes resulting from poorly controlled asthma.

GENETICS

- Children of asthmatics have higher incidence of asthma:

—6% to 7% risk if neither parent has asthma
—20% risk if one parent has asthma
—60% risk if both parents have asthma

- Several genes are known to be associated with the development of atopy and bronchial muscle responsiveness.

EPIDEMIOLOGY

- Most common chronic illness in children
- Death from asthma in children nearly tripled from 1980 to 1995, and incidence of death from asthma does not seem to correlate with severity.
- Wheezing in children is extremely common in the industrialized world (cumulative prevalence, 30% to 60%).
- In younger children, most episodes occur following viral infections.
- Over 50% of children who wheeze in early childhood stop wheezing by age 6 years.
- 14% of all young children (40% of those who wheeze during infancy) continue to wheeze.

COMPLICATIONS

- Morbidity

—Frequent hospitalizations and absence from school
—Psychologic impact of having a chronic illness
—Decline in lung function over time

PROGNOSIS

- With proper therapy and good adherence with treatment regimen: excellent

 Differential Diagnosis

INFECTIOUS

- Pneumonia
- Bronchiolitis
- Chlamydia infection
- Laryngotracheobronchitis
- Sinusitis

MECHANICAL

- Extrinsic airway compression
- Vascular ring
- Foreign body
- Vocal cord dysfunction
- Tracheobronchomalacia

MISCELLANEOUS

- Cystic fibrosis
- Bronchopulmonary dysplasia
- Pulmonary edema
- Gastroesophageal reflux (GER)
- Recurrent aspiration
- Bronchiolitis obliterans

 Data Gathering

HISTORY

Inquire about these symptoms: coughing, wheezing, shortness of breath, chest tightness

- Frequency of symptoms defines severity
- Precipitating factor (trigger)
- Response to bronchodilator or antiinflammatory medication

PATTERN OF SYMPTOMS

- Perennial versus seasonal
- Continuous versus acute
- Duration and frequency of episodes
- Diurnal variation/nocturnal symptoms

Do any of the following set off the breathing difficulty?

- Infections (upper respiratory, sinusitis)
- Exposure to:

—Dust (mites)
—Animal dander
—Pollen
—Mold

- Cold air or weather changes
- Exercise or play
- Environmental stimulants

—Cigarette smoke
—Strong odors
—Pollutants

- Emotional factors

—Laughing
—Crying
—Fear

- Drug intake

—Aspirin
—Nonsteroidal antiinflammatory drugs
—β-blockers

- Food additives
- Endocrine factors

—Menses
—Pregnancy
—Thyroid dysfunction

- Family history of asthma or atopy

REVIEW OF SYSTEMS

- Symptoms of complicating factors (GER, sinusitis, allergies)

—Dyspepsia, sour taste (GER)
—Throat clearing, purulent nasal discharge, halitosis, cephalalgia, or facial pain (sinusitis)
—Nasal itching, ("allergic salute"), eye rubbing, sneezing, watery nasal discharge (allergies)

IMPACT OF ASTHMA

- Number of hospitalizations/ICU admissions
- Number of ER visits/doctor's office visits
- Asthma attack frequency
- Number of missed school days/parent workdays
- Limitation on activity
- Number of courses of systemic steroids needed

ENVIRONMENTAL HISTORY

- Type of home
- Location of home (urban, suburban, rural)
- Heating system/air conditioning
- Use of humidifier
- Presence of molds, cockroaches, rodents
- Fireplace
- Carpeting
- Stuffed animals
- Pets
- Exposure to cigarette smoke

 ## Physical Examination

- Pulmonary examination may be normal when asymptomatic.
- Assess work of breathing

—Level of distress
—Intercostal/supraclavicular muscle retractions

- Chest shape (i.e., normal vs. barrel-shaped)
- Lung auscultation

—Wheezing
—End-expiratory involuntary cough
—Prolonged expiratory phase
—Crackles or coarse breath sounds
—Stridor (indicates extrathoracic airway obstruction)

- HEENT examination: signs of allergies or sinusitis

—Watery or itchy eyes
—Allergic shiners
—Dennie lines
—Nasal congestion
—Boggy nasal turbinates
—Nasal polyps
—Postnasal drip

- General examination: vital signs

—Blood pressure (pulsus paradoxus)
—Respiratory rate (tachypnea)

- Skin: evidence of eczema
- Extremities: digital clubbing (suggests alternative diagnosis)

PHYSICAL EXAMINATION TRICK

Forced exhalation maneuver to observe for wheezes or for precipitating coughing

 ## Laboratory Aids

TESTS

- Pulmonary function tests

—Essential for the assessment and ongoing care of children with asthma.
—Spirometry measures the degree of airway obstruction and the response to bronchodilators.
—Values obtained can measure absolute degree of airway obstruction.
—Serial values can follow progress of disease and response to treatment.
—Children as young as 3 years old can usually perform spirometry with practice.

- Provocational testing

—Exercise challenge: determines effect of exercise on triggering airway obstruction
—Cold air challenge: indirect test of airway hyperresponsiveness
—Methacholine challenge: a positive test supports the diagnosis of asthma; useful in cases where history is equivocal and pulmonary function test is normal; measures the degree of airway hyperreactivity

- Allergy evaluation

—Blood tests (eosinophil count, IgE level)
—Skin testing (best test for assessing allergen sensitivity)
—RAST testing (not as accurate as skin testing)
—Sputum/nasal examination for presence of eosinophilia

- Other studies

—GER evaluation
—pH probe
—Milk scan
—Barium swallow (confirms normal anatomy)

- Bronchoscopy to rule out:

—Anatomic malformations
—Foreign bodies
—Mucus plugging
—Vocal cord dysfunction

- Assess for aspiration (lipid-laden macrophages)

IMAGING

- Chest radiograph should usually be obtained at least once for all children to rule out congenital lung malformations or obvious vascular malformations. Findings can be normal. Common findings are peribronchial thickening, subsegmental atelectasis, and hyperinflation.
- Sinus CT is useful if symptoms suggest sinusitis.
- Chest CT should be performed if bronchiectasis or anatomic abnormality is suspected.

HOME TESTING

- Peak flow meter

—Measures peak flow rate (PEFR)
—Used with patients who have poor symptom recognition or labile asthma
—Dips in PEFR precede onset of clinical asthmatic symptoms.
—PEFR should be performed at least once a day

- PEFR values are divided into three zones:

—Green: 80% of baseline or higher
—Yellow: 50% to 80% of baseline
—Red: 50% of baseline
—Specific PEFR guidelines should be individualized for each patient based on the best measurement obtained during a 14-day period when the child is well.

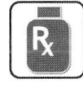 ## Therapy

DRUGS

Antiinflammatory Agents

- Indicated for all patients with asthma except for those with very infrequent and mild symptoms.
- Three classes of inflammatory agents described below
Corticosteroids
Most effective antiinflammatory agent
Preparations
Inhaled

—Reduce airway inflammation and hyperresponsiveness more than any other inhaled agent
—Inhibit production and release of cytokines and arachidonic acid—associated metabolites
—Enhance β-adrenoceptor responsiveness
—Side effects: oral thrush; may minimally affect growth velocity at moderate or high doses
—Dosage individualized to each patient
—Agents vary in topical potency and systemic bioavailability
—Available as pressurized metered dose inhaler (pMDI), dry powder inhaler (DPI), or nebulized as indicated below
—Fluticazone (44, 110, 220 μg/puff pMDI) (Flovent)
—Budesonide (200 μg/puff DPI; 250 and 500 μg vials for nebulizer) (Pulmicort)
—Beclomethasone (42, 84 μg/puff) (Beclovent, Vanceril)
—Triamcinolone (100 μg/puff) (Azmacort)
—Flunisolide (250 μg/puff) (Aerobid)

- Oral—used for asthma exacerbations or for severe asthma that cannot be otherwise controlled

—Exacerbations—prednisone 1–2 mg/kg per day 3 to 7 days or longer; usually tapered if more than 7 days of therapy required or if systemic steroids are used frequently
—Ongoing therapy—0.5 to 1 mg/kg per day daily or every other day for patients with severe asthma
—Undesirable Side-Effect Profile

Asthma

When used daily, assess bone density and for cataract formation at least yearly

- Intravenous

Methylprednisolone (Solumedrol) 1 mg/kg IV q6–12h until able to take oral medication

Leukotriene Modifiers

- Block the synthesis and/or action of leukotrienes
- 5-Lipoxygenase inhibitors; zileuton. May cause hepatic dysfunction.
- Leukotriene receptor antagonists; zafirlukast (10 mg; Accolate) and montelukast (4, 5, and 10 mg; Singulair)
- Indicated as monotherapy for mild or exercise-induced asthma and in combination with an inhaled corticosteroid for more effective symptom control or using a lower dose of inhaled corticosteroid

Mast-Cell Stabilizers

- Weak antiinflammatory agents
- Preparations

—Cromolyn sodium (Intal)
—Nedocromil sodium (Tilade)

- Decrease bronchial hyperresponsiveness
- Can be used prior to exercise for exercise-induced symptoms
- No significant side effects
- Inhaled

—Nebulizer
—MDI

Bronchodilators

- Relax airway smooth muscle
- Three classes described below

β2-Agonists

- Indication is for relief of acute bronchoconstriction (quick relief medicine)
- Used as needed in people with asthma who have breakthrough symptoms
- Used prior to exercise in exercise-induced bronchospasm
- Regular use or overuse associated with worsened control of asthma
- Routes

—Inhaled (most effective): metered dose inhaler or nebulizer
—Oral (least effective; most side effects)

- Preparations: Short-acting (effect lasts 4–6 hours):

—Albuterol (Ventolin, Proventil)
—Terbutaline (Brethaire, Brethine)
—Metoproterenol (Alupent)

- Preparation: Long-acting (lasts up to 12 hours)

—Salmeterol (Serevent)—available as pMDI and DPI
—Can be used daily in conjunction with antiinflammatory agent for improved symptom control

Theophylline

- Second line agent used when more conventional therapies are unsuccessful
- Indications

—Chronic, poorly controlled asthma
—Nocturnal asthma (if no GER)
—Adjunctive therapy with β2 drugs and steroids in hospitalized patients in selected cases

- Route: oral or IV
- Serum levels must be routinely monitored

—Therapeutic levels: 5 to 15 mg/mL
—Side effects are seen with increased levels.
—Many factors affect theophylline levels.
—Increased levels seen with:
  Erythromycin
  Ciprofloxacin
  Cimetidine
  Viral illnesses
  Fever
—Decreased levels seen with:
  Phenobarbital
  Phenytoin
  Rifampin

Anticholinergic Agents

- Adjunctive bronchodilator, may be useful in patients who only partially respond to β-agonists
- Preparations

—Ipratropium bromide MDI or ampule for nebulization (Atrovent)

MISCELLANEOUS DRUGS USED IN SEVERE CASES

Steroid-Sparing Agents

- Troleandomycin (Tao)
- Macrolide antibiotic
- Decreases clearance of corticosteroids, thus prolonging the effects of corticosteroids on the lung
- Lower corticosteroid dosing required

Methotrexate

- Potent immunosuppressive drug
- Needs further investigation in children

Cyclosporine

- Has been shown to have steroid-sparing effect in adult population with asthma
- Side effects are significant and may limit use.

Intravenous Immunoglobulin (IVIG)

- High-dose therapy under investigation
- MgSO4
- Used intravenously as a smooth muscle relaxer in severe acute asthma exacerbation

Helium

- May improve airflow in severe asthma
- Can improve ventilation and potentially oxygenation

IMMUNOTHERAPY

- Efficacy in asthma is controversial.
- Used only in select cases if medical management and environmental control measures are ineffective.

Duration of Therapy

- Antiinflammatory agents

—Use every day
—May be decreased in patients as asthma comes under long-standing control

- Bronchodilators

—Should be used as needed

EDUCATION/ENVIRONMENTAL CONTROL

- Patient and caregiver education is mandatory to establish provider/caregiver partnership and ensure adherence with treatment plan.
- Every patient/caregiver should be taught that asthma is a chronic, inflammatory condition that can be controlled with proper therapy.
- All medications should be explained and potential risks (side effects) and benefits reviewed.
- A written asthma management plan should be provided, outlining daily therapy and an "action plan" for managing exacerbations of asthma.

Environmental Counseling

—Avoid airborne irritants (tobacco smoke, wood stoves, noxious fumes).
—Minimize dust-mite exposure.
—Avoid using in-room humidifier or vaporizer.
—Minimize stuffed animals, quilts, books, and clutter.
—Use dust mite–proof coverings on mattresses, pillows, and box springs.
—Wash pillows, blankets, and sheets in hot water.
—Avoid molds by decreasing relative humidity to 50%.
—Remove pets from child's bedroom, and from house if patient is allergic to the animal.

DIET

- Avoid foods or food additives (if truly allergic).
- Food-induced asthma is uncommon.

Follow-Up

WHEN TO EXPECT IMPROVEMENT

• In acute asthma attacks, with appropriate therapy, improvement is usually seen within 24 to 48 hours.
• Long-term control of symptoms can usually be obtained within 2 to 4 weeks

SIGNS THAT MAY INDICATE PROBLEMS

• Increased symptoms (cough day or night, wheeze)
• Exercise limitations or symptoms during exercise
• Decrease in PEFR
• Increasing use of inhaled bronchodilators
• Subject not improving on enhanced home therapy

PITFALLS

• Not recognizing that asthma can manifest as chronic cough
• Reluctance to "label" child with having asthma (uses terms like reactive airways disease or bronchitis)
• Frequent antibiotic or cough medicine use to treat asthma symptoms
• "Recurrent pneumonias" many times are actually asthma exacerbations; subsegmental atelectasis on chest radiography misdiagnosed as an infiltrate
• Underreporting of asthma symptoms
• Poor adherence with therapy once symptoms are controlled
• Failure to properly use inhaled medications

—Inhaled medication use must be taught and reviewed at each visit.
—A fixed volume holding chamber should always be used with a pMDI, regardless of patient age.
—pMDIs should be refilled based on the number of doses used, not by estimating contents by shaking or spraying.

 Common Questions and Answers

Q: Will my child outgrow his or her asthma?
A: Family history and allergies affect the ultimate outcome. Wheezing during the first 3 years of life is extremely common, with 40% to 50% of all children wheezing at some time. Many of these children do not develop asthma and "outgrow" their illness by school age. Some patients develop asthma again as young adults.

Q: Can my child become dependent on asthma medications?
A: Children do not become "dependent" on these medications as they would with narcotic agents. Daily asthma medications are required to maintain airway patency and to control airway inflammation.

Q: Will my child be on medications for the rest of his or her life?
A: This depends on the severity of the asthma. The types, doses, and frequency of asthma medications will change over a patient's lifetime.

Q: Do inhaled steroids affect patient growth?
A: There is some transient and slight decrease in growth velocity seen in children who receive moderate-dose inhaled corticosteroids (approximately 0.5 mg/day). Ultimate height does not seem to be affected.

ICD-9-CM 493.01
BIBLIOGRAPHY

Crater SE, Platts-Mills TA. Searching for the cause of the increase in asthma. *Curr Opin Pediatr* 1998;10(6):594–599.

Hakonarson H, Grunstein MM. Management of childhood asthma. In: Barnes P, Grunstein MM, Leff A, et al, eds. *Asthma, vol 2.* New York: Raven Press 1997:1847–1868.

Kercsmar CM. Current trends in management of pediatric asthma. *Respiratory Care* 2003;48:194–205.

Liu AH, Szefler SJ. Advances in childhood asthma: hygiene hypothesis, natural history, and management. *J Allerg Clin Immunol* 2003;111:S785–S792.

National Asthma Education and Prevention Program. Expert Panel Report 2: *Guidelines for the diagnosis and management of asthma.* NIH-NHLBI publication. Washington, DC: US Government Printing Office, February 1997.

Reid MJ. Complicating features of asthma. *Pediatr Clin North Am* 1992;39:1327–1341.

Salvatoni A, et al. Inhaled corticosteroids in childhood asthma: Long-term effects on growth and adrenocortical function. *Paediatric Drugs* 2003;5:351–361.

Silverstein MD, Mair JE, Katusik SK, et al. School attendance and school performance: a population-based study of children with asthma. *J Pediatr* 2001;139(2):278–83.

Stempel DA. The pharmacologic management of childhood asthma. *Pediatr Clin North Am* 2003;50:609–629.

Turktas I, Ozkaya O, Bostanci I, et al. Safety of inhaled corticosteroid therapy in young children with asthma. *Ann Allergy Asthma Immunol* 2001;86(6):649–654.

Authors: Ronn E. Tanel
Russell G. Clayton Sr., 3rd edition

Ataxia

Database

DEFINITION

Ataxia is incoordination or clumsiness of movement. Caused by cerebellar, vestibular (inner ear), or proprioceptive sensory (large fiber/peripheral nerve; dorsal root ganglion; posterior column/spinal cord) dysfunction. Cerebellar dysfunction due to intoxication is the most common cause of ataxia in children.

- Appendicular ataxia affects limb movement and results from disease of the cerebellar hemispheres.
- Truncal ataxia, gait ataxia, dysarthria, and nystagmus often occur together and reflect dysfunction of cerebellar midline structures (vermis).

CLINICAL PRESENTATION

- Acute cerebellar ataxia following a benign viral infection is common in children.
- Chronic ataxia usually signals serious underlying pathology (tumor, metabolic, or hereditary disorder).

PATHOPHYSIOLOGY

- Unilateral cerebellar ataxia is produced by lesions of the ipsilateral cerebellum (Purkinje and granule cells in the cerebellar cortex, deep cerebellar nuclei) or its afferent or efferent connections.
- Lesions of the frontal cerebral cortex and the cerebellum may mimic a contralateral cerebellar problem.
- The cerebellum is sensitive to structural (e.g., tumor, stroke, malformation), infectious, or metabolic/toxic processes. It can also become the target of autoimmune phenomena or genetic defects.

EPIDEMIOLOGY

- About 1 in 1,000 children develop acute ataxia following Varicella infection
- The most common congenital cerebellar syndromes are caused by perinatal trauma and hypercoagulable or hemorrhagic vascular events ("ataxic cerebral palsy"). Fetal stroke is estimated to complicate 1 in 4,000 full-term births. The Dandy-Walker syndrome is a rarer cause of congenital cerebellar dysfunction.
- Cerebellar medulloblastomas represent 20% of pediatric primary brain tumors and are also associated with certain inherited disorders (ataxia-telangiectasia, basal cell nevus syndrome). Cerebellar astrocytomas, fourth ventricle ependymomas, and brainstem gliomas are also more common in children than in adults.
- Metabolic/heredodegenerative causes are rare.

—Ataxia telangiectasia incidence is about 1/100,000.
—Friedreich ataxia is 2–4/100,000.
—Ataxia with oculomotor apraxia occurrence is near 5/100,000.

GENETICS

Hereditary causes of chronic ataxia include the recessively inherited Friedreich ataxia, ataxia telangiectasia, and late-infantile/juvenile-onset forms of some inborn errors of metabolism (aminoacidopathies; Hexosaminidase A deficiency, abeta/hypobetalipoproteinemia, Wilson disease, mitochondrial diseases and peroxisomal disorders, childhood neuronal ceroid lipofuschinosis). Dominantly inherited episodic ataxia is seen in the pediatric age group. The dominantly inherited, progressive spinocerebellar ataxias (SCA types 2 and 7) occasionally present in infancy. Episodic ataxia may signal a disorder of pyruvate or ammonia metabolism

ASSOCIATED CONDITIONS

- Acute ataxia most often due to intoxication; association with opsoclonus-myoclonus syndrome may indicate underlying neuroblastoma/ ganglioneuroma. Isolated, transient "cerebellitis" frequently associated with EBV, varicella, and other viruses.
- Friedreich ataxia associated with cardiomyopathy, diabetes, scoliosis, pes cavus, and peripheral neuropathy.
- Ataxia telangiectasia associated with skin/conjunctival telangiectases, with frequent bronchopulmonary infection, and leukemia/lymphoma or other cancers.
- Mitochondrial disorders commonly feature short stature, seizures, retinopathy, heart block, myopathy, mental retardation.
- Langerhans cell histiocytosis and Wolfram syndrome manifest with diabetes insipidus.

Data Gathering

HISTORY

Establish acute versus chronic onset of ataxia to narrow the differential diagnosis.

- Acute ataxia, history directed to possible intoxication, head trauma, or migraine.
- History of episodic change in consciousness or convulsions point to seizure disorder (postictal ataxia).
- Recent varicella or other infection suggests postviral cerebellar ataxia, labyrinthitis, or Guillain-Barré syndrome (GBS) (see Guillain-Barré Syndrome)
- Congenital heart disease or other known circulatory disorder raises the possibility of cerebellar stroke.
- Irritability or progressive macrocrania—brain tumor.
- Family history of neurologic disease

Physical Examination

The neuroanatomic localization of the ataxia must be determined.

- Dysarthria and "drunken" movements; unless the brainstem is affected, consciousness is normal. Other signs include:

—Intentional tremor—oscillations seen (e.g., on finger-nose testing) when agonists and antagonists cocontract to orient limb movement.
—Disdiadochokinesia—impairment of rapid alternating movements.
—Titubation, truncal ataxia, and pathologic nystagmus-midline cerebellar or vestibular disease.
—Cranial nerve findings, especially third, sixth, or lower cranial nerves, point to possible brain tumor
—Asymmetric ataxia or weakness may signify tumor, stroke, or demyelinating disease.

- Sensory ataxia (disease of sensory ganglia or peripheral nerve) signs:

—Romberg sign—ataxia worsened by eye closure. Indicates proprioceptive, or vestibular dysfunction
—Areflexia—not seen in central causes of ataxia

- Toxic/metabolic causes—e.g., intoxications, postictal ataxia, and sleep drunkenness, usually alter consciousness.

Differential Diagnosis

Simple postural or resting tremor, chorea, athetosis, or proximal limb weakness may be mistakenly diagnosed as ataxia.

ACUTE ATAXIA

- Intoxication: Depressed mental status; toxicologic screen; medications at home
- Posttraumatic: History/physical findings
- Postinfectious: Acute cerebellar ataxia (with dysarthria, mild hypotonia)
- Paraneoplastic: Ataxia may precede opsoclonus/myoclonus due to neuroblastoma/ganglioneuroma
- Migraine: Resolves in hours; headache may precede ataxia
- Labyrinthitis: Fast phase of nystagmus is unidirectional
- Acute disseminated encephalomyelitis (ADEM): White matter changes on MRI or CT
- Acute polyneuropathy: GBS (areflexia, signs of sensory ataxia)
- Stroke: Focal deficits; abnormal imaging studies
- Postictal: Rapidly resolving ataxia with negative studies, slowing on EEG; history of convulsion
- Familial periodic ataxia: Family history
- Metabolic disorders: Pyruvate dysmetabolism (attacks provoked by febrile illness, associated lactic acidosis), biotinidase deficiency (associated seizures, skin rash)
- Acute ataxia: Can be a rare presentation of meningitis/encephalitis
- Psychogenic: "Astasia abasia" (variable effort; no pathologic nystagmus; characteristic gait is grossly unsteady, corrective steps before falling)

CHRONIC ATAXIA

- Brain tumor (esp. under 10 years): Associated cranial neuropathies, papilledema, headache, pyramidal tract signs
- Friedreich ataxia: Onset 5–15 years; other affected siblings, associated cardiomyopathy, diabetes, polyneuropathy, scoliosis, pes cavus
- Ataxia telangiectasia: Onset under 5 years; frequent bronchopulmonary infection, and leukemia/lymphoma (elevated alpha-fetoprotein)
- Ataxia with oculomotor apraxia type 1: Onset 2–18 years; associated polyneuropathy, chorea, cognitive difficulty (hypoalbumenemia, hypercholesterolemia)
- Leukodystrophy: Adrenoleukodystrophy, metachromatic leukodystrophy, Pelizaeus-Merzbacher disease (abnormal MRI signal in white matter)
- Other metabolic diseases: Niemann-Pick type C ("sea-blue" histiocytes on bone marrow biopsy); cerebrotendinous xanthomatosis (elevated serum cholestanol levels); Refsum disease (elevated serum phytanic acid; associated retinitis pigmentosa, hearing loss, polyneuropathy); juvenile-onset Tay-Sachs disease, neuraminidase deficiency (lysosomal disorders); maple syrup urine disease (MSUD), Hartnup disease (amino acid screen); familial coenzyme Q10 deficiency; familial vitamin E deficiency; cerebral folate transport disorder (low 5-MHTF in csf)
- Abetalipoproteinemia (hypocholesterolemia)
- Mitochondrial disease (retinopathy, sensorineural hearing loss, diabetes, growth delay, seizures, stroke-like episodes, myopathy, elevated pyruvate and lactate levels)

Congenital disorders of glycosylation.

- Thiamine deficiency (Wernicke encephalopathy) associated with malnutrition, TPN
- Celiac disease
- Hereditary ataxia: autosomal dominant, molecular diagnosis
- Long-term phenytoin use: Primarily adults
- Rare: Ataxic cerebral palsy, brain dysgenesis, Joubert syndrome, multiple sclerosis, Gerstmann-Straussler (familial; prion disease)

Laboratory Aids

- Toxicologic screen is usually a good initial screen in acute ataxia.
- Radiologic studies are necessary when intoxication has been ruled out (rule out tumor, stroke, demyelination); MRI is superior to CT for imaging the cerebellum, though contrast CT can rule out posterior fossa tumor.
- Spinal tap may reveal a few cells/mild increase in protein in benign acute cerebellar ataxia of childhood or in acute demyelinating encephalomyelitis.

- EEG if postictal ataxia is a possibility.
- Full work up for neuroblastoma in ataxia-opsoclonus/myoclonus includes body CT, serum ferritin, urine homovanillic/vanillylmandelic acid (HVA/VMA).
- Low cholesterol in chronic ataxia suggests abetalipoproteinemia; high cholesterol and low albumen suggest ataxia with oculomotor apraxia type 1.
- Elevated alpha-fetoprotein and decreased serum IgA suggest ataxia telangiectasia.
- Genetic tests for Friedreich ataxia, ataxia telangiectasia, ataxia with oculomotor apraxia type 1, and the dominantly inherited spinocerebellar ataxias type 1, 2, 3, 6, 7, 8, 10, 12, and 17 are available.
- Laboratory testing for mitochondrial ataxia includes urine organic acids, plasma or csf lactate and pyruvate, genetic testing on blood, muscle biopsy.

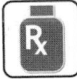

Therapy

- As indicated for any underlying condition; precautions and limitation of activity to decrease the chance of injury/aspiration
- Steroids (2 mg/kg IV prednisolone) and IVIG (400 mg/kg/day for 5 days) have been used for ADEM, though there is no proven benefit.
- Immunomodulatory therapies have been tried (plasmapheresis, IVIG) for paraneoplastic ataxia-opsoclonus/myoclonus, which may persist long after therapy for the tumor.
- Acetazolamide may be helpful for familial periodic ataxia; amantadine and buspirone may provide symptomatic relief in Friedreich ataxia; most drugs useful for tremor can be helpful for cerebellar tremor.
- Replacement therapies may stabilize or reverse ataxia in some conditions (deficiencies of vitamin E, thiamine, coenzyme Q10; biotin in biotinidase deficiency; folinic acid in cerebral folate transport disorder). Coenzyme Q10 and vitamin E supplementation have been shown to benefit the cardiomyopathy (but not the ataxia) of Friedreich ataxia

Follow-Up

- Acute postinfectious cerebellar ataxia usually resolves over days to weeks; if imaging studies show demyelination, recovery may take longer and the chance of recurrence may be higher.
- If initial studies in opsoclonus/myoclonus do not reveal a neoplasm, follow-up studies should be repeated.

PITFALLS

- Children with acute recurrent ataxia should be evaluated for ornithine transcarbamoylase deficiency, mitochondrial disorders, or one of the paroxysmal dyskinesias (ion channelopathies)

- Inadvertent intoxication with anticonvulsants may not be detected on routine toxin screen. Ask about carbamazepine, phenytoin.
- Symptoms of progressive herniation of the cerebellar tonsils in a child or adolescent with Arnold-Chiari type 1 malformation may mimic migraine. Head CT or MRI should be done on a child with ataxia and a headache.

Common Questions and Answers

Q: What intoxications are most likely to cause ataxia?
A: Benzodiazepines, the major anticonvulsants (except valproate), psychotropic medications, ethanol, tricyclics, antihistamines.

Q: How long can postinfectious cerebellar ataxia last?
A: Rarely, it may last for months, but usually improves during that time.

Q: What is the role of physical therapy for cerebellar ataxia?
A: Rhythmic, repetitive exercise; exercise for balance and coordination; and muscle conditioning exercise may improve level of performance in patients with ataxia. Vestibular compensation exercise may improve symptoms of dizziness or vertigo in patients with vestibular ataxia.

ICD-9-CM 334.3

BIBLIOGRAPHY

Connolly AM, Dodson WE, Prensky AL, et al. Course and outcome of acute cerebellar ataxia. *Ann Neurol* 1994;35:673–679.

Lodi R, et al. Antioxidant treatment improves in vivo cardiac and skeletal muscle bioenergetics in patients with Friedreich's ataxia. *Ann Neurol* 2001;49:590–596.

Mercuri E, et al. Cerebellar infarction and atrophy in infants and children with a history of premature birth. *Pediatr Radiol* 1997;27:139–143.

Moreira MC, et al. The gene mutated in ataxia-ocular apraxia 1 encodes the new HIT/Zn-finger protein aprataxin. *Nat Genet* 2001;29:189–193.

Perlman SL. Diagnostic evaluation of ataxic patients. In: Pulst SM, ed. *Genetics of Movement Disorders*. San Diego: Academic Press, 2003;254–267.

Ullrich NJ, Pomeroy SL. Pediatric brain tumors. *Neurol Clin* 2003;21:897–913.

Internet Information for Parents: National Ataxia Foundation website- http://www.ataxia.org.

Author: Susan Perlman

Atelectasis

Database

DEFINITION

- State of collapsed and airless alveoli
- May be subsegmental, segmental, or lobar, or may involve the entire lung
- A radiographic sign of an underlying disease and not a diagnosis unto itself

CAUSES

- Airway obstruction (resorption atelectasis)

—Most common cause for atelectasis in children
—Obstructed communication between alveoli and trachea

- Large airway obstruction:

—Intrinsic: Foreign-body aspiration, mucus plug, inflammatory tumor
—Extrinsic: Hilar adenopathy, mediastinal mass, congenital lung malformations

- Small airway obstruction:

—Altered mucociliary clearance: CNS depression, smoke inhalation, pain
—Acute infection: Bronchiolitis, pneumonia (respiratory infections are the most common cause of acute atelectasis)

- Mechanical compression of the pulmonary parenchyma or pleural space (compressive atelectasis)
- Intrathoracic compression: Pneumothorax, pleural effusion, lobar emphysema, intrathoracic tumors, cardiomegaly, diaphragmatic hernias
- Abdominal distension: Large intraabdominal tumors, hepatosplenomegaly, massive ascites, morbid obesity
- Decreased surface tension in the small airways and alveoli (adhesive atelectasis)

—Stems from surfactant deficiency
—Diffuse surfactant deficiency: Hyaline membrane disease, ARDS, smoke inhalation
—Localized surfactant deficiency: Acute radiation pneumonitis, pulmonary embolism

- Neuromuscular weakness (hypoventilation)

—Inherent weakness: Muscular dystrophy, spinal muscle atrophy, paralysis
—Acquired weakness: Postanesthesia (hypoventilation)

PATHOPHYSIOLOGY

- Reduced lung compliance
- Loss of alveoli (if extensive) may lead to hypoxia.
- Intrapulmonary shunting develops from hypoxia-induced pulmonary arterial vasoconstriction, which may lead to areas of ventilation/perfusion (V/Q) mismatch and further hypoxia.
- If atelectasis is extensive, pulmonary hypertension may develop.
- Atelectatic areas are prone to bacterial overgrowth.

GENETICS

- Depends on the underlying disease causing atelectasis

EPIDEMIOLOGY

- Depends on the underlying disease causing atelectasis
- Resorption atelectasis the most common form

COMPLICATIONS

- Recurrent infections
- Bronchiectasis
- Hemoptysis
- Abscess formation
- Fibrosis of the pulmonary parenchyma

PROGNOSIS

- Dependent on the underlying disease process

—In otherwise healthy individuals: Excellent

Differential Diagnosis

- Pneumonia

—Viral pneumonia versus subsegmental atelectasis
—Bacterial pneumonia versus segmental or lobar atelectasis

- Thymus (may be mistaken for atelectasis in an upper lobe)
- Congenital malformations (i.e., sequestration, bronchogenic cyst)
- Pleural effusion

Data Gathering

HISTORY

- Dependent on the underlying disease process
- May be asymptomatic
- Cough and/or wheeze can be present
- Dyspnea
- Chest pain

Special Questions

- Is the atelectasis acute, recurrent, or chronic in terms of its duration?
- Is there a history of asthma, chronic lung disease, or exposure to smoke or toxic fumes that would increase the risk for atelectasis?

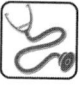

Physical Examination

- May be normal
- Tachypnea
- Rales or rhonchi
- The most specific sign is localized decrease or loss of breath sounds.
- Dullness to percussion if large area involved
- Tracheal deviation and shift of heart sounds toward atelectatic side
- Localized wheezes in cases of partial obstruction
- Cyanosis (seen when extensive atelectasis is present causing impairment of oxygenation and areas of V/Q mismatch)

Laboratory Aids

TESTS

Appropriate test is dependent on the underlying etiology

- Asthma

—Spirometry
—Sweat test (if CF suspected)

- Infection

—Cultures (sputum, blood, bronchoalveolar lavage fluid)
—Nasal washing (especially for viruses)
—PPD (when tuberculosis is suspected)

- Foreign body aspiration

—Bronchoscopy (to remove the obstructing agent)

- Immunodeficiency

—CBC with differential
—Immunoglobulins (IgG, IgA, IgM)
—HIV testing

- Congenital malformations

—CT scan of the chest (for lung malformation)
—Bronchoscopy (for H-type tracheoesophageal fistula [TEF] or bronchial stenosis)

Imaging

Chest Radiography

- Most important diagnostic tool
- Radiographic signs of atelectasis:

—Loss of lung volume from the affected lobe
—Compensatory hyperexpansion of the remaining lobes on the affected side
—Shift of interlobar fissures
—Elevation of diaphragm
—Mediastinal shift toward the affected side
—Approximation of ribs on the affected side

CT of Chest

- Confluence of bronchi and blood vessels converge toward the affected side
- Provides information in regard to precise location and extent of any obstructing process

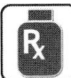 ## Therapy

- Treat underlying disease (i.e., removal of aspirated foreign body)
- Chest physical therapy with bronchodilators—usually for at least 1 month
- If no improvement with conservative therapy, a bronchoscopy with lavage to remove possible mucus plug is indicated (lavage may be with saline or in select cases, with recombinant human DNase)
- Surgery to remove the affected region should be considered when atelectasis occurs:

—Is chronic or recurrent
—Is unresponsive to therapy
—Focal bronchiectasis has developed
—When significant morbidity is seen

- Prevention of recurrent or future atelectasis: directed toward underlying cause, when applicable

 ## Follow-Up

WHEN TO EXPECT IMPROVEMENT

- 1 to 3 months in typical, uncomplicated cases

 ## Common Questions and Answers

Q: When is the optimal time for bronchoscopy?
A: There are no established criteria for when a bronchoscopy should be performed. A bronchoscopy should be done early in the course of illness when there is a high suspicion of a foreign body, significant respiratory distress is present, or if the atelectasis is extensive and conservative treatment is ineffective.

ICD-9-CM 518.0

BIBLIOGRAPHY

Birnkrant DJ, et al. Management of the respiratory complications of neuromuscular diseases in the pediatric intensive care unit. *J Child Neurol* 1999;14(3):139–143.

Greene R. Acute lobar collapse: adults and infants differ in important ways. *Crit Care Med* 1999;27(8):1677–1679.

Karlson KH. *Pediatric Respiratory Disease: Diagnosis and Treatment.* Philadelphia: WB Saunders, 1993:436–440.

Oermann CM, Moore RH. Foolers: things that look like pneumonia in children. *Semin Respir Infect* 1996;11:204–213.

Redding GJ. Atelectasis in childhood. *Pediatr Clin North Am* 1984;31:891–905.

Slattery DM, Waltz DA, Denham B, et al. Bronchoscopically administered recombinant human dnase for lobar atelectasis in cystic fibrosis. *Pediatr Pulmonol* 2001;31:383–388.

Woodring JH, Reed JC. Types and mechanisms of pulmonary atelectasis. *Thorac Imaging* 1996;11:92–108.

Author: Richard M. Kravitz

Atopic Dermatitis

 ## Database

DEFINITION

Atopic dermatitis or eczema is a chronic, recurrent, pruritic skin eruption seen in individuals with associated personal or family history of atopy—asthma, allergies, hay fever, or rhinitis. The disease is characterized by intermittent acute flares. It most commonly begins in infancy or early childhood.

CAUSES

- Etiology of atopic dermatitis is multifactorial, with genetic, environmental, physiologic, and immunologic factors.
- Decreased resistance to sensitization and increased viral and dermatophyte infections seen in these patients suggest decreased cell-mediated immunity.
- Patients often have elevated IgE levels and decreased chemotaxis of neutrophils.
- Up to 70% of patients have a family history, but the mode of inheritance is not well defined.

PATHOLOGY

- Histologic findings are dependent on the stage of atopic dermatitis—acute or chronic.
- Lymphocytes can be seen infiltrating the epidermis.
- The acute form shows spongiosis and intercellular edema that can lead to vesicle formation.
- The chronic form is characterized by epidermal psoriasiform hyperplasia and hyperkeratosis.

GENETICS

- There is a genetic trait seen in atopic dermatitis, with 30% to 70% of family members having atopy—allergies, asthma, eczema, or hay fever.
- The exact mode of inheritance is not well defined and appears to be multifactorial.

EPIDEMIOLOGY

- Atopic dermatitis is a common disease, occurring in up to 18% of children.
- Approximately 60% of patients with atopic dermatitis will develop it in the first year of life, and 30% between the ages of 1 and 5 years.
- A family history of atopy—allergies, asthma, eczema, or hay fever—is present in 30% to 70% of patients.
- Atopic dermatitis is usually worse in the winter.

COMPLICATIONS

- Decreased cell-mediated immunity and decreased chemotaxis can result in increased infection—viral, dermatophyte, and bacterial. Patients with atopic dermatitis have a high density of *Staphylococcus aureus* on their skin, and given the fissures and open excoriations, there is a risk of superinfection of these lesions.
- The decreased integrity of the skin can result in widely spread cutaneous infections such as herpes simplex infection, known as Kaposi varicelliform eruption or eczema herpeticum. Similar problems can also be seen with coxsackievirus or molluscum contagiosum and used to occur with vaccinia.
- Cataracts can be found in patients with atopic dermatitis.
- Overuse of potent topical steroids can result in hypopigmentation, telangiectasias, atrophy, and striae, as well as excess systemic absorption leading to hypothalamic-pituitary axis suppression and growth retardation.
- Early growth delay is not uncommon among children with atopic dermatitis, although later catch-up growth is generally seen. This may be related to various mechanisms including impaired growth hormone release. This growth delay can occur independent of topical steroid exposure.

 ## Differential Diagnosis

Diagnostic criteria have been established for atopic dermatitis. The differential diagnosis of atopic dermatitis includes:

- Severe seborrheic dermatitis
- Contact dermatitis
- Allergic or irritant, psoriasis
- Wiskott-Aldrich syndrome
- Histiocytosis X
- Acrodermatitis enteropathica
- Scabies
- Xerosis
- Hyper-IgE syndrome
- Metabolic deficiencies

—Carboxylase
—Prolidase deficiencies

 ## Data Gathering

HISTORY

- Age of onset
- Location
- Prior treatment
- Bathing habits
- Family history of atopy—allergies
- Asthma
- Eczema
- Hay fever

 ## Physical Examination

- Acute flares reveal weeping and crusted erythema.
- Chronic disease is characterized by hyperpigmentation or hypopigmentation, lichenification, and scaling.
- The distribution of the disease is dependent on age.

—During infancy to approximately 2 years of age, the disease is widespread and includes cheeks, forehead, scalp, and extensor surfaces.
—In children from approximately 3 to 11 years, the disease involves the more characteristic flexural sites with lichenification.
—The hands and face can also be involved.
—From adolescence to adulthood, the flexures, neck, hands, and feet are frequently involved, with the face and neck flaring occasionally.

- When the disease is severe, it can present as exfoliative erythroderma with diffuse scaling and erythema.
- Other associated findings include geographic tongue, Dennie-Morgan folds (infraorbital folds), pityriasis alba, (dry white patches), hyperlinear palms, facial pallor, infraorbital darkening, follicular accentuation, keratosis pilaris (dry, rough hair follicles on extensor surfaces of upper arms and thighs), and ichthyosis.

Special Questions

Excessive dryness exacerbates this disease; therefore, inquiry about bathing habits, frequency, and emollients is helpful.

Laboratory Aids

- No tests are diagnostic of atopic dermatitis.
- Biopsy can be helpful to rule out papulosquamous disease, such as psoriasis.
- IgE levels are often elevated. Cultures can help identify superinfection during acute flares and viral cultures, and Tzanck smear can identify complications of eczema herpeticum.
- Patch testing can help differentiate atopic dermatitis from contact dermatitis.

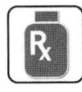

Therapy

- There is no cure for atopic dermatitis.
- Parents must understand that this is a chronic disease with intermittent flares and that control is the aim of treatment.
- Good skin care is critical to maintenance and includes use of mild soaps, frequent use of emollients, and avoidance of excessive bathing.
- Avoidance of irritants from the environment, such as wool sweaters or blankets, is recommended. Protective clothing at night to avoid scratching while sleeping is also helpful, as is trimming the nails.
- Antihistamines such as hydroxyzine or diphenhydramine may help to decrease itching.
- Topical steroids control inflammation and mid- to high-potency steroids can be used during acute flares, with tapering of steroids to milder potency when control is achieved. Once cleared, topical steroids can be held and substituted with emollients. Long-term use of steroids can lead to atrophy, telangiectasias, tachyphylaxis, and occasionally, stunting of growth.
- Oral antibiotics are indicated with superinfection of lesions, severe flares, or recalcitrant disease.
- Tacrolimus ointment and pimecrolimus cream are topical therapies recently approved for use in children 2 years of age and older. These are topical immunosuppressive calcineurin inhibitors that act to suppress T-cell function. Since these are not steroids, they are not atrophogenic and do not appear to alter hypothalamic-pituitary axis function. They may be especially useful for facial dermatitis where steroids are known to pose risks.

However, little is known regarding their long-term effects in children. Children who receive this medication should receive instructions for diligent sun protection and sunscreen use to minimize potentiation of sun damage. At the time of this publication, the US Food and Drug Administration (FDA) has announced a Public Health Advisory regarding the potential association of topical calcineurin inhibitors and lymphoma. This concern is based on animal data (mouse and monkey models) that very high doses (26–47x the maximum recommended human doses) used topically and systemically show a dose-dependent risk of lymphoma and skin cancer. In randomized controlled trials involving 38000 patients and postmarketing surveillance in 7 million patients, there is no evidence to suggest an increased risk for lymphoma or skin cancer at this time. Emollients, atopic skin care, and topical steroids are still considered first-line agents for the treatment of atopic dermatitis. Therefore, when calcineurin inhibitors are used, they may still be considered useful secondary options and used as short-term, intermittent therapies.
- The food and drug administration has required black boxwarnings and additional patient educational information regarding the possibility of increased lymphoma risks. This is based on evidence that systemic administration of these drugs in animals has been associated with malignancy. However, at this time, no evidence exists to suggest an increased risk for other cancers when using these agents, topically.
- However, at this time, no evidence in human exists to suggest an increased risk for lymphoma and other cancers when using these agent topically.
- Antivirals are needed for cases of eczema herpeticum. During acute flares with oozing and crusting and when there is superinfection with bacteria or herpes simplex virus, compresses can be helpful.
- Systemic steroids are generally not used because of the chronicity of atopic dermatitis, and are reserved for when control of the eruption is very difficult, and then use should be of short duration.
- Phototherapy with ultraviolet B can be used in patients with extensive disease resistant to other therapy.

Follow-Up

It should be emphasized to the parents that atopic dermatitis is a chronic disease and that good skin care is necessary to control disease activity. Up to 40%–50% of children will outgrow their atopic dermatitis after the age of 5 years.

Common Questions and Answers

Q: Will the child outgrow this?
A: Up to 40%–50% of children will outgrow their atopic dermatitis after the age of 5 years. In some patients, however, the disease will persist to variable extents throughout adulthood.

Q: When atopic dermatitis is controlled, is any treatment necessary?
A: Excessive dryness can exacerbate or flare disease; therefore, less use of soaps and frequent use of emollients are recommended.

Q: Do food hypersensitivities play a role in atopic dermatitis?
A: This is a debated issue. In general, the majority of patients are probably not adversely affected by foods. However, some individuals, particularly those unresponsive to routine therapy, may benefit from screening for food hypersensitivity and a trial of avoidance to any foods that test positive. The most common foods associated with exacerbation when an association can be made are eggs, milk, wheat, soy, peanuts, and fish.

ICD-9-CM 691.8

BIBLIOGRAPHY

Boguniewicz M. Advances in the understanding and treatment of atopic dermatitis. *Curr Opin Pediatr* 1997;9(6):577–581.

Burks AW, James JM, Hiegel A, et al. Atopic dermatitis and food hypersensitivity reactions. *J Pediatr* 1998;132(1):132–136.

Eichenfield LF, et al. Consensus conference on pediatric atopic dermatitis. *J Am Acad Dermatol* 2003;49(6):1088–1095.

Fitzpatrick TB, Eisen AZ, Wolfe K, et al. *Dermatology in General Medicine*. 4th Ed. New York: McGraw-Hill, 1993:1543–1564.

Hill DJ, Hosking CS. Emerging disease profiles in infants and young children with food allergy. *Pediatr Allergy Immunol* 1997;8(10 Suppl):21–26.

Oakes RC, Cox AD, Burgdorf WH. Atopic dermatitis: a review of diagnosis, pathogenesis, and management. *Clin Pediatr* 1983;22(7):467–475.

Stone KD. Atopic diseases of childhood. *Curr Opin Pediatr* 2003;15(5):495–511.

Author: Albert C. Yan

Atrial Septal Defect

 Database

DEFINITION

An opening in the atrial septum, other than a patent foramen ovale (PFO).

- Four major types of atrial septal defects (ASDs):

—Secundum ASD
—Primum ASD
—Sinus venosus ASD.
—Coronary sinus ASD

- A PFO usually does not cause a significant intracardiac shunt. A probe patent PFO can be found in up to 15% to 25% of normal hearts at pathologic examination.
- Secundum defects make up 60% to 70% of all ASDs; usually there is a shunt from the left atrium to the right atrium.
- Primum defects occur in about 30% of all ASDs. They are usually associated with a cleft mitral valve. This defect is the result of an abnormality of the endocardial cushions, and therefore is also referred to as an incomplete AV canal defect.
- Sinus venosus defects can be of the superior or inferior venal caval type and occur in about 5% to 10% of all ASDs. In ASDs of the superior venal caval type, the right pulmonary veins (usually right upper lobe) may drain anomalously to the superior vena cava or right atrium.
- Coronary sinus ASDs are rare and occur in <1% of all ASDs. They are often associated with absence of the coronary sinus and a persistent left SVC that joins the roof of the left atrium (also known as an "unroofed coronary sinus").

PREVALENCE

The incidence of ASD is difficult to determine. It occurs in 6%–10% of all cardiac anomalies encountered and is seen more frequently in females than males (2:1).

ASSOCIATED LESIONS

An ASD may be associated with partial or total anomalous pulmonary venous drainage, mitral valve anomalies, transposition of the great arteries or tricuspid atresia. Although usually occurring spontaneous, ASDs may occur as part of a syndrome (Holt-Oram [autosomal dominant]).

PATHOPHYSIOLOGY

A left-to-right shunt occurs through the ASD. For large defects this results in right atrial and right ventricular (RV) volume overload. There is usually increased pulmonary blood flow. The left-to-right shunt generally increases with time as pulmonary resistance drops and RV compliance normalizes. Moderate and large defects are associated with a Qp/Qs ratio of more than 2:1. The direction of atrial shunting is determined by the relative compliance of the RV and LV.

PROGNOSIS

- The prognosis of small ASDs seems excellent without specific therapy.
- Spontaneous closure of some small secundum ASDs can occur in up to 80% of infants in the first year of life. Isolated secundum ASDs of moderate and large size do not typically cause symptoms in most infants and children.
- Pulmonary hypertension is rare in childhood.
- Atrial flutter and fibrillation present in up to 13% of unoperated patients over 40 years of age.
- Bacterial endocarditis is rare in children with isolated ASD.
- Paradoxical emboli may occur, and should be considered in patients with cerebral or systemic emboli.

 Differential Diagnosis

- Ventricular septal defect
- Patent ductus arteriosus
- AV canal defect
- Valvar pulmonary stenosis

 Data Gathering

HISTORY

- Most infants are asymptomatic.
- Older children with moderate left-to-right shunts are often asymptomatic, but may have mild fatigue or dyspnea especially with exercise.
- Children with large left-to-right shunts may complain of fatigue and dyspnea, which may become noticeable when the child gets older.
- Growth failure is uncommon. Older patients with large atrial shunts may develop atrial arrhythmias.

 Physical Examination

- Inspection and palpation of the precordium are usually normal although older children with a large ASD may have a hyperdynamic precordium, RV heave and precordial bulge.
- Auscultation reveals three important features:

—Wide and "fixed" splitting of S2; splitting of S2 (A2 and P2 components) is caused by delay in emptying of a volume loaded right ventricle.
—A systolic ejection murmur at the upper left sternal border; murmur is caused by increase in blood flow across a normal pulmonary valve. It may be differentiated from the murmur of pulmonary stenosis because there is no click.
—A diastolic murmur at the lower sternal border, indicating a Qp/Qs ratio of at least 2:1. This murmur is caused by increased flow across the tricuspid valve.

 Laboratory Aids

ECG

Usually normal sinus rhythm with an rSR' (incomplete right bundle branch block pattern) in lead V1, indicating RV volume overload. First-degree AV block may be present. For larger shunts ECG may have evidence of right atrial enlargement. A late finding suggestive of pulmonary hypertension is right ventricular hypertrophy.

CXR

Cardiomegaly, increased pulmonary vascular markings, and a dilated pulmonary trunk are seen in patients with significant left-to-right shunts.

ECHO

A two-dimensional echo study is diagnostic; it reveals the location, size, and associated defect, if any. It may demonstrate dilated right-heart structures. Color Doppler generally permits visualization of the direction of shunt flow. Older children and adolescents may require transesophageal echo to best define the ASD.

CARDIAC CATHETERIZATION

Generally this procedure is unnecessary for diagnostic purposes. It is indicated when pulmonary vascular disease is suspected (determination of pulmonary vascular resistance) or for associated cardiac defects.

Atrial Septal Defect

 Therapy

Infants with congestive heart failure should be treated with digoxin and diuretics. Elective surgical repair is indicated for ASDs associated with large left-to-right shunts, cardiomegaly, or symptoms. The timing of the repair is usually deferred until 3 to 5 years of age. The mortality of surgical repair for an uncomplicated ASD approaches 0%. For most secundum ASDs, device closure of the defect can be done in the cardiac catheterization laboratory. Prevention of paradoxical emboli and cerebrovascular accidents are another possible indication for closure of ASDs or PFOs. Irreversible pulmonary hypertension from long-term left to right shunt usually does not occur until adolescence or young adulthood. Sinus venosus and ostium primum defects require elective surgery regardless of the defect size.

 Follow-Up

- Children with typical auscultation and ECG findings should undergo an echocardiographic evaluation to determine the location and size of the ASD.
- Children with ASDs should have regular follow-up to assess for signs of congestive heart failure or RV volume overload. Restriction on activity is unnecessary. SBE prophylaxis is not indicated in isolated secundum ASDs. Residual ASD after surgery is rare.
- SBE prophylaxis is indicated for the first 6 months (assuming no residual defect) after closure of a secundum defect.
- Complications related to surgery include:

—Sinus node dysfunction
—Venous obstruction (facial or pulmonary edema) may occur after a sinus venosus ASD repair.
—Postpericardiotomy syndrome, which manifests with nausea, vomiting, abdominal pain or fever, may occur a few weeks after surgical repair. Although a friction rub may not be present, CXR may demonstrate cardiomegaly, and echo may reveal a pericardial effusion.

 Common Questions and Answers

Q: When should a moderate secundum ASD be closed?
A: This can generally be electively performed in children prior to their starting grade school.

Q: What is the significance of a patient having gastrointestinal complaints (nausea and vomiting) 2–3 weeks after surgical closure of an ASD?
A: This may represent a pericardial effusion (postpericardiotomy syndrome).

ICD-9-CM 745.61

BIBLIOGRAPHY

Chang AC, Hanley FL, Wernovsky G, et al. *Pediatric Cardiac Intensive Care.* Baltimore: Williams & Wilkins 1998:207–211.

Garson A, Bricker J, McNamara D. *The Science and Practice of Pediatric Cardiology.* Philadelphia: Lea & Febiger 1990:1023–1036.

Horton SC, Bunch TJ. Patent foramen ovale and stroke. *Clin Proc* 2004;79(1):79–88.

Meijboom F, et al. The role of the atria in congenital heart disease. *Cardiol Clin* 2002;20(3):351–366.

Ohye RG, Bove EL. Advances in congenital heart surgery. *Curr Opin in Pediatr* 2001; 13(5):473–481.

Radzik D, Davignon A, van Doesburg K, et al. Predictive factors for spontaneous closure of atrial septal defect diagnosed in the first 3 months of life. *J Am Coll Cardiol* 1993;22: 851–853.

Rocchini AP. Pediatric cardiac catheterization. *Curr Opin in Cardiol* 2002;17(3):283–288.

Zanchetta M, et al. Role of intracardiac echocardiography in atrial septal abnormalities. *J Intervent Cardiol* 2003; 16(1):63–77.

Authors: Jonathan Fleenor
Song-Gui Yang, 2nd edition

Attention-Deficit/Hyperactivity Disorder

 Database

DEFINITION

Attention-deficit hyperactivity disorder (ADHD) is a chronic neurobehavioral disorder, characterized by an inability to control the levels of impulsivity, attention, or activity to the point of disrupting his/her ability to function in an academic, social and/or home setting. Diagnostic types and criteria:

- ADHD, Combined type—characterized by difficulties in inattention and hyperactivity or impulsivity
- ADHD, Predominantly inattentive type—characterized by inability to attend to a task for any significant period of time; daydreaming.
- ADHD, Predominantly hyperactive, impulsive type—characterized by high level of activity (above normal for age), trouble sitting still, impulsive behaviors (fights, dangerous choices), or difficulty following rules

DSM IV criteria:

- At least six of nine behaviors in inattention and/or hyperactivity/impulsivity domains.
- Presence in two or more settings (home, school, afterschool activities) for at least 6 months.
- Presence prior to age 7 years.
- Significant impairment in learning, occupational and/or social functioning.

ASSOCIATED CONDITIONS

- Motor coordination disorders, social skills deficits, enuresis and encopresis, oppositional defiant disorder (ODD, 35%), conduct disorder (CD, 26%), anxiety (26%), depression (18%), learning disabilities (LD, 12% to 60%)

COMPLICATIONS

- Lower educational attainment, higher rates of school failure, lower job ratings by employers, poor social skills, high rates of accidental injuries (motor vehicle accidents, falls), higher rates of sexual activity and tobacco use, conflicting evidence about rates of drug and alcohol use

PROGNOSIS

- 70% of children with ADHD will have symptoms as adults.
- 22% to 85% will continue to meet diagnostic criteria at adolescence.
- 4% to 50% of adults will still meet diagnostic criteria.
- Increased risk of antisocial personality disorder in adulthood.

 Differential Diagnosis

ENVIRONMENTAL

- Lead poisoning
- Iron-deficiency anemia
- Child abuse/neglect

- Parental psychopathology
- Inappropriate educational setting

DEVELOPMENTAL

- Normal behavior
- Cognitive impairment
- Giftedness
- Learning disability
- Autistic spectrum disorders
- Language or speech disorders

CONGENITAL

- Fragile X syndrome
- Fetal alcohol syndrome or effects

NEUROLOGIC

- Sensory impairment
- Seizure disorder

ENDOCRINE

- Thyroid disorders

TOXINS

- Substance abuse

MISCELLANEOUS

- Medication side effect
- Malnutrition
- Sleep apnea

PSYCHIATRIC

- Mood disorders
- Anxiety disorder
- Oppositional defiant disorder
- Posttraumatic stress disorder
- Adjustment disorder

 Data Gathering

HISTORY

- Why the parent is concerned, and what behaviors are the most difficult for the child and family.
- Ask the child's opinions about his/her own attention or activity level.

Question: Who initiated the evaluation?
Significance: There can be differences in the history if a teacher recommended the evaluation, but the family is reluctant to believe the teacher's report. Parents may minimize home behaviors in these settings.

Question: What activities hold the child's attention?
Significance: Most children, even those with ADHD, will be able to attend to things they enjoy, such as TV or video games.

Question: What activities do not hold the child's attention?
Significance: If there is only one subject area, for example, it could be that the work is at an inappropriate level, either too low or high. This could be a sign of either giftedness or a learning disability, respectively.

Question: Does the child have difficulty playing with other children?
Significance: Many children who are impulsive will be turned away by other children for not being able to follow the rules or for being too aggressive. A child, who has trouble academically, may be fine socially and vice-versa.

 Physical Examination

- Many children with developmental issues will have "soft" neurologic signs. These are often overflow movements to help them attend to or complete a task that is particularly challenging for them. These may include tongue twitching during sustained postures or opposite limb movement during rapid single limb tasks.

 Laboratory Aids

- Laboratory tests are rarely necessary when evaluating a child for ADHD; although they should be considered when clinically indicated. For example, thyroid function tests should be ordered when considering the diagnosis of thyroid dysfunction.
- The AAP practice guidelines recommend the usage of specific ADHD rating scales (such as the Vanderbilt assessment, Connor's Rating Scales or the Child Behavior Checklist) in various settings, including but not limited to home and school. Use of nonspecific scales is less useful in the diagnosis of ADHD.

Vanderbilt Assessment

- Standardized assessment for ADHD with screening for ODD, CD, depression and anxiety (uses DSM criteria for all except anxiety and depression)
- Has performance assessment section for parents and teachers
- Follow-up assessment form also includes section to provide more objective score on side effects
- Scale used in the AAP ADHD Tool Kit

Connor Rating Scale

- ADHD-specific rating scale
- Uses DSM criteria
- No screening of comorbid conditions, performance rating or side effect rating

Achenbach Child Behavior Checklist (CBCL)

- Assesses behavior of child, but does not use DSM criteria for ADHD
- Provides good screening for comorbid conditions
- Very comprehensive, but can be long for some families

Psychoeducational assessment

- IQ testing—intelligence testing can help in the diagnosis of LD and mental retardation (MR) as well as give some awareness of inattention or impulsivity in testing situations
- Achievement testing—important to make an accurate diagnosis of LD, but also helps in assessment of attention and activity level during testing

- Mental status and cognitive evaluations should be considered when applicable to help rule out other developmental and emotional conditions.
- Continuous performance tasks are not sensitive in diagnosing ADHD

All children being evaluated for ADHD should have their hearing and vision evaluated to ensure their inattention is not related to a hearing or vision problem.

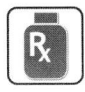 ## Therapy

- Help family understand the chronicity of ADHD
- Behavioral therapy: evidence for behavioral therapy alone is not very good, but in combination with stimulants there is evidence for its utility. Behavioral therapy is intended to help the family and school focus on positive behaviors
- Cognitive or play therapy: To address associated conditions such as depression or anxiety
- Group therapy: Can help with social skills and anger management skills.
- Support groups for parents and children can help decrease guilt and help in problem solving for difficult behaviors.
- Academic interventions can be a very important part of the treatment plan for a child with ADHD. All children with ADHD should have a 504 plan (also, known as an Individualized Education Plan or IEP), a federally mandated plan, which details educational accommodations for children who have medical conditions impacting their ability to perform in school
- 60% of patients with ADHD try complementary and alternative medicine—changes in diet, biofeedback, herbal supplements, and vision training often—without their provider's knowledge. There are no trials to support the effectiveness of these treatments

DRUGS

Stimulants—weight-based dosing is not effective because of differences in metabolism of these medications. Side effects are similar for all medications in this class. However, if a child has a side effect to one of the stimulants, the child will not necessarily have the same side effect with other stimulants. Side effects include: appetite suppression, weight loss, headache, stomach ache, behavioral rebound, and less commonly moodiness and tics.

Methylphenidate

- Ritalin and Methylin—short-acting (3 to 5 hours); usually requires multiple doses during the day.
- Ritalin SR, Metadate ER, Methylin ER—intermediate-acting (5 to 8 hours); cannot be chewed or cut in half, and the capsule must not be opened
- Ritalin LA, Metadate CD, and Concerta—long-acting (8 to 12 hours); can be given once a day; some children will need

a second dose or a dose of a short-acting stimulant in the afternoon; Metadate CD capsule can be opened and mixed with food.

Dextroamphetamine

Dexedrine—short-acting (4 to 6 hours); usually requires multiple doses a day; elixir no longer available.
Dexedrine spansules—long-acting (6 to 10 hours); can be mixed with food; some children will require a second dose of either a short or long-acting stimulant.

Mixed Amphetamine Salt

- Adderall (6 to 8 hours)—cannot break tablet; may require second dose of shorter acting stimulant or other medication.
- Adderall XR (8 to 12 hours)—can open capsule and mix with food; may require second dose of shorter-acting stimulant.

Nonstimulants (Second-Line Medications)

- Tricyclics—inhibit reuptake of norepinephrine and serotonin; onset of action for maximal response 4 to 6 weeks; need baseline ECG and repeat when changing doses and when at optimal dose to rule out arrhythmias. Must titrate off medication. Side effects: arrhythmia, lower seizure threshold, anticholinergic effects (dry mouth, constipation)
- Bupropion—blocks reuptake of norepinephrine and dopamine; can take 4 weeks to see full effects of medication; provides 24-hour coverage; more appropriate for adolescents; not approved for children less than 18 years old. Side effects: lowers seizure threshold; motor tics.
- Atomoxetine (Strattera)—selective norepinephrine reuptake inhibitor. Similar side effect profile to stimulants; 24-hour coverage; capsule must be swallowed. Not a controlled substance, so refills can be given, and can be called in to a pharmacy. Not approved for children less than 6 years old and often not covered by insurance unless a patient has failed stimulant medications first.
- Clonidine or Guanfacine—alpha-2 adrenergic agonists. Side effects: sedating (clonidine more than guanfacine), hypotension, depression; takes several weeks to see effect; usually dosed twice a day after titrating up to an optimal dose; used in children with tics without any increase in morbidity.

 ## Follow-Up

- Help family and school set target goals.
- Scales similar to those used for the initial assessment can be helpful for follow-up.
- During medication initiation or while changing medications, need to have frequent contact with families and school. This will facilitate titration to the appropriate dose.
- During the maintenance period, children should be seen 2–4 times per year.
- Children in families who decide not to use medications should be seen 2–4 times per year to follow behavior and help family monitor symptoms.

PITFALLS

- Incomplete evaluation missing learning disabilities, bipolar disorder
- Poor response to medication due to inadequate dosing; inadequate time to response (particularly for secondary medications); individual intolerance for medications

Common Questions and Answers

Q: Will my child outgrow this?
A: An estimated 30% to 70% of children with ADHD will continue to have symptoms as adults. The strategies used during childhood should work toward improving the child's awareness of how to maximize their strengths and utilize them to overcome their weaknesses.

Q: Will my child become addicted to the medications?
A: No, but as the child grows, he/she may need higher doses to achieve the same effect. Children with ADHD who are appropriately treated with stimulants are less likely to go on to become addicted to alcohol and other drugs than those who are not treated.
Q: Should my child take the ADHD medication every day?
A: Whether or not a child takes medication daily (i.e., including weekends and summer breaks) depends on the extent of symptoms and the settings where symptoms occur. Some children respond well to individualized attention at home and do not need to take medications on the weekends. Other children with ADHD have difficulty with socialization and benefit from being on medications year-round. Children should be evaluated routinely to make sure they are appropriately being medicated.

Q: When should I send the child to see a specialist?
A: The AAP clinical guidelines were developed to help general pediatricians manage children with ADHD. Children with other coexisting conditions are children that may not respond as well to stimulant medications alone and may benefit from seeing a specialist (developmental-behavioral pediatrician, psychiatrist, or neurologist). In addition, children who do not respond to stimulant medications or have significant side effects should be considered for referral to a specialist.

ICD-9-CM: 314.0

BIBLIOGRAPHY

Reiff MI, Stein MT. Attention-deficit/hyperactivity disorder evaluation and diagnosis: a practical approach in office practice. *Pediatr Clin North Am* 2003; 50(5):1019–1048.

Wender EH. Managing stimulant medication for attention-deficit/hyperactivity disorder. *Pediatr Rev* 2001;22:183–189.

Author: Nathaniel S. Beers

Atypical Mycobacterial Infections

 Database

DEFINITION

Atypical mycobacterial (ATM) infection refers to disease caused by Mycobacterium other than tuberculosis, bovis, and leprae, and usually involves *Mycobacterium avium-intracellulare, M. scrofulaceum, M. kansasii, M. fortuitum,* and *M. chelonae.* These diseases are also referred to as nontuberculous mycobacterial infections, environmental mycobacterial infections, and mycobacteria other than tuberculosis (MOTT) infections.

CAUSES

• The most common associated illness is unilateral chronic cervical adenopathy/adenitis in preschool-aged children.
• In adults, ATM infection may cause a chronic single pulmonary nodule or more extensive chronic lung disease.
• In children and adults infected with HIV, disseminated disease is common, yet it is not common in other acquired or congenital immunodeficiencies that affect T-cell function.
• Rarely, it may cause otitis/mastoiditis in immunocompetent children.
• Chronic skin, bone, or soft tissue infections may develop after trauma/surgery, usually with *M. chelonei* or *M. fortuitum* as the etiologic agents.
• Infections of indwelling central venous catheters appear to be on the increase.

—Colonization with these mycobacterium is common among older patients with cystic fibrosis. Whether these organisms play a pathogenic role in ongoing lung damage in this population is an area of intense study.

PATHOPHYSIOLOGY

• Organisms are ubiquitous in the environment: soil, fresh water, ocean water, home and hospital water, dust, and food (eggs, dairy products, meat).
• It is spread by aerosol inhalation or ingestion of contaminated food, dust, or water.
• Person-to-person spread has never been documented and is not a concern.

EPIDEMIOLOGY

• Eighty percent to 90% of cases of adenitis caused by ATM infection occur in preschool-aged children (ages 1 to 5 years).
• Early in the HIV epidemic, the incidence rate of disseminated disease in HIV-infected adults was approximately 40%; in HIV-infected children, 10% to 20%. This rate has decreased markedly in recent years through the routine use of prophylaxis and because of the improved immunologic function in HIV-infected individuals on newer antiretroviral agents.

COMPLICATIONS

• Chronic draining of infected cervical nodes
• Rarely, pulmonary disease or dissemination
• Chronic skin/bone infections
• Disseminated disease

PROGNOSIS

• For localized adenopathy: excellent
• For disseminated disease, generally treatable in the rare immunocompetent individual
• In patients with AIDS, treatable in terms of symptom relief, but requires lifelong therapy

 Differential Diagnosis

• For unilateral adenopathy/adenitis:

—Viral/bacterial adenitis-affected nodes are tender, warm, and erythematous; usually associated with upper respiratory symptoms and/or fever.
—Cat-scratch disease (contact with cat, usually kitten). Frequently, child will have scratch/puncture mark on arm. There are rarely any systemic signs/symptoms.

• Neoplastic disease

 Data Gathering

HISTORY

• Region of residence
• Recent travel
• Length of time of adenopathy, associated systemic symptoms
• Contact with cats (for differential of cat-scratch disease or toxoplasmosis)
• Systemic symptoms, such as fever and weight loss, make neoplastic disease more likely.
• Chronic cough would suggest *M. tuberculosis.*
• Recent upper respiratory symptoms/fever suggest viral or bacterial cause.

Physical Examination

- Most common: single or regional cervical adenopathy, 90% of the time, is unilateral, firm, not fixed, and not especially tender nor warm; occasionally, there is spontaneous drainage.
- Generalized adenopathy makes ATM disease unlikely.
- Systemic signs of infection are absent.
- Hepatosplenomegaly indicates other diagnosis, especially neoplastic disease or HIV-related illness.
- Normal nutritional status

 ## Laboratory Aids

- Specific PPD tests are not readily available at this time. Many children with ATM adenitis will have 5- to 10-mm reactions to standard PPD.
- Definitive diagnosis is made by isolation and identification of organism. The most frequently identified strains are: *M. avium-intracellulare*, *M. kansasii*, *M. chelonei*, *M. fortuitum*, and *M. scrofulaceum*.
- Normal chest radiograph
- In disseminated disease, cultures are positive from blood and bone marrow aspirates.

—Diagnosis using PCR assays under development. May be helpful on staining of biopsied material.

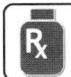 ## Therapy

- Complete surgical excision for isolated adenopathy secondary to ATM; chemotherapy unnecessary in most cases.
- For disseminated or pulmonary disease, or when complete surgical excision of an infected node is not possible, three- or four-drug treatment regimens based on sensitivity. Combinations generally include several of the following antibiotics: rifabutin, clarithromycin or azithromycin, ethambutol, ciprofloxacin, and amikacin. Newer antibiotics, such as mefloquine and moxifloxacin, may also have significant activity against atypical mycobacterial strains.

PREVENTION

For HIV-infected children with severe immunodeficiency, prophylaxis with daily clarithromycin or rifabutin, or once-weekly azithromycin, decreases the risk of development of disseminated disease.

 ## Follow-Up

Routine follow-up should be done for 1 year after excision to monitor for possible local/contralateral recurrence.

PITFALLS

Use of incision and drainage/aspiration for treatment of adenitis, which can lead to chronically draining node. Aspiration may be needed to make the original diagnosis, but total excision results in almost 100% cure rates.

 ## Common Questions and Answers

Q: Should all cases of cervical adenitis be tested for ATM?
A: The typical case of cervical adenitis, presenting with the usual prodrome, responds rapidly to appropriate oral or parenteral antibiotics, which would not be the case if ATM were the culprit. Certainly, a PPD test should be done on all children with cervical adenitis. If the node is aspirated, in addition to routine bacterial cultures, fluid should be sent for mycobacterial culture. Additionally, testing for cat-scratch disease should be part of the evaluation of all cases of cervical adenitis.

Q: Should patients with disease secondary to ATM undergo a chest radiograph?
A: Yes. Though uncommon, ATM-related pulmonary disease can be seen in children.

Q: If the node is excised, should oral therapy be instituted?
A: Most studies suggest that oral therapy is unnecessary following total excision.

ICD-9-CM 031.9

BIBLIOGRAPHY

Hazra R, Robsin CD, Perez-Atayde AR, et al. Lymphadenitis due to nontuberculous mycobacteria in children: presentation and response to therapy. *Clin Infect Dis* 1999;28:123–129.

McGarvey J, Bermudez LE. Pathogenesis of nontuberculous mycobacteria infections. *Clin Chest Med* 2002;23.

Olivier KN, Weber DJ, Wallace RJ Jr, et al. Nontuberculous Mycobacteria. I. Multicenter prevalence study in Cystic Fibrosis. *Am J Respir Crit Care Med* 2003;167:828–834.

Schaad UB, Votteler TP, McCracken GH, et al. Management of atypical mycobacterial lymphadenitis in childhood: a review based on 380 cases. *J Pediatr* 1979;95:356–360.

Starke Jr. Management of nontuberculous mycobacterial cervical adenitis. *Pediatr Infect Dis J* 2000;19:674–675.

Author: Richard M. Rutstein

Autism/Pervasive Developmental Disorder Spectrum

 Database

DEFINITION

Autism and pervasive developmental disorder (PDD) are neuropsychiatric syndromes characterized by:

- Delays/impairments in development of social, communication, play and behavioral skills
- Onset in first years of life
- Frequent association with mental retardation
- Increased risk of seizure disorder

Autism and PDD are a spectrum of related disorders including:

- Autistic Disorder—symptoms prior to age 3, impairments in: social relatedness, communication, play, restricted interests/activities
- PDD-NOS—subthreshold autism
- Asperger Syndrome—social deficits, restricted range of interests, relatively stronger language development, average to above average cognitive abilities
- Childhood disintegrative disorder—developmental deterioration after 24 months;
- Rett Syndrome—females, hand-washing/wringing movements, head growth deceleration before 48 months

EPIDEMIOLOGY

- Autistic disorder: prevalence—1–2 cases/1,000, 3–4:1, male:female ratio recent evidence prevalence may be increasing), females more likely to have more severe symptoms and be mentally retarded

—50% of cases exhibit severe to profound mental retardation
—30% of cases have mild to moderate mental retardation
—20% of cases have normal cognitive abilities

- PDD-NOS: Prevalence—5 cases/1,000
- Asperger syndrome: Prevalence—2–4 cases/1,000, more common in boys
- Rett disorder: Prevalence—0.83 cases/1,000 females
- Childhood disintegrative disorder: Prevalence—0.011 cases/1,000, occurs predominately in males, as of 1999, 106 cases reported.

ETIOLOGY

- No single cause of autism identified, syndrome likely has multiple etiologies; toxic factors are controversial, unimmune causes under research
- Twin genetic studies strongly implicate role of genetic factors
- Siblings of proband at higher risk
- Monozygotic twins have higher concordance rate than dizygotic twins
- Approximately 1/100 persons with autism exhibit fragile X anomaly
- Rate of autism in tuberous sclerosis elevated.

Disorders associated with PDD spectrum disorders:

- Prenatal: Toxemia, rubella, cytomegalovirus, toxoplasmosis
- Perinatal: Anoxia, trauma, hyperbilirubinemia
- Chromosomal: Angelman syndrome, ring chromosome 15, Prader-Willi syndrome, fragile X syndrome, trisomy 21, XYY syndrome, tuberous sclerosis
- Metabolic: Phenylketonuria, hyperthyroidism, histidinemia, lipidosis
- Congenital: Microcephaly, hydrocephalus, Dandy-Walker syndrome
- Acquired: Infantile spasms, meningitis, encephalitis

PRESENTING SIGNS/SYMPTOMS IN PDD SPECTRUM DISORDERS

- Delays/impairments in language development
- Rare cases present with "acquired epileptic aphasia" (paroxysmal EEG in sleep)
- Marked inability to initiate and sustain conversation (when speech is present)
- Cognitive delays
- Impairment in eye contact, facial expression, nonverbal social behaviors
- Lack of interest in or impairments in social interactions
- Impaired peer relationships
- Stereotypies (e.g., rocking, hand flapping)
- Restricted range of interests/activities
- Attachment to unusual objects, fascination with parts of objects
- Behavioral rigidity, distress with changes in routine
- Lack of spontaneous imaginary play appropriate to developmental level
- In Rett Disorder—scoliosis, breathing problems, seizures, motor problems

DIFFERENTIAL DIAGNOSIS IN PDD SPECTRUM DISORDERS

- Mental retardation—differs from PDD/autism in that communication, behavior, play, and social skills appropriate for developmental age.
- Deafness—delayed/absent oral language acquisition, behavioral difficulties/social skill deficits, if present, related to language delays
- Mixed receptive-expressive language disorder—language impairments not associated with qualitative deficits in social interactions or restrictive interests
- Selective mutism—developmentally appropriate communication in some social situations, no qualitative deficits in social interactions or restrictive interests

 Data Gathering

HISTORY

- Prenatal, neonatal, developmental, medical, family and social history essential
- Diagnosis based on significant impairments in: verbal/nonverbal communication, social skills, presence of restrictive/repetitive behaviors
- History of: absence of verbal or nonverbal communication joining parent and child's attention, stereotyped behavior, behavioral rigidity, tactile defensiveness, clumsiness, apraxia, epilepsy, poor appetite, narrow diet, and poor sleep frequently present.
- Essential to consider comorbidities of: attention problems, OCD traits, tics, anxiety, depression, epilepsy, mood instability, sleep problems, aggression, lack of fear, mistreatment of animals, and self-injury.

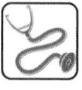 Physical Examination

- Evaluate for growth disturbance secondary to restrictive/obsessive eating
- Evaluate for self-injurious behavior
- Neurologic exam necessary to assess stereotypic behavior, involuntary movements, motor coordination abnormalities, mirror/overflow movements
- Ophthalmologic/audiologic evaluations to R/O visual or hearing deficits
- PE may suggest alternate (metabolic) disorders or underlying basis of autism

—Long, thin face, prominent ears—fragile X, (macroorchidism may not be present until after puberty)
—Pigmented lesions—neurocutaneous syndromes, hypopigmented macules/fibromas suggest tuberous sclerosis
—Microcephaly—TORCH infection, Angelman syndrome, Rett disorder
—Macrocephaly—neurocutaneous disorder, storage disease, hydrocephalus, or no identifiable cause
—Presence of spasticity, visual loss, ataxia—leukodystrophy

Autism/Pervasive Developmental Disorder Spectrum

 Laboratory Aids

- Neurodiagnostic tests not useful unless specific neurological disorders suspected
- Routine neuroimaging of limited diagnostic or practical value.

TESTS/SIGNIFICANCE

The following tests may be considered especially in children with significant mental retardation:

- EEG: 20% to 40% of autistic patients develop seizures
- Chromosome studies: Genetic counseling helpful
- Inborn error screen: Detects PKU, other amino acid disorders
- Head MRI/CT: Evaluation of structural CNS if focal neurological deficit, microcephaly/macrocephaly present
- TORCH titers: Evaluation of microcephaly
- Complete blood count: Evaluation of growth delay and/or pica
- Blood lead level: Rule out lead intoxication.
- Thyroid function tests: Rule out hyper/hypothyroidism.
- Audiogram/BAER: Recommended for children with speech and language delay

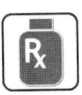 Therapy

MEDICAL MANAGEMENT

- Pharmacotherapy does not treat most core symptoms of autism
- Medication helps to treat comorbid symptoms and behaviors that interfere with a patient's ability to function at highest potential in educational and social activities
- Symptoms and medications to consider:

—Self-injurious behavior: Atypical (and typical) antipsychotics, Naltrexone
—Sleep disturbances: Melatonin, clonidine, Trazodone
—Seizures: Newer anticonvulsants, carbamazepine, phenytoin, valproate, barbiturates often worsen hyperactivity
—Hyperactivity/attention difficulties: Psychostimulants, Strattera, buproprion, venlafaxine, clonidine, guanfacine
—OCD symptoms/perseveration: SSRIs, Clomipramine
—Tic disorders: Guanfacine, clonidine, atypical/typical antipsychotics
—Depression: SSRIs, bupropion, Venlafaxine
—Anxiety: SSRIs, buspirone, venlafaxine, benzodiazepines (may increase disorganization)
—Aggression: Atypical antipsychotics, SSRIs, anticonvulsants

EDUCATIONAL, PSYCHOSOCIAL, AND MEDICAL MANAGEMENT

- Complete psychoeducational assessment and treatment plan for cognitive, developmental, adaptive, functional, communication, and social skills necessary

—Intensive educational/behavioral interventions should target acquisition of communicative, social, cognitive skills

- Early sustained structured behavioral intervention using applied behavior analysis (ABA) and behavior modification highly beneficial in many children
- Vocational training important for some adolescents and adults
- Consider social skills training for higher functioning patients
- Education and support for parents and siblings integral to treatment
- Psychotherapy not indicated to address core features of autism and PDD

PITFALLS

- Autism and the PDD spectrum disorders vary greatly in symptom presentation-discordancy among clinicians' diagnoses, and underdiagnoses and overdiagnoses of these disorders are common
- Symptom presentation differs at different stages of development
- Medication often not helpful; patients with PDD/autism often develop side effects
- Subclinical seizure types may be detected only on EEG

 Follow-Up

- Prognosis linked to cognitive ability & acquisition of social/communication skills
- If no language by 6 years, language development unlikely and outcome is poor
- Children with autism/PDD often require lifelong treatment and support

 Common Questions and Answers

Q: What are the chances of having a second child with autism?
A: In families with one child with autism the recurrence risk for subsequent children is 3% to 7%. This is in contrast to the risk in the general population, which is 0.1% to 0.2%.

Q: What is the value of brain imaging in autism?
A: MRI may help diagnose a heritable syndrome with genetic counseling implications (e.g., leukodystrophy, tuberous sclerosis), but is usually unhelpful in high-functioning cases.

ICD-9-CM 299

BIBLIOGRAPHY

Bryson SE, et al. Autism spectrum disorders: early detection, intervention, education and psychopharmacological management. *Can J Psychiatr* 2003;48(8):506–516.

Committee on Children with Disabilities: Technical Report: the pediatrician's role in the diagnosis and management of autistic spectrum disorder in children. *Pediatrics* 2001;107(5):E85.

University of North Carolina at Chapel Hill. Division TEACCH: Treatment and Education of Autistic and related Communication handicapped Children. www.teacch.com

Volkmar F, Cook EH Jr, Pomeroy J, et al. Practice parameters—autism and pervasive developmental disorders. *J Am Acad Child Adolesc Psych* 1999;38(12):32S–54S.

Walker DR, et al. Specifying PDD-NOS: a comparison of PDD-NOS, asperger syndrome and autism. *J Am Acad Child Adolesc Psych* 2004;43(2):172–180.

Author: Jeanne Greenblatt

Autoimmune Hemolytic Anemia

 ## Database

DEFINITION

Autoimmune hemolytic anemia (AIHA) is characterized by shortened red-cell survival that is caused by autoantibodies directed against red blood cells, with or without the participation of complement on the red-cell membrane.

CAUSES

- Idiopathic
- Passive transfer of maternal antibodies
- Secondary to an underlying disorder

—Infection: Viral [e.g., *Mycoplasma*, Epstein-Barr virus (EBV), cytomegalovirus (CMV), hepatitis, HIV] or bacterial (e.g., *Streptococcus*, typhoid fever, *Escherichia coli* septicemia)
—Drugs: Antimalarials, antipyretics, sulfonamides, penicillin, rifampin
—Hematologic disorders: Leukemia, lymphoma
—Immunopathic/autoimmune disorders: Lupus, mixed connective tissue disorders, Wiskott-Aldrich syndrome, ulcerative colitis, rheumatoid arthritis, scleroderma
—Tumors: Ovarian, carcinomas, thymomas, dermoid cysts

PATHOPHYSIOLOGY

- Warm autoantibodies

—Maximal activity of in vitro red-cell binding at 37°C
—IgG-class antibody sometimes with relative specificity for Rh erythrocyte antigens
—IgG-coated RBCs cleared—predominantly in the spleen by macrophages
—Complement not required for clearance, although complement fixation may contribute to clearance

- Cold autoantibodies (cold agglutinins)

—Maximal activity of in vitro red-cell binding at temperatures between 0°C and 30°C
—Almost always caused by IgM antibody with specificity for antigens of the i/I system on RBCs
—Anti-I antibodies characteristic of *Mycoplasma pneumoniae*-associated hemolysis
—Anti-i antibodies usually found in infectious mononucleosis
—IgM-coated RBCs are cleared primarily in the liver by hepatic macrophage C3b receptors.
—Hemolysis is complement-dependent.

- Paroxysmal cold hemoglobinuria (PCH)

—IgG autoantibody binds RBC at cooler areas of the body (i.e., extremities), causing irreversible binding of complement components (C3 and C4). When coated RBCs enter warmer areas of the body, IgG falls off and complement causes hemolysis (Donath-Landsteiner biphasic hemolysin).
—Unusual IgG antibody with anti-P specificity
—Most frequently found in children with viral infections (30%)

- Occurs at an incidence of about 1:50,000 to 80,000 persons per year
- Less common in children and adolescents than in adults
- No apparent racial or sexual preponderance (in childhood)
- Peak incidence in childhood is in first 4 years of life with warm AIHA.
- Mortality in pediatric series ranged from 9% to 19%.

COMPLICATIONS

Heart failure may be seen in severe anemia; requires aggressive supportive care. Morbidity is usually secondary to treatment (see Therapy section).

 ## Differential Diagnosis

- Defects intrinsic to RBC

—Membrane defects
—Enzyme defects
—Hemoglobin defects
—Congenital dyserythropoietic anemias
—Paroxysmal nocturnal hemoglobinuria

- Defects extrinsic to RBC

—Immune-mediated defects
—Isoimmune: Hemolytic disease of the newborn, blood-group incompatibility
—Autoimmune: See in Database section, Causes
—Drug-dependent red-cell antibodies
—Nonimmune mediated defects
—Idiopathic
—Secondary to an underlying disorder (i.e., hemolytic uremic syndrome [HUS], thrombotic thrombocytopenic purpura [TTP])
—Mechanical: march hemoglobinuria, heart valves

 ## Data Gathering

NATURAL HISTORY

- Acute disease

—Onset with rapid fall in hemoglobin level over hours to days
—Usual course: complete resolution of disease within 3 to 6 months
—Resolution more likely in children who present between 2 and 12 years of age

- Chronic disease

—Slower onset of anemia over weeks to months, with some having persistence of hemolysis or intermittent relapses
—More likely to be associated with underlying disorder
—More common in adults and children <2 years or >12 years of age

HISTORY

- Pallor
- Jaundice
- Dark urine
- Fever
- Weakness
- Dizziness
- Syncope
- Exercise intolerance

 ## Physical Examination

- Pallor
- Jaundice
- Splenomegaly
- Hepatomegaly
- Tachycardia, systolic flow murmur
- Orthostasis in acute onset

 ## Laboratory Aids

- CBC: Hb level decreased (occasionally, thrombocytopenia seen in Evans syndrome); MCV may be normal
- Reticulocyte count increased
- Peripheral smear: spherocytes, polychromasia, macrocytes, rouleaux formation
- Direct antiglobulin test (Coombs): positive

—Single most important test
—Warm AIHA will have IgG ± C3 positive
—Cold AIHA and PCH will have C3 positive

- Haptoglobin level decreased
- Indirect hyperbilirubinemia
- Elevated LDH
- Urinalysis: hemoglobinuria, increased urobilinogen
- Bone marrow aspiration—erythroid hyperplasia (to rule out leukemia or lymphoma associated with AIHA)
- Cold agglutinin titer: Positive (usually 1:64)
- Donath-Landsteiner test should be performed in cases of suspected PCH.

PITFALLS

A negative Coombs test can occur when small numbers of IgG or C3 molecules are present on the red-cell membrane (i.e., in cases of less severe hemolysis). Radiolabeled Coombs test or enzyme immunoassays are more sensitive diagnostic tests in these circumstances. Reticulocytopenia may occur in most severe cases where the antibody coats and removes reticulocytes.

Therapy

PATIENT MONITORING

- Hemoglobin level q4h to q12h (depending on severity)
- Reticulocyte count: Daily
- Spleen size: Daily
- Hemoglobinuria: Daily
- Coombs test: Weekly

BLOOD TRANSFUSION

- Indication

—Blood transfusion is indicated in cases of physiologic compromise from the anemia (usually only in severe acute onset) or with continued blood loss.

- Complications

—The blood bank may be unable to find compatible blood. In IgG-mediated disease, autoantibody is usually panreactive; therefore, you must use the least incompatible unit of blood. In cold agglutinin disease, you must prewarm all infusions to decrease IgM binding and must monitor for acute hemolysis during transfusion.

- Dose

—Use only a volume of blood sufficient to relieve compromise from anemia.

CORTICOSTEROIDS

- Indication

—In IgG-mediated disease, steroids have been shown to interfere with macrophage Fc and C3b receptors responsible for RBC destruction. They also have been shown to elute IgG Ab from the RBC surface (improving survival).
—In chronic warm AIHA, pulsed high-dose dexamethasone has been shown to be effective in some cases.

- Complications

—There are both short- and long-term side effects of steroids. Corticosteroids are generally not effective in cold agglutinin disease.

- Dose

—Start prednisone po/methylprednisolone IV at 2 mg/kg/day in divided doses. Tapering of steroids should begin once a therapeutic response is achieved (may take several weeks to months). Alternative treatments should be considered for patients unresponsive to steroids or who require high doses for maintenance of hemoglobin level.

- Goal

—The goal is initially to return to normal hemoglobin level with nontoxic levels of steroid, or no steroids. However, in some patients, the goal may be to achieve decreased hemolysis and a clinically asymptomatic state with minimal steroid side effects.

INTRAVENOUS IMMUNE GLOBULIN (IVIG)

- Indication

—IVIG may be useful in selected cases of immune hemolytic anemia unresponsive to steroids. The mechanism of action is not entirely clear.

- Complications

—The effect is usually temporary; retreatment may be required q3 to q4 weeks. There may be a risk of hepatitis C. IVIG is expensive.

- Dose

—Up to 1 g/kg/day for 5 days has been required to achieve a beneficial effect.

PLASMAPHERESIS/EXCHANGE TRANSFUSION

- Indication

—This treatment will slow the rate of hemolysis in severe disease.
—Indicated for AIHA associated with TTP

- Complications

—It is only of short-term benefit and is expensive.

- Dose

—The frequency and duration depend on response.

SPLENECTOMY

- Indication

—Patients unresponsive to medical management, who require moderate to high maintenance doses of steroids or who develop steroid intolerance may be candidates for splenectomy. It is not effective in cold agglutinin disease.

- The response rate is about 50% to 70%, with the majority only partial remissions.
- Complications

—There is a high morbidity rate for the surgical procedure and during the postoperative period.
—There is an increased risk of sepsis.

IMMUNOSUPPRESSIVE AGENTS (ANTIMETABOLITES AND ALKYLATING AGENTS)

- Indication

—When there is a clinically unacceptable degree of hemolysis that is refractory to steroids and splenectomy, immunosuppressive agents are indicated. Some have been effective in cold agglutinin disease.

- Complications

—There are varying side effects dependent on the agent used. Therefore, clinical indications must be strong and exposure to drug should be limited.

- Dose

—Adjusted to maintain WBC >2,000, ANC >1,000, and platelet count at 50,000 to 100,000 cells/mm^3

PROGNOSIS

Dependent on age, underlying disorder (if any), and response to therapy. See also in Data Gathering section, Natural History.

 Common Questions and Answers

Q: Will the anemia go away?
A: Children with cold autoantibodies tend to have short-lived illness, whereas children with warm antibodies often have a chronic clinical course characterized by periods of remissions and relapses.

Q: Is this contagious?
A: No. Another child may acquire the same viral illness; however, the body's response to produce an autoantibody is dependent on the individual patient.

ICD-9-CM 283.0

BIBLIOGRAPHY

Domen RE. An overview of immune hemolytic anemia. *Cleve Clin J Med* 1998;65(2):89–99.

Engelfriet CP, Overbeeke MAM, Kr., von dem Borne AEG. Autoimmune hemolytic anemia. *Semin Hematol* 1992;29(1):3–12.

Lanzkowsky P. Hemolytic anemia. In: Lanzkowsky P, ed. *Manual of Pediatric Hematology and Oncology.* New York: Churchill Livingstone, 2000:137–199.

Meyer O, Stahl D, Beckhove P, et al. Pulsed high-dose dexamethasone in chronic autoimmune hemolytic anemia. *Br J Haematol* 1997;98(4):860–862.

Ware RE, Rosse WF. Autoimmune hemolytic anemia. In: Nathan DG, Oski FA, eds. *Hematology of Infancy and Childhood.* 5th Ed. Philadelphia: WB Saunders, 1998:499–522.

Ware RE. Autoimmune hemolytic and thrombocytopenic disease in the adolescent patient. *Adolesc Med* 1999;10(3):377–384.

Author: Tammy I. Kang

Avascular (Aseptic) Necrosis of the Femoral Head (Hip)

 ## Database

DEFINITION

Avascular (aseptic) necrosis (AVN) results from the interruption of the blood supply of bone (either traumatic or nontraumatic occlusion). The femoral head is the most common site of AVN. When idiopathic AVN of the hip occurs in children, this is known as Perthes disease (See Perthes Disease).

CAUSES

- Traumatic

—After fracture
—After hip dislocation
—After slipped capital femoral epiphysis
—After casting, bracing, surgery

- Nontraumatic

——Idiopathic (older, after physeal closure); similar to adult AVN
—Idiopathic (younger, before physeal closure, Perthes disease)
—Caisson disease
—With sickle cell disease
—After septic arthritis
—With steroids or chemotherapy

PATHOPHYSIOLOGY

- Necrosis of bone with gradual return of blood supply
- Necrotic bone gradually resorbed and replaced by new bone

EPIDEMIOLOGY

- Variable, depending on cause

GENETICS

- Variable, depending on cause

COMPLICATIONS

- Decreased range of motion, pain, limping
- Osteoarthritis
- Physeal arrest with growth disturbance

PROGNOSIS

- Variable, depending on cause

 ## Differential Diagnosis

- Trauma

—Osteochondral fracture
—Impaction fracture
—Epiphyseal/physeal fracture

- Infection

—Osteomyelitis
—Septic arthritis

- Neoplastic process

—Epiphyseal tumors (chondroblastoma, Trevor disease, etc.)

- Rheumatologic processes

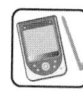 ## Data Gathering

HISTORY

- Onset (gradual or after traumatic event)
- Association with:

—-Trauma
—Medications (steroids or chemotherapy)
—Casting, splinting, surgery (iatrogenic)
—Pain, limping?
—Stiffness (decreased range of motion)

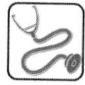 ## Physical Examination

- Gait

—Limping
—Antalgic gait (decreased)
—Trendelenburg gait

- Range of motion

—Flexion and extension
—Abduction and adduction
—Internal and external rotation

- Hip joint irritability (short arc rotation)
- Sign of other disease process (e.g., sickle cell disease)
- Physical examination trick

—Loss of internal rotation is usually the first and most affected loss of motion seen.

 ## Laboratory Aids

TESTS

Laboratory examinations should be normal in most forms of AVN of the femoral head. Exceptions:

—Sickle cell disease
—Septic arthritis
—Chemotherapy

IMAGING

- Usual

—Sclerosis
—Subchondral fracture
—Collapse
—Reossification
—Repair

- Variable

—Cysts
—Physeal growth arrest (young)
—Early osteoarthritis
—Subluxation

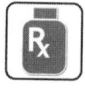 ## Therapy

DRUGS

- NSAIDs may be effective in decreasing associated inflammation.
- If associated with steroid use, discontinuation or elimination if appropriate

TREATMENT PRINCIPLES

- Maintain range of motion (physical therapy, traction, continuous passive motion).
- Contain the femoral head in the acetabulum (see Perthes Disease principles).
- Surgery

—Redirectional osteotomy
—Femoral or acetabular (see containment operations of Perthes)
—Core decompression to introduce new blood supply (older patient)

DURATION OF THERAPY

- Variable, depending on cause

DIET

- Thought not to alter disease process; recommend general balanced diet

Avascular (Aseptic) Necrosis of the Femoral Head (Hip)

 Follow-Up

WHEN TO EXPECT IMPROVEMENT

- Variable, depending on cause

SIGNS

- Subluxation
- Early osteoarthritis
- Growth arrest

PROGNOSIS

- Overall, good if mild involvement (usual) and patient is young
- See Prevention, below

PREVENTION

- Traumatic

—After fracture: Early anatomic reduction is key.
—After hip dislocation: Early reduction is key.
—After slipped capital femoral epiphysis: Associated with unstable grade 3 slips.
—After casting, bracing, surgery: Prevention is key.

- Nontraumatic

—Idiopathic (older, after physeal closure); similar to adult AVN
—Idiopathic Perthes (younger, before physeal closure); see Perthes Disease
—Caisson disease: rare now
—With sickle cell disease: good medical management is important
—After septic arthritis: early surgical drainage of hip key to prevention
—With steroids or chemotherapy: do not use unless no other alternatives

 Common Questions and Answers

Q: What type of medication is most often associated with AVN of the hip?
A: Steroids

Q: For AVN in children (Perthes disease of the hip, for example), is younger or older age associated with a better prognosis?
A: Younger age

ICD-9-CM

Legg Perthe 731.1

Avascular Necrosis 733.40

BIBLIOGRAPHY

Lahdes-Vasama T, Lamminen A, Merikanto J, et al. The value of MRI in early Perthes disease: An MRI study with a 2 year follow up. *Pediatr Radiol* 1997;27(6):517–522.

Roposch A, et al. Age at onset, extent of necrosis, and containment in Perthes disease. Results at maturity. *Archives of Orthopaedic & Trauma Surgery* 2003;123(2–3):68–73.

Sanders JO, Browne RH, Mooney JF, et al. Treatment of femoral fractures in children by pediatric orthopedists: results of a 1998 survey. *J Pediatr Orthop* 2001;21(4): 436–441.

Tokmakova KP, et al. Factors influencing the development of osteonecrosis in patients treated for slipped capital femoral epiphysis. *Journal of Bone & Joint Surgery (American Volume)*. 2003;85-A(5):798–801.

Tokmakova KP, et al. Mason DE. Factors influencing the development of osteonecrosis in patients treated for slipped capital femoral epiphysis. *Journal of Bone & Joint Surgery— (American Volume)*. 2003;85-A(5):798–801.

Weinstein SL. Legg-Calve-Perthes Syndrome. In: Morrissy RT, Weinstein SL, eds. *Lovell and Winter's Pediatric Orthopedics*. 5th Ed. Philadelphia: Lippincott Williams & Wilkins 2001:957–998.

Author: John P. Dormans

Babesiosis

 Database

DEFINITION

Human babesiosis is a tick-borne malaria-like illness characterized by fever, malaise, and hemolytic anemia. However, most infected individuals are asymptomatic.

CAUSES

- Human babesiosis is caused by the intraerythrocytic parasite of the *Babesia* genus.
- In the northeast United States, *Babesia microti* is transmitted by *Ixodes dammini*, the same tick responsible for Lyme disease.
- *Babesia divergens* is the responsible agent in Europe. WA-1 and MO-1 cause babesiosis in western United States and Missouri, respectively.
- Rarely, the disease has been acquired through transfusion of contaminated blood products or vertical transmission from mother to fetus.

PATHOPHYSIOLOGY

- A bite from an infected tick transmits the protozoa.
- The incubation period is usually 1 to 4 weeks but can be as long as 9 weeks.
- Infection of the erythrocyte causes membrane damage and lysis, which promotes adherence to the endothelium and microvascular stasis.
- The spleen plays an important role in decreasing the protozoal load through antibody production and filtering abnormally shaped infected red blood cells (RBCs).

EPIDEMIOLOGY

- The first human case in the United States was reported from California in 1966.
- The most severely affected are those who are at the extremes of age, functionally or anatomically asplenic, those with HIV, or otherwise immunocompromised.
- Transmission usually occurs in the summer and early fall.
- In the United States, most cases have been reported from the Northeast, Midwest, and the Pacific Coast. Endemic areas include Rhode Island, Massachusetts, and New York. There also have been cases from Maryland, Virginia, Georgia, Wisconsin, and Minnesota.

COMPLICATIONS

- Rarely fatal in the United States.
- Pancytopenia and overwhelming secondary bacterial sepsis may occur.
- Serious and fulminant complications have been described:

—Pulmonary edema and adult respiratory distress syndrome, often occuring after treatment has begun.
—Congestive heart failure
—Renal failure
—Hemophagocytic syndrome/disseminated intravascular coagulation
—Seizures/coma

- Those coinfected with Lyme disease are susceptible to more severe disease and complications.

ASSOCIATED ILLNESSES

It is estimated that 23% of patients have concurrent Lyme disease.

 Differential Diagnosis

- Infection
- Nonspecific viral syndrome
- Malaria

 Data Gathering

- Few patients recall a tick bite.
- Patients live in or have had recent travel to an endemic region.
- Initial symptoms are vague and may include progressive fatigue, malaise, headaches, and anorexia, accompanied by intermittent fevers as high as 40°C.
- Chills, myalgias, and arthralgias may follow these symptoms.
- Less common complaints include cough, sore throat, abdominal pain, and emotional lability.

 Physical Examination

- Fever is often the only finding.
- Mild conjunctival injection and pharyngeal erythema
- Some may have a mildly enlarged liver and/or splenomegaly.
- Jaundice or hematuria may also be seen.
- Petechiae and ecchymosis are rare.

 Laboratory Aids

SPECIFIC TESTS

- Giemsa- or Wright-stained thick and thin blood smears may demonstrate the intraerythrocytic ring form.
- Indirect immunofluorescent assay (IFA) is antigen-specific for B. microti and can be used when blood smears are negative. In general, a titer = 1:64 indicates exposure, and titers = 1:256 suggest acute infection. In endemic areas, the IFA test has a sensitivity of 91% and a specificity of 99%.
- Polymerase chain reaction (PCR) is highly specific.
- Isolation of the parasite can be done by intraperitoneal injection of a patient's blood into a golden hamster, but results takes weeks.

OTHER TESTS

Most of the abnormal routine tests are the result of hemolysis.

- Urinalysis: proteinuria, hemoglobinuria
- Complete blood count: normal leukocyte count/leukopenia, normocytic/ normochromic anemia, thrombocytopenia, and atypical lymphocytosis
- Possible positive Coombs test
- Elevated erythrocyte sedimentation rate
- Liver function tests: elevated bilirubin, lactate dehydrogenase, and liver transaminases

In asymptomatic patients, these tests are often normal.

FALSE NEGATIVES

- The blood smears may not demonstrate the protozoan at low levels of parasitemia.
- Serologic false positives for *B. micoti* include cross-reactivity with other *Babesia* species or malarial organisms.
- Theoretical serologic false positives for WA1: Rheumatoid factor, antinuclear antibody and antibody to *Toxoplasma gondii*.

Therapy

- Those with mild clinical disease usually recover without treatment.
- Asplenic, immunodeficient, or symptomatic patients should be treated with clindamycin and quinine.

—The dose of clindamycin is 20 to 40 mg/kg per day divided into three doses for 7 days.
—Quinine is dosed 10 to 25 mg/kg per day divided into three doses for 7 days.
—The combination of atovaquone and azithromycin have similar treatment effectiveness with fewer side effects than clindamycin and quinine in adults.
—The use of atovaquone and azithromycin has not been studied in the pediatric population and clindamycin and quinine are the recommended treatment choice for symptomatic children.

- For life-threatening infections, exchange transfusion has been successful.
- Progressive respiratory distress may require mechanical ventilation.

 ## Follow-Up

WHEN TO EXPECT IMPROVEMENT

- Those who are only mildly affected usually have resolution of their symptoms over a few weeks.
- For the severely affected and immunodeficient patients, the convalescent period may be as long as 18 months.
- In untreated asymptomatic individuals, parasitemia may persist for months to years

SIGNS TO WATCH FOR

- Respiratory distress, especially after treatment has begun
- Pancytopenia and lymphadenopathy: May indicate the development of hemophagocytic syndrome

PITFALLS

- Children who are from endemic areas and have an acute febrile illness may be misdiagnosed with a nonspecific viral illness.
- One should be suspicious for a coinfection with Lyme disease in those who are not responding to standard therapy.
- Delayed recognition of this uncommon disease may be life-threatening in the immunocompromised patient.
- In endemic areas, babesiosis should be considered in a post transfusion febrile illness in at risk populations.

PREVENTION

- Prevention begins with avoidance of tick bites.
- For most individuals, simple measures include wearing long-sleeved shirts and long pants, with pants tucked into the socks in tick-infested areas.
- Light clothing will make ticks easier to see.
- Spraying the bottoms of one's pants with a tick repellent may also be helpful.
- Children and dogs should be inspected for ticks after being outside.
- High-risk individuals may want to avoid endemic areas from May to September.
- Currently, there is no universal laboratory screening of blood products.
- No prophylaxis treatment after a tick bite is recommended.

 ## Common Questions and Answers

Q: How long does a tick have to be attached for infection to occur?
A: In general, successful transmission requires at least 24 hours of attachment.

Q: How should a tick be removed?
A: The tick should be grasped with forceps as close to its head as possible and pulled straight up. If possible, it should be saved for identification.

Q: Does infection confer lifetime immunity?
A: Reinfection is possible.

ICD-9-CM 088.82

BIBLIOGRAPHY

Aguero-Rosenfeld ME. Laboratory aspects of tick-borne diseases: lyme, human granulocytic ehrlichiosis and babesiosis. *Mount Sinai J Med* 2003;70:197–206.

American Academy of Pediatrics. Babesiosis. *Red Book: Report of the Committee of Infectious Diseases.* Washington, DC. American Academy of Pediatrics, 2000:181–182.

Bonoan JT, Johnson DH, Cunha BA. Life-threatening babesiosis in an asplenic patient treated with exchange transfusion, azithromycin, and atovaquone. *Heart Lung* 1998;27:424–428.

Boustani MR, Gelfand JA. Babesiosis. *Clin Infect Dis* 1996;22:611–615.

Krause PJ, et al. Persistent parasitemia after acute babesiosis. *N Engl J Med* 1998;339: 160–165.

Krause PJ, et al. Babesiosis: an underdiagnosed disease of children. *Pediatrics* 1992;89:1045–1048.

Krause PJ, et al. Comparison of PCR with blood smear and inoculation of small animals for diagnosis of Babesia microti parasitemia. *J Clin Microbiol* 1996;34:2791–2794.

Krause PJ, et al. Concurrent Lyme disease and babesiosis. Evidence for increased severity and duration of illness. *JAMA* 1996;275: 1657–1660.

Krause PJ. Babesiosis. *Med Clin North Am.* 2002;86:361–373.

McGinley-Smith DE. Tsao SS. Dermatoses from ticks. *J Am Acad Dermatol* 2003;49(3): 363–92, 393–396.

New DL, et al. Vertically transmitted babesiosis. *J Pediatr* 1997;131:163–164.

Author: Frances M. Nadel

Barotitis

 Database

DEFINITION

Barotrauma of the middle or inner ear, most often caused by scuba diving or flying.

PATHOPHYSIOLOGY

• The eustachian tube is responsible for equalizing pressure of the middle ear to the external ear and environment. Differences in the atmospheric pressure between the inner ear, middle ear, and the environment result in injury to the middle and/or inner ear. When ambient pressure decreases (e.g., airplane ascent) the tympanic membrane bulges outward and the eustachian tube vents the excess middle ear pressure. With a functioning eustachian tube, barotitis does not develop; the pressure is easily equalized. When ambient pressure increases (e.g., scuba diving, airplane descent) the tympanic membrane bulges inward and the eustachian tube resists inward flow of air to the middle ear. Even with a normally functioning eustachian tube, pressure equalization is difficult.
• Middle ear barotitis results in vascular engorgement, bleeding, and exudate formation.
• Inner ear barotrauma can cause labyrinthine window rupture.
• At a pressure differential of 60 mm Hg (greater ambient to middle ear pressure), subjective discomfort is reported. At a pressure differential of 90 mm Hg, the eustachian tube becomes "locked," because the palatal musculature is not strong enough to open the eustachian tube, and air is unable to enter the middle ear in order to allow for equalization of the pressure. The tympanic membrane can rupture at pressure differentials over 100 to 500 mm Hg.
• Barotitis is sometimes classified using Teed's classification of disease severity (see Physical Examination section).
• Nasal congestion has been shown to increase the likelihood of developing barotitis.

EPIDEMIOLOGY

• Significant disease is uncommon in commercial (pressurized) aircraft, although mild negative pressure of the middle ear is common after flying.
• Significant symptoms or injury can occur in scuba divers, and those who fly military aircraft and experience rapid altitude changes during tactical maneuvers.

COMPLICATIONS

• Vertigo
• Hearing loss
• Tympanic membrane rupture
• Oval or round window rupture
• Hemorrhage

PROGNOSIS

• Complete spontaneous resolution in mild cases
• Rarely, tympanotomy or tympanostomy is required to relieve pressure and pain, as well as prevent complications.
• Variable outcome for auditory and vestibular symptoms and injuries to the inner ear

 Differential Diagnosis

INFECTION

• Otitis media with effusion
• Acute otitis media

TRAUMA

• Blunt trauma to the tympanic membrane
• Exposure to extremely loud noise

HISTORY

The symptoms most likely reported by patients with barotrauma include:

• Ear pain, sensation of pressure, and decreased hearing

Symptoms of inner ear damage may include:

• Vestibular and/or auditory complaints.

Important questions to ask the patient include the following:

• Has the patient been on an airplane or scuba diving recently?
• Has the patient attended a "heavy metal" concert recently or been exposed to remarkably loud noises?
• Has the patient been "clapped" on the ears by another child?
• Has anyone inserted a foreign object, such as a Q-tip cotton swab into the ear?

 Physical Examination

Teed's classification to describe appearance of the tympanic membrane:

Grade 0: Normal

Grade 1: Retraction, redness in Shrapnell membrane and along manubrium

Grade 2: Retraction, with redness of entire eardrum

Grade 3: Grade 2 plus hemotympanum or clear exudate

Grade 4: Perforation of tympanic membrane

Also, assess for:

• Nystagmus
• Hearing loss

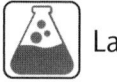 Laboratory Aids

TESTS

Hearing tests: Should be performed on all patients who have signs of barotrauma, and on patients with normal physical examinations but who are symptomatic.

RADIOGRAPHIC STUDIES

• Magnetic resonance imaging (MRI) of the inner ear: may be indicated in patients with vestibular symptoms or hearing loss to rule out inner ear damage.

Therapy

- Valsalva maneuver—blowing the nose while pinching the nostrils closed may be helpful when diving or descending and will force air into the middle ear via the eustachian tube, thereby equalizing the pressure between the middle ear and the environment.
- Swallowing, yawning, and chewing—can help to release pressure through the eustachian tube when ascending in an airplane or when returning to the water surface while scuba diving.
- Politzer bag—an instrument used for clearing pressure disequilibrium that has not improved with Valsalva maneuvers and a trial of decongestants (See Brown, 1994).
- Otovent—another instrument that can be used for treatment or prevention. Usage can be taught to children as young as 2 to 6 years of age.
- Tympanotomy or tympanostomy—may be required to relieve pressure in severe disease.
- Myringotomy—effective for the patient with excruciating pain or unrelenting eustachian tube dysfunction; best performed by an otorhinolaryngologist.

DRUGS

- Nasal decongestant sprays—have been reported to be helpful. The theory is that by constricting mucosal arterioles eustachian tube function is enhanced. Topical decongestants are used 1 hour prior to plane travel/diving and 1/2 hour prior to plane descent. One randomized control trial of oxymetazoline versus placebo found no difference between the two groups.
- Oral decongestants—may be helpful through the same physiologic pathway as topical agents. They should be initiated 1 to 2 days prior to the expected pressure change. There are 2 randomized control trials that suggest that oral decongestants may be effective; though a trial in children did not show a beneficial effect.
- Antihistamines—may also be helpful by reducing mucosal edema and enhancing the eustachian tube orifice. They can be used on the day of the expected pressure change.

 ## Follow-Up

- Pressure differential without damage to the middle or inner ear usually resolves within a few days of returning to normal atmospheric pressure.
- Barotitis that resulted in injury to the middle or inner ear has a variable rate of improvement; some damage is permanent (e.g., that to the organ of Corti), while other injury is reversible (e.g., that involving the tympanic membrane).

PREVENTION

- Travel in commercial aircraft will generally not result in severe barotitis.
- Most items in the Therapy section can be used as prevention: antihistamines, decongestants, and Valsalva maneuver.
- Ascend and descend gradually when scuba diving.

 ## Common Questions and Answers

Q: Is the Valsalva maneuver also effective on plane ascent?
A: Yes, creating even greater pressure in the middle ear by performing the Valsalva maneuver can overcome a resistant eustachian tube and result in sudden venting of increased middle ear pressure.

Q: Can children with otitis media travel in airplanes?
A: Yes, Weiss and Frost (1987) have shown that commercial air travel did not result in worsening of symptoms, and, in fact, the presence of otitis media with effusion seemed protective against barotitis.

Q: How can I minimize my child's ear pain when traveling in an airplane?
A: Have the child nurse, take a bottle, or eat during ascent and descent. This will result in pharyngeal movements that will repeatedly open the eustachian tube and equalize middle ear pressure to environmental pressure. Also, if the child is currently experiencing an upper respiratory infection, use of decongestants prior to flight may be helpful.

ICD-9-CM 993.0

BIBLIOGRAPHY

Buchanan BJ, et al. Pseudophedrine and air travel associated ear pain in children. *Arch Pediatr Adolesc Med* 1999;153:466–468.

Brown TP. Middle ear symptoms while flying: ways to prevent a severe outcome. *Postgrad Med* 1994;96:135–142.

Janvrin S. Middle ear pain and trauma during air travel. *Clin Evid* 2002;7:466–468.

Jones JS, et al. A double blind comparison between oral pseudophedrine and topical oxymetazoline in the prevention of barotrauma during air travel. *Am J Emerg Med* 1998;16:262–264.

Nakashima T, Itoh M, Sato M, et al. Auditory and vestibular disorders due to barotrauma. *Ann Otol Rhinol Laryngol* 1988;97:146–152.

Stangerup SE, Tjernstrom O, Klokker M, et al. Point prevalence of barotitis in children and adults after flight, and effect of autoinflation. *Aviat Space Environ Med* 1998;69(1):45–49.

Weiss MH, Frost O. May children with otitis media with effusion safely fly? *Clin Pediatr* 1987;26:567–568.

Author: Laura N. Sinai

Bell Palsy

 Database

DEFINITION

First described by Friedreich in 1798 and Powell in 1813, and later associated with the work of Sir Charles Bell (1820), Bell palsy has historically been regarded as an idiopathic facial paralysis limited to the VII cranial nerve. This "paralysis" may involve all of the modalities affected by VII:

- Mimetic facial movement
- Taste
- Cutaneous sensation
- Hearing acuity
- Lacrimation
- Salivation.

CAUSES

Idiopathic

- Pregnancy-related

Infectious

- Herpes simplex virus 1
- Human herpes virus 6
- Herpes Zoster (without Ramsay-Hunt syndrome)

Associated illnesses (can cause or be predisposed to an isolated facial nerve palsy, but are important to distinguish from a classic Bell palsy)

- Rubella
- Lyme disease (*Borrelia burgdorferi*)

—In Lyme neuropathy, early reports indicated a preponderance of tick bite histories involving the ipsilateral face, suggesting a retrograde migration of the spirochetes into the nerve and resultant nerve root/arachnoid irritation in at least some cases, as opposed to hematogenous dissemination and CNS penetration

- Epstein-Barr virus (EBV)
- Cytomegalovirus (CMV)
- Mumps
- Human immunodeficiency virus (HIV)
- *Mycoplasma pneumoniae*

COMPLICATIONS

- Corneal injury, due to decreased lacrimation and poor eye closure.
- Several sequelae, generally related to aberrant reinnervation of affected end organs, are observed after an episode of Bell palsy.
- Various synkinesias (an abnormal involuntary movement which accompanies a normally executed voluntary movement), including the Marin-Amat phenomenon (spontaneous eye closure with mouth opening, or its converse)
- Blepharospasm, hemifacial spasm, facial contractures
- The crocodile tears phenomenon (eating provokes ipsilateral tearing) results from crossed reinnervation between lacrimal and salivary parasympathetic fibers.

PROGNOSIS

- 60%–70% full recovery rate from isolated VIIth nerve palsy
- Signs of recovering function (generally improving control of mimetic movement) are typically apparent by the 3rd week after onset.
- Of those with less than total recovery, many will experience at least partial return to normal function; cosmetic results vary in this group.
- Outcome of idiopathic facial palsy as a pregnancy complication seems to be less favorable (around 55% full recovery).
- Up to 7% of patients may experience a second occurrence at some point in the future.

 Differential Diagnosis

TRAUMA

- Birth (especially forceps pressure to lateral face)
- Congenital facial palsies should not be regarded as Bell palsy, but rather symptomatic of some other cause.
- Temporal bone/petrous bone fractures
- Deep lacerations or trauma to parotid region

INFECTION

- Purulent otitis media/mastoiditis
- Basilar meningitis
- Petrositis (Gradenigo syndrome)
- Varicella-Zoster (Ramsay-Hunt syndrome)
- Syphilis
- Trichinosis
- Tuberculosis
- Leprosy

INFLAMMATORY

- Sarcoidosis
- Behcet disease
- Giant cell arteritis
- Polyarteritis nodosa
- Guillain-Barre syndrome
- Melkersson-Rosenthal Syndrome—rare neurologic disorder characterized by recurring facial paralysis, swelling of the face and lips (usually the upper lip), and the development of folds and furrows in the tongue

TUMORS

- Cerebello-pontine angle tumors, osteosarcomas, cholesteatomas, neurofibomas, lymphomas
- Hyperostosis cranialis interna, osteopetrosis

METABOLIC

- Diabetes (nerve ischemia), hyper-parathyroidism, hypothyroidism, porphyria

CONGENITAL/GENETIC

- Congenital absence or hypoplasia of depressor anguli oris muscle
- Mobius syndrome
- Chiari malformation
- Syringobulbia

 Data Gathering

HISTORY

- Mastoid or retroauricular pain ipsilateral to the side of developing symptoms (40%–50% of patients).
- Half of patients will have no clear sensory prodrome.
- Bell palsy often follows some identifiable infectious illness, such as viral URI symptoms, Mycoplasma pneumonia, or infectious mononucleosis. However, an identified antecedent illness is not requisite for the diagnosis.
- The onset is almost always rapid, with progression to a fairly constant state of unilateral paresis or paralysis within hours to 2 or 3 days.
- As the weakness progresses, the patient (and family members) may note:

—Difficulty with oral motor tasks (e.g., eating and drinking) due to inability to maintain mouth closure
—Inability to completely close the eye on the affected side (sometimes leading untrained observers to note an eyelid "droop" on the normal side, due to the contrast with normal eyelid closure and movements)
—Decreased lacrimation and eye itching and burning
—Hyperacusis
—Ipsilateral facial numbness (less commonly)
—Distortion of the taste of foods (dysgeusia)

- Bilateral symptoms (<1%) are distinctly rare, and suggest an alternative diagnosis, such as Guillain-Barre syndrome or other infectious, inflammatory, or metabolic diseases.

 Physical Examination

- Weakness of all muscles of mimetic facial movement is noted on the affected side.
- A classic feature of peripheral facial nerve palsies is symmetric weakness or paralysis or both upper (frontalis), mid (orbicularis oculi), and lower (orbicularis oris) muscles on both voluntary and involuntary mimetic movements. Having the patient wrinkle his/her forehead and raise his/her eyebrows, close his/her eyes tightly, and bare his/her teeth or smile, respectively, tests these.
- The examiner will typically note slow or absent spontaneous blinking on the affected side.
- Reflexes, such as the corneal reflex, should be decreased or absent on the affected side, but the consensual response on the unaffected side should be preserved.

- The sensory division of VII is tested by examining taste perception on the anterior tongue:

—This is done by applying ipsilaterally, swabs soaked in both a sugar solution and a salt solution to the anterolateral aspect of the tongue, without allowing for mouth closure and dispersion of the substances to the other side.

—Despite complaints of retroauricular pain and unilateral facial "numbness," abnormalities of cutaneous sensation typically are not verifiable by sensory testing in pure VII nerve palsies. The presence of true diminution of sensation should raise the question of other cranial nerve involvement (V).

- Examination of the external auditory canal on both sides is crucial.

—Vesicular lesions of the tympanic membrane suggests a Zoster-associated palsy (Ramsay-Hunt syndrome)

—Purulent otitis or evidence of trauma would mandate aggressive antibiotic treatment, as well as possible urgent surgical subspecialty evaluation and imaging of the temporal bone.

 ## Laboratory Aids

TESTS

Cases of uncomplicated VIIth nerve palsy require no workup.

Test: Serology for *Borrelia burgdorferi*
Significance: Recommended in all areas where Lyme disease is endemic. Lyme IgM titers are more sensitive for acute infection than IgG titers.

Test: Lumbar puncture and studies for cerebrospinal fluid (CSF) glucose, protein, cell count, culture
Significance: Recommended when signs of meningeal inflammation are present (e.g., nuchal rigidity, headache, fever, etc). A mild pleocytosis may be seen in Lyme disease.

RADIOGRAPHIC STUDIES

Test: Magnetic resonance imaging (MRI) of the head with gadolinium enhancement.
Significance: Recommended in cases of unusual presentation or progression, e.g., bilateral involvement, slow progression (over more than 1 week), or other cranial nerve findings. Several small series have proposed that gadolinium enhancement of the involved VII nerve predicts a slower or less optimal recovery.

OTHER STUDIES

Test: Audiologic testing (i.e., brainstem auditory evoked potentials, BAEP)
Significance: These modalities are only useful in distinguishing an isolated VII from a combined VII and VIII lesion (such as would be produced by a CPA tumor).

Test: Nerve conduction studies
Significance: In cases of later-than-expected recovery, nerve conduction studies may be of some limited value (evidence of nerve degeneration has been associated with a poorer prognosis for recovery).

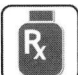 ## Therapy

- Eye protection and lubrication

—A significant risk for corneal injury is best managed by applying artificial tear solutions at least 3–4 times daily, and lubricating gels (e.g., Lacri-Lube) at night. Patching and protective eyewear, during both active play and sleep, is usually prescribed based upon the degree of remaining eyelid closure.

- Corticosteroids

—Prednisone—only considered within the first 72 hours of symptoms. Recommended dose: 1 mg/kg per day (maximum 30 mg) for 5 days, with or without a taper over the following 5 days.

- Acyclovir

—Most clearly indicated for the treatment of Ramsay-Hunt syndrome. It is also empirically used by some practitioners in standard Bell palsy management. Recommended dose: 20 mg/kg per day, divided into 5 times per day, for 10 days; maximum 400 mg, 5 times daily.

—Generally, any evidence of vesicular eruption in the ear canal or face should be treated promptly with acyclovir, as outcomes from VZV-associated palsies are reported to be worse in general.

—A great deal has been written about the use of corticosteroids, acyclovir or related antivirals, or both in the treatment of Bell palsy. However, clear evidence supporting the use of either therapy is lacking.

—Surgical decompression

—Previously, surgical decompression of the VIIth nerve had been proposed as a possible treatment in cases where recovery was delayed or the clinical course more severe. No clinical evidence to support the benefit of this strategy has emerged. Surgical decompression is best reserved for "other" cases of facial nerve palsy in which there is a definable syndrome of nerve compression due to extrinsic factors, such as exostoses, tumor, etc.

- Antibiotics

In areas where Lyme disease is endemic, many practitioners will begin treatment with oral antibiotics presumptively, while awaiting serologies (recall that the IgM titer is the most useful in the acute setting). See chapter on Lyme disease.

- Subspecialty consultation

—Generally, patients are referred if their recovery time is prolonged, or if there is a relapsing pattern, or other deviations form the expected course. However, the presence of other questionable cranial nerve involvement, recent trauma, meningeal symptoms, or neurologic findings (e.g., eye movement abnormalities, acute hemiparesis, etc.) should be viewed with great concern, and evaluated in an urgent-care setting.

PITFALLS

- The most important feature in diagnosis and management of Bell palsy is the distinction between a peripheral and a central VIIth nerve palsy.
- Identifying treatable causes of VIIth nerve palsy, e.g., Lyme Borreliosis and Ramsay-Hunt syndrome, is crucial for optimizing outcome and preventing comorbidities of these illnesses.
- The decision to defer medical imaging in the evaluation of a typical Bell palsy should be based upon a sound clinical history and physical examination. Unusual features should provoke thoughtful review and broader investigation where indicated.
- The decision to not treat a true idiopathic VIIth nerve palsy requires the strength of scientific conviction. Patients and families will often require explanation of this approach. In general, the avoidance of unnecessary exposure to antibiotics or corticosteroids should be viewed as a positive feature of this more conservative, evidence-based approach.

 ## Common Questions and Answers

Q: How does one differentiate between peripheral facial nerve palsy and a central nervous system lesion?
A: A critical step in diagnosis is the differentiation of peripheral from central (upper motor neuron) lesions. With upper motor neuron lesions (above the level of the VIIth nerve nucleus), there is preferential weakness of lower facial musculature, and sometimes differential paresis of voluntary versus spontaneous emotional mimetic movements.

Brainstem lesions, on the other hand, may produce a peripheral-appearing lesion, but almost always have involvement of other pathways and cranial nerve nuclei, e.g., ipsilateral lateral rectus palsy and contralateral somatic hemiplegia (Millard-Gruber syndrome).

ICD-9-CM CODE 351.0

BIBLIOGRAPHY

Axelsson S, et al. Outcome of treatment with valacyclovir and prednisone in patients with Bell's palsy. *Ann Otol Laryngol* 2003;112: 197–201.

Grose C, et al. Chickenpox and the geniculate ganglion: facial nerve palsy, Ramsay Hunt syndrome and acyclovir treatment. *Pediatr Inf Dis J* 2002;21:615–617.

Author: Stephen J. Falchek

Bezoars

 ## Database

DEFINITION

Bezoars are an accumulation of foreign material in the gastrointestinal tract. They are commonly divided into three categories, based upon the substance from which they are derived: vegetables, hair, and milk.

- The peak age of onset reported in the literature is 10 to 19 years.
- Ninety percent of patients reportedly are female.
- Documented over two millennia and has some medical value in some cultures.

CAUSES

Classification of bezoars is dependent on the most prominent substance from which they are formed including:

- Trichobezoars: Hair
- Phytobezoars: Indigestible fruit and vegetable matter
- Lactobezoars: Milk
- Less common materials include foreign bodies, gallstones, and medicines including vitamins, antacids, psyllium, sucralfate, cimetidine, and nifedipine.

 ## Differential Diagnosis

Any gastric foreign body can mimic a gastric mass and may present on palpation.

 ## Data Gathering

TRICHOBEZOARS

- Associated with trichotillomania and trichophagia; also may digest own hair but also rugs and animal hair.
- Retention of hair strands in the gastric folds
- Bezoars may become large, form a cast in the stomach leading to abdominal mass.
- Bezoar may extend through the pylorus into the small bowel. This "tail" may obstruct the papilla of Vater, leading to jaundice and pancreatitis.
- Presents with abdominal mass, crepitation over the stomach, iron-deficiency anemia. Parents report hair in the child's stool.
- Most cases of trichophagia do not result in bezoar formation.
- History of trichophagia is obtained in only 50% of cases.

PHYTOBEZOARS

- Most common form among adults
- Associated with gastric dysmotility and poor gastric emptying (either primary or following gastric surgery) and hypochlorhydria.
- Composed primarily of cellulose, hemicellulose, lignins, and tannins

LACTOBEZOARS (MILK)

Most often reported in premature, low-birth-weight infants (although there are reports in full-term infants and exclusively breast-fed infants)

- Factors contributing to lactobezoar formation include:

—Formulas with high casein content
—Early and rapid feeding advancement in small infants
—High-caloric-density formulas
—Formulas with high calcium/phosphate content
—Continuous tube feedings
—Altered gastric motility in low-birth-weight infants

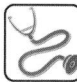 ## Physical Examination

HISTORY

Symptoms and signs of bezoar formation include:

- Pain
- Halitosis
- Nausea
- Vomiting
- Diarrhea
- Gastric ulceration
- Upper gastrointestinal bleeding and perforation
- Left upper quadrant (LUQ) mass

TRICHOBEZOARS

- Unusual patterns of balding
- Palpable LUQ mass in the abdomen is often detected.
- Hair found in the stool

PHYTOBEZOARS

Abdominal mass is palpable in less than half of patients.

Bezoars

 ## Laboratory Aids

- Iron-deficiency anemia
- Presence of steatorrhea or protein-losing enteropathy
- Plain abdominal radiography of the abdomen
- Upper gastrointestinal studies may identify and outline the mass.
- Endoscopy may provide the diagnosis of the specific type of bezoar.

 ## Therapy

TRICHOBEZOARS

Are difficult to remove and should not be removed endoscopically. The solution is surgical removal: they are normally too large, and hair is not dissolvable. Any trial to break the hairball may lead to metastatic migration and need of small intestinal surgery.

PHYTOBEZOARS

- Diet alteration
- Medications such as prokinetic agents to stimulate gastric motility
- Enzyme therapy to help dissolve the material
- N-Acetylcysteine treatment via nasogastric tube has been documented in one case report.
- Papain has shown to be approximately 87% effective. (Papain tablets are not currently available in the United States, so monosodium glutamate [MSG] dissolved in clear liquids has been used.) Complications of this therapy include the development of gastric ulceration and hypernatremia secondary to the high sodium content of MSG.
- Endoscopic fragmentation or extraction
- Surgical extraction

LACTOBEZOARS

- Withholding feedings for approximately 48 hours while the patient is sustained on IV fluids will resolve most lactobezoars.

 ## Common Questions and Answers

Q: What are some commonly used medications that can lead to bezoar formation?
A: Vitamins, antacids, psyllium, sucralfate, cimetidine, and nifedipine.

Q: What may place an infant at risk for formation of a bezoar?
A: The literature suggests that formulas with a high casein contact may be linked with lactobezoar formation. Other possible contributing factors include early and rapid feeding advancement in small infants, high-density formulas; formulas with high calcium/phosphate content, continuous tube feedings, and altered gastric motility in low-birth-weight infants.

ICD-9-CM 938

BIBLIOGRAPHY

Chen MK, Beierle EA. Gastrointestinal foreign bodies. *Pediatr Ann* 2001;30(12):736–742.

DuBose TM 5th, et al. Lactobezoars: a patient series and literature review. *Clin Pediatr* (Phila). 2001;40(11):603–606.

Lynch KA, et al. Gastric trichobezoar: an important cause of abdominal pain presenting to the pediatric emergency department. *Pediatr Emerg Care* 2003;19(5):343–347.

Phillips MR, et al. Gastric trichobezoar: case report and literature review. *Mayo Clin Proc* 1998;73(7):653–656.

Walker-Renard P. Update on the medicinal management of phytobezoars. *Am J Gastroenterol* 1993;88(10):1663–1666.

Author: Dror Wasserman

Biliary Atresia

 Database

DEFINITION

Biliary atresia is a progressive obliteration of the lumen of the extrahepatic (EHBA) and intrahepatic biliary duct systems of the liver.

PATHOPHYSIOLOGY

The etiology is unclear. Each of the following etiologies has been suggested but has never been substantiated:

- Environmental factors
- Viral infection (retrovirus 3, rotavirus, cytomegalovirus [CMV])
- Vascular insufficiency
- Genetic factors: ?HLA genotype
- Immune dysregulation in neonate affecting hepatobiliary system
- Pancreatic reflux
- Defective morphogenesis
—Features of ductal plate malformation have been noted in a subset of BA liver biopsies
—Laterality genes or JAG1 may play a role in some cases
- Multifactorial: For example, one might hypothesize that a viral infection occurring in the early neonatal period, in a genetically susceptible host, could trigger an immune reaction resulting in the progressive destruction of the biliary tree.

PATHOLOGY

Gross Anatomy

EHBA can affect all or any part of the extrahepatic biliary tree. When the affected portion is limited to the distal common bile duct, cystic duct, or gallbladder, the form is considered correctable because biliary drainage may be established. This situation occurs in less than 10% of patients. Coexisting anomalies are found in approximately 20% of patients. Some of the reported associations include:

- Absence of the inferior vena cava with azygous continuation
- Preduodenal portal vein and symmetric liver
- Malrotation
- Situs inversus
- Bronchial anomalies
- Multiple spleens (polysplenia)

—Other anomalies within the spectrum of heterotaxy, including structural congenital heart defects in a minority of patients

HISTOLOGY

The pathologic findings vary with stage of disease evolution. Extrahepatic biliary obstruction begins near the time of birth and progresses.

- Early in the course of the disease (approximately the first year), the liver biopsy shows cholestasis, interlobular bile duct proliferation, and a mononuclear infiltrate invading the periductal tissue. Bile plugs may be present within ducts. In addition, portal tracts are expanded by fibrosis, and some patients may already have well-established cirrhosis at the time of diagnosis.
- Later biopsies show degeneration and loss of bile ducts.
- If the biopsy is performed prior to 4 weeks of age, the pathology may be confused with other causes of neonatal cholestasis, such as giant-cell hepatitis.

GENETICS

- No clear genetic inheritance can be demonstrated, as indicated by discordance for both monozygotic and dizygotic twins.
- However, HLA-B12, HLA-A9-B5, and HLA-A28-B35 are found with a higher frequency in affected individuals.
- Human genes that determine laterality (ZIC3, LEFTB, and ACVR2B) and genes that affect bile duct development including HNF6 and JAG1 are all potentially important in pathogenesis of some cases.

EPIDEMIOLOGY

EHBA accounts for 25% to 30% of the cases of neonatal cholestasis and occurs with a frequency of 1 per 8,000 to 15,000 live births. It is the most common cause of neonatal jaundice for which surgery is indicated.

 Differential Diagnosis

The differential diagnosis includes all causes of neonatal cholestasis (NC).

EXTRAHEPATIC CAUSES OF NEONATAL CHOLESTASIS

- Biliary atresia
- Choledochal cyst
- Sclerosing cholangitis (?intrahepatic)
- Bile duct stenosis
- Anomalies of the choledochopancreaticoductal junction
- Spontaneous perforation of the common bile duct
- Obstructing neoplasia or stone
- Inspissated bile or mucus plug

INTRAHEPATIC DISORDERS OF NEONATAL CHOLESTASIS

Infection

- Sepsis
- Urinary tract infection (UTI)
- TORCH infections (Toxoplasma, Rubella, CMV, HSV)
- Coxsackie B virus, echovirus, adenovirus, enterovirus
- Viral hepatitis
- HIV
- EBV

Metabolic Abnormalities

- α1-Antitrypsin deficiency
- Cystic fibrosis
- Galactosemia
- Inborn errors of bile acid metabolism
- Hereditary fructose intolerance
- Zellweger syndrome
- Tyrosinemia
- Neonatal iron-storage disease (likely to present with liver failure)
- Citrin deficiency
- Respiratory chain disorders

Genetic Disorders

- Alagille syndrome (syndromic bile duct paucity)
- Trisomy 17, 18, 21 and Turner syndrome
- Progressive familial intrahepatic cholestasis

—FIC1 deficiency (Byler Syndrome)
—BSEP deficiency (PFIC2)
—MDR3 deficiency
—Benign recurrent intrahepatic cholestasis

- Dubin-Johnson syndrome
- Rotor syndrome

Drugs/Toxins

- Medications
- Total parenteral nutrition (TPN)

Systemic Disease

- Postshock
- Postasphyxia
- Congestive heart failure
- Panhypopituitarism

Other

- Idiopathic neonatal giant-cell hepatitis
- Nonsyndromic paucity of interlobular bile ducts

 Data Gathering

HISTORY

Typically, the patient is an otherwise healthy infant who develops jaundice within the first 90 days of life, and laboratory data demonstrate a conjugated hyperbilirubinemia.

 Physical Examination

- Jaundice is best visualized by examination of the hard palate, buccal mucosa, or sclera and may not be present until the bilirubin exceeds 5 to 7 mg/dL in the newborn period and 2 mg/dL in the older child.
- Acholic stools, hepatomegaly, and abnormal liver consistency are variable findings and do not need to be present to establish the diagnosis of biliary atresia.

 Laboratory Aids

- Conjugated hyperbilirubinemia is defined as a conjugated fraction greater than 2.0 mg/dL or a conjugated bilirubin greater than 15% of the total.

- Any child with a conjugated hyperbilirubinemia should undergo the following examinations:
—Fractionated bilirubin
—AST, ALT, Alkaline Phosphatase, GGT, total protein, albumin
—CBC, PT/PTT
—Bacterial cultures (blood, urine, and stool)
—Viral studies (hepatitis B, hepatitis C, Epstein-Barr virus [EBV], TORCH, HIV, adenovirus, enterovirus)
—α-1-Antitrypsin with Pi typing
—Urine and serum amino acids
—Urine organic acids
—Urine for reducing substance while the child is taking lactose-containing formula; if positive, assay of galactose-1-phosphate uridyl transferase activity
—X-ray studies to exclude evidence of congenital infections and Alagille syndrome (i.e., calcifications of brain and butterfly vertebrae), as indicated
—Eye examination for congenital infections
—Sweat chloride measurement
—Thyroid-function tests

OTHER STUDIES

- Abdominal ultrasound: Ultrasound is useful in ruling out biliary anomalies such as choledochal cyst, and also may identify laterality defects, such as polysplenia. Although ultrasound findings are not diagnostic of biliary atresia, the identification of a unique triangular or tubular echogenic density (the "triangular cord" sign), representing the fibrous cone of the bile duct remnant at the hepatic porta, may be significant. One recent study suggests that using a higher frequency (13 MHz rather than 7 MHz) ultrasound transducer may identify abnormalities in gallbladder size, wall thickness, and morphology that are characteristic of biliary atresia.
- Hepatobiliary scintigraphy.
- Liver biopsy
- Operative cholangiogram, if liver biopsy is suggestive of biliary obstruction.

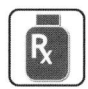 ## Therapy

- General approach
—Once the diagnosis of EHBA is established, a surgical drainage procedure is performed.
—Subsequent management is directed at providing nutrition and monitoring for common problems.
—Although surgical intervention is helpful, liver disease progresses and the majority of patients will ultimately require liver transplantation.
—Surgical drainage
—Correctable biliary atresia occurs in up to 10% of patients and is defined as obstruction limited to the distal common bile duct, cystic duct, and/or gallbladder. These patients may undergo a more limited operation linking the patent distal portion of the tree to the intestine, bypassing the obstruction.
—Noncorrectable biliary atresia occurs most frequently and is manifested as an absent

extrahepatic biliary tree. The standard surgical procedure is the hepatoportoenterostomy (Kasai procedure).
—Corticosteroids are used as an additional component of post-operative care
—Traditional Chinese medicine, kanzou (licorice root, glycyrrhizic acid), a hepatoprotective and cell-proliferative agent, have also been used
- Nutrition
—Malabsorption due to decreased concentration of bile acids within the duodenal lumen is common and leads to fat-soluble vitamin deficiency and malnutrition. Patients receive routine supplementation with vitamins A, D, E, and K. The diet should be enriched with medium-chain triglycerides to ensure adequate fat ingestion. Nasogastric tube feedings should be implemented if growth is inadequate.
- Prevention of cholangitis—During the first year of life most children are maintained on daily oral antibiotics to prevent infections from ascending into the liver.
- Pruritus is common and develops when there is increased serum bile acid concentration. Many approaches to treatment with only limited success have included ursodeoxycholic acid, antihistamines, cholestyramine, improved nutrition (e.g., nasogastric supplements), rifampin, phenobarbital, naloxone, and biliary diversion.
- Hyperlipidemia/xanthomas: Hyperlipidemia develops as a complication of chronic liver disease and can be treated with choleretic agents such as ursodeoxycholic acid as well as with improved nutrition.
- Ascites
—Spironolactone, chlorothiazide, and furosemide are commonly used diuretics. Acute changes in fluid balance or a rapid diuresis can be achieved by the use of furosemide in conjunction with albumin replacement

- Liver transplantation: indications for transplantation include life-threatening hemorrhage from portal hypertension, failure to thrive, intractable pruritus, and liver failure.

 ## Follow-Up

COMMON LONG-TERM PROBLEMS

- Poor growth
- Fat-soluble vitamin deficiency
- Cholangitis
- Portal hypertension
- Pruritus
- Progression of liver damage despite a surgical drainage procedure

The clinician should:

- Keep notes in a flowchart.
- Monitor growth parameters and fat-soluble vitamins.
- Monitor liver span, liver texture, and spleen size to follow progress of disease.
- Follow liver-function tests and CBC.
- Watch closely for cholangitis: the most important findings suggestive of cholangitis are fever and elevated transaminases and GGT levels.

PITFALLS

Because age at the time of surgical intervention is the most important determinant of outcome, a delay in diagnosis can be tragic. Surgery is successful in 86% of infants prior to 8 weeks, 36% of infants between 8 and 12 weeks, and only 20% for those over 12 weeks. Without surgical intervention, 50% to 80% of children will die (without liver transplantation) from biliary cirrhosis by age 1 year, and 90% to 100% will die by age 3 years.

 ## Common Questions and Answers

Q: When should a patient with neonatal jaundice have a fractionated bilirubin test?
A: If hyperbilirubinemia has not resolved by 4 to 6 weeks, fractionation should be performed to allow ample time for evaluation of neonatal cholestasis and the possible need for surgical intervention.

Q: What are the most important factors in success of the Kasi portoenterostomy?
A: The age at referral of the patient for evaluation and the experience of the center performing the procedure are the most important factors in determining surgical outcome.

Q: Can the physician prioritize the diagnostic evaluation?
A: In general, the answer is no. Because the diagnosis must be made as early as possible and because many tests are performed only in special laboratories, the full workup should be complete within a few days to 2 weeks, depending on the age of the child.

Q: What are the implications of long-term survival after a Kasai portoenterostomy?
A: In a single center report of 244 children operated on between 1979 and 1991, in King's College Hospital in the United Kingdom, 11% of adolescents were "cured" of their disease. On of the problems with the study were lack of follow-up on a large percentage of the cohort.

ICD-9-CM 751.61

BIBLIOGRAPHY

Haber BA, Lake A. Neonatal cholestatis. *Clin Perinatol* 1990;17:483–506.

Hadzic N, et al. Long-term survival following Kasi portoenterostomy: Is chronic liver disease inevitable? *J Pediatr Gastroenterol Nutr* 2003;37:430–433.

Karrer FM, Bensard DDM. Neonatal cholestasis. *Semin Pediatr Surg* 2000;(4):166–169.

Ohi R. Biliary atresia: a surgical perspective. *Clin Liver Dis* 2000;4:779–804.

Sokol RJ, et al. Pathogenesis and outcome of biliary atresia: Current concepts. *J Pediatr Gastroenterol Nutr* 2003;37:4–21.

Authors: Andrew E. Mulberg and Kathleen Loomes

Blastomycosis

 Database

DEFINITION

Blastomycosis is a systemic infection caused by the dimorphic soil fungus *Blastomyces dermatitidis*. Dimorphism is characterized by a mold phase (mycelial form) that grows at room temperature and a yeast form that grows at body temperature.

PATHOPHYSIOLOGY

• Infection is most commonly caused by inhalation of spores from *Blastomyces dermatitides*.
• Blastomycosis most commonly presents as a subacute pulmonary disease, but the clinical spectrum of the disease extends from asymptomatic to disseminated disease that involves the skin, bones, and genitourinary (GU) system.
• Inhalation of the fungus into the lung is followed by an inflammatory response with neutrophils and macrophages.

—Less common modes of acquiring the infection include: accidental inoculation, dog bites, conjugal transmission, and intrauterine transmission

EPIDEMIOLOGY

• Similar to other dimorphic fungi, *B. dermatitidis* is a soil saprophyte (mycelial form)
• No person-to-person transmission has been documented
• Infection is endemic in the United States in the southeast and central states and in the towns bordering the Great Lakes, with the highest incidence in Arkansas, Kentucky, Louisiana, Mississippi, North Carolina, Tennessee, and Wisconsin. Other reported areas of infection include parts of Canada (Ontario, Manitoba), Africa, India, and South America.

—Point-source outbreaks have been associated with occupational and recreational activities that occur in areas with moist soil and decaying vegetation such as along streams and rivers.

• Natural infection occurs only in two mammalian species: humans and dogs.
• Disease may be more severe and chronic in children with T-cell defects (especially HIV infection).
• Children account for 3% to 11% of cases of blastomycosis
• Incubation period estimated at 30 to 45 days

COMPLICATIONS

• Dissemination is the main complication of the infection occurring in up to 80% of children with blastomycosis.
• Systemic infection may be well advanced before symptoms are noted, making eradication more difficult. Long-term therapy and follow-up may be necessary.

PROGNOSIS

• Prior to the availability of antifungal medications, the mortality associated with blastomycosis was up to 90%.
• Appropriate treatment with antifungal medications result in excellent cure rates and mortality rates of less than 10%.
• The prognosis for chronic cutaneous disease is better than that for systemic disease.

ASSOCIATED ILLNESSES

• Pulmonary blastomycosis: most common form of infection by *Blastomyces* in children; can be acute, subacute, or chronic. Illness severity can vary greatly, from asymptomatic to presentations of upper respiratory tract infection, bronchitis, pleuritis, pneumonia, or severe respiratory distress.
• Cutaneous blastomycosis: Skin manifestations are variable and include nodules, verrucous lesions, subcutaneous abscesses, or ulcerations. Cutaneous disease occurs following pulmonary inoculation in most cases, but can also occur after direction inoculation into the skin.
• Disseminated blastomycosis: Usually begins as pulmonary infection, with subsequent spread to involve skin (most commonly), bone, GU tract, and central nervous system (CNS).

 Differential Diagnosis

• Acute bacterial infection
• Neoplasm
• Tuberculosis
• Other fungal infections causing pneumonia

 Data Gathering

HISTORY

• Children with acute pulmonary blastomycosis present with cough (may be productive), fever, chest pain, and malaise are the most common presenting symptoms. Children with chronic pulmonary disease present with chronic (greater than 2 weeks) nonproductive cough, pleuritic chest pain, poor appetite. There may also be a history of fever, chills, weight loss, fatigue, night sweats, or, rarely, hemoptysis.
• History of residence or travel to an endemic area

 Physical Examination

• Initial pulmonary infection may present with physical examination findings similar to those of bacterial pneumonia. Respiratory signs and symptoms often have resolved by the time cutaneous manifestations are apparent.
• Skin involvement appears as nodules, nodules with ulceration, and, finally, granulomatous lesions with advancing borders.
• Sites in disseminated disease include lung, skin, bone, GU tract, CNS, and, infrequently, liver and spleen, lymph nodes, thyroid, heart, adrenals, omentum, GI tract, muscles, and pancreas.
• Chest radiography commonly reveals consolidation of lobar consolidation. Cavitation, fibronodular patterns, and mass effect may also be seen.

Laboratory Aids

• Definitive diagnosis requires the growth of *B. dermatitidis* from a clinical specimen.

—Direct visualization of the yeast form may be performed on samples of sputum, urine, CSF, BAL sample, or tissue biopsy.

• Culture of the organism from samples can be performed and a DNA probe used to identify *B. dermatitidis*.
• Serologic tests lack sensitivity and specificity and are generally not helpful in establishing of blastomycosis.
• A negative serologic test does not rule out infection and a positive test should not be used as an indication to start treatment for *Blastomyces*.
• The most accurate serologic test is the enzyme immunoassay

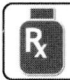

Therapy

• Mild or moderate disease pulmonary disease is treated with oral itraconazole. Alternative agents include ketoconazole or fluconazole
• Severe pulmonary disease, CNS or other severe infection should be treated with intravenous amphotericin B. Therapy for some patients may be switched to oral itraconazole after clinical stabilization with amphotericin B.
• The use of lipid formulations of amphotericin B has not been reported for CNS blastomycosis, but this treatment may be an alternative for patients unable to tolerate amphotericin B.
• Length of therapy is site-dependent: at least 6 months for pulmonary disease and at least 12 months for bone disease.

—Voriconazole, a new azole agent, and casponfungin, an echinocandin class antifungal, have in-vitro activity against *B. dermatitidis*.

PREVENTION

• No special precautions for hospitalized patients are indicated.
• The natural reservoir is undetermined.

ICD-9-CM 116.0

BIBLIOGRAPHY

American Academy of Pediatrics. Blastomycosis. In: Pickering L, ed. *2000 Red Book: Report of the Committee on Infectious Diseases*. 26th Ed. Elk Grove Village, IL: American Academy of Pediatrics 2003: 219–220.

Bradsher RW, et al. *Infect Dis Clin North Am* 2003;17(1):21–40.

Chapman SW, Bradsher RW, Campbell GD Jr, et al. Practice guidelines for the management of patients with blastomycosis. *Clin Infect Dis* 2000;30:679–683.

Chapman SW. Blastomyces dermatitis. In: Mondell GL, et al., eds. *Principles and Practice of Infectious Diseases*. 5th Ed. New York: Churchill Livingstone, 2000:2733–2746.

Maxon S, Jacobs RF. Community-acquired fungal pneumonia in children. *Semin Respir Infect* 1996;11(3):196–203.

Schutze G. Blastomycosis. In: Feigin RD, Cherry JD, eds. *Textbook of Pediatric Infectious Diseases*. 5th Ed. Philadelphia: WB Saunders, 2004:2560–2568.

Varkey B. Blastomycosis in children. *Semin Respir Infect* 1997;12(3):235–242.

Author: Theoklis Zaoutis

Blepharitis

 Database

DEFINITION

Blepharitis is inflammation or infection of the margins of the eyelid. The hallmark clinical features include redness, itching or burning, and crusting or scaling of the lid margins. Various types:

- Seborrheic blepharitis—notable for easy-to-remove, yellow, greasy scales along the eyelashes; occurs in conjunction with similar seborrheic scales of the eyebrow, scalp and external ears.
- Staphylococcal blepharitis—localized infection of the eyelid margin caused by *Staphylococcus aureus* or *S. epidermidis*. The hallmark features of staphylococcal-induced blepharitis are fibrinous, difficult-to-remove scales at the eyelash bases with concomitant inflammation of the lid margin, and occasionally loss of eyelashes.
- Mixed blepharitis—presence of a staphylococcal infection complicating seborrhea of the eyelids.
- Parasitic blepharitis—inflammation of the eyelids due to infestation by crab lice (*Pediculus pubis*) or head lice (*Pediculus capitis*).

PATHOPHYSIOLOGY

- There are several glands (meibomian glands, pilosebaceous glands of Zeis, and the apocrine glands of Moll) that exit along the eyelid margin. These glands produce the lipid component of tears.
- When these glands become infected or dysfunctional, the clinical features notable for blepharitis may occur.
- Spread of bacteria to the glands of Zeis or the meibomian glands can lead to development of a hordeolum or stye.
- Staphylococcal exotoxins can lead to conjunctivitis or keratitis.

EPIDEMIOLOGY

Atopic or allergic contact dermatitis as a cause of blepharitis occurs in up to 65% of patients.

COMPLICATIONS

- Loss of eyelashes (madarosis) from traction of hair due to rubbing
- Hordeolum (stye)
- Conjunctivitis
- Keratitis
- Chalazion

PROGNOSIS

- Blepharitis is frequently a chronic and relapsing process.
- With appropriate treatment, symptoms may resolve within a week.

 Differential Diagnosis

- Atopic or contact dermatitis
- Psoriasis
- Rosacea (usually accompanied by dilated telangiectasia of the blood vessels in the lid margins, cheeks, nose, and chin)
- Dacryostenosis
- Acute conjunctivitis (bacteria, viral, or allergic)

 Data Gathering

HISTORY

Ask about:

- History of previous inflammation of eyelid margins, or presence of symptoms for a prolonged period of time
- Pruritus
- Use of any medications or products (i.e., contacts lens, soaps, or makeup) used on or around the eye
- Frequent rubbing of the eye or contact with eyelids by hands
- Hand-washing practices
- Cleansing of eyelids
- Past medical and family histories of atopy
- Seasonal variation of symptoms (suggests allergic etiology)
- History of lice

 Physical Examination

- Evaluate eyelid margins and eyelashes for crust, erythema, loss of hair, and ulceration. With chronic infection, you may see thickening of the eyelid margin. With herpes simplex viral infection, you may see grouped vesicles along the eyelid.
- Evaluate remainder of eye, particularly the conjunctiva and sclera, for evidence of inflammation or infection.
- Examine the scalp and skin of the head for evidence of seborrhea, atopic dermatitis, contact dermatitis, louse infestation, or rosacea.

 Laboratory Aids

- Laboratory testing is only indicated in cases that do not respond to treatment.
- Bacterial or viral culture of the lid margins can be helpful in cases when the diagnosis is unclear, or in severe cases of blepharitis with ulceration.
- Giemsa staining of conjunctival scrapings—may show the presence of neutrophils, which is useful in cases where cultures do not conclusively show signs of infection.

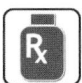 Therapy

- Eyelid margin cleansing twice daily is considered first-line therapy.

—First a warm compress should be placed over closed eyelids for 5 to 10 minutes to loosen debris.
—Next the eyelid margins should be cleansed with a dilute mixture of baby shampoo (brands that do not irritate the eyes) and water.
—Commercial eyelid cleansers are also available.

- In cases associated with seborrhea, treatment of the accompanying scalp and eyebrow involvement should be initiated with selenium sulfide shampoo once to twice a week, with manual removal of the crusting in those areas with a fine-toothed comb or soft bristle brush.
- More resistant cases or those that fail improve may be treated with application of a topical antibiotic ointment or solution with efficacy against staphylococcal species (e.g., bacitracin or erythromycin ophthalmic ointment) for 1 to 2 weeks.
- The most severe cases, particularly those associated with rosacea, may need to be treated with an oral antibiotic, such as a first generation cephalosporin or, in the case of rosacea, erythromycin or doxycycline (the latter in older adolescents).

—Contact lens use should be avoided until resolution of symptoms.

 Follow-Up

- Once symptoms have resolved, there is no need for routine follow-up of blepharitis.
- If symptoms begin to recur, encourage early initiation of eyelid hygiene with the soap and water wash.

PREVENTION

- Treat seborrheic dermatitis of scalp early.
- Discourage eye rubbing in patients.
- Encourage frequent hand washing for children.
- For children with allergic symptoms, oral antihistamines may decrease eye rubbing

 Common Questions and Answers

Q: Is blepharitis contagious?
A: Blepharitis is not spread to other family members. However, the bacteria that can cause the infection are frequently transmitted by hand contact, so frequent hand washing is recommended.

Q: Does blepharitis recur?
A: Blepharitis may recur. In cases of children with seborrhea and atopic dermatitis, treatment of these conditions may limit the frequency of flare-ups. Early eyelid hygiene may limit the severity of future recurrences.

ICD-9-CM 373.00

BIBLIOGRAPHY

Beltrani VS. Dermatologic disorders of the eyelids. *Immunol Allergy Clin North Am* 1997;17(1):103–129.

Denton P, Barequet IS, O'Brien TP. Ocular infections: update on therapy. Therapy of infectious blepharitis. *Ophthalmol Clin North Am* 1999;12(1):9–14.

Farpour B, McClellan KA. Diagnosis and management of chronic blepharokeratoconjunctivitis in children. [Journal Article] *J Pediatr Ophthalmol & Strabis* 2001;38(4):207–212.

Hara JH. The red eye: diagnosis and treatment. *Am Fam Physician* 1996;54(8):2423–2430.

Lemp MA. Contact lenses and associated anterior segment disorders: dry eye, blepharitis, and allergy. *Ophthalmol Clin North Am* 2003;16(3):463–469.

McCulley JP, Shine WE. Changing concepts in the diagnosis and management of blepharitis. [Review] [88 refs] [Journal Article. Review. Review, Tutorial] *Cornea* 2000;19(5):650–658.

Mourits MP, et al. Grotesque bilateral eyelid swelling as a symptom of Munchausen's syndrome. [Case Reports. Letter] *Br J Ophthalmol* 2001;85(11):1389–1390.

Nazir SA, et al. Ocular rosacea in childhood. *Am J Ophthalmol* 2004;137(1):138–144.

Shields SR. Managing eye disease in primary care: part 2. How to recognize and treat common eye problems. *Postgrad Med* 2000;108(5):83–96.

Author: Lee R. Atkinson-McEvoy

Bone Marrow and Stem Cell Transplantation

 Database

DEFINITION

Reconstitution of damaged, defective, or infiltrated bone marrow with IV infusion of hematopoietic progenitor (stem) cells from:

- The patient (autologous)
- An identical twin (syngeneic)
- A histocompatible donor (allogeneic)

INDICATIONS

- Accepted indications if a human leukocyte antigen (HLA) identical sibling is available:

—Acute lymphoblastic leukemia (ALL) in second complete remission (CR) and in certain patients in first CR (Philadelphia chromosome positive ALL)
—Acute myelogenous leukemia in first CR
—Chédiak-Higashi and other severe neutrophil defects
—Chronic myelogenous leukemia (CML) when in the chronic phase and within a year from time of diagnosis
—Congenital bone marrow failure syndromes
  —Diamond-Blackfan anemia (resistant to medical therapy)
  —Schwachman-Diamond syndrome (resistant to therapy)
—Fanconi anemia
—Juvenile myelomonocytic leukemia (formerly called JCML)
—Lymphoma after second CR
—Myelodysplastic syndromes
—Myelofibrosis
—Osteopetrosis
—Severe aplastic anemia
—SLE especially if unresponsive or intolerant to conventional medical therapy
—Severe combined immunodeficiency and other congenital immunodeficiencies
—Thalassemia major (treatment of choice in Italy)
—Wiskott-Aldrich syndrome

Autologous transplantation is an accepted treatment for lymphoma in second CR and for high-risk or Stage IV solid tumors in CR or very good partial response.
Tandem autologous peripheral stem cell transplants also are under investigation for treatment of high-risk neuroblastoma, PNET, brain tumors.

- BMT can lead to restoration of enzymatic activity in white cells and removal of accumulated substrates in affected tissues. In some diseases, such as adrenoleukodystrophy (childhood onset), it has been successful. In others, such Krabbe disease (infantile form), it has not been as successful.
Nonmyeloablative BMT is also being studied as an option for these patients. Of concern is that improvement in organ function has not always led to improvement in intellectual function.

DONOR SELECTION (IN ORDER OF PREFERENCE)

- Identical twin: The increased risk of relapse of leukemia is offset by decreased treatment-related mortality.
- HLA identical sibling
- Other family members

—Rarely (i.e., in 5% of families), a nonsibling relative who is phenotypically mismatched for one antigen will be found. Such transplantations have comparable results to HLA-identical sibling BMT.

- Haploidentical transplantations (2 or 3 HLA-antigen mismatch) have been performed but require depletion of T cells from the graft to avoid fatal graft-versus-host disease (GVHD). T-cell depletion can help prevent or ameliorate GVHD, but T-cell depletion can cause graft failure, delay in immunologic recovery, and/or loss of graft versus leukemia (GVL) effect. They are associated with a lower survival than conventional BMT.
- Unrelated donors

—The National Marrow Donor Program (NMDP) presently has over 2 million volunteers registered and maintains a cooperative search agreement with European registries. Over 60% of preliminary searches yield at least one potential donor, although this percentage is lower for minority patients.

- Autologous (either peripheral stem cells or bone marrow)

—Peripheral blood or bone marrow stem cells are provided by the patient in remission
—Gene-marking studies have shown that infused marrow containing tumor can contribute to relapse. Thus, one needs to ensure that the graft stem cells do not contain any viable tumor cells, so the stem cells undergo purging or positive selection prior to infusion into the recipient. However, these methods still need to be improved.

- Nonmyeloablative transplants

—Use less cytotoxic preparative regimens
—Require sufficient immunosuppression of host and a generous infusion of hematopoietic stem cells
—Leads to mixed chimerism
—Being pursued as an option in patients with nonhematologic malignancies

PREPARATIVE REGIMENS (CONDITIONING)

- The purpose of conditioning (either chemoradiotherapy or chemotherapy alone) is threefold:

—To provide immune suppression in order to avoid destruction of the allograft by residual, immunologically active cells in the host
—To destroy any residual cancer cells
—To provide space for the new bone marrow to grow

- Agents used primarily for immunosuppression:

—Cyclophosphamide
—Antithymocyte globulin (ATG)
—Alemtuzumab (Campath)

- Agents used primarily for antineoplastic effects or bone marrow ablation:

—Busulfan
—Cytarabine (ARA-C)
—Etoposide (VP-16)
—Carmustine (BCNU)
—Carboplatin
—Melphalan

- Agents used for both purposes:

—Total-body irradiation (TBI)
—Thiotepa

Note: Few randomized trials have compared one regimen to another. Choice depends on the disease being treated, the type of donor available, and previous treatment received.

STEM-CELL COLLECTION METHODS

- Conventional bone marrow

—Harvested from the posterior iliac crests under general anesthesia (alternative sites include anterior iliac crests, sternum).
—100 to 300 million stem cells per kilogram of the recipient's weight are harvested.
—T-cell depletion is performed on allografts to reduce risk of GVHD, but it increases risk of graft failure/rejection and of relapse in the patient with leukemia
—Average time to engraftment is 14 to 28 days for allograft and 12 to 21 days for autograft

- Peripheral blood stem-cell (PBSC) collections via apheresis

—Hematopoietic stem cells normally circulate in the peripheral blood in small numbers but can be mobilized by chemotherapy and/or growth factors (e.g., GM-CSF or G-CSF) and then phoresed and cryopreserved.
—PBSC transplants do not require general anesthesia to harvest stem cells.
—Previously used for autografts, successful allogeneic transplantations have now been performed with PBSCs.
—Autologous and allogeneic PBSC transplants have shorter time to engraftment than allogeneic bone marrow transplants, but have increased risk for more severe acute GVHD and chronic GVHD (but may have better GVL).
—Convincing survival advantage overall has not been demonstrated yet.
—Average time to engraftment is 14 to 15 days.

- Umbilical cord blood (UCB)

—A rich source of hematopoietic stem cells; even 45 mL of cord blood is sufficient to reconstitute the hematopoietic system of a child.
—Decreased incidence and severity of acute GVHD and chronic GVHD, but has longer engraftment time.
—Advantages: Abundant source of stem cells are harvested at no risk to the mother or fetus; UCB is cryopreserved and banked, so it is available on demand; can target minority populations; do not "lose" donors because of increased donor age, the donor's developing a new medical conditional or donor geographic relocation.

—Disadvantages: Limited number of hematopoietic stem cells in collected UCB may contribute to delay or failure of engraftment; future development of potential abnormal newborn's stem cells into adulthood; cannot collect additional donor stem cells for recipient experiencing graft failure; cannot collect donor lymphocytes for recipient who has relapsed.

TOXICITIES

- Chemoradiotherapy

—Universal: nausea/vomiting/diarrhea, alopecia, pancytopenia
—Possible and agent-specific:
  —TBI: skin erythema, parotitis
  —Cyclophosphamide: hemorrhagic cystitis, SIADH, cardiomyopathy
  —ATG: allergy, serum sickness
  —Busulfan: seizures, pulmonary fibrosis, bronzing of the skin
  —ARA-C: fever, neurologic symptoms, acute respiratory distress syndrome (ARDS)
  —VP-16: allergic reactions
  —BCNU: pulmonary fibrosis

- Graft failure

—Usually due to destruction of the graft by the immunologically active cells in the host
—Predisposing factors:
  —Previous blood transfusions
  —Less intensive high-dose preparative regimens
  —Use of methotrexate rather than cyclosporine to prevent GVHD
  —T-cell depletion of donor cells
—Can occur early (failure to engraft) or even after successful engraftment
—Rare in HLA-identical sibling transplantations
—Risk increases with unrelated donors (6%) or T-cell depletion (approximately 14% but depends on the degree of T-cell depletion and the use of ATG seems to decrease incidence of graft rejection markedly)
—Usually fatal

- Graft-versus-host disease (see chapter on GHVD)
- Infection: the major cause of nonrelapse mortality

—Immune dysfunction is caused by a period of severe myelosuppression immediately following stem cell transplant, lack of sustained transfer of clinically significant donor-derived B and T cell immunity, a capitulation of normal lymphoid ontogeny, and the effects of GVHD and its treatment.
—In the first month posttransplantation, bacterial and fungal infections predominate. Use of prophylactic broad-spectrum antibiotics and fluconazole during the time of severe myelosuppression has helped considerably.
—In the second and third months, viral infections predominate, which include cytomegalovirus (CMV), adenovirus, herpesvirus, varicella virus and polyomaviruses as well as PCP.
—After 3 months: herpes zoster and bacterial infections in patients with chronic GVHD

—Acyclovir prophylactically is used in patients who are HSV or VZV positive.

Gancyclovir is started prophylactically in CMV seropositive donors or recipients, and is started 100 days after transplant because of drug-related neutropenia

- Hepatic venoocclusive disease

—Clinical criteria met when two of the following are present:
  —Hepatomegaly and/or right upper quadrant pain
  —Hyperbilirubinemia (>2.0 mg/dL)
  —Greater than 5% weight gain and/or ascites
  —Incidence of approximately 25% (range, 1% to 54%) and mortality of 30% (range, 3% to 67%) have been reported.
  —Progressive hepatic failure and often renal failure develop in severely affected patients.
—Therapy is largely supportive. Currently, there is no definitive therapy.

- Interstitial pneumonitis

—Typically appears 40 to 80 days post-BMT as rapid-onset tachypnea, fever and hypoxia associated with bilateral interstitial infiltrates
—Common etiologies include:
  —CMV
  —Pneumocystis carinii
  —Idiopathic: when no bacterial, viral, fungal, or protozoan cause is identified. Radiation to the lungs probably plays a role in the development of "idiopathic" pneumonitis.

LATE COMPLICATIONS

- Endocrine
—Hypothyroidism: seen in approximately 20% of patients after TBI; rare after chemotherapy alone
—Growth hormone deficiency: seen in over half of patients receiving TBI
—Primary gonadal failure and absence of development of secondary sexual characteristics are common, especially if the recipient was prepubertal at the time of transplantation or received TBI.

- Infertility: Sterility is expected after TBI; fertility may be preserved after cyclophosphamide alone.
- Opthalmologic: Cataracts are seen in 40% of patients after TBI and in 20% after chemotherapy alone. A higher incidence is seen in those who also receive steroids.
- Dental: Poor calcification of teeth and root blunting have been seen. The defects are more severe in children younger than age 7 at transplantation.

- Renal
—Radiation nephritis
—Hemolytic uremic syndrome and thrombocytopenic purpura occur, especially during treatment with cyclosporine

Note: After T-depleted transplantations, the risk of fatal Epstein-Barr virus infection is significant.

- Secondary malignancies: Fifteen-year cumulative incidence rates are 20% and 6% after regimens with and without TBI, respectively.
- Recurrent leukemia—current treatment options include donor leukocyte infusions to induce GVL effect, nonmyeloablative "mini" transplants, or full allogeneic bone marrow transplant.
- Intellectual function: Few prospective studies published

 ## Common Questions and Answers

Q: When should I immunize a patient after transplantation?
A: At 1 year post-BMT, patients free of chronic GVHD should begin a primary immunization schedule with DPT and Salk polio, HiB, hepatitis B, pneumovax and prevnar. MMR or other live vaccines is usually given at 2 years post-BMT. Influenza vaccine should be given after 1 year and then annually.

Q: If my patient relapses after BMT, can a second BMT be done?
A: Previously, there were few therapeutic options for patients who relapsed less than 1 year post-BMT. Remissions after an infusion of buffy coat (containing T cells) from the patient's donor, called donor leukocyte infusion, can be achieved. Although the majority of successful infusions have been in patients with CML, success has also been seen in acute leukemia. Chronic GVHD will often result.

BIBLIOGRAPHY

Armitage JO. Bone marrow transplantation. *N Engl J Med* 1994;330:827–838.

Cutler C, Antin JH. Peripheral blood stem cells for allogeneic transplantation: A Review. *Stem Cells* 2001;19:108–117.

Laughlin MJ. Umbilical cord blood for allogeneic transplantation in children and adults. *Bone Marrow Transplantation* 2001;27:1–6.

Sanders JE. Bone marrow transplantation in pediatric oncology. In: Pizzo PA, Poplack DG, ed. *Principles and Practice of Pediatric Oncology.* 3rd Ed. Philadelphia: Lippincott Williams & Wilkins, 1997:357–373.

Sanders JE. Bone marrow transplantation for pediatric malignancies. *Ped Clin North Am* 1997;44(4):1005–1020.

Thomas ED. Bone marrow transplantation: A Review. *Seminars in Hematology* 1999;36(Suppl 7):95–103.

Author: Valerie I. Brown

Botulism

Database

DEFINITION

An illness produced by neurotoxins elaborated by *Clostridium botulinum,* which causes an acute, descending, flaccid paralysis. The neurotoxin may be ingested or absorbed from infected wounds, or ingested spores germinate, producing toxin. There are three types of illness:

- In infant botulism, ingested spores germinate and colonize the infant's colon and elaborate toxin.
- In adults, the patient ingests preformed toxin while eating improperly prepared or stored foodstuffs.
- In wound botulism, spores germinate in an infected wound and toxin is absorbed.

CAUSES

C. botulinum, the etiologic agent, is a gram-positive, spore-forming, obligate anaerobic bacteria that is found in soil throughout the world.

PATHOPHYSIOLOGY

- Neurotoxin is taken up by nerve endings and irreversibly blocks acetylcholine release in peripheral cholinergic synapses.
- Cranial nerves are usually affected first and most severely, leading to difficulty swallowing and loss of airway protective reflexes. Respiratory failure develops.
- Botulinum toxin does not cross the blood–brain barrier; therefore, the sensorium remains clear.
- Recovery occurs with the regeneration of terminal motor neurons and the formation of new motor end plates.
- Infants are particularly prone to colonic colonization with *C. botulinum.* When foods other than breast milk are introduced in breastfed infants, changes in flora may be especially important.

EPIDEMIOLOGY

- Infant botulism occurs in the first year of life, with more than 95% of cases reported in the first 6 months. Intestinal botulism is the most common form of human botulism in the United States, with over 100 cases reported annually.
- Infants are usually white, breastfed, and from middle-class families. Infants who have less than one bowel movement per day may be at increased risk. Cases are seen more frequently in rural and suburban areas.
- Most cases have been reported in California, Utah, and Pennsylvania.
- There often is a history of a recent change in feeding practice (addition of formula or solids or changing from breast- to bottle-feeding).
- Honey seems to be a particularly contaminated food and has been implicated in California. Corn syrup has also been reported to contain botulinum spores but much less frequently than honey and has been associated with significantly fewer cases of infant botulism.
- Breastfed infants get ill at an older age than do bottle-fed infants; all cases of sudden infant death syndrome (SIDS) associated with infant botulism have been in bottle-fed infants.
- Food-borne cases are usually associated with the use of home-processed foods—especially vegetables, fruits, and condiments.
- Wound botulism is very rare.

COMPLICATIONS

- The most serious and fatal complication is respiratory failure due to paralysis of the respiratory muscles.
- Bulbar dysfunction in infant botulism may lead to dehydration before presentation.
- The loss of airway protective reflexes can lead to aspiration and pneumonia.
- Constipation and urinary retention may precede the onset of paralysis and may complicate later management as well. Cases of severe *Clostridium difficile* enterocolitis with hypovolemia, hypotension and prolonged ICU stays have been reported in infants with botulism.
- The earliest symptoms in adults and older children may be visual changes, including blurred vision, loss of accommodation, and diplopia.
- SIADH and urinary tract infections have been reported in infants with infant botulism.

PROGNOSIS

Food-borne botulism carries a mortality rate of 20% to 25%. This rate is lower in patients younger than 20 years old (about 10%). Patients with a shorter incubation period usually have more severe involvement and a worse prognosis, probably related to an increased amount of toxin ingested.
If recognized early and treated aggressively, botulism carries a good prognosis, and complete recovery can be expected. Fatigability may persist for up to 1 year.
Infant botulism has an estimated mortality rate of less than 5% in hospitalized patients. Complete recovery can be expected when disease is recognized early and treated appropriately.

Differential Diagnosis

INFECTIONS

- In noninfants, bacterial sepsis, meningitis, poliomyelitis, tick paralysis, and diphtheric polyneuritis.
- In infants, sepsis and meningitis may present in a similar way.

—Absence of fever and a clear sensorium make sepsis and meningitis less likely.

NEUROLOGIC

- Myasthenia gravis usually spares the pupillary response, while it is fatigable in botulism, if not absent.
- In Werdnig-Hoffman disease (type I spinal muscle atrophy), facial muscles are spared.

DRUGS/TOXINS

Drug ingestions may lead to weakness and lethargy.

Data Gathering

HISTORY

- Usually constipation. With a progressive course of lethargy, weakness, and poor feeding.

—Occasionally, the progression may be quite rapid, and the abrupt onset of lethargy and weakness may suggest the diagnosis of bacterial sepsis or meningitis.

- Food-borne cases result in complaints of emesis in about 50% of patients.

—There may initially be complaints of diarrhea followed by constipation.
—The incubation period from ingestion to the onset of symptoms is usually 18 to 36 hours (range, a few hours to several days).
—Patients complain of weakness and dry mouth.
—Visual complaints include blurry vision, loss of accommodation, and diplopia.
—Patients may complain of dysphagia or dysarthria.
—Patients may have urinary retention.
—Fever is absent.
—Within 3 days, there is the onset of the characteristic descending, symmetrical paralysis. The cranial nerves are usually affected first.
—Mentation is clear, except for understandable anxiety and agitation.

Wound botulism has an incubation period of 4 to 14 days.

—Fever may or may not be present.
—Patients often report constipation but rarely nausea or vomiting.
—They may complain of unilateral sensory changes and of purulent discharge from the wound.

Physical Examination

- Older children and adults often appear alert and are afebrile.
- Ptosis, extraocular palsies, and fixed and dilated pupils are often the first signs of descending paralysis. Loss of airway protective reflexes and respiratory muscle weakness lead to respiratory failure.
- The triad of bulbar palsies, a lucid sensorium, and the absence of fever should prompt one to strongly consider the diagnosis of botulism.
- Infant botulism presents in a similar way. Patients are usually afebrile. They are usually weak, with decreased spontaneous activity at presentation. They have an expressionless (masklike) face, ptosis, a weak cry, poor head control, and generalized weakness and hypotonia.
- Pupils are often midposition initially and may be at least weakly reactive. The pupillary response is fatigable. The pupils become fixed and dilated for a period in many cases. Except for the symmetric, descending paralysis, the remainder of the physical examination is normal.
- Signs of autonomic instability include unexpected fluctuations in skin color, blood pressure, and heart rate.

Physical Examination

In infants, early in the course of the disease, pupillary and corneal reflexes may fatigue easily.

Laboratory Aids

TESTS

- Tests for the presence of toxin or the organism can be conducted on patient samples (serum, gastric aspirates, feces, or wound exudate) or suspected foodstuffs.
- Anaerobic cultures of a wound or the GI tract may yield the organism.
- Electromyography (EMG) shows a characteristic pattern of brief duration, sharp amplitude, overly abundant motor unit action potentials (brief short-acting potentials, BSAPs).
- EEG, MRI, and CT are nonspecific and usually normal in the absence of any complications.

Requirements for Testing

- Most tests for toxin and cultures are conducted by state health departments.
- The most common test performed is an assay for botulinum toxin in stool.
- Specimens must be shipped in sealed, break-proof, and leak-proof containers. Even small amounts of toxin, if inhaled or ingested, can lead to disease.
- Suspect foods should be shipped refrigerated and in their original containers if possible.

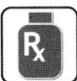

Emergency Care

- Good supportive care with emphasis on respiratory support, including intubation and mechanical ventilation when needed, is the most important consideration in emergency therapy.
- In suspected infant botulism, aminoglycoside antibiotics (e.g., gentamicin) should be avoided as they may produce an abrupt worsening of the weakness and ensuing respiratory failure.

Therapy

- All patients with suspected botulism should be admitted to the hospital and have continuous monitoring of their heart rate, respiratory rate, and oxygenation, as well as frequent assessment of their respiratory effort and airway protective reflexes.
- The mainstay of therapy is meticulous supportive care. Particular attention is paid to respiratory and nutritional needs.
- Endotracheal intubation may be necessary both for patients with frank respiratory failure and when airway protective reflexes are lost.
- Wounds should be explored and debrided and anaerobic cultures should be obtained.
- Cases of suspected toxin ingestion should be treated early with induced emesis and/or gastric lavage in an attempt to decrease toxin exposure.
- All cases should be reported to the state health department and the CDC.

DRUGS

- Antibiotics are not helpful in infant botulism.
- Prompt recognition of infant botulism and early treatment with human intravenous botulism immune globulin (BIG–IV) has been shown to decrease time to recovery and hospital discharge. The FDA approved the use of human BIG–IV for the treatment of infant botulism in 2003. Equine antitoxin is not recommended for infant botulism.
- Antibiotics are indicated only for documented complications such as pneumonia.
- Cathartics are not beneficial, and enemas may cause colonic distension and increased toxin absorption.
- Cases of botulism resulting from ingested toxin or wound infection should be treated with botulism equine trivalent antitoxin (ABE), available from the CDC. Antitoxin should not be administered to asymptomatic individuals who have only eaten suspect foods.
- Wound botulism should be treated with IV penicillin G 250,000 units/kg/day.

DURATION

- In wound botulism, antibiotics should be continued for 10 to 14 days.
- Supportive care should be continued until the patient is able to be weaned from respiratory support and begin PO feedings.

Follow-Up

The nadir of the paresis in infants is usually 1 to 2 weeks after presentation. Infants remain at their nadir for 1 to 3 weeks. Infants are ready for discharge when gag, suck, and swallow reflexes are adequate to protect against aspiration. In food-borne and wound botulism, recovery may be prolonged, with symptoms of fatigability persisting for up to 1 year.

PREVENTION

- Botulinum toxin is heat-labile; 5 minutes of boiling will destroy the toxin.
- Home-canned foods should be boiled for at least 10 minutes before serving.
- Spores are more resistant to heat. Home canners must use temperatures well above boiling to destroy spores effectively (120°C for 30 minutes). Pressure cookers are needed to achieve these conditions.

Common Questions and Answers

Q: Can infant botulism recur?
A: True recurrence in infant botulism has not been documented.

Q: Should antitoxin be given to persons who have ingested food that they think might be contaminated with botulinum toxin?
A: Since the antitoxin carries a significant risk of serum sickness, it should be given only to persons with neurologic symptoms.

Q: Where is antitoxin obtained?
A: Antitoxin may be obtained from the Centers for Disease Control and Prevention, Atlanta, Georgia; 404-639-3753 (days), 404-639-2888 (nights).

Q: Where is human BIG–IV obtained?
A: Human BIG–IV, which is produced from pooled human plasma from screened individuals may be obtained from the California Department of Health Services Infant Botulism Treatment and Prevention Program at 501-540-2646.

ICD-9-CM 005.1

BIBLIOGRAPHY

Infant botulism—New York City, 2001–2002. *MMWR Morby Mortal Wkly Rep* 52(2)24–26: 2003 Jan 17.

Muensterer OJ. Infant botulism. *Pediatr Rev* 2000;21(12):427.

Passaro DJ, et al. Wound botulism associated with black tar heroin among injecting drug users. *JAMA* 1998;279:859–863.

Shapiro RL, Hatheway C, Swerdlow DL. Botulism in the United States: A clinical and epidemiologic review. *Ann Intern Med* 1998;129:221–228.

Author: James M. Callahan

Brachial Plexus and Erb Palsy

 Database

DEFINITION

The brachial plexus is a network of nerves in the neck and shoulder, usually derived from the fifth cervical through the first thoracic nerve roots, consisting of anatomic structures termed trunks, divisions and cords, terminating in specific nerves to individual muscles of the shoulder girdle, arm, and hand. Lesions of the brachial plexus can result in:

• Motor impairment: Weakness, atrophy, and secondary joint contracture
• Sensory impairment: Dermatomal or peripheral nerve distribution
• Functional and cosmetic impairment, limb length discrepancy, chronic pain.

CLINICAL AND ANATOMIC RELATIONSHIPS

• 5th and 6th cervical (C5, C6) nerve roots fuse to form the upper trunk of the plexus.

—C5 impairment causes arm abduction (deltoid and supraspinatus) weakness, while C6 compromise causes weakness of external rotation of the shoulder (infraspinatus), elbow flexion (mainly biceps), and partial supination (supinator) weakness.
—If the lesion is at the C5, C6 root level or very proximal upper trunk, then winging of the scapula (serratus anterior) occurs. The biceps and brachioradialis deep tendon reflexes (DTRs) are depressed or absent.

• 7th cervical (C7) nerve root alone forms the middle trunk of the plexus and is largely responsible for weakness of elbow (triceps), wrist (extensor carpi ulnaris) and finger extension (extensor digitorum), and wrist flexion (flexor carpi radialis).
• 8th cervical (C8) and 1st thoracic (T1) nerve roots fuse to form the lower trunk of the plexus and innervate the intrinsic hand muscles responsible for grip and thumb opposition/abduction. The triceps DTR reflects the C7, C8 roots, but is difficult to obtain in newborns. The pectoralis DTR has the same distribution and is easier to elicit.

NEONATAL "OBSTETRIC" BRACHIAL PLEXUS INJURY

• Erb palsy is the most commonly encountered partial lesion of the plexus seen in children, accounting for approximately 73%–90% of all newborn cases, and occurs in approximately 1 to 4 per 1,000 live births. It involves the C5-6 and sometimes the C7 nerve roots and/or upper-middle trunks of the plexus.

—Risk factors: mainly large for gestational age (gestational diabetes), shoulder dystocia and having a prior infant with Erb palsy.
—Not all cases are due to a traumatic delivery; antepartum compressive causes are well described in a minority of cases.

• Full brachial plexus palsy occurs in approximately 20% neonatal cases and is the most severe form.
• Clinical categories of Erb palsy

(1) *Mild:* Approximately one-third of patients have a mild injury due to stretching of the myelin sheath of the nerve fibers.

(2) *Moderate:* Another third of babies are very weak to fully flaccid at birth due to disruption of axons within the nerve sheaths. This group appears initially like the mild one, but has slower recovery as the axons regrow and reconnect over several months.

Thus, two-thirds of all patients regain full strength and function, with half doing so rapidly (the mild group) and half more slowly (the moderate group).

(3) *Severe:* The remaining third is the most severely affected group, typically with a full flaccid paralysis at birth, no improvement at 2 weeks of age, less than antigravity arm abduction and elbow flexion at 3 months. Ultimately, there is limited to poor return of strength in arm abduction and elbow flexion/extension, with secondary contractures developing and chronic motor impairment.

Ipsilateral diaphragm weakness is seen in about 5%, due to phrenic nerve (C4, C5) compromise. Bilateral arm weakness, typically asymmetric in degree, is noted in about 10%. Torticollis is frequent and facial palsy is seen in about 10%. These do not carry an added unfavorable prognosis.
Associated subluxation of the cervical spine and related spinal cord injury is identified in up to 5% and requires urgent neurosurgical attention. This results in added neurologic deficit. Shoulder subluxation is an urgent orthopaedic issue.

• Klumpke palsy is rare, approximately in 2% of neonatal cases, and is due to C8-T1 nerve root avulsion.

—Risk factors: breech delivery and face presentation.
—Results in a weak hand grip and absent palmar grasp reflex, with preserved shoulder and arm strength. The prognosis is often limited, as root avulsion is more common than with an Erb lesion.

Inherited

• Neuralgic amyotrophy with predilection for the brachial plexus

—Autosomal-dominant inherited condition that maps to a chromosome 17q25.1 locus.
—Episodes of recurrent unilateral or bilateral brachial neuritis begin in childhood and are characterized by recurrent pain followed by weakness, with sensory impairment and absent reflexes.
—There may be mild lumbar involvement or dysmorphic features.
—Attacks are often triggered by recent infection or immunization. It remits spontaneously over weeks to months.

• Hereditary neuropathy with liability to pressure palsy is an autosomal-dominant inherited disorder

Inflammatory

• Postinfectious brachial neuritis:

—Reported following EBV, CMV, West Nile virus, and herpes zoster infection.
—Spontaneous recovery with supportive care is the rule.

• Postimmunization brachial neuritis:
Only the tetanus toxoid component of the DPT immunization has been clearly associated with brachial neuropathy in infants. It resolves fully, but may recur with future such immunizations.

Tumor

• Primary tumors of peripheral nerve in childhood are largely confined to neurofibromatosis.
• Secondary invasion of the brachial plexus from a local tumor, e.g., sarcoma.

 Differential Diagnosis

• Lesions of the brain and spinal cord can produce focal weakness in mainly one limb. Usually the ipsilateral leg will have at least mild findings to indicate a hemiparesis.
• Congenital malformations (Sprengel deformity) and contractures may mimic a BPP.
• Acute orthopaedic problems such as a fracture or a subluxation of the radial head
• Fascioscapulohumeral dystrophy

 Data Gathering

HISTORY

• Pregnancy and birth history, birth weight
• Trauma
• Recent viral infection
• Recent tetanus injection
• Family history; prior similar episodes that have resolved

PHYSICAL EVALUATION

• Testing of tone, strength, muscle bulk, joint range of motion, sensation, muscle stretch reflexes (DTRs) and elicited infant reflexes (Moro, asymmetric tonic neck response), diaphragm excursion, pupil size, pulses, and perfusion of the affected limb. Compare to the other side and the legs as well.
• Sensory loss is difficult to assess when only part of the plexus is impaired, because of overlap of dermatomes.
• Upper plexus lesion, such as Erb palsy (C5-6),

—Upper trunk of the plexus is compromised, typically from trauma, sometimes also with nerve root avulsion.
—Arm hangs limply at the shoulder, adducted and internally rotated, the elbow extended and the forearm pronated, wrist and fingers flexed ("waiter's tip posture").
—Hand grip is preserved.
—Sensory impairment is often present over the lateral deltoid.

—The biceps and brachioradialis muscle stretch reflexes are unelicitable.
—The triceps reflex is preserved (difficult to elicit in normal neonates). Testing the pectoralis reflex is preferred. The Moro reflex is asymmetric.

- Lower plexus lesion, such as Klumpke palsy (C8, T1),

—Compromise from trauma or an apical lung lesion.
—Elbow flexion, supination of the forearm, wrist and finger extension, and an odd cupped-hand position.

- Triceps jerk is often absent.
- Sensation may be impaired in the C8-T1 dermatomes.
- An ipsilateral Horner sign (ptosis and miosis) indicates T1 involvement.
- Complete plexus lesion: the entire upper limb and shoulder girdle is flaccid, anesthetic, and areflexic.
- Acute lesions often have severe pain.

 ## Laboratory Tests

IMAGING STUDIES

- Chest and arm x-ray

—Identifies subluxation of the spine or shoulder, fracture of the humerus or clavicle, and diaphragmatic palsy

- Magnetic resonance imaging (MRI)

—Images the cervical spinal cord, nerve roots, and plexus
—May be valuable in identifying the nature and extent of injury to the brachial plexus and with tumor lesions.
—There are occasional false-positive and negative findings for root avulsion and many plexus lesions are not apparent on MRI.

ELECTROPHYSIOLOGICAL TESTING

- Electromyography (EMG) and nerve conduction velocity studies (NCV) can confirm the localization of the lesion, and whether there has been axonal damage and repair.

 ## Therapy

Mild weakness will recover in most cases without special treatment.
For severe injury, with flaccid shoulder girdle

- Immobilization: babies with a fracture or who have significant pain should have the limb partly immobilized for 2 weeks, to allow for rest during the acute phase of pain.

—Cuff can be pinned to the midline of the jersey at the umbilicus level.

- Caregivers should be instructed in proper lifting and positioning techniques to avoid pressure at the axilla.

- Passive range of motion stretching (PROM) After 3 weeks, immobilization should be discontinued and gentle passive range of motion should be initiated under the supervision of a therapist.

—Fracture or shoulder subluxation needs to be excluded on x-ray before starting PROM.

- Regular visits to a pediatric occupational or physical therapist are necessary.
- Electrical muscle stimulation: External and implantable devices that directly stimulate muscle can potentially prevent atrophy, while awaiting nerve healing and reinnervation. It is not used routinely.

—Alternative therapies, such as acupuncture, have not been studied in any systematic way in this setting. Some parents believe it helps with recovery.

- Surgical issues: Important to identify as early as possible those babies who are not likely to spontaneously recover normal strength and function, so that a timely surgical referral can be considered.

—Serial exams between 1 and 6 months of age and sometimes EMG testing at 3 to 6 months can estimate prognosis.
—For the typical Erb palsy, return of biceps is the single most important prognostic factor in determining whether surgery is indicated.
—Return of external rotation of the shoulder and forearm supination best predicts full recovery of function.
—The critical window of time to consider surgical intervention is at 3 months when the deltoid-biceps remain flaccid and between 6 and 12 months when at least some early recovery of strength is seen. Primary repair of the nerve never results in full functional recovery. It is used when the natural history predicts a poor or limited outcome and an operation will restore some added functional strength.

- Good functional recovery is unlikely to occur spontaneously if by 6 months strength is still less than antigravity in elbow flexion, progress has plateaued, and there is little reinnervation on EMG.

 ## Follow-Up

- The newborn with BPP should be reevaluated at 2 weeks and if not nearly back to normal, then referred for weekly occupational or physical therapy and seen again at 3 months.
- When there is persisting weakness but with steady improvement between 2 weeks and 3 months, the patient is monitored closely with the above prognostic guidelines kept in mind and focusing on therapy to prevent development of contractures. The status at 3 to 6 months will predict whether full functional recovery is likely to occur spontaneously or whether an operation may be indicated.

PROGNOSIS

- Peripheral nerve stretch injury has the most favorable prognosis.
- Axonal disruption with preserved continuity of the nerve sheath (axonotmesis), can recover fully, but is more variable and tends to take longer as axonal regrowth is about 1 mm per day. If the nerve is ruptured and not in continuity (neurotmesis), the prognosis is very poor. Lesions of mixed and partial types can result in recovery occurring in phases. This is why observing the distribution and extent of recovery within the first 6 months is so critical.
- Nerve root avulsion from the spinal cord harbors the worst prognosis.
- Full recovery reported has been reported in 69% to 95% of patients, but has been defined variably in these studies. Probably one-third of Erb palsy patients have some degree of permanent functional impairment.
- Pure C5, C6 Erbs palsy patients do the best as a group.
- Prognosis is more guarded when C7 is involved.
- Involvement of the whole plexus or C8, T1 (Klumpkes palsy) distribution fares least well.

 ## Common Questions and Answers

Q: Will my baby get better?
A: The majority of babies gain full recovery, but this may take several weeks or months. S/he will need to be followed closely to monitor the progress and determine if any therapy or future testing will be necessary.

Q: What if my baby does not get better?
A: About one in three babies have poor or limited recovery in the first few months, in which case we would suggest consulting with a surgeon, to see if an operation to fix the nerve injury will enhance the recovery. In the older child with some functional use of the arm, there may be a role for latter surgery to release contractures, transfer tendons, or stabilize the shoulder joint.

ICD-9-CM 767.6, ERB PALSY

BIBLIOGRAPHY

Hoeksma AF, et al. Neurological recovery in obstetric brachial plexus injuries: an historical cohort study. *Dev Med Child Neurol* 2004;46:76–83.

Pondaag W, et al. Natural history of obstetric brachial plexus palsy: a systematic review. *Dev Med Child Neurol* 2004;46:138–144.

Semin Pediatr Neurol 2000 7 (1). This entire issue is devoted to the evaluation and management of brachial plexus injuries in the newborn and child.

Shenaq SM, et al. The surgical treatment of obstetric brachial plexus palsy. *Plast Reconstr Surg* 2004;113:54e–67e.

Author: Richard S. Finkel

Brain Abscess

Database

DEFINITION

A suppurative infection involving the brain parenchyma; it may be a single (or multiple) lesion.

CAUSES

- Bacteria are the most common causes of brain abscesses.
- *Streptococcus sp.* and *Staphylococcus sp.* are the two most commonly cultured microorganisms.
- Neonates may develop abscesses after a gram-negative meningitis (Proteus, Citrobacter and Enterobacter).
- A single organism is found in about 70% of patients.
- Anaerobic organisms are being found with increasing incidence with improved laboratory and culture techniques. Common pathogens are: Bacteroides, Peptostreptococcus, Fusobacterium, Propionibacterium, Actinomyces, Veillonella and Prevotella.
- No growth of a pathogen occurs in 30% of specimens.
- Parasitic infections are often caused by Taenia solium (neurocysticercosis).
- Fungi and protozoa are commonly found with immunocompromised patients.

PATHOPHYSIOLOGY

- Microorganisms enter the brain parenchyma by contiguous or hematogenous (metastasis) pathways.

LOCATION OF BRAIN ABSCESSES

- Cyanotic congenital heart disease patients tend to have abscesses within the middle meningeal artery distribution: frontal, parietal, and temporal lobes.
- Frontal abscesses are commonly seen with sinus and dental infections.
- Temporal, parietal, or cerebellar abscesses tend to occur with mastoid or otitis media infections.
- Brain abscesses can occur anywhere in the brain parenchyma regardless of a predisposing risk factor secondary to hematogenous metastasis.

PREDISPOSING RISK FACTORS

- Cyanotic congenital heart disease (CCHD)
- Otorhinolaryngologic infections such as sinusitis, mastoiditis and chronic otitis media
- Meningitis (especially with neonates)
- Penetrating head trauma
- Surgical manipulation of the brain (ventriculoperitoneal shunts, tumor removal, etc.)
- Esophageal manipulation (sclerotherapy or dilation)
- Cystic fibrosis
- Dental infections
- Lung infections
- Any site of infection (osteomyelitis, orbital, cellulitis, urinary tract infections, etc.)
- Patients who have traveled to endemic areas with neurocysticercosis (Latin America, parts of Africa, Asia, and the Indian subcontinent)
- Congenital or acquired immunocompromised patients
- No definitive etiology occurs in 30% of patients.

EPIDEMIOLOGY

- Approximately 1,500 to 2,500 cases (adults and pediatric combined) occur per year
- Males are affected more than females (2:1 male to female predominance).
- Average age of presentation is about 7 years of age.
- About 2% to 4% of children with cyanotic congenital heart disease will develop a brain abscess (tetralogy of Fallot being the most common).

COMPLICATIONS

- These arise from the location, size, and number of intracranial abscesses and can vary from SIADH, seizures, to focal neurologic deficits.

PROGNOSIS

- A high index of suspicion is required to diagnose a brain abscess. A delay in diagnosis or performing a lumbar puncture (LP) for suspected meningitis increases mortality and morbidity.
- With the advent of computed tomography (CT) and magnetic resonance imaging (MRI) scans, the mortality rate has dropped from 30% to <14%.
- Multiple abscesses, coma on presentation, less than 2 years of age, performance of an LP, and rupture of abscess into the ventricle carry a higher mortality rate. About 30% to 40% of patients will have some morbidity. This ranges from seizures, hemiparesis, focal neurologic deficits, hydrocephalus to cognitive/behavior problems.

Differential Diagnosis

- Infectious: Meningitis, encephalitis, subdural empyema, epidural abscess
- Vascular: Venous sinus thrombosis, migraine, cerebral infarct, cerebral hemorrhage
- Miscellaneous: Primary or secondary tumor, pseudotumor cerebri, hydrocephalus

Data Gathering

HISTORY

- It should be noted that the location of the brain abscess or abscesses will often influence the history of presentation and physical examination.
- Classic triad of fever, headache, and focal neurologic findings occurs in less than 30% of cases.
- Headache is the most common complaint.
- The average duration of symptoms prior to diagnosis is about 4 weeks.
- Vomiting and mental status changes can often be the presenting chief complaints.
- Neonates will often have a history of meningitis before developing a brain abscess.
- Questions should focus on acute or chronic otolaryngologic infections such as sinusitis, chronic otitis media, and mastoiditis, as well as a history of cholesteatomas.
- Cyanotic congenital heart disease (CCHD) should be determined, as well as a partially repaired CCHD.

Physical Examination

- Neonates may present with a full fontanel, increasing head circumference, seizures, or vomiting.
- Older children may have signs of a focal neurologic deficit, hemiparesis, or even papilledema.
- Meningeal symptoms occur in about 30% of patients.
- Ataxia may be found with cerebellar lesions.

Laboratory Aids

- CBC may be mildly elevated and less than 10% will show a left shift.
- Erythrocyte sedimentation rate (ESR) is a poor indicator of brain abscesses.
- Electrolytes may show low sodium, indicating SIADH.
- A lumbar puncture is contraindicated if any intracranial mass lesion is suspected, but if CSF is obtained, it may show a mild to moderate pleocytosis (20% of patients may have normal values); the opening pressure is always elevated; glucose may be decreased in 30% of patients; the protein is elevated in 70% of cases; and only 10% of cultures are positive, unless the abscess ruptures into the ventricles.

STUDIES

- CT and MRI scans are the studies of choice in diagnosing brain abscesses.
- Cranial ultrasound may be useful in premature neonatal cases.

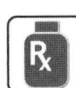
Therapy

- Broad-spectrum antibiotics should be started at the time of diagnosis until identification of the microorganism is determined. At that time, the antibiotics can be tailored to the offending microorganism.
- Most brain abscesses are surgically removed. A few may require CT-guided aspiration.
- When multiple abscesses are found on CT scan, one lesion should be aspirated to determine the identification of the microorganism.
- There are patients successfully managed with antibiotics alone.
- Antiparasitic medications are controversial in the treatment of neurocysticercosis.
- Antifungals should be considered with immunocompromised patients.
- The use of steroids is controversial.
- If a patient is manifesting signs and symptoms of increased intracranial pressure (Cushing triad: bradycardia, hypertension, and abnormal respirations) or if the patient is comatose and is unable to protect his/her airway, the patient should be intubated, hyperventilated, and given mannitol.
- Those patients with unknown predisposing factors should be evaluated by cardiology, dental, and otorhinolaryngology. Immunology should be considered in those children with significant medical histories of chronic infections.

Follow-Up

- Neonates and older patients may be discharged with home physical therapy and home nursing for intravenous antibiotics.
- Patients will need intravenous antibiotics for a total of 3 to 4 weeks. Some may require longer courses of antibiotics.
- Some children will need follow-up CT or MRI scans.
- Follow-up with neurosurgical, rehabilitation, and neurology clinics are usually required.

PREVENTION

- During recreational activities, wearing helmets may prevent penetrating head trauma.
- Preventive medicine: Dentistry and otorhinolaryngology

PITFALLS

- Not all patients with brain abscesses will have fevers.
- Failing to consider a brain abscess in a child with altered mental status, fevers, and meningismus
- Performing a lumbar puncture
- Failing to use contrast with the CT scan

Common Questions and Answers

Q: Do all brain abscesses require surgery?
A: No. Some will regress with antibiotics and follow-up with MRI.

Q: What is the best way to diagnose brain abscess?
A: MRI.

ICD-9-CM 324.0

BIBLIOGRAPHY

Calfee DP, Wispelwey B. Brain abscess. *Sem Neurol* 2000;20:353–360.

Cochrane DD. Brain abscess. *Pediatr Rev* 1999;20:209–214.

Jadavji T, Humphreys RP, Prober CG. Brain abscesses in infants and children. *Pediatr Infect Dis J* 1985;4:394–398.

Kaplan K. Brain abscess. In: Symposium on infections of the central nervous system. *Med Clin North Am* 1985;69:345–360.

Mitchell WG. Neurocysticercosis and acquired cerebral toxoplasmosis in children. *Semin Pediatr Neurol* 1999;6:267–277.

Renier D, Flandin C, Hirsch E, et al. Brain abscesses in neonates. *J Neurosurg* 1988;69:877–882.

Rennels MB, Woodward CL, Robinson WL, et al. Medical cure of apparent brain abscesses. *Pediatrics* 1983;72:220–224.

Saez-Llorens X. Brain abscess in children. *Sem Pediatr Infect Dis* 2003;14:108–114.

Saez-Llorens XJ, Umana MA, Odio CM, et al. Brain abscess in infants and children. *Pediatr Infect Dis J* 1989;8:449–458.

Sidaras D, et al. Neonatal brain abscess-potential pitfalls of CT scanning. *Childs Nerv Syst* 2003;19:57–59.

Author: Jeffrey P. Louie

Brain Injury—Traumatic

 Database

DEFINITION

Traumatic brain injury (TBI) is damage to the brain from accidental or nonaccidental trauma.

- Children >1 year—i.e., Glasgow Coma Score (GCS) <14, amnesia >15 minutes for event, and penetrating head injury
- Children <1 year—any loss of consciousness (LOC), protracted emesis, and suspected abuse
- Severe brain injury usually present with an initial GCS <9

EPIDEMIOLOGY

- Trauma is the number one cause of death of children >1 year. Head injury is the most common contributor to morbidity and mortality.
- Between 29,000 and 50,000 children in the United States less than 19 years old suffer permanent disability from TBI each year.
- Age-dependent mechanism of injury and pathophysiology

—<2 years old—nonaccidental trauma principle cause of TBI
—>2 years old—falls (~37%) most common cause of trauma.
—For severe TBI, nonaccidental trauma remains principal cause in young children.
—Motor vehicle accidents in older children, although penetrating injuries are becoming more common.

PATHOPHYSIOLOGY

Primary—focally applied forces, lacerations, penetration injuries, skull fractures. Contusions, intracerebral hematomas are uncommon. Epidurals, classic subdurals less than 10% in children.
Acceleration-deceleration/shearing forces—cervical spine injuries, diffuse axonal injury (DAI), nonaneurysmal subarachnoid hemorrhage, subdural hematoma from shear forces
Secondary—extension of injury to viable tissue/entire brain. Dysautoregulation of cerebral blood flow, neuroexitotoxicity and inflammatory mediators. CT or MRI signs of edema may progress over 3 to 5 days (see Treatment).

AGE-SPECIFIC PATHOPHYSIOLOGY

Infants and Toddlers

- Shear forces on the brain due to acceleration/deceleration avulses axons from their cell bodies (DAI); often compounded by tearing and bleeding of dural veins.
- Unmyelenation infant brain absorbs rather than transfers impact. Immature, distensible skull renders brain less likely to contuse or herniated, but more likely to sustain diffuse secondary injuries, with swelling.
- Subgaleal hematoma, cephalohematoma (below the periosteum), and caput succedaneum (confined to the superficial scalp) at birth don't predict brain injury.
- More severe birth trauma can result in subdural hematoma.
- Bilateral interhemispheric SDH suggests nonaccidental trauma.
- Diffuse injuries secondary to shaken impact syndrome can lead to cerebral swelling with secondary infarction and/or decreased central respiratory control, leading to apnea, hypoxia, and cerebral edema.
- Children <3 at risk of growing skull fracture when leptomeningeal cyst protrudes through a dural tear (late effect).
- Suspect nonaccidental trauma with growing skull fracture, if more than one cranial bone involved or if other injuries are present.

Older Children and Adolescents

- Still more subject to diffuse axonal injury (DAI) than adults due to incomplete myelination
- Projectile injuries in adolescent population
- Can result from nonaccidental trauma (usually with other stigmata of assault)

 Differential Diagnosis

Neurologic presentation varies in severity from a normal examination through coma similar to hypoxic-ischemic brain injuries (e.g., near-drowning), other causes of stupor/coma, seizure activity (postictal encephalopathy).

- Distinction between simple concussion, DAI, and hypoxic-ischemic injury may be difficult at initial presentation, becoming clear as clinical picture/neuroimaging evolves.

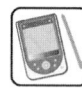 Data Gathering

HISTORY

- Eyewitness accounts are invaluable.
- Details of who was caring for the child
- Falls—Did loss of consciousness precede fall? Height of fall? Surface of impact?
- History of epilepsy, cardiac problems
- History of previous concussions (consider "second impact syndrome") or trauma
- Intoxications (of child, caregiver, others in the environment)
- Prior physical abuse and neglect?
- Restrained motor vehicle passenger? Angle of impact.
- How did patient act or change over time? Unresponsive? Confused? Headache? Visual changes? Vomiting? Seizure?

Emergent Management and Physical Examination

- Airway, Breathing, Circulation
- Prehospital stabilization—avoid hypoxemia and hypotension (strong, possibly modifiable, independent predictors of outcome in TBI)
- Cervical spine stabilization and clearance. In severe TBI entire spine stabilized.

—If necessary, orotracheal intubation with rapid sequence induction. Avoid hypotension.
—Hyperventilation may induce regional cerebral ischemia in children especially in first 24 hours.
—Increased ICP managed by bed elevation 30°, hypertonic fluids, sedation

- Hemodynamic stabilization (normal high systolic BP (~135) predictor of better outcome in TBI). [Median systolic BP = 90 mm Hg + (2 × age in years)]

—Hemodynamic instability indicative of systemic hemorrhage (abdomen, long bone fractures). Pericardial tamponade (narrow pulse pressure). Neurogenic shock.
—Hypotension late sign. Early: ↑HR, ↓ capillary refill, ↓ urine output
—Fluid resuscitate—consider hypertonic saline. Mounting evidence of improved outcomes especially with hemorrhagic shock and TBI. (Titrate continuous 3% saline infusion 0.1 – 1.0 mL/kg/hr)
—Fluid bolus may worsen intracranial hypertension (ICP)
—Considering monitoring intracranial pressure (ICP) to maintain <20 mm Hg) for abnormal admission CT scan, and GCS 3–8 after CPR, or normal CT and GCS 3–8, and posturing, or hypotension, or if serial neurologic exams precluded by sedation
—Maintenance of CPP above 50 positively influences outcome in TBI (MAP − ICP = CPP) especially in first 48 hours.

- A rapid neurologic exam repeated over time is instrumental in directing the patient's care.
- Secondary Survey: External evidence of head injury-deformities, ecchymoses (periorbital-orbital roof fracture; mastoid-petrous temporal fracture), lacerations, penetrations. CSF leak nasal/otic.
- Seizures—Ativan, 0.1–0.2 mg/kg IV @ 2mg/min or rectal Diastat 0.3–0.5 mg/kg if no IV access. Then load fosphenytoin 15–20 mg/kg IV. Important to treat to avoid increase in ICP, neurotoxicity and hypoxia.
- No evidence that seizure prophylaxis >1 week posttrauma prevents late seizures
- No evidence that steroids improve outcome
- Hypothermia may be protective, no difference in long-term outcome.
- No evidence for prophylactic use of mannitol, though it is effective for control of increased ICP
- Bolus doses 0.25 g/kg of body weight to 1 g/kg of body weight to goal ICP <20 mm Hg
- Hypertonic saline for increased ICP as above under fluid resuscitation.
- The postresuscitation GCS score should be recorded in all trauma patients.
- Involvement of neurosurgery with moderate GCS <13 injury, even if patient initially stable.
- Survival for children with severe TBI is greater when treated in Pediatric ICU.

Decompressive craniectomy may be considered given the following conditions:

- Diffuse cerebral swelling on cranial CT imaging
- Within 48 hours of injury
- No episodes of sustained ICP >40 mm Hg before surgery
- GCS >3 at some point subsequent to injury
- Secondary clinical deterioration
- Evolving cerebral herniation syndrome

Rapid Neurologic Exam in Trauma. Can derive some of these by observation. Note presence of neuromuscular blockers/sedation.

Level of arousal—awake, lethargic, stuporous, unresponsive
Resting posture—spontaneous restless, still normal, flexor, extensor
Respiration—in context of arousal and posture, hyperpnea or Cheyne-Stokes respiration
Response to stimulation—voice, pain (of earlobe to avoid spinal withdrawal response) note localization, withdrawal, posturing
Pupils—equal, anisocoria >1 mm, unequal/ sluggish pupil, unequal/wide/fixed pupil

Extraocular movements—disconjugate gaze nonlocalizing with drugs/trauma, 3rd nerve palsy uncal herniation sign, 4th nerve palsy common in head injuries, 6th nerve palsy from trauma or increased ICP.
Brainstem reflexes—Corneals (V & VII), oculocephalic if patient unable to cooperate with eye exam and cervical spine cleared. Avoid gag—raises ICP.
Muscle reflexes/motor examination— lateralizing signs may indicate contralateral hemispheric lesion, with ipsilateral dilated pupil may indicate uncal herniation.
Sensory—brief for four limbs/ spinal level if indicated

This exam should be repeated often according to the patient's level of acuity. A more detailed exam tailored to degree of arousal can be done as the patient is stabilized.

 ## Laboratory/Radiography Aids

- Unenhanced CT scan of the brain is the imaging study of choice for initial evaluation of a patient with suspected traumatic brain injury

—Abnormal CT—lesion density, midline shift, compression of cisterns, bone fragments

- MRI—useful for DAI (with a negative head CT) as well as showing small lesions (e.g., punctate contusions)
- In suspected cervical spine injury where patient is unresponsive, MRI of the spine to R/O noncontiguous unstable ligamentigous injury.
- Long-bone films if degree of injury is not consistent with history or history of fall from unclear height
- With CT scan showing normal brain/ventricular spaces: consider EEG and lumbar puncture if a nontraumatic etiology for altered mental status is suspected.
- In all patients with suspected traumatic brain injury, consider:

—CBC (infants can have a large amount of intracranial blood loss)
—PT/PTT (to evaluate a possible bleeding disorder as a possible preoperative laboratory test)
—Electrolytes
—Toxin screen

PROGNOSIS

- Presence of both hypoxemia and hypotension on arrival to ER bode poorly
- 24 hour GCS better predictor of outcome than post resuscitation, PRISM score also helpful
- GCS <3, poor prognosis unless secondary to epidural hematoma, rapid evacuation can minimize permanent deficits
- Diffuse white matter, subcortical gray or brainstem lesions on MRI portend long periods of coma and poorer outcome
- Somatosensory evoked potentials, (VEPS or BAEPs) are less sensitive but have high specificity in predicting neurologic outcome
- Degree of injury on head CT can be predictive (see Marshall Classification system for head CT)
- Patients who have sustained moderate-to-severe head injury (GCS of 13) often have academic difficulties, memory abnormalities, disinhibition
- Monitoring for cognitive difficulties, hyperactivity, seizures, hydrocephalus, movement disorders, paralysis, visual/hearing disturbance, headache; psychologists, neurologists, neurosurgeon, ophthalmologists, audiologists, and physical therapists may be helpful.
- Leptomeningeal cyst (especially in children <3 years old) almost always develops within 6 months of injury.
- Refer any patient with known skull fracture who manifests a new swelling in area of old fracture to neurosurgery for 3-D CT imaging of the head.
- Approximately 10% of patients with severe head injury will develop epilepsy.

ICD-9-CM 854.0

BIBLIOGRAPHY

Adelson PD, et al. Critical pathway for the treatment of established intracranial hypertension in pediatric traumatic brain injury. *Pediatr Crit Care Med* 2003;4(3 Suppl):S65–S67.

Pollack MM, et al. Pediatric risk of mortality (PRISM) score. *Crit Care Med* 1988;16:1110–1116.

Suspected cervical spine trauma. Reston (VA): American College of Radiology ACR; 2002.

White JR, et al. Predictors of outcome in severely head-injured children. *Crit Care Med* 2001;29:534–40.

Zink BJ. Traumatic brain injury outcome: concepts for emergency care. *Ann Emerg Med* 2001;37(3):318–332.

Authors: Karen LeComte
Todd Maugans, 3rd edition

Brain Tumor

 Database

DEFINITION

A brain tumor is a primary neoplasm arising in the central nervous system (CNS).

PATHOPHYSIOLOGY

- No specific causative agents are known, but there is an association with radiation, chemical exposure, other malignancies, familial/heritable diseases, immunosuppression (lymphoma).
- The majority of tumors are classified based on their histology. The most common:
- Glioma

—Arises from astrocytes (supportive tissue)
—>50% of childhood CNS tumors
—Ranges from benign or low grade (often in the cerebellum or optic pathway) to malignant or grade III to IV (in the cerebrum or brainstem)
—Locally recurrent and invasive when malignant

- Primitive neuroectodermal tumor (PNET)/medulloblastoma

—Malignant embryonal tumor arising from unknown cell type
—Comprises about 20% of childhood CNS tumors
—Most common malignant brain tumor in children
—Majority arise in the midline of the cerebellum (referred to as medulloblastoma)
—Predisposition for leptomeningeal dissemination

- Ependymoma

—Arises from ependymal cells that line the ventricular system
—Comprises about 5% to 10% of childhood CNS tumors
—Most commonly occurs in the fourth ventricle; may arise in the spinal cord
—Locally recurrent and invasive; spinal metastases rare at initial diagnosis

- Germ cell tumor

—Derived from totipotent germ cells
—3% to 5% of childhood CNS tumors
—Majority are located in the pineal or suprasellar region

- Rhabdoid or atypical teratoid tumor

—Rare embryonal tumor arising from unknown cell type; often misdiagnosed as PNET
—Comprises less than 3% of childhood CNS tumors
—Majority arise in children younger than 5 years of age
—Propensity to arise in the posterior fossa with frequent leptomeningeal dissemination; reported in association with malignant rhabdoid tumors of the kidney

- Craniopharyngioma

—6% to 9% of childhood CNS tumors

- Tumors of the choroid plexus
- Ganglioglioma
- Meningioma and hemangioblastoma, rare in children

GENETICS

- Not a heritable condition
- Primary CNS tumors are associated with several familial syndromes:

—Neurofibromatosis (NF) with optic pathway gliomas (NF1) and meningiomas (NF2)
—Tuberous sclerosis with gliomas and rarely ependymomas
—Li-Fraumeni syndrome with astrocytomas
—Von Hippel-Lindau with cerebellar hemangioblastoma
—Turcot syndrome with PNET

EPIDEMIOLOGY

- Most common solid neoplasm of childhood (second to leukemia in overall incidence)
- Incidence rising (about 2,000 new cases/year)
- 2.5 to 4 cases/100,000 children per year
- Peak incidence in children 7 years of age and younger
- Slight male predominance
- Majority arise infratentorially (within cerebellum or brainstem) in children 1 to 11 years of age
- Majority arise supratentorially in children <1 year of age

COMPLICATIONS

- Secondary to disease

—Increased intracranial pressure (ICP)
—Obstruction of cerebrospinal fluid (CSF) flow
—Requires immediate neurosurgical evaluation

- Secondary to radiotherapy

—Neurocognitive sequelae (age- and dose-related)
—Endocrinopathy (growth hormone deficiency, hypothyroidism, gonadal dysfunction)
—Risk of second malignancies (meningioma, glioma, sarcoma)

- Secondary to chemotherapy

—Risks associated with bone marrow suppression (infection, bleeding, anemia)
—Hearing loss
—Risk of secondary leukemia

PROGNOSIS

Dependent on histology of tumor, location, and extent of initial resection.

- Glioma

—Low grade: 70% to 90% 5-year event-free survival (EFS)
—High grade: 16% to 46% 5-year EFS
—Intrinsic pontine: median overall survival of 9 to 13 months from diagnosis

- Medulloblastoma

—60% to 90% survival at 5 years if localized, gross total resection achieved and >3 years old at diagnosis
—30% to 40% survival if disseminated

- Ependymoma

—50% to 70% survival at 5 years with total resection
—Less than 30% survival with subtotal resection

- Infants overall have a worse prognosis, possibly due to the limitations of therapy and/or the aggressiveness of the tumor.

 Differential Diagnosis

- Infection

—Cerebral abscess

- Tumors

—Metastatic tumor to brain uncommon with childhood solid tumors

- Trauma

—Hemorrhage unlikely to be confused with tumor

- Congenital

—Arteriovenous malformation
—Hamartoma
—Dysplastic brain

- Psychosocial

—Some patients with nausea, vomiting, or behavior changes are first diagnosed with psychiatric disorders, gastrointestinal disorders, failure to thrive, or anorexia nervosa prior to discovery of a brain tumor.

 Data Gathering

- Tumor location dictates symptoms and signs

HISTORY

Question: Headache and vomiting (particularly in the morning), irritable, lethargy?
Significance: Associated with increased intracranial pressure (ICP)

Question: Difficulty swallowing, slurred speech, and diplopia?
Significance: Brainstem tumor

Question: Visual field deficits (bumps into things)?
Significance: Optic tract lesion

Question: Focal weakness?
Significance: Pyramidal tract lesion

Question: Ataxia?
Significance: Cerebellar lesion

Question: Changes in behavior or school performance, new-onset seizures, weakness?
Significance: Supratentorial lesion

Question: Polyuria/polydipsia?
Significance: Hypothalamic/pituitary lesion

Question: Failure to thrive, emaciation, euphoria, and increased appetite in an infant?
Significance: Hypothalamic lesion (diencephalic syndrome)

Question: Back pain, extremity weakness, bowel/bladder dysfunction?
Significance: Spinal cord metastases (often seen with PNET/medulloblastoma and germ cell tumors)

 ## Physical Examination

Finding: Macrocephaly, bulging fontanelle, papilledema, impaired upgaze
Significance: Increased ICP

Finding: Focal deficit on neurologic examination
Significance: Localizes mass lesion

Finding: Isolated cranial nerve VI and VII palsies
Significance: Brainstem tumor

Finding: Ataxia, dysmetria
Significance: Cerebellar mass

Finding: Decrease visual acuity, visual field deficit, absent pupillary light response, strabismus
Significance: Optic tract tumor

Finding: Changes in cognitive function, mood, and affect
Significance: Supratentorial lesion

Finding: Impaired upgaze, convergence nystagmus, pupils respond to accommodation but poorly to light
Significance: Pineal lesion (Parinaud syndrome)

Finding: Signs of neurocutaneous disease (e.g., café-au-lait spots, Lisch nodules)
Significance: Syndrome like neurofibromatosis

 ## Laboratory Aids

IMAGING

Test: MRI with and without gadolinium enhancement
Significance: Gold standard for identification, localization, and characterization of tumor

Test: CT
Significance: Can be used as an initial study, but if negative with a high index of suspicion, follow with MRI. Useful to evaluate for hydrocephalus and hemorrhage.

STAGING OF TUMOR

Test: Postoperative head MRI within 24 to 48 hours
Significance: To determine residual disease before postoperative inflammatory changes are prominent

Test: Spine MRI; CSF cytology
Significance: Neuraxis staging for tumors with high risk of leptomeningeal dissemination

Test: α-Fetoprotein (AFP), quantitative β-HCG
Significance: Serum and CSF markers for germ cell tumors

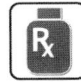 ## Therapy

SURGERY

• Both for histology and to attempt maximal tumor debulking; surgery should be performed by an experienced pediatric neurosurgeon
• Rarely indicated in intrinsic pontine (brainstem) glioma
• Ventriculoperitoneal (VP) shunt when needed for obstructive hydrocephalus (risk of peritoneal seeding minimal)

DRUGS

• Dexamethasone to control increased intracranial pressure (0.5 mg/kg divided q6h)
• Chemotherapy

—Drugs are most often used in combination
—Temozolamide for high-grade glioma
—Cisplatin, CCNU, vincristine for PNET/medulloblastoma
—Carboplatin, vincristine or 6-thioguanine, procarbazine, CCNU, vincristine for low-grade glioma

• New protocols currently under development

—High-dose chemotherapy with stem cell rescue for high-risk PNET/medulloblastoma
—Targeted therapies, angiogenesis inhibitors

RADIATION THERAPY (XRT)

• Volume and dose vary depending on histology.
• XRT to the tumor bed is used for most patients with brain tumors.
• Medulloblastoma/PNET patients need craniospinal XRT. The one exception is in infants and young children (<3 years of age) in whom cognitive deficits from XRT can be devastating.

DURATION OF THERAPY

• Radiation therapy: 6 weeks
• Chemotherapy: 1 to 2 years

POSSIBLE CONFLICTS WITH OTHER TREATMENTS

Chemotherapy can alter anticonvulsant levels.

 ## Follow-Up

• Neurologic deficits can take months to improve or stabilize with permanent deficit.
• Any relapse or worsening of symptoms must be evaluated for tumor recurrence.
• MRI every 3 months the first year, every 6 months for the next 2 years, and annually thereafter. Benefit of routine surveillance imaging is controversial.

PITFALLS

• New onset of psychoses should prompt imaging to rule out tumor.
• Even benign tumors may be life-threatening if their location precludes resection.
• Not referring the patient to a pediatric brain tumor/oncology center at diagnosis (preoperatively). This requires an experienced (pediatric) neurosurgeon.

 ## Common Questions and Answers

Q: Are my other children at risk for getting a brain tumor?
A: No (except in rare cases of certain familial syndromes).

Q: Did something I do cause this?
A: No. In addition, the claims made about high-power lines causing brain tumors or cancer are unproven.

ICD-9-CM 191.9

BIBLIOGRAPHY

Gurney JG, et al. Incidence of cancer in children in the United States. *Cancer* 1995;75:2186–2195.

Packer RJ. Brain tumors in children. *Arch Neurol* 1999;56:421–425.

Phillips PC, Grotzer MA. Brain tumors in children. In: Asbury AK, McKhann GM, McDonald WI, et al, eds. *Diseases of the Nervous System: Clinical Neuroscience and Therapeutic Principles.* 3rd Ed. Cambridge: Cambridge University Press, 2002:1448–1461.

Strother DR, et al. Tumors of the central nervous system. In: Pizzo PA, Poplack DG, eds. *Principles and Practice of Pediatric Oncology.* 4th Ed. Philadelphia: Lippincott Williams & Wilkins, 2002:751–824.

Valentino TL, et al. Pediatric brain tumors. *Pediatr Ann* 1997;26(10):579–587.

Author: Michael J. Fisher

Branchial Cleft Malformations

 Database

DEFINITION

• The fetal branchial apparatus is a foregut derivative and develops in the second fetal week.
• Five paired pharyngeal arches are separated by four endodermal pouches internally and four ectodermal clefts externally.
• Overgrowth of the second through fourth cleft creates the cervical sinus and occurs during weeks 4 and 5.
• Persistence of the cervical sinus produces a spectrum of cysts, sinus tracts, and fistulas.

CLASSIFICATION

• First branchial cleft anomalies

—Site: Anywhere from external auditory canal to angle of mandible, usually superior to or within parotid
—Fistula tract: External auditory canal

• Second branchial cleft anomalies

—Site: Ventral to anterior border of sternocleidomastoid muscle, lateral to carotid sheath, and dorsal to submandibular gland
—Fistula tract: Palatine tonsil

• Third branchial cleft anomalies

—Site: Posterior triangle in middle to lower left side of the neck near level of upper thyroid lobe
—Fistula: Upper lateral piriform sinus wall to lower lateral neck posterior to sternocleidomastoid muscle

• Fourth branchial cleft anomalies

—Site: Close association to thyroid gland and associated with clinical thyroiditis if cyst infected
—Fistula: Apex of piriform sinus to base of neck anterior to sternocleidomastoid muscle

GENETICS

• Familial history of branchial defects occasionally noted

EPIDEMIOLOGY

• Overwhelming majority of cysts in newborns and infants are developmental, whereas in children and adults they are inflammatory or neoplastic.
• Midline malformations are most often thyroglossal duct cysts or dermoids.
• Cysts occurring in the laterocervical region are usually branchial cleft malformations, the most common of these are derivatives of the second cleft, followed by those of the first cleft, of the fourth pouch and thymic cysts.
• Third and fourth branchial cleft anomalies are rare, with most presenting as sinus tracts rather than cysts.
• Suspect congenital anomaly in the clinical setting of recurrent infection.

COMPLICATIONS

• Cysts, sinus tracts, and fistulas can become recurrently infected (especially with abscess formation).
• Surgery is more difficult if there have been previous infections or previous surgery.
• Damage to facial, hypoglossal, and glossopharyngeal nerves or carotid artery can occur during surgical repair.
• Recurrence of the lesion is seen if not fully removed.
• Thyroiditis
• Parotiditis (more common in first branchial arch malformation)

PROGNOSIS

• If lesion completely excised: excellent. Many patients require multiple procedures.

 Differential Diagnosis

CONGENITAL

Anterior Triangle of Neck

• Thymic cyst

Midline and Anterior Triangle of Neck

• Ranula
• Laryngocele
• Sialocele
• Thyroglossal cyst
• Dermoid/teratomatous cyst
• Bronchogenic cyst

Posterior Triangle of Neck

• Lymphangioma
• Hemangioma

INFLAMMATORY

• Adenitis
• Granulomatous disease (sarcoidosis, tuberculosis)
• Lymphoepithelial cysts (HIV)
• Otorrhea
• Parotiditis
• Retropharyngeal abscess
• Thyroiditis

TUMORS

• Lymphoma
• Rhabdomyosarcoma
• Cystic Schwannoma (anterior triangle of neck)

Data Gathering

HISTORY

- Present since birth
- Recurrent neck infections
- Intermittent discharge from neck
- Fever
- Tenderness

Physical Examination

- Mass usually mobile
- Usually a single lesion
- Nonpulsatile
- Lesion usually nontender (unless actively infected)
- Assess for sites of drainage:

—At the anterior or posterior border of the sternocleidomastoid muscle
—In the posterior pharynx at the tonsillar fossa or piriform sinus

Laboratory Aids

Test: CBC with differential
Significance: Increased WBC with left shift seen with infection.

Test: Tuberculin test
Significance: To rule out tuberculosis

IMAGING

Test: Chest radiography
Significance: Assess for hilar adenopathy, suggesting a systemic process (such as tuberculosis or malignancy)

Test: Lateral neck radiography
Significance: Assess for airway compromise (not usually seen)

Test: Ultrasound
Significance: Help differentiate solid masses from cystic masses

Test: Fistulogram
Significance: Inject contrast into the fistula to delineate its course

Test: CT scan of neck
Significance: Superior spatial delineation and definition of anatomic compartment of the lesion

Test: MRI
Significance: More detailed soft tissue characterization and recognition of solid components within cystic masses

Therapy

DRUGS

- Antibiotics are indicated if the defect is infected.

CAUTERIZATION

- Cauterization with Trichloroacetic acid has been tried.

SURGERY

- Excision of the entire lesion
- Surgery should be delayed if infection present.

Follow-Up

- Postoperative follow-up as outpatient for wound inspection
- Observation for recurrence or reinfection

PITFALLS

- Lesion may recur if not completely excised.
- High incidence of reinfection if not properly treated.

Common Questions and Answers

Q: Can the cyst, fistula, or sinus recur?
A: Only a 3% recurrence rate is seen if the lesion is completely excised. A higher rate of recurrence is seen in cases of incomplete excision or with previous surgeries.

Q: Should the lesion be removed as soon as it is discovered?
A: The lesion should not be removed if there is an active infection present; treat the infection first and then schedule elective surgery.

ICD-9-CM 744.41

BIBLIOGRAPHY

Fourth branchial pouch sinus with recurrent deep cervical abscesses successfully treated with trichloroacetic acid cauterization. *Acta Otolaryngol* 2003;123(7):879–882.

Graham A. Development of the pharyngeal arches. *Am J Med Genet* 2003;119A(3): 251–256.

Huang RY, Damrose EJ, Alavi S, et al. Third branchial cleft anomaly presenting as a retropharyngeal abscess. *Int J Pediatr Otorhinolaryngol* 2000;54(2–3):167–172.

Karmody CS. Developmental anomalies of the neck. In: Bluestone CD, Stool S, Kenna M, eds. *Pediatric Otolaryngology*. 3rd Ed. Philadelphia: WB Saunders, 1996:1497–1511.

Langman's Medical Embryology. 6th Ed. Baltimore: Williams & Wilkins, 1990:298–327.

Lev S, Lev MH. Imaging of cystic lesions. *Radiol Clin North Am* 2000;38:1013–1027.

Lusk RP. Neck masses. In: Bluestone CD, Stool S, Kenna M, eds. *Pediatric Otolaryngology*, 3rd Ed. Philadelphia: WB Saunders, 1996:1488–1496.

McGuirt WF. The neck mass. *Med Clin North Am* 1999;83:219–234.

Nicollas R, et al. Congenital cysts and fistulas of the neck. *Int J Pediatr Otorhinolaryngol* 2000;55:117–124.

Nusbaum AO, et al. Recurrence of deep neck infection: a clinical indication of an underlying congenital lesion. *Arch Otolaryngol Head Neck Surg* 1999;125:1379–1382.

Authors: Anita Bhandari and Raezelle Zinman

Breast Abscess

 Database

DEFINITION

Breast abscess is an infection of the breast bud or tissue associated with localized pus and inflammation.
Mastitis is an infection of the breast tissue primarily observed during lactation.

CAUSES

• **Newborn infection:** *Staphylococcus aureus* (most common), group A or B streptococcus, and Gram-negative enteric bacteria, including *Escherichia coli*, *Pseudomonas aeruginosa*, *Proteus mirabilis*, Salmonella species.
• **Adolescent/adult infection:** *Staphylococcus aureus* (most common); *Escherichia coli*, *Pseudomonas aeruginosa*, *Mycobacterium tuberculosis*, *Neisseria gonorrhoeae*, and *Treponema pallidum* are infrequent pathogens.

PATHOPHYSIOLOGY

• **Newborns:** Trauma, breast hypertrophy from maternal hormone, or compromised host defenses enable spread of bacteria that are often colonized in the nasopharynx and umbilicus. The bacteria and/or its toxin, in turn, cause(s) subcutaneous destruction and loculated pus formation.
• **Adolescents/adults:** Trauma (e.g., sexual manipulation, nipple rings, tight-fitting bra, incorrect latching during breast feeding), contiguous spread of a local infection (e.g., mastitis, acne), or underlying structural abnormalities (e.g., mammary duct ectasia, epidermal cysts) cause breast tissue edema and destruction by bacteria and/or its toxin.
• When mastitis is associated with breast feeding, the inflammation inhibits milk release. The stasis of milk, in turn, promotes bacterial proliferation.

EPIDEMIOLOGY

• Affects primarily infants (peak age 1 to 6 weeks) and adolescents.
• Male to female ratio is 1:2 in neonates.
• Bilateral abscesses, seen among neonates, are rare.
• 5% to 11% of women with breastfeeding mastitis will develop a breast abscess.

COMPLICATIONS

• Cellulitis (most common; 5% to 10%)
• Abscess rupture with disseminated infection (e.g., bacteremia, pneumonia)
• Septicemia
• Toxin syndromes (e.g., toxic shock syndrome)
• Necrotizing fasciitis
• Scar formation from mammary gland destruction (associated with a reduced breast size after puberty)

PROGNOSIS

• Most children recover without any sequelae.
• Neonates more likely to have bilateral abscesses (<5% cases).
• Neonates have higher morbidity and complications.

 Differential Diagnosis

PHYSIOLOGIC CONDITIONS

• Breast engorgement (usually bilateral; absence of fever and erythema)
• Mastodynia (painful breast engorgement; associated with ovulatory cycles; cyclic pattern)

INFECTIOUS

• Cellulitis including mastitis (absence of a loculated breast mass)

TUMORS (RARE)

• Fibroadenomas
• Rhabdomyosarcoma
• Non-Hodgkin lymphoma
• Fibrocystic disease
• Intraductal papilloma
• Cystosarcoma phyllodes
• Hemangioma

TRAUMA

• Contusion (firm, tender, poorly defined mass)
• Hematoma (sharply defined mass with ecchymosis)
• Fat necrosis (firm, nontender, circumscribed, mobile mass)

MISCELLANEOUS

• Mondor disease (thrombophlebitis of the subcutaneous veins in the breast; presents with tenderness and pain; associated with trauma; spontaneously resolves)
• Vascular malformation

 Data Gathering

HISTORY

• Ask about history of breast trauma or manipulation, concomitant illness or infections, and patient's immunologic status.
• Constitutional symptoms including irritability and lethargy usually are absent unless the infection involves deeper tissue or the bloodstream (one-third of the cases).
• Salmonella infections present with gastrointestinal symptoms.

 Physical Examination

• Firm, tender breast mass with overlying erythema and warmth. Fluctuant mass may be present.
• Regional adenopathy
• Purulent nipple discharge (rare)
• Necrotizing fasciitis is distinguished from breast abscess by pain out of proportion of cutaneous signs, crepitation, or presence of straw-colored bullae.

 Laboratory Aids

Test: Gram stain and culture of nipple discharge, needle aspirate, and/or surgical incision and drainage.
Significance: Helps guide therapeutic decisions if a fluctuant mass or discharge is present.

Test: Blood culture
Significance: Useful in neonates. Consider full sepsis workup if patient is febrile and toxic appearing.

Test: Complete blood count (CBC)
Significance: Leukocytosis (>15,000 cells/mm^3) is present in one-half to two-thirds of patients.

Test: Surveillance cultures of nasopharynx and umbilicus
Significance: Consider in neonates to rule out colonization with *Staphylococcus aureus*.

RADIOGRAPHIC STUDIES

Test: Ultrasound
Significance: May be useful if fluctuant mass is suspected or if poor response to antimicrobial therapy.

Breast Abscess

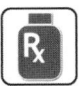 Therapy

Guided by clinical course as well as the pathogen isolate from a needle aspirate, surgical drainage, and/or nipple discharge. Outpatient therapy should be reserved for well-appearing adolescents who are able to tolerate oral therapy.

DRUGS

Neonatal Infection

• Parenteral β-lactamase-resistant anti-staphylococcal antibiotics (e.g., ceftriaxone 50–75 mg/kg/24 hr).
• Aminoglycosides (e.g., gentamicin 2.5 mg/kg/dose every 8 to 12 hours) should be included if the infant is ill-appearing or if the Gram stain reveals Gram-negative bacilli.

Adolescent Infection

• Parenteral antistaphylococcal antibiotics (e.g., nafcillin 50–100 mg/kg/24 hr; maximum 12 g/24 hr).
• Consider clindamycin (450–1,800 mg/24 hr orally with max dose 1.8 g/24 hr; 1,200–1,800 mg/24 hr parenterally with max dose 4.8 g/24 hr) in patients with penicillin allergies.
• Consider adding aminoglycosides in situations as described above.

Duration

• Usually for 10 to 14 days.
• Length of parenteral treatment is based on isolate and the clinical response. Oral agents may be used after a few days if a good clinical response occurs.

SURGERY

• Incision and drainage if a fluctuant mass is present.
• Surgical exploration is necessary if necrotizing fasciitis is suspected.

OTHER

• Warm compresses
• Analgesics (e.g., nonsteroidal antiinflammatory agent) help control the inflammation and pain in older children.
• Continuation of breast milk expression helps prevent engorgement and further milk stasis.

 Follow-Up

Clinical improvement should be evident after 48 hours of parenteral antibiotics.

SIGNS

• A poor or delayed clinical response to antibiotic therapy suggests a resistant organism, an unusual pathogen, or a different diagnosis.
• An evolving fluctuant mass warrants surgical intervention.
• Reaccumulation of fluctuant mass.
• Toxic appearance, prolonged fever, purulent discharge, or progressive erythema postoperatively.
• Crepitation associated with excessive pain and/or straw-colored bullae suggests necrotizing fasciitis.

PREVENTION

• Avoid breast manipulation (including piercing).
• Establish good breastfeeding techniques.
• Early recognition and treatment of mastitis.

PITFALLS

• Neonatal infections require prompt recognition, intervention, and identification of other involved sites to avoid poor outcome.
• Unrecognized fluctuant mass and its subsequent drainage will delay therapeutic response.
• Incidence of community-acquired methicillin resistant *Staphylococcus aureus* (MRSA) is increasing in some regions of the country.

 Common Questions and Answers

Q: How can you differentiate a breast abscess from mastitis?
A: Although both illnesses involve signs of inflammation (warmth, erythema, swelling, tenderness), a breast abscess is distinguished from mastitis by a firm, well-defined mass (with or without fluctuant material).

Q: Should a mother discontinue breastfeeding if she has a breast abscess?
A: Breastfeeding should be continued unless impeded by a surgical incision site or the overall clinical condition of the mother in order to avoid milk stasis.

Q: What is the role of homeopathic remedies (e.g., belladonna, *Phytolacca*) in the treatment of mastitis and breast abscess?
A: Currently, insufficient scientific evidence exists to support their routine use.

Q: Are anaerobic organisms common pathogens for breast abscesses?
A: No. Although anaerobic pathogens are isolated in up to 40% of infections, their role is controversial and therapy directed at them is unnecessary.

ICD-9-CM 611.0

BIBLIOGRAPHY

Barbosa-Cesnik C, et al. Lactation mastitis. *JAMA* 2003;289:1609–1612.

Bodemer C, Panhans A, Chretien-Marquet B, et al. Staphylococcal necrotizing fasciitis in the mammary region in childhood: a report of five cases. *J Pediatr* 1997;131:466–469.

Dixon JM. Repeated aspiration of breast abscesses in lactating women. *BMJ* 1988;297:1517–1518.

Greydanus DE, Parks DS, Farrell EG. Breast disorders in children and adolescents. *Pediatr Clin North Am* 1989;36:601–638.

Michie C, et al. The challenge of mastitis. *Arch of Dis in Childr* 2003;88:818–821.

Walsh M, McIntosh K. Neonatal mastitis. *Clin Pediatr* 1986;25:39–399.

Author: Charles A. Pohl

Breast-feeding

 Database

DEFINITION

Lactation is the process of milk secretion that begins during the sixth or seventh month of pregnancy.

Involution is the cessation of milk secretion that occurs when regular extraction of milk from the mammary gland ceases and prolactin is withdrawn.

Feeding positions:

Cradle rest—the infant's head rests in the mother's arm on the side that she will nurse from, and the infant's stomach is level with and facing the mother's stomach.
Football hold—the infant's head is in the mother's hand or on her forearm, with the infant's feet and legs tucked behind the mother's arm toward her back, like holding a football.
Cross-cradle—the mother's opposite hand (left hand for right breast and right hand for left breast) supports the back of the infant's head, neck and shoulders. The infant is on his/her side with the stomach facing the mother.
Side-lying—the mother is lying down on her side facing the infant who is also lying on his/her side.

PHYSIOLOGY

• Milk synthesis begins in the sixth or seventh month of pregnancy.
• With the delivery of the placenta at birth, estrogen and progesterone levels fall and prolactin levels rise, leading to increased milk synthesis.
• When the neonate is placed to the breast and begins suckling, the neuroendocrine reflex is triggered, causing oxytocin to be released. Oxytocin causes the cells that line the breast ducts to contract, expelling milk from alveoli into ducts and subareolar sinuses that empty into a nipple pore—this is known as the milk ejection or "let down" reflex. If milk is not expressed, the breast becomes engorged and milk production diminishes.
• Breast milk during the first several days after birth is primarily composed of *colostrum*. The onset of the production of *transitional milk* is usually described by mothers as the time when their milk "came in" and can occur anywhere from 2 to 5 days until 10 to14 days after birth. *Mature milk* usually begins at the end of the first week after birth.
• Mature milk is composed of *foremilk* (the milk first drawn during a feeding, which is usually low in fat content with more protein) and *hindmilk* (the milk that follows foremilk, which contains more fat and a higher caloric content). Foremilk is designed to quench the infant's thirst while hindmilk provides the nutritional content necessary for adequate growth. This is the reason it is important to emphasize adequate emptying of the breast with feedings.

• Successful breast feeding can be negatively affected by cesarean delivery. Medications given during cesarean delivery may also hinder milk production. Postoperative pain may make positioning of the infant more difficult.
• Breast milk from mothers of premature infants contains greater amounts of antibodies and nutrients than breast milk from mothers of term infants and may provide protection against infection and necrotizing enterocolitis.

EPIDEMIOLOGY

• In the United States in 2001, 69.5% of women report some breast feeding at birth, and 32.5% reported some breast feeding at 6 months.
• There are racial/ethnic differences in rates of breast feeding: African-American mothers are less likely (52.9% in hospital vs. 72.2% for whites and 73% for Hispanics) to breastfeed and tend to breastfeed for a shorter (21.9% at 6 months vs. 34.2% for whites and 32.8% for Hispanics) durations of time than white or Hispanic mothers.
• Breastfed infants have a decreased incidence of otitis media, diarrhea, respiratory infections, sudden infant death syndrome, and necrotizing enterocolitis.

COMPLICATIONS

Mother

• Engorgement
• Obstructed milk duct
• Mastitis
• Nipple pain: Multiple causes, but most commonly due to improper positioning of the infant at the breast and nipple candidiasis.
• Insufficient milk syndrome: Due to anatomic breast variations or medical illness (e.g., retained placenta), difficulty latch-on because of engorgement or positioning, and inappropriate infant feeding routines.

Infant

• Poor weight gain
• Jaundice
• Dehydration
• Hypernatremia

 Data Gathering

HISTORY

Question: How often and for how long does the baby nurse?
Significance: Infants feeding less than 8–12 times every 24 hours may have inadequate milk intake. Those who nurse for less that 10 minutes or greater than 50 minutes during the first few weeks of life may be receiving inadequate amounts of milk due to inadequate milk production or ineffective suckling, respectively.

Question: Does the mother have problems positioning the baby at the breast?
Significance: Poor positioning at the breast can lead to inadequate milk intake.

Question: Is the baby able to latch onto the breast, and does the baby have a strong suck when latched onto the breast?
Significance: Inability of the infant to latch on may result in inadequate milk intake.

Question: How many wet diapers per day is the baby having?
Significance: Failure to produce at least 6 adequate wet diapers per day by 4 days of age requires further investigation.

Question: Does the mother experience the sensation of "let down" when nursing?
Significance: The sensation of "let down" is a good indication that the infant has good position at the breast and is receiving milk; though some women who are successful at breastfeeding report that they never feel the "let down" sensation.

Question: Is the family using supplemental feedings?
Significance: Supplemental feedings may contribute to inadequate milk supply for mothers concerned that the baby isn't getting enough milk. In contrast, mothers who are adamant about breastfeeding may not recognize the need for supplemental feedings.

Question: Will the mother be returning to work soon?
Significance: Mothers planning to continue breastfeeding after returning to work may consider pumping and storing breastmilk for future use. Mothers wishing to discontinue breastfeeding upon returning to work should be informed about weaning to prevent problems with engorgement and leaking.

Question: Does the mother have social support for breastfeeding?
Significance: External supports contribute to the success of breastfeeding.

 Physical Examination

Finding: Weight.
Significance: To ensure that the infant has adequate weight gain. Weight loss of 7%–8% or more from birthweight, failure to surpass birthweight by 2 weeks of age, or failure to commence weight gain of approximately 25 to 30 g per day by 5 days of age warrants further investigation.

Finding: Jaundice.
Significance: May be prolonged or exaggerated if there is inadequate intake and delayed or inadequate stooling.

Finding: Oral thrush.
Significance: May cause or be due to nipple candidiasis, which often presents as nipple soreness.

Finding: Membranous cleft palate or other abnormalities of the mouth.
Significance: May result in inadequate milk intake and/or breastfeeding difficulties that can lead to poor weight gain and dehydration

Finding: Signs of dehydration.
Significance: Breastfed infants are at risk for hypernatremic dehydration that may be unrecognized by parents.

Finding: Direct observation of feeding.
Significance: Poor positioning at the breast or ineffective latch can lead to inadequate milk intake.

 Laboratory Aids

Test: Prefeeding and postfeeding weight.
Significance: Quantitative assessment of adequate milk intake at feedings.

Test: Electrolytes (if clinically indicated).
Significance: Breastfed infants are at risk for hypernatremic dehydration.

Test: Bilirubin level (if clinically indicated).
Significance: Breastfed infants are at risk for jaundice. May also be an indicator for inadequate nutritional status.

 Therapy

- Frequent and effective milk removal is essential for establishing and maintaining an adequate milk supply, as well as rest and hydration for the mother. Lactating mothers should continue to take their prenatal vitamins.
- Support: Breast-feeding mothers should be connected with local supports to enhance the likelihood of breast-feeding success. Potential resources include lactation consultants/specialists, local breast-feeding support groups (usually sponsored by hospitals), local La Leche League chapters (www.lalecheleague.org).
- Engorgement: Treatment includes reassurance that the symptoms will resolve, and regular emptying of the breast, either by frequent breast-feeding, if possible, pumping or manual expression. Warm showers and/or compresses may be effective to help express breast milk.
- Sore nipples: Usually due to improper position or latch-on technique or both. Prenatal and postnatal education help prevent this from occurring. When nipple trauma occurs that results in pain, expressed breast milk can be applied to the nipple to facilitate healing. Purified lanolin may also aid in the healing process. The underlying cause of the pain must be identified and addressed. Occasionally mothers may experience nipple candidiasis, which may be treated with topical antifungals effective against *Candida albicans*. Simultaneous treatment of the infant for oral Candidal infection is also recommended.

 Follow-Up

- Prevention of breast-feeding difficulties should include timely follow-up after hospital discharge. The American Academy of Pediatrics recommends that infants discharged less than 48 hours after delivery be seen by a pediatrician or other knowledgeable health care practitioner at 2 to 4 days of age.
- It is important for health care professionals to recognize maternal risk factors for breast-feeding problems, such as age greater than 37 years; lack of previous breast-feeding experience; cracked or bleeding nipples, or severe or persistent nipple pain; failure of milk to "come in" by 4 days postpartum.
- Infant risk factors for and signs of breast-feeding problems include: prematurity (including borderline premature infants born 36–37 weeks gestation); sleepy, nondemanding infant behavior and the need to be awakened for feedings; weight loss; not passing yellow, seedy stools by 4 days of age; less than 6 clear voids per day by 4 days of age; failure to surpass birthweight by 10–14 days of age; and poor weight gain.

Contraindications to Breastfeeding

- In the United States, mothers with HIV are advised not to breastfeed.
- Mothers newly diagnosed with infectious tuberculosis should not breastfeed until they have received 2 or more weeks of treatment.
- Infants with galactosemia should not breastfeed.
- Maternal medications that are contraindicated during breast-feeding include: Recreational drugs, bromocriptine, cyclophosphamide, cyclosporine, ergotamine, lithium, and methotrexate.

 Common Questions and Answers

Q: How do I know if my baby is getting any breast milk?
A: The infant will have rhythmical and deep suckling in short bursts separated by pauses. You will hear regular swallowing and usually see movement at the jaw angle. If the infant's cheeks are puckered inward or you hear clicking noises, the infant may not be latched on correctly.

Q: How often should I nurse my baby and how long should a nursing session last?
A: Newborns should not go longer than 2–3 hours between feedings during the daytime or 4 hours at night-time. A nursing session should last as long as possible, but generally 10 to 15 minutes per side once breast-feeding is well established. Newborns may need 20 to 30 minutes per side. Stopping a baby from nursing before he/she is finished may interrupt the supply-and-demand rhythm of breast-feeding. Shorter, timed nursing periods may not allow your infant the full benefits of breast milk and may lead to engorgement and other complications. If nursing sessions are too short (<10 minutes) or too long (>50 minutes) your infant may not be receiving enough milk due to ineffective suckling or low milk production.

Q: I want to give my infant breast milk when I return to work. When should I begin giving my infant expressed breast milk?
A: An ideal time to introduce your baby to expressed breast milk in a bottle is during the second month of life. Introduction of a bottle before 3–4 weeks of life can lead to "nipple confusion." Allowing the infant drink breast milk from a bottle will likely provide a smoother transition when you return to work.

Q: What is the "Baby Friendly Hospital Initiative?"
A: The Baby Friendly Hospital Initiative is an international program of the World Health Organization (WHO) and the United Nations Children's Fund (UNICEF) to recognize hospitals and birth centers that have made efforts to provide an environment that promotes and supports breast-feeding. For more information, see www.babyfriendlyusa.org.

BIBLIOGRAPHY

Lawrence RM, Lawrence RA. Given the benefits of breastfeeding, what contraindications exist? *Pediatr Clin North Am* 2001;48: 235–251.

Meek J. *American Academy of Pediatrics: New Mother's Guide to Breastfeeding.* New York, New York: Bantam Books; 2002.

Neifert MR. Prevention of breastfeeding tragedies. *Pediatr Clin North Am* 2001;48: 273–297.

Neville MC. Anatomy and physiology of lactation. *Pediatr Clin North Am* 2001;48: 13–34.

Prachniak GK. Common breastfeeding problems. *Obstet Gynecol Clin North Am* 2002;29:77–88.

Sinusas K, Gagliardi A. Initial management of breastfeeding. *Am Fam Physician* 2001;64: 981–988.

Wight NE. Management of common breastfeeding issues. *Pediatr Clin North Am* 2001;48:321–344.

Zembo CT. Breastfeeding. *Obstet Gynecol Clin North Am.* 2002;29:51–76.

Author: Ivor Braden Horn

Breast-Feeding Jaundice and Breast Milk Jaundice

 Database

DEFINITION

Early-onset breast-feeding jaundice (BFJ) and late-onset breast milk jaundice (BMJ) are the two major overlapping causes of jaundice in otherwise healthy breastfed infants.

- BFJ: Associated with inadequate breast-feeding; exaggerated early onset (3 to 5 days), physiologic, unconjugated hyperbilirubinemia (>12 mg/dL)
- BMJ: Associated with being fed breast milk; late onset (1 to 6 weeks), unconjugated hyperbilirubinemia (>10 mg/dL)

PATHOPHYSIOLOGY

Bilirubin is a breakdown product of hemoglobin and other heme-containing proteins. In newborns, the shorter lifespan of a larger number of erythrocytes, the immaturity of the bilirubin uptake and conjugation system in the liver, and the increased enterohepatic circulation (initiated by a more rapid hydrolysis of the conjugated bilirubin to the unconjugated form) contribute to hyperbilirubinemia and physiologic jaundice.

- BFJ: Inadequate intake of milk and calories with or without relative dehydration leading to increased intestinal bilirubin absorption and enterohepatic circulation
- BMJ: Several hypotheses proposed but remain unproven. Factors found in the milk of some mothers of infants with BMJ include:

—Pregnanediol isomer: Steroid metabolite of progesterone, competitive inhibitor of hepatic glucuronyl transferase
—Increased concentrations of nonesterified (free) fatty acids that inhibit hepatic glucuronyl transferase)
—Factors that increase enterohepatic circulation of bilirubin
—Also defects in bilirubin uridine diphosphate-glucuronosyltransferase gene (UGT1A1) may be associated with BMJ.

EPIDEMIOLOGY

- BFJ is likely to be the predominant cause of early-onset jaundice; however, often difficult to distinguish from jaundice related to other causes because of considerable overlap.
- BMJ affects 10% to 30% of breastfed newborns during the second to sixth weeks of life.

GENETICS

- BFJ: Subsequent siblings of infants with jaundice are more likely to develop jaundice
- BMJ: Mutations in the bilirubin uridine diphosphate-glucuronosyltransferase gene have been identified in a Japanese population and were felt to be associated with breast milk jaundice.

COMPLICATIONS

- BFJ and BMJ: Kernicterus (bilirubin encephalopathy; extremely rare), characterized acutely by opisthotonus and seizures, and on a more chronic basis by hearing loss, upward gaze palsy and cerebral palsy
- Cessation of breast-feeding
- Parental and health care provider anxiety

PROGNOSIS

- BFJ and BMJ: Excellent if hyperbilirubinemia identified and treated appropriately; however, both evaluation and treatment may contribute to interruption of breast-feeding and increased parental anxiety, leading to cessation of breast-feeding

 Differential Diagnosis

INFECTION

- Sepsis (jaundice is usually not the sole presenting sign)

HEMATOLOGIC

- Blood group incompatibility
- Rh incompatibility
- Erythrocyte enzyme defects [e.g., glucose-6-phosphate dehydrogenase (G6PD) deficiency]
- Erythrocyte membrane defects (e.g., hereditary spherocytosis)
- Polycythemia

GASTROINTESTINAL

- Intestinal obstruction (e.g., meconium ileus, Hirschprung disease, pyloric stenosis)

CONGENITAL

- Transient familial neonatal hyperbilirubinemia

METABOLIC

- Hypothyroidism
- Galactosemia
- Gilbert syndrome
- Crigler-Najjar syndrome

MISCELLANEOUS

- Dehydration
- Cephalohematoma
- Maternal oxytocin use

 Data Gathering

HISTORY

Question: How is early infant feeding?
Significance: Infrequent and difficult breastfeeding are predictors of breast-feeding jaundice. Many such infants have increased enterohepatic circulation and dehydration reflected by delayed passage of meconium and significant weight loss. Poor intake also delays stooling, which contributes to increased enterohepatic circulation of bilirubin.

Question: Is there a family history of jaundice in a sibling?
Significance: Prior history may indicate similar risk factors and genetic propensities for developing jaundice. Severe neonatal jaundice suggests familial or inherited hemolytic disease.

Question: Are there relatives with a history of anemia, gallbladder disease or splenectomy?
Significance: Hemolytic anemias constitute an inheritable cause of severe and prolonged jaundice.

Question: Are there maternal risk factors?
Significance: Maternal illness (e.g., diabetes) and medication use (e.g., oxytocin) are associated with jaundice. Infants born to mothers positive for Group B streptococcus are at increased risk for neonatal sepsis.

Question: Are there birth-related risk factors?
Significance: Sepsis should be included in the differential diagnosis for presence of fever, prolonged rupture of amniotic membranes or cloudy or malodorous amniotic fluid. Traumatic delivery, including the use of instruments such as forceps or vacuum, may result in jaundice because of associated bruising and cephalohematoma formation.

Question: When did jaundice become noticeable?
Significance: Jaundice before 24 hours of age suggests a hemolytic process or infection. Early jaundice beyond 24 hours is associated with BFJ while prolonged jaundice beyond 1–2 weeks suggests BMJ.

Question: How is the infant doing?
Significance: Infants with breast milk jaundice are in good health, vigorous, eating well and gaining weight.

 Physical Examination

Jaundice generally progresses from the face to the lower extremities in proportion to rising serum bilirubin concentrations.

Finding: Cephalohematoma, facial bruising
Significance: May contribute to hyperbilirubinemia

Finding: Increased respirations, cyanosis, grunting, nasal flaring, intercostal retractions
Significance: May suggest infection

Finding: Hepatosplenomegaly
Significance: Suggests infectious, metabolic or severe hemolytic causes of hyperbilirubinemia

Finding: Abdominal distension
Significance: Suggests intestinal obstruction

Finding: Dry mucus membranes and skin tenting
Significance: Consistent with dehydration and may contribute to BFJ

Finding: Well-appearing older infant who is gaining weight
Significance: Consistent with BMJ

Laboratory Aids

Generally, minimal laboratory evaluation is necessary in a healthy breastfed infant with mild to moderate jaundice in the absence of risk factors for other causes of jaundice. However, BFJ and BMJ are diagnoses of exclusion. The following tests should be considered depending on the clinical presentation:

Test: Total serum bilirubin
Significance: Quantification of bilirubin levels can assist in diagnosis and choice of therapy (e.g., phototherapy); bilirubin must be measured in all infants with very early jaundice <24 hours of age; serum bilirubin level recommended in all infants with persistent jaundice.

Test: Conjugated serum bilirubin
Significance: Elevated conjugated bilirubin (>1 mg/dL or 10% of total serum bilirubin) may indicate infection, biliary obstructive disease, cholestasis, metabolic disease or severe hemolysis.

Test: Maternal blood type and Rh status; and infant blood type and Coombs test from cord blood if indicated (mother's blood type is O and/or Rh is negative)
Significance: Identification of risk for hemolytic anemia from blood type and/or Rh incompatibility, with considerations for treatment at lower levels of total serum bilirubin.

Test: Complete blood count and smear
Significance: Assessment of the hematocrit will diagnose polycythemia or anemia, and the smear is helpful to look for signs of hemolysis. Decreases in hematocrit over time may reflect ongoing hemorrhage or hemolysis. An abnormal white cell count may indicate infection

Test: G6PD activity
Significance: G6PD deficiency is common worldwide and a rapid increase in bilirubin may occur later than in other types of hemolytic disease; risk of kernicterus seems to be higher in infants with G6PD deficiency, indicating consideration of treatment at lower levels of total serum bilirubin.

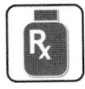

Therapy

Goal of therapy is to maintain the total serum bilirubin concentration at a level to minimize the risk of encephalopathy.

• BFJ: Increase frequency of breast-feeding to 10–12 times per day during the first 3 days of life.
• Supplement with formula if significant feeding problems or poor milk production.
• Phototherapy if serum bilirubin levels exceed the American Academy of Pediatrics recommended threshold levels for phototherapy for full term infants based upon infant's age in hours (i.e., implement phototherapy for infants 25–48 hours old if total serum bilirubin ≥15 mg/dL; 49–72 hours old if bilirubin ≥18 mg/dL; >72 hours old if bilirubin ≥20 mg/dL); for infants <24 hours, phototherapy is recommended if bilirubin > half of infant's age (in hours).
• Phototherapy may contribute to dehydration; therefore, it is essential to monitor hydration status.
• Consider partial exchange blood transfusion for infants 25–48 hours old and total serum bilirubin above 25 mg/dL and for infants ≥48 hours old and total serum bilirubin above 30 mg/dL. Exchange transfusion should be considered in conjunction with phototherapy.
• Home phototherapy poses less of an obstruction to effective breast-feeding than hospitalization, and may be an option in certain circumstances (i.e., stable social situation, treatable level in the absence of other risk factors, etc).

BMJ:

• Continue observation
• Refrain from complete or partial interruption of nursing and the feeding of formula
• If bilirubin >20 mg/dL and/or evidence of significant starvation or dehydration, consider supplementation with formula or interruption of breast-feeding temporarily and substitution with formula; and/or administration of phototherapy. Depending on the degree of dehydration, some infants may require intravenous fluid resuscitation.

SUPPORTIVE CARE

• BFJ and BMJ: Monitor serum bilirubin levels closely.
• BFJ: Lactation consultation
• BMJ: Close observation

DURATION OF THERAPY

• BFJ and BMJ: Continue treatment until serum bilirubin levels consistently within acceptable levels.

Follow-Up

WHEN TO EXPECT IMPROVEMENT

• BFJ: If phototherapy instituted, significant improvement in jaundice expected within 24 hours
• BMJ: After temporary interruption of breastfeeding for 24 to 48 hours

PROGNOSIS

• Generally excellent prognosis for BFJ and BMJ.
• Bilirubin encephalopathy (kernicterus) extremely rare if serum bilirubin ≤30 mg/dL in infants who are otherwise well.
• Increased risk for hyperbilirubinemia in subsequent siblings.

PITFALLS

• Visual assessment of jaundice may be inaccurate.
• Thresholds for starting phototherapy are lower for infants with hemolytic diseases, including G6PD deficiency and Rh incompatibility; and for premature infants and infants who are ill, because kernicterus occurs at lower levels of bilirubin than in newborns without these risk factors.
• Discharge follow-up at 48–72 hours of age, especially for breastfed infants, important to identify significant hyperbilirubinemia given decreasing duration of postpartum hospital stay

Common Questions and Answers

Q: Will my baby have developmental or neurologic problems afterwards?
A: Not from jaundice, if hyperbilirubinemia appropriately monitored and treated.

Q: Will exposure to sunlight decrease the level of jaundice?
A: Yes. However, avoid prolonged exposure and direct sunlight to avoid sunburn. Periodic indirect sunlight (e.g., exposure in a warm sunlit room) is sufficient.

Q: Should I stop breast-feeding?
A: The frequency of breast-feeding should be increased and appropriate lactation consultation obtained for BFJ. Early frequent breast-feeding can decrease the risk. For BMJ, temporary cessation of breast-feeding will lower the total serum bilirubin; however, this recommendation should be considered along with supplementation with formula and phototherapy only if total serum bilirubin is ≥20 mg/dL.

ICD-9-CM CODES

Breastmilk jaundice: 774.39

Neonatal physiologic hyperbilirubinemia: 774.6

BIBLIOGRAPHY

American Academy of Pediatrics Subcommittee on hyperbilirubinemia. Management of hyperbilirubinemia in the newborn 35 or more weeks of gestation. *Pediatrics* July 2004;114:297–316.

Gartner LM. Breast feeding and jaundice. *J Perinatol* 2001;21:S25–S29.

Hannon PR, et al. Persistence of maternal concerns surrounding neonatal jaundice. *Arch Pediatr Adolesc Med* 2001;155:1357–1363.

Hintz SR, et al. Serum bilirubin levels at 72 hours by selected characteristics in breastfed and formula-fed term infants delivered by cesarean section. *Acta Paediatr* 2001;90:776–781.

Author: John I. Takayama

Breath-Holding Spells

 Database

DEFINITION

Breath-holding spells (BHSs) are nonseizure events consisting of involuntary breath holding, which may be associated with loss of consciousness, color change, and tonic and/or clonic movements. Generally they are associated with an inciting event.

- BHSs are categorized as cyanotic or pallid, depending on the child's color during the event. Each type has a different pathophysiology.
- BHSs associated with tonic and/or clonic movements are termed complicated or severe breath-holding spells. True seizures associated with BHSs are called anoxic-epileptic seizures.

ETIOLOGY

Cyanotic

- Often triggered by a noxious stimulus (e.g., pain, fright, frustration or anger).
- Crying becomes interrupted during exhalation (a Valsalva maneuver), followed by cyanosis, and sometimes loss of consciousness.
- The combination of hypocapnia caused by crying, decreased cardiac output associated with a Valsalva maneuver during exhalation, and hypoxia leads to a cyanotic BHS.

Pallid

- Primarily caused by painful stimuli
- Generally not associated with crying
- Associated with a short period of asystole
- Likely due to autonomic dysfunction, specifically an excess vagal response to painful stimuli
- Anemia may play a role in the etiology of both types of BHSs, but the mechanism is unknown.

EPIDEMIOLOGY

- Approximately 5% of children will experience a BHS.
- No difference between genders.
- There is a positive family history for BHSs in 25% to 35% of children.
- Approximately 50% to 60% of BHS patients experience cyanotic BHSs, 20% to 30% have pallid BHSs, and 20% have both.
- Complicated BHSs may be seen in about 15% of children with BHSs
- Age of onset: first month of life to early childhood, with a peak between 6 and 24 months.
- Frequency peaks between 12 and 18 months, with up to several episodes per day, before episodes disappear by 4 to 6 years of age.

COMPLICATIONS

- There are no serious long-term sequelae associated with BHSs.
- Approximately 15% of children who experience pallid BHSs in early childhood may have syncopal episodes in later childhood or adolescence.
- Reports of deaths associated with BHSs exist, but are extremely rare and generally seen in children with other complex medical problems.

 Differential Diagnosis

NEUROLOGIC

- Seizures/epilepsy—only rarely associated with inciting stimuli

BEHAVIORAL

- Temper tantrums

PSYCHIATRIC

- Panic attacks—rarely occur in young children
- Munchausen syndrome by proxy

CARDIAC

- Long Q-T syndrome

 Data Gathering

HISTORY

Obtaining the historical features and details surrounding the event is crucial to making the diagnosis.

Question: Was there an inciting stimulus (pain, anger, frustration)?
Significance: BHSs are always associated with an inciting event.

Question: If the child had a seizure, in what sequence did the episode occur?
Significance: Children with complicated BHSs will have a seizure only after they have been breath holding. An event that begins with a seizure is unlikely to be a BHS.

Question: How do the parents respond to an episode?
Significance: Behavioral problems, such as temper tantrums, will worsen if the child experiences significant secondary gain.

Question: Is there a family history of BHSs?
Significance: 25% to 35% of children with BHSs have a positive family history.

Question: Is there a family history of syncope during exercise or sudden cardiac death?
Significance: Either of these two findings should raise concerns for Long Q-T syndrome.

 Physical Examination

Finding: Physical examination, including detailed neurological examination is normal
Significance: Any cardiac or neurologic abnormality should suggest an alternate diagnosis.

Laboratory Aids

Usually no tests are needed for uncomplicated BHS

Test: Complete blood count (CBC)
Significance: Iron-deficiency anemia is associated with some BHSs.

Test: Electrocardiogram (ECG)
Significance: Long Q-T syndrome is a potentially fatal cause of syncopal episodes. If the history is not classic for a BHS, an ECG should be performed.

Test: Electroencephalogram (EEG)
Significance: May be helpful in ruling out seizures if the history is not classic for a BHS

Test: Ocular compression with EEG/ECG
Significance: Children with BHSs often experience asystole and stereotypical EEG changes with ocular compression. However, the risk of retinal detachment and prolonged asystole requires that this only be performed by an experienced clinician, generally a neurologist, in a controlled setting with pediatric advanced life support available.

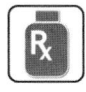

Therapy

- Inform parents that BHSs are unharmful, short episodes.
- Place the child in the lateral recumbent position during a spell.
- Prolonged unconsciousness (>1 minute) warrants emergency medical evaluation.
- Reassure parents that regular discipline should not be avoided for fear of provoking a BHS.
- In extremely rare, severe cases of pallid BHSs, pacemaker implantation has been used successfully to prevent asystole during a spell.

DRUGS

- Iron: has been shown to be effective in reducing frequency of BHSs, particularly in children with associated iron deficiency. However, some non-iron-deficient children have responded to iron therapy as well. The use of iron for children with BHSs who are not iron-deficient must be balanced against the risks of therapy. The usual dose of iron replacement is 4 to 6 mg/kg/day for 2 to 3 months or until the patient is iron replete.
- Atropine: Should be reserved for children with particularly severe or frequent BHSs. The dose is 0.01 mg/kg/day ÷ b.i.d., but no oral preparation is currently available in the United States.
- Anticonvulsants: Can be considered for children with prolonged anoxic-epileptic activity associated with BHSs. However, anticonvulsants have no effect on the BHSs.

Follow-Up

- Only limited follow-up is required.
- Follow-up visits should concentrate on reassuring and educating parents about the benign nature of BHSs.

PITFALLS

- If the history is classic for a BHS, avoid overexuberant laboratory evaluations
- If secondary gain related to the BHS is large, their frequency may increase
- Children experiencing a BHS almost never require cardiopulmonary resuscitation.

Common Questions and Answers

Q: Are breath-holding spells dangerous?
A: No. Although frightening to watch, BHSs are benign and do not result in any long-term sequelae.

Q: Should all patients with BHSs undergo laboratory evaluation?
A: Recent evidence does support an evaluation for iron-deficiency anemia, but further work-up (EEG, ECG) should be reserved for the unusual case without classic historical features.

Q: Should all children with BHSs receive iron therapy?
A: It is clear that any child with BHSs and iron-deficiency anemia should be treated with iron. However, evidence is less persuasive for children without underlying iron deficiency. In this situation, the risks and benefits of iron therapy for each patient must be considered

ICD-9-CM: 786.9

BIBLIOGRAPHY

Breningstall GN. Breath-holding spells. *Pediatr Neurol* 1996;14:91–97.

Daoud AS, Batieha A, Al-Sheyyab M, et al. Effectiveness of iron therapy on breath-holding spells. *J Pediatr* 1997; 130(4):547–550.

DiMario FJ. Prospective study of children with cyanotic and pallid breath-holding spells. *Pediatrics* 2001;107:165–169.

Evans OB. Breath-holding spells. *Pediatr Ann* 1997;26:410–414.

Kelly AM, et al. Breath-holding spells associated with significant bradycardia: successful treatment with permanent pacemaker implantation. *Pediatrics* 2001;108(3):698–702.

Lombroso CT, Lerman P. Breathholding spells (cyanotic and pallid infantile syncope). *Pediatrics* 1967;39(4):563–581.

Author: Paul S. Matz

Bronchiolitis

 Database

DEFINITION

Also see Respiratory Syncytial Virus
Acute lower respiratory tract infection
causing obstruction of the small to medium
conducting airways of the lung.

PATHOPHYSIOLOGY AND CAUSES

- Respiratory syncytial virus (RSV) is the
most common cause of this illness (50% to
90% of those infants hospitalized).
- Other agents associated:

—Human parainfluenza viruses, Influenza
virus, Adenovirus, Human metapneumovirus,
Rhinovirus, *Mycoplasma pneumoniae*
(in older children)

RSV is transmitted by:

—Close contact with infected secretions,
large particle aerosols, and fomites, leading to
—Self-inoculation of conjunctivae or nose
with infected hands
—Secretions remain infectious on
countertops and stethoscopes for up to
6 hours, rubber gloves for $1\frac{1}{2}$ hours, and on
hands or tissue for about 30 minutes

EPIDEMIOLOGY

- In the United States, occurs from late fall
through the winter and early spring. The RSV
epidemic season begins earlier in the
Southeastern United States, and in some
areas (e.g., Florida, Hawaii) can occur
throughout the year.
- RSV infects most children within the first
2 years of life; 57% of those hospitalized are
younger than 6 months.
- Mortality associated with primary RSV
infection in otherwise healthy children has
been estimated to be 3.1 deaths per 100,000
person years in infants less than 1 year of
age, and is approximately 1% to 3% among
children with underlying conditions.
- Risk factors for acquisition of RSV infection
- Patient groups at high risk of severe RSV
disease:

—Premature infants (<35 weeks' gestation)
—Infants <6 weeks of age at time of RSV
infection
—Congenital heart disease, chronic lung
disease, low birth weight, cystic fibrosis
—Compromised immune function (from
chemotherapy, transplant, congenital or
acquired immunodeficiencies)

PROGNOSIS

- For most previously healthy infants,
prognosis is good.
- Premature infants 32–35 weeks gestation
hospitalized for bronchiolitis have been
shown to have an increased number of
subsequent hospitalizations for respiratory
problems, a greater number of outpatient
visits, and an increased risk of sudden death

compared with those who were not
hospitalized for bronchiolitis.
- Mortality associated with primary RSV
infection in otherwise healthy infants is
0.005% to 0.02%.
- Up to 50% of infants with bronchiolitis
develop subsequent episodes of recurrent
wheezing until 11 years of age.
- Bronchiolitis obliterans may be a sequela in
a few patients infected with adenovirus or
mycoplasma pneumoniae.

 Differential Diagnosis

- Pneumonia (viral or bacterial)
- Asthma
- Gastroesophageal reflux (GER)
- Foreign body aspiration
- Exposure to noxious agents (chemicals,
fumes, toxins)
- Congestive heart failure
- Cystic fibrosis

INDICATIONS FOR HOSPITALIZATION

- Historical risk factors for severe disease

—<2 months of age
—Gestational age younger than 35 weeks
—Underlying cardiopulmonary disease (e.g.,
hemodynamically significant heart disease,
bronchopulmonary dysplasia)
—Immunodeficiency or other high-risk group
for developing severe disease

- Clinical risk factors for severe disease

—Presence of apnea, tachypnea (respiratory
rate >70/min), retractions, poor feeding,
pallor, lethargy or agitation (signs of
impending respiratory failure)
—Pulse oximetry <95% in room air
—Atelectasis on chest radiograph

 Data Gathering

HISTORY

Question: Rhinorrhea with clear to white
copious nasal secretions?
Significance: Characteristic of disease

Question: Coughing?
Significance: Initially hoarse cough for
3–5 days; Progresses to deep wet cough of
increased frequency

Question: Poor feeding?
Significance: Early sign of respiratory fatigue;
may lead to dehydration

Question: Restlessness or lethargy?
Significance: May indicate impending
respiratory failure (hypoxemia and/or
CO_2 retention)

Question: Apnea?
Significance: Can be sole presenting sign in
younger infants, or if respiratory distress is
present, suggests impending respiratory
failure

Question: Cyanosis/color change or increased
work of breathing?
Significance: Impending respiratory failure

 Physical Examination

- Interactive versus ill-appearing
- Paroxysmal cough (most common sign), not
associated with "whoop"
- Nasal flaring
- Nasal congestion with copious secretions
- Pattern of breathing: Presence or absence
of apnea or periodic breathing
- Tachypnea

Significance: >70/min is associated with
severe illness

- Nasal flaring and accessory muscle use
- Intercostal retractions (increased
resistance, decreased compliance); subcostal
retractions (hyperinflation)
- Thoracoabdominal asynchrony
- Hyperresonance to percussion
- Diffuse, high-pitched heterophonous
wheezing
- Prolonged expiratory phase
- Fine inspiratory crackles (may be heard in
both bronchiolitis and pneumonia)
- ± Diffuse rhonchi
- Signs of dehydration
- Low-grade fever
- Tachycardia
- Bradycardia associated with apnea
- Possible cyanosis of nailbeds and oral
mucosa
- Liver and spleen typically caudally
displaced by hyperinflated lungs

 Laboratory Aids

BLOOD TESTS

Test: Pulse oximetry

Test: Arterial blood gas

Test: RSV serology (acute and convalescent
serum samples)

RAPID VIRAL IDENTIFICATION

- Best samples for testing

—Nasopharyngeal aspirate
—Nasopharyngeal wash

- Adequate samples for testing

—Nasal swab
—Tracheal aspirate
—Bronchoalveolar lavage fluid

- Rapid tests

—Immunofluorescence (direct or indirect IFA)
—>85% sensitivity and specificity
—Results in 45 minutes

Enzyme immunoassay (EIA)

—60%–90% sensitivity
—70%–95% specificity
—Results in 15 to 30 minutes
—Does not require the presence of viable virus

VIRAL CULTURE

Test: Culture of nasopharynx
Significance: Considered "gold standard." May take up to 14 days for results

IMAGING

Chest radiography: findings include

- Hyperinflation, flattened diaphragms, peribronchial thickening, patchy or more extensive atelectasis, possible collapse of a segment or a lobe, diffuse interstitial infiltrates commonly seen

Therapy

GENERAL MANAGEMENT

- Most cases are mild and may be treated at home.

SUPPORTIVE OUTPATIENT MANAGEMENT

- Adequate fluid intake
- Maintenance of nasal airway patency:

—Short-term nasal decongestant
—Suction secretions with suction bulb

SUPPORTIVE INPATIENT MANAGEMENT

- Careful fluid hydration; deficit plus ~2/3 maintenance fluids

Supplemental Oxygen

- Given to any patient with hypoxemia
- Preferably warmed, humidified, by nasal cannula, head box or tent

MANAGEMENT TO OVERCOME AIRWAY OBSTRUCTION

Bronchodilators

- Some, but not all infants with bronchiolitis will improve clinically with bronchodilator administration. A trial of an aerosolized β-adrenergic agent with critical assessment to see if there is any relief of symptoms is reasonable.
- Infants with history of prior wheezing or familial history of asthma or atopy are more likely to respond to bronchodilators.
- Theophylline is not usually useful as a bronchodilator in bronchiolitis, and may potentially worsen GE reflux, if present.

Nebulized Epinephrine

- Potentially beneficial in infants with moderate to severe bronchiolitis. It has combined α- and β-receptor agonists.

- Both racemic epinephrine (0.1 mL/kg of 2.25% solution) and L-epinephrine have been studied separately and showed beneficial results compared with β-agonists.

Anticholinergic Agents

Ipratropium bromide has not been shown to be effective in the treatment of bronchiolitis.

Corticosteroids

- In previously healthy infants, corticosteroids are not routinely recommended.
- Effects of steroids may be greater in infants with more severe disease or impending respiratory failure.
- Use of inhaled corticosteroids does not decrease duration of symptoms or recurrence of cough and wheezing after acute bronchiolitis resolves.

Leukotriene Modifiers

- No studies have evaluated the use of leukotriene modifiers during the acute phase of bronchiolitis.

Mucolytics

- Recombinant human DNase and N-acetyl cysteine are not effective

Surfactant

- Shown to prevent progression of deterioration in lung mechanics in a small number of infants with respiratory failure requiring mechanical ventilation secondary to RSV bronchiolitis

Antibiotics

- Not usually indicated
- Other than otitis media, the incidence of concurrent serious bacterial infection (pneumonia, meningitis, sepsis) is <2% in healthy infants with no underlying disease who have RSV bronchiolitis.

Antiviral Agents (Ribavirin)
See Respiratory Syncytial Virus
Immunoprophylaxis
See Respiratory Syncytial Virus

- The major means of preventing bronchiolitis is strict observance of infection control, with frequent handwashing, avoidance of known ill contacts and crowded places during the winter months for infants at risk of severe disease, and if possible, avoidance of daycare and secondhand smoke during the bronchiolitis season.

Follow-Up

WHEN TO EXPECT IMPROVEMENT

- Most infants with no underlying disease improve within 3 to 5 days. In some, nasal congestion and cough may continue for 1 to 3 weeks. Premature infants and those with

underlying cardiopulmonary disease typically experience a protracted illness.
- Those who need mechanical ventilation may have difficulties with extubation due to excessive secretions and atelectasis.

SIGNS TO WATCH FOR

- Impending respiratory failure (increased work of breathing, retractions, hypoxemia, CO_2 retention, lethargy).
- Sudden deterioration suggesting atelectasis due to mucous plugging.
- Fatigue may occur in infants who have prolonged and extensive disease.
- Fatigue will manifest with increased pCO_2 and worsening hypoxemia.

PITFALLS

- Hypoxemia is common, so always follow oxygen saturation.
- In cases of clinical bronchiolitis, causes of false-negative ELISA tests:

—Poor quality of sample, sample contamination, insufficient sample, non-RSV bronchiolitis

Common Questions and Answers

Q: How did my child get bronchiolitis?
A: RSV bronchiolitis is a common, seasonal, lower respiratory tract infection that is easily transmissible.

Q: Can my child become reinfected?
A: Children can become reinfected with RSV bronchiolitis, and infection can occur more than once during the same respiratory season.

Q: Do patients with bronchiolitis need to be isolated?
A: RSV-positive patients need to be isolated with other RSV-positive patients and from uninfected patients. Patients receiving ribavirin should be kept in isolation.

ICD-9-CM 466.1

BIBLIOGRAPHY

Bertrand P, et al. Efficacy of nebulized epinephrine versus salbutamol in hospitalized infants with bronchiolitis. *Pediatr Pulmonol* 2001;31:284–288.

Hall CB. Respiratory syncytial virus and parainfluenza virus. *N Engl J Med* 2001;1917–1928.

Meissner HC, Long SS. Revised indications for the use of palivizumab and respiratory syncytial virus immune globulin intravenous for the prevention of respiratory syncytial virus infections. *Pediatrics* 2003;112:1447–1452.

Weisman LE. Populations at risk for developing respiratory syncytial virus and risk factors for respiratory syncytial virus severity: infants with predisposing conditions. *Pediatr Infec Dis J* 2003;22:S33–S39.

Author: Howard B. Panitch

Bronchopulmonary Dysplasia

 Database

DEFINITION

Subsequent improvements in the care of premature neonates have decreased incidence of severe bronchopulmonary dysplasia (BPD), as described by Northway, et al., and many authors have proposed refinement in the original definition, making the precise definition of BPD somewhat controversial.

PATHOPHYSIOLOGY

- Barotrauma is the result of positive-pressure applied to a surfactant-deficient lung, causing unequal pressures and thus unequal aeration of the tracheobronchial tree.
- Terminal bronchioles and alveolar ducts are prone to damage and rupture when subjected to higher than normal pressures.
- Ruptured bronchioles can lead to pulmonary interstitial emphysema (PIE), which increases the risk of BPD sixfold.
- Free radical damage is increased in premature lung, from hyperoxia and impaired antioxidant activity.

GENETICS

- Premature infants with a strong familial history of asthma and eczema are more likely to develop BPD.
- There is an association with HLA-A2.

EPIDEMIOLOGY

- Risk is inversely proportional to birth weight.
- Rare in infants weighing more than 1,500 g; common in infants weighing less than 1,000 g.
- Most common form of chronic lung disease in infancy.

COMPLICATIONS

- Prolonged intubation may cause subglottic stenosis and tracheomalacia.
- Pulmonary hypertension may occur as a result of vasculature damage and subsequent intimal proliferation, which may, in turn, produce right ventricular hypertrophy and, if severe enough, cor pulmonale.
- Pulmonary edema often occurs secondary to increased pulmonary capillary permeability and increased pulmonary pressures.
- Reactive airways, bronchospasm, and altered pulmonary mechanics due to a poorly compliant lung may result in abnormal pulmonary function testing and increased work of breathing.
- Malnutrition and growth failure may occur as a result of increased work of breathing and a subsequently high caloric expenditure.
- Impaired lung defenses result in an increased susceptibility to infection, especially respiratory syncytial virus (RSV).

PROGNOSIS

- Majority of survivors demonstrate slow, steady improvement.
- High death rate (17%–47%) for patients with severe disease requiring prolonged mechanical ventilation.
- Despite multiple and varied treatment modalities, none has shown significant impact on the long-term outcome of chronic BPD.
- BPD survivors often have long-term pulmonary sequelae including hyperinflation, reactive airways, and exercise intolerance.
- Even older children and young adults who were felt to be asymptomatic have been shown to have abnormal responsiveness to exercise.
- Newer technologies, in particular the use of high-frequency ventilation and the wide-spread use of exogenous surfactant, have definitely improved survival rates for premature infants; however, concomitant reduction in the incidence and severity of BPD has been difficult to demonstrate.

 Differential Diagnosis

- Asthma
- Bronchiolitis obliterans
- Congenital heart disease
- Cystic adenomatoid malformation
- Cystic fibrosis
- Idiopathic pulmonary fibrosis
- Infections
- Meconium aspiration syndrome
- Recurrent aspiration

 Data Gathering

HISTORY

- Maternal use of antenatal steroids?
- Gestational age, birth weight, APGAR score?
- Initial resuscitative efforts, need for intubation, use of surfactant, duration in intubation, type of ventilation, duration of supplemental oxygen therapy, and other factors? These may have influenced the type and degree of lung injury.
- Familial history of asthma, atopy, or other children with BPD?
- Social support structure?
- Any potentially exacerbating factors such as exposure to smoking?

 Physical Examination

- Review of systems to include careful assessment of work of breathing both at rest and during activity.
- Feeding and sleeping history, and a review of growth charts.
- Vitals to include respiratory rate and pulse oxymetry both at rest and with activity.
- Signs of pulmonary hypertension, including peripheral edema, hepatomegaly, and venous distension.

 Laboratory Aids

Test: Changes on chest radiography
Significance: Include hyperinflation, emphysema, cyst formation, pulmonary edema, fibrosis, and cardiovascular changes. The severity of these changes may help predict the severity of the disease.

Test: Electrocardiogram
Significance: Often followed serially to assess for right ventricular hypertrophy (RVH).

Test: Echocardiogram
Significance: Often a useful adjunct to follow those patients with RVH.

Test: Cardiac catheterization
Significance: Reserved for those patients with evidence of pulmonary hypertension and cardiac dysfunction.

Test: Pulmonary function testing
Significance: Often used to follow patients and evaluate responsiveness to interventions.

Test: Blood gases
Significance: Useful both in the acute and chronic management of BPD to follow the degree of hypoxia and hypercapnia.

Test: Bronchoscopy, barium swallow, PH probe, and sleep studies
Significance: May reveal other underlying conditions possibly contributing to pulmonary dysfunction.

 Therapy

DIURETICS

- Diuretics are used for treating pulmonary edema, often improving lung mechanics and gas exchange.
- Furosemide may have other nondiuretic benefits, including effects on prostaglandin synthesis, direct vasodilatation, and improved surfactant production.
- There are many side effects from long-term furosemide therapy including azotemia, ototoxicity, electrolyte abnormalities, excessive urinary calcium loss, osteopenia, and nephrocalcinosis.
- Thiazide diuretics, usually used in conjunction with a potassium-sparing diuretic such as spironolactone, are generally considered to be not as effective as furosemide.
- Routine monitoring of electrolytes recommended for patients on long-term diuretic therapy.
- Electrolyte supplementation often required with long-term diuretic usage.

BRONCHODILATORS

- Inhaled β-agonists are effective treatment for reversible bronchospasm, though the safety and efficacy of long-term usage of these agents has yet to be established.
- Albuterol is often the drug of choice, though longer acting agents often used as well.

- Muscarinic antagonists, such as ipratropium, may be useful adjuncts, especially in patients who are not significantly responsive to albuterol. Felt to work on large- and medium-sized airways.
- Cromolyn, though not a bronchodilator, is often used for its antiinflammatory effects and has a low side-effect profile.
- Methylxanthines, such as caffeine and theophylline, are often used in the treatment of apnea because of their effects on respiratory drive, also have a mild diuretic effect and help improve diaphragmatic contractility, making them a potentially useful adjunct in BPD as well.

PULMONARY VASODILATORS

Supplemental oxygen is an effective vasodilator and remains a mainstay of treatment for infants with either chronic or intermittent hypoxia.

STEROIDS

- Steroid usage in BPD is controversial.
- Increased risk for sepsis has probably been overstated.
- Often used successfully in short regimens to wean ventilatory support and hasten extubation.
- No long-term benefits of steroid therapy have been demonstrated, including reduced hospitalization, improved survival, or reduced incidence of BPD.
- Inhaled steroids may provide the desired antiinflammatory effects, without systemic side effects, making them attractive as both prevention and treatment, although their routine use in premature infants is an active area of investigation. Linear growth retardation has been a concern. Newer agents that can be nebulized are now available, improving drug delivery in small infants.

NUTRITION

- Infants with BPD may have increased caloric needs as much as 150 kcal/kg per day
- Premature and critically ill infants may be deficient in antioxidants such as vitamin A, vitamin E, and superoxide dismutase (SOD).
- Supplementation of vitamin A, vitamin E, and SOD at therapeutic and supratherapeutic levels have not yet shown to affect outcomes in BPD, though antioxidant supplementation remains an area of ongoing research.

 Follow-Up

- A multidisciplinary approach is recommended for all patients with moderate and severe BPD.
- Team may include primary care physician, pediatric pulmonologist, pediatric cardiologist, nutritionist, speech, respiratory, occupational, and physical therapists.
- Monitor growth and nutritional status.
- Monitor neurodevelopmental status, including NICU "high-risk" follow-up.

PREVENTION

- Antenatal steroids for all mothers with irreversible preterm labor, less than 35 weeks' gestation.
- Surfactant administration clearly improves mortality, though a reduction in the incidence or severity of BPD has been difficult to demonstrate.
- A change in ventilatory strategy toward "permissive hypercapnia," which favors the acceptance of lower pH and higher P_{CO_2} in exchange for lower peak inspiratory pressures and less barotrauma, has been widely adopted.
- High-frequency ventilation, with either oscillatory or jet technology, may prevent barotrauma, though has yet to be shown to affect the incidence or severity of BPD.
- Avoidance of pulmonary edema, including the prophylactic and early treatment of patent ductus arteriosis may be of benefit.
- Early nutritional support, including the supplementation of antioxidant vitamins and minerals at therapeutic and supratherapeutic levels, may be of benefit.

PITFALLS

- Ensure adequate calcium and phosphorus intake in patients at risk for hyperparathyroidism and ricketts.
- Patients less than 2 years old are candidates for RSV immune globulin prophylaxis, if not contraindicated.
- Patients older than 6 months are candidates for influenza vaccine, if not contraindicated.
- Chest physiotherapy may cause pathologic fractures in patients with osteopenia.

 Common Questions and Answers

Q: Will antibiotics help my child?
A: While some evidence suggests that infection with ureaplasm may be important in the pathogenesis of BPD, it remains to be seen whether or not treatment of this particular organism affects outcome. Excessive usage of antibiotics increases occurrence of antibiotic resistance.

Q: Which babies should get RSV immune globulin (Respigam or Synagis)?
A: Immunoprophylaxis has been recommended by the AAP Committee on Infectious Diseases for infants with BPD who are less than 2 years old at the onset of RSV season. Other premature infants may be candidates as well, regardless of their BPD status, according to their gestational age at birth and their age at the onset of RSV season. Those infants who were born at 28 weeks or less at the onset of RSV season and who are 12 months or less should receive immunoprophylaxis monthly for the entire RSV season. Those infants who were born between 29 and 32 weeks' gestation and who are 6 months old or younger at the beginning of RSV season should also receive immunoprophylaxis. Those in between 32 and 35 weeks may or may not be candidates depending on other risk factors, such as day-care attendance, exposure to tobacco smoke, and the number of other small children in the home.

Q: Will anti-RSV immunoprophylaxis prevent my baby from getting RSV?
A: It won't prevent RSV, but it will help your child's own immune system attack the virus.

Q: Will my child have asthma when he grows up?
A: Asthma occurs in over 50% of older children who survived BPD.

Q: What types of additional therapies can help my child?
A: Chest physiotherapy may be of benefit in infants with both early and late BPD, helping to mobilize secretions and to prevent atelectasis. Speech and occupational therapy may be of benefit as infants who have had prolonged intubation or other interventions that may have interfered with oral functioning may have some degree of oral-motor dysfunction and oral aversion. Other infants simply with increased work of breathing may have uncoordinated suck and swallow, making oral feedings difficult. Physical therapy may be of benefit to help infants with gross and fine motor delays, poor tone, and abnormal posture. Parents can learn many of the therapies in order to incorporate therapeutic exercises and positioning into their daily routines.

ICD-9-CM 770.7

BIBLIOGRAPHY

Bader D, Ramos AD, Lew CD, et al. Childhood sequelae of infant lung disease exercise and pulmonary function abnormalities after bronchopulmonary dysplasia. *J Pediatr* 1987; 10:693–699.

Bancalari E, et al. Bronchopulmonary dysplasia: changes in pathogenesis, epidemiology and definition. *Seminars in Neonatology* 2003;8(1):63–71.

Hageman JR. Neonatology Update. *The Pediatric Clinics of North America.* Philadelphia: WB Saunders, 1998.

Jobe AH, Ikegami M. Prevention of bronchopulmonary dysplasia. *Curr Opin Pediatr* 2001;13(2):124–129.

Northway WH Jr, Rosan RC, Porter DY. Pulmonary disease following respiratory therapy of hyaline membrane disease. *N Engl J Med* 1967;276:357–368.

Vaucher YE. Bronchopulmonary dysplasia: An enduring challenge. *Pediatrics in Review* 2002;23(10):349–358.

Author: John M. Good

Bruxism

 Database

DEFINITION

Bruxism is a nonfunctional grinding of the teeth. It is a poorly understood phenomenon with many suggested etiologies. It is usually a subconscious activity that can occur during the day or night. Clenching is a related condition that also is considered to be a nonfunctional habit. Nonfunctional (or "parafunctional") habits include mandibular movements not involved with normal chewing, swallowing, or speaking. Some examples of these include chewing pencils, nail, cheek, or lip biting.

INCIDENCE

• Bruxism may occur throughout life. Its frequency tends to peak up to the ages of 7 to 10 and thereafter decreases with age.
• Infants have been known to brux with the eruption of the first primary tooth. Bruxism may sometimes be temporarily or intermittently present, making diagnosis difficult.
• Incidence of bruxism in children has been reported to be from 5% to 88% (with most reports indicating an average of 15% to 30%)

ETIOLOGY

The exact cause of bruxism is not known, but several factors have been implicated:

• Dental (local) factors

—Occlusal interferences, including malocclusions, where teeth do not interdigitate smoothly
—"High" dental restorations (e.g., fillings or crowns)
—Intraoral irritation (e.g., sharp tooth cusp)
—Teething

• Psychological factors

—Nervous tension (related to stress, anger, and aggression)
—Personality disorders
—Mental retardation

• Systemic factors: Common

—Neuromuscular disorders (e.g., cerebral palsy)
—Brain injury
—Burn injuries

• Uncommon or rare

—Asthma
—Genetics
—Allergies
—Nutritional and vitamin deficiencies
—Intestinal parasites
—Endocrine disorders
—Restricted mobility of the cervical spine
—Mouth breathing

SIGNS/SYMPTOMS AND ASSOCIATED PROBLEMS

• Teeth

—Wear facets; abraded areas on teeth
—Extreme wear of the primary teeth is occasionally observed, but it is extremely rare that the pulp becomes exposed or nerve damage occurs
—Broken dental restorations
—Loosening of the teeth
—Exacerbation of preexisting periodontal disturbances (gingival inflammation and recession, alveolar bone loss)
—Tooth pain or sensitivity

• Muscular symptoms in any of the head and neck muscles—Most often seen in the lateral pterygoids, followed by the medial pterygoids and masseters

—Pain
—Trismus
—Spasm

• Headache (especially in the morning)
• Temporomandibular joint (TMJ) disorders

—Pain in the TMJ area
—Symptoms (pain, trismus, spasm) in the masticatory muscles
—Limited mandibular range of motion
—Degenerative changes in the TMJ (very rare, especially in children). The evidence equating bruxism as an etiologic factor in temporomandibular joint disorders is contradictory and insufficient to support active therapy on this basis.

• Grinding sounds, nocturnal and/or diurnal, which can be extremely distressing for parents and caregivers.

 Differential Diagnosis

• Dental problems
• Seizures
• Drug reaction
• Stress

 Therapy

• Treatment for bruxism is rarely indicated in children. Practical considerations include:

—Therapy is justified if damage to the permanent dentition or periodontal structures is observed (occasionally in adolescents)
—Treatment should be limited to the most simple and reversible measures. There are inadequate data to support the efficacy of irreversible treatment in children. (Irreversible approaches include selective tooth grinding and orthodontics.)

COMMONLY UTILIZED MODES OF TREATMENT

• Patient and family education

—Ensure that the bruxism itself does not become an issue generating stress for the child

• Behavior (habit) therapy
• Stress counseling

—Identify and address sources of stress
—Biofeedback exercises
—Counseling/psychotherapy
—Hypnosis

UNCOMMONLY UTILIZED MODES OF TREATMENT

• Plastic or vinyl bite guard
• Occlusal adjustment (selective tooth grinding to balance the bite)
• Dental restorations

—Treat and restore carious lesions
—Stainless steel crowns for extreme wear in primary teeth in order to stop tooth sensitivity and/or prevent pulpal exposure

RARELY UTILIZED MODES OF TREATMENT

- Physical therapy

—Warm compresses for muscle or TMJ symptoms
—Limit affected muscle activity (e.g., "do not open wide," "take very small bites," "do not chew gum")
—Ultrasound
—TENS
—Acupressure and/or acupuncture
—Correct cervical spine dysfunction (particularly head position)

- Medications

—Analgesic for symptoms
—Antiinflammatory (e.g., ibuprofen) for symptoms
—Muscle relaxants for symptoms
—Mild tranquilizers if anxiety plays an etiologic role

- Orthodontics

PROGNOSIS

Although the associated problems are well documented, there are no data that establish cause-and-effect relationships for bruxism in childhood continuing on into adulthood.

- Preschool children

—Bruxism typically ceases without therapeutic interventions.
—Associated problems are rare.

- School-age children

—Bruxism typically ceases without therapeutic interventions.
—Monitor for associated conditions without treatment.

- Adolescents

—More commonly benefit from therapeutic intervention.
—Associated problems may also require therapy (e.g., abrasion of teeth, muscular, TMJ symptoms).

- Special needs children

—The long-term prognosis for bruxism in special needs children is poor.
—Acute situations in children who are comatose or those who have suffered traumatic brain injuries or severe burns can be managed by the use of prefabricated bite blocks, or in rare cases, by the fabrication of custom-fitted mouth guards. These appliances are primarily used to prevent soft tissue damage from parafunctional habits such as lip, cheek, and tongue biting.

 Follow-Up

- Continue to monitor for significant associated problems.
- Intercede if damage to permanent dentition and/or periodontal structures is observed

 Common Questions and Answers

Q: How should bruxism in a preschool child be treated?
A: The great majority of bruxism in children stops without any therapy. Considering the controversial nature of treatment modalities, it is prudent to advise no treatment for childhood bruxism and to advise the parents that the condition is common and is usually outgrown.

Q: What about treating bruxism in adolescence?
A: Because damage to the permanent teeth or periodontal structures may have long-term consequences, bruxism in adolescence can be a concern. Still, treatment should be limited to the most simple and reversible approaches. Careful dental evaluation would be an important first step.

Q: Does damage to the primary teeth result in problems with the permanent teeth or with the TMJ?
A: There is no evidence that bruxism in children leads to problems during adolescence or later.

Q: Should custom-fitted mouth guards be fabricated for children with traumatic brain or burn injuries, who engage in lip or tongue biting?
A: The long-term prognosis for bruxism is often poor in these patients. For patients with transitory soft tissue injuries, conservative measures such as prefabricated bite-blocks to get through the acute stage should be tried first. Patients who exhibit chronic chewing may require the fabrication of custom-fitted mouth guards, which may require the use of deep sedation or general anesthesia procedures in order to construct the appliance. The risk of these procedures would need to be weighed against the benefit of the bite guard.

ICD-9-CM 306.8

BIBLIOGRAPHY

American Academy of Pediatric Dentistry. Guidelines on acquired temporomandibular disorders in infants, children and adolescents. *Reference manual 2002–03:Pediatric dentistry* 2003;24(7):103–107.

Ash M, Ramfjord S. Concepts of dysfunction. *Occlusion.* 4th Ed. Philadelphia: WB Saunders 1995:144–146.

Cash R. Bruxism in children: review of the literature. *J Pedodont* 1988;12:107–125.

Kieser JA, Groeneveld, HT. Relationship between juvenile bruxing and craiomandibular dysfunction. *J Oral Rehabil* 1998;25(9): 662–665.

Okeson J. Causes of functional disturbances in the masticatory system. *Management of temporomandibular disorders and occlusion.* 5th Ed. St. Louis: Mosby 2003:149–189.

Restrepo CC, et al. Effects of psychological techniques on bruxism in children with primary teeth. *J Oral Rehabil* 2001;28(4): 354–360.

Authors: Howard M. Rosenberg and Zuhair Sayany

Bulimia

 Database

DEFINITION

Bulimia nervosa is an eating disorder characterized by:

- Recurrent episodes of binge eating characterized by rapid consumption of large amounts of food in discrete periods of time, usually less than 2 hours.
- Accompanied by compensatory behavior such as self-induced vomiting, laxative, or diuretic use, strict dieting or vigorous exercise to induce weight loss.
- Minimum average of two binge-eating episodes per week for at least 3 months
- Feeling of lack of control over eating behavior during eating binges.
- Frenzied quality, often occurring alone and secretively.
- Associated feelings of guilt, anxiety, low self-esteem, and depression.
- Persistent overconcern with body shape and weight

PATHOPHYSIOLOGY

- Personality traits of low self-esteem, self-regulatory difficulties, frustration intolerance, and impaired ability to recognize and directly express feelings have been described in patients with bulimia nervosa.

GENETICS

Recent studies, including twin studies suggest that bulimia nervosa and binge-eating is familial.

EPIDEMIOLOGY

- Onset in late adolescence to early adulthood (range: 13 to 28 years of age)
- Females account for 85%–90% of cases
- Affects 1% to 3% of young females in Western countries
- Affects 4% to 10% of adolescent and college-age females
- Ten times more common than anorexia nervosa
- 83% have lifetime history of an anxiety disorder and 63% have a lifetime history of depression

COMPLICATIONS

Pulmonary

- Aspiration pneumonia
- Pneumomediastinum

Gastrointestinal

- Pancreatitis
- Parotid- or salivary-gland enlargement
- Gastric and esophageal irritation and gastroesophageal reflux
- Mallory-Weiss tears
- Paralytic ileus (due to laxative abuse and hypokalemia)
- Severe constipation (due to laxative abuse and subsequent dependence)

Metabolic

- Hypokalemia (due to laxative abuse or vomiting)
- Secondary cardiac dysrhythmias, myopathy, ileus
- Electrolyte imbalances, including hypomagnesemia,

—Acid, base disturbances

- Fluid imbalances
- Hyperamylasemia
- Edema (secondary to hypoproteinemia or renal sodium and water retention secondary to hypovolemia and secondary hyperaldosteronism)
- Bone loss (if amenorrhea; significantly more common in anorexia nervosa)

Dental

- Enamel erosion
- Caries and periodontal disease

PROGNOSIS

- Very low mortality: 0.3% (but may be underestimation secondary to poor follow-up in studies)
- Most have episodic course with trend toward improvement
- No studies of long-term prognosis in adolescents
- Adult studies: 5- to 10-year follow-up

—50% made full recovery
—30% relapsed
—20% still met full criteria for bulimia nervosa

- Poor prognostic indicators:

—Concomitant depression, personality disorder, or substance abuse
—Frequent vomiting
—History of substance abuse

- Good prognostic indicators:

—High motivation for treatment
—No concurrent disruptive psychopathology
—Good self-esteem

 Differential Diagnosis

Psychosocial

- Psychogenic vomiting
- Drug abuse

MISCELLANEOUS

- Gastrointestinal obstruction
- Hiatal hernia

 Data Gathering

HISTORY

Eating-Disorder Specific

- Eating habits
- Rituals, behaviors

- Body image
- Actual and desired weights, minimum and maximum weights
- Use of laxatives, diuretics, diet pills, emetics
- Presence of binge or purge behavior
- Menstrual history
- History of exercise

General

- Weakness or fatigue or hyperactivity
- Thirst, frequent urination
- Headaches
- Abdominal pain, fullness, bloating, or nausea
- Constipation or diarrhea

Psychiatric

- Mood disorder
- Substance abuse
- Anxiety
- Personality disorders
- Suicidal tendencies
- Low self-esteem
- Feelings of ineffectiveness

Family

- Medical and psychiatric histories

 Physical Examination

Finding: Vital signs
Significance: Check for hypotension

Finding: Weight
Significance: May be normal, overweight, or underweight

Finding: Edema of hands and feet
Significance: Evidence of low albumin or compensatory renal sodium and water retention

Finding: Calluses on knuckles or hands
Significance: Russell sign secondary to inducing vomiting

Finding: Erosion of dental enamel
Significance: Exposure to gastric juices secondary to frequent vomiting

Finding: Muscle cramps or weakness
Significance: Hypokalemia

SPECIAL QUESTIONS

- How much do you want to weigh?
- How do you control your weight?
- How do you feel about yourself?
- How often do you vomit, use diuretics or laxatives?

 Laboratory Aids

Perform a laboratory evaluation as part of the diagnostic workup. Laboratory evaluation is most useful for assessing complications. There is no diagnostic or confirmatory laboratory test for bulimia nervosa. Many patients have normal laboratory studies.

Test: CBC
Significance: Iron-deficiency anemia

Test: Electrolytes, including calcium, magnesium, and phosphate
Significance: Abnormalities may occur as a result of prolonged vomiting or use of laxatives

Test: BUN and creatinine
Significance: Renal function usually normal but BUN may be elevated secondary to dehydration or low secondary to protein loss.

Test: Glucose
Significance: Patient may be hypoglycemic

Test: Cholesterol, lipids
Significance: May be elevated in starvation states

Test: Amylase
Significance: Pancreatitis

Test: Total protein, albumin, prealbumin
Significance: Usually normal but may be low as evidence of malnutrition

Test: Liver function tests
Significance: Transaminases may be mildly elevated (up to twice normal)

Test: ESR
Significance: Almost invariably normal. If elevated consider occult organic process.

Test: HCO_3^-
Significance: Metabolic alkalosis from vomiting or metabolic acidosis if using laxatives

Test: Urine toxicology screen, optional
Significance: May be positive, as this disorder often is associated with substance abuse

Test: ECG with rhythm strip
Significance: May reveal U waves associated with hypokalemia

RADIOGRAPHIC STUDIES

- Consider upper GI series with small-bowel follow-through
- Consider DEXA scan if prolonged amenorrhea to evaluate bone density

OTHER DIAGNOSTIC AIDS

Eating disorder questionnaires—questionnaire assessments appear to be equivalent to diagnostic interview in diagnosing bulimia nervosa.

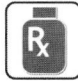

Therapy

- Hospitalize in cases of:

—Hypovolemia
—Severe electrolyte disturbances
—Intractable vomiting
—Acute psychiatric emergencies (e.g., suicidal ideation, acute psychosis)
—Medical complication of malnutrition (e.g., aspiration pneumonia, cardiac failure, pancreatitis, Mallory-Weiss syndrome, etc.)

—Comorbid diagnoses that interfere with the treatment of the eating disorder (e.g., severe depression, obsessive-compulsive disorder, severe family dysfunction)
—Failure of outpatient therapy

PSYCHOTHERAPY

- Outpatient therapy
- Cognitive behavioral therapy:

—More effective than interpersonal psychotherapy or behavioral therapy alone
—Helps patients determine other ways to cope with the feelings that precipitate purging and to try to correct maladaptive beliefs about body image.
—Cognitive behavioral therapy can also be done in a self-help format which may be as effective as the full intensive format

- Individual psychotherapy
- Family treatment (to help with dysfunctional family dynamics)
- Group therapy

DRUGS

- Antidepressants

—Decrease the binge-purge behavior
—Improve attitudes about eating
—Lessen preoccupation with food and weight
—Fluoxetine (Prozac), sertraline (Zoloft), desipramine, and fluvoxamine (Luvox) have been used with good results in patients with bulimia nervosa.
—Effect of antidepressant may diminish over time and patients may relapse when stopped.
  —Psychotherapy combined with antidepressant therapy appears to have the best outcome.
  —Response rate to alternative treatments after CBT and antidepressant first-line therapy is generally low
  —Few studies either of medication or psychotherapy have included patients under 18, so preferred therapy in these patients still uncertain.

- Stool softeners are often of little use for constipation; consider nonstimulating osmotic laxatives if severe.
- Ondansetron shown in one study to decrease vomiting frequency. It may help normalize the physiologic mechanism controlling satiation.

Other

Physical activity has been shown in one study to reduce the pursuit of thinness and to decrease binging/purging behavior.

Follow-Up

- Reduction in binge and purge episodes may take months or years.
- Behavioral and thought disorders associated with bulimia nervosa may be of long duration.

SIGNS

- Weight loss or major weight fluctuations
- Electrolyte abnormalities
- Muscle cramps
- Fatigue
- Depression or mood disturbance
- Willful behavior or acting out

PREVENTION

- Emphasize healthy self-esteem and body image during visits with preadolescents and adolescents.

PITFALLS

- During treatment, patients and their families may cause "splitting" of the hospital staff. To avoid this, always be supportive and maintain consistency in stating goals.

Common Questions and Answers

Q: How do I determine if a patient has anorexia with vomiting or bulimia?
A: The key feature of bulimia nervosa is the binge episode, which distinguishes it from anorexia nervosa. If there are not at least two binge eating episodes per week for at least 3 months, the diagnosis is not bulimia.

Q: What laboratory abnormalities should I look for in my patients with bulimia?
A: Electrolyte abnormalities, particularly hypokalemia. Patients may develop a hypochloremic metabolic alkalosis. If electrolytes are significantly abnormal, the patient should be hospitalized until they have normalized.

ICD-9-CM 133.6

BIBLIOGRAPHY

Agras WS, Walsh BT, Fairburn CG, et al. A multicenter comparison of cognitive-behavioral therapy and interpersonal psychotherapy for bulimia nervosa. *Arch Gen Psychiatry* 2000;57: 459–466.

Kaye WH, et al. Anorexia and bulimia nervosa. *Ann Rev Med* 2000;51:299–313.

Keel PK, et al. Assessment of eating disorders: comparison of interview and questionnaire data from a long-term follow-up study of bulimia nervosa. *J Psychosom Res* 2002;53:1043–1047.

Kreipe RE, Birndorf SA. Eating disorders in adolescent and young adults. *Med Clin North Am* 2000;84:1027–1049.

Mehler PS. Clinical practice. Bulimia nervosa. *NEJM* 2003;349:875–881.

Sundgot-Boregn J, et al. The effect of exercise, cognitive therapy, and nutritional counseling in treating bulimia nervosa. *Medicine and Science in Sports and Exercise* 2002;34:190–195.

Author: Nadja Peter

C1 Esterase Inhibitor Deficiency

 Database

DEFINITION

- C1 esterase inhibitor deficiency is a hereditary and acquired form of recurrent angioedema. The attacks are usually without urticaria.
- C1 esterase inhibitor deficiency has now been classified into a number of types including:

—Hereditary angioedema (HAE) type I (transmitted as autosomal dominant)
—HAE type II (transmitted as autosomal dominant)
—Acquired angioedema (AAE) type I
—AAE type II

- HAE type I accounts for approximately 85% of the C1 esterase deficiencies and is a genetic alteration that leads to impairment of mRNA transcription or translation and therefore, decreased enzyme synthesis.
- HAE type II is a genetic alteration that leads to production of an inactive protein.
- In acquired deficiency of C1 esterase inhibitor, there appears to be a normal ability to synthesize the enzyme; however, the enzyme is metabolized at an increased rate. This syndrome may be seen in patients with autoimmune diseases or malignancy and usually occurs after the fourth decade of life.
- AAE type I is a very rare syndrome usually associated with lymphoproliferative (usually B cell), carcinomas, autoimmune diseases, and paraproteinemias. Because of the other disease processes, complement-activating factors and idiotype-antiidiotype complexes act to increase consumption of C1 esterase inhibitor.
- AAE type II develops when an auto antibody is produced against the C1 esterase inhibitor protein. When these antibodies adhere to the C1 esterase molecule and conformational change occurs leading to decreased function or enhanced metabolism.
- AAE forms may be differentiated from HAE by genetic studies and serologically by significantly decreased C1q, C1r, C1s levels and decreased functional activity of the enzyme in AAE.

PATHOPHYSIOLOGY

- C1 esterase inhibitor is a single chain polypeptide with a molecular weight of 108 kd. The gene has been identified on chromosome 11 (11q12–q13.1)
- This protein inhibits the classic complement pathway by inhibiting activation of C2 and C4. In the fibrinolytic system, C1 esterase inhibitor inhibits formation of plasmin, the activation of C1r and C1s, and the formation of bradykinin from kininogen.
- With a deficiency of this enzyme, the classic complement system becomes activated along with fibrinolysis and kinin formation, which is felt to participate in the production of angioedema.
- Kinin is known to cause similar histologic lesions to histamine but without pruritus.
- The complement activation leads to production of C2b, a product that also has kinin-like activity, and bradykinin, a vasoactive peptide that may also participate in the formation of angioedema.

GENETICS

HAE type I and II are transmitted as autosomal dominant.

 Differential Diagnosis

- Immunoglobin E (IgE)-mediated

—Episodic angioedema
—Allergic reactions to food and drugs
—Physically induced angioedema

- Hypocomplementemic (hereditary angioedema)
- Idiosyncratic

—Nonsteroidal antiinflammatory drugs
—Other drugs

- Lupus erythematosus
- Idiopathic

 Data Gathering

HISTORY

Question: What is the presentation?
Significance: Patients with HAE usually present in the second decade of life with angioedema involving the subcutaneous tissues (mostly involving the extremities).

Question: What gastrointestinal effects are present?
Significance: Angioedema involving the gastrointestinal tract may lead to severe pain, vomiting, and diarrhea.

Question: Are there respiratory complications?
Significance: Two out of three patients will have orofacial or laryngeal swelling.

Question: Can there be hives?
Significance: The edema usually occurs without evidence of inflammation; however, episodes of urticaria have also been documented.

- The variability of clinical manifestations, even among individuals with the same genetic mutation, is striking, implicating nongenetic factors or other genes as possible mediators of clinical presentation.
- Emesis?
- Diarrhea?
- Hypotension from extravasation of plasma into the skin?
- Hemoconcentration?
- Azotemia?
- Central nervous system complaints including headache, hemiparesis, and seizures, may be triggered by trauma or stress.
- AAE presents in the same way but usually in the fourth decade of life, not associated with a familial history.

Physical Examination

Depending on the clinical features, angioedema causes pale, well-demarcated, tense, brawny, nonpruritic and nonpitting single or multiple localized swellings. These may involve the periorbital tissues, genitalia, face, tongue, lips, larynx, extremities, and gastrointestinal tract.

 ## Laboratory Aids

- C1 esterase inhibitor concentration
- C1 esterase inhibitor activity
- C4 concentration
- C1q concentration (usually lower in patients with AAE)

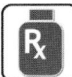 ## Therapy

- For these entities, therapy is divided into management of the acute attack maintenance therapy for HAE, and more specific interventions for those with AAE.
- During an acute episode, management focuses on adequate respiratory and fluid resuscitation, and the treatment of pain.
- In HAE, acute attacks are treated with replacement of the C1 esterase inhibitor with IV concentrates. Fresh frozen plasma may also be used.
- For prophylaxis, androgens (such as danazol and stanozolol) are used in postpubertal patients with HAE of both types.
- These androgens stimulate the synthesis of C1-INH, and, while the level of activity is not normalized, it is increased sufficiently to be clinically efficacious.
- In prepubertal children, androgens are used only in those with severe attacks or purified C1-INH if available.
- For those patients who do not tolerate androgens, tranexamic acid and ϵ-aminocaproic acid (antifibrinolytic inhibitors or plasmin activity) may be used, although they carry the risk of significant side effects.
- AAE type I requires an intensive search for malignancy, although this form of AAE occasionally appears before the development of clinical signs of the malignancy.
- Androgens are also effective in preventing attacks in individuals with this syndrome.
- AAE type II requires immunosuppression to decrease formation of the autoantibody.
- Androgen treatment has not led to good clinical response.

 ## Common Questions and Answers

Q: What are other causes of angioedema?
A: There are classic allergic reactions to food and drugs, physically induced angioedema, IgE-mediated episodic angioedema, idiosyncratic reactions to nonsteroidal antiinflammatory drugs (NSAIDs) and other drugs, lupus erythematosus, and idiopathic causes.

Q: What are the usual precipitating factors in causing reactions?
A: Recurrent episodes of angioedema, abdominal pain, nausea, vomiting occur, whether spontaneously or after local trauma, especially of the upper respiratory tract. Other causes include vigorous exercise, emotional stress, and with menstrual periods.

ICD-9-CM

Hereditary angioedema 277.6
Angioedema 955.1

BIBLIOGRAPHY

Buckley RH, Mathews KP. Common allergic skin diseases. *JAMA* 1982;248:2611.

Csepregi A, Nemesanszky E. Acquired C1 esterase inhibitor deficiency. *Ann Intern Med* 2000;133(10):838–839.

Green M. *Pediatric Diagnosis*. Philadelphia: WB Saunders, 1986.

Heymann WR. Acquired angioedema. *J Am Acad Dermatol* 1997;36:611–615.

Huston DP, Bressler RB. Urticaria and angioedema. *Med Clin North Am* 1992;76(4):805–840.

Kaplan AP. The pathogenic basis of angioedema and urticaria, recent advances. *Am J Med* 1981;70:755.

Oski FA, DeAngelis CD, Feign RD, et al. *Principles and Practice of Pediatrics*. Philadelphia: JB Lippincott, 1990.

Winnewisser J, Rossi M, Spath P, et al. Type I hereditary angio-oedema. *J Intern Med* 1997;241:39–46.

Zuraw BL. Urticaria, angioedema, and autoimmunity. *Clin Lab Med* 1997;17(3):559–569.

Author: Andrew E. Mulberg

Campylobacter Infections

 Database

DEFINITION

• *Campylobacter* species involved in human infections include *C. jejuni* (which causes enteritis), and *C. fetus* (implicated in systemic illness).
• *Campylobacter* is a motile, curved, microaerophilic, non–lactose-fermenting, gram-negative rod that requires oxygen and carbon dioxide for optimal growth.

PATHOPHYSIOLOGY

• *C. jejuni* adheres to epithelial cells and mucus, secretes cytotoxins (which play a role in the development of watery diarrhea), and induces an inflammatory ileocolitis.
• Enteritis, the best-known disease of *C. jejuni*, has been isolated more often than *Salmonella* or *Shigella*, with an incidence of 4% to 12% of diarrheal illness.
• Bacteremia, although uncommon, can occur, especially in the neonate and immunocompromised host; *C. fetus* is the species most likely to be isolated.
• *C. upsaliensis* has been identified in immunocompromised individuals and is usually associated with a self-limiting enteritis.

EPIDEMIOLOGY

• *Campylobacter* infections equal and perhaps exceed the number of cases of inflammatory enteritis as a result of other causes, with the highest attack rates observed in young children.
• Thirty percent to 100% of chickens, turkeys, and water fowl are infected asymptomatically in addition to swine, cattle, sheep, horses, rodents, and household pets (especially young). Contaminated water and milk sources also act as reservoirs for infections.
• Resistant strains are increasingly thought to be related to widespread use of antibiotics in agriculture.
• Transmission of disease is by the fecal-oral route from contaminated food and water or by direct contact with fecal material from animals or persons infected with the organism.
• Person-to-person transmission of *C. jejuni* has been reported when the index cases were young children who were incontinent of feces; vertical transmission from mother to neonate has also been reported.
• Asymptomatic hospital personnel or food handlers have not been implicated as sources.
• The peak rate of isolation occurs in the warmer months of the year (late summer, early fall).

COMPLICATIONS

• Postinfectious immunologic complications include reactive arthritis, Guillain-Barré syndrome (GBS), Reiter syndrome, and erythema nodosum.
• *C. jejuni* is the most frequently identified cause of GBS with serotypes O:19 and O:41, and is responsible for up to 40% of GBS cases.
• HLA-B27 antigen is associated with reactive arthropathy.
• Seizures may develop in young children with enteritis and high fevers.
• A typhoid-like syndrome and meningitis have also been reported in patients with *Campylobacter* infection.
• Spontaneous abortion, and hemolytic-uremic syndrome have been described with *C. upsaliensis*.

PROGNOSIS

• For patients with enteritis, the prognosis is very good, regardless of whether antibiotic treatment is given.

 Differential Diagnosis

Campylobacter infection should be considered in all patients with a diarrheal illness, especially those with a history of bloody or mucous stools, recurrent gastritis, or in immunocompromised hosts.

 Data Gathering

HISTORY

Question: Exposure to unpasteurized milk products?
Significance: Source of *Campylobacter* infection.

Question: Well water used?
Significance: Contaminated water serves as a reservoir.

Question: Inadequately cooked poultry?
Significance: Chickens are asymptomatic carriers.

Question: Fever, abdominal pain, bloody diarrhea?
Significance: Illness is characterized by fever, abdominal pain, and bloody diarrhea. Symptoms can last for 24 hours and be indistinguishable from a viral gastroenteritis, or can be relapsing, thus mimicking inflammatory bowel disease.

Question: Inflammatory ileocolitis?
Significance: The most common manifestation in children.

Question: Duration of symptoms?
Significance: Incubation period is 1 to 7 days and is usually self-limited by 5 to 7 days.

 Physical Examination

Finding: Abdominal pain, diarrhea, malaise, and fever.
Significance: Signs and symptoms of *C. jejuni* infection. If the infection establishes a chronic phase (20% of infected patients), symptoms may mimic inflammatory bowel disease and other immunoreactive complications such as reactive arthropathy, GBS, Reiter syndrome, and erythema nodosum may occur.

 Laboratory Aids

Test: Examination of fecal specimen for darting motility of *C. jejuni* by darkfield or phase-contrast microscopy
Significance: If examined within 2 hours of passage, it can permit presumptive diagnosis.

Test: Stool culture
Significance: Can be used, but selective media (Skirrow, Butzler, or campy-BAP) must be used to isolate *Campylobacter* species.

Test: DNA-based testing
Significance: Development of this diagnostic tool will improve the ability to detect and differentiate *Campylobacter* species much faster than the gold standard of stool culture.

 Therapy

• If treated early in the course of disease (less than 4 days), erythromycin or azithromycin for 5 to 7 days appears to be effective in eradicating the organism from the stool within 2 to 3 days.
• Ciprofloxacin, tetracycline, aminoglycosides, and imipenem are alternative antimicrobials if resistant or bacteremic strains are present.

Follow-Up

- Once treated, symptoms should improve in 2 to 3 days.
- In the untreated patient, the median excretion of organism is up to 2 to 3 weeks, and it was 3 months before all patients in one study were free of the organism. Asymptomatic carriage is uncommon.
- The expected course of treatment of *C. pylori* infection is variable since in vitro sensitivities are not reliable predictors of the response to treatment.

PREVENTION

- The importance of hand washing after contact with animals or animal products, proper cooling and storage of foods, pasteurization of milk, and chlorination of water supplies will decrease the overall risk for infection.
- In the hospital setting, enteric precautions are recommended for infected infants and children who are incontinent of stool and should be maintained until the patient receives at least 48 hours of antibiotic treatment.

PITFALLS

Not all bacterial colitis presents with blood- or mucus-appearing diarrhea. Therefore, suspicion should exist if the diarrhea is prolonged or environmental exposures pose a risk for developing infection.

 Common Questions and Answers

Q: Is treatment necessary if the child is asymptomatic by the time the *Campylobacter* is isolated as the pathogen causing the enteritis?
A: No treatment is needed in this situation. Therapy for symptomatic patients, although it may be of benefit, has not been proven efficacious.

Q: Are there any risks of *Campylobacter* infection to the pregnant patient?
A: Women infected symptomatically or asymptomatically may experience recurrent abortions or preterm deliveries. Life-threatening infections to the fetus or newborn are also possible.

Q: Can you develop immunity to *Campylobacter* infections?
A: Immunity to *C. jejuni* is acquired after one or more infections. For children living in endemic areas, effective natural immunity is as a result of significant repeated early exposure with a progressive decrease in the illness/infection ratio as age increases.

Q: What is the relationship between GBS and *C. jejuni* infection?
A: Many strains of *C. jejuni* have surface glycolipids that are similar to gangliosides, which are abundant in the central and peripheral nervous systems. Antibody formation from this infection binds to the gangliosides causing the demyelinating process characteristic of GBS.

ICD-9 CM 559.008.43

BIBLIOGRAPHY

Bereswill S, Kist M. Recent developments in Campylobacter pathogenesis. *Curr Opin Infect Dis* 2003;16(5):487–491.

Blaser MJ, Reller LB. Campylobacter enteritis. *N Engl J Med* 1981;305:1444–1452.

Bourke B, Chan VL, Sherman P. Campylobacter upsaliensis: waiting in the wings. *Clin Microbiol Rev* 1998;11:440–449.

Fields PI, Swerdlow DL. Campylobacter jejuni. *Clin Lab Med* 1999;19:489–504.

McCarthy N, Giesecke J. Incidence of Guillain-Barre syndrome following infection with Campylobacter jejuni. *Am J Epidemiol* 2001;153(6):610–614.

Peter G, Halsey NA, Marcuse EK, et al. Campylobacter infections. *2000 Red Book: Report of the Committee on Infectious Diseases.* 25th Ed. Elk Grove Village, IL: American Academy of Pediatrics, 2000:196–198.

Ruiz-Palacios G, Pickering LK. Campylobacter infections. In: Feigin RD, Cherry JD, eds. *Pediatric Infectious Diseases.* 3rd Ed. Philadelphia: WB Saunders, 1992:1073–1081.

Shea KM. Antibiotic resistance: what is the impact of agricultural uses of antibiotics on children's health? *Pediatr* 2003;112:253–258.

Tauxe RV, Hargrett-Bean N, Patton CM, et al. Campylobacter isolates in the United States, 1982–1986. *MMWR* 1987;37:10–25.

Thorson SM, Lohr JA, Dudley S, et al. Value of methylene blue examination, dark-field microscopy, and carbol-fuchsin Gram stain in the detection of Campylobacter enteritis. *J Pediatr* 1985;106:941–943.

Authors: Louis M. Bell
Philip V. Scribano, 3rd edition

Candidiasis

 Database

DEFINITION

Candidiasis represents a spectrum of diseases caused by *Candida* species (yeasts). In immunocomponent children, the majority of candidiasis is manifested as superficial mucosal (oropharyngeal candidiasis or thrush), and cutaneous (diaper dermatitis) infection. In immunocompromised children, Candida can cause invasive and disseminated disease. Candidasis is the most common fungal infection in hospitalized children.

ASSOCIATED DISEASES

Candida spp. may cause disease at any site.

Mucosal Candidiasis

• Oropharyngeal candidiasis (thrush) occurs in up to 40% of healthy newborns. Patches of white, curdish material are visible on the buccal and gingival mucosa. It may cause mouth pain and poor nursing. In older children, it is associated with the use of antibiotics or immunosuppressive drugs, conditions of endocrine or immune dysfunction, and malignancy.
• Candidal glossitis occurs secondarily to antibiotic therapy. The tongue is smooth and erythematous, and patients complain of glossodynia (painful tongue). Perlèche (angular cheilosis) results from chronic licking of the corners of the mouth and is characterized by fissuring, erythema, and pain.
• Esophageal candidiasis occurs in HIV-infected patients and those on immunosuppressive therapy; 30% have associated thrush.

Cutaneous Candidiasis

• Diaper dermatitis is most common during infancy as a result of predisposing factors found with diaper use.
• Intertriginous candidiasis is characterized by a confluent, erythematous, weeping rash with a scaling edge found at skin folds: axillae, groin, gluteal folds, intramammary region, interdigital spaces, and umbilicus. Predisposing factors in healthy patients include chronic moisture, recent antibiotic use, and obesity.

Vaginal Candidiasis

Characterized by vaginal discharge (curd-like or mucoid), pruritus, vulvar burning, and dysuria. Oral contraceptives, antibiotics, pregnancy, corticosteroids, and immunodeficiency are predisposing conditions. Classified as uncomplicated or complicated.

• Uncomplicated

—Ninety percent of patients

—Condition is mild to moderate; frequency is sporadic; organism is *C. albicans*; and the host is immunocompetent.

• Complicated

—Ten percent of patients
—Presence of any one of the following factors defines a complicated infection: severe, recurrent infection by non-*albicans Candida* species; or predisposing host factor.

• The reliability of self-diagnosis is poor (<50% correct); therefore, KOH/pH testing is suggested for diagnosis.

Congenital Candidiasis

Cutaneous infection acquired from contaminated amniotic fluid that is usually treated with topical antifungal agents and has an excellent prognosis.

Invasive Candidiasis

• Defined as candidemia and disseminated candidiasis
• Occurs in the immunocompromised host. Risk factors include:

—Prematurity, malignancy, immunodeficiency syndromes, and diabetes mellitus.
—Broad-spectrum antibiotic therapy, corticosteroids, chemotherapy, and hyperalimentation.
—Indwelling catheters, recent complex surgery, and organ transplantation.

• The most frequent sites of involvement are the GI tract, lungs, kidneys, liver, spleen, eyes, and brain. Fungal sepsis may occur. Peritoneal, urinary tract, and cardiac valve candidal infections are most often related to instrumentation or catheterization in the immunocompromised host.

Chronic Mucocutaneous Candidiasis

• Noninvasive infection of the skin, hair, mucus membranes, and nails
• Typically seen in the first year of life and almost all cases occur within the first decade
• Caused by a T-cell immunodeficiency resulting in a poor response to candidal antigens. Patients lack a delayed-type hypersensitivity reaction to intradermal injection of candidal antigens

EPIDEMIOLOGY

• Colonization of the oral mucosa, GI tract, respiratory tract, and vaginal mucosa is common in healthy children. Rates of colonization are substantially higher in hospitalized or chronically ill children.
• Eighty percent of vaginal candidiases are a result of *C. albicans*, the remainder are a result of other Candida species, including *C. glabrata* and *C. tropicalis*.

—While *C. albicans* was once the dominant species in invasive candidiasis, non-*albicans Candida* species are rapidly emerging as significant pathogens.
—Invasive candidiasis is associated with significant morbidity and mortality

COMPLICATIONS

• Persistent oropharyngeal candidiasis, especially in immunocompromised patients.
• Systemic dissemination (see above).

 Differential Diagnosis

• Oral lesions: aphthous stomatitis, acute necrotizing gingivitis, herpes gingivostomatitis, or other viral causes of stomatitis (e.g., coxsackievirus)
• Diaper dermatitis: atopic, seborrheic, bacterial, or occlusional
• Intertriginous infections: seborrheic and atopic dermatitides
• Vaginitis: *Neisseria gonorrheae, Trichomonas vaginalis, Chlamydia trachomatis, Gardnerella vaginalis, Bacteroides* spp., *Mycoplasma hominis, Peptostreptococcus*, and chemical or mechanical irritants
• Congenital candidiasis: viral infections (especially herpes viruses), bacterial infections, benign neonatal skin conditions
• Invasive candidiasis: bacterial infection or other fungal infection
• Chronic mucocutaneous candidiasis: HIV

 Data Gathering

HISTORY

Question: Is the infection recurrent?
Significance: In oral thrush, reinfection can occur from nipples, pacifiers, or toys (see Prevention and Pitfalls). In recurrent vaginitis, bacterial or non-*albicans Candida* species infections are possible.

Question: Recent antibiotic use?
Significance: Oral thrush often occurs in infants, but can occur in normal older children after treatment with systemic antibiotics.

Question: Are there predisposing conditions?
Significance: Oropharyngeal candidiasis in an immunocompromised host often requires oral azole (fluconazole) therapy. Systemic dissemination of infection is more likely with impaired immunity.

 Physical Examination

Finding: Oral lesions
Significance: Buccal or lingual mucosa, gingiva, and tongue lesions have a characteristic white, friable pseudomembrane that when scraped away reveals reddened, denuded, and sometimes ulcerated mucosa.

Finding: Rash
Significance: The rash of monilial diaper dermatitis is initially scattered. Erythematous papules progress and coalesce into a deeply erythematous, weeping, confluent rash with a scaling border and satellite lesions.

Laboratory Aids

LABORATORY STUDIES

Test: Direct light microscopic examination of specimen
Significance: KOH preparation (10% or 20% potassium hydroxide) allows visualization of the long, branching, hyphae of *C. albicans*. Vaginal pH remains normal (<4.5) with vaginal candidiasis.

Test: Fungal culture
Significance: However, the sensitivity of blood culture is only 50% to 60% in patients with invasive candidiasis.

OTHER STUDIES

Test: Dilated retinal examination (by an ophthalmologist)
Significance: Endophthalmitis, a sight-threatening complication, should be excluded in all patients with candidemia.

Test: CT scan and echocardiogram
Significance: Important to identify deep organ lesions (liver, spleen, brain, kidney, or heart) associated with disseminated infection.

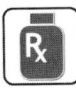 ## Therapy

Treatment of candidiasis is dependent on the site of infection, immune status of the host, and the risk of systemic dissemination.

OROPHARYNGEAL CANDIDIASIS

Oral Candidiasis

- Treat with nystatin suspension until 2 days after the lesions have cleared. Miconazole oral gel, while more effective, is not yet available in the United States.
- In older patients, nystatin as a swish-swallow suspension or in oral tablet form for >7 days is effective. Clotrimazole lozenges are also effective; 10 mg dissolved in mouth 5 times daily for 7 days.
- Gentian violet is no longer recommended for the treatment of oral candidiasis.
- Fluconazole and ketoconazole are effective for infections that are persistent or occur in immunocompromised hosts. Azole-resistant *C. albicans* has been described in HIV-infected individuals with recurrent infection.

Esophageal Candidiasis

- A therapeutic trial with fluconazole for patients with presumed esophageal candidiasis is a cost-effective alternative to endoscopy; symptoms should resolve within 7 days after the start of therapy. A 14- to 21-day course is recommended. Itraconazole solution and IV amphotericin B are acceptable alternatives.
- Patients with advanced AIDS commonly have recurrent infections and may benefit from chronic suppressive fluconazole therapy.

Cutaneous or Intertriginous Candidiasis and Candidal Diaper Dermatitis

Both are treated by keeping the area dry and using nystatin cream (100,000 units/g q.i.d.) until the rash has cleared. Topical regimens of clotrimazole 1%, miconazole 2%, ketoconazole 2%, and econazole 1% are also effective.

Vaginal Candidiasis

- Uncomplicated

—Topical agents are highly effective in uncomplicated infections (cure rates >80%): clotrimazole, miconazole, butoconazole, and terconazole (dose varies with 1-, 3-, or 7-day treatment).
—Oral agents are also effective: fluconazole (10 mg/kg up to 150 mg as a single-dose), ketoconazole (400 mg QID for 5 days), and itraconazole (200 mg bid for 1 day or 200 mg QID for 3 days).

- Complicated

—Extend antimycotic therapy to 7 to 14 days.
—Non-*albicans* species of *Candida* usually respond to topical boric acid (600 mg/day for 14 days). Azole-resistant *C. albicans* infections are extremely rare in the immunocompetent host.

- Recurrent (>4 episodes of proven infection during a 12-month period)

Recurrent vaginitis is usually as a result of azole-susceptible *C. albicans*. Induction therapy with 2 weeks of a topical or oral azole is followed by a maintenance regimen for 6 months. Suitable maintenance regimens include fluconazole (150 mg weekly), ketoconazole (100 mg daily), itraconazole (100 mg qod), or daily therapy with a topical azole.

Systemic or Disseminated Candidiasis

- Begin treatment in hospital as a result of severity of illness, underlying disease process, and need for the intravenous route of drug administration.
- Address predisposing factors (e.g., removal of indwelling catheters).
- Antifungal agents commonly used in children include amphotericin B, fluconazole, or the combination of fluconazole plus amphotericin B (with the amphotericin B administered for the first 5 to 6 days only).

Fluconazole may be used in those infected with a *Candida* species known to be a sensitive to be fluconazole-susceptible.

- Flucytosine could be considered in combination with amphotericin B for more severe infections.
- Lipid-based amphotericin B: 3 to 6 mg/kg IV per day. Appropriate for patients who are refractory to, intolerant of, or at high-risk of being intolerant of conventional amphotericin B preparations.

PREVENTION

- Sterilize bottle nipples and toys to prevent reinoculation of oral candidiasis.
- Avoid unnecessarily long courses of broad-spectrum antibiotics.
- Maintain intravenous catheters and catheter-skin insertion sites appropriately.

 ## Follow-Up

Follow-up is required only for disseminated/systemic candidiasis.

PITFALLS

- Failure to eliminate source of reinfection. Recurrent thrush in a breast-fed infant may indicate *C. albicans* colonization of the mother's nipples; this can be eliminated by treatment of the nipples with nystatin cream.
- Failure to consider that symptoms of persistent vaginitis may be caused by non-*albicans Candida* species or by bacteria (see Vaginitis).
- Failure to maintain a high index of suspicion for invasive candidiasis in an immunocompromised patient. Persistent fevers despite antibiotic therapy, diffuse rash, and visual complaints are important clues.

 ## Common Questions and Answers

Q: When should an older child with thrush be worked up for possible immunodeficiency?
A: Thrush in the older child is usually caused by recent antibiotic or steroid treatment. If no apparent cause is found, an immunologic evaluation that includes HIV testing, should be considered.

ICD-9-CM 112.9

BIBLIOGRAPHY

Hoppe JE. Treatment of oropharyngeal candidiasis and candidal diaper dermatitis in neonates and infants: review and reappraisal. *Pediatr Infect Dis J* 1997;16:885–894.

Hughes WT, Flynn PM. Candidiasis. In: Feigin RD, Cherry JD, eds. *Textbook of Pediatric Infectious Diseases*. 5th Ed. Philadelphia: WB Saunders, 2004:2569–2579.

Mermel LA, Farr BM, Sheretz RJ, et al. Guidelines for the management of intravascular catheter-related infections. *Clin Infect Dis* 2001;32:1249–1272.

Pappas PG, Rex JH, Sobel JD, et al. Guidelines for the treatment of candidiasis. *Clin Infect Dis* 2004;38:161–189.

Sobel JD, Faro S, Force RW, et al. Vulvovaginal candidiasis: epidemiologic, diagnostic, and therapeutic considerations. *Am J Obstet Gynecol* 1998;178:203–211.

Author: Theoklis Zaoutis

Carbon Monoxide Poisoning

 Database

DEFINITION

- Carbon monoxide (CO) is an odorless gas produced via incomplete combustion of carbonaceous fuels.
- Upon inhalation, some CO binds to hemoglobin to form carboxyhemoglobin.
- CO poisoning exists when carboxyhemoglobin and CO accumulation leads to impaired physiologic function.

PATHOPHYSIOLOGY

- Carboxyhemoglobin does not carry oxygen.
- Carboxyhemoglobin produces an allosteric leftward shift of the oxyhemoglobin dissociation curve.
- Carboxyhemoglobin elimination half-life:

—Approximately 4 hours in room air
—One to 2 hours in 100% oxygen
—Twenty minutes in 100% oxygen at 3 atmospheres

- CO interacts with cellular proteins leading to impaired mitochondrial function.
- CO poisoning may begin a cascade of inflammatory vasculitis within the central nervous system.

EPIDEMIOLOGY

- CO poisoning is the leading cause of death by intoxication within the United States.
- Over 15,000 CO exposures were reported to the American Association of Poison Control Centers in 2002, with over one-third of such exposures occurring to children.
- Seasonal cold weather leads to increases in incidence of exposure.
- Common sources of CO exposure include:

—automobile or boat exhaust
—smoke inhalation from house fires
—oil, gas, or kerosene space heaters or cooking stoves
—portable electrical generators and construction equipment, faulty home furnaces

- The solvent methylene chloride is metabolized to CO by the liver after ingestion, inhalation, or dermal absorption.

COMPLICATIONS

- Mild CO intoxication

—malaise, nausea, lightheadedness, headache, vomiting

- Moderate CO intoxication

—confusion, syncope, weakness, angina

- Severe CO intoxication

—seizure, coma, cardiac dysrhythmia, death

- Belated neurologic sequelae

—neurocognitive deficits, personality changes, Parkinsonism

PROGNOSIS

- Acute mortality appears to be as a result of carboxymyoglobin formation and ischemic ventricular dysrhythmia.
- Patients stable on presentation to medical care have a good prognosis for recovery.
- Delayed neurologic sequelae may manifest in as many as 10% to 40% of patients after a CO-mediated syncopal episode.

ASSOCIATED DISEASES

- Victims of house fires may suffer from thermal injury and/or cyanide poisoning.

 Differential Diagnosis

- Influenza
- Gastroenteritis
- Vasomotor syncope
- Asphyxia
- Stroke

 Data Gathering

HISTORY

Question: Health of family members?
Significance: CO is an environmental gas that often sickens multiple household members.

Question: Use of furnace or space heaters?
Significance: May suggest source of exposure.

Question: Time of exposure?
Significance: Carboxyhemoglobin levels must be interpreted with consideration to their timing.

Question: Duration of exposure?
Significance: Toxicity is related to both magnitude and duration of exposure.

Question: Loss of consciousness?
Significance: Syncope appears to be the best working predictor of delayed neurologic sequelae.

 Physical Examination

Finding: Soot on nasal mucosa
Significance: Suggests possibility of thermal pulmonary injury.

Finding: Hypotension
Significance: Suggests severe CO poisoning.

Finding: "Cherry red" skin
Significance: This "classic" sign is mostly a postmortem finding.

 Laboratory Aids

TESTS

Test: Co-oximetry
Significance: Allows quantitation of carboxyhemoglobin.

Test: Arterial blood gas
Significance: Allows accurate assessment of oxygenation.

Test: Hemoglobin quantitation
Significance: The percent carboxyhemoglobin concentration must be considered in relation to the total hemoglobin.

Test: Serum bicarbonate
Significance: A wide-anion gap metabolic acidosis suggests the accumulation of lactate, which may result from severe CO poisoning or concomitant cyanide poisoning.

Test: Creatine kinase
Significance: CO poisoning victims are susceptible to rhabdomyolysis.

Test: Neuroimaging
Significance: Not routinely helpful in acute management; globus pallidus and subcortical white matter changes may be seen after severe CO poisoning.

PITFALLS

- Pulse oximetry frequently overestimates the percentage of oxyhemoglobin.
- Smokers may have carboxyhemoglobin levels in excess of 10%.
- Hemolysis, or the presence of fetal hemoglobin, may lead to mild elevation of carboxyhemoglobin.
- In-hospital carboxyhemoglobin levels are not good at predicting risk of delayed neurologic sequelae.

Carbon Monoxide Poisoning

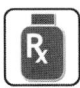 Therapy

- Recognize CO exposure
- Remove patient from source of CO
- Administer 100% oxygen at least until asymptomatic and carboxyhemoglobin level is less than 10%.
- Consider hyperbaric oxygen treatment referral to prevent delayed neurologic sequelae

Indications: loss of consciousness, seizures, pregnancy, persistent neurologic symptoms
Contraindications: concurrent illness or injury requiring ongoing acute care, unvented pneumothorax, lack of accessible hyperbaric oxygen chamber
Complications: barotitis media, tympanic membrane rupture, claustrophobic anxiety, seizure, pneumothorax

PITFALLS

- Failure to differentiate CO poisoning from winter viral illness
- Syncope may be hard to discern in young infants
- Undue delay in hyperbaric oxygen therapy, which is most effective in first 6 hours after exposure

 Follow-Up

- Delayed neurologic sequelae may develop 2 to 40 days after exposure

 Common Questions and Answers

Q: At what carboxyhemoglobin level should hyperbaric oxygen therapy be recommended?
A: In practice, most dissociation of carboxyhemoglobin occurs with administration of normal pressure oxygen before hyperbaric therapy can be administered. The advocated value of hyperbaric oxygen is to limit cerebral ischemic reperfusion injury in an effort to ameliorate delayed neurologic sequelae. Carboxyhemoglobin levels are not useful in this risk stratification, and the occurrence of syncope or seizure is used as a surrogate marker.

Q: In a household, which family member is at greatest risk of CO poisoning?
A: Smaller and younger children have greater minute ventilation rates and may attain higher carboxyhemoglobin concentrations at a given exposure level. It is unclear whether developing brain tissue is more susceptible to the deleterious effects of CO poisoning.

BIBLIOGRAPHY

Martin JD, Osterhoudt KC, Thom SR. Recognition and management of carbon monoxide poisoning in children. *Clin Ped Emerg Med* 2000;1:244–250.

Tomaszewski C. Carbon monoxide. In: Ford MD, Delaney KA, Ling LJ, Erickson T, eds. *Clinical Toxicology*. Philadelphia: WB Saunders, 2001:657–667.

Weaver LK, Hopkins RO, Chan KJ, et al. Hyperbaric oxygen for acute carbon monoxide poisoning. *New Engl J Med* 2002;347: 1057–1067.

Author: Kevin Osterhoudt

Cardiomyopathy

 Database

DEFINITION

Cardiomyopathy is defined as a disease of the myocardium. Originally used to describe myocardial disease not attributable to coronary artery disease (CAD), the definition has been revised to now refer to structural and functional abnormalities of the myocardium that are not secondary to hypertension, congenital heart disease, valvular abnormalities, or pulmonary vascular disease. There are three main classifications of cardiomyopathy:

- Dilated cardiomyopathy (DCM): The key finding in DCM is impairment of biventricular systolic function with predominant involvement of the left ventricle, which manifests as congestive heart failure.
- Hypertrophic cardiomyopathy (HCM): Historically, the classic definition has been asymmetric hypertrophy of the left ventricle with 20% to 25% of the patients exhibiting left ventricular (LV) outflow tract obstruction.
- Restrictive cardiomyopathy (RCM): This disease is defined as myocardial disease with impairment of ventricular filling as a result of decreased compliance from increased stiffness of the ventricle. Systolic function is generally preserved.

ETIOLOGY/PATHOPHYSIOLOGY

- DCM: There are many etiologies for DCM. This disease can occur as a finding associated with another disease or syndrome. These include inborn errors of fatty acid oxidation, disorders of mitochondrial oxidative phosphorylation, nutritional deficiencies, primary and secondary carnitine deficiency, and X-linked muscular dystrophies. Many of these disorders are familial and are genetically inherited. DCM can also occur as an end result of a disease process, such as toxin exposure (anthracyclines), infections (coxsackievirus B, echovirus, adenovirus), ischemic CAD (anomalous left coronary artery from the pulmonary artery, coronary aneurysms) and chronic tachyarrhythmias. Lastly, patients can also have idiopathic DCM. Regardless of the etiology, depressed systolic function and abnormally dilated ventricular chambers are the common features in all forms of DCM.
- HCM: The clinical manifestations of HCM can be explained by three distinct mechanisms: dynamic obstruction of the LV outflow tract, diastolic dysfunction, and mitral regurgitation.
- RCM: The causes of RCM include systemic lupus erythematosis, sarcoidosis, amyloidosis, infiltrative diseases (Gaucher disease, Hurler syndrome), storage diseases (Fabry disease), carcinoid syndrome, and radiation-induced fibrosis. There is also a familial form of RCM. This disease is manifest by increased stiffness of the myocardium leading to impairment of ventricular filling. Therefore, small increases in volume will cause a disproportionate increase in ventricular pressure.

GENETICS

- DCM: In familial DCM, autosomal dominant inheritance remains the most common pattern. Although no specific gene has been identified as the cause of familial DCM, six genes have been localized in different family cohorts. DCM has also been seen in association with diseases of X-linked inheritance, such as Duchenne and Beckermuscular dystrophy, and Barth syndrome. The last pattern of inheritance is through mitochondrial DNA, which can have varying scope and severity of disease by its differing penetrance.
- HCM: Approximately 90% of reported cases are considered to be inherited. Traditionally, HCM is inherited in an autosomal dominant pattern with incomplete penetrance. Mutations on chromosomes 1, 11, 14, and 15 have been implicated as major contributors to the development and progression of this disease.
- RCM: Idiopathic cases may have a familial occurrence and may be associated with a skeletal myopathy. An autosomal dominant form of the disease with variable penetrance has been associated with Noonan syndrome.

EPIDEMIOLOGY

- DCM: Differing studies have reported the incidence to range from 0.4 to 8.0 cases per 100,000 people with a prevalence of 36 cases per 100,000 people.
- HCM: Although the true prevalence is unknown, it is estimated to be 10 to 100 cases per 100,000 people.
- RCM: This is the least common form of cardiomyopathy.

COMPLICATIONS

- Congestive heart failure is common in all three forms of cardiomyopathy.
- Arrhythmias may be seen and are most often ventricular in origin.
- Thrombus formation can be seen in DCM as a result of the stasis of blood in a hypocontractile ventricle and, therefore, systemic or pulmonary emboli are possible.

PROGNOSIS

- DCM: In some studies, the survival rate at 1-year follow-up of those with DCM is 63% to 90% with a 5-year survival rate of 25% to 34%. A general rule for idiopathic DCM is that one-third of patients exhibit improved cardiac function, one-third of patients have stable cardiac dysfunction, and one-third of patients progress to significant cardiac dysfunction.
- HCM: Overall incidence of sudden death is 4% to 6% in children and adolescents, and as low as 1% in adults. Between the ages of 12 and 35 years and in young athletes, HCM is the most common cause of sudden death.
- RCM: The reported median survival in RCM is 1.4 years in children.

 Differential Diagnosis

- DCM: Children and young adults often present with symptoms that mimic other disease states. For example, abdominal distension, right upper quadrant pain, nausea, and anorexia indicate right heart failure but could be mistaken for hepatic or gallbladder disease. Wheezing, tachypnea, and dyspnea on exertion may be diagnosed as bronchitis or asthma. Cardiomegaly on chest radiograph may be mistaken for a large pericardial effusion.
- HCM: This disease must be differentiated from the LV hypertrophy that is seen in a well-trained athlete.
- RCM: Restrictive cardiomyopathy should be distinguished from constrictive pericarditis since the latter is usually a remediable process. A history of tuberculosis, trauma, or cardiac surgery may suggest constrictive pericarditis.

 Data Gathering

HISTORY

Question: Respiratory distress?
Significance: Left-sided congestive heart failure

Question: Irritability?
Significance: Left-sided congestive heart failure, pericardial effusion, palpitations, myocardial hypoperfusion/ischemia

Question: Diaphoresis?
Significance: Left-sided congestive heart failure or a tachyarrhythmia

Question: Gastrointestinal complaints (abdominal pain, nausea, emesis)?
Significance: Right-sided congestive heart failure, pericardial effusion, decreased systemic output

Question: Tachypnea with feeding, pallor, and poor weight gain?
Significance: Left-sided congestive heart failure

Question: Chest pain?
Significance: Myocardial hypoperfusion/ischemia, pericardial effusion, arrhythmia

Question: Syncope?
Significance: Inadequate cardiac output or arrhythmia

Question: Palpitations?
Significance: Arrhythmia

Question: Orthopnea, paroxysmal nocturnal dyspnea?
Significance: Left-sided congestive heart failure

Question: Peripheral edema?
Significance: Right-sided congestive heart failure

Question: Exercise intolerance?
Significance: Left-sided congestive heart failure, inadequate cardiac output, myocardial hypoperfusion/ischemia

Question: Mental status changes?
Significance: Systemic emboli, chronic hypoperfusion to the brain

Physical Examination

CARDIAC

Finding: DCM: tachycardia, cardiomegaly, hepatomegaly, S3, or S4 gallop
Significance: Evidence of congestive heart failure and decreased cardiac output.

Finding: HCM: Can be normal or have systolic murmur as a result of mitral regurgitation and/or LV outflow tract obstruction.
Significance: The presence of outflow tract obstruction produces a systolic ejection murmur of variable intensity related to the degree of obstruction; the murmur increases in intensity with Valsalva and decreases in magnitude with squatting. A parasternal or carotid thrill may be present.

Finding: RCM: Jugular venous pulse either fails to fall or rises during inspiration (Kussmaul sign), S3 or S4
Significance: Advanced cases may exhibit weak peripheral pulses as evidence of low cardiac output.

RESPIRATORY

Finding: Tachypnea, rales, dyspnea on exertion, paroxysmal nocturnal dyspnea, orthopnea, exercise intolerance
Significance: Left-sided congestive heart failure.

ABDOMINAL

Finding: Hepatomegaly, ascites, tenderness to palpation
Significance: Right-sided congestive heart failure.

EXTREMITIES

Finding: Peripheral edema in advanced cases
Significance: Right-sided congestive heart failure.

Laboratory Aids

NONSPECIFIC TESTS

Test: Chest radiograph
Significance: Cardiomegaly, pulmonary venous congestion, pulmonary edema, Kerley B lines, and pleural effusions; segmental atelectasis from compression of the bronchioles; skeletal abnormalities may be seen in certain syndromes

Test: Electrocardiogram
Significance: Sinus tachycardia, nonspecific ST-segment and T-wave changes, hypertrophy or enlargement of chambers (although generalized low voltages may be seen), ventricular and supraventricular tachyarrhythmias, atrioventricular block, localized Q waves

SPECIFIC TESTS

Test: Laboratory evaluation
Significance: In addition to routine inflammatory markers, specific tests should be obtained to establish the etiology. Metabolic: carnitine level, serum organic acids, urine organic and amino acids. Genetic: chromosomal analysis, genetic mutations of the dystrophin gene. Infectious: enterovirus, coxsackievirus A/B, hepatitis, cytomegalovirus, Eptein-Barr virus, Herpes simplex virus, human immunodeficiency virus.

Test: Echocardiography
Significance: Allows for measurement of systolic function, ventricular dimensions, outflow tract obstruction, and diastolic filling properties. This modality is the gold standard for diagnosing HCM; the three principal features seen are LV hypertrophy, intraventricular pressure gradient, and systolic anterior motion of the mitral valve.

Test: Cardiac catheterization
Significance: DCM: Rarely used as the primary diagnostic tool in this disease

Therapy

- DCM: Afterload reduction (enalapril, captopril), inotropic agents (milrinone, dobutamine, digoxin), aldactone (improves New York Heart Association [NYHA] functional class), anticoagulation to avoid embolic complications, antiarrhythmics as needed, β-adrenergic blockers (metoprolol, carvedilol), and at the time of diagnosis, a trial of intravenous gamma globulin and/or other immunomodulators (prednisone, azathioprine). Ventricular assist devices have been used in those with end-stage heart failure either as a bridge to recovery or to transplantation.
- HCM: β-Adrenergic blockers, calcium channel blockers, and disopyramide remain first-line medical therapy. Antiarrhythmics are also a mainstay of the medical regimen. If medical therapy is not effective, other options may include myotomy or myectomy and atrioventricular sequential pacing. There is no evidence that prophylactic medical treatment will reduce the risk of sudden death. The placement of an implantable cardioverter defibrillator (ICD) may be indicated.
- RCM: The mainstay of medical therapy is symptomatic treatment. Diuretics can be used with caution to treat venous congestion without reducing the ventricular filling pressure. Antiarrhythmics are used to treat the high incidence of atrial arrhythmias. ICDs have also been used to treat life-threatening ventricular arrhythmias. Anticoagulation is used as a result of the high risk of thrombus formation and embolic complications from hemostasis in the dilated atrium. Because of the natural history of this disease, most patients eventually require a cardiac transplant.
- Transplantation: Heart or heart-lung (if the pulmonary vascular resistance is elevated) transplantation may be necessary if all therapeutic endeavors prove to be futile.

Follow-Up

All of these patients require careful follow-up by a cardiologist in addition to their primary care physician to note any adverse alterations in their cardiovascular status. Patients should be referred for a transplant evaluation, as deemed clinically necessary.

PITFALLS

In the early stages of all three forms of cardiomyopathy, the symptoms are nonspecific and can mimic other disease processes. The cardiac examination can be completely normal; therefore, those patients that raise suspicion for this disease either by family history or clinical presentation should be carefully evaluated.

Common Questions and Answers

Q: Should family members be evaluated once a cardiomyopathy is diagnosed in a first-degree relative?
A: Yes. In some forms of cardiomyopathy, there is a strong genetic component and family members should be evaluated. Certainly, the diagnosis of acquired cardiomyopathy does not require evaluation of relatives.

Q: Does the cardiomyopathy of infants of diabetic mothers carry the same clinical course and outcome as that of patients with HCM?
A: No. The cardiomyopathy in these infants is usually benign and resolves within the first 6 months of life.

Q: What are the differentiating features of HCM and the benign physiologic hypertrophy of an athlete's heart?
A: Several criteria are used to make this distinction. For example, a familial history of HCM leads one to be suspicious of this entity. Studies have suggested specific echocardiographic LV dimensions to differentiate benign hypertrophy and HCM (i.e., a wall thickness of at least 15 mm or left ventricle cavity dimension <45 mm are more consistent with HCM). Also, echocardiographic evidence of abnormal mitral valve inflow is suggestive of HCM.

ICD-9-CM 425.4

BIBLIOGRAPHY

Ammash NM, Seward JB, Bailey KR, et al. Clinical profile and outcome of idiopathic restrictive cardiomyopathy. *Circulation* 2000;101(21):2490–2496.

Kelly DP, Strauss AW. Mechanisms of disease: inherited cardiomyopathies. *N Engl J Med* 1994;330(13):913–919.

Lipshultz SE, Sleeper LA, Towbin JA, et al. The incidence of pediatric cardiomyopathy in two regions of the United States. *N Engl J Med* 2003;348(17)1647–1655.

Towbin JA. Pediatric myocardial disease. *Pediatr Clin North Am* 1999;46(2):289–312.

Authors: P. Nelson Le
Timothy Hoffman, 3rd edition

Cat-Scratch Disease

 Database

DEFINITION

Cat-scratch disease (CSD) is a subacute, regional lymphadenitis syndrome that occurs following cutaneous inoculation. The majority of patients have had an identifiable contact with a cat, most notably in the form of a scratch or bite.

CAUSES

The etiologic agent for CSD is now referred to as *Bartonella henselae* (previously, *Rochalimaea henselae*), a pleomorphic gram-negative rod. Skin inoculation with the organism through cat contact is the typical mechanism of infection.

PATHOPHYSIOLOGY

Following infection, both the primary inoculation site and the affected lymph nodes show a characteristic central avascular necrotic area surrounded by lymphocytes with some giant cells and histiocytes. Involved nodes develop generalized enlargement, cortex thickening, and germinal-center hypertrophy. Progression leads to pus-filled sinuses within the affected nodes.

EPIDEMIOLOGY

- Occurs in patients of all ages, with 80% of cases being in those less than 21 years old
- Approximately 24,000 cases each year and likely represents the most common cause of chronic benign regional adenopathy
- More common when scratched by a cat less than 12 months of age

COMPLICATIONS

- Unilateral subacute or chronic tender nodes of the axillary, epitrochlear, and preauricular area support a diagnosis of CSD, especially in the face of a consistent cat contact.
- Regional lymphadenitis
- Parinaud oculoglandular syndrome. This occurs when the site of primary inoculation is the conjunctiva or eyelid. A mild to moderate conjunctivitis develops along with preauricular lymph nodes.
- Encephalopathy/encephalitis: may occur suddenly 2 to 6 weeks after the initial symptoms of CSD, and seizures may be the heralding symptom. Patients may become delirious and then comatose for several days before recovering. Spinal fluid is typically normal or shows minimal WBC and protein elevation. Recovery is generally complete.
- Systemic SCD will present as a fever of unknown etiology. Occasionally hepatosplenic involvement with multiple hypoechoic lesions will be found on abdominal ultrasound examination.
- Erythema nodosum: likely represents a delayed hypersensitivity reaction to the infection. Most often involves the subcutaneous fat of the legs and, at times, dorsum of arms, hands, and feet.
- Osteolytic bone lesions occur as a rare complication.
- Other rare complications include thrombotic thrombocytopenic purpura, erythema marginatum, mesenteric lymphadenitis, pneumonia, arthralgias, subacute iriditis, urethritis, lymphedema, thyroiditis, and anicteric hepatitis.

PROGNOSIS

Most patients with CSD have a benign course. Patients with significant complications such as encephalopathy, thrombocytopenic purpura, or bone lesions usually have a more prolonged course, but also have a good long-term prognosis.

 Differential Diagnosis

Most known causes of lymphadenopathy (see Neck Masses). Location of the abnormal lymph nodes may supply a strong clue.

 Data Gathering

HISTORY

Question: Cat contact?
Significance: The majority of patients have an antecedent cat contact.

Question: A skin rash?
Significance: May describe the appearance of a papule on the skin at the site of inoculation 3 to 5 days after the initial injury.

Question: Changes in rash?
Significance: This papule generally progresses through a vesicular and crusty stage.

Question: When did large lymph nodes appear?
Significance: Within 1 to 2 weeks, lymphadenopathy in the region of drainage may be noted.

Question: Other symptoms?
Significance: Mild associated symptoms of generalized achiness, malaise, anorexia may also be present. Fever is present in less than 10%.

 Physical Examination

- One or more red papules at the inoculation site may be detectable.
- The true sign of CSD (present in 10% of cases) is chronic or subacute lymphadenitis involving the first or second set of nodes draining the inoculation site.
- The groups affected, in decreasing order of frequency, are the axillary, cervical, submandibular, periauricular, epitrochlear, femoral, and inguinal lymph nodes.
- Usually tender with overlying erythema, warmth, and induration.
- Less than half become suppurative or form a sinus tract to the skin.

Laboratory Aids

Test: Direct fluorescence antibody testing
Significance: For detection of antibodies to *B. henselae*, conducted on serum samples at the Centers for Disease Control and Prevention. This test should be used to confirm a CSD diagnosis.

Test: Enzyme immunoassay
Significance: For detection of immunoglobin G (IgG) antibodies to *B. henselae*, also commercially available (Specialty Laboratories, Santa Monica, CA).

Test: Blood cultures
Significance: Using lysed or centrifuged blood may at times yield *B. henselae* growth from infected individuals in whom bacteremia is suspected.
Isolation of organism from skin lesions and nodal aspirates may be possible.

Therapy

- Antibiotic therapy for CSD is somewhat controversial. Many experts suggest conservative, symptomatic treatment only.
- Some experts still suggest the use of an oral antibiotic such as trimethoprim-sulfamethoxazole (TMP-SMX), 6 to 8 mg/kg of TMP b.i.d. to t.i.d. for 7 days.
- Alternatively, azithromycin 500 mg initially then 250 mg for a total of 5 days in patients more than 45.5 kg and 10 mg/kg on the first day and 5 mg/kg for the subsequent 4 days in children for uncomplicated CSD may be used. Percutaneous drainage of tender, fluctuant adenitis can provide relief of pain.
- For immunocompromised patients and those with severe disease (including encephalitis) gentamicin sulfate, 5 mg/kg per day divided q8h intramuscularly or intravenously, is recommended. The duration of treatment should be based on response.

PREVENTION

Measures to prevent CSD should be directed toward minimizing contact between infected cats and people. Keeping kittens and older cats indoors and avoiding rough play may decrease the likelihood of infection. Avoidance of stray animals and good local care of any sustained bite or scratch is essential.

Follow-Up

Most patients will have a benign course and can expect resolution of systemic symptoms in less than 2 weeks. Slow resolution of enlarged or painful lymph nodes will occur over weeks to months. As mentioned, percutaneous drainage of tender, fluctuant lymph nodes may be required to relieve pain. As stated previously, the course for patients with severe complications, including encephalitis, will be more prolonged, but without lasting sequelae.

Common Questions and Answers

Q: Can a sibling develop CSD from an infected patient?
A: No. Person-to-person transmission is not reported.

Q: Should the parents of a child with CSD get rid of the cat?
A: In general, this is not recommended. These animals are not ill. The capacity to transmit disease appears to be transient, and recurrent disease is rare.

ICD-9-CM 078.3

BIBLIOGRAPHY

Adal KA, Cockerell CJ, Petri WA. Cat-scratch disease, bacillary angiomatosis, and other infections due to Rochalimaea. *N Engl J Med* 1994;330:1509–1515.

Bass JW, Freitas BC, Freitas AD, et al. Prospective randomized double blind placebo-controlled evaluation of azithromycin for treatment of cat-scratch disease. *Pediatr Infect Dis J* 1998;17:447–452.

Carithers HA. Cat-scratch disease: an overview based on a study of 1,200 patients. *Am J Dis Child* 1985;139:1124–1133.

Carithers HA. Cat-scratch disease: acute encephalopathy and other neurologic manifestations. *Am J Dis Child* 1991;145:48–101.

Case records of the Massachusetts General Hospital. Weekly clinicopathological exercises. Case 1-1998. An 11-year-old boy with a seizure [clinical conference] [published erratum appears in *N Engl J Med* 1998;338(7):483]. *N Engl J Med* 1998;338(2):112–119.

Conrad DA. Treatment of cat-scratch disease. *Curr Opin Pediatr* 2001;13(1):56–59.

Heye S, Matthijs P, Wallon J, Van Campenhoudt M. Cat Scratch Disease Osteomyelitis. *Skeletal Radiol* 2003;32(1):49–51.

Jacobs RF, Schutze GE. Bartonella henselae as a cause of prolonged fever and fever of unknown origin in children. *Clin Infect Dis* 1998;26:80–84.

Kelly CS, Kelly RE Jr. Lymphadenopathy in children. *Pediatr Clin North Am* 1998;45(4):875–888.

Margileth AM. Antibiotic therapy for cat-scratch disease: clinical study of therapeutic outcome in 268 patients and a review of the literature. *Pediatr Infect Dis J* 1992;11:474–478.

Schutze GE. Diagnosis and treatment of Bortonella henselae infections. *Pediatr Infect Dis J* 2000;19(12):185–187.

Author: Louis M. Bell

Cataract

Database

DEFINITION

A cataract is any opacification of the normally clear crystalline lens of the eye. Some are small and nonprogressive and do not cause visual symptoms. Cataracts that are clinically significant and decrease visual acuity in children represent a major challenge.

CAUSES

- Of congenital cataracts, about one-third are inherited; one-third are associated with systemic genetic, metabolic, or maternal infectious disorders; and about one-third are idiopathic (cause unknown).
- A small number of cataracts are associated with other primary inherited ocular abnormalities.
- Developmental cataracts can result from metabolic disorders, toxic agents (steroids, radiation), and localized trauma.

PATHOPHYSIOLOGY

- Cataracts represent a derangement of the normal developmental growth of the crystalline fibers of the central lens nucleus or peripheral lens cortex, and the location of the opacity often suggests the gestational age at which they occurred.
- Cataracts are frequently classified according to their morphology or etiology.
- Dense central opacities of 3 mm or more usually produce substantial visual disability.

GENETICS

- Primary inherited congenital cataracts usually follow an autosomal-dominant mode of inheritance, but autosomal-recessive and X-linked–recessive varieties also occur. Multiple genes are involved in lens development, and numerous genetic loci have been identified.

EPIDEMIOLOGY

- Cataracts occur in as much as 0.4% of children and are estimated to cause between 10% and 40% of all blindness in children worldwide.

COMPLICATIONS

- Lack of removal of a visually significant cataract at the appropriate time leads to irreversible deprivation amblyopia, in which case no amount of surgery, optical correction, or amblyopia therapy is of benefit.
- Surgical removal of a cataract in children previously left the eye without a lens (aphakic) and unable to focus without some type of optical correction (spectacles or contact lenses). Unless rapid restoration of optical correction occurs, irreversible deprivation amblyopia may still occur after the cataract is removed, particularly if the cataract is unilateral. The aphakic pediatric eye is also more prone than an anatomically normal eye to elevated intraocular pressures (glaucoma) and early retinal detachments, either of which can cause permanent visual loss.
- More recently, intraocular lenses have become an accepted means of optical rehabilitation in children older than 2 years of age. Multicenter studies are underway to evaluate the use of intraocular lenses in younger children.

PROGNOSIS

- Prior to 1980, the majority of children treated for monocular cataracts had their best corrected vision only in the 20/200 to 20/800 range and children with bilateral cataracts obtained best corrected acuities in the 20/80 to 20/200 range.
- Earlier surgery, better surgical techniques, and rapid postsurgical optical correction now frequently afford corrected visual acuities of 20/40 to 20/200 for monocular cataracts and 20/40 or better for bilateral cataracts.
- Successful treatment of pediatric cataracts can be extremely difficult and intervention must occur very early in life in the case of congenital cataracts or as soon as possible in later-onset cataracts.
- Useful vision can be restored or obtained in newborns with unilateral cataracts if the surgery is completed within the first 6 weeks of life. After this time, visual restoration becomes progressively more difficult, again as a result of irreversible deprivation amblyopia.
- The prognosis for visual rehabilitation in children with bilateral congenital cataracts is slightly better, providing surgical removal and optical correction are accomplished early, preferably by 2 months of age.
- While later onset cataracts have a better prognosis because the visual system has developed to some degree, these children still require immediate evaluation and treatment.
- In all cases, the onset or presence of nystagmus before the cataract is removed is an ominous sign of poor outcome and adds further urgency to the need for surgical removal.
- Family compliance with both postsurgical optical correction and amblyopia treatment is critical and directly affects the child's ultimate visual outcome later in life.

Differential Diagnosis

The differential diagnosis of childhood cataracts is more concerned with the underlying cause of leukokoria ("white-pupil"), rather than the presence of some other entity, as the cataract itself is readily identified on examination by the ophthalmologist.

- Retinoblastoma, retinopathy of prematurity, juvenile retinoschisis, persistent hyperplastic primary vitreous, severe uveitis, and retinal detachment can all cause primary leukokoria or cause a cataract, which itself may produce leukokoria.

- Cataracts may also be an expression of a more severe, underlying systemic disease, which needs to be diagnosed to benefit the child's overall health.

ASSOCIATED DISEASES

- Maternal infections, such as the TORCH syndromes, especially congenital rubella.
- Metabolic and endocrine disorders such as galactosemia, neonatal hypoglycemia, and diabetes mellitus
- Fetal alcohol syndrome
- Chromosomal disorders, e.g., Down syndrome, trisomies 13 or 15, Turner syndrome
- Many craniofacial and mandibulofacial syndromes
- Dermatologic entities such as congenital ichthyosis, hereditary ectodermal dysplasia, and infantile poikiloderma
- Skeletal disorders such as Marfan and Conradi syndromes
- Renal disorders such as Lowe and Alport syndromes
- Neurofibromatosis
- Myotonic dystrophy
- Fabry disease and hypoparathyroidism
- Local ocular disorders, including aniridia, many of the anterior chamber dysgenesis syndromes, blunt or penetrating trauma, and diseases associated with ocular inflammation (chronic iritis or uveitis) such as juvenile rheumatoid arthritis.

Data Gathering

HISTORY

Question: Decreased visual responses?
Significance: Cataracts may decrease vision.

Question: Sun sensitivity or squinting in bright light?
Significance: Cataracts may cause glare and increase light sensitivity.

Question: Strabismus (ocular misalignment)?
Significance: Strabismus may indicate loss of vision in one eye.

Question: White pupil?
Significance: White pupil cataracts appear as a white object in or under the pupil.

Question: Unequal or abnormal pupillary reflections ("red eyes") with flash photography?
Significance: Cataract will block the standard red reflex.

Question: Nystagmus?
Significance: Nystagmus can be an ominous sign for the degree of vision loss.

Question: Careful family and prenatal history?
Significance: Up to one-third of congenital cataracts are inherited.

Question: Positive family history or known history of a disorder associated with cataracts?
Significance: See Associated Diseases.

Physical Examination

Finding: Decreased vision/visual acuity
Significance: Cataracts may cause decreased visual acuity.

Finding: Strabismus
Significance: May indicate loss of vision in one eye.

Finding: White pupil (leukokoria) on flashlight examination
Significance: Cataracts may appear as a white pupil.

Finding: Unequal, irregular, or poor red fundus reflections by direct ophthalmoscopy
Significance: Cataracts will interfere with seeing a red reflex.

Finding: Presence or absence of nystagmus
Significance: Nystagmus is a poor prognostic sign.

Finding: Bilaterality of disease
Significance: Bilateral cataracts are more likely to be secondary to systemic disease.

Finding: Size of globe ("eye ball")
Significance: Microphthalmia (small eye) suggests congenital cataracts.

Finding: Thorough physical examination for systemic syndromic findings
Significance: See Associated Diseases.

Laboratory Aids

- Complete ophthalmic evaluation, including slit-lamp biomicroscopy and fundus examination
- Ultrasonography if unable to visualize ocular structures behind the opacity
- Electrophysiologic analysis of the visual system
- A selective workup may be more indicated with bilateral cataracts and includes:

—TORCH titers, including syphilis
—Urine tests for reducing substance (galactosemia), protein, amino acids, and pH (Lowe syndrome)
—Blood glucose, calcium, phosphate
—Quantitative amino acids and RBC enzyme levels (galactokinase, gal-1-uridyltransferase)
—Genetic consultation, chromosome analysis, and ocular examination of parents and siblings

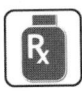

Therapy

- In the case of a monocular, small cataract, sometimes simple pharmacological pupillary dilatation of the affected eye and occlusion of the normal eye help to overcome mild amblyopia and preserve acceptable vision without surgical removal of the cataract. Glasses may or may not be of additional help.

- Small cataracts can progress, so nonsurgical treatments require close patient follow-up.
- Visually significant cataracts must be removed surgically. However, without optical correction of the operated, aphakic (lensless) eye, visual rehabilitation is impossible.
- Prior to age 2 years, optical correction of bilateral aphakia is most frequently accomplished with contact lenses or spectacles. In unilateral cataract cases, successful visual rehabilitation always requires extensive occlusion therapy to the normal eye for years. In these cases, optical correction of the unilateral aphakia is best obtained with a contact lens. Even when visual rehabilitation of monocular aphakia is successful, normal binocular vision with preserved depth perception is unlikely.
- In children older than 2 years, especially those with unilateral cataracts, intraocular lenses (IOLs) have, in appropriate cases, proved successful and are now being used frequently. They can afford faster visual rehabilitation and increased chances of normal binocular vision.
- Refractive corneal surgery for optical correction of aphakia is not indicated in children at this time.

Prevention

There is currently no known way to prevent congenital cataracts other than correcting any underlying metabolic abnormality. However, it is essential that all newborns (and all children) receive screening eye examinations by nurses, pediatricians, and family practitioners. In many parts of the world, early diagnosis and referral is still the limiting factor for a child's ultimate visual prognosis.

Follow-Up

- Without treatment, visually significant cataracts result in progressive visual loss. When opacity is present at birth or very early in life, the visual loss quickly becomes irreversible.
- Once surgical removal is performed and optical correction is started, the child, parents, and physician enter into an intensive and long rehabilitation period, lasting until visual maturity and stability are reached (usually around 7 to 10 years of age). After this point, yearly eye examinations are a minimum requirement.
- Parental and educational support services may be needed for those with residual visual handicap.
- Special local, state, and federal services for the visually handicapped and blind may be required, as not all children who have successful surgical results will have good vision.

Common Questions and Answers

Q: Is surgical removal of the cataract a visual cure?
A: No. Surgery is only the beginning of treatment, which also includes optical correction and amblyopia therapy.

Q: Once the cataract is removed, will intensive, extensive follow-up be needed?
A: Yes. The visual prognosis is directly related to postsurgical treatment compliance.

Q: Is the cataract easier to treat when the child is older?
A: No. Irreversible deprivation amblyopia develops as the child grows, precluding any chance for normal vision.

BIBLIOGRAPHY

Cheng KP. Pediatric cataracts. *Curr Opin Opthalmol* 1996;7(1):63–68.

Childhood cataracts and other lens disorders. In: Simon JW, et al., eds. *Pediatric Ophthalmology and Strabismus: Basic and Clinical Science Course. Section 6.* San Francisco: American Academy of Ophthalmology, 2003–2004:271–282.

Gimbel HV, Basti S, Ferensowicz M, et al. Results of bilateral cataract extraction with posterior chamber intraocular lens implantation in children. *Ophthalmology* 1997;104:1737–1743.

Lambert SR, Drack AV. Infantile cataracts. *Surv Ophthalmol* 1996;40:427–458.

Levin AV. Congenital eye anomalies *Pediatr Clin of North Am* 2003;50(1):55–76.

Taylor AL, Russell-Eggitt DI, Nischal KK, Lengyel D. The morphology and natural history of childhood cataracts. *Surv Opthalmol* 2003;48(2):125–144.

Wilson ME Jr, Trivedi RH, Hoxie JP, Bartholomew LR. Treatment outcomes of congenital monocular cataracts: the effects of surgical timing and patching compliance. *J Pediatr Ophthalmol Strabismus* 2003;40(6):323–329; quiz 353–354.

Zwann J, Mullaney PB, Awad AA, et al. Pediatric intraocular lens implantation: surgical results and complications in more than 300 cases. *Ophthalmology* 1998;105:112–119.

Authors: Gil Binenbaum and Brian J. Forbes

Cavernous Sinus Syndrome

 Database

DEFINITION

Cavernous sinus syndrome (CSS)—disease processes that localize to the cavernous sinus—a venous plexus that drains the face, mouth, tonsils, pharynx, nasal cavity, paranasal sinuses, orbit, middle ear, and parts of the cerebral cortex. Small lesions in this region may produce dramatic neurological signs.

CAUSES

- Infections include staphylococcus and streptococcus
- Aseptic venous thrombosis—sickle cell anemia, trauma, dehydration, vasculitis, pregnancy, oral contraceptives, congenital heart disease, inflammatory bowel disease and hypercoagulable states.
- Neoplasms—pituitary adenomas, meningiomas, craniopharyngioma, neuroma, chordoma, nasophyryngeal carcinomas.
- Carotid cavernous fistulas
- Nonspecific inflammation of cavernous sinus (idiopathic cavernous sinusitis, Tolosa-Hunt syndrome—a diagnosis of exclusion.

PATHOPHYSIOLOGY

- The cavernous sinus is located lateral to the pituitary gland and sella turcica, superior to the sphenoid sinus, and inferior to the optic chiasm.

—Within the cavernous sinus are the carotid artery, the pericarotid sympathetic fibers, and the abducens nerve (VI); within its lateral wall are the oculomotor nerve (III), the trochlear nerve (IV), and the ophthalmic and maxillary divisions of the trigeminal nerve (V1, V2).
—CSS is typically caused by septic or aseptic sinus thrombosis, neoplasm, or trauma. Acute obstruction by mass or thrombosis may progress rapidly if not diagnosed and treated quickly.

COMPLICATIONS

- Depends on the etiology of CSS. Septic CSS thrombosis and fungal infections may rapidly evolve to life-threatening sepsis and meningitis.
- Mucormycosis, usually seen in patients with diabetic ketoacidosis, is especially devastating.
- Carotid arteritis with resulting stenosis, occlusion, or embolism may occur, resulting in focal neurologic deficits.
- Aseptic CSS thrombosis may evolve to more extensive intracranial venous sinus thrombosis.
- Local spread of neoplasms will continue if not treated appropriately.

PROGNOSIS

Prognosis depends on the underlying etiology. Bacterial infections usually respond if diagnosed and treated promptly.

 Differential Diagnosis

Other disorders that may resemble CSS include:

- Orbital cellulitis
- Sphenoid sinusitis
- Thyroid eye disease
- Cavernous carotid aneurysm
- Orbital apex tumor
- Orbital pseudotumor
- Ocular migraine
- Ocular trauma

 Data Gathering

- First priority is to rule out septic cavernous sinus thrombosis, a life-threatening complication of infections of the face, sinuses, middle ear, teeth, and orbit.

—Infectious agents include S. aureus, S. pneumoniae, gram-negative rods, and anaerobes; Mucormycosis and Aspergillus in immunocompromised patients.

- Aseptic venous thrombosis has been associated with sickle cell anemia, trauma, dehydration, vasculitis, pregnancy, oral contraceptive use, congenital heart disease, inflammatory bowel disease, and hypercoagulable states.
- Neoplasms involving the cavernous sinus include pituitary adenomas, meningiomas, trigeminal schwannomas, craniopharyngiomas, lymphomas, neuromas, chordomas, chondrosarcomas, nasopharyngeal carcinomas, and very rarely teratomas. Neoplasms may present with diplopia, visual-field deficits, headache, or isolated cranial nerve deficits.
- The lateral extension of pituitary neoplasms into the cavernous sinus usually affects the third cranial nerve, with the fourth and sixth nerves less commonly involved. Rupture of a cystic craniopharyngioma may appear as acute CSS. Carotid-cavernous fistulas, often with a more chronic course, are direct high-flow shunts between the internal carotid artery and the cavernous sinus. Almost always sequelae of trauma, they may present with a history of ocular motility deficits, arterialization of conjunctival vessels, and a bruit usually heard best over the orbit.
- Nonspecific and idiopathic inflammation of the cavernous sinus, also called idiopathic cavernous sinusitis or Tolosa-Hunt syndrome, has been reported in patients as young as 3.5 years. This is a diagnosis of exclusion. However, magnetic resonance imaging (MRI) may show enlargement of the affected cavernous sinus with an adjacent soft tissue mass that resolves after treatment with steroids.

HISTORY

Question: Is there a history of a recent local infection?
Significance: Facial furuncle or cellulitis, sinusitis, dental infection, otitis, or orbital cellulitis may predispose to CSS.

Question: Are local or systemic symptoms present?
Significance: Fever, headache, eye pain, diplopia, and facial paresthesias may be present.

 Physical Examination

Finding: Conjunctival injection with lid swelling and proptosis
Significance: Signs of cavernous sinus venous congestion

Finding: Ptosis, anisocoria, ophthalmoparesis, and facial sensory changes
Significance: Signs of cranial nerve involvement

Finding: Horner syndrome
Significance: Sympathetic nerve fibers traveling with V1 may be affected. This usually occurs in conjunction with an abducens nerve (CN VI) palsy with an inability to abduct the eye.

Finding: Signs and symptoms begin unilaterally.
Significance: But may rapidly spread bilaterally.

Finding: The optic nerve and visual acuity are spared early in CSS.
Significance: But can be affected as it progresses.

Finding: Funduscopic findings include venous dilatation and hemorrhages.
Significance: Papilledema is rare in acute cavernous sinus disease.

Finding: Ocular bruit
Significance: May be heard in any acute CSS, but especially in carotid-cavernous fistula.

Finding: Signs of meningitis and systemic toxicity
Significance: These rapidly evolve if infections are untreated.

Laboratory Aids

Test: CBC, erythocyte sedimentation rate (ESR), PT/PTT, blood culture
Significance: Basic studies in any child with suspected acute CSS. Blood cultures are positive in 70% of cases of septic venous sinus thrombosis.

Test: Lumbar puncture (LP)
Significance: LP should be performed if there is no contraindication and infection is suspected. About 35% of patients with septic cavernous sinus thrombosis have CSF findings consistent with bacterial meningitis—excess neutrophils, increased protein and/or decreased glucose.

Test: MRI or CT
Significance: Any child with proptosis, cranial nerve findings, or an ocular bruit should have an urgent MRI or CT. MRI, with and without gadolinium, with special attention to the cavernous sinus and parasellar region, is the imaging study of choice. Magnetic resonance venography (MRV) may be helpful.

Test: Angiography
Significance: Diagnosis of carotid-cavernous fistulas require angiography.

Test: Nasopharyngeal biopsy and culture
Significance: Helpful if Mucormycosis or Aspergillus is suspected.

Test: ANA panel, ACE level, HIV test
Significance: Obtain before a diagnosis of Tolosa-Hunt syndrome (diagnosis of exclusion) is made.

 ## Emergency Care

Depending on the clinical condition of the patient and suspected etiology, emergency imaging, lumbar puncture, antibiotics and/or anticoagulation may be indicated.

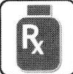 ## Therapy

For septic cavernous sinus thrombosis, broad-spectrum antibiotics (including coverage of penicillinase-resistant staphylococci and anaerobes) are begun immediately. Duration of therapy is usually 2 to 4 weeks beyond the resolution of symptoms.
Amphotericin B is given if Mucormycosis or *Aspergillus* is suspected.
Surgical drainage of the primary infection (i.e., sinusitis) may be indicated (avoiding surgical manipulation of the cavernous sinus itself).
Anticoagulation is controversial, but one study in adults found heparin reduced morbidity from septic cavernous sinus thrombosis.
Posttraumatic carotid-cavernous fistulas rarely close spontaneously; have been treated with endoarterial balloon embolization.
Consultation with a neuro-oncologist and a neurosurgeon are important for suspected neoplasms or surgical lesions.
Idiopathic cavernous sinusitis, a diagnosis of exclusion, responds to corticosteroids. Treatment should not be started until neoplasm and infection have been ruled out.

 ## Follow-Up

Septic cavernous sinus thrombosis may relapse or embolic abscesses may develop, 2 to 6 weeks after therapy has been stopped. Repeat MRI with gadolinium should be considered, especially if symptoms recur or new symptoms develop. Mortality remains 13% to 30%, and less than 40% of patients recover fully from cranial-nerve deficits. Patients with carotid-cavernous fistulas frequently have persistent cranial-nerve deficits even after embolization.
Idiopathic cavernous sinusitis responds to steroids, but relapses can be problematic. Clinical follow-up and serial MRI scans are indicated to rule out a low-grade neoplasm or fungal infection.

PREVENTION

Local bacterial infections—sinusitis, facial cellulitis, dental abscesses, otitis media, preseptal cellulitis, and orbital cellulitis—should be treated promptly. Patients with suspected hypercoagulable states should be evaluated fully; dehydration must be avoided in such patients and anticoagulation may be necessary.

PITFALLS

Ophthalmoplegic migraine or cluster headache must be distinguished from CSS by neuroimaging studies and history. Proptosis does not occur in migraine or cluster headache. Migraine is a diagnosis of exclusion, especially on first presentation. Acute infection and hemorrhage of the pituitary gland—pituitary apoplexy—may present with acute bilateral ophthalmoplegia and signs of acute pituitary insufficiency. This most commonly occurs with pituitary neoplasms, but may also occur in pregnant women at the time of delivery. Chronic granulomatous disorders such as sarcoid and tuberculosis may underlie CSS.

 ## Common Questions and Answers

Q: Will my child's eye movements return to normal?
A: In most cases, oculomotor nerves regain function as other signs improve, though they may take the longest to recover.

Q: Can more pain medicine be given?
A: There is often an attempt to balance side effects of sedation and hypoventilation against the need for pain control, especially when intracranial pressure is a concern.

BIBLIOGRAPHY

Cakirer S. MRI findings in Tolosa-Hunt syndrome before and after systemic corticosteroid therapy. *Eur J Radiol* 2003;45:83–90.

Eisenberg MB, Al-Mefty O, DeMonte F, Burson GT. Benign nonmeningeal tumors of the cavernous sinus. *Neurosurgery* 1999;44: 949–955.

Gallagher RM, Gross CW, Phillips CD. Suppurative intracranial complications of sinusitis. *Laryngoscope* 1998;108:1635–1642.

Keane JR. Cavernous sinus syndrome—analysis of 151 cases. *Arch Neurol* 1996;53: 967–971.

Liu GT, Volpe NJ, Galetta SL. *Neuro-Opthalmology: Diagnosis and Management*. Philadelphia: W.B. Saunders, 2001:550–561.

Authors: Dennis J. Dlugos and Sabrina E. Smith

Cavernous Transformation and Portal Vein Obstruction

 Database

DEFINITION

Major cause of prehepatic portal hypertension. Cavernous transformation is defined as the collection of collaterals that develop around an obstructed vessel. In pediatrics, the obstruction is most typically of the portal vein. In portal vein obstruction the main portal vein or splenic vein is obstructed anywhere along its course, between the hilum of the spleen and the porta hepatis.

PATHOPHYSIOLOGY

Asymptomatic splenomegaly or upper gastrointestinal hemorrhage, resulting from extrahepatic portal hypertension. Less commonly, the patient presents with ascites or failure to thrive. Fifty percent of portal vein obstructions are idiopathic. Identified etiologies include:

- Congenital vascular anomaly—portal vein malformation, webs or diaphragms within the portal vein.
- Clot resulting from a hypercoagulable states
- Clot from other etiologies—omphalitis, umbilical-vein catheterization, portal pyelophlebitis, intraabdominal sepsis, surgery near the porta hepatis, sepsis, cholangitis, dehydration, trauma
- Other causes for portal vein obstruction in older children include ascending pyelephlebitis from perforated appendicitis, primary peritonitis, cholangitis, and pancreatitis causing a splenic vein thrombosis and inflammatory bowel disease.

GENETICS

A genetic basis of this problem has not been identified although congenital abnormalities of the heart, major blood vessels, biliary tree, and renal system are often found.

EPIDEMIOLOGY

Most children with portal vein thrombosis present between birth and 15 years of age. Bleeding is more typical in patients presenting before 7 years of age; splenomegaly in the absence of symptoms is more typical for patients between ages 5 and 15.

DIAGNOSIS AND EVALUATION:

Clinical history and examination should concentrate on identifying possible etiologies predisposing to portal vein obstruction. Ultrasound remains the most useful imaging study especially with Doppler interrogation. Computed tomography (CT) or a magnetic resonance angiography can give additional information if needed.

COMPLICATIONS

- Variceal hemorrhage from the upper tract or from the perianal varices
- Splenomegaly with hypersplenism: thrombocytopenia, consumption coagulopathy, and leukopenia.
- Steatorrhea and protein-losing enteropathy occurs secondary to venous congestion of the intestinal mucosa.
- The degree of portal hypertension is variable and depends on the formation of spontaneous shunts that may decompress the portal hypertension. These auto-shunts may predispose to the development of complications such as hepatic encephalopathy or hepatopulmonary syndrome.
- The spleen can undergo autoinfarction resulting in intermittent episodes of pain.
- A large spleen is susceptible to traumatic rupture and spontaneous rupture may occur with infectious mononucleosis.

 Differential Diagnosis

The differential diagnosis must exclude other causes of splenomegaly and portal hypertension.

 Data Gathering

- Portal hypertension: spider nevi, prominence of abdominal veins, and splenomegaly.
- Bruising: prominent especially when there is a coexistent consumption of clotting factors.
- Normal liver palpation and percussion
- Ascites is rarely present.

HISTORY

Question: Other causes of splenomegaly?
Significance: Exposure to infectious mononucleosis, metabolic storage disease, and malignancy.

A history of prematurity and admission to neonatal intensive care unit (NICU) should alert the clinician to previous umbilical catheterization and increased risk of portal vein thrombosis.

 Physical Examination

Finding: Splenomegaly and possible hemorrhoids
Significance: The spleen is measured from the left anterior axillary line at the costal margin diagonally toward the umbilicus and inferiorly toward the iliac crest.

 Laboratory Aids

Test: CBC
Significance: Leukopenia and thrombocytopenia will be present if there is hypersplenism.

Test: AST/ALT/GGT
Significance: Should be normal

Test: PT/PTT
Significance: May be abnormal if malabsorption is present.

Test: Additional testing:

- Protein C
- Protein S
- Antithrombin III levels
- Factor V Leiden mutation
- Activated protein C resistance
- Lupus anticoagulation evaluation
- Anticardiolipin antibodies (IgA, IgG, IgM)
- Antinuclear antibody (ANA)
- Blood homocysteine
- Prothrombin 20-21-0 mutation
- Methylene tetrahydrofolate reductase mutation evaluation
- Factor Vlll coagulant
- Reptilase time
- Heparin cofactor ll
- Tissue plasminogen activator
- Plasminogen activator inhibitor-1
- Sticky platelet evaluation
- Paroxysmal nocturnal hemoglobinuria (genetics or flow cytometry evaluation).

Significance: Associated with hypercoagulable states.

Test: Ultrasound with Doppler
Significance: To examine portal vein flow and to identify collateral veins if there is cavernous transformation of the portal vein. The liver may be slightly small, but may be normal in texture.

Test: Liver biopsy
Significance: Exclude other etiologies. Not done as a routine.

Test: Upper endoscopy and sigmoidoscopy
Significance: To define extent of varices.

Test: Bone marrow examination
Significance: To determine if there is an underlying myeloproliferative disease.

Cavernous Transformation and Portal Vein Obstruction

 Therapy

Therapy is designed to manage variceal hemorrhage and to identify an underlying etiology to determine if the patient is at risk for additional venous thrombosis or malignancy. The therapy for gastrointestinal (GI) hemorrhage is:

1. Prophylactic variceal banding/sclerotherapy
2. β-blocker therapy in older children.
3. Rex shunt (mesenterico-left intrahepatic portal vein shunt) is created using the internal jugular vein, internal iliac vein, or the dilated coronary vein, which is used to connect the superior mesenteric vein and the umbilical portion of the left portal vein (in the liver). This restores the physiologic intrahepatic portal vein perfusion and avoids the consequences of long-term portosystemic shunting, especially hepatic encephalopathy.
4. Portosystemic shunts—These divert portal blood into the low-pressure systemic venous circulation and are classified into:

• Nonselective shunts: These communicate the entire portal venous system to a systemic venous circulation such as the mesocaval shunt, proximal splenorenal shunt, and portacaval shunts.
• Selective shunts: These divert the gastrosplenic portion of the portal venous flow into the left renal vein or the inferior vena cava. The most common selective shunt is the distal splenorenal shunt (also known as the Warren shunt).

Nonselective shunts divert more blood into the systemic venous system and patients are more likely to have encephalopathy.

 Follow-Up

Focus on growth parameters, early detection of malabsorption, presence of GI hemorrhage and nutritional intervention.

PITFALLS

The patient should be advised about activity restrictions as a result of splenomegaly. Spleen guards are recommended. Patient should be told to avoid medicines that interfere with platelet function. Medications that increase blood pressure are sometimes found in over the counter (OTC) cold medications (e.g., phenylephrine) can increase splanchnic pressures and may provoke variceal bleeds. Prior to long-distance flights, it may be prudent to endoscope patients to see if they have large varices that may bleed.

Aggressive contact sports are actively discouraged in children with hepatosplenomegaly.

 Common Questions and Answers

Q: What is the long-term prognosis?
A: Good. Upper GI hemorrhage becomes less problematic as the child becomes older. Shunting is rarely required. Most patients undergo prophylactic banding or sclerotherapy. If the liver function remains normal as in most cases, it is rare for encephalopathy to develop unless a large portosystemic is created.

Q: Should I restrict my child's activities?
A: Contact sports should be limited or a spleen guard used. Nonsteroidal antiinflammatory drugs (NSAIDs), including aspirin, should be avoided because of the risk of hemorrhage.

ICD-9-CM 747.49

BIBLIOGRAPHY

Fuchs J, Warmann S, Kardorff R, et al. Mesenterico-left portal vein bypass in children with congenital extrahepatic portal vein thrombosis: a unique curative approach. *J Pediatr Gastroenterol Nutr* 2003;36:213–216.

Mowat AP. *Liver Disorders in Childhood*. Boston: Butterworths, 1987.

Ryckman FC, Alonso MH. Portal hypertension: causes and management of portal hypertension in the pediatric population. *Clin Liver Dis* 2001;5(3).

Suchy F. *Liver Disease in Children*. 2nd Ed. Philadelphia: Lippincott Williams & Wilkins, 2001.

Authors: Vani Gopalareddy and John Tung

Celiac Disease

 Database

DEFINITION

Lifetime sensitivity to gliadin fraction of the wheat protein gluten, and related alcohol-soluble proteins (called prolamins) found in rye and barley. Celiac disease (CD) occurs in genetically susceptible individuals who ingest these proteins, leading to chronic intestinal inflammation, resulting in villous atrophy and flattening of the mucosa.
Other names: celiac sprue, nontropical sprue, and gluten-sensitive enteropathy.

CLINICAL PRESENTATION

• CD can present at any age from 6 months to 85 years of age, with peaks occurring during infancy up to 2 years age and young adulthood.
• CD has a wide spectrum of gastrointestinal and extraintestinal manifestations.
• The presentations of CD can be divided into the following six categories:

—Classic gastrointestinal form (80%):
  —Under the age of 2 years, after the introduction of gluten-containing foods in the diet.
  —Diarrhea
  —Failure to thrive
  —Fat-malabsorption
  —Wasting of muscles
  —Bloated abdomen
  —Unhappy behavior.
  —Explosive and foul-smelling stools
  —Vomiting
—Late-onset gastrointestinal form:
  —Recurrent abdominal pain
  —Constipation
  —Mild or intermittent diarrhea
  —Weight loss
  —Short stature.
—Extraintestinal form:
  —Musculoskeletal system: Idiopathic short stature (10%), arthritis, rickets, osteomalacia, osteoporosis (older patients)
  —Dental enamel defects: Caries of permanent dentition in all 4 quadrants (30%).
  —Skin: pathognomonic lesion, *Dermatitis herpetiformis* in 5% patients >15 years of age. The lesions are severely pruritic with erythematous blisters distributed symmetrically over the face, elbows, back, buttocks, and knees. Urticaria (hives) and psoriasis are also described.
  —Mucous membranes: Recurrent aphthous stomatitis.
  —Reproductive system: Delayed puberty, infertility, and spontaneous abortion.
  —Hematological system: Anemia (Iron, Vitamin B12, folic acid deficiency), easy bruising, bleeding (Vitamin K malabsorption)
  —Hepatic system: Cryptogenic hepatitis, autoimmune hepatitis, and chronic hypertransaminasemia.
  —Pancreatitis

—Central nervous system:
  —Epilepsy (20 times increased risk)
  —Depression
  —Dementia
  —Schizophrenia
  —Ataxia ("gluten-associated ataxia" as a result of cerebellar degeneration)
  —Migraine headaches
  —Behavioral changes: irritability, separation anxiety, emotional withdrawal and autistic-like behavior.
—Silent/asymptomatic celiac disease: Patients lack any gastrointestinal or extraintestinal signs and symptoms. They are usually identified through mass serologic screening or as a result of a proven CD in a first-degree relative. The small intestinal biopsy reveals mucosal damage in this group of individuals.
—Latent celiac disease: These patients have positive serology for the disease; however, the small intestine reveals normal histology. Over time, with further ingestion of gluten, it is believed that these individuals will develop CD.

Associated conditions: Patients with other autoimmune disorders are at substantially higher risk to have CD or to develop it in future: importantly diabetes type I.

Finally, some toddlers present with classic celiac disease on endoscopy and gluten challenge but after a few years they tolerate a gluten-containing diet with no endoscopic evidence of enteropathy. This is probably a form of transient protein intolerance, such as with milk protein intolerance.

PATHOPHYSIOLOGY

Small bowel biopsy is done by direct endoscopy with forceps
Features that characterize celiac disease are:

• Total villus atrophy (Severe case)
• Crypt hyperplasia
• Increased crypt cell mitosis
• Infiltration of lamina propria with excess lymphocytes (CD4 T cells mainly) and plasma cells.

EPIDEMIOLOGY

Prevalence: 1 in 120 to 300 persons in both Europe and North America.
Women more affected than men.

GENETICS

• There is a 5% to 15% concordance in first-degree relatives with celiac disease and 75% concordance in twins demonstrating the genetic causality.
• In addition, 90% of patients have the HLA-DQ2 molecule coded by the alleles DQA1*0501 and DQB1*0201 and 5% carry the HLA-DR4, DQ8 haplotype.

OTHER ASSOCIATED DISEASES

• Ankylosing spondylitis, scleroderma, systemic lupus erythematosus (SLE), Sjögren syndrome, and sarcoidosis.
• Addison disease, autoimmune thyroiditis, Graves disease, parathyroid adenoma, diabetes mellitus type I.
• Alopecia, atopic eczema, dermatitis herpetiformis, psoriasis.
• Mouth diseases such as cancer, lichen planus, and recurrent stomatitis.
• Inflammatory bowel disease and oropharyngeal cancers.
• Chronic active hepatitis, primary biliary cirrhosis, primary sclerosing cholangitis.
• Neurologic and behavioral disorders, epilepsy with posterior cerebellar calcification.
• Selective IgA deficiency.
• Chronic fibrosing alveolitis.
• Chromosomal anomalies such as Down and Turner syndrome.
• Cystic fibrosis.
• Alpha1-Antitrypsin deficiency.

 Differential Diagnosis

SMALL BOWEL VILLOUS ATROPHY

• Presumed infectious causes:

—Giardiasis
—Rotavirus
—Parasites
—Chronic gastroenteritis
—Postenteritis enteropathy
—Intractable diarrhea if infancy
—Tropical sprue
—Intestinal bacterial overgrowth
—Immunodeficiency syndromes (HIV).

• Presumed noninfectious:

—Celiac disease
—Milk or soy protein intolerance
—Protein—calorie malnutrition
—Eosinophilic gastroenteritis
—Autoimmune enteropathy
—Graft vs. host disease
—Collagenous sprue
—Peptic duodenitis
—Immunodeficiency syndromes
—Crohn disease
—Congenital enteropathies (microvillus inclusion disease, tufting enteropathy), bowel ischemia, radiation, chemotherapy

 Data Gathering

HISTORY

Question: Diet?
Significance: Determine the relationship between intake of gluten and symptoms. Find out the amount of wheat, rye, and barley.

Question: Growth pattern?
Significance: Most patients have short stature.

Question: Description of stools?
Significance: Stools tend to be explosive and foul-smelling.

Question: Description of behavior?
Significance: Patients tend to be irritable.

 ## Physical Examination

Finding: Growth pattern
Significance: Often have short stature

Finding: Classic presentation is large abdomen with wasted buttocks.
Significance: Many patients do not have that appearance.

DIAGNOSTIC TESTS FOR CD

1. Specific tests: Serology, histology and response to gluten free diet (GFD)
2. Nonspecific tests: Laboratory tests for vitamin and mineral deficiency states, tests of absorption (fecal fat, D-Xylose uptake), bone densitometry, Class II HLA genotyping (DQ2 and DQ8)

- Serology: Tissue transglutaminase antibody IgA (tTG IgA),
- Antireticulin antibody
- Antigliadin antibody IgA/ IgG (AGA IgA/ IgG)

Test: IgA quantification
Significance: Two percent of patients with celiac disease and 0.2% to 0.4% of general population are immunoglobin A (IgA)-deficient.

Test: Antigliadin antibody (AGA) IgA and IgG
Significance: Fifty percent to 90% with active celiac disease are positive. Unfortunately, many normal individuals without CD will have an elevated Ig G antigliadin antibody causing much confusion. Currently its use is restricted to the diagnostic workup of younger children <2 years of age who do not produce sufficient IgA and patients with IgA deficiency.

Test: Antireticulin antibody (AR) IgA
Significance: More specific but less sensitive than antigliadin Ab

Test: Tissue transglutaminase (tTG) IgA
Significance: The autoantigen responsible for the endomysial pattern is tissue transglutaminase (90% to 100% sensitive and specific). The tTG assay correlates well with AEA-IgA and biopsy. It is less expensive, rapid, and not a subjective test as opposed to AEA assay and is widely used. It has replaced antiendomysial antibodies as a serologic test.

BIOPSY

- Before a biopsy is done it is usual to check all the celiac antibodies as a screening test. With diagnosed patients AGA and tTG titers are useful monitoring tools for compliance and recovery.
- Should be performed on a regular diet.
- Reveals flattened villi with plasma cell infiltrate.

CBC

- Microcytic anemia as a result of iron deficiency is common in the absence of folic acid or Vitamin B12 deficiency

DIAGNOSIS

- Because AEA and tTG IgA are so specific for CD, some people have advocated treatment based on these antibodies alone. However the current standard is still to obtain a small bowel biopsy on a gluten-containing diet. Symptoms should resolve on a gluten-free diet with reversal of enteropathy on subsequent biopsy.
- Additional monitoring is done with symptoms and antibody testing.
- To diagnose transient gluten intolerance, a gluten challenge is carried out after an interval. There is no consensus as to when this should be performed.

TREATMENT

Gluten-free diet (GFD) with normalization of symptoms and enteropathy, which can take up to 6 months. Within 2 weeks of commencing GFD, 70% of patients will note symptomatic improvement.

COMPLICATIONS AND PROGNOSIS

Intestinal lymphoma has been reported in 10% to 15% of adult patients (>40 years of age) with CD who are noncompliant with GFD. Other complications include gastrointestinal malignancies including carcinoma, strictures, ulcerative jejunoileitis, splenic atrophy, and skeletal disorders.
Patients on strict GFD, there is very little risk of malignant lymphoma and other malignancies. Therefore, in patients with proven celiac disease it is advisable to remain on GFD for life.

Refractory CD

- It is a diagnosis of exclusion defined by persistent symptoms of malabsorption despite a strict GFD for at least 6 months with continued villus atrophy on duodenal biopsy.
- This should provoke a workup for other causes of villus atrophy.
- Refractory sprue affects 5% of patients with CD.
- Seventy-five percent of these patients harbor an abnormal clonal intraepithelial T-lymphocyte population, which is associated with a condition currently classified as cryptogenic enteropathy-associated T-cell lymphoma.

- Complications: Enteropathy-type intestinal T-cell lymphoma (EITCL), ulcerative jejunoileitis, and collagenous sprue.
- Treatment: Immunosupressants including corticosteroids, azathioprine, cyclosporin in addition to the GFD.

 ## Follow-Up

Compliance of patients can be monitored by the fall of AGA or tTG IgA antibodies with a gluten-free diet. This should be accompanied by improvement of presenting symptoms such as failure to thrive, diarrhea, and anemia.

 ## Common Questions and Answers

Q: Why do you do a gluten challenge when CD is a lifelong disease?
A: This is to exclude the diagnosis of transient gluten intolerance, which is more like a milk protein intolerance and disappears when the gut heals. In such patients, a gluten challenge is normal.

Q: Are oats included in the gluten-containing cereal?
A: Strictly speaking, wheat, rye, barley, and oats are more closely related in their development from the primitive grains such as rice, corn, sorghum, and millets, which do not activate celiac disease. Gluten-free means a diet devoid of all wheat, rye, barley, and oats but some adult studies have shown that ingestion of even up to 50 g of oats did not cause clear-cut histologic or clinical deterioration in celiac patients. It appears that of the four grains, oats is the least "toxic" to celiac patients.

Q: Can patients with CD drink beer?
A: Not if the beer is derived from barley, rye, wheat, or oats. However, they can drink light rum, white wine, and potato vodka.

ICD-9-CM 579.0

BIBLIOGRAPHY

Loftus CG, Murray JA. Celiac disease: diagnosis and management. *Hosp Phys* 2003;May:45–55.

McPherson RA. Advances in the laboratory diagnosis of celiac disease. *J Clin Lab Anal* 2001;15(3):105–107.

Pietzak MM. Celiac Disease: going against the grains. *Nutr Clin Prac* 2001;16:335–344.

Authors: Vani Gopalareddy and John Tung

Cellulitis

 Database

DEFINITION

- Inflammation/infection of the skin/subcutaneous tissues
- Often classified by body area involved:

—Periorbital
—Orbital
—Buccal
—Peritonsillar
—Extremity
—Breast
—Perianal
—Adenitis

CAUSES

- *Staphylococcus aureus*
- Group A β-hemolytic streptococci (*Streptococcus pyogenes*)
- *S. pneumoniae*: less common since advent of childhood vaccination with heptavalent pneumococcal conjugate vaccine (Prevnar)
- Group B streptococci, gram-negative bacilli: neonates
- *Haemophilus influenzae* type b: very rare now as a result of childhood immunization
- *Pseudomonas aeruginosa*, anaerobic bacteria: immunocompromised children
- *Pasteurella* species: from cat and dog bites
- *Eikenella corrodens*: from human bites

PATHOPHYSIOLOGY

- Most commonly secondary to local trauma

—Abrasions
—Lacerations
—Bite wounds
—Excoriated dermatitis, varicella
—Other breaches in the integument

- May develop secondary to local invasion or infection (e.g., sinusitis leading to orbital cellulitis).
- Hematogenous dissemination

EPIDEMIOLOGY

- The most common cause of cellulitis in children is *S. aureus* or *S. pyogenes* infection, which develops secondary to local trauma of the integument.
- Bacteremic disease, previously seen commonly when *H. influenzae* type b was prevalent, has now been surpassed by *S. pneumoniae*.
- Clinical failures with penicillin-resistant *S. pneumoniae* have not yet become a significant problem in cases of uncomplicated cellulitis.
- Methicillin-resistant *S. aureus* (MRSA) infections have risen dramatically in the past few years.

ASSOCIATED ILLNESSES

- Periorbital

—Usually secondary to local trauma
—Impetigo
—Varicella
—Eczema
—Hematogenous is very uncommon
—Rarely associated with infectious conjunctivitis

- Orbital

—Most commonly associated with severe sinusitis
—Much less commonly: dental abscess, trauma, hematogenous

- Buccal

—Same pathophysiology and epidemiology as periorbital cellulitis (excluding conjunctivitis)

- Peritonsillar

—Commonly secondary to severe group A β-hemolytic streptococcal pharyngitis
—Cellulitis may progress to a peritonsillar abscess

- Extremity

—Almost always secondary to local trauma

- Breast

—Usually with mastitis (most often in neonates)

- Perianal

—Seen in infants and young children
—Etiology: Group A Streptococcus
—Perianal pain, pruritus, and erythema; sometimes associated with bloody stools.

- Cellulitis-Adenitis Syndrome

—Uncommon infection seen in neonates and young infants
—Etiology: Group B Streptococcus, *S. aureus*, gram-negative bacilli
—Bacteremia and/or meningitis commonly associated

COMPLICATIONS

- Local as well as distant spread of infection is possible.
- Suppuration and abscess formation may occur (e.g., peritonsillar abscess).
- Extremity cellulitis may extend into the deep tissues to produce an arthritis or osteomyelitis, or it may extend proximally as a lymphangitis.
- Orbital cellulitis may be complicated by visual loss and/or cavernous sinus thrombosis.
- Prior to widespread immunization against *H. influenzae* type b, the bacteremia associated with facial cellulitis was commonly associated with pneumonia, meningitis, pericarditis, epiglottitis, as well as arthritis and osteomyelitis.

PROGNOSIS

- The prognosis for complete recovery is good as long as appropriate antimicrobials are administered in a timely fashion.

 Differential Diagnosis

- Allergic angioedema is the most common entity; it can usually be excluded by its lack of tenderness and the absence of fever.
- Contact dermatitis, similarly, is distinguished by its painlessness, pruritus, and the Koebner phenomenon (appearance of isomorphic lesions in the lines of scratching).
- A traumatic contusion may be mistaken for cellulitis, but the history should be confirmatory.
- Severe conjunctivitis may mimic periorbital cellulitis; conjunctival injection, chemosis, and discharge usually implicate conjunctivitis.
- "Popsicle panniculitis," a cold-induced fat injury to the cheeks of infants, may be almost indistinguishable from buccal cellulitis; a history of cold weather exposure, or ice or popsicle sucking should be sought.
- A primary eye malignancy (retinoblastoma), locally invasive tumor (rhabdomyosarcoma), or metastatic disease (neuroblastoma, leukemia, lymphoma), may simulate periorbital or orbital cellulitis.

 Data Gathering

HISTORY

Question: Is there an expanding, red, painful area of swelling?
Significance: This is the most common presentation.

Question: Are there associated, mild constitutional symptoms (with or without fever)?
Significance: Commonly associated with cellulitis.

Question: Is there a history of local trauma to the integument?
Significance: This is the clue to the portal of bacterial entry.

Question: Are there visual changes, or pain with (or limitation of) eye movements?
Significance: Worrisome for orbital cellulitis.

Question: Is there painful swallowing, pain with opening the mouth (trismus), muffled ("hot-potato") voice?
Significance: Classic presenting symptoms of peritonsillar cellulitis/abscess.

Physical Examination

Finding: Erythema, edema, tenderness, and warmth
Significance: The classic clinical findings of cellulitis.

Finding: Distinct demarcation of raised erythema
Significance: The classic description of erysipelas, a superficial cellulitis usually associated with *S. pyogenes*.

Finding: A red streak extending proximally from the extremity
Significance: Lymphangitis, which usually implies more serious involvement.

Finding: Regional adenopathy
Significance: Commonly associated with minor cellulitis. Occasionally complicated by lymphadenitis.

Laboratory Aids

Test: WBC count
Significance: May be normal or elevated.

Test: Blood culture
Significance: Blood cultures are rarely positive in most routine cases of cellulitis. Ill-appearing children, and children with extensive cases of cellulitis, however, should probably have a culture obtained.

Test: Wound culture
Significance: As resistance continues to rise, cultures should be sent from any site in which *S. aureus* is a suspected pathogen.

Test: X-ray studies
Significance: Sometimes helpful to rule out complications such as arthritis or osteomyelitis. Also useful in cases of suspected foreign bodies.

Test: Head CT scan
Significance: Important in orbital cellulitis to delineate extent of disease, and also in some cases when distinction from periorbital cellulitis is clinically difficult.

Therapy

- Most cases of uncomplicated, superficial cellulitis can be treated with oral antibiotics active against *Staphylococcus* and *Streptococcus* (e.g., amoxicillin-clavulanate, cephalexin, and erythromycin).
- For more severe infections, in which *S. aureus* is a suspected pathogen, clindamycin should be considered as empiric therapy; allergic patients should receive trimethoprim-sulfamethoxazole.
- Ill-appearing children or those with extensive cellulitic lesions require intravenous antibiotics.
- Initial intravenous therapy should be directed against *S. aureus* and *Streptococcus* (e.g., oxacillin, nafcillin, cefazolin, or ampicillin/sulbactam).
- As MRSA infections continue to rise, many experts now recommend clindamycin as initial parenteral therapy.
- Vancomycin should be used as empiric therapy for severe or rapidly progressive infections.
- If hematogenous dissemination is a strong possibility, an agent active against *H. influenzae* type b also should be added (e.g., ceftriaxone, cefotaxime).
- Infants ≤6 weeks of age should have gram-positive and gram-negative coverage (e.g., oxacillin/nafcillin and gentamicin, or oxacillin/nafcillin and cefotaxime) to cover the enterics as well.
- The duration of antibiotics (intravenous and oral) should generally be 7 to 10 days.
- Abscesses should be surgically drained.
- Bite wounds should have tetanus and rabies prophylaxis issues addressed.

Follow-Up

- Rapid, steady improvement should be expected.
- If daily improvement is not noted, inappropriate antimicrobial coverage, a deeper infection or abscess, or some other complication should be suspected (e.g., foreign body).

PREVENTION

- Good wound care can prevent most cases of cellulitis.
- Parents should be instructed to cleanse all wounds thoroughly with soap and water, then cover with a clean, dry cloth.
- Topical antibiotic ointment is optional.

PITFALLS

- Do not forget to consider the possibility of MRSA in all deep, invasive, or persistent infections (Clindamycin is recommended).
- Penicillin and amoxicillin are never good empiric choices for even superficial cellulitis (poor *S. aureus* coverage).

Common Questions and Answers

Q: Should MRSA only be considered in patients with risk factors, such as recent hospitalization, chronic illness, health care worker contact, and recent antibiotic use?
A: No, many patients do not have commonly identified risk factors.

Q: Is ophthalmology consultation necessary in all cases of periorbital cellulitis?
A: Ophthalmology consultation is not necessary in simple, uncomplicated cases of periorbital cellulitis that clearly have no associated proptosis, limitation in extraocular eye movement, or visual impairment that would suggest a more serious orbital cellulitis.

ICD-9-CM 682.9

BIBLIOGRAPHY

Berger-Sadow K, Chamberlain JM. Blood cultures in the evaluation of children with cellulitis. *Pediatrics* [serial online]. March 1998;101(3):e4.

Danik SB, Schwartz RA, Oleske JM. Cellulitis. *Cutis* 1999;64:157–164.

Eady EA, Cove JH. Staphylococcal resistance revisited: community-acquired methicillin resistant Staphylococcal aureus—an emerging problem for the management of skin and soft tissue infections. *Curr Opin Infect Dis* 2003; 16(2):103–124.

Givner LB. Periorbital versus orbital cellulitis. *Pediatr Infect Dis J* 2002;21(12):1157–1158.

Greenberg MF, Pollard ZF. The red eye in childhood. *Pediatr Clin N Am* 2003;50(1): 105–124.

Lee MC, Rios AM, Aten MF, et al. Management and outcome of children with skin and soft tissue abscesses caused by community-acquired methicillin resistant Staphylococcal aureus. *Pediatr Infect Dis J* 2004;23:123–127.

Santos-Juanes J, Medina A, Concha A, et al. Varicella complicated by group A streptococcal facial cellulitis. *J Am Acad Dermatol* 2001;45(5):770–772.

Sobol SE, Marchand J, Tewfik TL, et al. Orbital complications of sinusitis in children. *J Otolaryngol* 2002;31(3):131–136.

Starkey CR, Steele RW. Medical management of orbital cellulitis. *Pediatr Infect Dis J* 2001;20(10):1002–1005.

Author: Nicholas Tsarouhas

Cerebral Palsy

 Database

DEFINITION AND CLASSIFICATION

- Cerebral palsy (CP) is a nonprogressive motor impairment condition that results from damage to or dysfunction of the brain. Subtypes are defined by type of neurologic impairment and anatomic distribution:

—Spastic CP (pyramidal CP) (40%): increased deep tendon reflexes, sustained clonus, hypertonia, and the clasp-knife response
—Spastic diplegia—lower extremity involvement
—Spastic hemiplegia—one side of the body involved
—Spastic quadriplegia—total-body involvement.
—Dyskinetic CP (30%): fluctuating tone, rigidity total-body involvement by definition.

- Persistent primitive reflex patterns (e.g., asymmetric tonic neck reflex [ATNR], labyrinthine) often seen. Subtypes:

—Athetoid CP: slow writhing movements (or chorea: rapid, random, jerky movements),
—Dystonic CP: posturing of the head, trunk, and extremities. Ataxic CP (< 10%): characterized by cerebellar signs (ataxia, dysmetria, past-pointing, tremor, nystagmus) and abnormalities of voluntary movement
—Mixed CP (10%): two or more types codominant, most often spastic and dyskinetic

- Other CP (10%): criteria for CP met but specific subtype cannot be defined
- Extrapyramidal CP: sometimes applied to nonspastic types of CP as a group

EPIDEMIOLOGY

- Prevalence approximately 2 per 1,000
- Approximately 50% of cases are associated with prematurity.
- Increased incidence with multiple gestation (10% were twins in one study)
- Increased concordance among monozygotic versus dizygotic twins in some studies (not in others)
- Intrauterine growth retardation (IUGR) more common in CP than controls, especially for full-term infants in whom CP develops.
- Male/female ratio, 1.3:1
- Inconsistent correlation to maternal age, socioeconomic status, and parity
- Epidemiologic studies suggest that prenatal factors are more strongly associated with subsequent CP than perinatal or postnatal factors; however, individual risk factors are poorly predictive of subsequent CP in the individual child.
- Diagnosis of perinatal asphyxia requires evidence of multiorgan system hypoxic-ischemic insult and severe encephalopathy (e.g., neonatal seizures, severe hypotonia), and accounts for only about 9% of cases of CP.

ETIOLOGY

- In the majority of cases, etiology is not apparent. A more recently recognized perinatal factor is the presence of chorioamnionitis; mild or even subclinical cases may have increased association with CP.
- Epidemiologic studies indicate two types of vulnerability to CP: prematurity-related and IUGR-related.

—Prematurity-related: unique vulnerability of the periventricular white matter between 28 and 32 weeks of gestation results in periventricular leukomalacia.
—IUGR-related: in full-term infants, fetal abnormalities associated with central nervous system (CNS) dysgenesis, non-CNS malformation, teratogens, growth retardation, evidence of hypoxic-ischemic encephalopathy more often seen.

ASSOCIATED IMPAIRMENTS

- Sensory

—Sensorineural and conductive hearing loss
—Impairments of visual acuity
—Oculomotor dysfunction
—Strabismus
—Somatosensory impairments

- Cognitive

—Mental retardation (MR) in about 50%, especially in spastic quadriparesis
—High incidence of learning disabilities
—Attention deficit/hyperactivity disorder
—Sleep and behavioral disturbances

- Neurologic

—Seizures
—Hydrocephalus

- Musculoskeletal

—Contractures
—Hip subluxation/dislocation
—Scoliosis

- Cardiorespiratory

—Upper airway obstruction
—Aspiration pneumonitis
—Restrictive lung disease
—Secondary to thoracic deformity
—Reactive airway disease

- Gastrointestinal tract/nutrition

—Failure to thrive
—Gastroesophageal reflux
—Constipation
—Oral motor dysfunction/dysphagia

- Gastrourinary tract
- Neurogenic bladder
- Skin

—Decubitus ulcers

- Dental

—Caries
—Gingival hyperplasia
—Abnormalities of enamel (congenital)

 Differential Diagnosis

- Motor impairment syndromes related to spinal cord, lower motor neuron, peripheral nerve, primary muscular disease, or progressive disorders of the basal ganglia.
- Connective-tissue disorders (primary and secondary) resulting in musculoskeletal abnormalities (e.g., arthrogryposis multiplex, skeletal dysplasias)

 Data Gathering

HISTORY

Question: Prenatal history?
Significance: Exposure to toxins/drugs, infections or fever, HIV/STD risk, vaginal bleeding, abnormal fetal movement, preeclampsia (especially proteinuria), breech position, poor maternal weight gain, premature labor, fetal distress, IUGR, prenatal testing, placental disorders.

Question: Perinatal history?
Significance: Premature delivery, neonatal resuscitation, low Apgar scores (7 at 5 and 10 minutes), birth trauma, evidence of neonatal encephalopathy (seizures, severe hypotonia), complicated neonatal course (intraventricular hemorrhage, prolonged respiratory support, meningitis, sepsis, hyperbilirubinemia).

Question: Postnatal history?
Significance: Hospitalization for severe infection or trauma, periodic or persistent deterioration in function (suggests neurodegenerative/metabolic disease).

Question: Development?
Significance: Severe delay in motor milestones (e.g., not rolling at 7 months, not sitting at 8 months, not walking at 15 months) associated with persistent primitive reflexes (e.g., prominent tonic neck and labyrinthine responses at 1 year of age) and delayed or absent development of protective reactions (e.g., lateral prop at 7 months, parachute at 13 months). Associated delays in language, play, social, and adaptive behavior.

 Physical Examination

GENERAL

Finding: Respiratory pattern
Significance: Obstruction, aspiration risk, evidence of dysmorphism/pigmentary skin changes and growth abnormalities contribute to assessment of etiology.

Finding: Head circumference
Significance: To evaluate for microcephaly/macrocephaly/ hydrocephaly-growth velocity is important

Finding: Strabismus/cataracts/iris or retinal abnormalities
Significance: Either cranial nerve damage, muscle imbalance, metabolic disease, or congenital infection.

MUSCULOSKELETAL

Finding: Range of motion
Significance: Decreased with contractures

Finding: Leg-length discrepancy
Significance: Hip dislocation

Finding: Spinal curvature
Significance: Neuromuscular imbalance

NEUROLOGIC

Finding: In addition to formal examination, documentation of best level of visual motor/manipulative skills (e.g., able to run, transfer, hold a cup, etc.)
Significance: Helpful in following the course of the motor impairment.

Finding: Cranial nerves
Significance: Especially strabismus, speech and swallowing, vision and hearing.

Finding: Tone
Significance: Spasticity versus rigidity versus hypotonia

Finding: Strength
Significance: Often decreased

Finding: Clasp-knife response
Significance: Hyperactive deep tendon reflexes, and clonus in spasticity; Babinski reflex (extensor response to plantar stimulation)

Finding: Persistent primitive reflexes
Significance: CNS damage

Finding: Protective reactions
Significance: Head and trunk righting, prop reactions, parachute; cerebellar signs

Finding: Postural stability
Significance: Neuromuscular imbalance

Finding: Gait abnormalities, subtle seizures
Significance: Motor or CNS damage

 ## Laboratory Aids

Test: Hearing and vision
Significance: All in first year with regular follow-up examinations (identification of sensory deficits and clues to etiology)

Test: Brain imaging
Significance: Should be performed when hydrocephalus is suspected; frequently useful in determining etiology

Test: Genetic and metabolic studies
Significance: Indicated when the history and physical examination suggest a progressive or hereditary disorder

Test: Chest radiograph studies
Significance: Should be done routinely in spastic diparesis for hip dislocation;

usefulness of scoliosis films depends on physical findings

Test: Audiologic evaluation
Significance: Required for those with language delay or those who manifest hearing impairment

Test: Radionucleotide studies or pH probe
Significance: "Milk scan"; evaluate gastroesophageal reflux (GER), gastric emptying, aspiration

Test: Blood tests—chemistries, liver-function studies, cell counts
Significance: Evaluate nutritional/metabolic status, anticonvulsant levels

Test: Urodynamic studies
Significance: Spastic bladder, indicated in those with recurrent urinary tract infections or voiding dysfunction

Test: Sleep study
Significance: May disclose treatable obstructive sleep apnea in those with excessive somnolence or abnormal sleep-wake cycles

Test: Pulmonary-function studies
Significance: Helpful in documenting progressive restrictive pulmonary dysfunction (e.g., in severe scoliosis)

Test: EEG
Significance: Seizure disorder is suspected

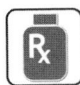 ## Therapy

- Family-centered care is directed toward optimizing function/minimizing handicap (habilitation).
- Interdisciplinary clinics: to provide multiple services (medical, surgical, therapy, etc.) coordinated with primary care physician.
- Therapy with intramuscular injections of botulinum toxin is used increasingly, though the therapy may need to be repeated every 3 to 5 months. Specific, concrete goals for the therapy should be established at initiation.
- Education services: recent emphasis on inclusion/mainstreaming; for many children, special education services are still required and appropriate.
- Physical, occupational, speech/language therapy, other allied health professionals: therapy provided in home, school, and hospital settings, directed primarily at improved functioning in the areas of mobility, self-care, and communication; orthodontists for braces.
- Social services: provided in a variety of contexts to aid in the coordination of care

 ## Follow-Up

- Requirements for follow-up vary greatly with the degree of disability and the scope of impairments. An interdisciplinary clinic setting may be more appropriate for a child with severe CP.

- Early referral to a pediatric orthopedist is indicated, especially for monitoring of early hip subluxation, which is best managed before progression to frank dislocation.
- Early referral for developmental assessment to establish need for early intervention, to optimize development, and to promote family coping

PITFALLS

- Overdiagnosis of CP in infants with spastic hypertonia (especially those born prematurely); normalization of tone/function may take up to 2 years.
- Slowly progressive neurogenerative disease may masquerade as CP.
- Cervical cord lesions may masquerade as quadriparetic spastic CP. Swallowing reflexes may be preserved; cognitive development is normal.
- Determination of ideal body weight may be complex in CP; growth standards according to CP type are under development.

 ## Common Questions and Answers

Q: Is severe clumsiness a form of CP?
A: Mild spastic diplegia or hemiplegia may present this way, but spasticity and contractures distinguish these from developmental coordination disorders.

Q: Do children with CP also have mental retardation?
A: Not necessarily; although 50% have mental retardation, it is not a part of the definition of CP.

Q: What about surgery for CP?
A: Spasticity in the lower extremities may be addressed directly with selective dorsal rhizotomy (interruption of afferent limb of stretch reflex arch). Otherwise, surgical therapy in CP is directed at associated conditions; many children with CP undergo orthopaedic procedures for hip dislocation, release of contractures, and scoliosis. Surgery for correction of strabismus or placement of a gastrostomy tube is commonly performed.

ICD-9-CM 343.9

BIBLIOGRAPHY

Ashwal S, Russman BS, Blasco PA, et al. Practice Parameter: diagnostic assessment of the child with cerebral palsy. Report of the Quality Standards Subcommittee of the American Academy of Neurology and the Practice Committee of the Child Neurology Society. *Neurology* 2004;62:851–863.

Online Information for Parents: United Cerebral Palsy Association, www.ucp.org.

Authors: Robert Harkam Mitchell
Louis Pelligrino, 2nd edition

Cervicitis

Database

DEFINITION

Cervicitis is infection of the endocervix resulting in inflammation leading to mucopurulent cervical discharge, edema, erythema, and friability of the cervix and endocervical canal.

CAUSES

In the majority of young women, no pathogen is isolated. Common identifiable causes include:

- *Chlamydia trachomatis*
- *Neisseria gonorrhoeae*
- *Herpesvirus hominis*
- *Trichomonas vaginalis*
- *Candida albicans*

ASSOCIATED DISEASES

The presence of other sexually transmitted diseases must be considered including:

- *T. vaginalis*
- Syphilis
- Hepatitis B
- HIV
- Bacterial vaginosis

EPIDEMIOLOGY

The true incidence of mucopurulent cervicitis is unknown; however, it is quite common. As many patients are asymptomatic and the interpretation and presence of the clinical signs is quite variable, many cases go undiagnosed.

COMPLICATIONS

The patient with endocervical infection is at risk for:

- Reinfection
- Other sexually transmitted diseases
- Pregnancy
- Symptomatic or asymptomatic upper genital tract disease with all its sequelae

—Tubo-ovarian abscess
—Infertility
—Ectopic pregnancy
—Chronic pelvic pain

PROGNOSIS

If treated appropriately, these patients are cured and have no sequelae from the infection.

Differential Diagnosis

- It is helpful to consider cervicitis /vaginitis as a single disease because the symptoms of these two entities are the same.
- Inflammation of the vulva, the urethra and/or bladder, the vagina, and the endocervical canal
- In patients presenting with abnormal menstrual bleeding, these infectious causes are common.

Data Gathering

HISTORY

Symptoms Consistent With But Not Diagnostic of Cervicitis

Question: Abnormal vaginal bleeding and/or discharge?
Significance: Inflamed cervix may bleed spontaneously or following sexual intercourse.

Question: Dysuria?
Significance: May indicate urethritis or bladder infection.

Question: Vulvar itching?
Significance: May be associated discharge from cervical inflammation or a coexisting vaginal infection.

Question: Dyspareunia?
Significance: Common complaint as a result of the sensitive cervix.

MEDICAL HISTORY

Important Questions of Women's Health Assessment But Not Diagnostic of Cervicitis

Question: Previous sexually transmitted disease (STD)?
Significance: Identifies patients at increased risk for reinfection.

Question: Last menstrual period?
Significance: Symptomatic infection often occurs within 7 days of the last menstrual period as a result of loss of the protective endocervical mucous plug.

Question: Birth control method?
Significance: Condoms are protective.

Question: Exposure to infected partner?
Significance: Identifies patient at increased risk.

Question: Gravity?

Question: Parity?

Physical Examination

ABDOMEN

Finding: No tenderness on palpation of the abdomen
Significance: Infection is limited to the cervix.

PELVIC

Finding: Mucopurulent discharge from the cervical os or yellow exudative discharge present on a cotton-tipped swab from the endocervical canal
Significance: Clinical evidence of cervical infection

Finding: No cervical motion or adnexal tenderness or masses
Significance: Pathology has not extended beyond the cervix to the upper genital tract

Finding: Friability of the exocervix.
Significance: Easily induced bleeding from the cervical canal, not to be confused with normal cervical ectopy (area of columnar epithelium around the cervical os presenting as a discrete, nonfriable, reddish circle)

Laboratory Aids

Test: Nucleic acid amplification tests done on the patient's urine offer the least invasive method to detect chlamydia and/or gonococcal infection. Cervical or vaginal swabs can also be used for nucleic acid amplification tests provided that there is no bleeding. Cervical swabs, vaginal swabs obtained by the health-care provider, and urine have similar sensitivity and specificity. Cervical cultures for chlamydia and gonorrhea will also identify the pathogen, but this requires a speculum examination.
Significance: Identifies the pathogen which is important for patient and partner treatment, and disease surveillance

Test: HSV culture if vesicular rash or ulcers are present
Significance: Important to identify the cause of the ulcers for treatment and patient counseling.

Test: Wet preparation or culture for *T. vaginalis*
Significance: Often coexisting infection when other STIs are idientified

Test: Potassium hydroxide preparation for budding hyphae
Significance: Test for *Candida*

Therapy

- Patients meeting the criteria for the clinical diagnosis for cervicitis or those in have a high likelihood of infection should receive therapy for *N. gonorrhoeae* and *C. trachomatis*. Treat other pathogens if clinically indicated or if documented by laboratory studies.
- Gonorrhea

—Ciprofloxacin, 500 mg PO, single dose
—Ofloxacin 400 mg PO, single dose
—Ceftriaxone, 125 mg IM, single dose

- *C. trachomatis*

—Azithromycin, 1 g PO, single dose
—Doxycycline, 100 mg PO b.i.d. for 7 days
—Erythromycin base 500 mg PO q.i.d. for 7 days

- *T. vaginalis*

—Metronidazole, 2 g PO single dose
—Metronidazole, 500 mg PO b.i.d. for 7 days

- *H. hominis*

—Acyclovir 400 mg PO t.i.d. for 7 to 10 days, or until resolution
—Acyclovir, 200 mg PO five times daily for 7 to 10 days, or until resolution
—Famciclovir 250 mg PO t.i.d. for 7 to 10 days, or until resolution
—Valciclovir 1 g PO b.i.d. for 7 to 10 days, or until resolution

- *C. albicans*

—Butoconazole 2% cream 5 g intravaginally for 3 days
—Butoconazole 2% cream 5 g (Butoconazole1 sustained release) single vaginal application
—Clotrimazole 1% cream, 5 g intravaginally for 7 to 14 days
—Clotrimazole 100 mg vaginal tablet, for 7 days
—Clotrimazole 500 mg vaginal tablet, single application
—Miconazole 2% cream, 5 g intravaginal for 7 days
—Fluconazole 150 mg PO single dose

 ## Follow-Up

The recommended treatment regimens have an excellent cure rate. The patient should have resolution of symptoms 3 to 5 days after starting therapy. Routine follow-up cultures are not necessary unless the patient remains symptomatic. Nucleic acid amplification tests done < 3 weeks following treatment can yield false-positive results as a result of persistence of dead organisms. Detection of an STI at follow-up is most likely as a result of reexposure and reinfection.

PITFALLS

Failure to recognize the importance of evaluating the internal pelvic organs by physical examination with the presenting symptoms of dysuria, vaginal discharge, or abnormal menstrual bleeding in the postpubertal female.

 ## Common Questions and Answers

Q: How much cervical motion tenderness is present in patients with cervicitis?
A: None. Patients with cervicitis have inflammation and infection of the cervix only. They do not have any evidence of peritoneal inflammation on physical examination. Therefore, patients with tenderness should be treated with the protocols recommended by the Centers for Disease Control and Prevention for pelvic inflammatory disease. This does not include the use of a single dose of azithromycin.

Q: Which partners should be referred for treatment?
A: Sex partners from the preceding 60 days should be referred for evaluation and treatment. Treatment is based on documented or presumptive etiologies.

ICD-9-CM 616.0

BIBLIOGRAPHY

American Academy of Pediatrics. Sexually transmitted diseases. In: Pickering LK, ed. *2003 Red Book: Report of the Committee on Infectious Diseases.* 26th Ed. Elk Grove Village, IL: American Academy of Pediatrics, 2003.

Holmes KK. Lower genital tract infections in women: cystitis, urethritis, vulvovaginitis, and cervicitis. In: Holmes KK, Mardh P, Sparling PF, et al., eds. *Sexually Transmitted Diseases.* 2nd Ed. New York: McGraw-Hill, 1990:527–545.

Neinstein LS. *Adolescent Health Care: A Practical Guide.* 4th Ed. Baltimore: Urban and Schwarzenberg, 2002.

U.S. Department of Health and Human Services. 2002 Guidelines for treatment of sexually transmitted diseases. *MMWR Morb Mortal Wkly Rep* 2002;51RR-6

Author: Jane Lavelle

Etiology of Infection

VULVITIS	VAGINITIS	CERVICITIS	URETHRITIS	CYSTITIS
Herpes simplex	Gardnerella	*C. trachomatis*	*C. trachomatis*	Coliforms
C. albicans	*C. albicans*	*N. gonorrhoeae*	*N. gonorrhoeae*	*S. sapprophyticus*
HPV	*T. vaginalis*	HSV	HSV	
C. albicans	*C. trachomatis*		*U. urealyticum*	
	Foreign body			
	N. gonorrhoeae			

Chancroid

 Database

DEFINITION/CAUSES

Infection with the gram-negative rod *Haemophilus ducreyi* resulting in necrotizing, painful genital ulcers which may be associated with regional lymphadenitis. Chancroid must be distinguished from the other causes of genital ulcers including syphilis, HSV, *Lymphogranuloma venereum*, and *Granuloma inguinale*. The most common etiologies for "genital ulcer syndrome" include syphilis, HSV, and chancroid.

PATHOPHYSIOLOGY

Trauma and abrasion allow the organism to penetrate the epidermis. Four to 7 days later, an erythematous, tender papule develops, which progresses to a pustule. The pustule ruptures after 2 to 3 days leaving a shallow ulcer with a necrotic, granulomatous base. The ulcers are shallow and have undermined edges.

ASSOCIATED DISEASES

• Associated with HIV transmission and infection
• Coinfection with syphilis and human herpesvirus can occur (10%).

EPIDEMIOLOGY

In 1999, there were 143 reported cases in the United States. It is probably underrecognized and underreported. In underdeveloped countries it is a major cause of genital ulcer syndrome in poorer countries. Importantly, it is a major cofactor in the transmission of HIV. Transmission occurs via sexual contact with an individual with an ulcer. It is seen more commonly in males.

COMPLICATIONS

• Draining bubo
• Coinfection with syphilis and HSV
• HIV infection

 Differential Diagnosis

• The "genital ulcer syndrome" is commonly caused by infection with *Treponema pallidum*, herpes simplex, or chancroid. More than one of these pathogens may be present in individual cases.
• Uncommon etiologies include:

—Trauma
—Fixed drug eruptions
—Lymphogranuloma venereum
—Inflammatory bowel disease
—Behçet syndrome

 Data Gathering

HISTORY

• Males usually present with symptoms referable to an ulcer.
• Females present with nonspecific symptoms such as dysuria, dyspareunia, vaginal discharge or rectal pain, or bleeding.

 Physical Examination

Classic findings include:

• Presence of an extremely painful ulcer with an irregular, undermined border and a gray, necrotic center.
• Males: Found on prepuce and coronal sulcus
• Females: Found on the vulva, cervix, and perianal area
• Inguinal lymphadenopathy, present in 50%, may spontaneously drain (bubo)
• Extragenital sites very rare, include the inner thigh area, breasts, fingers

 Laboratory Aids

Diagnosis is made by clinical findings and exclusion of other causes of genital ulcers. The following can be considered:

Test: Gram stain from the base of the ulcer
Significance: Gram stain may show short gram-negative bacilli in parallel "school of fish" arrangement. This finding does not compare favorably with culture proven or clinically diagnosed cases, and so routine use is not helpful.

Test: Cultures from the ulcer
Significance: H. ducreyi is a fastidious organism and requires specialized media and technique for successful isolation. Compared to newer amplification techniques, culture has been proven to be 75% sensitive. Culture is helpful in the face of treatment failure, and is useful for following trends in antimicrobial resistance. Currently it is the only method routinely available for the diagnosis of chancroid.

Test: DNA Amplification
Significance: A multiplex polymerase chain reaction (M-PCR) has been developed for simultaneous amplification of DNA targets form *H. ducreyi, T. pallidum,* and HSV, Types 1 and 2, which offers improved sensitivity when compared to culture. This technology is not routinely available, but offers the advantage of evaluating the patient for the major causes of "genital ulcer syndrome" simultaneously.

Test: Monoclonal antibody
Significance: Monoclonal antibody against the outer membrane protein of *H. ducreyi* using immunofluorescent antibody has also proven to be more sensitive than culture. This could provide easy, rapid inexpensive, sensitive testing, but it is not available currently.

Test: Culture for HSV, RPR
Significance: Evaluation for the common causes of genital ulcer syndrome should be done routinely

Test: HIV
Significance: Genital ulcers are a significant cofactor for HIV infection.

Therapy

- Azithromycin, 1 g PO
- Ceftriaxone, 250 mg IM
- Ciprofloxacin, 500 mg b.i.d. for 3 days (patients >18 years)
- Erythromycin base, 500 mg q.i.d. for 7 days

PREVENTION

- Condom use
- Partners should be treated whether or not symptoms are present.
- Patients should be evaluated for the presence of other sexually transmitted diseases.

 Follow-Up

- Patients are symptomatically improved within 48 to 72 hours.
- Ulcers themselves heal between 1 and 4 weeks.
- Lymphadenopathy may take longer to regress and may progress to fluctuance in spite of adequate therapy. Patients should be followed weekly until symptoms resolve.
- For patients who do not follow the typical course, consider other causes of genital ulcers, noncompliance, presence of a coexisting STD, especially HIV infection, and, rarely, presence of a resistant organism.
- Recent sexual partners (within the preceding 10 days) should be treated.

 Common Questions and Answers

Q: How do the ulcers of chancroid differ from those caused by herpes simplex and *T. pallidum*?
A: The ulcers caused by chancroid have irregular margins with deep undermined edges. They are very painful and occur singularly or in small numbers. Herpes simplex lesions occur as grouped vesicles that when ruptured leave behind painful shallow ulcers. The ulcers of syphilis are painless and solitary and have smooth margins surrounding a clean indurated base. However, accurate clinical diagnosis, even in experienced hands is difficult and thus should be supported by laboratory evaluation.

ICD-9-CM 099.0

BIBLIOGRAPHY

American Academy of Pediatrics. Sexually transmitted diseases. In: Pickering LK, ed. *2003 Red Book: Report of the Committee on Infectious Diseases.* 26th Ed. Elk Grove Village, IL: American Academy of Pediatrics, 2003.

Lewis DA. Chancroid: clinical manifestations, diagnosis and management. *J Sex Health and HIV* 2003;79:68–71.

Lewis DA. Diagnostic tests for chancroid. *J Sex Health and HIV* 2000;76:137–141.

Author: Jane Lavelle

Chickenpox (Varicella, Herpes Zoster)

 Database

DEFINITION

Varicella-zoster virus (VZV) is a herpesvirus. Only one strain is recognized. Humans are the only source of infection.

PATHOPHYSIOLOGY

- The virus can be demonstrated in the vesicular lesions by immunofluorescence, viral culture, and polymerase chain reaction (PCR) in specimens obtained from skin lesions, cheek and throat swabs, and organs such as brain, lung, and placenta, or cerebrospinal fluid.
- Humoral immunity is sometimes insufficient to provide protection. Severe varicella is due more to impairment of the cell-mediated immune response than to a defect in humoral immunity.
- Healthy children in whom a cell-mediated immune response develops after the varicella exanthem have mild primary VZV infection, whereas in immunodeficient children in whom VZV-specific lymphocytes fail to proliferate progressive disseminated varicella develops.

ASSOCIATED DISEASES/COMPLICATIONS OF VARICELLA INFECTION

- Secondary bacterial infection—especially virulent group A streptococcal infections and staphylococcal (drug resistance, an increasing problem)
- Varicella pneumonitis (more common in adults and infants)
- Gastrointestinal complications associated with viscous involvement, such as pancreatitis, appendicitis and hepatitis, idiopathic thrombocytopenia (ITP), and bleeding diathesis
- Nephritis
- Transverse myelitis
- Encephalitis, 60 cases per year pre-VZV vaccination
- Disseminated intravascular coagulation (hemorrhagic VZV)
- Individuals with AIDS may have chronic VZV
- Arthritis, which can become superinfected usually with *Staphylococcus aureus*
- Congenital varicella syndrome that occurs in the first or second trimester of pregnancy, characterized by limb atrophy and scarring of the extremity. Central nervous system and eye manifestations also occur.
- Death—1 to 2 deaths per week in the United States; between 1990 and 1994, varicella was the most common vaccine-preventable cause of death in individuals under 20 years of age. However, the impact of the universal immunization program has and b in 2003 but this number represents under reporting reduced this to 4 in year 2001.
- These complications are associated with significant morbidity and may occur irrespective of the use of acyclovir.

EPIDEMIOLOGY

- Person-to-person transmission occurs by direct contact with varicella or zoster and respiratory secretions.
- Varicella is most common during late winter and early spring, although in regions of high vaccine coverage this seasonality is now less pronounced.
- The introduction of an index case of varicella into a home results in transmission of the virus to susceptible persons and secondary cases of disease in 87% to 98% of susceptible persons.
- Secondary cases in this situation usually have more severe disease.
- Most reported cases occur between the ages of 5 and 9 years, although in areas of the United States, where many 1 to 4 year olds are in child care, this age group predominates with an increase in complications. Since 2002, regions where vaccine coverage is above 80% are experiencing increasing numbers of adolescents and adults with varicella secondary to having not been vaccinated and remaining susceptible.
- Lifelong immunity from natural disease is common, but symptomatic reinfections do occur; more common are asymptomatic reinfections, with a fourfold boost in antibody level.
- Immunocompromised individuals with either primary varicella or zoster are at risk for severe disease.
- Disease is also more severe in infants older than 3 months of age, adolescents, adults, those on oral and/or intravenous steroids or long-term aspirin therapy, or those with pulmonary disorders including asthma.
- Congenital varicella syndrome risk is about 2%, and is greatest from the 12th to 20th week.
- Incubation 10 to 21 days after contact; cases most contagious 2 days before the rash appears and until 5 days after lesions stop cropping (longer in immunocompromised patients).
- In varicella active surveillance sites, breakthrough varicella or reinfection with varicella now represents 48% of all reported varicella cases. The case definition reinfection VZV disease by the Council of State and Territorial Epidemiologists (CSTE) is a maculopapular-vesicular rash, which occurs in a vaccinated individual 6 weeks or more after vaccine. These rashes are atypical of varicella, are of shorter duration, usually have fewer lesions, are usually itchy, come in crops, and scab. Individuals with more than 50 lesions have been shown to transmit disease; however, it is less contagious (30%) than natural VZV (87%). Since many other rashes including insect bites, fleas, scabies, and enteroviral rashes among others have been demonstrated to be in the differential diagnosis; ideally the diagnosis needs to be verified by either PCR of the lesion and/or acute and convalescent serum immunoglobin (IgG) showing a rise in titer. To date only wild-type varicella has been identified from these confirmed cases of reinfection (breakthrough) VZV. Using these diagnostic tests the Centers for Disease Control and Prevention (CDC) active surveillance project in Philadelphia has demonstrated that 50% of what physicians thought might be a VZV reinfections is not.

 Differential Diagnosis

- With limited or mild rash, the differential diagnosis includes other causes of vesiculation such as:

—Coxsackie virus infection with hand, foot, and mouth disease
—Rickettsial pox
—*Molluocerm contagorm*
—*Pseudomonas* (in immunocompromised individuals)
—Eczema herpeticum
—Herpes zoster with dissemination
—Toxic epidermal necrosis, and various noninfectious vesicular conditions of the skin
—Scabies
—Insect bites
—Impetigo
—Drug reactions

 Data Gathering

HISTORY

Question: Time of year?
Significance: More common in winter and spring, although in regions of high vaccine coverage this seasonality is now less pronounced.

Question: Typical rash that has multiple stages identified?
Significance: Classic finding

Question: Does a history of not previously having had varicella usually make the diagnosis?
Significance: Varicella infection provides immunity, although recent studies have implicated 10% who may have had a previous history (although the initial diagnosis may not have been confirmed by a physician).

 Physical Examination

- The appearance of a typical rash that occurs in successive crops of macules, papules, and vesicles is distinctive; crops usually appear every 3 days.
- Vesicles may appear in the mouth, conjunctiva, vagina, and urethra.
- Some lesions may be secondarily infected.

Laboratory Aids

- Immunofluorescence of the vesicular fluid
- Culture of the vesicular fluid
- PCR of any tissue or vesicular fluid (reference labs include Dr. Philip LaRussa, NY, and Dr. Scott Schmid, CDC National Viral Hepatitis).
- The complement-fixation test is not reliable in determining immunity, and has been abandoned.

Test: Acute and convalescent sera for antibody testing by a number of assays, including enzyme immunoassay (EIA), immunofluorescence assay (IFA), latex agglutination (LA), fluorescent antibody to membrane antigen (FAMA), and, through the CDC laboratory group, ELISA, which is important in determining vaccine immunity. *Significance:* These tests can also be used to determine immunity.

The whole-cell EIA is better for immunity from "wild/natural" diseases.
The latex agglutination in commercial laboratories is not recommended for screening health-care workers.
The glycoprotein ELISA is more sensitive than the whole cell ELISA

Therapy

- Acyclovir, vidarabine, Famvir, foscarnet, and a number of antiviral agents—pending licensure—have been shown in clinical trials to be effective against VZV.
- Acyclovir is the drug of choice in children (FDA approved).
- Who benefits? Any child who is ill enough to warrant hospitalization and whose rash demonstrates new vesicle formation should be treated with acyclovir (IV dose is 1,500 mg/m^2 divided into three doses q8h).
- Consider oral acyclovir (80 mg/kg divided in four doses q6h) for children over 12 years of age, those with chronic cutaneous or pulmonary disorders, persons on short or intermittent corticosteroids or aerosolized corticosteroids, newborn infants, and selected immunocompromised persons at risk for severe varicella.
- Children with varicella should not receive salicylates because of the association with Reye syndrome. Acetaminophen may be used to control the fever. Nonsteroidal antiinflammatory drugs (NSAIDs) may increase complications from bacterial superinfection.
- In the era of a preventable disease, acyclovir should be considered before complications of varicella warrant hospitalization.

ISOLATION OF HOSPITALIZED PATIENTS

- Strict isolation for the duration of vesicular eruption (usually 5 days, longer in immunocompromised patients).

- Patients should be in negative-pressure rooms if possible.
- Exposed susceptible persons should be in strict isolation for 8 to 21 days after the onset of the rash in the index patient.
- Those who received varicella zoster immune globulin (VZIG) should be kept in isolation for 28 days after exposure.
- Immunocompromised patients who have zoster (localized or generalized) and normal patients with disseminated zoster should remain in strict isolation for the duration of the illness. For normal patients with localized zoster drainage and secretion, precautions are recommended until all lesions are crusted.

PREVENTION

- This is now a vaccine-preventable disease and is incorporated in the harmonized immunization schedule recommended by the AAP and ACIP since 1995, and is covered by the vaccine for children's program.
- The vaccine is recommended for routine immunization of all healthy susceptible children, adolescents, and adults.
- One dose (0.5 mL subcutaneously) is required for children 12 months to 13 years of age.
- Individuals over 13 years of age require two doses, 1 to 2 months apart.
- The vaccine is safe, with a <4% rash rate from immunization. Postlicensure surveillance has documented three incidences of transmission over 25 million doses.
- Duration of immunity from individuals followed in the clinical trials has shown that both humoral and cell-mediated immune responses persist for at least 10 years (U.S. data) and 20 years (Japanese data).
- The vaccine is not currently recommended for immunocompromised individuals, but there are studies in process. HIV positive children whose CD4 is 25% of normal value should get two doses of vaccine 1 to 3 months apart.
- Vaccine is available by protocol for acute lymphatic leukemia in remission.
- For those individuals who cannot receive VZV vaccine because of an immunocompromised state, varicella-susceptible pregnant women (until the VZV vaccine registry has data to make alternative recommendations), and newborns, VZIG would continue to be recommended.
- Varicella vaccine is recommended for postexposure prophylaxis within 5 days of a household exposure, or if an outbreak in a school is identified as soon as the local health authorities notify the parents.

Follow-Up

- In the postvaccine era, accurate diagnosis of "breakthrough/reinfection varicella" chickenpox varicella occurring more than 42 days after vaccine is crucial as it may point to lowered efficacy of improperly stored and administered VZV vaccine. Accurate diagnosis of VZV vaccine strain would be made by sending a PCR specimen to the CDC.

- For normal healthy individuals follow-up is not necessary.

PROGNOSIS

- 50 to 100 previously healthy children used to die each year (1 to 2 each week) from varicella. The impact of the universal varicella vaccination program has been that this has now been reduced to 4 deaths in 2001 (In 2003 the deaths including 3 children who were not vaccinate).
- For most children, this childhood exanthem is a benign disease that lasts 6 to 8 days.

Common Questions and Answers

Q: What do you do for a patient on corticosteroids who has not had VZV and is exposed to VZV?
A: These patients are immunosuppressed (if the dose of steroids is >0.2 mg/kg/day) and would require VZIG or treatment with acyclovir within 72 hours of developing VZV, if VZIG had not been administered.

Q: What about asthmatics on inhaled steroids? Can they be immunized safely and are they at risk of more severe varicella if not immunized?
A: Asthmatics on inhaled steroids can be immunized as the dose of inhaled steroids is not immunosuppressive. Recent data show that asthmatic children who are unimmunized do get more severe varicella.

Q: Is there any patient who should not receive VZV vaccine?
A: Yes. Immunosuppressed individuals, pregnant patients, and infants less than 1 year.

Q: How contagious is breakthrough (reinfections) varicella disease?
A: Surveillance studies have demonstrated that the secondary attach rate from breakthrough (reinfections) varicella is 30% in individuals with >50 lesions.

Q: If a child gets zoster, with wild-type or vaccine strain, should she or he be treated with antiviral drugs?
A: It depends on the symptoms—particularly pain. Pain with zoster is more common in adolescents than in children. Acyclovir and valacyclovir seem to be generally benign drugs.

ICD-9-CM 052.9

BIBLIOGRAPHY

Seward JF, Watson B, Petersen C, et al. Varicella disease after introduction of varicella vaccination in the United States, 1995–2000. *JAMA* 2002;287:606–611.

Watson B. Varicella—A vaccine-preventable disease? A review. *J Infect* 2002;00:1–6.

Author: Barbara Watson

Child Abuse—Physical

Database

DEFINITION

Injuries or illnesses that occur to children as a result of family dysfunction. In practice, child abuse is considered nonaccidental injury of children at the hands of their caregivers. Physical abuse is legally defined by state laws.

- Multifactorial etiology:

—Include societal, familial, and individual factors
—Associated with poverty, family stress, family isolation

- Associated problems:

—Domestic violence
—Sexual abuse
—Neglect
—Emotional abuse
—Juvenile delinquency
—Poverty
—Parental substance abuse, including alcohol

EPIDEMIOLOGY

- In 2000, there were 2.8 million referrals to child welfare agencies in the United States for child abuse and neglect.
- Approximately 500,000 substantiated cases are identified in the United States each year
- Almost 2,000 deaths per year, by conservative estimates
- Parents who were abused as children are at much greater risk for abusing their own children. It is estimated that 30% of abused children go on to be abusive parents.
- Domestic violence and child abuse have a 50% concurrence.

COMPLICATIONS

- Death
- Mental retardation
- Cerebral palsy
- Seizures
- Learning disabilities, school failure
- Emotional problems

PROGNOSIS

Varies greatly depending on injuries sustained, family problems, available support systems.

Differential Diagnosis

Varies depending on injuries sustained.

- Accidental injury
- Dermatologic disorders

—Mongolian spots
—Erythema multiforme
—Phytophotodermatitis

- Hematologic disorders

—Idiopathic thrombocytopenic purpura (ITP)

—Leukemia
—Hemophilia
—Vitamin K deficiency
—Disseminated intravascular coagulopathy (DIC)

- Cultural practices

—Cao gio (coining)—practice of rubbing the skin with a coin to alleviate various symptoms of illness
—Quat sha (spoon rubbing)

- Infection

—Sepsis
—Purpura fulminans with meningococcemia

- Genetic diseases

—Ehlers-Danlos
—Familial dysautonomia (with congenital indifference to pain)

- Vasculitis

—Henoch-Schonlein purpura

BURNS

- Accidental burns
- Infection

—Staphylococcal scalded skin syndrome
—Impetigo

- Dermatologic

—Phytophotodermatitis
—Stevens Johnson reaction
—Fixed drug eruption
—Epidermolysis bullosa
—Severe diaper dermatitis

FRACTURES

- Accidental injury
- Birth trauma
- Metabolic bone disease

—Osteogenesis imperfecta
—Copper deficiency
—Rickets

- Infection

—Congenital syphilis
—Osteomyelitis
—Moxibustion: Chinese folk remedy in which cones or balls of the moxa herb are burned on the skin at therapeutic points.

HEAD TRAUMA

- Accidental head injury
- Hematologic disorders

—Vitamin K deficiency (hemorrhagic disease of the newborn)
—Hemophilia

- Intracranial vascular abnormalities
- Infection
- Metabolic diseases

—Glutaric aciduria type I

Data Gathering

HISTORY

- A detailed history of injury is essential for comparing the mechanism provided by the historian to the injuries sustained.

The following historical features should raise the question of child abuse:

- History provided does not correlate with findings
- Child's development not compatible with mechanism described
- History of events changes with time
- Unexpected delay in seeking care
- No history of trauma is provided. In such cases, ask when the child was last well, and who was caring for the child at that time. This may be helpful in identifying when the child was injured, and by whom.
- Search for indications of family stress, isolation, substance abuse, and violence, including domestic violence.

Physical Examination

Always perform a complete examination in a well-lit room. Assess child for:

- Growth failure
- Bruises—any inflicted injury that lasts more than 24 hours constitutes significant injury
- Burns
- Oral injuries
- Palpable rib fractures
- Abdominal injuries
- Genital injuries
- Retinal hemorrhages—children with suspected inflicted head injury should have dilated eye examination by an ophthalmologist.
- Are the findings explained by any medical condition? Examples would include multiple bruises in a patient with a bleeding disorder (such as hemophilia) or long bone fractures in a patient with a metabolic bone disease (such as rickets).

Laboratory Aids

For children with bruising and/or bleeding:

Test: CBC, including a platelet count

Test: PT/PTT
Significance: Evaluate for hemophilia and other bleeding disorders

Test: Bleeding time/von Willebrand panel
Significance: Screen for von Willebrand disease

Test: Liver function tests
Significance: Evaluate for liver injury

Test: Amylase, lipase
Significance: Evaluate for pancreatic injury

Test: Urinalysis
Significance: Screen for genitourinary injury, abdominal trauma, or myoglobinuria

Test: Creatine kinase (if muscle injury or extensive soft tissue injury)
Significance: Evaluate for muscle injury, possible myoglobinuria

Test: Lumbar puncture
Significance: Evaluate for meningitis; identify bloody CSF

Test: Toxicology screen
Significance: If it is suspected that the child may have been poisoned

RADIOGRAPHIC STUDIES

- Skeletal survey: recommended for all children less than 2 years old and for some children 2 to 5 years old with suspected abusive injuries. Not generally used for children older than 5 years. Bony injuries highly suggestive of abuse include posterior rib, metaphyseal (also known as bucket handle or corner fractures), scapular, sternal, and spinous process fractures.
- Other chest radiographs: clavicle, long bone shaft, and linear skull fractures are common fractures and are sometimes related to abuse, but have low specificity for abuse.
- Radionuclide bone scan: serves as an adjunct to skeletal survey
- Computed tomography (CT) and magnetic resonance imaging (MRI): for suspected head, thoracic, or abdominal trauma. These should be considered for all children <1 year of age with other concerning/suspicious injuries. Subdural hemorrhage is a hallmark of inflicted head injury. Subdural hemorrhages associated with abuse can be located anywhere around the brain, but are often found in the posterior interhemispheric fissure.

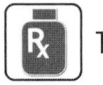 Therapy

- Report all suspected abuse to local child welfare agency.
- Report abuse to law enforcement when injuries warrant police investigation.
- Consult social worker.
- Subdural hemorrhages do not usually require surgical evacuation.

 Follow-Up

- Cases will be investigated by child welfare agents and/or the police.
- Need for foster care placement and/or ongoing supervision decided by child welfare investigators.
- Improvement of individual injuries varies according to the injury
- Family functioning may improve with intervention for some families, but may never improve for others. Changes in family functioning often require intensive, long-term intervention.

- Noncompliance with medical follow-up or additional injuries to child may indicate ongoing abuse, parental substance abuse, etc.

PREVENTION

- Much of what is considered prevention is actually early intervention in high-risk families.
- Primary prevention would include universal parenting education and home visitation for all families. Currently, families thought to be at risk for abuse are identified and offered services.
- Home visitation by nurses for first-time, low-income women has been shown to decrease the risk for child abuse.

PITFALLS

- Failing to consider abuse in the differential diagnosis of all pediatric trauma.
- Failing to consider abuse in the differential diagnosis of all infants and toddlers with mental status changes (especially apparent life-threatening events [ALTEs]), even in the absence of bruising.
- Failing to consider alternative medical diagnoses in children for whom you suspect abuse.
- Acute (<10 days) rib fractures are easily missed on plain films.

 Common Questions and Answers

Q: What are the signs of abusive head trauma (also known as shaken-baby syndrome)?
A: Abusive head trauma is a clinical diagnosis based on history, physical examination findings, and radiologic data. The hallmark of abusive head trauma is subdural hemorrhage, which is often a marker for diffuse, acceleration-deceleration brain injury. The majority of victims (80%) have retinal hemorrhages, which tend to be bilateral, multilayered, and sometimes severe. Some, but not all, children have old and/or new skeletal or skin injuries, although these are not needed to make the diagnosis.

Q: Are retinal hemorrhages pathognomonic for physical abuse?
A: No, retinal hemorrhages may be seen in a variety of diseases and in some newborn infants. They occur in approximately 30% of newborns delivered vaginally. In these children they usually resolve in a few days, but may rarely last for 5 to 6 weeks. Outside of the newborn period, severe inflicted injury is the leading cause of retinal hemorrhages in children. Retinal hemorrhages may also result from increased intracranial pressure, severe hypertension, carbon monoxide poisoning, meningitis, vasculitis, endocarditis, and coagulopathy. Severe, bilateral hemorrhages are almost always a result of abuse.

Q: When is a child-abuse report filed?
A: Whenever there is a suspicion, based on the history, physical examination, laboratory data, and/or psychosocial assessment, that a

child's injuries or illnesses were a result of abuse or neglect. Certainty regarding the diagnosis is not needed.

Q: Can I be held liable for reports that are made that are not substantiated?
A: No. Health-care workers who report suspected abuse "in good faith" are protected from civil and criminal litigation arising from allegations of false reports.

ICD-9-CM 995.81

BIBLIOGRAPHY

American Academy of Pediatrics, Committee on Child Abuse and Neglect. When inflicted skin injuries constitute child abuse. *Pediatrics* 2002;110:644–645.

American Academy of Pediatrics, Section on Radiology. Diagnostic imaging of child abuse. *Pediatrics* 2000;105:1345–1348.

Block RW. Child abuse-controversies and impostors. *Curr Probl Pediatr* 1999;29: 249–272.

Duhaime AC, Christian CW, Rorke LB, et al. Nonaccidental head injury in infants—the "shaken-baby syndrome." *N Engl J Med* 1998;338:1822–1829.

Helfer ME, Kempe RS. *The Battered Child.* 5th Ed. Chicago: University of Chicago Press, 1997.

Jenny C, Hymel KP, Ritzen A, et al. Analysis of missed cases of abusive head trauma. *JAMA* 1999;281:621–629.

Kleinman PK. *Diagnostic Imaging of Child Abuse.* St. Louis: Mosby Yearbook, 1998.

Olds D, Eckenrode J, Henderson CR, et al. Long-term effects of home visitation on maternal life course and child abuse and neglect: fifteen-year follow-up of a randomized trial. *JAMA* 1997;278:637–643.

Rubin DM, Christian CW, Bilaniuk LT, et al. Occult head injury in high-risk abused children. *Pediatrics* 2003;111:1382–1386.

Sugar NF, Taylor JA, Feldman KW. Bruises in infants and toddlers: those who don't cruise rarely bruise. *Arch Pediatr Adolesc Med* 1999; 153:399–403.

US Department of Health and Human Services. Administration on Children, Youth and Families. Child Maltreatment 2000. Washington, DC: US Government Printing Office; 2002.

Authors: Cindy W. Christian and Matthew Cox

Chlamydial Infections

 Database

DEFINITION

Chlamydiae are obligate intracellular bacteria responsible for pulmonary infections, ocular trachoma, sexually transmitted disease, and infections of the genital tract in the pediatric and adult population.
- The genus Chlamydia (Chlamydophila) has three species known to affect humans:
  —C. trachomatis (CT)
  —C. psittaci
  —C. pneumoniae (CP)
- All three species can produce the clinical manifestations of the so-called atypical or interstitial pneumonia.
- CT can cause afebrile pneumonia in 10% to 20% of infants born to infected mothers. Infected infants usually present prior to 2 months of age. Up to 50% of patients have a history of inclusion conjunctivitis.
- C. psittaci is mainly pathogenic for birds and occasionally affects humans, typically causing interstitial pneumonitis with associated fever, headache, malaise, and nausea.
- CP causes pneumonia, pharyngitis, sinusitis, and bronchitis in humans. Along with Mycoplasma pneumoniae, CP probably accounts for most of the community-acquired pneumonias (CAPs) in school-age children and adolescents.

EPIDEMIOLOGY

C. Trachomatis

There are at least 15 serologically distinct variants (serovars).
- This is the most common reportable sexually transmitted infection in the United States. The number of new infections exceeds 4 million annually.
- Rates of infection in adolescent girls are 15% to 20%.
- Twenty-three percent to 55% of all cases of nongonococcal urethritis in men are caused by CT.
- Up to 50% of men with gonorrhea may be coinfected with CT.
- CT is the most frequent cause of epididymitis in sexually active young men.
- CT pneumonia usually develops in infected infants under 2 months of age (2 weeks to 5 months).
- The contagiousness of pulmonary disease is unknown, but is considered low.
- Half of the neonates born to infected mothers via vaginal delivery will acquire CT.
  —Conjunctivitis may develop in 30% to 50%.
  —Pneumonia may develop in up to 30% of infants with nasopharyngeal infection.
- Ocular trachoma caused by serovars A, B, Ba, and C is the most common cause of preventable blindness in the world, but is rare in the United States.
- Incubation period: 5 to 14 days after delivery for conjunctivitis
- The possibility of sexual abuse should be considered in older infants and children with vaginal, urethral, or rectal CT.

C. Psittaci (Psittacosis/Ornithosis)

- Both healthy and sick birds can transmit the bacteria via the airborne route by their excrement or secretions.
- Important sources of human disease are parakeets, parrots, macaws, pigeons, and turkeys.
- Though usually rare in children, it should be considered in any child with environmental exposure who develops an atypical pneumonia. The incubation period is 7 to 14 days.

C. Pneumoniae

- CP is antigenically, morphologically, and genetically distinct from other chlamydiae.
- It is assumed to be transmitted from person to person through aerosolized respiratory secretions.
- Increased prevalence rates of CP specific antibody have been documented in school-age children, reaching 30% to 45% in adolescents.
- CP has recently been associated with atherosclerotic cardiovascular disease. Limited evidence associates CP with asthma and bronchospasm, Alzheimer disease, multiple sclerosis, Kawasaki disease, HIV and other immune disorders, malignancy, otitis media, and episodes of acute chest syndrome in patients with sickle cell disease.
- The majority of infections are mild or asymptomatic. Acute infection does not appear to vary by season. A carriage state has been detected in 2% to 5% of patients. Recurrent infection is common, especially in adults.
- Co-infection with other respiratory pathogens, especially M. pneumoniae and Streptococcus pneumoniae, is frequent.
- Incubation period: about 21 days.

COMPLICATIONS

- In very young infants, chlamydial pneumonia can lead to apnea or respiratory failure.
- Untreated infection can persist for weeks to months.
- Complications of psittacosis include myocarditis, hepatitis, pancreatitis, and secondary bacterial pneumonia.

PROGNOSIS

- In general, good
- Infection with CT has been associated with long-term respiratory sequelae, such as an increased incidence of reactive airway disease and abnormal pulmonary function tests.

 Differential Diagnosis

CHLAMYDIA TRACHOMATIS

- Viral respiratory pathogens:
  —Respiratory syncytial virus (RSV)
  —Adenovirus
  —Influenza A and B
  —Parainfluenza
- Other agents that can cause pneumonitis:
  —Cytomegalovirus
  —Pneumocystis carinii
  —Ureaplasma urealyticum
  —Bordetella pertussis

CHLAMYDIA PNEUMONIAE

- M. pneumoniae
- Influenza A and B
- Parainfluenza
- Adenovirus
- RSV
- Can resemble typical bacterial pneumonia
- Less frequently: C. psittaci, Coxiella burnetii, or Legionella pneumophila

 Data Gathering

HISTORY

C. Trachomatis

- Presents between 4 and 12 weeks of age
- Insidious onset
- Afebrile illness
- Rhinorrhea
- Repetitive cough
  —Staccato type in more than 50% of infants
  —Sometimes pertussis-like coughing spells
- Conjunctivitis in up to 50% of infants
- Mild-to-moderate respiratory distress

C. Pneumoniae

- Often insidious onset
- May manifest as pharyngitis, sinusitis, bronchitis, or pneumonia
- Fever
- Hoarseness
- Prolonged cough; can be productive
- Biphasic course

 Physical Examination

CHLAMYDIA TRACHOMATIS

- Afebrile
- Fifty percent of patients will have conjunctivitis with discharge (can be seen up to several weeks after birth)
- Rhinitis with mucoid discharge or nasal stuffiness, sometimes causing significant airway obstruction.
- Hypoxia frequently present
- Moderate tachypnea (50 to 60 breaths per minute)
- Frequent cough during examination
- Scattered rales on chest auscultation
- Wheezing is an uncommon finding.

C. PNEUMONIAE

- Patients may be asymptomatic or mildly to moderately ill.
- Cervical lymphadenopathy
- Postnasal discharge
- Nonexudative pharyngitis
- Wheezing, frequently without rales on chest auscultation

 Laboratory Aids

TESTS

C. Trachomatis

- Definitive diagnosis is by isolation of the organism in tissue culture. Confirmation is by microscopy of the characteristic inclusions by fluorescent antibody staining. Specimens are obtained from the nasopharynx, conjunctiva, vagina, or rectum. Dacron polyester–tipped swabs should be used for collection.

- FDA approved nucleic acid amplification methods such as polymerase chain reaction (PCR) and strand displacement amplification (SDA) and transcription mediated amplification (TMA) are more sensitive than cell culture and more specific and sensitive than DNA probe, direct fluorescent antibody (DFA), or enzyme immunoassay (EIA). These have also been approved for urine in both men and women making them useful noninvasive tests for adolescents.
- DNA probe, DFA, and EIA are the most common nonculture direct antigen-detection tests approved by the FDA. These are most sensitive (90%) and specific (95%) in conjunctival specimens. These methods can have false-positive results when used for vaginal or rectal specimens.
- Serum antibody detection can be performed by microimmunofluorescence (MIF). These are difficult to perform and are not widely available.
—Chlamydia-specific immunoglobin (IgM) titer of 1:32 or greater is diagnostic for CT pneumonia.
- Eosinophilia of 300 to 400/mm^3, hyperinflation, bilateral diffuse infiltrates on chest radiograph and elevation of IgM (>110 mg/dL) and IgG (>500 mg/dL) are indirect evidence that suggest CT pneumonia.
- Only culture should be used for sexual abuse or other forensic purposes.

C. Pneumoniae

- No reliable test is available commercially. Serologic testing is the primary laboratory means of diagnosis.
- The nasopharynx is the optimal site for recovery of CP. It has also been isolated from sputum and pleural fluid.
- The organism can be grown in tissue culture. Its presence can be detected by using PCR and a fluorescent antibody test. This method is not validated or FDA approved.
- Serologic diagnosis by MIF is the most sensitive and specific test. Evidence of acute infection:
—Fourfold elevation of IgG titers
—Specific IgM titer of 1:16 or greater
—Specific IgG titer of 1:512 or greater
- WBC count is usually normal.

Imaging

- Chest radiography
—C. trachomatis: the most consistent finding is hyperinflation with bilateral diffuse infiltrates
—C. pneumoniae: presents with focal to bilateral infiltrates; pleural effusions have been reported.

 ## Therapy

DRUGS

C. Trachomatis

- Erythromycin, 50 mg/kg per day divided q.i.d. for 14 days (therapy is effective in 80% to 90% of cases). Additional topical therapy is unnecessary. An association between oral erythromycin and infantile hypertrophic pyloric stenosis (IHPS) has been reported, in infants younger than 6 weeks of age. Parents should be informed of the possible risk of IHPS and its signs.
- If the patient does not tolerate erythromycin, oral sulfonamides may be used after the immediate neonatal period. Children older than 8 years can be treated with tetracycline, 25 to 50 mg/kg per day divided q.i.d. for 7 days.
- A single 1-g oral dose of azithromycin may be used in children who weigh at least 45 kg or who are at least 8 years old.
- In adults and adolescents, a single 1-g dose of azithromycin or doxycycline 100 mg b.i.d. orally for 7 days is first-line treatment.

C. Pneumoniae

- Erythromycin suspension, 50 mg/kg per day divided q.i.d. for 14 days. For adolescent patients, erythromycin 500 mg q.i.d. for 14 days or 250 mg q.i.d. for 21 days.
- An alternative for children over 9 years of age is doxycycline 100 mg b.i.d. for 14 days.
- Clarithromycin 15 mg/kg per day divided b.i.d. for 10 days was proven as effective as erythromycin.
- Azithromycin 10 mg/kg on day one (maximum, 500 mg) followed by 5 mg/kg days 2 to 5 (maximum, 250 mg) has been shown as efficacious as erythromycin in pediatric studies.
- Adolescents can be treated with doxycycline 100 mg b.i.d. for 14 to 21 days, tetracycline 250 mg q.i.d. for 14 to 21 days, azithromycin 1.5 g for 5 days, levofloxacin 500 mg/d orally or intravenously for 7 to 14 days or moxifloxacin 400 mg/d orally for 10 days.

 ## Follow-Up

- Slow recovery
- Cough and malaise may persist for several weeks.

PREVENTION

Adequate surveillance and treatment of CT colonizing the genital tract of pregnant women is the best way of preventing disease in the infant.

PITFALLS

C. Trachomatis

- Infection can occur in infants delivered by cesarean section, even without rupture of amniotic membranes.

- Ocular prophylaxis at birth does not reliably prevent C. conjunctivitis or extraocular infection, even if erythromycin ointment is used. Topical treatment alone is not recommended because it does not eradicate the nasopharyngeal colonization.
- Antibiotic treatment failure rate is about 20%. A second course of therapy is sometimes needed. Follow-up should be recommended

C. Pneumoniae

- Lack of a commercially reliable test for diagnosis. MIF is proven diagnostic in less than 50% of infected children. An increase in antibody titer may be delayed for several weeks after onset of symptoms. Early antimicrobial therapy may interfere with the development of detectable antibodies.
- Sometimes it is difficult to differentiate between infection and carrier state, and recent and past infection.
- Recurrent infections are common. Prolonged nasopharyngeal shedding can occur for months after acute disease.
- Isolation: standard precautions for both CP and CT
- Control measures: In infants infected with CT, the mother and her sexual partner should be treated. None for CP pneumonia.

 ## Common Questions and Answers

Q: If the mother has an untreated genital infection, should we treat the asymptomatic newborn?
A: Yes. The child should receive oral erythromycin for 14 days.

Q: Do we need to pursue the diagnosis of other sexually transmitted diseases?
A: Yes. Gonorrhea, syphilis, hepatitis B, and HIV infection need to be ruled out. If conjunctivitis is present, an ocular swab to exclude Neisseria gonorrhoeae infection must be included.

Q: When do we need to suspect CT pneumonia?
A: In any infant younger than 4 months of age who presents with cough, tachypnea, and rales on examination, when the chest radiograph shows bilateral infiltrates with hyperinflation.

ICD-9-CM 483.1

BIBLIOGRAPHY

American Academy of Pediatrics. 2003 Red Book: Report of the Committee on Infectious Diseases. Elk Grove Village, IL: American Academy of Pediatrics, 2003:235–243.

Centers for Disease Control and Prevention. Sexually transmitted disease guidelines 2002. MMWR Morbid Mortal Wkly Rep 2002;519 (No. RR-6)1–75.

Hamerschlag MR. Chlamydia trachomatis and chlamydia pneumoniae infections in children and adolescents. Pediatr Rev 2004;25(2): 43–51.

Author: Sumit Bhargava

Cholelithiasis

 Database

DEFINITION

Cholesterol and/or pigment stones in the gallbladder. Incidental or silent gallstones are detected more often in children. High-risk populations include pediatrics (sickle cell disease in newborns)

CAUSES

- Hemolytic disease (17% to 29% of children with sickle cell disease)
- Total parenteral nutrition
- Prematurity
- Necrotizing enterocolitis
- Cystic fibrosis
- Obesity
- Pregnancy
- Oral contraceptives
- Down syndrome

PATHOLOGY

- Bile is composed of five major components: water, bilirubin, cholesterol, pigments, and phospholipids and calcium salts. Stones are of two types: pigment and cholesterol stones. The formation of cholesterol stones is associated with sludge and cholesterol supersaturation. Other important factors include:

—Gallbladder stasis
—Excess lecithin
—Increased biliary mucus secretion
—Rapidity of nucleation time

- Total parenteral alimentation is associated with decrease in bile flow, stasis, sludge, and stone formation.
- Formation of gallstones secondary to ileal disease/resection reported in children and adults because of a decreased bile acid pool and cholesterol supersaturation of the bile.

EPIDEMIOLOGY

- Cholelithiasis is relatively uncommon in childhood; however, gallstones have even been detected in utero.
- Pigment stones are more prevalent in prepubertal children, whereas cholesterol stones are predominant in adolescence and adulthood.
- In males, the incidence of gallstones remains negligible throughout childhood and adolescence.
- Gallstones predominate in females where the incidence is 0.27% during ages 6 to 19 years and increases to 2.7% between the ages of 18 and 29.
- Canadian Eskimos and Native Africans have the lowest risk of cholelithiasis.
- Native Americans, Swedes, and Czechs have the highest risk.

SYMPTOMS

- Silent gallstones present coincidentally in infancy and preschool-age children.
- Classic symptoms of right-upper-quadrant (RUQ) pain (Murphy sign) and vomiting exist only in older children and adolescents.
- Younger children present with nonspecific symptoms, including obstructive jaundice.
- Fever is unusual in all age groups and often indicates the development of rare complications in children:

—Cholecystitis
—Choledocholithiasis
—Cholangitis
—Gallbladder perforation

- Pancreatitis develops in 8% of patients with gallstones and is the most common complication. Pancreatitis is more common in obese adolescents who have undergone rapid weight reduction, as reported in the adult population.

 Data Gathering

HISTORY

- Most gallstones are incidental findings on abdominal ultrasound and are clinically silent.
- Biliary colic, pancreatitis, obstructive jaundice, cholangitis, or other complications should be excluded.
- Intolerance to fatty food rarely exists in children.

The history should always include questions concerning:

- Previous episodes of RUQ abdominal pain
- Any risk factors for hemolysis
- History of prematurity and necrotizing enterocolitis
- Total parenteral nutrition
- Diuretic use
- Short gut syndrome/resection of the terminal ileum.

Physical Examination

- The physical examination may be completely normal or may uncover the acute abdomen of pancreatitis.
- Murphy sign (tenderness on palpation of the RUQ of the abdomen associated with inspiration) may be elicited in adolescents.

Laboratory Aids

TESTS

- Blood testing is usually unrewarding.
- Leukocytosis, elevation in liver enzymes, or elevated amylase/lipase may be detected.
- Abdominal radiography may show the presence of a gallstone; However 50% of these are radio-opaque.
- Ultrasound is the diagnostic procedure of choice—noninvasive with high sensitivity and specificity.
- Endoscopic retrograde cholangiopancreatography (ERCP) is especially good for evaluation of choledocholithiasis and removal of common bile duct stones.

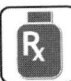

Therapy

- Children with asymptomatic gallstones should only be observed. During infancy, there is a chance for spontaneous stone dissolution, especially if cholelithiasis is linked to total parenteral nutrition (TPN). In children who are TPN-dependent: patients with short-bowel syndrome, pseudo-obstruction, and inflammatory bowel disease, gallstones should be removed.
- Cholecystectomy remains the procedure of choice in children with symptoms or in the presence of silent gallstones in older children.
- Laparoscopic cholecystectomy may decrease the length of the hospital stay and the extent of the required abdominal incision.
- Medical treatment for cholesterol gallstones in children may include chenodeoxycholic acid and ursodeoxycholic acid. However, this treatment is not recommended in the pediatric age group because of low success rate.
- Prevention of gallstone formation is done by treating underlying risk factors (small enteral feeds in addition to TPN, early pancreatic enzyme supplements in patients with cystic fibrosis, using alternative forms of contraception in high-risk populations, and weight control in obese infants and children with known hemolytic disease).
- Pigment stone formation increases with age. Cholecystectomy, even for the asymptomatic patient, is warranted. Sickle cell patients should have the gallbladder removed once stones are identified. This will decrease the risk of cholecystitis and other complications, and will also help to differentiate between biliary colic and sickle cell crisis.
- Patients with a history of cholecystitis are at increased risk for further episodes (69% will have biliary colic within 2 years, and 6% will require cholecystectomy).

Follow-Up

- Asymptomatic patients: Follow up every year with ultrasound; monitor for onset of symptoms.
- Symptomatic patients: consider cholecystectomy.

Common Questions and Answers

Q: Does my child with cystic fibrosis (CF) have a greater problem with gallstones?
A: Yes, children with CF may have more frequent development of gallstones than will normal children. Reports of gallstones while on ursodeoxycholic acid therapy have also been noted.

Q: Why does my child with sickle cell disease have gallstones?
A: Because the process involves breakdown of hemoglobin, which is then derived into bilirubin; this process may accelerate the formation of pigmented gallstones.

Q: If my child has repeated attacks of abdominal pain and there are gallstones in the gallbladder, should he or she have surgery? What kind?
A: Yes; in older adolescents, laparoscopic cholecystectomy is recommended. For younger children or infants, open cholecystectomy is the preferred choice of treatment.

ICD-9-CM 574.20

BIBLIOGRAPHY

Gertner M, Farmer DL. Laparoscopic cholecystecomy in a 16-day-old infant with chronic cholelithiasis. *J Pediatr Surg* 2004; 39(1):E17–19

Heubi JE, Lewis LG. Diseases of the gallbladder in infancy, childhood, and adolescence. In: Suchy F, eds. *Liver Diseases in Children*. Chicago: Mosby-Year Book, 1994: 609–621.

Irish MS, Pearl RH, Caty MG, et al. The approach to common abdominal diagnosis in infants and children. *Pediatr Clin North Am* 1998;45(4):729–772.

Kasirajan K, Obermeyer RJ, Kehris J, et al. Microinvasive laparoscopic cholecystectomy in pediatric patients. *J Laparoendosc Adv Surg Tech A* 1998;8(3):131–135.

Lobe TE. Cholelithiasis and cholecystitis in children. *Semin Pediatr Surg* 2000;9(4): 170–176.

Stringer MD, Taylor DR, Soloway RD. Gallstone composition: are children different? *J Pediatr* 2003;142(4):435–440.

Yusoff IF, Barkun JS, Barkun AN. Diagnosis and management of cholecystitis and cholangitis. *Gastroenterol Clin North Am* 2003;32(4):1145–1168.

Author: Dror Wasserman

Chronic Active Hepatitis

 Database

DEFINITION

Chronic active hepatitis is a continuing inflammation of the liver that may become cirrhotic. Features include inflammation not as a result of acute self-limiting infection or past drug exposure with raised transaminases and histologic evidence of hepatitis.

CAUSES

- Autoimmune liver disease
- Viral hepatitis
- Progressive familial intrahepatic cholestasis (PFIC) syndromes
- Congenital hepatic fibrosis
- Cystic fibrosis
- Metabolic disease:

—Mitochondrial disease
—Lysosomal storage
—Peroxisomal disease
—Lipid storage disease
—Glycogen storage disease
—Wilson disease and others

- Medications associated with liver disease

—Methotrexate
—Isoniazid
—Thioguanine
—6-mercaptopurine
—Valproate

- Liver disease associated with other chronic diseases:

—Cardiac disease
—ARPKD (autosomal recessive polycystic kidney disease)
—Diabetes mellitus
—Langerhan cell histiocytosis
—Immunodeficiency
—TPN cholestasis

PATHOPHYSIOLOGY

Pathology has been traditionally classified as chronic persistent hepatitis, chronic aggressive hepatitis, and chronic lobular hepatitis. The hepatocytes are damaged, with inflammatory cellular infiltration accompanied by liver regeneration.

Chronic Persistent Hepatitis

Minimal portal tract fibrosis, slightly widened portal tracts. The limiting plate is intact and inflammation does not extend beyond this. There is no bridging fibrosis between portal tracts.

Chronic Aggressive Hepatitis

Perilobular hepatitis, with inflammatory cells extending from portal tracts into parenchyma with fibrosis. Piecemeal necrosis is necrotic hepatocytes surrounded by lymphocytes and fibroblasts. In advanced disease, fibrosis bridges the portal tracts (bridging fibrosis). Cirrhosis occurs when there is loss of architecture as a result of fibrosis.

Chronic Lobular Hepatitis

Liver architecture is preserved with scattered changes of acute hepatitis with hepatocyte necrosis in the lobules (perivenular regions). These changes are most often associated with hepatitis B and non-A, non-B (NANB) hepatitis.

EPIDEMIOLOGY

This depends on the etiology of the underlying disease.

- Hepatitis B: common in immigrant children from Asia and Eastern Europe.
- Hepatitis C: common among those who had blood transfusions and blood products before screening became available; users of IV drugs and nasal cocaine users.
- Wilson disease present in older children and adults mainly.
- Autoimmune liver disease: in females and older children.
- Some patients have other autoimmune diseases associated with this such as diabetes, ulcerative colitis, autoimmune thyroiditis, and celiac disease.
- Methotrexate, 6 thioguanine: liver fibrosis and veno-occlusive disease.

 Differential Diagnosis

- Hepatomegaly:

—Elevated right-sided cardiac pressures, such as patients with Fontan operations, right-sided heart failure; respiratory diseases with lung hyperexpansion

- Splenomegaly:

—Blood malignancies
—Storage diseases
—Hematological disease with hemolysis
—Storage diseases with fat
—Glycogen and lipids.

- Jaundice: often confused with hyper-carotenemia.
- Elevated transaminases: consider nonhepatic sources such as skeletal muscles in myopathies; with jaundice consider hypopituitarism in infancy.
- Alkaline phosphatase: growing children and in rickets and may not indicate biliary obstruction.
- GGT: produced in choroids plexus, renal tubules, pancreatic and biliary ducts. Often elevated in patients on anti-epileptic drugs and in alcoholics.
- Abnormal coagulation: anticoagulant medications, bacterial overgrowth with malabsorption or dysfibrinogenemia.

 Data Gathering

HISTORY

- Preceding clinical signs and symptoms for at least 6 months and data gathering will require a complete medical history.

—History of blood transfusions
—Surgery
—Medications
—Foreign travel
—Social circumstances which predispose to liver diseases

- Symptoms of chronic illness can be nonspecific:

—Poor growth
—Intermittent jaundice
—Abdominal pain
—Bleeding
—Malabsorption
—Fever
—Amenorrhea
—Poor school achievement
—Itching

Variceal bleeding may be a presenting syndrome in patients with portal hypertension.

- A history of jaundice in infancy, family history of liver disease or autoimmune liver disease, blood transfusions, intravenous drug abuse, or multiple sexual partners can suggest an etiology of hepatitis.

 Physical Examination

- Stigmata of chronic liver disease are:

—Spider nevi
—Cutaneous shunts
—Palmar erythema
—Cyanosis (hepatopulmonary syndrome)
—Jaundice
—Itching
—Enlarged liver or small, shrunken liver
—Splenomegaly
—Ascites
—Rickets
—Mental changes
—Fetor associated with high ammonia

Laboratory Aids

TESTS

Laboratory Tests

- Albumin, creatinine, GGT, AST, ALT, bilirubin, PT, CBC, blood group, Coombs test.
- Serum ceruloplasmin, serum copper, 24-hour urine copper (penicillamine challenge), liver copper.
- Cholesterol, triglycerides elevated in cholestatic syndromes, glycogen storage, Alagille's disease, certain lysosomal disease, steatohepatitis.
- Immunoglobulins: IGG elevated in autoimmune liver disease.
- Autoantibodies: liver kidney microsomal, smooth muscle, pericytoplasmic antineutrophil (p-ANCA), antinuclear
- Virology: hepatitis B, hepatitis C, hepatitis D.
- α_1-Antitrypsin phenotype.
- Urinary succinylacetone: tyrosinemia.
- Urinary bile acids: bile acid synthetic defects and some progressive intrahepatic cholestatic syndromes.
- Sweat test and CF genotyping.
- Alpha-fetoprotein.

INVESTIGATIONS

- Chest radiograph.
- Ultrasound scan: focus on liver, spleen with Doppler flow studies.
- Liver biopsy.
- Percutaenous transhepatic cholangiography or endoscopic retrograde
- Cholangiopancreatography or magnetic retrograde cholangiopancreatography.
- Colonoscopy: sclerosing cholangitis: inflammatory bowel disease.
- Bone marrow aspirate: exclude Niemann-Pick type C or other storage disorders.
- Enzyme from white cells or cultured fibroblasts (skin biopsy): to exclude lysosomal storage disease, glycogen storage disease.
- Angiography: congenital or acquired venous or arterial malformations, assessment of portosystemic shunt
- Cardiac catheterization: to assess pulmonary hypertension and cardiac status.
- Microaggregate albumin scan: to assess hepatopulmonary syndrome and hepatic encephalopathy.
- Muscle biopsy: to assay respiratory chain enzymes in mitochondrial disorders.
- Genotyping: Wilson disease, cystic fibrosis and other.
- Liver biopsy.

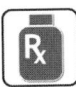 ## Therapy

The management of patients is that of the underlying diagnosis.

GENERAL MANAGEMENT

- Maintaining growth and development is of paramount importance to optimize the physical and mental well being of the patient.
- Fat-soluble vitamins (ADEK) given orally are poorly absorbed and levels must be monitored.
- Anthropometric parameters must be recorded, including skinfold thickness.
- Medium-chain triglyceride rich formulas can reduce fat malabsorption.
- Branched-chain amino acids may be useful in patients with hepatic encephalopathy.
- Ursodeoxycholic acid: choleretic
- Encourage bolus feedings and minimizing continuous feeding and TPN may reduce gallbladder sludge.
- Proactive involvement of the clinical psychologist and play therapist can help alleviate some of the problems, such as depression and fear.
- Aggressive weight management in patients with obesity/hypermetabolic syndrome with steatohepatitis.
- Chronic debilitating pruritus: indication for liver transplantation after failure of medical therapy.
- Treatment for pruritus includes:

—Antihistamines
—Cholestyramine
—Naltrexone
—Rifampicin
—Ursodeoxycholic acid

- Monitoring portal hypertension: assessment of portal flow on ultrasound and splenic size may provide some indication of disease progression.
- Treatment of recurrent cholangitis: may decelerate the progression of liver disease.
- Aggressive treatment for spontaneous bacterial peritonitis in patients with ascites: mortality rate between 55% and 78% and a recurrence rate of 69% after 1 year.
- Early referral to a liver transplant center.
- Complete immunization schedule including Hepatitis A

SPECIFIC MANAGEMENT

This depends on the underlying liver disease. Some diseases are progressive and not amenable to treatment and many patients will progress to end stage liver disease and the treatment for some of these will include liver transplantation.

 ## Common Questions and Answers

Q: What are the risks of providing very young patients with a liver transplant?
A: Although transplant in the very young is more difficult with the increased use of split liver techniques, outcomes of orthotopic liver transplantation (OLT) in infants have improved.

Q: Why should we be aggressive with vitamin supplementation?
A: There is significant malabsorption of vitamins A, D, E, and K. Vitamin D and E deficiencies are the most significant causing rickets and neuropathy.

Q: Oral supplements of vitamins are sometimes very difficult to administer in the very young. How can I overcome this problem?
A: It is common practice in some centers to give vitamins D and E as an intramuscular injection on a monthly basis, with levels done in between.

Q: Why do jaundiced children scratch?
A: It is the accumulation of bile salts that causes pruritus.

Q: Are the stigmata of chronic liver disease also seen in children?
A: It is very common to find spider nevi, liver palms, splenomegaly, cutaneous shunts, and clubbing.

ICD-9-CD

571.49 chronic active hepatitis
790.4 elevated LFTs
575.2 gallbladder obstruction/sludge
572.3 portal hypertension

BIBLIOGRAPHY

Geller SA. Hepatitis B and hepatitis C. *Clin Liver Dis* 2002;6(2):317–334.

Hardy S, Kleinman R. Cirrhosis and chronic liver failure. In: Suchy F, Sokol R, Balistreri W, eds. *Liver Disease in Children*. 2nd Ed. Philadelphia: Lippincott Williams & Wilkins, 2001:89–127.

The liver. In: Walker WA, Goulet O, Kleinman R, et al, eds. *Pediatric Gastrointestinal Disease*. 4th Ed. Hamilton, Ontario. B.C. Decker Inc, 2004;880–1311.

Authors: John Tung and Vani Gopalareddy

Chronic Diarrhea

 ## Database

DEFINITION

Diarrhea lasting more than 2 weeks, whereas acute diarrhea, generally caused by enteric pathogens, is self-limiting and duration of symptoms is less than 1 week. Stool output in excess of 200 g per day in children and adults, or 10 g per kg per day in infants is considered diarrhea.

PATHOPHYSIOLOGY

The major categories are osmotic and secretory. Inflammatory and motility disorders are smaller but important subcategories to consider. In many conditions, more that one process may be present.

- Osmotic diarrhea occurs when unabsorbable solute accumulates in the lumen of the small intestine and colon. This increases the intraluminal osmotic pressure and results in excessive fluid and electrolyte losses in stool. Osmotic diarrhea will improve with fasting. Osmotic diarrhea is usually related to malabsorption of dietary products or to the presence of congenital or acquired disaccharidase deficiency or glucose-galactose defects. See table, Differences Between Osmotic and Secretory Diarrhea
- Secretory diarrhea occurs when the net secretion of fluid and electrolyte is in excess of absorption in the intestine. The intestinal mucosa is normally very active in both of these processes. The diarrhea occurs independently of the osmotic load in the intestinal lumen and does not improve with fasting. The mechanisms for secretory diarrhea include the activation of intracellular mediators such as cyclic adenosine monophosphate (cAMP), cyclic guanosine monophosphate (cGMP), and calcium dependent channels. These mediators stimulate active chloride secretion from the crypt cells and inhibit the neutral coupled sodium chloride absorption.
- Inflammation in the intestine can cause an alteration in mucosal integrity resulting in exudative loss of mucus, blood, and/or protein. Increased permeability and altered mucosal surface area may affect absorption and result in diarrhea as a result of a malabsorptive process.
- Motility disorders will affect the intestinal transit time. Hypermotility will cause rapid transit through the intestine and hence, shorten the effective absorptive capacity of

the bowel. Hypomotility states such as stasis from bacterial overgrowth can lead to diarrhea. These processes can be a primary cause of diarrhea, but are more commonly associated with another pathologic process.

EPIDEMIOLOGY

Chronic diarrhea seen in the tropics and developing countries is more likely infectious in nature than in the United States. Gender and genetic factors do not play a significant role in most cases of chronic diarrhea.

COMPLICATIONS

The most common complications include:

- Dehydration
- Failure to thrive
- Electrolyte abnormalities

 ## Differential Diagnosis

The causes of chronic diarrhea differ depending on the age of the child.

- Infants younger than 1 year of age:

—Cow's-milk and/or soy protein intolerance
—Intractable diarrhea of infancy is associated with diffuse mucosal injury beginning prior to 6 months of age resulting in malabsorption and malnutrition.
—Protracted postinfectious diarrhea
—Microvillus inclusions disease
—Autoimmune enteropathy
—Hirschsprung disease with enterocolitis
—Transport defects (e.g., congenital chloridorrhea)
—Nutrient malabsorption (e.g., congenital glucose-galactose malabsorption and congenital lactase deficiency, sucrase-isomaltase deficiency.
—Cystic fibrosis
—AIDS enteropathy
—Primary immune defects
—Munchausen syndrome by proxy (factitious)

- Children between 1 and 5 years of age:

—Chronic nonspecific diarrhea of infancy (toddler's diarrhea)
—Postinfectious enteritis
—Giardiasis
—Eosinophilic gastroenteritis
—Sucrase-isomaltase deficiency
—Tumors (neuroblastoma, VIPoma with secretory diarrhea)
—Inflammatory bowel disease
—Celiac disease
—Cystic fibrosis

—Small bowel bacterial overgrowth
—AIDS enteropathy
—Factitious

- Children older than 5 years of age:

—Acquired lactose deficiency (early adolescent)
—Inflammatory bowel disease
—Constipation with (overflow) encopresis
—Irritable bowel syndrome (adolescent)
—Laxative abuse (adolescents)
—Giardiasis
—Tumors (neuroblastoma, VIPoma with secretory diarrhea)
—Primary bowel tumors (rare, adolescent)

 ## Data Gathering

HISTORY

- Dietary intake including the types of food and the occurrence of diarrhea in close relationship to specific foods (e.g., dairy products) may be diagnostic. The amount and type of liquid ingested may also be helpful in diagnosis.
- Evaluation of the stool pattern, including consistency, frequency, and appearance. The history of blood and mucus in stool is strongly suggestive of an inflammatory process.
- Nutritional status and growth parameters need to be assessed. The presence of growth failure or malnutrition has considerable implications compared with a child with normal growth and no history of weight loss.

 ## Physical Examination

- Nutritional status of the patient needs to be assessed. Comparing height, weight, and head circumference with normal standards and old measurements is extremely important.
- Anthropometric measurements are important in assessing loss of body fat and muscle mass.
- Peripheral edema, ascites, rash, dystrophic nails, alopecia, chronic chest findings, and pallor may all be indicative of nutritional deficiencies secondary to chronic diarrhea.
- A rectal examination may reveal stool impaction with overflow as the apparent cause of "uncontrolled diarrhea." Is there blood in the stool?
- Evidence of infection should be considered with symptoms such as fever, bloody diarrhea, and vital sign instability.

 ## Laboratory Aids

- Stool samples:

—Stool should be tested for occult blood and for the presence of fecal leukocytes, which indicate the presence of inflammation (usually colonic).

Table 1. Differences Between Osmotic and Secretory Diarrhea

	OSMOTIC	SECRETORY
Volume of stool	<200 mL/24 hr	>200 mL/24 hr
Response to fasting	Stops	Continues
Stool sodium	<70 mEq/L	>70 mEq/L
Reducing substances	Positive	Negative
Stool pH	<5	>6

—Stools pH and reducing substances: If stool is positive for reducing substances and/or the pH is less than 5.5, carbohydrate malabsorption with or without proximal small-bowel injury is likely. (Note: Sucrose is not a reducing substance. If sucrose malabsorption is suspected, stool sample has to be hydrolyzed with hydrochloric acid and heated before analysis.)

—A positive Sudan stain of the stool is indicative of fat malabsorption. However, a 72-hour fecal fat collection remains the gold standard to diagnose fat malabsorption. Stool for fecal elastase is now also available to assess fat malabsorption.

—Stool should be cultured for bacteria, ova and parasites, and viral organisms. *Clostridium difficile* toxins A and B are heat labile and stool must be kept cool during transport.

—Stool may be collected for electrolyte and osmolality measurements.

• Blood samples:

—Hemoglobin and RBC indices may show evidence of deficiencies in iron, vitamins, or other micronutrients.

—Prealbumin and albumin are good parameters of protein and overall nutritional status.

—Electrolytes may be helpful in the diagnostic process if significant changes exist in the Na+, Cl−, HCO3−.

—ESR, CRP can serve as markers for inflammatory conditions.

—Hormonal studies to assess for secretory tumors (VIP, gastrin, secretin, urine assay for 5-HT).

—In the evaluation for celiac disease, serum tissue transglutaminase antibody and antiendomysial antibodies has now replaced antigliadin as the screening antibody test of choice, so long as the total serum immunoglobin (IgA) is normal.

• Specialized studies:

—A D-xylose absorption test is helpful in screening for small-bowel injury. Timed serum D-xylose following oral ingestion is significantly lower in diseases causing diffuse mucosal damage to the small bowel, i.e., postviral enteropathy, celiac disease.

—A hydrogen breath test may be helpful in evaluating for the possibility of small bowel bacterial overgrowth. Lactose or sucrose hydrogen breath tests are done if lactose or sucrase-isomaltase is suspected, respectively.

—Viral serologies such as HIV and cytomegalovirus need to be considered in the immunocompromised host with diarrhea.

—Sweat chloride if cystic fibrosis is suspected.

—Plain x-ray studies are not usually helpful in the evaluation of chronic diarrhea. Upper gastrointestinal series with small bowel follow through may show partial small-bowel obstruction, strictures, or evidence of inflammatory bowel disease.

—Endoscopy with small-bowel biopsy and small-bowel aspirate for culture can be helpful in diagnosing certain congenital, immunologic, or infective causes of diarrhea.

Small-bowel disaccharidase studies will help detect carbohydrate malabsorption.

—Colonoscopy will diagnose colitis related to inflammatory bowel disease or infection.

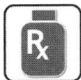 ## Therapy

• The first goal is to ensure adequate nutritional intake to permit normal growth and development.

• In cases in which infection is detected, appropriate antibiotic therapy should be initiated.

• In infants in whom the infection is severe or protracted in its course, a predigested (elemental or semielemental) formula may be necessary early in the recovery phase of the illness. These formulas tend to be much better tolerated and absorbed by the injured small bowel. Once the infant has shown good improvement, transition to a regular diet can be attempted. If the diarrhea is severe and oral nutrition appears inadequate, the formula can be given in a slow, continuous fashion via a nasogastric/nasojejunal tube. This again allows for better absorption of nutrients by the injured bowel.

• When the offending agent is identified as the cause of the diarrhea, e.g., cow's-milk protein, soy protein, lactose, or gluten, these agents should be promptly removed.

• In cases in which there is increased motility and thus rapid transit time, such as in chronic nonspecific diarrhea, alterations in the diet can be very helpful.

• Elimination of sorbitol-containing juices, which increases the osmotic load, and low-carbohydrate diet will help to lower the osmotic load delivered to the intestine. Furthermore, a high-fat diet will slow the intestinal transit time and increase the time available to absorb fluid, electrolytes, and nutrients from the intestinal tract.

• Certain causes of chronic diarrhea require specific therapy. Tumors, inflammatory bowel disease, or cystic fibrosis requires chronic and multifactorial treatment regimens to manage the underlying disease.

• Many causes of congenital diarrhea do not have specific therapy available and treatment is supportive. In the case of congenital microvillus inclusion disease atrophy leads to an intractable diarrhea, and the patient is supported with the use of hyperalimentation (HAL). No current treatment has been found to correct this entity. Patients eventually succumb to complications of long-term HAL. Small-bowel transplant remains experimental and should be offered only in select cases.

 ## Follow-Up

With many of the chronic and complicated causes of chronic diarrhea, the best markers to follow as indicators of disease activity tend to be growth and nutritional status. If the patient is able to thrive and grow, the disease is being well controlled.

PITFALLS

• Avoid the reinstitution of a regular diet too quickly following a severe and/or protracted insult to the gut since this may further exacerbate the diarrhea.

• The use of antimotility and antisecretory agents should be judicious and as an adjunct to other therapy, but not as the mainstay in the treatment regimen.

• In patients with cow's milk and/or soy allergy, rechallenge should be after 12 months of age and should be in a controlled environment in case anaphylaxis occurs.

 ## Common Questions and Answers

Q: In my infant with cow's milk allergy, when can he have cow's milk?
A: In patients with cow's milk and/or soy allergy, rechallenge should be after 12 months of age and should be in a controlled environment in case anaphylaxis occurs. If the testing is negative, ingestion of cow's milk can be recommended.

Q: What are the best markers for success in management of chronic diarrhea?
A: If weight and height normalize, the chances of continued malabsorption are unlikely.

Q: What are the best ways to diagnose celiac disease now?
A: The easiest way to diagnose celiac disease now includes blood testing called endomysial antibodies and transglutaminase. These tests have replaced the use of the gliadin antibodies. Additionally, there are genetic HLA markers that are also now available.

BIBLIOGRAPHY

Ali SA, Hill DR. Giardia intestinalis. *Curr Opin Infect Dis* 2003;16(5):453–460.

Baldassano RN, Liacouras CA. Chronic diarrhea, a practical approach for the pediatrician. *Pediatr Clin North Am* 1991; 38(3):667–686.

Guerrant RL, Bobak DA. Bacterial and protozoal gastroenteritis. *N Engl J Med* 1991;325:327–340.

Lee SD, Surawicz CM. Infectious causes of chronic diarrhea. *Gastroenterol Clin North Am* 2001;30(3):679–692.

Salvilahti E. Food-induced malabsorption syndromes. *J Pediatr Gastroenterol Nutr* 2000;30(Suppl):S61–66.

Smith MM, Lifshitz F. Excess fruit juice consumption as a contributing factor in nonorganic failure to thrive. *Pediatrics* 1994;93(3):438–443.

Vanderhoof JA. Chronic diarrhea. *Pediatr Rev* 1998;19(12):418–422.

Author: Edisio Semeao

Chronic Granulomatous Disease

 Database

DEFINITION

Chronic granulomatous disease is a rare inherited defect involving phagocytes. The defective phagocytes (neutrophils and monocytes) have a decreased or absent ability to generate reactive oxygen intermediates, leaving the host susceptible to recurrent bacterial and fungal infections.

PATHOPHYSIOLOGY

- Associated defects involve the NADPH oxidase complex of the neutrophil.
- Neutrophils in chronic granulomatous disease have an impaired ability to combat infection via an impaired respiratory burst.
- The NADPH oxidase complex is composed of four subunits, any of which may be defective in chronic granulomatous disease.

—Sixty percent of patients with chronic granulomatous disease have a defect in the gp91-phox subunit, which is inherited in an X-linked manner.
—Thirty-three percent of patients have a defect in the p47-phox subunit, which is inherited in an autosomal-recessive manner.
—Defects occur less frequently in the p22-phox and p67-phox subunits.

GENETICS

- Gene mutations may occur spontaneously and are inherited as an X-linked variant, or autosomal-recessive variant.
- Mutations may occur in any one of the four subunits of the neutrophil NADPH oxidase complex:

EPIDEMIOLOGY

- Prevalence: approximately 1 in 500,000 individuals

COMPLICATIONS

These patients have an increased susceptibility to bacterial and fungal infections that usually are not pathogenic in normal hosts

- Recurrent skin infections
- Sepsis
- Chronic lung disease (secondary to recurrent infections)
- Chronic liver disease (secondary to recurrent infections)
- Chronic osteomyelitis of large and small bones
- Malabsorption
- Systemic and discoid lupus erythematosus: increased incidence in female carriers

The diagnosis of chronic granulomatous disease should be considered in patients with:

- Recurrent lymphadenitis
- Staphylococcal hepatic abscess
- *Aspergillus* or *Nocardia* pneumonia
- *Serratia marcescens* osteomyelitis
- Infections with *Pseudomonas cepacia*
- *Salmonella* sepsis
- Perirectal abscesses
- Brain abscesses

PROGNOSIS

Survival beyond the fourth decade is common. Bone marrow transplantation is curative.

 Differential Diagnosis

INFECTIOUS

Infections are related to the immune deficiency.

GENETIC/METABOLIC

- Leukocyte glucose-6-phosphate dehydrogenase deficiency
- Myeloperoxidase deficiency
- Humoral immune deficiencies
- Complement deficiencies

COMMON CAUSES

- Chronic granulomatous disease is not acquired; it is inherited as an X-linked variant or as an autosomal variant.

 Data Gathering

HISTORY

Question: At what age did the patient present?
Significance: Patients with chronic granulomatous disease usually present before 2 years of age with marked lymphadenopathy, hepatosplenomegaly, draining lymph nodes, and pneumonias.

Question: What is the infecting organism?
Significance: Patients with chronic granulomatous disease tend to develop infections with unusual organisms, such as *S. aureus*, *S. epidermidis*, *S. marcescens*, Pseudomonas, *Escherichia coli*, Candida, Aspergillus, Nocardia, and Salmonella.

Question: Are there other affected family members?
Significance: Chronic granulomatous disease is inherited in an X-linked and autosomal-recessive pattern. Therefore, there may be other affected family members.

Question: Does the mother have lupus?
Significance: There is a higher incidence of lupus in females who are carriers for chronic granulomatous disease.

 Physical Examination

Finding: Skin abscess or boils
Significance: Patients with chronic granulomatous disease develop frequent skin infections.

Finding: Mucous membrane and perirectal infections
Significance: Patients with chronic granulomatous disease commonly develop infections at mucous membrane and epidermal junctions, especially in the perirectal area.

Finding: Lymphadenopathy
Significance: Patients with chronic granulomatous disease commonly develop lymphadenopathy and draining lymph nodes.

Finding: Hepatosplenomegaly
Significance: Hepatosplenomegaly is a common finding in patients with chronic granulomatous disease.

Finding: Abnormal lung examination
Significance: Pulmonary disease is common in patients with chronic granulomatous disease.

Chronic Granulomatous Disease

 ## Laboratory Aids

APPROACH TO THE PATIENT

- General goal: Decide whether the patient's type of infections (osteomyelitis, perirectal abscess, etc.) and infecting organisms are consistent with the diagnosis of chronic granulomatous disease.
- Order a nitroblue tetrazolium (NBT) test.
- If abnormal, initiate sulfamethoxazole/ trimethoprim prophylaxis.

Test: The NBT
Significance: The NBT is the most widely available test for chronic granulomatous disease. Neutrophils from normal individuals can reduce the dye, resulting in a color change. Neutrophils from patients with chronic granulomatous disease cannot reduce the dye, and it remains colorless. Neutrophils and monocytes from patients with chronic granulomatous disease have an impaired hexose monophosphate shunt. Therefore, they have a decreased conversion of NADP to NADPH, and a decreased oxidative burst, which results in an inability to reduce the NBT in this study.

Test: The 2,7-dichlorofluorescin (DCF)
Significance: DCF can directly measure the production of hydrogen peroxide utilizing a fluorescent label and flow cytometry. Patients with chronic granulomatous disease have decreased hydrogen peroxide production.

Test: Immunoblotting
Significance: Immunoblotting can be used to quantify the amount of each NADPH subunit present.

ISSUES FOR REFERRAL

Factors that may help alert you to make a referral include:

- A new diagnosis of chronic granulomatous disease: Immunologists can assist with antibiotic prophylaxis and with parameters for when to seek medical attention, and they can help identify which genetic variant is responsible for the patient's disease.
- Pregnant carrier for chronic granulomatous disease: Immunologists can help with prenatal diagnosis. Furthermore, some centers may consider in utero bone marrow transplantation for an affected fetus.
- Fever or suspected infection: Patients with chronic granulomatous disease tend to develop infections in unusual sites with unusual organisms. An immunologist can help with the evaluation and appropriate antibiotic coverage.

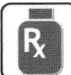 ## Therapy

- Antibiotic prophylaxis: Trimethoprim-sulfamethoxazole is the antibiotic of choice, because both components are concentrated in the neutrophil, and for its bacterial spectrum.
- Recombinant interferon-γ: This is reserved for patients with severe disease. This therapy may decrease the incidence of infection.
- Bone marrow transplant: Chronic granulomatous disease has been cured in patients with matched transplants.
- Acute infections:

—Broad-spectrum intravenous antibiotics: There should be a low threshold to start this therapy. Severe infections should be treated with broad-spectrum intravenous antibiotics until an organism is identified. Good initial antibiotics include intravenous penicillins, aminoglycosides, and antipseudomonal antibiotics.
—Amphotericin B: This should not be withheld if a fungal infection is suspected, or if the patient's clinical status is deteriorating despite broad-spectrum antibiotics.
—Leukocyte transfusions: These are reserved for severe infections, and efficacy is controversial.

 ## Follow-Up

Chronic granulomatous disease is a lifelong disease. These patients tend to develop chronic lung disease; therefore, pulmonary function studies should be followed at least annually. Liver disease is also common; therefore, liver function studies should also be followed at least annually. Female carriers should be observed for signs of lupus erythematosus.

 ## Common Questions and Answers

Q: How do you interpret an NBT test reported as 50% of normal?
A: This is generally consistent with a carrier state. The carrier is not at increased risk for infection. However, carrier females have an increased risk of developing lupus.

Q: What do the infecting organisms have in common?
A: Patients with chronic granulomatous disease are most susceptible to catalase-positive organisms.

Q: Are all chronic granulomatous disease patients with fever admitted automatically?
A: No. It is true that these patients are more prone to invasive and systemic infections, but these patients are not admitted with every febrile episode (especially if there is evidence of a minor bacterial or viral infection). However, subtle signs of an invasive infection must be taken very seriously, and these patients are certainly admitted.

Q: Can a prenatal diagnosis be made?
A: Yes. However, currently this can only be done in a limited number of research laboratories, and the testing is not commercially available. Testing involves chorionic villus sampling, and it can be done only on families in which the specific mutation has been mapped.

ICD-9-CM 288.1

BIBLIOGRAPHY

Horwitz ME, Barrett AJ, Brown MR, et al. Treatment of chronic granulomatous disease with nonmyeloablative conditioning and a T-cell-depleted hematopoietic allograft. *N Engl J Med* 2001;344(12):881–888.

Jirapongsananuruk O, Malech HL, Kuhns DB, et al. Diagnostic paradigm for evaluation of male patients with chronic granulomatous disease, based on the dihydrorhodamine 123 assay. *J Allergy Clin Immunol* 2003;111(2):374–379.

Kamani N, Douglas SD. Natural history of chronic granulomatous disease. *Diagn Clin Immunol* 1988;5:314–317.

Schappi MG, Klein NJ, Lindley KJ, et al. The nature of colitis in chronic granulomatous disease. *J Pediatr Gastroenterol Nutr* 2003; 36(5):623–631.

Authors: Mathew Fogg
Christopher A. Smith, 3rd edition

Cirrhosis

Database

DEFINITION

Cirrhosis is the end stage of progressive hepatic fibrosis and regenerative nodule formation that may occur as a result of many different liver diseases. In its advanced form it is irreversible and often requires liver transplantation for survival of the patient.

PATHOPHYSIOLOGY

- Cirrhosis is a dynamic process that perpetuates even after the initial insult has ceased.
- Hepatocellular injury (of any cause) leads to cell death or necrosis.
- In response to such injury, hepatocytes and their supportive cells deposit an abnormally thick and dense extracellular connective tissue matrix leading to fibrosis.
- Fibrosis distorts liver architecture and shunts blood flow.
- Poor blood flow to focal areas causes ischemia and thus further cellular injury.
- As the volume of normally vascularized liver tissue decreases, compensatory growth of liver tissue occurs to form regenerative nodules.
- Regenerative nodules further impede blood flow by compression of blood vessels.
- The cycle continues as fibrosis and nodule formation perpetuate further necrosis.
- The resultant altered blood flow in the liver also leads to portal hypertension and its associated complications.

CAUSES

In children, a wide range of causes of hepatocellular injury may result in cirrhosis.

- Biliary

—Extrahepatic biliary atresia
—Choledochal cyst
—Tumors
—Common bile duct and biliary lithiasis
—Alagille syndrome
—Biliary hypoplasia
—Primary familial intrahepatic cholestasis (PFIC)
—Sclerosing cholangitis
—Graft-vs.-host disease
—Drugs (e.g., trimethoprim-sulfamethoxazole)
—Langerhans cell histiocytosis

- Hepatic

—Neonatal hepatitis, including TORCH infections
—Viral—hepatitis B, C, D, EBV, CMV
—Autoimmune hepatitis
—Nonalcoholic steatohepatitis (NASH), associated with obesity
—Drugs/toxins and alcohol

- Genetic/metabolic

—Cystic fibrosis
—α_1-Antitrypsin deficiency
—Metal storage defects—Wilson disease, iron storage disorders (hemochromatosis)
—Carbohydrate defects—galactosemia, hereditary fructose intolerance, glycogen storage III and IV
—Amino acid defects—tyrosinemia, urea cycle disorders
—Lipid storage diseases—Gaucher's disease, Niemann-Pick type C
—Mitochondrial disorders—fatty acid β-oxidation defects, respiratory chain defects
—Peroxisomal disorders—Zellweger's syndrome
—Porphyrias—Erythropoietic protoporphyria

- Vascular

—Budd-Chiari syndrome
—Veno-occlusive disease
—Congestive heart failure

GENETICS

HLA markers have been identified in several disorders, including sclerosing cholangitis and hemochromatosis. However, no specific markers correlate with cirrhosis.

EPIDEMIOLOGY

Based on the varying etiologies, no specific epidemiologic pattern can be identified.

COMPLICATIONS

- Malnutrition and growth failure
- Malabsorption (diarrhea, steatorrhea, fat-soluble vitamin deficiencies)
- Portal hypertension and variceal bleeding
- Chronic gastritis, peptic ulcer disease, gastroesophageal reflux
- Ascites
- Encephalopathy
- Hypersplenism (associated with anemia, thrombocytopenia, and neutropenia)
- Anemia (GI blood loss, hemolysis, iron/folate deficiency, malnutrition, dilution)
- Coagulopathy
- Hepatopulmonary syndrome (hypoxemia, cyanosis, dyspnea, digital clubbing)
- Hepatorenal syndrome (rapidly progressive renal failure in patients with cirrhosis)
- Bacterial infections, spontaneous bacterial peritonitis
- Hepatocellular carcinoma

PROGNOSIS

- The prognosis for cirrhosis leading to decompensation depends on the underlying cause.
- Knowledge of the natural history of particular disease states is of value (e.g., tyrosinemia and biliary atresia).
- Most available liver tests have poor predictive value until liver decompensation has occurred.
- Poor prognostic features in children include prolonged prothrombin time unresponsive to vitamin K, ascites, malnutrition, low plasma cholesterol, elevated bilirubin level, partial thromboplastin time prolonged by more than 20 seconds, and presence of hepatorenal syndrome.

Data Gathering

CLINICAL PRESENTATION

- Compensated (latent) cirrhosis—asymptomatic, with no signs or symptoms of liver disease. Discovered incidentally either during routine physical examinations with an enlarged liver and/or palpable spleen, or as a result of an investigation for an unrelated condition.
- Decompensated (active) cirrhosis—as cirrhosis progresses, overt signs and symptoms may occur including failure to thrive, muscle weakness, fatigue, fever, jaundice, edema, abdominal pain, ascites, and steatorrhea. This stage may also present with acute, precipitous liver failure or a life-threatening complication such as an esophageal variceal hemorrhage.

HISTORY

Based on the varying etiologic agents, one should elicit pertinent historical features characteristic of each specific problem as detailed:

- Exposure to hepatitis, antecedent viral illnesses
- Exposure to hepatotoxins
- Family history of genetic, metabolic, or autoimmune diseases
- Neurologic problems, deteriorating school performance, depression (Wilson disease)

Physical Examination

- General—poor growth, malnutrition, fever, cachexia
- Skin—jaundice, flushing, pallor, cyanosis, palmar erythema, spider angiomata, easy bruising
- Abdomen—ascites (distension, fluid wave, shifting dullness), caput medusa, splenomegaly, rectal varices, hepatomegaly, or a shrunken liver
- Extremities—digital clubbing, hypertrophic osteoarthropathy, muscle wasting
- Endocrine—gynecomastia, testicular atrophy, delayed puberty
- CNS—asterixis, positive Babinski sign, mental status changes, hyperreflexia, muscle wasting

Laboratory Aids

TESTS

These tests focus on determining the etiology and the severity of liver disease prior to a liver biopsy.

- Tests of liver cell injury—alanine aminotransferase, aspartate aminotransferase, lactic dehydrogenase
- Tests of synthetic function—albumin and other serum proteins, prothrombin time, ammonia, plasma and urine amino acids, serum lipids and lipoproteins, cholesterol and triglycerides
- Tests of cholestasis—fractionated bilirubin, alkaline phosphatase, γ-glutamyltransferase, 5'-nucleotidase, serum and urine bile acids
- Tests of fibrosis—are being investigated but not yet available; possible markers include serum levels of procollagen III peptide, laminin, hyaluronate, and type IV collagen
- Miscellaneous disease-specific serum tests

—Viral serologies—TORCH, hepatitis B, C, EBV, CMV
—Wilson disease—ceruloplasmin, serum and urine cooper, and slit-lamp exam for Kaiser-Fleischer rings
—α_1-Antitrypsin deficiency—α_1-antitrypsin serum level and protease inhibitor (Pi) phenotype
—Autoimmune hepatitis—sedimentation rate, autoantibodies, immunoglobulins
—Hemochromatosis—serum iron, total iron binding capacity, ferritin
—Metabolic/genetic—fasting blood sugar, lactate, pyruvate, uric acid, sweat test, carnitine, CPK, porphyrins, serum amino acids, urine organic acids, urine reducing substances, urine succinylacetone, fatty acid degeneration products

IMAGING

- Ultrasound with Doppler images—evaluates for anatomic variation or obstruction of the biliary tree, presence of ascites, portal hypertension and vascular obstruction.
- Hepatobiliary radioisotope scanning—assess for biliary excretion in neonatal cholestasis.
- Cholangiography (ERCP, MRCP, intraoperative)—assess for extrahepatic biliary disease (stones, choledochal cyst, sclerosing cholangitis).

LIVER BIOPSY

- Percutaneous needle biopsy, intraoperative wedge biopsy, transjugular liver biopsy
- Confirm the presence, type, and degree of activity of cirrhosis.
- Various hepatic diseases that progress to cirrhosis have characteristic histologic findings. However, the process of cirrhosis may obscure the nature of the original insult, rendering morphologic and histologic classifications unhelpful.

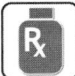 ## Therapy

MEDICAL

- Fat-soluble vitamin supplementation—vitamins A, D, E, and K
- Diuretic therapy (furosemide, spironolactone, chlorothiazide) for patients with ascites
- Albumin infusions for patients with refractory ascites
- β-Blockers have been shown to decrease portal pressure and reduce the risk of variceal bleeding in adults
- Antibiotics if suspicious of spontaneous bacterial peritonitis (avoid nephrotoxic agents)
- Lactulose and neomycin are used for patients with hepatic encephalopathy

NUTRITION

Malnutrition is common in chronic liver diseases because of several metabolic derangements, fat malabsorption, anorexia, and increased energy requirements. Adequate caloric intake is critical and often will require supplemental nocturnal nasogastric tube feedings. Some of the dietary fat should be provided as medium-chain triglycerides which do not require bile for absorption. Fat-soluble vitamins should be supplemented. Careful attention must also be paid to fluid and electrolyte balance; sodium restriction may be necessary in the presence of ascites.

SURGERY AND PROCEDURES

- Endoscopic variceal band ligation or sclerotherapy for GI bleeding
- Paracentesis for refractory ascites or diagnosis of spontaneous bacterial peritonitis
- Porta-systemic shunt placement (surgical or radiologic TIPS procedure) for uncontrolled portal hypertension
- Liver transplantation for decompensated cirrhosis

 ## Follow-Up

Close monitoring and management of any complications of chronic liver disease.

 ## Common Questions and Answers

Q: Will my child with cystic fibrosis develop cirrhosis?
A: The medical literature cites a 5% to 20% incidence of cirrhosis in children with cystic fibrosis. Many factors seem to relate to the development of cirrhosis in these children, but the genetic type of cystic fibrosis does not seem to be a cause.

Q: Will every child with cirrhosis need a liver transplant?
A: Most children who develop cirrhosis from causes such as biliary atresia or metabolic disease will ultimately require a liver transplant.

ICD-9-CD 571.0

BIBLIOGRAPHY

Hardy S, Kleinman RE. Cirrhosis and chronic liver failure. In: Suchy FJ, Sokol RJ, Balistreri WF, eds. *Liver Disease in Children*. Philadelphia: Lippincott Williams & Wilkins, 2001:89–127.

Kelly DA. Current results and evolving indications for liver transplantation in children. *J Pediatr Gastroenterol Nutr* 1998; 27(2):1214.

Molleston JP, White F, Techman J, et al. Obese children with steatohepatitis can develop cirrhosis in childhood. *Amer J Gastroenterol* 2002;97(9):2460–2462.

Poupon R, Chazouilleres O, Poupon RE. Chronic cholestatic diseases. *J Hepatol* 2000;32(Suppl 1):129.

Shepherd R. Complications and management of chronic liver disease. In: Kelly DA, eds. *Diseases of the Liver and Biliary System in Children*. London: Blackwell Science, 1999: 189–210.

Authors: Rose C. Graham-Maar
Lynette A. Gillis, 3rd edition

Cleft Lip and Palate

 Database

DEFINITION

A cleft lip (CL) is a deformity of the upper lip that may include a discontinuity of vermilion, skin, muscle, and mucosa, as well as the underlying gingiva and bone. It can be unilateral or bilateral. A complete cleft extends into the nose, while an incomplete cleft has at least some bridge of intact tissue separating the oral and nasal cavities. A cleft palate (CP) usually represents a visible separation between the two halves of the roof of the mouth, involving mucosa, muscle, and often the bones of the hard palate. A submucous CP has intact mucosa, but the underlying muscle and bone are at least partially divided.

ETIOLOGY

• Cleft lip may result from failure of the medial nasal and maxillary processes to join in utero, or possibly from lack of adequate mesenchymal reinforcement, leading to subsequent breakdown and separation. CP results from failure of the palatal shelves to fuse.
• Lower-than-expected incidence of CL and CP has been noted with prenatal dietary supplementation with folic acid and vitamin B6. Folic acid supplementation has also been clearly associated with a decreased incidence of neural tube defects.

PATHOPHYSIOLOGY

Muscle fibers are atrophic and disorganized in the region of the cleft, and mitochondrial abnormalities are noted at the cleft margins by histochemical and electromyographic studies.

ETIOLOGY AND GENETICS

• One-third of patients with CL and/or CP have a positive family history; positive family history is noted twice as often in CL with or without CP as in CP alone.
• Although a number of recognized patterns of malformation that include CL and/or CP may be caused by exposure to teratogens such as alcohol, anticonvulsants, and isotretinoin, there is little evidence linking isolated clefts to exposure to any single teratogenic agent. One notable exception is the anticonvulsant phenytoin, the use of which during pregnancy has been associated with a 10-fold increase in the incidence of CL.

• The incidence of CL in infants born to mothers who smoke during pregnancy is twice that of those born to nonsmoking mothers.
• Among patients with clefts of the secondary palate alone, those syndromes associated with microdeletions of chromosome 22q11.2 (velocardiofacial syndrome, DiGeorge syndrome, and conotruncal anomaly face syndrome) are currently the most common syndromic diagnoses.
• Inheritance is autosomal dominant with considerable variability in phenotypic expression, which may include facial dysmorphism, developmental delay, cardiovascular anomalies, immunologic abnormalities, CP, and velopharyngeal dysfunction.
• The next most common syndrome associated with palatal clefts is Stickler syndrome, characterized by autosomal dominance, CP, epicanthal folds, flat facies, severe myopia, retinal detachment, and glaucoma, caused by a mutation of the gene for type 2 collagen (chromosome 12q).
• Other syndromes linked to specific chromosomal abnormalities include Van der Woude (autosomal dominant, CP and/or CL, lower lip pits, 1q32), and Smith-Lemli-Opitz (defect in cholesterol synthesis, 7q34).
• The majority of clefts are nonsyndromic and may be either multifactorial in origin or the result of changes at a major single-gene locus.

EPIDEMIOLOGY

• Incidence of CL with or without CP is 1 in 700 births.
• Racial heterogeneity noted in CL and CP (Asians, 2.1 in 1,000 births; whites, 1 in 1,000; blacks, 0.41 in 1,000)
• Isolated CP is in 1 in 2,000 births across races.
• Bilateral CL is associated with CP in 86% of cases, and unilateral CL is associated with CP in 68% of cases.
• CL/CP is more common on the left side, particularly in boys.
• Incidence of CL with or without CP increases with parental (especially paternal) age greater than 30 years. Some association with low socioeconomic class may be nutrition-related.

COMPLICATIONS

• Airway obstruction and feeding disorders, particularly with Pierre Robin sequence (micrognathia, glossoptosis, airway obstruction, with or without CP)
• Chronic otitis media
• Speech problems, including hypernasality and articulation errors
• Associated malformations
• About one-third of patients with CP have associated anomalies, with isolated having the highest
• Central nervous system, cardiac, and urinary tract malformations and clubfoot are commonly associated with clefting.

 Data Gathering

HISTORY

Prenatal exposure to alcohol, cigarettes, phenytoin, isotretinoin; family history of CL or CP, or speech problems in first-degree relative

 Physical Examination

• Incomplete or complete cleft of lip, alveolus, hard and soft palate, or uvula. Soft palate and uvula clefts are always midline, while lip, alveolar, and hard palatal clefts can be unilateral or bilateral.
• A bifid uvula may indicate a submucous cleft.
• A small mandible and retropositioned tongue may indicate a risk for airway obstruction (Pierre Robin sequence).
• Look for associated anomalies of the face, heart, and extremities that may indicate a clefting syndrome.

TRICKS

Examine the palate from the top of the patient, with the head in your lap, using a tongue depressor and flashlight. Palpate the posterior hard palate for a possible notch in the bone. Palpate the gums and maxilla for a possible notch in the floor of the nose.

 Laboratory Aids

The following tests should be performed if indicated by history and physical examination:

• Complete ophthalmologic examination to check for myopia, glaucoma, retinal detachment
• Pulse oximetry to check for desaturation while feeding or while supine
• Polysomnography to distinguish central from obstructive apnea
• Increased serum 7-dehydrocholesterol and decreased serum cholesterol to rule out Smith-Lemli-Opitz syndrome
• Karyotype to rule out specific genetic abnormalities
• Fluorescence in situ hybridization (FISH) to rule out a chromosome 22q11.2 deletion
• Echocardiography, renal ultrasound, IV pyelography if indicated

Cleft Lip and Palate

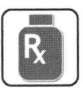 Therapy

NEONATAL

Airway management, prone positioning if tongue is causing airway obstruction. Cleft patients may have significant feeding problems because of inability to generate negative intraoral pressure necessary to feed efficiently. Premie nipples with enlarged or cross-cut openings, or soft plastic squeezable bottles, can facilitate milk flow. Poor weight gain may necessitate nasogastric tube feedings.

SURGICAL

• Significant airway obstruction and desaturation in the neonatal period refractory to prone positioning may indicate the need for a tongue-lip adhesion, release of the floor of the mouth musculature, mandibular distraction, or tracheostomy.
• Wide clefts of the lip may benefit from preliminary lip adhesion at 2 to 3 months of age. Timing of definitive lip repair varies from 2 to 6 months of age.
• Palate repair is generally done prior to 1 year of age to decrease speech and language difficulties.
• Otitis media is more common with CP, and bilateral myringotomy tubes can be inserted at the time of cleft repair.
• Correction of secondary deformities may include lip scar revision, cleft nasal deformity correction (infancy to adulthood), alveolar bone grafts (usually when permanent canines are erupting), pharyngoplasty for soft palate–velopharyngeal incompetence, closure of palatal fistulas, and orthognathic surgery for severe jaw deformities.

ORTHODONTICS

May include obturators to facilitate feeding and speech, nasal molding and palatal repositioning prior to lip and palate repair, palatal expansion prior to bone grafting, conventional orthodontics (appliances, prosthetic teeth, bridgework), and preorthognathic surgery manipulation of the dentition.

 Follow-Up

MULTIDISCIPLINARY TEAM

• Pediatrician
• Plastic surgeon
• Speech pathologist
• Orthodontist
• Pediatric dentist
• Psychologist
• Social worker
• Nurse practitioner
• Anthropologist (facial growth specialist)
• Geneticist
• Support groups

POTENTIAL PROBLEMS

• Hypernasal resonance and nasal air emission during speech may indicate velopharyngeal incompetence or palatal fistula. Up to 30% of patients may require additional palatal or pharyngeal surgery following initial palate repair.
• Multiple ear infections may require prolonged use of myringotomy tubes to prevent hearing impairment. Audiograms should be obtained regularly.
• Delays in speech and language development may require detailed evaluation, early intervention programs, and speech therapy.
• Poor dentition, occlusal problems (crossbite), gingivitis, and crowding have been noted.
• Behavior disorders and psychosocial adjustment disorders may require attention.

PROGNOSIS

Good, for normal growth and development with long-term follow-up by a multidisciplinary team and with good parental support

PITFALLS

• Failure to diagnose airway obstruction in infants with Pierre Robin sequence may lead to failure to thrive or, in severe cases, in death.
• Failure to diagnose associated anomalies may lead to missed syndromes and inaccurate genetic counseling.
• A submucous CP can be easily missed until hypernasal speech is noted later in life.

 Common Questions and Answers

FOR NONSYNDROMIC CL WITH OR WITHOUT CP

Q: What is our risk of having a second child with a cleft, if neither of us has a cleft?
A: Two percent.

Q: What is my child's risk of later having a child with a cleft?
A: Four percent.

Q: What is our risk of having a third child with a cleft, if we have two affected children, but neither of us is affected?
A: Nine percent.

Q: What is our risk of having a second child with a cleft, if one of us also has a cleft?
A: Seventeen percent.

FOR NONSYNDROMIC ISOLATED CP

Q: What is our risk of having a second child with a cleft, if neither of us has a cleft?
A: Two percent.

Q: What is my child's risk of later having a child with a cleft?
A: Six percent.

Q: What is our risk of having a third child with a cleft, if we have two affected children, but neither of us is affected?
A: One percent.

Q: What is our risk of having a second child with a cleft, if one of us also has a cleft?
A: Fifteen percent.

Q: Will my child look normal?
A: All CL repairs will leave some type of permanent scar, with potential asymmetry that may benefit from later additional lip scar revision. The goal is to create a lip that does not attract undue attention. The nose is often the most difficult to correct, because of asymmetry in cartilage and skin contour.

Q: Will my child speak normally?
A: Most children will achieve velopharyngeal competence and normal speech, but may require additional speech therapy to achieve this goal.

ICD-9-CM 749.10, 749.20

BIBLIOGRAPHY

Kaufman FL. Managing the cleft lip and palate patient. *Pediatr Clin North Am* 1991;38(5):1127–1147.

Mulliken JB, Wu JK, Padwa BL. Repair of bilateral cleft lip: review, revisions, and reflections. *J Craniofac Surg* 2003;14(5):609–620.

Murray JC. Gene/environment causes of cleft lip and/or palate. *Clin Genet* 2002;61(4):248–256.

Redford-Badwal DA, Mabry K, Frassinelli JD. Impact of cleft lip and/or palate on nutritional health and oral-motor development. *Dent Clin North Am* 2003;47(2):305–317.

Strong EB, Buckmiller LM. Management of the cleft palate. *Facial Plast Surg North Am* 2001;9(1):15–25.

Witt PD, Marsh JL. Advances in assessing outcome of surgical repair of cleft lip and cleft palate. *Plast Reconstr Surg* 1997;100(7):1907–1917.

Authors: Richard E. Kirschner, Christine A. Carman-Dillon, and David W. Low

Clubfoot

 Database

DEFINITION

Clubfoot is a congenital or neuromuscular deformity in which the hindfoot is fixed in equinus and varus and the forefoot is fixed in varus and often cavus.

CAUSES

• Most cases are idiopathic (multifactorial inheritance pattern with significant environmental influence).
• Infrequently, neuromuscular imbalance may underlie the deformity (cerebral palsy, myelomeningocele, lipomas of the cord, caudal or sacral agenesis, polio, arthrogryposis, fetal alcohol syndrome).

PATHOPHYSIOLOGY

• Many anatomic abnormalities have been postulated as causing clubfoot: anomalous or deficient muscles, myoblasts, mast cells, abnormal primary bone formation, joint and muscle contractures, vascular anomalies (absent dorsalis pedis artery), nerve anomalies, and abnormalities of the fibrous connective tissue.
• Interruption of the development of the embryonic foot has also been suggested.

EPIDEMIOLOGY

• Prevalence is 1 to 1.4 per 1,000 live births, but can vary among different ethnic groups.
• The risk of deformity increases by 20 to 30 times where there is an affected first-degree relative. Male:female ratio is 2:1.

 Differential Diagnosis

• Distinguish other deformities of the foot:
—Metatarsus adductus or varus (heel is in neutral position)
—Calcaneovalgus (foot is in valgus)
—Vertical talus (foot is in valgus, heel in equinovalgus)
—Many children with clubfoot also have tibial torsion.

 Data Gathering

HISTORY

• Family history of clubfoot (3%)
• Onset of deformity (congenital or developmental)

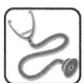 Physical Examination

Careful examination is called for, especially of:

• The neuromuscular system for neuromuscular etiologies such as lumbosacral sinuses, dimples, and lipomas
• The hips for hip dysplasia
• The neck for torticollis

PHYSICAL EXAMINATION TRICKS

Push the foot into a corrected position. Is the deformity fully correctable? Overcorrectable?

 Laboratory Aids

• X-ray studies (after 3 months of age)
• Tarsal bones are poorly ossified in the newborn, therefore diagnosis is clinical.
• At 3 to 6 months of age, anteroposterior (AP) and lateral x-ray films in dorsiflexion (maximal correction) may help in defining residual deformity. The beam should be focused on the hindfoot for both the AP and lateral x-rays, as the measured angles will be hindfoot angles.
• Decreased talocalcaneal angle on the AP and lateral views (25 degrees or less) confirm persistent deformity.
• Medial displacement of the cuboid on the calcaneus and persistent plantar flexion of the forefoot on the hindfoot (talar to first metatarsal angle) indicate more complex deformities.

 Emergency Care

• Care can begin in the first week after birth.

 Therapy

• Initial treatment is serial (weekly) manipulation and casting.
• Taping may be useful for treatment of the infant requiring ICU care; access to the feet should be maintained for blood tests.
• Failure to correct the deformity completely by manipulation within 3 to 9 months requires surgical treatment.
• Long-leg serial casting by the Ponseti technique improves results so that in most clubfeet little more than heel cord lengthening is required.

Follow-Up

- Realignment of the deformity is the goal and should be achieved at surgery or by casting.
- Most surgeons cast the feet for 3 months postoperatively.
- Some brace the feet for 6 months. With the Ponseti technique bars and shoes are recommended full time for 3 months and nights for 3 years to maintain the correction.
- Remember, the cause of the deformity is not corrected. Only the alignment of the bones and lengthening of the soft tissues are corrected.
- Depending on the severity of the deformity all corrected clubfeet can be expected to demonstrate varying amounts of: calf narrowing and weakness, ankle and subtalar stiffness, a difference between the feet of one to two shoe sizes and even a leg-length discrepancy.
- There also will be decreased ankle and subtalar motion as compared to the normal.
- Adolescent children with clubfeet often will get leg cramps and will tire easily while doing sports.

—Recurrence of heel cord tightness is common, especially during periods of rapid growth. Additional heel cord stretching, casting and infrequently, additional surgery may be needed.

- All true recurrences should lead to further evaluation for neuromuscular or syndromic causes that might have been missed in the infant.

 ## Common Questions and Answers

Q: How can a rigid clubfoot be distinguished from a positional clubfoot?
A: During initial evaluation of the child, it is important to assess the amount of flexibility in a clubfoot. This can be most easily done by flexing the hip to 90 degrees, flexing the knee to 90 degrees, and then gently trying to turn the forefoot into a straight position lined up with the thigh. If the foot easily spins around into a normal position, it can be assumed that this is a flexible or positional clubfoot. If deformity persists, this is a rigid deformity. If possible, the examining physician should palpate the heel to see if the os calcis comes out of its equinus position filling the heel pad. In some children, particularly with a rocker bottom sole, the heel pad looks as if it is in the correct position, but the os calcis remains in equinus with the posterior aspect of the os calcis proximal to the heel pad.

Q: What percentage of clubfeet are successfully treated by casting?
A: To some extent, the amount of success depends on how much correction is desired. Occasionally, cast correction will provide a partial correction. Some feet, after casting, can be held in the corrected position, only to spin back to the clubfoot deformity when released. Positional clubfeet are likely to improve with casting in perhaps 80% of cases. Rigid clubfeet are much less likely to be corrected by casting. The success rate in the rigid feet is likely to be about 10% to 20%.

Q: What will be the permanent disability of a congenital clubfoot deformity?
A: While casting and surgical correction of a congenital clubfoot can realign the bones, the surgery does little to correct the underlying neuromuscular problems. As a result, all children with rigid clubfeet are likely to have a leg-length inequality (usually less than 1.5 inches), a smaller foot (usually one to two sizes), calf narrowing that cannot be significantly improved with exercise, and joint stiffness (ankle, subtalar, and midfoot). Even children with optimal realignment of the deformity will notice their inability to perform gymnastic activities or running activities requiring normal range of motion of the ankle and foot. Many will complain of the inability to keep up with their peer group during adolescent and young adult sports activities.

Q: How soon should an infant with congenital clubfoot be referred to an orthopaedic surgeon?
A: If casting is to be even partially successful, cast treatment should begin within the first week or two of life. Clearly, medical and life-threatening conditions will take precedence over the treatment of the clubfoot. Access to the feet for IV or blood studies will interfere with a casting regimen. Casting should begin as soon as is practical. It may even be possible to begin taping of the foot as an alternative to casting, which will still allow IV access to the feet. Referral to an orthopaedic surgeon should therefore follow as soon as is practical.

ICD-9-CM 754.70

BIBLIOGRAPHY

Hamel J, Becker W. Sonographic assessment of clubfoot deformity in young children. *J Pediatr Orthop B* 1996;5(4):279–286.

Johnston CE II, Hobatho MC, Baker KJ, et al. Three-dimensional analysis of clubfoot deformity by computed tomography. *J Pediatr Orthop B* 1995;4(1):39–48.

Napiontek M. Clinical and radiographic appearance of congenital talipes equinovarus after successful nonoperative treatment. *J Pediatr Orthop* 1996;16(1):67–72.

Ponseti I. Treatment of congenital clubfoot. *J Bone Joint Surg* 1992;74(3):448–454.

Roye BD, Hyman J, Roye DP Jr. Congenital idiopathic talipes equinovarus. *Pediatr Rev* 2004;25(4):124–130.

Scherl SA. Common lower extremity problems in children. *Pediatr Rev* 2004;25(2):52–62.

Yamamoto H, Muneta T, Morita S. Nonsurgical treatment of congenital clubfoot with manipulation, cast, and modified Denis Browne splint. *J Pediatr Orthop* 1998;18(4):538–542.

Author: Richard S. Davidson

Coarctation of Aorta

 Database

DEFINITION

Discrete stenosis of the upper thoracic aorta, usually just opposite the site of insertion of the ductus arteriosus (juxtaductal). A segment of tubular hypoplasia and/or a remnant of ductal tissue gives rise to a prominent posterior infolding ("the posterior shelf"). The hemodynamic lesion is most often discrete, but may be long-segment or tortuous in nature. It is usually juxtaductal but may occur in other sites (e.g., the abdominal aorta). The prevalence of other associations (bicuspid aortic valve) and long-term complications (hypertension) indicate the possibility that this lesion is part of a broader spectrum arteriopathy.

PATHOPHYSIOLOGY

- Decreased systemic blood flow to lower extremities after ductal closure
- Increased resistance to left ventricular (LV) outflow causes LV hypertrophy. Relative underperfusion of the renal vessels, baroreceptors, and multiple other mechanisms combine to induce a compensatory systolic hypertension.
- If the coarctation is severe, LV dysfunction and congestive heart failure result, with low cardiac output and increased LV end-diastolic pressure.
- Decreased myocardial perfusion may be present in cases of very low output.

GENETICS

- Multifactorial; occurs in 35% of patients with Turner syndrome (XO)
- Has been described in cases of monozygotic twins
- Many studies document the prevalence of a microdeletion at 22q11 in patients with arch anomalies and ventricular septal defects.

EPIDEMIOLOGY

Approximately 6% to 8% of patients with congenital heart disease have coarctation. Male predominance with male:female ratio of 1.5 to 4.0:1.

COMPLICATIONS AND ASSOCIATED FINDINGS

- Shock, if severe untreated obstruction
- Congestive heart failure, if severe untreated obstruction
- Systemic hypertension, before and after intervention
- Intracranial aneurysms
- Mesenteric ischemia
- Paraplegia

PROGNOSIS

Untreated coarctation has a poor natural history with the onset of congestive heart failure, especially in those patients with other intracardiac malformations. Claudication is common in older children with previously undiscovered coarctation. Generally, the short-term prognosis following successful intervention for isolated coarctation in infancy or childhood is excellent. Procedure related mortality in every modern series is very near zero. Clinical conditions that may affect long-term prognosis after repair of coarctation include:

- Residual or recurrent coarctation
- Hypertension (rest and exercise)
- Aortic aneurysm (associated with repair technique)
- Associated intracardiac lesions
- Intracranial aneurysms
- Occurrence or progression of aortic valve disease
- Premature coronary arterial and cerebrovascular disease

ASSOCIATED LESIONS

- Bicuspid aortic valve occurs in 85% of patients with coarctation.
- Patent ductus arteriosus (PDA)
- Ventricular septal defect (VSD)
- Valvar or subvalvar aortic stenosis
- Mitral stenosis: often associated with structural mitral valve abnormalities (i.e., supravalvar mitral ring, thickening of mitral leaflet, single papillary muscle with parachute deformity, or short dysplastic chordae tendinae)
- Shone syndrome: multiple left-sided obstructive lesions, including mitral stenosis, subaortic obstruction, aortic valve stenosis, and coarctation
- Berry aneurysm of the circle of Willis
- Renal artery stenosis associated with abdominal coarctation

 Differential Diagnosis

- Other left-sided heart obstructive lesions
- Hypoplastic left heart syndrome
- Cardiomyopathy and/or myocarditis
- Critical aortic stenosis (aortic obstruction to a degree that adequate systemic perfusion depends on patency of the ductus arteriosus)

 Data Gathering

HISTORY

There are two typical patterns for the clinical presentation of coarctation:

- An infant with congestive heart failure or shock—a small, pale, irritable child in respiratory distress. Typically precipitated by ductal closure, this presentation is more common in infants with coarctation and other intracardiac malformations (20% to 30%).

—Poor feeding
—Dyspnea
—Diaphoresis
—Poor weight gain
—Oliguria

- An otherwise asymptomatic child with systolic hypertension and/or a heart murmur (70% to 80%)

—Lower extremity claudication
—Headaches

 Physical Examination

- Tachypnea and tachycardia
- Discrepant arterial pulses and systolic blood pressure in the upper and lower extremities
- Weak "thready" pulses
- Grades 2 to 3/6 systolic ejection murmur
- Gallop rhythm in an infant with congestive heart failure
- Ejection click of a bicuspid aortic valve

—The most important finding: decreased or absent lower extremity pulses. Are pulses present? Is there a delay between the brachial and femoral pulses?

1. Heart murmur: best heard at the upper left sternal border, at the base and radiating to the left interscapular area posteriorly

An infant with severe coarctation and a PDA may have "differential cyanosis." The lower part of the body appears cyanotic because the descending aortic flow is provided by the right ventricle through the PDA (see Postductal Saturation).

 Laboratory Aids

- ECG: Right ventricular hypertrophy is usually present in symptomatic infants. ECG is often normal in children. LV hypertrophy is apparent with more severe coarctation or coarctation of longer standing.
- Chest radiograph: in the infant, moderate-to-severe cardiomegaly with increased pulmonary vascular markings (PVM). In an asymptomatic child, the heart size is often normal with normal PVM. Rib notching may be seen in older children secondary to erosion of the ribs by dilated intercostal collateral vessels.
- Echocardiography: localization, degree of coarctation, and associated findings (PDA, arch hypoplasia). Assessment of associated left-sided obstruction (severity of which may be underestimated in patients with congestive heart failure, low cardiac output, or the presence of a PDA): mitral valve abnormality, LV outflow obstruction, and aortic stenosis (bicuspid aortic valve)
- MRI: clearly defines the location and severity of coarctation. Is useful for serial follow-up postoperatively (especially aortic aneurysms)
- Cardiac catheterization and angiography: usually not indicated unless there are further questions to be answered and/or a planned intervention.

Therapy

MEDICAL

For the sick neonate who presents with severe congestive heart failure or shock (ductal-dependent left-sided obstructive lesion):

- Prostaglandin infusion: 0.05 μg/kg per minute (anticipating adverse effects including apnea)
- Inotropic support
- Diuretics for pulmonary venous hypertension or pulmonary edema
- Surgical intervention should follow as soon as possible.

For the asymptomatic child, elective repair and assessment of hypertension are appropriate; however, aggressive antihypertensive pharmacotherapy may not be indicated.

SURGICAL

Infancy

- Surgical repair of severe coarctation and coarctation associated with intracardiac anomalies
- The surgical mortality rate for infants with coarctation and a large VSD ranges from 5% to 15% and is higher for children with more complex intracardiac anomalies.

Childhood

- Elective coarctation repair between ages 18 months to 3 years in asymptomatic children without severe upper extremity hypertension. Later repair is associated with an increased risk of sustained hypertension and other late complications.

Types of Surgical Repair

- End-to-end anastomosis
- Subclavian flap aortoplasty
- Prosthetic patch aortoplasty
- Bypass graft

Nonsurgical Option

- Percutaneous balloon angioplasty of native coarctation in infants and children is pursued in some centers. Others find controversy with concern about rates of recurrent stenosis, hypertension, and aneurysm formation.

POSTOPERATIVE COMPLICATIONS

- Bleeding
- Postcoarctectomy syndrome/mesenteric arteritis
- Paradoxical hypertension
- Spinal cord ischemia (0.4%)
- Residual coarctation
- Chylothorax
- Stridor
- Diaphragm paralysis
- Subclavian steal
- Aortic aneurysm or dissection

 Follow-Up

- Reexamine every 12 months with four-extremity pulse and blood pressure assessment.
- Residual or recurrent coarctation (7% to 60%); occurs most commonly in those patients requiring repair in infancy and can depend on the technical details or specific method of surgical intervention (e.g., higher incidence with patch aortoplasty and coarctation ridge resection); some centers delay percutaneous balloon angioplasty of residual or recurrent lesions until 2 months postoperatively.
- Persistent systemic hypertension; most common in patients whose coarctation repair is delayed beyond late childhood
- Aortic aneurysm formation
- Intracranial aneurysms and/or cerebrovascular accidents
- Antibiotic prophylaxis to prevent endocarditis or endarteritis
- May have hypertension with exercise, even if normotensive at rest
- Exercise-induced hypertension without anatomic stenosis may respond to β-blocker therapy.

PITFALLS

- The most reliable clinical findings to diagnose native, residual, or recurrent coarctation are the presence of pressure differences in the upper and lower extremities and decreased or absent femoral pulses. Palpable pulses do not exclude coarctation. What one palpates is pulse pressure, not absolute systolic pressure.
- Four-extremity blood pressure measurement is very important in assessing infants and children with possible congenital heart disease. Proper cuff size must be used.

 Common Questions and Answers

Q: When is the most appropriate time to perform surgical repair of simple coarctation?
A: Recommendations vary regarding the age at which asymptomatic children (without severe upper extremity hypertension) should undergo intervention. Advances in technique no longer require patients to be "grown" to a threshold size or weight, and there is increasing evidence that severity and incidence of late complications correlate directly with older age at repair. While some authors mention 3 to 5 years of age, others recommend repair as early as 18 months to 2 years.

Q: What is the incidence of systemic hypertension after surgical repair of coarctation?
A: Greatly depends on age at repair, surgical method or technique, length of follow-up interval, and how one defines or measures hypertension. In no situation is the answer zero, and this important complication is one

of several reasons patients require lifelong detailed follow-up. One year after a technically perfect repair via resection with end-to-end anastomosis, the patient operated on in early childhood is unlikely to have hypertension at rest. However, 20 years further along, a patient of older age at repair is quite likely to have significant hypertension on exercise stress testing.

ICD-9-CM 747.10

BIBLIOGRAPHY

Bogers AJ, Simoons ML. Aortic valve and aortic arch pathology after coarctation repair: magnetic resonance angiographic study of 100 patients. *Mayo Clin Proc* 2003 Dec;78(12): 1491–1499.

Brickner ME, Hillis LD, Lange RA. Congenital heart disease in adults. First of two parts. *N Engl J Med* 2000;342(4):256–263.

Celermajer DS, Greaves K. Survivors of coarctation repair: fixed but not cured. *Heart* 2002;88(2):113–114.

Connolly HM, Huston J 3rd, Brown RD Jr, et al. Intracranial aneurysms in patients with coarctation of the aorta: a prospective. *Heart* 2003;89(9):1074–1077.

Hernandez-Gonzalez M, Solorio S, Conde-Carmona I, et al. Coarctation of the aorta: natural history and outcome after surgical treatment. *Q J Med* 1999;92(7): 365–371.

Munayer J, David F, et al. Intraluminal aortoplasty vs. surgical aortic resection in congenital aortic coarctation. A clinical random study in pediatric patients. *Arch Med Res* 2003;34(4):305–310.

Rao PS, Jureidini SB, Balfour IC, Singh GK, Chen SC. Severe aortic coarctation in infants less than 3 months: successful palliation by balloon angioplasty. *J Invasive Cardiol* 2003;15(4):202–208.

Roos-Hesselink JW, Scholzel BE, Heijdra RJ, et al. Long-term follow-up of patients after coarctation of the aorta repair. *Am J Cardiol* 2002;89(5):541–547.

Younoszai AK, Reddy VM, Hanley FL, Brook MM. Intermediate term follow-up of the end-to-side aortic anastomosis for coarctation of the aorta. *Ann Thorac Surg* 2002;74(5): 1631–1634.

Author: Geoffrey Bird

Coccidioidomycosis

 ## Database

DEFINITION

Coccidioidomycosis is an infection caused by the dimorphic fungus *Coccidioides immitis*.

PATHOPHYSIOLOGY

- Inhalation of arthrospores from disturbed, arid soil is the major route of infection.
- Sixty percent of acute infections are subclinical (asymptomatic).
- Most patients have infection limited to a localized area of lung and hilar nodes after mounting an intense inflammatory response with granuloma formation.
- Dissemination occurs in a minority of patients via lymphatic or hematologic spread.
- The course of illness is highly variable and dependent on host immune response and amount of exposure. HIV-infected patients and other patients with immunosuppression as a result of T-lymphocyte dysfunction (lymphoma, organ transplantation) are particularly susceptible to severe forms of pulmonary and extrapulmonary coccidioidomycosis.

EPIDEMIOLOGY

- *C. immitis* is found in the soil and is endemic in the southwestern United States (west Texas, New Mexico, Arizona, California), northern Mexico, and parts of South and Central America. Up to one-third of the population in endemic areas has been infected.
- There is no person-to-person spread.
- The average incubation period is 10 to 16 days (range 1 to 4 weeks).
- Primary infection is most commonly seen in the summer and fall months.

COMPLICATIONS

- Localized complications of primary pulmonary infection are infrequent and include pleural effusions and pericarditis.
- Approximately 5% of lung infections result in residual pulmonary sequelae, usually nodules or abscess cavities. One third of these cavities spontaneously resolve within 2 years. Hemoptysis and rupture of the abscess, with formation of an empyema, are potential complications in patients with unresolved cavities.
- Risk factors for disseminated coccidioidomycosis include immunosuppression, male gender, extremes of age (neonates and elderly), African or Filipino descent, and pregnancy.
- Extrapulmonary dissemination usually develops within a year after the initial infection, but may appear much later if immunity is impaired (e.g., HIV infection, malignancy, immunosuppressive therapy).
- Hydrocephalus may occur with CNS involvement.

PROGNOSIS

- Most infections are asymptomatic (60%) or mild (35%) and self-limited.
- Primary infection of the lungs is usually self-limited, with a course of illness lasting 1 to 3 weeks; complications (see above) may prolong the course.
- Dissemination is infrequent (see above for risk factors). Morbidity and mortality have improved with use of antifungal therapy, but immunocompromised patients still have a poor prognosis after the development of disseminated infection. The mortality rate is 70% in HIV-infected patients with diffuse pulmonary coccidioidomycosis.
- Meningitis, untreated, is nearly always fatal within 2 years of diagnosis.

ASSOCIATED DISEASES

- Primary pulmonary infection is usually asymptomatic.
- Symptomatic pulmonary infection is characterized by cough, chest pain, and fever. Rash, myalgias, and arthralgias may be present. Chronic pulmonary lesions are rare in children (see Complications).
- Extrapulmonary dissemination is rare and usually involves the skin, skeletal system, and CNS.
- Primary cutaneous coccidioidomycosis occurs by direct inoculation of the skin (trauma). A relatively painless, indurated nodule with occasional central ulceration develops at the site of injury. Regional lymphadenopathy is often present.
- Secondary cutaneous coccidioidomycosis occurs by hematogenous spread to the skin. Lesions range from superficial maculopapular lesions to verrucous ulcers. Lesions can occur anywhere but are most common along the nasolabial fold.
- Osteomyelitis is subacute or chronic and frequently involves more than one bone (40%). Common sites are the hands, feet, ribs, and vertebrae.
- Meningitis develops within 6 months of initial infection. Hydrocephalus is a common complication. CNS vasculitis and intracerebral abscesses are rare.

 ## Differential Diagnosis

- Other pulmonary mycoses (e.g., *Histoplasma capsulatum*, *Aspergillus fumigatus*, and *Blastomyces dermatitidis*)
- *Mycobacterium tuberculosis* (lung or CSF)
- *Mycoplasma pneumoniae*
- Influenza and other viral infections that present as bronchopneumonia

 ## Data Gathering

HISTORY

- Travel or residence in an endemic area is typical. Risk factors for disseminated infection should be sought.
- Fever, dry or productive cough, and pleuritic chest pain suggest pulmonary infection.
- Hemoptysis, although rare in children, is reported in 15% of adults with symptomatic pulmonary infection.
- Trauma precedes primary cutaneous disease.
- Myalgias, arthralgias, chills, night sweats, and anorexia suggest systemic dissemination.
- Headache, vomiting, and altered mental status suggest meningitis.

 ## Physical Examination

- Most infections (60%) are asymptomatic.
- Signs of pneumonia and pleural effusions are often present with symptomatic pulmonary infection.
- Indurated nodules and regional lymphadenopathy are seen with primary cutaneous infection.
- Erythematous maculopapular rash suggests secondary cutaneous involvement and is seen in 50% of symptomatic children. It is usually limited to the lower trunk and thighs, but may be diffuse.
- Erythema nodosum occurs later in the course of infection. Erythema nodosum correlates with the development of cell-mediated immunity and is associated with a low incidence of dissemination.
- Chorioretinal lesions are present in up to 40% of patients with disseminated disease.
- Stridor is present with infection of the subglottic tissues.
- Signs of increased intracranial pressure are seen with CNS infection. Classic signs of meningeal irritation are usually absent.

Laboratory Aids

DIRECT EXAMINATION AND CULTURE

- Cytologic examination of bronchoalveolar fluid is diagnostic in only about one-third of persons and is less sensitive than culture. Visualization of large spherules is possible in stained specimens of sputum, tracheal aspirates, urine, or tissue biopsy. They are rarely seen in CSF.
- The organisms can be detected by culture in experienced laboratories. The yield is highest from purulent material. The yield from other sources, such as pleural fluid, blood, and gastric aspirates is lower.

SKIN TESTING

- Coccidioidin or spherulin intradermal skin test is positive (delayed type hypersensitivity; >5 mm induration) within 2 weeks of symptom onset (range 2 days to 4 weeks). Recent conversion is diagnostic; reactivity persists after infection, thereby limiting its usefulness as a diagnostic test for acute infections.
- Skin tests are often negative in progressive or disseminated disease and in immunocompromised patients.

SEROLOGIC STUDIES

- C. immitis–specific immunoglobin (IgM) antibody is detectable in 75% of patients 1 to 3 weeks after symptom onset and usually is absent after 6 months. False-positive results are seen in 15% of patients with cystic fibrosis.
- IgG is detected by the complement fixation (CF) assay from serum or CSF. It is positive in 50% of patients at 4 weeks and 83% at 3 months following symptomatic primary infection. In general, higher titers reflect more extensive infection and rising CF antibody concentrations are associated with worsening disease.
- Hematologic findings include elevated ESR, leukocytosis, and, eosinophilia (in 10%).

OTHER STUDIES

- CSF findings in meningitis include hypoglycorrhachia and pleocytosis with mononuclear cell predominance.

RADIOLOGIC STUDIES

- Chest x-ray may reveal well-circumscribed nodules, lobar or patchy pulmonary infiltrates, pleural effusions, cavitary lesions, and hilar adenopathy.
- X-rays of involved bones may reveal lytic lesions. Scintigraphy of bone is more sensitive for the diagnosis of osteomyelitis.

 ## Therapy

- Uncomplicated or minor disease is self-limited and should not be treated with antifungal therapy (>95% of cases).
- Treatment of uncomplicated respiratory infection is recommended for infants, pregnant women, and patients with continuous fever for >1 month, >10% weight loss, extensive or progressive pulmonary disease, negative skin test results, or immunodeficiency (either from HIV or as a result of immunosuppressive medications). Use either oral fluconazole or itraconazole for 3 to 6 months.
- Surgical debridement is used for localized and persistent lesions in bone and lung.
- Diffuse pneumonia: Start therapy with amphotericin B and replace with oral fluconazole or itraconazole when clinical improvement is demonstrated. The total length of therapy should be at least 1 year, and for patients with severe immunodeficiency, oral azole therapy should be continued as secondary prophylaxis.
- Disseminated infection, nonmeningeal: Treat with oral fluconazole or itraconazole. Amphotericin B is alternative therapy, especially if lesions worsen or are at critical locations, such as the vertebral column. The duration of therapy may be longer than for those with pneumonia only.
- Meningitis: Oral fluconazole is preferred (800 to 1,000 mg/day). Itraconazole (400 to 600 mg/day) is also effective. Therapy should be continued indefinitely.
- Intrathecal amphotericin B may be useful in CNS infections
- Voriconazole, a new azole agent, and casponfungin, an echinocandin class antifungal, have in-vitro activity against C. immitis.

PREVENTION

Infection Control

- No special isolation or precautions for the hospitalized patient.
- Contaminated dressings from skin lesions should be handled and discarded with care.
- Preventive efforts are aimed at dust control and trials to eliminate organisms from soil.
- Avoidance of field activities or travel in highly endemic areas is recommended for children with a negative skin test.

PITFALLS

- Skin test in disseminated disease may be negative.
- Clinicians in endemic areas should maintain a high level of clinical suspicion.
- Diagnosis in nonendemic areas may be missed as a result of low clinical suspicion or missed travel history.

 ## Common Questions and Answers

Q: Do all patients with symptomatic primary respiratory infection as a result of C. immitis require treatment?
A: No, since >95% of initial pulmonary infections are self-limited, treatment is not always required. Patients with concurrent risk factors (e.g., HIV infection, organ transplant, or high doses of corticosteroids) or evidence of unusually severe infections should always be treated. Factors suggesting increased severity of infection include weight loss of >10%, night sweats, infiltrates involving more than half of one lung or portions of both lungs, complement fixation antibody to C. immitis >1:16, and failure to develop dermal hypersensitivity of coccidioidal antigens.

Q: How should pregnant women with coccidioidomycosis be managed?
A: Diagnosis of primary infection during the third trimester of pregnancy or immediately in the postpartum period should raise consideration for treatment. During pregnancy, amphotericin B is the treatment of choice because fluconazole and other azole antifungals are likely teratogenic.

ICD-9-CM 114.9

BIBLIOGRAPHY

Deresinski SC. Coccidioidomycosis: efficacy of new agents and future prospects. Curr Opin Infect Dis 2001;14(6):693–696.

Dosanjh A, Theodore J, Pappagianis D. Probable false positive coccidioidal serologic results in patients with cystic fibrosis. Pediatr Transplant 1998;2:313–317.

Galgiani JN, Ampel NM, Catanzaro A, et al. Practice guidelines for the treatment of coccidioidomycosis. Clin Infect Dis 2000;30: 658–661.

Galgiani JN, Catanzaro A, Cloud GA, et al. Comparison of oral fluconazole and itraconazole for progressive, nonmeningeal coccidioidomycosis: a randomized, double-blind trial. Ann Intern Med 2000;133:676–686.

Galgiani JN. Coccidioides immitis. In: Mandell GL, Bennett JE, Dolin R, eds. Principles and Practice of Infectious Diseases. 5th Ed. New York: Churchill Livingstone, 2000:2746–2757.

Shehab ZM. Coccidioidomycosis. In: Feigin RD, Cherry JD, eds. Textbook of Pediatric Infectious Diseases. 5th Ed. Philadelphia: WB Saunders, 2004:2580–2591.

Stevens DA. Coccidioidomycosis. N Engl J Med 1995;332:1077–1082.

Authors: Theoklis Zaoutis and Samir S. Shah

Colic

Database

DEFINITION

A poorly defined and incompletely understood state of prolonged or excessive crying in young infants who are otherwise well.

- No standard definition of this phenomenon
- Best definition available: more than 3 hours a day of irritability, fussing, or crying on more than 3 days in any 1 week during the first 3 to 4 months of life in an infant who is otherwise healthy and well fed. Some add the criterion of crying for the duration of 3 weeks or more.
- Crying is not qualitatively different, but quantitatively. It is considerably more than the average.
- Lack of a firm, standard definition means that varying groups of subjects have been studied, and limits our certainty as to causes of prolonged crying and as to effectiveness of management plans.

PATHOPHYSIOLOGY

- No single cause is always found.
- Typically, the problem lies in the interaction between factors in the infant and the environment at a unique time of biological vulnerability.

a. In the infant there is a normal physiologic or temperamental predisposition to be more sensitive, irritable, intense, less rhythmical, or harder to soothe than average for the age.
b. Parents generally have not yet learned how to read the infant's individual needs correctly and respond appropriately. They may be manipulating the infant in ways that increase rather than decrease the amount of crying.
c. This interaction takes place at a time when the immature central nervous system makes the infant temporarily more vulnerable to the disorganizing effects of this poor fit.

- Colic generally occurs in the absence of any abnormality in the infant or the parents, but rather when the parents have not yet learned to interact harmoniously with the infant.
- There is no evidence that the bowel is at fault; flatus is more likely to be the result of the crying than the cause.
- Psychosocial risk factors, such as poor support for the mother and various stressors, are probably more common than in noncolicky infants, but they are not necessary.
- When such external factors are present, they seem to exert their effects by reducing the parent's ability to respond appropriately to the infant.
- Physical problems in the infant, such as milk allergy or gastric reflux, probably account for no more than 10% of all prolonged crying at this time, and would exclude an infant from this diagnosis of colic, which requires that the infant be physically well.

GENETICS

No genetic influence has been discovered, but it has not been investigated. Temperamental traits are known to be largely inborn, however.

EPIDEMIOLOGY

- Colic typically begins shortly after a baby comes home from a newborn nursery.
- It can last until 3 to 4 months of age if not successfully managed.
- If excessive crying lasts after 4 months, other diagnoses should be considered.

COMPLICATIONS

- Excessive crying does not turn into any other condition, but the factors that caused it may contribute to sleep problems and other behavioral concerns in the infant after the colic has gone.
- Parents are usually exasperated by it.
- The most serious outcome is that, as a result of parental exasperation, the infant may be physically abused.
- The infant is likely to be overfed.

PROGNOSIS

Without intervention this prolonged crying usually diminishes somewhere around 3 to 4 months. Some recent studies have reported a variety of possible long term outcomes such as continued aversive temperaments, more behavior problems, and diminished parental self-confidence. More investigations with attention to methodological details are needed to clarify these matters. Particularly deserving attention is the possible pathogenic role of the physician in incorrectly informing the parents that there is something physically wrong with the infant.

Differential Diagnosis

- Normal crying: Average, normal infants cry about 2 hours a day at 2 weeks of age, just under 3 hours at 6 weeks, and then decrease to about 1 hour by 12 weeks. Normal crying, like colic, tends to occur predominantly in the evening and can vary from day to day.
- Prolonged or excessive crying from physical causes:

—Faulty feeding techniques: overfeeding or underfeeding and inadequate burping or sucking
—Physical problems in the infant: acute disorders such as otitis media, intestinal cramping with diarrhea, corneal abrasion, and incarcerated hernia; or chronic ones such as gastroesophageal reflux
—Cow's milk allergy, lactose intolerance, or transmission of irritating substances such as caffeine via breast milk

Data Gathering

HISTORY

- Define symptoms: intensity, duration, and frequency of crying. Some parents complain more than others about the crying.
- Ask parents to describe a typical day.

—Description of a typical day or keeping a crying diary is helpful.
—This will give insights into the daily routine, feeding, rest, interpretive skills, and responses of the parents.

- Ask parents to describe and demonstrate their soothing techniques.
- Information on the baby's temperament can be obtained by asking the parents to describe the baby's typical reaction patterns to stimuli.
- Medical history should include concerns about the pregnancy and the newborn period, anxieties related to parents' own experiences as children or with previous children, and the quality of family supports and other stressors.

Physical Examination

- No findings are expected if the child has colic. However, examination should always be performed to reassure both parents and physician.
- Attempts at management over the telephone without a physical examination are likely to be unsuccessful.

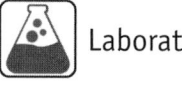
Laboratory Aids

No tests are indicated unless specifically suggested by history or physical examination.

Colic

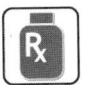

Therapy

- The most effective form of treatment at present is counseling the parents about the interaction. It should consist of these main points:

—The infant is not sick. Crying may be persistent, but there is no evidence of a physical problem. There is no proof the infant is having pain, just distress. Avoid iatrogenic problems caused by suggesting that something is wrong with the infant. The infant is probably overaroused and tired.

—Education about infant crying. Parents need to know how much normal infants cry and how they vary in sensitivity, irritability, and soothability. The way parents react to their infants can affect the amount of crying. Parents often do not understand that a common reason for infant crying is fatigue and a need to be left alone.

—The excessive crying can be reduced. Parents have to learn to tune in more sensitively to infants' needs and to be more appropriately and effectively responsive to them.

- Basic strategy: Soothe more, as by a pacifier, repetitive sound, or a hot water bottle, and stimulate less by decreasing the picking up, holding, and feeding the infant when it is not appropriate. Contrary to popular opinion, there is no evidence that there is a better behavioral outcome at the present or later from the parents' always responding immediately to every cry.

—A quiet environment, correction of any faulty feeding techniques, and a minimum of unnecessary handling without changing the composition of the feedings. Pertinent psychosocial issues should be dealt with.

- Expression of optimism by the pediatrician about the immediate outcome is justified and in itself improves chances of success. Simply saying that the colic will be gone by 3 to 4 months of age is not comforting and may be quite the opposite.
- Extra carrying does not help.
- Drugs, such as phenobarbital or diphenhydramine, are seldom necessary. Some observers have reported beneficial effects, when used for a week or two in conjunction with counseling, but these results have not as yet been subjected to double-blind studies. Simethicone has not been shown to be helpful. Herbal teas should not be recommended because of their varied and often unknown contents.
- Formula changes are frequently attempted by physicians hoping for a simple solution, but they rarely are effective. Sometimes they seem to be helpful for a few days, only to cease being so soon after that.
- Almost any procedure done with conviction is likely to be followed by a temporary reduction in crying because of the placebo effect.

- The normal trend toward diminished crying over time has given some forms of treatment an undeserved reputation of effectiveness.

Follow-Up

- It is important to keep in close touch with parents of an excessively fussy baby. Telephone contact every 2 to 3 days is essential until improvement. Reexamination is rarely needed.
- Standard pediatric textbooks state that little can be done to change the pattern. However, several studies report that colic can be sharply reduced within 2 to 3 days if management such as that described above is used. Some infants take longer, but virtually all respond to suitable management.

PREVENTION

No study has yet demonstrated any certain way of preventing this prolonged or excessive crying. Methods that are likely to be helpful are education of all parents about infant crying and soothing, informing them of the expected average number of hours per day. Most parents do not know that one of the commonest reasons for an infant to cry is fatigue, and that stimulation at these times is not helpful. Dealing with various pertinent parental anxieties when they occur should be undertaken.

PITFALLS

Numerous pitfalls await the unprepared physician:

- Overdiagnosing the condition of the infant or caregiving inadequacies of parents
- Overtreatment of the infant with changes of feedings, medications, and various inappropriate procedures such as enemas and rectal manipulations. Despite the widely held, popular view that cow's milk allergy is a principal reason for excessive crying, no study of acceptable double-blind design has demonstrated its occurrence in infants who are free of respiratory, gastrointestinal, or cutaneous manifestations of allergy.
- Unnecessary laboratory tests
- Colic is defined as a pattern of recurring episodes of crying. Other explanations should be carefully considered first for an acute bout of crying.

The physician should be wary of enthusiastic reports in the popular press or the medical literature that "at last there is a cure for colic." Certainty is not easily achieved in an area in which there is such a problem with definitions and with methodological problems like achieving truly double-blind trials.

Common Questions and Answers

Q: What is wrong with my baby? What can we do to relieve the pain? Why is he/she so gassy? How do you know that it is not as a result of an allergy? Shouldn't we strengthen the formula? You mean it's all my fault? Will this ever stop? What will he/she be like later?
A: All the answers are to be found above.

ICD-9-CM 789.0

BIBLIOGRAPHY

Carey WB. "Colic": prolonged or excessive crying in young infants. In: Levine MD, Carey WB, Crocker AC, eds. Developmental-Behavioral Pediatrics. 3rd Ed. Philadelphia: WB Saunders, 1999.

Carey WB. The effectiveness of parent counseling in managing colic. Pediatrics 1994;94:333–334.

Lester BM, Barr RG. Colic and excessive crying. 105th Ross Conference on Pediatric Research Columbus, OH: Ross Products Division, Abbott Laboratories, 1997.

St. James-Roberts I. Summary: What do we know? What are the implications of the findings for practitioners? What do we need to know? In: Barr RG, St. James-Roberts I, Keefe MR, eds. New Evidence on Unexplained Early Infant Crying: Its Origins, Nature and Management. Johnson & Johnson Pediatric Institute, 2001:327–333.

Van IJzendoorn MH, Hubbard FOA. Are infant crying and maternal responsiveness during the first year related to infant-mother attachment at 15 months? The Signal, Newsletter of the World Association for Infant Mental Health, 2001:1–12.

Wessel MA, Cobb JC, Jackson EB, et al. Paroxysmal fussing in infants, sometimes called "colic." Pediatrics 1954;14:421–434.

Author: William B. Carey

Common Variable Immunodeficiency

 Database

DEFINITION

Common variable immunodeficiency (CVID) is a heterogeneous immunodeficiency syndrome characterized by hypogammaglobulinemia, recurrent infections, and a wide spectrum of immunologic abnormalities, including autoimmune disease, inflammatory conditions, and the development of lymphomas. It is a common primary immunodeficiency. Other terminology for this disease includes:

- Acquired hypogammaglobulinemia
- Adult-onset hypogammaglobulinemia
- Dysgammaglobulinemia
- Common variable hypogammaglobulinemia

Diagnosis of exclusion, requiring decreased immunoglobulins of at least two isotypes (IgG, IgA and/or IgM) at two standard deviations below the normal mean for age.

ETIOLOGY

- The primary immunologic defect(s) leading to this syndrome is (are) unknown, but B-cell defect is likely. Multiple defects have been associated with CVID including: lack of somatic mutation within variable region genes, lack of memory B cells, mutation in ICOS
- Hypogammaglobulinemia is the main characteristic.
- Most patients have impaired immunoglobulin and specific antibody production despite normal
- B-lymphocyte numbers. An increased proportion of immature B cells is often present.
- Functional defects of both B and T lymphocytes occur.

GENETICS

- Some evidence for potential susceptibility locus on 6p21 (proximal part of MHC locus).
- Some families have a pattern consistent with autosomal-recessive inheritance.
- Immunoglobin A (IgA) deficiency more likely in offspring of parents with CVID (mothers more likely to transmit).
- Incidence of IgA deficiency, autoimmune disease, malignancies increased in family members of patients with CVID.

EPIDEMIOLOGY

- Incidence is estimated to be 1 in 25,000 to 1 in 66,000 in the general population.
- Can present at any age, but usually seen in the second to third decade of life. CVID has been described in patients as young as 6 months.
- Diagnosis is usually made several years after the onset of recurrent infections (pneumonia, sinusitis, otitis).
- A subgroup of children has been described in which the onset of disease was most often before 5 years of age. This group was characterized by a relapsing and remitting course in which autoimmune disease predominated.
- About 20% to 25% of patients with CVID have one or more autoimmune conditions at the time of diagnosis.

COMPLICATIONS

- Autoimmune disease in 20% of CVID patients. Most common are autoimmune hemolytic anemia (AHA) and idiopathic thrombocytopenia purpura (ITP).
- GI complications include chronic diarrhea, malabsorption, and weight loss. Inflammatory bowel disease and *Helicobacter pylori* infection have also been observed.
- Granulomatous infiltrations may mimic sarcoidosis.
- Lymphoproliferative disease: overall risk is 8% to 10%. The most common are lymphomas, usually non-Hodgkin lymphoma, well differentiated, mostly Epstein-Barr virus (EBV) negative.
- Chronic sinusitis and lung disease with abnormal pulmonary function tests (PFTs).
- Progressive decline in T-lymphocyte function.

 Differential Diagnosis

- Other primary antibody-deficiency disorders: X-linked agammaglobulinemia and transient hypogammaglobulinemia of infancy
- Severe malabsorption with protein-losing enteropathy
- HIV infection
- Chronic lung disease: cystic fibrosis, immotile cilia syndrome, and α_1-antitrypsin deficiency
- Primary autoimmune diseases: immune thrombocytopenic purpura (ITP), autoimmune hemolytic anemia (AIHA), systemic lupus erythematosus (SLE), and thyroiditis

 Data Gathering

HISTORY

- Recurrent sinopulmonary infections, especially sinusitis and pneumonias, with encapsulated bacteria
- Autoimmune diseases such as AIHA, ITP, thyroid disease, and chronic active hepatitis
- Persistent diarrhea of infectious (e.g., *Giardia lamblia*) or noninfectious etiologies
- Severe or unusual viral infections with herpes simplex, cytomegalovirus (CMV), and varicella, such as pneumonitis, hepatitis, or encephalitis. Chronic meningoencephalitis can be seen with enteroviral infection.

 Physical Examination

- Evaluation should focus on the presence of infection.
- Thirty percent of patients will have lymphadenopathy and/or splenomegaly.

Laboratory Aids

TESTS

- IgG, IgA, IgM, and IgE below age-appropriate norms
- CBC with differential: examine smear for evidence of hemolysis in AIHA.
- Autoimmune antibody screen: ANA, autoantibody panel
- Stool culture for bacteria and ova/parasites to evaluate chronic diarrhea
- Isohemagglutinins as well as functional antibody titers to bacterial antigens such as tetanus, diphtheria, and pneumococcus are usually low to absent.
- Spirometry may be helpful in following chronic lung disease.
- Mitogen/antigen stimulation studies will help assess lymphocyte function.
- T- and B-lymphocyte enumeration by flow cytometry
- Absent B lymphocytes suggests X-linked agammaglobulinemia (XLA) rather than CVID.
- Appropriate cultures based on site of infection

IMAGING

Chest radiograph and sinus x-ray studies/CT scans may be warranted for evaluation of chronic disease.

DIAGNOSTIC PROCEDURES

- GI endoscopy with biopsies for cases of idiopathic persistent diarrhea
- Lymph node biopsy in suspected malignancy

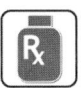

Therapy

- Appropriate antibiotics for acute infections. Prophylactic antibiotics may be helpful in chronic/recurrent infections.
- Monthly IV immunoglobulin (IVIG) replacement: nadir IgG levels should be greater than 300 mg/dL.
- Cautious use of corticosteroids may be necessary in the treatment of GI and autoimmune manifestations.

Follow-Up

- Close and frequent follow-up is warranted for patients with severe, recurrent symptoms. It may be as frequent as monthly, depending on symptoms.
- Signs and symptoms suggesting malignancy (e.g., persistent adenopathy in absence of infection, significant weight loss, or abdominal mass) should be evaluated expeditiously.

Common Questions and Answers

Q: What is the life expectancy of patients with the diagnosis of CVID?
A: Since the clinical presentations and symptoms are variable, it is difficult to predict the life expectancy in individual patients. The availability of IVIG, in addition to antibiotic therapy, has greatly improved the outlook for these patients. However, despite adequate therapy, a large percentage of patients with CVID have a progressive decline in immune function. Major morbidity and mortality usually result from the associated complications of malignancy, chronic lung disease, and severe autoimmune disease. Lymphoma is the major cause of death followed by complications of chronic pulmonary disease. In one study, the mortality is estimated between 23% and 27% over a median follow-up of 7 years (0 to 25 years). The 20-year survival rate after diagnosis for males is 64% and for females 67% versus 92% and 94%, respectively, for the general population.

Q: Do children differ in their presentation compared with adults?
A: In a subgroup of children with CVID, autoimmune disease may be the major clinical problem rather than infections.

Q: Should patients with CVID receive live viral vaccines?
A: In general, patients receiving IVIG therapy do not require any vaccinations. Live viral vaccines should be avoided in these patients, especially if they have deteriorating immune function.

Q: Can CVID be diagnosed prenatally?
A: Since there are no clear genetic inheritance patterns, prenatal diagnosis is unavailable.

ICD-9-CM 279.06

BIBLIOGRAPHY

Ballow, M. Primary immunodeficiency disorders: antibody deficiencies. *J Allergy Clin Immunol* 2002;109(9):581–591.

Cunningham-Rundles C. Common variable immunodeficiency. *Curr Allergy Asthma Rep* 2001;1:421–429.

Cunningham-Rundles, C. Immune deficiency: office evaluation and treatment. *All Asthma Proc* 2003;24(6):409–415.

de Asis ML, Iqbal S, Sicklick M. Analysis of a family obtaining three members with common variable immunodeficiency. *Ann Allergy Asthma Immunol* 1996;76(6):527–529.

Eisenstein EM, Sneller MC. Common variable immunodeficiency: diagnosis and management. *Ann Allergy* 1994;73:285–294.

Simonte S, Cunningham-Rundles, C. Update on primary immunodeficiency: defects of lymphocytes. *Clin Immunol* 2003;109: 109–118.

Sneller MC, Strober W, Eisenstein E, et al. New insights in common variable immunodeficiency. *Ann Intern Med* 1993;118:720–730.

Winkelstein JA, et al., eds. *Patient and Family Handbook for the Primary Immune Deficiency Diseases*. 2nd Ed. Immune Deficiency Foundation, 1993.

Yocum MW, Kelso JM. Common variable immunodeficiency: the disorder and treatment. *Mayo Clin Proc* 1991;66:83–96.

Author: Elena Perez

Complement Deficiency

 Database

DEFINITION

Complement consists of more than 30 plasma and cell membrane proteins that function as cofactors in defense against pathogenic microbes and in the generation of many immunopathogenic disorders. Biologic actions include:

- Cytolysis: destruction of cells by disrupting cell membrane
- Opsonization of organisms, which facilitates phagocytosis
- Inflammation by generation of peptides, which can upregulate chemotaxis and can cause vasodilatation
- Clearance of immune complexes and apoptotic cells
- Interaction and augmentation of adaptive immune response

PATHOPHYSIOLOGY

- Three pathways—the classic, the alternative, and the mannan-binding lectin, that converge on same terminal pathway—the membrane attack complex
- Classic pathway requires antibody for initiation, although alternative and mannan-binding lectin pathways can be activated independent of antibody
- Complement deficiencies may be primary or secondary
- Secondary deficiencies of complement are usually as a result of a consumptive or decreased productive state:

—Newborn state
—Malnutrition, anorexia nervosa
—Liver cirrhosis
—Reye syndrome
—Nephrotic syndrome

See table, Complement Deficiency and Related Clinical Problems.

GENETICS

- Deficiencies of either pathway are usually autosomal-recessive traits.
- Properdin deficiency is X-linked
- C1 inhibitor deficiency is autosomal dominant.
- Heterozygotes are usually phenotypically normal.

EPIDEMIOLOGY

Prevalence of known primary immunodeficiency is 1 per 100,000. Complement accounts for approximately 2% of all primary immunodeficiencies.

SYMPTOMS/COMPLICATIONS

Deficiencies can lead to:

- Recurrent infection
- Immune complex disease
- Autoimmunity

 Differential Diagnosis

Humoral deficits such as immunoglobulin deficiency or dysfunction; consumptive process such as sepsis

 Data Gathering

HISTORY

Indications for evaluating complement system

- SLE, juvenile rheumatoid arthritis (JRA), or other immune complex disease
- Recurrent pyogenic infections
- Second episode of bacteremia at any age
- Second episode of meningococcal meningitis or gonococcal arthritis
- Recurrent angioedema
- Pneumococcal bacteremia after infancy

Physical Examination

- Failure to thrive
- Scars from various infections
- Joint destruction

 ## Laboratory Aids

- CH50: to assess integrity of classical pathway. It is the quantity of serum required to lyse 50% of an aliquot of antibody-sensitized sheep RBC. Handling of the specimen is paramount because complement components are thermolabile, and a common cause of an abnormal value is improper handling. Procedure may require use of dry ice.
- APH50: to assess integrity of alternate pathway
- C3, C4, and other individual components based on clinical history

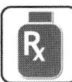 ## Therapy

- Fresh-frozen plasma for acute severe infections
- Aggressive workup and management of infections
- Prophylactic antibiotics may be useful for recurrent infections.
- Immunization for pneumococci, *Haemophilus influenzae*, and *Neisseria meningitidis* for patient and household members
- Close monitoring for onset of autoimmune disease
- Study other family members for genetic counseling.

PITFALLS

- Special care is required for the proper handling of blood test to prevent falsely low values.
- Sometimes the complement cascade can be activated and consume the complement factor, leading to the improper diagnosis of a complement deficiency.

Common Questions and Answers

Q: How common are complement deficiencies?
A: Very uncommon. They account for 2% of all immunodeficiencies.

Q: When should I evaluate for a complement deficiency?
A: Any child with recurrent sinopulmonary infections or more than one episode of a Neisserial infection.

ICD-9-CM 279.3

BIBLIOGRAPHY

Berger M, Frank MM. The serum complement system. In: Stiehm ER, ed. *Immunologic Disorders in Infants and Children*. 3rd Ed. Philadelphia: WB Saunders, 1989:97–115.

Bonilla FA, Geha RS. Primary immunodeficiency diseases. [erratum appears in *J Allergy Clin Immunol* 2003 Aug;112(2): 267]. *J Allergy Clin Immunol* 2003; 111(Suppl 2):S571–S581.

Colten HR. Complement deficiences. *Annu Rev Immunol* 1992;10:809–834.

Ernst T, Spath PJ, Aebi C, et al. Screening for complement deficiency in bacterial meningitis. *Acta Paediatr* 1997;86(9): 1009–1010.

Frank MM. Complement deficiencies. *Pediatr Clin North Am* 2000;47(6):1339–1354.

Frank MM. Detection of complement in relation to disease. *J Allergy Clin Immunol* 1992;89:641–648.

Frieri M. Complement-related diseases. *Allergy Asthma Proc* 2002;23(5):319–24.

Walport MJ. Complement: first of two parts. *N Engl J Med* 2001;344(14):1058–1066.

Walport MJ. Complement: second of two parts. *N Engl J Med* 2001;344(15):1140–1144.

Authors: Erin E. McGintee
Michelle M. Klinek, 3rd edition

Complement Deficiency and Related Clinical Problems

DEFICIENCY	CLINICAL MANIFESTATIONS
C1(qrs), C2, C4	Systemic lupus erythematosus (SLE), vasculitis, glomerulonephritis, pyogenic infections
C3	Glomerulonephritis, pyogenic infections, Neisserial infections, immune complex disease
C1 inhibitor	Hereditary angioedema
Factor H, I	Hemolytic uremic syndrome, glomerulonephritis
Properdin	Neisserial infections
Factor B, D	Neisserial infections
MBL, MASP	Repeated infections, accelerated course of SLE, rheumatoid arthritis
C5, C6, C7, C8, C9	Disseminated neisserial infections
CD55, CD59	Paroxysmal nocturnal hemoglobinuria

Concussion

 ## Database

DEFINITION

Concussion is an alteration of consciousness secondary to head trauma, which may or may not involve a loss of consciousness. Symptoms of concussion can be categorized into early and late symptoms.

- Early symptoms most commonly include confusion and amnesia but also include headache, dizziness/vertigo, and nausea/vomiting, and are expected to resolve in minutes to hours.
- Late symptoms evolve over days to weeks after the injury and include persistent low-grade headache, poor attention, memory difficulties, easy fatigability, photo-/phonophobia, anxiety, and sleep disturbance. Late symptoms are most prominent after repeated concussive injury.
- A grading scale has been established in sports medicine to determine the severity of injury:

Grade 1: (a) transient confusion, (b) no loss of consciousness, (c) mental status changes resolve in less than 15 minutes.

Grade 2: (a) transient confusion, (b) no loss of consciousness, (c) mental status changes longer more than 15 minutes.

Grade 3: any loss of consciousness, either brief or prolonged.

PATHOPHYSIOLOGY

The brain is buoyed in the cranium by cerebrospinal fluid (CSF), which surrounds it and acts as protective insulation from the hard bone. In acceleration-deceleration accidents the brain continues to experience forward momentum and slams against hard bone. The temporal and frontal lobes of the brain are particularly prone to injury by this mechanism because of their location inside the skull.

Depressed level of consciousness is thought to be the result of rotational stretch injury to the dorsal aspect of the brainstem where the reticular activating system lies. The injuries are usually mild and rarely visible on MRI scans.

EPIDEMIOLOGY

Concussions per 1,000 athlete exposures:

- Sports played with helmets

—Ice hockey 0.27
—Football 0.25
—Men's lacrosse 0.19
—Women's softball 0.11

- Sports played without helmets

—Men's soccer 0.25
—Women's soccer 0.24
—Field hockey 0.20
—Wrestling 0.20

COMPLICATIONS

- Concussion

—Confusion
—Alteration of consciousness
—Headaches and vomiting
—May also be symptoms of more serious complications of head injury

- Serious head injury

—Contusion (brain bruise)
—Epidural bleed (from tearing of arteries that feed the membranous covering of the brain)
—Subdural bleed (tearing of the veins that drain blood from the brain)
—Intraparenchymal bleeds (bleeds in the brain tissue itself)

These may occur with or without fracturing the skull.

PROGNOSIS

- In general the prognosis is excellent but depends on the severity of the injury.
- The typical adult patient with a concussion will recover to baseline function in 6 to 12 weeks.
- Athletes and children usually recover in 48 hours. However, children with previous head injury, learning difficulties, or neurologic, psychiatric, or family problems may continue to show significant ongoing problems at 3 months.
- Chronic headaches, persistent difficulty with short- and long-term memory and episodic confusion are common sequelae of the cumulative damage that occurs with repeated concussive injuries.

 ## Data Gathering

HISTORY

Sideline Evaluation: Mental Status

Question: What happened?
Significance: Insight into injury

Question: Orientation?
Significance: Person, place, and time should be known if mental status is normal

Question: Concentration (backward digits/months)?
Significance: A higher-level test of brain function

Question: Memory?
Significance: If patient can recall five objects at 5 minutes, recent events, and the president's name, then memory is fine.

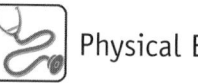 ## Physical Examination

NEUROLOGIC EXAMINATION

- Cranial nerves: equally reactive pupils, conjugate eye movements, full visual fields, symmetric grimace, normal speech.
- Motor: moves all four extremities, normal and symmetric strength
- Sensory: intact and symmetric light touch, no paresthesias
- Coordination, agility: finger-to-nose-to-finger, rapid alternating movements (finger tapping, toe tapping), heel/toe/tandem gait
- Exertional provocative tests: 5 push-ups, 5 sit-ups, 5 knee bends, 40-yard sprint; look for change in exam

 ## Laboratory Aids

BLOOD

Blood tests are not useful for diagnosing concussion.

IMAGING

- Computed tomogram of the head (HCT) is essential to rule out intracranial bleeding in grade 3 concussions.
- Magnetic resonance imaging (MRI) may be necessary in patients experiencing long-term effects of repeated head injury.

Concussion

Therapy

MEDICAL

Medical intervention is dependent on the grade of concussion. In athletic competition the following guidelines apply:

- **Grade 1**

—Remove from contest.

Examine the patient immediately and at 5 minutes postinjury.

—The patient may return to the contest if all postconcussive symptoms clear within 15 minutes.
—A second grade 1 concussion in the same contest eliminates the player from competition that day. If asymptomatic for 1 week, the player may return to competition.

- **Grade 2**

—Remove from contest and disallow return to competition that day.
—Examine patient frequently for signs of evolving intracranial pathology (e.g., intracranial hemorrhage).
—Follow-up examination by a trained physician on the day after injury.
—Head CT or MRI should be performed in instances where the postconcussive symptoms persist or worsen after injury.
—The patient may return to competition if asymptomatic for 1 week and a physician has performed a neurologic examination.
—Following a second grade 2 concussion players should not return to play until they have been asymptomatic for at least 2 weeks.

- **Grade 3**

—Transport the injured player to the nearest emergency room by ambulance with cervical spine immobilization.
—A thorough neurologic examination should be performed with the appropriate neuroimaging (HCT or MRI).
—Hospitalization is indicated if any signs of pathology are detected on physical exam, on neuroimaging, or if the mental status remains abnormal.
—If the findings are normal at the time of initial medical evaluation, the patient may return home with explicit written instructions on observation.
—Neurologic status should be assessed daily until all symptoms have stabilized or resolved.
—Prolonged unconsciousness, persistent mental status alterations, worsening postconcussive symptoms, or abnormalities on neurologic examination require urgent neurosurgical evaluation or transfer to a trauma center.

—After brief (seconds) grade 3 concussions the patient may return to competition only after being asymptomatic for 1 week. After prolonged (minutes) grade 3 concussions the patient should be withheld from play for at least 2 asymptomatic weeks.
—Following a second grade 3 concussion, the patient should be withheld from play for at least 1 asymptomatic month.
—Neuroimaging is recommended for any postconcussive symptoms that persist or worsen for over 1 week.
—Any abnormality of neuroimaging consistent with brain swelling, contusion, or other intracranial pathology should result in termination of the athletic season and return to play in the future should be seriously discouraged.

SURGICAL

- Neurosurgical evaluation or transfer to a trauma center should be considered for symptoms of prolonged unconsciousness, persistent mental status alterations, worsening postconcussive symptoms, or abnormalities on neurologic examination.

Follow-Up

- **Grade 1**

—Examinations are required at 0 and 5 minutes after injury

- **Grade 2**

—Frequent examinations are required immediately after injury to assess for signs of evolving intracranial pathology (e.g., intracranial hemorrhages).
—Follow-up examination by a trained physician on the day following the injury.

- **Grade 3**

—A trained physician should see the patient on a daily basis until all symptoms have stabilized or resolved.
—Neuroimaging is recommended for any postconcussive symptoms that persist or worsen for over 1 week.

Signs to watch for:

- First 24 hours: Worsening of headache, depression of mental status, increased confusion, photophobia, or blurred or double vision.
- First week: Insidious worsening of symptoms (continued nausea and vomiting past first 24 hours, dizziness, photophobia, or blurred or double vision); emotional liability or mental status changes.
- Prevention: Rest and fluids for the first 24 hours after injury. Avoid exertion and reinjury.

Common Questions and Answers

Q: Should athletes with two or more grade 3 concussions be allowed to resume team play?
A: Brain injury from concussions is cumulative; even with normal neuroimaging results the athlete should be discouraged from returning to the sport.

Q: What is second-impact syndrome?
A: Second-impact syndrome is the result of second concussion injury while an individual is still symptomatic from a first concussion. In this syndrome the athlete suffers malignant brain swelling as a result of vascular engorgement.

Q: What are some symptoms of postconcussion syndrome in children?
A: Hyperactivity, impulsivity, and aggressive behaviors were once thought to be the pediatric manifestations of postconcussive syndrome, but these were most likely premorbid conditions. In reality, children experience the same constellation of symptoms as adults, with depression, dizziness, headaches, and memory problems being the most common.

ICD-9-CM

850.1 Brief

850.2 Moderate

850.3 Prolonged

BIBLIOGRAPHY

Bijur P, Haslum M, et al. Cognitive outcomes of multiple mild head injuries in children. *J Dev Behav Pediatr* 1996;17(3):183–185.

Hinton-Bayre AD, Geffen G. Severity of sports-related concussion and neuropsychological test performance. *Neurology* 2002;59(7):1068–1070.

Kelly JP, Rosenberg JH. Diagnosis and management of concussion in sports. *Neurology* 1997;48:575–580.

Kushner D. Mild traumatic brain injury: toward understanding manifestations and treatment. *Arch Intern Med* 1998;158(15):1617–1624.

McCrea M, Kelly JP, et al. Standardized assessment of concussion in football players. *Neurology* 1997;48:586–588.

McCrea M, Guskiewicz KM, Marshall SW, et al. Acute effects and recovery time following concussion in collegiate football players: the NCAA Concussion Study. *JAMA* 2003;290(19):2556–25563.

Ponsford J, Willmott C, Rothwel A, et al. Cognitive and behavioral outcome following mild traumatic head injury in children. *J Head Trauma Rehabil* 1999;14(4):360–372.

Report of the Quality Standards Subcommittee. Practice parameter: the management of concussion in sports. *Neurology* 1997;48:581–585.

Author: Daniel Licht

Condyloma (Condyloma Acuminata)

 ## Database

DEFINITION

Members of the Papovaviridae family, the human papillomaviruses cause warts of the skin and mucous membranes. Exophytic venereal warts or condylomata acuminata are caused by human papillomavirus (HPV) types 6 and 11. HPV types 6 and 11 are associated with squamous cell carcinoma of the external genitalia. Virus types 16, 18, 31, 33, and 35 typically cause subclinical infection in the anogenital region and have been associated with intraepithelial genital carcinomas. Warts can be found on the external genitalia, and the urethra, vagina, cervix, anus, and mouth.

PATHOPHYSIOLOGY

- Transmission is primarily through sexual contact.
- It can also be acquired during the birth process.
- Transmission from nongenital sites occurs rarely.
- The incubation period is variable and ranges from 3 months to several years.
- The virus is trophic for epithelial cells and infects the basal layer of actively dividing cells.
- Infection results in koilocytosis and nuclear atypia. These changes may progress to severe dysplasia and CIS (carcinoma in situ).
- Recurrence is common

EPIDEMIOLOGY

- HPV infection is not a reportable disease.
- It is the most common viral STD.
- A minimum of 10% to 20% of sexually active women are infected with HPV.
- Genital warts and HPV infection are diseases of young adults 16 to 25 years of age.

PROGNOSIS

Therapy will not eradicate the virus; thus, HPV causes recurrent disease.

ASSOCIATED DISEASES

- Laryngeal papillomas
- Other sexually transmitted diseases

 ## Differential Diagnosis

- Condyloma lata
- Molluscum contagiosum
- Pink pearly papules or hypertrophic papillae of the penis
- Lipomas
- Fibromas
- Adenomas

 ## Data Gathering

HISTORY

- Most patients have no symptoms.
- Presence of warts
- Vaginal, urethral, or anal discharge, bleeding, local pain
- Dysuria
- Pruritus

 ## Physical Examination

- Warts appear as soft, sessile tumors with surfaces ranging from smooth to rough with many finger-like projections.
- HPV may also cause flat keratotic plaques that project only slightly with a hyperpigmented surface and are difficult to identify without the addition of acetic acid.
- Subclinical infection is common, causing many foci of epithelial hyperplasia invisible to the examiner.
- In males, infection is found on the penis, urethra, scrotum, and perianal areas.
- In females, infection involves the urethra, vagina, cervix, and perianal area.
- Diagnosis is made by visual inspection of the anogenital region and/or Pap smear.

 ## Laboratory Aids

- Application of 3% to 5% acetic acid for 5 minutes causes lesions to appear white and thus more readily apparent and can help with the detection of cervical disease.
- Tissue specimens may show koilocytosis typical for HPV infection.
- Colposcopy aids the diagnosis of cervical lesions.
- No cultures are available currently, but PCR is commercially available.

Therapy

- To date, no therapy exists that eradicates the virus. Recurrences are likely a result of reinfection.
- Most patients require a course of therapy rather than a single treatment.
- Lesions on mucosal surfaces respond better to topical treatments.
- All available therapies have equal efficacy in eradicating warts, ranging from 22% to 94%, with the significant rate of relapse of 25% within 3 months (see table, Treatment for External Warts).

—Consider size, location, number of warts, previous treatment, and patient preference.
—Also consider patient preference, expense, and side effects.
—Patients with extensive lesions should be referred to physicians who routinely treat these lesions.

TREATMENT

- External: see table below
- Meatal: cryotherapy or podophyllin
- Anal: cryotherapy or TCA
- Vaginal: TCA
- Cervical: Refer to an expert.

PREVENTION

- Condom use may diminish transmission.
- Examine partners; treat those infected.

Patient education, http;//www.ashastd.org

Follow-Up

- Follow up should continue until the warts have disappeared.
- Patients should return for recurrent disease.
- Latent infection and recurrent disease are common.

Common Questions and Answers

Q: What treatment is indicated during pregnancy?
A: Most experts recommend surgical removal if necessary. Podophyllin is absolutely contraindicated.

Q: Should partners of patients with genital warts be referred for examination?
A: Recurrence is as a result of reactivation of the virus; reinfection plays no role. Partner may benefit from an examination to evaluate for the presence of warts, and for education and counseling. There is no information regarding prophylaxis to prevent infection so treatment for this is not indicated. The majority of partners have subclinical infection. Female partners/patients should follow the routine recommendations for Pap smear screening.

Q: Are genital warts in children always indicative of sexual abuse?
A: No. The HPV virus has an incubation period of many months. Thus, warts transmitted to infants at the time of birth may not become clinically apparent for 1 to 2 years. Whether the incubation period can be longer than this remains unknown. Thus, maternal history and, potentially, examination are both important factors. However, all children with anogenital warts should be carefully evaluated by experienced clinicians for child abuse. It is possible that caregivers may transmit the virus to children through close but nonsexual contact; thus, this history is also important in older children.

ICD-9-CM 078.0

BIBLIOGRAPHY

Brentjens MH, Yeung-Yue KA, Lee PC, Tyring SK. Human papillomavirus: a review. *Dermatol Clin* 2002;20(2):315–331.

Emans SJ, Goldstein DP. Human papillomavirus (HPV) and human immunodeficiency virus (HIV). In: Emans SJ, Goldstein DP, eds. *Pediatric and Adolescent Gynecology*. 4th Ed. Boston: Little, Brown, 1998:385–410.

Gunter J. Genital and perianal warts: new treatment opportunities for human papillomavirus infection. *Am J Obstet Gynecol* 2003;189(3 Suppl):S3–11.

Neinstein LS. Adolescent health care: a practical guide. 4th ed. Baltimore: Urban and Schwarzenberg, 2002.

Oriel D. Genital human papillomavirus infection. In: Holmes KK, Mardh P, Sparling PF, et al., eds. Sexually transmitted diseases. 2nd ed. New York: McGraw-Hill, 1990: 433–441.

U.S. Department of Health and Human Services. 2002 Guidelines for treatment of sexually transmitted diseases. *MMWR Morb Mortal Wkly Rep* 2002;51(RR-6).

Author: Jane Lavelle

Treatment for External Warts

MEDICATION	PROCEDURE	SIDE EFFECT
Podofilox 0.5%	Patient applies medicine with a cotton swab b.i.d. for 3 days. After 4 days, it is repeated as necessary for four cycles. The area for treatment should not exceed 10 cm2 and total drug should not exceed 0.5 mL/d.	Local
Imiquimod 5% cream	Patients applies cream at bedtime 3 times per week for up to 16 weeks. It is washed off after 6–10 hours.	Local
Podophyllin 10%–25%	A practitioner applies a small amount to each wart and allows it to air dry. It is washed off 1–4 hours later. Dose is limited to 0.5 mL per treatment, to avoid systemic toxicity.	Local
Trichloroacetic acid (TCA) 80%–90%	The practitioner aplies this sparingly to each wart directly. Talc is applied to remove unreacted acid. It is washed off after 4 hours	Local
Laser surgical excision	Requires special equipment and training; often requires general anesthesia; controlled tissue destruction	Local
Cryotherapy	Liquid nitrogen or cryoprobe is used every two weeks	Local

Congenital Hepatic Fibrosis

 Database

DEFINITION

Congenital hepatic fibrosis (CHF) is an inherited, noncirrhotic liver disease associated with cystic disease of the kidneys. Prominent clinical features include:

—portal hypertension
—increased risk of ascending cholangitis.

Liver biopsy shows the classic lesion of ductal plate malformation
Patients are typically divided into two group presentations:

—infancy with severe renal disease (autosomal-recessive polycystic kidney disease, ARPKD), associated with high mortality. In survivors, liver biopsy reflects CHF.
—childhood with symptoms of liver disease predominating and more mild renal disease

The relationship of ARPKD to CHF is controversial, but many believe that these two developmental disorders of the liver and kidneys represent a single disease entity.

EPIDEMIOLOGY

The incidence of ARPKD is 1 per 4,000 to 1 per 8,000 live births.

GENETICS

- Inheritance is autosomal recessive in most families.
- The gene (PKHD1) causing ARPKD/CHF has been identified and the locus has been mapped to chromosome 6p21-p12. The gene is large consisting of at least 86 exons extending over 469kb of genomic DNA. It is expressed at high levels in fetal and adult kidneys and at lower levels in the liver and pancreas.
- Mutations of the PKHD1 gene include frameshift, nonsense, and out of frame splicing alterations that are consistent with a loss of function mechanism.
- Two frequent truncating mutations found by liquid chromatography are 9689delA and 5896insA.
- Disease may result from loss of function of the PKHD1 gene product.
- The PKHD1 product is a protein called polyductin or fibrocystin, predicted to be a membrane protein that may be a cell surface receptor or secreted protein with enzymatic activity. Further studies will be needed to identify the biologic function of polyductin and to determine how mutations of the protein cause disease.

PATHOPHYSIOLOGY

- Ductal plate malformation is a characteristic histologic lesion of the liver, implying a disturbance of the normal formation of the bile ducts. Hallmarks on pathology include:

—persistence of the ductal plate
—increased numbers of large and abnormally shaped duct elements
—increased amounts of noninflammatory fibrosis in the portal tracts
—normal appearance of hepatocytes and lobular architecture

- Some studies suggest that the primary defect in ARPKD may be linked to ciliary dysfunction. Mutations of the PKHD1 gene may result in defective polyductin or fibrocystin that in turn affect renal ciliary function.
- PKHD1-gene products are members of a novel class of proteins that belong to a family of proteins involved in regulation of cell proliferation and cellular adhesion and repulsion, and share structural features with hepatocyte growth-factor receptor and plexins. Enhanced deposition of fibrillin-1 has been observed in portal connective tissue and fibrous septa in cases of congenital hepatic fibrosis.
- Developmental abnormalities involve the liver and kidneys, and less commonly, the vasculature and the heart.
- Portal hypertension is thought to result from the fibrosis in the portal tracts, as well as, in some patients, from portal vein abnormalities.

 Data Gathering

HISTORY

- CHF most commonly presents with hematemesis or melena, generally between the ages of 5 and 13 years.
- Patients may present with fever and jaundice (cholangitis) or, rarely, with signs of liver failure.
- The majority has hepatosplenomegaly or GI bleeding within the first decade.

 Physical Examination

- Firm, enlarged liver with a prominent left lobe
- Splenomegaly
- Kidneys may be palpable.

 Laboratory Aids

BLOOD TESTS

- Thrombocytopenia and leukopenia associated with hypersplenism
- Liver enzymes and bilirubin are typically normal; transaminases may be mildly elevated in some patients.
- Usually hepatic synthetic functions (albumin, PT) are normal.
- May see elevated BUN and creatinine with renal involvement.
- Rapid mutation screening method for ARPKD can detect the two frequent truncating mutations: 9689delA and 5896insA.

IMAGING

- Ultrasound with Doppler:

—increased echogenicity
—splenomegaly
—evidence of portal hypertension

- Angiography: may show duplication of intrahepatic branches of the portal vein
- Renal ultrasound and IVP: minor abnormalities in up to 70% of patients

LIVER BIOPSY

- Characteristic histology of ductal plate malformation
- Send specimen for bacterial culture to exclude cholangitis.

COMPLICATIONS

- Portal hypertension with hypersplenism and variceal bleeding
- Cholangitis
- Renal and/or hepatic failure
- Associated vascular anomalies in the liver and brain
- Increased risk of hepatocellular or cholangiocarcinoma
- May be associated with congenital heart disease
- Systemic hypertension as a result of renal involvement
- Rare associations between CHF and severe pulmonary hypertension, as well as septo-optic dysplasia

Differential Diagnosis

- Varies with presentation. Usually differential diagnosis is that of cirrhosis but liver histology is highly characteristic.

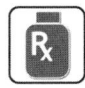

Therapy

- Suspected cholangitis should be managed with liver biopsy, culture, and appropriate antibiotics. Some patients with chronic cholangitis may require antibiotic prophylaxis.
- Choleretic agents, including ursodeoxycholic acid, are used in bile stasis and refractory cholangitis.
- Prophylactic sclerotherapy provides relief from variceal hemorrhage in many cases.
- Portosystemic shunting may be required.
- Liver transplant may be indicated for chronic cholangitis, recurrent bleeding, or progressive hepatic disease.

Follow-Up

- Watch for recurrent upper gastrointestinal tract bleeding.
- Morbidity occurs mainly from portal hypertension and cholangitis. A study by Khan revealed complications from CHF in 79% of children who underwent renal transplant for ARPKD.
- Mortality often results from ascending cholangitis associated with sepsis and hepatic failure.
- Mortality related to CHF may account for up to 80% of deaths in those with ARPKD who underwent renal transplantation.
- Those presenting in infancy may develop chronic renal failure.
- The prognosis is good when the disease presents in older children.

Common Questions and Answers

Q: Will other children of mine be affected?
A: Maybe. The inheritance pattern is autosomal recessive, with the possibility of an affected sibling being 1:4.

Q: Is my child at increased risk if he or she contracts viral hepatitis?
A: Yes, the underlying liver disease places these patients at increased risk. They should be immunized against hepatitis A and B.

Q: If my child has a fever, does he or she need to be seen by a doctor?
A: Yes. Patients with CHF who have fever without an obvious source should be evaluated for possible cholangitis, at least by obtaining a blood culture and liver enzymes.

ICD-9-CM 571.5

BIBLIOGRAPHY

Desmet VJ. Congenital diseases of the intrahepatic bile ducts: variations on the theme "ductal plate malformation". *Hepatology* 1992;16(4):1069–1083.

Igarashi P, Somlo S. Genetics and pathogenesis of polycystic kidney disease. *J Am Soc Nephr* 2002;13(9):1–21.

Khan K. Morbidity from congenital hepatic fibrosis after renal transplantation for autosomal recessive polycystic kidney disease. *Am J Transplant* 2002;2(4):360–365.

Kikuchi Y. A rare case of congenital hepatic fibrosis with severe pulmonary hypertension in an adolescent. *Pediatr Neurol* 2001; 43(3):319–322.

Lamireau T. Abnormal hepatic expression of fibrillin-1 in children with cholestasis. *Am J Surg Path* 2002;26(5):637–646.

Minami K. Septo-optic dysplasia with congenital hepatic fibrosis. *Pediatr Neurol* 2003;29(2):157–159.

Mucher G, Becker J, Knapp M, et al. Fine mapping of the autosomal recessive polycystic kidney disease locus (PKHD1) and the genes MUT, RDS, CSNK2b, and GSTA1 at 6p21. 1-p12. *Genomics* 1998;48(1):40–45.

Perisic VN. Long-term studies on congenital hepatic fibrosis in children. *Acta Paediatr* 1995;84:695–696.

Rossetti S. A complete mutation screen of PKHD1 in autosomal-recessive polycystic kidney disease (ARPKD) pedigrees. *Kidney Int* 2003;64(2):391–403.

Author: J. Fernando del Rosario

Congenital Hypothyroidism

 Database

DEFINITION

- Primary thyroid failure that is present at birth

PATHOPHYSIOLOGY

- Thyroid gland malformation

—Agenesis: absent thyroid gland
—Dysgenesis: ectopic (e.g., sublingual) or incorrectly formed (e.g., hemigland) thyroid

- Dyshormonogenesis

—Fifteen known defects of thyroxine (T4) synthesis, including those in iodide transport and iodide organification

- Transient hypothyroidism

—Maternal ingestion of antithyroid drugs
—Transplacental transfer of maternal antithyroid antibodies (can be transient or permanent damage)
—Exposure to high levels of iodine (povidone) in neonatal period

GENETICS

- Dysgenesis is usually sporadic.

—Familial occurrence in 2%.
—Mutations have been found in the TSH-receptor gene and in the transcription factors PAX-8, TTF-1 and TTF-2.

- Dyshormonogenesis is inherited in an autosomal-recessive pattern. Most commonly:

—Chromosome 2p: Mutations in the thyroid peroxidase (TPO) gene result in partial or complete loss of iodide organification function.
—Chromosome 19p: Mutations in the sodium-iodide symporter gene result in an inability to maintain the normal thyroid-to-plasma iodine concentration difference.

- Down syndrome neonates have lower T4 (left-shifted normal distribution) and mildly elevated TSH concentrations, suggesting a mild hypothyroid state.

EPIDEMIOLOGY

- Worldwide, the incidence of congenital hypothyroidism is 1 in 3,000 to 4,000 births; in North America, it is 1 in 3,700.
- Male:female ratio is 1:2 to 3.
- Eighty percent dysgenesis or agenesis; 20% dyshormonogenesis
- Racial differences: prevalence in black infants about one-third that in whites.
- Higher prevalence of congenital hypothyroidism in low birth weight (<2,000 g) and macrosomic (≥4,500 g) babies.

COMPLICATIONS

- If untreated:

—Severe mental retardation (cretinism)
—Poor motor development
—Poor growth

- Children with hypothyroidism as part of hypopituitarism do not seem to be as significantly affected by their low thyroid hormone levels as do those with primary hypothyroidism.

PROGNOSIS

Excellent, if treatment is started within the first 4 weeks of life. Level of T4 at birth is an important indicator of long-term sequelae.

 Differential Diagnosis

- Developmental

—Transient hypothyroxinemia in the first weeks of life in premature babies

- Metabolic

—Sick euthyroid syndrome in severely ill neonates

- Secondary or tertiary

—Panhypopituitarism
—Congenital isolated central hypothyroidism (a "hot spot" mutation in the TSH-β gene)
—Central congenital hypothyroidism as a result of maternal Graves disease during pregnancy (estimated incidence 1:35,000; hypothesized to indicate impaired maturation of the fetal hypothalamic-pituitary-thyroid system from a hyperthyroid fetal environment)

- Genetic

—Thyroid-binding globulin (TBG) deficiency (X-linked recessive)

- Environmental

—Iodine exposure (e.g., delivery by cesarean section, surgery in the neonatal period)
—Maternal iodine deficiency
—Maternal ingestion of antithyroid drugs or lithium

- Immunologic

—Transfer of maternal antithyroid and TSH-receptor blocking antibodies

 Data Gathering

Most children are diagnosed by the neonatal screening program.

- Five percent to 10% false-negative rate
- Neonatal screening protocols differ state to state, whether they screen T4 levels, TSH levels, or both
- Beware in severely ill neonates who are transferred from one unit or hospital to another that sending off the state screen is

not overlooked! If missed by the state screening procedure, the findings below are seen within the first 2 months of life.

HISTORY

- Symptoms that may relate to hypothyroidism:

—Prolonged jaundice
—Poor feeding
—Constipation
—Sedate or placid child
—Poor linear growth

- Family history of thyroid disorders:

—Autoimmune thyroid disease
—Vague histories of "mild hypothyroidism" not requiring treatment are often found in families with TBG deficiency.

- Maternal medications
- Birth history
- Results of the newborn screen

 Physical Examination

- Signs that may relate to hypothyroidism:

—Hypothermia
—Large fontanelles (especially posterior) with wide cranial sutures
—Coarse facial features, including macroglossia
—Hoarse cry
—Hypotonia
—Delayed deep tendon reflex release
—Distended abdomen
—Umbilical hernia

- Examine for possible goiter; helpful tricks:

—Inspect the base of the tongue for an ectopic gland.
—While supporting the posterior neck and occiput, allow the infant's head to hang back over a parent's arm or examination table. This will extend the neck and allow better visualization of the anterior region.

 Laboratory Aids

TESTS

Neonatal Screening Program (Filter Card)

- Methods vary from state to state; screen for T4 and then run TSH levels on the lowest tenth percentile of that day's T4 values OR screen for TSH elevations.
- Abnormal results on state screen should prompt immediate examination and confirmatory tests.
- Delayed TSH elevations in very low birth weight (VLBW) babies, especially those with iodine exposure, and babies with congenital cardiac anomalies may need rescreening for diagnosis of their hypothyroidism.

CONFIRMATORY TESTS

- Serum T4 and TSH are preferable to a repeated filter screen, which may result in delayed diagnosis and treatment.
- If abnormalities in binding are suspected, also check TBG level and free T4 level or triiodothyronine T3 resin uptake.
- Free T4 level is the most sensitive indicator of secondary or tertiary hypothyroidism (hypopituitarism).

ANTENATAL TESTS

- Fetal goiter can be detected by prenatal ultrasound.
- Reference ranges for third trimester amniotic fluid concentrations of TSH, total and free T4 have been established for diagnosis of fetal hypothyroidism among those with goiters. Otherwise, cordocentesis is needed to biochemically assess fetal thyroid status.

IMAGING

- ^{123}I or technetium thyroid scan will define gland anatomy (agenesis, dysgenesis, or ectopic gland).
- ^{123}I scan with perchlorate washout may also help to identify dyshormonogenesis (especially organification defects).
- ^{123}I scan must be obtained prior to the initiation of thyroxine replacement therapy. If this significantly delays the commencement of treatment, defer scanning until brain growth is complete (2 years of age), when a period off medication can be more safely pursued.
- Ultrasonagraphy can also evaluate thyroid anatomy (but not dyshormonogenesis), and does not require deferment of treatment.

FALSE POSITIVES

- Blood specimens obtained before 48 hours of life may have "elevated" TSH as a result of the normal postnatal surge.
- TBG deficiency: total T4 is low, but TSH is normal. Especially consider in males (X-linked).

 Therapy

DRUGS

- L-thyroxine

—10 to 15 mcg/kg per day once a day. Titrate dose to keep T4 in the upper range of normal.
—TSH levels may not come into the normal range for several weeks, even with good T4 values.
—A minority of infants have variable pituitary-thyroid hormone resistance, with relatively elevated serum levels of TSH for their free T4 that improves with age.
—Starting dose of 50 mcg daily (12 to 17 mcg/kg per day) may provide more rapid normalization (free T4 by 3 days and TSH by 2 weeks).

DURATION

- Lifelong
- If medication is started without imaging studies and diagnosis is not clear-cut, can stop L-thyroxine following completion of brain growth (2 to 3 years of age). Reevaluate need for continued supplementation after a 6-week trial off.

DIET

- No restrictions
- Soy formulas may interfere with absorption of L-thyroxine.

 Follow-Up

WHEN TO EXPECT IMPROVEMENT

- Most children are asymptomatic at diagnosis.
- Parents may note an increase in activity, improvement in feeding, and increase in urination and bowel movements soon after starting treatment.

SIGNS TO WATCH FOR

Poor growth and low T4 and elevated TSH values suggest poor compliance or undertreatment.

NEUROPSYCHOLOGICAL SEQUELAE

- Although IQ scores are predominantly in the normal range, subtle impairments in language and motor skills and specific learning disabilities may occur despite early treatment.
- Neurocognitive evaluation and rehabilitation should be provided.
- Maternal hypothyroxinemia during early gestation can also lead to neurodevelopmental delays if not corrected during pregnancy.

PITFALLS

- X-linked TBG deficiency: low total T4, normal TSH, and normal free T4. Diagnose with low TBG level or high T3 resin uptake. No treatment is necessary!
- Panhypopituitarism: low T4 and low or low-normal TSH because of the loss of the negative feedback loop. Screen with free T4. Treat with L-thyroxine as would primary hypothyroidism, and investigate for other pituitary hormone deficiencies.

 Common Questions and Answers

Q: Will my child be retarded?
A: It depends on when the diagnosis was made and how quickly treatment was started. Some long-term studies have suggested an increase in learning disabilities when compared with siblings, even in patients treated within the first 4 weeks of life.

Q: What if I forget a dose?
A: Give it as soon as you remember. If it is the next day, give two doses.

Q: How do I give this medicine to my baby?
A: L-thyroxine is only available in tablet form. Crush the tablet between two spoons and dissolve the powder in a small amount of formula or breast milk, which you offer to the baby at the start of a feeding to ensure complete ingestion.

Q: Are there side effects from the medication?
A: None. The tablet contains only the hormone that your child's thyroid is not making. It is synthetically produced, so there are no infectious risks.

Q: Should the transient hypothyroxinemia of prematurity be treated with L-thyroxine?
A: Severe hypothyroxinemia in preterm infants has been associated with increased problems in neurologic and mental development later in childhood, but causality has not been established. A randomized, placebo-controlled, double-blind trial of thyroxine supplementation in 200 infants born before 30 weeks' gestation, revealed no improvement in mental, motor, or neurologic outcome at 2 years of age, though higher developmental testing was seen for those born before 27 weeks' gestation.

ICD-9-CM 243

BIBLIOGRAPHY

Bubuteishvili L, Garel C, Czernichow P, Leger J. Thyroid abnormalities by ultrasonography in neonates with congenital hypothyroidism. *J Pediatr.* 2003;143:759–764.

Fisher DA, Schoen EJ, La Franchi S, et al. The hypothalamic-pituitary-thyroid negative feedback control axis in children with treated congenital hypothyroidism. *J Clin Endocrinol Metab* 2000;85:2722–2727.

Kempers MJ, van Tijn DA, van Trotsenburg AS, et al. Central congenital hypothyroidism due to gestational hyperthyroidism: detection where prevention failed. *J Clin Endocrinol Metab* 2003;88:5851–5857.

Larson C, Hermos R, Delaney A, Daley D, Mitchell M. Risk factors associated with delayed thyrotropin elevations in congenital hypothyroidism. *J Pediatr* 2003;143:587–591.

Oerbeck B, Sundet K, Kase BF, Heyerdahl S. Congenital hypothyroidism: influence of disease severity and L-thyroxine treatment on intellectual, motor, and school-associated outcomes in young adults. *Pediatrics* 2003;112:923–930.

Selva KA, Mandel SH, Rien L, et al. Initial treatment dose of L-thyroxine in congenital hypothyroidism. *J Pediatr* 2002;141:786–792.

Van Trotsenburg AS, Vulsma T, van Santen HM, Cheung W, de Vijlder JJ. Lower neonatal screening thyroxine concentrations in Down syndrome newborns. *J Clin Endocrinol Metab* 2003;88:1512–1515.

Author: Adda Grimberg

Congestive Heart Failure

Database

DEFINITION

Congestive heart failure (CHF) is the pathophysiologic state in which the heart is unable to pump sufficient blood to meet the metabolic demands of the body.

ETIOLOGY

- Low cardiac output CHF
—Cardiomyopathy
—Severe atrioventricular (AV) valve regurgitation
- High cardiac output CHF
—Left-to-right shunt (atrial septal defect [ASD], ventricular septal defect [VSD], patent ductus arteriosus [PDA])
—Arteriovenous malformation (AVM)
—Anemia and other noncardiovascular causes

MANIFESTATIONS

- Right heart failure
—Hepatomegaly; jugular venous distension; edema; right ventricular/parasternal heave
- Left heart failure
—Tachypnea; pulmonary edema; orthopnea; shock/poor systemic perfusion; diffuse or displaced point of maximal impulse (PMI)
- Nonspecific manifestations:
—Exercise intolerance; poor feeding, gastrointestinal symptoms

CAUSES

In Utero

- Arrhythmias: supraventricular (SVT) or ventricular tachycardia (VT), complete heart block (CHB)
- Volume overload: AV valve regurgitation, AVM
- Primary myocardial disease: cardiomyopathy (dilated, hypertrophic), myocarditis
- Anemia: Rh isoimmune disease, thalassemia, twin-twin transfusion
- Premature closure of the ductus arteriosus or foramen ovale

In Neonates

- Myocardial dysfunction: asphyxia, sepsis, myocarditis, hypoglycemia, acidosis, cardiomyopathy (dilated, hypertrophic, ventricular noncompaction), ischemia (anomalous left coronary artery from the pulmonary artery), metabolic defects (carnitine deficiency, other inborn errors of metabolism) or pressure overload (aortic stenosis, coarctation of the aorta)
- Volume overload: large ASD, large VSD, moderate to large PDA, truncus arteriosus, aortopulmonary window, total anomalous pulmonary venous return, AVM
- Arrhythmias: SVT, VT, or CHB
- Left-heart inlet obstruction: mitral stenosis, cor triatriatum, pulmonary venous obstruction

In Infants

- Myocardial dysfunction: cardiomyopathy (dilated, hypertrophic, restrictive, ventricular noncompaction), endocardial fibroelastosis, metabolic disease, mitochondrial disease, glycogen storage disease, myocarditis, Kawasaki disease, anomalous left coronary artery from the pulmonary artery, or chronic pressure overload (aortic stenosis, coarctation of the aorta)
- Volume overload: ASD, VSD, PDA, common AV canal defect, partial anomalous pulmonary venous return
- Secondary causes: renal disease resulting in volume overload or electrolyte disturbances, hypertension, hypothyroidism, sepsis
- Arrhythmias: SVT, VT, or CHB
- Pericardial effusion as a result of systemic lupus erythematosus (SLE), juvenile rheumatoid arthritis (JRA), other inflammatory diseases, postpericardiotomy syndrome

In Childhood and Adolescence

- Unrepaired congenital heart disease (CHD) with volume and/or pressure overload
- Repaired CHD with a residual defect that results in volume and/or pressure overload
- Acquired heart disease: pericarditis, myocarditis, endocarditis, acute rheumatic fever
- Cor pulmonale: pulmonary hypertension, Eisenmenger syndrome, chronic obstructive pulmonary disease
- Cardiomyopathy as a result of primary myocardial disease (dilated, hypertrophic, restrictive, ventricular noncompaction), anthracycline chemotherapeutic agents, sickle cell anemia, thalassemia, neuromuscular disease (Duchenne or Becker muscular dystrophy)

Differential Diagnosis

- Tachycardia
—Fever; dehydration; anemia; SVT or VT; hyperthyroidism; pericardial effusion
- Tachypnea
—Respiratory disease or infection; pulmonary venous obstruction; acidosis (metabolic disease, poisoning); pneumothorax or pleural effusion
- Edema
—Hypoalbuminemia; systemic inflammatory conditions; hypothyroidism
- Sepsis
- Hepatomegaly
—Liver disease; storage disease; extramedullary hematopoiesis

Data Gathering

HISTORY

Infants and Neonates

- Prolonged feedings associated with tachypnea, retractions, and diaphoresis
- Emesis, inadequate caloric intake, and failure to thrive
- Irritability with feeding and frequent respiratory infections
- Orthopnea: distress when supine
- Family history of heart failure or sudden unexpected death at a young age

Childhood and Adolescence

- Exercise intolerance with exertional dyspnea
- Palpitations or chest pain
- Chronic cough, wheezing, orthopnea, fatigue, weakness, anorexia, nausea, and edema
- Weight loss secondary to anorexia, nausea, and increased metabolic demands
- Weight gain secondary to fluid retention
- Family history of heart failure or sudden unexpected death at a young age

Physical Examination

INFANTS AND NEONATES

- Tachycardia
- Gallop
- Murmur of outflow tract obstruction, increased flow, AV valve regurgitation, VSD, or semilunar valve incompetence
- Systolic ejection click
- Abnormal second heart sound (fixed split, loud P2)
- Tachypnea
- Wheezing
- Crackles
- Nasal flaring, grunting, retractions
- Abdominal or cranial bruit
- Hepatomegaly and/or splenomegaly
- Edema (periorbital)
- Cool and/or mottled extremities
- Poor capillary refill
- Weak pulses

CHILDHOOD AND ADOLESCENCE

- Tachycardia
- Gallop
- Murmur of outflow tract obstruction, increased flow, AV valve regurgitation, VSD, or semilunar valve incompetence
- Loud second heart sound (P2 component)
- Hyperactive precordium, displaced PMI
- Tachypnea
- Cool and pale extremities, with cyanosis and poor capillary refill
- Jugular venous distension
- Wheezing ("cardiac asthma")
- Hepatomegaly and/or splenomegaly
- Edema (periorbital or peripheral)
- Pulsus alternans
- Pulsus paradoxus
- Evaluation of mucus membranes, skin, and extremities for manifestations of Kawasaki disease, rheumatic fever, and endocarditis

Laboratory Aids

TESTS

Chest Radiograph

- Cardiomegaly, increased pulmonary vascular markings, hyperinflation, pleural effusion, Kerley-B lines

Electrocardiography

- Abnormal P-waves and nonspecific ST-T wave changes

- Ischemia
- Hypertrophy (cardiomyopathy, congenital heart disease, storage disease)
- Heart block (1st, 2nd, or 3rd degree) or tachyarrhythmia
- Identify diagnoses with characteristic ECG findings, such as anomalous left coronary artery from the pulmonary artery (lateral Q waves and T wave inversion, acute ischemic changes), pericarditis (diffuse ST segment changes)

Echocardiography

- Rule out CHD, identify coronary artery origins
- Assessment of cardiac function

Cardiac Catheterization

- Delineation of cardiac hemodynamics and anatomy (used only in selected cases)
- Cardiac biopsy may be helpful in the diagnosis of myocarditis, storage disease, or cardiomyopathy.
- Electrophysiology study to identify arrhythmia
- Intervention may also be performed during a diagnostic procedure.

Other Laboratory Abnormalities

- Blood gas: metabolic acidosis with elevated lactate
- Chemistry: hyponatremia, either dilutional or as a result of chronic diuretic therapy
- Blood counts: anemia, leukocytosis, or leukopenia (viral myocarditis)
- Erythrocyte sedimentation rate elevation (rheumatic fever, Kawasaki disease)
- B-type natriuretic peptide elevation
- Urine: proteinuria, high urine specific gravity, microscopic hematuria
- Evaluation as to the cause of cardiomyopathy may also include pyruvate, amino acid quantification, urine organic acids, carnitine, selenium, acylcarnitine, liver function tests, and viral studies.

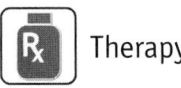 Therapy

TREATMENT OF UNDERLYING CAUSE

- Anticongestive and antiarrhythmic medical therapy or radiofrequency catheter ablation for arrhythmias
- Interventional cardiac catheterization (balloon dilation of aortic or pulmonary valve stenosis, coil embolization of PDA, device closure of ASD)
- Carnitine replacement therapy for patients with carnitine deficiency
- Targeted medical treatment for endocarditis, myocarditis, anemia, acute rheumatic fever, Kawasaki disease, or hypertension
- Surgical management of congenital heart disease
- Administration of antiarrhythmic agents to the mother has been used to control congestive heart failure in the fetus secondary to an arrhythmia
- Control of chronic inflammatory conditions, such as SLE or JRA

MANAGEMENT

- Assessment of degree of illness
—If perfusion is compromised or acidosis is present, ICU care is necessary
—In "compensated" heart failure is related to a left-to-right shunt, myocarditis, or anemia, inpatient treatment may be needed
—Many outpatients diagnosed with congenital heart disease or a mild cardiomyopathy may not require inpatient treatment
- Acute Management
—General measures: activity restriction, oxygen as needed, tube feedings to spare infants of the metabolic demands of feeding, increased caloric intake, limit of salt intake in some cases
—Drainage of pericardial effusion
—Inotropic agents (digoxin, milrinone, dobutamine)
—Diuretics (furosemide, spironolactone, bumetanide, metolazone)
—Nesiritide (synthetic B-type natriuretic peptide) in refractory cases
—Mechanical support (intubation, extracorporeal membrane oxygenation [ECMO], left ventricular assist device [VAD])
- Chronic therapy
—Digoxin
—Diuretics
—Afterload reducing agents (angiotensin-converting enzyme inhibitors, milrinone)
—Antagonism of activated neurohormonal systems (angiotensin-converting enzyme inhibitors, spironolatone, β-blockers)
—Anticoagulation and antiplatelet therapy for restrictive or severe dilated cardiomyopathy
—Biventricular pacing/cardiac resynchronization therapy
—Heart and heart/lung transplantation

 Follow-Up

- Depends on the etiology and degree of CHF
- For patients with heart failure symptoms as a result of pericardial effusion, anemia, or a treated metabolic disorder, long-term follow-up may be unnecessary.

PREVENTION

- Intravenous immunoglobulin (IVIG) for myocarditis or Kawasaki disease
- Limited use of anthracycline chemotherapeutic agents in cancer therapy
- Prompt treatment of streptococcal pharyngitis to prevent rheumatic fever
- Antibiotic prophylaxis, when indicated, to prevent infective endocarditis

PITFALLS

- In patients with CHF as a result of a large left-to-right shunt, long-term spontaneous clinical improvement of symptoms with a decrease in murmur intensity may indicate the development of pulmonary vascular disease (Eisenmenger syndrome) before cyanosis develops.
- Patients with a VSD can develop a right ventricular muscle bundle or subaortic membrane, even if the VSD closes spontaneously. Some patients with a VSD

develop prolapse of an aortic valve cusp with subsequent aortic insufficiency.
- Care must be used during the administration of oxygen to the infant with undiagnosed heart disease. In patients with ductal dependent lesions, oxygen can increase the PaO_2 and result in metabolic acidosis by increasing pulmonary blood flow and decreasing systemic blood flow.

 Common Questions and Answers

Q: My child has a large VSD and is taking digoxin and furosemide. Should I take salt out of his or her diet?
A: No. Excessive salt restriction is seldom enforceable and is not necessary. A no-added-salt diet is sufficient.

Q: What is the importance of tachycardia and bradycardia in heart failure?
A: Tachycardia limits diastolic filling time and may result in decreased cardiac output. However, bradycardia may be poorly tolerated in patients with heart failure and a relatively fixed stroke volume who are dependent on heart rate to maintain an appropriate cardiac output.

Q: What are the major causes of death in heart failure patients?
A: Ventricular arrhythmias are the most common cause of sudden death in children with ventricular dysfunction. Other causes include myocardial infarction as a result of thromboembolism and progressive worsening of low cardiac output syndrome.

Q: My patient has a normal blood pressure, but the cardiologist says more angiotensin-converting enzyme inhibition is needed. Why?
A: By decreasing the blood pressure as much as possible, short of causing dizziness or syncope, the work of the heart and myocardial oxygen consumption may be reduced. Reduction of the systemic blood pressure also reduces the amount of left-to-right shunting through a VSD, PDA, or aortopulmonary window by equilibrating the systemic and pulmonary vascular resistances.

ICD-9-CM 437.8

BIBLIOGRAPHY

Bristow MR. Beta-adrenergic receptor blockade in chronic heart failure. *Circulation* 2000;101:558–8–569.

Burch M, Runciman M. Dilated cardiomyopathy. *Arch Dis Child* 1996;74(6): 479–9–481.

Kay JD, Colan SD, Graham Jr TP. Congestive heart failure in pediatric patients. *Am Heart J* 2001;142(5):923–928.

Shaddy RE. Optimizing treatment for chronic congestive heart failure in children. *Crit Care Med* 2001;29(10 Suppl):S237–S240.

Towbin JA, Bowles JA: The failing heart. *Nature* 2002;415(10):227–233.

Woods WA. Care of children who have had surgery for congenital heart disease. *Am J Emerg Med* 2003;21(4):318–327.

Author: Jondavid Menteer

Conjunctivitis

Database

DEFINITION

Conjunctivitis is an inflammatory process involving the external membrane of the eye or the conjunctiva that is manifested by redness and edema of the conjunctiva, frequently with associated discharge.

PATHOPHYSIOLOGY

A bacterial, viral, allergic, or toxic activation of the inflammatory response that causes dilation and exudation from conjunctival blood vessels or conjunctivitis.

PATHOLOGY

- Dilated conjunctival capillaries with leukocytic infiltration and edema of conjunctiva and substantia propria.
- In children with competent lymphocyte function (>3 months of age), visible conjunctival aggregates of lymphoid tissue (follicles) or smaller infiltrates of inflammatory cells (papillae) may develop.

GENETICS

There is no clear genetic profile.

EPIDEMIOLOGY

- Viral conjunctivitis is extremely common and highly contagious. Adenovirus is the common cause of viral conjunctivitis.
- Conjunctivitis is also caused by bacteria (staphylococci, streptococci, and *Haemophilus*) and serious complications of these are rare.
- Ophthalmia neonatorum or neonatal conjunctivitis remains a significant cause of blindness worldwide.
- *Chlamydia*, herpes simplex, and chemicals such as silver nitrate are other causes of conjunctivitis.

COMPLICATIONS

- Significant complications are extremely rare for common bacterial, viral, or allergic conjunctivitis.
- Blindness may result from untreated neonatal conjunctivitis.

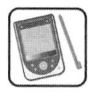 Differential Diagnosis

FOR NEONATAL CONJUNCTIVITIS

- Chemical conjunctivitis

—Noninfectious, mild, self-limited
—Result of silver nitrate or povidone iodine administration

- Birth trauma

—Unilateral, often with associated eyelid contusion
—History of forceps use or difficult delivery

- Congenital glaucoma

—Mild conjunctival redness, minimal discharge
—Look for enlarged eye, cloudy cornea, tearing, and photophobia

- Nasolacrimal duct obstruction

—Unilateral or bilateral discharge
—May be clear to mucopurulent with reflux from nasolacrimal sac
—The conjunctiva is usually white and nonerythematous

FOR ALL CONJUNCTIVITIS

- Episcleritis

—Presents as a red eye and consists of inflammation of the thick loose connective tissue, which lies between the clear conjunctiva and the white appearing stroma of the sclera.
—Rare disease in childhood and can be associated with rheumatologic disease.

- Scleritits

—Presents as a red eye. More severe disease involving inflammation of the sclera.
—Rare disease in childhood and associated with systemic disease. Requires oral or intravenous steroids.

- Preseptal cellulitis

—Early eyelid edema/erythema
—Looks like conjunctivitis, especially in young children, with the difficulty of examination
—Motility deficit, proptosis, decreased vision, afferent pupillary defect are consistent with orbital cellulitis.

- Keratitis

—Keratitis signifies corneal infection and may have associated conjunctivitis.
—Primary herpes keratitis is associated with vesicular eyelid rash and pain.
—Consult an ophthalmologist for specific treatment. Bacterial keratitis may be caused by staphylococci, streptococci, and Pseudomonas; Lyme spirochete; or vitamin A deficiency.

- Iritis

—Frequently unilateral, with or without a history of trauma
—Photophobia, decreased vision, and constant pain (except if associated with juvenile rheumatoid arthritis)
—A contagious history is rare.
—Consult an ophthalmologist for full evaluation, including pupillary dilation.

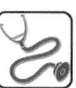 Data Gathering

HISTORY

- Type I ophthalmia neonatorum (<60 days of age)

—Acute perinatal conjunctivitis with purulent discharge.

- Type 2 ophthalmia neonatorum

—"Pink eye"
—Red, watery eyes with acute onset, with or without upper respiratory tract infection
—Often, history of similar infection in siblings or contacts
—Usually viral, occasionally bacterial, commonly self-limited

Classically, a complaint of itching in an older child is associated with red eyes is often a result of some noninfectious offending agent such as an allergen or a chemical exposure.

Physical Examination

- Discharge ranges from clear, watery (often viral) to mucopurulent (often bacterial).
- Conjunctiva is inflamed and edematous.
- May have eyelid swelling or submandibular or preauricular lymphadenopathy.
- Cornea is clear.
- Vision, pupils, and motility are normal.
- Refer to an ophthalmologist if vesicular rash is present on eyelids and corneal changes are present, as the condition may be caused by herpes simplex.

Laboratory Aids

TESTS

- Gram stain of discharge (always in ophthalmia neonatorum):

—Gonococcus (GC): gram-negative intracellular diplococcus
—Polymorphonuclear leukocytes without bacteria likely chemical (neonatal) or viral conjunctivitis
—*Chlamydia*: intracytoplasmic, paranuclear inclusion bodies on Gram stain and basophilic intracytoplasmic inclusion bodies, PMLs, and lymphocytes on Giemsa stain

- Culture

—Thayer-Martin test for GC
—Blood agar, chocolate agar for bacterial
—Viral cultures for herpesvirus and adenovirus are not clinically useful.
—*Chlamydia* culture techniques are not widely available.

- Immunofluorescence staining

—May be useful in identifying Chlamydia infection.

Therapy

- GC: Ceftriaxone, 28 to 50 mg/kg/day IV q8–12h and ocular irrigation followed by topical 0.5% erythromycin or 1.0% tetracycline ophthalmic ointments q.i.d. for 14 days. Also treat for *Chlamydia* as below.
- *Chlamydia*: Oral erythromycin syrup, 12.5 mg/kg/day in four doses for 14 days. Topical 0.5% erythromycin or 1.0% tetracycline ophthalmic ointment q.i.d. both eyes for 14 days above. (providone-iodine 1.25% ophthalmic drops q.i.d. can be used if other antibiotics are not readily available)
- Bacterial: Empiric antibiotic treatment if bacterial infection is suspected, including erythromycin 0.5%, levofloxacin 0.5%, tetracycline 1% ointment, or polymyxin B solution four times a day.
- Herpes simplex: Topical trifluorothymidine (viroptic solution), nine times a day for at least 14 days with or without systemic acyclovir (IV solution)
- Allergic: Remove offending allergen (if possible). Mild symptoms can be treated with artificial tears (make sure tears are preservative free). A new class of topical mast cell stabilizers such as olopatadine twice a day is effective for more involved cases.
- Chemical

—Close observation only
—Self-limited

- Viral or epidemic keratoconjunctivitis

—Cool compresses
—No specific antiadenovirus treatment is available.

Follow-Up

- Daily follow-up is necessary for GC, *Chlamydia*, and herpes simplex virus.
- For epidemic viral conjunctivitis, frequency is dictated by severity (daily to weekly).
- For allergic conjunctivitis, follow-up can be made after a few weeks of treatment.

NATURAL HISTORY

- GC conjunctivitis is benign if recognized early, and devastating if misdiagnosed or delayed.
- *Chlamydia* chronic infection leads to scarring and corneal opacity; chlamydial pneumonia develops in 20% of these patients.
- Viral: usually benign course, but may rarely lead to conjunctival scarring.
- HSV may lead to significant visual loss from recurrence and corneal scarring, even with proper therapy.

PITFALLS

- Failure to diagnose GC conjunctivitis may lead to corneal perforation.
- Recommending no follow-up routinely

—Follow atypical conjunctivitis closely until a more serious disease can be excluded.
—A nonresponsive or worsening condition needs ophthalmic consultation.

- Treating any red eye with steroids

—Activates or accelerates unrecognized HSV infection
—Chronic administration may raise intraocular pressure or cause cataracts.

- Chronic use of empiric broad-spectrum antibiotics for self-limited conjunctivitis promotes bacterial resistance.
- It is critical to rule out GC infection because of the destructive nature of eye disease and associated systemic infection.

Common Questions and Answers

Q: Is conjunctivitis contagious?
A: All infectious conjunctivitis is contagious, but to varying degrees. Viral or epidemic keratoconjunctivitis (EKC) is the most contagious. Careful handling of secretions, tissues, towels, bed linens, and strict hand washing usually prevent spread. Wipe surfaces with isopropyl alcohol or dilute bleach to prevent recontamination. GC, *Chlamydia*, and HSV can be transmitted through infected discharge or secretions, but this is less common. The most common source is the infected birth canal.

Q: Should the patient with "pink eye" (non-GC, non-*Chlamydia*, non-HSV conjunctivitis) be treated with empiric antibiotics?
A: Empiric treatment with topical antibiotics can cause harm in the case of sulfa-containing compounds. Antibiotic toxicity, including Stevens-Johnson reactions, can occur from sulfa antibiotics, and use of antibiotics long term promotes selection of resistant strains of bacteria. Empiric treatment also increases manipulation of the infected eye and thus increases the risk of spread.

Q: How long is the patient with "pink eye" (non-GC, non-*Chlamydia*, non-HSV conjunctivitis) contagious and when can the patient return to school?
A: The organism can be recovered from the eye for up 2 weeks after onset of symptoms, demonstrating that patients are infectious during this time. Practically, children should probably be kept out of school for at least 1 week.

ICD-9-CM 372.30

BIBLIOGRAPHY

Bielory L, Mongia A. Current opinion of immunotherapy for ocular allergy. *Curr Opin Allergy Clin Immunol* 2002;2(5):447–452.

Crede CSF. Reports from the obstetrical clinic in Leipzig: prevention of eye inflammation in the newborn. *Am J Dis Child* 1971;121:3–4.

Greenberg MF, Pollard ZF. The red eye in childhood. *Pediatric Clinics of North America* 2003;50(1):105–124.

Isenberg SJ, et al. A controlled trial of providone-iodine to treat infectious conjunctivitis in children. *Am J Ophthalmol* 2002;134(5):861–868.

Lepage P, Bogaerts J, Kestelyn P, et al. Single-dose cefoxamine intramuscularly cures gonococcal ophthalmia neonatorum. *Br J Ophthalmol* 1988;72:518–520.

Rietveld RP, van Weert HC, ter Riet G, Bindels PJ. Diagnostic impact of signs and symptoms in acute infectious conjunctivitis: systematic literature search. *BMJ* 2003;327(7418):789.

Strauss EC, Foster CS. Atopic ocular disease. *Ophthalmol Clin N Am* 2002;15(1):1–5.

Trocme SD, Sra KK. Spectrum of ocular allergy. *Curr Opin Allergy Clin Immunol* 2002;2(5):423–427.

Authors: Brian J. R. Forbes and William R. Katowitz

Constipation

Database

DEFINITION

Passage of infrequent bowel movements, which may be hard or painful. May refer to a decrease in frequency of bowel movements compared with the patient's usual bowel pattern. Constipation can result in pain, rectal bleeding, and encopresis or soiling.

CAUSES

• Most patients will have idiopathic or functional constipation with no identifiable cause.

—There is usually an acute event followed by chronicity.

• Intentional or unintentional withholding of stool passage may result in hard stools, anal pain, and fissures that perpetuate and lead to constipation.

—Rectal dilatation, decreased sensation of the urge to defecate, shortening of the anal canal, decreased tone of the external anal sphincter, and leaking or encopresis can result

• Precipitating events include the following:

—Transition from breast milk to cow's milk in infants
—Power struggle in toddlers
—Refusal to use toilets outside the home
—Streptococcal infection of the anus and perianal area
—Transient viral illness (diarrhea followed by constipation)
—Zealous toilet training

• Constipation also can be caused by anatomic anomalies in the lower gastrointestinal (GI) tract, decreased propulsion, impaired rectal sensation (primary or secondary), or a functional outlet obstruction (muscular spastic levator ani or impaired relaxation of the puborectalis).
• Neurologic causes:

—Abnormalities of the myenteric plexus
—Intestinal pseudo-obstruction
—Congenital aganglionosis
—Intestinal neuronal dysplasia
—Muscular diseases (familial and nonfamilial visceral myopathies)
—Lesions of the spinal cord result in loss of rectal tone and sensation and reduced anal closure, affecting the sacral reflex center (e.g., myelomeningocele, spina bifida occulta, tethered cord).

• Anatomic disorders of anus and rectum (stricture, stenosis, mass, ectopic anus, imperforate anus)
• Endocrine abnormalities (hypothyroidism), drugs, electrolyte abnormalities

PATHOPHYSIOLOGY

• Retention of stool allows water to move out of stool, increasing size and firmness.
• Decreased motility will lead to retention of stool. See Causes.

GENETICS

Often a family history of motility disturbances or constipation can be found. Several genes have recently been identified that are associated with Hirschsprung disease.

COMPLICATIONS

• Anal fissures: Infrequent hard stools can cause a tear of the anal mucosa, causing pain and withholding.
• Encopresis: Chronic constipation leads to progressive rectal dilatation and decreased rectal sensation. Fecal impaction results in secondary soiling or encopresis.
• Intestinal obstruction: manifests as vomiting, abdominal pain, and constipation, with abdominal x-ray (AXR) films showing intestinal obstruction and presence of large amounts of stool.
• Sigmoid volvulus: A chronically constipated child may present with symptoms of acute abdomen, fever, tender abdomen, and palpable mass. AXR shows obstruction in the colon. Barium enema may be both diagnostic as well as therapeutic by achieving reduction.

PROGNOSIS

• For functional constipation, the success rate is variable (45% to 90%), depending on the treatment and follow-up. Presence of abdominal pain at the time of presentation, close follow-up, and use of mineral oil are good prognostic factors. Presence of soiling, use of Senokot, and lack of follow-up were associated with failure and recurrences.

Differential Diagnosis

• Hirschsprung disease: congenital aganglionic megacolon (i.e., the absence of ganglion cells)
• Neuromuscular causes: tethered spinal cord, spinal muscular atrophy
• Anal abnormalities: anteriorly displaced anus, ectopic anus, imperforate anus
• Endocrine abnormalities: hypothyroidism and hyperparathyroidism
• Electrolyte imbalance: hypokalemia, hyponatremia, hypomagnesemia, hypercalcemia
• Lead ingestion: can present with anemia, constipation, and abdominal pain
• Infant botulism: constipation, aphonia, and weakness in a previously well infant
• Meconium ileus: cystic fibrosis can present with inspissated stool at birth
• Abdomino-pelvic mass: can cause constipation by pressure (e.g., distended bladder or pelvic tumor); pregnancy can also cause constipation.
• Chronic intestinal pseudo-obstruction syndrome: can present with abdominal distention, diarrhea, and constipation; usually a diagnosis of exclusion
• Surgical conditions: malrotation, congenital intestinal bands, intestinal stenoses, acquired colonic strictures resulting from inflammatory bowel disease (IBD), necrotizing enterocolitis (NEC), pyloric stenosis

• Drugs: calcium supplements, iron, barium, opiates, anticholinergic agents; always get a careful drug history to avoid missing drug-related constipation.

Data Gathering

HISTORY

Question: What is the timing of the passage of meconium?
Significance: If it is delayed for more than 48 hours, consider Hirschsprung disease.

Question: Is the child able to pass a bowel movement unaided by a suppository or enema?
Significance: If rectal stimulation is required for passage of a bowel movement, think of Hirschsprung's disease or habituation to rectal stimulation.

Question: What are the size, frequency, and consistency of bowel movements?
Significance: One to three normal (in size and consistency) painless bowel movements may be passed every 1 to 3 days. The size of bowel movements reflects the caliber of the colon.

Question: Does the child experience frequent urination, bed wetting, or urinary tract infections?
Significance: These are seen frequently with chronic constipation.

Question: Is there soiling?
Significance: Soiling occurs if the stool is impacted or with nerve damage involving the anus.

Question: Is there presence of rectal sensation?
Significance: Patients with long-standing constipation or withholding who develop a dilated rectum will often lose the sensation of rectal distention.

Question: Is there a history of painful bowel movements or rectal fissure?
Significance: This could be the cause of withholding secondary to fear of painful bowel movements. Some children are too busy playing to take the time to have a bowel movement. Some children do not want to use the toilet in school because of hygiene issues.

Question: Is the child experiencing any stressful events (e.g., new sibling, death in family)?
Significance: Stress can precipitate stool withholding, leading to constipation.

Question: Does the child have an unsteady or clumsy gait?
Significance: This may suggest neuromuscular problems.

Question: Did the child experience difficult toilet training?
Significance: Some children with encopresis have a history of difficult toilet training.

Question: What is the diet history for fluid, milk, caffeine, and fiber intake?
Significance: Excessive amounts of milk (calcium) and caffeine may be constipating in some individuals. Diets low in fiber and fluid can cause constipation.

Physical Examination

- General: Look for evidence of systemic illness.
- Abdomen: Abdominal distension (indicative of the presence of stool or gas), presence of stool masses (size, location), distended bladder and bowel sounds (may be decreased in intestinal pseudo-obstruction).
- Rectal examination:
—Perianal soiling
—Size and position of anus (may suggest imperforate or ectopic anus)
—Presence of skin tags and fissures
—Perianal or anal erythema (streptococcal proctitis)
—Evidence of child abuse.
On digital examination, assess anal tone (in functional constipation, anal tone is decreased; Hirschsprung disease may cause the anal canal to appear very long and tight); amount and consistency of stool size of rectum (dilated rectum suggestive of chronic constipation; tight and empty anus suggestive of Hirschsprung disease) presence of blood. Absence of anal wink suggests neurologic abnormalities.
- Neurologic examination: Check reflexes in the lower extremities.
- Back: Check for sacral dimple, tuft of hair (suggestive of underlying sacral abnormality), flat buttocks, and patulous anus.

PITFALLS

- "Grunting baby syndrome": Infants with this syndrome cry, scream, and draw up their legs during a bowel movement. They respond to rectal distention by contracting their pelvic floor. This is not constipation.
- Always rule out an organic cause for constipation.
- In patients with chronic medical conditions, look for medications that could cause constipation.

Laboratory Aids

TESTS

- Abdominal x-ray study: Look for presence and location of stool and evidence of bowel obstruction.
- Barium enema: An unprepped study is useful to diagnose Hirschsprung's disease. A prepped study is useful to diagnose a stricture. Most patients with constipation will not require this test.

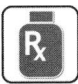

Therapy

TREATMENT OF FUNCTIONAL CONSTIPATION

- Disimpaction: If patient is impacted, then a series of three to five hypertonic phosphate enemas may be required for initial disimpaction, depending on the amount of retained stool. Significant anecdotal use of the milk and molasses enema has also been successful for this purpose. In general, children over 2 to 3 years of age require adult-size enemas although younger children should get pediatric-size enemas.
- Evacuation: Following rectal disimpaction, evacuation of the bowel can be achieved by using polyethylene glycol solution (Go-Lytely), given orally or via nasogastric tube over 6 to 8 hours until the effluent is clear. Alternatively, Miralax (a similar medication) can be used on a daily basis to achieve evacuation over 1 to 2 weeks. Doses are given in 8 ounces of water once or twice a day.
- Maintenance stool softeners: Infants up to 1 year of age may be given lactulose or Maltsupex (barley malt—1 tsp/8 oz of formula) up to several times a day. Children over 1 year of age may get lactulose or Miralax to soften the stools. Mineral oil or Kondremul are often added as adjunctive lubricants to aid in the passage of stool but contraindicated in children less than 12 to 15 months.
- Rescue stimulant laxatives: Bisocodyl or senna may be used as a stimulant laxative for short periods of time. Long-term use has been associated with colonic nerve damage in adults.
- Diet: A high-fiber diet is recommended (toddler: 10 to 12 g/day; school-aged: 12 to 16 g/day; adolescent: 16 to 20 g/day). Fiber should be increased gradually to minimize side effects of flatulence. For some patients, caffeine and excessive milk-product intake (>16 oz/day of milk) may be constipating.
- Fluid intake: High fluid intake is important.
- Toilet sitting: regular toilet sitting twice a day for 10 minutes, preferably after meals, is necessary to help retrain the bowel.
- Calendar: It is important to keep a record of stools, accidents, toilet sitting, and medication intake. It is hard for parents to remember details, which may be important in identifying causes of failure.
- Education about constipation, the importance of adhering to all of the components of treatment, and frequent follow up visits are critical to success of therapy.
- Biofeedback can be helpful in patients who fail conventional therapy and who have the following abnormalities on anorectal manometry: decreased sensory threshold to rectal distention, paradoxical contraction of the external anal sphincter, and puborectalis muscle during simulated defecation.

TREATMENT OF COMPLICATIONS

- Encopresis (soiling or diarrhea): Abdominal x-ray film shows large amounts of stool in the colon, including a dilated rectum. Disimpaction or clean-out, followed by treatment of constipation, is recommended.
- Intestinal obstruction: vomiting, abdominal pain, and constipation. AXR film shows intestinal obstruction. Make NPO, give IV fluids, and rule out an acute abdomen. Then give enemas and clear out stool from below. Never give oral laxatives or a polyethylene glycol solution in a case of obstruction.
- Sigmoid volvulus: chronically constipated child with symptoms of acute abdomen, fever, tender abdomen, and palpable mass. AXR shows obstruction in the colon. Contrast enema may reveal and possibly reduce a volvulus.

Follow-Up

- Schedule regular visits to make sure therapy is maintained.
- Have parents call as soon as problems develop.
- Once patient is doing well, decrease the frequency of visits.
- Compliance and good follow-up are key to successful management of constipation.

PREVENTION

- Dietary measures: high-fiber diet, plenty of fluids, avoidance of excessive caffeine intake, plus regular physical activity.

Common Questions and Answers

Q: When is constipation an emergency?
A: When intestinal obstruction, sigmoid volvulus, or Hirschsprung enterocolitis occur.

Q: Does Miralax have a taste?
A: Miralax advantages include its lack of taste, smell or odor and can be mixed in any liquid.

ICD-9-CM 564.0

BIBLIOGRAPHY

Abi-Hanna A, Lake AM. Constipation and encopresis in childhood. *Pediatr Rev* 1998;19(1):23–30, quiz 31.

Baker SS, Liptak GS, Colletti RB, et al. Constipation in infants and children: evaluation and treatment: a medical position statement of the North American Society for Pediatric Gastroenterology and Nutrition. *J Pediatr Gastroenterol Nutr* 1999;29:612–626.

Castoglia PT. Constipation in children. *J Pediatr Health Care* 2001;15(4):200–202.

Lewis LG, Rudolph CD. Practical approach to defecation disorders in children. *Pediatr Ann* 1997;26:4260–4268.

Loening-Baucke V. Encopresis and soiling. *Pediatr Gastroenterol* 1996;43:1279–1297.

Pashankar D, Loening-Baucke V, Bishop W. Safety of polyethylene glycol 3350 for the treatment of chronic constipation in children. *Arch Pediatr Adolesc Med* 2003;157:661–664.

Youssef N, et al. Dose response of PEG 3350 for the treatment of childhood fecal impaction. *J Pediatr* 2002;141(3):410–415.

Authors: Rose C. Graham-Maar and Maria R. Mascarenhas

Contact Dermatitis

 Database

DEFINITION

Contact dermatitis is an eczematous eruption that may result from two different processes: direct irritation to the skin or a delayed hypersensitivity reaction to a contact allergen. Diaper rash is a common form of contact dermatitis (see Diaper Dermatitis)

PATHOPHYSIOLOGY

• Direct irritation to the skin commonly results from harsh soaps, acids, certain foods, saliva, urine, and feces. It does not involve an immunologic response.
• Allergic contact dermatitis first requires exposure and sensitization to an antigen. This sensitization phase lasts at least 5 to 7 days. Repeat exposure to allergens can lead to a dermatitis in 6 to 18 hours, which peaks in 3 to 5 days and can last up to 3 weeks if untreated. Common allergens resulting in delayed hypersensitivity reactions include

—Vinyl
—Cosmetics
—Preservatives
—Fragrances
—Dyes
—Metals (particularly nickel)
—Topical medications
—Plasticizers in rubber products
—Poison ivy

• A strong allergen such as poison ivy may cause sensitization in one exposure, whereas weaker allergens may take multiple exposures.
• Both processes results in nonspecific findings of intracellular edema and inflammation, indistinguishable from other forms of eczema

GENETICS

Susceptibility to certain contact allergens for delayed hypersensitivity is in part genetically determined. In the past, it was thought that atopic children had a decreased incidence of contact dermatitis, however recent studies have suggested that it may actually be a predisposing factor.

EPIDEMIOLOGY

Contact dermatitis can occur at any age, although young infant skin is more easily irritated by a primary irritant, but seems to be less likely to develop a delayed hypersensitivity response. It is very common problem, for example most children develop diaper dermatitis, (a form of contact dermatitis) before 1 year of age.

COMPLICATIONS

Generally, there are no long-term complications, although secondary bacterial infections may occur. Exposure to certain substances, such as latex, can cause reactions ranging from a mild contact dermatitis to life threatening anaphylaxis.

PROGNOSIS

Complete resolution can be expected after elimination of further exposure to the allergen.

DIFFERENTIAL DIAGNOSIS

• Infection

—Impetigo and cellulitis (bacterial infections of the skin, usually caused by Staphylococcus or Streptococcus, with characteristic yellow, crusty lesion)
—Scabies: Skin lesions from itching and topical therapies may resemble atopic dermatitis.

• Tumors

—Letterer-Siwe (or Langerhans cell histiocytosis) is an uncommon disease that may present with a rash that begins with a scaly erythematous eruption on the scalp, behind the ears, or in the intertriginous regions, and is differentiated by the presence of small reddish-brown papules or vesicles, purpuric lesions, hepatosplenomegaly, and adenopathy.

• Metabolic

—Acrodermatitis enteropathica (deficiency of zinc, in addition to vesiculobullous lesions of the hands and feet, and surrounding mouth and diaper areas). These patients have failure to thrive, diarrhea, alopecia, and frequent bacterial and candidal infections.

• Immunologic

—Atopic dermatitis usually affects infants at a later onset, is very pruritic, and is often accompanied by a family history of atopy.
—Seborrheic dermatitis: erythematous, scaly, or crusting lesions that are characteristically yellow or salmon-colored and greasy; it tends to involve the scalp, face, and postauricular and intertriginous areas.
—Nummular eczema, named for its characteristic "coin-like" lesions that develop on areas of dry skin, usually begins as tiny papules and vesicles.
—Psoriasis (known for its silvery adherent scale and underlying reddish hue; these lesions have well-delineated margins and usually affect the scalp, extensor surfaces, and genital regions. Guttate (teardrop-shaped) psoriasis is often seen after bacterial and viral infections (especially streptococcal).

 Data Gathering

HISTORY

• The diagnosis is made by determining contact of an offending allergen with the areas of skin involved.
• Obtaining the history of offending allergens is often difficult.
• Depending on the distribution of skin involved, particular allergens may be specifically asked about.
• For many contact dermatitis, long term and repeated exposure rather than recent exposure is significant.
• Having the patient keep a diary may provide clues to other allergens as inciting agents.

 Physical Examination

• Diagnosis is determined by the recognition of the erythematous, edematous, and papular-vesicular eczematous lesions and the distribution of the rash. The vesicles often rupture, leaving a crust.
• Contact dermatitis commonly shows sharp delimitation or bizarre asymmetric distributions.
• Rashes localized to one area (such as face and dorsum of the feet) and those with discrete borders and shapes suggest a contact dermatitis.
• Determining the distribution of the rash may give clues to the etiology. Areas where clothes contact the skin, such as wrist or waist, may suggest detergent or flame-retardant allergies; eruptions on the face and hands suggest a soap dermatitis. Rash on the earlobes or near the umbilicus suggest a nickel allergy. A perioral rash is often from older children repeated licking their lips.
• A perineal rash in an adolescence may be a result of the use of perfumed creams or powders, feminine hygiene sprays, or douches. Vulvar skin is irritated more easily than thigh or vaginal skin. Feminine hygiene sprays can lead to either an irritant reaction from the propellant or an allergic contact reaction from perfumes in the spray.
• It is not often possible to differentiate irritant from allergic contact dermatitis by physical examination. Furthermore, pruritis may lead to scratching and secondary infection in both, further confusing the diagnosis. Chronic irritant and allergic dermatitis will result in lichenification (thickening) of the skin.

Laboratory Aids

TESTS

The patch test is the controlled exposure of an antigen to the skin. It should be used only to confirm a suspected allergen. After removal of the patch (generally 48 hours) the skin is examined 20 to 60 minutes later for erythema, papules, vesicles, or bullae.

PITFALLS

- The patch test may be falsely positive if done during times when the skin is acutely inflamed or if it is performed too closely to the previously existing dermatitis.
- The patch test is not well standardized. Most physicians now use adult concentrations of allergens on children.
- The patch test should not be done while the patient is on antihistamines.

 ## Therapy

- Mainstay therapy is determining to the irritant or allergen and eliminating future exposure. This may require education regarding potential sources and using a barrier between the allergen and the skin.
- Application of cool compresses can be helpful.
- Topical corticosteroids will help with the pruritus but will not accelerate resolution of the rash.
- For a short period (1 to 2 weeks), stronger fluorinated topical corticosteroids can be used in areas other than the face, axillae, and groin. The skin of these areas is thinner and more susceptible to side effects from the steroids. A weak steroid cream such as hydrocortisone should be used instead.
- The therapy should be continued for as long as the rash is present. Systemic antihistamines are generally not necessary for treating contact dermatitis, but can be considered if puritis is extreme.
- In severe cases (over 10% of body surface), systemic corticosteroids may be used for a short course, with a tapering course to avoid a rebound of the dermatitis.
- Use of lotions with potential topical sensitizers, such as benzocaine and antihistamines, should be avoided.
- For instances of chronic contact dermatitis, the new topical immunosuppressants, such as tacrolimus and pimecrolimus have been suggested as alternatives to prolonged use of topical corticosteroid.

FOLLOW-UP

- Follow-up depends on the severity of the dermatitis and elimination of continued exposure to the allergen.
- Generally, improvement is seen in 5 to 7 days.

PREVENTION

Prevention is the only approach to reduce the incidence of contact dermatitis. Desensitization, using systemic administration of the allergen, is not effective.

 ## Common Questions and Answers

Q: Can the fluid from blisters caused by poison ivy spread the rash to other parts of the body?
A: The contents of the vesicles and bullae from rhus dermatitis are not contagious. After exposure to poison ivy is eliminated, new lesions appear because of the variable sensitivity of various areas of the body to the allergen.

Q: After making lemonade at a picnic on the beach, my child developed a red, blistering rash on his face. What was the cause?
A: An interesting contact dermatitis comes from exposure to plant psoralens and ultraviolet light (sunlight). Called phytophotodermatitis, the plants that can cause this include: lime and lemons, celery, dill, parsnip, and carrot juices.
It has been confused with child abuse in the past.

Q: Is it possible to avoid contact dermatitis using protective clothing or skin barrier creams?
A: Proper fitting protective gloves and clothing are a highly effective means of decreasing irritant exposure. However, gloves permeable to irritants, such as organic solvents, may even increase the exposure to the irritant. Rubber gloves are contraindicated in individuals with immediate and delayed type allergy to latex and rubber additives. The use of skin protective creams such as skin moisturizers, have not been well studied and have limited usefulness.

Q: How does saliva cause a perioral rash in some children's is there something unusual in the saliva that is causing this?
A: "Liplicker's dermatitis" demonstrates the fact that with excessive exposure, even substances that normally wouldn't cause a rash can be quite irritating.

ICD-9-CM 692.9

BIBLIOGRAPHY

Akhavan A, Cohen SR. The relationship between atopic dermatitis and contact dermatitis. *Clin Dermatol* 2003;21(2): 158–162.

Beltrani VS, Beltrani VP. Contact dermatitis. *Ann Allergy Asthma Immunol* 1997;78: 160–173.

Friedlander SF. Contact dermatitis. *Pediatr Rev* 1998;19:166–171.

Weston WL, Bruckner, A. Allergic contact Dermatitis. *Pediatr Clin N Am* 2000;47:4.

Author: Robert Kamei

Contraception

Database

DEFINITION

- Contraception is the prevention of conception or pregnancy.
- The "ideal" contraceptive is 100%, has no side effects, can be easily reversed, and can be easily used by adolescents.

CLASSES OF CONTRACEPTIVES AND THEIR HEALTH BENEFITS

- Abstinence
—Refraining from vaginal or anal intercourse
—Only "ideal" contraceptive
—Refusal, negotiation, and planning skills are necessary for the adolescent to successfully employ this method.
—Most effective way to prevent transmission of HIV, viral hepatitis, syphilis, *Neisseria gonorrhoeae*, and *Chlamydia trachomatis*.
- Barrier methods to sperm entry (male and female condoms, diaphragm)
—Male condoms are 86% effective with typical use. The female condom and diaphragm with spermicide are 79% and 80% effective, respectively.
—Proper use of the male and female condoms can prevent spread of HIV, viral hepatitis, syphilis, *N. gonorrhoeae*, and *C. trachomatis*. Condoms are not reliably effective in preventing the acquisition of herpes simplex virus (HSV) or human papillomavirus (HPV).
- Spermicidal agents (foam, film, vaginal inserts)
—Nonoxynal-9 is the active agent most widely used.
—73% effective in preventing pregnancy with typical use.
—Reduced transmission of *C. trachomatis* and *N. gonorrhoeae*
—Spermicides used with condoms will increase overall efficacy to 93% with typical use.
—Hormonal agents (oral contraceptive pills [OCPs], transdermal patch, vaginal ring, injectable, and emergency contraception)
- OCPs
—Categories of OCPs include fixed-dose combination pills, combination phasic pills, and the progestin-only "mini" pill.
—Monophasic and triphasic combination pills contain a fixed dose of estrogen, and a fixed or varying dose of progestin, respectively.
—Estrogen/progestin combined OCPs are 94% to 97% effective in preventing pregnancy with typical use (99.9% effective with perfect use). They are effectively used to treat problems, including dysfunctional uterine bleeding and polycystic ovary syndrome.
—The progestin-only mini-pill contains progesterone only.
—The mini-pill is 99.7% effective in preventing pregnancy.
- Transdermal patch—contains ethinyl estradiol and norelgestromin. Each patch is left in place for 7 days and changed weekly allowing 1 patch-free week per month to allow menses to occur; efficacy is comparable to OCPs; convenient as a result of a once

weekly change. Patch may be less effective in women weighing >90 kg
Vaginal ring—a soft, flexible, polymer ring containing ethinyl estradiol and etonogesterel that is inserted into the vagina for 3 weeks and then removed for 1 week to allow menses to occur.
Benefits include once a month insertion, avoidance of first pass liver effects, and lower hormone doses.
- Injectable hormonal methods
Depo-medroxyprogesterone acetate (Depo-Provera) is an effective contraceptive that is administered intramuscularly once every 3 months. The benefit of the injectable methods is that they require no daily maintenance on the part of the teenaged woman giving them typical use efficiency rates comparable to OCPs.
- Intrauterine devices, Norplant, tubal ligation, vasectomy, withdrawal, and biofeedback in general are not recommended for the vast majority of teenagers because of increased side effects, irreversibility, high failure rates, or difficult maintenance.
- Emergency contraception—also called postcoital contraception, is a safe method of contraception that employs either combination or progestin-only OCPs.
—Combination pills, containing estrogen and progestin, can reduce the risk of pregnancy by 75% after unprotected intercourse, if taken in correct doses within 72 hours.
—The progesterone-only method may reduce the risk of pregnancy by 85% if taken with 48 hours of unprotected intercourse.

COMPLICATIONS

Barrier Methods

- Latex allergy: Patients may use polyurethane rather than latex condoms.
- Breakage or permeability: Oil-based lubricants and most intravaginal medications used with latex condoms will increase the risks of these complications. Animal skin condoms are permeable to viral pathogens.
- Irritation, urinary tract infections, and toxic shock syndrome (if left in place longer than 24 hours) may be seen with diaphragm use.

Spermicides

- Local irritation or allergic reaction

Hormonal Contraceptives

- Mortality from gynecologic and related causes of 15- to 19-year-olds was 7.0 (per 100,000 women per year) if no fertility control measures were used, 0.3 in nonsmoking OCP users, and 2.2 in smoking OCP users.
- Minor side effects of combination OCPs include menstrual spotting, nausea, breast changes, fluid retention, leukorrhea, minor headache, and depression.
- Thromboembolic events and liver disease are extremely rare in nonsmoking adolescents using estrogen-containing OCPs. Patients experiencing severe and sudden head, chest, abdominal, or leg pain, sudden change in

vision, severe depression, and jaundice should contact their health provider immediately.
- Contraindications to combination OCPs include history of thromboembolic event, structural heart disease, breast cancer, pregnancy, liver problems, migraine headaches, prolonged immobilization, or severe hypertension. Caution should be taken when prescribing combination OCPs to adolescents with undiagnosed abnormal uterine bleeding, less than 3 weeks postpartum, use of drugs that affect liver enzymes, and gallbladder disease.
- Minor side effects of progestin only methods include weight gain, rapid hair turnover, and menstrual irregularities.
- Depo-medroxyprogesterone acetate has been shown to reduce bone mineral density in several studies. Since adolescence is the period of peak bone mass accretion, there is some concern that its use during adolescence may increase the risk for osteopenia or osteoporosis later in life. Until more studies are available, it is probably advisable to avoid its use in those women at high risk of osteoporosis, such as women with anorexia nervosa or chronic renal failure.
- Nausea and/or vomiting occur in most patients using emergency contraception or "doubling up" on OCPs.

PROGNOSIS

- Within 3 months of OCP use, only 44% to 45% of patients remain compliant. After 1 year, only 33% are compliant.

Data Gathering

HISTORY

General considerations in method selection include the following:
- What is the teen's sexual history?
- Is sexual activity spontaneous or planned?
- Does the patient feel that she/he can be compliant with a daily pill or barrier methods?
- Does the patient require absolute confidentiality?
- Is the patient comfortable inserting a diaphragm or applying a condom?
- Does the patient have open communication with his/her partner?
- Does the patient desire pregnancy? Does his/her partner?
- Are there any other barriers to compliance with the chosen contraceptive method?

Physical Examination

- Obtain baseline weight and blood pressure.
- It is not absolutely necessary to perform a pelvic examination on young women initiating hormonal contraception. Biannual screening for sexually transmitted infections and regular Papanicolou smears ideally occur with any sexually active woman.

Contraception

 ## Laboratory Aids

- Pregnancy test prior to initiating hormonal contraceptives
- Lipid profile if there is a family history of sudden death or cardiovascular disease

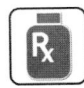 ## Therapy

BARRIER METHODS

- Trained personnel can teach the proper technique for application of the diaphragm, and male and female condoms.

SPERMICIDES

- These must be inserted near the time of intercourse; some formulations require 10 to 15 minutes for activation, and most have an unpleasant taste.
- Trained office personnel can teach the proper technique for insertion.

ORAL CONTRACEPTIVE PILLS (OCPS)

- OCP monthly packages contain 3 weeks of hormone, followed by 1 week of placebo.
- Menstruation begins after 2 or 3 days of placebo.
- OCPs are taken as a daily pill, preferably at the same time every day (at night with food, to minimize nausea).
- OCPs are usually started on the first Sunday after the menstrual period begins.
- Instructions for missed pills should be explained and given to all adolescents initiating OCPs.
- OCPs may not offer protection during the first cycle; therefore, a back-up barrier method should be used.
- Fertility returns, on average, 2 to 3 months after discontinuation. 1% to 2% of patients will experience a delay in fertility for up to 1 year.

OTHER HORMONAL AGENTS

- Depo-Provera is given intramuscularly in the deltoid or gluteus maximus.
- Each shot has a 3-month duration, with subsequent shots occurring every 12 weeks.
- The initial shot should be given within 5 days after the start of the last menstrual period.
- Depo-Provera offers contraceptive protection immediately.
- Fertility (and ovulatory cycles) should return within 6 months of the last injection.

EMERGENCY CONTRACEPTION

- The Yuzpe regimen is safe and well studied. It consists of two fixed-dose combination pills containing at least 35μg of estrogen each, taken within 72 hours of unprotected intercourse. This is followed by 2 additional pills in 12 hours.
- This dose of estrogen will almost always cause nausea and vomiting; therefore, pretreatment with an antiemetic is recommended.

- The FDA has approved two prepackaged preparations: Preven (similar to Yuzpe regimen) and Plan B (progestin only).
- The progestin only method may be taken as 1.5 mg levonorgesterel once or 0.75 mg of levonorgesterel twice 12 hours apart.

DRUG INTERACTIONS

- Drugs that activate the cytochrome P-450 enzyme will diminish the efficacy of hormonal contraceptives. This is of greatest concern with low-dose preparations and can be remedied by using higher doses.
- Drugs that diminish hormonal contraceptive effects include phenobarbital, carbemazepine, primidone, rifampin, griseofulvin, and tetracyclines (including doxycycline). Hormonal contraceptives can increase levels of phenytoins, benzodiazepines, antidepressants, corticosteroids, beta-blockers, theophylline, and alcohol. Hormonal contraceptives can decrease the efficacy of acetaminophen, oral anticoagulants, hypoglycemics, and methyldopa.
- Practitioners should refer to the *Physician's Desk Reference* for any question about drug interactions.

 ## Follow-Up

- Patients using hormonal contraceptives should be seen within 6 weeks to 3 months of initiation to evaluate compliance and side effects.
- Blood pressure should be monitored at every visit.

PREVENTION

- Inform patients that only male and female condoms offer some protection from HIV, Hepatitis B, gonorrheal, chlamydial, or trichomonal infection. They offer very limited protection from HPV or HSV, which are transmitted through skin to skin contact. Encourage the consistent use of latex condoms.
- Patients using OCPs must be strongly encouraged to cease tobacco use. Methods of treating nicotine dependence should be employed if indicated.

PITFALLS

- Advising teenagers to abstain from all forms of physical intimacy may be counterproductive in the context of their psychosocial development.
- Contraceptive use may lead to patients' discontinuing use of condoms. Providers should emphasize at every visit that only condoms protect against STDs.
- Practitioners who are reluctant to use of contraceptives in adolescents should balance the risks of pregnancy with that of the contraceptive method. OCPs are among the most extensively studied and safest medications prescribed for adolescents.

 ## Common Questions and Answers

Q: My patient asks for confidentiality regarding contraception. Should I comply?
A: Yes, teenagers have the right to confidentiality regarding contraception and treatment of STDs. Every state has a law or provision for confidential access to contraceptive services. Importantly, it may be in the patient's best interest to have a caring adult involved. Which adult and how he/she is involved should be negotiated with the adolescent.

Q: The FDA recently approved mifepristone (Mifeprex) for use in the United States. Is it a safe to use in adolescents?
A: Mifepristone, commonly known as RU-486, is used to end an early pregnancy. No age restrictions were described by the FDA; however, as an abortifacient, the use of Mifeprex is subject to state-by-state parental notification or consent statutes.

Q: One of my patients has asked me to preprescribe emergency contraception for her. Is this something that I should do?
A: Studies done thus far have shown that use of emergency contraception is safe. In fact, there are no absolute contraindications to using progestin-only emergency contraception. Since unprotected sexual encounters often take place at a time when women do not have access to their health-care providers, like evenings or weekends, advanced prescription is of benefit for many women.

Q: What should I tell my patient if she misses a dose of her oral contraceptive?
A: If she has missed 1 pill, she should take it as soon as she remembers; then take the next pill at the regular time. If she has missed 2 doses, she should take two when she remembers, and then 2 the next day. She should use a back-up method during the cycle in which she had to "double up." If she has missed 3 or more pills, she will probably menstruate. After discarding the last pack, she should start a new pack on the first Sunday after the start of her next period. She is not protected during the remainder of this cycle.

ICD-9-CM
Family planning advice V025.09
Oral prescription V025.01
Other agents V025.02

BIBLIOGRAPHY

Hatcher RA, Trussell J, Stewart F, et al. *Contraceptive Technology*, 17th Ed. New York: Ardent Media, Inc., 1998.

Pettinato A, Emans SJ. New contraceptive methods: update 2003. *Curr Opin Pediatr* 2003;15:362–369.

Polaneczky M. Adolescent contraception. *Opin Obstet Gynecol* 1998;10:213–219.

Rimsza M. Counseling the adolescent about contraception. *Pediatr Rev* 2003;24:162–169.

Westhoff C. Emergency contraception. *N Engl J Med* 2003;349:1830–1835.

Authors: Daniel H. Reirden and Jonathan R. Pletcher

Cor Pulmonale

 Database

DEFINITION

Cor pulmonale is right ventricular (RV) failure secondary to an altered cardiopulmonary process, resulting in excessive pulmonary artery pressure and resistance (PVR). Cor pulmonale is not the result of a primary congenital heart defect.

CAUSES

- Parenchymal lung disease (most common)
- Chronic obstructive pulmonary disease

—Cystic fibrosis
—Asthma

- Restrictive lung disease

—Infectious
—Pulmonary toxins
—Pulmonary fibrosis
—Bronchopulmonary dysplasia (combined)

- Upper airway diseases
- Tonsillar/adenoidal hypertrophy
- Syndromes (Down, Treacher Collins)
- Neuromuscular disorders
- Duchenne muscular dystrophy
- Pulmonary vascular abnormalities
- Collagen vascular diseases
- Pulmonary veno-occlusive disease
- Pulmonary thromboembolism
- Chest wall deformities
- Primary pulmonary hypertension (PPHN)

PATHOPHYSIOLOGY

Chronic hypoxia is the principal factor, resulting in a cascade of endothelial dysfunction with pulmonary vasoconstriction, followed by the development of pulmonary hypertension. A variety of vasoactive mediators may be responsible for the effect on vasomotor tone. Alveolar hypoventilation, hypoxemia, hypercarbia, and acidemia all result in increased RV afterload and decreased RV systolic function.

EPIDEMIOLOGY

Cor pulmonale may be found at any age, but is typically as a result of a long-standing pulmonary process. PPHN is most often diagnosed in the second or third decade of life. There is a female predominance, and it is often diagnosed during pregnancy.

COMPLICATIONS

Aside from the underlying lung process, the chronic hypoxia results in anemia, polycythemia, decreased systemic oxygen delivery, and RV failure secondary to the inability of the RV to handle the excessive afterload.

PROGNOSIS

Patients with reversible lung disease usually have a better prognosis. Patients with cor pulmonale are at risk for sudden death because of the inability to augment cardiac output with exercise secondary to a relatively fixed PVR. Numerous medical therapies and lung transplantation may improve long-term survival.

 Differential Diagnosis

Congenital heart disease with pulmonary hypertension and right-to-left shunting (Eisenmenger syndrome) should be ruled out.

 Data Gathering

HISTORY

- Fatigue
- Dizziness
- Syncope
- Exercise intolerance
- Chest pain (secondary to RV ischemia)
- Palpitations
- Hemoptysis

 Physical Examination

- Tachycardia
- Parasternal RV impulse
- Cyanosis may be evident.
- Hepatomegaly, jugular venous distention, peripheral edema
- A loud, narrowly split or single second heart sound (P2), gallop, holosystolic murmur right of the sternum (tricuspid regurgitation), and diastolic murmur at the left upper sternal border (pulmonary insufficiency)

 Laboratory Aids

NONSPECIFIC TESTS

- ECG: may show right atrial enlargement, RV hypertrophy, and T-wave inversion
- Decreased PaO_2, increased $PaCO_2$, and a compensatory metabolic alkalosis
- Polycythemia may be consistent with chronic hypoxemia.
- Chest radiograph: cardiomegaly from RV dilation and main pulmonary artery enlargement
- Echocardiography: RV dilation, RV hypertrophy, pulmonic insufficiency, and if tricuspid regurgitation is present, an RV pressure can be estimated.
- Cardiac catheterization, although invasive, remains the gold standard.

Therapy

- The primary goal is reduction of the abnormally elevated pulmonary artery pressure and the RV workload.
- If at all possible, address the primary etiology (e.g., tonsillectomy/adenoidectomy in a patient with obstructive upper airway disease).
- Oxygen (nocturnal oxygen)
- Diuretics (if pulmonary congestion)
- Bronchodilators (theophylline)
- Digoxin (may improve RV contractility)
- Anticoagulants
- Pulmonary vasodilators

—Nitric oxide
—Prostacyclin
—Calcium channel blockers
—Sildenafil

- Atrial septostomy (in select cases, may improve cardiac output at the expense of hypoxemia)
- Lung or heart-lung transplantation

 Follow-Up

PROGNOSIS

Long-term survival is variable and depends on the age at onset of pulmonary changes and the underlying conditions (e.g., Down syndrome) that may adversely affect survival. Death often occurs in the second or third decade of life.

PITFALLS

In newborns, the RV muscle mass is comparable to the left ventricle. RV failure from pulmonary hypertension is rare in newborns. RV failure in newborns is usually a consequence of hypoxemia, ischemia, and metabolic acidosis (e.g., persistent fetal circulation).

 Common Questions and Answers

Q: Is cardiac catheterization indicated in all patients with cor pulmonale?
A: Yes. While a great deal of information can be learned from echocardiography, direct pulmonary artery pressure/resistance measurements require an invasive procedure. In addition, assessment of the reactivity of the pulmonary vascular bed to various agents (oxygen, prostacyclin, and calcium channel blockers) is best performed in the catheterization laboratory.

Q: Is nocturnal oxygen therapy beneficial?
A: Nocturnal oxygen has been speculated to delay the progression of cor pulmonale in some select patients with obstructive sleep hypoxemia.

ICD-9-CM 416.9

Chronic 415.0

BIBLIOGRAPHY

Bandla HP, Davis SH, Hopkins NE. Lipoid pneumonia: a silent complication of mineral oil aspiration. *Pediatrics* 1999;103(2):E19.

Brouillette RT, Fernback SK, Hunt CE. Obstructive sleep apnea in infants and children. *J Pediatr* 1982;100:31.

Perkin RM, Anas NG. Pulmonary hypertension in pediatric patients. *J Pediatr* 1984;105:511.

Wessel DL, Adatia I, Thompson JE, et al. Delivery and monitoring of inhaled nitric oxide in patients with pulmonary hypertension. *Crit Care Med* 1994;22(6):930–938.

Author: Mitchell I. Cohen

Costochondritis

 Database

 Differential Diagnosis

 Data Gathering

DEFINITION

Costochondritis is chest pain that emanates from a costal cartilage and is reproducible on compression of that cartilage.

PATHOPHYSIOLOGY

- Inflammation of unknown etiology (histologic examination is usually normal).
- Infection

—Complication of median sternotomy
—Can present months to years after surgery (the costal cartilage is avascular, making it vulnerable to infection if it has been exposed, injured, or denuded of perichondrium)
—Occurs by spread from adjacent osteomyelitis or may arise de novo during surgery
—Bacterial
   —*Staphylococcus aureus* (especially after thoracic surgery)
   —Salmonella (in sickle cell disease)
   —*Escherichia coli*
   —Pseudomonas species
   —Klebsiella species
—Fungal
   —Aspergillus flavus
   —*Candida albicans*
—Post-trauma

EPIDEMIOLOGY

- Costochondritis accounts for 10% to 31% of all pediatric chest pain.
- Peak age for chest pain in children is 12 to 14 years.
- Incidence of sternal wound infections following median sternotomy is 0.1% to 1.6%.

PROGNOSIS

- Inflammatory costochondritis: excellent
- Infectious costochondritis: prognosis relates to:

—Underlying clinical condition of the patient (e.g., immunocompromised, postradiation therapy for cancer, postcardiac surgery)
—Extent of surgery required to reconstruct the area damaged by the infection

ETIOLOGIES

- Cardiovascular

—Myocardial infarction
—Pericarditis
—Pericardial effusion
—Myocarditis
—Endocarditis
—Cardiomyopathy
—Premature ventricular contractions
—Supraventricular tachycardia
—Dissecting aneurysm

- Pulmonary

—Asthma
—Exercise-induced bronchospasm
—Pneumonia
—Pleural effusion
—Pneumothorax
—Pulmonary embolism

- Gastrointestinal

—Gastroesophageal reflux
—Esophagitis
—Gastritis
—Achalasia

- Mechanical

—Muscle strain
—Stress fractures
—Precordial catch syndrome
—Trauma

- Rheumatologic

—Rheumatoid arthritis
—Ankylosing spondylitis

- Oncologic

—Rhabdomyosarcoma
—Leukemia
—Ewing sarcoma

- Miscellaneous

—Tietze syndrome
—Psychogenic chest pain
—Breast tissue pain (both sexes)

HISTORY

Inflammatory Costochondritis

- Pain usually preceded by exercise or an upper respiratory tract infection
- Description of pain:

—Usually sharp
—Affects the anterior chest wall
—Localized or radiates to the back or abdomen
—Usually unilateral (left side greater than right side)

- The fourth to sixth costochondral junction is the usual site of pain.
- Motion of the arm and shoulder on the affected side elicits the pain.
- Girls are affected more often than are boys.

Tietze Syndrome

- Onset is usually abrupt, but can be gradual.
- Believed to be caused by a minor trauma, though etiology is unknown
- Description of pain:

—Radiates to arms or shoulder
—May last up to several weeks
—Swelling at the sternochondral junction may persist for several months to years.

- Usually affects the second or third costochondral joint
- Pain is aggravated by sneezing, coughing, deep inspiration, or twisting motions of the chest. No differences in frequency between sexes

Infectious Costochondritis

- Slow, insidious course
- Usually unimpressive clinical symptomatology

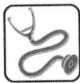 ## Physical Examination

- Usually normal
- Inspect for evidence of trauma, scars, bruising, and swelling.
- Palpation and percussion of the costochondral and costosternal junctions should reproduce and localize the pain.
- In Tietze syndrome, spindle-shaped swelling is visible at the sternochondral junction.

 ## Laboratory Aids

TESTS

- WBC not helpful (even when infection present)
- ECG (may be helpful if cardiac etiology is being considered)

IMAGING

- Radiologic studies (chest radiography, CT) usually not helpful
- Gallium scan

—May be useful in some cases of infectious origin
—Not highly specific
—May show increased radionuclide uptakeNo evidence of osteomyelitis of the sternum in most cases

- Technetium bone scan

—Not highly specific

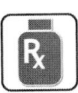 ## Therapy

INFLAMMATORY COSTOCHONDRITIS

- Antiinflammatory and analgesic agents
- Reassurance
- If pain disturbs normal activities and sports, infiltration with local anesthetic may prove useful.

INFECTIOUS COSTOCHONDRITIS

- Prolonged course of IV antibiotics
- Prompt surgical resection of all involved cartilage
- Reconstructive surgery with muscular flaps should be done.

 ## Follow-Up

WHEN TO EXPECT IMPROVEMENT

- Inflammatory costochondritis

—Long-lasting condition
—Follow-up once a year is recommended.

- Infectious costochondritis

—Long-term follow-up after surgery is mandatory.

PITFALLS

- Inflammatory costochondritis

—Important cause of school absence
—Adolescents tend to limit physical activity unnecessarily for long periods.
—Restriction of activities is usually not required.
—Most adolescents still worry about cardiac problems, even after the diagnosis has been made.

- Infectious costochondritis

—Long-term IV antibiotics alone do not resolve the problem; surgical resection and repair also are required.
—There is a tendency for the infection to spread to adjacent costal cartilages and across the sternum to the contralateral chest wall.
—In general, avoid costochondral junctions when performing surgical procedures in the chest (e.g., chest-tube placement).

 ## Common Questions and Answers

Q: Am I having or will I have a heart attack?
A: Chest pain does not imply a heart problem. This pain arises from the chest wall; there is no risk of a myocardial infarction. A cardiac etiology to chest pain in an adolescent is usually uncommon.

Q: Is costochondritis related to arthritis?
A: There is no relation to any form of arthritis.

ICD-9-CM 733.6

BIBLIOGRAPHY

Brown RT, Jamil K. Costochondritis in adolescents: a follow-up study. *Clin Pediatr* 1993;32:499–500.

Fraz M. *Pediatric Respiratory Disease: Diagnosis and Treatment*. Philadelphia: WB Saunders, 1993:162–172.

Kocis KC. Chest pain in pediatrics. *Pediatr Clin North Am* 1999;46:189–203.

Mendelson G, Mendelson H, Horowitz SF, et al. Can 99mtechnetium methylene diphosphate bone scans objectively document costochondritis? *Chest* 1997;111:1600–1602.

Selbst DM. Chest pain in children: consultation with the specialist. *Pediatr Rev* 1997;18:169–173.

Author: Richard M. Kravitz

Crohn Disease

 Database

DEFINITION

Crohn disease (CD) is a chronic inflammatory bowel disease that can affect any part of the gastrointestinal tract.

CAUSES

- Multifactorial, see Pathophysiology

PATHOPHYSIOLOGY

- Interaction and combination of environmental factors, genetic susceptibility, host's intestinal flora, and yet unspecified triggering factor leads to a dysregulated immune response, causing chronic intestinal inflammation.
- Patients with CARD15 mutation have dysregulated response to bacterial products, which changes innate low grade to a high-grade inflammatory response.
- Initially, T helper-1 lymphocyte pathway is activated, causing inflammatory cytokines to generate microscopic inflammation, which infiltrates all layers of intestine with cryptitis or crypt abscesses, and distortion of crypt architecture.
- Macroscopically the intestinal wall is edematous, mesentery may be thickened, local lymph nodes enlarged, and fat extends from the mesentery and "creeps" over the serosal surface.
- Granulomas are found in 20% to 40% of biopsies and if found are pathognomonic.
- Normal bowel can exist in continuity with affected bowel (skip areas).

GENETICS

- First-degree relatives have a 5% to 25% higher risk than normal population.
- Family members of patients with Crohn disease have increased risk for both Crohn disease and ulcerative colitis.
- Offspring and siblings have an 8% risk of developing inflammatory bowel disease (IBD).
- Concordance in monozygotic twins is 44.4% versus 3.8% in dizygotic twins.
- Susceptibility regions located on different chromosomes (6,12,16).
- CARD15 mutation is present in approximately 14% to 18% of patients.

EPIDEMIOLOGY

- The incidence rate in children is 4.56 per 100,000 in North America.
- More than a third of patients first present in childhood or adolescence.
- Family history is present in 30% of patients under 30 years old.
- Males and females are equally affected in adulthood, although in childhood it is slightly more predominant in males (M:F = 1.6:1).
- Highest incidence in the Caucasian population.

COMPLICATIONS

- Intestinal obstruction as a result of strictures, or adhesions
- Abscess or phlegmon formation
- Enteroenteric, enterovesical, enterovaginal, and enterocutaneous fistulas
- Perforation
- Gallstones, kidney stones
- Intestinal lymphoma, colon cancer
- Malabsorption resulting in deficiency (e.g., vitamin B12 and bile salt deficiency, iron deficiency)
- Massive hemorrhage is rare (1%).
- Growth failure is frequent; final height is reduced and puberty is delayed in Crohn disease affecting prepubertal children.
- Osteopenia and osteoporosis secondary to inflammation, nutritional deficiency, and therapeutic side effects (corticosteroids)
- Toxic megacolon is a rare but serious complication.

 Differential Diagnosis

- Ulcerative colitis
- Appendicitis
- Infection:

—Mycobacterium tuberculosis
—Salmonellae
—Shigella dysenteriae
—Campylobacter jejunii
—Aeromonas sp.
—Yersinia entercolitica
—Clostridium difficile
—Escherichia coli
—Giardia lamblia
—Cryptosporidium
—Strongyloides

- Hemolytic-uremic syndrome
- Henoch-Schönlein purpura
- Irritable bowel syndrome
- Peptic ulcer disease
- Autoimmune enteropathy, immunodeficiency
- Cow's milk protein allergy
- Small intestinal lymphoma

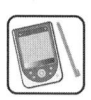 Data Gathering

HISTORY

- Frequency of signs and symptoms

—Weight loss, 85%
—Diarrhea, 80%
—Abdominal pain, 85%
—Fever, 40%
—Rectal bleeding, 50%
—Growth failure, 35%
—Nausea and vomiting, 25%
—Rectal disease, 25%
—Extraintestinal signs, 25%
—Perianal disease, 25%

- Symptoms depend on the intestinal site of disease activity.
- Sites most often affected in decreasing frequency are terminal ileum, right colon, isolated colon, proximal small bowel, and upper gastrointestinal (GI) tract (stomach, duodenum, esophagus).

SPECIAL CONCERNS

- Chronic diarrhea
- Weight loss
- Growth failure (careful charting of recent growth parameters, especially growth velocities from school or medical records, is essential.)
- Delayed puberty
- Recent travel (enteric infections)
- Antibiotic use (Clostridium difficile)
- Family history of IBD
- Extraintestinal disease:

—Arthritis
—Erythema nodosum
—Pyoderma gangrenosum
—Mouth ulcers
—Episcleritis
—Uveitis
—Thromboembolic disease
—Vasculitis
—Renal stones
—Amyloidosis
—Sclerosing cholangitis
—Pancreatitis

 Physical Examination

- Growth delay and weight loss, delayed puberty
- Abdominal examination:

—Hyperactive bowel sounds
—Right lower quadrant (RLQ) mass and tenderness
—Palpable thickened loop of intestine

- Rectal and perianal examination: skin tag, fissure, fistula, and abscess

 Laboratory Aids

TESTS

Laboratory Tests

- Complete blood count (CBC): microcytic anemia as a result of iron-deficiency, normocytic anemia as a result of chronic disease, macrocytosis suggesting nutrient deficiency: iron, B12, folate, zinc
- Erythrocyte sedimentation rate, C-reactive protein, fecal calprotectin (disease activity)
- Electrolytes (hydration, renal function)
- Transaminases, alkaline phosphatase, γ-glutamyl transpeptidase (hepatobiliary disease)
- Stool for occult blood and presence of white cells
- Stool cultures, Clostridium difficile toxin A and B
- Perinuclear anti-neutrophil cytoplasmic antibody (pANCA) and anti-Saccharomyces cerevisiae antibody (ASCA) may be helpful in differentiation between types of IBD

IMAGING

- Consider plain abdominal radiograph in acute presentation to rule out obstruction or perforation.
- Barium upper GI and small bowel follow-through; to evaluate extent of disease in small bowel not accessible to endoscopy.
- Barium enema has been replaced by colonoscopy in acute colitis; useful in evaluation of complications such as strictures and fistulas.
- CT scan and ultrasound useful for evaluation of complications (abscess, phlegmon).
- Magnetic resonance imaging, and abdominal ultrasound are increasingly being used for assessment of disease extent and activity.
- Colonoscopy and upper endoscopy with multiple biopsies are the gold standard tests for initial evaluation and diagnosis of Crohn disease.
- Video capsule endoscopy can be used to access small bowel not visualized at the time of endoscopy.

 Therapy

DRUGS

- The goal of therapy is resolution of all symptoms, appropriate growth, and good quality of life. The therapy is used in a step-wise fashion.
- Several 5-aminosalicylic acid (5-ASA) preparations are being used according to their intestinal site of activation as a result of their anti-inflammatory properties:
—Asacol (terminal ileum, colon) 50 to 100 mg/kg per day (maximum 4.8 g per day for active disease and 3.2 g per day to maintain remission)
—Pentasa (duodenum, jejunum, ileum, colon), 50 to 100 mg/kg per day (maximum, 4 g per day for active disease and 3 g per day to maintain remission)
—Colasal (6.75 g per day, can be given to small children as liquid preparation)
—Rowasa, 4-g enemas and 500-mg suppositories qd–b.i.d. PR
- Corticosteroids can control intestinal inflammation (1 to 2 mg/kg per day oral prednisone (maximum, 60 mg). Initially, patient is treated for several weeks and tapered off within several weeks. Topical hydrocortisone is useful in localized left-sided colonic disease and is available in liquid and foam enemas. Corticosteroid with controlled ileal release, budesonide (9 mg per day) is available but no pediatric data or indications exist.
- Nutritional therapy is frequently used in Europe and Canada as a first-line therapy:
—Elemental and polymeric diet reported to be effective in inducing remission in active disease
—To correct growth failure an increase in caloric intake is recommended and can be given as overnight nasogastric feeding if oral supplements are not tolerated.
- Azathioprine, 2.0 to 3.0 mg/kg per day, and its metabolite 6-mercaptopurine, 1.0 to

1.5 mg/kg per day are used for the immunomodulatory properties in patients who are unresponsive to corticosteroids, or dependent on them, and for perianal disease. Adverse events include liver toxicity, and leukopenia (frequent laboratory follow up is necessary and white cell count should be maintained greater than 3 to 4 × 109/L and platelets greater than 100 × 109/L.
- Methotrexate, 15 to 25 mg IM q week.
- Other immunomodulatory therapy infrequently used: cyclosporine, tacrolimus (FK-506), thalidomide etc.
- Antibiotics
—Metronidazole (15 mg/kg/d)
—Ciprofloxacin (20 mg/kg/d).
- Infliximab, a biologic, chimeric anti-tumor necrosis factor-α antibody (5 mg/kg IV infusion, given q 2 to 3 months, after initial 3-dose induction therapy at 0, 2, and 6 weeks) for severe and fistulizing disease unresponsive to other therapy.
- Other biologic therapy currently in clinical trials.
- Complementary therapy (probiotics, pre-biotics).

SURGERY

Surgery is used in patients with localized disease unresponsive to other therapy, intractable bleeding, stricturizing disease especially in case of proximal intestinal dilatation, and perforation. There are several types of procedures available: strictureplasty, abscess drainage, and intestinal resection (side to side anastomosis is widely accepted method). Most of these procedures are performed laparoscopically, which reduces recovery time.
Surgery is not curative and postoperative recurrence at the site of anastomosis is common.

 Follow-Up

- The morbidity of this disease is high. The majority of patients experience recurring disease.
- In adults, 55% of patients will have mild-to-severe disease at any one time, with the remainder in remission.
- Most patients have good general health in between disease and go on to lead productive lives.
- Carcinoma surveillance is necessary on regular basis.
- After 5 and 20 years of disease, the probability of survival is 98% and 89% of expected survival, respectively.
- Death is a rare complication (2.4% in a large series).

 Common Questions and Answers

Q: Should the diet of patients with Crohn disease be restricted?

A: Adequate nutrition is very important, especially in children with Crohn disease. Balanced nutrition is required to assure appropriate growth and development. The only foods not recommended are poorly digestible vegetables (if eaten raw), nuts, and popcorn, which can cause obstruction in the narrowed, inflamed intestine. Patients with secondary lactose intolerance should use lactase supplements, or avoid milk products although ensuring adequate calories and calcium intake.

Q: What is the cause of Crohn disease?
A: Both genetic and environmental factors are important in the development of Crohn disease. Possible environmental factors include aseptic environment in the first few years of life, lack of breast-feeding, frequent use of antibiotics or aspirin, and diet.

Q: Where can I learn more about Crohn disease?
A: The Crohn and Colitis Foundation of America (CCFA at www.CCFA.org) is a nonprofit organization dedicated to the care of people with Crohn disease and ulcerative colitis.

Q: What new therapies will be used in the near future?
A: Biologic agents, which use our recently improved knowledge of the immune system, either to downregulate inflammatory mediators or upregulate immunomodulatory mediators. It is hoped that this new class of therapies will greatly improve our care of people with Crohn disease.

ICD-9-CM 558.9

BIBLIOGRAPHY

Cabre E, Gassull MA. Nutritional and metabolic issues in inflammatory bowel disease. *Curr Opin Clin Nutr Metab Care* 2003;6(5):569–576.

Hildebrand H, Karlberg J, Kristiansson B. Longitudinal growth in children with IBD. *J Pediatr Gastroenterol Nutr* 1994;18(2): 165–173.

Mamula P, Markowitz JE, Baldassano RN. Inflammatory bowel disease in early childhood and adolescence: special considerations. *Gastroenterol Clin N Am* 2003;32(3):967–995.

Navarro F, Hanauer SB. Treatment of inflammatory bowel disease: safety and tolerability issues. *Am J Gastroenterol* 2003;98(12 Suppl):S18–S23.

Seidman E, Leleiko N, Ament M, et al. Nutritional issues in pediatric inflammatory bowel disease. *J Pediatr Gastroenterol Nutr* 1991;12:424.

Spray C, Debelle GD, Murphy MS. Current diagnosis, management and morbidity in paediatric inflammatory bowel disease. *Acta Paediatr* 2001;90(4):400–405.

Authors: Douglas Jacobstein, Robert Baldassano, and Petar Mamula

Croup (Laryngotracheobronchitis)

 Database

DEFINITION

- Croup (laryngotracheobronchitis) is an acute viral infection classically characterized by a triad of symptoms: a barking cough, inspiratory stridor, and hoarseness that result from variable degrees of subglottic edema and inflammation.
- Spasmodic croup is characterized as recurrent, acute onset of inspiratory stridor and barking cough, usually occurring at night for several hours and quickly resolving. It can recur over several nights in a single episode and occur several times a year.

ETIOLOGY

- Human parainfluenza virus type 1, most commonly identified
- Human parainfluenza virus types 2 and 3
- Respiratory syncytial virus (RSV)
- Human metapneumovirus
- Adenovirus
- Influenza viruses A and B
- Enteroviruses
- *Mycoplasma pneumoniae* (rare)

EPIDEMIOLOGY

- Annual incidence: 1.5% to 6% of children less than 6 years old
- Most commonly occurs in the first 3 years of life (6 to 36 months)
- Peak incidence: second year of life (60 per 1,000)
- The male:female ratio is 3:2.
- Most prevalent in the late fall and winter

Severity Score of Croup Patients

INDICATOR OF SEVERITY OF ILLNESS	SCORE
Inspiratory stridor	
None	0
At rest, with stethoscope	1
At rest, without stethoscope	2
Retractions	
None	0
Mild	1
Moderate	2
Severe	3
Air entry	
Normal	0
Decreased	1
Severely decreased	2
Cyanosis	
None	0
With agitation	4
At rest	5
Level of consciousness	
Normal	0
Altered mental status	5
Mild croup	0–3
Moderate to severe croup	>3

- Fewer children require hospitalization than previously

COMPLICATIONS

- Poor oral intake/dehydration
- Hypoxia
- Upper airway obstruction
- Respiratory failure (rare)

PROGNOSIS

- The vast majority of patients do not require hospitalization.
- Almost all patients go on to complete recovery.

 Differential Diagnosis

CONGENITAL

- Tracheoesophageal fistula
- Foregut duplication
- Laryngomalacia
- Tracheomalacia
- Vocal cord paralysis
- Arnold-Chiari malformation
- Vascular ring
- Laryngeal web

INFECTIOUS

- Epiglottis (although less common since universal HiB vaccine)
- Bacterial tracheitis
- Retropharyngeal abscess
- Adenotonsillitis
- Diphtheria
- Pneumonia
- Ulcerative laryngitis

ENVIRONMENTAL

- Foreign-body aspiration
- Caustic material ingestion (very alkaline products)
- Smoke inhalation

TRAUMATIC

- Subglottic edema/stenosis post intubation
- Laryngeal or subglottic hematoma
- Laryngeal fracture

TUMORS

- Papillomatosis
- Hemangioma
- Cystic hygroma
- Lymphoma
- Rhabdomyosarcoma
- Thymoma
- Teratoma
- Thyroglossal duct cyst
- Branchial cleft cyst

GENETIC/METABOLIC

- Hypocalcemia

ALLERGIC/INFLAMMATORY

- Asthma
- Angioneurotic edema (anaphylaxis)
- Microaspiration secondary to gastroesophageal reflux

 Data Gathering

HISTORY

Question: How long have the symptoms been present? Is the process acute or chronic?
Significance: Croup is an acute illness.

Question: Any fever?
Significance: Croup is often associated with fever. If no fever, consider foreign-body or caustic ingestions.

Question: When did the stridor begin or occur?
Significance: If the child awakens at night, this supports the diagnosis of croup. If the child is playing at the onset of stridor, consider foreign-body aspiration.

Question: How have the symptoms progressed?
Significance: Ask about the prodrome of upper respiratory tract symptoms, sore throat, change in quality of voice, dysphagia/drooling (consider peritonsillar or retropharyngeal abscess, epiglottitis), dysphonia, particular position of comfort.

Question: Is there a history of previous airway problems or recurrent stridor?
Significance: Recurrence or a prolonged history should lead one to consider subglottic stenosis, gastroesophageal reflux or spasmodic croup.

 Physical Examination

- In general, children with croup are often anxious and ill-appearing. Allow them to sit in a comfortable position and in their caregiver's (parent's) lap, which may reduce the agitation provoked by examination.
- It is important initially to assess level of consciousness, irritability, color, and respiratory distress.
- Vital signs: Check for pulsus paradoxus (large inspiratory drop in systolic blood pressure because of a fall in pleural pressure secondary to airway obstruction).
- What is the preferred position? Sitting in a tripod position with the neck extended to "sniff" is concerning for epiglottis.
- Assess work of breathing, including respiratory rate, nasal flaring, retractions, abdominal breathing, and head bobbing.
- Assess air entry into the chest.
- Listen for audible stridor at rest (biphasic stridor is particularly concerning for impending respiratory failure).
- Listen for the presence of wheezing, which may indicate lower respiratory tract involvement.
- Observe for drooling.

- Assess the quality of the voice.
- The presence of a neck mass is concerning for bacterial infection.
- Bruising of the neck may be suggestive of trauma.
- The Croup Score (as developed by Westley et al. and modified by Super et al.) is utilized by many clinicians to describe the severity of symptoms (see table, Severity Score of Croup Patients). It is probably the best-validated scoring system in croup that will demonstrate change in clinical status after intervention.

 ## Laboratory Aids

LABORATORY TESTS

- In general, laboratory tests are not required to make this diagnosis.
- Blood testing, such as arterial blood gas or complete blood count with differential, is not helpful in diagnosing croup. In fact, the pain and fear of testing will likely heighten the child's anxiety and worsen respiratory distress.

RADIOGRAPHIC STUDIES

Anteroposterior and lateral view x-rays of the neck: the anteroposterior view classically demonstrates the "steeple" sign in patients with croup. The lateral view is useful in ruling out epiglottis, retropharyngeal cellulitis/abscess (fullness or free air in the retropharyngeal space), and a radiopaque foreign body. Generally, croup is a clinical diagnosis and x-rays will rarely be needed.

OTHER PROCEDURES

Pulse oximetry: helpful for children in respiratory distress to determine if hypoxia is present.

 ## Emergency Care

- Racemic epinephrine (see below)
- The need for endotracheal intubation is very rare.

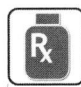 ## Therapy

- Most do well with conservative management at home or, much less commonly, after a short stay in the emergency department.
- In the child with impending respiratory failure, prompt intubation and direct visualization of the airway in the operating room is imperative. Do not wait for x-rays to confirm a diagnosis.
- Steroids: Utilized in the outpatient and inpatient settings, steroids have resulted in dramatic reduction in the number of admissions and length of hospital stays in patients with croup.

—Dexamethasone (half-life 36 to 54 hours) is given intramuscularly (IM) or orally in the setting of moderate-to-severe croup (croup score >or equal to 3). A few studies have shown that a single dose of 0.15 mg/kg is as effective as 0.6 mg/kg, although there are not a sufficient number of studies to date to firmly recommend a change of dosage. There is no evidence to support multiple doses. Oral dexamethasone is the most cost-effective steroid treatment available.
—Budesonide given via nebulizer at a dose of 2 mg administered every 12 hours has been shown in recent studies to be as effective as dexamethasone in reducing symptoms. It has less systemic absorption compared to dexamethasone, with maximum deposition of drug in the upper airway. Though widely accepted, budesonide is not as readily used as dexamethasone because it is much more expensive.
—Racemic epinephrine: A nebulized racemic epinephrine treatment offers immediate reduction in swelling of the laryngeal airway in children who present in extreme respiratory distress or in whom humidified air does not improve stridor (croup score >3) after 20 to 30 minutes. Dose: 0.5 mL of 2.25% solution (D- and L-isomers) in 2.5 mL normal saline delivered via nebulizer as needed.
—L-epinephrine: If racemic epinephrine is not available, 5 cc of L-epinephrine 1:10,000 delivered via nebulizer is effective.

 ## Follow-Up

- In most cases, the illness is self-limited, lasting 3 to 5 days.
- A "rebound phenomenon" with worsening of stridor and respiratory distress after initial relief with the racemic epinephrine treatment may be seen up to 2 hours posttreatment in some patients. Several studies have shown that children can be safely discharged 3 to 4 hours after racemic epinephrine treatment.

PITFALLS

Recurrent croup may signal an underlying anatomic problem. In younger children (infants), congenital anomalies and gastroesophageal reflux are more likely contributors.

 ## Common Questions and Answers

Q: Why is humidity not listed as a recommended treatment for a patient presenting with croup?
A: Humidified air delivered in the hospital or at home has been used in the management of croup for a long time. Most of the evidence has been anecdotal. In the last year the first randomized controlled trial of mist in the ED setting showed no improvement in symptoms in patients with moderate croup.

Q: Should all children with croup receive steroids?
A: Steroids are now the first line treatment for croup. Meta-analysis of the available literature strongly supports the use of dexamethasone (oral or IM) or nebulized budesonide for children with moderate-to-severe croup scores.

Q: Do children who receive racemic epinephrine for croup require hospitalization?
A: No. Several studies have shown that after a 3- to 4-hour period of observation and dexamethasone, children can be safely discharged home. Any rebound effects should occur within the first 2 hours.

Q: Can dexamethasone be given via nebulizer?
A: Nebulized dexamethasone performed no better than placebo at improving clinical symptoms. The oral route is optimal as it is inexpensive and the least noxious to the young patient.

Q: Can I just give my patient prednisolone syrup instead of dexamethasone?
A: The bioavailability of steroids is excellent, whether IM or orally administered. The half-life of dexamethasone is much longer (36 to 54 hours) than that of prednisone (12 to 36 hours). With croup, many patients have poor oral intake exacerbated by respiratory distress. If oral intake can be assured, dexamethasone at 0.15 mg/kg or 0.6 mg/kg (as a single dose for croup has been proven to be inexpensive and effective. There are no studies evaluating the effectiveness or dosing of prednisolone in croup.

Q: Why is budesonide dosed every 12 hours?
A: Like much of our clinical practice, dosing guidelines are based on what successful studies utilized. Every-12-hour dosing is an interval used in asthma management that has been extrapolated to croup.

ICD-9-CM 464.4

BIBLIOGRAPHY

Brown JC. The management of croup. *Br Med Bull* 2002;61:189–202.

Donaldson D, Poleski D, Knipple E, et al. Intramuscular versus oral dexamethasone for the treatment of moderate-to-severe croup: a randomized, double-blind trial. *Acad Emerg Med* 2003;10:16–21.

Neto GM, Kentab O, Klassen TP, Osmond MH. A randomized controlled trial of mist in the acute treatment of moderate croup. *Acad Emerg Med* 2002;9:873–879.

Russell K, Wiebe N, Saenz A, et al. Glucocorticoids for croup (Cochrane Review). In: *The Cochrane Library*. Chichester, UK: John Wiley & Sons, Ltd, 2004.

Westley CR, Cotton EK, Brooks JG. Nebulized racemic epinephrine by IPPB for the treatment of croup. *Am J Dis Child* 1978;132:484–487.

Author: Shannon Connor Phillips

Cryptococcal Infections

Database

DEFINITION

Cryptococcosis, an opportunistic fungal infection caused by *Cryptococcus neoformans*, may involve several organ systems, including the central nervous system (CNS), lungs, bones, visceral organs, and skin.

PATHOPHYSIOLOGY

• Primary infection occurs through the inhalation of aerosolized soil particles containing the yeast forms. The skin and gastrointestinal (GI) tract are also portals of entry.
• Protective immune response requires specific T-cell–mediated immunity.
• CNS involvement with *C. neoformans* results from hematogenous dissemination.

EPIDEMIOLOGY

• Infection occasionally occurs in normal hosts.
• Occurs in 5% to 15% of HIV-infected adults, usually with CD4+ lymphocyte counts <50 cells/mm^3. It is less common in HIV-infected children, occurring in 0.8% to 2.3% of cases. The infection rate in children reflects their lower exposure to sources of *C. neoformans*. The overall seroprevalence is 0% in neonates and 4.1% in school-aged children, compared to 69% in adults.
• 1% to 3% of solid organ transplant recipients develop *C. neoformans* infections
• There is no person-to-person spread of the infection.

COMPLICATIONS

• CNS involvement occurs in approximately three-fourths of patients.
• Pulmonary, cutaneous, and bone involvement may occur (see Associated Diseases).
• In solid organ transplant patients, those receiving tacrolimus immunosuppression are less likely to have CNS involvement and more likely to have skin, soft tissue, or osteoarticular involvement.

PROGNOSIS

• Survival is good with early treatment but, in HIV-infected patients, relapse rates are high (see Prevention).
• Up to 40% of patients with cryptococcal meningitis have residual neurologic deficits.
• In the normal host with cryptococcal meningitis, patients with serum or CSF cryptococcal titers >1:32 or CSF WBCs <20/mm^3 have a worse prognosis. In HIV-infected patients, it is unclear whether the magnitude of titers affects outcome.
• In HIV-infected patients with cryptococcal meningitis, poor prognostic factors include the presence of hyponatremia, concomitant growth of *C. neoformans* from another site, increased intracranial pressure, and any

alteration of mental status. Placement of a ventricular shunt has not been shown to improve mortality.
• Patients with isolated pulmonary or cutaneous disease have a favorable prognosis.

ASSOCIATED DISEASES

• *C. neoformans* is the most common cause of fungal meningitis in the United States
• Disseminated infection occurs more commonly among immunocompromised hosts.
• Concurrent *Pneumocystis carinii* pneumonia was detected in 13% of adults with cryptococcal meningitis.
• Pulmonary involvement is asymptomatic in up to 50% of cases and disease may be either focal or widespread.
• Bone involvement occurs in 10% of cases of disseminated cryptococcal infection.
• Cutaneous involvement mimics acne-type eruptions that ulcerate and results from hematogenous spread of the organism or from direct extension of bone infection.

Differential Diagnosis

• Although cryptococcosis occurs most commonly in HIV-infected patients with low CD4+ lymphocyte counts, the diagnosis warrants consideration in all febrile immunocompromised children (e.g., solid organ transplant, leukemia)
• Meningitis: Viruses and *Mycobacterium tuberculosis*.
• Pneumonia: Other pulmonary mycoses, including aspergillosis, histoplasmosis, and blastomycosis. Also consider *Mycoplasma pneumoniae* and *M. tuberculosis*.
• Bone: Osteogenic sarcoma.
• Cutaneous: Molluscum contagiosum, HSV infection, pyoderma gangrenosum, and cellulitis

Data Gathering

HISTORY

• Cryptococcal meningitis may present as either an indolent infection or acute illness.
• Symptoms of cryptococcal meningitis include headache, malaise, and low-grade fever. Nausea, vomiting, altered mentation, and photophobia are less common. Stiff neck, focal neurologic symptoms (e.g., decreased hearing, facial nerve palsy, or diplopia), and seizures are rare.
• Primary pulmonary cryptococcal disease is not well described in children because most cases are disseminated at the time of diagnosis. Fifty percent of adults have cough or chest pain, and fewer have sputum production, weight loss, fever, and hemoptysis.
• In immunocompromised hosts, the onset of infection is more rapid and the course more severe. Pulmonary involvement is minimal when dissemination occurs quickly.

Physical Examination

None of the presenting signs of cryptococcal infection are sufficiently characteristic to distinguish it from other infections, particularly in immunocompromised patients.

• CNS involvement: Nuchal rigidity, photophobia, and focal neurologic deficits.
• Respiratory tract involvement: Cough, tachypnea, grunting, and subcostal or intercostal retractions. Decreased breath sounds or dullness to percussion may be present or the lung exam may be normal.
• Cutaneous manifestations: Erythematous or verrucous papules, nodules, pustules, acneiform lesions, ulcers, abscesses, or granulomas. Lesions can occur anywhere on the body but are found most often on the face and neck.
• Mucocutaneous findings are present in 10% to 15% of cases of disseminated disease.

Laboratory Aids

TESTS

Test: Lumbar puncture
Significance: Diagnose cryptococcal meningitis.

• CSF should be sent for cell count and differential; protein; glucose; cultures for bacterial, fungal, and viral pathogens; India ink stain; and cryptococcal antigen.
• Examination of the CSF reveals <500 WBCs/mm^3 (usually <100 WBCs/mm^3), mostly mononuclear leukocytes, with minimal changes in protein. CSF glucose is <50 mg/dL in approximately 65% of patients.
• Budding yeast are seen on India ink stain in 50% of cases.
• CSF cultures are positive in approximately 90% of patients.
• The latex agglutination test for cryptococcal polysaccharide antigen is specific, sensitive, and rapid. Titers ≥1:4 suggest the diagnosis of cryptococcal infection if appropriate controls (to exclude the presence of rheumatoid factor or other nonspecific agglutinins) are negative.
• HIV-infected patients with pneumonia and CD4+ T-lymphocyte counts <200 cells/mm^3 should be evaluated with sputum fungal culture, blood fungal culture, and a serum cryptococcal antigen test. A lumbar puncture to exclude the possibility of occult meningitis should be considered. If any test is positive for *C. neoformans*, then a lumbar puncture should be performed to exclude cryptococcal meningitis.

Test: Blood culture and serum cryptococcal antigen titers
Significance: Diagnose disseminated cryptococcal infection.

Test: Sputum culture
Significance: Diagnose cryptococcal pneumonia.

Test: Skin or bone biopsy
Significance: Diagnose cutaneous or osteoarticular cryptococcal infection.

Test: HIV testing
Significance: Evaluation for immunodeficiencies, including HIV, is warranted in any patient with cryptococcosis.

Test: Complete blood count with differential
Significance: May reveal hypereosinophilia (absolute eosinophil count $>1,500/mm^3$)

Test: Serum electrolytes
Significance: Detect hyponatremia, a complication of cryptococcal meningitis.

RADIOGRAPHIC IMAGING

Test: Chest radiograph (PA and lateral)
Significance: Nodules, diffuse infiltrates, and pleural effusions may be seen in cryptococcal pneumonia.

Test: Head CT
Significance: May demonstrate granulomatous lesions or elevated ICP.

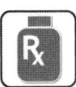 ## Therapy

Clinical management depends on extent of disease and immune status of the host.

PULMONARY AND EXTRAPULMONARY DISEASE, HIV-NEGATIVE

• A normal host with isolated pulmonary nodules does not need treatment if the serum cryptococcal antigen is negative and the patient is asymptomatic.
• Patients with extensive pulmonary disease or evidence of extrapulmonary disease require treatment.
• Fluconazole (PO; 6 to 12 mg/kg per day, max. 400 mg) for 6 to 12 months. Alternative regimen: itraconazole (PO; 4 to 10 mg/kg per day, max. 400 mg) for 6 to 12 months; or amphotericin B (IV; 0.7 to 1 mg/kg per day) for 3 to 6 months.
• HIV-negative, immunocompromised hosts with pulmonary or extrapulmonary disease and those with severe symptoms are treated with amphotericin B in the same fashion as patients with CNS disease.
• Due to the high rate of relapse in immunocompromised patients, maintenance therapy with fluconazole should continue as long as the patient is immunocompromised (see Prevention).

CNS DISEASE, HIV-NEGATIVE

• Induction/consolidation: amphotericin B plus flucytosine (PO; 100 to 150 mg/kg per day divided every 6 hours) for 2 weeks, then fluconazole (PO; see above for dosing) for a minimum of 10 weeks. Alternative regimen: amphotericin B plus flucytosine for 6 to 10 weeks.

PULMONARY AND EXTRAPULMONARY DISEASE, HIV-INFECTED

• Fluconazole (PO) lifelong. Alternative regimen: itraconazole (PO) lifelong.
• Consider surgical debridement for patients with persistent or refractory pulmonary or bone lesions.

CNS DISEASE, HIV-INFECTED

• Induction/consolidation: Amphotericin B (IV) plus flucytosine (PO) for at least 2 weeks, followed by fluconazole PO lifelong. Alternate regimen: fluconazole plus flucytosine for 6 weeks followed by fluconazole or itraconazole lifelong (see above for dosing).
• Intrathecal amphotericin B is very toxic but may be used in refractory cases.
• HIV-infected patients require continuation of antifungal drugs indefinitely because of the high recurrence rate of cryptococcosis.
• Lipid formulation of amphotericin B (IV; 3 to 6 mg/kg per day) may be substituted for amphotericin B.
• Flucytosine is used only in combination with amphotericin B and not as a single agent because of the rapid emergence of drug resistance.
• Itraconazole for IV administration is available but there are insufficient data to guide its current use. Voriconazole, a new triazole antifungal agent, demonstrates excellent in vitro activity against *C. neoformans* but requires clinical study. Caspofungin, a new echinocandin antifungal agent, is not active against *C. neoformans*.

 ## Follow-Up

Follow-up is important as a result of the risk of relapse. Patients should be seen at 3-month intervals for 12 to 18 months following treatment, with cultures obtained for fungal isolation. Immunocompromised patients should be evaluated every 2 to 3 months, even while on suppressive therapy, to monitor clinically for relapse.

• Repeat lumbar punctures documenting a decrease in CSF cryptococcal antigen and sterility of culture are useful in evaluating response to treatment. During therapy for acute meningitis, an unchanged or increased titer of CSF antigen correlates with clinical and microbiologic failure to respond to treatment. Serum antigen titers are not helpful for this purpose.
• Evaluate patients with cryptococcal meningitis for neurologic sequelae.
• HIV-infected patients require lifelong suppressive antifungal therapy (see Prevention).

PREVENTION

• The dramatic reduction of cryptococcal infections since the introduction of potent antiretroviral therapy suggests that the best prophylaxis for cryptococcosis is effective treatment of HIV.
• In HIV-infected patients with low CD4+ lymphocyte counts, relapse rates are 100% without maintenance antifungal therapy, 18% to 25% with amphotericin B or itraconazole, and 2% to 3% with fluconazole.
• Prophylaxis with fluconazole is also effective in preventing new onset cryptococcal disease.
• Cryptococcal meningitis occurred once (0.4%) among 231 HIV-infected children receiving fluconazole 200 mg three times weekly.
• There is no consensus on the duration of fluconazole therapy after acute therapy in HIV-negative immunocompromised patients. Most experts provide suppressive antifungal therapy for at least 1 year after the completion of acute treatment and then reassess its ongoing use based on the level of current immunosuppression.

 ## Common Questions and Answers

Q: What are the sources of *Cryptococcus* in nature?
A: Pigeon droppings and soil. Naturally acquired infections occur in lower mammals, especially cats. However, neither animal-to-human nor human-to-human infections have been reported.

Q: Should all children with *Cryptococcus* be evaluated for immunodeficiency?
A: Yes.

ICD-9-CD 117.5

BIBLIOGRAPHY

Harrison TS. Cryptococcus neoformans and cryptococcosis. *J Infect* 2000;41:12–17.

Perfect JR, Casadevall A. Cryptococcosis. *Infect Dis Clin N Am* 2002;16(4):837–74.

Powderly WG. Current approach to the acute management of cryptococcal infections. *J Infect* 2000;41(1):18–22.

Author: Samir S. Shah

Cryptorchidism

 ## Database

DEFINITION

An undescended testis is one that does not remain at the bottom of the scrotum after the cremaster muscle has been fatigued by overstretching. This is commonly confused with a retractile testis, one that may not always lie in the scrotum, but that will stay in the bottom of the scrotum after overstretching the cremaster.

CAUSES

• A multifactorial mechanism of occurrence involving two types of theories have been postulated:

—Hypogonadotropic hypogonadism
—Abnormal mechanical factors (gubernaculum, epididymis, genitofemoral nerve innervation, intraabdominal pressure)

• While boys with undescended testes do have abnormal attachment of the gubernaculum, the mechanical theories do not consistently explain the testis histology found in cryptorchidism.
• Many boys with cryptorchidism have lower morning urinary LH and a decreased LH/FSH response to GnRH, corresponding to the abnormal germ cell development in both the undescended and contralateral descended testis.
• The normal initial postnatal gonadotropin surge at 60 to 90 days is absent or blunted in some boys with cryptorchidism. Without this surge, Leydig cells do not proliferate, testosterone does not increase, germ cells do not mature, and infertility may result. This suggests that a mild endocrinopathy is responsible and cryptorchidism may be a variant of hypogonadotropic hypogonadism.
• Secondary undescended testes can occur after inguinal surgery, either a result of scar tissue or difficulty in diagnosing an undescended testis in a young boy with a hernia.

PATHOLOGY

• The undescended testis fails to show normal maturation at both 3 months and 5 years.

—At 3 months, the fetal gonocytes are transformed into adult dark spermatogonia.
—At 5 years, the adult dark spermatogonia become primary spermatocytes.
—Both of these steps are abnormal in the undescended testis, and to a lesser extent, the contralateral descended testis.
—Previous beliefs that the undescended testis was normal between birth and 1 year are incorrect, since they were derived from counts of all germ cells without taking into account whether maturation was occurring.
—After 2 years of age, thermal effects on the testis being left out of position are seen independent of the endocrinologic effects.

GENETICS

Of boys with undescended testes, 4% of their fathers and 6% to 10% of their brothers also had undescended testes. Androgen receptor gene mutations are not linked to isolated cryptorchidism. Abnormalities in HOXA10, HOXA11, INSL3, and the LGR8/GREAT receptor genes are being investigated in patients with cryptorchidism.

EPIDEMIOLOGY

• 3% of full-term boys have cryptorchidism.
• This percentage falls to 1% by 3 months.
• Normal descent occurs during the 7th month of gestation.
• The majority of testes that will spontaneously descend do so by 3 months of age, possibly as a result of the gonadotropin surge that is responsible for maturation of the germ cells.
• Therefore, patients with undescended testes should be referred for surgical evaluation no later than 3 months of age.
• There are two peaks for detection of undescended testes: at birth, and at 5 to 7 years of age. The latter group probably represents those patients with low undescended testes that become apparent with linear growth. Bilateral undescended testes occur in 10% of patients with undescended testicles. Unilateral anorchia is found in 5% of patients. Patients with Prune Belly, Klinefelter, Noonan, and Prader-Willi syndromes have undescended testes.

 ## Differential Diagnosis

• Retractile testes are commonly confused with undescended testes. The key to distinguishing them from undescended testes is the physical exam. All retractile and many undescended testes can be delivered into the scrotum. The retractile testis will stay in the scrotum after the cremaster muscle has been overstretched. The low undescended testis will immediately pop back to its undescended position after being released.
• Atrophic or "vanishing" testes are found anywhere along the normal path to the scrotum. They are believed to be a result of neonatal vascular ischemia. The contralateral testis can be hypertrophied in these boys, but this is not a reliable diagnostic sign.
• Upon evaluation, 80% of nonpalpable testes are present in either the abdomen or in the inguinal canal. A child with bilateral nonpalpable testes should have an endocrine evaluation to rule out anorchia or intersex.
• Cryptorchidism associated with hypospadias should also raise the possibility of intersex states, which occurs in 30% to 40% of patients, mainly consisting of defects in gonadotropin or testosterone synthesis.

 ## Data Gathering

HISTORY

• Prematurity
• Exogenous maternal hormones (used in infertility treatments)
• Use of oral contraceptives
• Central nervous system lesions
• Previous inguinal surgery
• Family history for urologic abnormalities
• Neonatal deaths
• Precocious puberty
• Infertility
• Consanguinity

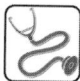 ## Physical Examination

• The undescended testis may be found at the upper scrotum, in the superficial inguinal pouch, or in the inguinal canal. For treatment purposes, the main distinction that needs to be made is whether or not the testis is palpable.
• The patient should be examined supine in the frogleg position with both legs free.

—With warmed hands, check the size, location, and texture of the contralateral descended testis.
—Begin the examination of the undescended testis at the anterior superior iliac spine.
—Sweep the groin from lateral to medial with the nondominant hand.
—Once the testis is palpated, grasp it with the dominant hand, and continue to sweep the testis toward the scrotum with the other hand.
—With a combination of sweeping and pulling, it is sometimes possible to bring the testis to the scrotum.
—Maintain the position of the testis in the scrotum for a minute, so that the cremaster muscle is fatigued.
—Release the testis, and if it remains in place, it is a retractile testis.
—If it immediately pops back, it is an undescended testis.

• For the difficult-to-examine patient (chubby 6-month-olds or obese youths), the sitting cross-legged position can help relax the cremaster. Wetting the fingers of the nondominant hand with lubricating jelly or soap can increase the sensitivity of the fingers in palpating the small, mobile testis.

Laboratory Aids

TESTS

- For the typical patient with a unilateral palpable or nonpalpable undescended testis, no further laboratory evaluation is necessary.
- For the patient with bilateral undescended testis, with one testis palpable, no further workup is necessary.
- The patient with bilateral nonpalpable testes should have a chromosomal and endocrinologic evaluation, as should the patient with one or two undescended testes and hypospadias.
- If the patient has bilateral nonpalpable testes and is younger than 3 months of age, serum LH, FSH, and testosterone will determine whether testes are present.
- After that age, hCG stimulation will result in a measurable serum testosterone if testes are present. A failure to respond to hCG stimulation in combination with elevated LH/FSH levels is consistent with anorchia.

IMAGING

Ultrasound, CT, and MRI can detect testes in the inguinal region, but this is also the region where they are most easily palpable. They are only 50% accurate in showing intraabdominal testes. Imaging is rarely necessary preoperatively, since for nonpalpable testes, exam under anesthesia, open inguinal exploration, or laparoscopy is necessary to confirm the presence of testes.

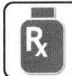 ## Therapy

HORMONAL THERAPY

- This is widely used in Europe for inducing descent of undescended testes. Both GnRH and hCG are used, with success rates of 30% to 50%. Treatment is most successful for low undescended testes, but there is a 25% relapse rate.
- For these reasons, as well as the fact that GnRH and hCG are not approved for this indication in the United States, most therapy in the United States aimed at bringing the testis down to the scrotum is surgical (orchiopexy).
- The use of hormonal therapy after orchiopexy to improve semen analyses in high-risk patients is in its preliminary stages of investigation in Europe and the United States

SURGICAL THERAPY

Goals in bringing the testis into the scrotum:

- Prevent ongoing thermal damage to the testis.
- Treat the associated hernia sac.
- Prevent testis torsion/injury against the pubic bone.
- Achieve a good cosmetic result/avoid psychological effects of empty scrotum.
- Show the older child how to perform testicular self-exam for cancer.

PROGNOSIS

- Surgery cannot reverse the maturational failure of the undescended testis, but it can prevent ongoing thermal injury.
- Parents are often concerned about future fertility.

—In patients who have undergone orchiopexy at an early age, it appears that 90% of boys with unilateral cryptorchidism and 64% with bilateral cryptorchidism will achieve paternity.
—Patients who are interested in their risk for infertility may have a semen analysis performed at age 18.

- Surgery also has no effect on the increased risk of testicular cancer (annual age-adjusted increase from 2 to 3 to 49/100,000), but it can make the testis easier to examine.

—Approximately 15% of tumors arise in the contralateral descended testis.
—All patients should be taught proper monthly testicular self-exam at the time of puberty. Some patients with cryptorchidism are at a higher risk of cancer (prune belly syndrome, ambiguous genitalia, karyotypic abnormalities, or the post-pubertal boy).

 ## Follow-Up

After successful orchiopexy, patients are examined at 6 to 12 months to check on testicular size and position. They are rechecked at puberty to explain the technique and need for monthly testis self-exam concerning early recognition of testis cancer. Patients with retractile testes should be examined annually until age 7 because about 5% will be found to have a testis out of the scrotum.

 ## Common Questions and Answers

Q: If there is only one testicle in the scrotum, will fertility be affected?
A: In general, the outlook for paternity is good in a patient with only one descended testicle. Paternity is more significantly affected with a history of two undescended testicles.

Q: Why do patients with retractile testes require follow up?
A: The ability to distinguish between retractile and undescended testes can be difficult in some patients. Some of the patients will be found to have true undescended testes as they grow.

ICD-9-CM 752.51

BIBLIOGRAPHY

Berkowitz GS, Lapinski RH, Dolgin SE, et al. Prevalence and natural history of cryptorchidism. *Pediatrics* 1993;92:44–49.

Callaghan P. Undescended testis. *Pediatr Rev* 2000;21:395.

Kogan S, Hadziselimovic F, Howards SS, et al. Pediatric andrology. In: Gillenwater JY, Grayhack JT, Howards SS, et al., eds. *Adult and Pediatric Urology*. 4th Ed. Mosby: St. Louis, 2002.

Lee PA, Coughlin MT. Fertility after bilateral cryptorchidism. Evaluation by paternity, hormone, and semen data. *Horm Res* 2001;55(1):28–32.

Pyorala S, Huttunen N-P, Uhari M, et al. A review and meta-analysis of hormonal treatment of cryptorchidism. *J Clin Endocrinol Metab* 1995;80:2795–2799.

Schneck FX, Bellinger MF. Abnormalities of the testes and scrotum and their surgical management. In: Walsh PC, Retik AB, Vaughn ED, et al., eds. *Campbell's Urology*. 8th Ed. Philadelphia: WB Saunders, 2002.

Authors: Hsi-Yang Wu and Thomas F. Kolon

Cryptosporidiosis

 Database

DEFINITION

In an immunocompetent patient, disease is manifested as a self-limiting gastroenteritis. However, immunocompromised patients can develop protracted severe gastroenteritis, which can lead to severe wasting and ultimately death.

CAUSES

Most commonly, gastrointestinal illness is caused by ingestion of the oocysts of *Cryptosporidium parvum*; a coccidian protozoa that is frequently found in the feces of animals (mammals, birds and reptiles) as well as some insects.

PATHOLOGY/PATHOPHYSIOLOGY

- Transmission occurs when oocysts contaminating food or water are ingested or, more commonly, through fecal-oral transmission from person to person.
- The infectious dose for humans is low, estimated at less than 10 oocysts. The incubation period is approximately 2 to 14 days with a median of 7 days and oocyst shedding may occur for weeks to months.
- Invasion of intestinal epithelial cells of the upper gastrointestinal tract leads to a secretory diarrhea. The exact mechanism by which this occurs is still unclear.

EPIDEMIOLOGY

- Typically children under 5 years of age are most often affected. Severe disease is usually seen in the immunocompromised, such as patients with impaired cell-mediated immunity (in particular those who are HIV positive or taking immunosuppressive medications), those with immunoglobulin deficiencies, as well as interferon-γ deficiencies.
- A significant seasonality has been reported, with peaks occurring in North America during the late summer and early fall.
- Outbreaks have been associated with swimming pools, lakes, water recreation parks, drinking water supplies, day camps, unpasteurized apple cider, exposure to farm animals, and day-care attendance. The oocyst form is resistant to chlorination therefore properly functioning water filtration systems are necessary to remove the parasite.
- Other risk factors include exposure to dogs, cats, deer, cockroaches, and traveling abroad.

COMPLICATIONS

- In immunocompromised patients, infection can lead to severe protracted diarrhea with malnutrition and wasting. Biliary tract disease and systemic dissemination such as pulmonary disease can also be seen in the immunocompromised.

PROGNOSIS

- For immunocompetent hosts, gastrointestinal disease is self-limited usually lasting 10 to 14 days. Supportive therapy is usually all that is necessary.
- For immunocompromised patients, diarrhea can be severe, debilitating, and often life-threatening. Aggressive supportive therapy is usually required along with a trial of antimicrobial therapy. Unfortunately, there are no agents that are uniformly effective against *Cryptosporidium parvum*.

 Differential Diagnosis

INFECTIOUS

- Viral gastroenteritis including but not limited to:

—Rotavirus
—Adenovirus
—Astrovirus
—Norwalk
—Cytomegalovirus (CMV)

- Bacterial gastroenteritis including but not limited to:

—*Salmonella*
—*Shigella*
—*Yersinia*
—*Campylobacter*
—*Aeromonas*
—*Plesiomonas*
—Enterotoxigenic *Escherichia coli*
—*Vibrio cholerae*

- Parasitic gastroenteritis including but not limited to:

—*Giardia*
—*Entamoeba*
—*Cyclospora*
—*Isospora*
—*Microsporidia*
—*Dientamoeba fragilis*
—*Blastocystis hominis*
—*Clostridium difficile* enterocolitis

NONINFECTIOUS

- Allergic
- Autoimmune
- Anatomic
- Endocrine
- Iatrogenic/medications
- Inflammatory bowel disease
- Malabsorption
- Neoplastic

 Data Gathering

HISTORY

- Onset: Acute onset of watery nonbloody diarrhea, crampy abdominal pain, low-grade fever, and occasionally nausea and vomiting.
- Exposure: Exposure to ill contacts, public swimming pools, lakes or wave parks, animals, day-care attendance, travel history, dietary history such as consumption of unpasteurized beverages and drinking water supply.
- Evidence of immunosuppression: Immunosuppression secondary to disease or medication as well as exposure to immunosuppressed individuals in the household or, if patient is old enough, through occupation.

 Laboratory Aids

Test: Modified acid fast stain
Significance: Diagnosis is made by observing the 4- to 5-μm cysts in preserved stool specimens. Immunofluorescent antibody (with microscopy) or rapid (3 minute) direct antigen detection tests (enzyme immunoassay; EIA) are also available. False positives and negatives may occur with the EIA test and should by confirmed with microscopy. Because of intermittent shedding, stool specimens should be performed three times on alternate days to exclude the diagnosis.

Test: Must specifically request that the microbiology lab test for this organism.
Significance: A recent national survey of clinical laboratories revealed only 5% routinely tested for *C. parvum*.

Test: Sputum specimen
Significance: For respiratory infections, diagnosis is made by finding the oocysts in sputum specimens.

Test: H and E staining of small intestinal biopsies
Significance: May show the organism protruding from the microvillus border of enterocytes.

Therapy

- Fluid and electrolyte replacement. For protracted cases, patients will eventually require hyperalimentation.
- Nitazoxanide oral suspension has been licensed by the FDA for treatment of children with the disease. A 3 day course is recommended. Dosage for children 1 to 3 years old is 100 mg b.i.d., for children 4 to 11 years old, 200 mg b.i.d. and for adults, 500 mg BID. The antibiotic paromomycin, an aminoglycoside, alone or in combination with azithromycin has not been shown to decrease symptoms or parasite excretion in the feces. For immunosuppressed patients, oral administration of human immune globulin or bovine colostrum has been shown to be beneficial. Improving the CD4 cell count in HIV + patients with antiretroviral therapy can improve the course of cryptosporidal disease in these patients. Some patients have been shown to have improvement in their clinical symptoms with the gastrointestinal hormone octreotide. The dosage is 300 to 500 g three times a day.
- *Cryptosporidium* is on the CDC recommended reporting list of infectious diseases; however, not all states in the United States mandate reporting *Cryptosporidium*.

 ## Follow-Up

- Since the oocysts can be shed in the stool for a long time after clinical resolution, it is not necessary to check follow-up convalescent stools. However, it is important to realize that asymptomatic patients can still transmit the infection to household and day-care contacts.
- Requiring patients whose diarrhea has resolved to have a negative stool test for *Cryptosporidium* before reentry to day care has not been evaluated as an outbreak control measure. Repeated testing is expensive.

PREVENTION

- Isolation of hospitalized patient

—Contact precautions (e.g., gown and gloves for all patient contact) are recommended for the length of the hospital stay. If possible, a single bedroom would be optimal so that a bathroom does not need to be shared.

- Community prevention

—Public water supplies should be adequately filtered in order to ensure oocyst removal.
—Communities that do not use filtration systems are at increased risk for outbreaks, the most recent of which was the Milwaukee epidemic, in which an estimated 400,000 people were affected.
—Homeowners with well water should consider installing drinking water filtration systems.
—Sources of drinking water should be protected from possible fecal contamination.
—Garden hoses should not be used to provide drinking water.
—All juices should be pasteurized. *Cryptosporidium* has been shown to survive in unpasteurized apple cider for up to 4 weeks.
—Symptomatic patients should not be allowed to swim in public pools.
—Good hand washing after contact with animals.

- Control measures

—Hand washing especially after changing diapers.
—Separation of diapering and food handling areas.
—Disinfection of diapering areas after each use, frequent (at least twice daily) disinfection of toys, tabletops, and high chairs during outbreaks is recommended.
—Oocysts can survive for long periods and are resistant to many disinfectants such as pine oil, cresylic acid, ethanol, n-propanol, isopropanol, Lysol, phenol, iodophors, aldehydes, benzalkonium chloride, and quaternary ammonia compounds. Exposure of oocysts to 5.25% sodium hypochloride (full-strength bleach) will destroy infectivity after 10 minutes. However, normally used concentrations of bleach have been shown to be poor disinfectants for *Cryptosporidium*. And 3% hydrogen peroxide is felt to be more effective and is recommended for outbreak control; 5% ammonia is also effective; however, it has a strong odor and if mixed accidentally with chlorine containing solutions (such as bleach) can produce hazardous chlorine gas.
—Temporarily excluding or, if possible, cohorting symptomatic children. Since fecal shedding can be quite prolonged, it is generally recommended that once symptoms have resolved children should be allowed to return to their regular settings.

- During an outbreak, screening should be considered for children and caregivers who are in a household or in close contact with immunocompromised persons.
- Swimming pools found to be contaminated with *Cryptosporidium* require closing and hyperchlorination. The level of chlorination required to kill *Cryptosporidium* oocysts is approximately 640 times greater than that required to kill *Giardia* cysts. Maintaining this level of chlorination is not feasible and, therefore, swimming in public pools places an immunocompromised patient at increased risk.

PITFALLS

- Not considering the diagnosis in patients with acute diarrhea.
- Not sending the appropriate number of stool specimens to exclude the diagnosis.
- Assuming the microbiology lab will routinely test for *C. parvum*.
- Forgetting to test for other parasites if *C. parvum* is found in the stool.

 ## Common Questions and Answers

Q: For whom should cryptosporidiosis as a differential diagnosis be considered?
A: For anyone with acute onset of watery diarrhea with any of the mentioned risk factors.

Q: When is it safe for a child with *Cryptosporidium* to return to day care?
A: When the diarrhea has resolved.

ICD-9-CM 559.007.4

BIBLIOGRAPHY

American Academy of Pediatrics. Cryptosporidium. *2003 Red Book: Report of the Committee on Infectious Diseases.* 26th Ed. Elk Grove Village, IL: American Academy of Pediatrics, 2003:255–256.

Chappell CL, Okhuysen PC. Cryptosporidiosis. *Curr Opin Infect Dis* 2002;15(5):523–527.

Cordel RL, Addiss DG. Cryptosporidiosis in child care settings: a review of the literature and recommendations for prevention and control. *Pediatr Infect Dis* 1994;13:310–317.

LaVia W. Parasitic gastroenteritis. *Pediatr Ann* 1994(23):556–560.

Outbreak of cryptosporidiosis at a day camp. *MMWR Morb Mortal Wkly Rep* 1996;45(21):442–444.

Outbreaks of *Escherichia coli* 0157:H7 infection and cryptosporidiosis associated with drinking unpasteurized apple cider. *MMWR Morb Mortal Wkly Rep* 1997;46(1):4–8.

Author: Jane M. Gould

Cushing Syndrome (Adrenal Excess)

 Database

DEFINITION

Cushing syndrome is a state of excess cortisol secretion by the adrenal cortex. This may be associated with excess production of other adrenal hormones, such as androgens and mineralocorticoids.

PATHOPHYSIOLOGY

- Cushing disease—pituitary ACTH oversecretion, usually due to pituitary adenoma, with resultant bilateral adrenal hyperplasia.
- Adrenal tumors
- Adrenal adenomas—benign tumors which secrete mainly cortisol
- Adrenal cortical carcinomas—usually large, rapidly growing tumors, which produce a variety of hormones including cortisol and androgens.
- Ectopic ACTH production—a rare cause of Cushing syndrome (CS) in pediatrics. Small-cell carcinoma, pheochromocytomas, medullary thyroid carcinoma, and carcinoid tumors can all secrete ectopic ACTH.
- Exogenous steroids—Iatrogenic CS is the most common cause in pediatrics. CS can be caused by chronic systemic, topical, or intranasal steroid, or ACTH use.

EPIDEMIOLOGY

- Incidence

—0.1 to 0.5 new pediatric cases per million population per year
—Ten times more common in adults

- Gender

—Cushing disease—female predominance
—Adrenocortical carcinoma—female predominance

- Age

—Cushing disease—most common cause of endogenous Cushing syndrome, accounting for 80% of Cushing syndrome in adults and children greater than 7 years of age.
—Adrenal tumor—adrenocortical carcinomas account for more than 50% of Cushing syndrome in children less than age 7. These tumors are less common in adults and children older than 7 years of age.

COMPLICATIONS

- Growth arrest
- Obesity
- Pubertal arrest
- Glucose intolerance
- Osteoporosis
- Adrenal carcinomas—metastatic spread

PROGNOSIS

- The prognosis for cure is good with Cushing disease and adrenal adenoma.
- The prognosis for adrenal carcinoma is poor because of the frequency of micrometastases and high recurrence rate.

 Differential Diagnosis

- Cushing disease

—Pituitary ACTH oversecretion

- Adrenal tumors

—Adrenal adenomas
—Adrenal cortical carcinomas

- Exogenous glucocorticoid treatment

 Data Gathering

HISTORY

- Weight gain, gradual onset
- Weakness and fatigue
- Emotional or mental changes
- Use of oral, topical, inhaled, or intranasal steroids

 Physical Examination

Finding: Growth arrest
Significance: Most consistent finding

Finding: Obesity
Significance: Cervicodorsal fat (localized: moon facies, truncal obesity)

Finding: Thin skin with striae, facial plethora
Significance: Sign of cortisol excess

Finding: Hirsutism, acne
Significance: Sex hormone effect

Finding: Pubertal arrest/menstrual disorders
Significance: Common finding

Finding: Hypertension
Significance: Mineralocorticoid effect

Finding: Bruising
Significance: Capillary friability

Finding: Hyperpigmentation
Significance: ACTH effect

Finding: Virilization/feminization
Significance: Sex hormone effect

 Laboratory Aids

DIAGNOSTIC TESTS

Test: Midnight salivary cortisol level >0.35 mcg/dL. Patients are instructed to collect saliva by chewing a commercially available cotton swab at midnight. It provides a convenient, first-line diagnostic test.
Significance: Establishes hypercortisolism

Test: Urinary 24-hour free cortisol greater than 90 μg/24 hour. Correct for creatinine and surface area. Two or three separate collections are preferable.
Significance: Establishes the diagnosis of hypercortisolism

Test: Urinary 24-hour 17-hydroxysteroids greater than 6 mg/g creatinine
Significance: Establishes the diagnosis of hypercortisolism

Test: Overnight dexamethasone suppression test (15 μg/kg)
Significance: Screening only; 8:00 a.m. plasma cortisol >5 μg/L suggests hypercortisolism

Test: Loss of diurnal variation of plasma cortisol in older children.
Significance: Normally, the 11:00 p.m. cortisol is less than 50% of 8:00 a.m. value. The majority of patients with Cushing syndrome have mean elevated plasma cortisol, without diurnal variation.

DIFFERENTIATE CAUSES

Test: random ACTH level
Significance: Cushing disease: increased ACTH with increased cortisol level. Adrenal tumor: low ACTH and increased cortisol.

Test: Androgen levels
Significance: Often high in adrenocortical carcinoma. Androgen levels are low in benign, cortisol-secreting adenomas.

Test: Dexamethasone suppression tests. Low dose dexamethasone (30 μg/kg per day) divided q6h PO × 2 days, followed by high dose (120 μg/kg per day) divided q6h PO × 2 days. Collect 24-hour urine for cortisol and 17-hydroxysteroids throughout.
Significance: Non-Cushing states usually suppress urinary-free cortisol and 17 hydroxysteroids to 50% to 90% of baseline values after low dose.

- Majority of pituitary tumors suppressible after high dose.
- Adrenal source: Hypercortisolism will not suppress.

TUMOR LOCATION

Test: Pituitary MRI with gadolinium
Significance: May demonstrate a pituitary adenoma.

Test: Abdominal CT/MRI
Significance: Will demonstrate adrenal carcinoma, adrenal adenomas, or bilateral hyperplasia/nodules resulting from Cushing disease.

Test: Cavernous sinus sampling for ACTH
Significance: Will help to lateralize pituitary microadenomas.

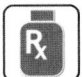 ## Therapy

CUSHING DISEASE

- Transphenoidal pituitary surgery

—70% to 80% success, may be less in some series
—Perioperative glucocorticoid replacement required
—Postoperative complications can include transient diabetes insipidus, and rarely, hypopituitarism or permanent DI.

- Pituitary radiation—6 to 18 months for effect

—Remission in 45% to 85% of individuals
—Remission rate improved if combined with o,p′DDD
—Hypopituitarism is the most common side effect.

- Bilateral adrenalectomy

—Indicated in patients with bilateral micronodular disease or in patients with Cushing disease who fail surgery or radiotherapy
—High rate of surgical complications
—May result in Nelson syndrome—pituitary adenoma growth and hyperpigmentation, long-term glucocorticoid and mineralocorticoid replacement.

- Drug therapy

—Ketoconazole—inhibits multiple adrenal enzymes
—o,p′DDD—adrenolytic agent
—Metyrapone—11-hydroxylase inhibitor
—Aminoglutethimide—20,22-desmolase inhibitor
—Trilostane—3β-hydroxysteroid dehydrogenase inhibitor
—RU-486—Glucocorticoid receptor antagonist
—Drug combinations may lower individual doses and lessen side effects

ADRENAL TUMOR

—Aggressive surgical resection
—Chemotherapy for carcinoma: Cytoxan, Adriamycin, 5-FU, MTX

- Drug therapy to control hypercortisolism

—o,p′DDD at high doses—may improve recurrence risk in patients with complete tumor resection. In those with residual or recurrent disease, it may improve hypercortisolism, but not survival

- Glucocorticoid and possibly mineralocorticoid replacement.

 ## Follow-Up

- Chronic glucocorticoid replacement 10 to 12 mg/m^2 day divided as b.i.d. to t.i.d. until recovery of hypothalamic/pituitary function (6 to 12 months). Parents should be taught to triple the dose for stress, fever, illness, or vomiting. Injectable hydrocortisone should be given for emergency use. Taper corticosteroid treatment gradually.
- Reassess 24-hour urinary cortisol/ketosteroid secretion during the first week after treatment and at 6 weeks.
- In the week after effective pituitary surgery, cortisol should be undetectable and ACTH less than 5 pg/mL, 24 hours after last hydrocortisone dose. Stimulation and suppression tests are performed 6 weeks postsurgery (holding hydrocortisone dose).
- Frequent follow-up to monitor for recurrence. Monitor for cortisol withdrawal symptoms, hypopituitarism. Consider medical treatment for persistent hypercortisolism.

PITFALLS

- False-positive tests for hypercortisolism

—Stress—lack of suppression
—Depression
—Anorexia
—Primary glucocorticoid resistance

- False-negative tests

—Incomplete urine collection
—Periodic or intermittent cortisol hypersecretion
—Slow metabolism of dexamethasone

- Aberrant renal metabolism
- Repeat if suspicion is strong

 ## Common Questions and Answers

Q: What clinical features help distinguish patients with pituitary Cushing disease from patients with adrenal tumors?
A: Cushing syndrome and hyperpigmentation suggests an ACTH effect. Cushing syndrome and virilization suggests adrenal carcinoma.

Q: What physical characteristics most clearly differentiate children with exogenous obesity from those with Cushing syndrome?
A: Exogenous obesity is associated with robust linear growth while Cushing syndrome is associated with growth failure.

ICD-9-CM 255

BIBLIOGRAPHY

Arnaldi G, Angeli A, Atkinson AB, et al. Diagnosis and complications of Cushing's Syndrome: a consensus statement. *J Clin Endocrinol Metab* 2003;88:5593–5602.

Boscaro M, Barzon L, Fallo F, et al. Cushing's syndrome. *Lancet* 2001;357(9258):783–791.

Cacciari E, Cicognani A, Pirazzoli P, et al. Adrenocortical tumours in children: our experience with nine cases. *Acta Endocrinol Suppl (Copenh)* 1986;279:264–274.

Gomez MT, Malozowski S, Winterer J, et al. Urinary free cortisol values in normal children and adolescents. *J Pediatr* 1991;118(2):256–258.

Leinung MC, Kane LA, Scheithauer BW, et al. Long term-follow-up of transsphenoidal surgery for the treatment of Cushing's disease in childhood. *J Clin Endocrinol Metab* 1995;80(8):2475–2479.

Magiakou MA, Chrousos GP. Cushing's syndrome in children and adolescents: current diagnostic and therapeutic strategies. *J Endocrinol Investigation* 2002;25:181–194.

Papanicolaou DA, Yanovski JA, Cutler GB JR, et al. A single midnight serum cortisol measurement distinguishes Cushing's syndrome from pseudo-Cushing states. *J Clin Endocrinol Metab* 1998;83(4):1163–1167.

Putignano P, Toja P, Dubini A, et al. Midnight salivary cortisol versus urinary free and midnight serum cortisol as screening tests for Cushing's syndrome. *J. Clin Endocrinol Metab* 2003;88(9):4153–4157.

Yanovski JA, Cutler GB JR, Chrousos GP, et al. The dexamethasone-suppressed corticotropin-releasing hormone stimulation test differentiates mild Cushing's disease from normal physiology. *J Clin Endocrinol Metab* 1998;83(2):348–352.

Yanovski JA, Friedman TC, Nieman LK, et al. Inferior petrosal sinus AVP in patients with Cushing's syndrome. *Clin Endocrinol* 1997;47(2):199–206.

Authors: Lorraine Katz and J. Nina Ham

Cutaneous Larva Migrans

 Database

DEFINITION

Infestation of the epidermis by the infectious larvae of certain nematodes. Humans are accidental hosts, with the primary hosts being dogs and cats.

CAUSES

- Most common organism is the dog or cat hookworm, *Ancylostoma braziliense*.
- Other species include *A. canium, Uncinaria stenocephala*, and *Bunostomum phlebotomum*.

PATHOPHYSIOLOGY

- Humans are accidental hosts.
- Filariform larvae penetrate the epidermis either through hair follicles or fissures or through intact skin with the use of proteases.
- Diagnosis is usually clinical. Organisms rarely recovered from biopsy and antibody titers unreliable because symptoms are a result of hypersensitivity to the organism or its excreta, and immunity usually does not develop.

ASSOCIATED DISEASES

- Most common manifestation is an intensely pruritic, linear, reddened, elevated, serpiginous skin lesion known as a "creeping eruption."
- Most common complication is secondary bacterial infection of the involved skin.
- Rare cases of a peripheral eosinophilia with pulmonary infiltrates (Loffler syndrome) occur when dermal penetration by the larvae occurs and the bloodstream is invaded.

EPIDEMIOLOGY

- Contracted from contaminated soil.
- Worldwide distribution, but most frequent in warmer climates, including the Caribbean, Africa, South America, Southeast Asia, and Southeastern United States.
- Occupational exposures occur from crawling under buildings, such as plumbers and pipe-fitters.

Route of Spread

- Primary host (dog or cat) passes eggs to ground through feces.
- Warm, sandy soil acts as an incubator.
- Eggs mature into rhabditiform larvae (noninfectious), which molt in 5 days to filariform larvae (infectious).
- Incubation period from infection to symptoms usually 7 to 10 days, although can range up to several months.

COMPLICATIONS

- Most common complication is secondary bacterial infection of the skin. Self-limited disease—if untreated, larvae die within 2 to 8 weeks but may persist for up to 1 year.
- Rarely, the larvae can invade the dermis and, subsequently, the bloodstream, leading to a peripheral eosinophilia and pulmonary infiltrates (Loffler syndrome).

PROGNOSIS

- This is a self-limited disease and without treatment will resolve when the larvae die.
- There is a 98% response rate to topical thiabendazole, 97% cure rate with ivermectin, and an 89% response rate reported with oral thiabendazole.

 Differential Diagnosis

- Cutaneous larva migrans should be considered in anyone with an intensely pruritic, raised, serpiginous, linear cutaneous eruption.

—Hookworm infections (*Strongyloides stercoralis, U. stenocephala, B. phlebotomum, Gnathostoma spinigerum*)
—Free living nematodes (*Pelodera strongyloides*), and insect larvae.
—Other cutaneous eruptions that may mimic cutaneous larva migrans include erythema chronicum migrans of Lyme disease, jelly fish stings, and photosensitivity.

 Data Gathering

HISTORY

Question: What is the incubation period?
Significance: Usual time from infection to symptoms is 7 to 10 days but may last for up to several months.

Question: Is there a rash?
Significance: It is intensely pruritic, raised, serpiginous, and linear. Most commonly located on feet, buttocks, and abdomen. Also found on face, extremities, and genitalia.

Question: Is there pruritus?
Significance: Symptoms typically begin with some tingling in the affected area with the development of the typical rash with intense pruritus.

Question: How fast does rash spread?
Significance: Rash typically lengthens by 2 to 3 cm daily.

Question: Where does one obtain this infection?
Significance: Most frequently contracted from beaches in tropical countries where dogs are frequently found.

Physical Examination

The classic rash is described as erythematous, raised, serpiginous rash. It also may begin as vesicular. Tracks under the skin reflect the course of the larvae. The active end is not part of the track.

 Laboratory Aids

Test: Biopsy
Significance: Not indicated since it rarely yields organisms

Test: Serologic testing
Significance: Not helpful; diagnosis based on clinical presentation

 Therapy

• First-line treatment is topical thiabendazole, supplied as a 10% suspension of 500 mg/5 mL applied four times per day for 10 days.
• Alternatively, oral thiabendazole in a dose of 25 to 50 mg/kg per day q12h for 2 days. Not well tolerated.
• Ivermectin 12 mg in a single dose. May repeat if symptoms persist.
• Albendazole, not approved for use in the United States, is available in other countries and is administered as 400 mg/day for 3 days in adults.

 Follow-Up

• Symptoms persist for 8 weeks but up to 1 year in untreated patients.
• Those with extensive involvement should be seen after treatment to be certain of improvement in symptoms.

 Common Questions and Answers

Q: Can children spread the infection to each other?
A: The usual spread of infection is from direct contact with the larvae. Spread from one individual to another usually does not occur.

ICD-9-CM 126.9

BIBLIOGRAPHY

Blackwell V, Vega-Lopez F. Cutaneous larva migrans: clinical features and management of 44 cases presenting in the returning traveller. *Br J Dermatol* 2001;145:434–437.

Bouchaud O, ne Houze S, Schiemann R, et al. Cutaneous larva migrans in travelers: a prospective study, with assessment of therapy with ivermectin. *Clin Infect Dis* 2000;31:493–498.

Brenner MA, Patel MB. Cutaneous larva migrans: the creeping eruption. *Cutis* 2003;72(2):111–115.

Caumes E. Treatment of cutaneous larva migrans. *Clin Infect Dis* 2000;30(5):811–814.

Van den Enden E, Stevens A, Van Gompel A. Treatment of cutaneous larva migrans. *N Engl J Med* 1998;339(17):1246–1247.

Authors: Jason Newland and Louis M. Bell

Cyclospora

 Database

DEFINITION

Cyclospora catayensis, a parasite, causes a diarrheal illness first described in humans in 1977.

PATHOPHYSIOLOGY

- Infected patients excrete unsporulated oocysts in their stool.
- Sporulation then occurs days to weeks after release into the environment.
- Ingestion of sporulated oocysts occurs and sporozoites are released that invade the intestinal epithelial cells.
- Sporozoites develop into trophozoites, which undergo schizogony and form merozoites.
- Merozoites may develop into macro- or microgametes, which become fertilized resulting in oocysts.
- Entire life cycle is completed in the host.

EPIDEMIOLOGY

- Infection occurs through the consumption of contaminated food and water.
- Transmission does not occur through person-to-person spread.
- Worldwide distribution with areas of endemic infection (Nepal, Peru, Haiti)
- Incubation period is between 1 and 11 days with an average of 7 days.
- People living in endemic areas have a shorter illness or may be asymptomatic carriers.
- In the United States infection occurs primarily in spring and summer.
- Outbreaks have been associated with the consumption of raspberries, mesclun (young salad greens), and basil.
- *Cyclospora* is an opportunistic infection in HIV patients.

COMPLICATIONS

- Dehydration and weight loss are the most common complications.

—Severe, prolonged diarrhea may lead to dehydration.
—Malabsorption of D-xylose and excretion of fecal fat occurs leading to weight loss.

- May cause ascending biliary tract disease in AIDS patients
- Rare-associated complications:

—Guillain Barre syndrome
—Reiter syndrome

PROGNOSIS

- Most cases are self-limited.
- Diarrhea may last up to 3 months in untreated patients who obtained the parasite in a foreign country endemic with vyclospora.
- In the United States outbreaks, the average duration of diarrhea ranged from 10 to 24 days.
- Relapses may occur in untreated patients.
- Patients with HIV have more severe and prolonged diarrhea, which may recur.

 Differential Diagnosis

CRYPTOSPORIDIUM

- Outbreaks associated with contaminated water sources (municipal pools)
- Person-to person-transmission may occur
- Clinically indistinguishable from *cyclospora*

ISOSPORA BELLI

- Outbreaks associated with food and water
- Clinically indistinguishable from *cyclospora*

MICROSPORIDIUM

- Oubreaks associated with contaminated water sources
- Chronic diarrhea occurs in immunocompromised patients, especially HIV
- Fever is uncommon

GIARDIA LAMBLIA

- Community epidemics associated primarily with contaminated water sources
- Person-to-person transmission may occur and have led to outbreaks in day-care centers
- Clinical presentation may vary from occasional acute watery diarrhea to a severe, protracted diarrheal illness

VIRAL GASTROENTERITIS

- Rotavirus
- Adenovirus 40/41

BACTERIAL GASTROENTERITIS

- *Clostridium dificile*
- *Vibrio cholera* and noncholera *Vibrio* species
- *Escheria coli*, especially toxin-producing strains
- *Shigella* species
- *Salmonella* species
- *Yersinia enterocolitica*
- *Campylobacter* species

Data Gathering

HISTORY

Question: Is fever associated?
Significance: Fever is present in approximately 25% to 50% of cases.

Question: Is there a clinical prodrome?
Significance: Acute onset of diarrhea is typical, but a flu-like prodrome may occur.

Question: What is the nature of the diarrhea?
Significance: Profuse, nonbloody, watery diarrhea that may be foul-smelling

Question: What other symptoms are experienced?
Significance: Abdominal cramping, fatigue, anorexia, and vomiting

Question: What foods have been consumed in past 2 weeks?
Significance: Illness has been attributed to contaminated raspberries, mesclun, and basil.

Physical Examination

Finding: Dehydration
Due to profuse diarrhea signs of dehydration (tachycardia, dry mucous membranes, sunken eyes, poor skin turgor, and weight loss) may be present.

Laboratory Aids

Test: Ova and parasites with modified acid fast staining
Significance: Identification of *cyclospora, isospora* and *cryptosporidium*

Test: Ova and parasites
Significance: Identify common protozoans including *Giardia*

Test: *Cryptosporidium* and *Giardia* antigen test
Significance: Immunoassay with high sensitivity and specificity

Test: Electron microscopy of stool
Significance: Gold standard for diagnosing *microsporidia*

Test: Bacterial stool cultures
Significance: Identify common bacterial pathogens

Test: Stool for *Clostridium dificile* A and B toxin
Significance: Identify a common cause of diarrhea.

Test: Electrolytes, BUN, creatinine
Significance: Determine extent of dehydration

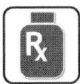
Therapy

- Immunocompetent patient

—Trimethoprim (5mg/kg per dosage)-sulfamethoxazole twice daily for 7 to 10 days

- HIV patient

—Trimethoprim-sulfamethoxazole four times daily for 10 days and then prophylactic dosing three times per week to prevent relapse.
—Based on severity of dehydration treatment may be indicated with intravenous fluids.

PREVENTION

- Fresh produce, especially raspberries, should be washed thoroughly prior to being eaten, which still may not entirely eliminate the risk of transmission.

Follow-Up

- Infected patients need to be observed closely for dehydration.
- Relapse may occur in the HIV patients so close follow up is essential.

Common Questions and Answers

Q: Does routine ova and parasites detect *cyclospora*?
A: Rarely, therefore modified acid fast staining must be performed to improve the laboratories ability to detect the oocysts.

Q: Can person to person transmission occur in *cyclospora* illness?
A: No. It takes days to weeks for oocysts to sporulate and become infectious.

ICD-9-CM 007.9

BIBLIOGRAPHY

American Academy of Pediatrics. Cyclospora. In: Pickering LK, ed. *2003 Red Book: Report of the Committee on Infectious Diseases*. 26th Ed. Elk Grove Village, IL: American Academy of Pediatrics, 2003:258.

Atkins JT, Cleary TG. Cryptosporidiosis, cyclospora infection, isosporiasis, and microsporidiosis. In: Feigin RD, Cherry JD, Demmler GJ, Kaplan SL, eds. *Textbook of Pediatric Infectious Diseases*. 4th Ed. Philadelphia: WB Saunders, 2004:2687–2707.

Herwaldt BL. Cyclospora cayetanensis: a review, focusing on the outbreaks of cyclosporiasis in the 1990s. *Clin Infec Dis* 2000;31:1040–1057.

Keystone JS, Kozarsky P. Isospora beli, sarcocystis species, bloastocystis hominis, and Cyclospora. In: Mandell GL, Douglas RG, Bennett JE, eds. *Principles and Practice of Infectious Diseases*. 4th Ed. New York: Churchill Livingstone, 2001:2915–2920.

Author: Jason Newland

Cystic Fibrosis

 Database

DEFINITION

Cystic fibrosis (CF) is an inherited, autosomal-recessive disorder, characterized by chronic obstructive lung disease, pancreatic exocrine insufficiency, and elevated sweat chloride concentration.

PATHOPHYSIOLOGY

- CF transmembrane conductance regulator (CFTR)

—Membrane glycoprotein, which functions as a cyclic adenosine monophosphate (AMP)-activated chloride channel at the apical surface of epithelial cells.
—An abnormality in CFTR results in defective chloride conductance.
—May have other roles in the regulation of membrane channels and the pH of intracellular organelles.

- In the respiratory system

—Lungs are morphologically normal at birth.
—Increased viscosity of mucus
—Early bacterial colonization despite a robust neutrophilic inflammatory response.
—Mucus plugging and atelectasis
—Bronchiectasis

- In the gastrointestinal tract

—Exocrine pancreatic insufficiency
—Focal biliary cirrhosis of the liver
—Hypoplasia of the gallbladder

GENETICS

- CFTR gene

—Located on the long arm of chromosome 7
—Most common mutation results in deletion of phenylalanine at position 508 in the CFTR glycoprotein. This δ508 mutation occurs in almost 70% of CF patients.
—Over 1,000 mutations have been reported in the CFTR gene.

EPIDEMIOLOGY

- Most common lethal inherited disease in the Caucasian population
- Carrier frequency of mutations in the CFTR gene

—1:29 in Caucasians
—1:49 in Hispanics
—1:53 in Native Americans
—1:62 in African Americans
—1:90 in Asians

- Incidence of CF

—1:3,300 in Caucasians
—1:9,500 in Hispanics
—1:11,200 in Native Americans
—1:15,300 in African Americans
—1:32,100 in Asians

COMPLICATIONS

- Respiratory complications

—Recurrent bronchitis and pneumonia
—Atelectasis
—Bronchiectasis
—Pneumothorax
—Hemoptysis
—Chronic sinusitis and nasal polyps

- Gastrointestinal complications

—Pancreatic insufficiency in 85% to 90% of CF patients
—Patients usually have steatorrhea, poor growth, and nutritional status
—Decreased levels of vitamins A, E, D, and K
—Rectal prolapse
—Ten percent to 15% of patients have meconium ileus
—Distal intestinal obstruction syndrome
—Clinically significant focal biliary cirrhosis hepatobiliary disease in 5% of CF patients
—Esophageal varices
—Splenomegaly
—Hypersplenism
—Cholestasis

- Reproductive complications:

—Sterility in 98% of the males as a result of absence or atresia of the vas deferens
—Slight decrease in fertility for females secondary to abnormalities of cervical mucus.

- Endocrine complications:

—CF-related diabetes occurs with increasing frequency in CF adolescents and adults.

PROGNOSIS

- Median survival is approximately 30 years of age.
- Variable course of the disease

 Differential Diagnosis

PULMONARY

- Recurrent pneumonia or bronchitis
- Asthma
- Aspiration pneumonia

GASTROINTESTINAL

- Failure to thrive
- Celiac disease
- Protein-losing enteropathy

OTHER

- Metabolic alkalosis
- Immune deficiency

 Data Gathering

HISTORY

Question: Have there been respiratory symptoms?

Significance: The most common presenting respiratory symptoms:

- Chronic cough
- Recurrent pneumonia
- Nasal polyps
- Chronic pansinusitis

Question: Have there been gastrointestinal symptoms?
Significance: Most common presenting gastrointestinal symptoms:

- Meconium ileus (15% to 20% of patients present with this symptom).
- Pancreatic insufficiency occurs in 85% of patients.
- In infants, fat malabsorption may lead to failure to thrive.
- In older patients, pancreatitis
- Rectal prolapse

—Occurs in 2% of the patients
—Must consider CF until proven otherwise
—Commonly seen between 1 and 5 years

- Meconium ileus equivalent:

—Distal obstruction of the small intestine
—Seen in older children and adults

Question: Evidence of heat intolerance?
Significance: In summer, increased sweating may lead to dehydration with hyponatremia or hypochloremic metabolic alkalosis.

 Physical Examination

Findings: Respiratory findings
Significance:

- Frequent cough, often productive of mucopurulent sputum
- Rhonchi
- Crackles
- Hyperresonance to percussion
- Nasal polyposis

Findings: Other common findings:

- Digital clubbing
- Hepatosplenomegaly in patients with cirrhosis
- Growth retardation
- Hypertrophic osteoarthropathy
- Delayed puberty

 Laboratory Aids

Test: Sweat test
Significance: Keystone for the diagnosis of CF; sweat chloride greater than 60 mEq/L is abnormal.

Other causes of elevated sweat chloride:

- Malnutrition
- Adrenal insufficiency
- Nephrogenic diabetes insipidus
- Ectodermal dysplasia
- Fucosidosis
- Hypogammaglobulinemia

- False-negatives seen in:

—CF Patients with edema

Test: Mutation analysis
Significance: Can detect over 90% of the CF patients. Failure to identify two mutations reduces, but does not eliminate the possibility of CF.

Collection methods include blood samples or cheek brushings.

Test: Sputum culture
Significance: Frequently recovered organisms include:

- *Haemophilus influenzae*
- *Staphylococcus aureus*
- *Pseudomonas aeruginosa* (nonmucoid and mucoid)
- *Burkholderia cepacia*
- *Stenotrophomonas maltophilia*
- *Aspergillus species*

Test: Pulmonary function tests
Significance: Usually reveals obstructive lung disease, although some patients may have a restrictive pattern.

Test: Analysis of stimulated pancreatic secretions
Significance: Degree of pancreatic exocrine deficiency

Test: 72-hour fecal fat measurement
Significance: Fat malabsorption

Test: Stool trypsin levels
Significance: Correlates with pancreatic insufficiency in infants

IMAGING

- Chest radiology

  —Typical features include:
  —Hyperinflation
  —Peribronchial thickening
  —Atelectasis
  —Bronchiectasis

- CT scan

—Early bronchiectasis

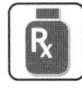 Therapy

DRUGS

- Antibiotic therapy (based on sputum culture results)

—Oral antibiotics
  —Cephalexin
  —Cefaclor
  —Trimethoprim-sulfamethoxazole
  —Ciprofloxacin
—Inhaled
  —Tobramycin or colistin in selected patients
—Intravenous antibiotics
  —To treat *S. aureus* consider oxacillin, ticarcillin with clavulanic acid, or vancomycin.

—To treat *P. aeruginosa* and *B. cepacia* consider aminoglycoside plus ticarcillin, ceftazidime, or piperacillin.
—Severe cases with resistant strains may benefit from imipenem or meropenem.
—Synergistic antibiotic studies should be performed in patients with multiresistant organisms.

CLEARANCE OF PULMONARY SECRETIONS

- Chest physiotherapy with postural drainage and vibrations given manually, or with high-frequency oscillatory vest device. Adjunct therapy such as Flutter valve or PEP mask may also be used.
- Bronchodilator: aerosol or MDI

—β^2-agonist

- Mucolytics

—*N*-acetylcysteine
—RhDNase

- Antiinflammatory

—Cromolyn sodium
—Steroid (inhaled or short-term oral)

LIVER DISEASE

- Patients with cholestasis may benefit from therapy with ursodeoxycholic acid
- Pancreatic enzyme replacement therapy:

—Used in CF patients who are pancreatic insufficient
—Dosage adjusted for frequency and character of the stools and for growth pattern
—Generic substitutes are not bioequivalent to name brands
—The maximum recommended dose is 2,500 units of lipase/kg per meal

- Vitamin supplements:

—Multivitamin supplement
—Fat-soluble vitamins (usually E and K)

DIET

- High-calorie diet with added salt

DURATION

- Usually lifelong nutritional support required
- Duration of antibiotic therapy is controversial; more frequent use is required as pulmonary function deteriorates

 Follow-Up

CARE PLAN

- Specialized care should be at a CF center
- Frequency of visits depends on severity of illness; usually every 2 to 3 months

PROGNOSIS

- Current median survival is approximately 30 years

- The median survival has been increasing for the past 4 decades, although the rate of increase in age has slowed in the past decade.

PREVENTION

- Prepregnancy carrier detection

PITFALLS

- Most common pitfall is failure to diagnose.
- Not uncommon to delay making the diagnosis in patients with mild symptoms.

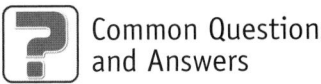 Common Questions and Answers

Q: Should relatives be tested?
A: All siblings should have a sweat test.

Q: How well will a child with CF do?
A: The course of the illness is variable. It is difficult to predict the course of disease in an individual.

Q: How should borderline sweat test be interpreted?
A: Borderline sweat tests should always be correlated with other findings such as physical examination, sputum cultures, pulmonary function, radiographic findings, nutritional evaluation, mutation analysis.

ICD-9-CM 277.0

BIBLIOGRAPHY

Baumer JH. Evidence based guidelines for the performance of the sweat test for the investigation of cystic fibrosis in the UK. *Arch Dis Child* 2003;88(12):1126–1127.

Davis PB, Drumm M, Konstan MW. Cystic fibrosis. *Am J Respir Crit Care Med* 1996:1229–1256.

Dezateux C, Walters S, Balfour-Lynn I. Inhaled corticosteroids for cystic fibrosis. *Cochrane Database Syst Rev* 2000;2:CD001915.

Farrell MH. Farrell PM. Newborn screening for cystic fibrosis: ensuring more good than harm *J Pediatr* 2003;143(6):707–712.

Quittner AL. Measurement of quality of life in cystic fibrosis. *Curr Opin Pulmon Med* 1998;4(6):326–331.

Ryan G, Mukhopadhyay S, Singh M. Nebulised anti-pseudomonal antibiotics for cystic fibrosis. *Cochrane Database Syst Rev* 2000;2:CD001021.

Ryan G, Mukhopadhyay S, Singh M. Nebulised anti-pseudomonal antibiotics for cystic fibrosis. *Cochrane Database Syst Rev* 2000;3:CD001021.

Smyth A, Walters S. Prophylactic antibiotics for cystic fibrosis. *Cochrane Database of Cochrane Database Syst Rev* 2000;2:CD001021.

Yankaskas JR, Marshall BC, Sufian B, et al. Cystic fibrosis adult care: consensus conference report. *Chest* 2004;125:1S–39S.

Author: Thomas F. Scanlin

Cytomegalovirus Infection

 Database

DEFINITION

Cytomegalovirus (CMV) is a ubiquitous double-stranded DNA virus that is a member of the herpesvirus family. Establishes latency in peripheral mononuclear cells.

PATHOPHYSIOLOGY

Infection leads to intranuclear inclusions with massive enlargement of cells. Almost any organ may become infected with CMV in severe disseminated infection.

EPIDEMIOLOGY

- Seroprevalence varies with socioeconomic status; 50% of middle and 80% of lower socioeconomic status adults are seropositive.
- Increased rates of primary infection are seen in early childhood, adolescence, and childbearing years.
- Transmission may occur by contact with infected respiratory secretions, urine, or breast milk, sexual contact, solid organ transplantation, or transfusion of infective blood products.

COMPLICATIONS/PROGNOSIS

Varies with nature of infection (see Associated Diseases).

ASSOCIATED DISEASES

Congenital Infection

- Occurs in 1% of newborns.
- Ten percent of infected infants are symptomatic at birth, with severe cytomegalic inclusion disease characterized by growth retardation, hepatosplenomegaly, thrombocytopenia, and CNS involvement.
- Ten percent to 20% of infants who are asymptomatically infected at birth will develop long-term sequelae.
- CMV is the most common cause of congenital deafness.

Mononucleosis Syndrome

CMV can cause a mononucleosis-like syndrome similar to that caused by Epstein-Barr Virus (EBV) infection

- The most common symptoms are malaise (67%) and fever (50%). Approximately 70% of patients will have abnormal liver function tests.
- Pharyngitis and splenomegaly are less common and less severe than observed with EBV-induced mononucleosis.

Interstitial Pneumonitis

- Primarily seen in immunosuppressed children and adults.
- Usually begins with fever and nonproductive cough, but may progress to dyspnea and severe hypoxia over 1 to 2 weeks.

- Mild, self-limited pneumonitis may occur in immunocompetent patients.

Retinitis

- Seen in approximately 30% of infants with symptomatic congenital infection.
- May complicate CMV disease in patients with severe immunodeficiency.

Hepatitis

- Occurs in healthy individuals with primary infections and immunosuppressed patients with either primary or reactivated disease.
- Characterized by mildly elevated liver function studies, mild hepatomegaly, and fever.
- Jaundice and severe hepatitis uncommon.

Gastrointestinal Disease

- Severely immunosuppressed patients may experience esophagitis, gastritis, colitis, or pancreatitis.

CNS Disease

- Commonly seen in infants with symptomatic congenital infection.
- Characterized by microcephaly, periventricular calcifications, seizures, developmental delay, and sensorineural hearing loss.
- Encephalitis or meningoencephalitis may occur postnatally in either healthy or immunocompromised patients.

 Differential Diagnosis

CONGENITAL INFECTION

- Congenital rubella syndrome
- Toxoplasmosis
- Syphilis
- Neonatal herpes simplex virus
- HIV
- Enteroviral infection

MONONUCLEOSIS SYNDROME

- EBV infection
- Toxoplasmosis
- Hepatitis A or B infection

INTERSTITIAL PNEUMONITIS

- Respiratory syncytial virus
- Adenovirus
- Measles
- Varicella
- Pneumocystis carinii
- Chlamydia
- Mycoplasma
- Fungal
- Drug/toxin-induced pneumonitis

RETINITIS

- Ocular toxoplasmosis
- Candidal retinitis
- Syphilis
- Herpes simplex virus

HEPATITIS

- EBV infection
- Hepatitis A, B, or C infection
- Enterovirus
- Adenovirus
- Herpes simplex virus
- Drug/toxin-induced

GASTROINTESTINAL DISEASE

- Herpes simplex virus
- Adenovirus
- Salmonella
- Shigella
- Campylobacter
- Yersinia
- C. difficile
- Giardia
- Cryptosporidium

CNS DISEASE

- Congenital disease (see Congenital Infection, above)
- Meningoencephalitis in immunocompetent host: herpes simplex virus, EBV, varicella-zoster virus, enterovirus, arbovirus
- Meningoencephalitis in immunocompromised host: in addition to organisms listed previously, differential diagnosis should include HIV encephalitis, fungal meningitis (due to Cryptococcus, Candida, Aspergillus, Histoplasma), toxoplasmosis.

 Data Gathering

HISTORY

Question: Day-care attendance?
Significance: Increased risk of infection

Question: Recent blood transfusion?
Significance: Transfusion-associated CMV

Question: Use of immunosuppressive medications?
Significance: Increased use of serious infection

Question: Prolonged fever?
Significance: Mononucleosis-like syndrome

Question: Blurred vision?
Significance: CMV retinitis

Question: Cough, dyspnea, wheezing?
Significance: CMV pneumonitis

Question: Vomiting, abdominal pain, diarrhea (watery or bloody)?
Significance: CMV colitis

Physical Examination

Finding: Microcephaly
Significance: Congenital infection

Finding: White, perivascular retinal infiltrates and hemorrhage
Significance: Retinitis

Finding: Deafness (may require audiogram, brainstem evoked auditory responses, etc.)
Significance: Congenital infection

Finding: Photophobia, headache, nuchal rigidity
Significance: Meningitis

Finding: Tachypnea, rales
Significance: Pneumonitis

Finding: Hepatomegaly and/or splenomegaly
Significance: Mononucleosis-like syndrome

Finding: Rash
Significance: Petechiae, purpura, "blueberry muffin" lesions, rubelliform rash

Finding: Adenopathy
Significance: Mononucleosis-like syndrome

Laboratory Aids

Test: Viral culture
Significance: Virus may be isolated from nasopharyngeal/oropharyngeal secretions, urine, stool, white blood cells. Isolation of virus may take up to 4 weeks.

Test: Shell-vial assay
Significance: Enhanced viral culture through the use of centrifugation. Allows detection of virus 24 to 72 hours after inoculation.

Test: Direct immunofluorescence
Significance: Detection of CMV-infected cells in specimens from biopsy or bronchoalveolar lavage.

Test: Quantitative antigenemia assay
Significance: Detection of circulating CMV-infected mononuclear cells by indirect immunofluorescence. In an immunocompromised patient, may monitor response to therapy or identify viral reactivation.

Test: DNA hybridization
Significance: Detection of viral nucleic acid in tissue specimens

Test: Histologic examination
Significance: Presence of typical enlarged cells with intranuclear inclusions ("owl's-eye" nuclear inclusion)

Test: Serology
Significance: ELISA or indirect fluorescent antibody assay to detect the presence of CMV IgM or IgG. CMV IgM usually persists for 6 weeks following primary infection although may persist up to 6 months.

PITFALLS

• As a result of frequency of asymptomatic shedding, mere isolation of virus does not necessarily establish an etiologic association.
• Severely immunocompromised patients who are actively infected with CMV may be seronegative.
• Fourfold rise in CMV IgG not diagnostic of primary infection. Increased antibody titers may occur with reactivation.
• False-positive detection of CMV IgM may occur as a result of production of cross-reactive antibodies.
• Congenital CMV infection should be established by viral isolation from urine or nasopharyngeal secretions within the first 2 weeks of life.

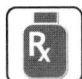

Therapy

DRUGS

• Ganciclovir will suppress viral replication but not eradicate virus (virostatic agent).

—Indications: CMV chorioretinitis in immunocompromised patients; tissue diagnosis (hepatitis, enteritis, pneumonitis) of CMV infection or isolation of CMV from buffy coat of immunocompromised patient; may consider for neonate with documented CNS disease to prevent progressive postnatal hearing loss.
—Side effects: neutropenia (~50%), thrombocytopenia (~5%)

• Foscarnet—virostatic agent

—Indications: CMV chorioretinitis, pneumonitis, hepatitis, enteritis (biopsy-proven) in an immunocompromised patient who has failed to improve on ganciclovir therapy or has experienced significant bone marrow toxicity related to ganciclovir use
—Side effects: renal impairment (25%), headache (25%), seizures (10%)

PREVENTION

• Drainage and secretion, and pregnant women precautions should be instituted for hospitalized patients known to be shedding CMV.
• Seriously ill neonates should receive blood products from CMV-negative donors.
• CMV-seronegative solid organ or bone marrow transplantation recipients should receive organs (and all blood products) from CMV-negative donors whenever possible.
• Controversy exists over role of hyperimmune globulin to prevent disseminated CMV disease in CMV-negative recipient of CMV-positive transplantation.

Common Questions and Answers

Q: Should children with congenital CMV infection be excluded from day-care settings?
A: No. As a result of the high frequency of shedding of CMV in the urine and saliva of asymptomatic children, especially under 2 years of age, exclusion from out-of-home care is not justified for any child known to be infected with CMV. Careful attention to hygienic practices, especially hand washing, is important.

ICD-9-CM 078.5

BIBLIOGRAPHY

Boppana SR, Pass RF, Britt WJ, et al. Symptomatic congenital cytomegalovirus infection. *Pediatr Infect Dis J* 1992;11:93–99.

Brown HL, Abernathy MP. Cytomegalovirus infection. *Semin Perinatol* 1998;22(4): 260–266.

Cullen A, Brown S, Cafferkey M, et al. Current use of the TORCH screen in the diagnosis of congenital infection. *J Infect* 1998;36(2): 185–188.

Demmler GJ. Acquired cytomegalovirus infections. In: Feigin RD, Cherry JD, eds. *Textbook of Pediatric Infectious Diseases*, 3rd Ed. Philadelphia: WB Saunders 1992:1532–1547.

Demmler GJ. Congenital cytomegalovirus infection. *Semin Pediatr Neurol* 1994;1(1):36–42.

Fowler KB, Stagno S, Pass RF, et al. The outcome of congenital cytomegalovirus infection in relation to maternal antibody status. *N Engl J Med* 1992;326(10):663–667.

Kimberlin DW, Lin CY, Sanchez PJ, et al. Effect of ganciclovir therapy on hearing in symptomatic congenital cytomegalovirus diseases involving the central nervous system: a randomized controlled trial. *J Pediatr*, 2003:143:16–25.

Wreghitt TG, Teare EL, Devi SR, Rice P. Cytomegalovirus infection in immunocompetent patients. *Clin Infect Dis* 2003;27:1603–1606.

Author: Susan E. Coffin

Daytime Incontinence

 Database

DEFINITIONS

- Enuresis—the expulsion of urine beyond the age of anticipated control, generally thought to be 5 years.
- Incontinence—the involuntary leakage of urine in a child older than 5 years.
- Voiding dysfunction—a dysfunction of the lower urinary tract without a recognized organic cause, generally in the form of bladder–sphincter discoordination.

CAUSES

- Neurogenic bladder (e.g., myelomeningocele)
- Anatomic anomalies (e.g., ectopic ureter)
- Obstructive uropathy (e.g., posterior urethral valves)
- Bladder irritability caused by urinary tract infection
- Constipation
- Increased urinary output/polyuria
- Infrequent or deferred voiding
- Overactive bladder
- Low functional bladder capacity, with detrusor instability during filling
- Temperamental factors (short attention span, inattentiveness to body signals) in children who ignore the urge to void
- Developmental differences in age at which toilet training is achieved
- Vaginal reflux with subsequent leakage of urine

EPIDEMIOLOGY

- Of all children who wet, 10% have only daytime wetting, 75% wet only at night, and 15% wet during the day and at night.
- Studies in children 6 to 7 years of age have shown that 3.1% of girls and 2.1% of boys had an episode of wetting at least once per week.
- Spontaneous cure rate of 14% per year without treatment.

GENETICS

- Only anecdotal relationships have been seen in functional daytime incontinence, unlike studies showing genetic tendencies in nocturnal enuresis.
- Increased rates of daytime wetting have been reported in urofacial (Ochoa) syndrome, an autosomal-recessive condition, and Williams syndrome.

COMPLICATIONS

- Local irritation and inflammation of the perineum
- Functional daytime incontinence is primarily a social problem that affects children's self-esteem and interactions with peers.

ASSOCIATED PROBLEMS

- Constipation
- Nocturnal enuresis
- Urinary tract infections
- Vesicoureteral reflux is seen more frequently in children with voiding dysfunction as a result of elevated detrusor pressures that overcome a marginal vesicoureteral junction.

 Differential Diagnosis

- Urinary tract infection
- Constipation
- Normal developmental variations in toilet training
- Neurogenic bladder
- Spinal cord abnormality
- Giggle incontinence
- Genitourinary tract abnormality (posterior urethral valve, ectopic ureter)
- Vaginal reflux
- Benign increased urinary frequency (pollakiuria)
- Sexual abuse

 Data Gathering

HISTORY

- Onset (primary versus secondary)
- Frequency of voiding
- Frequency and degree of wetting
- Presence or absence of any dry interval
- Signs of urgency; use of hold maneuvers, waiting until the last minute to void
- Description of stream (strong/weak; continuous/interrupted)
- Straining or pushing during voiding
- Frequency and description of bowel movements
- History of soiling
- History of urinary tract infections, vesicoureteral reflux
- ADD/ADHD, learning disabilities, or developmental delays
- Level of concern on part of child/family
- Medications
- Quality and quantity of fluid intake
- Other medical conditions

 Physical Examination

- Focused PE

—Abdomen—signs of constipation; distended bladder
—Rectal—if constipation is suspected
—Spine—sacral abnormalities
—Genitalia—labial adhesions, erythema, phimosis, stenosis, urethritis
—Neurologic—sensation, reflexes, and gait

 Laboratory Aids

TESTS

- First a.m. urinalysis to check concentrating ability, rule out occult renal disease
- Urine culture to rule out infection

IMAGING

- Renal and bladder ultrasound in children who wet with a history of urinary tract infections and in children with persistent wetting despite regular voiding.
- Kidneys, ureter, and bladder (KUB) x-ray if history/exam suggestive of constipation
- Further imaging generally not indicated if history, PE and previous radiographic studies are normal.

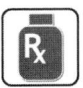

Therapy

MEDICAL/ BEHAVIORAL

• Aggressive management of bowels so that child is passing at least one soft BM daily (see Constipation)
• Place child on a timed elimination schedule, with voids every 2 to 3 hours and time to defecate at least once/day
• Positive reinforcement for regular voiding
• Avoid acidic/diuretic beverages (caffeine, carbonation, chocolate, citrus)
• Hydration
• Local management of perineal irritation/ vulvovaginitis to ensure comfort during voiding
• Girls with postvoid dribbling as a result of vaginal reflux should void with their legs wide apart, sitting backward on the toilet when possible, to minimize backflow of urine into the vagina. Wipe after standing up.

PHARMACOLOGIC

If child continues to wet in spite of medical/ behavioral management, a trial on an anticholinergic medication may be indicated. Extended-release formulations may be tolerated better than short-acting preparations. Common side effects include dry mouth and decreased diaphoresis with flushing. Some patients note blurred vision, dizziness and constipation.

• Oxybutynin (Ditropan/Ditropan XL); 5 to 15 mg/day
• Tolterodine (Detrol/Detrol LA); 2 to 4 mg/day
• Hyoscyamine (Levbid); 0.75 to 1.5 mg/day

REFERRAL TO PEDIATRIC UROLOGIST

When wetting is refractory to behavioral and standard pharmacologic treatment, child may benefit from:

• Urodynamic study to assess for detrusor instability
• Biofeedback training to learn appropriate relaxation during voiding

Follow-Up

• Spontaneous cure rate of 14% per year without treatment

PITFALLS

• Failure to recognize and manage constipation, before attempting to manage wetting
• Failure of anticholinergic medication in children with significant postvoid residuals or with constipation
• Use of anticholinergic medications in children with benign frequency of childhood is generally ineffective.
• Increased risk of urinary tract infections when child is placed on anticholinergic, as a result of infrequent voiding/incomplete emptying

Common Questions and Answers

Q: What findings can distinguish functional incontinence from an ectopic ureter?
A: An ectopic ureter usually empties below the sphincter or elsewhere such as in the vagina. Therefore, these girls wet all the time with no dry period. They do not have symptoms such as urgency. Since, in most cases, the ureter draining the kidney is duplicated, an ultrasound or intravenous pyelogram (IVP) may provide more information.

Q: What is benign urinary frequency?
A: This condition, commonly seen in both genders around 4 to 5 years of age, is thought to be secondary to stress. It is episodic and may develop temporally after a stressful event such as the beginning of school or an illness in the family. These children may urinate frequently but they do not wet. At night the problem usually disappears. A urinalysis and urine culture are required to exclude organic pathology.

ICD-9-CM 788.30

BIBLIOGRAPHY

Abidari JM, Shortliffe LM. Urinary incontinence in girls. *Urol Clin North Am* 2002;29:661–675.

Bauer S. Special considerations of the overactive bladder in children. *Urology* 2002;60(Suppl)1:43–48.

Curran MJ, Kaefer M, Peters C, Logigian E, Bauer SB. The overactive bladder in childhood: long-term results with conservative management. *J Urol* 2000; 163:574–577.

Loening-Baucke V. Urinary incontinence and urinary tract infection and their resolution with treatment of chronic constipation of childhood. *Pediatrics* 1997;100:228–231.

Rushton H. Wetting and functional voiding disorders. *Urol Clin North Am* 1995;22:75–93.

Saedi N, Schulman SL. Natural history of voiding dysfunction. *Pediatr Nephrol* 2003; 18:894–897.

Wiener JS, Scales MT, Hampton J, et al. Long-term efficacy of simple behavioral therapy for daytime wetting in children. *J Urol* 2000;164:786–790.

Authors: Amanda Berry and Seth Schulman

Dehydration

 Database

DEFINITION

- Dehydration is a negative balance of body fluid, usually expressed as a percentage of body weight. Mild, moderate, and severe dehydration correspond to deficits of <5%, 5% to 10%, and >10%, respectively.
- Dehydration is classified into three types based on the serum sodium concentration: isotonic (Na 130 to 150 mmol/L), hypotonic (Na <130 mmol/L), and hypertonic (Na >150 mmol/L).

PATHOPHYSIOLOGY

Dehydration is caused by either excessive fluid losses or inadequate intake. Some conditions leading to dehydration include:

- Gastrointestinal losses—vomiting, diarrhea (most common cause of dehydration in pediatric patients)
- Renal losses—diabetes mellitus, diabetes insipidus, diuretic agents
- Insensible losses—sweating, fever, tachypnea, increased ambient temperature, large burns
- Poor oral intake—stomatitis, pharyngitis, anorexia, oral trauma, altered mental status
- Note that infants and debilitated patients are at particular risk as a result of lack of ability to satisfy their thirst freely.

EPIDEMIOLOGY

Approximately 10% of children in the United States with acute gastroenteritis develop at least mild dehydration. Although it accounts for 10% of all nonsurgical hospital admissions for children under 5 years of age, up to 90% of cases can be managed on an outpatient basis.

COMPLICATIONS

- Severe dehydration may lead to hypovolemic shock and acute renal failure.
- Hyponatremia is associated with hypotonia, hypothermia, and seizures.
- Overly rapid correction of hypernatremia can produce cerebral edema.

PROGNOSIS

Excellent with appropriate rehydration therapy.

 Data Gathering

HISTORY

Question: Frequency and duration of emesis and/or diarrhea?
Significance: This will give a rough estimate of risk of dehydration.

Question: Amount and type of liquids taken?
Significance: If there were large quantities of water, be alert for hypotonic dehydration. If excessive electrolyte solution used for hydration, may have hypertonic dehydration.

Question: Frequency and quantity of urination (may be difficult to estimate in infants with diarrhea)?
Significance: Decreased urination indicates possibility of dehydration.

Question: Fever?
Significance: Fever increases insensible water loss.

Question: Exertion or heat exposure?
Significance: Increases insensible water loss.

 Physical Examination

Acute change in weight is the best indicator of the fluid deficit. If the child's recent preillness weight is not available for comparison, a reasonable estimate of the degree of dehydration may be made from physical findings.

Finding: General appearance
Significance: Lethargy, irritability, thirst

Finding: Vital signs
Significance: Tachycardia; orthostatic increase in heart rate or hypotension; hyperpnea

Finding: Skin
Significance: Prolonged capillary refill at fingertip (<2 seconds is normal in warm environment); mottling; poor turgor

Finding: Eyes
Significance: Decreased or absent tears; sunken eyes

Finding: Mucous membranes
Significance: Dry or parched

Finding: Anterior fontanelle
Significance: Sunken

DIAGNOSTIC PITFALLS

- Physical signs generally appear when the deficit is at least 2% to 3%.
- No single finding is pathognomonic of dehydration. A reasonable guideline is that the presence of three or more findings indicates at least mild dehydration. The number and severity of physical signs increase with the degree of dehydration.
- Urine output decreases early in the course of dehydration, and a history of decreased urination is a nonspecific finding.
- Capillary refill time is a specific indicator, but may be falsely prolonged by cool ambient temperature (<20°C [<68°F]). It is not affected by fever.
- Children with a deficit greater than 15% will show signs of cardiovascular instability such as severe tachycardia and hypotension.
- Physical findings may be more significant for a given degree of dehydration in children with hyponatremia, leading to overestimation of the deficit. Conversely, the clinical picture is reported to be somewhat moderated in hypernatremia.

 Laboratory Aids

Diagnosis of dehydration is best made on clinical grounds. The following laboratory tests are sometimes helpful adjuncts.

Test: Serum sodium
Significance: Classifies type of dehydration. Hyponatremia and hypernatremia are uncommon (<5% of cases). Measure sodium levels in cases of clinically severe disease, or if risk factors are present (e.g., young infant, history of excessive free water intake, children with significant neurologic impairment limiting their ability to regulate their own intake).

Test: Rapid glucose test or serum glucose
Significance: To detect hypoglycemia as a result of prolonged fasting.

Test: Urine specific gravity
Significance: This is elevated early in dehydration, but may not become elevated at all in young infants or children with sickle cell disease.

Test: Serum bicarbonate
Significance: This is frequently low with diarrheal illness, even in the absence of dehydration. Useful to detect significant acidosis when dehydration is clinically severe.

Test: Blood urea nitrogen (BUN)
Significance: Rises only late in dehydration in children.

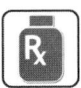 ## Therapy

ORAL REHYDRATION THERAPY (ORT)

Most children can be successfully managed with ORT.

- Use rehydration solution containing 2% to 2.5% glucose and 75 to 90 mmol/L Na (e.g., WHO solution), or 45 to 50 mmol/L Na (e.g., Pedialyte [Ross Laboratories, Columbus, OH], Infalyte, [Mead Johnson, Evansville, IN]).
- Replace entire deficit in 4 to 6 hours—for mild dehydration, 50 mL/kg; for moderate to severe dehydration, 80 to 100 mL/kg. Include ongoing losses, approximately 5 mL/kg for each diarrheal stool.
- Begin with slow administration, with strict limits when vomiting is present—5 mL every 1 to 2 minutes. For infants, use a syringe or spoon rather than a bottle. After 1 hour, if the oral liquids have been tolerated, increase the volume and rate.
- Have the child's caregiver participate in giving the fluids, and provide education regarding fluid replacement and signs of dehydration.
- Monitor weight, intake and output, and clinical signs. Failure of ORT includes intractable vomiting, clinical deterioration, or lack of improvement after 4 hours.

INTRAVENOUS FLUID THERAPY

Intravenous fluids are required when ORT fails or is contraindicated, such as in severe dehydration or shock, poor gag or suck, depressed mental status, preterm infant, severe hypernatremia (Na >160 mmol/L), suspected surgical abdomen.

- Administer intravenous bolus of normal saline or Ringer lactate, 20 mL/kg, over 10 to 30 minutes. Repeat as needed to restore cardiovascular stability. Avoid dextrose-containing solutions for boluses except to correct documented hypoglycemia.
- Calculate maintenance fluid requirements: 100 mL/kg for the first 10 kg, plus 50 mL/kg for the next 10 kg, plus 20 mL/kg over 20 kg.
- Calculate fluid deficit based on clinical estimate or known weight loss. For isotonic or hypotonic dehydration, give one-third to one-half normal saline with 5% dextrose, at a rate to provide maintenance and replace deficit over 24 hours. For hypertonic dehydration, replace deficit over 48 hours, using one-fifth to one-fourth normal saline with 5% dextrose.
- Monitor weight, intake and output, and clinical signs. With hypernatremia, measure serum sodium every 4 to 6 hours; do not exceed rate of fall of 1 mmol/L per hour.
- For mild to moderate isonatremic dehydration, rapid replacement of deficit over 2 to 6 hours may be possible. Give normal saline, or one-half normal saline with 2.5% dextrose, at a rate to replace the estimated deficit at a rate of 25 to 40 cc/kg per hour.

 ## Follow-Up

After rehydration, children with ongoing losses, as in gastroenteritis, should receive a maintenance solution in addition to regular feedings to maintain a positive fluid balance. Recommend 5 to 10 mL/kg for each diarrheal stool. Avoid clear liquids with excessive glucose, such as fruit juices, punches, and soft drinks, as these can promote osmotic fluid losses in the stool. In infants less than 6 months old, do not give large amounts of plain water, which can lead to hyponatremia.

PREVENTION

Many cases of frank dehydration may be prevented by early institution of adequate oral maintenance fluid therapy in children with gastroenteritis, with particular attention to replacement of ongoing stool losses and slow administration of fluids to children with vomiting. Use of appropriate solutions is essential to prevent electrolyte disturbance and worsening of diarrhea.

 ## Common Questions and Answers

Q: How can an oral rehydration solution be prepared at home?
A: An acceptable rehydration solution (2.2% glucose, 70 mmol Na/L) can be prepared with the following: half teaspoon of table salt, half teaspoon of baking soda, and 1 cup of orange juice, added to 3 cups of water. For maintenance solution, decrease the table salt to a quarter teaspoon.

Q: Can commercially available maintenance solutions be used for rehydration as well as maintenance?
A: Data suggest that reduced-osmolarity maintenance solutions, with a sodium concentration of 45 to 50 mmol/L, are equally effective for rehydration as solutions with a higher sodium content.

Q: How can oral rehydration solution be made more palatable?
A: Rehydration solutions may be more palatable if iced, or flavored with apple or orange juice (1 part juice to 4 parts rehydration solution) or unsweetened Kool-Aid powder (2.5 mL powder per 240 mL of solution).

ICD-9-CM 276.5

BIBLIOGRAPHY

American Academy of Pediatrics Provisional Committee on Quality Improvement, Subcommittee on Acute Gastroenteritis. Practice parameter: the management of acute gastroenteritis in young children. *Pediatrics* 1996;97:424–436.

Armon K, Stephenson T, MacFaul R, et al. An evidence and consensus based guideline for acute diarrhea management. *Arch Dis Child* 2001;85(2):132–142.

Armon K, Stephenson T, MacFaul R, Eccleston P, Werneke U. An evidence and consensus based guideline for acute diarrhoea management: practice guideline. Review. [Review, Academic] *Arch Dis Child* 2001;85(2):132–142.

CHOICE Study Group. Multicenter, randomized, double-blind clinical trial to evaluate the efficacy and safety of a reduced osmolarity oral rehydration salts solution in children with acute watery diarrhea. *Pediatrics* 2001;107(4):613–618.

Farthing MJ. Oral rehydration: an evolving solution. *J Pediatr Gastroenterol Nutr* 2002;34 Suppl 1:S64–S67.

Gorelick MH, Shaw KN, Murphy KO. Validity and reliability of clinical signs in the diagnosis of dehydration in children. *Pediatrics* 1997;99(5):e6.

Gorelick MH. Rapid IV rehydration in the emergency department: a systematic review. PEM-Database. Org. Available at http://researchinpem.homestead.com/files/rapid_iv_hydration_23.07.doc Accessed February 17, 2004.

Kallen RJ. The management of diarrheal dehydration in infants using parenteral fluids. *Pediatr Clin North Am* 1990;37:265–286.

Roberts KB. Fluid and electrolytes: parenteral fluid therapy. *Pediatr Rev* 2001;22(11): 380–387.

Author: Marc H. Gorelick

Dermatomyositis/Polymyositis

 Database

DEFINITION

The dermatomyositis/polymyositis complex includes a number of conditions in which muscle becomes damaged by a nonsuppurative lymphocytic inflammatory process. Juvenile dermatomyositis (JDM) is the most common seen in the pediatric population.

DIAGNOSTIC CRITERIA FOR JDM

Diagnosis requires the presence of the pathognomonic rash plus three additional criteria.

- Progressive symmetric weakness of proximal muscles
- Dermatitis-heliotrope rash over eyelids, Gottron papules over extensor surfaces of joints
- Elevated serum level of muscle enzymes
- Electromyograph (EMG) findings of myopathy and denervation
- Biopsy demonstration of inflammatory myositis
- Although not a criterion, T2-weighted MRI is useful in establishing active myositis.

PATHOPHYSIOLOGY

- Unknown
- Several potential mechanisms include the following:

—Abnormal cell-mediated immunity
—Immune-complex formation
—Immunodeficiency
—Infection
—Toxoplasma gondii
—Coxsackievirus B
—Others

EPIDEMIOLOGY

- Incidence: 1:200,000
- The average age of onset is 7 years
- Overall male:female ratio is 1.0:1.7; however, equal in children under 10 years of age

COMPLICATIONS

- Myositis
- Rash
- Arthritis
- Calcinosis
- Raynaud syndrome
- Dysphagia and dysphonia
- Restrictive lung disease and aspiration pneumonia
- Myocarditis (rare)
- Gastrointestinal tract vasculitis
- Osteoporosis
- Joint contractures
- Skin infections

PROGNOSIS

- Normal to good, 65% to 80%
- Minimal atrophy and joint contractures, 24%
- Calcinosis, 20% to 40%
- Wheelchair dependent, 5%
- Death, 7% to 10%

 Differential Diagnosis

POSTINFECTIOUS

- Influenza A and B, coxsackievirus B, schistosomiasis, trypanosomiasis, toxoplasmosis
- Bacterial/pyomyositis-focal

MYOSITIS WITH OTHER CONNECTIVE TISSUE DISEASES

- Overlap with JRA
- Mixed connective tissue disease
- Systemic lupus erythematosus

CHILDHOOD NEUROMUSCULAR DISEASES

If no rash, consider:

- Muscular dystrophy
- Congenital myopathies
- Metabolic disorders

—Glycogen storage disease
—Carnitine deficiency
—Myoadenylate deaminase

- Neurogenic atrophies

—Spinal muscular atrophy and anterior horn
—Peripheral nerve dysfunction

- Neuromuscular transmission disorders
- Inclusion body myositis

 Data Gathering

HISTORY

Question: Fever?
Significance: Evidence of systemic illness

Question: Anorexia and weight loss?
Significance: Gastrointestinal involvement

Question: Fatigue?
Significance: Sign of muscle weakness

Question: Weakness?
Significance: Difficulty rising from floor, climbing stairs, swallowing, regurgitation through nose

Question: Dysphonia?
Significance: Sign of muscle weakness

Question: Rash?
Significance: Clue to diagnosis

 Physical Examination

Finding: Muscle weakness
Significance: Proximal and symmetric tenderness strength

- 0—no contractility
- 1—contracts, no joint movement
- 2—full range of motion (FROM) without gravity
- 3—FROM against gravity
- 4—complete ROM with some resistance
- 5—normal

Finding: Rash
Significance: 75% have pathognomonic rash, which usually appears several weeks after muscle weakness.

Finding: Facial rash
Significance: Violaceous, heliotropic changes over eyelids

Finding: Extremities
Significance: Gottron papules over extensor surfaces

Finding: Nail-fold telangiectasia
Significance: Simultaneous dilated loops, dropout, and arborized capillary loops

PHYSICAL EXAMINATION TRICKS

- Gower sign: Inability to rise from floor without using hands
- Use ophthalmoscope to examine nail-fold for telangiectasia
- Objective measure of strength: duration of straight leg raise (normal = 20 seconds)

Laboratory Aids

Test: Autoantibodies
Significance:

- Normal RF, complement, and double-stranded DNA (dsDNA)
- ANA: 10% to 50%
- PM-1: 60% adult polymyositis; however, rare in children
- Jo-1: associated with interstitial lung disease

Test: Muscle enzymes
Significance:

- Elevated in 95% cases
- Creatine kinase
- AST
- Aldolase
- LDH

PATHOLOGY

- Skeletal muscle

—Group atrophy or perifascicular myopathy
—Variation in fiber size as a result of concomitant degeneration and regeneration
—Inflammatory exudate in perivascular distribution
—Necrotizing vasculitis of arterioles, capillaries, and venules; probably as a result of immune complex deposition

- Skin

—Epidermal atrophy
—Vascular dilatation
—Lymphocyte infiltration of the dermis

ELECTROMYOGRAPHY

- Myopathic motor units
- Denervation potentials
- High-frequency repetitive discharges
- Do not biopsy same muscle used for EMG

MRI

- Inflamed muscles are identified by signal enhancement
- Useful to direct biopsy

BARIUM SWALLOW

- To identify palatal or proximal esophageal weakness

PULMONARY FUNCTION TESTS/PEAK FLOW

- To evaluate pulmonary musculature and interstitial lung disease

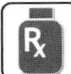 Therapy

PHYSICAL THERAPY/OCCUPATIONAL THERAPY

- Initially to maintain ROM
- Strengthening only after acute inflammation resolves

DRUGS

- 2 mg/kg of steroids per day for 1 month, taper over 2 years
- Intravenous gamma globulin, controversial, efficacious for rash
- Plaquenil, particularly useful for the rash
- Methotrexate, PO, SC, or IV, avoid IM, which may alter serum levels of muscle enzymes
- Cyclosporine

SUPPORTIVE CARE

- Monitor for swallowing difficulty
- Respiratory compromise/occasionally requires mechanical ventilation
- Treatment of calcinosis may include colchicine, diltiazem, and alendronate

 Follow-Up

- Function
- Muscle strength
- Joint ROM
- Development of calcinosis
- Muscle enzyme levels

PITFALLS

- Steroid-induced myopathy
- Insidious onset
- Proximal and distal muscles, often large muscle groups such as hip flexors
- Normal serum muscle enzymes
- Minimal myopathic changes on EMG
- Type II fiber atrophy on muscle biopsy

 Common Questions and Answers

Q: Is it mandatory to perform a muscle biopsy to confirm the diagnosis?
A: No.

Q: How long should you treat with prednisone?
A: The usual practice is 2 years minimum.

Q: Is there an associated risk of malignancy as for adults with this disorder?
A: No.

ICD-9-CM 710.3

BIBLIOGRAPHY

Cawkwell GM. Inflammatory myositis in children, including differential diagnosis. *Curr Opin Rheumatol* 2000;12:430–434.

Cron RQ, Sharma S, Sherry DD. Current treatment by United States and Canadian pediatric rheumatologists. *J Rheumatol* 1999;26:2036–2038.

Huber AM, Lang B, LeBlanc CM, et al. Medium- and long-term functional outcomes in a multicenter cohort of children with juvenile dermatomyositis. *Arthritis Rheum* 2000;43:541–549.

Kimball AB, Summers RM, Turner M, et al. Magnetic resonance imaging detection of occult skin and subcutaneous abnormalities in juvenile dermatomyositis. Implications for diagnosis and therapy. *Arthritis Rheum* 2000;43:1866–1873.

Mukamel M, Horev G, Mimouni M. New insight into calcinosis of juvenile dermatomyositis: a study of composition and treatment. *J Pediatr* 2001;138:763–766.

Pachman LM. Juvenile dermatomyositis: immunogenetics, pathophysiology, and disease expression. *Rheum Dis Clin North Am* 2002;28:579–602.

Ramanan AV, Feldman BM. Clinical features and outcomes of juvenile dermatomyositis and other childhood onset myositis syndromes. *Rheum Dis Clin North Am* 2002;28:833–857.

Reed AM, Lopez M. Juvenile dermatomyositis: recognition and treatment. *Paediatr Drugs* 2002;4:315–321.

Reed AM, Ytterberg SR. Genetic and environmental risk factors for idiopathic inflammatory myopathies. *Rheum Dis Clin North Am* 2002;28:891–916.

Rider LG, Miller FW. Idiopathic inflammatory muscle disease: clinical aspects. *Baillieres Best Pract Res Clin Rheumatol* 2000;14:37–54.

Wargula JC. Update on juvenile dermatomyositis: new advances in understanding its etiopathogenesis. *Curr Opin Rheumatol* 2003;15:595–601.

Author: Randy Q. Cron

Developmental Disabilities

 Database

DEFINITION

Developmental Delay is a descriptive term, not a specific diagnosis, composed of many disorders and encompassing a broad category of etiologies. The term describes any situation in which a child is not meeting age appropriate milestones as expected in one or more streams of development. These streams of development include gross motor, fine motor, receptive and expressive language, adaptive and social. The key feature is that the rate of progress has been slow over time in the area(s) of delay.

PATHOPHYSIOLOGY

This is highly variable depending on etiology, which can include genetic, familial, metabolic, infectious, endocrinologic, traumatic, anatomic brain malformations, environmental toxins, and degenerative disorders as causes. These disorders often result in some neurologic or neuromuscular injury causing the delay. In many cases etiology is never determined.
Prevalence of this group of disorders may vary depending on how inclusive the definition. The milder delays are quite common and can be found in any pediatric practice. Some disorders in this grouping are more prevalent in boys. The long-term outcome depends on the severity and type of delay, with the more involved children usually having lifelong disability.

ASSOCIATED FINDINGS

- There are numerous associated findings including, seizures, sensory impairments, feeding disorders, psychiatric disorders (especially depression), and behavioral disorders.
- Having a child with significant developmental delays also can add stress to the family in terms of time, finances, and emotions.

 Differential Diagnosis

The differential can be extensive and may become more evident with further workup. Broad diagnoses include:

- Mental retardation
- Developmental language disorder
- Autism
- Learning disability
- Cerebral palsy
- Attention deficit hyperactivity disorder
- Significant visual or hearing impairment
- Degenerative disorders

- Specific etiologies are too numerous to list completely but a partial list of the more common causes would include:
  —Genetic/familial
    —Fragile X Syndrome
    —Trisomy 21 (Down syndrome)
    —Other chromosomal abnormalities
    —Tuberous sclerosis
    —Neurofibromatosis
    —Phenylketonuria
    —Muscular dystrophy
  —Nervous system anomalies
    —Hydrocephalus
    —Lissencephaly
    —Spina bifida
    —Seizures
  —Infections
    —Prenatal cytomegalovirus,
    —Rubella,
    —Toxoplasmosis,
    —HIV
    —Postnatal bacterial meningitis,
    —Neonatal herpes simplex
  —Endocrinological
    —Congenital hypothyroidism
  —Environmental
    —Heavy metal poisoning such as lead
    —In utero drug or alcohol exposure
  —Trauma/injury
    —Closed head trauma
    —Asphyxia
    —Stroke
    —Perinatal cerebral hemorrhages

 Data Gathering

HISTORY

A complete and detailed history is needed including:

Question: Pregnancy history?
Significance:

- Maternal age and parity
- Maternal complications (including infections and exposures)
- Medications/drugs used
- Tobacco or alcohol used, along with quantities
- Fetal activity

Question: Birth history?
Significance:

- Gestational age
- Birth weight
- Route of delivery
- Maternal or fetal complications/distress
- Apgar scores

Question: General health?
Significance:

Significant illnesses, hospitalizations or surgeries

- Accidents or injuries
- Hearing and vision status
- Medications used
- Known exposures to toxins
- Any new or unusual symptoms

Question: Developmental history?
Significance:

- Current developmental achievement in each stream of development
- Age when developmental milestones were achieved
- Any loss of skills
- Where parents think their child is functioning developmentally

Question: Educational history?
Significance:

- Type of schooling and services received, if any
- Any previous educational/developmental testing

Question: Behavioral history?
Significance:

- Any perseverative or stereotypical behaviors
- Interaction skills
- Attention and activity level

Question: Family history?
Significance: Anyone with developmental delays, neurologic disorders, syndromes, consanguinity

 Physical Examination

A complete physical examination including growth perimeters is needed looking for etiology. Key features to include are:

Finding: Observation of interactions and behavior
Significance: Any atypical behaviors and general impression

Finding: Head circumference
Significance: Looking for macro- or microcephaly

Finding: Skin exam
Significance: Looking for neurocutaneous lesions

Finding: Major or minor dysmorphic features
Significance: Any indication of a syndrome or anatomic malformation

Finding: Neurologic examination
Significance: Looking for cranial nerve deficits, neuromuscular status, reflexes, balance and coordination and any soft signs

DEVELOPMENTAL TESTING

Although considerable information will already be available on history and observation, a more formal developmental screening or testing should be done. Possible office tests would be the Denver Developmental Screening Test, the CAT/CLAMS, or the ELM. The latter test is basically for language screening. Referral to a specialist or a multidisciplinary team for more detailed testing would be indicated when delay is suspected.

LABORATORY TESTS

There is no specific laboratory test battery for general developmental delays. The testing needs to be tailored to the individual situation based on the history and physical examination. A high index of suspicion should be maintained for any associated findings and delays in the other streams of development. Listed below are some of the more common studies ordered for developmental delay workup.

Test: Audiologic
Significance: Hearing should be checked in any child with speech and language and/or cognitive delays.

Test: Genetic testing
Significance: Warranted for any dysmorphic features, a family history of delays or genetic disorder. A karyotype and Fragile X DNA should be considered particularly for significant cognitive delays.

Test: Metabolic tests
Significance: Tests such as quantitative plasma amino acids, quantitative urine organic acids, lactate, pyruvate or ammonia should be considered if there is any loss of skills or indication of a metabolic disorder.

Test: Thyroid function tests
Significance: Most infants will have had screening for hypothyroidism shortly after birth. This should be rechecked if symptoms indicate.

Test: Electroencephalogram
Significance: An EEG should be considered if there is any concern about seizures.

Test: Head MRI
Significance: Consider a head MRI for head abnormalities, significant neurological findings, loss of skills or for workup of a specific disorder such as trauma or leukodystrophy.

Test: Subspecialists:
Significance: Referral to other medical specialists may also be indicated. These specialists may include developmental pediatrics, neurology, genetics, orthopaedics or ophthalmology.

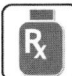 Therapy

• Therapy should include appropriately treating any medical conditions and associated findings, for example, anticonvulsants for seizures or hearing aids when appropriate for hearing impairment. In addition, traditional therapy has included early intervention or special education services specifically addressing the areas of delay.
• Therapy could include physical therapists, occupational therapists, speech/language therapists, special educators, psychologists, and audiologists depending on the needs of the child.

 Follow-Up

• General pediatric care for well-child visits and to monitor any underlying medical conditions is indicated.
• These children need ongoing monitoring of their therapy and educational programs to ensure that it is still meeting their individual needs, as these needs change over time.
• The families will also need ongoing counseling and support in dealing with a child having special needs.

PREVENTION

There is no known prevention of developmental delays, although prevention of some of the underlying etiologies is possible.

PITFALLS

• Children with behavioral problems may also be masking developmental delays.
• Children with delays in one stream of development may also have delays in other areas of development. For example, language delay may be an indication of general cognitive delays.
• Hearing impairment may present as a delay in development

 Common Questions and Answers

Q: When do you test a child for delays?
A: A child can have developmental assessments at any age, including infancy. Making a specific diagnosis, for example, level of mental retardation, may need to wait until the child is older.

Q: When can a child start receiving services?
A: Children who qualify can receive therapy services starting at birth and in some cases extending up to 21 years of age.

Q: The parents are raising a concern about delays but the general impression in the office is that the child is doing OK. What should be done next?
A: Parents or grandparents may be the first to express concerns, especially in a child with milder delays. A more detailed developmental history and more formal developmental screening or testing would be indicated as an initial step.

ICD-9-CM: 315.9

BIBLIOGRAPHY

Battaglia A, Carey JC. Diagnostic evaluation of developmental delay/mental retardation: An overview. *Am J Med Genet* 2003;117C(1):3–14.

Gilbride KE. Developmental testing. *Pediatr Rev* 1995;16:338–345.

Johnson CP, Blasco PA. Infant growth and development. *Pediatr Rev* 1997;18:224–242.

Levy SE, Hyman SL. Pediatric assessment of the child with developmental delay. *Pediatr Clin North Am* 1993;40:465–477.

Liptak GS. The pediatrician's role in caring for the developmentally disabled child. *Pediatr Rev* 1996;17:203–210.

Mendola P, Selevan SG, Gutter S, Rice D. Environmental factors associated with a spectrum of neurodevelopmental deficits. *Ment Retard Devel Disab Res Rev* 2002;8(3): 188–97.

Simms MD, Shum RL. Preschool children who have atypical patterns of development. *Pediatr Rev* 2000;21:147–158.

Author: Rita Panoscha

Developmental Dysplasia of the Hip

 Database

DEFINITION

A range of congenital hip disorders: from mild acetabular dysplasia to dislocation of the femoral head from the acetabulum.

CAUSES

Mechanical Factors

- Breech position
- Oligohydramnios
- Packing phenomenon (e.g., first-born child)
- Postnatal positioning (e.g., swaddling in extension and adduction)

Laxity or Genetic Factors

- Female
- Family history ($\sim$ 20%)
- Certain ethnic groups
- Generalized ligamentous laxity

PATHOLOGY

Due to mechanical forces, abnormal growth, or underlying laxity, the spatial and biomechanical relationship between the femoral head and the acetabulum is altered.

EPIDEMIOLOGY

Incidence of hip dysplasia is 0.5% to 2% of live births; however, true dislocation occurs in 0.1% to 0.2% of live births.

GENETICS

Many patients are first-born females, with familial history of affected first-degree relative.

COMPLICATIONS

- When congenital hip dysplasia results in hip subluxation or dislocation, complaints include limp, pain, and accelerated degenerative disease of the hip.
- Avascular necrosis of the femoral head is a complication of treatment.

 Differential Diagnosis

- Infection
- Spastic hip dislocation as a result of cerebral palsy, closed head injury, or anoxic brain injury.

 Data Gathering

HISTORY

Question: Breech delivery?
Significance: Much higher incidence of developmental dysplasia of the hip in breech delivery.

Question: Familial history of hip dysplasia?
Significance: 10% to 20% of patients have familial history.

 Physical Examination

- Infants are tested with the Ortolani and Barlow tests. These maneuvers involve feeling a "clunk" with either gentle reduction of the dislocated femoral head with abduction and anterior force (Ortolani) or gentle dislocation or an unstable femoral head with adduction with posterior force (Barlow).
- Check neck for torticollis, metatarsus adductus, and other "packaging" abnormalities.
- Check for an abnormal sacral dimple.
- Although a baby with a dislocated hip may have asymmetric thigh or gluteal folds, many babies with normal hips have such asymmetry
- Children older than 4 to 6 months may have a negative Ortolani but have limited abduction on the affected hip. Galeazzi sign may be positive (comparing the femoral lengths by flexing the hip and knee in the supine position).
- Walking-age children may have a Trendelenburg gait (lurching to the side) and a leg length inequality.

PHYSICAL EXAMINATION TRICKS

- The infant should be as relaxed as possible—preferably sleeping. Check the hips first—once the baby is active or crying it is difficult to get a good exam.
- The infant should be examined on a firm surface. The pelvis is stabilized with the opposite hand.

Laboratory Aids

IMAGING

Test: X-ray studies
Significance: Generally not very useful prior to 4 to 6 months, and may appear normal because of difficulty determining hip/acetabulum relation in cartilaginous femoral head.

Test: Hip ultrasound
Significance: Can determine hip laxity, subluxation, dislocation, reducibility, presence of interposed tissue, and status of the acetabulum.

FALSE POSITIVES

Hip "clicks" will be present in 10% of infants; only a small percentage will have hip dysplasia.

PITFALLS

• Examination may be normal initially. Consequently, hip evaluation should be performed as part of infant physical examination through 12 months of age.
• Many babies have "clicks" when their hips or knees are manipulated. These high-pitched snapping sensations should not be mistaken for the instability felt on a properly performed Ortolani or Barlow test.

Therapy

• Triple diaper: No longer considered to be effective treatment. Expensive for parents.
• Pavlik harness: Up to 95% effective if used prior to 6 months of age. Harness is worn 24 hours per day. Exam or ultrasound should be performed 2 to 3 weeks after initiating the harness for a dislocated hip to prove that the hip is reduced in the harness. Adjust straps every 3 weeks to accommodate growth. After 6 consecutive weeks of treatment, reassess with physical examination and/or ultrasound. Wean if hip is then stable. Complications include avascular necrosis of proximal femur, femoral nerve palsy (resolves spontaneously), skin irritation.
• Closed or open reduction: For patients who present after 6 months of age.

Follow-Up

WHEN TO EXPECT IMPROVEMENT

• Usually after about 6 weeks of treatment in the Pavlik harness.

SIGNS TO WATCH FOR

• A plain radiograph (AP pelvis x-ray) is performed at 6 and 12 months. Measure the acetabular index and check for subluxation or dislocation. Depending on the presence of residual dysplasia, later annual visits may be appropriate.

PROGNOSIS

If diagnosed in infancy, prognosis is generally excellent.

PITFALLS

• Missed early diagnosis can result in more complicated management and less favorable outcome.
• Missing an associated syndrome or condition (e.g., tethered cord, arthrogryposis).
• Mistaking a "click" for instability.

Common Questions and Answers

Q: Why is follow-up needed if the looseness disappears on examination?
A: Follow-up examinations and radiographs periodically detect late instability or acetabular dysplasia.

Q: How effective is the Pavlik harness if used within the first 4 months of life?
A: In patients with reducible hip dysplasia, the current success rate of the Pavlik harness is about 95%.

ICD-9-CM 755.63

BIBLIOGRAPHY

American Academy of Pediatrics. Clinical practice guideline: early detection of developmental dysplasia of the hip (AC0001). *Pediatrics* 2000;105(4):896–905.

Aronsson DD, Goldberg MJ, Kling TF, et al. Developmental dysplasia of the hip. *Pediatrics* 1994;94:201–212.

Bauchner H. Developmental dysplasia of the hip (DDH): an evolving science. *Arch Dis Child* 2000;83(3):202.

Bialik V, Bialik GM, Blazer S, et al. Developmental dysplasia of the hip: a new approach to incidence. *Pediatrics* 1999;103:93–99.

Bond CD, Hennrikus WL, Della Maggiore E. Prospective evaluation of newborn soft tissue hip clicks with ultrasound. *J Pediatr Orthop* 1997;17:199–201.

Clegg J, Bache CE, Raut VV. Financial justification for routine ultrasound screening of the neonatal hip. *J Bone Joint Surg* 1999;81B:852–857.

Goldberg MJ. Early detection of developmental hip dysplasia: synopsis of the AAP Clinical Practice Guidelines. *Pediatr Rev* 2001;22(4):131–134.

Guille JT, Pizzutillo PD, MacEwen GD. Development dysplasia of the hip from birth to six months. *Journal of the American Academy of Orthopaedic Surgeons* 2000;8(4):232–242.

Hadlow V. Neonatal screening for congenital dislocation of the hip: a prospective 21-year surgery. *J Bone Joint Surg* 1988;70B:740–743.

Hubbard AM. Imaging of pediatric hip disorders. *Radiol Clin North Am* 2001;39(4):721–732.

Murray KA, Crim JR. Radiographic imaging for treatment and follow-up of developmental dysplasia of the hip. *Sem Ultrasound, CTMR* 2001;22(4):306–340.

Tredwell S, Bell H. Efficacy of neonatal hip examination. *J Pediatr Orthop* 1981;1:61–65.

Vitale MG, Skaggs DL. Developmental dysplasia of the hip from six months to four years of age. *Journal of the American Academy of Orthopaedic Surgeons* 2001;9(6):401–411.

Wynne-Davies R. Acetabular dysplasia and familial joint laxity: two etiological factors in congenital dislocation of the hip: a review of 589 patients and their families. *J Bone Joint Surg* 1970;52:704–716.

Author: John M. Flynn

Diabetes Insipidus

 Database

DEFINITION

Polyuria and polydipsia caused by inability to produce or respond to antidiuretic hormone (ADH) also called arginine vasopressin.

CAUSES

Insufficient ADH Secretion

- Traumatic or postsurgical
- Nonaccidental injury in children
- Related to tumor invasion of posterior pituitary:
- Extension from anterior pituitary/suprasellar: optic glioma, rarely adenomas
- Hypothalamic: germinoma, craniopharyngioma, meningioma
- Lymphoma
- Granulomas: histiocytosis X, sarcoidosis
- Metastatic carcinoma
- Post-severe ischemic or hypoxic injury to the brain
- Familial (autosomal dominant)
- Congenital malformation of central nervous system
- Infection
- Viral encephalitis
- Meningitis
- Tuberculosis
- Increased metabolic clearance of ADH (gestational diabetes insipidus)
- Drug- or toxin-related: snake venom, tetrodotoxin
- Autoimmune disorders; hypophysitis
- Psychogenic: excessive water drinking
- Idiopathic: must observe for many years to exclude slow-growing tumors

Unresponsive to ADH

- Familial or "nephrogenic" (X-linked dominant and autosomal-recessive forms)
- Tumor-related
- Urinary tract obstruction, especially in utero
- Renal medullary cystic disease
- Electrolyte disturbances: hypokalemia, hypercalcemia (hypercalciuria)
- Drugs: usually reversible

—Diuretics
—Diphenylhydantoin
—Reserpine
—Cisplatin
—Rifampin
—Lithium: may become permanent
—Demeclocycline
—Ethanol
—Chlorpromazine
—Volatile anesthetics
—Foscarnet
—Amphotericin B

- Loss of the medullary concentrating gradient as a result of excessive free water intake relative to solute intake

PATHOPHYSIOLOGY

- ADH stimulates the formation of cyclic adenosine monophosphate (cAMP) in the renal collecting ducts, thereby increasing water permeability and increasing reabsorption of free water.
- Lack of ADH effect results in urinary loss of free water.
- Patients with an intact thirst mechanism drink copiously (polydipsia) to compensate for free water loss.
- If the thirst mechanism is not present or if access to free water is limited (e.g., infants or vomiting), severe dehydration can occur.

GENETICS

- Rare cases of autosomal-dominant transmission of ADH deficiency
- Nephrogenic diabetes insipidus (DI) is usually familial (autosomal recessive or dominant and X-linked)

EPIDEMIOLOGY (AGE-RELATED)

Because most cases are secondary to another disease, the incidence depends on the primary causes.

COMPLICATIONS

- Without treatment and without access to water:
- Hypernatremia
- Dehydration
- Coma
- When overdosed with water:

—Hyponatremia
—Seizures
—Cerebral edema

PROGNOSIS

- Generally good, but depends on the primary cause

 Differential Diagnosis

- Psychogenic polydipsia
- Abnormal thirst mechanism (dipsogenic DI)
- Hypernatremic dehydration
- Diabetes mellitus
- Polyuric renal failure (e.g., renal tubulopathy)
- Hypercalcemia
- Adrenal insufficiency
- Cerebral salt wasting

 Data Gathering

HISTORY

Question: Is the child growing normally?
Significance: Abnormal growth can be a sign of DI.

Question: Does the patient wake up during the night to drink or void? If so, what does the patient prefer to drink?
Significance: True DI is associated with polyuria throughout the day and night. Enuresis may be the first sign in a child who previously acquired bladder control. Patients, including infants, prefer water to other liquids such as juice, soda, or milk.

Question: How many hours can the patient go without drinking?
Significance: Patients with complete DI do not voluntarily stop drinking for more than 1 to 2 hours, unless the thirst mechanism is also abnormal.

Question: Does the child drink everything he can including bath and toilet water?
Significance: Patients with DI have such overwhelming thirst, they will drink anything.

Question: Volume of urine output in a day (not just frequency of urination)?
Significance: The daily volume of urine can be as high as 4 to 10 L. Younger or dehydrated children with DI tend to make less urine daily than older or hydrated children with DI.

Question: Familial history of DI?
Significance: Nephrogenic DI will typically affect maternal uncles during infancy and mothers may have a mild form.

Question: Has the child had frequent episodes of dehydration requiring medical attention?
Significance: Families may disregard the polydipsia as normal behavior. Repeated episodes of severe dehydration can damage the brain.

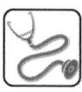 Physical Examination

Finding: Signs of dehydration
Significance: DI is typically associated with dry, pale skin and mucous membranes. Because this is hyperosmolar dehydration the patient may not look as severely dehydrated as she is.

Finding: Complete neurologic examination
Significance: Check for impaired visual fields that can be the first sign of brain tumor.

 Laboratory Aids

SPECIFIC TESTS

Test: Morning urinary osmolality with simultaneous serum sodium and serum osmolality.
Significance: If urine osmolality is at least two times higher than serum osmolality, patient does not have complete DI, but may still have partial DI.

Test: Water-deprivation test
Significance: Though definitive, it requires admission to the hospital for controlled testing under the close supervision of a pediatric endocrinologist. Patient fails test if either:

- Urinary osmolality cannot concentrate more than twice serum osmolality at the same time that serum osmolality exceeds 305 mOsm/kg
- Serum osmolality exceeds 305 mOsm/kg at any time
- Patient loses more than 5% of body weight and becomes symptomatic from hypovolemia
- Once patient fails the water deprivation test, a dose of aqueous vasopressin should be given followed by close monitoring of urinary osmolality to document responsiveness to ADH.
- Never attempt a water deprivation trial at home.

NONSPECIFIC TEST

Test: Urinary specific gravity
Significance: Insufficient by itself and nondiagnostic during a water deprivation test.

IMAGING

Test: MRI of the head
Significance: To confirm the "bright spot" normally seen in the posterior pituitary and to search for tumors. Its absence is not pathognomonic of DI.

HOME TESTING

Test: 24-hour urine collection
Significance: To obtain accurate urinary volume while patient has free access to water.

Do not restrict water intake unless the patient is in the hospital under close surveillance!

 ## Therapy

DRUGS

- DDAVP: intranasal spray or oral tablets
- Aqueous vasopressin: subcutaneous

—Comes as 4 mcg/mL solution and doses range from 0.05mcg up to 1mcg subcutaneously twice daily. Titrate dose as you would with DDAVP

- Duration of action of DDAVP is variable from patient to patient. Titration and frequency of dosing should be made by the family under the supervision of an endocrinologist.
- Control of DI in infants is more difficult because these patients may increase fluid intake as a result of hunger or increase caloric intake as a result of thirst, thereby causing an imbalance between free water intake and output. Some infants can be treated with diluted formula—the volume and frequency of feedings will be increased, but intake of free water will better match urine output. Strict record keeping of intake/output and accurate daily weighing are usually necessary for infants or patients without an intact thirst

mechanism. All infants with DI must be treated by people experienced with DI of infancy.
- Nephrogenic DI may be treated with diuretics and solute restriction as these patients are resistant to DDAVP.

SIDE EFFECTS OF DDAVP

- Facial flushing
- Increase in blood pressure
- Headache
- Nasal congestion
- Hyponatremia: caused by water overdose (intoxication), not by overdose of drug. Taking a higher dose of DDAVP will generally extend the period of antidiuresis but will not cause hyponatremia. Drinking too much water in the setting of antidiuresis causes hyponatremia. Water intoxication most often occurs in antidiuresed patients who also are on intravenous fluids, lack an intact thirst mechanism, or have psychogenic polydipsia.

DURATION

Lifelong generally. Some tumors regress with radiation, allowing recovery of ADH secretion.

DIET

- Patients with an intact thirst mechanism should drink only when thirsty.
- Patients without an intact thirst mechanism should drink only a carefully calculated fluid volume.

POSSIBLE CONFLICTS WITH OTHER TREATMENTS

Nasal congestion or gastrointestinal illness can affect the absorption of DDAVP administered.

 ## Follow-Up

Depends on the patient and underlying disease causing DI.

WHEN TO EXPECT IMPROVEMENT

- Effects of DDAVP are immediate.
- Most cases of DI are lifelong. One exception is DI that occurs during the 7 to 10 days immediately after neurosurgery, since this postsurgical DI may resolve spontaneously within 1 to 2 weeks after surgery.

SIGNS TO WATCH FOR

- Lethargy
- Somnolence
- Irritability
- Hyperpyrexia
- Any sign of dehydration
- Seizures

PITFALLS

- Management of patients without an intact thirst mechanism and of newborns is difficult.
- Patients with psychogenic polydipsia may fail a water deprivation test because prolonged excessive water intake can wash out the renal medullary gradient required for concentrating the urine.
- Surreptitious water intake during water deprivation test.
- Idiopathic, acquired DI can be as a result of slowly growing brain tumors not visible on the initial MRI.

 ## Common Questions and Answers

Q: In a patient with intact thirst mechanism and partial DI is the use of DDAVP necessary?
A: No, as long as the patient has constant access to free water.

Q: How does therapy of DI affect daily life? Is it easily integrated into normal activity and eating patterns?
A: DDAVP is used in a patient with intact thirst mechanism to facilitate the daily routine as well as to allow patients to sleep without the need to void frequently during the night.

Q: Is there a longer acting preparation or an implantable pump for dosing?
A: The longest-acting form of ADH is an injected medication and can have effects for 3 days, increasing the risks of hyponatremia. Home use of the nasal spray or tablets, therefore, is easier and safer than the use of injections.

ICD-9-CM 253.5

BIBLIOGRAPHY

Kirchlechner V, Koller DY, Seidl R, et al. Treatment of nephrogenic diabetes insipidus with hydrochlorothiazide and amiloride. *Arch Dis Child* 1999;80(6):548–552.

Leger J, Velasquez A, Garel C, et al. Thickened pituitary stalk on magnetic resonance imaging in children with central diabetes insipidus. *J Clin Endocrinol Metab* 1999;84(6): 1954–1960.

Mootha SL, Barkovich AJ, Grumbach MM, et al. Idiopathic hypothalamic diabetes insipidus, pituitary stalk thickening, and the occult intracranial germinoma in children and adolescents. *J Clin Endocrinol Metab* 1997; 82(5):1362–1367.

Robertson GL. Diabetes insipidus. *Endocrinol Metab Clin North Am* 1995;24(3):549–572.

Siegel AJ, Baldessarini RJ, Klepser MB, et al. Primary and drug-induced disorders of water homeostasis in psychiatric patients: principles of diagnosis and management. *Harv Res Psychiatry* 1998;6(4):190–200.

Author: Paul S. Thornton

Diabetes Mellitus

 Database

DEFINITION

Diabetes mellitus (DM) is a disorder of absolute or relative insulin deficiency that results in disruptions in normal energy storage and metabolism. This causes impaired glucose tolerance, hyperglycemia, ketosis, and acidosis, which can ultimately lead to dehydration, shock, and death.

CAUSES

- Type 1 DM: In genetically susceptible individuals, an environmental trigger (believed viral) causes an autoimmune-mediated destruction of pancreatic β-cells, leading to absolute insulin deficiency.
- Type 2 DM: Insulin resistance (peripheral) in susceptible individuals (impaired β-cell function) leads to relative insulin deficiency.

PATHOLOGY (TYPE 1 DM)

- Induction of expression of DR antigens on β-cell surface following viral infection.
- Recruitment of cytotoxic lymphocytes.
- Production of anti-insulin and anti-islet-cell antibodies (GAD65, ICA512)
- Progressive loss of β-cell mass and insulin supply as a result of inflammatory process, resulting in insulin deficiency.

EPIDEMIOLOGY

- Most common endocrine/metabolic disorder of childhood
- Type 1 DM: More common in Caucasians of Northern European descent

—Prevalence of type 1 DM in youth 0 to 19 years in the United States about 1.7/1,000
—Annual U.S. incidence is about 19/100,000 in children 10 to 19 years of age
—Incidence of type 1 DM rising, especially in younger children, ~3% per year

- Type 2 DM: More common in African-Americans, Latino, and Native Americans, usually with strong family history

—Incidence of type 2 DM increasing rapidly, may be as high as 8% to 46% of new cases of diabetes in youth
—Estimated prevalence of type 2 DM in youth of 4.1/1,000
—Estimated prevalence of impaired glucose tolearance in youth of 1.8/1,000

GENETICS

- Susceptibility for type 1 DM associated with HLA region of chromosome 6 fivefold greater risk with MHC antigen types DR3 and DR4
- Genetic defect in type 2 DM unknown
- Maturity-onset diabetes of youth (MODY) is a family of autosomal-dominant syndromes caused by mutations of genes involved in the regulation of pancreatic development or insulin secretion; the syndromes represent a small minority of non-type 1 diabetes in children.

COMPLICATIONS

- Diabetic ketoacidosis (DKA): profound metabolic derangement characterized by hyperglycemia, ketosis, and acidosis, leading to osmotic diuresis, dehydration, shock, and death
- Hypoglycemia—severe events may result in neurocognitive dysfunction, coma, seizure
- Long-term effects:

—Nephropathy—microalbuminuria, hypertension, proteinuria, chronic renal failure
—Retinopathy—microvascular proliferation, visual loss
—Neuropathy—progressive diminution of nerve conduction velocity
—Vasculopathy—accelerated atherosclerosis, large-vessel disease
—Embryopathy—infants of diabetic mothers at increased risk of birth defects
—Growth failure (Mauriac syndrome) and delayed sexual maturation
—Rate of development of chronic complications related to degree of metabolic control
—Comorbidities of type 1 DM are increased risk of other auto-immune disorders: thyroiditis, adrenal insufficiency, celiac disease

 Differential Diagnosis

- Urinary tract infection (polyuria)
- Renal glycosuria
- Hypercalcemia (polyuria, weight loss)
- Chronic illness (weight loss, malaise)
- Stress-related hyperglycemia
- Drug-induced hyperglycemia (steroids)
- Psychogenic polydipsia
- Pneumonia (in DKA)
- Sepsis (in DKA)
- Acute abdominal event (in DKA)

 Data Gathering

HISTORY

Question: Polyuria, nocturia, enuresis?
Significance: Related to hyperglycemia.

Question: Polydipsia?
Significance: Increased thirst follows polyuria and dehydration.

Question: Polyphagia?
Significance: Increased appetite related to loss of calories from glucosuria.

Question: Weight loss, poor growth?
Significance: Dehydration, loss of calories

Question: Malaise, weakness?
Significance: Electrolyte disturbance and acidosis.

Question: Changes in behavior, school performance?
Significance: Chronic illness.

 Physical Examination

- Usually normal in type 1 DM, but weight loss may be present
- Obesity and acanthosis nigricans (hypertrophic skin pigmentation of the neck and skin folds) in type 2 DM
- In DKA, signs of dehydration and acidosis (Kussmaul respirations)

 Laboratory Aids

- Diagnosis based on blood glucose (BG) level: fasting BG ≥126, random BG ≥200 mg/dL, or 2-hour BG ≥200 on oral glucose tolerance test.
- Other categories of glucose disorders: Impaired glucose tolerance, defined as 2-hour BG between 140 and 200 on oral glucose tolerance test; and impaired fasting glucose, defined as fasting BG 100 to 125.
- Glycosuria, ketonuria (latter is variable in type 2 DM)
- Hemoglobin A1c (gives approximation of average blood glucose level over previous 2 to 3 months)

Test: Measurement of GAD65 and other autoantibodies
Significance: may help differentiate type 1 from type 2 DM.

Therapy

• Insulin

—Usually given in combination of short-acting and long-acting preparations b.i.d. to q.i.d.
—Total daily dose (TDD) usually about 0.7 to 1.2 U/kg per day, less during "honeymoon period."
—"Split-mixed regimen": two-thirds of TDD in morning (one-third of that as short-acting and two-thirds long-acting), and one-third of TDD in evening (with one-half of that as short-acting and one-half as long-acting, either as one injection at dinner or split between dinner and bedtime).
—"Basal/bolus regimen": approximately one-half of TDD given as one injection of very long-acting insulin, and bolus doses of short-acting insulin given for meals and snacks based on BG and carbohdrate content of meals. This may be given via multiple injections or via continuous subcutaneous insulin infusion (insulin pump therapy)

• Oral antidiabetic agents may be effective in type 2 DM
• Sulfonylureas: increase endogenous insulin production and release
• Biguanides: reduce hepatic glucose production
• Thiazolidinediones: improve peripheral insulin sensitivity
• α-Glucosidase inhibitors: competitively inhibit intestinal glucose absorption

DIET

Guidelines for meal content:

• 20% of daily calories from breakfast and lunch
• 30% from dinner
• 10% from snacks evenly spaced between meals and before bedtime
• Balance of source of calories is important:

—55% from carbohydrates (of which 70% complex)
—30% from fats
—15% from protein

• Carbohydrate "counting" for those on basal/bolus therapy or insulin pumps
• Weight reduction/stabilization critical for most children with type 2 diabetes

EXERCISE

• Regular exercise helps to reduce insulin requirements and reduce blood glucose, by increasing insulin sensitivity, in both type 1 and type 2 DM.
• Regular aerobic activity critical in management of type 2 diabetes

HOME MONITORING

• Checking blood glucose before meals and snacks, with symptoms of hypoglycemia, after exercise, and with intercurrent illness
• Checking urine for ketones whenever blood glucose more than 240 mg/dL or during intercurrent illnesses.

Follow-Up

• Regular appointments with diabetes specialist every 3 months to assess growth and development and trouble-shoot management problems
• Meetings with nutritionist periodically to reassess meal plan
• Meetings with psychologist as needed to address psychosocial and family stressors
• Monitoring of HbA1c every 3 months to assess long-term control and compliance
• Yearly urine samples for microalbuminuria
• Yearly ophthalmologic examination to evaluate retinopathy
• Yearly cholesterol profile to evaluate hyperlipidemia
• Yearly T4, TSH, anti-tissue transglutaminase IgA for thyroiditis and celiac disease

Common Questions and Answers

Q: What is the "honeymoon period"?
A: The period of "remission" following initial stabilization of metabolism with exogenous insulin. It is marked by the presence of residual endogenous insulin secretion; insulin doses usually drop to 0.5 U/kg per day or less. The honeymoon phase usually lasts weeks to months, but may persist 1 to 2 years.

Q: What is the risk of diabetes in a sibling or child of a person with type 1 DM?
A: It is 5% to 10% in first-degree relatives (siblings, offspring), 40% to 50% in identical twins.

Q: What are the goals of glucose control?
A: HbA1c <7.0 %; fasting blood glucose 70 to 120 mg/dL; postprandial blood glucose <180 mg/dL; avoidance of episodes of hypoglycemia; maintenance of a reasonably nonrestrictive lifestyle and psychological adjustment.

Q: Does having diabetes necessarily mean that one will develop the long-term complications?
A: The Diabetes Control and Complications Trial showed that intensive management and tight control (average blood sugar <140 mg/dL) reduces the risk of complications (retinopathy, nephropathy, and neuropathy) by 50% to 75%.

ICD-9-CM 250.0

BIBLIOGRAPHY

American Diabetes Association. Standards of medical care for patients with diabetes mellitus. *Diabetes Care* 1994;17:616–623.

American Diabetes Association. Type 2 diabetes in children and adolescents. *Pediatrics* 2000;105:671–680.

Dabelea D, Pettitt DJ, Jones KL, et al. Type 2 diabetes mellitus in children and adolescents: an emerging problem. *Endocrinol Metab Clin North Am* 1999;28:709–730.

Diabetes Control and Complications Trial Research Group. The effect of intensive treatment of diabetes on the development and progression of long-term complications in insulin-dependent diabetes mellitus. *N Engl J Med* 1993;329:977–986.

Kaufman FR. Diabetes in children and adolescents: areas of controversy. *Med Clin North Am* 1998;82:721–738.

Laffel LM, Vangsness L, Connell A, Goebel-Fabbri A, Butler D, Anderson BJ. Impact of ambulatory, family-focused teamwork intervention on glycemic control in youth with type 1 diabetes *J Pediatr* 2003;142(4):409–416.

Sperling M. Diabetes mellitus. In: Sperling M, ed. *Clinical Pediatric Endocrinology.* Philadelphia: WB Saunders, 1996:229–263.

Svoren BM, Butler D, Levine BS, Anderson BJ, Laffel LM. Reducing acute adverse outcomes in youths with type 1 diabetes: a randomized, controlled trial. *Pediatrics* 2003;112(4): 914–922.

Weiss R, Dufour S, Taksali SE, et al. Prediabetes in obese youth: a syndrome of impaired glucose tolerance, severe insulin resistance, and altered myocellular and abdominal fat partitioning *Lancet* 2003;362(9388):951–957.

Authors: Kristen Calcagni and Stuart A. Weinzimer

Diabetic Ketoacidosis

 Database

DEFINITION

- State of severe metabolic derangement that occurs in patients with insulin-dependent diabetes mellitus secondary to insulin deficiency and stress hormone excess.
- Hyperglycemia (blood glucose >200 mg/dL)
- Ketonemia (>3 mmol in serum) or ketonuria
- Acidosis (pH <7.3 or HCO_3 <15 mEq/L)

CAUSE/PATHOLOGY

- Insulin deficiency and excess of the counter-regulatory hormones glucagon, cortisol, and epinephrine lead to increased glucose production, impaired peripheral glucose utilization, increased proteolysis and lipolysis.
- Glycogenolysis and gluconeogenesis lead to hyperglycemia.
- Lipolysis and ketone production lead to metabolic acidosis.
- Hyperosmolar state leads to osmotic diuresis, dehydration, and electrolyte loss.

EPIDEMIOLOGY

- 15% to 67% of DKA at diabetes onset; higher percentage in children under 4 years and in families with lower socioeconomic status (SES).
- Risk of DKA in established type 1 diabetes is 1% to 10% per patient per year, increased risk in children with poor metabolic control, previous episodes of DKA, adolescent girls, and families with lower SES
- Annual hospitalization rates for DKA for new and established type 1 diabetes around 10/100,000 children per year
- 65% of all hospital admissions in diabetic children under 19 years old

COMPLICATIONS

- Cardiovascular collapse

—Caused by osmotic diuresis and dehydration
—Treated with prompt initiation of fluid resuscitation

- Overwhelming acidosis

—From ketoacid accumulation
—Treated with insulin infusion, sodium bicarbonate infusion if necessary

- Hypoglycemia from insufficient dextrose supplementation, treated by increasing dextrose
- Hypokalemia

—Caused by loss of potassium in the urine and correction of acidosis with insulin
—Treated by intravenous potassium supplementation

- Cerebral edema

—Most serious complication of DKA and most frequent cause of death

—Rapid changes in serum osmolality lead to influx of water into brain tissue
—Occurs 6 to 18 hours after initiation of therapy, often as patient is clinically improving
—Heralded as headache, change in mental status, or abnormal neurological signs
—May progress rapidly to brain herniation and death
—Treatment is supportive, aimed at reducing intracranial pressure with intravenous mannitol and mechanical hyperventilation

PROGNOSIS

- Mortality of DKA in children approximately 0.2% to 0.3%
- Most common cause of death (>50%) in diabetic children
- 57% to 87% of mortality in DKA is a result of cerebral edema

 Differential Diagnosis

- Gastroenteritis
- Severe intraabdominal process (e.g., ulcer, pancreatitis, appendicitis)
- Urinary tract infection
- Pneumonia
- Stress hyperglycemia
- Hypercalcemia
- Salicylate ingestion
- Inborn error of metabolism
- Nonketotic hyperosmolar coma

 Data Gathering

HISTORY

Question: Polyuria, polydipsia, and polyphagia with weight loss?
Significance: Symptom of hyperosmolar state.

Question: Nausea, vomiting, abdominal pain?
Significance: Related to acidosis and electrolyte disturbance.

Question: Changes in breathing patterns (Kussmaul respirations)?
Significance: Related to acidosis and respiratory correction.

Question: Precipitating event, such as an intercurrent illness or psychosocial stress?
Significance: Increased need for insulin in these states.

 Physical Examination

Finding: Vital signs—tachycardia, hypotension
Significance: Seen with dehydration

Finding: Dry mucous membranes, sunken eyes, poor skin turgor, poor distal perfusion, weak pulses
Significance: Dehydration

Finding: Fruity odor to breath
Significance: Ketosis

Finding: Deep, sighing, hyperpneic (Kussmaul) respirations
Significance: Respiratory compensation for primary acid-base disturbance

Finding: Abdominal tenderness
Significance: Related to ketosis, acidosis

Finding: Altered mental status, lethargy, obtundation
Significance: Acidosis, dehydration, and hyperosmolarity

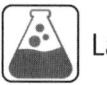 Laboratory Aids

Test: Glucose more than 200 mg/dL
Significance: Indicates insulin deficiency

Test: Urinalysis—glycosuria and ketonuria
Significance: Glucose level exceeds renal threshold

Test: Sodium—serum levels low; from electrolyte losses and artifact of hyperlipidemia; actual Na level = measured Na + 1.6 × [(glucose − 200)/100]
Significance: Severity of dehydration

Test: Potassium—serum levels may be elevated, normal, or low; total body is potassium-depleted.
Significance: Potassium depletion from osmotic diuresis. Serum level is dependent on degree of acidosis and dehydration.

Test: Bicarbonate less than 15 mEq/L
Significance: Metabolic acidosis

Test: Phosphate—low, secondary to osmotic diuresis
Significance: may contribute to poor oxygen delivery to peripheral tissues

Test: ABG—low pH (<7.3), low pCO_2, and low HCO_3
Significance: Metabolic acidosis

Test: CBC—elevated WBC count even in the absence of infection
Significance: Stress reaction

Therapy

- Resuscitation

—Assess adequacy of airway and breathing.
—Restore circulation if necessary with normal saline bolus of 10 to 20 mL/kg, repeat as needed
—Cannot gauge hydration status initially by urine output because of osmotic diuresis.
—Avoid excessive fluid resuscitation—too-rapid correction of hyperosmolarity increases risk of cerebral edema. However, shock must be treated aggressively.

- Monitoring

—ICU admission for infants, toddlers, initial pH <7.0, hemodynamic or neurological instability
—ECG monitoring for hypokalemia or hyperkalemia
—Serial neurological examinations q1h, with special attention to headache, declining mental status, any neurological symptoms
—Hourly blood sugars
—pH and electrolytes q1–2h until stable

- Fluids

—Assume at least 7% to 10% dehydration, 15% in infants.
—Replacement fluids should have tonicity >$\frac{1}{2}$ normal saline, rate of administration calculated to rehydrate evenly over 48 hours
—Urinary losses should not be added to the calculation of replacement fluids

- Electrolytes

—Assume Na and K losses of approximately 5 to 10 mEq/kg.
—Hyponatremia will correct as fluids and insulin are given.
—Continued drop in Na is associated with increased risk of cerebral edema.
—Replace potassium as an equal mixture with chloride and phosphate; initial K+ concentration should be 40 mEq/L; if hypokalemic on presentation, may require higher potassium replacement given through central IV; if hyperkalemic on presentation, defer potassium administration until urine output is documented.

- Acidosis

—Usually corrects once adequate insulin and fluids are given.
—Most patients will not need alkali therapy; bicarbonate use may be associated with hypokalemia, delayed time to recovery, and increased central nervous system acidosis
—Severely acidotic patients (arterial pH < 6.9) or those with inadequate respiratory compensation ($pCO_2 > (1.5 \times [HCO_3]) + 8$) may benefit from judicious use (slow infusion, 1 to 2 mEq/kg, given over 1 to 2 hours

- Insulin

—Prompt initiation critical in terminating ongoing ketone and acid production.
—Initial dose is 0.1 U/kg per hour as continuous intravenous infusion.
—Do not give subcutaneously in DKA, as skin perfusion may be suboptimal.
—Aim to lower serum glucose by 50 to 100 mg/dL per hour. If glucose levels are dropping quickly, slow the fall with dextrose rather than reduce the insulin dose

- Glucose

—Add 5% dextrose to intravenous stock when blood glucose <300 mg/dL
—Change to 10% dextrose when blood glucose <200 mg/dL

- Duration

—Stop infusion when pH >7.3, HCO_3 >15, glucose <300, and patient is tolerating oral fluids.

- Convert to subcutaneous therapy by adding up total insulin given over 24 hours and dividing into two to four injections or return to usual home regimen of insulin with frequent monitoring and extra insulin as needed.

Follow-Up

- New diabetic patients should be followed closely after hospital discharge to assess adequacy of insulin regimen.
- Children with recurrent DKA should be evaluated for treatment failure (family dysfunction, knowledge deficits).

PREVENTION

- Timely referral for children with symptoms of polyuria, polydipsia, and weight loss.
- Surveillance with frequent blood sugar and urine ketone monitoring, supplemental insulin dosing; phone contact with pediatrician or endocrinologist should avert almost all episodes of DKA in children known to have diabetes.
- Psychological or family counseling may be required for children with recurrent episodes of DKA associated with poor adherence to diabetes management or known insulin omission.

Common Questions and Answers

Q: What are the usual triggers for DKA?
A: Intercurrent illnesses, such as gastroenteritis, urinary tract infections, pneumonia; psychosocial stressors; failure to take insulin on schedule.

Q: Does an episode of DKA mean that the insulin regimen is inadequate?
A: DKA always implies insulin deficiency; insulin regimen may be adequate when child is well, but additional stresses of illness or psychosocial factors often require supplemental insulin.

ICD-9-CM 250.1

BIBLIOGRAPHY

Dunger DB, Sperling MA, Acerini CL, et al. and the European Society for Paediatric Endocrinology/Lawson Wilkins Pediatric Endocrine Society. European Society for Paediatric Endocrinology/Lawson Wilkins Pediatric Endocrine Society consensus statement on diabetic ketoacidosis in children and adolescents. *Pediatrics* 2004;113(2): e133–140.

Glaser N, Barnett P, McCaslin I, et al. Risk factors for cerebral edema in children with diabetic ketoacidosis. *N Engl J Med* 2001;344:264–269.

Green SM, Rothrock SG, Ho JD, et al. Failure of adjuvant bicarbonate to improve outcome in severe pediatric diabetic ketoacidosis. *Ann Emerg Med* 1998;31:41–48.

Harris G, Fiordalisi I. Physiologic management of diabetic ketoacidemia. *Arch Pediatr Adolesc Med* 1994;148:1046–1052.

Kaufman FR. Diabetes in children and adolescents: areas of controversy. *Med Clin North Am* 1998;82(4):721–738.

Krane E. Diabetic ketoacidosis: biochemistry, physiology, treatment, and prevention. *Pediatr Clin North Am* 1987;34(4):935–960.

Marcin JP, Glaser N, Barnett P, McCaslin I, et al. and the American Academy of Pediatrics/The Pediatric Emergency Medicine Collaborative Research Commitee. Factors associated with adverse outcomes in children with diabetic ketoacidosis-related cerebral edema. *J Pediatr* 2002;141(6):793–797.

Rosenbloom A, Hanas R. Diabetic ketoacidosis (DKA): treatment guidelines. *Clin Pediatr* 1996;35:261–266.

Author: Stuart A. Weinzimer

Diaper Rash

 Database

DEFINITION

Commonly known as diaper or nappy rash, it is a collection of dermatoses defined by its etiology and distribution.

PATHOPHYSIOLOGY

Diaper rashes are the result of several different processes, alone and in combination:

- Friction: Rubbing of wet diapers against exposed skin areas such as the inner surface of the thighs, genitals, buttocks, abdomen results in an erythematous, shiny rash that spares the intertriginous areas.
- Irritation: Confined to the exposed areas under the diaper, sparing the intertriginous areas, secondary to irritants such as feces/urine, cleaning materials.
- Allergic: Contact allergies may be the result of detergents, topical medicines.
- Atopic: Usually later onset in infants, is pruritic and is often accompanied by a familial history of atopy.
- Seborrhea: Typical yellow-salmon-colored greasy rash especially affecting the intertriginous areas, and may be seen in other areas such as the scalp, face, neck, and flexural areas.
- Candidal: Especially common during or immediately after antibiotic administration, this rash is beefy red, with a raised sharp margin, and characteristic pinpoint erythematous, satellite lesions.

GENETICS

Dependent on the individual causes of diaper dermatitis, such as predisposition for atopy or other allergic-based rashes.

EPIDEMIOLOGY

This dermatitis is by definition exclusive to individuals wearing diapers, and generally resolves when diapers are no longer worn. It is estimated to affect approximately 7% to 35% of the infant population at any given time and is most commonly found in the 9 to 12 month age group.

COMPLICATIONS

Generally none, although secondary bacterial or fungal infections may lead to ulceration. Severe bacterial superinfections in newborns or immune-compromised infants can lead to sepsis.

PROGNOSIS

Diaper rash usually resolves with good skin care. It completely resolves once the child is potty trained and out of diapers.

 Differential Diagnosis

Although any rash under a diaper can be considered a diaper rash, the following are other diseases that may present on the skin of the anogenital region but are not common causes of diaper dermatitis.

- Infection

—Congenital syphilis: Less commonly seen now because of maternal screening, this infection may manifest with a macular, papular, or bullous lesion in the diaper area. The palms and soles may also reveal lesions.
—HIV infection: May first present with erosive and ulcerated lesions, especially in the gluteal cleft. May be associated with other infections such as cytomegalovirus or herpes, may be pruritic. Other findings such as anemia, hepatosplenomegaly are often present.
—Scabies, herpes virus, varicella

- Tumors

—Letterer-Siwe (Langerhans cell histiocytosis) may present as a diaper rash with small reddish-brown papules or vesicles.

- Metabolic

—Acrodermatitis enteropathica: Deficiency of zinc. In addition to vesiculobullous lesions of the hands and feet and surrounding mouth and diaper areas, these patients have failure to thrive, diarrhea, alopecia, and frequent bacterial and candidal infections.
—Biotin deficiency:

- Immunologic

—Psoriasis: Although unusual, may affect the diaper area with dark red, well-marginated plaques with silvery scales. Other areas of the body are usually similarly affected.

- Other

—Granuloma gluteal infantum, the etiology is not well understood, probably an inflammatory response to a variety of irritants. Results in discrete red painless nodules up to 4 cm in size.
—Child abuse, epidermolysis bullosa

 Data Gathering

HISTORY

Question: Any skin disorders at other sites?
Significance: Skin disorders such as atopic dermatitis or seborrhea located elsewhere on the body suggest involvement in the diaper area as well.

Question: Use of medications (especially oral antibiotics, or topical medications)?
Significance: Medications can directly affect the diaper area, or leave it more susceptible to rashes. Oral antibiotics change the normal bowel and skin flora, and may cause diarrhea, which can irritate the skin. Topical medications such as steroid ointments may change the appearance of the rash, or may cause changes in the skin (such as thinning). Some fungal creams contain sensitizers, such as ethylenediamine hydrochloride.

Question: Use of detergents or soaps on skin or clothes?
Significance: These substances are often not recognized by parents as containing irritants (such as perfumes) which can damage the skin, leaving it susceptible to diaper rash.

Question: Any current medical problems (such as diarrhea) which might irritate the skin?
Significance: Many medical problems manifest themselves in the skin, and may affect the diaper rash.

Question: Review skin care techniques: what is put on the skin and how is it used?
Significance: Parents often think a diaper rash represents poor hygiene, and as a result increase the cleaning of the area around the rash. Depending on how it is done and what is used, this cleaning may instead result in further irritation and damage to the skin.

Physical Examination

Finding: Location of the rash should be carefully noted.
Significance: Is it predominately in the exposed surfaces (contact, friction) or in the intertriginous areas (seborrhea, candidal)?

Finding: The margins of the rash should be inspected for satellite lesions.
Significance: Candida classically has satellite lesions.

Finding: Appearance of lesions
Significance: The lesion is dry or moist appearing (candidal); if it has a shiny parchment paper-like appearance (friction or atopic dermatitis).

Finding: A thorough examination of other areas of skin (e.g., looking for atopic or seborrheic dermatitis).
Significance: May give clues to the underlying skin of the diaper area and determine etiological factors of the rash.

 ## Laboratory Aids

Almost always a clinical diagnosis. Candidal infections may be verified by skin scraping and viewed with potassium hydroxide under a microscope. Other etiologies should be considered with resistant diaper rash and may rarely require skin biopsy.

 ## Therapy

Proper skin care is the primary treatment modality. When soiled, the skin should be gently washed with a mild soap and patted dry or air-dried. The diaper should be kept off and the rash exposed to air as much as possible. Any moderate to severe rash will invariably be secondarily infected with *Candida* and should be treated with topical nystatin, miconazole, or clotrimazole. If the skin is very inflamed and especially if there is evidence of contact, atopic, or seborrheic dermatitis, a small amount of topical corticosteroid cream (such as 1% hydrocortisone) can be used for a few days. Although gentle skin care techniques should be permanently adopted, the use of topical antifungal medication and ointments should be continued until the rash completely resolves. Steroid medications should be stopped after a few days, when the intense acute inflammation has improved. Sucrafate has been used topically in severe situations, it acts as a physical barrier and may neutralize bile acids and pepsin. It should be considered in children with ostomies who are prone to diaper rashes.

 ## Follow-Up

With proper treatment, the rash should be noticeably better within 4 to 7 days. Failure of resolution of rash indicates that another dermatologic process may be complicating the diaper rash.

PREVENTION

Proper skin care with gentle cleaning and mild soap should be used. Superabsorbent diapers may be suggested, along with frequent diaper changes. Barrier creams such as zinc oxide may help protect the skin from external irritants after resolution of the rash.

PITFALLS

General pitfall to avoid is the use of laboratory aids to help diagnose this disorder, because it is almost always a clinical diagnosis. Topical steroid used alone may worsen a candidal infection.

- Often the caretaker believes the rash is a result of inadequate cleansing of the skin and, subsequently, attempts to wash the skin more. This additionally irritates and exacerbates the rash. Topicals that strongly adhere to the skin do not need to be scrubbed completely off before putting on another treatment.
- Steroids marketed by drug companies in combination with antifungal creams are often more potent than necessary. In addition, the action of topical steroids is potentiated when used under "occlusion" (the diaper). When topical steroids are used, they are best given as a separate prescription that can be stopped at an earlier time (usually when the rash starts to improve) than the antifungal medication.
- Talcum powder can worsen the irritation, and may be aspirated by both baby and caretaker. Its use should be discouraged.
- If a candidal diaper infection is resistant to treatment, and thrush (monilia infection of the mouth) is present, oral nystatin may be added q.i.d. Since an infected mother may reinoculate her infant, an evaluation of the mother for candidal infections of the nipples could be considered. In severe cases, a short course of oral fluconazole may be necessary.
- Severe cases of diaper rash may be complicated by bacterial infections and oral antibiotics may be considered.

 ## Common Questions and Answers

Q: Should I switch from cloth to disposable diapers (or vice versa)?
A: This is controversial, although there are some studies that indicate that the superabsorbent disposable diapers may be better for controlling diaper rashes. Cloth diapers used with plastic overpants probably irritate the skin more because they trap moisture against the skin. Frequent changing of diapers is very helpful, along with not wearing diapers at all when practical.

Q: Is the diaper rash as a result of not keeping the skin clean enough?
A: Although the combination of stool and urine may release enzymes that help break down skin integrity, probably more harmful to skin is vigorous and frequent scrubbing with relatively abrasive materials on the macerated, easily damaged skin typically found in the diaper area. This rough cleaning allows introduction of bacteria and yeast into the skin and results in a diaper rash. Parent should be advised to use soft cleaning materials (such as cotton balls) to gently clean stool from the diaper area. It is not usually necessary to clean the skin of urine every time, rather patting the infant dry with a soft cloth and then replacing the diaper is all that is generally required.

ICD-9-CM 691

BIBLIOGRAPHY

Boiko S. Making rash decisions in the diaper area. *Pediatr Ann* 2000;29(1):50–56.

Friedlander SF. Contact dermatitis. *Pediatr Rev* 1998;19:166–171.

Kazaks EL, Lane AT. Diaper dermatitis. *Pediatr Clin N Am* 2000;47(4):900–919.

Singalavanija S, Frieden I. Diaper dermatitis. *Pediatr Rev* 1995;16:142–147.

Wong LD, Brantly D, Clutter LB, et al. Diapering choices: a critical review of the issues. *Pediatr Nurs* 1992;18:41–54.

Author: Robert Kamei

Diaphragmatic Hernia (Congenital)

 Database

DEFINITION

- Herniation of abdominal contents into the thoracic cavity through an opening in the diaphragm causing varying degree of pulmonary hypoplasia
- Two types of congenital diaphragmatic hernia (CDH)
—Bochdalek hernia (posterolateral location)
—Morgagni hernia (retrosternal location)

CAUSES

- True cause: unknown
- Diaphragm forms between 7 and 10 weeks of gestation
- Diaphragm is composed of two parts:
—Pleuroperitoneal folds attach to the chest wall, develop a muscular lining, and become the lateral and dorsal portions of the diaphragm.
—Septum transversum, which becomes the central tendon of the diaphragm.
- Anything that interferes with the formation of the diaphragm allows an abdominal hernia to develop.
- Bochdalek hernia develops when:
—Midgut returns to the abdominal cavity prematurely or diaphragmatic development is delayed.
—Bowel is trapped in the thoracic cavity, preventing the pleuroperitoneal folds from connecting with the thoracic wall.
—This allows a communication to exist between the thoracic and abdominal cavities.
- Morgagni hernia develops when:
—A defect develops in the septum transversum

PATHOPHYSIOLOGY

- Bochdalek hernia
—Usually occurs on the left side (left-sided pleuroperitoneal folds close later than the right)
—Bilateral lung hypoplasia (ipsilateral lung hypoplasia worse than contralateral side)
—Lung abnormal in respect to: morphology, differentiation and maturation
—Abnormal morphology of pulmonary arteries (suggesting primary vascular hypoplasia)
—Possible surfactant deficiency
—Bowel in the thoracic cavity
- Morgagni hernia
—Usually occurs on the right side (left-sided defects are covered by the heart)
—Hernia can contain: liver, bowel, and omentum
—Less lung hypoplasia seen than with Bochdalek hernias

EPIDEMIOLOGY

- Bochdalek hernia
—Accounts for 90% of cases of congenital diaphragmatic hernias
—Incidence: in 1/2,000 to 1/5,000 live births
—80% to 90% of cases on the left side (2% bilateral)
—More common in males

—40% of cases associated with some type of congenital malformation:
—chromosomal abnormalities in 5% to 16% of cases (e.g., Turner syndrome, trisomy 18 and 13, Fryn syndrome)
—congenital heart disease in 10% to 35% of cases
—Others: neurologic defects (hydrocephalus, spina bifida, anencephaly), digestive, IUGR
- Morgagni hernia
—Accounts for 2% of all diaphragmatic hernias; more common in females

GENETICS

- Estimated 2% recurrence rate in first-degree relatives

COMPLICATIONS

- Bochdalek hernia
—Pulmonary hypoplasia
—Persistent fetal circulation
—Pulmonary hypertension
—Right to left shunt
—Pulmonary insufficiency
—Death
- Morgagni hernia
—10% incidence of strangulation of the bowel if not repaired

 Differential Diagnosis

PULMONARY

- Pulmonary cysts
- Cystic adenomatoid malformation
- Pneumatocele
- Congenital lobar emphysema
- Pulmonary sequestration
- Eventration of the diaphragm
- Hiatal hernia
- Laryngotracheal obstruction
- Atelectasis
- Pneumothorax
- Anterior mediastinal mass
- Pneumonia
- Pleural effusion

CARDIAC

- Dextrocardia
- Congenital heart disease

 Data Gathering

HISTORY

Question: Bochdalek hernia?
Significance: Presents at birth; patient frequently presents in severe cardiopulmonary distress.

Question: Morgagni hernia?
Significance: Usually asymptomatic. If symptomatic, usually presents later in life. May have complaints of: vague abdominal discomfort, vomiting, failure to thrive, chest pain, dyspnea, cough, and recurrent respiratory infections.

 Physical Examination

Finding: Bochdalek hernia
Significance: Symptoms are critical in the first 72 hours:

- Severe respiratory distress
- Cyanosis
- Tachypnea
- Decreased breath sounds on the affected side
- Hyperresonance to percussion on the affected side
- Asymmetry of the chest wall (enlarged on the affected side)
- Increased anterior-posterior diameter of the chest
- Occasional bowel sounds heard in the chest
- Tachycardia
- Cardiac point of maximal impulse shifted away from the affected side
- Scaphoid abdomen (abdominal contents in thoracic cavity)

Finding: Morgagni hernia
Significance: Examination may be normal

 Laboratory Aids

TESTS

Test: Arterial blood gas
Significance:

- pO_2 shows evidence of severe hypoxia
- pCO_2 elevated
- pH, bicarbonate, lactate: reveal significant acidosis (both respiratory and metabolic)

IMAGING

Test: Chest radiograph
Significance:

- Bochdalek hernia
—Mediastinal structures shifted away from the affected side
—Heart shifted away from the affected side
—Decreased lung volumes (ipsilateral lung more than contralateral lung)
—Atelectasis of the contralateral lung
—Unable to visualize the diaphragm on the ipsilateral side
—Loops of bowel in the thoracic cavity
—In left-sided hernias, a nasogastric tube inserted into the stomach will be seen in the thoracic cavity
—Abdominal bowel is usually gasless
- Morgagni hernia
—A mass is seen in the anterior mediastinum: may be solid or gas-filled.

Test: Echocardiogram
Significance: Assessment of the degree of pulmonary hypertension and exclusion of congenital heart defect

Diaphragmatic Hernia (Congenital)

Test: Ventilation/perfusion scan
Significance: Decreased ventilation and perfusion in the hypoplastic lung

Test: Fetal ultrasound
Significance: Abdominal viscera in the thoracic cavity; polyhydramnios

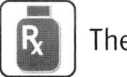 Therapy

• Bochdalek hernia
—Physiologic emergency requiring resuscitation and early stabilization of the patient:
—ET tube placement, minimal bag mask ventilation
—Oxygenation; preductal saturation of greater than 85%
—Ventilation: permissive hypercapnia has been shown to be the preferred strategy
—Correction of acidosis; pH >7.3
—Normalization of blood pressure
—Decompression of the intrathoracic bowel (placement of a nasogastric tube to low suction allows the bowel to decompress, thus letting the ipsilateral hypoplastic lung expand)
—Surgical repair of the defect:
—Decreased morbidity and mortality if the patient can be stabilized prior to surgical repair
—ECMO (extracorporeal membrane oxygenation)
—May prove useful in the perioperative management:
—Preoperative: for patient stabilization
—Postoperative: to allow the lungs to fully expand after the compressing intrathoracic bowel has been removed
—Other: nitric oxide, high-frequency ventilation, liquid ventilation
—Fetal surgical interventions:
—Fetal tracheal occlusion in some fetuses might improve lung growth and development
—Consider in severe cases of CDH when diagnosis is made early enough in gestation (i.e., 24 to 28 weeks' gestation)
• Morgagni hernia
—Surgical repair is indicated, even if the patient is asymptomatic, as a result of the high rate of strangulation of the intrathoracic bowel (10%).

 Follow-Up

WHEN TO EXPECT IMPROVEMENT

Dependent on the extent of pulmonary hypoplasia and pulmonary hypertension.

SIGNS TO WATCH FOR

• The development of pulmonary hypertension in the postoperative period
• Rapid development of hypoxia is associated with the development of a pneumothorax.

PROGNOSIS

• Bochdalek hernias:
—Dependent on the degree of pulmonary hyperplasia and pulmonary hypertension:
—If patient survives the perioperative period: 55% to 65% survival (up to 90% in the most advanced centers)
—Poor prognostic factors:
—Polyhydramnios in utero
—Liver herniation into the thorax
—Fetal stomach in the thoracic cavity
—Fetal lung area to head circumference ratio less then 1.0
—Early presentation (i.e., presenting in the first 6 hours versus after 24 hours)
—Presence of cardiac and chromosomal abnormalities
—Persistent elevated pCO_2 and decreased pO_2
—Low birth weight and APGAR score in 5 minutes
• Morgagni hernias: excellent

PITFALLS

• Bochdalek hernias
—Not being able to stabilize the patient (suggestive of severe pulmonary hypoplasia and/or pulmonary hypertension)
—Iatrogenic injury to hypoplastic lungs; aggressive ventilation causing barotrauma
—Delay in getting the patient to an appropriate medical center
—Not recognizing other congenital malformations or chromosomal abnormalities that may affect the patient's ultimate outcome or that would represent a contraindication for surgical repair (e.g., Trisomy 18)
• Morgagni hernias
—Not considering the diagnosis when abnormalities seen on chest radiograph

LONG-TERM SEQUELAE

• Pulmonary
—Chronic lung disease (60%)
—Diminished perfusion in the hypoplastic lung with progressive improvement in ventilation seen on ventilation/perfusion scan
—Lung function in CDH survivors: spirometry may be normal or indicate mild airway obstruction, slightly reduced lung volumes, normal total lung capacity (TLC) and diffusion capacity
—Recurrent respiratory infections
• Gastrointestinal/nutrition
—Gastroesophageal reflux and delayed gastric emptying (62% to 81%): may need surgical repair
—Oral aversion (as a result of prolonged intubation and delay in development of the swallowing reflex)
—Failure to thrive: may need tube feeding
• Neurodevelopmental
—Developmental delays in the first 2 years
—Motor delays tend to improve
—Hearing loss
—Hypotonia
• Chest wall
—Increased incidence of pectus deformity and scoliosis
• Reoccurrence of hernia

 Common Questions and Answers

Q: What is the long-term pulmonary function in survivors of Bochdalek hernias?
A: Dependent on the degree of pulmonary hypoplasia; pulmonary function testing shows evidence of both obstructive and/or restrictive lung disease. Decreased perfusion on the affected side.

Q: What is the optimal time for surgical repair in neonates with Bochdalek hernias?
A: Delayed surgical repair until the patient is stabilized, avoidance of hyperventilation and alkalization, and pressure-limited ventilation have been shown to significantly decrease mortality in neonates who meet ECMO criteria (up to 90%).

ICD-9-CM 553.3

BIBLIOGRAPHY

Bohn D. Congenital diaphragmatic hernia. *Am J Respir Crit Care Med* 2002;166:911–915.

Congenital Diaphragmatic Hernia Study Group. Estimating disease severity of congenital diaphragmatic hernia in the first 5 minutes of life. *J Pediatr Surg* 2001;36(1):141–145.

Downard CD, Jaksic T, Garza JJ, et al. Analysis of an improved survival rate for congenital diaphragmatic hernia. *J Pediatr Surg* 2003;38(5):729–732.

Flake AW, Crobleholme TM, Johnson MP, et al. Treatment of severe congenital diaphragmatic hernia by fetal tracheal occlusion: clinical experience with fifteen cases. *Am J Obstet Gynecol* 2000;183(5):1059–1066.

Geer JJ, Babiuk RP, Thebaud B. Etiology of congenital diaphragmatic hernia: the retinoid hypothesis. *Pediatr Res* 2003;53(5):726–730.

Ijsselstjin H, Tibboel D. The lungs in congenital diaphragmatic hernia: Do we understand? *Pediatr Pulmonol* 1998;26:204–218.

Katz AL, Wiswell TE, Baumgart S. Contemporary controversies in the management of congenital diaphragmatic hernia. *Clin Perinatol* 1998;25(1):219–248.

Marven SS, Smith CM, Chapman J, et al. Pulmonary function, exercise performance and growth in survivors of congenital diaphragmatic hernia. *Arch Dis Child* 1998;78:137–142.

Muratore CS, Wilson JM. Congenital diaphragmatic hernia: Where we are and where do we go from here? *Semin Perinatol* 2000;24(6):418–428.

Walsh DS, Adzick NS. Fetal surgical intervention. *Am J Perinatol* 2000;17(6):277–283.

Author: Gordana Lovrekovic

Diarrhea, Functional

 ## Database

DEFINITION

Daily painless recurrent passage of three or more large unformed stools, for more than 4 weeks, with onset between 6 and 36 months. The child is normally active and growing and there is no failure to thrive (if caloric intake is adequate) or passage of stools during sleep.

Also known as toddler's diarrhea, chronic nonspecific diarrhea, and irritable colon of childhood.

CAUSES

• Nutritional factors:

—Excessive consumption of fruit juice (increased sorbitol, fructose) leading to carbohydrate intolerance.
—Diet that is high in fluid but low in fat and fiber.

• Motility disorder, i.e., variant of irritable bowel syndrome of infancy.

PATHOPHYSIOLOGY

• Diarrhea is often preceded by acute gastroenteritis or other viral infection that results in dietary restrictions. Increased oral fluids, including juices are used to compensate for stool losses and prevent dehydration.
• Carbohydrate malabsorption causing osmotic diarrhea
• Capacity of small intestine to absorb fructose is limited. Foods that contain equivalent amounts of fructose and glucose are more readily absorbed because of the additive effect of a glucose-dependent fructose cotransport mechanism. An excess of fructose over glucose will result in fructose malabsorption by the small intestine.
• Sorbitol is nonabsorbable and inhibits fructose absorption and may cause gastrointestinal symptoms.
• Excessive intake of juices high in sorbitol and those with a high fructose to glucose ratio will result in fructose malabsorption and gastrointestinal symptoms.
• Colonic function: possibly, there is a disruption of colonic ability to ferment unabsorbed carbohydrates into short chain fatty acids (SCFA) which maintain colonic function and prevent colon-based diarrhea.
• Motility disorder:

—Persistence of immature bowel motility pattern. Failure of initiation of normal postprandial delayed gastric emptying and rapid transit as a result of persistence of small-bowel fasting motility pattern.
—Meals with high dietary fat delay gastric emptying. This protective mechanism is lost with high-fluid, low-fat meals.

• Low-fiber diet: Dietary fiber (pectin) serves as bulking agent

GENETICS

Family members often report nonspecific gastrointestinal complaints or functional bowel disorders.

EPIDEMIOLOGY

It is the most common cause of prolonged diarrhea without failure to thrive (FTT) in children in the developed world.

PROGNOSIS

Generally good. Carbohydrate-containing fluids contribute to unbalanced nutrition, nonorganic failure to thrive, and also to short stature and obesity.

 ## Differential Diagnosis

All causes of chronic diarrhea should be considered:

• Infection:

—Intestinal: bacterial, viral, fungal (giardiasis*, cryptosporidiosis*)
—Nonintestinal: Urinary tract infection

• Pancreatic: cystic fibrosis*, Shwachman-Diamond syndrome, Johannson-Blizzard syndrome, chronic pancreatitis
• Bile acid disorders: chronic cholestasis, terminal ileum disease, bacterial overgrowth*
• Carbohydrate malabsorption: Post infectious-secondary lactose intolerance, sucrase-isomaltase deficiency
• Immunologic: celiac disease*, cow's and soy protein intolerance*, food allergy* (multiple), immunodeficiency, AIDS enteropathy
• Miscellaneous: antibiotics, laxatives, fecal retention constipation*, abetalipoproteinemia, inflammatory bowel disease, short bowel syndrome, hormone secreting tumors like vasoactive intestinal peptide (VIP)-oma, neuroblastoma, Munchausen-by-proxy.

*More common conditions to be considered (Most of the diseases listed above cause morbidity and malnutrition. A thorough clinical history, a simple physical examination and limited number of laboratory tests should make an obvious diagnosis of functional diarrhea. It is not a diagnosis of exclusion.)

 ## Data Gathering

HISTORY

Question: Nutritional history?
Significance: Essential with attention to the "four F's": fiber, fluid, fat, and fruit juices

Question: Diarrhea?
Significance: For a toddler it may not be abnormal to have more than three soft and occasionally loose stools a day with visible food remnants.

Question: Stool characteristics?
Significance: Stools foul smelling and contain undigested food particles, with shortened colonic transit time. Presence of blood or mucus suggests another diagnosis.

Question: Timing of diarrhea?
Significance: No stools passed at night and typically the first stool of the day is large and has better consistency than those occurring later on in the day.

Question: Are other children affected?
Significance: Presence of other affected family members or day-care mates makes infectious etiology more likely.

 ## Physical Examination

Normal, children are healthy appearing, eat well, and are growing normally, although weight might be influenced by the dietary measures.

 ## Laboratory Aids

Test: Stool tests and culture
Significance: Negative for white blood cells, blood, and pathogens

Test: Infectious workup
Significance: Negative

Test: Breath hydrogen tests?
Significance: Usually of limited benefit.

Test: Complete blood count (CBC) normal
Significance: No anemia

Test: Serum electrolytes normal
Significance: No dehydration

Therapy

Reassurance on underlying gastrointestinal diseases and normalization of diet.

DIET

- The child's feeding pattern should be normalized according to the "four F's":

—Overconsumption of fruit juices should be discouraged, especially those that contain sorbitol and a high fructose-to-glucose ratio (apple juice for example).
—Fiber intake should be normalized by introduction of whole meal bread and fruits.
—Increase dietary fat to at least 35% to 40% of total energy intake. Substitution of low-fat milk with whole milk may be sufficient.
—Restrict fluid intake to less than 150 cc/kg per day, and fruit juices to less than 12 oz per day.
—Improvement occurs within a few days to a couple of weeks after initiating the above therapy. Parental reassurance is confirmed by good response to dietary therapy.

PREVENTION

Vicious cycle may be initiated after acute gastroenteritis and food restrictions. Parents should be instructed to give an oral rehydration solution (ORS) and resume normal feeding early.

MEDICATIONS

Loperamide is effective in normalizing bowel patterns but only as long as it is given. Medications seem unwarranted for a condition with mostly nutritional etiology that does not hamper growth.

REFERRAL

- Failure of response to the above therapy
- Weight loss despite adequate intake
- Presence of other symptoms like anorexia, irritability, fever, and vomiting
- Blood and mucus in diarrhea

TESTS TO PREPARE FOR CONSULTATION

- Sweat chloride
- Celiac disease panel (antiendomysial antibodies, tissue transglutaminase antibodies, with IgA serum levels)
- Serum albumin
- ESR
- Stool Sudan III stain for fecal fat.

SPECIAL INSIGHTS

- Good history is required because all the illnesses in the differential diagnosis are associated with morbidity, if diagnosis is delayed.
- Consider constipation, if diarrhea alternates with normal or hard stools. KUB will show colonic fecal retention.
- Need to make follow-up phone call to parents within a few days of instituting diet. If no improvement within a week despite good compliance with dietary recommendations, then rethink diagnosis and consider referral to a specialist.
- Improvement with dietary changes confirms the diagnosis and also reassures the parents.

Common Questions and Answers

Q: Is growth normal in a patient with toddler's diarrhea?
A: Growth is usually normal; weight may be mildly influenced by the prior dietary practices and measures, and failure to thrive has also been reported recently.

Q: What are the components of a successful treatment plan?
A: Attention to the "four F's": decreased fruit juice intake, increased fat intake, decreased fluid, and increased fiber intake

Q: When should care by a pediatric gastroenterologist be sought?
A: If no response after 2 weeks of compliance with dietary therapy, growth delay or other gastrointestinal or systemic complaints

ICD-9-CM 787.91564.5 (functional diarrhea)

BIBLIOGRAPHY

Dennison BA. Fruit juice consumption by infants and children: a review. *J Am Coll Nutr* 1996;15 (5 suppl):4S–11S.

Hamdi I, Dodge JA. Toddler diarrhea: observations on the effects of aspirin and loperamide. *J Pediatr Gastroenterol Nutr* 1985;4:362–365.

Hoekstra JH. Toddler diarrhea: more a nutritional disorder than a disease. *Arch Dis Child* 1998;79(1):2–5.

Hoekstra JH, Van den Aker JHL, Kneepkens CMF, et al. Evaluation of $^{13}CO_2$ breath tests for the detection of fructose malabsorption. *J Lab Clin Med* 1996;127(3):303–309.

Huffman S. Toddler's diarrhea. *J Pediatr Health Care* 1999;13(1):32–33.

Kneepkens CMF, Hoekstra JH. Chronic nonspecific diarrhea of childhood. *Pediatr Clin North Am* 1996;43:375–390.

Lifshitz F, Ament ME, Kleinman RE, et al. Role of juice carbohydrate malabsorption in chronic nonspecific diarrhea in children. *J Pediatr* 1992;120:825–829.

Rasquin-Weber A, Hyman PE, Cucchiara S, et al. Childhood functional gastrointestinal disorders. *Gut* 1999;45(supp II):II60–II68.

Authors: Vered Yehezkely-Schildkraut and Raanan Shamir

DiGeorge Syndrome

 ## Database

DEFINITION

DiGeorge syndrome is characterized by thymic and parathyroid aplasia or hypoplasia, cardiac outflow tract abnormalities, cleft palate, velopharyngeal insufficiency, and facial dysmorphism.

- T-cell immunodeficiency is observed in 80% of children with DiGeorge syndrome.
- Patients with complete DiGeorge syndrome have a severe T-cell defect.
- Partial DiGeorge syndrome occurs when the immune system is intact.

PATHOPHYSIOLOGY

DiGeorge syndrome is believed to be a developmental defect of the third and fourth pharyngeal arches.

GENETICS

- Heterogeneous
- Some reported cases of autosomal dominant, autosomal recessive, and X-linked modes of inheritance
- Most common associated chromosomal abnormalities are microdeletions of 22q11.2.

COMPLICATIONS

In the newborn period, patients present with hypocalcemic tetany, manifestation of cardiac abnormality, and recurrent infections. Later on, patients present more commonly with neurologic and developmental or behavioral issues.

PROGNOSIS

Prolonged survival is seen in most patients after the spontaneous improvement of T-cell numbers and function. Patients with complete DiGeorge syndrome may have more severe and persistent T-cell dysfunction. Complications may include an increase in autoimmune phenomena and neurologic sequelae.

 ## Data Gathering

HISTORY

- Neonatal hypocalcemia secondary to hypoparathyroidism
- Recurrent infections: diarrhea, candidiasis, respiratory infections, PCP
- Heart murmurs
- Cardiac defects, particularly interrupted aortic arch, septal defects, tetralogy of Fallot, and truncus arteriosus.
- Failure to thrive

 ## Physical Examination

Finding:

- Facial dysmorphism—micrognathia; low, rotated ears; "fish-shaped mouth"; short philtrum, anteverted nares, and hypertelorism
- Cleft lip and palate
- Heart murmur
- Hydronephrosis
- Colobomas
- CNS malformations
- Major immunologic features present at birth:

—Lymphopenia
—T-cell dysfunction
—Antibody levels and function are variable

 ## Laboratory Aids

Test: Chest radiograph study
Significance: To evaluate for cardiac malformation and also for the presence of a thymic shadow

Test: CBC with differential
Significance: Immediately after birth, a lymphocyte count of <1,200/mm³ is suspicious.

Test: Serum levels of calcium and parathormone
Significance: Evaluation of parathyroid function.

Test: Lymphocyte markers
Significance: To determine absolute numbers of T and B cells and their subsets

Test: Mitogen studies
Significance: To study the functional abilities of T and B cells. In DiGeorge syndrome, you may see a variably depressed response to phytohemagglutinin, concanavalin A, and pokeweed mitogen.

Test: Quantitative immunoglobulins (IgG, IgA, IgM, and IgE)
Significance: Often the humoral system will be abnormal if there is helper T-cell dysfunction.

Test: FISH (fluorescence in situ hybridization) for 22q11 deletion
Significance: Most common chromosomal defect.

Therapy

Depending on the defects or deficiencies the child manifests, some of the following issues may need to be addressed:

- Cardiology for the cardiac malformations
- Otolaryngology and feeding specialist for cleft palate
- Endocrinology for follow-up of hypoparathyroidism
- Speech and cognitive intervention for speech delay
- Immunology to monitor T-cell disorder and recurrent infections
- Severe immunodeficiency may require matched sibling bone marrow transplant or thymic transplant

SPECIAL CONSIDERATION WITH INFECTIONS

Children with the complete DiGeorge syndrome are at increased risk of morbidity and mortality from viral infections either from vaccines such as oral polio or natural infections such as varicella. It is advisable to:

- Avoid live viral vaccines in cases of T-cell dysfunction. These patients may need intravenous immunoglobulins to provide protection from infections.
- Consider varicella immune globulin in a patient either with unknown humoral immunity status or definitive humoral abnormalities. Intravenous acyclovir may be necessary if varicella develops and patient has a low T-cell count or abnormal mitogens.

SPECIAL CONSIDERATION WITH BLOOD TRANSFUSIONS

Because these patients are at risk for graft-versus-host disease, it is best to use cytomegalovirus-negative, irradiated blood.

 Common Questions and Answers

Q: Is there a definitive test to distinguish between partial and complete DiGeorge syndrome?
A: Over time, patients with partial DiGeorge syndrome will reconstitute their T cells and acquire improved function based on mitogen and antigen studies.

ICD-9-CM 279.11
BIBLIOGRAPHY

Ballow M, O'Neil KM. Approach to the patient with recurrent infections. In: Adkinson NF, Yunginger JW, BUsse WW, Bochner BS, Holgate ST, Simons FER, eds. *Middleton's Allergy Principles and Practice*. 6th Ed. Philadelphia: Mosby Inc, 2003:1057–1058.

Notarangelo LD. T cell immunodeficiencies. In: Leung DYM, Sampson HA, Geha RS, Szefler SJ, eds. *Pediatric Allergy Principles and Practice*. St. Louis, MO: Mosby Inc, 2003:104–105.

Perez E, Sullivan KE. Chromosome 22q11.2 deletion syndrome (DiGeorge and velocardiofacial syndromes). *Curr Opin Pediatr* 2002;14:678–683.

Radford DJ. The DiGeorge syndrome and the heart. *Curr Opin Pediatr* 1991;3:828–831.

Sullivan KE. DiGeorge syndrome/chromosome 22q11.2 deletion syndrome. *Curr All Asthma Rep* 2001;1(5):438–444.

Authors: Erin E. McGintee
Michelle M. Klinek, 3rd edition

Diphtheria

 Database

DEFINITION

Diphtheria is an acute infectious disease caused by *Corynebacterium diphtheriae* and affects primarily the membranes of the upper respiratory tract with the formation of a gray-white pseudomembrane.

CAUSES

The causative organism, *C. diphtheriae*, is a gram-positive pleomorphic bacillus.

PATHOPHYSIOLOGY

The initial entry site for *C. diphtheriae* is via airborne respiratory droplets, typically the nose or mouth, but occasionally the ocular surface, genital mucous membranes, or preexisting skin lesions. Following 2 to 4 days of incubation at one of these sites, the bacteria elaborates toxin. Locally, the toxin induces formation of a necrotic coagulation of the mucous membranes (pseudomembrane) with underlying tissue edema. Respiratory compromise may ensue. Elaborated exotoxin may also have profound effects on the heart, nerves, and kidneys in the form of myocarditis, demyelination, and tubular necrosis, respectively.

EPIDEMIOLOGY

- The single known reservoir for *C. diphtheriae* is humans; disease is acquired by contact with either a carrier or a diseased person.
- Though the disease is distributed throughout the world, it is endemic primarily in developing regions of Africa, Asia, and South America. In the Western world, the incidence of diphtheria has changed dramatically in the past 50 to 75 years, as a result of the widespread use of diphtheria toxoid after World War II. The incidence has declined steadily and is now a rare occurrence.
- Recent outbreaks have occurred, most notably in the new independent states of the former Soviet Union, and supply additional evidence that disease occurs among the socioeconomically disadvantaged living in crowded conditions.
- The majority of cases occur during the cooler autumn and winter months in individuals younger than 15 years of age who are unimmunized.

ASSOCIATED ILLNESSES

- Respiratory tract diphtheria:

—Nasal diphtheria starts with mild rhinorrhea that gradually becomes serosanguineous, then mucopurulent, and often malodorous. This form occurs most often in infants.
—Tonsillar and pharyngeal diphtheria begins with anorexia, malaise, low-grade fever, and pharyngitis. A membrane appears within 1 to 2 days. Cervical lymphadenitis and edema of the cervical soft tissues may be severe. Disease course varies with extent of toxin elaboration and membrane production. Respiratory and cardiovascular collapse may occur.
—Laryngeal diphtheria most often represents extension of a pharyngeal infection and clinically presents as typical croup. Acute airway obstruction may occur, and in severe cases the membrane may invade the entire tracheobronchial tree.
—Cutaneous diphtheria occurs in warmer tropical regions. It is characterized by chronic nonhealing ulcers with gray membrane and may serve as a reservoir in endemic and epidemic areas of respiratory diphtheria.

- Other sites: rarely vulvovaginal, conjunctival, or aural forms occur.

COMPLICATIONS

- Cardiac toxicity: myocarditis may develop secondary to elaborated toxin anytime between the first and sixth week of illness. Though cardiac failure can occur, the majority of cases are transient.
- Neurologic toxicity again occurs secondary to toxin elaboration and mainly reflects bilateral motor involvement.
- Paralysis of the soft palate is most common, but ocular paralysis, diaphragm paralysis, peripheral neuropathy of the extremities, and loss of deep tendon reflexes also occur.
- The frequency of all complications, including those listed above, increases with increasing time between symptom onset and antitoxin administration and also with extent of membrane formation.

PROGNOSIS

- Most strongly dependent on the immunization status of the host. Those without prior adequate immunization have significantly higher morbidity and mortality.
- Delay in onset of treatment also increases mortality. When appropriate treatment has been administered on day 1 of illness, mortality may be as low as 1%. When treatment has been delayed until day 4, the mortality rate is up to 20-fold higher.
- Organism virulence: toxigenic strains are associated with more severe disease and a poorer prognosis.
- Location of membrane: laryngeal diphtheria has a higher mortality owing to airway obstruction.
- A megakaryocytic thrombocytopenia and WBC <25,000 are associated with poor outcome.

 Differential Diagnosis

- Nasal diphtheria can present much like the common cold, nasal foreign body, sinusitis, adenoiditis, or snuffles (congenital syphilis).
- Tonsillar or pharyngeal diphtheria may be confused with streptococcal pharyngitis, infectious mononucleosis, primary herpetic tonsillitis, thrush, Vincent angina, posttonsillectomy faucial membranes, or the oropharyngeal involvement caused by toxoplasmosis, cytomegalovirus, tularemia, and salmonellosis.
- Laryngeal diphtheria: differential diagnosis includes croup, acute epiglottitis, aspirated foreign body, peripharyngeal and retropharyngeal abscess, laryngeal papillomas, or other masses.

 Data Gathering

HISTORY

Question: Exposure?
Significance: Exposure to an individual with diphtheria is not necessarily elicited because contact with an asymptomatic carrier may be the only source of infection.

Question: Incubation period?
Significance: The incubation period is 1 to 6 days. Respiratory diphtheria, depending on the site of infection, may begin with nasal discharge alone or with pharyngitis accompanied by mild systemic symptoms. Progression of symptoms thereafter occurs as outlined above (see Associated Illnesses).

 Physical Examination

Finding: Nasal discharge, nasal or pharyngeal membrane, heart rate out of proportion to body temperature, respiratory distress, stridor, cough, hoarseness, palatal paralysis, neck swelling, and cervical lymphadenitis. Attempts to remove any membrane present will result in bleeding.
Significance: Classic findings.

Finding: Conjunctival diphtheria
Significance: Gives palpebral conjunctival involvement with a red, edematous, membranous appearance.

Finding: Aural diphtheria
Significance: Presents as otitis externa with a purulent, malodorous discharge.

Finding: Cutaneous diphtheria
Significance: See Associated Illnesses.

SPECIAL QUESTIONS

Previous diphtheria immunization history, diphtheria exposure.

Diphtheria

Laboratory Aids

Test: Diagnosis should be on clinical grounds.
Significance: Delay in treatment increases morbidity and mortality.

Test: Culture of material from the membrane or beneath the membrane should be attempted.
Significance: If a strain of *C. diphtheriae* is isolated, additional testing for presence or absence of toxin production should be conducted by a laboratory prepared to conduct an animal neutralization test or, alternatively, neutralization (with antitoxin) in tissue culture.

Test: Examination of a methylene blue-stained lesion
Significance: Metachromatic granules can be helpful, if performed by an experienced technician.

Test: Fluorescent antibody testing and counterimmunoelectrophoresis
Significance: Previously performed in state laboratories; no longer widely available.

Therapy

DIPHTHERIA ANTITOXIN (DAT)

DAT antiserum, produced in horses, must be administered as soon as possible as follows. (Note: For patients with known horse serum sensitivity, a test dose should be administered first, and if positive, the patient should be desensitized.)

- Pharyngeal or laryngeal disease of <48 hours; duration, 20,000 to 40,000 units IV
- Nasopharyngeal lesions, 40,000 to 60,000 units IV
- Extensive disease of 3 or more days' duration or diffuse neck swelling, 80,000 to 100,000 units IV

ANTIBIOTIC THERAPY

- Antibiotic therapy should be used in addition to DAT, not in place of it, as follows:
- Respiratory diphtheria

—Penicillin G
—Aqueous crystalline, 100,000 to 150,000 U/kg per day in four divided doses × 14 days
—Procaine, 25,000 to 50,000 U/kg per day in two divided doses × 14 days or
—Erythromycin, 40 to 50 mg/kg (maximum 2 g per day) PO or parenterally × 14 days

- Cutaneous diphtheria: requires local care of the lesion with soap and water and administration of antimicrobials for 10 days.

PREVENTION

Active immunization with diphtheria toxoid is the cornerstone of population-based diphtheria prevention. The current recommendations from the Advisory Committee on Immunization Practices (ACIP) of the CDC are:

- Ages 2 months to 7 years: five doses of diphtheria vaccine, the first three given as DTP vaccine 0.5 mL IM at 2-month intervals beginning at 2 months of age. The fourth dose should be either DTaP or DTP at 15 to 18 months of age, and a fifth dose of DTaP or DTP at 4 to 6 years of age.
- Age >7 years: primary immunization of those >7 years should be conducted with adult-type diphtheria and tetanus toxoids, adsorbed (Td) with two doses given IM at least 4 weeks apart and a booster dose 1 year later.
- Booster doses of Td should be given at 10-year intervals to all immunized individuals. Isolation of patients with diphtheria is required until culture from the site of infection is negative on three consecutive specimens.

Follow-Up

- In mild cases of diphtheria, after membrane sloughs off in 7 to 10 days, recovery is usually uneventful.
- In more severe cases, recovery may be slower and serious complications can occur.

Common Questions and Answers

Q: Are there currently places in the world in which diphtheria is a problem?
A: Yes. A diphtheria epidemic began in 1990 in Russia, spread in 1991 to Ukraine, and during 1993 and 1994 spread to the remaining new independent states of the former Soviet Union. During 1994, provisional totals of 47,802 cases (39,907 in Russia) and 1,746 deaths as a result of diphtheria were reported throughout the new independent states.

Q: What is the incidence of diphtheria in the United States?
A: From 1980 to 1993, only 40 cases of diphtheria were reported in the United States, an average of three per year (all respiratory disease).

Q: What precautions should be taken by travelers to areas of the world with diphtheria outbreaks?
A: The ACIP recommends that travelers to such areas should be up-to-date for diphtheria immunization. Infants traveling to areas in which diphtheria is endemic or epidemic should receive three doses of DTP or DT before travel.

ICD-9-CD 032.9

BIBLIOGRAPHY

Bisgard KM, Hardy IR, Popovic T, et al. Respiratory diphtheria in the United States, 1980 through 1995. *Am J Public Health* 1998;88(5):787–791.

Enhanced surveillance of non-toxigenic Corynebacterium diphtheriae infections. *CDR Weekly* 1996;6(4):29–32.

Feigin RD, Stechenberg BW, Strandgaard BH. Diphtheria. In: Feigin RD, Cherry JD, eds. *Textbook of Pediatric Infectious Diseases.* 3rd Ed. Philadelphia: WB Saunders, 1992:1110–1115.

Galazka A. The changing epidemiology of diphtheria in the vaccine era. *J Infect Dis* 2000;181(suppl 1):52–59.

MacGregor RR. Corynebacterium diphtheriae. In: Mandell GL, Douglas RG Jr, Bennett JE, eds. *Principles and Practice of Infectious Diseases.* 3rd Ed. New York: Churchill Livingstone, 1990:1574–1581.

Nekrassova LS, Chudnaya LM, Marievskiv F, et al. Epidemic diphtheria in Ukraine, 1991–1997. *J Infect Dis* 2000;181 (suppl 1):335–340.

Toxigenic Corynebacterium diphtheriae—Northern Plains Indian Community, August–October 1996. *MMWR Morb Mortal Weekly Rep* 1997;46(22):506–510.

Author: Louis M. Bell

Diskitis

 ## Database

DEFINITION

- Benign, self-limited inflammatory process of an intervertebral disk

CAUSES

- Idiopathic or initiated by low-grade infection

PATHOLOGY

- Probably of infectious etiology by an indolent organism
- Usually none identified; occasionally *Staphylococcus aureus*, Moraxella, or the Enterobacteriaceae are cultured.

EPIDEMIOLOGY

- Over half of cases occur in children younger than 4 years old.
- Peak incidence is between 1 and 3 years of age.

GENETICS

- No specific predispositions identified

COMPLICATIONS

- Occasionally, scoliosis or kyphosis
- Rarely, facet joint degenerative disease

 ## Differential Diagnosis

- Infection

—Vertebral osteomyelitis (Staphylococcus, Salmonella, etc.)
—Potts disease (tuberculous spondylitis)

- Environmental trauma

—Fracture
—Disk herniation

- Tumors

—Osteoid osteoma

- Vascular

—Avascular necrosis of vertebral body

- Congenital

—Spondylolisthesis

- Immunologic

—Ankylosing spondylitis

- Miscellaneous

—Scheuermann disease (osteochondritis of the vertebral bodies)

 ## Data Gathering

HISTORY

- Uncomfortable child?
- Refuses to walk?
- History of fever?
- Back or abdominal pain?
- Symptoms are of short duration prior to presentation?

 ## Physical Examination

- Usually, rigid posture and pain elicited on movement
- Focal tenderness to palpation
- Most common locations: L4–5 and L3–4

 ## Laboratory Aids

TESTS

- PPD
- WBC
- ESR
- Blood cultures

IMAGING

Test: Plain x-ray studies
Significance: Usually normal, though may demonstrate disk narrowing as illness progresses.

Test: Bone scan
Significance: Demonstrates increased uptake at affected area.

Test: MRI
Significance: Useful in atypical situations to confirm location of pathology (demonstrates disk edema).

Therapy

DRUGS

- Usually, quite responsive to NSAIDs
- Rarely, antibiotics are indicated.

DURATION

- Follow CBC and ESR.
- Continue treatment until child is asymptomatic.

PHYSICAL AND OCCUPATIONAL THERAPY

- Patient should be immobilized during acute period.
- Casting may be required.

DIET

- No special changes

 ## Follow-Up

WHEN TO EXPECT IMPROVEMENT

Most patients are asymptomatic in 6 to 8 weeks.

SIGNS TO WATCH FOR

- Recurrence of symptoms as a result of reactivation of the disease
- Progressive loss of disk height
- Destruction of adjacent vertebral bodies

PROGNOSIS

- Usually, excellent
- Scoliosis can occur
- Rarely, facet joint symptoms occur years later.

PITFALLS

- Difficulty separating early vertebral body osteomyelitis from diskitis

 ## Common Questions and Answers

Q: When is a biopsy and tissue culture indicated?
A: If there is bony destruction of adjacent vertebral bodies or if clinical course is prolonged.

Q: When are antibiotics indicated?
A: Obviously in situations with positive cultures, or if course is atypical or prolonged.

ICD-9-CM 722.90

BIBLIOGRAPHY

Brown R, Hussain M, McHugh K, et al. Discitis in young children. *J Bone Joint Surg* 2001;83:106–111.

Early SD, Kay RM, Tolo VT. Childhood diskitis. *J Am Acad Orthop Surg* 2003;11:413–420.

Fernandez M, Carrol CL, Baker CJ. Discitis and vertebral osteomyelitis in children: an 18-year review. *Pediatrics* 2000;105:1299–1304.

Garron E, Viehweger E, Launay F, et al. Nontuberculous spondylodiscitis in children. *J Pediatr Orthop* 2002;22:321–328.

King HA. Back pain in children. *Orthop Clin North Am* 1999;30:467–474.

Mahboubi S, Morris MC. Imaging of spinal infections in children. *Radiol Clin North Am* 2001;39:215–222.

Author: Randy Q. Cron

Disseminated Intravascular Coagulation

 ## Database

DEFINITION

Disseminated intravascular coagulation (DIC) is a syndrome characterized by diffuse fibrin deposition in the microvasculature, consumption of coagulation factors, and endogenous generation of thrombin and plasmin in an uncontrolled fashion usually leading to significant bleeding.

PATHOPHYSIOLOGY/PATHOLOGY

- DIC is not a disorder in itself, but occurs as a result of various initiating events.
- DIC is characterized by microvascular hemorrhage and thrombosis.
- DIC may be acute (e.g., meningococcemia) or chronic (e.g., malignancy/leukemia).
- DIC most likely initiated through tissue factor (extrinsic) pathway.
- Most common causes are sepsis (particularly gram-negative sepsis), hypotensive shock, and trauma (particularly head trauma).
- Exact mechanism of DIC is unclear, but in most cases, tissue damage leads to the release of clot-promoting material. Also, all means of anticoagulation are impaired and fibrin is not adequately removed because endogenous fibrinolysis is suppressed by high plasma levels of plasminogen activator inhibitor-1 (PAI-1). The principal cytokine mediator appears to be IL-6.
- Procoagulant factors released in the blood may initiate DIC in acute promyelocytic leukemia.
- Endotoxins released during infections cause activation of coagulation factor XII, endothelial injury, platelet aggregation, and inhibition of fibrinolysis.

- The following disease processes can cause DIC:

—Infections
—Bacterial/septic shock
—Meningococcemia
—Gram-negative and -positive sepsis (e.g., group B streptococcus)
—Parasites—malaria
—Fungal—Aspergillus
—Rickettsial—Rocky Mountain spotted fever
—Viral

- Tissue injury
- Massive head trauma
- Multiple fractures with fat emboli
- Crush injuries
- Profound shock or asphyxia
- Hypothermia or hyperthermia
- Massive burns
- Malignancies

—Acute promyelocytic leukemia
—Acute monoblastic or monocytic leukemia
—Metastatic carcinomas or other widespread malignancies (e.g., neuroblastoma)

- Obstetric causes

—Intrauterine fetal death
—Amniotic fluid embolism
—Abruptio placentae
—Gastrointestinal

- Fulminant hepatitis
- Reye syndrome
- Severe inflammatory bowel disease
- Neonatal

—Necrotizing enterocolitis
—Congenital viral infections
—Group B streptococcus infection
—Erythroblastosis fetalis
—Small for gestational age newborn

- Miscellaneous

—Acute hemolytic transfusion reaction
—Kasabach-Merritt syndrome
—Snake bite or insect bite
—Severe thrombotic thrombocytopenic purpura
—Hemolytic uremic syndrome
—Homozygous protein C deficiency (purpura fulminans)
—Severe graft rejection
—Severe collagen vascular disease
—Heparin-induced thrombosis
—Infusion of activated prothrombin complex concentrate
—VP shunt
—Kawasaki disease

EPIDEMIOLOGY

- Exact incidence not known.
- Most commonly secondary to infections.
- Snakebite may be most common cause worldwide.

COMPLICATIONS

- Hemorrhage

—Pulmonary
—Intracranial
　　—Renal failure
　　—Multiorgan system failure

PROGNOSIS

- Poor unless underlying disease is treated.
- The intensity and duration of DIC depend on the degree of activation of the coagulation system, liver function, blood flow, and the ability to reverse underlying etiology that has led to DIC.

 ## Differential Diagnosis

- Prolonged bleeding from venipuncture sites.
- Coagulopathy of liver disease
- Vitamin K deficiency
- Pathologic fibrinolysis
- Microangiopathic disease, e.g., thrombotic thrombocytopenic purpura
- Effects of cardiopulmonary bypass

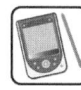 ## Data Gathering

HISTORY

- Presence of one of the underlying conditions listed above (see Causes)
- Abrupt onset of bleeding
- Prolonged bleeding from venipuncture sites
- Bleeding from multiple sites, especially venipunctures, cut-down sites, mucous membranes, skin, GI tract, and GU tract
- Pulmonary or intracranial hemorrhage
- Major organ dysfunction—pulmonary, renal, hepatic
- Oliguria

Disseminated Intravascular Coagulation

 ## Physical Examination

- Signs of underlying disease.
- Generally a very toxic-appearing patient.
- Ecchymosis and petechiae.
- Bleeding from previously intact venipuncture sites.
- Skin infarctions (purpura fulminans) secondary to thrombosis of dermal vessels.
- Pulmonary hemorrhage, gastrointestinal bleeding, bleeding from surgical wounds, hematuria.
- Intraperitoneal and pleural hemorrhages.

 ## Laboratory Aids

- There is no single test that can reliably diagnose DIC.
- All these tests should be checked every 4 to 8 hours because they change rapidly.

Test: CBC
Significance: Decreased platelet count, often earliest abnormality.

Test: Peripheral smear
Significance: Schistocytes, microspherocytes (50% of cases).

Test: PT, PTT, and thrombin time
Significance: Prolonged

Test: Fibrinogen
Significance: Decreased

Test: Fibrin degradation products or fibrin split products
Significance: Increased

Test: Soluble fibrin monomer complexes (D-dimers)
Significance: Increased; most sensitive marker for DIC

Test: Antithrombin III or protein C levels
Significance: Decreased

Test: Factor VIII and V
Significance: Decreased; factor VIII is normal in coagulopathy of liver disease.

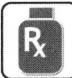 ## Therapy

- Treat the underlying disorder.
- Cryoprecipitate, platelets, and fresh frozen plasma to control bleeding.
- Fresh frozen plasma also replaces anticoagulants—protein C and S.
- Heparin used for management of purpura fulminans as a result of meningococcemia.
- Routine use of heparin for DIC is controversial. It has been used in chronic DIC, arterial thromboses, or large-vessel venous thromboses.
- AT III and protein C concentrates at supraphysiologic dosing have been used rarely but currently are under investigation.

SUPPORTIVE CARE

- Manage other organ system failure.

ICD-9-CM 286.6

BIBLIOGRAPHY

Levi M, deJonge E, van der Poll T, et al. Novel approaches to the management of disseminated intravascular coagulopathy. *Crit Care Med* 2000;28 (9 suppl):S20–S24.

Levi M, ten Cate H. Current concepts: disseminated intravascular coagulopathy. *N Engl J Med* 1999;341(8):586–592.

Monagle P, Andrew M. Acquired disorders of hemostasis. In: Nathan DG, Orkin SH, Ginsburg D, Look AT, eds. *Nathan and Oski's Hematology of Infancy and Childhood.* 6th Ed. Philadelphia: WB Saunders, 2003: 1597–1630.

Richey ME, Gilstrap LC, 3rd, Ramin SM. Management of disseminated intravascular coagulopathy. *Clin Obstet Gynecol* 1995;38:514–520.

ten Cate H, Schoenmakers SH, Franco R, et al. Microvascular coagulopathy and disseminated intravascular coagulation. *Crit Care Med* 2001;29:S95–S97; discussion S97–S98.

Wintrobe M. *Wintrobe's Clinical Hematology,* vol 2. 10th Ed. Baltimore: Lippincott Williams & Wilkins, 1998:1480–1493.

Authors: Don E. Eslin
Valerie Brown, 3rd edition

Down (Trisomy 21) Syndrome

Database

DEFINITION AND FEATURES

- Syndrome consisting of multiple abnormalities, including hypotonia, flat facies, up-slanting palpebral fissures, and small ears
- First described by John Langdon Down in 1866
- Trisomy chromosome 21
- Multiple abnormalities found in Down syndrome:
—Congenital heart disease (40% to 50%; most not symptomatic as newborn)
—Atrioventricular (AV) canal (60% of those with congenital heart disease)
—Ventriculoseptal defect (VSD)
—Patent ductus arteriosus (PDA)
—Atrioseptal defect (ASD)
—Aberrant subclavian artery
—Tetralogy of Fallot
    —Hearing loss (66% to 75%): sensorineural and conductive
    —Strabismus (33% to 45%)
    —Nystagmus (15% to 35%)
    —Fine lens opacities (by slit-lamp examination 59%), cataracts (1% to 15%)
    —Refractive errors (50%)
    —Nasolacrimal duct stenosis
    —Delayed tooth eruption
    —Tracheoesophageal fistula
    —Gastrointestinal atresia (12%)
    —Meckel diverticulum
    —Hirschsprung disease (less than 1%)
    —Imperforate anus
    —Renal malformations
    —Hypospadias (5%)
    —Cryptorchidism (5% to 50%)
    —Thyroid disease (15%): congenital hypothyroidism, hyperthyroidism
    —Transient myeloproliferative disorder, neonatal (leukemoid reaction)
    —Neonatal polycythemia
    —Leukemia (less than 1%; 10 to 30 times greater risk than general population)
    —Retinoblastoma and testicular germ-cell tumors (slightly greater risk than general population)
    —Infertility, especially in males
    —Obesity
    —Alopecia areata (10% to 15%)
    —Seizures (5% to 10%), usually myoclonic
    —Alzheimer disease (nearly all over age 40 years)
    —Mild to moderate mental retardation (IQ range 25 to 70)
    —Dry, hyperkeratotic skin (75%)

EPIDEMIOLOGY

- Incidence: 1/600 to 1/800 live births although incidence varies with maternal age
- 1/1,500 for maternal ages 15 to 29 years
- 1/800 for maternal ages 30 to 34 years
- 1/270 for maternal ages 35 to 39 years
- 1/100 for maternal ages 40 to 44 years
- Male:female ratio is 1.3:1
- Best recognized and most frequent chromosomal syndrome of humans
- One of the three most common autosomal trisomies in humans (others are trisomy 18 and 13)

- Most common autosomal chromosomal abnormality causing mental retardation
- More than 50% of trisomy 21 fetuses are spontaneously aborted in early pregnancy

GENETICS

- 94% to 97% of cases are a result of chromosomal nondisjunction (failure to segregate during meiosis) in the maternal DNA
- Less than 5% of cases are as a result of paternal nondisjunction
- 2.4% of live births are mosaic (nondisjunction occurs after conception; two cell lines are present); generally less severely affected
- Remainder a result of translocations between chromosome 21 and 14 [t(14q21q)]; rarely between 21 and 13 or 15; 50% of translocations are sporadic de novo events; 50% result from balanced translocations in one parent.

COMPLICATIONS

- Serous otitis media (50% to 70%)
- Conjunctivitis (frequent)
- Sinusitis
- Tonsillar and adenoidal hypertrophy
- Obstructive airway disease with associated sleep apnea (33% to 75%), cor pulmonale
- Obstructive bowel disease (12%, newborn period)
- Constipation (as a result of low tone and decreased gross motor mobility)
- Subluxation of the hips (secondary to ligamentous laxity)
- Atlantoaxial instability (10% to 20%; secondary to ligamentous laxity, which is most severe prior to age 10 years)

PROGNOSIS

- Dependent on the associated findings
- Life expectancy is mildly decreased, with many living into the sixth decade.
- Alzheimer disease affects approximately 15% after the fourth decade.
- Recurrence is approximately 1% if parents are not translocation carriers.
- As adults, the majority of patients with Down syndrome can work in supported positions.

Data Gathering

HISTORY

- Check for previous history of infant with Down syndrome in the family.
- Ask about growth and developmental status.
- Ask about feeding problems.
- Ask about snoring, signs of sleep apnea (e.g., restless sleep).
- Ask about stool habits.
- Ask about hearing concerns.

Physical Examination

The phenotype is variable from person to person.

General: Short stature; hypotonia (80% to 100%), with an open mouth and a protruding tongue; midface hypoplasia.
Head: Brachycephaly with a flattened occiput, microcephaly, false fontanel (95%).
Eyes: Up-slanting palpebral fissures (98%), inner epicanthal folds, Brushfield spots (speckling of the iris), fine lens opacities on slit-lamp examination, cataracts, refractive error, strabismus, nystagmus.
Ears: Small, prominent; low set; overfolding of upper helix; small canals with difficulty visualizing tympanic membranes.
Nose: Small (85%); flat nasal bridge.
Tongue: Relative but not true macroglossia (tongue mass is normal); fissuring.
Mouth: High-arched or abnormal palate.
Teeth: Missing (50%), small, hypoplastic; irregular placement.
Neck: In infancy, excess skin at the nape; short appearance; occasionally webbed.
Lungs: Check for signs of infection or congestive heart failure.
Heart: Assess for murmur, arrhythmia, cyanosis.
Abdomen: In neonate, distension may be present as a result of obstruction or atresia; diastasis recti.
Genital: In adolescents, straight pubic hair; in males, small penis, cryptorchidism.
Extremities: Hands, broad with short metacarpals and phalanges; fifth finger with hypoplasia of the midphalanx (60%) and clinodactyly (50%); simian crease (single transverse palmar crease) in approximately 50%; wide gap between the first and second toes (96%); syndactyly of second and third toes; hyperflexibility of joints. A newborn with a simian crease has a 1 in 60 chance of having Down syndrome.
Skin: Cutis marmorata (43%); in older children, hyperkeratotic dry skin (75%); fine, soft, sparse hair.

Laboratory Aids

Test: Second Trimester Prenatal "Triple Screen" Test (Alpha-fetoprotein (AFP), unconjugated estriol and human chorionic gonadotropin (hCG)
Significance: The screen is performed at 15 to 18 weeks. These three serum markers together can detect approximately 60% of the pregnancies affected by trisomy 21, with a false positive of about 5%. A positive test is an indication for karyotyping with amniocentesis.

Test: First Trimester Maternal Serum Screening (pregnancy-associated plasma protein A and free β-human chorionic gonadotropin)
Significance: While second trimester screening has been the standard in the United States, first trimester screening is becoming popular if done with first trimester ultrasound measurement of nuchal translucency (see Radiographic Studies below). When these two tests are conducted together, it has been shown in multiple studies to have higher sensitivity than second trimester prenatal screens (91% versus 70%).

Test: Prenatal karyotyping via amniocentesis (16 to 18 weeks' gestation) or chorionic villus sampling (9 to 11 weeks' gestation).
Significance: This is performed for any woman who presents with a positive "triple screen." In addition, because this test fails to detect 10% to 15% of Down syndrome in older women, amniocentesis is typically offered to all women >35 years.

Test: Chromosomal karyotype on cultured lymphocytes from peripheral blood
Significance: May be performed postnatally for confirmation if there is a clinical suspicion of Down syndrome.

Test: Tissue sample other than blood (usually skin)
Significance: To check for mosaicism.

Test: CBC
Significance: In the newborn period to check for polycythemia and transient myeloproliferative disorder; Down syndrome patients may have an increased mean corpuscular volume (MCV) on CBC, making the diagnosis iron-deficiency anemia difficult; repeat in adolescence.

Test: Thyroid-function tests
Significance: To rule out hypo- or hyperthyroidism.

RADIOGRAPHIC STUDIES

Test: First trimester ultrasound measurement of nuchal translucency
Significance: Increasingly popular prenatal screen for Down syndrome, performed in the first trimester along with maternal serum screening (see Laboratory Aids above).

Test: Fetal ultrasound
Significance: May show polyhydramnios if bowel obstruction is present. A thickened nuchal fold is associated with an increased risk for Down syndrome.

Test: Echocardiography and chest x-ray study
Significance: Done in the first month of life to rule out cardiac disease.

Test: Lateral cervical spine x-ray studies in flexion, neutral, and extension
Significance: To rule out atlantoaxial instability, defined as greater than 5-mm space between atlas and odontoid process of the axis. Important measures include (a) the atlantodens interval (ADI; normal <4.5 mm), which is the distance between the posterior surface of the anterior arch of C1 and the anterior surface of the dens; (b) the neural canal width (NCW; normal ≥14 mm), which is the distance between the posterior surface of the dens and the anterior surface of the posterior arch of C1; and (c) the distance of subluxation at the occipitoatlantal joint, which is normally ≥7 mm.

OTHER STUDIES

Test: Electrocardiogram (ECG)
Significance: Done within the first month of life to rule out cardiac disease.

Test: Auditory brainstem response
Significance: Done within the first 3 months of life to rule out hearing loss.

Therapy

Not applicable except for treatments specific to complications/associated illnesses.

Follow-Up

GROWTH AND DEVELOPMENT
Specific growth charts for Down syndrome are available; average age for acquiring developmental milestones differs from normal population; late closure of fontanelles; consider early intervention program for hypotonia and developmental delay.

GENETICS
Genetic counseling recommended.

CARDIAC
Early evaluation in newborn period, with follow-up until the presence or absence of disease is evident; subacute bacterial endocarditis prophylaxis for patients with certain types of cardiac disease.

OPHTHALMOLOGIC
Early evaluation for cataracts and glaucoma; with visit by 6 months to the ophthalmologist, and then every 2 years.

EAR, NOSE, AND THROAT (ENT)/AUDIOLOGIC
Annual audiologic evaluation in the first 3 years of life, then every other year; ENT referral to visualize tympanic membranes with microscopic otoscope if small narrow external canals.

ORTHOPAEDIC
Screen for atlantoaxial instability with x-ray studies in preschool years, then every decade. Prior to participation in contact sports (e.g., Special Olympics), must evaluate for atlantoaxial instability.

ENDOCRINE
Thyroid-function tests in newborn period, age 6 months and 12 months, then yearly.

OTHER
Many organizations (e.g., Down Syndrome International) are available to families of children with Down syndrome.

PITFALLS
• Caution with endotracheal intubation if absence or presence of atlantoaxial instability is not known to avoid spinal cord injury, which may be seen in rare cases.
• Hearing loss may be misinterpreted as a behavioral problem.
• Care with atropine and pilocarpine use for ophthalmologic evaluation because of cholinergic hypersensitivity that may be seen.

Common Questions and Answers

Q: Why was Down syndrome referred to as mongolism in the past?

A: There was a mistaken notion about a racial cause for this syndrome as a result of the facial appearance, which was thought to be similar to that of those from Mongoloid origin.

Q: Do all children with Down syndrome have mental retardation?
A: No. Though all persons with nonmosaic Down syndrome have some degree of cognitive disability, some have IQs greater than 70 and are not considered to have mental retardation.

Q: Do children with this syndrome have an increased susceptibility to infection?
A: The literature on this subject is unclear and has been subject to debate. Midface hypoplasia may contribute to an increased incidence of ear, sinus, and nasolacrimal duct infections. There may be an increased risk of lower respiratory tract infection for children with unrepaired heart disease.

Q: Can a normal cardiac examination rule out the presence of a cardiac anomaly?
A: No. The American Academy of Pediatrics recommends that all patients with Down syndrome should have a cardiology consultation within the first month of life. Timely surgery may be necessary to prevent serious complications.

Q: Are patients with atlantoaxial instability symptomatic?
A: No, most are asymptomatic, but symptoms of cord compression may be seen in 1% to 2% of patients.

Q: I have seen growth charts for Down syndrome patients that allow for plotting of lengths, heights, and weights. Are there special growth charts available for plotting head circumference?
A: Yes. If appropriate growth charts are not used for plotting head circumference, head growth may appear abnormal. Head circumference growth charts are available through the Internet: http://www.growthcharts.com.

ICD-9-CM 758.0

BIBLIOGRAPHY

American Academy of Pediatrics. Health supervision for children with Down syndrome. *Pediatrics* 2001;107:442–449.

Bahado-Singh R, Cheng CC, Matta P, Small M, Mahoney MJ. Combined serum and ultrasound screening for detection of fetal aneuploidy. *Sem Perinatol* 2003;27(2):145–151.

Brockmeyer D. Down syndrome and craniovertebral instability. Topic review and treatment recommendations. *Pediatr Neurosurg* 1999;31:71–77.

Canick JA, Saller DN Jr, Lambert-Messerlian GM. Prenatal screening for Down syndrome: current and future methods. *Clin Lab Med* 2003;23(2):395–411.

Cronk C, Crocker AC, Pueschel SM, et al. Growth charts for children with Down syndrome: 1 month to 18 years of age. *Pediatrics* 1988;81:102–110.

Authors: Esther K. Chung and Karen P. Zimmer

Dysfunctional Uterine Bleeding

 ## Database

DEFINITION

- Endometrial bleeding beyond the range of normal menses, with normal defined as duration of 2 to 8 days, occurring every 21 to 40 days, with blood loss of 20 to 80 mL/cycle.
- Dysfunctional uterine bleeding (DUB) can vary in presentation from heavy, long menses followed by long periods of amenorrhea to short, heavy menses occurring every 1 to 2 weeks.
- Most commonly results from anovulatory cycles, which are secondary to an immature hypothalamic-pituitary-ovarian axis.

PATHOPHYSIOLOGY

In most cases of DUB presenting within 2 years of menarche, anovulation (failure to ovulate) results in absence of the corpus luteum. Without the secretory effect of progesterone from the corpus luteum, endometrial proliferation continues as a result of unopposed estrogen.

- The thickened endometrium eventually outgrows support from the basal endometrium, resulting in sloughing of the highest endometrial levels. Alternatively, cyclic estrogen withdrawal may occur, which will lead to sloughing of the endometrium in the absence of progesterone.
- As subsequent levels of endometrium are shed, bleeding increases. Profuse bleeding can result when the basal endometrium is exposed.

GENETICS

- Familial history of anovulatory cycles is common.
- Patients with disorders such as blood dyscrasias and polycystic ovary syndrome (PCOS) usually have familial histories including these disorders.

COMPLICATIONS

- Mild to severe anemia resulting from blood loss

 ## Differential Diagnosis

Approximately 80% of abnormal uterine bleeding in adolescents can be attributed to anovulatory cycles. However, it is important to rule out other causes for irregular or heavy vaginal bleeding.

PREGNANCY

- Should be considered and ruled out in every patient, regardless of patient's reported sexual history
- Ectopic pregnancy
- Threatened abortion, incomplete abortion
- Placenta previa
- Hydatiform mole

INFECTION

- Vaginitis (e.g., trichomonas)
- Cervicitis or endometritis (e.g., gonorrhea or chlamydia)
- Pelvic inflammatory disease

HEMATOLOGIC

- Bleeding disorders often present as heavy periods from time of menarche
- Thrombocytopenia (e.g., immune thrombocytopenic purpura [ITP], leukemia)
- Platelet dysfunction
- Coagulation defect (e.g., von Willebrand disease)

ENDOCRINOLOGIC

- Thyroid disease, especially hypothyroidism
- Hyperprolactinemia
- Polycystic ovarian syndrome
- Adrenal disorders

TRAUMA

- Laceration to vagina to cervix

FOREIGN BODY

- Usually associated with strong, foul odor

MEDICATIONS

- Direct affect on hemostasis (e.g., coumadin, chemotherapeutic agents)
- Hormonal effects (e.g., oral contraceptives, Depo-Provera)

SYSTEMIC DISEASE

- Disruption of hypothalamic-pituitary-ovarian axis
- Other examples include: systemic lupus erythematosis, chronic renal failure

PRIMARY GYNECOLOGIC

- Endometriosis
- Uterine polyps, submucosal myomas
- Hemangioma, arteriovenous malformation

 ## Data Gathering

HISTORY

Question: When did the abnormal bleeding begin? How much bleeding occurs?
Significance: Assessing the amount and site of bleeding will help to determine the nature and extent of the problem. It is important to know how much bleeding has occurred to know if the patient is at risk for hemodynamic instability.

Question: When was the onset of menarche? What are typical menstrual cycles with respect to interval between cycles and amount of bleeding?
Significance: The pattern of DUB in relation to the menstrual cycle can help guide the diagnostic workup. Normal cyclic intervals with increased bleeding during each cycle

may suggest a bleeding disorder, normal with bleeding between cycles may suggest infection or foreign body, and abnormal with no cycle regularity may suggest anovulatory cycles, endocrinopathy, or hormonal contraception.

Question: Cramping?
Significance: The presence of cramping suggests ovulation and the presence of progesterone. Anovulatory cycles are thus less likely.

Question: Time lapse between menarche and onset of DUB?
Significance: Increased time lapse between menarche and the onset of DUB lessens the likelihood of anovulatory cycles.

Question: Bruising history?
Significance: Easy bruisability, epistaxis, and/or bleeding gums may be suggestive of a bleeding disorder.

Question: Is there a family history of thyroid disease, bleeding disorder, PCOS, or DUB?
Significance: A family history of any of the above will help guide the laboratory workup.

 ## Physical Examination

- Patients with DUB will often have a normal physical exam.
- Assess vital signs, including orthostatic blood pressures, for signs of cardiac instability resulting from severe blood loss.
- Assess sexual maturity rating (SMR, or Tanner stage). Menarche usually does not occur before SMR 3, so bleeding before this stage suggests a nonmenstrual source of bleeding.
- Look for signs of androgen excess (e.g., hirsutism, acne), which may be reflective of disrupted ovulatory function.
- Bitemporal hemianopsia is suggestive of a pituitary adenoma leading to hyperprolactinemia.
- Only one-third of adolescents with hyperprolactinemia will experience galactorrhea.
- Assess for evidence of thyroid disease, hematologic disorder (e.g., bruising, petechiae), or systemic disease (e.g., poor nutritional status).
- Pelvic examination can help determine source of bleeding. Bimanual examination can assess for ovarian or uterine masses, signs of PID, or signs of pregnancy.

 ## Laboratory Aids

TESTS

Test: Urine or serum β-HCG should be obtained, regardless of sexual history.

Significance: Urine β-HCG testing can reliably detect pregnancy as early as 2 weeks postconception; however, it may be positive for up to 2 weeks following an abortion.

Test: Complete Blood Count
Significance: Degree of anemia guides treatment plan. Assess for thrombocytopenia.

Test: For *C. trachomatis* and *N. gonorrhea*, obtain cervical cultures or use nucleic acid amplification tests (e.g., polymerase chain reaction) on urine or cervical swabs. Also, wet mount to identify trichomonas or white blood cells.
Significance: To identify presence of STDs.

Test: Consider prolactin level and thyroid function tests.
Significance: Hyperprolactinemia can have several causes, including pituitary microadenoma, and result in amenorrhea or DUB.

Test: PT, PTT, von Willebrand factor
Significance: To assess for hematologic causes of bleeding.

Test: LH and FSH. Androgen levels, including testosterone (total and free), dehydroepiandrosterone sulfate (DHEAS), androstenedione.
Significance: Abnormal levels are supportive of PCOS.

RADIOGRAPHIC IMAGING

Test: Pelvic ultrasound
Significance: Indicated when ectopic pregnancy is suspected. Should be considered when a pelvic mass is felt, uterine anomaly is being considered, or bimanual examination cannot be completed.

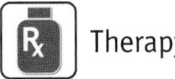 Therapy

- If DUB is attributed to anovulatory cycles, or if a complete workup fails to yield a diagnosis, treatment is guided by the severity of DUB and the presence of active bleeding.
- For mild DUB (inconvenient, unpredictable bleeding, and the patient has a normal hemoglobin):

—Reassurance until ovulatory cycles resume. Encourage maintenance of a menstrual calendar with follow-up in 3 to 6 months.
—Iron supplementation
—If inconvenience and anxiety are unresponsive to reassurance, hormonal therapy with a daily combined oral contraceptive pill (OCP) should be considered to regulate menstrual cycle. If estrogen is contraindicated, may use medroxyprogesterone acetate (Provera), 10 mg daily for 7 days every 35 to 40 days.

- For moderate DUB (irregular, prolonged, heavy bleeding with a hemoglobin >10 g/dL):

—Hormonal therapy, as described previously.
—Menstrual calendar with follow-up every 1 to 3 months

- For severe DUB (heavy, prolonged bleeding with a hemoglobin <10 g/dL), treatment depends on the presence of active bleeding.
- If not actively bleeding, hemodynamically stable patients can be started on OCPs, iron supplementation, and have follow-up in 1 to 2 months.
- In the presence of active bleeding:

—Hormonal therapy, using combined OCP containing higher dose of estrogen (50 mcg ethinyl estradiol).
—One pill q.i.d. until bleeding stops, followed by pill taper (q.i.d. × 4 days, t.i.d. × 3 days, b.i.d. × 2 weeks, then 1 pill daily). Switch to lower dose pill (30 to 35 mcg) after taper complete.
—Antiemetic therapy necessary for high doses of estrogen.
—Hospitalization of patient during treatment if severe anemia (Hb <7 g/dL), if hemodynamically unstable, or compliance concerns.
—Blood transfusion as necessary
—If patient unstable and unable to tolerate oral pill regimen, can give IV conjugated estrogen every 4 hours for 24 hours to stop bleeding. Add OCP with progesterone as soon as patient able to tolerate oral regimen, in order to prevent excessive withdrawal bleed.

- Iron supplementation
- Dilatation and curettage rarely necessary, although may be needed if hormonal therapy fails.

POSSIBLE SIDE EFFECTS

- Estrogen, given in high doses, will cause nausea and/or vomiting. An appropriate antiemetic should be used for prophylaxis against these symptoms.
- High-dose estrogen can have vascular side effects and should be used with caution in patients particularly at risk for vascular events (e.g., patients with a history of lupus, strokes, or thrombotic phenomena; and those who smoke cigarettes). In these cases, consult a gynecologist for an alternative progesterone-only therapy.

 Follow-Up

WHEN TO EXPECT IMPROVEMENT

- Bleeding usually tapers after the first few doses of hormone therapy.
- After 6 to 12 months have passed, and the patient does not wish to remain on OCPs, a trial off of medication might reveal normal ovulatory cycles.
- DUB persists for 2 years in 60% of patients, 4 years in 50%, and up to 10 years in 30%.

PITFALLS

- Neglecting to perform testing for pregnancy in an adolescent who denies sexual activity.
- Neglecting to consider a retained foreign body (e.g., tampon)

- If there is a prolonged course of DUB, consider PCOS, thyroid disease, or other endocrinopathy.

 Common Questions and Answers

Q: If most girls have anovulatory cycles, why do only some present with DUB?
A: Most girls do have an irregular menstrual cycle during the first 2 years after menarche. However, in a majority of those girls, the negative-feedback system of estrogen will lead to cyclic endometrial shedding in an anovulatory pattern.

Q: If DUB from anovulatory cycles is caused by lack of progesterone, why does the initial treatment of severe DUB with active bleeding involve large doses of estrogen?
A: Estrogen has procoagulation effects that promote hemostasis (e.g., effects on platelet aggregation and levels of fibrinogen and clotting factors). In addition, severe DUB can lead to an exposed endometrial base that bleeds profusely. For progesterone to exhibit its secretory effects, the endometrium in that area must be restored by estrogen.

Q: When hormonal therapy fails, and the basal endometrium continues to bleed, how does a dilation and curettage act as the final treatment?
A: The curettage removes any remaining bleeding vessels and stimulates local prostaglandins to create a uterine contracture that inhibits bleeding. This is rarely needed in adolescent patients, as they usually respond to hormonal therapy.

ICD-9-CM 626.8

BIBLIOGRAPHY

Bravender T, Emans SJ. Menstrual disorders: dysfunctional uterine bleeding. *Pediatr Clin North Am* 1999;46:545–553.

Emans SJ, Laufer MR, Goldstein DP. *Pediatric and Adolescent Gynecology*. 4th Ed. Philadelphia: Lippincott-Raven, 1998.

Levine LJ, Catallozzi M, Schwarz DF. An adolescent with vaginal bleeding. *Pediatr Case Rev* 2003;3:83–90.

Mitan LA, Slap GB. Dysfunctional uterine bleeding. In: Neinstein LS, ed. *Adolescent Health Care: A Practical Guide*. 4th Ed. Philadelphia: Lippincott Williams & Wilkins, 2002.

Munro MG. Dysfunctional uterine bleeding: advances in diagnosis and treatment. *Curr Opin Obstet and Gyn* 2001;13(5):475–489.

Rimsza ME. Dysfunctional uterine bleeding. *Pediatr Rev* 2002;23:227–232.

Rimsza ME. Dysfunctional uterine bleeding [erratum appears in *Pediatr Rev* 2002 Sep;23](9). *Pediatr Rev* 2002;23(7):227–33.

Authors: Leonard J. Levine and Jonathan R. Pletcher

Dysmenorrhea

 Database

DEFINITION

- Pain and discomfort during menses that is uterine in origin.
- Categorized as primary if there is no pathological cause, and secondary if a pathological cause is identified.

PREDISPOSING FACTORS

- Younger age at menarche
- Increased duration and/or amount of menstrual flow
- Cigarette smoking
- Possibly low fish consumption

COMPLICATIONS

- Dysmenorrhea is a common cause of school and work absenteeism, with school absenteeism rates reported between 17% and 52%.
- Complications of secondary dysmenorrhea depend on the underlying cause. Infertility is a notable complication of many of these underlying causes (e.g., pelvic inflammatory disease).

PROGNOSIS

- Less than one-third of adolescent women with dysmenorrhea seek advice and/or treatment from a health care provider, therefore many teens are untreated or inadequately treated.
- Most patients with primary dysmenorrhea respond well to standard medical treatment. Secondary dysmenorrhea should be considered if a patient does not respond to therapy.
- The prognosis of secondary dysmenorrhea depends on the underlying cause. Many of these causes can be effectively treated if identified.

 Differential Diagnosis

GENITOURINARY

- Endometriosis
- Ovarian or paratubal cyst
- Mullerian anomalies
- Obstructive genital outflow tract anomalies
- Pelvic adhesions
- Ectopic pregnancy
- Miscarriage
- Cervical stricture/stenosis

INFECTIOUS

- Pelvic Inflammatory Disease (PID)
- Pelvic abscess
- Appendicitis
- Giardiasis

TUMORS

- Neoplasm (i,e., uterine leiomyomata)
- Lymphoma

GASTROINTESTINAL

- Inflammatory bowel disease
- Constipation
- Lactose intolerance
- Malrotation
- Irritable bowel syndrome

MISCELLANEOUS

- Psychogenic
- Musculoskeletal pain
- Acute intermittent porphyria

 Data Gathering

HISTORY

Question: How severe is the pain and when does it occur?
Significance: Primary and secondary dysmenorrhea can cause severe pain. However, 10% of patients with severe dysmenorrhea have a secondary cause. Pain from primary dysmenorrhea is most likely to begin with the onset of, or 1 to 2 days after, menstruation whereas pain from secondary dysmenorrhea typically begins 1 to 2 days before the menstrual cycle begins. Also, primary dysmenorrhea typically does not begin until 6 to 12 months after menses have started, corresponding to the onset of ovulatory cycles.

Question: Is there any fever associated with the pain?
Significance: Fever in relation to pain should raise the suspicion of an underlying cause, such as PID or a pelvic abscess.

Question: Are there any systemic symptoms associated with the pain?
Significance: Systemic symptoms during menses are sometimes seen with primary dysmenorrhea as a result of the effect of prostaglandins. These symptoms can include decreased appetite, nausea, vomiting, diarrhea, headache, back pain, muscle aches, dizziness, flushing, and disordered or volatile mood. Weight loss or any systemic symptoms that are particularly severe or persist beyond menses should raise the level of suspicion for secondary dysmenorrhea.

Question: Is there any vaginal discharge?
Significance: This is suspicious for pelvic inflammatory disease.

Question: What is the past medical and surgical history?
Significance: A chronic medical condition can suggest other causes for pelvic pain. Prior abdominal surgery should raise concern for pelvic adhesions.

Question: What medications have been used by the patient to treat her dysmenorrhea?
Significance: Pain unresponsive to medical therapy is more likely to be a result of secondary dysmenorrhea.

Question: Is there a family history of pelvic pain or endometriosis?
Significance: A family history of pelvic pain or endometriosis should raise the suspicion for endometriosis.

Question: What is the patient's sexual history?
Significance: A history of unprotected sex would raise suspicion for intrauterine or ectopic pregnancy and/or sexually transmitted infections (STI). It is important to ask if the teen has had previous STIs or pregnancies.

Question: Has the teen missed school or work secondary to pain?
Significance: This is common and may help you determine the severity of the pain and the impact it is having on the teen's life.

 Physical Examination

Finding: The complete physical examination is normal.
Significance: This may suggest primary amenorrhea.

Finding: Pelvic mass
Significance: May be seen with pregnancy, and ovarian or uterine tumors.

Finding: Vaginal discharge
Significance: May be seen with PID and/or STIs.

Finding: Acute abdomen
Significance: Suggests pelvic pain from other cause such as obstruction or appendicitis

Finding: Weight loss
Significance: Concerning for other, potentially serious causes of pain such as inflammatory bowel disease or neoplasm.

 Laboratory Aids

Typically not needed since most cases of primary dysmenorrhea are easily diagnosed by history and physical. If secondary dysmenorrhea is suspected, further laboratory testing may be warranted.

Test: Vaginal/cervical cultures
Significance: Should be done if STIs are suspected

Test: Urine HCG
Significance: Should be performed if pregnancy is suspected or if the patient has amenorrhea

Dysmenorrhea

RADIOGRAPHIC STUDIES

Test: Pelvic ultrasound
Significance: Indicated if there is a pelvic mass, a suspicion of a congenital anomaly, or if dysmenorrhea is unresponsive to 6 months of medical treatment.

DIAGNOSTIC SURGERY

Test: Laparoscopy
Significance: Consider if patient is unresponsive to 6 months of medical therapy.

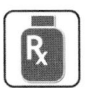 Therapy

Treatment of secondary dysmenorrhea is specific to the underlying disease. The following apply to treatment of primary dysmenorrhea.

DRUGS

Nonsteroidal anti-inflammatory medications (NSAIDs)—best to initiate 1 to 2 days before menstrual cycle begins. The most common side effect is gastrointestinal irritation. Use with caution in patients with gastrointestinal ulcers or renal disease.

- Ibuprofen: 200 to 600 mg every 6 hours as needed. Commonly used as first-line medication. Side effects include GI irritation or bleeding, rashes and granulocytopenia.
- Naproxen sodium: 440 to 550 mg as loading dose, followed by 220 to 275 mg every 8 hours as needed. Commonly used as first-line medication. Side effects include GI irritation or bleeding, thrombocytopenia, drowsiness, tinnitus.
- Mefenamic acid: 500 mg as loading dose followed by 250 mg every 6 hours as needed.
- Safety and efficacy have not been determined in children less than 14 years old. Should not use for more than one week at a time. Can be useful as a second-line therapy—has effect on already synthesized prostaglandins. Possible side effects include pancytopenia, gastrointestinal effects, drowsiness and renal toxicity.
- Rofecoxib—50 mg once per day as needed for up to 5 days. Safety and efficacy not established in children less than 18 years of age. Second-line therapy. Possible side effects include gastrointestinal effects, neurologic effects such as dizziness or fatigue, and cardiac effects such as hypertension.
- Combined oral contraceptives—Not firmly established as effective treatment although commonly used. Typically initiated if a patient has no or inadequate response to treatment with NSAIDs after 3 months. Treatment has additional benefit of providing contraception in sexually active adolescent. Side effects can include thromboembolic events, hypertension, nausea, headaches, irregular bleeding and mood changes.
- Depot medroxyprogesterone acetate (DMPA)—A long acting, injectable contraception (given once every 3 months). Theoretically improves dysmenorrhea by

inhibiting ovulation. Side effects can include amenorrhea, abnormal uterine bleeding, weight gain, hair loss and headaches.

Dietary Supplements

Magnesium aspartate—Given 1 to 3 times daily as a dietary supplement. Two randomized controlled trials have shown a decrease in pain over a 5- to 6-month period as compared to placebo. Other studies have shown no difference. Not first-line treatment. Thiamine—100 mg daily; large randomized control trial showed that pain was better controlled after 60 days than placebo. Not a first-line treatment.

NONPHARMACOLOGICAL THERAPY

These therapies may be considered as an adjunct to pharmacologic therapy or for a patient who is opposed to the use of pharmacologic therapy. In general, there is limited or mixed evidence on the effectiveness of these options. Risks and benefits should be weighed carefully.

- Smoking cessation—limited evidence of effectiveness; however intervention would clearly improve overall health.
- Exercise—limited evidence from a small study suggests that 30 minutes of exercise 3 times per week can be effective.
- Transcutaneous nerve stimulation (TENS)—evidence is mixed with some studies showing that high frequency TENS may be effective but other studies show no effect.
- Topical heat application with hot water bottle or heat patch—limited evidence that this may be effective.
- Acupuncture—limited evidence that this may be effective.
- Muscle relaxation exercises—insufficient evidence that this is effective. Low risk to patient.
- Laparoscopic uterine nerve ablation and laparoscopic presacral neurectomy—very limited evidence suggesting that these may be effective.

 Follow-Up

- Patients should be followed every 3 months unless symptoms have abated, or there is a significant worsening or change.
- If no response to adequate trial of NSAIDs and combined oral contraceptives, secondary dysmenorrhea should be suspected and referral to gynecologist should be initiated.

PITFALLS

- Failure to obtain a thorough history and physical with attention to signs and symptoms of secondary dysmenorrhea can lead to misdiagnosis.
- Adolescents should be aggressively managed in order to minimize school and work absenteeism. Failure to adequately respond to treatment should prompt referral to a specialist.

Common Questions and Answers

Q: What is the best approach to treatment of the adolescent with primary dysmenorrhea?
A: The mainstay of therapy is treatment with NSAIDs (presuming the patient has no contraindications to taking them). If there is inadequate response to NSAID therapy after 3 menstrual cycles, treatment with combined oral contraceptives should be considered for at least 3 additional menstrual cycles.

Q: When should one suspect secondary dysmenorrhea?
A: If the patient shows inadequate response to treatment after 6 months of therapy with NSAIDs and/or combined oral contraceptive pills (see previous question); if the history is not typical for primary dysmenorrhea; if there is a history of vaginal discharge or fevers accompanying the pain; if there is a family history of endometriosis; if the pain is chronic and noncyclic, or is particularly severe; if menses are irregular or absent; or if there are any physical exam findings which indicate a secondary cause.

Q: When should a pelvic examination be performed in the evaluation of dysmenorrhea?
A: If there is any suspicion of secondary dysmenorrhea; and as normally indicated in sexually active adolescents (within the first 3 years after initial coitus, no later than age 21 and earlier if any concern for STI). An adolescent who is not sexually active and has a history and physical strongly suggestive of primary dysmenorrhea does not need a pelvic exam at initial evaluation.

Q: When should referral to a gynecologist be initiated?
A: If secondary dysmenorrhea is suspected because of the patient's history and/or physical or if there is an inadequate response to 6 months of treatment.

BIBLIOGRAPHY

Davis AR, Westhoff CL. Primary dysmenorrhea in adolescent girls and treatment with oral contraceptives. *J Pediatr Adolesc Gynecol* 2001;14:3–8.

Proctor M, Farquhar C. Dysmenorrhoea. *Clin Evid* 2002:1639–1653.

Author: Lee Ann Savio Beers

Ehrlichiosis

 Database

DEFINITION

A zoonotic infection caused by four microorganisms of the genus Ehrlichia. The two most common clinically described infections are human monocytic ehrlichiosis (HME) caused by *Ehrlichia chaffeensis* and human granulocytic ehrlichiosis (HGE) caused by Anaplasma phagocytophila. Another organism, *E. ewingii*, has been described and is clinically indistinguishable from HGE. A fourth species, E. sennetsu, causes a mononucleosis-like syndrome, has been found in Japan and Malaysia. The genus Ehrlichia is found within the family Rickettsiaceae.

CAUSES

- HME and HGE are both carried by tick vectors.
- HME is thought to be transmitted by Amblyomma americanum, the lone star tick
- The vector for HGE is believed to be Ixodes scapularis, a deer tick, or Dermacentor variabilis, a brown dog tick.

GEOGRAPHIC DISTRIBUTION

- HGE is typically found in the following areas: northern Midwest, costal regions of the eastern and northeastern United States.
- HME is typically found in the southern to southeastern United States
- HGE and HME have been found in California and from Rhode Island to Florida.

PATHOPHYSIOLOGY

- Obligate intracellular, pleomorphic, coccobacillary bacteria
- Transmission to a human by a tick vector
- Incubation period ranges from 1 to 21 days
- HME infects mononuclear phagocytes, while HGE infects granulocytes
- The Ehrlichia reside within a leukocyte phagosome (called a morula), where the bacteria divide by binary fission and produce microcolonies.
- The infected cell is destroyed by the morula, thus releasing more organisms into the phagocyte system.

GENERAL EPIDEMIOLOGY OF EHRLICHIOSIS

- Most patients are infected during April through September, the months of greatest tick and human outdoor activity.
- HME and HGE have been found in Europe.

EPIDEMIOLOGY OF HME

- Males are more often infected (57%).
- Average age is 6.7 (range 7 months to 13.7 years).
- Most infected children reside in rural areas.
- HME is found in similar states where Rocky Mountain spotted fever (RMSF) occurs.
- Data from Georgia demonstrated that ehrlichiosis was more common than RMSF, with an incidence of 5.3 per 100,000.

EPIDEMIOLOGY

- Prevalence and incidence are not known.
- The majority of HGE infections have occurred in states where Lyme disease is very prevalent: Wisconsin, Minnesota, and Connecticut.
- Congential transmission of HGE has been described.

COMPLICATIONS

Neurologic Sequelae

- Headache, described as severe
- Mental status changes
- Seizures
- Coma
- Focal neurologic findings
- Cognitive learning deficits

Hematologic

- Disseminated intravascular coagulopathy (DIC)
- Thrombocytopenia
- Leukopenia
- Lymphopenia
- Anemia

Gastrointestinal

- Gastrointestinal hemorrhage
- Elevated liver enzymes
- Hepatosplenomegaly

Respiratory

- Pulmonary hemorrhage
- Interstitial pneumonia
- Pleural effusions
- Noncardiogenic pulmonary edema

Infectious

- Fungal superinfection
- Nosocomial infections
- Opportunistic infections

Renal

- Renal failure
- Proteinuria
- Hematuria

Cardiac

- Cardiomegaly
- Cardiac murmurs

Metabolic

- Hyponatremia

PROGNOSIS

- The majority of patients are hospitalized (>60%).
- Case fatality for HME is 2% to 5%, HGE is 7% to 10%.
- Elevated BUN and creatinine have been associated with a more severe course.
- Children appear to have an excellent outcome.

—Blood, renal, and liver abnormalities resolve in 1 to 2 weeks after initiating antibiotics.

- Cognitive and behavioral problems have been reported.
- Neuropathy has also been described.

 Differential Diagnosis

TICK-BORNE INFECTION

- RMSF, tularemia, relapsing fever, Lyme disease, Colorado tick fever, and babesiosis

INFECTION

- Toxic shock syndrome, Kawasaki disease, meningococcemia, pyelonephritis, gastroenteritis, hepatitis, leptospirosis, EBV, influenza, CMV, enterovirus, streptococcus throat

MISCELLANEOUS

- Leukemia, idiopathic thrombocytopenia purpura (ITP), hemolytic uremic syndrome (HUS)

 Data Gathering

HISTORY AND PRESENTING SYMPTOMS

- Tick-bite history or exposure to wooded areas that are endemic for tick-borne diseases is very helpful.
- Classic presentation is described as fevers, headache, and myalgias, followed by the development of a progressive leukopenia, thrombocytopenia, and anemia.
- Fevers are found in all children.
- Rash occurs in about 66% of patients and is pleomorphic. It has been described as macular, maculopapular, petechial, erythematous, vesicular, scarlet form or in a combination. The distribution is usually located on the trunk and on the extremities.
- Myalgia is found in the majority of children.
- Severe headache is often described.
- Abdominal pain, vomiting, anorexia, and diarrhea are often elicited.
- Arthralgia
- Cough and sore throat is often described.

 Physical Examination

- Mental status changes/irritability
- Nuchal rigidity
- Cardiac murmur (II/VI systolic ejection murmur at the LLSB)
- Hepatosplenomegaly
- Poor perfusion with hypotension (shock) has been described in a few children as a presenting symptom.
- Conjunctival or throat injection
- Rash as described

Laboratory Aids

- CBC with differential (with smear)

—Thrombocytopenia, <150,000/mm^3 (77%–92% incidence)
—Lymphopenia, <1,500/mm^3 (75%)
—Leukopenia, <4,000/mm^3 (58% to 68%)
—Anemia, Hct <30% (38% to 42%)
—Intracytoplasmic morulae within leukocytes (10% to 80%)

- Electrolytes with BUN and creatinine

—Hyponatremia (33% to 65%)

- Liver function tests

—Elevated ALT, >55 U/L (90%)

- Coagulation labs, type, and cross as indicated
- Cerebrospinal fluid (CSF)

—Leukocytosis, with an average cell count of 100/mm^3
—Lymphocytic predominance
—Elevated protein and borderline low glucose
—Microbiology cultures are negative.
—Ehrlichia morulae (intraleukocytoplasmic Ehrlichia microorganisms) have been described on CSF smears.

- Bone marrows are usually hypercellular, but normocellularity and hypocellularity have also been found.

SERUM STUDIES

- Serum titers for both HGE and HME have been developed.
- Titers are available through state health departments, at the CDC or a reference laboratory.
- Acute and convalescent antibody titers of *Ehrlichia* (a fourfold rise or fall is considered positive), obtained 2 to 4 weeks apart.
- An acute antibody titer of ≥1:64 is considered diagnostic.
- Polymerase chain reaction (PCR) has been developed and shows promise.
- The detection of intraleukocytoplasmic *Ehrlichia* microcolonies (morulae) on peripheral blood monocytes or granulocytes is diagnostic.

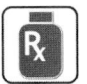

Therapy

- Supportive care and medical management
- Volume and blood pressure medications as needed
- Intubation for respiratory failure
- Dialysis for renal failure
- Platelets for thrombocytopenia
- Packed red blood cells for anemia
- Fresh frozen plasma, cryoprecipitate, and vitamin K for DIC
- Antifungal or antibiotics for secondary infections

DRUGS

- Doxycycline either oral or intravenous is the drug of choice regardless of the age of the child who is severely ill: children less than eight years of age, 4.4 mg/kg per day (maximum of 100 mg per dose) divided q 12 hours for 1 week, while in children older than 8 years of age, the dose is 100 mg q 12 hours for 1 week.
- Rifampin has been reported to be an effective antibiotic for children less than 8 years of age who are less toxic, but who are experiencing an HGE infection. The dose is 20 mg/kg per day divided q 12 for 5 to 10 days.
- Treatment for a minimum of 5 to 10 days and should continue for 3 days after defervescence.
- Doxycycline is a tetracycline and long-term use has been associated with permanent dental staining and enamel hypoplasia. Short courses, such as those for ehrlichiosis, are unlikely to cause noticeable dental staining. Other side effects of doxycycline are photosensitivity, hepatotoxicity, nausea, and pseudotumor cerebri.
- Unlike Lyme disease, amoxicillin or ceftriaxone have not been shown to be effective for the treatment of ehrlichiosis.

PREVENTION

- Avoid tick-infested areas.
- Clothes should cover arms and legs.
- Tick repellents, but use with caution in young children.
- A thorough body search should always be done after returning from a tick-infested area. If a tick is found, the area should be cleaned with a disinfectant. To remove the tick, grasp the tick at the point of origin with forceps; staying as close to the skin as possible. Applying steady, even pressure, the tick is slowly pulled off the skin. Once the tick is removed, the skin should be cleaned with a disinfectant.
- Instruct parents to seek medical attention only if symptoms develop.
- No vaccine is available.

PITFALLS

- Simultaneous infections have been documented with ehrlichiosis and Lyme disease; therefore, in patients diagnosed with ehrlichiosis, Lyme titers should also be measured to determine if there is a dual infection. One study from Wisconsin documented a 12% coinfection rate.
- Other coinfections with ehrlichiosis have also been documented with either Rocky Mountain spotted fever or babesiosis.
- Failing to consider the diagnosis of ehrlichiosis or a delay in treatment pending confirmatory serum titers.

Common Questions and Answers

Q: If a tick is removed from my child, should antibiotics be started?
A: Unlike Lyme disease, this has yet to be defined. Antibiotics should be started if a child becomes symptomatic.

Q: What is the most common chief complaint in children with ehrlichiosis?
A: Intense unremitting headache. In patients with fever, headache and flu-like illness in the spring to early fall, consider the diagnosis. Laboratory abnormalities of leukopenia, thrombocytopenia and hepatitis should lead to presumptive therapy until the diagnosis is clear.

ICD-9-CM 066.8

BIBLIOGRAPHY

American Academy of Pediatrics. Ehrlichiosis (human). In: Pickering LK, eds. *2004 Red Book: Report of the Committee on Infectious Disease*, 26th Ed. Elk Grove Village, IL: American Academy of Pediatrics, 2004:226–268.

Barton LB, Rathmore MH, Dawson JE. Infection with Ehrlichia in childhood. *J Pediatr* 1992;120:998–1001.

Berry DS, Miller S, Hooke JA, et al. Ehrlichial meningitis with cerebrospinal fluid morulae. *Pediatr Infect Dis J* 1999;18:552–555.

Buller RS, Arens M, Hmiel P, et al. Ehrlichia ewingii, a newly recognized agent of human ehrlichiosis. *N Engl J Med* 1999;341:148–155.

Dumler JS, Bakken JS. Ehrlichial diseases of humans: emerging tick-borne infections. *Clin Infect Dis* 1995;20:1102–1110.

Fichtenbaum CJ, Peterson LR, Weil GT. Ehrlichiosis presenting as a life-threatening illness with features of the toxic shock syndrome. *Am J Med* 1993;95:351–357.

Harkess JR, Ewing SA, Brumit T, et al. Ehrlichiosis in children. *Pediatrics* 1991;87:199–203.

Horowitz HW, Kilchevsky E, Haber S, et al. Perinatal transmission of the agent of human granulocytic ehrlichiosis. *N Engl J Med* 1999;339:375–378.

Jacobs RF, Schultze GE. Ehrlichiosis in children. *J Pediatr* 1997;131:184–192.

Krause PJ, et al. Successful treatment of human granulocytic ehrlichiosis in children using rifampin. *Pediatrics* 2003,e252–e253.

Lantos P, Krause PJ. Ehrlichiosis in children. *Sem Infect Dis* 2002;13:249–256.

Nadelman RB, Horowitz HW, Heish T, et al. Simultaneous human granulocytic ehrlichiosis and Lyme borreliosis. *N Engl J Med* 1997; 337:27–30.

Nadelman RB, Nowakoski J, Fish D, et al. Prophylaxis with single dose doxycycline for the prevention of Lyme disease after an Ixodes scapularis tick bite. *N Engl J Med* 2001;345:79–84.

Schutze GE, Jacobs RF. Human monocytic ehrlichiosis in children. *Pediatrics* 1997;100:e10

Author: Jeffrey P. Louie

Encephalitis

Database

DEFINITION

Encephalitis is inflammation of the brain parenchyma due to infection. Meningoencephalitis is inflammation of the brain and the meninges.

PATHOPHYSIOLOGY

- Direct or delayed (postinfectious) reaction by the immune system to a virus, bacteria, fungus, or parasite
- Organisms enter the CNS via the systemic circulation, direct inoculation (trauma), or neural pathways (rabies, herpes simplex virus [HSV]).
- Infiltration of inflammatory cells into the CNS with release of cytokines
- Inclusion bodies (intranuclear; HSV, subacute sclerosing panencephalitis [SSPE], viral, intracytoplasmic; rabies), CSF, and serology changes

EPIDEMIOLOGY

- Incidence varies with age, geographic location, and season
- The most common causes of encephalitis are viruses

—Summer (enteroviruses)
—Summer and fall (Western and Eastern equine, St. Louis, La Crosse and West Nile encephalitis.)
—Winter (varicella)

- Nonviral causes (tuberculosis, Lyme disease, toxoplasmosis, cat-scratch disease, rickettsial disease, tick-borne infections) are sometimes associated with specific environmental or geographic exposure.
- The most common cause of sporadic encephalitis is HSV (rabies and HIV also occur in all seasons).

COMPLICATIONS

Seizure disorders, focal or generalized, quadriparesis/hemiparesis, ataxia, learning disabilities, and aphasias can result from encephalitis.

PROGNOSIS

Outcome ranges from complete recovery to coma, persistent vegetative state, and death.

Differential Diagnosis

Several toxic, metabolic, vascular, or epileptic syndromes may resemble encephalitis:

- Ingestions
- Hypothyroid crisis
- Acute electrolyte disturbance, especially hyponatremia
- Reye syndrome

- Noninfectious encephalitides, triggered by immunization or infection include acute hemorrhagic leukoencephalitis and acute disseminated encephalomyelitis (associated *Mycoplasma*, EBV, or other infection), in context of acute rheumatic fever (rare)
- Intracranial hemorrhage
- Pituitary infarction
- Acute obstructive hydrocephalus or ventriculoperitoneal shunt obstruction
- Sinus thrombosis
- Subdural empyema
- Cerebral vasculitis, stroke or septic embolization (endocarditis)
- Brain abscess or subdural empyema
- Malignant hyperthermia
- Status epilepticus
- Other considerations include bacterial meningitis (*Neisseria meningitidis*, *Haemophilus influenzae* type b, group B *streptococcus* in the neonate, *Escherichia coli* in the neonate).
- Diagnosis of specific causes of true encephalitis depends on geographic location, age, and clinical and associated laboratory findings
- Microbes to consider:

—Herpes viruses (in the child and adult, herpes has preference for the medial temporal lobe)
—Lyme disease; possible coinfection with ehrlichiosis, babesiosis
—Varicella (postinfectious or primary varicella infection)
—Cat-scratch and rickettsial diseases
—Leptospirosis
—Tuberculosis
—Fungal (cryptosporidiosis)
—Parasitic (amoebae, toxoplasma, schistosoma, cysticercosis)
—Toxoplasma

- Meningitis:

—Meningitis may cause secondary parenchymal inflammation of the brain
—Mental status changes are more prominent in primary encephalitis compared with meningitis

Data Gathering

HISTORY

- Ask about a viral prodrome with symptoms such as upper respiratory infection, cough, coryza, malaise, anorexia, decreased enteral intake, diarrhea, nausea, and vomiting.
- Encephalitis is often heralded by headaches, photophobia, a stiff neck, increased sleeping, change in mental status, irritability, confusion, hallucinations, and seizures.
- Prodromal symptoms can range from hours to weeks; seizures or sudden lapse of consciousness are uncommon as initial symptoms of encephalitis
- Inquire about recent travel history, pets, tick or mosquito bites.

Physical Examination

- Hypertension, bradycardia, or apnea may suggest impending herniation due to brain swelling.
- Neck: The patient may have meningismus and positive Kernig and Brudzinski signs.
- Adenopathy (mycobacterium, cat-scratch encephalitis)
- Chest: Signs of pneumonia, rales, rhonchi (especially mycobacteria, *Mycoplasma*, influenza)
- Abdomen: Hepatosplenomegaly
- Skin: May show various types of rashes, from petechial (Rickettsial infection, meningococcemia) to an erythematous or papular rashes (especially Lyme, enteroviridae).
- Neurologic examination: Mental status ranging from mild confusion to delirium with hallucinations to stupor and coma.
- Aphasia (suggestive of herpes) is distinguished from psychomotor slowing by prominence of grammatic errors and dysarthria with normal alertness.
- Cranial nerve examination may reveal papilledema, nystagmus.
- Increased muscle tone, pathologic deep tendon reflexes, Babinski sign, clonus, or ataxia (especially varicella) may be encountered.
- Flaccid paralysis, or a "poliolike" syndrome has been seen with the West Nile Virus.

PITFALLS

A CSF sample without any RBCs does not rule out herpes simplex.

- Never assume that a CSF pleocytosis is secondary to seizures. Institute antiviral and/or antibacterial therapy promptly; it can always be discontinued once an organism is identified or cultures are negative.
- Children with immunodeficiency are at higher risk for fungal meningoencephalitis, which may be missed unless appropriate studies are sent.
- Amebic infection of the brain should be considered in children with exposure to fresh water sources.
- Cysticercosis is common in tropical and underdeveloped areas. Ring-enhancing lesions may point to this diagnosis or to toxoplasmosis.

Laboratory Aids

TESTS

Laboratory testing strategies depend on the severity of symptoms.

Radiologic

• CT or MRI of the brain with and without contrast medium should be performed urgently to rule out surgically remediable conditions (empyema, abscess).
• Typical changes in encephalitis include parenchymal, meningeal, and focal or diffuse enhancement of the brain. (HSV has a preference for the medial temporal lobe.)
• Hydrocephalus, obstructive or communicating, may occur weeks following the encephalitis.

Spinal Tap

A CSF spinal tap should be deferred until airway, gas exchange, and circulation has been stabilized. Thereafter, lumbar puncture should be deferred if (a) there is papilledema, or (b) if imaging shows subfalcine herniation (left-to-right shift of lateral ventricles), cerebral edema, obstructive hydrocephalus (lateral ventricles large, fourth ventricle relatively small), or central herniation (asymmetry or effacement of fourth ventricle/basilar cystern).

Lumbar Puncture

If there is no papilledema or radiologic evidence for increased intracranial pressure, a lumbar puncture should be performed

• Opening pressure is frequently elevated.
• Pleocytosis is lymphocytic if viral, and usually neutrophilic if bacterial.
• Protein will be increased, glucose variably decreased, and RBCs may be present (particularly in HSV).
• CSF should be sent for bacterial and viral culture. Fungal culture if suspected.
• If HSV is suspected, PCR should be obtained. Other PCR-based tests on CSF, including assays for the Lyme spirochete, enteroviruses and West Nile virus, may be considered.
• Gram stain and acid-fast bacillus, cryptococcal antigen, and yeast tests also should be ordered.
• State or local departments of health are often helpful in planning and handling extended virologic studies

Other Routine Tests

• Blood electrolytes, BUN, glucose, calcium, magnesium, phosphorus, blood count with differential, blood and urine culture, and toxicology screen
• EEG, particularly if HSV is suspected; periodic lateralizing epileptiform discharges (PLEDs) are suggestive, but not diagnostic, of herpes.
• Continuous EEG monitoring for comatose patients with known seizures
• PPD if CSF or other signs suggest the possibility of Mycobacterium

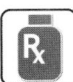
Therapy

• General: Patients with encephalitis frequently require ICU care with cardiorespiratory support. Mini-dose subcutaneous heparin is standard for prophylaxis of intravascular thrombosis in acutely ill adults, but is untested in the pediatric age group. Early involvement of physical and occupational therapy is important.
• Treatment of intracranial hypertension includes mannitol and hyperventilation, usually with assistance from intensivists or neurology/neurosurgery consultants; these measures should be reserved for situations in which vital or neurologic signs indicate impending herniation. Intracranial pressure monitoring is not routinely indicated.
• Antiinfective agents: Depending upon severity of the illness and clinicians' level of suspicion, initial treatment could include antibacterial and antiviral agents (acyclovir: monitor renal function) until the cause becomes clear or cultures are negative.
• Confirmed-HSV encephalitis: Infants—Acyclovir 20 mg/kg every 8 hours for 21 days; older children: 10 mg/kg every 8 hours, 10–14 days.
• CMV: Consider ganciclovir or foscarnet
• HIV encephalitis: Consider zidovudine, didanosine, ritonavir.
• SSPE (diagnosed by spinal fluid titers): Consider isoprinosine
• Fluids: Avoidance of fluid overload, which may exacerbate cerebral edema, requires strict attention to fluid/osmotic balance. Normal saline is preferred; electrolytes are closely monitored, anticipating possible SIADH or diabetes insipidus.
• Anticonvulsants are reserved for clinical or electrographic evidence of seizure/epileptic activity; usual choices include lorazepam, phenytoin, phenobarbital, and carbamazepine. Treatment of PLEDs without associated convulsions is controversial. Potential side-effects and sedation from anticonvulsants should be considered in this decision.
• Consultation with an infectious disease specialist, neurologist, or neurosurgeon may be helpful.

Follow-Up

The outcome from encephalitis varies greatly and depends on age and degree of CNS involvement. Physical and occupational therapy should be consulted early in the course. Neuropsychologic testing is helpful to identify cognitive deficits and to maximize the patient's recovery.

PREVENTION

• Completion of routine immunizations (varicella) and routine hygiene (hand washing) are the best preventive measures.
• Other measures should be taken according to the infection (e.g., skin testing contacts in cases of tuberculosis).
• Isolation of hospitalized patient: depends on organism suspected. Airborne, droplet, and contact precautions are frequently used together during the first 24 hours, pending a more specific diagnosis from cultures. The hospital infectious disease department will determine type and duration of isolation and whether family members need to be treated.

Common Question and Answer

Q: My child has been diagnosed with encephalitis; will he be mentally retarded?
A: The complications following encephalitis vary greatly from severe mental retardation and cerebral palsy to full recovery. There is a correlation between degree of brain destruction and outcome. However, children frequently recover better than adults with a similar degree of illness.

ICD-9-CM 323.9

BIBLIOGRAPHY

Bonthius D, Karacay B. Meningitis and encephalitis in children: an update. *Neurologic Clinics* 2002;20:1013–1038.

Patient Information: National Center for Infectious Diseases website-http://www.cdc.gov/ncidod/

Redington J, Tyler K. Viral infections of the nervous system, 2002: update on diagnosis and treatment. *Arch of Neurol* 2002;59: 712–718.

Sampathkumar P. West Nile Virus: epidemiology, clinical presentation, diagnosis, and prevention. *Mayo Clin Proc* 2003;78:1137–1144.

Author: A.G. Christina Bergqvist

Encopresis

 Database

DEFINITION

Encopresis is the repeated passage of feces into inappropriate places (usually clothing or floor) after the age of 4 years without any organic cause. Most commonly associated with constipation and functional fecal retention. A second subtype is functional nonretentive fecal incontinence that refers to encopresis in the absence of constipation, and structural or inflammatory diseases (also known as solitary or nonretentive encopresis).

PATHOPHYSIOLOGY

• Chronic constipation with fecal impaction results in overflow incontinence and reduced sensation secondary to rectal distension. The pattern of holding fecal matter, leading to chronic constipation and overflow incontinence, may result from a variety of etiologies, such as a painful experience from a fissure, difficult toilet training or refusal to use school bathrooms. However, the history often does not reveal a triggering event.

—The chronic constipation leads to a dilated rectum, decreased rectal sensation, shortening of the anal canal and decreased anal sphincter tone in some patients.
—Findings on anorectal manometry include increased rectal sensory threshold and paradoxical contraction of the external anal sphincter during attempts at defecation (known as anismus).

• Functional nonretentive fecal incontinence occurs in children without constipation. The soiling may be a manifestation of an emotional disturbance and they may be associated to specific triggers (person or place) or may represent an impulsive action triggered by unconscious anger. In some cases it may represent a primary rectal sensation disorder that interferes with the child's ability to contract the external anal sphincter in response to stool in the rectum.

GENETICS

Monozygotic twins have a fourfold higher incidence than do dizygotic twins.

EPIDEMIOLOGY

The reported ratio of boys to girls ranges from 2:1 up to 6:1. There is no association with family size, ordinal position in the family, age of parents, or socioeconomic status.

COMPLICATIONS

• Social problems
• Urinary tract infections, especially in girls
• Abdominal discomfort
• Decreased appetite

 Differential Diagnosis

The physician must determine if stool leakage is due to functional constipation or an underlying anatomic, metabolic, or neurologic abnormality. Fecal incontinence may be secondary to diarrheal diseases or defective neuromuscular control, such as in children with spinal defects.

• Neuromuscular: Spinal cord tumor, tethered spinal cord, meningomyelocele
• Anal abnormalities: Anteriorly displaced anus, ectopic anus
• Inflammatory: Proctitis (infectious or ulcerative), fistula secondary to Crohn disease
• Stricture (after necrotizing enterocolitis or inflammatory bowel disease)
• Abdominal pelvic mass (sacral teratoma, meningomyelocele)
• Hypotonia (cerebral palsy, amyotonia congenita, familial visceral myopathy)
• Hirschsprung disease (constipation common, fecal incontinence rarely seen)
• Postsurgical repair of imperforate anus or Hirschprung disease
• Endocrine: Hypothyroidism, panhypopituitarism, diabetes mellitus
• Constipating drugs: Opiates, calcium supplements, psychotropics

 Data Gathering

HISTORY

• Toileting habits:

—Is there a history of constipation? Frequency and size of bowel movements (large diameter bowel movements are common in children with encopresis associated with functional fecal retention)
—History of bowel movements that obstruct the toilet and/or history of chronic abdominal pain relieved by enemas or laxatives
—Retentive posturing: Avoiding defecation by contraction of pelvic floor, squeezing the buttocks together (leg scissoring, crossing the legs, standing on tip toes)

• Irritability, abdominal cramps, decreased appetite (symptoms improve after passage of large stool)
• Onset: Elicit history of triggering events (perianal infection, diet changes, toilet training, avoidance of school bathrooms, sexual abuse or other stressful events)
• History of enuresis (secondary daytime enuresis common in patients with megarectum compressing the bladder)
• Timing in the neonatal period of meconium passage, as well as past surgeries, medical history, and medications, are relevant.
• Unsteady or clumsy gait may suggest a neuromuscular disorder
• Children with nonretentive fecal soiling do not have any history of constipation and have daily bowel movements

 Physical Examination

• Encopresis with functional fecal retention

—Fecal mass palpable in 40% of patients, fecal soiling in the perianal region
—Dilated rectum but a normally positioned anus.
—The anal sphincter tone can be normal or slightly decreased and the anal canal is usually shorter than normal.

• Nonretentive fecal incontinence

—No palpable fecal mass, normal size rectum, normal sphincter length

• Examination should include deep tendon reflexes, anal wink, rectal examination, and documentation of normal growth.
• In patients with extreme fear of anal examination a perianal inspection should be attempted and a plain radiograph of the abdomen obtained to establish a fecal impaction. In children who fear painful defecation the necessity of a rectal examination remains debatable.

 Laboratory Aids

• No laboratory tests are needed if both the history and physical examination are consistent with functional constipation and associated encopresis. If the patient's history or physical is atypical and a systemic disorder is suspected, appropriate diagnostic tests should be done.
• Abdominal x-ray is often necessary for patients who refuse a rectal exam, or when a rectal impaction is not palpable on abdominal exam (obese patients).
• Referral to a gastroenterologist for anorectal manometry is often a useful adjunctive modality for patients who are recalcitrant to standard management.

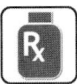
Therapy

Management combines pharmacology, behavioral modification, and dietary alterations.

- Pharmacology

—Remove fecal impaction with cathartic regimens, including laxatives. Choices include magnesium citrate, milk of magnesia or high dose Miralax (1.5 gm/kg per day) combined with a stimulant laxative like Senna or docusate. Although some authors favor the use of enemas, they should be avoided for toddlers and school-age children with fear of anal manipulation.
—Stool softeners: Miralax (0.75 mg/kg per day) is the preferred agent due to its palatability and lack of taste. Milk of magnesia (0.5–1 mL/kg per day) is a good option. Mineral oil can also be used.

- Behavior modification

—Decrease family stress.
—Have the child sit on toilet for 5 to 10 minutes 1 to 2 times per day (ideally after a meal, tailored to the age of the child).
—Delay toilet training if the child is in diapers (to reduce stress).
—Motivate
—Biofeedback (reserved for very difficult cases)

- Diet

—High-fiber diet
—Adequate fluid

- Patients with nonretentive fecal incontinence usually require referral to a mental health professional for more intensive behavioral intervention.

Follow-Up

The first follow-up is at 2 weeks to ensure compliance and success with the initial management. If the fecal impaction has been successfully removed, a reward system is started. The patient is followed at monthly intervals to ensure motivation and to be supportive. Treatment with stool softeners is needed until behavior and diet have improved and until rectal dilatation has resolved. Medication is often needed for 6 months or longer.

PITFALLS

- Parents may misconstrue stool-withholding behavior as an attempt to defecate.
- Parents think that their child's soiling is deliberate. They do not understand that the child can neither feel the passage of stool nor prevent it. The usual urge to defecate, which comes from stretching of the ampulla and internal anal sphincter, is not felt because the rectal ampulla is massively distended.
- Patients or their parents often stop stool softeners as soon as a normal stool pattern starts. If therapy has been ended prematurely, the patient's constipation and encopresis returns immediately, because rectal tone is still poor and no other behavior or dietary modifications have been made.

Common Questions and Answers

Q: Is the medicine addictive?
A: Stool softeners rather than cathartics are chosen for long-term therapy because the colon does not become dependent.

Q: Will my child become sick if this problem is not resolved?
A: Most children with chronic constipation and encopresis grow well and do not develop other health problems. The major problems are social and should be taken seriously. Social development is crucial for the school-aged child.

ICD-9-CM 787.6

BIBLIOGRAPHY

Brooks RC, et al. Review of the treatment literature for encopresis, functional constipation, and stool-toileting refusal. *Ann Behav Med* 2000;2:260–267.

Di Lorenzo C, Benninga MA. Pathophysiology of pediatric fecal incontinence. *Gastroenterology* 2004;126(1 Suppl 2): S33–S40.

Griffiths DM. The physiology of continence: idiopathic fecal constipation and soiling. *Semin Pediatr Surg* 2002;11:67–74.

Kuhn BR, et al. Treatment guidelines for primary nonretentive encopresis and stool toileting refusal. *Am Fam Physician* 1999;59:2171–8, 2184–2186.

Loening-Baucke V. Encopresis. *Curr Opin Pediatr* 2002;14:570–575.

Loening-Baucke V. Functional fecal retention with encopresis in childhood. *J Pediatr Gastroenterol Nutr* 2004;38:79–84.

Rasquin-Weber A, et al. Childhood functional gastrointestinal disorders. *Gut* 1999;45 (Suppl II):II60–II68

Author: Victor M. Pineiro-Carrero

Endocarditis

Database

DEFINITION

Infective endocarditis is microbial infection of the endocardium of the heart.

PATHOGENESIS

- Infective endocarditis is primarily seen in patients with preexisting heart disease (congenital or acquired) who develop bacteremia with organisms that are likely to cause infection.
- Intravenous drug abusers and patients with indwelling intravenous catheters may develop endocarditis even in the absence of prior heart disease.
- Local turbulence secondary to the cardiovascular abnormality is thought to result in damage of the endocardial surface.

—The development of a fibrin and platelet network occurs in which bacteria can then become entrapped, causing infection.

- Bacteremia can be a complication of focal infection (e.g., pneumonia, cellulitis, or urinary tract infection) or can be associated with various dental and surgical procedures. Bacteremia, however, can occur spontaneously and has been documented with usual activities such as chewing hard candy and brushing teeth.

MICROORGANISMS

- Gram-positive cocci account for 90% of culture-positive endocarditis.

—α-Hemolytic streptococci (*Streptococcus viridans*) are responsible for most cases of endocarditis in all age groups.
—Staphylococci (*S. aureus* and coagulase-negative *staphylococci*) are the second largest group.
—Other organisms that can cause endocarditis are β-hemolytic *streptococci*, *pneumococci*, enterococci, *Pseudomonas* species, the HACEK bacteria, *Neisseria* species, and *Candida* species.

- Approximately 5% of endocarditis cases are reported as culture-negative.

EPIDEMIOLOGY

- Infective endocarditis is relatively uncommon. Studies have reported incidences between 1 in 1,280 and 1 in 4,500 of all pediatric hospital admissions.
- The overall incidence of endocarditis appears to have decreased with the advent of antibiotics. One might expect, however, an increase in incidence with better survival of patients with congenital heart disease and the wide and often prolonged use of central vascular catheters.

COMPLICATIONS

Despite improvements in diagnosis and treatment of endocarditis, it continues to be a disease with significant morbidity and mortality (approximately 10%).

- Cardiac

—Damage to the valve leaflets may result in valvar regurgitation, heart failure, or conduction abnormalities.

- Embolic

—Embolic events can occur to multiple organ systems (central nervous system, kidneys, spleen, skin, lungs).

PROGNOSIS

If diagnosed in a timely fashion and appropriate therapy is instituted, prognosis is relatively good for bacterial endocarditis. Fungal endocarditis, however, is associated with a higher morbidity and mortality.

Differential Diagnosis

- Other infections (e.g., acute rheumatic fever)
- Malignancy
- Connective tissue disorders

Data Gathering

HISTORY

Fever, malaise, anorexia, weight loss, symptoms of heart failure, arthralgia, neurologic symptoms, gastrointestinal symptoms, chest pain. Occasionally, a recent infection, dental visit or surgical procedure can be identified.

Physical Examination

- General

—Fever (usually low grade with α-hemolytic streptococci and high grade with *S. aureus*), petechiae (occurring in one-third of cases)

- Embolic or immunologic phenomena

—Splinter hemorrhages, retinal hemorrhages, Osler nodes (painful), Janeway lesions (painless), splenomegaly (occurring in about half of cases), clubbing, arthralgia, and arthritis

- Cardiac

—New or change in heart murmur, signs of congestive heart failure

- Neurologic

—Neurologic symptoms can be seen on the basis of central nervous system emboli and hemorrhage, and can sometimes mimic the picture of an abscess, aseptic meningitis, or cerebral infarct.

Laboratory Aids

TESTS

Blood Cultures

- Blood culture is the most important diagnostic test for endocarditis.
- Blood cultures are positive in 85% to 90% of the reported cases of endocarditis
- Three to five sets of blood cultures should be obtained from different sites during the first 24 hours of suspected endocarditis.
- As large a volume as clinically reasonable should be collected.
- The bacteremia of endocarditis is continuous; therefore, it is not necessary to wait to obtain the blood cultures during a fever spike.

Nonspecific Laboratory Data

Elevated ESR (80%), anemia (44%), positive rheumatoid factor (38%), hematuria (35%), leukocytosis, and decreased complement.

Electrocardiogram

- New-onset ECG abnormalities such as AV block (even first degree) may represent conduction system and myocardial involvement from invasive disease.

Echocardiography

- Transthoracic echocardiography is a valuable noninvasive technique in the identification of vegetations.
- The sensitivity and specificity of transthoracic echocardiography, however, is not 100%; therefore, a negative echocardiogram does not rule out endocarditis.
- Transesophageal echocardiography, especially in older or obese patients, provides better visualization of smaller vegetations that may not be readily seen using transthoracic imaging.
- In patients with an inconclusive transthoracic study but a high index of suspicion for endocarditis, transesophageal echocardiography is recommended.

PITFALLS

- The absence of vegetation(s) by echocardiography does not rule out endocarditis.
- In patients with a prosthetic valve, echocardiography is not always helpful, as there is frequently artifact from the prosthetic valve. Abnormal movements of the valve leaflets may suggest vegetation.
- The ESR may remain elevated for some time, even after cessation of bacteremia.

Therapy

- General

—Rest, antipyretics, optimal nutrition and hydration, careful dental hygiene

- Antibiotics

—Prolonged therapy (at least 4 weeks) with intravenous antibiotics is needed. The choice of antibiotic(s) and the duration of antibiotic treatment depend on the infecting organism and its sensitivity pattern. For fungal SBE, intravenous therapy is given for a minimum of 6 to 8 weeks.

- Surgery: Potential indications for surgical therapy (mostly adult data)

—Severe/worsening congestive heart failure with/without embolization or persistent infection
—Aortic valve disease with unstable hemodynamics
—Failing medical therapy
—Large, mobile vegetations
—Fungal endocarditis

Follow-Up

Repeat blood cultures should be obtained after a few days of antibiotic or antifungal therapy to ensure the eradication of bacteria. After completion of a full course of antibiotics, blood cultures should be again obtained in the first 2 months after discontinuation of therapy.

PREVENTION

- Dental hygiene
- Minimal use of central lines
- Correction of the cardiovascular anomaly by surgery or interventional catheterization techniques
- SBE Prophylaxis

SBE PROPHYLAXIS (AHA RECOMMENDATIONS, 1997)

For Dental, Oral, Respiratory Tract, or Esophageal Procedures

- Amoxicillin (50 mg/kg orally 1 hour before procedure; maximum, 2.0 g). If unable to take oral medications, ampicillin (same dose) may be given 30 minutes before the procedure.
- Clindamycin (20 mg/kg orally 1 hour before procedure or same dose IV within 30 minutes of the procedure; maximum, 600 mg) may be used if the patient is allergic to penicillin.

For Genitourinary/Gastrointestinal (Excluding Esophageal) Procedures

- High-risk patients: Ampicillin (50 mg/kg; maximum, 2.0 g IM/IV) plus gentamicin 1.5 mg/kg (maximum, 120 mg) within 30 minutes of starting procedure; 6 hours later, 25 mg/kg IV ampicillin (maximum, 1 g) or amoxicillin 25 mg/kg/PO (maximum, 1 g). Vancomycin plus gentamicin may be used for patients allergic to amoxicillin/ampicillin.
- Moderate-risk patients: Amoxicillin (50 mg/kg/PO; maximum, 2.0 g) 1 hour prior to the procedure, or ampicillin 50 mg/kg IM/IV (maximum, 2.0 g) within 30 minutes of starting the procedure. Vancomycin may be used for patients allergic to amoxicillin/ampicillin.

Cardiac Conditions That Require SBE Prophylaxis

- High-risk group: Prosthetic valves, previous SBE, cyanotic heart disease, surgically constructed shunts or conduits
- Moderate-risk group: most other congenital heart disease, acquired valvar disease (e.g., rheumatic valvar disease), hypertrophic cardiomyopathy, mitral valve prolapse with regurgitation or thickened leaflets

Cardiac Lesions That Do Not Require SBE Prophylaxis

- Isolated secundum atrial septal defect
- Surgically repaired patent ductus arteriosus
- Ventricular septal defect and atrial septal defect beyond 6 months (without residual)
- Previous coronary artery bypass surgery
- Mitral valve prolapse without regurgitation
- Previous Kawasaki syndrome without valvar dysfunction
- Rheumatic fever without valvar dysfunction
- Pacemakers and defibrillators

Procedures That Require SBE Prophylaxis

- Tonsillectomy, adenoidectomy, surgery of respiratory mucosa, rigid bronchoscopy
- Sclerotherapy for esophageal varices, esophageal dilation, biliary tract and intestinal surgery, endoscopic retrograde cholangiography
- Prostatic surgery, cytoscopy, urethral dilation
- Dental extractions, periodontal procedures, dental implant, endodontic procedures, dental cleaning, intraligamentary injections, initial placements of orthodontic bands, subgingival placement of antibiotic fibers/strips

Procedures That Do Not Require SBE Prophylaxis

These may be recommended in high-risk patients.

- Endotracheal intubation, flexible bronchoscopy, ear tubes, transesophageal echocardiography, GI endoscopy
- Vaginal hysterectomy, vaginal delivery, cesarean section, urethral catheterization, uterine dilation and curettage, abortion, sterilization, intrauterine devices
- Cardiac catheterization
- Circumcision
- Shedding of primary teeth

Common Questions and Answers

Q: I forgot to give my child antibiotics prior to the procedure. Should I give him a dose afterward?
A: In regard to preventing endocarditis, no data exist on the benefit of administering antibiotics after a procedure.

Q: My child has an innocent heart murmur. Does he need SBE prophylaxis?
A: SBE prophylaxis is not indicated.

Q: My child needs SBE prophylaxis in the appropriate setting and she just fell and scraped her knee. Does she need antibiotics to prevent a heart infection?
A: SBE prophylaxis is not indicated.

ICD-9-CM

421.9-Active or Subacute

421.0-Bacterial

BIBLIOGRAPHY

Dajani AS, Taubert KA, Wilson W, et al. Prevention of bacterial endocarditis: recommendations by the American Heart Association. *JAMA* 1997;277:1794–1801.

Milazzo AS Jr, Li JS. Bacterial endocarditis in infants and children. *Pediatric Infectious Disease Journal* 2001;20(8):799–801.

Steinberger J, Moller JH, Berry JM, et al. Echocardiographic diagnosis of heart disease in apparently healthy adolescents. *Pediatrics* 2000;105(4):815–818.

Author: Zev Jacobson

Enuresis

 Database

DEFINITION

Involuntary urination after age of expected bladder control, generally reserved for children 6 years or older.

- Generally refers to nocturnal enuresis or bedwetting—urinary incontinence only at night
- May include small group of children incontinent of urine during daytime as well as nighttime
- Primary enuresis: never continent of urine during timeframe considered (daytime, nocturnal or both)
- Secondary enuresis: had continent period of at least 6 months then relapse of enuresis
- Majority (80%) of nocturnal enuresis is primary.

Prevalence

- Female: Male ratio is 3:1
- At age 5, 15% of children have primary nocturnal enuresis
- Approximately 15% of children with enuresis spontaneously remit each year such that by age 10 only 5% still have nocturnal enuresis
- Frequency, severity, longevity of primary nocturnal enuresis increases with positive family history
- Approximately 1% of adolescents have nocturnal enuresis

GENETICS

- No specific genetic abnormality described
- Incidence:

—43% to 47% if one parent was enuretic
—15% if neither parents was enuretic
—Twice as high in monozygotic twins as dizygotic twins

CAUSES

- Primary nocturnal enuresis

—Underlying treatable cause is uncommon
—Any condition causing polyuria
—Theories include:
  —Deep sleep with failure of signal of increased bladder pressure to reach consciousness
  —Maturational delay with bladder emptying at lower volume secondary to small bladder capacity
  —Failure to decrease urinary volume at night compared to dry peers.

- Diurnal enuresis—day and night

—As above
—Urinary reflux into vagina with seepage after conclusion of voiding
—Abnormal insertion of ureter into urethra or vagina
—Incontinence with increased abdominal pressure (laughing, coughing, increased intravesicular pressure)

- Secondary enuresis

—Any condition causing polyuria
—Urinary tract infection
—Encopresis
—Emotional stress or trauma including physical and sexual abuse, divorce, depression, new sibling, household moving, new school

Secondary complications:

- Physical

—Vulvovaginitis
—Diaper dermatitis

- Emotional

—Embarrassment
—Poor self-esteem
—Reluctance to sleep out with peers or nonimmediate family
—Depression

 Differential Diagnosis

- UTI/urethritis
- Obstipation/constipation
- Water intoxication
- Diabetes mellitus
- Diabetes insipidus
- Sickle cell disease
- Nephritis/nephrosis
- Anatomic abnormalities of the urinary tract
- Sleep disorders
- Depression
- Anxiety
- Medications (sedatives, soporifics, antihistamines, diuretics, caffeine, methylxanthines)
- Spinal cord disease
- Cognitive disorders
- Seizure disorders
- Legitimate safety issues in going to bathroom alone
- Substandard living conditions (cold bathrooms, poor facilities)

 Data Gathering

HISTORY

- Onset—primary versus secondary
- Nocturnal versus diurnal
- Has there ever been dry period even if only for weeks
- Frequency
- Pattern of urination

—Constantly wetting pants (dribbling)
—Frequent small urine
—Dysuria
—Frequency
—Hesitancy
—Dry when sleeping out

- Past medical history

—Obstipation, constipation, stool incontinence
—Behavioral, developmental history
—Toilet training history
—Medications
—Neurologic symptoms
—Other medical problems

- Family history

—One parent or two
—Is child aware?

- Social history

—For whom is this a problem—parent or child?
—Effect on child
  —Can he or she sleep out without embarrassment?
  —Teasing at school
  —Emotional effect

- Social changes

—Divorce
—New significant other for parent
—New sibling
—Household move
—Change in school
—Death or illness in family
—Other change in home environment

- Intervention

—What has been attempted—treatment or punishment?
—How effective?

 Physical Examination

- Vital signs
- Growth parameters and pattern
- Neurologic examination with fundoscopy—rule out intracranial pressure
- Abdominal examination—rule out masses especially renal mass
- Genitalia—rule out adhesions, vulvo-vaginitis, balanitis, stenosis, foreign bodies
- Urinary stream
- Rectal examination—tone, peri-anal sensation, anal wink
- Spine—bony defects, cutaneous signs of underlying defects
- Neurologic examination—gait, tone, sensory, motor, DTR's, cremasteric reflex

Laboratory Aids

TESTS

- Urinalysis

—Specific gravity
—Glucose
—Protein
—Blood
—? first morning void for specific gravity and protein

- Urine culture

—Usually not necessary if no symptoms

Imaging

- Rarely necessary in primary enuresis
- Only if suggestion of anatomic or functional abnormality of GU system
- Consider renal ultrasound, voiding cystourethrogram, radionucleotide renal scan

Therapy

- Specific therapy to address specific anatomic, infectious, or functional renal problems
- If the problem is affecting only the parents and the child is not affected, the treatment should be education and support for the parents

—Prognosis for self resolution
—Benign nature
—Available interventions if child becomes concerned

- Avoid all negative interventions
- Fluid restriction before bed—controversial

—May create arguments with parents
—Success rate low

- Retention training, bladder stretching exercises—controversial
- Cognitive behavioral interventions
  —Formal programs developed and used by pediatric psychologists
    —High rate of success
    —Involve frequent practice and rewards for voiding procedures
  —Positive reinforcement for dry nights
  —Use of praise, stickers, token economies

- Bell and pad alarm systems

—Most effective of behavioral interventions
—More effective in conjunction with formal behavioral program
—High relapse rate after remission and cessation of alarm usage
—Second remission very frequent with reintroduction of alarm system
—Second relapse rare
—Hypnotism
—Appears to work by increasing subconscious awareness of bladder pressure during sleep allowing increased awareness during sleep of intravesicular pressure

—Use of bell and pad alarm may increase success rate

- Avoid medication intervention before age 6–8 years

- Medication

—Desmopressin (DDAVP)
—Can be used intermittently only on sleep out nights
—Effective in 70% of primary nocturnal enuresis (PNE)
—If used chronically must monitor electrolytes and fluid status appropriately
—Available in nasal spray and tablets
—Imipramine

- Tricyclic antidepressant

—80% effective
—No longer 1st or 2nd line choice for benign condition due to risk of QTc prolongation and controversial risk of sudden cardiac death, risk of ingestion in siblings
—Oxybutynin
    —Used in patients with documented detrusser instability

Follow-Up

- Prognosis for resolution is 99% without treatment
- Spontaneous resolution is approximately 15% per year after age 5

PITFALLS

- Decision to treat is a balance of the effect on the child of nontreatment (social, emotional) with the potential side-effects of medication
- Laboratory evaluation rarely yields specific diagnosis. Balance risks and costs with unlikelihood of yield. Evaluation should generally involve no more than urinalysis.

Common Questions and Answers

Q: Do the medications cure the enuresis?
A: None of the medications cure the problem. DDAVP increases reabsorption of water in the kidney resulting in decreased bladder volumes. Tricyclic antidepressants cause urinary retention by the noradrenergic effects on bladder contraction and detrusser relaxation. Oxybutynin decreases detrusser irritability resulting in larger bladder capacity before emptying. The medications result in nonemptying of the bladder during sleep, but has not affected the underlying cause. Any resolution that occurs after cessation of medication treatment is probably from the natural resolution of the problem with age

Q: Isn't it important to cure the enuresis when the parents bring it up as a problem?
A: Developmental resolution of nocturnal enuresis occurs at a range of ages and in almost all cases resolves spontaneously. The most important historical point is who does this problem affect. If the child is not affected by the enuresis and it is only the parents who desire a cure, the important intervention is to educate them on the natural history of the problem, and to let them know about the available interventions and their success rates for when the child desires a cure.

Q: Are there any other interventions available only on sleep out nights?
A: One helpful tip is to allow the child to take a sleeping bag on sleep outs. Inside the sleeping bag is a pull-up. When the child gets into the sleeping bag he or she can change into the pull-up without anyone knowing. In the morning he or she puts his underwear back on leaving the damp pull up in the sleeping bag. His/her parent can take it out when he or she gets home.

ICD-9-CM 788.30

BIBLIOGRAPHY

Bosson S, Lyth N. Nocturnal enuresis. *Clinical Evidence* 2002;(7):341–348.

Butler RJ. The body-worn alarm in the treatment of childhood enuresis. *Br J Clin Pract* 1990;44:237–241.

Devlin JB. Predicting treatment outcome in nocturnal enuresis. *Arch Dis Child* 1990;65:1158–1161.

Essen J. Nocturnal enuresis in childhood. *Dev Med Child Neurol* 1976;18:577–589.

Forsythe WI. Enuresis and spontaneous cure rate: Study of 1129 enuretics. *Arch Dis Child* 1974;49:259–263.

Glazener CM, et al. Tricyclic and related drugs for nocturnal enuresis in children. *Cochrane Database of Systematic Reviews* 2003;(3): CD002117.

Jalkut MW. Enuresis. *Ped Clin NA* 2001;48:6:1461–1488.

Meadow R. Childhood enuresis. *BMJ* 1970;4:787–789.

Moffatt ME. Desmopressin acetate and nocturnal enuresis: How much do we know. *Pediatrics* 1993;92:420–425.

Starfield B. Increase in functional bladder capacity and improvements in enuresis. *J Pediatr* 1968;72:483–487.

Wille S. Comparison of Desmopressin and enuresis alarm for nocturnal enuresis. *Arch Dis Child* 1986;61:30–33.

Author: Eugene R. Hershorin

Epiglottitis

 Database

DEFINITION

Epiglottitis is an acute, life-threatening bacterial infection consisting of cellulitis and edema of the epiglottis, aryepiglottic folds, arytenoids and hypopharynx, resulting in narrowing of the glottic opening.

CAUSES AND PATHOPHYSIOLOGY

• Etiologic agents include: *Haemophilus influenzae,* nontypable and type B (accounted for >90% of cases prior to the introduction of HiB vaccine), *Staphylococcus aureus, Streptococcus pneumoniae, Streptococcus pyogenes* (group A β-hemolytic streptococcus), and group C and G β-hemolytic streptococcus (rare). *Candida albicans* may be an etiologic agent in immunocompromised patients. *Pasteurella multocida* has been implicated in a few cases after exposure to nasopharyngeal secretions from a cat. There have been recent reports of epiglottitis due to *Neisseria meningitidis.*
• The inhaled anesthetic, sevoflurane, has been implicated in a few cases of epiglottitis.
• Erythema and edema of the uvula, aryepiglottic folds, arytenoids, epiglottis, and vocal cords include an exudate rich in neutrophils and fibrin, which usually proceed to organization and fibrous scarring.

EPIDEMIOLOGY

• Disease due to *H. influenzae* type B occurs most often between the ages of 2 and 7 years (overall range: infancy to adulthood).
• Epiglottitis and other invasive disease secondary to *H. influenzae* have been reduced by 98% since the introduction of the conjugate vaccines in 1989 (approved at 15 months) and 1990 (approved at 2, 4, and 6 months).
• Nontypable *H. influenzae* now appears to be a more common cause of invasive disease than type B.
• Incidence of epiglottitis due to any organism has declined substantially (e.g., 20.9/100,000 per year to 0.9/100,000 per year from 1987 to 1996 in Sweden)
• Year-round occurrence
• Affects males and females equally
• All geographic areas
• Rare in populations in which the peak incidence of meningitis is shifted toward infancy (i.e., Alaskan Eskimos, Native Americans)
• Occasional secondary cases in households or daycare centers
• May be more frequent in children with sickle cell anemia, asplenia, immunoglobulin defects, or hematologic malignancies (e.g., leukemia)
• Disease due to *S. pyogenes* occurs most often in early school-age children during the winter and early spring, and has now been seen as a complication of varicella infection.

COMPLICATIONS

• Without prompt medical intervention, complete airway obstruction leading to respiratory arrest, hypoxia, and death
• Necrotizing cervical fasciitis (rarely)
• Therapeutic complications include: Aspiration, endotracheal tube dislodgment and extubation, tracheal erosion or irritation, pneumomediastinum, pneumothorax, and pulmonary edema.
• Complications of *H. influenzae* type B bacteremia include: Septic shock, pneumonia, cervical lymphadenopathy, and, rarely, arthritis and pericarditis.

PROGNOSIS

• Mortality is estimated to be 8% in hospital series.
• Virtually all cases in which arrest occurred prior to transfer to tertiary center resulted in fatality.

 Differential Diagnosis

• Viral laryngotracheobronchitis (croup) with or without secondary bacterial tracheitis
• Severe parainfluenza or influenza infection
• Uvulitis
• Peritonsillar, retropharyngeal or lingual abscess
• Foreign-body aspiration in a child with an upper respiratory infection
• Upper respiratory infection, including croup, in a child with a congenital or acquired airway problem (e.g., premature infant with subglottic stenosis, laryngeal web, vascular ring, tracheal stenosis)
• Diphtheria: Rare in the United States
• Laryngeal infections, including laryngeal tuberculosis

 Data Gathering

HISTORY

• Abrupt onset of high fever (39°C to 40°C), sore throat, and dysphagia
• Very limited or no prodrome of mild upper respiratory illness
• Rapid onset of toxicity and respiratory distress
• Cough and hoarseness are late symptoms, if they occur at all.
• Time from onset of symptoms to presentation with progressive respiratory distress is generally less than 12 hours.
• Has the child been immunized against *H. influenzae* type B?
• How does the child prefer to sit or position him or herself? (i.e., sitting upright, leaning forward with chin hyperextended)
• Exposure to cats

 Physical Examination

• Extremely anxious appearance
• Child prefers to remain sitting up.
• Child often leaning forward with chin hyperextended to maintain airway
• Slow and labored respiratory effort
• Drooling is seen as a manifestation of dysphagia.
• Inspiratory stridor, retractions, and late cyanosis
• Diagnosis can be suspected on history and observation of child's appearance alone.
• Do *not* attempt to examine the throat if epiglottitis is a serious consideration.

 Laboratory Aids

TESTS

• Complete blood count (CBC): Increased white blood cell count with left shift
• Cultures of blood (positive in up to 90%) and epiglottis (only performed in the operating room): May be positive for the causative organism.

RADIOGRAPHIC STUDIES

• Lateral neck radiograph: showing characteristic "thumb sign" of edematous epiglottis, with narrowing of the posterior airway and ballooning of the hypopharynx (should not be performed until "airway team" is in place)

 Therapy

• Airway management: Maintain child upright, *never supine*. Personnel experienced in airway management should accompany the child at all times, including during transport and in radiology.
• Rapid assembly of a team, which should include an anesthesiologist, an otolaryngologist, and a pediatrician, if possible.
• Allow the child to assume his or her most comfortable position (usually in the mother's arms/lap).
• Oxygen by mask or blown by face
• Transport to operating room as soon as possible for anesthesia and intubation, followed by positive pressure ventilation as necessary.
• Institute intravenous catheterization and blood collection, and culturing of epiglottis only after the airway is secured.
• Perform emergent cricothyrotomy if obstruction occurs prior to controlled airway management.
• Use fluid resuscitation in cases of septic shock.

DRUGS

- Empiric antibiotic coverage to include gram-positive cocci and β-lactamase-producing *H. influenzae* type B. Duration of therapy: 7 to 10 days for all but staphylococcal disease (14 to 21 days). Switch may be made to oral medication after extubation and resumption of feeding.
- Cefuroxime: 150 mg/kg per day divided every 8 hours
- Ampicillin/sulbactam: 200 mg/kg per day divided every 6 hours
- Chloramphenicol: 75 to 100 mg/kg per day divided every 6 hours
- Ampicillin: 100 to 200 mg/kg per day divided every 6 hours for non-β-lactamase-producing *H. influenzae* type B (approximately 80% of isolates)
- Penicillin: 100,000 to 200,000 U/kg per day divided every 4 to 6 hours for streptococcal disease
- Oxacillin: 100 to 200 mg/kg per day for staphylococcal disease

 Follow-Up

- Extubation is usually possible within 24 to 48 hours. Criteria include: Decreased erythema and edema of the epiglottis upon direct inspection, and development of an air leak around the endotracheal tube.
- Defervescence is usually prompt after initiation of appropriate antimicrobial therapy.

PREVENTION

- Rifampin: 20 mg/kg per day in a single dose for 4 days to eradicate *H. influenzae* type B colonization (see *Control Measures*)
- Universal immunization with *H. influenzae* type B capsular polysaccharide, conjugate vaccines at 2, 4, and 6 months, with booster at 12 to 18 months

ISOLATION OF HOSPITALIZED PATIENT

Droplet precautions should be continued for at least 24 hours from the initiation of effective therapy.

CONTROL MEASURES

- Prophylaxis for *H. influenzae* type B index case and susceptible children in household, child care setting, and intimate contacts

PITFALLS

- A radiograph is indicated only when the diagnosis is in doubt, and should not delay airway management.
- Blood collection should be avoided until the airway has been secured, so as not to upset the child unnecessarily.
- Failure to ensure appropriate airway management prior to any other interventions, including laryngeal examination, radiographs, and laboratory studies

 Common Questions and Answers

Q: What is the incidence of epiglottitis since the introduction of conjugate vaccines against *H. influenzae* type B?
A: Because *H. influenzae* type B caused 90% of epiglottitis, and the incidence of all invasive disease due to *H. influenzae* type B has decreased by 98% in children under 5 years of age, it is estimated that the incidence of epiglottitis has been reduced by almost 90%.

Q: Have there been reports of epiglottitis caused by *H. influenzae* type B after complete vaccination?
A: Yes, several cases due to *H. influenzae* type B have been reported in the US and abroad after partial and complete vaccination. Therefore, even a history of having received a full vaccination series does not eliminate the possibility of HiB-associated epiglottitis.

Q: How many cases of invasive disease due to *H. influenzae* type B occur in children with inadequate vaccination?
A: During 1994 and 1995, 47% of children under 4 years of age were too young (aged 5 months or younger) to have completed a primary series for HiB vaccine. Among children old enough to have been fully vaccinated, 63% of those developing disease were undervaccinated, and the remainder (37%) had completed a primary series in which vaccine failed. In a recent report from Australia 34/412 (8%) cases of invasive HiB disease (including epiglottitis) were reported as vaccine failures. Therefore, HiB cannot be ruled out as a cause of epiglottitis in a fully vaccinated child although the overwhelming majority of cases occur in unvaccinated children.

Q: Should a fully vaccinated child who develops invasive disease due to H. influenzae type B be tested for an underlying immunodeficiency?
A: Probably. In one study, about one-third of children diagnosed with invasive disease due to *H. influenzae* type B were found to have a previously undiagnosed immunoglobulin deficiency.

Q: Can epiglottitis recur?
A: Yes, but rarely.

Q: Are corticosteroids of any value in the management of epiglottitis?
A: There appears to be no benefit.

ICD-9-CM 464.30

BIBLIOGRAPHY

American Academy of Pediatrics. *Haemophilus influenzae* infections. In: Pickering LK, ed. *Red Book 2003: Report of the Committee on Infectious Diseases,* 26th Ed. Elk Grove, IL: American Academy of Pediatrics, 293–301.

Garpenholt O, et al. Epiglottitis in Sweden before and after introduction of vaccination against *Haemophilus influenzae* type B. *Pediatr Infect Dis J* 1999;18:490–493.

Grodin M. Epiglottitis. *J Emerg Med* 1983;1:13–19.

Heath PT, et al. Non-type b *Haemophilus influenzae* disease: clinical and epidemiologic characteristics in the *Haemophilus influenzae* type b vaccine era. *Pediatr Infect Dis J* 2001;20:300–305.

Hickerson SL, Kirby RS, Wheeler JG, et al. Epiglottitis: a 9-year case review. *South Med J* 1996;89:487–490.

Midwinter KI, Hodgson D, Yardley M, et al. Paediatric epiglottitis: the influence of the *Haemophilus influenzae* B vaccine, a ten-year review in the Sheffield region. *Clin Otolaryngol & Allied Sci* 1999;24:447–448.

Stroud RH, Friedman NR. An update on inflammatory disorders of the pediatric airway: epiglottitis, croup, and tracheitis. *Am J Otolaryngol* 2001;22(4):268–275.

Wenger JK. Supraglottitis and Group A Streptococcus. *Pediatr Infect Dis J* 1997;16:1005–1007.

Author: Mark L. Bagarazzi

Epstein-Barr Virus (Infectious Mononucleosis)

 Database

DEFINITION

Epstein-Barr virus (EBV) is a double-stranded DNA virus, and was implicated as the causative agent for infectious mononucleosis by 1968.

PATHOPHYSIOLOGY

- EBV replicates initially in the oropharyngeal epithelium.
- Selective infection of B lymphocytes occurs.
- The clinical syndrome of infectious mononucleosis results from proliferation of cells in the tonsils, lymph nodes, and spleen.
- Nonspecific humoral immune responses include the formation of heterophile antibodies and autoantibodies.
- Specific antibodies to EBV antigens are produced.
- Despite humoral responses, cellular immunity is responsible for controlling EBV infection.
- Latent, lifelong infection of B lymphocytes occurs.
- Latent virus can be reactivated during periods of immunosuppression.

EPIDEMIOLOGY

- Worldwide distribution
- Humans are the only known reservoir.
- EBV spreads between individuals in saliva, and occasionally via blood transfusions.
- The incubation period is 30 to 50 days.
- Antibodies to EBV are almost universally present in adult populations.
- Populations with a high population density or low socioeconomic status usually become primarily affected within the first 3 years of life.
- In developed countries, acquisition of EBV is biphasic

—The initial peak in incidence occurs before the age of 5 years.
—The second peak occurs during adolescence, coinciding with an increased frequency of intimate oral contacts.

COMPLICATIONS

- Dehydration

—Severe pharyngitis often limits fluid intake.
—Is the most common problem requiring hospitalization

- Streptococcal pharyngitis

—Between 5% and 25% of patients with acute EBV infection may have concomitant group A streptococcal pharyngitis.

- Antibiotic-induced rash

—Morbilliform in appearance
—Most common after administration of ampicillin or amoxicillin
—Rare association with penicillin
—Usually benign, resolves with discontinuation of the aminopenicillin

- Splenic rupture

—Incidence of approximately 1 in 1,000 patients
—More common in males
—Half of the cases of splenic rupture are spontaneous; half follow blunt trauma.

- Airway obstruction

—May result from massive lymphoid hyperplasia and mucosal edema

PROGNOSIS

- Most patients with primary EBV infection will recover uneventfully in 1 to 4 weeks.
- Long-lasting immunity generally ensues.
- Prognosis of patients with unusual manifestations of EBV infection depends on the severity of the illness and the organ system involved.
- Patients with inherited or acquired immunodeficiency are at higher risk of complications and neoplasms.

ASSOCIATED ILLNESSES

- Subclinical infection

—The majority of EBV infections in children, and even in adolescents, are clinically inapparent.
—Mild, nonspecific symptoms may include coryza, diarrhea, and/or fever.
—Immunologic seroconversion does occur.

- Infectious mononucleosis ("glandular fever")

—Most commonly observed with late primary acquisition of EBV
—The classically defined illness is characterized by:
—Fatigue
—Malaise
—Fever
—Tonsillopharyngitis (often exudative)
—Lymphadenopathy
—Splenomegaly
—Usually associated with increased numbers of atypical lymphocytes in the peripheral blood

- Rare illnesses of the nervous system have been reported:

—Guillain-Barré syndrome
—Bell's palsy
—Aseptic meningitis
—Meningoencephalitis
—Peripheral and/or optic neuritis

- Hematologic disorders have been reported in rare association with EBV:

—Aplastic anemia
—Hemolytic anemia
—Hemolytic-uremic syndrome

- Other illnesses associated with EBV in case reports:

—Hepatitis
—Pancreatitis
—Myocarditis
—Mesenteric adenitis
—Orchitis
—Genital ulcerative disease

- Congenital infection

—Primary EBV infection during pregnancy is uncommon.
—Although rare, TORCH-like congenital defects may conceivably be linked to EBV.

- Lymphoproliferative disorders

—EBV is suspected of occasionally playing a role in the etiology of the lymphoproliferative disorders:
—Burkitt lymphoma
—Nasopharyngeal carcinoma
—Lymphoma and non-Hodgkin lymphoma (in immunocompromised children)
—Virus-associated hemophagocytic syndrome
—Lymphomatoid granulomatosis
—Posttransplant lymphoproliferative disorders (PTLD)

- Chronic fatigue syndrome

—EBV, as well as many other infectious and environmental agents, have been proposed to contribute to this vague clinical syndrome.

 Differential Diagnosis

- Infectious mononucleosis is an illness with characteristic clinical features caused by EBV. Other causes of the infectious mononucleosis syndrome include:

—Adenovirus
—Cytomegalovirus
—Human herpes virus-6
—Human immunodeficiency virus
—Rubella
—Toxoplasma gondii

 Data Gathering

HISTORY

- A prodrome may occur:

—Commonly lasts 2 to 5 days
—Malaise, fatigue, ± fever

- In the acute phase the following features are common:

—Fever—begins abruptly and lasts 1 to 2 weeks
—Fatigue
—Malaise
—Anorexia
—Sore throat

"Swollen glands"

- Young children are more likely to have a rash or abdominal pain.

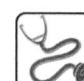 Physical Examination

- Tonsillopharyngitis

—May be exudative and mimic streptococcal pharyngitis
—Often accompanied by palatal petechiae

- Lymphadenopathy

—Occurs in 90%
—Most prominent in cervical chains
—May be diffuse
—Usually nontender, nonerythematous, and discrete

- Hepatosplenomegaly

—Splenomegaly occurs in over half of cases.
—Even if not palpable, splenomegaly may be demonstrated on ultrasound.
—Most prominent in second to fourth week of illness
—Hepatomegaly is less common

 Laboratory Aids

TESTS

- CBC with differential

—Leukocyte count up to 20,000/mm^3
—Lymphocytosis
—Atypical lymphocytes often comprise more than 10% of total leukocyte count.
—Thrombocytopenia may occur.

- Liver enzymes

—Mild hepatitis often is found.
—Jaundice is rare.

- "Monospot" (mononucleosis rapid slide agglutination test for heterophile antibodies)

—Detects heterophile antibodies (nonspecific IgM antibodies to unrelated antigens)
—Often negative in children less than 4 years of age
—Detects 90% of cases in adolescents and adults

- EBV serology

—Typically reserved for heterophile-negative patients or children less than 4 years of age where strong clinical suspicion persists
—Antibodies detected by indirect immunofluorescence or ELISA techniques
—Acute or past infection can usually be detected and differentiated.

- Other technology

—Tissue culture of EBV is difficult and therefore not clinically useful.
—Polymerase chain reaction (PCR) may detect EBV genetic material.
—Real-time PCR may quantify the amount of EBV genome present. This is useful in patients with PTLD.

False Positives

- CBC

—Atypical lymphocyte counts greater than 10% of the total leukocyte count also occur with cytomegalovirus and toxoplasmosis infections.

- Monospot

—False-positive tests are infrequent.
—Heterophile antibodies are also produced in serum sickness and neoplastic processes.
—Heterophile antibodies may persist for months after acute infection and be indicative of past illness.

PITFALLS

- Heterophile antibodies may not appear early in the illness.
- Up to 10% of patients with acute EBV infection may have no heterophile response 3 weeks into the illness.
- The heterophile response is less common in infants and children and should not be used in children less than 4 years of age.

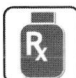 Therapy

- Supportive care and symptomatic treatment will be sufficient for most cases of primary EBV infection.
- Acetaminophen or ibuprofen will reduce fever and provide analgesia.
- Oral, and sometimes IV, rehydration is often indicated.
- Corticosteroids (prednisone, 1 mg/kg per day divided into two doses) may reduce swelling of lymphoid tissues (see Common Questions and Answers)

—Indicated for patients with impending airway obstruction
—May be considered for patients with severe tonsillopharyngitis requiring IV hydration
—May be considered for patients with rare, life-threatening manifestations of EBV infection, such as hepatitis, aplastic anemia, and CNS dysfunction

- Acyclovir has not been shown to provide clinical benefit.
- Patients with PTLD should have immunosuppression reduced.

PREVENTION

- No vaccine is clinically available.
- Hospitalized patients need not be isolated when rigorous hand washing is employed.
- Restriction of intimate contact with immunosuppressed individuals may be advisable.
- Patients with recent EBV infection, either proven or suspected, should not donate blood.

 Follow-Up

- Immunocompetent individuals usually recover uneventfully in 1 to 4 weeks.
- Recovery is often biphasic, with a worsening of symptoms after a period of improvement.
- Splenomegaly may persist for weeks after primary infection (see Common Questions and Answers).
- Fatigue may persist months after recovery.

 Common Questions and Answers

Q: Should all patients with infectious mononucleosis be given corticosteroids?
A: Even though children may feel tired, weak, and ill, symptomatic EBV infection is most often self-limited and requires only symptomatic care. Long-term effects from the use of steroids to treat EBV are not known. EBV has been linked to certain lymphoproliferative disorders, and theoretical risks to modulating the host immune response with corticosteroids have been proposed.

Q: How long after infectious mononucleosis may a patient return to athletic activity?
A: Over half of patients with "mono" will have a boggy, enlarged spleen. This enlarged spleen is prone to rupture even if it is not palpable. All athletic activity should be restricted until no evidence exists for a clinically enlarged or tender spleen. If this criterion is met, and the patient feels subjectively better, light (noncontact) activities may be resumed. Return to contact sports is not advised until at least 4 to 6 weeks after resolution of all signs and symptoms of illness. Some experts recommend ultrasound study of the spleen before a return to heavy contact sports such as rugby, football, lacrosse, and hockey.

ICD-9-CM 075

BIBLIOGRAPHY

Hickey SM, Strasburger VC. What every pediatrician should know about infectious mononucleosis and adolescents. *Pediatr Clin North Am* 1997;44:1541–1556.

Jenson HB. Acute complications of Epstein-Barr virus infectious mononucleosis. *Curr Opin Pediatr* 2000;12:263–268.

Leach CT, Sumaya CV. Epstein-Barr Virus. In: Feigin RD, et al, eds. *Textbook of Pediatric Infectious Diseases.* 4th Ed. Philadelphia: WB Saunders, 2004:1932–1956.

Macsween KF, Crawford DH. Epstein-Barr virus-recent advances. *The Lancet Infect Dis* 2003;3(3):131–140.

Okano M. Overview and problematic standpoints of severe chronic active Epstein-Barr virus infection syndrome. *Crit Rev Oncol-Hematol* 2002;44(3):273–278.

Peter J, Ray CG. Infectious mononucleosis. *Pediatr Rev* 1998;19:276–279.

Sullivan KE. DiGeorge syndrome/chromosome 22q11.2 deletion syndrome. *Curr Allergy & Asthma Rep* 2001;1(5):438–444.

Authors: Jason Newland and Kevin C. Osterhoudt

Erythema Multiforme

 Database

DEFINITION

Erythema multiforme (EM) is an acute self-limited cutaneous eruption with many different or multiform lesions. It is characterized classically as a target or iris lesion, but can appear as erythematous macules, papules, vesicles, and bullae with mucosal involvement. There are many triggers of EM, which is thought to encompass a spectrum of disease from relatively mild disease (EM minor) to severe forms with more than one mucosal surface involved (EM major or Stevens-Johnson syndrome). Some authors include toxic epidermal necrolysis (TEN) as the most severe form of EM, characterized by widespread erythema, bullae, and sloughing of large sheets of skin, with significant morbidity and mortality. However, some debate exists as to whether classic EM minor may represent an entity altogether separate from Stevens-Johnson and toxic epidermal necrolysis.

CAUSES

- The major causes of EM, which is thought to be an immune-mediated reaction, include drugs such as sulfa, penicillin, and phenytoin, and infections such as herpes simplex virus and Mycoplasma.
- There are a host of other etiologic factors, including exposure to various chemicals and tumors. The eruption usually occurs 1 to 2 weeks after the initial exposure.
- Often the causative factor is not identified.
- Recurrent EM is generally secondary to herpes simplex virus.
- EM major is commnly associated with drugs, it can be seen in mycoplasma infection

GENETICS

Although simultaneous cases in family members have been reported, the disease is not genetic.

PATHOLOGY

The pathologic findings vary according to the lesion examined. Biopsy reveals necrosis of keratinocytes to varying degrees, depending on the clinical lesion biopsied. There is moderate-to-severe papillary dermal edema with mild-to-moderate perivascular dermal infiltrate composed predominantly of mononuclear cells and also some eosinophils (particularly if drug-related). Subepidermal blistering may be seen. Extravasated blood cells are found, but there is no evidence of vasculitis. Hydropic degeneration of the basement membrane also can be seen, as can epidermal spongiosis.

EPIDEMIOLOGY

- Erythema multiforme is seen in approximately 1% of all dermatology patients and has an equal incidence in men and women. (Some studies suggest a slightly higher incidence of EM minor in women.)
- The disease occurs predominantly in young adults and is believed by some to occur more frequently in spring and summer, with the more severe form of EM major occurring in the winter.

COMPLICATIONS

- Erythema multiforme minor is generally self-limited, with rare complications.
- In EM major, mucosal involvement can lead to stricture formation of the urethra, trachea, and esophagus, as well as conjunctivitis, corneal erosions, and, rarely, blindness.
- Pneumonitis, nephritis, hepatitis, and infection are other reported complications.
- In TEN, mortality and morbidity are high, with death occurring from sepsis.

 Differential Diagnosis

Classic presentation with targetoid lesions and mucosal involvement is generally not a diagnostic challenge; however, given the many forms of presentation, the diagnosis of EM can be difficult. The differential diagnosis can be extensive, depending on the presentation, and includes:

- Viral exanthem
- Bullous impetigo
- Staphylococcal scalded-skin syndrome
- Bullous pemphigoid
- Urticaria
- Urticarial vasculitis
- Systemic lupus erythematosus
- Serum sickness
- Pemphigus vulgaris
- Secondary syphilis
- Chickenpox
- Rocky Mountain spotted fever
- Acute neutrophilic dermatosis
- Lyme disease
- Fixed drug eruption

 Data Gathering

HISTORY

The cutaneous findings are sometimes preceded by a prodrome with fever and malaise. A careful drug and exposure history, as well as any signs or symptoms of infection or herpetic lesions, may reveal the etiologic cause. Inquire in detail about the patient's drug history, over-the-counter preparations, and signs or symptoms of infection or herpetic lesions.

Physical Examination

- Erythema multiforme classically appears as target lesions characterized by a dark, dusky center surrounded by a pale zone and then a zone of erythema. The lesions are typically acrally distributed.
- The lesions occur in many forms and can appear as red macules, papules, urticarial lesions, or vesicles and bullae.
- Oral involvement is typically seen. Mucosal involvement with superficial denudation can also occur in the eyes, nasopharyngeal mucosal, or anogenital region.

 ## Laboratory Aids

TESTS

- There are no diagnostic laboratory tests; however, biopsy is often helpful, and other tests may help identify a cause.
- A WBC count with differential, looking for eosinophilia, may help identify a drug as causative.
- Cultures to evaluate for herpes or chest x-ray studies to evaluate for pneumonia or infectious cause of EM
- Cold agglutinins associated with Mycoplasma
- Antistreptolysin-O titers and leukocytosis may identify a particular infectious cause.
- ESR may be elevated, but is nonspecific.

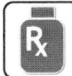 ## Therapy

MILD FORMS

- Mild forms of EM resolve spontaneously without scarring and require only supportive therapy, including antihistamine or topical steroid for pruritus associated with the lesions.
- Oral lesions are often painful, and oral preparations to swish and spit, made of diphenhydramine or viscous lidocaine, may provide relief.
- Treatment of the underlying process is helpful (e.g., acyclovir for herpes simplex virus-associated cases).

ERYTHEMA MULTIFORME MAJOR

- May be life-threatening and can require hospitalization
- Supportive care, ophthalmology consultation, monitoring of fluid and electrolyte balance, and vigilant observation for infection are necessary.
- Antibiotics, analgesics, and local care including compresses with acetic acid soaks or saline will help decrease the incidence of infection.
- The use of systemic steroids is controversial, but when helpful, they are given early in the course of disease for approximately 2 weeks when there is no contraindication, such as infection.

TOXIC EPIDERMAL NECROLYSIS

- High associated mortality is often secondary to infection.
- Care is ideally at a burn center, with careful attention to infection and to fluids and electrolytes.
- Antibiotics, local compresses with acetic acid, or saline can help prevent superinfection.
- The use of systemic steroids is controversial, and is most effective when started early. The benefits and risks, including infection, must be weighed.
- Some recent reports demonstrated that 0.5–1 gm/kg/day IVIG given over 3 to 5 days provided rapid improvement with little to no adverse effects in adult patients with toxic epidermal necrolysis.

 ## Follow-Up

- Mild forms of EM are acute and self-limited, with lesions resolving in 2 to 4 weeks, with postinflammatory hyperpigmentation or hypopigmentation.
- Sequelae due to mucosal scarring can occur.
- Severe forms of EM major or TEN have associated morbidity and mortality.
- When recurrent, EM is often associated with herpes simplex virus.

ICD-9-CM 695.1

BIBLIOGRAPHY

Ayangco L, Rogers RS, III. Oral manifestations of erythema multiforme. *Dermatol Clin* 2003;21(1):195–205.

Duvic M. Erythema multiforme. *Dermatol Clin* 1983;1(2):493–496.

Huff JC, Weston WL, Tonnessen MG. Erythema multiforme: a critical review of characteristics, diagnostic criteria and causes. *J Am Acad Dermatol* 1983;8(6):763–775.

Lever WF, Schaumberg-Lever G. *Histopathology of the Skin.* 7th Ed. Philadelphia: Lippincott, 1990.

Metry DW, et al. Use of intravenous immunoglobulin in children with stevens-johnson syndrome and toxic epidermal necrolysis: seven cases and review of the literature. *Pediatrics* 2003;112(6 Pt 1): 1430–1436.

Weston WL, Badgett JT. Urticaria. *Pediatr Rev* 1998;19(7):240–244.

Author: Albert C. Yan

Erythema Nodosum

 ## Database

DEFINITION

Erythema nodosum is a delayed, cell-mediated hypersensitivity syndrome characterized by red, tender, nodular lesions that are usually on the pretibial surface of the legs and occasionally on other areas of the skin where subcutaneous fat is present.

CAUSES

- Thought to be a result of a host hypersensitivity immune response to circulating immune complexes secondary to infectious and/or inflammatory stimuli, which then results in chronic injury to the blood vessels of the reticular dermis and subcutaneous fat
- There are many associated triggering/underlying diseases:

—In children
  —Streptococcal infection and tubercular infection are the most common causes.
—In older patients
  —*Streptococcus* and sarcoidosis are most common.
  —Drugs (oral contraceptives, sulfonamides, iodides/bromides, phenytoin)
  —Infection (streptococcal infection, tuberculosis, psittacosis, histoplasmosis, yersiniosis, lymphogranuloma venereum, cat-scratch disease, coccidioidomycosis, upper respiratory infection)

- Systemic (sarcoidosis, inflammatory bowel disease, Hodgkin disease, Behçet disease)
- Pregnancy

PATHOLOGY

- Septal panniculitis: Lymphocytic perivascular infiltrate in the dermis; lymphocytes and neutrophils in the fibrous septa in the subcutaneous fat
- In older lesions, histiocytes, giant cells, and occasionally plasma cells are seen.
- No fat-cell destruction or vasculitis is present.

EPIDEMIOLOGY

- Girls are affected more often than boys.
- Most cases seen in the third decade, but not uncommon after age 10
- Greatest seasonal incidence in spring and fall

 ## Differential Diagnosis

- Infection

—Erysipelas/cellulitis
—Superficial or deep thrombophlebitis
—Erythema induratum (nodular vasculitis)
—Deep fungal infection
—Angiitis

- Environmental (poisons)
- Tumors
- Trauma: Accidental trauma or child abuse
- Bruise
- Palmoplantar hidradenitis
- Metabolic

—Panniculitis secondary to pancreatic disease
—Congenital

- Immunologic

—Major insect bite reaction
—Psychosocial

- Sarcoidosis
- Polyarteritis nodosa
- Granuloma annulare
- Miscellaneous
- Weber-Christian (thighs and trunk) lesions may suppurate and heal with atrophy/localized depression.

PROGNOSIS

- Most individual lesions will completely resolve in 10 to 14 days.
- In general, erythema nodosum resolves in 3 to 6 weeks with or without treatment, unless the underlying cause is a chronic infection or systemic disorder.
- Aching of legs and swelling of ankles may persist for weeks; rarely, symptoms may persist for up to 2 years.
- In children, the recurrence rate is 4% to 10% and is often associated with repeated streptococcal infection.

 ## Data Gathering

HISTORY

- In over 50% of patients, a history of arthralgia is noted 2 to 8 weeks prior.
- Prodromal symptoms of fatigue/malaise or upper respiratory infection precedes by 1 to 3 weeks.
- Patients often present with pain and tenderness of extremities, sometimes to the point of difficulty in ambulation.

 ## Physical Examination

- Red, often tender, nodules on anterior lower legs, 2 to 6 cm in diameter
- Overlying skin is normal except for erythema.
- Initially, lesions are bright to deep red with palpable warmth.
- Later, lesions develop a brownish red or violaceous, bruise-like appearance.
- Smaller lesions are slope-shouldered nodules.
- Larger lesions are flat-topped plaques.

SPECIAL QUESTIONS

- Medication history (oral contraceptives, sulfonamides, iodides/bromides)
- Last menses (erythema nodosum is seen in pregnancy)
- History of diarrhea (inflammatory bowel disease or infectious diarrhea)
- TB exposure

PHYSICAL EXAMINATION TRICKS

- Erythema nodosum never ulcerates or suppurates.
- Usually, there are fewer than six lesions at a time.
- As a rule, both legs are affected.

Erythema Nodosum

 Laboratory Aids

TESTS

- Throat culture
- Antistreptolysin-O titer
- PPD
- CBC
- ESR
- Stool culture, if history of diarrhea
- Serologic testing, if yersiniosis, histoplasmosis, or coccidioidomycosis suspected
- Chest x-ray study, if diagnosis is in doubt
- Excisional biopsy specimen for histopathology, bacterial and fungal cultures is helpful

False Positives

Bilateral hilar adenopathy may also be seen with sarcoidosis, coccidioidomycosis, histoplasmosis, TB, streptococcal infection, or lymphomatosis.

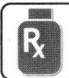 Therapy

- Identification and treatment of underlying cause
- Bed rest and leg elevation

DRUGS

- Salicylates or other NSAIDs, such as ibuprofen, naproxen or indomethacin
- Potassium iodide, 300 mg PO t.i.d. for 3 to 4 weeks, especially for cases diagnosed early in course
- Corticosteroids are effective, but rarely necessary.
- Duration: 2 to 4 weeks

 Follow-Up

WHEN TO EXPECT IMPROVEMENT

- Within 2 to 3 days
- Return visit in 1 week

SIGNS TO WATCH FOR

If lesions recur after cessation of treatment, underlying infection may worsen as well.

 Common Question and Answer

Q: Will the lesions leave a scar?
A: Erythema nodosum virtually always heals without scarring.

ICD-9-CM 695.2

BIBLIOGRAPHY

Gonzalez-Gay MA, et al. Erythema nodosum: a clinical approach. *Clin & Exper Rheumatol* 2001;19(4):365–368.

Hurwitz S. *Clinical Pediatric Dermatology: A Textbook of Skin Disorders of Childhood and Adolescence.* 2nd Ed. Philadelphia: WB Saunders, 1993.

Pettersson T. Sarcoid and erythema nodosum arthropathies. *Best Practice & Research in Clinical Rheumatology* 2000;14(3):461–476.

Author: Albert C. Yan

Ewing Sarcoma

 Database

DEFINITION

Ewing sarcoma is the second most common malignant bone tumor in children and adolescents. It represents a family of tumors, including Ewing sarcoma of bone, extraosseus Ewing sarcoma (arises in soft tissue adjacent to bone), and peripheral neuroectodermal tumor (PNET) of bone or soft tissue. The cause of Ewing sarcoma is unknown.

PATHOLOGY

- One of the "small round blue" cell tumors of childhood
- In approximately 90% of cases, the specific translocations t(11;22) and the minority t(21;22) can be detected by polymerase chain reaction methods. These translocations lead to the fusion of the EWS gene on chromosome 22 with genes that encode for transcription factors (FLI1 on chromosome 11, ERG on chromosome 21).
- Often a large soft tissue component is present.
- Necrosis and hemorrhage are common.
- The PNET variant has more neural differentiation.

GENETICS

- Majority of cases occur sporadically
- Not associated with familial cancer syndromes

EPIDEMIOLOGY

- Second most common malignant bone tumor of children and young adults
- Approximately 110 new cases are diagnosed in the United States each year.
- Sixty-four percent occur in the second decade of life.
- More common in males than in females
- Ninety-six percent of cases in Caucasian population; extremely rare in Asians and blacks
- Associations (rare): Skeletal anomalies (endochondroma, aneurysmal bone cyst), genitourinary anomalies (hypospadias, duplicated renal collecting system), Down syndrome, hereditary retinoblastoma

COMPLICATIONS

- Pathologic fracture
- Cord compression secondary to vertebral involvement
- Metastatic spread is seen in 20% at diagnosis. Sites include lung, bone, and bone marrow; liver and lymph nodes are less often involved.

PROGNOSIS

- Overall, 50% to 70% of patients will be disease-free at 5 years from diagnosis.
- Late metastases may occur so that survival rates decrease to 50% 10 years from diagnosis.
- Favorable prognostic features

—Localized disease
—Primary site: Distal bone, rib
—Tumor size less than 100 mL or 8 to 10 cm
—Age less than 10 years
—Histologic response to chemotherapy: no viable tumor at time of surgical resection
—Presence of the type 1 EWS-FLI1 gene fusion transcript

- Unfavorable prognostic features

—Metastatic disease at diagnosis, especially involving bone or bone marrow (<30% disease-free survival)
—Primary site: Pelvis
—Elevated LDH
—Presence of neural differentiation
—Presence of mutations in the tumor tissue of the tumor suppressor gene P53 or the cell proliferation nuclear antigen Ki-67

 Differential Diagnosis

- Malignant

—Osteosarcoma
—Neuroblastoma
—Non-Hodgkin lymphoma
—Rhabdomyosarcoma

- Nonmalignant

—Osteomyelitis
—Trauma/fracture
—Langerhans cell histiocytosis (eosinophilic granuloma)
—Benign bone tumor (giant-cell tumor) or cyst

 Data Gathering

HISTORY

- Presenting symptoms and their frequency of occurrence:

—Local pain (85%)
—Local swelling (60%)
—Fever (30%)
—Paraplegia, back pain (2%)

- Systemic symptoms (fever, weight loss) are more common among patients with metastatic disease
- Delay between first symptom and diagnosis is quite common; the duration of symptoms ranges from 4 weeks to 4 years, with an average of 9 months

 Physical Examination

- Can develop in any bone of the body, with equal involvement of flat and long bones (unlike osteosarcoma, which arises more commonly in long bones)
- Distribution of primary sites include the following:

—Extremities (53%): usually begins in the midshaft; lower extremities affected more than upper extremities
—Central axis (47%): Pelvis (45%), chest wall (34%), spine or paravertebral (12%), head or neck (9%)

- Extraskeletal Ewing sarcoma is rare; however, it can be found in the majority of soft tissue regions of the body

 Laboratory Aids

TESTS

Laboratory Tests

- CBC
- Serum LDH is often elevated at diagnosis
- Electrolytes, liver and renal function tests, serum calcium, phosphorus in anticipation of starting chemotherapy

Imaging and Other Tests

To evaluate primary site and confirm diagnosis:

- X-ray (bony destruction with "onion skin" appearance most often seen)
- CT scan or, preferably, MRI scan
- 99m-Tc-diphosphonate bone scan
- Biopsy: Biopsy should be performed by an experienced physician so as to avoid contamination of the tumor site or removal of insufficient tissue to make the diagnosis. In addition to routine morphologic and immunohistochemical stain assessments, analysis of tumor chromosomes by traditional cytogenetics, fluorescent in situ hybridization, or reverse transcriptase PCR is helpful in making the diagnosis and may provide information regarding prognosis. Because of the importance of these studies, consultation with a pediatric oncologist before the biopsy is strongly encouraged.

To evaluate for evidence of distant metastases (present in 20% of patients at diagnosis):

- Chest radiograph and CT scan
- 99m-Tc-diphosphonate bone scan
- Bilateral aspiration and biopsy of iliac bone marrow

Therapy

- Therapy is a multimodal approach based on location and extent of disease.

—Surgery
—Chemotherapy: Common agents used include vincristine, dactinomycin, cyclophosphamide, doxorubicin, etoposide, and ifosfamide. Other agents such as irinotecan are being investigated.
—Radiation therapy: Used in all patients except those with completely resected tumors.

- All patients with localized disease at diagnosis also have tumor cells outside the primary site that cannot be detected by standard measures; chemotherapy is therefore essential for cure.
- Duration of therapy depends on location and extent of disease.
- The surgical trend is toward less radical surgery, with limb preservation. Limb salvage surgery is the primary goal but the decision is based on the probability of obtaining a wide margin and the tumor response to chemotherapy.
- Most children are treated according to large cooperative group protocols at pediatric oncology centers.
- Treatment is characterized by significant side effects, including increased susceptibility to infection, severe mucositis, and poor nutritional status.
- Most patients require placement of an indwelling central venous catheter for the duration of their therapy.
- Experimental therapies such as high-dose chemotherapy with stem cell rescue, immunotherapy (vaccination with fusion-gene peptide products) and antiangiogenic therapies are being investigated in clinical trials for patients with high-risk or relapsed disease.

Follow-Up

WHEN TO EXPECT IMPROVEMENT

All patients with Ewing sarcoma require approximately 30 to 48 weeks of chemotherapy to prevent recurrence in the original site of tumor or distant spread. However, some improvement in signs and symptoms is usually seen within the first several weeks of therapy.

ACUTE EFFECTS OF THERAPY

Therapy for Ewing sarcoma is intensive. Patients can expect many of the following side effects:

- Frequent admissions to the hospital for chemotherapy or complications of the therapy
- Complications from bone marrow, suppressive effects of chemotherapy, or radiotherapy:

—Anemia: Blood transfusions are usually necessary; erythropoietin (a stimulator of erythropoiesis) may be given to reduce the number of transfusions required.
—Thrombocytopenia: Platelet transfusions are often necessary to reduce the risk of serious bleeding.
—Neutropenia: Increased risk of bacterial and fungal infections; G-CSF (granulocyte colony-stimulating factor) is usually administered daily following chemotherapy to shorten the duration of neutropenia.

- Complications from the gastrointestinal side effects of chemotherapy or radiotherapy:

—Nausea and vomiting; relieved with ondansetron and other antiemetic agents
—Malnutrition secondary to reduced appetite and mucosal ulcerations; nutritional supplements (oral, nasogastric, gastrostomy tube or parenteral) may be necessary.
—Complications from radiotherapy
—Skin erythema or breakdown
—Pathologic fracture or poor function

LATE EFFECTS OF THERAPY

Therapy for Ewing sarcoma is intensive, and is associated with significant long-term adverse effects. Regular follow-up with a pediatric oncologist is strongly recommended. These late effects of therapy include the following:

- Cardiomyopathy

—Anthracyclines (doxorubicin) weaken cardiac muscle, leading to reduced left ventricular function many years after therapy.
—Approximately 5% of patients receiving cumulative doses of doxorubicin greater than 500 mg/m^2 will develop congestive heart failure.
—Radiation to the heart can lower the cumulative dose threshold to 300 mg/m^2.
—Any patient who has received an anthracycline should be cautioned against initiating strenuous physical activity without adequate preparation.
—Pregnant women who have received anthracyclines in the past should inform their obstetrician so that appropriate cardiac assessment can be completed prior to vaginal delivery.

- Kidney and bladder damage

—Urinalysis should be performed to detect hemorrhagic cystitis or tubular damage with spilling of sugar, protein, and phosphate into the urine.
—Blood pressure should be monitored in patients who received irradiation to the kidneys; vascular damage and hypertension may develop many years after therapy.

- Infertility and delayed puberty

—Reduced or absent gonadal function is related to high doses of alkylating agents (cyclophosphamide, ifosfamide): males are at high risk of azoospermia; females may be fertile, but are at risk for premature menopause.
—Low-dose estrogen therapy with oral contraceptive medications may be necessary for amenorrheic women.

- Second malignant neoplasms

—Sarcomas may occur within the radiation field.
—Myelodysplastic syndromes and acute myeloid leukemia may occur secondary to chemotherapy (cyclophosphamide, ifosfamide, etoposide).

- Growth abnormalities/functional defects at the primary site

—Radiation doses greater than 20 Gy will cause growth retardation in prepubertal children.
—Scoliosis can occur if the vertebrae are involved in the radiation field.
—Risk for pathologic fractures or aseptic necrosis of joints remains elevated.

Common Questions and Answers

Q: At what time point is a child with Ewing sarcoma considered cured?
A: Typically, cure is measured as 5-year survival without evidence of disease. However, late relapses or second tumors do occur in children with Ewing sarcoma.

Q: Should a Ewing sarcoma be completely resected at the time of diagnosis?
A: Most times, this is not recommended, as Ewing sarcoma is very sensitive to chemotherapy, facilitating an improved delayed surgical resection.

ICD-9-CM 170.4

BIBLIOGRAPHY

Grier HE. The Ewing family of tumors: Ewing sarcoma and primitive neuroectodermal tumors. *Pediatr Clin North Am* 1997;44(4): 991–1004.

Kennedy JG, et al. Ewing sarcoma: current concepts in diagnosis and treatment. *Curr Opin Pediatr* 2003;15:53–57.

Rodriquez-Galindo C, et al. Treatment of Ewing sarcoma family of tumors: current status and outlook for the future. *Med Pediatr Oncol* 2003;40:276–287.

Author: Kara M. Kelly

Exstrophy of the Bladder

 Database

 Physical Examination

 Laboratory Aids

DEFINITION

Exstrophy of the bladder is an anomaly in which the open bladder is part of the anterior abdominal wall. Bladder exstrophy presents as part of a complex of anomalies including male and female epispadias and wide separation of the pubis symphysis. The most severe variant of this complex is cloacal exstrophy where there is a large omphalocele, split bladder, imperforate anus, shortened colon and multiple upper urinary tract and limb anomalies.

Embryology

• Normal development: The cloacal membrane is located at the caudal end of the infraumbilical abdominal wall by 2 weeks gestation. Mesenchyme from the primitive streak migrates between the layers of the cloacal membrane to reinforce the abdominal wall as the cloacal membrane regresses.
• Bladder exstrophy: Pathogenesis is still unclear but represents an error in embryogenesis. It is proposed that an abnormal overdevelopment of the cloacal membrane prevents medial migration of the mesenchymal tissue and normal lower abdominal wall development. Because the membrane lacks reinforcement, it ruptures. The timing of this rupture determines the variant of the exstrophy-epispadias complex. In bladder exstrophy, rupture of the membrane occurs after the urorectal septum has descended.
• Cloacal exstrophy: Abnormally large cloacal membrane ruptures prior to division of the cloaca by the urorectum septum.

EPIDEMIOLOGY

• Incidence estimated between 1 in 10,000 to 1 in 50,000 live births.
• Male to female ratio for classic bladder exstrophy is between 2 and 4:1.
• Risk of second affected family member is 3.6%.
• Risk of bladder exstrophy in offspring of individuals with bladder exstrophy and epispadias is 1 in 70 births (500-fold greater than the general population).
• Cloacal exstrophy is exceedingly rare with an incidence of 1 in 200,000 births (incidence continues to decrease due to prenatal diagnosis and termination).

BLADDER EXSTROPHY

• All cases of exstrophy have widening of the symphysis pubis caused by outward rotation of the innominate bones.
• Triangular defect caused by premature rupture of the abnormal cloacal membrane is occupied by the exstrophied bladder and posterior urethra and bounded by the umbilicus superiorly, the two separated pubic bones laterally and the anus inferiorly
• The distance between the umbilicus and anus is shortened in exstrophy.
• Indirect inguinal hernia and incarceration are common in boys.
• Perineum is short and broad with the compromised pelvic support structures.
• Male genital anomalies

—Penis in boys with exstrophy is short and wide.
—Corpora cavernosa are short and widely separated.
—Marked dorsal chordee causes upward curvature of the penis with a short urethral plate.
—Epispadias is present when the urethral meatus is located on the dorsum at the penopubic junction. In rare cases epispadias is present in the absence of bladder exstrophy.

• Female genital anomalies

—Overall less complex
—Mons pubis is displaced laterally with bifid clitoris.
—Vagina and introitus are displaced anteriorly.
—Uterus and vagina may be duplicated.
—Epispadias may be less obvious.

• Urinary defects

—Bladder mucosa at birth usually appears normal. Ectopic bowel mucosa or polyp may be present in rare exstrophy variants.
—Exstrophic bladder may exhibit maturational delay that improves following closure.
—Upper urinary tract is usually normal.
—Horseshoe, pelvic, hypoplastic, solitary, or dysplastic kidney occasionally occurs.
—100% of children with exstrophy have vesicoureteral reflux requiring correction.

CLOACAL EXSTROPHY

• Two halves of the exstrophied bladder separated by an exstrophied ileocecal bowel segment that represents the hindgut.
• Prolapsed ileum superiorly, and blind-ending colon stump inferiorly.
• Imperforate anus
• Bifid vagina and uterine abnormalities likely.
• Large omphalocele usually present.
• Upper urinary tract anomalies seen in up to 70% of children.
• Vertebral and neurologic abnormalities present in over 50% of children.

IMAGING

• Prenatal sonographic findings by 20 weeks consistent with absence of a normal fluid-filled bladder, an anterior abdominal mass increasing in size, low-set umbilicus and wide pubic ramus are suggestive of bladder exstrophy.
• Radionuclide scans and ultrasound are required to confirm prenatal findings and diagnose associated anomalies in the neonatal period.
• Prospective parents of children with bladder exstrophy should be counseled as to excellent overall prognosis and favorable long-term outcome with early intervention by a pediatric urologist.

Therapy

- Postnatal and nursery care
- Umbilical cord tied with 2–0 silk to avoid traumatizing the bladder mucosa with an umbilical clamp.
- Bladder covered with plastic wrap to prevent mucosa from sticking to clothing or diapers.
- Occasional warm saline irrigations.
- Immediate transfer to an appropriate center for evaluation by a pediatric urologist and surgical correction.
- Surgical treatment

—Goals:
  —Provide urinary continence and preserve renal function.
  —Surgically reconstruct the male penis to provide an erection straight enough for vaginal penetration and upright voiding.
—Complete primary repair of exstrophy (CPRE):
  —Bladder closure, bladder neck reconstruction and epispadias repair completed in a single procedure. Procedure may be performed with or without bilateral posterior iliac and anterior innominate osteotomy.
  —May be postponed until 4 to 6 weeks of age to allow maternal bonding and to facilitate surgical planning to include orthopaedic and pediatric urologic support
  —Regaining popularity as initial approach in neonates.
  —Total penile disassembly involves total mobilization of the urethra to its ventral position without tension, and the bladder and urethra are closed in continuity.
  —Prophylactic antibiotic therapy should be continued in all children until antireflux procedure is completed or until vesicoureteral reflux resolves.
  —Practical advantage of allowing more normal bladder cycling that may facilitate bladder development.
—Staged closure of bladder exstrophy:
  —In the early neonatal period, bladder, posterior urethra and abdominal wall closure is performed with or without osteotomy.
  —Epispadias repair at 6 months to 1 year of age.
  —Bladder neck reconstruction with an antireflux procedure delayed until 3.5 to 4 years to facilitate adequate bladder growth and development.

—Results and complications:
  —For complete primary repair of exstrophy:
    —Daytime continence and volitional voiding in up to 86% (early results)
    —Additional bladder neck surgery to gain continence is often required.
    —No upper urinary tract changes or hydronephrosis in more than 80% of patients.
  —For staged closure:
    —Daytime continence and volitional voiding in 60% to 74% following bladder neck surgery (long-term follow-up).
    —Bladder capacity is a strong predictor of continence.
    —Minimal risk for upper urinary tract changes or hydronephrosis.
  —For epispadias repair:
    —Cosmetic and functional success with a straight penis with erections ranges from 60% to 95%
    —Urethral strictures and urethrocutaneous fistula are the most common complications of epispadias repair seen in up to 25% of patients.
  —Complications for both types of closures:
    —Dehiscence, stone formation, and hydronephrosis requiring urethral dilation or vesicostomy may occur. Patients must be followed carefully.
    —Initial closure success very important for continence.
      —Second attempt at closure delayed 6 months.
      —Expectation for continence decreases with each closure attempt.
    —Failed bladder neck repair in 20% to 50% may require further reconstruction.
    —Adenocarcinoma of the bladder occurs in patients with exstrophy 400 times more commonly than in the normal population. This disease is not reported in adults who have had bladder closure after infancy.
—Fertility and pregnancy:
  —Sexual function and libido in exstrophy patients is normal following successful reconstruction.
  —Up to 87% of boys have erections following epispadias repair.
  —Retrograde and small volume ejaculation should be expected.
  —Successful impregnation has been achieved with assisted reproductive techniques.
  —Pregnancy is commonly achieved in women with bladder exstrophy but uterine and cervical prolapse are common following pregnancy. Cesarean section is recommended in females completing reconstruction.

BIBLIOGRAPHY

Gearhart JP. The bladder exstrophy-epispadias-cloacal exstrophy complex. In: Gearhart Rink, Mouriquand, eds. *Pediatric Urology*. Philadelphia: WB Saunders, 2001:511.

Grady RW, et al. Complete primary closure of bladder exstrophy. Epispadias and bladder exstrophy repair. *Urol Clin North Am* 1999;26(1):95–109.

Poli-Merol ML, et al. New basic science concepts in the treatment of classic bladder exstrophy. *Urology* 2002;60(5):749–755.

Stein R, Thuroff JW. Hypospadias and bladder exstrophy. *Curr Opin Urol* 2002;12(3):195–200.

Authors: Aseem Shukla and Douglas Canning

Fetal Alcohol Syndrome

 Database

DEFINITION

Pattern of physical, behavioral, and cognitive abnormalities in individuals exposed to alcohol in utero.

DIAGNOSTIC CATEGORIES (INSTITUTE OF MEDICINE)

Fetal alcohol syndrome (FAS) with confirmed maternal exposure to alcohol (see below)*

- Characteristic facial anomalies
- Growth retardation
- Central nervous system (CNS) neurodevelopmental abnormalities

FAS without confirmed maternal exposure

- As above

Partial FAS with confirmed exposure

- Confirmed maternal alcohol exposure
- Characteristic facial anomalies
- Either growth retardation, CNS abnormalities, or unexplained behavior/cognitive abnormalities

Alcohol-Related Birth Defects (ARBD)

- Confirmed maternal alcohol exposure
- Birth defects

Alcohol-related neurodevelopmental disorder (ARND)

- Confirmed maternal alcohol exposure
- Either CNS abnormalities or unexplained behavior/cognitive abnormalities
- *Confirmed maternal exposure to alcohol as evidenced by: Substantial regular intake or heavy episodic drinking as evidenced by frequent episodes of intoxication, development of tolerance or withdrawal, social or legal problems related to drinking, engaging in physically hazardous behavior while drinking, or alcohol-related medical problems, e.g., hepatic disease
- Note: Some leading dysmorphologists prefer not to use the terms ARBD and ARND. See discussion below (Common Questions and Answers).

DIAGNOSTIC FINDINGS

Facial Anomalies

- Short palpebral fissures
- Premaxillary features (thin upper lip, flat/smooth philtrum, flat midface)
- Ptosis
- Short, upturned nose
- Ptosis and short, upturned nose are not mentioned in IOM criteria, but are commonly seen in children with FAS.

Growth Retardation (At Least One for Diagnosis)

- Low birth weight for gestation
- Growth retardation despite adequate nutrition
- Low weight relative to height

CNS Neurodevelopmental Abnormalities (At Least One for Diagnosis)

- Microcephaly at birth
- Structural brain abnormalities (e.g., agenesis of corpus callosum, cerebellar hypoplasia)
- Neurologic hard or soft signs (e.g., impaired fine motor skills, neurosensory hearing loss, poor tandem gait, poor eye-hand coordination)

Unexplained Behavior or Cognitive Abnormalities

- Learning difficulties
- Poor school performance
- Poor impulse control
- Problems in social perception
- Deficits in higher level receptive and expressive language
- Poor abstract reasoning
- Poor math skills
- Impaired memory, attention, or judgment

Birth Defects

- Cardiac (30%): Atrial septal defect (ASD), ventricular septal defect (VSD) (most common), aberrant great vessels, tetralogy of Fallot (TOF)
- Skeletal (18%): Clinodactyly, camptodactyly, nail dysplasia, radioulnar synostosis
- Renal: Hydronephrosis, renal agenesis, hypoplastic kidney
- Ocular: Strabismus, retinal vascular tortuosity, abnormal corneal curvature
- Auditory: Hearing loss (conductive—75% of children with FAS; neurosensory—less common)
- Others

PATHOPHYSIOLOGY

Alcohol and its metabolite, acetaldehyde, are embryotoxic and teratogenic, capable of reducing fetal growth and inducing malformations during critical periods in the development of the fetus. Pathophysiology may involve increased susceptibility to cell damage by free radicals in the developing tissues, leading to cell death or decreased cellular proliferation. Exposure in the first trimester affects organogenesis and craniofacial development, resulting in characteristic facial features and birth defects. Exposure at varying times can cause CNS neurodevelopmental effects, because brain formation and neuronal maturation occur throughout pregnancy. Exposure also causes pre- and postnatal growth retardation, probably by inhibiting protein and DNA synthesis.

EPIDEMIOLOGY

Incidence of FAS, alcohol-related birth defect (ARBD), and alcohol-related neurodevelopmental disorder (ARND) range widely from 0.3 to 5 per 1,000 live births. Higher rates reported among selected subgroups, e.g., African Americans and Native Americans, probably relate to lower socioeconomic status rather than race.

GENETICS

Genetic factors contribute to variable susceptibility of individuals to FAS. Evidence: Concordance of FAS is higher in monozygotic than dizygotic twins; differential sensitivities to in utero alcohol exposure in different strains of mice.
(Other factors that contribute to variable susceptibility include: maternal age/parity, nutritional status, use of other drugs.)

PROGNOSIS

- Fifty percent are mentally retarded (IQ <70). Average IQ in individuals with FAS is in the 60s (mild MR); however, a wide range of IQ exists, from 16 to 115.
- Sixty-two percent have severe behavioral problems, even if a normal IQ exists.
- The major disabilities of FAS caused by the neurocognitive/neurobehavioral effects lead to poor academic performance, legal problems, employment difficulties, and secondary mental health problems.

 Differential Diagnosis

BY PHYSICAL FEATURES

- Aarskog syndrome
- Williams syndrome
- Noonan syndrome
- Dubowitz syndrome
- Bloom syndrome
- Fetal hydantoin syndrome
- Maternal phenylketonuria fetal effects

BY NEUROBEHAVIORAL FEATURES

- Fragile X syndrome
- 22q11 deletion syndromes
- Turner syndrome
- Opitz syndrome

Data Gathering

HISTORY

- Birth history, birth and subsequent growth parameters (weight, height, head circumference)
- Medical history
- Maternal history for alcohol use (binge drinking, average number of drinks per day, timing in pregnancy) and other drug use
- Learning/behavior problems

—Infancy
  —May or may not have EtOH withdrawal as newborn
  —Irritable, irregular sleep, poor feeding, hypotonia, delayed motor function
—Preschool and school age
  —Hyperactive?
  —Slow verbal learning?
  —Slow visual-spatial learning?
  —Poor abstract thinking (planning and organizing)?
  —Perseverates (can't abandon ineffective strategies)?
  —Attention problems?
  —Difficulty with peer interactions?
—Adolescence and adulthood:
  —Substance abuse?
  —Criminal behavior?
  —Unable to work?
  —Unable to live independently?

Q: Are siblings affected?
A: Usually younger siblings are affected more severely; if older sibling wasn't previously diagnosed, and shows signs of alcohol-related effects, he/she will also need evaluation and services.

Q: Is child in a high-risk living situation? Who is the caregiver?
A: Keep in mind that external influences such as poverty, unstable home environment, poor emotional support, or educational resources contribute to behavioral problems.

 ## Physical Examination

- Weight, height, head circumference

—Microcephaly persists throughout life
—Some catch-up growth occurs in adolescence, especially in girls, but adult height attained remains lower than expected for parental height.

- Facial examination (short palpebral fissures, ptosis, flat midface, upturned nose, smooth philtrum, thin upper lip)

—Facial features become less prominent in adolescence and adulthood

- Complete PE, including neurologic exam

—Look for associated defects of the heart, skeletal system

 ## Laboratory Aids

- No laboratory marker exists for FAS.
- Consider chromosome studies if diagnosis is unclear.
- Other laboratory tests as indicated by the child's specific medical problems.

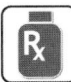 ## Therapy

The role of the pediatrician is early identification (with help from specialists) resulting in early intervention and appropriate referrals:

- To social and educational resources in the community to support family and child
- For comprehensive neuropsychologic evaluation (IQ, achievement, executive function, memory, adaptive function, language, reasoning and judgment, behavior)
- For ophthalmologic examination (consider routine screening prior to school, then every 2 years)
- For hearing test [consider brainstem auditory evoked response (BAER) at 6–12 months]

 ## Follow-Up

- Growth and nutrition in infancy since failure to thrive is a common problem.
- Regular evaluations of vision and hearing, because these problems occur at a high rate.
- As indicated by other medical/psychological problems.

PREVENTION

FAS is preventable if women of childbearing age abstain from alcohol prior to conception and throughout pregnancy. Recent FAS prevention research has focused on finding and treating women who drink during pregnancy, e.g., using a screening questionnaire to assess problem drinking in women, and then intervening at a level determined by the level of drinking.

 ## Common Questions and Answers

Q: What is FAE (fetal alcohol effect)?
A: FAE originally described abnormalities seen in animal studies, then was adopted by clinicians, being widely used to refer to behavioral and cognitive problems in children exposed to alcohol in utero without the typical diagnostic features. Because of lack of diagnostic criteria for FAE, and the imprecise use of this term, IOM replaced FAE with the terms alcohol-related neurodevelopmental disorder (ARND) and alcohol-related birth defects (ARBD).

Use of these terms (ARND and ARBD) is also controversial in that they imply that confirmed maternal alcohol exposure is causative of the associated abnormalities, which at present is not proven. In summarizing the problem list for an individual who may not meet the criteria for FAS or partial FAS, some leading dysmorphologists recommend listing the elements separately without attribution, rather than using the confusing terms FAE or ARND/ARBD. [e.g., Impression: (1) Prenatal alcohol exposure, (mild, moderate, or severe), (2) cleft lip and palate, complete bilateral, (3) cognitive deficit (mild, moderate, or severe).]

Q: How much alcohol does it take to produce damage?
A: Clinically significant effects are more common in children whose mothers consume five or more drinks per occasion per week. (Peak blood alcohol level is more important than a lower sustained blood alcohol level.) However, no minimum safe level of alcohol consumption has been determined.

Q: Do most children with FAS have ADHD?
A: Although hyperactivity appears to be common in FAS, many of these children are misdiagnosed as having ADHD. Instead of difficulty focusing and sustaining attention, children with FAS often have difficulty shifting attention from one task to another. Use of stimulant medication is not routinely supported, although a small proportion may respond to stimulant medication in educational settings.

ICD-9-CM 760.71

BIBLIOGRAPHY

Aase JM, Jones KL, Clarren SK. Do we need the term "FAE"? *Pediatrics* 1995;95:428–430.

Abel EL. *Fetal Alcohol Abuse Syndrome.* New York: Plenum Press, 1998.

American Academy of Pediatrics. Fetal alcohol syndrome and alcohol-related neurodevelopmental disorders. *Pediatrics* 2000;106:358–361.

Dorris M. *The Broken Cord.* New York: Harper Collins, 1990.

Institute of Medicine. *Fetal Alcohol Syndrome, Diagnosis, Epidemiology, Prevention, and Treatment.* Washington DC: National Academy of Sciences, 1996.

National Institute on Alcohol Abuse and Alcoholism. Fetal alcohol exposure and the brain. *Alcohol Alert* December 2000;50.

Thackray HM, Tifft C. Fetal alcohol syndrome. *Pediatr Rev* 2001;22:47–55.

Author: Janet M. Li-Tempest

Floppy Infant Syndrome

 ## Database

DEFINITION

"Floppy infant" implies generalized hypotonia presenting at birth or early in life with decreased movement, decreased resistance to movement, or increased joint laxity. Transient hypotonia occurs in nonneurologic illnesses in infants; it is a nonspecific sign that may also suggest central nervous system (CNS), lower motor neuron, peripheral nerve, primary muscle, endocrine, or metabolic disease.

GENETICS

• Many heritable disorders, feature infantile, hypotonia including those with autosomal dominant, autosomal recessive, x-linked, and nonmendelian inheritance patterns

COMPLICATIONS

• Respiratory insufficiency/recurrent pneumonia
• Orthopaedic deformities
• Poor nutritional status

ASSOCIATED ILLNESSES

• Metabolic disorders
• Hip dislocation, contractures, and joint laxity
• Sucking and swallowing difficulties
• Seizure disorders
• Developmental/motor delay

 ## Differential Diagnosis

NONPARALYTIC HYPOTONIA

• Benign congenital hypotonia—transient hypotonia without dysmorphology or weakness. Affected infants may exhibit mild motor delay, but no other neurologic, physical, or laboratory abnormalities. By definition, prognosis is good.
• Connective tissue disorders

—Ehlers-Danlos syndrome
—Marfan syndrome
—Osteogenesis imperfecta
—Chondrodysplasia
—Benign joint laxity

• Metabolic/systemic disorders

—Sepsis
—Trauma
—Malnutrition
—Drug intoxication (maternal sedative, analgesic, and/or anesthetic exposure)
—Gastrointestinal disease (obstruction, bleed, malabsorption)
—Congenital heart disease
—Endocrinopathies (hypothyroidism)
—Renal tubular acidosis
—Rickets
—Hypercalcemia
—Cystic fibrosis

—Organic acidemias
—Glycogen storage disease
—Mucopolysaccharidoses

• Disorders involving the cerebral cortex, cerebellum, brainstem

—Congenital malformations (lissencephaly, holoprosencephaly)
—Hypoxic ischemic encephalopathy
—Intracranial hemorrhage
—Infections (meningitis, encephalitis)
—Trauma
—Metabolic encephalopathies
—Hypoxic-ischemic encephalopathies
—Chromosomal disorders (Prader-Willi and Down syndromes)
—Developmental disturbance (neuronal migration disorders)
—Sphingolipidoses

• Disorders involving spinal cord

—Myelodysplasias (meningomyeloceles, diplomyelia, diastematomyelia)
—Traumatic injury

PARALYTIC HYPOTONIA

Paralytic causes must be considered in floppy infants whose physical examination reveals significant and usually persistent motor weakness and decreased or absent deep tendon reflexes. Differential diagnosis in this category involves disorders of the anterior horn cell, peripheral nerve, neuromuscular junction, and of the muscle itself.

• Disorders of the anterior horn cell

—Spinal muscle atrophy (Werdnig-Hoffmann disease)
—Neurogenic arthrogryposis multiplex congenita
—Glycogen storage disease type II (Pompe disease)
—Neonatal poliomyelitis (possibly other enteroviruses)

• Disorders of peripheral nerve

—Dejerine-Sottas disease
—Guillain-Barre syndrome
—Familial dysautonomia (Riley-Day syndrome)
—Congenital hypomyelination neuropathy
—Leukodystrophies (Krabbe's disease and metachromatic leukodystrophy)
—Leigh disease

• Disorders of neuromuscular junction

—Myasthenia gravis (congenital and neonatal transient)
—Toxic-metabolic defects (hypermagnesemia, antibiotics [especially aminoglycosides], nondepolarizing neuromuscular blockers)
—Infantile botulism

• Disorders of muscle

—Congenital structural myopathies such as central core disease; nemaline, centronuclear, and myotubular myopathy
—Congenital myotonic dystrophy
—Congenital muscular dystrophy (many subtypes)
—Metabolic myopathies (mitochondrial disorders, glycosylation disorders, lipid storage disease, many others)

PITFALLS

• Virtually any acute illness in infancy may present with decreased tone and/or weakness.
• Prader Willi often presents as paralytic hypotonia in newborns or young infants.
• Hypermagnesemia is a common cause of hypotonia and apnea in newborn. Monitoring in the intensive care nursery should be considered. When there is a history of intrapartum maternal magnesium administration.

 ## Data Gathering

HISTORY

Important factors in the history may be categorized according to the child's chronologic development, with the prenatal period and delivery, the neonatal period, and later infancy considered individually.

• Prenatal period and delivery

—Prenatal period
    —Family history
    —Parental consanguinity
    —Maternal illness
    —Drug/teratogen exposure
    —Polyhydramnios
    —Fetal movements
    —Gestational maturity
—Delivery
    —Trauma
    —Hypoxia/anoxia
    —Shortened umbilical cord
    —Apgar scores

• Neonatal period

—Infections, recent illnesses, medications
—Seizures
—Apnea

• Later infancy

—Delayed motor milestones
—Delayed social, fine motor, or language milestones
—Feeding difficulties

Physical Examination

- General physical examination

—Presence or absence of dysmorphology
—Infants with neuromuscular disease are typically alert as opposed to those with CNS disease, who typically display a depressed level of consciousness
—Abnormal head size and/or shape (brain disease)
—High arched palate (neuromuscular disorders)
—Tongue fasciculations (anterior horn cell disease)
—Large tongue (storage disorders)
—Ophthalmologic examination may reveal cataracts (peroxisomal disorders), pigmentary retinopathy (peroxisomal disorders), lens dislocation (rare metabolic disorders),
—Visceral enlargement (storage disorders)
—Arthrogryposis (central, neuromuscular, or connective tissue disorders)
—Joint laxity (connective tissue disorders)

- Neurologic Examination

—Muscle tone
   —Hypotonic infants typically exhibit abnormal posture (abduction, external rotation of legs, flaccid extension of the arms) and prominent head lag on pull to sit maneuver.
   —Generalized hypotonia with increased tone in the thumb adductors, wrist pronators, and hip adductors is often noted in early cerebral palsy.
   —Posture and tone should be noted in the supine position, in ventral suspension, and with traction. The elbow of the hypotonic infant typically extends beyond the midsternum with ease (scarf sign).
—Strength
   —Weakness may be reflected by a low-pitched, progressively weakening cry.
   —Decreased expression indicates facial weakness (myotonic dystrophy, congenital muscular dystrophy, congenital myopathies)
   —Ptosis and ophthalmoplegia (myasthenic syndromes, congenital myopathies, and congenital muscular dystrophies)
   —Regional differences in strength often suggest certain disorders or syndromes. SMA initially spares muscles of the face, diaphragm, and pelvic sphincters. Neuropathies typically present with weakness of distal limb muscles and sparing of proximal muscles. Myasthenic syndromes affect bulbar and oculomotor muscles preferentially.
   —Fatigability (progressive weakness with exertion), a cardinal feature of the myasthenic syndromes, may also occur in other neuromuscular diseases of infancy.
—Reflexes
   —Increased deep tendon reflexes imply central dysfunction
   —In myopathic diseases, deep tendon reflexes are diminished in proportion to the degree of weakness

—Absent reflexes in the setting of minimal weakness is typical of neuropathic disease.

Laboratory Aids

TESTS

- Initial noninvasive tests may include electrolytes (including calcium and magnesium), thyroid function tests, creatine kinase (CK), and arterial blood gas. Appropriate tests to eliminate infectious etiology should be performed (blood/urine/CSF cultures).
- Laboratory testing should be directed toward identifying an inborn error of metabolism if complex multisystem involvement is suggested. Assays for uric acid, ammonia and lactate (blood, urine, CSF), quantitative analysis of amino acids (blood, urine), organic acid and acylcarnitine profiles (blood), as well as assays of very long chain fatty acids (plasma) are among those tests to be considered.
- The karyotype will reveal chromosomal duplications, deletions, and trisomies.

—Fluorescent in-situ hybridization probes may indicate microdeletions and disomies.
—Methylation studies and direct mutation analyses may disclose a variety of diagnoses.

- Appropriate imaging studies (CT, MRI) may disclose structural malformations in infants presenting with central hypotonia.
- Administration of an anticholinesterase medication in suspected myasthenic syndrome may provide rapid diagnosis.
- Stool samples should be evaluated for Clostridium when botulism is suspected.
- Electromyography (EMG) and nerve conduction velocity (NCV) are useful tools in assessing disorders affecting the lower motor unit. These tests are particularly helpful in localizing the site of involvement in the motor unit.
- Muscle ultrasonography can contribute to the differential diagnosis of neuromuscular diseases, but does not allow a definitive diagnosis.
- Muscle biopsy is the gold standard in the diagnosis of congenital myopathies and muscular dystrophies.

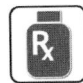

Therapy

- Anticipate respiratory insufficiency in infants with paralytic hypotonia. Chest physical therapy, suctioning, prophylactic antibiotics, bronchodilators, and supplemental oxygen may be helpful. Intermittent positive pressure devices and endotracheal intubation with total respiratory assist in severe cases or concomitant pulmonary illness.
- Feeding and swallowing difficulties may necessitate nutritional supplementation and/or feeding tube placement. Infants with

significant gastroesophageal reflux may require Nissen fundoplication.
- Underlying toxic or metabolic causes should be addressed and treated appropriately.
- Anticholinesterase medications may be required in the treatment of myasthenic syndromes.
- Intravenous immunoglobulin and plasmapheresis have been used in the treatment of infants with Guillain-Barré syndrome.
- Physical therapy may help maintain maximum muscle function and reduce secondary deformities.

Follow-Up

- Orthopaedic consultation to evaluate hips and contractures. Surgical intervention in later childhood to correct primary as well as secondary deformities.
- In noncomplicated infantile hypotonia (without weakness or dysmorphology), benign congenital hypotonia must be considered and limited evaluation may be undertaken.
- Watchful waiting may be appropriate in infants whose motor skills are progressing and who exhibit normal development in other areas.

PITFALLS

- EMG and NCV in the newborn and young infant are difficult to perform and interpret.
- Values change quickly with normal development and variation is high. As a result, these tests are only valuable when performed by experienced individuals.

Common Questions and Answers

Q: By what age should one expect resolution of benign congenital hypotonia?
A: Hypotonia has typically resolved by the time the infant is walking, which may be delayed to 18 months.

Q: What clinical sign can help distinguish between SMA and infantile botulism?
A: Tongue fasciculations (seen in SMA). Also, decreased pupillary light reflex in botulism.

ICD-9-CM 781.9

BIBLIOGRAPHY

Johnston H. The floppy weak infant revisited. *Brain & Development* 2003;25:155–158.

Prasad A, Prasad C. The floppy infant: contribution of genetic and metabolic disorders. *Brain & Development* 2003;(27):457–476.

Riggs J, et al. Congenital myopathies/dystrophies. *Neurologic Clinics* 2003;21(4):779–794.

Author: Michael Andrew Ferguson

Food Allergy

 Database

DEFINITION

A food allergy is an adverse immunologic response to food proteins.
There are excellent discussions of cutaneous and respiratory food hypersensitivities elsewhere and this chapter will focus on gastrointestinal aspects.

CAUSES

Oral tolerance to food proteins develops through T cell anergy or induction of regulatory T cells. Food hypersensitivity develops when oral tolerance fails to develop or breaks down. Gastrointestinal food hypersensitivity reactions may be classified as follows:

- IgE mediated—T cells induce B cells to produce IgE antibodies that initially bind on the surface of mast cells; reexposure to the food protein causes a release of histamine and other chemical mediators that produce the allergic symptoms:
—Urticaria
—Angioedema
—Immediate GI reactions
—Oral allergy syndrome
—Rhinitis
—Anaphylaxis
—Symptoms of nausea, abdominal pain, colic, vomiting develop within 2 hours of ingesting offending foods, and diarrhea develops within 2 to 6 hrs.
- NonIgE mediated (cell-mediated) food allergy is due to T cells reacting to protein by inducing eosinophilic inflammation and increased vascular permeability. These mediators lead to subacute and chronic responses affecting primarily the gastrointestinal tract.
—Cell-mediated hypersensitivity conditions include:
    —Dietary protein enterocolitis
    —Proctitis and enteropathy
    —Celiac disease.
- Some reactions fall into a mixed IgE and nonIgE (cell-mediated) category including atopic dermatitis, eosinophilic gastroenteropathies. Allergic gastritis and gastroenteropathy are characterized by eosinophilic infiltration of the intestinal wall, occasionally deep to the serosa.
—Thickening of the bowel wall may lead to obstruction
—If serosal, ascites.
—Allergic eosinophilic gastritis associated with:
    —Vomiting
    —Gastric bleeding
    —Abdominal pain
    —Anorexia
    —Failure to thrive. Gastric outlet obstruction may mimic pyloric stenosis.
    —Weight loss is a key feature of eosinophilic gastroenteropathy, and some infants have a large protein losing enteropathy component causing low serum albumin and hypogammaglobulinemia.
—Eosinophilic esophagitis:
    —Dysphagia
    —Intermittent vomiting
    —Food refusal
    —Abdominal pain
    —Irritability
    —Failure to respond to reflux medication. Skin and RAST tests are often negative. Patients may respond to hypoallergenic formulas; older patients may require free amino acid formulas.

Epidemiology and Risk Factors

- Food allergies affect about 5% to 8% of children <3 years of age.
- Nearly 2.5% of infants have hypersensitivity reactions to cow milk during the first year, however most outgrow this by 5 years of age.
- Population-based studies reveal a prevalence egg allergy in 2.6% by age 2½ yr.
- Most common food allergies: milk, egg, soy, peanut, wheat and fish. In adults, the most common food allergens are peanuts, tree nuts, fish, and shellfish.
- Anaphylaxis to food is the most common cause of anaphylactic reactions treated in emergency departments in the United States. Food allergy is present in 37% of children with moderate to severe atopic dermatitis.
- About 6% of asthmatic children in a pulmonary clinic will have food-induced wheezing.

Complications

- Food protein allergy can cause:
—Nausea
—Anorexia
—Vomiting
—Diarrhea
—Poor growth
—Protein losing enteropathy
—Anemia
—Cutaneous food sensitivity reactions include:
    —Urticaria
    —Angioedema
    —Atopic dermatitis
    —Contact dermatitis
    —Dermatitis herpetiformis.

	ILLNESS	SYMPTOMS	DIAGNOSIS
IgE mediated	Anaphylaxis	Rapid onset; nausea and vomiting, abdominal pain, +/− diarrhea, other organ systems involvement–skin, respiratory system.	History, + skin prick or RAST test; oral challenge only in monitored setting with emergency access and under stringent protocol.
IgE mediated	Oral allergy syndrome (children and adults)	Mild pruritus, angioedema of lips and oropharynx; sense of tightness in throat; rare systemic symptoms.	History, + skin prick tests; oral challenge + with fresh foods and—with cooked foods
IgE &/or cell mediated	Allergic eosinophilic gastroenteritis	Failure to thrive, weight loss, abdominal pain, irritability, early satiety, intermittent vomiting, protein losing enteropathy, edema, ascites.	History, + skin prick; endoscopy with biopsy; elimination diet, recurrence with rechallenge.
IgE &/or cell mediated	Allergic eosinophilic esophagitis	Gastroesophageal reflux (GER) with failure to respond to medications, vomiting, dysphagia, intermittent abdominal pain, irritability.	History, endoscopy with biopsy, elimination diet with rechallenge. Poor correlation of skin tests to causative proteins. Serum eosinophils high in some.
Cell mediated	Allergic proctocolitis 'breast milk colitis' (infants)	Bloody stool, melena in first few months of life; no diarrhea or failure to thrive (FTT).	Elimination of food (cow milk) clears bleeding in 72 hr; reexposure causes recurrence. RAST /skin prick NOT helpful.
Cell mediated	Allergic enterocolitis, (infants)	Severe symptoms, vomiting 1 to 3 hrs after meal, diarrhea +/− blood, abdominal distention, failure to thrive, dehydration, hypotension.	Elimination of protein clears symptoms in 1 to 3 days. Skin prick/RAST NOT helpful.
Cell mediated	Food protein-induced enteropathy (infants)	Diarrhea, steatorrhea, abdominal distention, flatulence, FTT or weight loss, nausea/vomiting; oral ulcers	Endoscopy with biopsy; elimination diet resolves symptoms. Similar symptoms to celiac, but resolves by 2 years of age.
Cell mediated	Celiac disease (infant to adults)	Diarrhea, steatorrhea, FTT, abdominal distention, flatulence, weight loss, nausea/vomiting; oral ulcers	Endoscopic biopsy; gluten-free diet resolves symptoms. Antigliadin and TTG antibodies; HLA-DQ2 and DQ8 are found.

Respiratory food hypersensitivity reactions:
- Rhinoconjunctivitis
- Asthma
- Heiner syndrome, a rare food-induced pulmonary hemosiderosis

Prognosis

Generally good, once the offending food antigens are removed from the diet and assure nutrients in the diet are adequate.

 ## Differential Diagnosis

Symptoms vary depending upon the individual and the type of food hypersensitivity. Rectal bleeding may be caused by proctocolitis or enterocolitis secondary to food allergies. Other disease processes that may cause rectal bleeding include:
- Anal fissures or tears
- Infection or inflammatory bowel disease
- Hirschsprung enterocolitis
- Polyps
- Meckel diverticulum
- Arteriovenous malformation

Vomiting may be caused by food hypersensitivity or other illnesses such as:
- Gastritis from other causes—Crohn disease, *H. pylori*
- Intestinal obstruction
—Pyloric stenosis (nonbilious)
—Duodenal web
—If bilious emesis, rule out malrotation with volvulus or other distal obstruction.
- Infection
—Viral
—Giardia
- Neurologic problems
- Systemic infections including urinary tract infections

Excessive eosinophils are found systemically or in tissues in other conditions such as:
- Inflammatory bowel disease
- Parasitic infection
- Celiac disease or autoimmune enteropathy
- Drug reaction
- Hypereosinophilic syndrome
- Malignancy
- Collagen vascular disease

 ## Laboratory Aids

Depending on clinical presentation and patient symptoms, appropriate laboratory investigation may include the following:
1. CBC with differential:
   a. Anemia in patients with enteropathy
   b. Eosinophilia in patients with eosinophilic gastritis or enteropathy.
2. Serum IgE:
   a. Elevated in IgE-mediated hypersensitivities, and in 50% of those with allergic eosinophilic gastritis.
3. Albumin:
   a. Low with protein-losing enteropathies associated with allergic (mixed)

eosinophilic gastroenterocolitis, and non-IgE-mediated protein enterocolitis
4. Radioallergosorbent tests, or "RAST" serum testing:
   a. May be helpful in IgE-mediated illness
   b. Many false positives
   c. CAP fluorescent enzyme immunoassay (FEIA) provide more useful positive and negative predictive values.
      i. High specificity, and positive predictive values of 95% to 100% for egg, milk and peanut have been developed.
      ii. RAST studies should NOT be performed on patients with enterocolitis syndrome, as they may cause life-threatening reactions.
5. In children suspected of IgE-mediated disease:
   a. Prick/puncture skin test (PST) have replaced scratch tests.
      i. Negative skin tests in children greater than 1 year have high negative predictive accuracy, thereby excluding IgE-mediated food allergy. Positive predictive accuracy is lower, about 50%.
      ii. In children less than 1 year, the negative predictive accuracy is lower, about 80% to 85%.
6. Patch skin testing:
   a. May be used to evaluate for mixed (IgE/non-IgE)-mediated or cell-mediated sensitivities. Standards for interpretation and methods for reliability are under development.
7. Double-blinded, placebo-controlled food challenges:
   a. Gold standard for diagnosis of food allergy, but are impractical in most clinical settings. These are utilized when the probability of food allergy is low and may be unsafe in patients with convincing histories of severe allergic reaction and evidence of IgE antibody to the specific food.
8. Elimination diets should be done with care
   a. May lack critical nutrients.
   b. Oral rechallenge should be carefully planned, since a more severe reaction may ensue after a food has been temporarily removed.
   c. When there is a history of acute reactions, challenges should be performed by an allergist, with access to emergency medication and equipment.

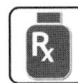 ## Therapy

For anaphylaxis, full monitoring of vital signs, epinephrine if significant respiratory or cardio-vascular symptoms. Antihistamines (diphen-hydramine) may be given for milder symptoms. Treatment of nonanaphylactic food allergies:
- Removal of the offending food agent from the diet
- Severe eosinophilic gastroenteropathies:
—Systemic steroids
—Hydrolyzed or elemental formulas.

—Anti-IgE and other forms of immunotherapy
—Probiotics have shown in one Finnish study to be effective in the prevention of early atopic dermatitis in high-risk children.
—Probiotics such as Lactobacillus GG may decrease hypersensitivity reactions to food antigens, and diminish intestinal inflammation in patients with atopic eczema and food allergy by promoting endogenous intestinal barrier mechanisms.

 ## Follow-Up

- Tolerance to allergens usually develops over time.
- IgE-mediated disease may persist longer.

 ## Common Questions and Answers

Q: What are common allergens?
A: The most common allergens to which children are sensitive are milk, egg, soy, wheat, fish and nuts.

Q: Do you recommend elimination diets?
A: Only in extreme circumstances because they can result in nutrient deficient diets and malnutrition without identifying the offending allergen. Double-blinded food challenges are a better method to identify the offending agent.

ICD-558.3

BIBLIOGRAPHY

Bock SA. Pediatric food allergy: diagnostic evaluation. *Pediatrics* 2003;111(6):1638–1644.

Burks W. Pediatric food allergy: skin manifestations of food allergy. *Pediatrics* 2003;111(6):1617–1624.

Eggesbo M. The prevalence of allergy to egg: a population-based study in young children. *Allergy* 2001;56:403–411.

John MJ. Pediatric food allergy: respiratory manifestations of food allergy. *Pediatrics* 2003;111(6):1625–1630.

Sampson HA, Anderson JA. Summary and recommendations: Classification of gastrointestinal manifestations due to immunoligic reactions to foods in infants and young children. *J Pediatr Gastroenterol and Nutr* 2000;30(Suppl 1):S87–S94.

Sampson HA. Anaphylaxis and emergency treatment. *Pediatrics* 2003;111(6):1601–1608.

Sampson HA. Food allergy. *J Allerg and Clin Immunol* 2003;111(2):(Suppl) S540–7.

Sicherer SH. Symposium: pediatric food allergy. *Pediatrics* 2003;111(6):1591–1594.

Sicherer SH. Pediatric food allergy: clinical aspects of gastrointestinal food allergy in childhood. *Pediatrics* 2003;111(6):1609–1616.

Authors: Linda Muir, Christopher Justinich, and Stephen McGeady

Food Poisoning or Foodborne Illness

 Database

DEFINITION

Rapid onset of diarrhea, vomiting, and/or fever from 1 to 96 hours after the ingestion of contaminated food.

CAUSES

Variety of bacteria and/or toxins: Most common are *Campylobacter, Salmonella* (nontyphoid), and *E. coli* 0157:H7 or by a group of viruses called *Calcivirus*.

ETIOLOGY

Important clues to determining the etiology are:

- History of food consumption
- Incubation period
- Duration of the resultant illness
- Predominant clinical symptoms, and
- Population involved in the outbreak.

PATHOLOGY

- Ingestion of preformed toxin
- Elaboration of toxin from bacteria into the gastrointestinal tract
- Direct invasion of mucosa by bacteria

EPIDEMIOLOGY

Approximately 500 outbreaks of food-borne disease are reported each year in the United States.

 Differential Diagnosis

INFECTION

- Parenteral infections

—Upper respiratory tract
—Urinary tract infections
—Otitis media

- *Escherichia coli* (Non 0157:H7)
- *Vibrio*
- *Clostridium difficile*
- *Yersinia enterocolitica*
- *Aeromonas hydrophilia*
- *Giardia lamblia*
- *Entamoeba histolytica*
- *Rotavirus*
- *Campylobacter jejuni*, most common
- *Listerosis*
- *Vibriosis*
- *Yersinia*

FOOD INTOLERANCE/FOOD ALLERGIES

- Cow's milk protein allergy
- Carbohydrate intolerance (most common is lactose)

MISCELLANEOUS

- Use of antibiotics
- Malnutrition

—Altered mucosal structure
—Defective disaccharidase activity
—Abnormal motility

DIETARY MANIPULATIONS

- Hyperosmolar formulas
- Food additives (dyes, processing materials, coloring)
- Caffeine
- Overfeeding
- Low fat intakes (especially during recovery phase)
- Excessive fluids

 Data Gathering

HISTORY

- Outbreak of illness following ingestion of a meal
- Others in family with similar symptoms
- Time of onset of vomiting after ingestion—relates to type of bacterial toxins (see the table Clinical Aspects of Food Poisoning in Section VIII)
- *E. coli, Campylobacter*, and *Salmonella* are more frequent in summer months

 Physical Examination

- See the table, Clinical Aspects of Food Poisoning in Section VIII
- Botulism

—Severity related to host susceptibility and to amount of toxin ingested
—Disease may be so mild that consultation is not obtained; in other cases, it is fatal within a few hours.
—Generalized hypotonia
—Absent deep tendon reflexes
—Dilated, reactive pupils
—Poor suck
—Decreased to absent gag reflex
—Ptosis

 Laboratory Aids

TESTS

- Isolation of the organism from stools and the suspected food
- Demonstrating the toxin in the suspected food
- Identifying 10^5 organisms per gram of suspected food
- Finding 10^6 organisms or spores per gram of patient's stool or vomitus
- Lesions on the hands of food handlers may be the source of contamination and should be cultured.

Botulism

- Toxin in stools is diagnostic.
- Stool culture for *Clostridium botulinum*
- Electromyography with repetitive stimulation
- Lumbar puncture to exclude other diagnoses

Enterohemorrhagic series *E. coli* 0157:H7

- Latex agglutination test

 Therapy

- No specific treatment
- Intramuscular antiemetics
- If clinically dehydrated, rehydration can be accomplished in 4 to 6 hours, using an oral solution containing 75 to 90 mEq Na/L.
- IV fluids for patients unable to be rehydrated via the oral route (because of ileus, circulatory failure, CNS complications), or with stool losses greater than 10 mL/kg per hour
- Most foods (except for lactose) should be tolerated in the pediatric patient recovering from food poisoning.
- The BRATT diet (bananas, rice, applesauce, toast, tea) is inappropriate for the management of acute diarrheal episodes, because of low calorie, protein, and fat contents.
- A balanced, varied diet, providing easily digestible, complex carbohydrates, will promote increased stool consistency.

DRUGS

Antibiotics

Salmonella (Nontyphoid)

- Not used in patients with uncomplicated gastroenteritis
- Does not shorten the duration of the disease
- Can prolong the duration of excretion of *Salmonella* organisms
- Antimicrobial therapy is warranted for *Salmonella* gastroenteritis occurring in patients with an increased risk of invasive disease and other complications:

—Infants under 3 months of age
—Patients with malignancies
—Hemoglobinopathies
—AIDS
—Recipients of immunosuppressive therapy
—Persons with chronic gastrointestinal tract disease
—Patients with severe colitis

- Ampicillin, amoxicillin, trimethoprim-sulfamethoxazole, cefotaxime, or ceftriaxone is recommended for susceptible strains in patients for whom therapy is recommended.

Botulism

- Supportive care
- Monitor cardiac and respiratory function.
- Endotracheal intubation and assisted ventilation
- Avoid aminoglycosides.

 Follow-Up

PROGNOSIS

- Most gastroenteritis secondary to food poisoning is mild and self-limited.
- Recovery is complete in 2 to 5 days in most individuals.
- In the very young, the prognosis is more guarded, because these patients can become dehydrated quickly.
- Once the patient has survived the paralytic phase of botulism, the outlook for complete recovery is excellent.

PREVENTION

- Parenteral vaccines are not recommended for use in children.
- Botulism in infants, 1 year:

—Wash objects placed in infants' mouths (pacifiers, toys, etc.).
—Wash or peel skin of fruits and vegetables.
—Avoid honey.

FOODBORNE DISEASES AND CONDITIONS DESIGNATED AS NOTIFIABLE AT THE NATIONAL LEVEL—UNITED STATES 2003

Notifiable BACTERIAL Foodborne Diseases and Conditions

- Anthrax
- Botulism
- *Brucellosis*
- Cholera
- Enterohemorrhagic *Escherichia coli*
- Hemolytic uremic syndrome, postdiarrheal
- *Listeriosis*
- *Salmonellosis* (other than S. *Typhi*)
- *Shigellosis*
- Typhoid fever (S. *Typhi* and S. *Paratyphi* infections)

Notifiable VIRAL Foodborne Diseases and Conditions

- Hepatitis A

Notifiable PARASITIC Foodborne Diseases and Conditions

- *Cryptosporidiosis*
- *Cyclosporiasis*
- *Giardiasis*
- *Trichinellosis*

In the United States, additional reporting requirements may be mandated by state and territorial laws and regulations. Details on specific state reporting requirements are available from state health departments and from the Council of State and Territorial Epidemiologist (http://www.cste.org/nndss/reportingrequirements.htm or Phone number: 770-458-3811)

 Common Questions and Answers

Q: What are the most common causes of food poisoning?
A: Bacteria (*Campylobacter, Salmonella* (nontyphoid), and *E. coli* O157:H7).

Q: How are the signs and symptoms of food poisoning different from a viral gastroenteritis?
A: The signs and symptoms of food poisoning and gastroenteritis are similar in that the patient displays diarrhea, vomiting, and fever. Usually, food poisoning occurs after ingestion of a meal, at which time several people can be affected.

Q: Which foods are most likely to be contaminated?
A: Dairy products that are not refrigerated properly and meat that is not cooked at high enough temperatures.

ICD-9-CM 005.9

BIBLIOGRAPHY

Gastroenterosis. In Pickering L & Snyder JD. *Nelson Textbook of Pediatrics.* 16th Ed. Philadelphia: WB Saunders. 2000, 767–768.

Morbidity and Mortality Weekly Report, CDC. *Diagnosis and Management of Foodborne Illnesses.* 2004;53:RR–4.

Salmonella infections, staphylococcal infections. *2003 Red Book: Report of the Committee on Infectious Diseases.* 26th Ed. Elk Grove Village, IL: American Academy of Pediatrics, 2003, p 810.

Authors: Samuel Maldonado and Andrew E. Mulberg

Frostbite

 Database

DEFINITION

Frostbite is localized injury of the epidermis and underlying tissue resulting from exposure to extreme cold, or contact with extremely cold objects. Distal extremities and unprotected areas (e.g., fingers, toes, ears, nose and chin) are most commonly affected. Frostbite is classified according to severity:

- Superficial, first degree: Partial skin freezing
- Superficial, second degree: Full-thickness skin freezing
- Deep, third degree: Full-thickness skin and subcutaneous tissue freezing
- Deep, fourth degree: Full-thickness skin, subcutaneous tissue, muscle, tendon and bone freezing

A new classification of frostbite severity at day 0 has been proposed based on findings that correlate the extent of the frostbite with the outcome of the involved body part along with the results of bone scans. The 4 degrees of severity are defined as:

- First degree—leads to recovery
- Second degree—leads to soft tissue amputation
- Third degree—leads to bone amputation
- Fourth degree—leads to large amputation with systemic effects

PATHOPHYSIOLOGY

- Tissue damage and cell death result from the initial freeze injury and the inflammatory response that occurs with rewarming.
- Direct cellular damage can occur from frostbite. As the temperature of freezing tissue approaches –2°C, extracellular ice crystals form and cause increased osmotic pressure in the interstitium. This leads to cellular dehydration. As freezing continues, these shrinking, hyperosmolar cells die due to abnormal intracellular electrolyte concentrations. With rapid freezing, intracellular ice crystal formation occurs, resulting in immediate cell death.
- Indirect cellular damage results from progressive microvascular insult. Initial tissue response to extreme cold exposure is vasoconstriction. Blood flow to the extremities is reduced as freezing continues. Ice crystals form in the plasma, blood viscosity increases, and cessation of circulation occurs in the distal extremities, resulting in hypoxia and tissue damage.
- Oxygen-free radicals and inflammatory mediators, especially prostaglandin F2 and thromboxane A2, contribute to tissue injury following rewarming and reperfusion of the damaged tissue.

COMPLICATIONS

- Amputations
- Arthritis
- Changes in skin color
- Chronic pain
- Digital deformities
- Gangrene
- Growth plate abnormalities (only in children)
- Hyperesthesias
- Neuropathy
- Rhabdomyolysis
- Squamous cell carcinoma (rare)
- Tetanus
- Tissue loss
- Wound infection

PROGNOSIS

- Dependent on degree of cold injury
- Favorable indicators: sensation in affected area, healthy-appearing skin color, blisters filled with clear fluid
- Unfavorable indicators: cyanosis, blood-filled blisters, unhealthy-appearing skin

 Differential Diagnosis

- Frostnip: Mild form of cold injury with pallor and painful, tingling sensation. Warming of the cold tissue results in no tissue damage.
- Hypothermia
- Thermal injury: Easily excluded based on history, but can result from warming techniques.

 Data Gathering

HISTORY

Special Questions

- Was there prolonged exposure to cold environment? In frostbite, there is typically a history of prolonged cold exposure.
- Was there contact with a cold object, especially metal? Metal will drain heat from skin through conduction and increase the risk of frostbite.
- What was the timing and duration of exposure?
- Was there any treatment prior to presentation?

Symptoms depend on severity:

- Superficial, first degree: Transient tingling, stinging, and burning followed by throbbing and aching with possible hyperhidrosis
- Superficial, second degree: Numbness with vasomotor disturbances in more severe cases
- Deep, third degree: No sensation initially, followed by shooting pains, burning, throbbing, and aching
- Deep, fourth degree: Absent sensation and muscle function, pain, and joint discomfort

 Physical Examination

- Superficial, first degree: Waxy appearance, erythema, and edema of involved area without blister formation.
- Superficial, second degree: Erythema, significant edema, blisters with clear fluid within 6 to 24 hours. Desquamation may occur with eschar formation 7 to 14 days after initial injury.
- Deep, third degree: Hemorrhagic blisters, necrosis of the skin and subcutaneous tissues, skin discoloration in 5 to 10 days.
- Deep, fourth degree: Initially, little edema with cyanosis or mottling; eventually, complete necrosis, then becomes black, dry, and mummifies; occasionally results in self-amputation.

 Laboratory Aids

TESTS

Laboratory tests usually are not necessary but may be indicated when infection is suspected.

RADIOGRAPHIC STUDIES

- No diagnostic studies done immediately after rewarming can accurately predict the amount of nonviable tissue.
- Radionucleotide angiography with 99m-Tc-pertechnetate or bone scanning with 99m-Tc-methylene diphosphonate 1 to 2 weeks after initial injury is advocated by some to assess tissue viability in cases of third- and fourth-degree frostbite.
- MRI and magnetic resonance angiography are being advocated by some as superior techniques. These techniques allow direct visualization of occluded vessels and tissue giving a more clear-cut demarcation of ischemic tissue injury. This may allow for earlier surgical intervention.

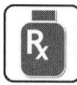 Therapy

IMMEDIATE

- Do not rub the area; this may cause mechanical injury.
- Do not expose the area to direct heat; this may cause burn injury.
- Remove wet clothing and constricting jewelry.

MEDICAL CARE

- Check core temperature to rule out hypothermia, which would need to be addressed first.
- Rapid rewarming in warm water (40° to 42°C) for 15 to 45 minutes. Do not rewarm slowly. Rewarming is complete when skin is soft and sensation returns. Usually this is all that is needed for superficial, first-degree frostbite.

- Apply dry, sterile dressings to affected areas and between frostbitten toes and fingers.
- Drain clear-fluid blisters (thromboxane-containing) to avoid ongoing tissue injury.
- Leave hemorrhagic blisters intact to avoid infection.
- Elevate affected parts to minimize edema.
- Daily hydrotherapy with hexachlorophene or povidone-iodine added to the water.
- Topical application of aloe vera to debrided blisters and intact hemorrhagic blisters to minimize further thromboxane synthesis.
- Tetanus prophylaxis: dT or DT/DTaP, depending on age, and tetanus immunoglobulin if patient is not fully immunized.
- NSAIDs are recommended by some to prevent prostaglandin-induced platelet aggregation and vasoconstriction.
- Analgesics, as indicated.
- Antibiotics: Given prophylactically by some, while others recommend waiting for signs of infection.
- High-protein, high-calorie diet to promote healing.
- Prohibit nicotine because of vasoconstrictive properties.
- Physical therapy after edema resolves.

SURGICAL CARE

- Conservative surgical intervention is recommended because it usually takes 6 to 8 weeks for injured tissue to declare viability.
- Escharotomy is performed on digits with impaired circulation or movement.
- Fasciotomy is performed if significant edema causes a compartment syndrome.
- Early amputation and debridement with closure of the wound site are necessary for uncontrolled infection.
- Debridement of mummified tissue is performed after 1 to 3 months.

FUTURE TREATMENT

Experimental work is being done to identify agents that interrupt vasoconstriction, cell injury, and vascular stasis, and those that inhibit prostaglandins and free radicals.

 Follow-Up

WHEN TO EXPECT IMPROVEMENT

- Superficial, first-degree frostbite heals in a few weeks.
- More severe frostbite needs to be followed closely for signs of infection.
- Physical therapy and rehabilitation are needed with severe frostbite.

PREVENTION

- Avoid prolonged cold exposure whenever possible.
- Dress appropriately for cold weather. Dress in layers: Undergarments should be made of material that absorbs perspiration and prevents heat loss, and outer garments should be windproof and water repellent/proof. Cover head, ears, and neck. Mittens help to conserve heat better than gloves. Footwear should be water repellent and insulated.

PITFALLS

- Refreezing after thawing leads to increased injury.
- Rubbing tissue that is frostbitten increases injury through mechanical injury.

 Common Questions and Answers

Q: What type of clothing can protect my child from getting frostbite?
A: Dress your child in layers of clothes. Their outer garments should be waterproof and windproof and make sure he or she is wearing a hat, scarf, and mittens.

Q: I live in Buffalo, New York, where the winters are very cold and the wind chill factor is often below zero. My children like playing outside, especially in the snow. How can I prevent them from getting frostbite?
A: Since there is a risk of frostbite with a wind chill factor of −25°C, try to encourage indoor play when the temperature dips this low. It is important to have the children come inside frequently during the winter months to warm up, and for you to check for signs of cold injury.

Q: My family members are avid skiers. While traveling in Europe last winter I purchased a protective emollient that was sold there. Can the protective emollients prevent frostbite if used on the face and exposed areas while skiing?
A: No, research has shown that the use of "protective" emollients and creams leads to a false sense of safety and leads to an increased risk of frostbite. This is thought to be mostly due to the lack of using more efficient protective measures when the emollients and creams are used.

Q: If my child has had frostbite in the past, can she or he get it again?
A: Yes, children who have had a previous frostbite injury are at increased risk for repeat injury, especially in the location of previous damage. Appropriate clothing and limitation of cold exposure should be strictly enforced.

Q: To prevent frostbite, is there a temperature below which I should not let my child go out to play?
A: Though body tissue freezes more quickly at lower temperatures, the degree of damage from frostbite is related to the length of time tissue remains frozen. Therefore, the amount of time spent outside during cold weather should never be prolonged.

Q: How can I tell if my child has frostbite or just cold fingers?
A: Cold fingers are red and may be painful but do not become numb or white. Frostbitten fingers are painful, white, and waxy prior to rewarming and turn red with rewarming. The sequential development of digital blanching, occasional cyanosis, and erythema of the fingers or toes following cold exposure and subsequent rewarming is known as Raynaud phenomenon. All types of cold injury should be treated by immersing the fingers in warm water for 15 to 45 minutes. If blisters form or there is no sensation in the fingers, medical care is needed.

Q: If I suspect frostbite in my child and we are outdoors without access to warm water, are there any options for treatment?
A: Of course you and your child should go indoors as soon as possible. If that is not possible, you can start to thaw your child's body part by using your body as a warmer, by placing the exposed body part under your armpit and keeping it there until further care can be initiated. Before starting the rewarming process you must be sure refreezing will not recur.

Q: When should I call the doctor?
A: The doctor should be called if, after rewarming, the skin is not soft and/or sensation does not return to normal. Call the doctor immediately if the skin is discolored and cold, blisters develop during rewarming, or there are signs of infection, such as the appearance of red streaks leading from the affected area, pus accumulation, or fever.

Q: Is frostnip the same thing as frostbite?
A: No, frostnip is the mildest form of cold injury that commonly occurs on exposed parts of the body, such as the fingers, nose, and ears. The symptoms of frostnip are numbness and pallor of the involved body parts. Warming of these areas is the only treatment that is needed, and there is no associated tissue damage.

ICD-9-CM 991.3

BIBLIOGRAPHY

Biem J, et al. Out of the cold: management of hypothermia and frostbite. *CMAJ* 2003;168(3):305–311.

Bracker MD. Environmental and thermal injury. *Clin Sports Med* 1992;2:419–436.

Britt LD, et al. New horizons in management of hypothermia and frostbite injury. *Surg Clin North Am* 1991;71:345–370.

Cauchy E, et al. Retrospective study of 70 cases of severe frostbite lesions: a proposed new classification scheme. *Wilderness Environ Med* 2001;12:248–255.

DeGroot DW, et al. Epidemiology of U.S. Army cold weather injuries, 1980–1999. *Aviat Space Environ Med* 2003;74:564–570.

Holmer I. Work in the cold: review of methods for assessment of cold exposure. *Int Arch Occup Environ Health* 1993;65:147–155.

Lehmuskallio E. Emollients in the prevention of frostbite. *Int J Circumpolar Health* 2000;59:122–130.

Murphy J, et al. Frostbite: pathogenesis and treatment. *J Trauma* 2000;48:171–185.

Author: Denise A. Salerno

Functional Diarrhea of Infancy

 ## Database

DEFINITION

Daily painless recurrent passage of three or more large unformed stools, for more than 4 weeks, with onset between 6 and 36 months. The child is normally active and growing and there is no failure to thrive (if caloric intake is adequate) or passage of stools during sleep. Also known as toddler's diarrhea, chronic nonspecific diarrhea and irritable colon of childhood.

CAUSES

• *Nutritional factors:*

—Excessive consumption of fruit juice (increased sorbitol, fructose) leading to carbohydrate intolerance.
—Diet that is high in fluid but low in fat and fiber.

• *Motility disorder,* i.e., variant of irritable bowel syndrome of infancy.

PATHOPHYSIOLOGY

• Diarrhea is often preceded by acute gastroenteritis or other viral infection that results in dietary restrictions. Increased oral fluids, including juices are used to compensate for stool losses and prevent dehydration.
• Carbohydrate malabsorption causing osmotic diarrhea
• Capacity of small intestine to absorb fructose is limited. Foods that contain equivalent amounts of fructose and glucose are more readily absorbed because of the additive effect of a glucose-dependent fructose cotransport mechanism. An excess of fructose over glucose will result in fructose malabsorption by the small intestine.
• Sorbitol is nonabsorbable and inhibits fructose absorption and may cause gastrointestinal symptoms.
• Excessive intake of juices high in sorbitol and those with a high fructose to glucose ratio will result in fructose malabsorption and gastrointestinal symptoms.
• Colonic function: possibly, there is a disruption of colonic ability to ferment unabsorbed carbohydrates into short chain fatty acids (SCFA) which maintain colonic function and prevent colon-based diarrhea.
• Motility disorder:

—Persistence of immature bowel motility pattern. Failure of initiation of normal postprandial delayed gastric emptying and rapid transit due to persistence of small-bowel fasting motility pattern.
—Meals with high dietary fat delay gastric emptying. This protective mechanism is lost with high-fluid, low-fat meals.

• Low-fiber diet: Dietary fiber (pectin) serves as bulking agent

GENETICS

Family members often report nonspecific gastrointestinal complaints or functional bowel disorders.

EPIDEMIOLOGY

It is the most common cause of prolonged diarrhea without failure to thrive (FTT) in children in the developed world.

PROGNOSIS

Generally good. Carbohydrate-containing fluids contribute to unbalanced nutrition, non-organic failure to thrive, and also to short stature and obesity.

 ## Differential Diagnosis

All causes of chronic diarrhea should be considered:

• Infection:

—Intestinal: bacterial, viral, fungal (giardiasis*, cryptosporidiosis*)
—Nonintestinal: Urinary tract infection

• Pancreatic: cystic fibrosis*, Shwachman-Diamond syndrome, Johannson-Blizzard syndrome, chronic pancreatitis
• Bile acid disorders: chronic cholestasis, terminal ileum disease, bacterial overgrowth*
• Carbohydrate malabsorption: Post infectious-secondary lactose intolerance, sucrase-isomaltase deficiency
• Immunologic: celiac disease*, cow's and soy protein intolerance*, food allergy* (multiple), immunodeficiency, AIDS enteropathy
• Miscellaneous: antibiotics, laxatives, fecal retention constipation*, abetalipoproteinemia, inflammatory bowel disease, short bowel syndrome, hormone secreting tumors like vasoactive intestinal peptide (VIP)-oma, neuroblastoma, Munchausen-by-proxy.

*—**More common conditions to be considered** Most of the diseases listed above cause morbidity and malnutrition. A thorough clinical history, a simple physical examination and limited number of laboratory tests should make an obvious diagnosis of functional diarrhea. It is not a diagnosis of exclusion.

 ## Data Gathering

HISTORY

Question: Nutritional history?
Significance: Essential with attention to the "four Fs": fiber, fluid, fat, and fruit juices

Question: Diarrhea?
Significance: For a toddler it may not be abnormal to have more than three soft and occasionally loose stools a day with visible food remnants.

Question: Stool characteristics?
Significance: Stools foul smelling and contain undigested food particles, with shortened colonic transit time. Presence of blood or mucus suggests another diagnosis.

Question: Timing of diarrhea?
Significance: No stools passed at night and typically the first stool of the day is large and has better consistency than those occurring later on in the day.

Question: Are other children affected?
Significance: Presence of other affected family members or day-care mates makes infectious etiology more likely.

 ## Physical Examination

Normal, children are healthy appearing, eat well, and are growing normally, although weight might be influenced by the dietary measures.

 ## Laboratory Aids

Test: Stool tests and culture
Significance: Negative for white blood cells, blood and pathogens

Test: Infectious workup
Significance: Negative

Test: Breath hydrogen tests?
Significance: Usually of limited benefit.

Test: Complete blood count (CBC) normal
Significance: No anemia

Test: Serum electrolytes normal
Significance: No dehydration

Therapy

Reassurance on underlying gastrointestinal diseases and normalization of diet.

DIET

• The child's feeding pattern should be normalized according to the "four Fs":

—Overconsumption of fruit juices should be discouraged, especially those that contain sorbitol and a high fructose-to-glucose ratio (apple juice for example).
—Fiber intake should be normalized by introduction of whole meal bread and fruits.
—Increase dietary fat to at least 35% to 40% of total energy intake. Substitution of low-fat milk with whole milk may be sufficient.
—Restrict fluid intake to less than 150 cc/kg/day, and fruit juices to less than 12oz/day.
—Improvement occurs within a few days to a couple of weeks after initiating the above therapy. Parental reassurance is confirmed by good response to dietary therapy.

PREVENTION

Vicious cycle may be initiated after acute gastroenteritis and food restrictions. Parents should be instructed to give an oral rehydration solution (ORS) and resume normal feeding early.

MEDICATIONS

Loperamide is effective in normalizing bowel patterns but only as long as they are given. Medications seem unwarranted for a condition with mostly nutritional etiology that does not hamper growth.

REFERRAL

• Failure of response to the above therapy
• Weight loss despite adequate intake
• Presence of other symptoms like anorexia, irritability, fever, and vomiting
• Blood and mucus in diarrhea

TESTS TO PREPARE FOR CONSULTATION

• Sweat chloride
• Celiac disease panel (antiendomysial antibodies, tissue transglutaminase antibodies, with IgA serum levels)
• Serum albumin
• ESR
• Stool Sudan III stain for fecal fat.

SPECIAL INSIGHTS

• Good history is required because all the illnesses in the differential diagnosis are associated with morbidity, if diagnosis is delayed.
• Consider constipation, if diarrhea alternates with normal or hard stools. KUB will show colonic fecal retention.
• Need to make follow-up phone call to parents within a few days of instituting diet. If no improvement within a week despite good compliance with dietary recommendations, then rethink diagnosis and consider referral to a specialist.
• Improvement with dietary changes confirms the diagnosis and also reassures the parents.

Common Questions and Answers

Q: Is growth normal in a patient with toddler's diarrhea?
A: Growth is usually normal; weight may be mildly influenced by the prior dietary practices and measures, and failure to thrive has also been reported recently.

Q: What are the components of a successful treatment plan?
A: Attention to the "four Fs": decreased fruit juice intake, increased fat intake, decreased fluid, and increased fiber intake

Q: When should care by a pediatric gastroenterologist be sought?
A: If no response after 2 weeks of compliance with dietary therapy, growth delay or other gastrointestinal or systemic complaints

ICD-9-CM 787.91

564.5 (Functional Diarrhea)

BIBLIOGRAPHY

Dennison BA. Fruit juice consumption by infants and children: a review. *J Am Coll Nutr* 1996;15(5 suppl):4S–11S.

Ghishan FK. Chronic Diarrhea. In: Behrman RE, Kliegman RM, Jenson HB, eds. *Nelson Textbook of Pediatrics*. Philadelphia: Saunders, 2004:1276–83.

Hamdi I, Dodge JA. Toddler diarrhea: observations on the effects of aspirin and loperamide. *J Pediatr Gastroenterol Nutr* 1985;4:362–365.

Hoekstra JH. Toddler diarrhea: more a nutritional disorder than a disease. *Arch Dis Child* 1998;79(1):2–5.

Hoekstra JH, Van den Aker JHL, Kneepkens CMF, et al. Evaluation of $^{13}CO_2$ breath tests for the detection of fructose malabsorption. *J Lab Clin Med* 1996;127(3):303–309.

Huffman S. Toddler's diarrhea. *J Pediatr Health Care* 1999;13(1):32–33.

Kneepkens CMF, Hoekstra JH. Chronic nonspecific diarrhea of childhood. *Pediatr Clin North Am* 1996;43:375–390.

Lifshitz F, Ament ME, Kleinman RE, et al. Role of juice carbohydrate malabsorption in chronic nonspecific diarrhea in children. *J Pediatr* 1992;120:825–829.

Rasquin-Weber A, Hyman PE, Cucchiara S, et al. Childhood functional gastrointestinal disorders. *Gut* 1999;45(supp II):II60–II68.

Authors: Vered Yehezkely-Schildkraut and Raanan Shamir

Fungal Skin Infections (Dermatophyte Infections, Candidiasis, and Tinea Versicolor)

Database

DEFINITION
• Superficial mycoses (fungal infection) involving the skin, hair, or nails usually characterized by scaling, erythema and/or change in skin pigmentation.

ETIOLOGY
• Dermatophyte infections
—Tinea capitis: >90% *Trichophyton tonsurans* in North America; *Microsporum canis* is a predominant organism in other geographic regions.
—Nonhairy sites: *M. canis, T. tonsurans, T. rubrum, M. audouinii*
• Candidiasis: Usually *Candida albicans*
• Tinea versicolor: *Malassezia furfur* (also called *Pityrosporum ovale*)

PATHOPHYSIOLOGY
• Fungal elements penetrate skin, hair shaft, or nail.
• Predisposing factors may include moisture, macerated skin, and immune compromise.
• Fungistatic fatty acids in sebum after puberty may offer protection against tinea capitis.
• Host immune response is usually able to contain infection.
• Inflammatory response is variable; highly inflammatory forms may lead to pustular lesions and kerion (a large inflammatory mass) formation.

GENETICS
• Frequency and severity of infection are possibly determined by unclear genetic factors.
• Increased glycogen granules in the normal skin of patients with tinea versicolor suggest an underlying disorder or genetic predisposition.

EPIDEMIOLOGY
• Dermatophyte infections
—Etiology varies by geographic region.
—Tinea capitis is most common in prepubertal children and African-American children, with a peak age of about 4 years. Incidence has increased over the past decade.
—Tinea corporis is usually seen in younger children; tinea cruris, tinea pedis, and *onychomycosis* are uncommon in preadolescent children.
—Fomites and pets may be a source of infection. Cats and dogs are a major source of *M. canis*.
• Candidiasis: Vast majority of infants colonized with *C. albicans*.
• Tinea versicolor: Usually seen in adolescents and young adults

COMPLICATIONS
• Dermatophyte infections
• Secondary bacterial infection (which may obscure the diagnosis of dermatophyte infection)
• Kerion may lead to scarring alopecia.
• Candidiasis
—Scarring in severe disease
—Fungemia in immunocompromised host

Differential Diagnosis

• Dermatophyte infections
—Dermatologic conditions
—Tinea capitis: Seborrheic dermatitis, psoriasis, alopecia areata, trichotillomania, folliculitis, impetigo, atopic dermatitis
—Tinea corporis: Herald patch of pityriasis rosea, nummular eczema, psoriasis, contact dermatitis, tinea versicolor, granuloma annulare
—Systemic diseases: Cutaneous T-cell lymphoma, histiocytosis, primary skin cancer, sarcoid
• Candidiasis
—Dermatologic conditions: Contact dermatitis, seborrheic dermatitis, atopic dermatitis, bacterial infection
—Systemic diseases: Acrodermatitis enteropathica, histiocytosis
• Tinea versicolor
—Dermatologic conditions: pityriasis alba, postinflammatory hypopigmentation, vitiligo, seborrheic dermatitis, pityriasis rosea

PROGNOSIS
• Relapses and recurrences are not uncommon.
• Areas with a significant inflammatory component may lead to scarring and permanent alopecia.

Data Gathering

HISTORY
• Onset is usually gradual, except for candidal diaper rash, which is often abrupt
• Usually pruritic
• Contacts including exposure to pets
• Immunocompromised state
• Medications

Physical Examination

DERMATOPHYTE INFECTIONS
• Tinea corporis:
—Skin lesions usually annular, hence the term ringworm; may be flesh-colored, erythematous, or violet to brown in color
—Highly inflammatory forms may be frankly pustular.
—Lesions may occur anywhere on the body.
• Tinea capitis may have various presentations:
—Round to oval patches of alopecia with erythema
—Seborrheic dermatitis-like pattern with minimal or no alopecia
—Follicular pustules with crusting, resembling bacterial folliculitis
—Boggy, tender plaque with follicular pustules (kerion)
—Diffusely, dry scalp

—Presence of occipital lymphadenopathy may be more likely in tinea capitis.
• Onychomycosis
—White, yellow, or silvery discoloration of lateral border or distal portion of nail
—Nail eventually becomes discolored, thickened, and deformed.
—Affects toes more often than fingers
• Candidiasis
—Diffuse erythema (often "beefy" red)
—Raised edge with a sharp margin
—Pustulovesicular, satellite lesions
—Prefers dark, warm, moist environments; favors skin folds/creases (axillae, groin, below the breasts, and in infants, the diaper area)
• Tinea versicolor
—Scaling, oval macular patches
—Hypo or hyperpigmented, depending on sunlight exposure and complexion
—Distributed on upper trunk, neck, and proximal arms (high amount of sebum and free fatty acids, which the organism requires); occasionally occurs on the face

Laboratory Aids

TESTS
Diagnosis is usually made by characteristic lesions; if in doubt, may do Wood's lamp examination, potassium hydroxide (KOH) preparation, or fungal culture.

Wood's Lamp Examination (Short-Wave Ultraviolet Light)
• Examine in a completely darkened room.
• Dermatophytes: Hair infections caused by *Microsporum* species will give a green fluorescence but *Trichophyton* does not fluoresce; not helpful for skin or nail infections.
• Tinea versicolor: Yellow, coppery-orange, or bronze fluorescence.

KOH Preparation
• Clean the site with alcohol.
• Scrape the lesion along the scaling edge with a blade; obtain material from hair follicles and crusts.
• Place material on glass slide with one drop of 10% KOH.
• Warm the slide gently or let it sit for 30 minutes.
• Place a cover slip on the slide.
• Examine the slide under the microscope at low power under low light. Look for the following findings:
—Dermatophytes: Arthrospores around or within hair shaft; long branching hyphae for skin infections
—*Candidiasis*: Budding yeast, pseudohyphae
—Tinea versicolor: Hyphae and spores ("spaghetti and meatballs")

Fungal Culture
• Obtain a specimen with scalpel blade as described above.
• For the scalp, a sample obtained by rubbing a toothbrush over the dry scalp or area of concern can be plated on the appropriate media.

Fungal Skin Infections (Dermatophyte Infections, Candidiasis, and Tinea Versicolor)

- Results are available in several weeks.
- Some laboratories offer susceptibilities in addition to identification of fungus.
- It may be difficult to distinguish normal skin colonization from infection.

 Therapy

DRUGS

Dermatophyte Infections

- Tinea capitis
—First line: Griseofulvin 15 to 25 mg/kg once daily, taken with high-fat food (e.g., milk or ice cream) for 6 to 12 weeks; concomitant therapy of 2.5% selenium sulfide shampoo twice weekly will suppress viable spores and decrease spread. Side effects include vomiting, diarrhea, headache and photosensitivity.
—Second line: Itraconazole 3 to 5 mg/kg once daily for 4 to 6 weeks. May also use terbinafine 3 to 6 mg/kg per day for 2 to 4 weeks. May be associated with hepatic failure; should not be used in patients with underlying liver disease. Strongly consider liver enzymes before and during treatment.
- Tinea capitis with kerion: Treat as tinea capitis; may require oral steroids if significant inflammation is present.
- Tinea corporis
—Drug of choice: Topical imidazole (clotrimazole 1%, ketokonazole 2%) or terbinafine 1% cream applied twice daily for 2 to 4 weeks.
—Oral griseofulvin 15 to 25 mg/kg per day for 4 weeks may be used for persistent or extensive involvement.
- Onychomycosis
—Itraconazole in weekly pulses for 3 to 4 months is effective; 200 mg twice daily for 7 days, then off for 3 weeks.
—Terbinafine 3 to 6 mg/kg per day for 6 to 12 weeks. May be associated with hepatic failure; should not be used in patients with underlying liver disease. Strongly consider liver enzymes before and during treatment.

Candidiasis

- Topical nystatin cream or ointment three to four times daily for 7 to 10 days.
- Oral fluconazole (6 mg/kg on day 1 then 3 mg/kg daily for 2 weeks) may be used if poor response to topical therapy.

Tinea Versicolor

- Selenium sulfide 2.5% applied to the affected skin for 10 minutes. Wash off thoroughly. Monthly applications may help prevent recurrences.
- Topical imidazoles are effective but more expensive.
- Oral ketoconazole 200 to 400 mg per day for 5 to 10 days, or itraconazole 200 mg per day for 5 to 7 days may be used if extensive, recurrent, or persistent.

POSSIBLE CONFLICTS WITH OTHER TREATMENTS

Many antifungals have drug interactions. Consult a reference (e.g., *Physician's Desk Reference*) when prescribing them to a patient already on medication.

 Follow-Up

WHEN TO EXPECT IMPROVEMENT

- Dermatophyte: Inflammation should improve within several days, but may take several weeks to completely resolve; nail infections may take 6 to 12 months to show improvement.
- Candidal skin lesions improve within 24 to 48 hours and resolve by 1 week.
- Tinea versicolor may take weeks to improve; repigmentation may take months and requires exposure to sunlight.

SIGNS TO WATCH FOR

- Watch for signs of secondary bacterial infection.
- Highly inflammatory lesions may require systemic steroids.

PREVENTION

- Children should be discouraged from sharing clothing (especially hats).
- Hair utensils and hats should be washed in hot, soapy water at the onset of therapy.
- Pets should be watched and treated early for any suspicious lesions.
- Isolation of the hospitalized patient is not necessary.

PITFALLS

- Tinea capitis requires systemic therapy.
- Application of topical steroids will decrease inflammation and may mask infection ("tinea incognito"). Use only mild steroids, if necessary.
- Repeated infection may indicate a source that needs to be diagnosed and treated (e.g., family member or pet).
- Systemic therapies associated with elevated hepatic enzymes and hepatic failure. Terbinafine should not be used in patients with underlying liver disease.

 Common Questions and Answers

Q: What is the role of topical and systemic steroids in the treatment of dermatophyte infections?
A: Topical corticosteroids may be helpful with antifungal therapy to reduce inflammation for skin infections. Only mildly potent steroids should be used. Combination products containing a potent corticosteroid and an antifungal should be avoided, especially in the diaper area, where absorption may be increased. For tinea capitis, significant inflammation and kerion formation may benefit from a short course of systemic

steroids. Reducing the inflammation with steroids may help prevent scarring alopecia.

Q: What can be done to prevent recurrent tinea versicolor in an adolescent?
A: *M. furfur* is a ubiquitous organism and is present on the skin of postpubertal individuals. Humid environments, excessive sweating, and unclear genetic factors result in infection. Recurrences are common and can be prevented by monthly application of selenium sulfide 2.5%.

Q: What is the role of the newer antifungal agents in the treatment of tinea capitis?
A: Griseofulvin has long been considered the gold standard for the treatment of tinea capitis due to its efficacy and safety profile. Development of resistance to griseofulvin has required the use of larger doses and longer courses. This increases the likelihood of noncompliance and treatment failures. In addition, longer courses increase the cost of griseofulvin therapy. The newer antifungals, terbinafine and itraconazole offer some advantages over griseofulvin. Concentration of these drugs in nails and hair may allow for shorter courses of therapy, with improved compliance and lower cost than griseofulvin. Fluconazole has also been used for treatment of dermatophyte infections. It is available in a liquid formulation and is already FDA approved for treatment of candidal infections in children. Although still considered by many to be the preferred drug for tinea capitis, griseofulvin is likely to be replaced by these newer antifungals as experience with their use increases.

ICD-9-CM

Dermatophyte 110.9

Candidiasis 112.9

Tinea Versicolor 111.0

BIBLIOGRAPHY

Elewski BE. Tinea capitis: a current perspective. *J Am Acad Dermatol* 2000;42:1–20.

Friedlander SF. The evolving role of itraconazole, fluconazole and terbinafine in the treatment of tinea capitis. *Pediatr Infect Dis J* 1999;18:205–210.

Goldgeier M. Fungal infections of the skin, hair and nails. *Pediatr Ann* 1993;22:253–259.

Gupta AK, et al. The efficacy and safety of terbinafine in children. *Dermatologic Clinics* 2003;21:511–520.

Gupta AK, et al. The use of fluconazole to treat superficial fungal infections in children. *Dermatologic Clinics* 2003;21:537–542.

Skin disorders due to fungi. In: Hurwitz S. *Clinical Pediatric Dermatology*. 2nd Ed. Philadelphia: WB Saunders, 1993; 372–390.

Author: William R. Graessle

Gastritis

Database

DEFINITION

Gastritis is microscopic inflammation of the mucosa of the stomach. It is the most common cause of upper gastrointestinal tract hemorrhage in older children.

CAUSES

- *Helicobacter pylori* (children more likely to have more severe gastritis, specifically located in antrum of stomach)
- Physiologic stress (e.g., in central nervous system [CNS] disease, intensive care unit [ICU] patients, overwhelming sepsis)
- Major surgery, severe burns, renal, liver, respiratory failure, severe trauma
- Idiopathic
- Caustic ingestions (e.g., lye, strong acids, pine oil)
- Drug-induced (e.g., nonsteroidal antiinflammatory drugs [NSAIDs], steroids, valproate). More rarely, iron, calcium salts, potassium chloride, and antibiotics.
- Ethanol
- Protein sensitivity (e.g., cow's milk protein allergy), allergic enteropathy
- Eosinophilic gastroenteritis
- Crohn disease (up to 40% of Crohn patients have gastroduodenal involvement; gastric Crohn may manifest as highly focal, non *H. pylori*, nongranulomatous gastritis)
- Infection (e.g., tuberculosis, *H. pylori*, cytomegalovirus, parasites)

Less Common Causes

- Radiation
- Hypertrophic gastritis (Ménétrier disease)
- Autoimmune gastritis
- Zollinger-Ellison syndrome
- Vascular injury
- Direct trauma (nasogastric tubes)

EPIDEMIOLOGY

- One of the most frequent GI diagnoses
- 8 out of every 1,000 people
- >2% ICU patients have heavy bleeding secondary to gastritis

COMPLICATIONS

- Bleeding (from mild to hemorrhagic)
- When gastritis caused by acid/alkali ingestions, outlet obstruction may result from prepyloric strictures (4 to 8 weeks after ingestion)

Differential Diagnosis of Epigastric Abdominal Pain

- Gastroesophageal reflux with esophagitis
- Peptic ulcer disease
- Biliary tract disorders
- Pancreatitis
- Inflammatory bowel disease
- Genitourinary pathology (renal stones, infection)
- Nonulcer dyspepsia
- Functional pain

Data Gathering

HISTORY

- Epigastric pain
- Abdominal indigestion
- Nausea
- Vomiting postprandially
- Vomiting blood or coffee-ground like material
- Diarrhea
- Dark or black stools (or bright red blood per rectum, if bleeding is brisk and intestinal transit time is short)
- Irritability
- Poor feeding and weight loss
- Less often: chest pain, hematemesis, or melena

Physical Examination

- Epigastric tenderness upper left quadrant
- Normal bowel sounds

Laboratory Aids

TESTS

- Heme-test all stools.
- Anemia with other signs of chronic blood loss on CBC (e.g., microcytosis, low reticulocyte count)
- *H. pylori* identification

—Noninvasive *H. pylori* tests, including antibody (from serum, whole blood, saliva, or urine), antigen (from stool), or urea breath testing (UBT). The UBT and stool antigen tests are more reliable and sensitive than antibody testing; serologic testing is not recommended. Rapid urease test from gastric biopsy specimen for *H. pylori*

—Silver stain, Genta stain, modified Giemsa stain, or cresyl violet stain of gastric biopsy for *H. pylori*

—Culture of homogenized gastric biopsy for *H. pylori* (difficult to perform outside of research setting)

PROCEDURES

- Upper endoscopy with biopsies: sensitivity greatest
- Findings that may be seen on upper endoscopy:

—Edema around small ulcers
—Thickened hyperemic mucosa
—Atrophic mucosa
—Antral micronodules (represent lymphoid follicles) commonly seen in *H. pylori* infected children

- When endoscopy not available, upper GI radiography
- Chest x-ray may detect free abdominal air secondary to perforated ulcer (rare)

Gastritis

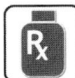 **Therapy**

DRUGS

• Antacids or H2 blockers to maintain gastric pH greater than 4–5

—Ranitidine, 2 to 3 mg/kg/dose b.i.d. to t.i.d. in children
—Cimetidine, 10 mg/kg/dose q.i.d. (can be used prophylactically for hospitalized patients at risk for bleeding)
—Famotidine, 0.5 to 2 mg/kg per day divided twice
—Omeprazole, lansoprazole, rabeprazole, esomeprazole

• Misoprostol may reduce risk of the progression of gastritis to ulcers in NSAID patients.
• Discontinue NSAIDs.

DIET

• Benefit of changes in diet is inconclusive.
• Eliminate alcohol, tobacco, and caffeine.
• For stress gastritis with hemorrhage, provide vigilant supportive care with close monitoring of hemodynamics, fluids, and electrolytes

H. PYLORI

—Triple therapy with proton pump inhibitor, i.e., PPI plus amoxicillin and clarithromycin
—If eradication is unsuccessful, quadruple therapy is recommended, including bismuth (of note, may need to avoid bismuth subsalicylate and choose instead bismuth subcitrate), metronidazole, a proton pump inhibitor, and another antibiotic (either amoxicillin, clarithromycin, or tetracycline) for 7–14 days.
—Drug regimens change frequently, and only tested regimens should be used.

 Follow-Up

• Monitor for hemoccult-positive stools.
• Follow complete blood counts.
• May elect to repeat endoscopy in severe cases.

PITFALLS

• Many antacids are not palatable to children and can lead to diarrhea or constipation. Prolonged use of large doses of aluminum hydroxide containing antacids may lead to phosphate depletion and aluminum-related CNS toxicity (particularly in patients with renal disease).
• Cimetidine may be associated with drug-drug interactions when given to patients receiving other medicines metabolized by the cytochrome P-450 system (e.g., theophylline).
• Significant gastritis relapse rates for children who remain infected with *H. pylori*
• If *H. pylori* eradication is attempted, it is important to use a tested regimen. Untested substitutions in the triple or quadruple regimens should be avoided.

 Common Questions and Answers

Q: Will a bland diet help to resolve gastritis?
A: Dietary changes have not been shown to affect the natural course of gastritis.

Q: What is *Helicobacter pylori*?
A: *H. pylori* is a bacterium frequently found in the gastric mucosa of patients with gastritis and peptic ulcer disease, and can be diagnosed by a variety of means, often including a combination of upper endoscopy and urea breath tests. Relapse rates for gastritis secondary to this cause are high (when the infection is left untreated). It is important to treat only confirmed *H. pylori* infections, not to treat on suspicion of infection.

ICD-9-CM 558.9

BIBLIOGRAPHY

Drumm B, et al. *Helicobacter pylori* infection in children: a consensus statement. European Paediatric Task Force on Helicobacter pylori. *J Pediatr Gastroenterol Nutr* 2000;30(2): 207–213.

Malaty HM. *Helicobacter pylori* infection and eradication in pediatric patients. *Paediatr Drugs* 2000;2(5):357–365.

Weinstein, W M. Emerging gastritides. *Curr Gastroenterol Rep* 2001;3(6):523–527.

Zheng P-Y, Jones NL. Recent advances in *Helicobacter pylori* infection in children: from the petri dish to the playground. *Can J Gastro* 2003;17:448–454.

Zimmermann AE, et al. A review of omeprazole use in the treatment of acid-related disorders in children. *Clin Ther* 2001;23(5):660–679.

Author: Kathleen Graham Lomax

ICD9 CODE	DESCRIPTION
535	Gastritis and duodenitis
535.0	Acute gastritis
535.00	Acute gastritis (without mention of hemorrhage)
535.01	Acute gastritis with hemorrhage
535.1	Atrophic gastritis
535.10	Atrophic gastritis (without mention of hemorrhage)
535.11	Atrophic gastritis with hemorrhage
535.4	Other specified gastritis
535.40	Other specified gastritis (without mention of hemorrhage)
535.41	Other specified gastritis with hemorrhage
535.5	Unspecified gastritis and gastroduodenitis
535.50	Unspecified gastritis and gastroduodenitis (without mention of hemorrhage)
535.51	Unspecified Gastritis and gastroduodenitis with hemorrhage
041.86	Helicobacter pylori (*H. pylori*) infection

Gastroesophageal Reflux

 Database

DEFINITION

Gastroesophageal reflux is an effortless regurgitation of gastric contents. Gastroesophageal reflux (GER) occurs physiologically at all ages, and most episodes are brief and asymptomatic. It is important to identify the rare child with pathologic reflux, to perform the appropriate diagnostic studies, and to start effective therapy.

• GER is divided into a pathologic and a physiologic process. Physiologic reflux (the normal GER of infancy) is the more common form. Most infants eventually outgrow the symptoms by the end of the first year of life. Pathologic reflux is defined by increased number of reflux episodes according to age-accepted norms and often includes complications such as esophagitis, esophageal stricture, failure to thrive, or chronic/recurrent respiratory tract disease.
• Signs/symptoms of complicated GER:

—Irritability
—Chest/abdominal pain
—Heartburn
—Blood loss
—Dysphagia
—Food refusal
—Cough, wheezing
—Obstructive apnea
—Dysphonia
—Aspiration pneumonia.
—Other complications that are suspected include chronic or recurrent otitis media and sinusitis. GER may be asymptomatic and still carry the risk of complications.

 Differential Diagnosis

Not all pediatric vomiting is reflux. Other causes of vomiting include:

• Infection

—Gastroenteritis
—Urinary tract infection
—Sepsis

• Neurologic

—Meningitis/encephalitis
—Intracranial injury
—Brain tumor
—Hydrocephalus
—Subdural hematoma

• Metabolic

—Uremia
—Aminoacidopathies
—Adrenal hyperplasia
—Phenylketonuria
—Galactosemia

• Food intolerance

—Milk/soy protein allergy
—Celiac disease

• Anatomic malformation

—Gastric-outlet obstruction
—Pyloric stenosis
—Volvulus/malrotation
—Esophageal atresia
—Meconium ileus
—Enteral duplications
—Intussusception
—Trichobezoar

DRUGS THAT AFFECT LOWER ESOPHAGEAL SPHINCTER PRESSURE

• Nitrates
• Nicotine
• Narcotics
• Caffeine
• Theophylline
• Anticholinergic
• Estrogen
• Somatostatin
• Prostaglandins

 Data Gathering

HISTORY

GER in the Infant

• Pay attention to feeding volume and frequency in addition to weight gain and FTT and irritability.
• Should identify episodes of pneumonia, obstructive apnea, chronic cough, laryngitis, stridor, and wheezing.
• Should identify additional signs/symptoms to suggest formula allergy (rash, diarrhea, hematochezia, irritability, FTT).
• Should exclude evidence of bowel obstruction (bilious emesis, polyhydramnios during pregnancy).
• If the vomiting is atypical or associated with other signs/symptoms, it is important to rule out infection, metabolic disease, or neurologic disease.

Special Questions

• Presence of polyhydramnios or bilious emesis?
• Family history of metabolic disease?
• Family history of allergies/atopy?
• Perinatal asphyxia (and other neurologic disorders)?
• History of prematurity?

GER in the Older Child

• Identify typical adult GERD complaints (chest pain, heartburn, regurgitation, dysphagia) but recognize that children describe discomfort poorly (isolated abdominal pain).
• Identify episodes of pneumonia, choking, chronic cough, laryngitis, stridor, and wheezing.
• Should consider evidence suggesting food allergy (rash, diarrhea, growth failure, reactive airways disease).

Special Questions

• Family history of GERD?
• Family history of allergies/atopy?

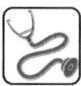 Physical Examination

• May be normal
• Growth failure
• Blood in the stool
• Reactive airways disease and other manifestations of pulmonary complications
• Anemia
• Erosive dental (molar) disease

 Laboratory Aids

TESTS

Diagnosis of GER is made clinically. Testing is needed to identify potential causes or complications. Evaluation should include:

• Stool hemoccult
• Growth parameters

Radiographic Studies

• Barium swallow or upper GI series; tracheoesophageal fistulogram
• Chest radiography
• Milk scan/gastric emptying study
• Salivagram

pH Probe

The gold standard for the evaluation of reflux; represents 24 hours of patient's life and attempts to correlate acid GER with symptoms

• Simple (single-channel)
• Double-channel
• Combined pH/multichannel intraluminal impedance (MII); new technology that allows detection of both acid and nonacid GER events; normative data pending; will surpass standard pH monitoring as gold standard test
• pH/Thermistor (apnea) study

Endoscopy

• Esophagogastroduodenoscopy (EGD)
• Laryngoscopy
• Bronchoscopy

Manometric Studies

• Esophageal manometry
• Antroduodenal manometry

Therapy

Several modes of therapy are available, depending on the severity, duration of reflux, and complications. The treatment should be individualized and should consider cost effectiveness.

Conservative Therapy

- Small frequent feeds
- Thickening of the feeds (approximately 1 tablespoon cereal/ounce of formula)
- Positioning: Head elevation
- Consider use of a hypoallergenic formula for patients with associated food allergy
- Dietary restrictions in older child: Caffeine, chocolate, acidic/spicy food, peppermint

Pharmacologic Therapy

- H2 blockers—for initial therapy of pain, esophagitis or respiratory complications; low incidence of side effects and few medication interactions

—Ranitidine (Zantac), 2 to 3 mg/kg per dose bid to t.i.d.
—Famotidine (Pepcid), 0.3 to 0.5 mg/kg per dose b.i.d.

- Proton pump inhibitors (PPIs)—for symptoms refractory to H2 blockers or severe esophagitis; uncommon side-effects include headache, abdominal pain, and diarrhea

—Omeprazole (Prilosec): 1.5 to 3.5 mg/kg per day divided b.i.d.
—Lansoprazole (Prevacid): <10 kg, 7.5 mg daily; 10–30 kg, 15 mg 1 to 2 times a day; >30 kg, 30 mg 1 to 2 times a day

- Prokinetics—as adjunctive therapy for more severe GER complications or emesis; there is no single drug that has optimal prokinetic effect and minimal side effects

—Metoclopramide (Reglan), 0.1 mg/kg per dose q.i.d.; may cause dystonia or oculogyric crisis
—Cisapride use has been aborted in the United States but a limited access program is available for special situations

- Antacids

—Require multiple dosing, carry risk of diarrhea and aluminum toxicity, and may also lead to malabsorption of other medications

- Mucosal protective agents

—Sucralfate (Carafate): For erosive esophagitis; maximally effective at pH 4 and on mucosal lesions

SURGERY AND REFLUX

- Fundoplication—The goal of surgery is to increase lower esophageal sphincter tone by wrapping a portion of the gastric fundus around the lower esophagus to provide for a more effective barrier to GER. Variations may include the addition of a gastric-emptying procedure (i.e., pyloroplasty) or gastrostomy placement.
- The indications for surgery include failure of aggressive medical management in patients with severe complications (i.e., esophageal stricture, large and symptomatic hiatal hernia, high-grade intestinal metaplastic changes, as in Barrett esophagus).
- Complications of fundoplication include intractable retching, bowel obstruction, dumping syndrome, dysphagia, paraesophageal hernia, and wrap failure with recurrent GER. The surgery has greater morbidity associated with it in the cohort of children with severe physical and mental disabilities.

Common Questions and Answers

Q: How long will my baby suffer with GER?
A: Most infantile reflux resolve by 9 to 12 months of age but symptoms may persist up to 24 months. If GER continues after 2 to 3 years, it is more likely to clinically behave as adult GERD.

Q: Should all babies with reflux be treated with medication?
A: No. Conservative treatments such as thickened feedings, frequent small feeds, and upright head position should be attempted first.

Q: What are the long-term effects of giving my child antireflux medications?
A: Although the effect of long-term acid suppression remains unknown, most medications used to treat GER are quite safe. One must also recognize that untreated reflux has the potential to lead to serious complications, so when considering safety, the option of not treating reflux may be the more dangerous course of action.

ICD-9-CM 530.81

BIBLIOGRAPHY

Boyle JT, et al. Do children with gastroesophageal reflux become adults with gastroesophageal reflux? What is the role of acid suppression in children. *J Pediatr Gastroenterol Nutr* 2003;37(Suppl 1): S65–S68.

Colletti RB, Di Lorenzo C. Overview of pediatric gastroesophageal reflux disease and proton pump inhibitor. *J Pediatr Gastroenterol Nutr* 2003;37(Suppl 1):S7–S11.

Israel DM, Hassall E. Omeprazole and other proton pump inhibitors: pharmacology, efficacy and safety, with special reference to use in children. *J Pediatr Gastroenterol Nutr* 1998;27:568–579.

Jolley S, Halpem L, Tunnell W, et al. The risk of sudden infant death from gastroesophageal reflux. *J Pediatr Surg* 1991;26:691–696.

McGuirt WF Jr. Gastroesophageal reflux and the upper airway. *Pediatr Clin North Am* 2003;50(2):487–502.

Orenstein SR. Gastroesophageal reflux. *Curr Probl Pediatr* 1991;5:193–241.

Orenstein SR. Gastroesophageal reflux. In: Wyllie R, Hyams J, eds. *Pediatric Gastrointestinal Diseases.* Philadelphia: WB Saunders, 1993:337–369.

Pashankar D, Blair GK, Israel DM, et al. Omeprazole maintenance therapy for gastroesophageal reflux disease after failure of fundoplication. *J Pediatr Gastroenterol Nutr* 2000;32:145–149.

Spitz L, et al. Gastroesophageal reflux. *Semin Pediatr Surg* 2003;12(4):237–240.

Vandenplas Y, and the ESPGHAN cisapride panel. Current pediatric indications for cisapride. *J Pediatr Gastroenterol Nutr* 2000;31:480–489.

Authors: Stephen E. Shaffer
Dror Wasserman, 3rd edition

German Measles (Third Disease Rubella)

 Database

DEFINITION

Rubella is derived from Latin, meaning "little red," and was initially considered a variant of measles. Infection is characterized by mild symptoms (often subclinical), with an erythematous rash progressing from head to toes. Prevention of congenital rubella syndrome (see below) is the main objective of vaccination programs.

CAUSE

Rubella virus is classified in the togavirus family as from the genus *Rubivirus*.

• It is an RNA virus with a single antigenic type.
• It was first isolated in 1962 by Parkman and Weller.

PATHOPHYSIOLOGY

• Respiratory transmission
• Replication in the nasopharynx and regional lymph nodes
• Viremia 5 to 7 days after exposure with spread of the virus throughout the body
• In congenital rubella syndrome (CRS), transplanted infection of the fetus occurs during viremia.

EPIDEMIOLOGY

• Spread person to person via airborne transmission; a worldwide infection
• In temperate regions, incidence peaks in the late winter and early spring.
• Infection is most contagious when rash is erupting. However, the virus may be shed, beginning 7 days before the rash to 14 days after.
• Infants with CRS may shed virus for up to 1 year.
• In the prevaccine era, the incidence of infection in the United States was approximately 58 per 100,000 population.
• Currently, fewer than 1,000 cases per year are reported. In 2002, 18 cases were reported to the Centers for Disease Control and Prevention (CDC).
• Infection occurs equally in the following age groups: under 5 years, 5 to 19 years, and 20 to 39 years.
• CRS was reported rarely during the 1980s, with fewer than five cases annually. From 1990 to 1991, approximately 30 cases were reported annually. In 2002, only 1 case was reported to the CDC.
• The rubella vaccine was licensed in 1969.

COMPLICATIONS

Complications tend to occur in adults, and most are uncommon. They include:

• Arthritis or arthralgia

—Occurs in 70% of adult women, lasting up to 1 month
—Usually affects small joints

• Encephalitis

—1 in 5,000 cases
—May be associated with mortality

• Bleeding

—1 in 3,000 cases
—Occurs in children more than in adults

• Thrombocytopenia is commonly noted.

—Rarely see orchitis and neuritis

• CRS

—In 1964, there were 20,000 newborns with CRS.
—Rubella infection in early gestation can lead to fetal death, premature delivery, and congenital defects.
—The severity of defects is worse the earlier in gestation the infection occurs.
—Eighty-five percent of infants are affected if infection occurs in the first trimester.
—Defects are rare if infection occurs after the 20th week.
—Common defects of CRS include:
  —Deafness: The most common defect
  —Ophthalmologic defects: cataracts, glaucoma, microphthalmia
  —Cardiac defects: patent ductus, arteriosus, ventricular septal defect, pulmonic stenosis, coarctation of the aorta
  —Neurologic defects: Mental retardation, microcephalism
—Some manifestations of CRS (diabetes mellitus, progressive encephalopathy) may be delayed for years.

PROGNOSIS

• Quite good. As many as 50% of infections are asymptomatic.
• Rubella infection in a pregnant woman can be devastating for the infant (see above).

ASSOCIATED DISEASES

• Congenital rubella syndrome (see Complications, above)

 Differential Diagnosis

Infections that are sometimes confused with rubella include:

• Modified measles
• Scarlet fever
• Roseola
• Erythema infectiosum (fifth disease, parvovirus B19 infection)
• Enteroviral infections
• Infectious mononucleosis
• Drug eruptions

 Data Gathering

HISTORY

• In children, the prodrome is not often recognized.
• In adults, a 1- to 5-day prodrome of low-grade fever, malaise, and cervical adenopathy may precede the rash.
• Inquire about immunizations and exposures.

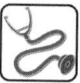 Physical Examination

• The rash begins on the face, and then progresses to the trunk and extremities. The rash does not usually coalesce, and lasts for 3 days.
• Adenopathies, especially postauricular, posterior cervical, and suboccipital, are commonly noted, along with conjunctivitis.
• Arthralgia/arthritis may be seen in adolescents and adults.

 Laboratory Aids

• Viral isolation from throat or urine
• A fourfold or greater rise in specific rubella antibodies, IgG, or a single IgM antibody is diagnostic.

Therapy

- Supportive care

PREVENTION

- The rubella vaccine was licensed in 1969. The current strain of the vaccine (RA 27/3, developed at the Wistar Institute in Philadelphia) was licensed in 1979 and has replaced all other strains.
- Immunity occurs in 95% of vaccines and is thought to be lifelong.
- The vaccine virus is not communicable, except in breast-feedings. Persons who are immunodeficient (except HIV infection) should not receive the vaccine.

PITFALLS

- Not ensuring full vaccination for preschool-aged children
- If suspicious of rubella, it should be reported to the local public health authorities.

Common Questions and Answers

Q: While pregnancy is a contraindication to rubella vaccination, if a pregnant woman is inadvertently vaccinated, will there be harm to the fetus?
A: Data collected since 1979 by the CDC show no evidence of CRS in 321 susceptible women who were vaccinated while pregnant.

Q: Is there any evidence that the MMR vaccine causes autism spectrum disorder (ASD)?
A: No. A systematic review by Wilson et al in 2003, revealed no difference in the rates of ASD and the MMR vaccine in children who were vaccinated and those who were not.

ICD-CM 056.9

BIBLIOGRAPHY

American Academy of Pediatrics. Rubella. In: Peter G, ed. *2000 Red Book: Report of the Committee on Infectious Diseases.* 25th Ed. Elk Grove Village, IL: American Academy of Pediatrics, 1994:406–412.

Atkinson W, Furphy L, et al. *Epidemiology and Prevention of Vaccine-Preventable Diseases,* 2nd Ed. Bethesda, MD: Centers for Disease Control and Prevention, 1995.

Plotkin SA. Rubella vaccine. In: Plotkin SA, Mortimer EA, eds. *Vaccines.* Philadelphia: WB Saunders, 1988:235–262.

Wilson K, et al. Association of autistic spectrum disorder and the measles, mumps, and rubella vaccine: a systematic review of current epidemiological evidence. *Arch Pediatr and Adolesc Med* 2003;157:628–634.

Zimmerman L, Reef SE. Incidence of congenital rubella syndrome at a hospital serving a predominantly Hispanic population, El Paso, Texas. *Pediatrics* 2001;107(3):E40.

Author: Louis M. Bell

Giardiasis

Database

DEFINITION

Giardia is the symptomatic infection of the duodenum and jejunum with the flagellated protozoon *Giardia lamblia*.

PATHOPHYSIOLOGY

- *Giardia lamblia* is not a normal inhabitant of the upper small intestine and a frequent cause of diarrhea throughout the world. The life cycle has a multiplying intraduodenal trophozoite responsible for the clinical illness and an excreted cyst stage responsible for the transmission of infection.
- Infection occurs after cyst ingestion from fecally contaminated water or by direct fecal-oral transmission in poor sanitary conditions.

GENETICS

- No confirmed predisposition
- Blood group A, certain human leukocyte antigen alleles are risk factors.

EPIDEMIOLOGY

- Most commonly diagnosed enteric protozoal infection in the United States.
- Most infected individuals are asymptomatic.
- There is a bimodal age distribution of clinical presentation, with peaks at ages 0 to 5 years and 31 to 40 years.
- Direct person-to-person transmission accounts for the very high prevalence rates over the past decade.

—High prevalence rates have recently been reported in patients with cystic fibrosis as well as Crohn disease.
—It is the most common nonopportunistic protozoan in AIDS patients.

COMPLICATIONS

- Malabsorption syndrome
- Steatorrhea
- Lactose deficiency
- Deficiencies of iron, folic acid, and vitamins A, B_{12}, and E
- Protein-losing enteropathy
- Urticaria
- Arthralgia
- Growth retardation

PATHOLOGY AND PATHOGENESIS

- Mucosal lesions vary from normal to subtotal villus atrophy with crypt hyperplasia and proliferation of intraepithelial and lamina propria lymphocytes. Trophozoite may be seen on biopsies as an S-like curled shape on longitudinal sections. Certain factors that could possibly be related to pathogenesis are:

—Small bowel bacterial overgrowth
—Deconjugation of intraluminal bile salts
—Breast milk that has anti-*Giardia* properties may be related to free fatty acids cleaved from milk triglyceride by a bile salt-stimulated lipase present in human milk

- *Giardia* also exhibits antigenic variation over the course of an infection.

PROGNOSIS

- Remains good for symptomatic patients
- Combination therapy with two medications has been successful when repeated courses of a single drug have failed.

Differential Diagnosis

- Celiac disease
- Cystic fibrosis
- Lactose intolerance

Data Gathering

HISTORY

- Exposure to well water
- Living in endemic area
- Asymptomatic infection can occur
- Common manifestations are watery, foul-smelling diarrhea without blood, abdominal cramps, bloating, anorexia, dyspepsia and nausea.
- A chronic course is associated with weight loss, abdominal distension, anorexia, and flatulence.
- Malabsorption syndrome may include steatorrhea; secondary lactase deficiency; deficiencies of iron, folic acid, vitamins A, B_{12}, and E; and protein-losing enteropathy.

Physical Examination

- Abdominal distension
- Urticaria
- Arthralgia

Laboratory Aids

- Stool microscopy for detection of cysts and/or trophozoite
- A commercial ELISA test for detection of *Giardia lamblia* antigen in stools is available.
- In the case of strong suspicion of giardiasis, but in which there are three negative stool samples, a small intestinal sample may be obtained from the duodenum. A duodenal biopsy specimen appears to be the most sensitive. Consideration of empiric antiparasitic therapy may be recommended in endemic areas.
- If immunodeficiency is suspected, check immune function, especially IgA.

Therapy

DRUGS

- Metronidazole is the most effective and best tolerated. Dose: 15 mg/kg per day divided t.i.d. for 7 days
- Furazolidone has lower efficacy but is better tolerated and is available in liquid suspension.
- For recurrent infection, combination therapy of metronidazole and quinacrine is used.
- Asymptomatic giardiasis, in the absence of risk factors, should not be treated.

INFECTION CONTROL

- Maintenance of good sanitary conditions
- Family members and close contacts should be examined and treated if necessary.
- Examine the water source in endemic areas.

Follow-Up

- The incubation period is usually 1 to 2 weeks.
- Reinfection is common if the source is not eradicated.
- If symptoms persist, with negative diagnostic studies, consider an alternative etiology or another enteropathogen.

Common Questions and Answers

Q: Where is a likely place that the infection occurs?
A: Well water is a common place.

Q: What do I do if I suspect *Giardia*, but the stool sample is negative?
A: Three samples are needed. If you are in an endemic area, you may choose to treat empirically.

ICD-9-CM 007.1

BIBLIOGRAPHY

Ali SA, Hill DR. Giardia intestinalis. *Curr Opin Infect Dis* 2003;16(5):453–460.

Farthing MJ, et al. Natural history of *Giardia* infection of infants and children in rural Guatemala and its impact on physical growth. *Am J Clin Nutr* 1986;43:395–405.

Fraser D. Epidemiology of *Giardia Lamblia* and Cryptosporidium infections in childhood. *Isr J Med Sci* 1994;30(5–6):356–361.

Hanson KL, Cartwright CP. Use of an enzyme immunoassay does not eliminate the need to analyze multiple stool specimens for sensitive detection of *Giardia Lamblia*. *J Clin Microbio* 2001;39(2):474–777

Nash TE, Ohl CA, Thomas E, et al. Treatment of patients with refractory giardiasis. *Clin Infect Dis* 2001;33(1):22–28.

Okhuysen PC. Traveler's diarrhea due to intestinal protozoa. *Clin Infect Dis* 2001;33(1):110–114.

Thielman NM, Guerrant RL. Persistent diarrhea in the returned traveler. *Infect Dis Clin North Am* 1998;12(2):489–501.

Walker-Smith JA. Post-infective diarrhea. *Curr Opin Infect Dis* 2001;14(5):567–571.

Author: Helen Anita John-Kelly

Gingivitis

Database

DEFINITION

Gingivitis is a reversible or chronic inflammation of the gum tissue margin surrounding the teeth. Symptoms may include bleeding, swelling, ulceration, and pain. Gingivitis is usually mild and asymptomatic. Some degree of gingivitis is usually associated with the onset of puberty. An intact gingival epithelium and salivary secretions that continuously flush the crevices with serum components protective against infection are the oral cavity's best defense against gingivitis and early periodontal disease.

ETIOLOGY

- Poor dental hygiene
- Caries
- Bacterial plaque, calcified and uncalcified
- Mouth breathing
- Orthodontic appliances
- Malocclusion
- Crowded teeth
- Erupting teeth margins
- Poor nutrition: Vitamin deficiencies (e.g., vitamin C deficiency), diet low in coarse detergent-like foods (e.g., raw carrots, celery, apples), high prevalence of anaerobic microflora
- Infections: Herpes simplex virus (HSV) type I, *candida albicans*, HIV, bacterial pathogens
- Drugs: phenytoin, cyclosporine, nifedipine, exogenous hormones (e.g., oral contraceptive pills)
- Trauma

PREDISPOSING CONDITIONS

- Behavioral factors: Smoking, stress, alcohol consumption
- Pregnancy
- Diabetes mellitus
- Chronic renal failure
- Immunologic deficiency (HIV, Chediak-Higashi, cyclic neutropenia)
- Histiocytosis X
- Scleroderma
- Secondary hyperparathyroidism
- Neurologic problems: Cerebral palsy, mental retardation, seizures. Routine dental care is often difficult due to poor cooperation and is often complicated by gingival hyperplasia caused by phenytoin.

PATHOPHYSIOLOGY

- Bacteria and food deposits adherent to the teeth (plaque) may accumulate, eroding the area where the gum and teeth meet.
- Incomplete dental care over time may result in this margin becoming inflamed with loss of integrity of vascular membrane, increased bleeding and low grade infections.
- Inflammation may be more severe in children with altered immune function.
- If allowed to progress, the connective tissue attachment of the teeth and the root surface may become involved, resulting in irreversible periodontal disease.
- Microscopic changes include edema, exudate, ulceration, and proliferation of the epithelium surrounding the tooth.

EPIDEMIOLOGY

- Affects more than 90% of children between the ages of 4 and 13 years, although it is generally low grade.
- Thirteen percent to 40% of children 6 to 36 months of age have eruption gingivitis, which commonly resolves after teeth erupt.
- Boys have more severe and prevalent gingivitis until the early teens.
- Peak incidence is in adolescence, probably due to hormonal influences and inconsistent dental hygiene.

COMPLICATIONS

- Periodontal disease
- Osteomyelitis
- Tooth decay
- Sepsis, particularly in patients who are immunocompromised

PROGNOSIS

- Good oral hygiene may reverse mild-to-moderate gingivitis within several months.
- Periodontal disease is not reversible; therefore, prevention is essential.

Differential Diagnosis

INFECTIOUS

- Abscess

TRAUMATIC

- Food impaction
- Orthodontic appliances
- Self-inflicted minor injury

HEMATOLOGIC

- Gingival bleeding due to hemophilia (factor VIII or IX deficiency)
- Thrombocytopenia

IMMUNOLOGIC

- Neutrophil disorders
- Leukemia
- HIV
- Graft versus host (infiltrative gingivitis)

MISCELLANEOUS

- Gingival hyperplasia due to medications, including phenytoin and nifedipine

Data Gathering

HISTORY

Question: Is there any bleeding along the gum line with routine brushing and flossing?
Significance: This is very common with gingivitis.

Question: Is there any gingival pain, spontaneous bleeding, or loose teeth?
Significance: All of the above may be seen with gingival disease, but one must consider other diagnoses.

Question: Are any dental appliances worn by the patient?
Significance: Orthodontic equipment makes gingiva more difficult to clean, and reactive tissue growth is more common.

Question: Are any regular medications taken?
Significance: Phenytoin may result in gingival hyperplasia, and chemotherapeutic agents, exogenous hormone therapy and calcium channel blockers may result in gingivitis.

Question: Has the patient undergone pubertal changes?
Significance: Pubertal changes seem to worsen gingival inflammation.

- Review significant medical history, ask about bleeding disorders and immunodeficiency.
- Review the diet of the child to assess for nutritional deficiencies.
- Review the frequency of dental care visits and the home dental hygiene regimen.

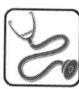

Physical Examination

- Examine the face and neck for signs of swelling, erythema, and warmth, which may be signs of more extensive bacterial infection.
- Evaluate the gingival tissue for erythema, swelling, ulceration, fluctuance, or drainage.
- Evaluate the teeth for caries, fractures, looseness, malocclusion, pain, and plaque.
- Assess the patient's oral hygiene technique in the office. This is the single largest contributor to gingivitis.

Laboratory Aids

TESTS

- Complete blood count with differential: If there is a concern for excess bleeding that may be due to thrombocytopenia or pancytopenia
- Blood culture: If there is a concern for sepsis complicating the picture
- Direct fluorescent antibody testing for HSV-1: If herpes is suspected (stomatitis is usually present); swab the base of a stoma/vesicle and smear on a slide.
- Biopsy is rarely necessary.

Radiographic Studies

Panoramic or individual tooth radiographic imaging is important to assess the bones for evidence of periodontal extension of the gingivitis in the more significant cases.

 Therapy

MILD GINGIVITIS

- Mechanical plaque removal
- Careful daily dental hygiene, including meticulous brushing and flossing

MODERATE-TO-SEVERE GINGIVITIS

- Care as outlined for mild gingivitis
- Should be evaluated by a pedodontist (if available) or by a general dentist
- Mouth rinses for plaque inhibition (e.g., chlorhexidine 0.12%)
- Irrigation devices
- Sonic toothbrushes
- Gingivectomies in cases of overgrowth to permit better cleaning
- Antibiotics to cover mouth flora organisms in the more severe cases when bacterial superinfection is suspected

 Follow-Up

- Routine dental care with professional cleaning and plaque removal is recommended for all children and adults.
- Appliances to keep gingival growth contained may be used in certain cases.

PREVENTION

- Consistent daily oral hygiene. For infants: gum massage, washcloth to remove plaque; in young children: assistance with brushing with a small amount of fluoridated toothpaste; in school-aged children: supervise brushing and assist if necessary.
- Fluorides: Supplements are appropriate if the water supply is not fluoridated.
- Sealants: Adherent plastic coating applied to the pits and fissures of the permanent teeth to provide a mechanical barrier
- Begin regular dental checkups every 6 months at 3 years of age. Children with gingival overgrowth, HIV, or ongoing chemotherapy need visits to the dentist every 3 months to ensure good hygiene. Routine daily care may be inconsistent and often impossible in children with motor and cognitive limitations; these children also need more frequent visits to the dentist.
- Mouth guards for competitive sports
- Counseling about dangers of smoking and contributions of alcohol use to poor oral health

PITFALLS

Success in preventing and treating gingivitis requires consistent daily care, which is often very difficult in children and adolescents.

 Common Questions and Answers

Q: Are there differences among toothpastes and prevention of gingivitis?
A: Yes. A study demonstrated that stabilized stannous fluoride toothpaste is effective in preventing gingivitis. When essential oil mouthwashes (e.g., Listerine) are added, there is additional reduction in the amount of gingivitis noted.

Q: What dietary changes may improve gingival health?
A: Avoiding frequent carbohydrate intake may reduce gingivitis. Carbonated beverages, sugared chewing gum, and candy often adhere to teeth. When daily dental care is inconsistent, plaque formation is increased and gingivitis is much more likely.

Q: Why do children generally not have the significant periodontal disease that adults get?
A: No one knows for sure; however, it is known that the gingiva of the primary dentition is rounder and thicker and contains more blood vessels and less connective tissue. Whether these differences mask disease or are helpful is unclear.

Q: When can we make the most impact in oral self-care?
A: It is mentioned over and over in the dental literature that oral care habits are already formed by adolescence, stressing the importance of patterning this behavior early in life. If children see this as a part of daily life like any other routine, it will be more consistent.

Q: Why is smoking associated with gingival disease?
A: Nicotine inhibits function of phagocytes and neutrophils, reduces bone mineralization, impairs vascularization and reduces antibody production. Smokers do not respond as well as nonsmokers to surgical and nonsurgical treatment.

ICD-9-CM 523.1

BIBLIOGRAPHY

Abrams RG, Romberg E. Gingivitis in children with malnutrition. *J Clin Pediatric Dentistry* 1999;23(3):189–194.

Beiswanger BB, McClanahan SF, Bartizek RD, et al. The comparative efficacy of stabilized stannous fluoride dentifrice, peroxide/baking soda dentifrice and essential oil mouthrinse for the prevention of gingivitis. *J Clin Dentistry* 1997;8(2):46–53.

Clerehugh V, Tugnait A. Diagnosis and management of periodontal diseases in children and adolescents. *Periodontol* 2001;26:146–168.

Eaton KA, Rimini FM, Zak E, et al. The effects of a 0.12% chlorhexidine-digluconate-containing mouthrinse versus a placebo on plaque and gingival inflammation over a 3-month period. A multicentre study carried out in general dental practices. *J Clin Periodontal* 1997;24(3):189–197.

Griffen AL, Goepferd SJ. Preventive oral health care for the infant, child, and adolescent. *Pediatr Clin North Am* 1991;38(5):1209–1226.

Kallio PJ. Health promotion and behavioral approaches in the prevention of periodontal disease in children and adolescents. *Periodontol* 2001;26:135–145.

Kinane DF, et al. Etiopathogenesis of periodontitis in children and adolescents. *Periodontol* 2001;26:54–91.

Jenkins WM, Papapanou PN. Epidemiology of periodontal disease in children and adolescents. *Periodontol* 2001;26:16–32.

McDonald RE, Avery DR, Weddell JA. Gingivitis and periodontal disease. *Dentistry for the Child and Adolescent*, 6th Ed. St. Louis: Mosby-Year Book, 1994:455–502.

Ramberg P, Axelsson P, Lindhe J. Plaque formation at healthy and inflamed gingival sites in young individuals. *J Clin Periodontol* 1995;22(1):85–88.

Author: Shannon Connor Phillips

Glaucoma (Congenital)

 Database

DEFINITION

Congenital glaucoma is the improper development of the drainage system for aqueous humor, leading to elevated intraocular pressure with enlargement of the eye and damage to the optic nerve.

CAUSES

• Aqueous humor, a clear fluid produced by the ciliary body at the posterior base of the iris, passes through the pupil and exits through the trabecular meshwork and Schlemm canal, which are located at the junction of the cornea and the anterior iris.
• Outflow blockage of the aqueous causes the pressure to build in the eye, resulting in enlargement of the eye in younger children and destruction of fibers of the optic nerve in children with abnormally high intraocular pressures.

PATHOPHYSIOLOGY

• Primary congenital glaucoma caused by structural abnormalities of the aqueous outflow mechanism, which includes the trabecular meshwork, iris, and cornea
• Secondary glaucoma may be associated with systemic abnormalities such as Lowe syndrome, aniridia, rubella, Sturge-Weber
• Glaucoma may also be acquired secondary to an ocular abnormality such as cataract

EPIDEMIOLOGY/GENETICS

• 1:10,000 births
• 2:5 female to male ratio
• Seventy percent bilaterally affected
• Primary congenital glaucoma accounts for approximately one-half of all cases of glaucoma in children.

COMPLICATIONS

If glaucoma is undetected or uncontrollable, then severe visual impairment or blindness is the likely result.
If glaucoma is controlled, the following are relatively common:

• Unrecognized and untreated amblyopia (the most serious threat to child's vision)
• High degrees of myopia
• Anisometropia (difference in refractive error between fellow eyes)
• Buphthalmos and corneal scarring

PROGNOSIS

Guarded; even if pressure is well controlled, the child must be carefully followed for amblyopia, abnormal refractive errors, and recurrence of glaucoma.

ASSOCIATED DISEASES

Aniridia, Sturge-Weber, neurofibromatosis, Marfan syndrome, Pierre Robin syndrome, homocystinuria, Lowe syndrome, rubella, chromosomal abnormalities, persistent hyperplastic, primary vitreous

 Differential Diagnosis

• Excessive tearing, most commonly due to nasolacrimal duct obstruction
• Megalocornea

—May be associated with high myopia
—Often familial

• Corneal haze
• Birth trauma, forceps
• Congenital corneal dystrophies, developmental anomalies, intrauterine inflammation (rubella, syphilis), mucopolysaccharidoses, cystinosis

 Data Gathering

HISTORY

Question: Is there tearing, light sensitivity, or lid squeezing?
Significance: Epiphora (tearing), photophobia (light sensitivity), and blepharospasm (lid squeezing) may be present due to corneal edema from increased intraocular pressure.

 Physical Examination

• General signs of many systemic syndromes associated with glaucoma (neurofibromatosis, Sturge-Weber)
• Corneal enlargement (11 mm suspicious in patients younger than 1 year)
• Corneal haze from edema and/or scarring, often seen with acute ruptures in Descemet membrane
• Myopia, often extreme degrees
• Optic nerve cupping develops rapidly in infants but may be reversible with control of glaucoma in very young children.

INTRAOCULAR PRESSURE MEASUREMENT

• An awake child is ideal; use bottle or breast to quiet along with low lighting.
• If examination under anesthesia is needed, check intraocular pressure as soon as possible after induction, as intraocular pressure drops with anesthetic agents.

CORNEAL INSPECTION

• Diameter measure with calipers

—Normal newborn, 10.0 to 10.5 mm
—Over 11.5 mm suspicious
—Watch for asymmetry.

• Clarity

—Haze may be due to edema or breaks in Descemet membrane (called Haab striae).

• Refractive error

—High myopia common
—Useful as an office measure of change over time

• Optic disc assessment

—Cupping of nerve head is an early sign.
—May reverse with good intraocular pressure control

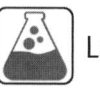 Laboratory Aids

TESTS

• Gonioscopy: Evaluation of anterior chamber angle (between iris and cornea)

—In trabeculodysgenesis, the insertion of the iris into the corneoscleral angle is often flat or concave.
—Iris defects may suggest the type of abnormality causing glaucoma.
—Abnormal iris vessels may influence the surgical plan.

• Ultrasound: Axial length using A-scan

—Eye usually abnormally long for age
—Longitudinal data very useful in determining continued presence of glaucoma

Therapy

IMMEDIATE

• Medical treatment for glaucoma in children is usually a temporizing measure prior to surgical intervention.
• In other types of glaucoma, medical treatment involves the use of the same medications as those used in adults, such as beta-blockers, adrenergic agents, and carbonic anhydrase inhibitors. In general, miotics are not used because they may cause a paradoxical rise in intraocular pressure.

SURGICAL PROCEDURES

• Goniotomy/trabeculotomy: Both of these procedures open portions of Schlemm canal (goniotomy approaches Schlemm canal from inside the eye and trabeculotomy from the outside) into the anterior chamber, allowing easier outflow of aqueous humor to the subconjunctival space.
• Trabeculectomy: This is similar to trabeculotomy but includes excision of a small portion of Schlemm canal and the trabecular meshwork.
• Seton procedures: Various devices are inserted from the subconjunctival space into the anterior chamber, allowing free flow of aqueous humor from the eye.
• Cyclodestructive procedures: Procedures involving destruction of the ciliary body (which produces aqueous humor) decrease aqueous production.
• Iridectomy: If the mechanism of glaucoma is limited outflow of aqueous humor from posterior to iris through the pupil, then removal of a portion of the iris may eliminate obstruction.

 ## Follow-Up

EARLY POSTOPERATIVE

• Postoperative steroids and cycloplegic drops are essential to prevent adhesions due to inflammation and to decrease pain.
• Corneal edema clears slowly, but intraocular pressure quickly falls if surgery is successful.
• For young infants, examination under anesthesia may be required frequently in the first 3 to 4 years of life to ensure adequate control of intraocular pressure.
• Contact with social services for blind and visually handicapped individuals must be made for children even if they are only suspected of being visually impaired. Encourage families to make the contact even when the child may be too young to provide objective data on the extent of visual handicap.

PITFALLS

• Even when pressure is well controlled and amblyopia treatment is undertaken vigorously, the child is still at high risk for visual impairment.
• The child and parents must understand that glaucoma may recur at any point and that continued, long-term surveillance is essential.
• Ensure that potential systemic medicines do not raise intraocular pressure.

 ## Common Questions and Answers

Q: Can glaucoma be painful?
A: If the ocular pressure rises quickly (hours), pain occurs frequently. Very high intraocular pressures may be present without pain if they occur slowly (months to years).

Q: Can glaucoma occur after eye trauma?
A: Yes. This is a very common cause of glaucoma and may be asymptomatic, thus requiring periodic follow-up ophthalmic examinations for early detection and treatment.

ICD-9-CM 743.20

BIBLIOGRAPHY

Beck AD. Diagnosis and management of pediatric glaucoma. *Ophthalmol Clin North Am* 2001;14(3):501–512.

Dickens CJ, Hoskins HD. Developmental glaucoma. In: Isenberg SJ, ed. *The Eye in Infancy.* 2nd Ed. Chicago: Yearbook Medical, 1994:318–335.

Mandal AK, et al. Outcome of surgery on infants younger than 1 month with congenital glaucoma. *Ophthalmology* 2003;110(10): 1909–1915.

Russell-Eggitt I. Childhood glaucoma. In: Taylor D, eds. *Paediatric Ophthalmology.* 2nd Ed. Oxford: Blackwell Science, 1997:477–497.

Shields MB. Primary congenital glaucoma. In: Shields MB, eds. *Textbook of glaucoma.* Baltimore: Williams & Wilkins, 1992:220–234.

Author: Monte D. Mills and *Graham E. Quinn, 3rd edition*

Glomerulonephritis

 Database

DEFINITION

- Glomerulonephritis (GN) presents with hematuria, oliguria, hypertension, and volume overload.
- Acute GN (AGN) is associated with inflammation and proliferation of the glomerular tuft. AGN may be rapidly progressive (RPGN).
- Chronic GN (CGN) implies that permanent damage has occurred.

PATHOPHYSIOLOGY

Causes

- Low serum complement level: Systemic diseases

—Vasculitis and autoimmune disease, e.g., systemic lupus erythematosus (SLE)
—Subacute bacterial endocarditis (SBE)
—Shunt nephritis
—Cryoglobulinemia

- Low serum complement level: Renal diseases

—Acute poststreptococcal GN (APSGN)
—Membranoproliferative glomerulonephritis (types 1, 2, and 3)

- Normal serum complement level: Systemic diseases

—Polyarteritis nodose group
—Wegener vasculitis
—Henoch-Schönlein purpura
—Hypersensitivity vasculitis
—Visceral abscess

- Normal serum complement level: Renal diseases

—IgA nephropathy
—Idiopathic rapidly progressive glomerulonephritis
—Immune-complex disease
—Pauci-immune glomerulonephritis

PATHOLOGY

In APSGN light microscopy reveals enlarged swollen glomerular tufts, mesangial and epithelial cell proliferation, with polymorphonuclear cell infiltration. There is granular deposition of C3 and IgG on immunofluorescence, and electron-dense subepithelial deposits or humps on electron microscopy. The histology varies in CGN and depends on the cause. RPGN is associated with crescent formation.

EPIDEMIOLOGY

- APSGN can occur in all ages but is most frequent in boys between 5 and 15 years.
- Incidence of APSGN in the United States has declined in the last two decades.
- CGN occurs more often at the end of the first decade of life and in adults.
- Genetic predisposition

—Familial GN (e.g., Alport syndrome, X-linked)
—Autoimmune diseases (e.g., SLE, familial)

COMPLICATIONS

- Acute renal failure
- Hyperkalemia
- Hypertension
- Volume overload (congestive cardiac failure, pulmonary edema, hypertension)
- Chronic renal failure

PROGNOSIS

- Prognosis is excellent in APSGN and variable for other causes of GN in childhood.

 Differential Diagnosis

- Acute postinfectious GN (Lancefield group A β-hemolytic streptococci, pneumococcus, *Mycoplasma*, mumps, Epstein-Barr virus)
- Infection related (hepatitis B and C, syphilis)
- IgA nephropathy
- Membranoproliferative GN
- Autoimmune GN (e.g., SLE)
- Familial GN
- Acute interstitial nephritis
- Hemolytic uremic syndrome
- Pyelonephritis

 Data Gathering

HISTORY

- Macroscopic hematuria (coke-colored urine)
- Sore throat
- Impetigo
- A prior URI of at least 1 week or skin lesions in the proceeding 3 to 4 weeks suggests APSGN.
- An upper respiratory infection URI in the proceeding few days suggests IgA nephropathy.
- Reduced urine output
- Dyspnea, fatigue, lethargy
- Headache
- Seizures (hypertensive encephalopathy)
- Symptoms of a systemic disease such as fever, rash (especially on the buttocks and legs posteriorly), arthralgia, and weight loss

Special Questions

Establish the time relationship between a sore throat and the AGN. The onset of APSGN is usually associated with a time delay of more than 1 week.

 Physical Examination

Look for:

- Hypertension
- Pallor
- Signs of volume overload (edema, jugular venous distention, hepatomegaly, basal pulmonary crepitation, and a triple cardiac rhythm)
- Impetigo or ecthyma (pyoderma)
- Signs of vasculitis such as rash, loss of fingertip pulp space tissue, Raynaud, and vascular thrombosis
- Signs of a systemic disorder (see vasculitis above)
- Signs of chronic renal insufficiency such as short stature, pallor, sallowness, edema, excoriations, pericardial friction rub, pulmonary rales and effusion, uriniferous breath, asterixis, myoclonus, and neuropathy

 Laboratory Aids

TESTS

- Throat culture for β-hemolytic streptococcus (positive in 15% to 20% with APSGN)
- Microscopy of the urine for crenated RBCs and RBC casts; CBC is normal in AGN; with chronic renal insufficiency a normocytic normochromic or hypochromic microcytic anemia is found.
- Serum chemistries will reflect the degree of renal failure (raised serum urea and creatinine). The serum potassium and phosphate will be elevated and the calcium decreased.
- ASOT (antistreptolysin O) titer. Positive in 60% of patients with APSGN.
- Streptozyme test. A mixed antigen test for β-hemolytic streptococcus. Together, the ASOT plus streptozyme tests have greater than 85% sensitivity.
- Complement C3 serum level will be low in APSGN and in other causes of GN as detailed above.
- ECG to assess ventricular size and for hyperkalemia.

Imaging

CXR to look for pulmonary edema and cardiac size.
Renal ultrasound if presentation or course not typical of APSGN. The ultrasound is to assess the size and parenchymal texture.

PITFALLS

- Look for and treat hyperkalemia.
- To control seizures treat the hypertension; anticonvulsants have a secondary role.
- Monitor the degree of renal failure.
- Home testing: Blood pressure monitoring may be required.

 ## Therapy

DIET

Restricted fluid, sodium, potassium, and phosphate are initially required.

DRUGS

The following may be required:

- Loop diuretics (furosemide) for volume, blood pressure, and potassium control
- Antihypertensive agents; vasodilators such as calcium channel blockers (nifedipine, isradipine, amlodipine) and loop diuretics are useful as first-line agents; intravenous hydralazine, labetalol, nicardipine, or nitroprusside may be required to treat severe refractory hypertension.
- Serum potassium-lowering agents (Kayexalate, furosemide, bicarbonate, insulin/glucose, salbutamol). Intravenous calcium is used to stabilize the myocardium in severe hyperkalemia.
- Phosphate binders
- Immunosuppressive agents such as prednisone, cyclophosphamide, and sometimes azathioprine are used in the treatment of vasculitis-associated GN, membranoproliferative GN, and RPGN. Plasmapheresis may be used to treat RPGN. Penicillin is used in APSGN but does not affect the course of the disease.

DURATION

APSGN is a self-limiting disease. Acute therapy is usually sufficient. The therapy of CGN depends on the underlying disease process, may include immunosuppressives and, ultimately, the management of CRF.

 ## Follow-Up

Drug doses may need modification if conflicts with other treatments arise. In APSGN improvement usually occurs within 3 to 7 days, hypertension is not sustained and macroscopic hematuria is transient. Watch for ongoing oliguria, unresolved hypertension, increasing proteinuria, or progressive azotemia.

PITFALLS

- Not checking a serum potassium level stat.
- Not recognizing fluid overload.
- Not recognizing the severity and type of renal failure.

 ## Common Questions and Answers

Q: When does the complement return to normal?
A: Hemolytic complement levels (C3) return to normal within a 6- to 8-week period in APSGN. Persistently low C3 levels suggest a cause other than APSGN.

Q: What are the indications for renal biopsy in AGN?
A: Patients in whom there is sustained hypertension, ongoing or progressive azotemia, or persistent proteinuria of more than 1.5 g/d should be biopsied.

ICD-9-CM 580.9

BIBLIOGRAPHY

Clark G, White RH, Glasgow EF, et al. Post-streptococcal glomerulonephritis in children: clinicopathological correlations and long-term prognosis. *Pediatr Nephrol* 1988;2:381–388.

Cole B, Salinas-Madrigal L. Acute proliferative glomerulonephritis and crescentic glomerulonephritis. In: Barratt TM, Avner ED, Harmon WE, eds. *Pediatric Nephrology*. 4th Ed. Baltimore: Williams & Wilkins, 1999:669–689.

Couser WG, Johnson RJ. Post infectious glomerulonephritis. In: Neilson EG, Couser WG, eds. *Immunologic Renal Diseases*. Philadelphia: Lippincott-Raven, 2001:899–929.

Jordan S, Lemire JM. Acute glomerulonephritis. Diagnosis and treatment. *Pediatr Clin North Am* 1982;29:857–873.

Madaio MP, Harrington JT. The diagnosis of acute glomerulonephritis. *N Engl J Med* 1984;309:1299–1302.

Author: Kevin E.C. Meyers

Glucose-6-Phosphate Dehydrogenase Deficiency

 Database

DEFINITION

Deficiency of the enzyme glucose-6-phosphate dehydrogenase (G6PD) in the red blood cell, which may result in a hemolytic anemia. There are several types G6PD genetic mutations that result either in deficient enzyme production or in production of an enzyme with diminished activity.

• Although the majority of patients with G6PD deficiency are never anemic and have mild to no hemolysis, the classic manifestation is acute hemolytic anemia.
• (AHA) World Health Organization (WHO) classification

—Class 1: Congenital nonspherocytic hemolytic anemia: a rare form manifesting itself with chronic hemolysis without exposure to oxidative stressors. Most patients have a mild-to-moderate anemia, although some patients are transfusion dependent. Can present with neonatal jaundice, hemolytic anemia, or a secondary manifestation of the chronic hemolysis (e.g., gallstones). Splenomegaly is present in 40% of patients. Affected individuals tend to be white males of Northern European background.
—Class 2: Severe deficiency (<5% detectable enzyme activity): Oxidative stress-induced hemolysis only. The prototype is G6PD-Mediterranean. Because of severe deficiency, all RBCs are sensitive to stressors, and hemolysis may be severe and persistent.
—Class 3: Mild deficiency (approximately 10% enzyme activity): The most common type of G6PD deficiency. Acute hemolytic anemia is uncommon and occurs only with stressors. The prototype is G6PD A-(African or of African descent). Because the enzyme is present and active in young RBCs, the hemolysis preferentially affects older cells and is milder and self-limited (i.e., all cells produced in response to the anemia have adequate G6PD levels).
—Class 4: Nondeficient variant: no symptoms, even during oxidant stressors, e.g., G6PD A (variant with normal activity); 20% to 40% allelic frequency in Africans.

• Deficient neonates may have hyperbilirubinemia out of proportion to their anemia. In severe subtypes, this may lead to kernicterus. Elevated bilirubin is only partially due to the hemolysis; the liver plays a role as well.

PATHOPHYSIOLOGY

• G6PD is necessary for the prevention of cell damage during oxidative stress and is critically important in red blood cells because of continuous oxidant stress (from O_2 metabolism) and because anuclear RBCs cannot synthesize more enzyme, unlike cells in other tissues.

• Red blood cells lose G6PD activity throughout their lifespan, so older cells are more prone to oxidative hemolysis.
• The normal RBC life span of approximately 120 days is unaffected in unstressed states, even with severe enzyme deficiency, but may be shortened during oxidant stress.
• G6PD-deficient RBCs are destroyed via intravascular hemolysis upon exposure to the oxidative stressor, and acute hemolytic anemia results.
• Oxidant stressors include infections (bacterial, viral, hepatitis) and chemical (mothballs, antimalarials, some sulfonamides, methylene blue, and others).
• Hemolysis usually follows stressor by 1 to 3 days and the nadir occurs 8 to 10 days postexposure. It is therefore necessary to obtain hemoglobins for over a week after the initial exposure.
• Favism, a severe hemolytic anemia in patients with G6PD deficiency related to fava bean ingestion.
• Normal G6PD activity is 7 to 10 IU/g hemoglobin.

GENETICS

• G6PD gene is on the X chromosome (Xq28).
• Males express the enzyme (mutant or normal) from their single X chromosome (hemizygotes). Females inheriting two deficient X chromosomes are considered homozygotes (rare) and are more severely affected than are female heterozygotes. Heterozygote females show variable intermediate expression because of random X inactivation (the Lyon hypothesis).

EPIDEMIOLOGY

• G6PD is the most common of all clinically significant enzyme defects.
• Because it is X-linked it primarily affects males.
• Discovered in 1958 while studying individuals who developed hemolytic anemia when exposed to primaquine, an antimalarial drug
• Over 300 biochemical variants of G6PD have been identified, affecting almost 400 million people worldwide.
• The frequency of different G6PD mutations varies from population to population:

—Africans: 20% to 40% of African X-chromosomes are G6PD A (a mutant enzyme with normal activity).
—Sardinians (some regions): 30% have G6PD-Mediterranean.
—Saudi Arabians: 13% have G6PD deficiency.
—African-Americans: 10%–15% have G6PD A- (a mutant enzyme with decreased activity; see below).
—The high incidence of mutant genes in some regions may relate to a survival advantage conferred against malarial infection (*Plasmodium falciparum*).

COMPLICATIONS

Neonates can be at risk for hyperbilirubinemia requiring treatment.
Severe life-threatening anemia may result after exposure to an oxidant stressor.

PROGNOSIS

• For those with the milder forms, the prognosis is excellent.
• Can cause significant morbidity, but rarely mortality, in those with the more severe forms.

 Differential Diagnosis

Intravascular hemolysis is very rare in children, but other causes include:

• Acute hemolytic transfusion reactions (Coombs test is positive)
• Microangiopathic hemolytic disease, such as hemolytic uremic syndrome, thrombotic thrombocytopenic purpura, and prosthetic cardiac valves
• Physical trauma (e.g., March hemoglobinuria); severe burns (uncommon)
• Other inherited RBC enzyme deficiencies
• Paroxysmal nocturnal hemoglobinuria

Extravascular hemolysis can also be confused with G6PD deficiency and includes:

• Hereditary spherocytosis (spherocytes) seen on smear or detected by osmotic fragility testing
• Autoimmune hemolysis and delayed hemolytic transfusion reactions (both Coombs-positive)
• Hemoglobinopathies (e.g., sickle cell anemia; often apparent from peripheral smear). Having G6PD deficiency and a hemoglobinopathy does not worsen either disease.
• Hypersplenism or severe liver disease
• Gilbert disease may present with intermittent jaundice and indirect hyperbilirubinemia after infections.

Data Gathering

HISTORY

Question: Fatigue, irritability or malaise?
Significance: Symptoms of anemia

Question: Dark urine ("coca-cola," or tea-colored)?
Significance: May follow moderate-to-severe hemolysis.

Question: Requiring phototherapy in newborn period
Significance: Hyperbilirubinemia due to hemolysis

Question: Recent drug, chemical, or food (fava bean) exposures?
Significance: May precipitate moderate-to-severe hemolysis.

Question: Family history of intermittent jaundice splenectomy, cholecystectomy, or blood transfusion.
Significance: Inherited condition

Question: Ethnicity?
Significance: May help determine type/severity of disease.

 ## Physical Examination

Finding: Tachycardia, a flow murmur, or pallor.
Significance: Signs of anemia

Finding: Jaundice or scleral icterus
Significance: Signs of hemolysis

 ## Laboratory Aids

TESTS

• CBC usually reveals a normochromic normocytic anemia with an appropriate reticulocytosis. Hemoglobin can drop precipitously and should be monitored closely until stable or a trend upward is seen. Checking a single hemoglobin the day of exposure to the stressor is not sufficient.
• Peripheral blood smear often shows bizarre RBC morphology with marked anisocytosis and poikilocytosis. Can see schistocytes, hemighost cells (uneven distribution of hemoglobin), bite cells, blister cells, and occasional Heinz bodies (on supravital staining).
• Hemoglobinemia can be seen in the plasma (pink-red supernatant) or may be measured as free serum hemoglobin.
• Hemoglobinuria occurs once hemoglobin-binding sites in the plasma (haptoglobin and hemopexin) are saturated and may be visible as hematuria or detected on routine urinalysis.
• Free serum haptoglobin levels decrease.
• Direct and indirect Coombs tests should be done to exclude autoimmune hemolytic anemia. They should be negative in G6PD deficiency.
• Plasma indirect bilirubin, LDH, and AST may be elevated, and hemosiderin may be found in the urine several days after hemolysis. LFTs should be normal.
• Renal functions should be obtained to rule out TTP and HUS.

Diagnostic Tests

• Rapid and relatively simple screening tests for G6PD activity in RBCs are available but are qualitative and will therefore not pick up all female heterozygotes who have a measurable but low enzyme level.
• It is necessary to confirm a deficiency or diagnose a suspected heterozygote with a test to quantify G6PD activity. Normal G6PD activity is 7 to 10 IU/g hemoglobin. This will accurately detect deficiency in males and homozygous females with no recent hemolysis and will be helpful with heterozygous women.

PITFALLS

• Measured enzyme levels will be higher immediately after an acute hemolytic event because younger RBCs (reticulocytes) with normal levels of G6PD will have replaced the older, more deficient population. Screening tests may be falsely negative during this time. The most cost-effective approach is to defer screening until 1 to 2 weeks after the resolution of hemolysis.
• Heterozygote female detection: Two RBC populations exist because of mosaicism from random X-inactivation. On average, one half are normal and one-half are deficient, but there may be variability. Therefore, quantitative results could be unreliable in extreme cases which makes family counseling difficult.

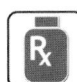 ## Therapy

• Removal of the oxidant stressor is of primary importance. Discontinue the suspected drug and/or treat the infection. In class 3 and 4 patients, essential drug therapy may be continued while monitoring for signs of severe hemolysis.
• Transfusion is rarely necessary (except in some type 1 and 2 deficiencies), but any patient who is symptomatic with anemia, or has a low hemoglobin and signs of ongoing brisk hemolysis should be transfused immediately with packed RBCs.
• Supportive care, evaluation of renal function (risk of acute tubular necrosis with brisk hemolysis), and monitoring degree of anemia and ongoing hemolysis are important.
• For the affected neonate, one should monitor the bilirubin closely and start phototherapy early. If necessary, an exchange transfusion should be performed. Phenobarbital has shown some success in decreasing the bilirubin level. Early discharge is not recommended in infants with jaundice and known risk for having G6PD deficiency.

 ## Follow-Up

The majority of G6PD-deficient individuals remain asymptomatic. When hemolysis does occur, it tends to be self-limited and resolves spontaneously, with a return to normal hemoglobin levels in 2 to 6 weeks. The development of renal failure is extremely rare in children, even with massive hemolysis and hemoglobinuria.

PREVENTION

• Avoidance of drugs and toxins known to cause hemolysis is the best prevention.
• Education regarding drug avoidance, signs and symptoms of hemolysis, and family and genetic counseling should be provided.

 ## Common Questions and Answers

Q: Do I need to follow a special diet or avoid medications if I have G6PD deficiency?
A: Though most patients will have no symptoms of their disease, certain medications may cause transient hemolytic anemia, and these should be avoided. When prescribing medications, your physician and pharmacist should know about your G6PD deficiency, but most necessary medications are safe and well tolerated. People with severe variants of the deficiency should also avoid fava beans, but otherwise no dietary restrictions are necessary.

Q: Do I need to know which variant of G6PD deficiency I have?
A: It may be clear which variant you are likely to have based on your clinical symptoms and ethnic background.

Q: Should my family be screened if someone has G6PD deficiency?
A: In families of patients with G6PD deficiency, screening members may help provide meaningful genetic counseling to female carriers and affected but asymptomatic males.

Q: How does G6PD affect sickle cell anemia and vice versa?
A: Having sickle cell disease is somewhat protective in patients with G6PD A-deficiency, because their RBC population is young and therefore higher in enzyme activity. On the other hand, G6PD has no affect on the clinical characteristics of sickle cell disease.

ICD-9-CM 282.2

BIBLIOGRAPHY

Beutler E. G6PD deficiency. *Blood* 1994;84:3613–3636.

Beutler E. Study of glucose-6-phosphate dehydrogenase: history and molecular biology. *Am J Hematol* 1993;42:53–58.

Mason PJ. New insights into G6PDF deficiency. *Br J Haematol* 1996;94(Suppl 4):585–591.

Author: Leslie Raffini

Goiter

Database

DEFINITION

Goiter is enlargement of the thyroid gland.

GENETICS

- The multinodular goiter 1 (MNG1) locus was identified on chromosome 14q by linkage analysis in one large Canadian family and on chromosome Xp22 in an Italian family. Other genes implicated in simple goiter formation include thyroglobulin, TSH-receptor, and Na^+/I^- symporter. Thyroid peroxidase (TPO) mutations lead to iodide organification defects and goitrous congenital hypothyroidism. Apart from genetic factors, twin and family studies show a modest to major contribution of environmental factors, especially iodine deficiency and cigarette smoking.
- Autoimmune goiters, such as chronic lymphocytic thyroiditis (CLT), occur in children with a genetic predisposition.
- Thyroid cancers are usually sporadic. Medullary carcinoma can be familial (autosomal dominant) as part of multiple endocrine neoplasia (MEN)-2A and -2B, or as isolated malignancy.

EPIDEMIOLOGY

- The most common cause of pediatric goiter in the United States is CLT.
- Prevalence of goiter in the United States is 3%–7%, though the incidence is much higher in regions of iodine deficiency.
- Thyroid cancers comprise 0.5%–1.5% of all malignancies in children and adolescents.
- Thyroid tumors and autoimmune thyroid disease are both more common in females than males.

COMPLICATIONS

- Depending on gland size, goiters can produce a mass effect on midline neck structures. If the goiter is intrathoracic, it may cause pleural effusions or chylothorax.
- Typically, the child is euthyroid, but clinical hypothyroidism or hyperthyroidism may result from certain types of goiters.
- Therapy for thyroid cancer may induce permanent hypothyroidism.

PROGNOSIS

- Depends on the cause of the goiter.
- Thyroid cancers usually follow an indolent course with excellent prognosis, especially the well-differentiated follicular cell carcinoma. Mortality is most common in medullary and undifferentiated carcinomas, which are relatively rare in children.

Differential Diagnosis

- Immunologic

—Chronic lymphocytic thyroiditis (often referred to as Hashimoto thyroiditis)
—Graves disease
—Amyloid deposition (familial Mediterranean fever, juvenile rheumatoid arthritis)

- Infectious

—Acute suppurative thyroiditis (most often *Streptococcus pyogenes*, *Staphylococcus aureus*, and *Streptococcus pneumoniae*)
—Subacute thyroiditis (often viral)

- Environmental

—Goitrogens: Iodide, lithium, amiodarone, oral contraceptives, perchlorate, cabbage, soybeans, cassava, thiocyanate in tobacco smoke (smoking is especially goitrogenic in iodine-deficient areas)
—Iodine deficiency (exacerbated by pregnancy)

- Neoplastic

—Thyroid adenoma/carcinoma
—Follicular adenoma: Benign
—Follicular, papillary, or mixed carcinoma: Well differentiated; follicular 90%
—Medullary carcinoma: 4%–10% as part of the MEN-2 syndrome
—TSH-secreting adenoma
—Lymphoma
—Liposarcoma of the thyroid (extremely rare)

- Congenital

—Ectopic gland
—Unilateral agenesis of gland
—Dyshormonogenesis
—Thyroxine resistance

- Miscellaneous

—Simple colloid goiter
—Multinodular goiter

Data Gathering

HISTORY

- Symptoms of hypothyroidism or hyperthyroidism

—Hypothyroidism: Increase in sedentary behavior, lethargy, weight gain, constipation, cold intolerance, dry skin and/or hair, hair loss
—Hyperthyroidism: Hyperactivity, irritability, difficulty concentrating or focusing in school, hyperphagia, weight loss, diarrhea, heat intolerance

- Careful dietary and medication history
- History of head, neck, or chest irradiation is associated with increased risk of carcinoma.
- Family history of thyroid carcinoma or MEN syndrome

Physical Examination

- Inspect, palpate, and auscultate the neck.

—Neck extension aids inspection.
—Palpation is best performed standing behind the child. Determine if the thyroid is diffusely enlarged or asymmetric, evaluate gland firmness, and assess for any nodularity. Check for cervical lymphadenopathy.
—Auscultate with the stethoscope diaphragm (while patient holds his/her breath) for a bruit, which is indicative of the hyperthyroidism-associated hypervascularity.

- Pain on palpation suggests acute inflammation.
- Careful examination for signs of hypothyroidism or hyperthyroidism: Pulse, linear growth and weight pattern, sexual development, deep tendon reflexes, skin

Procedure

Have patient drink water during inspection of gland. Isthmus of thyroid is just below the cricoid cartilage.

Laboratory Aids

TESTS

- Thyroid function tests: Total T4 and TSH comprise the best screen for hypo- or hyperthyroidism.
- T_3-RIA in cases of suspected hyperthyroidism (note: RIA, which measures total T_3, and not resin uptake, which indirectly assesses thyroid hormonebinding capacity!)
- In cases of suspected CLT: Antithyroglobulin and antimicrosomal (antiperoxidase) antibodies
- In cases of suspected Graves disease: Thyroid-stimulating immunoglobulins (or TSH-receptor antibodies)
- Fine-needle aspiration biopsy is not a commonly used procedure in children and should be considered only in the evaluation of low-risk or purely cystic thyroid nodules. Of all solitary thyroid nodules, the percent that is malignant is much higher in the pediatric age group than in adults.
- Calcitonin levels: Elevated in 75% of patients with medullary carcinoma

Imaging

- Ultrasound is useful in determining the number, size, and nature (cystic, solid, or mixed) of nodules.
- ^{123}I thyroid scans should be done in cases of solitary nodules to establish whether or not the nodule concentrates iodide. "Cold" nodules (no I uptake) are suggestive of neoplasia and require immediate evaluation by a pediatric endocrinologist and surgeon.

- Barium swallow studies can reveal a fistulous tract between the left piriform sinus and the left thyroid lobe in children with recurrent acute suppurative thyroiditis. Such fistulas are amenable to surgical resection.

False Positives

- Fat neck: Adipose tissue, large sternocleidomastoid muscles
- Thyroglossal duct cysts
- Nonthyroidal neoplasms: Lymphoma, teratoma, hygroma, ganglioneuroma

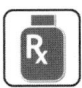 ## Therapy

Therapy is dictated by the cause of the goiter. Surgery solely to decrease the size of a goiter is indicated only if adjacent structures are compressed.

CANCER

- Surgery is recommended for a nonfunctioning nodule if there is a history of radiation, rapid growth of a firm nodule, satellite lymph nodes, evidence of impingement on other neck structures, or evidence of distant metastases.
- The affected lobe is removed and sent for frozen section; if this is suspicious, a total thyroidectomy should be performed.
- Following surgery, ^{131}I therapy is administered if a follow-up iodine scan reveals any residual tissue or metastases.
- Suppressive doses of exogenous thyroid hormone are then given to maintain TSH levels below 2 μIU/mL.
- Thyroglobulin levels are useful as markers of thyroid tissue; calcitonin level serves as tumor marker for medullary carcinoma.
- Some advocate subtotal thyroidectomy, no irradiation, and suppressive T_4 treatment.

DRUGS

L-thyroxine is indicated for the treatment of goiters with hypothyroidism. In cases of goiter with hyperthyroidism, initial treatment consists of antithyroid drugs (propylthiouracil or methimazole). Please see sections on hypothyroidism and Graves disease for further details.

DURATION

Depends on the cause of the goiter

DIET

Depends on the cause of the goiter. The incidence of iodine deficiency (endemic) goiter has greatly declined since the addition of potassium iodide to table salt. Iodide can also be added to communal drinking water or administered as an iodized oil in isolated rural areas.

POSSIBLE CONFLICTS

In the case of manic-depressive patients on lithium and cardiac patients on amiodarone, medication-induced thyroid abnormalities can be a significant problem that should be addressed by the endocrinologist and appropriate subspecialist.

 ## Follow-Up

- The potential for goiter regression depends on its cause. Goiters associated with CLT and Graves disease may or may not decrease in size with treatment.
- A goiter patient who is clinically and biochemically euthyroid still requires careful follow-up for the detection of the early signs of developing thyroid dysfunction.
- Potential complications of thyroid surgery include laryngeal nerve damage and hypoparathyroidism.

PITFALLS

Failure to work up solitary thyroid nodules aggressively; remember, incidence of malignancy in these nodules in children is 15% to 40% (less in adults).

 ## Common Questions and Answers

Q: Does a bigger thyroid gland mean increased thyroid functioning?
A: Goiters can be euthyroid, hypothyroid, or hyperthyroid, depending on cause.

Q: Will the goiter decrease in size with treatment?
A: This again depends on the cause of the goiter. For example, correction of an elevated TSH in CLT with treatment can result in goiter shrinkage. In iodine-deficient states, treatment will cause the early hyperplastic goiter to regress.

Q: Does a bigger thyroid gland mean cancer?
A: Most pediatric goiters are benign, and thyroid cancers often are detected as solitary nodules within an otherwise normal gland (in children with solitary nodules, up to 40% are carcinomas). Patients with a history of goiter or benign nodules/adenomas have an increased risk of developing thyroid cancer.

Q: Does thyroid cancer usually present with hyperthyroidism?
A: No. The usual chief complaint is a solitary, hard, painless nodule in a euthyroid patient.

Q: Is there an increased risk of thyroid cancer from diagnostic x-rays (chest x-rays, lateral neck films)?
A: Routine diagnostic x-rays should fall well below the levels of radiation thought to increase risk of thyroid neoplasia. During more prolonged radiologic procedures that might expose the thyroid to higher doses of radiation, a lead neck shield is used.

Q: Should prophylactic thyroidectomy be performed in children identified genetically as having familial medullary carcinoma?
A: Yes, due to the poorer prognosis associated with development of this cancer.

ICD-9-CM 240.9

BIBLIOGRAPHY

Aghini-Lombardi F, Antonangeli Z, Martino E, et al. The spectrum of thyroid disorders in an iodine-deficient community: the Pescopagano survey. *J Clin Endocrinol Metab* 1999;84: 561–566.

Alsanea O, Clark OH. Familial thyroid cancer. *Curr Opin Oncol* 2001;13:44–51.

American Academy of Pediatrics Committee on Environmental Health. Risk of ionizing radiation exposure to children: a subject review. *Pediatr* 1998;101:717–719.

Capon F, Tacconelli A, Giardina E, et al. Mapping of a dominant form of multinodular goiter to chromosome Xp22. *Am J Hum Genet* 2000;67:1004–1007.

Delange FM. Control of iodine deficiency in Western and Central Europe. *Central Europ J Public Health* 2003;11:120–123.

Feinmesser R, Lubin E, Segal K, et al. Carcinoma of the thyroid in children—a review. *J Pediatr Endocrinol Metab* 1997;10:561–568.

From G, Mellemgaard A, Knudson N, et al. Review of thyroid cancer cases among patients with previous benign thyroid disorders. *Thyroid* 2000;10:697–700.

Hegedus L, et al. Management of simple nodular goiter: current status and future perspectives. *Endocrine Rev* 2003;24:102–132.

Knudsen N, et al. Risk factors for goiter and thyroid nodules. *Thyroid* 2002;12:879–888.

Rios A, et al. Risk factors for malignancy in multinodular goitres. *Eur J Surg Oncol* 2004;30:58–62.

Wang C, Crapo LM. The epidemiology of thyroid disease and the implications for screening. *Endocrinol Metab Clin N Amer* 1997;26:189–218.

Yeh SD, La Quaglia MP. 131I therapy for pediatric thyroid cancer. *Semin Pediatr Surg* 1997;6:128–133.

Zimmerman D. Thyroid neoplasia in children. *Curr Opin Pediatr* 1997;9:413–418.

Zimmermann MB, et al. New reference values for thyroid volume by ultrasound in iodine-sufficient schoolchildren: a World Health Organization/Nutrition for Health and Development Iodine Deficiency Study Group Report. *Amer J Clin Nutr* 2004;79:231–237.

Author: Adda Grimberg

Gonococcal Infections

 Database

DEFINITION

Neisseria gonorrhoeae, an aerobic gram-negative diplococcus, is the etiologic agent of gonorrhea. In the United States, over 1 million new infections are diagnosed each year, usually in sexually active adolescents or adults.

PATHOPHYSIOLOGY

- Transmission results from contact with infected mucous membranes and secretions, usually through sexual activity, parturition, and (very rarely) household contact in prepubertal children.
- The risk of male-to-female transmission is 50% per episode of vaginal intercourse; the risk of female-to-male transmission is approximately 20% per episode. Rectal intercourse is also an effective mode of transmission, but orogenital contact is not.
- Incubation period is 2 to 5 days.
- Immunity is not induced by infection.

ASSOCIATED DISEASES

Pediatric gonococcal infections can be categorized by age group: neonates, prepubertal children, and sexually active adolescents.

- Neonatal gonococcal diseases include ophthalmia neonatorum, scalp abscess (complication of fetal scalp monitoring), and, rarely, vaginitis or systemic disease with arthritis, bacteremia, funisitis, or meningitis.
- Prepubertal gonococcal disease usually occurs in the genital tract. Vaginitis is the most common manifestation. Pelvic inflammatory disease (PID), perihepatitis, urethritis, proctitis, and pharyngitis rarely occur. Sexual abuse must be considered when genital, rectal, or pharyngeal gonococcal infections occur in prepubertal children (see Pitfalls, below).
- Sexually active adolescents have a spectrum of gonococcal disease similar to adults. Orogenital contact may lead to pharyngitis. Asymptomatic or symptomatic anorectal infection occurs in both sexes. In females, genital tract infection may be asymptomatic or cause urethritis, vaginitis, and endocervicitis. Ascending genital tract infection may lead to PID and perihepatitis. In males, acute urethritis is the predominant manifestation. Epididymitis occurs infrequently.

EPIDEMIOLOGY

- In the United States, the highest attack rates occur in 15- to 24-year-old women and men.
- Gonorrhea is the most common STD found in sexually abused children.

- Gonococcal conjunctivitis, though rare in adults, occurs by autoinoculation of infected secretions in patients with anogenital infection.
- PID occurs in 10% to 20% of women with endocervical gonococcal infection.

COMPLICATIONS

- Gonococcal infection during pregnancy

—Gonococcal PID is associated with spontaneous abortion, preterm labor, and perinatal infant mortality.

- Ophthalmia neonatorum

—Gonococcal ophthalmia neonatorum may rapidly progress to corneal ulceration and perforation, with subsequent scarring and blindness.

- Pelvic inflammatory disease

—Endometritis, salpingitis, tuboovarian abscess, and pelvic peritonitis occur as a consequence of untreated vaginal disease.
—Scarring secondary to salpingitis causes sterility in up to 20% of women with a single infection and up to 50% of women after three episodes of infection.
—A woman's risk of ectopic pregnancy increases sevenfold after one episode of PID.

- In males, rare complications include periurethral abscess, acute prostatitis, seminal vesiculitis, and urethral strictures.
- Disseminated disease

—Occurs via hematogenous dissemination of infection.
—Patients with multiple episodes of disseminated gonococcal infection should be tested for complement deficiency.
—In neonates, arthritis is the most frequent systemic manifestation of gonococcal disease. Symptoms develop 1 to 4 weeks after delivery. Involvement of multiple joints is typical, and most of these infants have no evidence of ophthalmia neonatorum.
—In older children and adolescents, septic arthritis (one joint) and a characteristic syndrome of polyarthritis (multiple joints)—dermatitis are predominant manifestations.
—Gonococcal meningitis, endocarditis, and osteomyelitis are very rare in children.

PROGNOSIS

- Good prognosis depends on early diagnosis and effective treatment of infection prior to progression.
- Prognosis has also been improved by treating all forms of infection with a third-generation cephalosporin due to the increased prevalence of penicillin-resistant *N. gonorrhoeae*.

 Differential Diagnosis

- Ophthalmia neonatorum: Other causes of neonatal conjunctivitis include *C. trachomatis*, *S. aureus*, *S. pneumoniae*, *Haemophilus* species, and HSV.
- Scalp infection: Gonococcal scalp abscesses may be difficult to distinguish from abscesses caused by staphylococcal species, group B *Streptococcus*, *H. influenzae*, *Enterobacteriaceae*, and HSV.
- Vaginitis: In the prepubertal child, other causes include chemical or environmental irritants, pinworms, foreign body, and infections (i.e., streptococci, other bacteria, *Trichomonas vaginalis*). In cases of sexual abuse, *C. trachomatis* and syphilis may occur.
- Genitourinary tract infection: In adolescents, other causes include *C. trachomatis*, syphilis, and *T. vaginalis*.
- Arthritis: Other bacterial causes of septic arthritis, Reiter syndrome, and reactive arthritis.
- Abdominal pain: Ectopic pregnancy, appendicitis, cholecystitis, and urinary tract infection.

 Data Gathering

HISTORY

Question: Premature or prolonged rupture of membranes (or fetal scalp monitoring)?
Significance: These are risk factors for conjunctival infection caused by *N. gonorrhoeae*. Fetal scalp monitoring places the infant at risk for gonococcal scalp abscess.

Question: Vaginal itching and discharge?
Significance: Signs and symptoms of vaginitis. Prepubertal gonorrheal vaginitis is typically a mild disease that rarely causes ascending or disseminated infection. In adolescents, estrogenization protects the vagina from infection. Instead, the vagina serves as a conduit for cervical exudate.

Question: Purulent urethral discharge and dysuria without urgency or frequency?
Significance: Urethritis.

Question: Abdominal pain?
Significance: Ascending infection is characterized by diffuse lower quadrant abdominal pain, which may cause significant discomfort with ambulation. Low back pain, dyspareunia, and abnormal vaginal bleeding occasionally occur. Fever, chills, nausea, and vomiting may be present. Acute perihepatitis (Fitz-Hugh-Curtis syndrome) causes right upper quadrant pain and results from direct extension of infection from the fallopian tube to the liver capsule.

Question: Symptoms of pharyngitis, arthritis, dermatitis, meningitis, or endocarditis?
Significance: Gonococcal infections may occur outside the genitourinary tract.

Gonococcal Infections

Physical Examination

Finding: Neonatal ophthalmia
Significance: Typical findings include bilateral eyelid edema, chemosis, and copious purulent discharge. Onset may be on the first day of life, if prolonged rupture of membranes has occurred, or as late as several weeks of age.

Finding: Neonatal scalp abscess
Significance: Complication of fetal scalp monitoring.

Finding: Cervical motion tenderness
Significance: Signs of PID include cervical motion tenderness, pelvic adnexal tenderness (usually bilateral), and lower or right upper quadrant abdominal pain (with perihepatitis).

Finding: Purulent vaginal discharge
Significance: Common in both cervicitis and urethritis. Associated bacterial vaginosis may be noted.

Laboratory Aids

Test: Gram stain and culture of infected exudate or body fluid
Significance: Intracellular Gram-negative diplococci on Gram stain. Confirmation depends on isolation of *N. gonorrhoeae* from culture. The specimens are inoculated onto Thayer-Martin or chocolate blood agar-based media at room temperature, and promptly incubated in an enriched CO_2 environment. In suspected sexual abuse, genital, rectal, and pharyngeal cultures should be collected

Test: STD panel
Significance: Test for other sexually transmitted diseases in the child in whom sexual abuse is suspected or when evaluating the sexually active adolescent. This includes testing for *C. trachomatis*, syphilis, *T. vaginalis*, and HIV.

Test: Nonculture gonococcal tests
Significance: DNA amplification by polymerase chain reaction or ligase chain reaction (LCR) are comparable to culture in sensitivity and specificity but should NOT be used in investigations of possible sexual abuse (due to the possibility of false-positive results). In nonabuse cases, LCR may be performed on freshly voided urine (95% sensitivity; 100% specificity) and self-administered introital swabs.

Test: CBC, ESR, and C-reactive protein
Significance: Leukocytosis and elevated ESR and C-reactive protein occur in two thirds of patients with PID.

Test: Pelvic ultrasound
Significance: May detect ectopic pregnancy and in PID reveals thick, dilated fallopian tubes or tuboovarian abscess.

Test: Synovial fluid cell count and culture
Significance: In septic gonococcal arthritis, synovial fluid has >50,000 WBC/mm³ and the synovial fluid culture is positive, while the blood culture is usually negative. In arthritis-dermatitis syndrome, the synovial fluid contains <20,000 WBC/mm³, and the synovial fluid culture is sterile, while the blood culture is positive.

Therapy

• Neonate: Hospitalize and obtain appropriate cultures (blood, CSF, conjunctival, or other site of infection).

—Ophthalmia neonatorum: Ceftriaxone, 25 to 50 mg/kg IV or IM (single dose; maximum, 125 mg); alternate for infants with hyperbilirubinemia is cefotaxime 100 mg/kg IV or IM (single dose).
—Neonates with gonococcal ophthalmia also require eye irrigation with sterile saline at presentation and at frequent intervals until the mucopurulent drainage has ceased.
—Disseminated infection: Ceftriaxone daily or cefotaxime b.i.d. for 7 days; continue treatment for 10 to 14 days for meningitis.

• Older children and adolescents:

—Uncomplicated gonococcal infection: A single IM dose of ceftriaxone (50 mg/kg; maximum 1 g), or an oral dose of ciprofloxacin (500 mg), ofloxacin (400 mg), or azithromycin (20 mg/kg; maximum, 1 g). Follow with a treatment regimen for *C. trachomatis*.
—PID: See *Pediatric Red Book 2003* for treatment regimens.
—Disseminated gonococcal infection: Ceftriaxone for 7 days (arthritis), 14 days (meningitis), or 28 days (endocarditis). For arthritis add erythromycin, azithromycin, or doxycycline for 7 days. For meningitis or endocarditis add erythromycin for 7 days.

Follow-Up

INFECTION CONTROL

• Neonatal ophthalmia: Routine use of prophylactic ophthalmic ointment is mandatory in the United States. Instillation of ointment in both eyes occurs immediately after birth; choice of drugs includes 1% silver nitrate, 1% tetracycline, and 0.5% erythromycin ophthalmic ointments.
• Sexual contacts of persons with gonorrhea should be counseled and treated.
• Evaluate for concurrent infection with other STDs, including syphilis, *C. trachomatis*, *T. vaginalis*, and HIV. Patients beyond the neonatal period should be treated presumptively for *C. trachomatis* infection.
• Routine screening cervical cultures should be performed at the first prenatal visit; repeat at term if high risk.
• All cases of gonorrhea must be reported to public health officials.

ISOLATION OF HOSPITALIZED PATIENT

• Contact isolation precautions for all patients with gonococcal disease in the neonatal and prepubescent age groups are recommended; no special policies are recommended for other patients.

PITFALLS

• Failure to consider the diagnosis of sexual abuse in a child with a gonococcal infection beyond the neonatal period. Cases of transmission via nonsexual contact have been reported (i.e., from freshly infected towels, or other fomites, or by digital transmission from an infected caregiver) but cannot be assumed without first excluding sexual abuse.
• Using DNA amplification methods instead of culture to diagnose infection in cases of suspected abuse.
• Failure to differentiate *N. gonorrhoeae* by culture from other *Neisseria* species, especially in prepubertal children, due to the underlying question of child sexual abuse.
• Failure to consider the diagnosis of acute gonococcal perihepatitis in females with right upper quadrant pain.
• Classic findings of fever, leukocytosis, and elevated ESR or C-reactive protein are absent in one-third of patients with laparoscopically documented PID.

ICD-9-CM 098.0

BIBLIOGRAPHY

American Academy of Pediatrics. Pelvic inflammatory disease. In: Pickering LK, eds. *2003 Red Book: Report of the Committee on Infectious Diseases.* 26th Ed. Elk Grove Village, IL: American Academy of Pediatrics, 2003: 468–472.

Darville T. Gonorrhea. *Pediatr Rev* 1999;20: 125–128.

Hollier LM, Workowski K. Treatment of sexually transmitted diseases in women. *Obstetrics & Gynecol Clin North Am* 2002;30(4):751–775.

Ingram DM, Miller WC, Schoenbach VJ et al. Risk assessment for gonococcal and chlamydial infections in young children undergoing evaluation for sexual abuse. *Pediatrics* 2001;107(5):e73.

Koumans EH, Johnson RE, Knapp JS et al. Laboratory testing for *Neisseria gonorrhoeae* by recently introduced nonculture tests: a performance review with clinical and public health considerations. *Clin Infect Dis* 1998;27:1171–1180.

Lieberman JM. *Neisseria gonorrhoeae*. In: Long SS, Pickering LK, Prober CG, eds. *Principles and Practice of Pediatric Infectious Disease.* New York: Churchill Livingstone, 2003:756–762.

Moran J. Gonorrhoea. *Clinical Evidence* 2002;(7):1437–1444.

Sparling PF, Handsfield HH. *Neisseria gonorrhoeae*. In: Mandell GL, Bennett JE, Dolin R, eds. *Principles and Practice of Infectious Diseases.* Philadelphia: Churchill Livingstone, 2000:2242–2258.

Author: Samir S. Shah

Graft Versus Host Disease

 Database

DEFINITION

Graft versus host disease (GVHD) is a multiorgan inflammatory process that develops when immunologically competent T lymphocytes from a histoincompatible donor are infused into an immunocompromised host who is unable to reject the donor T cells. It is divided into acute and chronic forms and is caused by:

- Bone marrow transplantation (BMT)
- Transfusion of nonirradiated blood products (e.g., products containing viable T lymphocytes) to congenitally immunodeficient hosts or to acquired immunodeficient hosts that develop from high-dose therapies that require BMT for hematopoietic recovery.
- Transfusion of nonirradiated blood products from a donor who is homozygous for one of the recipient's human leukocyte antigen (HLA) haplotypes (usually first or second degree relative).
- Intrauterine maternofetal transfusions and exchange transfusions in neonates
- Solid organ grafts that contain viable T cells (e.g., small bowel transplants)
- Acute GVHD develops within 100 days following allogeneic stem cell transplant.
- Chronic GVHD develops 100 to 500 days following allogeneic stem cell transplant.
- Chronic GVHD is divided into three subsets based on onset:

—Progressive onset-extension of acute GVHD
—Quiescent onset occurs after resolution of acute GVHD
—De Novo onset no prior acute GVHD

PATHOPHYSIOLOGY

- Need three conditions to be met before GVHD can develop:

—The graft must contain immunocompetent cells
—The host must possess important transplantation alloantigens that are lacking in the donor graft, so the host appears foreign to the graft and is capable of stimulating it antigenically.
—The host itself must be incapable of mounting an effective immune reaction against the graft.

EPIDEMIOLOGY

- Overall, acute GVHD occurs in 30% to 60% of matched-related donor transplants, and chronic GVHD occurs in 27% to 50% of sibling matched-related donor transplants, 42% to 72% of matched-related donor transplants, 42% to 72% matched unrelated donor transplants, and 54% to 70% of allogeneic peripheral blood stem cell transplants.
- Chronic GVHD is the most common late complication of allogeneic stem cell transplantation

- The major risk factor is HLA disparity. GVHD is most common in unrelated donor marrow transplants and absent in identical twin transplants.
- Other risk factors include:

—Type of GVHD prophylaxis and history of herpes virus infection in the donor or the recipient
—Prior pregnancies in the marrow donor (which give rise to allosensitization)
—Older donor or recipient age
—Gender mismatch
—Vigorous T-cell depletion decreases the incidence of both acute and chronic GVHD
—Prior acute GVHD increases the risk of developing chronic GVHD

COMPLICATIONS

- Mortality from GVHD after BMT is usually related to infection.
- Rarely, patients die of hepatic failure or abdominal catastrophe.
- In transfusion-associated GVHD, the major cause of death is bone marrow aplasia (usually does not respond to immunotherapy) due to destruction of the host's marrow by donor lymphocytes.

PROGNOSIS

- Acute GVHD is graded on a scale from I to IV with percent of total body surface involved (skin), volume of diarrhea (gut), and/or elevation of serum bilirubin (liver).
- Grade I GVHD only involves one organ, usually the skin
- Patients with grade I GVHD do not have a survival different from those without GVHD.
- Grade II GVHD involves more than one organ; patient can have nausea/vomiting, anorexia, and food intolerance; confirmed by EGD biopsy.
- Grade III GVHD is severe and has multiorgan involvement.
- Patients with grade IV GVHD have a survival of only 10%–15% as do patients with progressive chronic GVHD (defined as acute GVHD, which does not resolve followed by chronic GVHD).

 Differential Diagnosis

ACUTE GVHD

- Skin: Dermal changes from chemoradiotherapy, drug reaction, viral exanthem
- Liver: Hepatic venoocclusive disease (VOD), elevations of liver function tests due to total parenteral nutrition, drug toxicity or infection, especially bacterial sepsis and cytomegalovirus
- Gastrointestinal: Diarrhea secondary to the BMT preparative regimen and infectious causes, especially *Clostridium difficile* and cytomegalovirus

 Data Gathering

HISTORY

Acute GVHD

Question: Rash? Itching?
Significance: Pruritus can precede the rash, which in BMT appears as the patient's blood counts are beginning to rise (median time of onset is 19 days posttransplant), and it is usually the first manifestation of acute GVHD. In transfusion-induced GVHD, symptoms usually start 1 week after the transfusion.

Question: Jaundice? Diarrhea? Abdominal pain? Intestinal bleeding?
Significance: GVHD in distal small bowel/colon. Unusual for involvement to precede skin disease

Question: Anorexia? Nausea? Vomiting? Dyspepsia?
Significance: GVHD proximal to distal small bowel.

Chronic GVHD

Question: Dry eyes? Dry mouth?
Significance: Be sure to ask if the patient forms saliva or tears because sicca syndrome can develop.

Question: Dysphagia?
Significance: Complaints of difficulty swallowing or retrosternal pain may be due to esophageal strictures.

Question: Blurry vision? Eye irritation? Photophobia? Eye pain?
Significance: Keratoconjunctivitis

Question: Sensitive to mint, spicy foods or tomatoes?
Significance: Mucosal involvement of GVHD

Question: Weight loss?
Significance: GI tract involvement of GVHD

Question: Dyspnea? Wheezing? Cough?
Significance: Bronchiolitis obliterans

Question: Frequent infections?
Significance: GVHD leads to profound immunodeficiency, functional asplenia and can have variable IgG levels. Patients with chronic GVHD are at high risk for pneumococcal sepsis, PCP, invasive fungal infections.

 Physical Examination

Acute GVHD/Transfusion-associated GVHD

Finding: Skin
Significance: Often begins as erythema of the palms, soles, and ears. The rash can become confluent erythroderma, and in the most severe cases can lead to bulla formation and even denudation reminiscent of burn injuries.

Finding: Liver
Significance: Jaundice can be seen but painful hepatomegaly, ascites, and rapid weight gain are atypical and are more often seen in VOD.

Chronic GVHD

Characterized as limited (localized skin involvement or hepatic dysfunction) or extensive (diffuse skin and/or multiorgan involvement with a much worse prognosis).

Finding: Skin
Significance: Hyper- or hypopigmentation, patchy erythema, scaling, lichenoid and sclerodermatous changes can be seen. The skin is involved in almost every patient.

Finding: Alopecia
Significance: Scalp and body hair can be thin and fragile

Finding: Nails
Significance: Vertical ridging and fragile

Finding: Whitish lace-like plaques on cheeks or tongue (resembles lichen planus) or ulcerations that are painful
Significance: Mucosal involvement of GVHD or thrush so should do biopsy for viral and fungal cultures.

Finding: Joints
Significance: Swelling can be seen: A detailed range of motion examination is crucial because contractures can be found in the absence of joint swelling.

 Laboratory Aids

The diagnosis of GVHD is often made on clinical grounds.

Test: Laboratory
Significance: In hepatic GVHD isolated elevations of transaminases can be seen without hyperbilirubinemia. In more severe cases, a cholestatic picture is seen. Howell-Jolly bodies can be seen on peripheral blood smear in the functional asplenia of chronic GVHD. Occasionally, patients will have cytopenias, or eosinophilia.

Test: Pulmonary function tests
Significance: Evidence of bronchiolitis obliterans or pulmonary fibrosis

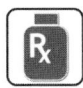 Therapy

The best therapy is prevention and includes γ-irradiation of all cellular blood products for patient at risk. Also important in the BMT setting are:

• Selection of a histocompatible donor
• Immunosuppressive therapy with the combination of cyclosporine and methotrexate is the gold standard.
• Steroids, usually in combination with cyclosporine or tacrolimus, have been used

for those patients who cannot tolerate methotrexate.

Treatment of established acute GVHD includes:

• Steroids at a dose of 2 mg/kg per day for 2 weeks followed by a taper over several months
• Cyclosporine or tacrolimus in those patients who did not receive it as prophylaxis
• Antithymocyte globulin (ATG) for steroid-resistant patients
• Mycophenolate mofetil (MMF), daclizumab (zenopax) and rapamycin are used as second line drugs.
• Infliximab (Remicade) and visilizumab (Nuvion) are other options for treatment of acute GVHD.

Options in treatment of chronic GVHD include:

• Steroids either alone or in combination with cyclosporine, MMF, daclizumab, or tacrolimus. Because many patients require treatment for months, the goal is alternate day therapy (e.g., steroids alternating with cyclosporine).
• Psoralen plus ultraviolet A (PUVA) is of some benefit in skin GVHD.
• Tacrolimus ointment has been effective in some patients with chronic GVHD to reduce pruritis and/or erythema of the skin.
• Oral beclomethasone has been used for treatment of gastrointestinal GVHD.
• IVIG for patients with low serum IgG levels.
• Manage patient's symptoms, e.g., lubricate dry skin with petroleum jelly, protect skin from injury, avoid sunburn, use artificial tears for sicca syndrome, and treat electrolytes imbalances for muscular aches and cramps.

 Follow-Up

• Acute GVHD: The institution of steroid therapy should lead to improvement within days in those patients who are destined to respond. However, gastrointestinal symptoms are notoriously slow to respond.
• Chronic GVHD: Acute GVHD, which merges directly into chronic GVHD, is termed progressive and has an extremely poor prognosis (approximately 10% survival at 5 years post-BMT). Thrombocytopenia is another poor prognostic factor. Such patients usually die of infection.
• Of note, patients with limited chronic GVHD have a decreased rate of relapse of leukemia and an increased survival rate.

PITFALLS

• Do not immunize a patient with a live vaccine if he or she has chronic GVHD. This may result in symptomatic infection.
• Take sudden high fevers seriously in a patient with GVHD. Overwhelming bacterial sepsis is not infrequent. Patients with chronic GVHD are often functionally asplenic (even if Howell-Jolly bodies are not seen on peripheral blood smear) and have profound immune function impairment.

 Common Questions and Answers

Q: If a child gets acute GVHD does that mean that he or she will get chronic GVHD?
A: No. Approximately 30% of patients less than 10 years of age who receive an HLA identical sibling BMT will get acute GVHD, whereas only 13% will develop chronic GVHD. Of note, chronic GVHD can develop in a patient who did not have acute GVHD. This is termed de novo and is much more favorable than progressive chronic GVHD.

Q: Do patients with severe chronic GVHD all die?
A: No. Occasionally the GVHD will "burn out." This is rare, and the process by which it happens is not understood.

BIBLIOGRAPHY

Burt RK, et al. How to identify graft versus host disease. *Contemporary Oncology* 1993;9:19–34.

Carpenter PA, Sanders JE. Steroid-refractory graft vs. host disease: past, present and future. *Pediatr Transplantation* 2003; 7(Suppl 3):19–31.

Ferrara JLM, Levy R, Chao NJ. Pathophysiologic Mechanism of Acute GVHD. *Biology of Blood and Marrow Transplantation* 1999;5:347–356.

Gaziev D, Galimberti M, Lucarelli G, et al. Chronic G-V-H disease: is there an alternative to the conventional treatment? *Bone Marrow Transplantation* 2000;25:689–696.

Lazarus HM, Vogelsang GB, Rowe JM. Prevention and treatment of acute GVH disease: the old and the new. A report from the Eastern Cooperative Oncology Group (ECOG). *Bone Marrow Transplantation* 1997;19:577–600.

Shivadansani RA, Haluska FG, Dock NL, et al. Brief report: graft-versus-host disease associated with transfusion of blood from unrelated HLA-homozygous donors. *NEJM* 1993;328:766–770.

Vogelsang GB. How I treat chronic graft versus host disease. *Blood* 2001;27(5):1196–1201.

Author: Valerie I. Brown

Graves Disease

Database

DEFINITION

Multisystem autoimmune disorder that presents with the classic triad of hyperthyroidism (goiter), exophthalmos, dermopathy (rare in children)

PATHOPHYSIOLOGY

• Autoimmune process that includes production of immunoglobulins against antigens in the thyroid, orbital tissue, and dermis.
• IgG_1 anti-TSH receptor-autoantibody (thyroid-stimulating immunoglobulin; TSI) activates the receptor, resulting in constitutive stimulation; thyroid follicular cells hyperfunction, leading to increased production and release of thyroid hormone.
• Fetal and neonatal hyperthyroidism can be caused by transplacental passage of maternal thyroid-stimulating immunoglobulins, activating Gs protein mutations (McCune-Albright syndrome) and activating TSH-receptor mutations.

EPIDEMIOLOGY

• 10%–15% of all childhood thyroid disorders.
• Incidence increases with age, peaking in adolescence and the third to fourth decade.
• Male: female ratio 1:4–5

COMPLICATIONS

• Endocrine disturbances: delayed/early puberty, menstrual irregularity, hypercalcemia
• Ophthalmologic: 3%–5% of patients develop severe ophthalmopathy, including eye muscle dysfunction and optic neuropathy, requiring specific treatment by an ophthalmologist. Pediatric ophthalmologic findings are more common but usually less severe than in adults.
• Bone: Hyperthyroidism leads to high bone turnover, with osteopenia common at the time of diagnosis. Bone mass corrects with treatment of the Graves disease and return to euthyroid status.
• Fetal/neonatal: IUGR, nonimmune hydrops fetalis, craniosynostosis, intrauterine death, goiter that complicates labor and possibly precipitates life-threatening airway obstruction at delivery, hyperkinesis, FTT, diarrhea, vomiting, cardiac failure and arrhythmias, systemic and pulmonary hypertension, hepatosplenomegaly, jaundice, hyperviscosity syndrome, thrombocytopenia

PROGNOSIS

• Good, if compliant with treatment.
• Mortality in severe thyrotoxicosis is possible from cardiac arrhythmias or cardiac failure.
• Spontaneous remission occurs in up to 25% of children after 2 years and 50% by 4.5 years. Relapse is not uncommon (3%–40%).
• Neonatal hyperthyroidism remits by 48 weeks, and commonly by 20 weeks.

Differential Diagnosis

For other causes of hyperthyroidism, see Goiter

INFECTIOUS

• Acute suppurative thyroiditis (transient thyroxine elevations).
• Subacute thyroiditis after viral illness (also transient hyperthyroidism).

ENVIRONMENTAL

• Thyroid hormone ingestion
• Ingestion of excess iodine (escape from Wolff-Chaikoff effect due to impaired autoregulation)

TUMORS (ALL RARE IN CHILDHOOD)

• TSH-producing pituitary adenoma
• Thyroid adenoma/hyperfunctioning autonomous thyroid nodule (most pediatric cases are euthyroid; incidence of nodule hyperfunctioning rises with increasing patient age).
• Thyroid carcinoma (rarely presents with hyperthyroidism)

CONGENITAL

• Neonatal Graves disease (transplacental antibody transfer from mothers with Graves disease or chronic thyroiditis)

Data Gathering

HISTORY

Question: Growth acceleration? May also be associated with precocious puberty
Significance: Hyperthyroidism can accelerate the bone age (developmental tempo).

Question: Declining school performance?
Significance: Mind racing, difficulty concentrating; may be mistaken for attention deficit/hyperactivity disorder.

Question: Any symptoms of hyperthyroidism and their duration?
Significance: If child complains of these symptoms, evaluate for possible hyperthyroidism

• Restlessness, emotional lability, and nervousness
• Fine tremor
• Insomnia and disturbed sleep pattern; may result in daytime fatigue
• Weight loss, despite increased appetite
• Palpitations and even chest pain with minimal exertion or at rest; diminished exercise tolerance
• Heat intolerance
• Diarrhea
• Muscle weakness (proximal)
• Plummer nails (separation of nail from nail bed)
• Menstrual irregularities
• Increased urination.

Question: Notice any thyroid gland enlargement? What is its duration? Tenderness?
Significance: Goiter can be a presenting sign of Graves. Tenderness suggests an infectious etiology.

Question: Bulging of the eyes or change in facial appearance? Increased staring? Change in vision?
Significance: Exophthalmos due to retroorbital immune depositions are a hallmark of Graves disease.

Question: Familial history of thyroid disease?
Significance: Increased incidence of Graves disease in families with positive history.

Physical Examination

Finding: Accelerated growth, or height above that expected by genetic potential
Significance: Due to bone age advancement.

Finding: Symmetrically enlarged, smooth, nontender goiter
Significance: More than 95% of cases

Finding: Auscultate the thyroid gland for bruit while patient holds his/her breath
Significance: Due to glandular hyperperfusion associated with hyperthyroidism.

Finding: Resting tachycardia with widened pulse pressure; hyperdynamic precordium
Significance: Cardiac effects of excessive thyroid hormone.

Finding: Slightly elevated temperature
Significance: Thyroid hormone is the main controller of basal metabolic rate and a positive modulator for catecholamine-induced thermogenesis.

Finding: Lid lag/stare; exophthalmos and proptosis
Significance: Severe ophthalmopathy is rare.

Finding: Fine tremor especially visible in hands and tongue
Significance: Occurs in about 60% of children with Graves disease

Finding: Proximal muscle weakness
Significance: Common but seldom severe

Finding: Exaggerated deep tendon reflexes
Significance: Variable

Finding: Skin warmth and moisture
Significance: Heat intolerance and excessive sweating occur in more than 30% of children.

Laboratory Aids

TESTS

Test: Total or free T4
Significance: Elevated

Test: T3 RIA
Significance: Elevated (T3 RIA, as direct measurement of T3, and not T3 RU, which indirectly evaluates thyroid hormone binding capacity).

Test: TSH
Significance: Significantly suppressed or undetectable

Graves Disease

Test: TSI titer
Significance: Positive in 90% of children

IMAGING

Test: I-123 scan
Significance: Usually not necessary to diagnose Graves disease, show diffuse increased uptake at 6 and 24 hours. If palpation suggests a nodule, however, a scan may be useful to reveal a "hot" nodule within a suppressed gland.

FALSE POSITIVES

• Elevated total T4 can also occur in conditions of increased protein binding, but does not signify hyperthyroidism.

—Increased estrogen states (e.g., pregnancy and oral contraceptive use) lead to augmented hepatic thyroid binding globulin (TBG) production
—Familial dysalbuminemic hyperthyroxinemia: mutation affecting the binding affinity leads to increased protein-bound pool

 Therapy

DRUGS

• First line of therapy in children
• Medications block thyroid hormone synthesis but not the release of already existing hormone.
• Antithyroid medications (thiourea derivatives): 65% to 95% effective

—Methimazole
—Propylthiouracil (PTU)

• Propranolol or atenolol: Block β-adrenergic related symptoms; should be used in conjunction with antithyroid medications at the initiation of treatment and whenever cardiac symptoms are prominent.
• Duration of treatment

—Antithyroid medications can be weaned and potentially discontinued after 2 to 3 years of therapy, depending on the patient's course.
—Beta-blockers: used until T4/T3 levels are under control (approximately 6 weeks).

• Other therapies should be considered in patients who are unresponsive to drug therapy, who have significant side effects from drug therapy, or who are chronically noncompliant.

I-131 ABLATION THERAPY

• 90% to 100% effective; safe and definitive, with predictable outcome
• Results in permanent hypothyroidism requiring lifelong thyroxine replacement

SUBTOTAL THYROIDECTOMY

• 80%–100% effective; rapid and definitive
• Expensive and invasive, with risk of significant complications
• Lifelong thyroxine replacement needed

POSSIBLE CONFLICTS

• Antihistamines and cold medications may exacerbate sympathetic nervous system symptoms.
• Treatment for severe ophthalmopathy: must refer to an ophthalmologist
—Three options: high-dose glucocorticoids, orbital radiotherapy, surgical orbital decompression
—Rehabilitative surgery involving the eye muscles or eyelids is commonly needed following ophthalmopathy treatment.

• Radioiodine ablation may exacerbate the ophthalmopathy, but this effect can be prevented with concomitant glucocorticoid administration.

 Follow-Up

WHEN TO EXPECT IMPROVEMENT

• Propranolol or atenolol should result in rapid relief of symptoms of sympathetic hyperactivity.
• 4 to 6 weeks of medical treatment should result in normalization of T4/T3 levels, though TSH may remain suppressed due to persistent underlying TSI activity.
• Duration and type of treatment depends on remission and relapse pattern.

SIGNS TO WATCH FOR

• Side effects of medications: Agranulocytosis (in 0.2–0.5%), rash (the most common side effect), gastrointestinal upset, headache, transient transaminitis/hepatitis with PTU, vasculitis with PTU (frequently associated with pANCA titers)

PITFALLS

• Discontinuation of antithyroid drugs because of low T4 values while TSH is still suppressed, reflecting continued TSI activity, will likely result in relapse. Antithyroid medication dose should be decreased or L-thyroxine should be added.
• Failure to recognize thyroid storm—an endocrinologic medical emergency.

 Common Questions and Answers

Q: Does hyperthyroidism mean my child has thyroid cancer?
A: No. The vast majority of pediatric thyroid cancers are euthyroid because even well-differentiated carcinomas synthesize thyroid hormone much less efficiently than does normal tissue.

Q: Does Graves disease lead to thyroid cancer?
A: No, though controversy surrounds the role of TSH and the closely related TSH-receptor antibodies of Graves disease in thyroid cancer incidence and aggressiveness. There is an increased incidence of benign thyroid adenoma from 0.6%–1.9% after use of I-131 ablation.

Q: Does hyperthyroidism affect long-term growth or final adult height?
A: No. Hyperthyroidism can cause tall stature and acceleration of skeletal maturity but does not typically affect final adult height.

Q: Should routine white blood cell counts be monitored while on antithyroid medications due to the risk of agranulocytosis?
A: No. Routine monitoring is not cost-effective due to the acuity and rarity of agranulocytosis. However, white blood cell counts should be checked whenever a patient on antithyroid medication develops a fever.

Q: Will the ophthalmopathy correct with antithyroid treatment?
A: Not necessarily. It may require specific intervention by an ophthalmologist.

Q: Sometimes my child's thyroid gland seems to get bigger and smaller even though the medication has not changed. Has anything been identified that exacerbates Graves disease?
A: Seasonal allergic rhinitis was found to not only induce antigen-specific IgE, but also stimulate increased serum antithyroid autoantibody concentrations among patients with Graves disease.

Q: Can mothers breast-feed while treated for Graves disease?
A: Yes. PTU has a lower milk/serum concentration ratio than methimazole (0.1 and 1.0, respectively). Three of 11 infants exclusively breast-fed by women on 300 to 750 mg daily PTU had high TSHs; of these three, one was just above the normal range and the other two completely corrected while the mother was still being medicated.

ICD-9-CM 242.0

BIBLIOGRAPHY

Bartalena L, Pinchera A, Marcocci C. Management of Graves' ophthalmopathy: reality and perspectives. *Endocr Rev* 2000;21:168–199.

Cooper DS. Antithyroid drugs in the management of patients with Graves' disease: an evidence-based approach to therapeutic controversies. *J Clin Endocrinol Metab* 2003;88:3474–3481.

Lippe BM, Landau EM, Kaplan SA. Hyperthyroidism in children treated with long term medical therapy: twenty-five percent remission every two years. *J Clin Endocrinol Metab* 1987;64:1241–1245.

Momotani N, Yamashita R, Makino F, et al. Thyroid function in wholly breast-feeding infants whose mothers take high doses of propylthiouracil. *Clin Endocrinol* 2000;53: 177–181.

Raza J, Hindmarsh PC, Brook CG. Thyrotoxicosis in children: thirty years' experience. *Acta Paediatr* 1999;88: 937–941.

Ringold DA, et al. Further evidence for a strong genetic influence on the development of autoimmune thyroid disease: the California twin study. *Thyroid* 2002;12:647–653.

Author: Adda Grimberg

Growth Hormone Deficiency

 Database

DEFINITION

Growth hormone (GH) deficiency is a lack of growth hormone synthesis, release, or effect.

CAUSES

- Idiopathic (the most common form)
- Congenital

—Congenital absence of the pituitary (empty sella syndrome)
—Deletion of the GH gene in familial isolated GH deficiency
—Familial panhypopituitarism
—Growth hormone receptor defect (Laron syndrome)
—Postgrowth hormone receptor defect
—In association with other midline defects: cleft lip, cleft palate, septooptic dysplasia, holoprosencephaly, male microphallus

- Acquired

—Trauma: Perinatal insult, birth trauma, surgical resection of pituitary gland, surgical damage to pituitary stalk, child abuse
—Infection: Viral encephalitis, bacterial or fungal infection, tuberculosis
—Vascular: Pituitary infarction, pituitary aneurysm
—Pituitary or hypothalamic irradiation
—Chemotherapy
—Tumors: Craniopharyngioma, glioma, pinealoma, primitive neuroectodermal tumor (PNET; medulloblastoma)
—Histiocytosis involving the pituitary gland or sella turcica
—Sarcoidosis
—Psychosocial dwarfism

PATHOPHYSIOLOGY

Lacking GH decreases levels of insulin-like growth factor I (IGF-I), a protein that acts on cartilage to stimulate linear growth.

GENETICS

—Spontaneous
—Autosomal recessive
—Autosomal dominant
—X-linked forms

EPIDEMIOLOGY (AGE-RELATED)

- Incidence in the United States is 1 per 4,000
- Males are more commonly diagnosed than females
- Two peak ages of diagnosis:

—Less than 1 year of age, usually because of associated hypoglycemia
—After 4 years of age, usually because of poor linear growth

COMPLICATIONS

- Short stature
- Lack of self-esteem due to the short stature
- Delay in pubertal changes (sexual characteristics and growth spurt) due to delayed bone age
- Hypoglycemia (in the newborn period)
- Osteopenia

PROGNOSIS

Excellent

 Differential Diagnosis

- Constitutional delay of growth and adolescence
- Familial short stature
- Malnutrition
- Intrauterine growth retardation
- Renal failure
- Inflammatory bowel disease
- Celiac sprue
- Hypo- or achondroplasia, or other skeletal dysplasia
- Turner syndrome
- Russell-Silver syndrome
- Prader-Willi syndrome and other genetic syndromes
- Cystic fibrosis
- Congenital heart disease
- Hypothyroidism
- Hypercortisolism

 Data Gathering

HISTORY

Question: Complications during pregnancy or delivery?
Significance: Growth failure associated with congenital GH deficiency manifests by third trimester; however, you must exclude maternal factors causing late intrauterine growth retardation such as oligohydramnios.

Question: Birth weight?
Significance: Birth weight is usually normal but birth length below the fifth percentile; length-for-weight at birth will be low.

Question: Hypoglycemia during infancy (the first months of life)?
Significance: GH is important to maintain euglycemia in the first months of life.

Question: Plot previous lengths/heights and characterize growth pattern (velocity)?
Significance: Growth velocity will be low, but the GH-deficient infant may not drop below the third percentile for length until the end of the first year of life.

Question: Signs/symptoms of systemic illness or chronic disease?
Significance: Vomiting, polyuria, loose stools, food-provoked gastrointestinal distress, etc., may suggest a cause other than GH deficiency.

Question: Heights of family members?
Significance: Measure both parents' heights whenever the family history reveals a man below 5′4″ or a woman below 4′11″ tall.

Question: Family timing of pubertal development: age at menarche or pubertal growth spurt?
Significance: Constitutional delay of growth and development tends to occur in multiple close family members.

Question: Document patient's growth pattern and heights of family members?
Significance: Measure height and weight of siblings whenever practical; always review prior growth records for the patient and siblings.

SPECIAL QUESTIONS

Question: Do girls with short stature who, as a result of a growth work-up, are discovered to have a form of Turner syndrome show classic features of Turner syndrome?
Significance: These girls show more subtle features of Turner syndrome such as wide-spaced breasts, scoliosis, marked short stature, and commonly delayed puberty. Rarely do such girls show a webbed neck, or lymph edema.

 Physical Examination

- Measure accurate weight and height with wall stadiometer
- Look for signs of syndromes, chronic disease, or malnutrition
- Evaluate Tanner stages of pubertal development
- Check males for micropenis (especially newborns)

Finding: Observe body habitus
Significance: Classic GH-deficient patient has:

- Protrusion of the frontal bones (frontal bossing)
- Midline facial defects such as poor development of nasal bridge and single central maxillary incisor
- Thin hair
- Poor nail growth
- High-pitched voice
- Truncal obesity and relative adiposity
- Cherubic facies

Finding: Observe dental development
Significance: Typically delayed

PROCEDURE

- Calculate dental age based on tooth eruption
- Quantify penile and testicular sizes:

—Small penis in congenital GH deficiency
—Testicular size (volume using Prader beads)

- Palpate for submucosal cleft palate
- Test visual fields
- Calculate growth velocity between growth measurements

Laboratory Aids

SPECIFIC TESTS

Test: Growth factors
Significance: IGF-I and IGFBP-3 (insulin-like growth factor binding protein-3) production is regulated directly by GH

Test: GH provocative testing.
Significance: A random GH level is generally of minimal value to diagnose GH deficiency because beyond the neonatal period, GH is only secreted in brief pulses during deep sleep (at night).

NONSPECIFIC TESTS

Growth factors and the following general tests should be used to screen for common causes of poor growth before embarking on GH provocative testing.

- CBC with differential
- Sedimentation rate: Looking for inflammatory processes
- Hepatic and renal function tests
- Chromosomes in females (to exclude Turner syndrome)
- Thyroid function tests

IMAGING

- Bone age: Radiography of left hand and wrist
- If proven to be GH deficient, use head MRI to look for central nervous system tumor or anomaly of the hypothalamus/pituitary

REQUIREMENTS FOR TESTING

All blood tests, except GH provocative testing, do not require any form of preparation.

 ## Therapy

DRUGS

- Recombinant human growth hormone (rhGH) by subcutaneous injection daily
- Nutropin depot (long-acting rhGH preparation)—discontinued production in 2004.
- Recombinant human GH-releasing hormone (rhGHRH) by subcutaneous injection
- IGF-1 therapy for the rare cases of GH resistance

DURATION OF THERAPY

- In children and adolescents:

—Until growth velocity drops to 2.5 cm per year
—Once puberty is complete

- In adulthood:

—GH-deficient adults may benefit from lifelong rhGH therapy due to its effects on body composition, lipids, bone density, and general sense of well-being

—Patient should again undergo GH provocative testing (off rhGH therapy)

DIET

Unrestricted

POSSIBLE CONFLICTS

Usually not given in cancer patients until 1 year has elapsed without recurrence

 ## Follow-Up

Every 3 months by an endocrinologist

WHEN TO EXPECT IMPROVEMENT

- Immediate effect on hypoglycemia
- Growth velocity improves within 3 to 6 months

SIGNS TO WATCH FOR

- Pseudotumor cerebri (headache, vision problems)
- Slipped capital femoral epiphysis (SCFE)
- Theoretically, increased risk of leukemia (though most studies suggest no significant increased risk)
- In adults, edema and carpal tunnel syndrome, but uncommon in children

PITFALLS

- Children with constitutional or pubertal delay show poor growth prior to starting puberty mimicking GH deficiency
- GH provocative testing may yield false-positive or false-negative results. 20% of normal children will fail at least one GH provocative test; obese but otherwise normal children are more likely to fail provocative GH testing.
- Malnutrition can cause low IGF-I.
- Psychosocial deprivation mimics GH deficiency. Such deprived patients may have low growth factors and respond poorly to GH provocative testing.
- rhGH therapy is associated with idiopathic intracranial hypertension (pseudotumor cerebri). This side effect is often transient, is usually reversible when the rhGH dose is decreased, and does not require cessation of therapy in all cases.
- Carefully evaluate any limp and knee or hip pain in patients on rhGH therapy because these symptoms may hail the onset of SCFE. SCFE mandates orthopedic consultation.
- There has been a slightly increased incidence of leukemia in rhGH-treated children. It is controversial whether this is due to rhGH or predisposing factors in these children (e.g., selection bias when studying children with growth failure).

 ## Common Questions and Answers

Q: Does growth hormone increase adult height in patients with familial short stature?
A: Clinical studies have shown that rhGH may improve final adult height in some children, however the results are unpredictable. The FDA added severe idiopathic short stature as an approved indication for hGH therapy, but controversy still exists.

Q: Does growth hormone cause tumors?
A: Clinical studies have not confirmed an association.

ICD-9-CM 253.3

BIBLIOGRAPHY

Botero D, Lifshitz F. Intrauterine growth retardation and long-term effects on growth. *Curr Opin Pediatr* 1999;11(4):340–347.

Clayton PE, Cohen P, Tanaka T, et al. Diagnosis of growth hormone deficiency in childhood. On behalf of the Growth Hormone Research Society. *Horm Res* 2000;53(Suppl 3):30.

Clayton PE, Cowell CT. Safety issues in children and adolescents during growth hormone therapy—a review. *Growth Hormone IGF Res* 2000;10(6):306–317.

Hintz RL, Attie KM Baptista J, et al. Effect of growth hormone treatment on adult height of children with idiopathic short stature. Genentech Collaborative Group. Multicenter study. Randomized controlled trial. *N Engl J Med* 1999;340(7):502–507.

Hintz RL. Approaches to the diagnosis and management of growth failure. *Pediatr Ann* 2000;29(9):537–538.

Rosenfeld RG. Transition from pediatric to adult care for growth hormone deficiency. *J Pediatr Endocrinol Metab* 2003;16(Suppl 3): 645–649.

Author: Craig A. Alter

Guillain-Barré Syndrome

 Database

DEFINITION

Guillain-Barré syndrome (GBS) is an acquired inflammatory demyelinating polyradiculoneuropathy. Inflammation of the peripheral nerves and nerve roots causes progressive weakness in the limbs, face, and respiratory muscles. Autonomic and sensory disturbance occurs. Stocking-glove distribution sensory loss may extend proximally.

CAUSES

• Follows viral infection in over 50% of cases. Cytomagalovirus (CMV), Epstein Barr virus (EBV), varicella-zoster virus (VZV), acute human immunodeficiency virus (HIV) infection, and others.
• Also associated with bacterial infection (especially *Campylobacter jejuni*), surgery, and vaccination.
• Tetanus toxoid is the only currently used vaccination with a clear link to GBS risk. Often, no precipitating event can be identified.

PATHOPHYSIOLOGY

Inflammatory cell-mediated and humeral-mediated immune mechanisms play a role in segmental demyelination on nerve biopsy; lymphocytes and macrophages participate in myelin destruction. Axonal variants of GBS have axonal degeneration without demyelination and minimal inflammatory infiltrate. Circulating antiganglioside antibodies (GM1, GM2, GQ1B, etc.) found in many cases suggests a molecular mimicry mechanism stimulated by infection.

ASSOCIATED DISEASES

• GBS is seen in a higher-than-expected rate in patients with sarcoidosis, systemic lupus erythematosis, lymphoma, HIV infection, Lyme disease, and solid tumors.
• Complications include respiratory failure, hypo or hypertension, urinary retention, aspiration, pain syndromes, deep venous thrombosis, infection susceptibility, muscle atrophy, joint contractures, and pressure ulcers.

EPIDEMIOLOGY

Overall yearly incidence rate of 0.6 to 1.9 cases per 100,000. Of 95 reported pediatric GBS patients, 45 were age 1 to 5, 36 were age 6 to 10, and 14 were age 11 to 15.

GENETICS

Genetic factors may influence susceptibility to GBS, and recent literature suggests particular subtypes of GBS are more common among certain HLA types. No data indicate an increase in GBS among first-order relatives.

PROGNOSIS

• 85% have a good recovery; ultimate functional recovery depends on the degree of axonal injury, which can be predicted from electrodiagnostic studies in adults.
• A recent study suggests that in children, there is no significant difference in recovery among demyelinating and axonal subtypes at 12 months.
• Early prognosticators include the severity of weakness at the disease nadir and fulminance of onset.
• Overall prognosis in children is better than adults.
• Death from early respiratory failure, autonomic instability, or other complications occurs in 3%–6%.

 Differential Diagnosis

• Myasthenia gravis
• Botulism
• Intoxication (heavy metals, organophosphates, etc.)
• Myopathy
• Poliomyelitis and other acute (viral) motor neuron disease
• Acute cerebellar ataxia
• Transverse myelitis
• Chronic inflammatory demyelinating polyneuropathy (CIDP)
• Vasculitic neuropathy
• Diphtheric neuropathy (rare)
• Porphyric neuropathy
• Locked-in state
• Psychogenic weakness/'astasia-abasia'

 Data Gathering

GBS has a variety of clinical presentations—index of suspicion is critical. Typical features are progressive motor weakness and areflexia, often following distal sensory changes. Common presentations include decreased ambulation (or crawling in toddlers), facial weakness, back pain, or sensory changes in the extremities. Acuity depends on the degree of respiratory involvement. Once respiratory status has been established and stabilized, attention should be directed to managing autonomic dysfunction, weakness, and pain. Close monitoring is required for dysautonomic symptoms; including arrhythmias, blood pressure lability/orthostatic hypotension, ileus, and urinary retention.

HISTORY

Question: Problems walking?
Significance: Most patients first note leg weakness or gait instability that progresses over days to weeks.

Question: Diminished finger and toe sensation?
Significance: Paresthesias and pain frequently appear early in the course. Sensory changes classically occur in a stocking-glove distribution and progress proximally.

Question: Recent fever, upper respiratory infection, or diarrhea?
Significance: Two-thirds of patients will report symptoms of an antecedent infection. The average interval between the infectious prodrome and GBS is 11 days, with a range of 7–21 days. Fever is generally not present at neurologic symptom onset.

Question: Respiratory problems?
Significance: Weakness may lead to respiratory paralysis in 20%–30% of children with GBS. Respiratory symptoms are rarely presenting complaints.

 Physical Examination

Finding: Weakness and sensory changes
Significance: Typical signs of GBS, classically with distal greater than proximal involvement. A proximal predominance of symptoms does not preclude the diagnosis.

Finding: Deep tendon reflexes are lost
Significance: Typical sign of GBS, though it may not occur until several days into the illness.

Finding: Respiratory difficulty, measured as decreased vital capacity, maximum inspiratory(PiMax) and expiratory(PeMax) pressures.
Significance: Respiratory failure leads to intubation in up to 10% of patients. Bulbar weakness and poor airway protection can also necessitate intubation. Impending respiratory failure can often be unpredictable, and blood gas determination is not a useful indicator of neuromuscular respiratory failure until intubation is imminent. If close monitoring of vital capacity, inspiratory or expiratory pressures suggest >30% decline in 24 hours, monitor patient in ICU.

Finding: Bilateral facial weakness
Significance: Occurs in up to 50% of cases.

Finding: "Floppy infant"
Significance: Neonates and infants may present as floppy infants.

Laboratory Aids

Test: Lumbar puncture
Significance: Nearly all patients have elevated cerebrospinal fluid protein after the first week of symptoms. Minimal pleocytosis (<10 WBC/mm³), comprised largely of mononuclear leukocytes, may occur but disappears in subsequent weeks.

Test: Electrodiagnosis
Significance: EMG findings can support the diagnosis of GBS and are often helpful when clinical or cerebrospinal fluid findings are ambiguous. EMG is abnormal in 50% of patients in the first 2 weeks and in 85% of patients afterwards. Features of demyelinating neuropathy include slowing of motor conduction, motor conduction block, prolonged distal motor latencies, and abnormalities of F waves. At presentation, conduction studies can frequently be normal.

Test: MRI of the spine (with gadolinium)
Significance: MRI should be performed if the clinical presentation is suspicious for a spinal cord compression syndrome (ie: paraparesis). Spinal nerve root enhancement on MRI can support the diagnosis of GBS.

Test: In atypical cases, consider heavy metal screen, HIV titer, Lyme titer, porphyria screen, acetylcholine receptor antibodies.
Significance: See Differential Diagnosis.

Test: IgA level should be considered if the child has a history of frequent pulmonary infections.
Significance: IgA deficiency would be a contraindication for IVIG therapy, due to anaphylaxis risk.

Emergency Care

The key elements of the emergency care of patients with GBS center around respiratory management, and deciding upon the need for hospitalization to monitor and treat possible progressive symptoms. Other potential concerns include heart block, hypotension, urinary retention, and neuropathic pain.

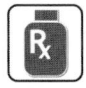
Therapy

A combination of supportive therapy and immunotherapy are the mainstays of treatment for patients with GBS.

- Regular monitoring of vital capacity; strongly consider intubation if vital capacity reaches less than 50% normal.
- Intravenous immunoglobulin (IVIG) and plasmapheresis have equivalent efficacy as first line immunotherapy. Combination of the two therapies has not proven more effective than either monotherapy alone. Complications and discontinuation of therapy are less common with IVIG.

- Most large randomized studies in GBS have been with adults, but pediatric studies have shown both modalities are well tolerated and yield similar results. Practice guidelines regarding immunotherapy in GBS exist for adults and are noted below.
- IVIG should be given at 0.4 g/kg (body wt) for 5 consecutive days, and initiated in ambulatory patients within 2 to 4 weeks of symptom onset.
- Plasmapheresis requires placement of a central pheresis catheter. Total plasma exchange volume of 200 to 250 mL/kg divided in 3 to 5 treatments over 7 to 14 days. Therapy initiation is recommended within 4 weeks of symptom onset for nonambulatory patients and 2 weeks for ambulatory patients.
- Corticosteroids have not been shown to be helpful as monotherapy or in combination with IVIG, and are not recommended.
- Management in an intensive care unit is often required. Respiratory vital capacity, maximum inspiratory and expiratory pressures should be frequently monitored. Elective intubation should be performed when the vital capacity falls below 10 mL/kg or less than 50% of expected normal. A 30% decline in VC, PiMax and PeMax are highly correlative with progression to respiratory failure.
- Close monitoring with telemetry and frequent blood pressures.
- Avoid contractures with lower extremity splinting and early passive range of motion. Aggressive PT and OT are essential for good outcomes.
- Particular attention should be given to preventing secondary compressive neuropathies.
- Pain from nerve root inflammation is common in GBS and should be treated aggressively.
- No known prevention measures.

Follow-Up

- First improvement typically begins 2 to 3 weeks after onset of symptoms but may not occur for 1 to 2 months in some patients.
- Improvement continues for up to 2 years.

PITFALLS

- Respiratory failure may occur quickly.
- Approximately 10% of patients present with a GBS variant. These include pure motor GBS, pharyngeal-cervical-brachial weakness, paraparetic form, ataxic form or Miller-Fisher syndrome (ophthalmoplegia, ataxia, and areflexia, associated with anti-GQ1B antibodies in the CSF), acute dysautonomia.
- Gait instability may mistakenly be interpreted as psychogenic early in the course of GBS.
- Treat hypertension cautiously; catastrophic, refractory hypotension may ensue.
- Although the loss of deep tendon reflexes is considered a hallmark of the disease, reflexes may be preserved in early stages of illness.

- Though distal onset of symptoms (motor and sensory) is the classic presentation, proximal symptoms may predominate early in the course of illness.
- Check for reflexes in patients with bilateral Bell palsy. Close observation for further development of symptoms or signs of GBS.

Common Questions and Answers

Q: Is GBS contagious?
A: No.

Q: Will I get GBS again?
A: Acute relapses occur in 1%–5% of patients in large series. Chronic inflammatory demyelinating polyradiculoneuropathy (CIDP) can begin with a rapid onset of weakness indistinguishable from GBS.

Q: Do all cases require hospitalization and immunomodulatory treatment?
A: It is reasonable to observe some youngsters who have mild, nondisabling sensory symptoms on an outpatient basis, though hospitalization and pharmacologic intervention is the usual default strategy. Treatment related fluctuations (worsening after completion of immunotherapy) can occur in up to 10% of patients and may require repeated treatment.

ICD-9-CM 357.0

BIBLIOGRAPHY

Abd-Allah SA, Jansen PW, Ashwal S, et al. Intravenous immunoglobulins as therapy for pediatric Guillain-Barre syndrome. *J Child Neurol* 1997;12(6):376–380.

Hahn AF. Guillain-Barre syndrome. *Lancet* 1998;352(9128):635–641.

Hughes RA, et al. Practice parameter: immunotherapy for Guillain-Barre syndrome: report of the Quality Standards Subcommittee of the American Academy of Neurology. *Neurology* 2003;61(6):736–740.

Lawn ND, et al. Anticipating mechanical ventilation in Guillain-Barre syndrome. *Arch Neurol* 2001;58(6):893–898.

Parent Intenet Information: Guillain-Barre Syndrome Foundation International- http://www.gbsfi.com.

Tekgul H, et al. Outcome of axonal and demyelinating forms of Guillain-Barre syndrome in children. *Pediatr Neurol* 2003;28(4):295–299.

Authors: James Boyd
Ann Poduri, 3rd edition

Gynecomastia

Database

DEFINITION

Any visible or palpable proliferation of breast glandular tissue, unilateral or bilateral, due to an increase in estrogen action relative to androgen action at the level of the breast.

ETIOLOGY

Physiologic

- Neonatal: Transient palpable breast tissue developing in newborns due to the high estrogen levels in the feto-placental unit. This condition resolves as estrogen levels decline.
- Pubertal: Benign transient gynecomastia occurring in otherwise healthy adolescent males. Breast tissue in pubertal gynecomastia measuring less than 4 cm in diameter has a high likelihood of spontaneous regression.
- Involutional: Breast enlargement occurring in elderly men.

Pathologic

- Drug-induced

—Hormones: Estrogen, androgens, gonadotropins, anabolic steroids, growth hormone, antiandrogens and estrogen-containing cosmetics, foods, hair products and herbal remedies.
—Antiinfective agents: Ethionamide, isoniazid, ketoconazole, metronidazole
—Antiulcer drugs: Cimetidine, ranitidine, omeprazole
—Chemotherapeutic agents: Alkylating agents, methotrexate, vinca alkaloids
—Cardiovascular agents: Amiodarone, captopril, digitoxin, diltiazem, enalapril, methyldopa, nifedipine, reserpine, spironolactone, verapamil
—Psychotropic agents: Diazepam, haloperidol, phenothiazines, tricyclic antidepressants
—Drugs of abuse: Alcohol, amphetamines, heroin, marijuana, methadone
—Miscellaneous: Metoclopramide, phenytoin, penicillamine, theophylline, gabapentin

- Hypogonadism: Primary or secondary
- Tumors: Testicular, adrenal, ectopic hCG-producing tumors
- Chronic disease: Hyperthyroidism, renal failure, liver disease, malnutrition with refeeding, HIV infection
- Congenital disorders: Klinefelter syndrome, vanishing testes syndrome (also known as anorchia, gonadal agenesis, or testicular regression), androgen resistance syndromes, true hermaphroditism, excessive peripheral tissue aromatase
- Acquired testicular failure: Viral orchitis, trauma, granulomatous disease or castration
- Chest wall trauma
- Intercostal nerve damage following surgery or herpes zoster
- Psychological stress
- Spinal cord injury

PATHOPHYSIOLOGY

Any situation that leads to an increase in the net effect of estrogen action relative to androgen action at the level of the breast may lead to gynecomastia. These situations could include:

- Increased estrogen concentration (endogenous or exogenous)
- Normal estrogen levels with decreased androgen concentrations
- Congenital reduction in estrogen receptors
- Pharmacologic blockade of androgen receptors
- Increased breast or peripheral tissue aromatase (aromatase converts androgens to estrogens)
- Testicular dysfunction
- High serum gonadotropins or increased sex hormone-binding globulin
- Elevated estrogen levels lead to proliferation of the ducts and surrounding mesenchymal tissue resulting in breast enlargement.

GENETICS

Gynecomastia is occasionally familial, following X-linked or sex-limited autosomal-dominant patterns.

EPIDEMIOLOGY

- Two peaks in age distribution occur in the pediatric population: in the neonatal period and in puberty.
- Neonatal gynecomastia occurs in 60%–90% of all newborns.
- 40% of boys develop transient gynecomastia (measuring ≥0.5 cm) during puberty.
- Peak incidence for pubertal gynecomastia in males at 14 years (range 10–16 years).

COMPLICATIONS

- Physical pain, which may interfere with sports
- Psychological stress
- Embarrassment
- Skin erosion of the nipple due to rubbing against clothing
- Breast cancer: patients with Klinefelter syndrome have a 16-fold increased risk of breast cancer; other causes of gynecomastia are not associated with an increased risk of breast cancer

PROGNOSIS

- Overall, good
- Pubertal gynecomastia: 75% disappears spontaneously within 2 years, and 90% within 3 years.
- Neonatal gynecomastia usually resolves within the first year of life.

Differential Diagnosis

INFECTIOUS

- Breast abscess

NEOPLASTIC

- Breast neoplasm
- Neurofibroma
- Lymphangioma
- Lipoma
- Neuroblastoma metastasis

TRAUMA

- Hematoma

MISCELLANEOUS

- Pseudogynecomastia: Excessive adipose tissue only; no discrete subareolar tissue
- Dermoid cyst

Data Gathering

HISTORY

Question: Time of onset relative to puberty?
Significance: Genitalia development will be present for at least 6 months before onset of breast development.

Question: Rate of progression?
Significance: Rapidly enlarging, painful gynecomastia with acute onset is more concerning than long-standing enlargement.

Question: Drug exposures, including alcohol and substance abuse?
Significance: Marijuana and heroin addiction may cause gynecomastia.

Question: Exposure to exogenous estrogen?
Significance: Gynecomastia in a prepubertal boy could suggest direct exposure to exogenous estrogens or indirect exposure from an adult.

Question: Symptoms suggestive of hyperthyroidism?
Significance: 30% of young men with hyperthyroidism develop gynecomastia.

Question: Symptoms suggestive of liver disease, such as cirrhosis?
Significance: Liver disease may alter the estrogen-androgen ratio causing gynecomastia. Damaged hepatic cells may lose the ability to inactivate estrogens. Impaired hepatic removal of androstenedione from the bloodstream provides more androstenedione for the periperal conversion to estrogen. Liver disease may result in the elevation of sex-steroid-binding globulin, which reduces circulating free testosterone.

Question: Symptoms suggestive of neoplastic disease?
Significance: In patients <10 years of age, consider pituitary, adrenal or testicular tumor. Liver tumors may cause gynecomastia due to increased aromatization of circulating adrenal androgens or by secretion of chorionic gonadotropins.

Question: Symptoms suggestive of hypogonadism, such as decreased libido, decreased erectile function, or infertility? *Significance:* These symptoms may suggest an abnormal estrogen to androgen ratio.

 ## Physical Examination

- Assess height, weight, growth velocity, and blood pressure.
- Assess for malnourishment. Malnourishment may result in hepatic dysfunction causing higher estrogen to androgen ratio.

Finding: Perform a complete breast examination.
Significance: With patient in the supine position, grasp the breast between the thumb and forefinger and move digits toward the nipple: look for a firm, rubbery, mobile, disk-like mound of tissue arising concentrically below the nipple and areola. Measure the diameter of the disk of glandular tissue. Asymmetry and tenderness are common.

Finding: Pseudogynecomastia
Significance: If pseudogynecomastia (fatty enlargement of breasts) is present, no glandular disk will be palpable.

Finding: Check for galactorrhea.
Significance: Seen with drug ingestion and pituitary tumor.

Finding: Determine if macrogynecomastia (disk diameter >5 cm with a secondary mound above the level of the breast) is present.
Significance: Macrogynecomastia may be physiologic or pathologic, and is unlikely to regress.

 ## Laboratory Aids

- None indicated for pubertal and neonatal gynecomastia.
- Renal, hepatic, and/or thyroid function tests if indicated.

Test: Karyotype
Significance: To rule out Klinefelter syndrome, if suspected.

Test: Luteinizing hormone (LH), follicle stimulating hormone (FSH), estradiol, testosterone, dehydroepiandrosterone (DHEA), and human chorionic gonadotropin (hCG).
Significance: To determine if hypogonadism, precocious puberty, testicular tumor or adrenal tumor could be present. An isolated elevated estradiol level in an otherwise normal prepubertal boy may suggest direct or indirect exogenous estrogen exposure.

Test: Prolactin level
Significance: To rule out a prolactin-secreting pituitary tumor. If galactorrhea present or if decreased testosterone with decreased or normal LH.

Test: Bone age (radiograph of the left hand and wrist)
Significance: Elevated estrogens may accelerate skeletal maturation

Test: Testicular ultrasound
Significance: To rule out testicular tumor, of elevated hCG, elevated estradiol or asymmetric testes on physical examination.

Test: Chest x-ray with abdominal computed tomography imaging (CT)
Significance: If hCG elevated and testicular ultrasound is normal to rule out extragonadal germ cell tumor or hCG-secreting nontrophoblastic neoplasm.

Test: Adrenal CT or magnetic resonance imaging (MRI)
Significance: To rule out adrenal neoplasm, if estradiol elevated, DHEA elevated, LH decreased or normal, and testicular ultrasound normal

Test: Skull x-ray, brain MRI, or CT
Significance: If pituitary tumor is suspected.

 ## Therapy

- Reassurance for patients with pubertal gynecomastia measuring less than 4 cm. Treatment guidelines are variable for gynecomastia measuring 4 to 5 cm. Surgical consultation in these patients should be considered.
- Reexamine at 3-month intervals.
- Discontinue any drugs known to induce gynecomastia and follow up in 1 month.
- Correct any underlying disorders (hyperthyroidism, malnutrition, etc.).

DRUGS

- The effectiveness of drugs in the treatment of gynecomastia has been difficult to evaluate due to the high prevalence of spontaneous regression.
- Generally, drug therapy should proceed under the guidance of an endocrinologist.

—Tamoxifen (as unlabeled or investigational use) and testolactone

- If gynecomastia has been present for more than 1 year, pharmacologic therapy is of little benefit.
- Surgery is the therapy of choice for macrogynecomastia, or persistent gynecomastia resistant to medical therapy.

Ultrasound-assisted liposuction has emerged as a new alternative surgical option.

 ## Follow-Up

- Watch for signs of psychological stress.
- Watch for symptoms of chronic disease, abnormal physical changes.

- Mistaking pseudogynecomastia (i.e., fatty enlargement of the breasts) for true gynecomastia
- Overlooking a potentially drug-related etiology. Drug-related gynecomastia is usually reversible if diagnosed within 1 year of onset.

 ## Common Questions and Answers

Q: When should a patient with gynecomastia be referred to a specialist?
A: If macrogynecomastia is present, if there is an abnormal hormonal workup or an abnormal imaging study, or if there is an abnormal rate of progression.

Q: For how long does neonatal gynecomastia persist?
A: Studies of healthy term infants have shown that the diameter of the breast tissue may actually increase during the first 2 weeks of life. The breast tissue then decreases to an average diameter of 10 mm until about 4 to 6 months of age. The breast tissue of female infants is generally larger and may persist longer than in males. Occasionally, the breast tissue will fail to regress and remain after the first year of life.

Q: How is gynecomastia distinguished from breast cancer?
A: Breast cancer usually presents as a unilateral, eccentric hard or firm mass that is fixed to underlying tissues. Associated findings can include dimpling of the skin, retraction of the nipple, nipple discharge, or axillary lymphadenopathy. The incidence of breast cancer in the pediatric population is extremely low. Less than 0.1% of all breast cancers occur in patients less than 20 years of age. Benign tumors, such as fibroadenomas, are much more common than malignant breast tumors.

Q: Has the incidence of gynecomastia increased?
A: As the prevalence of childhood and adolescent obesity has increased, the presence of pseudogynecomastia has also increased. If glandular tissue is not present, pseudogynecomastia should be treated with diet and exercise.

ICD-9-CM 611.1

BIBLIOGRAPHY

Felner EI, White PC. Prepubertal gynecomastia: indirect exposure to estrogen cream. *Pediatrics* 2000;105:e55.

Lazala C, Saenger P. Pubertal gynecomastia. *J Pediatr Endocrin & Metabol* 2002;15(5):553–560.

Mahoney CP. Adolescent gynecomastia: differential diagnosis and management. *Pediatr Clin North Am* 1990;37:1389–1404.

Author: Julie A. Boom

Hand-Foot-and-Mouth Disease

Database

DEFINITION

Hand-foot-and-mouth disease is a viral illness with the characteristic clinical features of:

- Vesiculoulcerative stomatitis
- Papular or vesicular exanthem on the hands and/or the feet
- Mild constitutional symptoms such as fever and malaise

CAUSES

Coxsackie A16 virus is the most common causative agent. Occasionally, hand-foot-and-mouth disease results from infection with:

- Coxsackie viruses A5, A7, A9, A10, A16, B1, and B3
- Enterovirus 71
- Other enteroviruses
- Herpesviruses

PATHOPHYSIOLOGY

- Enteroviruses are acquired by the oral or respiratory route.
- Lymphatic invasion leads to viremia and spread to secondary sites.
- Viremia ceases with antibody production.
- Direct inoculation of the extremities from oral lesions has been suggested in regard to hand-foot-and-mouth disease.

EPIDEMIOLOGY

- In temperate climates hand-foot-and-mouth disease is most common in the summer and fall (a pattern common to many of the enterovirus infections).
- Spread primarily by fecal contamination and contact. Oral and respiratory secretions may also transmit the virus.
- Incubation period is 4 to 6 days.
- Highly contagious, afflicting up to one half of those exposed.
- Close household contacts are particularly susceptible.
- May occur as an isolated case or in an epidemic distribution
- Most common in children under 5 years, but may affect adults.

COMPLICATIONS

- Hand-foot-and-mouth disease is usually self-limited and uncomplicated, resolving within 10 days.
- Dehydration is the most frequent morbid complication:

—Oral ulcerations are painful and interfere with feeding.
—Infants and children are at highest risk.

- Rare reports of other complications include:

—Neurologic complications such as aseptic meningitis, encephalitis, and a polio-like paralytic disorder
—Pneumonia
—Myocarditis
—A possible association with first trimester spontaneous abortions in previously infected women

PROGNOSIS

- In the vast majority of instances hand-foot-and-mouth disease will resolve quickly requiring only supportive care.
- Young children bear the closest scrutiny because they suffer the greatest morbidity.
- Careful history and examination should distinguish those individuals with the rare aforementioned complications.
- Rare cases may recur at intervals for up to 1 year.

Differential Diagnosis

Few infectious diseases have such characteristic clinical findings. Oral ulcerations followed by lesions on the distal extremities are virtually pathognomonic. The most difficult diagnostic dilemmas may be early in the disease course when isolated oral lesions predominate.

- Herpangina

—Also caused by Coxsackie A viruses
—Associated with higher fever
—Usually limited to the posterior oropharynx

- Herpetic gingivostomatitis

—Most common cause of stomatitis in children
—Associated with higher fever
—More frequently associated with lymphadenopathy
—Gingival involvement severe
—Aphthous ulcers
—Generally occurs without fever or upper respiratory symptoms
—Does not occur in "outbreaks"

- Stevens-Johnson syndrome

—Ulcerations frequently coalesce
—Usually affects other mucous membranes
—Often appears with separate cutaneous manifestations

- The "Boston exanthem"

—Caused by echovirus 16
—Mild febrile illness with a macular rash on the palms and soles occurring at time of or after defervescence
—Oral lesions absent

Data Gathering

HISTORY

Question: History of ill contacts?
Significance: Incubation period may be up to 1 week.

Question: Any fever, pain, or other symptoms?
Significance: A mild prodrome occasionally precedes the characteristic enanthem and exanthem by 1 or 2 days: low-grade fever (usually near 38.3°C), malaise, sore mouth, anorexia, coryza, diarrhea, abdominal pain.

Question: Bone pain?
Significance: Bone and joint aches infrequently accompany this illness.

Question: Lesions in mouth?
Significance: Oral lesions typically occur shortly before the hand and foot manifestations.

Question: Anyone in family sick?
Significance: Family members or close contacts are often similarly affected.

Question: Hydration status?
Significance: Determine quality and amount of oral intake, quality and amount of urine output, recent weight loss, duration of symptoms.

Physical Examination

Finding: Enanthem
Significance:

- Oral lesions begin as small, red papules.
- Papules quickly evolve to small vesicles on an erythematous base.
- Lesions progress to ulcerations.
- Tongue, buccal mucosa, palate, gingiva, uvula, and/or tonsillar pillars may be involved.
- Usually 2 to 10 lesions.
- Oral lesions may persist up to 1 week.

Finding: Exanthem
Significance:

- Less consistently present than oral lesions (occur in one-fourth to two-thirds of patients)
- Maculopapular eruptions progress to vesicles.
- Rarely tender or pruritic
- Most frequent on the dorsal aspects of fingers and toes
- May also occur on the palms, soles, arms, legs, buttocks, and face

Finding: Adenopathy
Significance: Enlarged anterior cervical, or submandibular nodes are present in one-fourth of cases.

Hand-Foot-and-Mouth Disease

Finding: Other
Significance: Attention should be given to the patient's vital signs, general appearance, and respiratory, cardiac, and neurologic functioning to help identify the rare patient with a threatening complication of hand-foot-and-mouth disease.

 Laboratory Aids

Test: Physical examination
Significance: Hand-foot-and-mouth disease has rather unique clinical features and a relatively benign course. Laboratory confirmation of the diagnosis is seldom needed or indicated.

Test: Culture
Significance: Causative viruses may be cultured from many sites:

- Oral ulcers
- Cutaneous vesicles
- Nasopharyngeal swabs
- Stool (isolation of an enterovirus from the stool does not confirm it to be the cause of disease; such a result must be paired with clinical suspicion or serologic findings)
- Cerebrospinal fluid (in cases where meningoencephalitis is suspected)

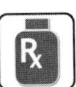 Therapy

- Most cases will spontaneously resolve and require no therapy other than parental reassurance.
- Acetaminophen may relieve malaise and minor discomfort associated with the oral ulcers. It also may be used as an antipyretic in those children with fever.
- Dietary adjustments often improve oral intake and prevent or relieve dehydration:

—Avoid spicy or acidic foods.
—Provide cool or iced liquids in small quantities frequently.

- Symptomatic relief from particularly painful oral ulcers may be accomplished by application of a topical antihistamine or anesthetic directly to the sores (see Common Questions and Answers, below).
- Dehydration should be treated when present. Intravenous fluids may be required in the more severe cases, especially in infants and young children.
- Good supportive care is generally sufficient to treat most complications.

PREVENTION

- Frequent hand washing, especially after changing diapers, and good personal hygiene are the most useful means to prevent spread of enteroviral illnesses.
- Enteric precautions should be maintained with all hospitalized patients.
- The prodromal and enanthem periods appear to be the most contagious; however, some carriers of Coxsackie A16 may shed virus in the stool 3 months after infection (see Common Questions and Answers, below).

 Follow-Up

- Hand-foot-and-mouth disease generally resolves spontaneously within 1 week after diagnosis.
- Small children must be followed closely for signs of dehydration.
- The extremely rare complication of myocarditis has been reported to result in at least two fatalities.
- Some patients may become asymptomatic carriers

 Common Questions and Answers

Q: What is in the "magic mouthwash" often used to relieve the pain of stomatitis?
A: Many health care providers will prescribe a "magic mouthwash" for symptomatic relief of oral ulcers, pharyngitis, and teething pain. The most common such treatment consists of an aluminum hydroxide/magnesium hydroxide gel suspension and diphenhydramine elixir (12.5 mg/5 mL) in a 1:1 formulation. It can be applied directly to the sores with a cotton swab or a small syringe before meals. Note: some people will have a reaction to topical diphenhydramine.

Q: Should lidocaine be used topically for symptomatic relief of oral ulcers?
A: The routine use of lidocaine in this situation is not recommended. Lidocaine is an effective topical anesthetic and comes in a 2% viscous suspension. In practice, the pain relief is short-lived, which encourages frequent administration. Lidocaine is absorbed from the mucous membranes (bypassing first-pass liver metabolism) and has been frequently reported to cause poisoning of the cardiovascular and central nervous system. Both pediatric and adult fatalities have occurred. The use of topical viscous lidocaine should be reserved for use by physicians knowledgeable regarding its proper dosage and potential side effects, and by educated, compliant parents or caregivers.

Q: When may children with hand-foot-and-mouth disease return to school?
A: This is a matter of some controversy for this highly contagious, but relatively benign, condition. However, good hygiene will greatly reduce viral transmission. And affected patients are contagious often before the diagnosis is made. Most now suggest isolation from school or day-care contacts while febrile and/or while the enanthem persists. As mentioned, some may shed the virus in their stool for months after symptoms have resolved (again stressing the need for good personal hygiene).

ICD-9-CM 074.3

BIBLIOGRAPHY

Cherry JD. Enteroviruses and parechoviruses. In: Feigin RD, et al, eds. *Textbook of Pediatric Infectious Diseases.* 4th Ed. Philadelphia: WB Saunders, 2004:1984–2041.

Robinson CR, Doane FW, Rhoades AJ. Report of an outbreak of febrile illness with pharyngeal lesions and exanthem: Toronto, 1957-isolation of coxsackie virus. *Can Med Assoc J* 1958;79:615–621.

Scott LA, Stone MS. Viral exanthems. *Dermatology Online Journal* 2003;9(3):4.

Slavin KA, Frieden IJ. Picture of the month: hand-foot-and-mouth disease. *Arch Pediatr Adolesc Med* 1998;152:505–506.

Authors: Jason Newland and Kevin C. Osterhoudt

Hantavirus/Hantapulmonary Syndrome

 Database

DEFINITION

Hantapulmonary syndrome (HPS) is a disease in humans due to a Hantavirus and acquired from certain chronically infected rodent species. When acquired by humans, it results in a syndrome characterized by a flu-like illness followed by rapidly progressive cardiac and respiratory failure with a high mortality.

CAUSE

Original human outbreak recognized in Southwest United States was caused by the Sin nombre strain of Hantavirus transmitted from chronically infected deer mice (*Peromyscus maniculatus*). Subsequent cases were recognized throughout the ubiquitous distribution of the deer mouse. Since then, additional strains of Hantavirus have been recognized each with a unique rodent host. The resulting human cases of HPS have now been identified from Canada to Argentina.

EPIDEMIOLOGY

- The host rodent develops a chronic nonfatal infection and excretes virus in urine, feces, and saliva.
- Humans acquire the infection by inhaling virus-contaminated airborne particles from the dried rodent excreta. Typically, this occurs when sweeping or otherwise disturbing a rodent-infested building.
- Human cases are more common in the spring and summer and also in years when the population of the rodent host has increased.
- Nosocomial transmission has been observed only with the Andes strain in Argentina, never in the United States.
- In the United States, HPS has occurred primarily in young healthy adults, although in South America a larger proportion of cases are in children.

PATHOLOGY/PATHOPHYSIOLOGY

- Pathophysiologic changes of most importance are myocardial depression resulting in shock and alveolar capillary leak pulmonary edema resulting in hypoxia.
- The cardiac dysfunction is characterized by a falling cardiac output, increased systemic vascular resistance and normal or low pulmonary artery wedge pressure.
- The pulmonary alveoli are flooded with fluid devoid of red cells but with a protein content similar to serum.

 Differential Diagnosis

- Pneumonic plague
- Influenza
- Bacterial sepsis, especially that caused by *pneumococcus* and other streptococci
- Other causes of shock and pneumonia or shock and pulmonary edema

 Data Gathering

The clinical symptoms, physical findings and laboratory findings progress in sequence. Early suspicion of the syndrome allows the clinician to prepare for that phase of the illness characterized by the rapid onset of respiratory failure and shock.

HISTORY

Question: Fever and myalgia?
Significance: Usually severe, characterize the prodromal phase lasting 3 to 6 days.

Question: Gastrointestinal complaints?
Significance: Frequently prominent including combinations of nausea, vomiting, diarrhea, or abdominal pain.

Question: Headache?
Significance: Is present in over one-half of patients.

Question: Cough?
Significance: Uncommon at the onset of the prodrome but heralds the onset of dyspnea and tachypnea, which is then followed by the rapid progression of cardiorespiratory failure.

Question: Coryza and sore throat?
Significance: Rarely part of the prodrome.

Question: A history of activities that might expose the patient to airborne virus-contaminated particles should be sought.
Significance: HPS acquired by inhalation on airborne particles.

 Physical Examination

Tachycardia and hypotension as late findings.

Finding: Fever
Significance: During the prodromal phase, fever is the only finding.

Finding: Cough
Significance: With the onset of the cardiopulmonary phase, there is cough and dyspnea associated with the production of frequently copious amounts of nonpurulent material.

 Laboratory Aids

TESTS

Test: Platelet count
Significance: The platelet count falls on serial testing during the prodromal phase and may be the only laboratory abnormality.

- In addition to leukocytosis, myelocytes and immunoblasts appear in the peripheral blood.
- Liver function tests are mildly abnormal.
- Hypoxemia accompanies the onset of the cardiopulmonary phase.
- Diagnostic serology demonstrates IgM antibody present at the time of clinical presentation.

IMAGING

Test: Chest radiograph
Significance: During the prodrome, chest radiography is normal. With the onset of cardiopulmonary symptoms, chest radiography will show evidence of interstitial fluid manifested by Kerley B lines, hilar indistinctness, and peribronchial cuffing. Alveolar flooding and pleural effusions develop in severe cases. Heart size remains normal.

PITFALLS

- The diagnosis depends on serologic testing, which can take some time.
- Lacking serologic confirmation, one mostly depends on clinical history and serial hematologic tests.
- In anticipation of the rapid progression of the cardiopulmonary phase, it is preferable to have the patient closely observed in the hospital.

 Therapy

Because of the rapid progression of the cardiorespiratory failure, all patients with HPS should be managed in an intensive care setting with a pulmonary artery catheter to guide therapy.

- Oxygen, intubation, and mechanical ventilation are frequently needed.
- Use fluids cautiously in view of the capillary leak.
- If the patient develops hypotension, an inotropic agent such as dobutamine should be added; if the patient continues to be hypotensive on maximal doses of dobutamine, vasopressors can be added to maintain blood pressure.
- Use empiric antibiotics because serologic tests confirming HPS are usually delayed and the differential diagnosis includes sepsis from a variety of antibiotic responsive organisms.

- Extracorporeal membrane oxygenation has been used for patients who fail to respond to maximal inotropic and ventilatory support.
- To date, antiviral agents have not been shown to be beneficial.

PREVENTION

- Universal precautions are appropriate in caring for persons with HPS; person-to-person transmission has been demonstrated only with the Andes strain in the Southern Hemisphere, not in the United States.
- Preventing infection depends on avoiding contact with airborne particles contaminated by rodent excreta.
- Eliminate rodents and seal off rodent access into the house.
- Reduce rodent shelter and food sources in the immediate vicinity of the home by cutting brush, removing trash, and storing grain and animal feed in rodent-proof containers.
- Wearing gloves, clean up rodent-contaminated areas by spraying nests and droppings with household disinfectants or dilute bleach, and sealing material in bags for burning or burial.
- Ventilate closed areas before initiating cleanup.

 Follow-Up

WHEN TO EXPECT IMPROVEMENT

- Patients who survive the shock phase typically then diurese fluid, which has been third spaced. Recovery is then generally rapid.
- Easy fatigability and mild pulmonary function abnormalities may persist.

PITFALLS

Recognizing the prodrome of HPS is difficult and requires a careful history, evaluation of the risk of exposure, and rapid access to testing.

 Common Questions and Answers

Q: What should I do if I find a dead mouse indoors?
A: Identify if it is a house mouse or a species that could be infected with Hantavirus. If the latter, assume that it is infected and dispose of as described previously and then seal off rodent access to the home and eliminate any still left inside.

Q: What should I do if I find what look like rodent droppings?
A: Clean up with gloves and disinfectant as noted here. Then use traps to catch and identify the rodents involved and proceed as in the answer to the previous question.

Q: Could a patient have HPS without knowing it?
A: In the United States, asymptotic HPS infections would appear to be uncommon based on serum screening of household contacts of cases and other populations at high risk, which show only infrequent evidence of prior infection.

ICD-9-CM 518.89;09.81

BIBLIOGRAPHY

All about hantavirus Web page: http//www.cdc.gov/ncidod/diseases/hanta/hps/index.htm

Butler JC, Peters CJ. Hantaviruses and hantavirus pulmonary syndrome. *Clin Infect Dis* 1994;19:387–395.

Duchin JS, et al. Hantavirus pulmonary syndrome: a clinical description of 17 patients with a newly recognized disease. *N Engl J Med* 1994;330:949–955.

Graziano KL, Tempest B. Hantavirus pulmonary syndrome: a zebra worth knowing. *American Family Physician* 2002;66(6):1015–1020.

Hallin GW, et al. Cardiopulmonary manifestations of hantavirus pulmonary syndrome. *Crit Care Med* 1996;24:252–258.

Khan AS, Young JC. Hantavirus pulmonary syndrome: at the crossroads. *Curr Opin Infect Dis* 2002;14(2):205–209.

Author: Bruce Tempest

Headache and Migraine

 Database

DEFINITIONS

Primary headache

- Has no underlying condition (migraine, tension headache, and cluster headache).

Secondary headache

- Is symptomatic of a specific cranial, oral, dental, or cervical pathologic process (e.g., trauma or tumor).

Temporal Patterns and Differential Diagnosis of Headache

Temporal patterns help distinguish migraine from tension headache, and from secondary headache.

- Pattern 1: Acute-first severe headache

—Upper respiratory tract infection, meningitis, cocaine, substance abuse

Medication induced

- Medication (methylphenidate, oral, steroids, psychotropic drugs, analgesics, cardiovascular agents); non hypertension; hydrocephalus, subarachnoid hemorrhage, intracranial hemorrhage, ventriculoperitoneal shunt malfunction

- Pattern 2: Chronic-progressive headache

—Brain tumor, brain abscess, hydrocephalus, vascular malformation, hematoma, chronic meningitis (Lyme disease), sinus thrombosis, pseudotumor cerebri (idiopathic intracranial hypertension), medication, depression, anemia, rheumatologic diseases

- Pattern 3: Acute, recurrent headache

—Migraine, cluster headache

- Pattern 4: Chronic or daily headache

—Medication overuse, substance abuse, rebound headache, caffeine, sinusitis, occipital neuralgia, temporomandibular joint syndrome, orthostatic headache, postLP headache, other systemic disease, posttraumatic, sleep disorder, depression, anxiety, other psychiatric illness, and tension headache

- Pattern 5: Mixed headache

—Migraine superimposed tension headache
—Diagnosis of Migraine

Migraine Criteria

Five or more headache attacks that:

Last 1–48 hours (compared with a shorter duration in adults)
Have at least two of the following features:

Bilateral (more common in children) or unilateral (frontal/temporal) location
Pulsating quality
Moderate to severe intensity
Aggravated by routine physical activities

—Are accompanied by at least one of the following:

—Nausea and/or vomiting or photophobia and/or phonophobia (do not occur simultaneously in adults)

70%—positive family history of migraine, especially those with classic migraine

MIGRAINE TYPES

Migraine in children can be divided into three groups:

- Migraine with aura—classic migraine: Spots, colors, image distortions, or visual scotoma.
- Migraine without aura—the majority of migraines: Mood changes or withdrawal from activity and sensitivity to light and sound.
- Migraine variants

—Hemiplegic or ophthalmoplegic migraine
—Hemianesthesia migraine
—Basilar migraine: Vertigo, diplopia, ataxia, visual field deficits
—Alice in Wonderland syndrome: distortions of vision, space, and/or time (e.g., micropsia, metamorphopsia, sensory hallucinations).
—Confusion migraine: Impaired sensorium, agitation, and lethargy, may progress to stupor.
—Benign paroxysmal vertigo, cyclic vomiting, and abdominal migraine are of uncertain relation to migraine.

EPIDEMIOLOGY OF MIGRAINE

Prevalence of headaches increases toward 80% by age 15. Migraines may start at age 6–7. 3% to 5% of prepubertal children affected. Female: male ratio increases to 2:1 among teenagers.

PATHOPHYSIOLOGY OF MIGRAINE

The current model of migraine involves a cycle of vasodilation, and perivascular inflammation, subject to humoral, circadian, and hormonal influences and involvement of bioactive amines such as serotonin and substance P. Interplay of genetic, environmental (e.g., sleep, diet), hormonal (e.g., menstruation), and emotional (e.g., peer or family conflicts) factors help make this a complex clinical problem.

 Data Gathering

HISTORY

- Clarify temporal pattern, location, duration, and intensity. Inquire about the time of onset, associated symptoms, precipitating and ameliorating factors, response to therapy, and family history.
- The following questions may be included on a written questionnaire prior to the visit.

1) Do you have more than one type of headache?
2) Since they started, have your headaches gotten worse or stayed the same?
3) How would you describe the pain (pounding, squeezing, stabbing, or something else)?
4) Do the headaches occur at any special time of day?
5) Do they wake you up from sleep?
6) What do you do during the headaches?
7) Do you have any thoughts about what is causing your headaches?

- Migraine typically fits the acute-recurrent headache pattern (Pattern 3). Nausea, vomiting, photophobia, phonophobia, and transitory neurologic disturbances are more suggestive of migraine.
- Tension headache usually presents as the chronic-nonprogressive headache pattern (Pattern 4). Often bilateral "band-like," diffuse, dull, and of mild to moderate intensity.
- Mixed headache pattern (Pattern 5) refers to migraine superimposed on tension headache.

 Physical Examination

- Review vital signs and anthropometric data (height, weight, and head circumference).
- Obesity—pseudotumor or sleep apnea syndrome? Resting tachycardia—anemia?
- Hypertension may underlie headache.
- Skin changes consistent with neurocutaneous syndrome. Individuals with neurofibromatosis commonly experience migraine, and are also at risk for intracranial mass.
- Auscultation for bruits over the supraclavicular areas, neck, temporal and occipital areas- arteritis, vascular malformation, or abnormal blood flow through a tumor.
- Examination for sinus tenderness, limitation of jaw excursion, or occipital trigger points
- Conclusive funduscopic exam may require pharmacologic dilatation or ophthalmologic consultation. Benign drusen may blur the disc margins, giving the (false) appearance of papilledema. Look for obscuration of blood vessels as they cross the disc boundary, radially oriented splinter hemorrhages, and loss of the light-reflective sheen of the retina approaching the disc margin. The presence of venous pulsations, best seen at the origin or branch points of the wider, darker veins within the disc margins, definitively excludes intracranial hypertension (except in patients with glaucoma).
- Neurologic examination should be normal in primary headache syndromes (migraine, tension), except perhaps during a complicated migraine. Stiff neck, head tilt, decreased alertness, abnormal eye movements, asymmetric deep tendon reflexes, asymmetric motor weakness or sensory deficit, ataxia, and gait disturbance may signal stroke, hemorrhage, tumor, or demyelination.

Laboratory Aids

Test: Neuroimaging studies (CT or MRI)
Significance: Emergency evaluation should concentrate on identifying acute processes that require emergent intervention. These include subarachnoid hemorrhage, meningitis, and mass lesions causing elevated intracranial pressure that may lead to herniation. Emergent neuroimaging should be performed for

- Acute first episode of severe headache ("worst headache of my life")
- Headaches or vomiting in the morning
- Headache worse in supine position
- Focal neurologic symptoms with or between episodes
- Cognitive decline
- New, abnormal neurologic exam findings (papilledema, hemiparesis, ataxia, asymmetric reflexes, abnormal eye movements, alteration of consciousness, nuchal rigidity)
- Presence of ventriculoperitoneal shunt

CT should be used in the emergent setting if there is any suspicion for subarachnoid hemorrhage, but otherwise MRI is generally preferred. Neuroimaging is not necessarily warranted in patients with acute-recurrent or chronic-nonprogressive headache (Patterns 3 and 4) who have a normal neurologic exam.

Test: EEG
Significance: Though 10% of children with migraine may show nonspecific abnormalities, there is no role for electroencephalography (EEG) in routine testing of individuals with headache.

Test: Lumbar puncture
Significance: Lumbar puncture (following CT) considered in chronic, progressive headache (Pattern 2) in a nonfebrile patient, even when chronic migraine or tension headache is (statistically) more likely. In addition to chronic meningitis (e.g., CNS Lyme disease), diagnostic considerations include subarachnoid hemorrhage, sinus thrombosis, and pseudotumor cerebri. Measured opening pressure with patient recumbent to rule out pseudotumor cerebri (where CSF analysis otherwise is normal).

Test: Others
Significance: Sinus films or CT if symptoms point to sinusitis. Sphenoid sinusitis may produce unremitting, chronic frontal headache. Migraine may mimic sinusitis and vice versa. Chronic anemia may be associated with headache.

Management of Migraine (and Tension Headache)

The management of migraine should include the following:

- Education and reassurance of both the patient and parents, emphasizing the absence of sinus, muscle, or spine disease, the episodic nature of migraine and the genetic and environmental factors.
- Review expectations of therapy—medicines help 60%–70% of the time.

- Patient to keep a headache record to identify possible triggers
- Address comorbid depression, anxiety, and substance abuse, and other medical conditions that may influence migraines—orthostatic intolerance, nocturnal hypoventilation, asthma, diabetes, gut or rheumatologic conditions.
- Outline a clear therapeutic plan.

—Nonpharmocologic approaches include avoiding triggers (caffeine, disrupted sleep, skipped meals, volatile chemicals, analgesic overuse, and dietary precipitants). Resolution of analgesic-induced rebound headache, if present, may require a few weeks. Other therapies include relaxation techniques, stress management, and biofeedback.
—Pharmocologic treatment.
—Acute treatment: The first line is ibuprofen (10 mg/kg). Antiemetics for nausea and vomiting also enhance the effectiveness of other analgesics. Drugs containing isometheptene (Midrin) and butalbital (Fiorinal) may aggravate headaches. "Triptans" are not currently FDA-approved for use in children. Trials in children demonstrate excellent safety profiles. In children who are unresponsive to conventional analgesics or antiemetics: sumatriptan (Imitrex), 25 mg oral tablets or a 20 mg nasal spray; rizatriptan (Maxalt, Maxalt-MLT) 5–10 mg tablets or oral dissolving wafers; and zolmitriptan (Zomig) 2.5–5 mg tablets or oral dissolving wafers. Not suggested in patients with complicated or basilar migraine. A nonoral route of administration (such as subcutaneous injection, or nasal spray [sumatriptan]) may be necessary.
—Status migrainosus: Migraine lasting more than 72 hours. The "Raskin protocol" (DHE-Dihydroergotamine; Linder modification) for ages 12–16 may be initiated in the emergency room or inpatient setting. Premedication with metoclopramide 0.2 mg/kg is given orally 30 minutes before a test dose of intravenous dihydroergotamine (DHE-45) 0.2 mg. This sequence is repeated every 6 hours for up to 12 doses or until the pain abates. Intravenous valproate 500 mg is similar in effectiveness to dihydroergotamine/metoclopramide for status migrainosus. Whether corticosteroids are effective in treating status migrainosus remains controversial. Narcotics often seem to lose efficacy rapidly, requiring doses that soon cause more sedation than pain relief. Addictive and rebound potentials are also of concern.
—Prophylaxis: Strategy is to start medication at a low dose, and then to increase weekly or biweekly toward a target maximum until headaches relent or side effects supervene. Beta-blockers (propranolol and nadolol) are discouraged in the setting of asthma, depression, or diabetes. Tricyclic agents (amitriptyline, nortriptyline) may benefit individuals with insomnia or depression. Anticonvulsants (topiramate, valproic acid) may benefit individuals with epilepsy. Cyproheptadine (Periactin), an antihistamine/antiserotonin agents are often used in younger adolescents (10–12 year old).

 ## Common Questions and Answers

Q: When should migraine be treated prophylactically?
A: More than 10 headache days per month or more than two severe attacks/month (i.e., leading to missed school or social life etc.) constitutes a relative indication for prophylaxis.

Q: What about allergy and headache?
A: Many believe that headache may represent a symptom of hypersensitivity. Headache in the setting of allergic rhinitis/asthma may be due to associated sinusitis/sinus congestion, side effect of treatment (especially theophylline), or muscle tension.

Q: At what age can migraine begin?
A: Even 2- to 3-year-olds may present with headache or "migraine equivalent" symptoms: episodic vomiting, episodic ataxia that improves after sleep.

ICD-9-CM 346.9

BIBLIOGRAPHY

Annequin D, Tournaire B, Massiou H. Migraine and headache in childhood and adolescence. *Pediatr Clin North Am* 2000;47(3):617–631.

Holden EW, Levy JD, Deichmann MM, et al. Practice parameter: Evaluation of children and adolescents with recurrent headaches. *Neurology* 2002;59:490–498.

Lewis DW. Migraine headaches in the adolescent. *Adolescent medicine state of the art reviews* 2002;13(3):413–432.

Linder SL. Treatment of childhood headache with dihydroergotamine mesylate. *Headache* 1994;34:578–580.

Rothner AD, et al. Chronic nonprogressive headaches in children and adolescents. *Semin Pediatr Neurol* 2001;8(1):34–39.

Singh BV, Roach ES. Diagnosis and management of headaches in children. *Pediatr Rev* 1998;19:132–135.

Winner P, Rothner DA. *Headache in Children and Adolescents*. Hamilton (ON): BC Decker Inc, 2001.

Authors: Yang Mao-Draayer
Ann Poduri, 3rd edition

Heat Stroke and Related Illness

Database

DEFINITION

Heat stroke results from an imbalance between heat production, absorption, and dissipation. This can result from excessive body heat generation and storage without appropriate dissipation, high ambient temperature, low radiation or convective heat loss, decreased evaporation, medical predisposition, behavioral abnormality, inability to respond to need for environmental change or intervention, or inadequate fluid (water and/or salt) replacement in response to ongoing losses through sweat or gastrointestinal disturbance. Heat illness encompasses a spectrum of heat-related disease processes.

PREDISPOSING CONDITIONS

• Environmental predisposition: Hot and humid without wind, heat wave, hot indoor environment, lack of air conditioning. Social isolation, inability to care for self or entrapment in closed space (car, trunk) (internal automobile temperature in sunlight with poor ventilation can reach 131–172°F—largest temperature increase within first 15 minutes).
• Medical: Cardiac disease, diabetes mellitus, diabetes insipidus, hyperthyroidism, parkinsonism, dehydration (gastroenteritis, diuretics, poor fluid intake), vascular disease, skin and sweat gland abnormalities (scleredema, cystic fibrosis, sun burned or scarred skin), malignancy, concurrent febrile illness, obesity, fatigue, anorexia nervosa, previous occurrence of heat illness.
• Drugs/medications
—Anticholinergics (inhibit perspiration)
—Beta-blockers (unable to increase cardiac output)
—Diuretics
—Ephedrine
—Phenothiazines
—Psychiatric medications (butyrophenones, phenothiazines)
—Drugs of abuse: Hallucinogens, cocaine, ecstasy
—Salicylates
—Sympathomimetics
—MAO inhibitors
—Lithium
—Antihistamines
—Ethanol
• Behaviors
—Lack of recognition of risk factors or warning signs
—Overexertion
—Athletics
—Inappropriate clothing: heavy, dark, tight-fitting, overbundling
—Lack of acclimatization and conditioning
—Inadequate fluid intake
—Children in enclosed space (interior, trunk) within motor vehicle

PATHOPHYSIOLOGY

• Heat production is increased 10 to 20 times by strenuous exercise.

• When environmental temperature is greater than body temperature, body gains heat by conduction and radiation and can lose heat by evaporation.
• Primary means of heat dissipation is evaporation, though conduction and convection may contribute. Radiation only occurs if ambient environmental temperature less than body temperature.
—With high humidity or little air movement, effectiveness of evaporative heat loss is decreased.

ASSOCIATED DISEASES

• Heat tetany: Paresthesias and carpopedal spasm help to distinguish tetany from heat cramps
• Heat syncope: Alteration of consciousness (dizziness, syncope) at end of strenuous or upright event.
• Heat edema: Swollen feet and ankles (vascular leak, orthostatic pooling).
• Heat exhaustion (prostration): Relatively slow onset, water and/or salt depletion. Clinically copious perspiration with headache, nausea, vomiting, malaise, myalgias, pallor, light headedness, visual disturbances, syncope, temperature 38° to 40°C, dehydration, electrolyte imbalance, hemoconcentration. Can evolve into heat stroke.
• Heat stroke: Core body temperature greater than 40°C with altered mental status ranging from confusion, disorientation, incoherent speech to delirium, decerebrate posturing, seizure, and coma. May have acute, sudden onset (80%), or slower onset (minutes to hours, 20%). Hypotension with widened pulse pressure, tachycardia, and hyperventilation. Classic heat stroke is associated with dry skin and prolonged exposure to elevated temperatures at rest (elderly and small children). Exertional heat stroke may present with dry skin or profuse sweating.

COMPLICATIONS

• Heat exhaustion: Hypovolemia, hyponatremia, hypernatremia, hypochloremia. Progression to heat stroke.
• Heat stroke: Hypokalemia, hyperkalemia, hypocalcemia and mild acid base disorders can occur. Seizures (especially with therapeutic cooling), adult respiratory distress syndrome (ARDS), acute renal, liver, cardiac failure, pulmonary edema, rhabdomyolysis (may be delayed 2 to 3 days), disseminated intravascular coagulation (DIC), coma, death. Severe dehydration if sweating occurred. May have persistent neurologic dysfunction (cerebellar, hemiparesis, dementia).

PROGNOSIS

• Heat illness (heat rash, edema, cramps, tetany, syncope, exhaustion): Rapid recovery with supportive care
• Heat stroke: Poor prognosis if not recognized and aggressively managed. Morbidity and mortality directly proportional to the rapidity with which cooling therapy is initiated. Eleven heat stroke deaths in children trapped in car trunks were reported in the United States between July–August 1998.

Differential Diagnosis

• Heat cramps: Rhabdomyolysis, tetany
• Heat edema: Thrombophlebitis, lymphedema, congestive heart failure
• Heat stroke: CNS process with fever (CVA, meningitis, encephalitis), other infections, anticholinergic poisoning (dilated pupils), drug-induced (medication, recreational), temperature rise, severe dehydration. Chills suggest febrile illness, not heat stroke.

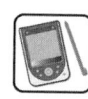

Data Gathering

HISTORY

Question: Initial temperature, if taken at scene?
Significance: The initial temperature can alert one to the potential for and extent of heat-related illness. If the first temperature is not obtained until after cooling interventions, extent of illness may not be fully appreciated, and appropriate therapy may be delayed.

Question: Cooling maneuvers en route to hospital?
Significance: A lower temperature may falsely reassure or mislead caregivers.

Question: History of CNS dysfunction?
Significance: A history of CNS dysfunction in conjunction with an environment consistent with or predisposing conditions conducive to development of heat-related illness should lead one to a presumptive diagnosis of heat stroke.

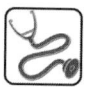

Physical Examination

Finding: Heat exhaustion
Significance: Weakness, lethargy, thirst, malaise, diminished ability to work or play, headache, nausea, vomiting, myalgias, pale skin, dizziness, visual disturbances, syncope, mild CNS dysfunction, impaired judgment, cramps, vertigo, hypotension, tachycardia, hyperventilation, paresthesias, agitation, incoordination, psychosis, temperature less than 40°C, sweating, environmental exposure and activity. No coma or seizures.

Finding: Heat stroke
Significance: Temperature more than 40.5°C (may be cooler due to prehospital maneuvers), with or without hot, dry (classic), or clammy (exercise-induced) skin, pink or ashen color, weakness, nausea, vomiting, anorexia, headache, dizziness, confusion, drowsiness, irritability, CNS dysfunction, euphoria, combativeness, abrupt or impending alteration of consciousness, obtundation, tachycardia, hypotension or normotension with wide pulse pressure, tachypnea, ataxia, posturing, incontinence, seizures, coma, purpura, or petechia. Two-thirds with constricted pupils. May have

muscle rigidity with tonic contractions and dystonia that mimic seizures.

Finding: Temperature measurement (continuous is best)
Significance:

- Esophageal thermometry probably the best
- Deep rectal thermometry a good approximation of core temperature
- Tympanic temperature reasonable estimation of CNS temperature
- Oral temperature not as useful due to mouth breathing and hyperventilation
- Axillary temperature unreliable, especially with cooling maneuvers

Laboratory Aids

Tests only to confirm diagnosis, evaluate extent of injury, or rule out other processes as treatment should be empiric.

- Heat cramps. Decreased serum and urine sodium and chloride; BUN normal or slightly increased
- Heat exhaustion: May see hyponatremia (salt loss) or hypernatremia (water loss), hypochloremia, low urine sodium and chloride, hemoconcentration. Differentiated from heat stroke by lack of significant liver function test abnormalities.
- Heat stroke: Blood chemistries: NaCl normal or high, hypokalemia, increased BUN/CR; hypophosphatemia, hypomagnesemia, hypocalcemia; lactate high; hypoglycemia. Hematologic: CBC (hemoconcentration, leukocytosis, thrombocytosis), coagulation profile for DIC (more likely in exertional than classic heat stroke): PT/PTT, fibrin split products, fibrinogen, malaria evaluation (thick smear), hematuria. Others: LFTs (AST and ALT markedly abnormal and useful to distinguish heat stroke from heat exhaustion), CPK (rhabdomyolysis), ABG (classic heat stroke: respiratory alkalosis and hypokalemia early; lactic acidosis later; exertional heat stroke: lactic acidosis), U/A (casts, brownish color proteinuria, microscopic hematuria, myoglobinuria), CSF, ECG, CXR.

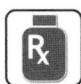
Therapy

- Rapid recognition and cooling imperative
- Specific therapy:
—Heat cramps: Rest, salt and water replacement
—Heat syncope: Self-limited as return to horizontal position is treatment; rest and fluids, salted liquids
—Heat exhaustion: Clinical findings (HR, BP, orthostatic changes, urine output) should direct therapy. Most treated as outpatient with rapid recovery (older patients or those with preexisting illnesses may require hospitalization); rest, rehydration, cooling; mild case: oral electrolyte solution (0.1–0.2% saline = approximately 1/4 to 1/2 teaspoon table salt in 1 quart of water); if CNS/GI

dysfunction (nausea, vomiting, inability to drink); IV (0.5% [similar to sweat losses] to 0.9% normal saline solution [NSS]); avoid rapid overcorrection of hypernatremia (treat as with hypernatremic dehydration); if hyponatremic seizures, treat slowly with 3% saline at approximately 5 mL/kg.
—Heat stroke: Immediate cooling and support of cardiovascular system. Remove clothing from patient and remove the patient from hot environment; use air conditioning, open vehicle for transport if possible; esophageal or rectal temperature probe (continuous temperature measurements); cooling should ideally approach 0.1° to 0.2°C per minute; slow cooling down at 38.5° to 39°C to avoid overshoot; cooling options (ice bath; cold water bath (15° to 16°C) as effective as ice bath without discomfort, shivering or vasoconstriction), massage with ice (this decreases the shivering response), ice packs to neck, groin, axilla, wet sheet over patient, moisten skin with water spray, convection increase (fan) to increase evaporative cooling, cooling blankets, cool/ice water lavage (peritoneum, rectum, gastric), cold to room temperature IV fluids, inotropes (as below) cardiopulmonary bypass, extracorporeal membrane oxygenation.

NONSPECIFIC

- Heat stroke: Treat empirically, and then rule out other causes of presentation. ABCs including securing airway as indicated, supplemental oxygen delivery.
—Fluid replacement: Usually only modest fluid requirements (patients often normovolemic with a distributive shock presentation due to vasodilatation; cooling redistributes volume from periphery to core; aggressive fluid resuscitation can lead to fluid overload and pulmonary edema). IV 0.9% NSS or Ringer's lactate solution. Ensure that patient is not hypoglycemic.

MEDICATIONS

Antipyretics are not useful because intact hypothalamus is required for action. Avoid anticholinergic drugs (atropine), which can inhibit sweating. May require inotropic support in addition to fluid support (dobutamine, isoproterenol, lower dose dopamine). Avoid inotropes with primarily alpha agonist characteristics, as vasoconstriction will interfere with heat dispersion. Dantrolene is not effective.

PREVENTION

- Recognize and intervene for those at risk in conditions that predispose to heat illness
- Recognize changes (medical or physical conditions, medications) that increase risk of heat illness
- Avoid enclosed spaces (children in closed cars)
- Limit physical activity, keep cool, use shaded areas. Adaption to warmer climates may take 8–10 exposures of 30–45 minutes each daily or every other day.
- Air conditioning or fans all or part of hot days

- Cool or tepid baths
- Increase fluid intake prior to exercise (400–600 mL in hour prior to exercise in adults), scheduled (not solely based on thirst) fluid replacement during strenuous activity (100–250 mL every 10–15 minutes); cool water and large volumes increase gastric emptying (high osmolality and carbohydrate content decreases gastric emptying), do not usually need glucose
- Fluid replacement during exercise that mimics losses. Carbohydrate concentration of 6% to 8% maximum to avoid delayed gastric emptying
- Loose (avoid occlusive), light-colored clothing, protective hat
- Acclimatization, gradual conditioning to hotter environment (7–14 days)
- Liberal dietary sodium: Avoid sodium chloride tablets: hypernatremia and potassium depletion, gastric irritant, delayed gastric emptying
- Frequently flex leg muscles when standing and avoid prolonged standing in hot environments
- Avoid caffeine and alcohol

Common Questions and Answers

Q: How can one distinguish between heat exhaustion and heat stroke?
A: If CNS abnormalities are present, temperature is greater than 40.6°C and liver function tests (ALT, AST) are markedly elevated, the patient is likely to have heat stroke.

Q: When should heat stroke be suspected?
A: Suspect heat stroke in a patient with or without sweating who demonstrates alterations of CNS function in environment that would be conducive to heat illness.

Q: Does the presence or absence of sweating help with the diagnosis of heat exhaustion versus heat stroke?
A: No. Sweating will be present with heat exhaustion and may or may not be present with heat stroke.

Q: Are children at increased risk of heat illness?
A: Yes, they have a number of predisposing factors: greater surface area to body mass ratio than adults, production of more metabolic heat per kilogram of body weight, slower rate of sweating than adults, temperature when sweating starts is higher, lower cardiac output at a given metabolic rate than adults, rate of acclimatization is slower, thirst response is blunted and access to fluids may be limited. In addition, ability to react or change the environment may be limited in children.

ICD-9-CM 992.0

BIBLIOGRAPHY

Bouchama A, Knochel JP. Heat stroke. *N Engl J Med* 2002;346(25):1978–1988.

Bytomski JR, Squire DL. Heat illness in children. *Curr Sports Med Rep* 2003;2:320–324.

Authors: Paige Wright and George A. Woodward

Hemangioma (Vascular Nevi)

 Database

DEFINITION

- Hemangiomas are nonmalignant neoplasms consisting of vascular endothelial cells
- Vascular malformations: Capillaries, veins, lymphatics, or arteries that underwent errors of morphogenesis (i.e., hamartomas); includes port-wine stains (nevus flammeus) and arteriovenous malformations (AVMs). The lesion is classified by the predominant vessel type present.
- Salmon patches (nevus simplex): distended dermal capillaries (nevus simplex, telangiectatic nevus).

PATHOPHYSIOLOGY

- Hemangiomas: Appear in first few weeks of life, growing rapidly in first 6 to 12 months of life, followed by a static period, and then involute. Lesions are made up of proliferating endothelial cells. Markers for angiogenesis are found in lesions. Recent investigations suggest that cells may have placental rather than fetal origin.
- Vascular malformations: Grow proportionally with the affected individual. Congenital, by definition, may not become apparent until adolescence or adulthood. Port-wine stains are apparent at birth. Port-wine stains are capillary vascular malformations. Lesions are dysplastic vessels without endothelial proliferation.
- Salmon patches: grow proportionally with affected individual. Lesion consists of distended dermal vessels.

Salmon Patches

- No genetic association

EPIDEMIOLOGY

Hemangiomas

- Female to male ratio of 3:1
- Increased incidence with prematurity
- 10×increased incidence if chorionic villus sampling was performed during pregnancy
- 10% of white infants are affected, 1.4% of black infants are affected
- 80% are single lesions
- 60% are found on head and neck
- 25% are found on the trunk

Vascular Malformations

- Port-wine stains and lymphatic malformations each have a female to male ratio of 1:1
- Venous malformations may occur in any body tissue including bone

Salmon Patches

- Found in 30%–40% of all newborns

COMPLICATIONS

Hemangiomas

- Local ulceration, bleeding, superinfection
- Obstruction of important structures including airway, GI tract, eye (even small periorbital lesions have been associated with astigmatism secondary to pressure on the globe).
- Multiple cutaneous hemangiomas may be associated with visceral hemangiomas, including liver, lung, and GI tract. Rarely, the meninges, brain, spinal cord, pancreas, spleen, or adrenals may be involved. Hemangiomas in these organs can result in significant functional impairment.
- Disseminated neonatal hemangiomatosis may be associated with high morbidity and mortality.
- High output cardiac failure
- Iron-deficiency anemia
- Liver lesions, particularly associated with high mortality
- Kasabach-Merritt syndrome: Platelet trapping, coagulopathy, thrombocytopenia; now generally felt only to occur with kaposiform hemangioendothelioma or tufted angiomas (clinically similar to hemangioma but histologically distinct); 20%–30% mortality.
- Rarely cause skeletal overgrowth secondary to increased blood flow

Vascular Malformations

- Port-wine stains can signal underlying developmental defects especially of the central nervous system and spine; may be associated with deep underlying venous malformations. arteriovenous (AV) malformations can lead to "steal" causing ischemic necrosis, pain, and increased cardiac output; frequently associated with skeletal abnormalities including hypertrophy (low flow) or destruction (high flow).
- Localized or disseminated intravascular coagulopathy possible, but uncommon
- Infection and bleeding into the lesion are potential problems with lymphatic malformations.
- Airway compromise can occur with head and neck lymphatic malformations (cystic hygroma).

PROGNOSIS

- Hemangiomas: Excellent if cutaneous alone. Association with other syndromes or visceral involvement worsens prognosis significantly. Superficial scarring varies but can be significant, especially with large lesions of the face.
- Vascular malformations: Varied depending on type of malformation, location, and associated syndromes.
- Salmon patches: Excellent.

 Differential Diagnosis

INFECTION

- Bacillary angiomatosis

TUMORS

- Glomus tumor
- Tufted angioma
- Kaposiform hemangioendothelioma
- Angioendothelioma
- Sarcoma

CONGENITAL

- Verrucous hemangioma

MISCELLANEOUS

- Pyogenic granuloma
- Angiokeratomas

APPROACH TO THE PATIENT

The single determination that the primary care provider must make is whether or not specialist referral is necessary. The following situations require specialist consultation:

- Multiple hemangiomas in "beard distribution" frequently associated with airway hemangiomas, patients with such lesions require direct visualization of the airway
- Patients with noisy breathing and multiple cutaneous hemangiomas in any distribution should be evaluated for airway involvement, especially when respiratory symptoms appear in the first weeks to months of life, when there is rapid hemangioma growth.
- Patients with multiple cutaneous lesions are at risk for visceral involvement. Patient should be referred for imaging studies to assess concealed involvement. Those with hepatic hemangiomas must be monitored very closely as they carry a high mortality rate.
- Those with disfiguring lesions (usually facial) or periorbital lesions should be referred to dermatology or plastic surgery and ophthalmology for treatment.
- Hemangiomas over the spine, especially in lumbosacral region, require further investigation for spinal dysraphism, tethered cord, and other anomalies.
- Lesions that interfere with function (e.g., periorbital, obstructing ear canal, anogenital region) must be treated aggressively.
- All vascular malformations (venous, arterial, lymphatic and mixed type) should be followed by the appropriate specialist.

 Data Gathering

HISTORY

Question: When did the skin finding appear and has it changed in size?
Significance: Hemangiomas are present in first few weeks of life, but often inapparent at birth. They grow rapidly in the first year of life. Vascular malformations are present at birth, though sometimes not noted until adolescence or adulthood. Sudden growth can occur in association with trauma, puberty and other factors. Salmon patches are noted at birth and tend to grow with the patient.

Physical Examination

Hemangiomas

Finding: Lesion with raised, bright red-pink color, sharply demarcated border, stippled surface—hence the term strawberry hemangioma
Significance: Young lesion in superficial dermis

Finding: Lesion is bluish in color, raised with smooth overlying skin.
Significance: Young lesion in lower dermis or subcutaneous tissue

Finding: Combination of above findings
Significance: Superficial and deep components can be combined in a single lesion.

Finding: Lesion develops gray or white areas, usually centrally located, which spread toward periphery
Significance: Involuting hemangioma

Vascular Malformations

Finding: Apparent at birth, pink-to-red sharply demarcated macule, possibly slightly raised, darkens with age, may develop papules over time
Significance: Port-wine stains

Finding: New lesion in adolescence or adulthood usually soft, easily compressed, and emptied of blood
Significance: Although congenital, vascular malformations other than port-wine stains may appear later in life.

Finding: Port-wine stains including first distribution of the trigeminal nerve
Significance: May reflect presence of anomalies of the choroid plexus and leptomeninges: Sturge-Weber. Specialist referral is often very helpful to determine the need for a brain imaging study.

Salmon Patches

Finding: Salmon patches
Significance: Often have more than one lesion; 80% on nape of neck, 45% on eyelids, 33% on glabella.

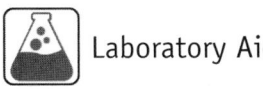

Laboratory Aids

RADIOGRAPHIC STUDIES

Hemangiomas

• Occasionally necessary to differentiate hemangiomas from vascular malformations
• Ultrasound: Useful to delineate visceral involvement with hemangioma
• Head magnetic resonance imaging (MRI): performed to rule out anomalies of the choroid plexus and leptomeninges (Sturge-Weber); serious consideration when port-wine stains include first distribution of the trigeminal nerve. Lesions in second and third distribution of trigeminal nerve do not have this risk.

• MRI of spine: Performed for hemangiomas overlying spine, especially when lumbosacral, to rule out spinal dysraphism. In young infants, ultrasound can be performed in place of MRI.

Vascular Malformations

Contrast venography and catheter arteriography—important in preoperative setting
Color flow Doppler and MRI—can be complementary modalities to fully characterize complex lesions.
MRI—optimal for assessing deep extension of neck lesions, such as cystic hygromas

Salmon Patches

None

Emergency Care

• Respiratory compromise can occur with rapidly growing airway hemangioma. Immediate ear, nose and throat specialist (ENT) involvement is a must.
• Respiratory compromise can also occur with cystic hygroma (lymphatic malformation) in the neck.
• Consumptive coagulopathy can occur with large lesions.
• High output cardiac failure can occur with hepatic hemangiomas and arteriovenous malformations.

Therapy

Hemangiomas

• For bleeding: Direct pressure
• For ulceration: Observation or wet compresses and topical antibacterials
• For ulceration that is difficult to manage: Pulse dye laser, corticosteroids
• For infection: Intravenous antibiotics for cellulitis, topical antibiotics with dressing changes for mild involvement
• Treatment is necessary for lesions that interfere with critical structures (e.g., eye, airway, GI tract) or for serious symptoms, such as consumptive coagulopathy. No therapy indicated in 95%.
• Intralesional or systemic steroids
• Interferon-α-2a or 2b for critically ill steroid-nonresponders
• Liquid nitrogen occasionally beneficial, some authors are revisiting sclerotherapy
• Laser therapy beneficial for superficial lesions only
• Surgical resection utilized infrequently

Vascular Malformations

• Port-wine stain: Cosmetic camouflage or laser therapy. Flashlamp pulsed dye laser therapy is being continuously improved in terms of quality of outcome and decreased complications as different types of lasers are developed and tested. Multiple laser

treatment sessions at 2- to 3-month intervals are usually necessary. Early treatment is advocated because of better outcome, especially children under 1 year of age.
• Venous and arterial malformations are usually treated with sclerotherapy and surgical resection.

Follow-Up

Hemangiomas

• 50% will spontaneously resolve by 5 years; 70% will spontaneously resolve by 7 years; 90% will spontaneously resolve by 9 to 12 years.
• Up to 40% of children are left with residual skin changes, including atrophy, redundant skin, discoloration, telangiectasias, and scarring.

Vascular Malformations

• No spontaneous resolution of lesions

Salmon Patches

• 50% on nape of neck and 95% of others spontaneously resolve.
• Tendency toward erythema in affected area may persist after lesions resolve.

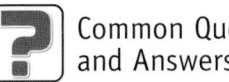

Common Questions and Answers

Q: What will happen to my child's hemangioma?
A: Expect it to enlarge, get a bluish or grayish hue, and then get smaller. In the first year of life, it may enlarge at a rate more rapid than the rest of the child's growth. After that time it will involute, and should resolve by 9 to 12 years of age; most resolve much earlier.

Q: What are the problems of the involuting hemangioma?
A: Infection and ulceration.

Q: What happens to the "stork bite" on the back of the neck?
A: A salmon patch in the nuchal region (also known as Unna nevus) persists in up to 50% of affected people. Some fade but still may be seen when vessels dilate, such as with crying or fever.

ICD-9-CM CODES

Port wine stain 757.32

Hemangioma 228.0

BIBLIOGRAPHY

Brown RL, Azizkhan RG. Pediatric head and neck lesions [tutorial]. *Pediatr Clin North Am* 1998;45:889–905.

Metry D, Hebert A. Benign cutaneous vascular tumors of infancy: when to worry, what to do. *Arch Dermatol* 2000;136:905–914.

Author: Laura N. Sinai

Hemolytic Disease of the Newborn

Database

DEFINITION

Hemolytic disease of the newborn is hemolytic anemia occurring in the newborn due to passive transfer of maternal antibodies (IgG) against fetal red cells.

CAUSES

- Most severe disease due to Rh (D) antigen sensitization
- A and B antigens may also be responsible.
- 1% of cases due to other antigens.
- Other antigens: Kell, Duffy, C, E, and c

PATHOPHYSIOLOGY

- Rh alloimmunization results from passage of fetal red blood cells that express surface Rh (D) antigen across the placenta into the circulation of an Rh-negative mother.
- The passage of fetal Rh positive cells occurs as a result of transplacental hemorrhage
- Initial exposure results in production of maternal IgM antibodies, which do not cross the placenta. This is followed by production of IgG antibodies, which can cross the placenta. On subsequent exposures there is a rapid production of anti-D antibodies
- Rh-negative mothers may have initial sensitization due to transfusion or previous pregnancy.
- Anti-D IgG produced in the maternal circulation crosses the placenta and coats fetal red blood cells (RBC). These cells are then destroyed in reticuloendothelial system, primarily the fetal spleen
- Alloimmunization may lead to severe anemia, hydrops, and hyperbilirubinemia.
- Extramedullary hematopoiesis in the fetal liver and spleen occurs as a response to fetal anemia leading to severe hepatosplenomegaly.
- ABO isoimmunization, usually in case of type O mothers with type A or B fetus, results in a clinically milder hemolysis.

EPIDEMIOLOGY

- 15% of Caucasians are Rh-negative (dd)
- 48% are heterozygous (Dd)
- 35% are homozygous (DD)
- Prevalence of Rh-positive fetus in Rh-negative mother: 15%
- Incidence of Rh hemolytic disease: 6–7/1,000 live births
- Of all Rh-sensitized pregnancies:

—50% require no treatment
—31% require treatment after a full-term delivery
—10% delivered early and require exchange transfusion
—9% require intrauterine transfusion

- Reasons for spectrum of clinical severity:

—Rh immunization rarely occurs in first pregnancy
—Many subsequent infants may be Rh-negative

—Only a fraction of women at risk develop antibodies
—50% of cases of ABO disease occur in first pregnancy

COMPLICATIONS

- Hydrops fetalis
- Still births
- Neonatal hyperbilirubinemia and kernicterus
- Fetal anemia

PROGNOSIS

Approximately half the infants have minimal anemia and hyperbilirubinemia and require either no treatment or only phototherapy.

- One fourth will require exchange transfusions.
- Hydropic infants have high mortality.

Differential Diagnosis

- Neonatal hyperbilirubinemia

—ABO incompatibility
—Galactosemia
—G6PD deficiency
—Hypothyroidism
—Pyruvate kinase deficiency
—Crigler-Najjar syndrome
—α-Thalassemia
—Gilbert syndrome
—Spherocytosis
—Breast-milk jaundice

- Hydrops fetalis

—Hematologic: α-thalassemia, severe G6PD deficiency, twin-to-twin transfusion
—Cardiac: Hypoplastic left heart syndrome, myocarditis, endocardial fibroelastosis, heart block
—Congenital infections: Parvovirus, syphilis, cytomegalovirus (CMV), rubella
—Renal: Renal vein thrombosis, urinary tract obstruction, nephrosis
—Placental: Umbilical vein thrombosis, true knot of umbilical cord
—Miscellaneous: Trisomy 13, 18, 21, triploidy, aneuploidy, diaphragmatic hernia

Data Gathering

HISTORY

- Previous stillbirths, abortions?
- Neonatal hyperbilirubinemia requiring therapy in previous pregnancy?
- Exposure of mother to blood products?
- Father's ABO and Rh type?
- Rh immune globulin given after previous pregnancy or abortion?

Physical Examination

- Pallor, tachycardia, tachypnea due to congestive heart failure (CHF) secondary to severe anemia

—Jaundice developing within 24 hours of birth

- Usually no jaundice at birth
- Generalized edema in cases with severe anemia and hydrops
- Massive hepatosplenomegaly in severe cases
- Milder cases manifest with neonatal hyperbilirubinemia only.
- ABO incompatibility usually manifests jaundice at 24 hours.

Laboratory Aids

ANTENATAL

- ABO and Rh type of all mothers at first prenatal visit
- Zygosity of the father—if the father is Rh+ homozygous, then all children will be Rh positive; if the father is heterozygous, then only 50% of children will be Rh+.
- Fetal Rh D genotyping can be performed on maternal plasma during second trimester.
- Monitor antibody titer by indirect Coombs test in Rh-negative mothers starting at 20 weeks.
- Amniocentesis if maternal antibody titer more than 1:8 at any time
- Spectrophotometric assessment of bilirubin concentration in amniotic fluid
- Amniotic fluid values in Liley's zone 3 and high zone 2 indicative of severe fetal disease (Liley's test measures optical density in amniotic fluid as an indicator for bilirubin levels; do not use for Kell sensitization as it is not a reliable indicator of severity of disease in these patients.)
- Fetal blood sampling in severe cases to assess degree of anemia

NEONATAL

- Cord blood ABO and Rh types
- Cord blood hemoglobin (Hb), hematocrit (Hct), bilirubin (direct and indirect), reticulocyte count
- Direct Coombs test on cord blood—will be positive in immune hemolytic disease
- Indirect Coombs test on cord blood for passively transferred antibody
- Identification of antibody after elution from RBC
- Peripheral smear: Nucleated RBC (spherocytes in ABO disease)

Therapy

- In severely affected fetuses where early delivery is not possible due to lung immaturity, intrauterine intravascular transfusion (IUIVT) is the therapy of choice. Risks of IUIVT include fetal loss (2%), premature labor and rupture of membranes, chorioamnionitis, fetal bradycardia, cord laceration, fetomaternal hemorrhage.
- Early delivery and subsequent resuscitation may be required in severe Rh isoimmunization.
- Phototherapy to start as soon as possible
- Exchange transfusion removes sensitized fetal RBC and circulating bilirubin and is indicated:

—To correct anemia in severely anemic infants
—To prevent or correct hyperbilirubinemia
—To remove circulating antibodies

- Indications for early exchange transfusion:

—Cord blood bilirubin more than 4.5 mg/dL and cord blood Hb less than 10 g/dL
—Bilirubin rising at rate more than 1 mg/dL per hour despite optimal phototherapy
—Indirect bilirubin greater than or equal to 20 mg/dL or rising to reach that level
—Lower indirect bilirubin levels are used in preterm or high-risk Infants
—Hb between 11 and 13 g/dL and bilirubin rising at rate more than 0.5 mg/dL per hour despite optimal phototherapy

- In hydropic infants, immediate partial exchange may be needed to correct anemia and CHF.
- Double-volume exchanges may be needed for hyperbilirubinemia.
- Selection of blood for exchange transfusion:

—As fresh as possible, CMV-safe, and irradiated
—For Rh disease (if prepared before delivery): Type O Rh-negative crossmatched against mother's blood; after delivery then O negative crossmatched against infant
—For ABO disease: Type O Rh-negative or Rh-compatible crossmatched against mother and infant

- Risks of exchange transfusion include prolonged neutropenia, thrombocytopenia, late anemia, metabolic abnormalities, arrhythmias, thrombosis, death
- Some studies indicate that administration of IVIG to the neonate diminishes hemolysis and may prevent the need for exchange transfusion

- Most infants with ABO incompatibility require no treatment or phototherapy only.
- Some infants with milder Rh isoimmunization may only have exaggerated physiologic anemia at 12 weeks.
- Avoid drugs that interfere with bilirubin metabolism or its binding to albumin (sulfonamides, caffeine, sodium benzoate).
- Infants who had hemolytic disease of the newborn are at risk for late anemia due to reticulocytopenia related to persistent high titers of circulating maternal antibody. They should have weekly Hct measured during the first few months of life.

ANTENATAL MANAGEMENT

- Rh immunoglobulin at a dose of 300 μg for the following:

—Unsensitized Rh-negative mother at 28 weeks' gestation and within 72 hours of delivery
—Unimmunized Rh-negative mothers who have undergone spontaneous or therapeutic abortions
—After ruptured tubal pregnancies in Rh-negative mothers

- If previous stillbirth or hydrops and fetus high risk after amniocentesis, plan early delivery
- Careful fetal monitoring and induction of pulmonary maturation
- If fetus is too immature for delivery, then intrauterine transfusions every 10 to 14 days are needed.

 Follow-Up

- Weekly Hct especially for patients who had exchange transfusion
- Watch for exaggerated physiologic anemia at 12 weeks.
- Assess for neurologic damage.

PREVENTION

Rh hemolytic disease can be prevented by administration of Rh Immune globulin to the Rh-negative women after any exposure to Rh positive blood and prophylactically during pregnancy.

 Common Questions and Answers

Q: Does the condition become worse with each pregnancy?
A: Yes, if the mother is not treated with Rh immunoglobulin after each Rh-positive pregnancy or abortion.

Q: Can maternal blood be used to transfuse the affected baby?
A: It can be used as a lifesaving measure in a situation when there is no other suitable blood available for the baby.

ICD-9-CM 774.6

BIBLIOGRAPHY

Bennebroek J. Diagnosis and treatment of severe alloimmunization. *Vox Sang* 1994;67(Suppl 3):235–238.

Bowman JM. Antenatal suppression of Rh alloimmunization. *Clin Obstet Gynecol* 1991;34(2):296–303.

Koenig JM. Evaluation and treatment of erythroblastosis fetalis in the neonate. In: Christensen RD, ed. *Hematologic Problems of the Neonate*. Philadelphia: WB Saunders, 2000:185–207.

Nathan DG, Oski FA, eds. *Hematology of Infancy and Childhood*. Vol 1. 5th Ed. Philadelphia: WB Saunders, 1998:53–78.

Whittle MJ. Rhesus hemolytic disease. *Arch Dis Child* 1992;67(1 spec no):65–68.

Authors: Tammy I. Kang and Sadhna M. Shankar, 2nd edition

Hemolytic Uremic Syndrome

 Database

DEFINITION

The hemolytic uremic syndrome (HUS) is a heterogeneous group of similar entities defined by microangiopathic hemolytic anemia, thrombocytopenia, and acute renal failure. HUS is the most common cause of acute renal failure in childhood.

- Enteropathic (verotoxin, typical, diarrhea-associated) form accounts for greater than 90% of pediatric cases and is characterized by the sudden onset of hemolytic anemia, thrombocytopenia, and acute renal failure after a prodromal illness of acute gastroenteritis, usually with bloody diarrhea.
- Nonenteropathic (atypical) form represents a heterogeneous group of disorders, including inherited HUS (e.g., mutations in complement regulatory pathways, chiefly factor H mutations), *Streptococcus pneumoniae*-related HUS, and HUS associated with pregnancy, oral contraceptives, cyclosporine, antitumor drugs, or malignancy.

GENETICS

Mutations have been reported in the complement regulatory protein factor H in both sporadic and familial HUS, with mutations identified in 10%–20% of cases. Mutations in other complement regulators (membrane cofactor protein CD46) have also been associated with familiar HUS.

EPIDEMIOLOGY

HUS has been reported throughout the world.

Typical

- Enteropathic HUS tends to occur in the summer months, and epidemics have been reported in day-care centers and nursing homes.
- Nonenteropathic HUS occurs mainly in older infants and young children, usually between 6 months and 4 years of age.
- The Shiga toxin producing *E. coli* is found in the intestine of beef cattle. Ground beef may be contaminated throughout with Shiga toxin. If a hamburger is inadequately cooked, infection may ensue.
- In reported outbreaks, the frequency of bloody diarrhea has ranged from 35%–90%.

Atypical

Nonenteropathic HUS has no seasonal variation and may occur at any age.

COMPLICATIONS

Gastrointestinal

- Acute colitis is usually transient.
- Complications include rectal prolapse, toxic megacolon, bowel wall necrosis, intussusception, perforation, and stricture.

- Pancreatic involvement may result in pancreatitis or insulin-dependent diabetes mellitus.

Central Nervous System

- Most patients have mild CNS symptoms that include irritability, lethargy, and behavioral changes.
- Major symptoms such as stupor, coma, seizures, cortical blindness, posturing, and hallucinations occur in 20%–40% of patients.
- Thrombotic or hemorrhagic stroke may occur.
- The risk of seizures is associated with hyponatremia.

PROGNOSIS

Enteropathic HUS

- Improved supportive care and a better understanding of the complications of enteropathic HUS have resulted in a decrease in mortality to an acute fatality rate of 4% to 12%.
- Approximately 25% of survivors demonstrate long-term renal sequelae after enteropathic HUS, such as proteinuria and hypertension; they should be evaluated regularly for many years.
- Persistence of proteinuria after 1 year is a poor prognostic sign and warrants additional evaluation.
- Recurrences of enteropathic HUS are exceedingly uncommon.
- Chronic renal insufficiency occurs in 4% to 9%. Children who do develop end stage renal disease are good candidates for kidney transplantation.

Nonenteropathic HUS

- In general, patients with nonenteropathic HUS have a worse prognosis.
- Neurologic symptoms are seen more commonly.
- Hypertension is common during the initial illness and prolonged antihypertensive treatment is required.
- Recurrences have been reported both before and after renal transplantation.
- In familial HUS, relapse, end-stage renal disease, and death are common.

 Differential Diagnosis

- Infectious causes such as *Shigella*, Salmonella, *Campylobacter, Yersinia enterocolitica, C. difficile,* and *Entamoeba histolytica*
- During the gastrointestinal prodrome, it may be difficult to distinguish HUS from appendicitis, inflammatory bowel disease, diverticulosis, or intussusception.
- Thrombotic thrombocytopenic purpura (TTP) shares many features with HUS.
- Sepsis with disseminated intravascular coagulation may present with acute renal failure and a microangiopathic process.

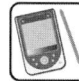 Data Gathering

HISTORY

Question: Gastrointestinal prodrome?
Significance: Affected children with enteropathic HUS are usually healthy before the initiation of the gastrointestinal prodrome. The diarrhea is usually watery or bloody and is associated with abdominal discomfort.

Question: Duration?
Significance: The prodrome lasts from 1 to 15 days and often improves before onset of the triad of features inherent to HUS.

Question: Symptoms of pneumonia?
Significance: Streptococcus pneumoniae associated HUS is associated with severe disease.

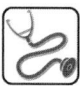 Physical Examination

- Pallor and petechiae
- Dehydration secondary to the gastroenteritis
- Pneumonia
- May have volume overload secondary to oligoanuric renal failure
- Peripheral edema, congestive heart failure, and hypertension may be present.
- Mild neurologic changes of irritability or behavioral changes

SPECIAL QUESTIONS

Finding: Recent hamburger ingestion.
Significance: Many cases of typical HUS have been associated with inadequately cooked hamburger meat. Epidemics have been reported in fast-food restaurant customers.

Finding: Consumption of unpasteurized milk, cheese, or cider.
Significance: May contain *E. coli* or Shiga toxins.

 Laboratory Aids

HEMATOLOGIC

Test: CBC
Significance: The microangiopathic hemolytic anemia may be mild or severe. Leukocytosis is often seen in typical HUS.

Test: Reticulocytes
Significance: Repeated exacerbations of the hemolysis may occur for days or weeks.

Test: Blood smear
Significance: Fragmented red blood cells or schistocytes

Test: Markers of hemolysis
Significance: Elevated lactic dehydrogenase, unconjugated bilirubin, and reticulocyte count are additional evidence of ongoing hemolysis.

Test: Platelets
Significance: The thrombocytopenia may also last for days or weeks.

Test: PT-PTT
Significance: Coagulation studies usually show increased fibrin degradation products with normal prothrombin and partial thromboplastin times.

Test: T-antigen
Significance: Request specific testing when *pneumococcus*-induced HUS is suspected, as current blood banking techniques do not routinely test for the presence of the T-antigen.

RENAL

Test: Renal function
Significance: Elevated creatinine and BUN

Test: Electrolytes
Significance: Elevated levels of potassium, phosphorus, hydrogen ion, and uric acid; decreased concentrations of sodium, calcium, and bicarbonate

Test: Urinalysis
Significance: Microscopic hematuria; varying degrees of proteinuria; macroscopic hematuria and RBC casts may be present.

GASTROINTESTINAL

Test: Electrolytes
Significance: Decreased serum potassium

Test: Liver function tests
Significance: Albumen decreased; liver function tests are usually normal.

Test: Amylase, lipase
Significance: Pancreatic involvement may result in hyperglycemia and elevated concentrations of serum amylase and lipase. Exocrine pancreatitis is difficult to evaluate since amylase and lipase are normally cleared by the kidneys.

MICROBIOLOGY

Test: Stool
Significance: All bloody stool samples should be screened for *E. coli* 0157:H7. Since the rate of recovery of the organism may decline rapidly after the first 6 days of illness, stool cultures should be obtained as early in the course of illness as possible. The local health department should be notified of any isolates.

Test: Verotoxins
Significance: Serologic evidence of verotoxin may be diagnostic.

IMAGING

Test: Plain film of the abdomen
Significance: Often demonstrates colonic distension. Look for free air as evidence of bowel perforation.

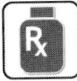 Therapy

- Supportive therapy
—Fluid and electrolyte
—Volume resuscitation initially
—In a euvolemic patient, fluids should provide replacement of ongoing losses with meticulous attention to urine output.
—Hyponatremia is common.
—If the patient is fluid overloaded, fluid intake should be restricted accordingly.
- Dialysis
—If medical management fails to correct hypertension, hyperkalemia, hyperphosphatemia, and severe metabolic acidosis, dialysis or hemofiltration may be indicated. Dialysis is required in one-half to one-third of patients.
- Anemia
—Transfusion of packed red blood cells if the hemoglobin concentration falls below 6.0 to 7.0 g/dL or if there is evidence of cardiac dysfunction. The transfusions should be given slowly since blood pressure occasionally increases during transfusions.
—Platelet transfusions should be reserved for patients with active bleeding or in preparation for an invasive procedure.
—Antibiotics are not prescribed routinely because there is evidence the antimicrobials may increase verotoxin release. Antimotility agents have also been associated with more severe disease and should be avoided.
—Nutrition must be maintained and may require total parenteral nutrition if the intestine is nonfunctional. The degree of renal insufficiency will dictate the need for potassium and phosphorus restriction.
- Specific therapy
—Therapies have not proven to be helpful: plasmapheresis, fresh frozen plasma, intravenous immunoglobulin, heparin, antibiotics, aspirin, vitamin E for enteropathic HUS.
—Plasmapheresis has been specifically advocated for nonenteropathic HUS

 Follow-Up

WHEN TO EXPECT IMPROVEMENT

- Resolution is usually heralded by a rise in platelet count and a gradual decrease in the frequency of blood transfusions.
- During the recovery phase patients may require folic acid and iron supplementation.
- Anuria rarely lasts more than 2 weeks. In general, a longer duration of anuria is a poor prognostic feature.
- Children who sustain structural neurologic damage during the acute phase of HUS may have residual impairment, but there is tremendous potential for improvement and recovery.
- Pancreatic insufficiency may persist requiring long-term insulin therapy beyond resolution of the acute illness.

PREVENTION

Most cases of typical HUS can be avoided by thoroughly cooking all hamburger-containing foods. Other sources of contaminated foods include unpasteurized apple cider or milk.

 Common Questions and Answers

Q: What are some predictors of the severity of enteropathic HUS?
A: Predictors include an elevated white cell count, a severe gastrointestinal prodrome, anuria early in the course of illness, and age under 2 years.

Q: In a patient with nonenteropathic HUS, what is the chance other siblings will be affected?
A: Familial HUS due to factor H deficiency may be autosomal dominant or recessive.

Q: How many patients with gastroenteritis from *E. coli* 0157:H7 will develop HUS?
A: 10% to 20%

Q: What should the family tell the day-care staff and neighbors?
A: If the patient has enteropathic HUS, contacts should be informed that any episodes of gastroenteritis merit close follow-up for evidence of anemia, thrombocytopenia, and renal insufficiency. No prophylaxis is indicated. Exclusion of infected children from day-care centers until two consecutive stool cultures are negative for *E. coli* 0157:H7 has been shown to prevent additional transmission.

ICD-9-CM 283.11

BIBLIOGRAPHY

Boyce TG, Swerdlow DL, Griffin PM. Current concepts: *Escherichia coli* 0157:H7 and the hemolytic-uremic syndrome. *N Engl J Med* 1995;333:364–368.

Constantinescu AR, et al. Non-enteropathic hemolytic uremic syndrome: causes and short-term course. *Am J Kidney Dis* 2004;43:976–982.

Eriksson KJ, et al. Acute neurology and neurophysiology of haemolytic-uraemic syndrome. *Arch Dis Child* 2001;84(5):434–435.

Garg AX, et al. Long-term renal prognosis of diarrhea-associated hemolytic uremic syndrome: a systematic review, meta-analysis, and meta-regression. *JAMA* 2003;290:1360–1370.

Kaplan BS, Meyers KE, Schulman SL. The pathogenesis and treatment of hemolytic uremic syndrome. *J Am Soc Nephrol* 1998;9:1126–1133.

Zipfel PF, et al. Genetic screening in haemolytic uraemic syndrome. *Curr Opin Nephrol Hypertens* 2003;12:653–657.

Author: Mary B. Leonard

Hemophilia

 Database

DEFINITION

Hereditary bleeding disorder caused by the absence, severe deficiency, or defective functioning of plasma coagulation factors VIII (hemophilia A) or IX (hemophilia B) inherited in an X-linked manner.

PATHOPHYSIOLOGY

- Both factors VIII and IX are crucial for normal thrombin generation via the intrinsic pathway. The absence of either protein (or level <25%) severely impairs the ability to generate thrombin and fibrin.
- Hemophilia patients do not bleed more rapidly; rather there is delayed formation of an abnormal clot.
- The friable clot formed has a tendency to ooze and rebleed.
- In closed spaces (e.g., joint), bleeding stops by tamponade; in open spaces (e.g., iliopsoas muscle, open wounds), significant amounts of blood may be lost.
- Repeated joint hemorrhages lead to synovial thickening and joint cartilage erosion. Joint space becomes narrowed and eventually fuses.

GENETICS

- X-linked recessive disorder
- Carrier status and prenatal testing available
- Hemophilia A:
—Inversion in the factor VIII gene resulting from an intrachromosomal recombination accounts for 40%–50% of all severe hemophilia A gene abnormalities; detectable by direct gene mutation analysis.
—In families with an unknown mutation, a coagulation-based assay comparing the level of factor VIII with von Willebrand factor can be used to identify carriers.
—Accuracy of screening: 90%
- Hemophilia B (Christmas disease):
—Factor IX genetic mutations are easily identified due to the small size of the factor IX gene.
—Majority of factor IX gene defects are due to single-base pair substitutions, which can be identified in nearly all affected individuals and carriers

EPIDEMIOLOGY

- Most common severe inherited bleeding disorder.
- Distribution
—Hemophilia A: 80%–85%
—Hemophilia B: 10%–15%
- Incidence:
—Hemophilia A: 1 per 5,000 male births
—Hemophilia B: 1 per 30,000 male births
- No geographic or ethnic associations

COMPLICATIONS

- Complications of disease
—Hemophilic arthropathy: Joint contractures, limited range of motion, and chronic pain

—Intracranial bleeding (can occur without known trauma in severe hemophilia)
—Compartment syndrome
—Airway compromise due to bleeds in the pharynx, tongue, or neck
—Life-threatening hemorrhage due to gastrointestinal, posttraumatic or perioperative bleeds
- Complications of therapy
—Viral transmission (HIV, hepatitis B and C) through clotting factor concentrates derived from pooled plasma preparations (>22,000 donors per lot)
—Inhibitors: Antibodies against factor VIII or IX, which can inactivate infused factor
—Anaphylaxis: Continued factor IX replacement in severe factor IX-deficient patients with inhibitors may lead to anaphylaxis
—Thromboembolic disease: Use of prothrombin complex concentrates has been associated with thrombus formation, thromboembolic events, and myocardial infarctions in children

 Differential Diagnosis

- Prolonged PTT associated with increased bleeding tendency
—von Willebrand disease
—"Acquired hemophilia" due to development of an inhibitory antibody to factor VIII or IX
—Hereditary factor XI deficiency
—Afibrinogenemia
- Prolonged PTT without increased bleeding tendency
—Factor XII deficiency
—High molecular weight kininogen deficiency
—Prekallikrein deficiency
—Antiphospholipid antibody (lupus anticoagulant)
—Heparin artifact

 Data Gathering

HISTORY

Question: Family history?
Significance: Familial history of hemophilia in male offspring of female blood relatives is present in 30%–40% of cases.

Question: Pattern of bleeding?
Significance: Characterized by easy, excessive, and palpable bruising with normal activity, spontaneous joint and muscle hemorrhages, and prolonged and potentially fatal hemorrhage after trauma or surgery.

Question: Age of onset of bleeding?
Significance: Bleeding events occur frequently when the child begins to crawl and walk or with the eruption of teeth.

Question: Location of hemarthroses?
Significance: Large weight bearing joints are most often involved: knees, elbows, ankles, shoulders, and hips.

 Physical Examination

- Acute hemarthrosis: Limitation of range of motion of the joint, warmth, swelling, tenderness
- Chronic joint: Crepitus, decreased range of motion, proximal muscle weakness; typically occurs in knees, ankles, elbows
- Intramuscular hematomas: Often little seen on exam; vague feeling of pain with motion
- Discrepancy in limb circumference is often the earliest sign of intramuscular hematoma
- Distal extremity neurovascular compromise can be a sign of compartment syndrome from bleeding into forearm or calf muscles.

 Laboratory Aids

TESTS

Test: Prothrombin time (PT), activated partial thromboplastin time (PTT), fibrinogen or thrombin time, platelet count, and von Willebrand studies
Significance: Initial screening studies if bleeding disorder is suspected.

Test: Assay for factor VIII and factor IX levels
Significance:

- Less than 1%: severe hemophilia. Most common, characterized by spontaneous bleeding; hemarthroses and deep-tissue hemorrhages; will need frequent factor replacement therapy.
- 1% to 5%: Moderate hemophilia. Gross bleeding following mild to moderate trauma; some hemarthrosis; seldom-spontaneous hemorrhage.
- 5% to 25%: Mild hemophilia. Rare bleeding; requires factor replacement therapy only with significant trauma or surgery.

PITFALLS

- Neonates have a physiologic reduction in the vitamin K-dependent factors, including factor IX, making a determination of the degree of factor IX deficiency difficult in the neonatal period
- Delivery-related stress and other neonatal problems may cause a transient elevation of factor VIII levels.
- Poor venipuncture technique can artifactually shorten or normalize the PTT.

 Emergency Care

LIFE-THREATENING HEMORRHAGES

- Central nervous system bleeding
- Bleeding into and around the airway
- Exsanguinating hemorrhage
- Prompt therapy with clotting factor concentrate should occur immediately and prior to any diagnostic procedures.

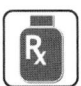 ## Therapy

ACUTE BLEEDING EPISODES

Factor Replacement

- Factor VIII replacement products
—Recombinant, nonplasma-derived factor VIII
—Plasma-derived, monoclonal antibody-purified factor VIII concentrate; heat or solvent detergent treated for viral inactivation
—Cryoprecipitate (rarely used today)
- Factor IX replacement products
—Recombinant, nonplasma-derived factor IX
—Plasma-derived, immunoaffinity-purified factor IX concentrate; heat or solvent detergent treated for viral inactivation
- Prothrombin complex concentrate (PCC): Crude plasma fraction, which contains variable amounts of activated factors II, VII, IX, and X; heat treated for viral inactivation.
- Rarely used: Fresh frozen plasma

Calculation of Dose

- Factor VIII dose (units) = % desired rise in plasma factor VIII × body weight (kg) × 0.5
- Factor IX dose = % desired rise in factor IX level × body weight (kg)

Target Factor Levels

- 30%–40% for 24–48 hours for most joint bleeds
- 70%–100% repeated over 12–48 hours for large muscle bleeds
- 100% maintained over 10–14 days for life-threatening bleeds or major surgery

DDAVP

- Synthetic vasopressin analog that stimulates release of endogenous factor VIII and von Willebrand factor
- Only suitable for patients with mild or moderate factor VIII deficiency who have shown a response to DDAVP in a trial
- Tachyphylaxis may occur with repeated dosing.
- Hyponatremia may occur in patients receiving repeated doses. Fluid restriction and close monitoring of urine output and serum electrolytes minimize risk of hyponatremic seizure.

Antifibrinolytic Therapy

- Antifibrinolytic therapy is used to stabilize a clot by inhibiting the normal process of clot lysis by the fibrinolytic system.
- Agents used for the treatment of oral hemorrhages and to minimize bleeding from dental procedures
- Epsilon aminocaproic acid (Amicar)—50–100 mg/kg per dose PO every 6 hours (max. 5 g per dose), or tranexamic acid (Cyklokapron)—25 mg/kg per dose PO every 8 hours (max. 1.5 g per dose)

Immobilization

- Splints, casts, crutches, and/or bed rest
- Prolonged immobilization may reduce recovery of joint range of motion; initiation of physical therapy with factor coverage is recommended, particularly after joint surgery

SPECIAL BLEEDING SITUATIONS

Intracranial Hemorrhage

- Significant bleeding can occur despite the absence of external bruising
- Factor replacement to 100% should be administered immediately
- CT scan of the head is useful but may be negative early in a bleed

Major Surgery

- Factor replacement to 100% pre and postoperatively
- Regular dosing of factor for a minimum of 1 week postoperatively, even in mild hemophilia

Compartment Syndrome

- Bleeding within the fascial compartments of muscles
- Most often occurs in the forearm and calf
- Neurovascular compromise can lead to Volkmann contracture

Iliopsoas Bleed

- Lower abdominal or upper thigh pain may be first symptom
- Examination is notable for inability to extend hip with preservation of internal and external rotation (allows distinction from hemarthrosis of hip joint)
- Diagnosis confirmed by ultrasound or CT scan
- Large volume of blood can be lost into the retroperitoneal space. Hemoglobin should be monitored.

Oral Bleeding/Epistaxis

- Constant pressure for 15 to 20 minutes
- ε-Aminocaproic acid or tranexamic acid
- Topical thrombin directly to the site of bleeding

Dental Care

- Significant dental procedures (e.g., tooth extraction) should be performed by a dentist with experience in treating hemophilia patients and preferably in a hospital setting where hematology consultation is available.
- Factor replacement is required pre- and postprocedure.

LACERATIONS

- Sutures should be avoided when possible.
- If sutures are required, factor replacement is necessary at time of placement and removal.

Hematuria

- Increased fluid intake and bed rest as initial treatment
- If hematuria persists 24 to 48 hours, 30% to 40% factor replacement
- Prednisone in HIV-negative patients

 ## Follow-Up

Patients should be followed regularly at a comprehensive hemophilia treatment center, in which care is coordinated by a team including the pediatric hematologist, nurse coordinator, social worker, psychologist, physical therapist, dentist, orthopaedic surgeon, and financial counselor.

PREVENTION

Prophylaxis

- Primary prophylaxis: Regular dosing in patients with no complications to prevent chronic joint damage. Typically initiated prior to 1 year of age.
- Secondary prophylaxis: Regular dosing in patients with target joints to prevent additional damage and facilitate healing and rehabilitation

 ## Common Questions and Answers

Q: Are there any medications contraindicated in a child with hemophilia?
A: Aspirin should not be given, as it interferes with platelet function. Nonsteroidal antiinflammatory agents cause a milder effect on platelets, and should also be avoided when possible.

ICD-9-CM 286.0

BIBLIOGRAPHY

DiMichele D, Neufeld EJ. Hemophilia: A new approach to an old disease. *Heme/Oncol Clin North Am* 1998;12:1315–1341.

Manco-Johnson MJ, et al. Advances in care of children with hemophilia. *Semin Thromb Hemost* 2003;29:585–594.

Mannucci PM, Tuddenham EGD. The hemophilias: Progress and problems. *Semin Hematol* 1999;36:104–117.

Montgomery RR, et al. Hemophilia and von Willebrand Disease. In: Roberts HR. Choice of replacement therapy for hemophilia. *J Thromb Haemost* 2003;1:595.

Authors: Don E. Eslin
Jane E. Minturn, 3rd edition

Hemoptysis

 ## Database

DEFINITION

It is the coughing up of blood from the respiratory tract. The term comes from the Greek words *haima*, meaning *blood* and *ptysis*, meaning *spitting*. The amount varies from mild to massive, which can cause hypoxia or exsanguination.

CAUSES

- Cavitary infections (e.g., tuberculosis, abscess, histoplasmosis)
- Tumors (lymphomas)
- Trauma (pulmonary contusion, bronchoscopy, airway manipulation)
- Congenital heart disease with large collateral vessels
- Foreign body aspiration
- Pneumonia
- Hemorrhagic diathesis including anticoagulant therapy
- H-type tracheoesophageal fistula
- Cystic fibrosis
- Tracheostomy-related complications
- Bronchiectasis
- Factitious hemoptysis

PATHOPHYSIOLOGY

- Related to the underlying pulmonary disease
- The vascular origin of hemoptysis is from two sites—pulmonary arteries or bronchial arteries.

EPIDEMIOLOGY

- Large series of pediatric patients with massive hemoptysis have not been described.
- Most instances of massive hemoptysis occur in older children.

COMPLICATIONS

- Respiratory insufficiency
- Hypovolemic shock

 ## Differential Diagnosis

- Infections: Pneumonia, pulmonary abscess, tuberculosis
- Pulmonary disease: Cystic fibrosis, bronchiectasis, foreign body, arteriovenous malformation, congenital lung malformation, pulmonary emboli, pulmonary hemosiderosis
- Cardiovascular disease
- Collagen vascular disease: Lupus, vasculitis, Goodpasture disease
- Trauma
- Coagulation disorder
- Munchausen syndrome
- Bronchogenic neoplasms
- Complications: Anemia, pneumonia

 ## Data Gathering

HISTORY

- Familial history of pulmonary disease or bleeding disorder?
- Exposure to environmental toxins?
- Exposure to tuberculosis?
- Drug use: Cocaine, marijuana?

Question: Recurrent episodes of hemoptysis with significant spectrum production and cyst formation on chest x-ray?
Significance: Suggests a diagnosis of bronchiectasis

Question: Acute pleuritic chest pain?
Significance: Raises the possibility of pulmonary embolism with infarction or some other pleurally based lesion. A pleural friction rub may be present.

 ## Physical Examination

Finding: Pleural friction rub
Significance: May be associated with pulmonary embolism

Finding: Pulmonary hypertension
Significance: Raises the diagnostic possibilities of primary pulmonary hypertension, mitral stenosis, and Eisenmenger syndrome

Finding: Localized wheeze over a major lobar airway
Significance: Suggests an intramural lesion such as a foreign body or carcinoma

Finding: Presence of a murmur over the lung fields
Significance: May suggest pulmonary arteriovenous malformation

Laboratory Aids

Test: Complete blood count, reticulocyte count, and coagulation profile
Significance: May reveal the volume of blood loss, chronicity, and evidence of bleeding diathesis

Test: Sputum and PPD
Significance: Tuberculosis is suspected.

Test: Drug screen
Significance: If appropriate

Test: Chest x-ray both AP and lateral
Significance: May reveal pleural effusion, bronchiectasis, foreign bodies, or consolidation

Test: Flexible fiberoptic bronchoscopy
Significance: Usually performed to localize the site of bleeding and at times may be therapeutic (e.g., in foreign body removal). Fiberoptic bronchoscopy performed acutely (during hemoptysis or within 48 hours after) is more likely to visualize and stop active bleeding or its site than delayed bronchoscopy.

Test: CT
Significance: Useful when chest radiographs and fiberoptic bronchoscopy are normal. High-resolution CT may identify source of bleeding especially if bronchiectasis and arteriovenous malformation are suspected.

Test: Angiogram
Significance: Used to detect bleeding from arteriovascular malformation.

Test: Ventilation-perfusion scans
Significance: An important study in patients suspected of having hemoptysis from pulmonary embolism or infarct

 Therapy

- Initial management should follow the lines of basic life support.
- Support intravascular volume by packed red blood cells or fresh frozen plasma.
- Methods used to stop localized bleeding include tamponade with balloon-tipped catheters, ice water lavage, catheter-directed umbilication, intravenous pitressin, and surgical resection. The last option is usually reserved for most difficult cases such as extensive collateralization of bronchial arteries or arteriovenous malformations not responsive to embolization. The most effective nonsurgical treatment is bronchial artery embolization. Some newer techniques include endoscopic instillation of fibrinogen-thrombin and endobronchial argon plasma coagulation.

PROGNOSIS

It depends on the etiology and the nature of hemoptysis. Immediate management of airway central decreases the morbidity and mortality.

ICD-9-CM 786.3

BIBLIOGRAPHY

De Gracia J. Use of endoscopic fibrinogen-thrombin in the treatment of severe hemoptysis. *Respir Med* 2003;97(7):790–795.

Gong H Jr, Salvatierra C. Clinical efficacy of early and delayed fiberoptic bronchoscopy in patients with hemoptysis. *Am Rev Respir Dis* 1981;124:221.

Jean-Baptiste E. Clinical assessment and management of massive hemoptysis. *Crit Care Med* 2000;28(5):1642–1647.

Thompson AB, Teschler H, Rennard SI. Pathogenesis, evaluation and therapy for massive hemoptysis. *Clin Chest Med* 1992;13(1):69–82.

Author: Helen Anita John-Kelly

Henoch-Schönlein Purpura

Database

DEFINITION

- Henoch-Schönlein purpura (HSP) is an immunologically mediated, nonthrombocytopenic, purpuric, and systemic vasculitis involving the small blood vessels of the skin, gastrointestinal (GI) tract, joints, and kidneys.
- Defined by the presence of two of the following:

—Palpable purpura
—Age of onset less than 20 years
—Abdominal pain
—Granulocytic infiltration of vessel walls

- In children, only palpable purpura with normal platelet count need be documented.
- While most children do have purpura, colicky abdominal pain and arthritis, up to one-half may present with symptoms other than purpura.

PATHOPHYSIOLOGY

- No single etiologic agent has been identified.
- Most cases associated with preceding upper respiratory infections, usually group A β-hemolytic streptococci. A recent study shows a significant association with *B. henselae*. Also reported following infections with parvovirus, adenovirus, Hepatitis A virus, *Helicobacter pylori*, and *Mycoplasma pneumoniae*. Parvovirus B19 previously proposed, but evidence is inconclusive.
- Also reported after drug ingestion (e.g., thiazides) and insect bites.
- Capillaries, arterioles, and venules are affected in HSP as opposed to polyarteritis nodosa, Wegener and systemic lupus erythematosus (SLE), where small arteries are affected.
- Immunofluorescent microscopy shows granular deposits of IgA1, C3, and fibrin.
- Biopsy of the involved kidneys shows endocapillary proliferative glomerulonephritis involving endothelial and mesangial cells. Crescent formation may also be present. IgA, IgG, C3, and fibrin are commonly found in the mesangial regions.

EPIDEMIOLOGY

- Incidence of 13.5 cases per 100,000 school-aged children per year (90% of patients are younger than 10 years old)
- Slightly more common in males—male to female ratio of 58:42 in 1 study
- Year-round occurrence, but more common in Spring, Winter, and Fall.
- Epidemics or clusters are rare.
- Most common in Caucasians, Japanese, and Native Americans. Low incidence in blacks, both in Africa and North America.

COMPLICATIONS

- Persistent hypertension

- End-stage kidney disease (acute or as a late sequela)
- Intussusception (most common gastrointestinal [GI] complication; affecting 1% to 5% of patients)
- Protein-losing enteropathy
- Hemorrhagic pancreatitis
- Hydrops of the gallbladder
- Strictures of the esophagus and ileus
- Bowel perforations, ischemia and infarctions
- Pseudomembranous colitis
- Appendicitis
- Skin necrosis
- Subarachnoid, subdural, and cortical hemorrhage and infarction
- Peripheral mono and polyneuropathies (Guillain-Barré syndrome)
- Pulmonary hemorrhage (uncommon, but may result in death)
- Torsion of the testis and appendix testes, and priapism
- Scrotal swelling and pain

PROGNOSIS

- Generally excellent: the majority (>60%) of children are better within 4 weeks of the onset
- Better prognosis associated with younger age
- Recurrence within the first 6 weeks in up to 33%
- Most have only one to three episodes of purpura; however, a few will continue to experience symptoms for months or years. These patients have a poor prognosis and are more likely to develop severe nephritis.
- Gastrointestinal tract disease accounts for the most significant morbidity in the short term.
- Renal involvement is the cause of the most serious long-term morbidity. Microscopic hematuria alone or with mild proteinuria generally has a good outcome. A nephritic and nephrotic combination is more guarded, and those patients with a high percentage of crescent formation do less well.

Differential Diagnosis

- Petechial and purpuric rashes seen in thrombocytopenia from:

—Idiopathic thrombocytopenic purpura (ITP)
—Sepsis/infection: Meningococcemia, Rocky Mountain spotted fever
—Leukemia
—Hemolytic uremic syndrome (HUS)
—Coagulopathies

- Vasculitic rashes may result from primary and secondary vasculitides:

—Polyarteritis nodosa
—Wegener granulomatosis
—Infection-related
—Connective tissue diseases (e.g., SLE), Berger disease (IgA nephropathy): glomerulonephritis similar to HSP both clinically and immunologically, but not associated with the skin, GI, or joint

manifestations of HSP streptococcal glomerulonephritis
—Infantile acute hemorrhagic edema: Vasculitis that presents with urticarial or maculopapular rash that then becomes purpuric. It is differentiated from HSP in that it usually affects children from 4 months to 2 years of age, is more common in the Winter, and is not associated with systemic symptoms. On biopsy, IgA deposits are not a consistent finding as they are with HSP.
—Rheumatoid arthritis
—Rheumatic fever

Data Gathering

HISTORY

Question: Previous disease?
Significance: Especially infections such as hepatitis, URI, and streptococcal infections

Question: Abdominal pain?
Significance: Pain is the most common GI symptom. Two-thirds of children have GI symptoms. Emesis and melena are also reported.

Question: Transient, nondeforming, nonmigratory arthritis of knees, ankles, wrists, elbows, and digits?
Significance: Frequent problem, most common in knees and ankles.

Question: Presence of testicular pain or scrotal swelling, headache, cough, edema of the ankles or periorbital region, and hematuria?
Significance: Vasculitic lesion in the associated system

Physical Examination

Finding: Particular attention to blood pressure.
Significance: Hypertension is common.

Finding: Low-grade fever.
Significance: In 50% of the cases.

Finding: Rash that is petechial or purpuric in a pressure-dependent, symmetric distribution, usually around the lateral malleoli of the ankles, on the ventral surfaces of the feet and on the buttocks.
Significance: Purpura may be briefly preceded by maculopapular or urticarial lesions.

Finding: Joints should be examined for swelling and limitation of motion.
Significance: Redness and warmth are not common. Symptoms precede the rash by up to 2 weeks in 25% of patients.

Finding: Nonpitting subcutaneous edema of the scalp, periorbital region, hands, and feet is often noted.
Significance: Generalized edema is more common in children under 3 years of age. May lead to acute hemorrhagic edema, now considered to be a variant of HSP

Henoch-Schönlein Purpura

Finding: Abdomen is often tender to palpation, but without rebound tenderness. Hepatosplenomegaly may be found. Because intussusception and appendicitis are possible complications, serial examinations may be necessary to determine if radiographic studies are indicated.
Significance: Abdominal symptoms may precede the rash by up to 2 weeks.

Finding: Orchitis, where affected testicle may be tender and swollen. Swelling and bruising may be noted on the scrotum.
Significance: Testicular torsion has also been reported in HSP and may mimic orchitis.

Finding: Neurologic changes
Significance: CNS involvement may present with headaches, seizures, or behavioral changes.

 ## Laboratory Aids

There are no definitive tests to confirm the diagnosis of HSP.

Test: Complete blood count (CBC)
Significance: Normal platelet count differentiates from thrombocytopenic purpura. Hemoglobin is usually normal; leukocytosis; eosinophilia especially may be present.

Test: Erythrocyte sedimentation rate (ESR)
Significance: Normal or elevated

Test: Prothrombin (PT) and partial thromboplastin time (PTT)
Significance: Normal

Test: IgA
Significance: Often elevated in the acute phase of illness, with normal or increased IgG and IgM

Test: C3
Significance: Normal (decreased in poststreptococcal glomerulonephritis and SLE)

Test: Antinuclear antibody
Significance: Negative (elevated in SLE)

Test: Throat swab for group A β-hemolytic streptococci
Significance: Positive in up to 75% of cases

Test: Serum basic/comprehensive chemistries
Significance: Elevated BUN and creatinine, and decreased protein and albumin are seen with renal involvement

Test: Urinalysis
Significance: Gross hematuria and proteinuria are present in many patients. Proteinuria alone is rare. Microscopic blood, RBCs, WBCs, and casts suggest glomerulonephritis.

Test: Stool guaiac
Significance: GI involvement may present as guaiac positive stools, bloody stools or melena. Important to have a low suspicion for intussusception which is a known complication of HSP.

Test: Renal biopsy
Significance: With severe renal failure, a biopsy should be performed to determine the extent of disease

Test: Skin biopsy
Significance: Direct Immunofluorescence for IgA helpful in confirming the diagnosis

RADIOGRAPHIC STUDIES

Test: Chest radiograph
Significance: May show interstitial lung disease

Test: Abdominal ultrasound
Significance: Barium enemas are NOT indicated for suspected intussusception. They will not reduce the ilio-ileal intussusception common to HSP (idiopathic intussusception is usually ilio-colic in location) and may damage or perforate the inflamed bowel.

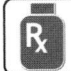 ## Therapy

HSP usually resolve spontaneously without specific therapy.

• Analgesics and NSAIDs may be used for control of joint pain and inflammation, but salicylates and other agents that affect platelet function should be avoided if GI bleeding is present.
• Steroids are used for painful cutaneous edema, arthritis, and abdominal pain (2 mg/kg per day of prednisone until clinical resolution); however, steroids have not been shown to affect purpura or to decrease duration of disease or frequency of recurrences.
• No consensus on management of GI and renal involvement. Oral prednisone at 2 mg/kg per day has shown faster resolution of abdominal pain, while other studies indicate the symptoms will resolve similarly without intervention.
• The majority will improve spontaneously. Treatment should be considered for children at high risk for chronic renal insufficiency or failure (those presenting with nephrotic syndrome or renal insufficiency).
• More than 50% crescentic glomerulonephritis on renal biopsy has a greater risk of future renal failure. Such cases should be considered for aggressive therapy with pulse or oral steroids and/or immunosuppressants (azathioprine, cyclophosphamide, cyclosporine) or plasmapheresis, IVIG, danazol, or fish oil.
• Treatment of hypertension may delay or prevent progression of renal disease in patients with glomerulonephritis.

 ## Follow-Up

• Patients should be seen weekly during the acute illness. Visits should include history and physical examination, along with blood pressure measurement and urinalysis.

• All patients, even those who did not present with renal involvement, should have urine checked for blood weekly for 6 months, and then monthly for 3 years as deterioration of renal function has been observed years after presentation in some patients.
• Women with a history of HSP should be monitored for proteinuria and hypertension during pregnancy

 ## Common Questions and Answers

Q: When should I consider hospitalization?
A: Often it is not necessary. Severe complications may require admission. These include GI hemorrhage, protein-losing enteropathy requiring total parenteral nutrition (TPN), decreased glomerular filtration rate (GFR) or hypertension, and pulmonary hemorrhage.

Q: Is there a role for prophylactic penicillin?
A: In patients with frequent relapses, where group A β-hemolytic streptococci is often the inciting agent, administration of penicillin may be helpful.

Q: Who are Henoch and Schönlein?
A: The clinical finding of joint pain associated with purpura was named "purpura rheumatica" in 1837 by Schönlein. Henoch, a student of Schönlein's, later described the association of GI and renal involvement. However, the first report was by Heberden in 1801. Of note, it has been speculated that Mozart, whose symptoms included fever, vomiting, exanthem, arthritis, anasarca, and coma, died of HSP.

ICD-9-CM 287.0

BIBLIOGRAPHY

Ayoub EM, et al. Role of *Bartonella henselae* in the etiology of Henoch-Schönlein purpura. *Pediatr Infect Dis J* 2002;21:28–31.

Davin JC, Weening JJ. Henoch Schönlein purpura nephritis: an update. *Eur J Pediatr* 2001;160:689–695.

Dillon MJ. Henoch-Schönlein purpura (treatment and outcome). *Cleve Clin J Med* 2002;69(Suppl 2):SII121–SII123.

Heegaard ED, Taaning EB. Parvovirus B19 and parvovirus V9 are not associated with Henoch-Schönlein purpura in children. *Pediatr Infect Dis J* 2002;21:31–34.

Kraft DM, et al. Henoch-Schönlein purpura: a review. *Am Fam Physician* 1999;58:405–408.

Piette WW. What is Schönlein-Henoch purpura, and why should we care? *Arch Dermatol* 1997;133:515–518.

Saulsbury FT. Henoch-Schönlein purpura. *Curr Opin Rheumatol* 2001;13:35–40.

Saulsbury FT. Epidemiology of Henoch-Schönlein purpura. *Cleve Clin J Med* 2002;69(Suppl 2):SII87–SII89.

Author: Blaze Robert Gusic

Hepatic Encephalopathy

 Database

DEFINITION

Disordered brain dysfunction that occurs as a consequence of acute hepatocyte failure.

CAUSES

- Gastrointestinal hemorrhage (secondary to varices, ulcers, gastritis, any source of gastrointestinal hemorrhage)
- Intracranial hemorrhage (secondary to coagulopathy from liver disease-related deficiency of coagulation factors)
- Infections, including spontaneous bacterial peritonitis
- Dehydration (often secondary to aggressive diuresis)
- Administration of sedatives (benzodiazepines and barbiturates)
- Placement of a porta-systemic shunt—surgical or transjugular intrahepatic portosystemic shunt (TIPS) procedure

PATHOPHYSIOLOGY

The appearance of hepatic encephalopathy (HE) depends on the interactions of three factors:

- Porta-systemic shunting: Shunting can occur around the liver through collateral vessels or through the liver as the blood passes by damaged or necrotic hepatocytes.
- Changes in the blood–brain barrier: Increased permeability of blood–brain barrier has been demonstrated with increased uptake of markers (e.g., horseradish peroxidase) during acute liver failure. Toxic metabolites of liver failure (ammonia and mercaptans) have been shown to increase blood–brain barrier permeability.
- Interactions of toxic metabolites with the CNS

—Ammonia hypothesis:
  —Ammonia, produced by the bacterial metabolism of amino acids, is usually detoxified in the liver by the urea cycle. Measures to decrease dietary protein and decrease serum ammonia (e.g., lactulose and neomycin) can improve the clinical status in HE.
  —Ammonia does not correlate with the stage of HE, and is not the sole mediator of HE.
—False neurotransmitter hypothesis:
  —Excessive production of brain "false" inhibitory neurotransmitters (serotonin and octopamine) that are usually not found in the brain or systemic circulation, and a deficiency of excitatory neurotransmitters (dopamine and norepinephrine).
—γ-Aminobutyric acid (GABA) inhibitory neurotransmitter hypothesis
  —GABA is an inhibitory neurotransmitter produced in the brain by decarboxylation of glutamic acid. GABA, benzodiazepines, and barbiturates activate the GABA receptor in the brain. Increased GABA-like agents and endogenous benzodiazepines are produced from intestinal bacterial metabolism, reaching the brain and promoting inhibitory neurotransmission.
—Synergistic neurotoxin hypothesis: HE may result from the combined accumulation of several neurotoxins, each of which alone would be insufficient to cause HE. These would include substances such as ammonia, mercaptans, short- and medium-chain fatty acids. This occurs in the setting of incomplete detoxification of potentially neurotoxic intestinal metabolites (secondary to impaired hepatocyte function and porta-systemic shunting) and increased permeability of the blood–brain barrier.

 Differential Diagnosis

- Infection: Meningitis, encephalitis
- Tumors: Intracranial lesions
- Trauma: Cerebral hemorrhage, cerebral hematoma
- Metabolic: Inborn errors of metabolism, lactic acidemias, urea cycle deficiencies
- Immunologic: AIDS dementia

 Data Gathering

HISTORY

Question: Alteration in mental status and personality?
Significance: Classic feature. Often first noted by family members or a child's teacher.

 Physical Examination

Central nervous system manifestations—the initial manifestations can be very subtle, especially in children.
Four clinical stages of hepatic coma are described, based on changes in conscious intellectual functioning and behavior. Any neurologic function can be impaired in HE.

- Changes in consciousness: Hypersomnia, reversal of sleep patterns, slowing of speech, and eventually coma.
- Personality changes: Irritability, inattentiveness, apathy, childishness, regressive behaviors, emotional outbursts. Any child with acute onset of combative or irrational behavior in the classroom should be evaluated for HE.
- Intellectual deterioration: Worsening of school performance secondary to inattentiveness and confusion.
- Constructional apraxia: A defect in visual spatial skills, demonstrated with age-appropriate tasks, such as writing, drawing, and coloring.
- Neuromuscular dysfunction: Muscle tone and deep-tendon reflexes may be exaggerated in early HE, but in later stages the muscles become flaccid and reflexes disappear.

- Signs of end-stage liver failure: Varices, ascites, spider angiomata, palmar erythema, caput medusa.
- Asterixis: Ask the patient to stand with both arms raised horizontally in front of him, wrists dorsiflexed, and fingers held apart for at least 15 seconds. A flapping tremor of the fingers and wrists will be present with voluntary movement, but absent at rest. This is characteristic of HE, although it may also be seen with uremia, respiratory failure, and congestive heart failure.

STAGES

Four clinical stages of HE are described. These are useful for assessing HE in older patients, but have less value in assessing neonates and younger children, especially in the early stages of HE.

Stage I: Alert, irritable, sleep rhythm reversal, poor handwriting, inattentive to tasks, slowness of mentation.

Stage II: Lethargic, confused, combative, inappropriate behavior, disorientation, mood swings, tremor, asterixis.

Stage III: Stuporous but arousable, marked confusion, delirious, hyperreflexia, positive Babinski sign.

Stage IV: Comatose, no motor activity, decerebrate or decorticate, may respond to painful stimuli.

 Laboratory Aids

TESTS

- No specific lab test, including serum ammonia, correlates well with the stage of HE.
- EEG: May show a slowing from the normal alpha frequency to the delta range. Nonspecific and may be seen in other disease processes.
- Visual evoked potentials: May become more useful than EEGs.
- Neuropsychiatric testing: Must be age-appropriate testing. In older children, can use subtraction of serial sevens, number connection test, handwriting, and event recall. In younger children, can use task of coloring within the lines, if this is a skill that the child had previously developed.

IMAGING

- Head CT scan: Assess for signs of increased intracranial pressure or cerebral edema. These do not help with diagnosis but may indicate severity of encephalopathy and suggest prognosis.
- Proton magnetic resonance spectroscopy: Characteristic changes have been identified in HE. Has not yet proven helpful in diagnosing subclinical HE.

Emergency Care

HE necessitates immediate hospital admission, usually to an intensive care unit, for close observation. It is imperative to promptly identify and treat any precipitating factor of HE.

 ## Therapy

SUPPORTIVE CARE

• Fluids and electrolyte monitoring, vital signs, paying close attention to development of infection (respiratory, urinary).
• Avoid administration of sedatives, which can worsen or confound the clinical neurologic status in HE.
• Frequent, repeated neurologic examinations. The clinical course typically fluctuates in HE, and patients can deteriorate within hours or days.

DRUGS

• Lactulose, a nonabsorbable disaccharide that is metabolized by colonic bacteria, which results in acidified fecal contents (pH <6.0) that trap ammonia. Lactulose has also been shown to change colonic flora, increasing *Lactobacillus* species. Complications include diarrhea and dehydration.
• Neomycin reduces the amount of bacterial urease available by directly suppressing ammonia-forming bacteria. Systemically absorbed and long-term use has been associated with ototoxicity.
• Acidifying enemas (lactulose or lactitol) can help lower serum ammonia, and are helpful after a GI bleed.
• Flumazenil, a benzodiazepine receptor antagonist, can block the GABA receptor in the brain, and result in temporary reversal of the electrophysiologic and clinical abnormalities in HE. Results are conflicting, and require randomized controlled trials.
• Branched-chain amino acids (BCAAs) may reverse the altered ratio of branched-chain to aromatic amino acids, and decrease muscle protein breakdown. Conflicting results in adults with chronic encephalopathy.
• Levodopa and bromocriptine, a dopamine agonist, have resulted in temporary reversal of HE in a few patients.

DIET

• Avoid hypoglycemia, which can further aggravate HE.
• Protein restriction is recommended during acute HE to avoid further increases in ammonia levels.
• In children, need to balance protein restriction, which can result in growth failure.

SURGERY

• Placement of a portosystemic shunt before the onset of the acute development of neurologic deterioration may suggest that the shunt is not allowing enough circulation through the liver. Reversal of the shunt, by either surgical or balloon occlusion, may improve the clinical picture.
• Liver transplantation

 ## Follow-Up

WHEN TO EXPECT IMPROVEMENT

Often, improvement (a change in the level of HE by 1 or 2 stages) is seen 2 to 3 days after initiation of therapy.

SIGNS TO WATCH FOR

• Progression of neurologic status through the stages of HE. Passage through the stages of HE can be very rapid (e.g., in fulminant hepatic failure) or more gradual in the setting of chronic liver disease.

PROGNOSIS

Depends to some degree on stage of encephalopathy. Prognosis is better if a precipitating factor can be promptly identified and treated effectively. Orthotopic liver transplantation should be performed in children with severe and worsening encephalopathy before the development of radiographically apparent cerebral edema. Cerebral edema with brainstem herniation is the major cause of mortality (frequency between 25% and 81% in various studies) in patients with fulminant hepatic failure in stage III or IV. Patients with HE and underlying chronic liver disease have a much lower incidence of cerebral edema. In one study, on multiple logistic regression analysis, presence of GI hemorrhage ($p = .005$), degree of coma ($p = .02$), and serum bilirubin level ($p = 0.025$) were identified as independent predictors of mortality.

 ## Common Questions and Answers

Q: My child has chronic liver failure and has experienced two episodes of hepatic encephalopathy managed in the ICU. Is there any special diet I should be providing him?
A: Because dietary intake of protein can lead to accumulation of nitrogenous waste that can accumulate into ammonia, it is best to keep your child on a low-protein diet.

ICD-9-CM 572.2

BIBLIOGRAPHY

Butterworth RF. Complications of cirrhosis III: hepatic encephalopathy. *J Hepatol* 2000;32(Suppl 1):171.

Hawkins RA, Mans AM. Brain metabolism in hepatic encephalopathy and hyperammonemia. In: Felipo V, Grisola S, eds. *Cirrhosis, Hyperammonemia, and Hepatic Encephalopathy*. New York: Plenum, 1994:13–19.

Jones EA. Pathogenesis of hepatic encephalopathy. *Clin Liver Dis* 2000;4(2):467.

Riordan SM, Williams R. Treatment of hepatic encephalopathy. *N Engl J Med* 1997;337(26):1921.

Rodes J. Clinical manifestations and therapy of hepatic encephalopathy. In: Felipo V, Grisola S, eds. *Cirrhosis, Hyperammonemia, and Hepatic Encephalopathy*. New York: Plenum, 1994:39–44.

Suchy FJ, Sokol RJ, Balistreri WF. *Liver Disease in Children*. Philadelphia: Lippincott, Williams & Wilkins, 2001.

Authors: Andrew E. Mulberg and Lynette Gillis

Hereditary Spherocytosis

 Database

DEFINITION

Hemolytic anemia with shortened red cell survival due to selective trapping of osmotically fragile spherocytic red blood cells in the spleen secondary to an inherent defect of the red cell membrane.

PATHOPHYSIOLOGY

The most common spectrin and/or ankyrin deficiency of two major proteins of the erythrocyte membrane skeleton. The membrane skeletal defect results in red cell membrane instability and loss of membrane surface. The sequelae are as follows:

• Loss of cell surface area relative to volume (spherocytosis) causing a decrease in cellular deformability.
• The spleen detains and "conditions" the nondeformable spherocytic red cells.
• Conditioning of cells involves depletion of ATP, increased glycolysis, increased influx and efflux of sodium, and loss of membrane lipid.
• Ultimately, the events lead to premature red cell destruction.

GENETICS

• Approximately 75% of cases are inherited in an autosomal-dominant pattern.
• The other 25% are autosomal-recessive forms, dominant disease with reduced penetrance, or new mutations.

EPIDEMIOLOGY

• Most common in people of Northern European extraction (about 1:2,000)

COMPLICATIONS

• Gallstones: Most common complication of hereditary spherocytosis (HS), pigment stones can lead to cholecystitis and/or biliary obstruction.
• Cholelithiasis in HS manifests in second and third decades of life.
• Aplastic crises: Can result in severe life-threatening anemia. Often caused by parvovirus B19 infection.
• Hyperhemolysis: Increased red cell destruction, often precipitated by infection.
• Postsplenectomy sepsis: Lower risk of infection if postponed until 4 to 5 years of age, and immunized with pneumococcal vaccine (50%–70% sepsis due to *Streptococcus pneumoniae*)
• Folate deficiency: Caused by insufficient dietary intake of folic acid for increased bone marrow requirement.
• Other rare complications: Gout, indolent leg ulcers, or chronic erythematous dermatitis on legs.

PROGNOSIS

Severity of disease is extremely variable ranging from extremely mild to severe anemia.

 Differential Diagnosis

• Hemolysis secondary to intrinsic RBC defects

—Membrane defects secondary to inherited disorders of membrane skeleton (hereditary spherocytosis and elliptocytosis) and red cell cation permeability and volume (stomatocytosis and xerocytosis)
—Enzyme defects: Embden-Meyerhof pathway (i.e., pyruvate kinase deficiency) and hexose monophosphate pathway (i.e., G6PD deficiency)
—Hemoglobin defects: Heme
—congenital erythropoietic porphyria; globin, qualitative (e.g., HbS, C, H, M) or quantitative (e.g., thalassemias)
—Congenital dyserythropoietic anemias

• Hemolysis secondary to extracorpuscular RBC defects

—Immune-mediated (important in differential because spherocytes are present on smear): isoimmune (e.g., hemolytic disease of the newborn, blood group incompatibility) and autoimmune (e.g., cold agglutinin disease, warm auto immune hemolytic anemia)
—Nonimmune-mediated: Idiopathic and secondary to underlying disorder (e.g., HUS, TTP)

 Data Gathering

HISTORY

Question: Fatigue?
Significance: Sign of anemia

Question: Jaundice, scleral icterus, dark urine?
Significance: Signs of hemolysis

Question: Requiring phototherapy in newborn period?
Significance: Hyperbilirubinemia due to hemolysis (50% of cases)

Question: Positive familial history (for disease, gallstones, or splenectomy)?
Significance: Autosomal-dominant inheritance

 Physical Examination

Finding: Splenomegaly, icterus/jaundice, pallor
Significance: All increased with hemolysis

Finding: Linear growth, weight gain, and sexual development may be delayed
Significance: Delayed growth is indication for splenectomy.

 Laboratory Aids

Test: CBC
Significance: Mild to moderate anemia; MCV usually normal; MCHC elevated (useful screening test with high specificity)

Test: Reticulocyte count
Significance: Level usually >6%; often accompanied with an elevated red blood cell distribution width (RDW).

Test: Indirect hyperbilirubinemia
Significance: Present in 50% to 60% of cases

Test: Peripheral smear
Significance: Microspherocytes, polychromasia

Test: Coombs test
Significance: Negative. Important differential test in a patient with hemolytic anemia

Test: Urinalysis
Significance: Hemoglobinuria, increased urobilinogen

SPECIAL TESTS

Test: Osmotic fragility (most useful test in diagnosis)
Significance: Spherocytes are more fragile; therefore, less resistant to osmotic stress and lyse in higher concentration of saline than normal red cells. This test can result in a false negative, especially in newborns whose red blood cells may be more dehydrated. It is important to use an age-matched control if possible.

 Emergency Care

A patient with hereditary spherocytosis may become extremely anemic during an aplastic crisis, hyperhemolysis or folic acid deficiency, requiring transfusion.

Therapy

- Folic acid supplement
- Penicillin prophylaxis (if splenectomized)
- Pneumococcal and *H. influenza* B vaccines (if splenectomized)

SPLENECTOMY

- High response rate (most patients normalize their blood counts)
- Indications: Moderate-to-severe anemia with significant hemolysis resulting in transfusion dependence, decreased exercise tolerance, skeletal deformities, or delayed growth.
- Complications: Risk of postsplenectomy sepsis

CHOLECYSTECTOMY

- Indications: Symptomatic gallbladder disease. Sometimes done concomitantly with splenectomy if gallstones evident by ultrasound.
- Complications: Morbidity of surgical procedure and postoperative period.

 Follow-Up

- Physical examination: Splenomegaly, follow growth curves closely
- CBC with reticulocyte count as needed—if patient develops fatigue, pallor, increased jaundice
- Penicillin prophylaxis if splenectomy

PITFALLS

- False-negative osmotic fragility tests can occur in several situations; therefore, index of suspicion must be high to follow the clinical course and repeat test (e.g., in neonatal period, during megaloblastic crisis, and recovery from aplastic crisis after transfusion).
- 20%–25% of HS patients have normal unincubated osmotic fragility (incubated test almost always positive; therefore, may need both).
- Spherocytes are often present in immune-mediated hemolysis.

 Common Questions and Answers

Q: Will my child require blood transfusions?
A: It depends on the clinical severity of his/her disease.

Q: If a parent has HS, how should the newborn be followed?
A: The infant has a 50% chance of having HS. In infants with HS the CBC is usually normal in the first 72 hours of life but then drops because of an inability to mount an appropriate erythropoietic response to increased destruction. Therefore, infants at risk should have a CBC with reticulocyte count after 72 hours. These infants also need to be monitored more closely for hyperbilirubinemia.

Q: What are the risks and benefits of splenectomy:
A: Splenectomy is almost always successful in ameliorating anemia, but adds the risk of postsplenectomy infections.

ICD-9-CM 282.0

BIBLIOGRAPHY

Becker PS, Lux SE. Disorders of the red cell membrane. In: Nathan DG, Oski FA, eds. *Hematology of Infancy and Childhood.* 5th Ed. Philadelphia: WB Saunders, 1998:578–601.

Delhommeau F, Cynober T, Schischmanoff P, et al. Natural history of hereditary spherocytosis during the first year of life. *Blood* 2000;95(2):393–397.

Hassoun H, Palek J. Hereditary spherocytosis: a review of the clinical and molecular aspects of the disease. *Blood Rev* 1996;10:129–147.

Michaels LA, Cohen AR, Huaquing Z, et al. Screening for hereditary spherocytosis by use of automated erythrocyte indexes. *J Pediatr* 1997;130(6):957–960.

Miraglia delGiudice E, et al. High frequency of de novo mutations in ankyrin gene (ANK1) in children with hereditary spherocytosis. *J Pediatr* 1998;132(1):117–120.

Shah S, Vega R. Hereditary spherocytosis. *Pediatrics in Review* 2004;25(5):168–172.

Author: Leslie Raffini

Heroin Intoxication

 ## Database

DEFINITION

- Heroin is a semisynthetic derivative of opium.
- The opioid family includes:

—Drugs that occur naturally in opium (from the poppy plant)
—Codeine
—Morphine
—Semisynthetic derivatives (e.g., hydromorphone, oxycodone)
—Synthetic compounds (e.g., meperidine, methadone)

PHARMACOLOGY/PATHOPHYSIOLOGY

- Well-absorbed from GI tract, nasal mucosa, pulmonary capillaries, and subcutaneous and intramuscular injection sites
- Oral dose less potent than parenteral because of first-pass hepatic metabolism
- IV heroin peaks in less than 1 minute; intranasal and IM heroin peak in 3 to 5 minutes
- Very lipid soluble; crosses blood–brain barrier within 15 to 20 seconds
- Extensive distribution into skeletal muscle, kidneys, liver, intestine, lungs, spleen, brain, and placenta
- Rapidly crosses the placenta, entering fetal tissues within 1 hour
- Crosses into breast milk in quantities sufficient to cause addiction
- Excreted in urine as morphine
- Receptor types

—Mu (or OP3)
—Located in CNS, GI tract, sensory nerve endings
—Effect: Analgesia, euphoria, respiratory depression, physical dependence, gastrointestinal dysmotility, miosis, pruritus, bradycardia
—Kappa (or OP2)
—Located in CNS
—Effect: Analgesia, miosis, diuresis, dysphoria
—Delta (or OP1)
—Located in CNS
—Effect: Spinal analgesia, modulation of mu receptors/dopaminergic neurons

EPIDEMIOLOGY

Neonatal

- Prevalence of fetal exposure <1% to 3.7%
- Fetal exposure commonly involves polysubstance abuse
- 60% to 80% of heroin exposed infants develop withdrawal—dependent on maternal dosing and length of use

Adolescents

- Use peaked among American adolescents in the 1970s and then declined.
- Use is increasing again because a more pure product allows for smoking or snorting as well as injecting.

- Most use experimentally or intermittently; few become addicted and use daily.

Overdose

- Up to one-third of heroin users experience nonfatal overdose.
- The majority occur in the home and with other people present.

Deaths

- Most heroin deaths occur when the drug is administered intravenously.
- Most deaths in patients in their late 20s or 30s with significant drug dependence.
- Multiple drug use is common in heroin-related deaths.

COMPLICATIONS

Intoxication/Overdose

- Respiratory arrest
- Noncardiogenic pulmonary edema
- CNS depression/coma
- Hypotension
- Aspiration pneumonia

Pregnancy

- No known teratogenic effects
- Poor prenatal care
- Preterm labor
- Premature rupture of membranes
- Breech presentation
- Antepartum hemorrhage
- Toxemia
- Anemia
- Uterine irritability
- Infection (e.g., HIV, Hep B)
- Infantile dependence

Naloxone Use

- May precipitate withdrawal syndrome in opioid-dependent patients
- Symptoms: Agitation, hypertension, tachycardia, emesis
- See below for dosing recommendations
- May cause acute severe withdrawal in infants born to addicted mothers

PROGNOSIS

Neonatal

- Long-term morbidity from neonatal heroin dependence unclear due to confounding variables (e.g., developmental environment)

Intoxication/Overdose

- With adequate early treatment, patients with uncomplicated overdoses do well—key is to prevent respiratory arrest

Addiction

- Dependent on involvement in other risky behaviors (polydrug use, high-risk sexual practices, school failure, delinquency, etc.)
- Longer treatment likely produces a better outcome
- Majority relapse; require lifetime of therapy

 ## Differential Diagnosis

NEONATAL EXPOSURE

- Sepsis
- Hypoglycemia
- Central nervous system abnormality
- Metabolic disorder
- Withdrawal from other maternal drug use

INTOXICATION/OVERDOSE

- Other pharmacologic agents:

—Clonidine
—Sedative-hypnotics
—Barbiturates
—Antipsychotics
—GHB

- Hypoglycemia
- Hypothermia
- Hypoxia
- Heatstroke
- Pontine or subarachnoid hemorrhage

 ## Data Gathering

HISTORY

Neonate

- Maternal history of heroin or other drug use
- Extent of prenatal care
- Time from most recent use to delivery
- Breast-feeding

Older Child/Adolescent

- History of heroin use
- Observed overdose
- Found in setting consistent with possible drug use

 ## Physical Examination

NEONATE WITH IN UTERO EXPOSURE

- Prematurity
- Low birth weight
- Perinatal depression with 5-minute Apgar <5
- Hypotonia

INTOXICATION/OVERDOSE

- Classic toxidrome

—Depressed level of consciousness
—Very decreased respiratory effort
—Miotic pupils
—± Diminished bowel sounds

- More severe overdose
  —Bradycardia
  —Hypotension

WITHDRAWAL

Early Signs (8–24 Hours)

- Anxiety
- Restlessness
- Insomnia
- Yawning
- Rhinorrhea
- Lacrimation
- Diaphoresis
- Stomach cramps
- Mydriasis

Late Signs (Up to 3 Days)

- Tremor
- Muscle spasms
- Vomiting
- Diarrhea
- Hypertension
- Tachycardia
- Fever
- Chills
- Piloerection
- Seizures

Additional Neonatal Withdrawal Signs and Symptoms

- Hyperirritability
- Hypertonicity
- Posturing
- Exaggerated startle
- Tachypnea
- Hyperpyrexia
- Poor suck/swallow coordination
- High-pitched cry
- Poor weight gain

 Laboratory Aids

- Therapy should not be withheld pending laboratory results
- Urine toxicology screen (heroin easily detected)
- Serum toxicology screen for acetaminophen level, etc., if suspect polydrug use
- Serum tests to rule out other etiologies, if needed (e.g., glucose)
- Meconium testing in neonates

 Therapy

INTOXICATION/OVERDOSE

- Start with the airway, breathing, circulation (ABCs)
- Antidote is naloxone (Narcan)
- Assessment of respiratory status/adequacy of ventilation
- If adequate respiratory effort, observe until normal level of consciousness

—Consider naloxone as diagnostic challenge

- If inadequate respiratory effort:

—Bag-valve-mask ventilation
—Intravenous naloxone (or subcutaneous, intramuscular, endotracheal)
—0.1 mg/kg if <20 kg; 2 mg if >20 kg. Can repeat to 10 mg total dose
—If suspect dependence, start with lower dose (0.4 mg amp)
—If no response to large dose, question diagnosis of heroin toxicity—heroin exquisitely sensitive to naloxone

—Naloxone loses efficacy in 20 to 40 minutes; may need repeat dosing
—Can give as continuous infusion if necessary; dosing recommendations vary
—One method: two-thirds of effective dose given over 1 hour with gradual wean
—Endotracheal intubation if no response to naloxone in 5 to 10 minutes, or other reason for invasive airway management

- Observe in ED for minimum 2 to 3 hours for respiratory status stabilization
- Consider chest x-ray

WITHDRAWAL

- Standard treatment methadone maintenance (adolescents/adults)

—Blocks euphoria and prevents withdrawal symptoms
—Patients generally treated in established methadone maintenance programs
—Stabilize with 20 to 40 mg per day ; wean by 2 to 5 mg per week over several months
—Adjust wean if signs of withdrawal appear

- Clonidine (0.2 mg q4–6h for 7 to 10 days) can control acute withdrawal symptoms
- Diazepam (10–15 mg q4–6h for 3 to 4 days), an alternative to clonidine
- Rapid and ultrarapid detoxification (using opioid antagonist with or without general anesthesia) a possibility in selected patients; research ongoing

—Should be used only by experienced team with appropriate resources

- In neonates:

—Paregoric (0.4 mg/mL) not recommended due to high alcohol content (45%) and toxic compounds such as camphor, anise oil, benzoic acid, and glycerin
—Tincture of opium (10 mg/mL) best diluted 25-fold to a concentration equal to paregoric (0.4 mg/mL)
—0.1 mL/kg (2 drops/kg) q4h; increase 0.1 mL/kg q4h as needed to control symptoms. After 3 to 5 days, wean dose by 0.1 ml/kg per day. Observe infant for 3 to 5 days after stopping therapy.
—May need IV morphine in severe cases
—Methadone has been used occasionally
—Clonidine gaining favor for use in infants; pharmacokinetic data are not available.
—Phenobarbital is not a first-choice agent due to long half-life, CNS depression, induction of drug metabolism, and rapid tolerance to sedative effect.

 Follow-Up

- Developmental follow-up for exposed neonates
- Most patients with overdose warrant hospitalization
- Social services and referral to substance abuse program
- Consider referral for testing for HIV, hepatitis B and C

Common Questions and Answers

Q: Is nalmefene an appropriate substitute for naloxone in a heroin overdose?
A: Nalmefene, a long-acting specific narcotic antagonist, has not proved to be as effective as naloxone in a randomized, double-blind trial. It also may result in prolonged, dangerous withdrawal. It therefore has limited usefulness in this setting.

BIBLIOGRAPHY

AAP Policy Statement. Neonatal drug withdrawal. *Pediatrics* 1998;101(6):1079–1088.

Alderman EM. Opiates. *Pediatr Rev* 1997;18(4):122–126.

Bauer CR. Perinatal effects of prenatal drug exposure. *Clin Perinatol* 1999;26(1):87–106.

Bishai R, Koren G. Maternal and obstetric effects of prenatal drug exposure. *Clin Perinatol* 1999;26(1):75–86.

Chamberlain JM, Klein BL. A comprehensive review of naloxone for the emergency physician. *Am J Emerg Med* 1994;12(6):650–660.

Gonzalez G, et al. Treatment of heroin (diamorphine) addiction: current approaches and future prospects. *Drugs* 2002;62(9):1331–1343.

Hans SL. Demographic and psychosocial characteristics of substance-abusing pregnant women. *Clin Perinatol* 1999;26(1):55–74.

Johnson K, et al. Treatment of neonatal abstinence syndrome. *Arch Dis Child* 2003;88:F2–F5.

Kandall SR. Treatment strategies for drug-exposed neonates. *Clin Perinatol* 1999;26(1):231–244.

Nelson LS. Opioids. In: Goldfrank LR, ed. *Goldfrank's Toxicologic Emergencies.* 6th Ed. Stamford: Appleton & Lange, 1998:975–995.

O'Connor PG, Kosten TR. Rapid and ultrarapid opioid detoxification techniques. *JAMA* 1998;279(3):229–234.

Sporer KA. Acute heroin overdose. *Ann Intern Med* 1999;130(7):584–590.

Tarabar AF, Nelson LS. The resurgence and abuse of heroin by children in the United States. *Current Opinion in Pediatrics* 2003;15(2):210–215.

Authors: Cynthia J. Mollen and Thomas J. Mollen

Herpes Simplex Virus (HSV)

 Database

DEFINITION

Herpes simplex virus (HSV) is a moderately large double-stranded DNA virus. There are two serologically distinguishable subtypes: HSV-1 and HSV-2. HSV produces a wide spectrum of illness ranging from fever blisters to fatal viral encephalitis.

PATHOPHYSIOLOGY

- Initial viral replication occurs at the portal.
- Vesicular fluid contains infected epithelial cells.
- After primary HSV infection, the virus remains latent in sensory neural ganglia innervating portions of the skin or mucous membranes originally involved. The virus can be reactivated by an appropriate stimulus such as sunlight or immune suppression.
- HSV can be replicated easily in the laboratory in tissue cultures.

EPIDEMIOLOGY

- HSV-1 usually causes infections of the upper torso, head, and neck.
- HSV-2 usually causes genital infection. However, both forms of HSV can infect either oral or genital cells and thus the virus type is not a reliable indicator of the anatomic site of infection.
- Neonatal HSV infections are acquired from maternal strains and 75%–85% are caused by HSV-2.
- After the neonatal period, HSV-1 infections predominate and 40%–60% of children are seropositive for HSV-1 by age 5 years.
- During puberty and early adolescence, the prevalence of HSV-2 increases and 20%–35% of adults are seropositive for HSV-2.
- Route of spread is usually by close bodily contact or trauma such as teething or a break in the skin.
- Incubation period is 2 to 12 days (average, 6 days).

ASSOCIATED DISEASES

- Neonatal infection is usually acquired from the maternal genitourinary tract and causes serious disease with high mortality and morbidity.
- Gingivostomatitis is the most common form of HSV primary infection in children.
- HSV Encephalitis accounts for 2%–5% of all encephalitis in the United States.

 Differential Diagnosis

- Neonatal HSV infection must be distinguished from viral or bacterial sepsis especially in the first 4 weeks of life.
- HSV infection should be considered in all neonates with vesicular rash, chorioretinitis, microcephaly, or hepatosplenomegaly. It must be distinguished from other congenital viral infections such as rubella or CMV.
- Herpes gingivostomatitis must be distinguished from herpangina, an enteroviral infection usually presenting as posterior pharyngeal ulcers, and sometimes as hand-foot-and-mouth disease.
- HSV encephalitis must be distinguished from other viral encephalitis and from the HSV-induced aseptic meningitis syndrome, which is a complication of primary genital infection.
- HSV vulvovaginitis must be distinguished from chancroid and syphilis. Syphilis lesions are usually nonpainful hard ulcers. Chancroid lesions are multiple purulent ulcers from which *Haemophilus ducreyi* can be cultured.

 Data Gathering

HISTORY

Neonatal Infection

- HSV-2, the most common cause of neonatal infection, is usually acquired from maternal labial lesions, but a history of previous or current genital HSV infection is only present in 20% to 30% of mothers who deliver infected infants. HSV-2 can be transmitted to the infant without rupture of the amniotic membranes or after delivery by cesarean section.
- HSV-1 can be transmitted to a neonate by any adult with active herpes labialis.
- A vesicular rash or bullae are present at birth or within a few days in almost all infants.
- Disseminated infection (32% of cases) involves the liver, lungs, adrenals, and sometimes the central nervous system (CNS).
- Localized CNS infection (33% of cases) presents with irritability, bulging fontanelle, or seizures.
- Localized skin, eye, or mouth infection (35% of cases) present with rash alone, or keratitis or chorioretinitis.

Gingivostomatitis

- Fever and irritability precede the development of vesicular lesions on the lips, gingiva, and tongue. The vesicles then break down and become gray ulcers that are friable and bleed easily.
- Children refuse to drink because of the mouth pain and are at risk of dehydration.
- The child usually starts to improve in 3 to 5 days and recovers in 14 days.
- Latent virus causes recurrent stomatitis or labiitis.

Encephalitis

- The illness begins with fever malaise and irritability that lasts 1 to 7 days and progresses to mental status changes, seizures, and coma. Meningeal signs are not common.
- Patients can develop hemiparesis, cranial nerve palsy, and visual field defects.
- No presence of oral or genital lesions
- It is the result of a primary infection in 30% of cases and recurrent in 70%.

Vulvovaginitis

- 35% to 50% of patients with the first episode of genital herpes will be able to give a history of genital HSV infection in their contact.
- The primary illness is characterized by fever, headache, malaise, and myalgias. Local genital symptoms include severe pain, itching, dysuria, vaginal or urethral discharge, and tender inguinal adenopathy. The genital lesions begin as vesicles and progress to ulcers before they crust over.
- Lesions last for 2 to 3 weeks.
- An aseptic meningitis syndrome occurs in 1% to 35% of cases. Patients will have fever, headache, meningismus, and photophobia.
- Latent virus causes recurrent episodes, which are painful but less severe than in primary infections.

 Laboratory Aids

NEONATAL INFECTION

- Samples for viral culture should be obtained from the eyes, oropharynx, and rectum.
- PCR testing of the CSF is the test of choice for diagnosing CNS disease.
- Cells from the base of freshly unroofed vesicles can be smeared on a slide for monoclonal antibody immunofluorescence.
- Serologic tests are not useful for diagnosis of maternal or neonatal herpes during the acute phase of the disease.

ENCEPHALITIS

- Cerebrospinal fluid (CSF) reveals a pleocytosis with up to 2,000 WBC/mm^3 and usually over 60% of the cells are lymphocytes.
- In an atraumatic lumbar puncture red blood cells, indicating hemorrhagic necrosis occur in 75% to 85% of cases.
- CSF protein is elevated (median, 80 mg/dL).
- HSV almost never grows from CSF. It can be identified by PCR
- Electroencephalogram (EEG) can reveal a "typical pattern" of unilateral or bilateral focal spikes.
- CT or MRI may show enhancement in the temporal areas.

Gingivostomatitis

- Physicians usually make this diagnosis clinically since it is so common in young children.

VULVOVAGINITIS

- A viral culture of the vesicle is the gold standard. Sensitivity is 94% for early lesions and decreases to 27% for crusted lesions.
- Immunofluorescence of infected cells is a more rapid diagnostic test and has a sensitivity of 78% to 88%.

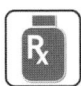 Therapy

NEONATAL INFECTION

Intravenous acyclovir (60 mg/kg per day in 3 divided doses) is the drug of choice. The recommended minimal duration of therapy is 14 days (if the disease is limited to the skin, eye, and mouth), and 21 days if disease is disseminated or involves the CNS. Infants with ocular involvement due to HSV infection should receive a topical ophthalmic drug (1% to 2% trifluridine, 1% iododeoxyuridine, or 3% vidarabine) in addition to parenteral antiviral therapy.

ENCEPHALITIS

Intravenous acyclovir (30 mg/kg per day) 3 times a day for 21 days is appropriate therapy for HSV encephalitis beyond the neonatal period. In addition to parenteral antiviral therapy, appropriate management of fluids, intracranial pressure, and seizures is essential.

GINGIVOSTOMATITIS

Most patients are managed with symptomatic therapy including antipyretics and oral fluids like popsicles. Oral anesthetics can be harmful and result in self-injury when children chew on anesthetized lips. Oral acyclovir (15 mg/kg 5 times a day) has been beneficial in reducing duration of lesions and symptoms. Patients with frequent or severe recurrences may benefit from oral acyclovir at onset of symptoms.

VULVOVAGINITIS

Acyclovir (Zovirax) is the appropriate therapy for genital herpes infection. Oral acyclovir is used for patients with primary genital HSV infection. Intravenous acyclovir is used for patients with severe local or systemic or complications like aseptic meningitis syndrome.

 Follow-Up

PREVENTION

- Neonatal infection

—The risk of HSV infection in an infant born vaginally to a mother with a first-episode primary genital infection is high (33% to 50%).
—The risk to an infant born to a mother with recurrent HSV infection at delivery is much lower (3% to 5%).
—Cesarean section in a mother with active genital herpes at the time of delivery is the main way to prevent neonatal infection. However, this does not prevent all cases, because 60% to 80% of mothers of infected infants are asymptomatic or have unrecognized infection.

- Postnatal infection

—Universal body substance precaution policies
—Adults with oral herpes must be particularly careful to use appropriate hygiene.
—Wrestlers with skin lesions suggestive of herpes
—Patients with genital lesions from HSV should not have intercourse until the lesions heal.
—Condoms can prevent the spread of virus.

PROGNOSIS

- Neonatal infection

—Overall mortality from untreated neonatal HSV infection is 50% and only 26% of survivors are normal.
—Infants with disseminated disease or localized CNS disease have the worst prognosis to 67%.
—The major sequelae in survivors are brain damage, seizures, and blindness.

 Common Questions and Answers

Q: What about recurrent cutaneous eruptions in a neonate? Should they be treated?
A: The need for retreatment of infants with recurrent skin lesions is undetermined and under study. Because of concerns about silent CNS recurrent infection, some experts recommend acyclovir, 80 mg/kg/day in 3 doses. Maximum 1000 mg revaluate in one year. One needs to look for neutropenia, which will occur in 25% of patients.

Q: Is prophylactic therapy for recurrent herpes genitalia helpful? When is it indicated?
A: Antiviral therapy has minimal effect on recurrent genital herpes. Oral acyclovir initiated within 2 days of onset of symptoms shortens the course. Topical acyclovir is not helpful.

Q: What steps should be taken in the nursery for an infant born to an HSV-positive mother?
A: Neonates with documented perinatal exposure to HSV may be in the incubation phase of infection and should be observed carefully. Infants of mothers with active HSV should be isolated if they have been delivered vaginally or by cesarean section after membranes were ruptured for more than 4 to 6 hours. The risk of HSV infection in possibly exposed infants (e.g., those born to a mother with a history of recurrent genital herpes) is low, and isolation is not necessary.

Q: Is a repeat lumbar puncture necessary at the end of therapy for neonates or for children with HSV encephalitis?
A: Some experts recommend repeating the lumbar puncture at the end of the planned course of therapy to determine whether the virus is still present by PCR assay. If there is a positive test, prolonging therapy may be considered.

ICD-9-CM 054.9

BIBLIOGRAPHY

American Academy of Pediatrics. Herpes Simplex. In: Pickering LK, ed. *2003 Red Book: Report of the Committee on Infectious Diseases.* 26th Ed. Elk Grove Village, IL: American Academy of Pediatrics, 2003:344–352.

Arvin A. Herpes Simplex Viruses 1 and 2. In: Feigin RD, Cherry JD, Demmler GJ, Kaplan SL, eds. *Textbook of Pediatric Infectious Diseases.* 4th Ed. Philadelphia: WB Saunders, 2004: 1884–1912.

Kimberlin DW, et al. Safety and efficacy of high-dose intravenous acyclovir in the management of neonatal herpes simplex virus infections. *Pediatrics* 2001;108(2):230–238.

Sanchez PJ. Viral infections of the fetus and neonate. In: Feigin RD, et al, eds. *Textbook of Pediatric Infectious Diseases.* 4th Ed. Philadelphia: WB Saunders, 2004:866–909.

Authors: Jason Newland and Louis M. Bell

Hiccups

 Database

DEFINITION

- Known medically as singultus, from the Latin "singult" (a sob or speech punctuated by sobs), hiccups are a result of involuntary spasm of the diaphragm and intercostal muscles, leading to inspiration and abrupt closure of the glottis. Hiccups affect nearly everyone at one time or another.

CAUSES

- Hiccup bouts may be precipitated by a number of benign causes including:

—Gastric distension: Aerophagia, ingestion of excessive food, carbonated beverages or alcohol, and gastric insufflation during endoscopy
—Changes in the ambient or gastrointestinal temperature: Cold showers, ingestion of hot or cold beverages, moving from cold to hot environment, or vice versa
—Sudden excitement or stress
—Tobacco use

- Persistent and intractable hiccups have many causes, which can be characterized as psychogenic, organic, or idiopathic:
- Psychogenic

—Stress
—Conversion reactions
—Anorexia nervosa
—Malingering
—Personality disorders

- Organic

—Central nervous system disorders: Ventriculoperitoneal (VP) shunts, hydrocephalus, arteriovenous (AV) malformations, stroke, temporal arteritis, central nervous system (CNS) trauma, encephalitis, meningitis, brain abscess
—Peripheral nervous system disturbances: Irritation of the phrenic or vagus nerve, from a variety of causes, including:
—Goiter, tumors or cysts of the neck, hiatal hernia, esophagitis, pneumonia, bronchitis, asthma, mediastinal lymphadenopathy, pericarditis, peptic ulcer disease, pancreatitis, inflammatory bowel disease, appendicitis, cholecystitis, and renal and hepatic disorders (stones or infections)
—Infectious etiologies: Sepsis, influenza, herpes zoster, malaria and tuberculosis
—Metabolic or pharmacologic causes: Anesthesia, methylprednisolone, barbiturates, diazepam, methyldopa, uremia, hypocalcemia, and hyponatremia

PATHOPHYSIOLOGY

- Hiccups serve no physiologic function and are often simply a benign affliction.
- A hiccup reflex arc has been postulated, although the exact anatomic mechanism remains unknown. The arc consists of:

—The afferent limb: Phrenic and vagus nerves, the pharyngeal plexus from C2 to C4 and the thoracic sympathetic chain from T6 to T12
—The efferent limb: Phrenic nerve to the diaphragm and the external intercostal nerves to the intercostal muscles
—A central connection: a nonspecific location incorporating the medulla but independent of the respiratory center, the hypothalamus, and the phrenic nerve nuclei

- Hiccups have negligible effect on ventilation and usually involve only unilateral diaphragmatic contraction, most frequently on the left.
- Hiccups serve no respiratory function, despite activation of inspiratory musculature far more than during normal respiration.

EPIDEMIOLOGY

- There is no male or female predominance for hiccup bouts; however, persistent and intractable hiccups have been shown to have a greater frequency in males, and are seen predominantly in adults.
- There is no racial, geographic, seasonal, or socioeconomic variability.
- Fetal hiccups are common in the third trimester of pregnancy.

COMPLICATIONS

Adverse effects that have been associated with intractable hiccups include malnutrition and dehydration, weight loss, insomnia, fatigue and psychological stress. Rarely, cardiac dysrhythmia, reflux esophagitis, pulmonary edema from the negative pressure and even death may occur.

PROGNOSIS

- Self-limited and resolves without complications
- Usually terminate within hours.
- Hiccup bouts may last up to 48 hours. Persistent hiccups last from 48 hours up to 1 month, and intractable hiccups last for longer than 1 month.

 Differential Diagnosis

- Hiccups are not often mistaken for any other entity
- The differential diagnosis for persistent and intractable hiccups is outlined above (see Definition)

 Data Gathering

HISTORY

- Severity, duration, and characteristics of hiccups?
- Medication and alcohol use?
- Hiccups persisting during sleep suggests an organic etiology.

 Physical Examination

Finding: Head and neck examination
Significance: May reveal evidence of trauma, foreign body in the ear, nuchal rigidity, masses, cervical lymphadenopathy, or an enlarged thyroid.

Finding: Assess the chest.
Significance: Evidence of pneumonia, bronchitis, or pericarditis

Finding: Assess the abdomen.
Significance: Evidence of appendicitis, intestinal obstruction, ruptured viscus, pancreatitis, or hepatobiliary disease

Finding: Neurologic examination
Significance: Evidence of trauma, meningitis, encephalitis, VP shunt malfunction, or neoplasm

 Laboratory Aids

Tests should be chosen based on historical and physical findings.

- Complete Blood Count (CBC)
- Renal function and electrolytes
- Liver function tests (LFTs) and calcium
- Toxicology screen and blood gas

RADIOGRAPHIC STUDIES

Test: Chest x-ray
Significance: May rule out phrenic, vagal, and diaphragmatic irritation by pulmonary, cardiac, and mediastinal abnormalities.

Therapy

- Directed at the underlying disease.
- If etiology is unknown, empiric therapy may be necessary.

DRUGS

- Studies confined to adult populations. Pharmaceuticals rarely recommended for children.
- Chlorpromazine widely used in adults in IV preparations. Intramuscular haloperidol has also been effective in adults.
- Anticonvulsants, including diphenylhydantoin, valproic acid, and carbamazepine reported effective.
- Combination of cisapride, omeprazole, and baclofen has been reported to be effective and is considered the mainstay for idiopathic chronic hiccups.
- Gabapentin has been shown to be effective as a substitute for baclofen or as an additional agent in the above regimen.

NONPHARMACOLOGIC MODALITIES

- Interruption of respiratory function: Sneezing, coughing, breath holding, hyperventilation, sudden pain or fright, and even positive airway pressure ventilation.
- Disruption of phrenic nerve transmission: Tapping over the fifth cervical vertebra, ice applied to the skin over the area of the phrenic nerve, and even transecting the phrenic nerve.
- Behavioral modification and hypnosis.
- Acupuncture: Reported to be successful in treatment of persistent hiccups.
- Nasopharyngeal stimulation: Traction of the tongue, stimulation of the pharynx with a cotton swab, lifting the uvula with a spoon.
- Old-fashioned home remedies such as sipping ice water, swallowing granulated sugar, drinking water from the far side of a glass or through a paper towel, and biting on a lemon.

Follow-Up

No specific follow-up is indicated unless a specific organic cause has been identified.

PREVENTION

Avoid precipitating factors.

PITFALLS

Failure to recognize a serious underlying condition and assigning the label of idiopathic or psychogenic hiccups to an otherwise serious illness

Common Questions and Answers

Q: Does breathing into a paper bag really work?
A: As a fall in PCO_2 can increase frequency of hiccups, rebreathing air will increase PCO_2 and thus terminate hiccups.

Q: Will hiccups harm my baby?
A: Hiccups alone are harmless. If they are truly persistent, intractable, or disrupt sleep, they may have the side effects as mentioned. Premature babies have been observed to spend 2.5% of their time having hiccups.

Q: Is there an association between gastroesophageal reflux and hiccups?
A: Hiccups can be caused by esophageal irritation from gastroesophageal reflux disease, and chronic hiccups have been linked to reflux esophagitis.

ICD-9-CM 786.8

BIBLIOGRAPHY

Kahrilas PJ, Shi G. Why do we hiccup? *Gut* 1997;41(5):712–713.

Lierz, P. Anesthesia as therapy for persistent hiccups. *Anesth Analg* 2002;95:494–495.

Peleg R, Schvartzman P. Hiccup. *J Fam Pract* 1996;42:424.

Petroiano G, Hein G, Petroiano A, et al. Idiopathic chronic hiccup: combination therapy with cisapride, omeprazole and baclofen. *Clin Ther* 1997;19:1031–1038.

Petroianu G, Hein G, Stegmeier-Petroianu, et al. Gabapentin "add-on therapy" for idiopathic chronic hiccup. *J Clin Gastroenterol* 2000;30(3):321–324.

Rousseau P. Hiccups. *South Med J* 1995;88(2):175–181.

Schiff E, et al. Acupuncture therapy for persistent hiccups. *Am J Med Sci* 2002;323:166–168.

Viera AJ, Sullivan SA. Remedies for prolonged hiccups. *Am Fam Physician* 2001;63:1664–1668.

Author: Blaze Robert Gusic

Hirschsprung Disease

 Database

DEFINITION

- Intestinal abnormality of abnormal innervation of the distal bowel beginning at the anus and extending proximately for a variable distance, causing partial or complete intestinal obstruction, difficulty in passing stools, and in some cases enterocolitis.
- Also known as congenital megacolon and was first reported by Harold Hirschsprung in 1887.
- Present as complete obstruction, delayed passage of meconium, "chronic constipation," or enterocolitis.

PATHOPHYSIOLOGY

- Basic histologic finding is the absence of Meissner and Auerbach plexuses, hypertrophied nerve bundles between the circular and the longitudinal muscles and in the submucosa.
- Defect considered as a failure of caudal migration of the neural crest cells.

GENETICS

- Possible gene loci at chromosomes 3p21, 10q11, and 19q12. Approximately 5% of patients with Hirschsprung disease have mutations in the Endothelin signaling pathway.

EPIDEMIOLOGY

- Most common cause of lower intestinal obstruction in neonates: 1 in 5,000 births
- Overall ratio of male:female patients is 2.8:1; in long-segment disease, it is 2.8:1, and in total colonic aganglionosis, it is 2.2:1.
- Familial incidence in total colonic aganglionosis: 75% of cases, rectosigmoid involved; 14%, descending colon involved; 8%, colon involved; 3%, small bowel affected.
- Syndromic and nonsyndromic Hirschsprung disease. In the former there are other congenital anomalies (30% of cases), whereas in the latter it occurs as an isolated trait.

ASSOCIATED DISEASES

In 3% of the patients, there has been an association with Down syndrome, cardiac anomalies, and coexistent multiple neuroblastomas. More recently there have been case reports of neurologic disorders associated in children with Hirschsprung disease.
Another study reveals upper gut dysmotility in patients with Hirschsprung disease and its allied disorders in adults.

 Differential Diagnosis

CHRONIC CONSTIPATION

 Data Gathering

HISTORY

Question: Age of presentation
Significance: 80% of the time patients present in the neonatal period.

Question: Typical symptoms
Significance: Failure to pass meconium by 48 hours of life; delayed passage of meconium after 24 hours of life; history of constipation; history of chronic laxative use, abdominal distension, bilious vomiting, diarrhea in 22% of patients.

Question: Growth pattern
Significance: Neonates usually have normal weight, but growth retardation may occur when the disease is severe.

Question: Type of stools
Significance: Children with Hirschsprung disease usually have small volume and small diameter stools. Some may have overflow diarrhea as well.

 Physical Examination

Finding: On rectal examination, the sphincter tone is usually normal or increased.
Significance: Removal of the finger may be followed by explosive diarrhea; transition zone is usually not felt in infants less than 2 months of age.

Finding: Stool in rectum.
Significance: In most instances, especially in older children, the rectum is empty.

Finding: Anemia?
Significance: Patients are usually anemic due to chronic blood loss from the large bowel secondary to infection.

 Laboratory Aids

TESTS

Test: Complete blood count
Significance: Anemia, leukocytosis in the presence of enterocolitis.

Test: Plain film of abdomen
Significance: May show distended loops of colon. Small bowel air is usually present in the bowel proximal to the obstruction. Diffuse intestinal pneumatosis has been reported as a rare presentation.

Test: Barium enema
Significance: Useful but not diagnostic; transition zone is a funnel-shaped area of intestine with normal distal area and dilated proximal area. Barium enema reveals large mucosal pattern, prominently thickened folds, and irregular margins secondary to ulceration. Significant delay in excretion of barium should also raise one's suspicion for Hirschsprung disease.

Test: Anorectal manometry
Significance: Diagnostic but usually reserved for those cases causing diagnostic difficulties, as in the ultrashort segment disease.

Test: Biopsy
Significance: Suction biopsy should be done approximately 2–4 cm from the anal verge depending on the age of the patient. The biopsies must have adequate submucosa to demonstrate neurofibrils detected using acetylcholinesterase as a stain. With the absence of ganglion cells, biopsy is diagnostic. If the suction biopsies are not conclusive, a full-thickness biopsy is mandatory.

COMPLICATIONS

Enterocolitis is the most important complication:

- Secondary to obstruction causing an increase in intraluminal pressure and decreased intramural capillary blood flow.
- Affects the protective mucosal barrier enabling fecal breakdown products, bacteria, and toxins, to enter into the bloodstream.
- Usually present with fever, diarrhea, and frequent, bloody, bilious vomiting.

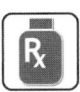 Therapy

- Stabilizing treatment is fluid resuscitation, nasogastric decompression, broad-spectrum antibiotics, and saline enemas.
- The initial operation is a defunctionalizing colostomy or an ileostomy for total colonic aganglionosis. This is performed to avoid the hazards of enterocolitis. If the child has already developed enterocolitis, colostomy is deferred until the general condition improves.
- Definitive surgery is performed 6 months to a year after the initial colostomy. The various surgical procedures performed are:

—Endorectal pull-through: Widely used. Basic principle is to strip the aganglionic rectum of its mucosa and then to bring normally innervated colon through the residual rectal muscular cuff, thereby bypassing the abnormal bowel from within. Advantages: Sphincter function is preserved and minimal danger of injury to pelvis.
—Retrorectal transanal pull-through (Duhamel procedure): The normally innervated bowel is brought behind the abnormally innervated rectum approximately 1 to 2 cm above the pectinate line and an end-to-side anastomosis is performed. This procedure creates a neorectum with the anterior one-half having normal sensory receptors and a posterior one-half with normal propulsion. Advantages: Reduces pelvic dissection to a minimum and retains the sensory pathway of rectal reflexes. Disadvantages: Incontinence if anastomosis is too low and obstructive symptoms if anastomosis is too high, or if the aganglionic segment is too long.

- Other procedures include the Soave (endorectal pull-through).
- In total colonic aganglionosis, the modified Lester Martin technique is performed. It involves the anastomosis of the cecum and ascending colon as an onlay patch graft in the more distal normal small bowel, which is then pulled through the amputated rectum that has been stripped of its mucosa and a primary anastomosis is performed.
- Laparoscopy-assisted abdominoperineal pull-through has shown good intermediate results and the more recent transanal pullthrough is promising. Long-term results are awaited.

PITFALLS

Early recognition is of utmost importance in reducing the morbidity and mortality of Hirschsprung disease.
Fecal incontinence could occur after surgery.

 Follow-Up

Most children are followed on a regular basis for the first decade after surgery.

 Common Questions and Answers

Q: Will the bowel movements be normal after surgery?
A: Studies have shown that 83% of children have three or fewer stools per day at a mean follow-up of 4.1 ± 2.5 years.

Q: Are laxatives required after surgery?
A: In about 20% of children some sort of laxative therapy or rectal irrigation may be required.

ICD-9-CM 751.3

BIBLIOGRAPHY

Abi-Hanna A, Lake AM. Constipation and encopresis in childhood. *Pediatr Rev* 1998;19(1):23–30.

Diseth TH, Egeland T, Emblein R. Effects of anal invasive treatment and incontinence on mental health and psychosocial functioning of adolescents with Hirschsprung disease and low anorectal anomalies. *J Pediatr Surg* 1998;33(3):468–475.

Hsieh WS, Yang PH, Huang CS, et al. Hirschsprung disease presenting with diffuse intestinal pneumatosis in a neonate. *Acta Paediatr Taiwan* 2000;41(6):336–338.

Jona JZ. Personal experience with 50 laparoscopic procedures for Hirschsprung disease in infants and children. *Pediatr Endosurg Techn* 2001;5:75.

Lyonnet S, Bolino A, Pelet A, et al. A gene for Hirschsprung disease maps to the proximal long arm of chromosome 10. *Nature Genet* 1993;4(4):346–501.

Shahar E, Shinawi M. Neurocristopathies presenting with neurologic abnormalities associated with Hirschsprung's disease. *Pediatr Neurol* 2003;28(5):385–391.

So HB, Becker JM, Schwartz DL, et al. Eighteen years' experience with neonatal Hirschsprung disease treated by endorectal pull-through without colostomy. *J Pediatr Surg* 1998;33(5):673–675.

Swenson O. Hirschsprung's disease: a review. *Pediatrics* 2002;109(5):914–918.

Teitelbaum DH, Cilley RE, Sherman NJ, et al. A decade of experience with the primary pull-through for Hirschsprung disease in the newborn period: a multicenter analysis of outcomes. *Ann Surg* 2000;232(3):372–380.

Teitelbaum DH, Coran AG. Primary pull-through for Hirschsprung's disease. *Seminars in Neonatology* 2003;8(3):233–241.

Tomita R, et al. Upper gut motility of Hirschsprung disease and its allied disorders in adults. *Hepatogastroenterology* 2003;50(54):1959–1962.

Van der Zee DC, Bax KN. One-stage Duhamel-Martin procedure for Hirschsprung disease: a 5-year follow-up study. *J Pediatr Surg* 2000;35(10):1434–1436.

Authors: Helen Anita John-Kelly and Andrew E. Mulberg

Histiocytosis

Database

DEFINITION
Clinical conditions resulting from or associated with proliferation of the mononuclear phagocytic system.

CLASSIFICATION
- Dendritic cell-related disorders (e.g., Langerhans cell histiocytosis)
- Macrophage-related disorders (e.g., hemophagocytic lymphohistiocytosis)
- Malignant histiocytic disorders

LANGERHANS CELL HISTIOCYTOSIS

Database

DEFINITION
- Reactive disorder of unknown etiology in which cells similar to Langerhans cells of the skin cause damage to organs by excessive production of cytokines and prostaglandins
- Previously known as histiocytosis X, eosinophilic granuloma, Hand-Schüller-Christian syndrome, Letterer-Siwe disease, and Hashimoto Pritzker syndrome

EPIDEMIOLOGY
- Incidence: 4–5.4 cases per million children are diagnosed each year.

COMPLICATIONS
- Single-system disease
—Some patients with bone involvement will have a chronic remitting and relapsing course.
- Multisystem disease
—Approximately 20% risk of fatal progression, especially in patients with liver, bone marrow or lung involvement and a slow response to initial therapy.
—Risk of diabetes insipidus, especially in patients with orbital, facial bone or sinus based lesions
—Chronic disabilities including pulmonary fibrosis, hepatic fibrosis, deafness, orthopaedic problems, short stature, permanent ataxia, neurocognitive deficits or poor dentition.

PROGNOSIS
- Majority of patients have no recurrence.
- Approximately 20%–35% of patients with single system disease will have a remitting and relapsing course.
- Tendency for the disease to "burn out" by the end of childhood. Approximately 5% will continue to have exacerbations as adults.
- 30%–50% of patients with multisystem disease will not respond to initial therapy and are at a higher risk for death.
- For patients with liver, bone marrow, or lung involvement who have not responded to initial therapy, the risk for fatal outcome is approximately 75%.

Differential Diagnosis

- Other histiocytic disorders:
—Hemophagocytic lymphohistiocytosis
—Sinus histiocytosis with massive lymphadenopathy (cervical nodes grossly enlarged)
—Malignant histiocytosis
- Bone/soft tissue lesions:
—Metastatic neuroblastoma
—Osteosarcoma
—Ewing sarcoma
—Rhabdomyosarcoma
—Craniopharyngioma
—Acute leukemias
—Burkitt lymphoma
- Organomegaly/pancytopenia:
—Acute leukemias
—Metastatic neuroblastoma

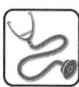

Data Gathering

HISTORY
- Swelling or pain, from soft tissue or bone lesion
- Persistent otitis
- Early loss of teeth
- Failure to thrive
- Bloody diarrhea
- Fever of unknown origin
- Anorexia
- Polydipsia or polyuria (diabetes insipidus from posterior pituitary gland involvement)
- Dyspnea
- Persistent cough
- History of spontaneous pneumothorax

Physical Examination

Growth: Height, weight, and head circumference <5%.
Skin: Brownish red papules often involving creases, seborrheic dermatitis of the scalp ("cradle cap"), purpura, petechial rash especially at areas of skin contact (e.g., top of diaper)
Ears: Otorrhea, deafness
Head: Skull swelling or mass, often very tender to palpation
Teeth: Gingivitis, "floating teeth"
Eyes: Orbital swelling, cranial nerve palsies
Lungs: Tachypnea, intercostal retractions
GI: Hepatosplenomegaly, ascites, edema, jaundice. Stool with blood or mucus
Neuro: Ataxia

Laboratory Aids

MANDATORY INITIAL INVESTIGATIONS
- Biopsy of affected area to establish the diagnosis
- CBC with differential
- PT, PTT, fibrinogen
- Electrolytes, liver function tests

- Chest x-ray
- Skeletal survey (radionuclide bone scan is not as sensitive as the skeletal radiograph survey in most patients)
- Test urine osmolarity in early morning as a screen for diabetes insipidus

OTHER INVESTIGATIONS
- Pulmonary involvement: High-resolution chest CT scan, pulmonary function tests, bronchoalveolar lavage to exclude infection
- Colon involvement: Endoscopic biopsy of small and large colon
- Liver dysfunction: Hepatic ultrasound, liver biopsy (to exclude sclerosing cholangitis)
- Neurologic involvement: MRI brain with gadolinium
- Diabetes insipidus: Endocrine evaluation including water deprivation test, evaluation of anterior pituitary hormone production, MRI brain with gadolinium
- Gingival involvement, loose teeth: panoramic dental radiography, CT scan of mandible and maxilla
- Aural involvement, deafness: Audiogram, ENT evaluation, MRI brain with gadolinium
- Bone involvement: FDG-PET scan may be more sensitive than radionuclide bone scan

Therapy

SINGLE SYSTEM
- Observation
- Local therapy
—Surgery
—Intralesional steroids (bone lesions)
—Radiotherapy is not recommended unless there is compromise to vital structures (optic nerve, spinal cord)
—Topical nitrogen mustard for refractory skin lesions
- Systemic therapy
—Low-dose chemotherapy is used for some patients with multifocal bone disease or multiply recurrent single bone lesions.
—Indomethacin may be effective for refractory bone lesions for both its analgesic and antiprostaglandin effects.

MULTISYSTEM
- Chemotherapy: Often a 6- to 12-month course; most commonly used agents: prednisone, vinblastine, methotrexate, and 6-mercaptopurine; etoposide and 2-chlorodeoxyadenosine also have activity in this disease.
- Immunotherapy: Cyclosporin A, antithymocyte globulin
- Radiation therapy
- Allogeneic stem cell transplantation for high-risk patients with organ dysfunction
- Intranasal DDAVP is generally permanently recommended for the management of diabetes insipidus as the posterior pituitary dysfunction is rarely reversible with systemic therapy.
- Most patients are treated at pediatric oncology centers. There is an international clinical trial in progress to identify the most effective treatment strategies.

Common Question and Answer

Q: Is Langerhans cell histiocytosis a form of cancer?
A: Although the abnormal Langerhans cells have been found to be derived from a single cell (i.e., monoclonal), the natural history of the disease is not typical of a malignant disorder, and therefore it is not classified as a type of cancer.

HEMOPHAGOCYTIC LYMPHOHISTIOCYTOSIS

Database

DEFINITION
Reactive disorder characterized by hypercytokinemia and organ accumulation of phagocytic histiocytes:

- Primary (also known as familial erythrophagocytic lymphohistiocytosis)
—Immunodysregulatory disorder
—Most episodes are triggered by infection
- Infection associated:
—Microorganisms implicated include: Epstein-Barr virus (EBV) (especially in cases from Asia), cytomegalovirus, herpes simplex virus, human herpes virus 6, varicella-zoster virus, parvovirus B19, human immuno-deficiency virus (HIV), adenovirus, tuberculosis, brucellosis, typhoid fever, leishmaniasis

GENETICS
- Primary:
—Autosomal recessive
—History of consanguinity may exist
—Familial history frequently negative
- Infection associated:
—Sporadic

EPIDEMIOLOGY
- Primary:
—Incidence: 1.2 cases per million children are diagnosed each year
—Males and females equally affected
—70% present in the first year of life
—Occurs in all races
- Infection associated:
—Incidence variable
—Patients often have an underlying immuno-deficiency disorder or are medically immuno-suppressed (e.g., cancer chemotherapy)

PROGNOSIS
- Primary:
—Usually fatal secondary to bleeding, infection (usually gram-negative sepsis) or progressive cerebral damage from CNS involvement
—Untreated the median survival is 2 to 3 months, 12% live more than 6 months
—Allogeneic stem cell transplantation has resulted in long-term survivors; a recent clinical trial reported the 3-year survival after stem cell transplantation was 62%.
- Infection associated:
—Mortality rates; immunocompromised 40%, immunocompetent 20%

—Improved recovery in cases associated with bacterial infections; EBV-associated has the worst prognosis

Differential Diagnosis

- Langerhans cell histiocytosis
- Sepsis with disseminated intravascular coagulation
- Syphilis
- Leishmaniasis
- Encephalitis
- Hepatitis
- Acute monoblastic leukemia
- Malignant histiocytosis
- Systemic juvenile rheumatoid arthritis
- Degenerative cerebral disorders
- Severe combined immunodeficiency disorder
- X-linked lymphoproliferative syndrome
- Chediak-Higashi syndrome

Data Gathering

HISTORY
Question: History of a rapid progression of symptoms or a viral prodrome for 2 to 6 weeks followed by constitutional symptoms, especially fever?
Significance: Evidence of systemic involvement

Question: Irritability, seizures, vomiting?
Significance: CNS involvement

Physical Examination

- Fever
- Splenomegaly
- Hepatomegaly
- Lymphadenopathy
- Seizure, irritability, bulging fontanel, neck stiffness, cranial nerve palsy, hypertonia or hypotonia, blindness, hemiplegia, coma and increased intracranial pressure

Laboratory Aids

Test: CBC with differential
Significance: Thrombocytopenia extent, neutropenia (neutrophils)

Test: Fibrinogen, prothrombin time, activated partial thromboplastin time
Significance: Low fibrinogen (<1.5 g/L), prolonged PT and aPTT

Test: Serum triglycerides, bilirubin, AST, ALT
Significance: Triglycerides classically very high; other liver function tests may be elevated

Test: Bone marrow aspirate/biopsy
Significance: Activated histiocytes with hemophagocytosis, particularly of erythrocytes

Test: Liver biopsy
Significance: Prominent histiocytes, many with hemophagocytosis

Test: Cerebrospinal fluid cell count

Significance: Moderate pleocytosis (5–50 × 10^6/L) with mainly lymphocytes

Therapy

The initial goals of treatment are to suppress the severe inflammation and to eradicate the pathogen-infected antigen-presenting cells. In patients with the inherited form, the next goal should be to replace the defective immune effector cells with normal functioning ones.

- Primary
—Cytotoxic drugs, etoposide, intrathecal methotrexate, corticosteroids, are the treatment of choice. An international clinical trial is in progress to identify the most effective treatment strategies.
—Allogeneic stem cell transplantation is necessary for cure
—Immunosuppressive therapy: Cyclosporin A, antithymocyte globulin, chloroquine
—Plasmapheresis or exchange blood transfusions
- Infection associated
—Withdrawal of immunosuppression if possible
—Antimicrobial therapy (as sole treatment in mild cases only)
—Corticosteroids
—Intravenous immunoglobulin
—Plasmapheresis
—For patients with uncontrolled fever, progressive pancytopenia, DIC, or impending organ failure, cytotoxic therapy (as used for primary hemophagocytic lymphohistiocytosis) should be instituted.

Common Questions and Answers

Q: How does one differentiate between the primary (inherited) and secondary (infection associated) forms of hemophagocytic lymphohistiocytosis?
A: There is no specific laboratory test that distinguishes the two entities. In general, diagnosis before age 2 years is strongly suggestive of primary hemophagocytic lymphohistiocytosis, whereas diagnosis after the age of 8 years is more consistent with a diagnosis of secondary hemophagocytic lymphohistiocytosis. Clinical judgment should be used to decide on treatment for those children aged 2 to 8 years.

ICD-9-CM 277.8

BIBLIOGRAPHY

Arico M, Egeler RM. Clinical aspects of Langerhans cell histiocytosis. *Hematol Oncol Clin North Am* 1998;12:247–258.

Janka G, Schneider EM. Modern management of children with haemophagocytic lymphohistiocytosis. *Br J Haematol* 2004;124:4–14.

Author: Kara M. Kelly

Histoplasmosis

 Database

DEFINITION

A spectrum of illness, ranging from primary pulmonary to disseminated infection, caused by the dimorphic fungus *Histoplasma capsulatum*.

CAUSES

• Inhalation of *Histoplasma capsulatum* spores
• The dimorphic fungus exists in mycelial form in the environment at 25°C and in yeast form in tissues at 37°C.

PATHOPHYSIOLOGY

• Micronidia or mycelial fragments inhaled into alveoli and transform to yeast phase.
• Phagocytosis followed by lymphatic and hematogenous spread.
• T-cell response follows in 10 to 21 days after infection; number of T-suppressor cells decreases while number of T-helper cells increase, resulting in delayed-type hypersensitivity.
• Localized mononuclear cell infiltrates may develop into a tuberculoid granuloma with multinucleated giant cells.
• Lesions can undergo caseation necrosis, fibrosis and, ultimately, calcification.
• Lesions usually localized to the lungs, though dissemination can occur.

EPIDEMIOLOGY

• Histoplasmosis is the most common systemic fungal infection in the United States.
• Organism has been found in nitrogen-rich soil contaminated by animal droppings, especially those of bats and birds.
• Outbreaks reported in pigeon breeders or cleaners of chicken coops, explorers of caves with bats, and populations living close to construction.
• Endemic in the eastern and central United States, specifically in the St. Laurence, Mississippi and Ohio River valleys, the Rio Grande, Texas, Oklahoma, Kansas, Pennsylvania, Maryland, and Virginia.
• 80% to 90% of adults in endemic areas are skin test positive.
• No human-to-human or animal-to-human transmission.
• The incubation period is variable, between 1 to 3 weeks.
• Severity of symptoms depends on the immunologic status of the host and the size of the inoculum.
• Asymptomatic in 50% to 95% of cases
• With heavy inoculum, 50%–100% develop symptoms. Of these, 80% develop flu-like symptoms: fever, chills, headache, myalgia, anorexia, nonproductive cough, pleuritic chest pain, lasting about a week. 10%–20% develop pericarditis, arthritis or erythema nodosum, resolving after a few weeks.
• Risk factors for severe disease (progressive disseminated histoplasmosis, PDH) include very old and very young (less than 2 years)

age, and cellular immunocompromise, e.g., AIDS.

COMPLICATIONS

In general, complications are rare, and usually indicate disseminated disease.
Symptoms include:
—Prolonged fever, malaise, cough, weight loss, hepatosplenomegaly, diarrhea. Patients may also develop disseminated intravascular coagulopathy, adult respiratory distress syndrome, renal failure, endocarditis, Addison disease

• Disseminated disease can involve:
—Skin
—Eyes (uveitis)
—Liver
—Spleen
—Adrenal glands (adrenal insufficiency)
—Bone marrow
—Heart
—Central nervous system (meninigitis)

Other complications include:
—Tracheobronchial compression
—Mediastinal granuloma formation or fibrosing mediastinitis
—Fistula formation
—Pericarditis
—Obstruction of the superior vena cava, esophagus or pulmonary arteries
—Chronic cavitary pulmonary disease very similar to tuberculosis

 Differential Diagnosis

• Infections
—Pneumonia (viral, bacterial)
—Influenza and other viral syndromes
—Tuberculosis
—Other fungal diseases: aspergillosis, blastomycosis, coccidiomycosis
—Sarcoidosis
• Malignancy

 Data Gathering

HISTORY

Question: Environmental exposures: Pigeon breeding, construction, cave exploration, travel in endemic areas?
Significance: Epidemiologically suggestive of histoplasmosis.

Question: Upper respiratory symptoms, low grade fever, cough, pleuritic chest pain?
Significance: Suggestive of mild disease lasting 1 to 5 days

Question: Arthritis, more severe chest pain, skin lesions?
Significance: Suggestive of pericarditis or pleural effusion, moderate disease lasting approximately 15 days

Question: High fever, night sweats, weight loss, cough, chest pain, shortness of breath, hoarseness lasting more than 2 to 3 weeks?
Significance: Suggestive of disseminated disease and underlying immune suppression

Question: Chronic cough, dyspnea, disabling respiratory dysfunction?
Significance: Suggestive of chronic cavitary pulmonary disease

 Physical Examination

Finding: Flu-like signs and symptoms
Significance: Common presentations, mild disease
• Fever
• Cough
• Physical examination may be normal

Finding: Less usual manifestations
Significance: Suggestive of moderate or disseminated disease
• Hepatosplenomegaly
• Adenopathy
• Pneumonitis
• Skin lesions (erythema nodosum)
• Pericardial friction rub
• Pallor, petechiae
• Central nervous system findings

 Laboratory Aids

Test: Culture of the organism in sputum, tissue specimens, peripheral blood or bone marrow
Significance: Definitive method of diagnosis, but requires 2 to 6 weeks. Sputum cultures are negative in most patients with mild disease. Cultures positive in two-third of patients with cavitary disease and one-third of patients with noncavitary disease. In PDH in patients with AIDS, bone marrow and blood cultures are positive in 80% to 90% of patients, and bronchoscopic cultures are positive in 80% to 90% of patients with abnormal chest radiographs.

Test: Identification of organism by microscopy
Significance: Histologic identification from sputum, blood (buffy coat-50% positive in PDH), bone marrow, biopsy specimens, and/or cerebrospinal fluid. Staining methods: Hematoxylin and eosin (H&E), Wright, Giemsa, periodic acid-Schiff (PAS). Gomori methenamine silver (GMS) more likely to detect sparse organisms.

Test: Skin testing
Significance: A positive delayed hypersensitivity reaction (48 hours) to the histoplasmin test may become reactive 2 to 6 weeks after infection. This test is not recommended for diagnostic purposes in adults; it is very often indicative of past infection in endemic areas (see Epidemiology). In children less than 5 years, only 0.5% from endemic areas are skin test positive. 50% of immunocompromised patients may have false-negative skin tests. False positives occur in blastomycosis and coccidiomycosis. Skin testing can falsely elevate antibody levels in 15%–25% of patients. Skin tests are not available in the United States and are no longer recommended.

Test: Radioimmune and hemagglutinin assays for *H. capsulatum* antigen
Significance: Radioimmunassay is a specific, sensitive and rapid method for diagnosing PDH. Hemagglutinin is found in urine or blood in 50%–90% of patients with PDH (with urine being more sensitive), and in bronchoalveolar lavage fluid in 70% of AIDS patients with pulmonary histoplasmosis. Antigen tests are generally useful only in the first month of infection, but can persist for much longer in AIDS patients. Antigen levels decrease with treatment, and can increase again with relapse. DNA probes are being increasingly used.

Test: Serologic studies for antibodies.
Significance: Titers become positive 4–6 weeks after infection, peak at 2–3 months and decline over a period of 2–5 years. Positive titers in 90% of patients with symptomatic disease. False positives in patients with coccidiomycosis, blastomycosis, tuberculosis and paracoccidiomycosis. False negatives in immunocompromised patients with PDH.

Test: Complement fixation
Significance: A single titer 1:32 (1:8 in nonendemic areas) is diagnostic; a four-fold increase in titers is diagnostic. This test is more sensitive than the immunodiffusion test, which is more specific.

Test: Precipitating antibodies by immunodiffusion
Significance: H band suggests active infection, M band less specific, presence of H and M bands highly diagnostic

Test: Evaluation for meningitis
Significance: Relative sensitivities:
—Stain of cerebrospinal fluid (CSF), <10%
—Culture CSF, 20%–60%
—Antigen CSF, 40%–70%
—Antibody CSF, 60%–80%
—Meningeal or brain biopsy, 50%–80%

IMAGING

Test: Chest radiograph
Significance: Normal in 75% of patients with histoplasmosis, 25%–50% of immunocompromised patients with disseminated disease

- Most common radiologic changes include:
—Small 2- to 5-mm infiltrates in the lung bases
—Lobar or diffuse infiltrates
—Enlarged or calcified hilar nodes
—Buckshot calcifications seen in patients with large inoculum
—Cavitary lesions
—Pleural effusions in 10% of chest radiographs in adults
—Calcified nodules in the liver and spleen

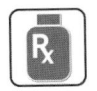 Therapy

DRUGS

- The uncomplicated cases of primary histoplasmosis of the lungs may not require drug therapy

- Patients with more severe or disseminated disease or the immunocompromised require treatment with antifungal agents. Treatment regimens can vary.
—Amphotericin B, 0.5 to 1.0 mg/kg per day IV for 4–6 weeks, or 35 mg/kg, total. Recommended for disseminated disease or patients with respiratory compromise and hypoxemia
—Milder disease: For the following drugs, interactions with other drugs are common; consult a drug interaction database or reference before prescribing. Limited or no information about use in newborn infants, and, in the case of ketoconazole, children under 2 years, is available.
—Ketoconazole, 3.3 to 6.6 mg/kg per day PO (400 mg per day initially, then 200 mg per day is maximum dose) for 3 to 6 months. Should be used with caution in patients receiving H2 blockers, because absorption is decreased in achlorhydric state. Levels can also be reduced by rifampin and phenytoin.
—Fluconazole, 6 to 12 mg/kg per day PO (400–800 mg per day is maximum dose) for 3–6 months. Reduced dose may also be given IV. Achieves levels in CSF.
—Itraconazole, 5 to 10 mg/kg per day PO (400 mg/d is maximum dose) for 3 to 6 months. May also be given IV. Although not approved for use in children, effective in the treatment of HIV patients with histoplasmosis. Does not achieve levels in CSF.
—In patients with AIDS, lifelong suppressive therapy is recommended
—Adjunct therapy with corticosteroids may be added in patients with life threatening airway obstruction secondary to hilar adenopathy
—Prophylaxis: considered for patients with AIDS, low CD4 counts and who live in endemic areas

 Follow-Up

WHEN TO EXPECT IMPROVEMENT

- In mild-to-moderate cases not requiring drug therapy, usually 1 to 2 weeks
- In cases requiring therapy, improvement is usually noted within 2 weeks.
- Response to therapy is more variable in AIDS patients

PROGNOSIS

- In most cases, prognosis is excellent.
- 90% mortality within 3 months in patients with acute disseminated histoplasmosis if left untreated.
- High relapse in AIDS patients if not treated with chronic suppressive therapy

PITFALLS

Can be difficult to distinguish between active disease and previous exposure in patients from endemic regions. Skin testing not recommended for adults in endemic regions, and may cause false-positive serology. May be confused with tuberculosis and other fungal diseases. Isolated pulmonary nodule on CXR may be difficult to distinguish from malignancy

PREVENTION & CONTROL MEASURES

- Investigation for the common source of infection in outbreaks. Limit exposure to soil and dust from areas contaminated with bat and bird droppings
- For occupational exposure to *H. capsulatum* contaminated soil
—Use of wetting agents to prevent aerosolization of contaminated dust
—NIOSH approved respirators, gloves and dispensable clothing. (see NIOSH web site in Reference section)
- Isolation of the hospitalized patient
—Standard precautions recommended

 Common Questions and Answers

Q: What are the most common clinical presentations of histoplasmosis?
A: Asymtomatic, mild primary pulmonary (1–2 weeks), moderate (2–3 weeks), disseminated, and cavitary

Q: How is histoplasmosis best diagnosed?
A: Skin test generally not useful; culture and serologic testing recommended

Q: Does histoplasmosis need to be treated with antifungal therapy?
A: Mild primary disease—no; more severe or disseminated disease—yes

Q: How can histoplasmosis be prevented?
A: Prevention can only be achieved by controlling the environmental factors in the affected areas; there are no vaccines for the prevention of histoplasmosis.

Q: Do patients with histoplasmosis need to be isolated?
A: No isolation of infected patients is required.

ICD-9-CM 115.90

BIBLIOGRAPHY

Afghani B, Marks MI. Other fungal infections: Histoplasmosis. In: Taussig L, Landau L, eds. *Textbook of Pediatric Respiratory Medicine.* Mosby: St. Louis, 1999:753–755.

American Academy of Pediatrics. Histoplasmosis. In: Pickering LK, ed. *2003 Red Book: Report of the Committee on Infectious Diseases.* 26th Ed. Elk Grove Village, IL: Academy of Pediatrics, 2003:353–356.

Maxson S, Jacobs RF. Community acquired fungal pneumonia in children. *Semin Respir Infect* 1996;11:196–203.

National Institute for Occupational Safety and Health (NIOSH) web site: http://www.cdc.gov/niosh/html

Walsh TJ, Gonzalez C, Lyman CA, et al. Invasive fungal infections in children: recent advances in diagnosis and treatment. *Adv Pediatr Infect Dis* 1996;11:187–290.

Wheat LJ. Current diagnosis of histoplasmosis. *Trends in Microbiology* 2003;11:488–494.

Wheat LJ. Histoplasmosis. *Infect Dis Clin N Am* 2003;17:1–19.

Author: Julian L. Allen

Hodgkin Lymphoma

 Database

DEFINITION

A malignant enlargement of lymph nodes characterized by a pleomorphic cellular infiltrate with multinucleated giant cells (Reed-Sternberg cells).

PATHOPHYSIOLOGY

- Exact cause unknown
- Reed-Sternberg cells are the malignant cells of Hodgkin lymphoma; however, their normal counterparts have not been definitively identified. They may originate from activated B or T lymphocytes or from an antigen-presenting cell. Histologically, Reed-Sternberg cells are dispersed among apparently normal reactive cells including lymphocytes, plasma cells, and eosinophils.
- The Rye classification histologically divides the disease into four categories: Lymphocyte predominant, mixed cellularity, lymphocyte depleted, and nodular sclerosis. The most common subtype in children is nodular sclerosis (approximately 50% of cases).
- Unicentric in origin with contiguous spread from one chain of lymph nodes to another.

GENETICS

- Familial clustering suggests the role of both genetic and environmental factors in pathogenesis:

—Three- to sevenfold increased risk of disease among siblings, in families where twins are concordant
—Reports in parent-child pairs have been noted

EPIDEMIOLOGY

- Incidence shows bimodal age distribution:

—Early peak, before adolescence in developing countries, mid to late 20s in United States
—Second peak, late adulthood >50 years of age
—Childhood cases, rare before 5 years of age, males > females less than 10 years of age, more common in white race >15 years of age

- Infections with Epstein-Barr virus, cytomegalovirus, and herpesvirus 6 may play role in transmission of disease

—Patients with history of EBV infection have a threefold increased risk of disease

- Male predominance

COMPLICATIONS

- Acute toxicity of treatment

—Radiation effects are generally reversible and not serious. They are a function of total dose and volume irradiated and includes erythema with or without hyperpigmentation of involved skin, nausea, fatigue, and possibly myelosuppression. Lhermitte syndrome, a sensation of "electric shock"

radiating down the back into the extremities, may occasionally be seen.
—Chemotherapy regimens will cause nausea, vomiting, and reversible alopecia to some degree. Transfusions may be required for anemia and thrombocytopenia. Each individual agent also has a list of toxicities that must be reviewed before using alone or in combination. Most important of these include cardiac toxicity with Adriamycin, neurotoxicity with vincristine, and pulmonary toxicity with bleomycin.

- Infection

—Most common dose-limiting acute toxicity of chemotherapy is myelosuppression. Patients may have to be admitted for antibiotics if fever develops during neutropenia. Prophylactic antibiotics and vaccines have reduced the incidence of serious bacterial infections in the splenectomized host.

PROGNOSIS

- With current therapy including chemotherapy and/or radiation, five-year disease-free survival ranges from:

—88%–100% in low stage disease
—54%–94% in advanced stage disease

 Differential Diagnosis

- Infection is most common cause for acute lymphadenopathy

—Bacterial (*Staphylococcus aureus*, β-hemolytic streptococcus, TB, atypical mycobacterium)
—Other (EBV, CMV, cat-scratch disease, toxoplasmosis, HIV, histoplasmosis)

- Malignancy is more common with chronic adenopathy.

—Non-Hodgkin lymphoma, neuroblastoma, leukemia, rhabdomyosarcoma

- Mediastinal masses divided anatomically:

—Anterior: Lymphoid and thyroid tumors, bronchogenic cysts, aneurysms, lipomas
—Middle: Lymphoid tumors, angiomas, pericardial cysts, teratomas, esophageal lesions, hernias
—Posterior: Neurogenic tumors, cysts, thoracic meningocele, sarcomas

 Data Gathering

HISTORY

- Signs/symptoms

—Fatigue, anorexia, weight loss in one-third of patients
—"B" symptoms (part of staging classification) include one of the following:
—Unexplained fever with temp >38°C for at least 3 days

—Unexplained weight loss >10% body weight in previous 6 months
—Drenching night sweats
—"A" disease (asymptomatic)
—Pruritis or pain that worsens with ingestion of alcohol seen in some patients

- History relative to possible EBV or HIV infection should be recorded as well as any history suggesting immunodeficiency

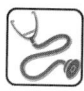 Physical Examination

- Painless lymphadenopathy most common

—Nodes are usually firmer and less mobile than inflammatory nodes, cervical chain most frequently involved

- Mediastinal mass in two-thirds of patients, may cause nonproductive cough or difficulty breathing
- Hepatosplenomegaly and bone tenderness in advanced stages
- Unusual signs and symptoms: Nephrotic syndrome, dermatomyositis, and acute dysautonomia

 Laboratory Aids

- CBC, ESR
- Liver and renal function studies
- Baseline thyroid functions (preradiotherapy)
- Baseline electrocardiogram, echocardiogram
- Baseline pulmonary function tests (preradiotherapy and/or bleomycin)

PATHOLOGY

- Lymph node biopsy for definitive diagnosis

RADIOLOGIC STUDIES

- Chest x-ray (PA and lateral), looks for mediastinal mass
- CT scan (chest, abdomen, pelvis), to rule out disseminated disease
- CT or MRI of spine (if bony tenderness or symptoms of cord compression suspected)

SPECIAL TESTS

- Bone marrow biopsy
- Gallium scan (detects residual disease in the mediastinum) or petscan
- Bone scan (evaluates bone involvement, optional)
- Lymphangiogram (evaluates retroperitoneal adenopathy, optional)

STAGING

- Staging laparotomy is indicated in patients with equivocal abdominal findings from clinical staging or in patients with radiotherapy treatment only.

—I: Involvement of a single lymph node region (I) or of a single extralymphatic organ or site (IE) by direct extension

—II: Involvement of two or more lymph node regions on the same side of the diaphragm (II) or localized involvement of an extralymphatic organ or site and one or more lymph node regions on the same side of the diaphragm (IIE)
—III: Involvement of lymph node regions on both sides of the diaphragm (III), which may be accompanied by involvement of the spleen (IIIS) or by localized involvement of an extra-lymphatic organ or site (IIIE) or both (IIIES)
—IV: Diffuse or disseminated involvement of one or more extralymphatic organs or tissues with or without associated lymph node involvement

- Staging is further subclassified "A" or "B" according to absence or presence of symptoms (listed above), respectively.

RISK GROUPS:

- Low risk

—IA-IIA, no bulk mediastinum
—No extranodal extension or B symptoms
—Two or fewer involved regions

- Intermediate risk

—IA-IIA with bulk mediastinum or extranodal extension or more than 3 involved nodal sites
—IB-IIB-IIIA

- High Risk

—IIIB, IVA-B

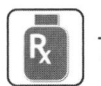

Therapy

RADIOTHERAPY (XRT)

- Exquisitely responsive to XRT
- Decisions to use XRT based on patient age, tumor burden, and potential complications
- Standard dose XRT, 2,000 cGy–2,500 cGy given to all involved areas
- Doses administered in fractions, 150–200 cGy per day, 5 times a week

CHEMOTHERAPY

Multiple agents allow different mechanisms of action (to circumvent resistance) and nonoverlapping toxicities so that full doses can be given.

- MOPP: mechlorethamine + vincristine (Oncovin) + procarbazine + prednisone (high degree of infertility in male patients who received this hybrid)
- COPP: cyclophosphamide substituted for mechlorethamine in MOPP (favored over MOPP, less AML)
- COMP: methotrexate substituted for procarbazine in COPP
- ABVD: doxorubicin (Adriamycin) + bleomycin + vinblastine + dacarbazine
- DBVE: doxorubicin + bleomycin + vincristine + etoposide
- DBVE-PC: DBVE + prednisone and cyclophosphamide
- Each cycle consists of 21–28 days, dependent on toxicity. Some regimens alternate therapy (i.e., MOPP alternating with ABVD), or use growth factor support to intensify schedule.

- Stages IA, IIA

—Attained full growth; no unfavorable signs: standard-dose XRT alone
—Still growing, bulky disease, or E lesions: (see staging) low dose XRT + 2 to 4 courses multiagent chemotherapy

- Stages IB, IIB, IIIA/B, IVA/B

—Attained full growth; no unfavorable signs: Combined modality therapy with three to five courses multiagent chemotherapy + low-dose XRT
—Still growing or large mediastinal mass: Low-dose XRT + chemotherapy (same as above)

Follow-Up

- Office visits monthly with CBC
- CT scan of involved areas every 3 months for first 2 years, then every 6 months for 3 years
- Relapse of disease usually occurs within first 3 years. Some may relapse as late as 10 years after initial diagnosis.
- Special studies as needed for toxicity-related complications. For example:

—Yearly thyroid function tests if history of irradiation
—Regular self breast examination for females treated with chest radiation
—Mammograms beginning by the age of 25 or 10 years postchest radiation (whichever is last) in females
—Regular electrocardiograms, echocardiograms and Holter monitors if treated with radiation and/or anthracyclines
—Regular pulmonary function tests if treated with radiation and/or bleomycin

LATE EFFECTS

- Radiation
—Pulmonary damage (radiation-induced)—pneumonitis, pulmonary fibrosis, decreased pulmonary function, pneumothorax
—Cardiac damage (XRT-induced)—cardiomyopathy resulting in CHF, pericarditis, valvular damage, coronary heart disease, and myocardial infarction
—Radiation nephritis
—Radiation-induced ovarian damage can be avoided by performing oophoropexy during laparotomy.
—Hypothyroidism, hyperthyroidism, thyroid nodules, thyroid cancer.
—Growth retardation with high doses of XRT (>3,500 cGy), resulting in a disproportionate alteration in sitting height versus standing height. Risk is highest during active bone growth (under 6 years of age and puberty).
—Secondary malignant neoplasms are a major concern in selecting therapy. One study showed the risk of second neoplasm 15 years after diagnosis was 7%, with breast cancer as the most common solid tumor. Other secondary neoplasms associated with treatment are thyroid and skin carcinomas, brain tumor, and malignant fibrous histiocytoma.

- Chemotherapy

—Pulmonary damage (bleomycin): Pulmonary fibrosis, decreased pulmonary function
—Cardiac damage (adriamycin): Cardiomyopathy resulting in CHF, arrhythmias with conduction defects, pericarditis
—Azoospermia induced by alkylating agents is almost always permanent in postpubertal boys
—Amenorrhea occurs in 20% of patients less than 25 years using the MOPP regimen.
—Secondary malignant neoplasms—the risk of developing leukemia (AML) is highest when both radiotherapy and alkylating agents are used.

- Laparotomy, splenectomy

—Obstruction, sepsis

Common Questions and Answers

Q: Is my child at risk for other cancers?
A: Yes. Although the incidence is low, children with Hodgkin disease are primarily at risk for cancers resulting from their treatment. Breast cancer is the most common solid tumor and can occur decades after therapy. Therefore, long-term follow-up is essential.

Q: Will my child be infertile following treatment?
A: It depends on the therapy he/she received. Certain chemotherapy agents are associated with a higher risk of infertility (alkylating agents). Radiation to the gonads is also associated with infertility.

BIBLIOGRAPHY

Bhatia S, Robinson LL, Oberlin O, et al. Breast cancer and other second neoplasms after childhood Hodgkin's disease. *N Engl J Med* 1996;334:745–751.

Hudson MM, Donaldson SS. Hodgkin disease. In: Pizzo PA, Poplack DG, eds. *Principles and Practice of Pediatric Oncology.* 4th Ed. Philadelphia: JB Lippincott, 2002:637–660.

Mack TM, Cozen W, Shibata DK, et al. Concordance for Hodgkin's disease in identical twins suggesting genetic susceptibility to the young-adult form of the disease. *N Engl J Med* 1995;332:413–418.

Murphy SB, et al. Results of little or no treatment for lymphocyte-predominant Hodgkin disease in children and adolescents. *J Pediatr Hematol/Oncol* 2003;25(9):684–687.

Ruymann FB, et al. Late Effects Study Group. High risk of subsequent neoplasms continues with extended follow-up of childhood Hodgkin's disease: report from the Late Effects Study Group. *J Clinical Oncol* 2003;21(23):4386–4394.

Smith RS, et al. Prognostic factors for children with Hodgkin's disease treated with combined-modality therapy. *J Clinical Oncol* 2003;21(10):2026–2033.

Author: Jill P. Ginsberg

Human Immunodeficiency Virus Infection

 Database

DEFINITION

• HIV-1 and HIV-2 are the etiologic agents of HIV infection and the acquired immunodeficiency syndrome (AIDS).
• HIV infection is a lifelong disease.
• For most infected individuals, a long clinically asymptomatic period (5–15 years in adults, frequently shorter in children), is followed by the development of generalized nonspecific signs and symptoms (weight loss, adenopathy, hepatosplenomegaly) and mild clinical immunodeficiency.
• Eventually, after progressive immunologic deterioration, patients are susceptible to a wide variety of opportunistic infections and cancers, which represent the clinical syndrome known as AIDS.

EPIDEMIOLOGY

• HIV infection is transmitted via:

—Sexual contact: Male to female transmission more efficient than female to male; anal receptive sex more likely to transmit than vaginal sex.
—Exposure to infected blood:
—Breast milk: The overall risk of breast-feeding is about 15%. In countries where breast-feeding is the norm, up to 40% of perinatally acquired HIV infections occur through breast-feeding.
—Perinatally, either in utero or during labor and delivery. Of perinatally infected infants, 5%–20% are believed infected in utero; the rest acquire the infection around the time of birth. The risk of an HIV-infected mother giving birth to an infected infant is approximately 20%, with increased rate of transmission for women with low CD4 counts or higher viral titers, and for those who were previously diagnosed with AIDS. In addition, vaginal delivery, especially with rupture of membranes longer than 8 hours, appears to increase the risk of infant infection. The presence of untreated STDs, chorioamnionitis, and prematurity also all increase the risk of mother-to-child transmission of HIV.

• HIV is not believed to be transmitted by:

—Bites
—Sharing utensils, bathrooms, bathtubs
—Exposure to urine, feces, vomitus (except where these fluids may be grossly contaminated with blood, and even then transmission is rare, if at all)
—Casual contact in the home, school, or day-care center

COMPLICATIONS

• *Pneumocystis carinii* pneumonia (PCP): With a peak age of 3–9 months, PCP is the most common early fatal illness in HIV-infected children. In infancy, the mortality is 30%–50% for the acute episode. A high index of suspicion is necessary for prompt diagnosis (by lavage) and initiation of therapy. 40% of new cases of HIV-related pediatric PCP involve infants not previously recognized as HIV-infected.
• Lymphocytic interstitial pneumonitis (LIP): Frequently asymptomatic, LIP can lead to slow onset of chronic respiratory symptoms. LIP causes a distinctive diffuse reticulonodular pattern on chest radiographs. Usually diagnosed between 2 and 4 years of age, LIP is related to dysfunctional immune response to EBV infection. Definitive diagnosis is made by lung biopsy. For symptomatic patients, prednisone is effective.
• Recurrent invasive bacterial infections: The risk of bacteremia is approximately 10% per year in HIV-infected children. Pneumococcal bacteremia is the most common invasive bacterial disease.
• Progressive encephalopathy: Generally diagnosed between 9 and 18 months of age, the hallmark is progressive loss of developmental milestones or neurologic dysfunction.
• Disseminated *Mycobacterium avium-intracellulare* (DMAC): DMAC occurs in older children, usually >5 years of age, with severe immunodeficiency (CD4 ≤100). Symptoms include prolonged fevers, abdominal pain, anorexia, and diarrhea.
• *Candida* esophagitis: As with DMAC, seen in older children with severe immunodeficiency. Patients usually present with dysphagia or chest pain. Oral thrush is noted on examination. Diagnosis suggested by findings on barium swallow. Definitive diagnosis made by biopsy.
• Disseminated CMV disease: Retinitis less common in HIV-infected children than in adults. CMV may also cause pulmonary disease, colitis, and hepatitis.
• HIV-related cancers: Non-Hodgkin lymphoma is the most common cancer, with primary site usually located in the CNS.
• Other organ dysfunction associated with HIV-infection in children: Cardiomyopathy, hepatitis, renal disease, thrombocytopenia/ITP.

PROGNOSIS

Prior to the advent of aggressive combination therapies, data suggested a bimodal survival curve, with 25% of perinatally infected infants developing early symptomatic disease, with an AIDS diagnosis by 1 to 2 years of life and frequently dying by 3 years of age. The remaining 75% have a delayed onset of symptoms, usually after 5 years of age, and the median survival of this group was to 8 to 12 years old. Since the use of a combination of three or more drugs have become standard, morbidity and mortality are both greatly decreased. The median survival is now clearly into late adolescence/adulthood. In addition, the incidence of new opportunistic infections (AIDS signal illnesses) has decreased greatly, as have hospital admissions.

 Differential Diagnosis

• Neoplastic disease: Lymphoma, leukemia, histiocytosis X
• Infectious: Congenital/perinatal CMV, toxoplasmosis, congenital syphilis, acquired Epstein-Barr virus (EBV)
• Congenital immunodeficiency syndromes: Wiskott-Aldrich syndrome, chronic granulomatous disease

 Data Gathering

HISTORY

• Parental risk factors? (Prematurity, PROM, HIV testing in the mother)
• Intravenous drug use?
• Noninjectable drug use?
• Sexually transmitted diseases, especially syphilis?
• Bisexuality?
• Transfusions before 1986?
• Frequent infections?
• Sinopulmonary infections?
• Recurrent pneumonia/invasive bacterial disease?
• Severe acute pneumonia (PCP)?
• Recurrent or resistant thrush, especially after 12 months of age?
• Congenital syphilis?
• Presence of STDs in an adolescent?
• Acquired microcephaly?
• Progressive encephalopathy, loss of developmental milestones?
• History of ITP/thrombocytopenia?
• Failure to thrive?
• Recurrent/chronic diarrhea?
• Recurrent/chronic enlargement of parotid gland?

 Physical Examination

May be entirely normal in the first few months of life; 90% will have some physical findings by age 2. The most common findings are:

• Adenopathy, generalized
• Hepatosplenomegaly
• Failure to thrive
• Recurrent/resistant thrush, especially after 1 year of age
• Recurrent or chronic parotitis

Laboratory Aids

Test: ELISA antibody screen
Significance: For children over 18 months of age, repeatedly reactive ELISA antibody screen, followed by confirmation with Western blot analysis, is diagnostic of HIV infection. Any positive test should always be repeated before a definitive diagnosis is discussed with family. In first year of life, positive HIV ELISA and Western blot antibody tests simply confirm maternal infection, because the antibody test is IgG based, and maternal anti-HIV antibodies readily cross placenta. Maternal antibodies may remain detectable until 15 months of age.

Test: HIV blood culture and/or PCR DNA testing
Significance: Most reliable way of diagnosing HIV infection in infancy. The PCR test has slightly more false positives and false negatives; the blood culture is more expensive, takes longer to run, and is technically more difficult. Both tests have sensitivities and specificities greater than 95% when performed after 4 weeks of age.

Test: Elevated IgG levels
Significance: First observed immune abnormality noted in HIV-infected infants, generally reaching twice the normal values by 9 months of age.

Test: CD4 counts
Significance: Obtained at diagnosis and every 1 to 3 months. Results need to be evaluated on the basis of age-adjusted normal values. Absolute CD4 counts are elevated in childhood, with normal median values greater than 3,000/mm^3 in the first year of life, which then gradually decline with age, reaching values comparable with adult levels (800 to 1,000/mm^3) by age 7.

Test: Quantitative viral RNA PCR assays
Significance: Termed "viral loads," results are reported in a range from "undetectable," usually less than 40 copies/mL, to upper values of over 10 million. Long-term prognosis is closely related to viral loads. Viral loads that remain over 100,000 are associated with poor short-term (2 to 5 year) outcomes.

Test: Neurologic evaluation, with psychometric testing, and an initial CAT scan/MRI screening for cerebral atrophy.
Significance: Should be repeated at yearly intervals.

Test: Postimmunization antibody levels
Significance: Assess B cell function.

Other frequent lab abnormalities include thrombocytopenia, anemia, and elevated liver enzymes.

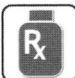 ## Therapy

- Immunizations: All infected children receive standard childhood immunizations, pneumococcal conjugate vaccine. Infected children should receive yearly influenza A/B immunizations and the pneumococcal vaccine at age 2. Symptomatic children should not receive the varicella vaccine, and those with severely low CD4 counts should not receive the MMR.
- Antiretroviral therapy: Specific combination antiretroviral therapy delays progression of illness, promotes improved growth, and improves neurologic outcome. The standard of care now involves the administration of combination (usually three or more drugs) therapy. The most potent agents are those that inhibit viral protease (termed protease inhibitors). Drug regimens are complex, with as many as nine doses of medication a day. Adherence to prescribed schedules is critical. When patients miss even 10%–20% of doses, the durability of response is short.
- Immune enhancement

—Passive: Recent studies suggest that monthly gamma globulin infusions decrease, somewhat, febrile episodes and pneumococcal bacteremia. The children who benefit the most are those not on antibiotic prophylaxis for PCP or otitis media.
—Prophylaxis: One of the major advances in the care of HIV-infected children and adults has been the ability to offer prophylaxis against the most common opportunistic infections.

PREVENTION

- HIV infection is almost completely preventable. Educational efforts aimed at achieving a change in behavior is a key component of HIV-directed work.
- It is now possible to significantly decrease the risk to newborns of HIV-infected women. Prenatal ZDV therapy, followed by continuous IV ZDV therapy during labor, and treatment of the infant for the first 6 weeks of life have been shown to decrease the risk of HIV infection in the infant from 20% to 8%. With the newer combination therapies, and delivery via elective cesarean section for selected cases, perinatal transmissions rates have now fallen below 2% to 3% in HIV-specialty care sites.

 ## Follow-Up

Psychosocial support for the family is critical. Because of the complexity of, and the rapidly changing, therapies available to treat pediatric HIV-infection, all infected patients should be comanaged with an HIV specialty care site.

PITFALLS

The result of failing to screen for HIV infection is the inability to offer antiretroviral therapy for pregnant women, therefore possibly preventing infant infection, and also the inability to prescribe PCP prophylaxis to infected newborns.

 ## Common Question and Answer

Q: Once the HIV-exposed infant has seroreverted to antibody negative status, how sure are we that he/she is uninfected?
A: With today's technology, if the child has also been PCR and/or HIV blood culture negative at least twice, and is clinically well, the chance that the child still harbors HIV is very low and appears to be less than 1 per 5,000. The child should continue to be followed by a health care provider aware of his/her past HIV antibody status. If clinical conditions warrant, retesting would be an option at a later date.

BIBLIOGRAPHY

Perinatal HIV Guidelines Working Group. PHS Task Force recommendations for use of antiretroviral drugs in pregnant HIV-1 infected women for maternal health and interventions to reduce perinatal transmission in the United States. Revised January, 2004. Available and updated, on line, at http://AIDSinfo.NIH.gov

Working Group on Antiretroviral Therapy and Medical Management of HIV-1 infected children. Guidelines for the use of antiretroviral agents in pediatric HIV infection. Available, and updated, on line, at http://www.hivatis.org. Accessed January, 2004.

Author: Richard M. Rutstein

Hydrocephalus

Database

DEFINITION

Hydrocephalus is the accumulation of cerebrospinal fluid (CSF) in the ventricles and subarachnoid spaces, leading to their enlargement. The overall head size often enlarges in response, depending on age and etiology.

CAUSES

• Intraventricular hemorrhage (related to prematurity or trauma) may result in a blood clot, meningeal adhesions, or granular ependymitis.
• Tumors or cysts of any histologic type located near the foramina or the aqueduct, or within the ventricular system, e.g., hypothalamic hamartoma, subarachnoid cysts.
• Infection (meningitis) can lead to leptomeningeal adhesions and granulations.
• Developmental

—Chiari malformation, type II (associated with myelomeningocele; brain migrational disorders; small posterior fossa; inferior displacement of medulla and cerebellar vermis; kinking of the brainstem; aqueductal stenosis; beaking of the tectum)
—Dandy-Walker malformation (absence of cerebellar vermis, small cerebellar hemispheres, enlarged posterior fossa, often with cystic fourth ventricle)
—X-linked and autosomal dominant hydrocephalus, the former is often associated with aqueductal stenosis and mutations in L1CAM on Xq28.
—Sporadic primary aqueductal stenosis
—Dysmorphic syndromes (e.g., Apert syndrome, Cockayne syndrome, Crouzon syndrome, Pfeiffer syndrome, trisomy 13, trisomy 21)
—Alexander disease
—Mucopolysaccharidoses (e.g., type VI, Maroteaux-Lamy)
—Migrational disorders/congenital muscular dystrophies (e.g., Miller-Diecker, Muscle-Eye-Brain disease, Fukuyama congenital muscular dystrophy, Walker-Warburg syndrome)
—Achondroplasia
—Neurocutaneous syndromes (e.g., neurofibromatosis type 1, rare)
—Idiopathic

PATHOPHYSIOLOGY

• Functions of CSF: Physical cushion for brain and spine, nutrition, clearance of waste products.
• Normal pathway of CSF: Choroid plexus and interstitial fluid (sources), lateral ventricles, foramina of Monro, third ventricle, aqueduct of Sylvius, fourth ventricle, foramina of Luschka and Magendie, subarachnoid space, arachnoid villi and venous circulation.
• Hydrocephalus often involves obstruction to CSF flow or inadequate reabsorption, even in the rare case of choroid plexus papilloma (overproduction of CSF).

• Noncommunicating (obstructive) hydrocephalus: The obstruction is in the ventricular system.
• Communicating hydrocephalus: The problem is outside of the ventricular system; generally there is a problem with reabsorption.
• Although the noncommunicating/communicating distinction has been fundamental in the literature, it has no prognostic significance; the value of the distinction concerns choice of a site for palliative drainage, and etiologic considerations.

COMPLICATIONS

• Acute hydrocephalus—herniation syndromes may be fatal
• Chronic hydrocephalus

—Macrocephaly
—Spastic paraparesis may lead to gait and motor problems.
—Developmental delay
—Premature sexual development

Differential Diagnosis

• Other causes of macrocephaly:

—Familial macrocephaly
—Pericerebral effusions
—Congenital anomalies of intra or extracerebral veins
—Tumors, intracranial cysts
—Primary megalencephaly, hemimegalencephaly
—GM2 gangliosidosis
—Some leukodystrophies (e.g., Alexander disease, Canavan disease)
—Head-sparing intrauterine growth retardation (relative macrocephaly)
—Rapid catch-up growth following prolonged malnutrition

• Other causes of ventriculomegaly, typically with normal head circumference, include brain atrophy and chronic ethanol or corticosteroid exposure (reversible)
• In "benign external hydrocephalus," both the ventricles and extraaxial CSF spaces are proportionately enlarged, and macrocephaly is common. A better name for this entity might be "benign extra-axial collections of infancy" since they are almost always asymptomatic and resolve spontaneously.

Data Gathering

HISTORY

• Hydrocephalus is common among preterm neonates.
• Infants and children may also present to the primary pediatrician with new-onset hydrocephalus.
• Presenting concerns, especially in infants, include:

—Behavioral changes (especially decreased feeding and increased somnolence or irritability)
—Enlarging head (most often revealed by serial head circumference measurements)
—Vomiting

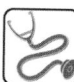
Physical Examination

• Vital signs: The Cushing triad (hypertension, bradycardia, respiratory irregularities), due to increased intracranial pressure, may be present in acute hydrocephalus, especially in advanced cases (generally not in infants prior to fusion of the sutures).
• Increasing head circumference in infants. Fullness of the anterior fontanelle is neither sensitive nor specific, but should be noted.
• Mental status: Irritability in infants, behavioral changes in children (acute or chronic)
• Cranial nerves: Parinaud syndrome (setting-sun sign, paralysis of upward gaze), papilledema or optic atrophy, visual changes (chronic only)
• Motor: Spastic paraparesis in chronic hydrocephalus
• Reflexes: Increased in chronic hydrocephalus

Laboratory Aids

TESTS

Imaging

• Head ultrasound

—Standard screening test for neonates with suspected hydrocephalus or intraventricular hemorrhage
—The anterior fontanelle must be patent for this test.
—Shows size of ventricles and presence or absence of blood; associated structures and anomalies.

• Unenhanced CT of the brain

—Mainly used in infants and children whose anterior fontanelles have closed and following shunt procedures.
—Advantage compared to ultrasound: Better visualization of fourth ventricle/brainstem, calcifications; standardized technique and better availability than ultrasound, especially in the emergency room setting.

• Magnetic resonance imaging

—Definitive test for analyzing brain anatomy.
—Can identify posterior fossa developmental malformations—Chiari and Dandy-Walker.
—Not indicated in acute hydrocephalus, especially when patient is unstable.

Therapy

ACUTE INTERVENTIONS

Neurosurgeons' use of therapeutic lumbar or ventricular puncture has decreased in recent years. These procedures must be weighed against risk of herniation (decreased when sutures are open).

VENTRICULAR SHUNT

- Indication: Progressive hydrocephalus
- Contraindications: Active central nervous system infection, active intraventricular hemorrhage, and poor overall prognosis
- Components: Ventricular catheter, reservoir (target of "shunt taps"), valve, distal catheter
- Distal sites: The peritoneum is the most common choice; pleura, ureter, venous system, and right atrium are other options.
- Approach: Typically performed as standard open procedure, but endoscopic procedures are available in some centers.
- Complications:

—Obstruction is the most common, approximately 60% revision rate in first year; presents with same signs and symptoms as hydrocephalus
—Infections occur at a rate of ~5% per shunt manipulation and rarely present before 2 weeks or after 2 months relative to shunt operation; low-grade persistent fever and signs and symptoms of shunt malfunction predominate; rarely present with wound infections of following sepsis.
—Siphon effect: Drop in ventricular pressure on sitting or standing due to negative pressure in shunt system; newer shunt systems, such as the Delta valve and Orbis Sigma valve, are designed to minimize the siphon effect, but the efficacy of their antisiphon mechanisms compared to the performance of standard differential pressure valves has been questioned; the siphon effect is less of a problem in infants and younger children due to the short distance between head and abdomen.

THIRD VENTRICLE FENESTRATION (THIRD VENTRICULOSTOMY)

- Background: An old procedure that had fallen out of favor with development of modern shunt systems
- Current status: New endoscopic techniques make this procedure useful in selected cases.
- Indications: Noncommunicating hydrocephalus is clearest indication, but this procedure has had some success in cases of pineal/tectal tumors and myelomeningocele.
- Complications: Overall rate of serious complications is 9.4%, these include infection, CSF leak, neurologic deficit, extraparenchymal hemorrhage; rare risk of damage to the basilar artery.

- Pitfall: Do not assume hydrocephalus is "cured." Although most failures occur shortly after procedure, delayed, unrecognized failures have resulted in death from acute hydrocephalus-related herniation.

FETAL MYELOMENINGOCELE REPAIR

- Has reduced the incidence of shunt-dependent hydrocephalus in the first year of life when performed in fetuses up to 25 weeks gestation and when myelomeningocele is at L3 spinal level or lower.

Follow-Up

- When the etiology or need for shunt placement may not be clear, it is important to follow clinical status, head circumference, and ventricular size (by head ultrasound or CT).
- Chronic hydrocephalus is often accompanied by spastic paraparesis, visual problems, and developmental delay.
- Most interventions are supportive, including physical therapy, occupational therapy, and orthopaedic therapies for spasticity; interdisciplinary cerebral palsy clinics can be critical in providing easy access to these resources. Special education programs may be appropriate for children with severe developmental delay.

PROGNOSIS

- Depending on the severity and etiology of hydrocephalus, efficacy of treatment, and the presence or absence of concomitant neurologic disorders, the outcome may vary widely from normal neurologic development to severe impairment or death.
- Children with shunted hydrocephalus and myelomeningocele typically have normal overall intelligence, but tend to have long-term difficulties with language development and school performance.

PITFALLS

- It is important for long-term patients in intensive care nurseries to have head circumferences recorded at least twice weekly. Macrocephaly is not always obvious on visual inspection.
- Absence of papilledema does not exclude chronic increased intracranial pressure.

—Head CT often will not show developmental malformations that may accompany hydrocephalus. MRI is the imaging procedure of choice.
—Timing of shunt placement is critical and problematic: Sometimes watchful waiting can obviate the procedure, while waiting too long may worsen permanent brain damage.

Common Questions and Answers

Q: When does an infant need a head ultrasound?
A: Any infant whose head circumference increases by more than a quartile on the growth chart. Preterm infants below a certain gestational age or birth weight (varies from hospital to hospital) should all receive screening head ultrasounds while in the intensive care nursery.

Q: When should an infant or child receive an MRI first rather than an ultrasound or CT?
A: Although MRI may be superior in many cases, the logistics of ordering the proper sequences and the need for sedation or anesthesia for long studies must be strongly considered. Consultation with a neurologist or neurosurgeon is generally advised.

Q: What is the workup for shunt obstruction and shunt infection?
A: Symptoms and signs of increased intracranial pressure should lead to a neurosurgical evaluation; frequently acquired studies include head CT (to assess ventricular size and placement of ventricular catheter), and shunt series (plain films of the entire shunt system to check for disruptions) and a tap of the shunt reservoir to ascertain pressures and patency. Fever is the most important indication for a shunt infection evaluation (shunt tap with CSF cell count, protein, glucose, Gram stain, and culture). Often patients will be evaluated for both complications.

ICD-9-CM 741.0

BIBLIOGRAPHY

Drake JM, et al. CSF shunts 50 years on—past, present and future. *Childs Nerv Syst* 2000;16(10–11):800–804.

Li V. Methods and complications in surgical cerebrospinal fluid shunting. *Neurosurg Clin N Am* 2001;12(4):685–693.

Parent Internet Information: National Hydrocephalus Foundation-http://www.nhfonline.org

Partington MD. Congenital hydrocephalus. *Neurosurg Clin N Am* 2001;12(4):737–742.

Tulipan N, et al. The effect of intrauterine myelomeningocele repair on the incidence of shunt-dependent hydrocephalus. *Pediatr Neurosurg* 2003;38(1):27–33.

Vachha B, Adams R. Language differences in young children with myelomeningocele and shunted hydrocephalus. *Pediatr Neurosurg* 2003;39(4):184–189.

Author: Peter B. Kang

Hydronephrosis

 Database

DEFINITIONS

• Hydronephrosis: Dilation of the renal pelvis (pelviectasis) and calyces (caliectasis) due to excess urine in the collecting system of the kidney
• Hydroureteronephrosis: Dilation of the renal collecting system and the ureter to the level of the bladder

ETIOLOGIES

• Ureteropelvic junction (UPJ) obstruction: Hydronephrosis caused by either an intrinsic narrowing of the UPJ or external compression of the UPJ from accessory renal vessels. For more information see Ureteropelvic Junction Obstruction.
• Ureterovesical junction (UVJ) obstruction: Hydroureteronephrosis caused by either an intrinsic narrowing or an aperistaltic segment of distal ureter. These are also called megaureters. These ureters enter the bladder in a normal position on the trigone.
• Vesicoureteral reflux (VUR): The reflux of urine from the bladder into the ureter during filling or voiding. In primary reflux (grades I–V depending on the severity) it is due to an insufficient flap valve type mechanism at the ureterovesical junction. Hydroureterone-phrosis is usually seen only with higher grades of reflux (grades III–V) or secondary reflux. Secondary reflux is reflux in the presence of an abnormal bladder, in which the reflux is often due to high storage or voiding pressures within the bladder. Secondary reflux is not graded.
• Ureterocele: Hydroureteronephrosis due to obstruction of the ureter from a cystic dilation of the intravesical portion of the distal ureter. These are most often associated with the upper pole ureter in a duplicated collecting system. They are less frequently associated with a single system.
• The ureterocele is further classified as intravesical (contained completely within the bladder) or ectopic (extending down the bladder neck and often into the urethra).
• Ectopic ureter: A ureter that drains into an abnormal location away from the trigone. The hydroureteronephrosis can be the upper pole ureter of a duplicated collecting system or a single system. Ectopic ureters can drain at various sites along the lower urinary tract depending on the sex of the child. In boys they can drain into the bladder neck, prostatic urethra, vas deferens, seminal vesicle or epididymis. In girls they can drain into the bladder neck, urethra, introitus, and vagina. The ectopic locations often require passage through the bladder neck or urogenital diaphragm, which produces obstruction of the distal ureter.
• Urolithiasis: Obstructing calculi often produce dilation of the urinary tract proximal to its location. Stone disease is rare in infancy except in preterm infants who receive

furosemide. The hydronephrosis is usually associated with renal colic.
• Posterior urethral valves (PUV): Hydroureteronephrosis, nearly always bilateral, produced by outflow obstruction of the bladder from valve leaflets in the prostatic urethra. Since both kidneys are affected, there is a significant risk of chronic renal insufficiency and development of end-stage renal disease.
• Triad syndrome (TS): Hydroureteronephrosis, often with massively dilated ureters, and a large bladder. The disorder is also known as prune belly syndrome or Eagle-Barrett syndrome. These boys have a triad of hypoplastic abdominal wall musculature (leading to a prune-like appearance), bilateral undescended testes, and a dilated urinary tract. Many have associated urethral atresia, which imparts a worse prognosis for renal function. The exact cause of TS remains elusive. There is a significant risk of renal insufficiency in these patients. A similar syndrome may occur in girls with a prune-like appearance to the abdomen and anomalies of the urogenital tract; however, it is very rare.
• Other rare causes—retrocaval ureter, pelvic tumor, ureteral valves, and cloacal malformation with hydrocolpos.

EPIDEMIOLOGY

• Incidence of genitourinary abnormalities noted on routine prenatal ultrasound is 0.2%.
• 87% of these are antenatally detected hydronephrosis/hydroureteronephrosis.
• 5% of fetuses with hydronephrosis are due to UPJ obstruction.
• Perinatal mortality associated with hydronephrosis has ranged from 13% to 72%, but is most strongly correlated with the presence of chromosomal abnormalities, multiple system abnormalities, detection earlier in gestation, oligohydramnios, and evidence of infravesical obstruction.
• PUV and TS account for 6% of cases.

 Differential Diagnosis

• Cystic renal tumor—most commonly Wilms tumor. These should be distinguished from hydronephrosis by ultrasound or CT scanning.
• Multicystic dysplastic kidney—can be difficult to distinguish from severe hydronephrosis with marked parenchymal thinning. A renal scan will show no function or perfusion with a multicystic dysplastic kidney.

 Data Gathering

HISTORY

Newborns

• Antenatal hydronephrosis: Presence of hydronephrosis or hydroureteronephrosis.

• If unilateral, severity of hydronephrosis and the status of contralateral kidney.
• If bilateral, presence of bladder wall thickening, bladder enlargement, bladder emptying, or a dilated posterior urethra (keyhole sign) may indicate PUV or TS.
• If oligohydramnios is present, pulmonary hypoplasia is a concern. The presence of oligohydramnios, increased renal echogenicity, and cystic changes in the kidneys are indicators of poor renal function and dysplasia.

Older Children

• History of urinary tract infections or gross hematuria
• General health and growth (poor growth with chronic renal insufficiency or acidosis)
• Daytime incontinence, poor urinary stream, or symptoms of voiding dysfunction may be an indicator of bladder dysfunction due to PUV.
• History of episodic abdominal (which may not lateralize well), flank, or back pain in the presence of hydronephrosis is often due to symptomatic UPJ obstruction (see Ureteropelvic Junction Obstruction).

 Physical Examination

• Neonate: Signs of oligohydramnios (Potter facies, lateral patellar dimples, clubfeet, and other limb deformities) and respiratory distress.
• Palpable abdominal mass. Palpable walnut-sized bladder (PUV). Patent urachus. Ascites.
• Development of abdominal wall musculature (wrinkled prune-like appearance in TS).

Older Children

• Presence of abdominal mass. Abdominal or flank tenderness.

 Laboratory Aids

LABORATORY TESTS

Newborn

• Hydronephrosis or hydroureteronephrosis with a normal contralateral kidney does not require any immediate laboratory testing.
• If both kidneys are affected or a solitary kidney is affected, there is a need for serial assessments of renal function (serum electrolytes and creatinine).

Older Children

• Urinalysis to detect hematuria or pyuria. Culture if infection is suspected.
• In cases where both kidneys are affected or there is a solitary kidney, renal function should be evaluated.

IMAGING

Antenatally hydronephrosis

- Infants with antenatally detected hydronephrosis typically are evaluated with three imaging studies:

—Renal/bladder ultrasound
—Voiding cystourethrogram
—Renal scan

- The timing can be elective for a unilateral lesion with a normal contralateral kidney, but if both kidneys are affected or a solitary kidney is involved, then prompt evaluation of the newborn should be undertaken.
- Renal/bladder ultrasound

—Because of a period of relative oliguria of a newborn in the first 24 to 48 hours of life, an ultrasound may underestimate the degree of hydronephrosis during this time and thus should be postponed until the infant is at least 48 hours old. This should not preclude evaluating an infant during this time as long as a study is repeated in 4 to 6 weeks.
—In cases where both kidneys were affected or there is a solitary affected kidney, the evaluation should not be delayed. Ultrasound of the kidneys should reveal the severity of dilation of the renal pelvis and calyces, changes in the amount and echogenicity of the parenchyma, and presence of cortical cysts. The evaluation of the full bladder is important as well. It will show dilated distal ureters, which may indicate a UVJ obstruction, VUR, or hydroureteronephrosis from PUV or TS.

- Voiding cystourethrogram (VCUG)

—Evaluates for the presence of VUR
—Allows for the grading of the severity of reflux as well
—The shape of the bladder, presence of diverticulum, and trabeculations may indicate hypertrophy from PUV, neurogenic bladder dysfunction, or voiding dysfunction (in older children).
—Test can be delayed until after discharge from the nursery unless there is concern about posterior urethral valves, in which case it should be performed in the early postnatal period.

- Renal scan: This study can quantify the differential renal function or the amount each kidney contributes to overall renal function (the normal differential function is 50%+/−5% for each kidney). The two most commonly used radionuclides are 3-mercaptoacetyl triglycine (MAG-3) and diethylenetriamine pentaacetic acid (DTPA). MAG-3 is the best choice for infants and babies. In addition to the ability to detect diminished function, if there is poor drainage of the affected kidney, furosemide is given to wash out the radiotracer. The time for washing out half of the accumulated radiotracer ($T_{1/2}$) is often given in the report. A prompt $T_{1/2}$ (less than 10 minutes) is indicative of a nonobstructed kidney. A slower $T_{1/2}$ may be indicative of obstruction when it is greater than 20 minutes. An intermediate $T_{1/2}$ (10 to 20 minutes) is indeterminate for obstruction. Many factors affect the $T_{1/2}$ making it less reliable for indicating obstruction. These factors include the hydration status, presence of VUR, and the overall function of the kidney (very poorly functioning kidneys have a poor response to diuretics).

- Intravenous pyelogram (IVP)

—This study is most useful for evaluating the anatomy of the kidney and the ureters.
—Also a useful test for evaluating an older child with intermittent symptoms of abdominal or flank pain
—Can be diagnostic of an intermittent UPJ obstruction as the cause of the child's pain

- CT scan: Most commonly done in cases where the hydronephrosis is symptomatic. A noncontrast spiral CT is the most sensitive way to detect stones, as even stones radiolucent on plain films (uric acid) will be detected by CT.
- MRI: Currently has a limited role in evaluating hydronephrosis, but contrast-enhanced MRI is currently being studied as an alternative to renal scans and ultrasound in the evaluation of hydronephrosis.

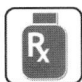 Therapy

- Neonates with hydronephrosis are started on prophylactic antibiotics (1/4 to 1/2 the therapeutic dose given once a day) of amoxicillin. When the baby is 2 months old the antibiotic can be changed to trimethoprim/sulfamethoxazole or nitrofurantoin.
- UPJ obstruction: After initial evaluation, the infants are usually followed with serial studies, either ultrasound or renal scans, depending on the degree of functional impairment, the severity of the hydronephrosis, and the pattern of drainage on the renal scan. Fmore information see Ureteropelvic Junction Obstruction.
- UVJ obstruction: After initial evaluation these children are followed with serial studies as with UPJ obstruction. These lesions are much less common than UPJ obstruction and the majority of the time the affected kidneys have normal function and can be followed conservatively. If the function of the kidney is significantly diminished (differential function of 35%–40%), surgical treatment of the obstruction is indicated.
- Vesicoureteral reflux: Infants with reflux are kept on prophylactic antibiotics. In the absence of breakthrough infections they are reevaluated annually. If persistent high-grade reflux continues or breakthrough infections are a problem, surgical correction is performed. For more information see Vesicoureteral Reflux.
- Ureterocele/ Ectopic ureter: Since these are obstructive lesions, they are generally treated surgically early in life at the time of diagnosis

- Posterior urethral valves (PUV): Full-term infants undergo cystoscopic valve ablation, whereas preterm infants may require a temporary vesicostomy until endoscopic treatment is feasible. These boys require careful follow-up from a pediatric urologist and nephrologist as they grow up. For more information see Posterior Urethral Valves.
- Triad syndrome (TS): Typically these boys will undergo bilateral orchiopexy with or without an abdominoplasty depending on the severity of the hypoplasia of the abdominal wall during the first 6 to 12 months of life.

 Common Questions and Answers

Q: If my baby has hydronephrosis affecting only one kidney, will he need a kidney transplant?
A: In the absence of oligohydramnios and bilateral hydroureteronephrosis, it would be a very rare event that a child would develop renal failure requiring transplantation.

Q: My unborn baby has hydronephrosis in only one kidney, and the other kidney is normal. What are the chances that it is a UPJ obstruction?
A: The chances are about 45% that isolated hydronephrosis will be due to a UPJ obstruction.

Q: My male unborn baby has bilateral hydronephrosis but a "normal" bladder. Is there still a chance that he has PUV?
A: Yes. Although it is less likely to be due to PUV than if a thick-walled, enlarged, poorly emptying bladder were seen, prenatal ultrasonography is operator dependent and can miss dilated ureters or bladder abnormalities.

BIBLIOGRAPHY

Carr MC. Anomalies and surgery of the ureteropelvic junction in children. In: Walsh PC, et al., eds. *Campbell's Urology.* 8th Ed. Philadelphia: WB Saunders, 2002:1995–2006.

Cooper CS, et al. Antenatal hydronephrosis: evaluation and outcome. *Curr Urol Rep* 2002;(3):131–138.

Schlussel RN, Retik AB. Ectopic ureter, ureterocele, and other anomalies of the ureter. In: Walsh PC, et al, eds. *Campbell's Urology.* 8th Ed. Philadelphia: WB Saunders, 2002:2007–2052.

Authors: J. Christopher Austin and Michael C. Carr

Hyperimmunoglobulinemia E Syndrome

 Database

DEFINITION

Hyperimmunoglobulinemia E syndrome is a rare disorder characterized by markedly elevated serum IgE levels, chronic eczematoid dermatitis, and recurrent infections.

PATHOPHYSIOLOGY

The syndrome is poorly understood and the following abnormalities have been noted in subgroups of patients:

- Phagocytic: Impaired chemotaxis
- T cell: Impaired proliferative response to antigens
- B cell: Variable heterogeneity of ability to form antibodies to antigens

GENETICS

- The genetic defect in hyperimmunoglobulinemia E is unknown
- The disorder is inherited in an autosomal dominant manner with incomplete penetrance

 Differential Diagnosis

- Atopic dermatitis
- Wiskott-Aldrich syndrome
- Chronic granulomatous disease

 Data Gathering

HISTORY

- Recurrent infection: Subcutaneous abscesses, pneumonia, pneumatoceles, otitis media, sinusitis
- Organisms that cause infection: *Staphylococcus aureus*, *Candida*, *Haemophilus influenzae*, *Streptococcus pneumoniae*, group A streptococcus
- Severe eczematoid dermatitis as early as 1 week of age
- Delayed shedding of primary teeth

 Physical Examination

- Coarse facial features, prominent forehead, broad nasal bridge, prominent nose
- Growth retardation can occur with recurrent illnesses.
- Osteoporosis complicated by recurrent fractures

 Laboratory Aids

TEST

- Eosinophilia: Peripheral eosinophils, >500 cells/mL
- Quantitative immunoglobulins: IgG, IgA, IgM usually normal, but IgE elevated, usually >5,000 IU/mL
- IgE antibodies against *S. aureus*
- Functional antibodies to diphtheria, tetanus, HIB, and *pneumococcus* results are variable, but there is a subgroup of patients who are unable to mount an appropriate antibody response to these antigens.
- Pulmonary function tests to evaluate extent of lung disease from infections such as pneumatoceles

Therapy

- Supportive, based on clinical and laboratory findings
- Lifelong use of antistaphylococcal therapy (i.e., dicloxacillin or Augmentin at therapeutic doses)
- Surgical intervention for management of pneumatoceles for drainage or secondary to compression of nearby parenchyma
- IVIG as replacement therapy for abnormal functional antibodies is usually given at 400 g/kg on a monthly basis.

 Follow-Up

Long-term outcome is unknown; it depends on a timely diagnosis that allows for close monitoring and aggressive treatment of infections. Sequelae from recurrent infections such as pneumonias and pneumatoceles can result in a debilitating course. An increased chance of malignancy has been reported in some cases.

 Common Question and Answer

Q: Is this disease also referred to as Job syndrome?
A: Yes, because Job suffered from difficulties with boils and other skin manifestations.

ICD-9-CM 279.3 (UNSPECIFIED)

BIBLIOGRAPHY

Buckley RH. The hyper-IgE syndrome. *Clin Rev Allergy Immunol* 2001;20:139–154.

Erlewyn-Lajeunesse MDS. Hyperimmunoglobulin-E syndrome with recurrent infection: A review of current opinion and treatment. *Pediatr Allergy Immunol* 2000;11:133–141.

Lavoie A, Rottern M, Grodofsky MD, et al. Anti-staphylococcus aureus IgE antibodies for diagnosis of hyperimmunoglobulinemia E-recurrent infection syndrome in infancy. *Am J Dis Child* 1989;143:38–104.

Leung DYM, Geha RS. Clinical and immunologic aspects of the hyperimmunoglobulin E syndrome. *Hematol Oncol Clin North Am* 1988;2(1):81–97.

Marone G, Florio G, Triggiani M, et al. Mechanisms of IgE elevation in HIV-1 infection. *Crit Rev Immunol* 2000;20(6):477–496.

Saini SS, MacGlashan D. How IgE upregulates the allergic response. *Curr Opin Immunol* 2002;14(6):694–697.

Sheerin KA, Buckley RH. Antibody response to protein, polysaccharide, and 0x174 antigens of the hyperimmunoglobulinemia E syndrome. *J Allergy Clin Immunol* 1991;87(4):803–811.

Authors: Erin E. McGintee
Michelle M. Klinek, 3rd edition

Hyperinsulinism/Hypoglycemia

 Database

DEFINITION

Hyperinsulinism (HI) is a disorder of dysregulated insulin secretion characterized by excessive and/or inappropriate insulin secretion resulting in hypoglycemia.

CAUSES

Mutations in four genes that lead to defects in early signaling events in beta cells have now been identified in patients with HI: genes coding for either of the two subunits of the beta cell KATP channel (SUR1, sulfonylurea receptor; Kir6.2, inwardly rectifying potassium channel), glucokinase (GK), and glutamate dehydrogenase (GLUD-1). These mutations result in uncoupling of insulin secretion from the glucose-sensing machinery of the pancreatic beta cell, and inappropriate insulin secretion even in the face of low blood glucose. The most common and severe forms of HI arise from SUR1 and/or Kir6.2 mutations, which can manifest in focal or diffuse disease. A transient form of HI has been associated with perinatal stress small for gestational age (SGA) birth weight, maternal hypertension, precipitous delivery, or hypoxia, but the mechanism responsible for this form of HI has not been elucidated.

PATHOLOGY

The histologic appearance of the pancreases from children affected with HI due to mutations in the KATP channel can be subdivided into two major forms:

- Diffuse HI, in which abnormally large islet cell nuclei are found diffusely throughout the pancreas.
- Focal HI, generally easily recognized as a discrete region of adenomatous hyperplasia, with a surrounding normal-appearing pancreas.
- Normal histology can also be found in cases of HI.

GENETICS

- Autosomal recessive mutations of KATP channel genes (SUR1, Kir6.2) at chromosomal locus 11p14–15.1 resulting in diffuse involvement throughout the pancreas (diffuse HI).
- Autosomal dominant mutations of SUR1.
- A nonmendelian mode of inheritance through loss of heterozygosity for maternal 11p and expression of paternally-transmitted KATP channel mutation (either SUR1or Kir6.2) on the paternal allele. The loss of maternally expressed tumor suppressor genes creates the first "hit," and expression of a mutant paternal allele creates the second "hit," resulting in clonal expansion of abnormally regulated beta cells, focal areas of adenomatosis (focal HI).
- Autosomal dominant mutations of glucokinase (GK): Activating mutation in the glucokinase gene.

- Autosomal dominant mutations of glutamate dehydrogenase (GLUD-1): Known as hyperinsulinism/hyperammonemia syndrome due to activating mutations of glutamate dehydrogenase (GDH) enzyme at regulatory guanosine triphosphate (GTP)-binding site.

EPIDEMIOLOGY

- Most common cause of persistent or recurrent hypoglycemia in children beyond the immediate neonatal period.
- Annual incidence estimated at about 1:40,000–50,000 live births.
- May be as high as 1:2,500 in select populations (Saudi Arabians, Ashkenazi Jews).

COMPLICATIONS

- Severe refractory hypoglycemia
- Cognitive deficits, especially short-term memory, visual-motor integration, and arithmetic skills
- Seizures
- Coma
- Permanent brain damage
- Glucose intolerance or frank diabetes mellitus after treatment

PROGNOSIS

- Historically, more than 50% patients sustained severe brain damage from hypoglycemia.
- Today the prognosis is somewhat more favorable, provided hypoglycemia is avoided.
- Glucose intolerance: Diabetes may develop later in life, especially postpancreatectomy.

 Differential Diagnosis

- Sepsis
- Congenital heart disease
- Infant of diabetic mother (IDM)
- Beckwith-Wiedemann syndrome (BWS)
- Panhypopituitarism
- Respiratory distress syndrome
- Erythroblastosis fetalis
- Other inborn errors of metabolism

 Data Gathering

HISTORY

Symptoms of Hypoglycemia in the Infant

- Poor feeding
- Hypotonia
- Lethargy
- Cyanosis
- Tachypnea
- Tremors
- Seizures
- Early-morning irritability that responds to feeding

 Physical Examination

Finding: Macrosomia
Significance: Suggests HI due to mutations in the KATP channel.

Finding: Small for gestational age
Significance: Suggests transient HI.

Finding: Macroglossia, umbilical hernia, visceromegaly
Significance: These findings suggest BWS, making hyperinsulinism less likely

Finding: Normal palate and genitalia
Significance: Cleft palate or micropenis suggests hypopituitarism.

 Laboratory Aids

Finding: Inappropriately elevated insulin level ($>2\ \mu$U/mL on newer assays) at time of hypoglycemia
Significance: Indicates uncoupling of insulin secretion from serum glucose concentration.

Finding: Suppressed levels of free fatty acids and ketones at time of hypoglycemia:

- Free fatty acid level <0.5 mM
- β-Hydroxybutyrate level <1.1 mM

Significance: Indirect signs of excessive insulin action.

Finding: Glycemic response to glucagon (blood sugar rise >30 mg/dL) at time of hypoglycemia
Significance: Sign of inappropriately stored glycogen at time of hypoglycemia (sign of excessive insulin action).

Finding: Suppressed insulin-like growth factor binding protein-1 (IGFBP-1) level
Significance: IGFBP-1 production is inhibited by insulin (sign of excessive insulin action).

Finding: Elevated ammonia levels
Significance: Suggests hyperinsulinism/ hyperammonemia syndrome.

Finding: Normal growth hormone, cortisol, and thyroxine levels
Significance: Excludes hypopituitarism.

Therapy

- The major goal is prevention of brain damage by controlling blood glucose

—Parenteral dextrose infusions to stabilize blood sugar acutely:
  —For an acute hypoglycemic event give a bolus of 2 to 3 mL/kg of 10% dextrose (0.2–0.3g/kg).
  —For maintenance use glucose infusion rates of 8 to 10 mg/kg per minute (some HI patients may need up to 25 mg/kg per minute).
—Supplemental oral or nasogastric/G tube feeds.
—Diazoxide, a suppressant of insulin secretion, at 5 to 15 mg/kg per day divided q12h (most patients with KATP HI do not respond to diazoxide).
—Octreotide, a long-acting somatostatin analog, at 5 to 20 μg/kg per day divided q6h or given by continuous subcutaneous infusion.
—Glucagon, at 1.0 mg per day by continuous intravenous infusion, may stabilize blood glucose levels in preparation for surgery.
—Subtotal pancreatectomy in those children refractory to medical therapy or in those with focal lesions.

- Diet:

—Frequent feedings and avoidance of long fasts.
—Avoidance of protein loads in those with hyperinsulinism/hyperammonemia, as high-protein diets may stimulate insulin secretion.

 ## Follow-Up

- Home blood glucose monitoring, especially with longer fasts or intercurrent illnesses.
- Hospitalizations for intravenous glucose infusions may be necessary during intercurrent illnesses with vomiting.
- Follow-up fasting studies may be needed to evaluate safety and/or disease regression.
- Close observation of linear growth is necessary, because octreotide can suppress GH secretion.

 ## Common Questions and Answers

Q: What is the chance of hyperinsulinism in the sibling of an affected child?
A: Twenty-five percent in the autosomal-recessive type; as high as 50% in the autosomal-dominant type.

Q: How low and for how long can glucose go before brain damage occurs?
A: The definition of hypoglycemia has been the subject of controversy in pediatrics but activation of glucose counterregulatory systems occurs when blood glucose levels reach the 65 to 70 mg/dL range; symptoms of hypoglycemia present at the 50 to 55 mg/dL level and cognitive dysfunction occurs when blood glucose levels are in the 45 to 50 mg/dL range. Taking these data into account blood glucose concentration should be maintained greater than 60 mg/dL. The duration of hypoglycemia necessary for brain damage to occur is unknown.

Q: What is the chance that it will eventually resolve without surgery?
A: Only approximately 40%–50% of cases are controlled with medication alone. Patients with mutations in SUR1 and/or Kir6.2 genes may be more likely to require surgery, and in those patients with focal disease, surgery may be curative.

ICD-9-CM 251.1

BIBLIOGRAPHY

De Lonlay P, Fournet J-C, Rahier J, et al. Somatic deletion of the imprinted 11p15 region in sporadic persistent hyperinsulinemic hypoglycemia of infancy is specific of focal adenomatous hyperplasia and endorses partial pancreatectomy. *J Clin Invest* 1997;100: 802–807.

Dunne MJ, et al. Hyperinsulinism in infancy: from basic science to clinical disease. *Physiol Rev* 2004;84:239–275.

Ferry RJ, Kelly A, Grimberg A, et al. Insulin responses to peripheral intravenous and intrahepatic arterial calcium stimulation in diffuse vs. focal forms of congenital hyperinsulinism due to mutations of the SUR1 sulfonylurea receptor. *J Pediatr* 2000;137: 239–246.

Glaser B, Kesavan P, Heyman M, et al. Familial hyperinsulinism caused by an activating glucokinase mutation. *N Engl J Med* 1998;338(4):226–230.

Grimberg A, Ferry RJ, Kelly A, et al. Dysregulation of insulin secretion in children with congenital hyperinsulinism due to sulfonylurea receptor mutations. *Diabetes* 2001;50:322–328.

Nestorowicz A, Inagaki N, Gonoi T, et al. A nonsense mutation in the inward rectifier potassium channel gene, Kir6.2, is associated with familial hyperinsulinism. *Diabetes* 1997;46:1743–1748.

Stanley CA, Baker L. Hyperinsulinism in infants and children: Diagnosis and therapy. *Adv Pediatr* 1976;23:315–355.

Stanley CA, Lieu YK, Hsu BY, et al. Hyperinsulinism and hyperammonemia in infants with regulatory mutations of the glutamate dehydrogenase gene. *N Engl J Med* 1998;338:1352–1357.

Stanley CA. Hyperinsulinism in infants and children. *Pediatr Clin North Am* 1997;44:363–374.

Suchi M, et al. Histopathology of congenital hyperinsulinism: retrospective study with genotype correlations. *Pediatr Dev Pathol* 2003;6(4):322–333.

Thornton PS, Satin-Smith MS, Herrold K, et al. Familial hyperinsulinism with apparent autosomal dominant inheritance: clinical and genetic differences from the autosomal recessive variant. *J Pediatr* 1998;132:9–14.

Weinzimer SA, Stanley CA, Berry GT, et al. A syndrome of congenital hyperinsulinism and hyperammonemia. *J Pediatr* 1997;130: 661–664.

Authors: Diva D. De León and SA Weinzimer

Hyperlipidemia

 Database

DEFINITION

Elevations of serum cholesterol, triglycerides, and lipoprotein. Total cholesterol consists of very low-density lipoprotein (VLDL), low-density lipoprotein (LDL), and high-density lipoprotein (HDL).

- Normal serum concentrations:

—Total cholesterol: 170 mg/dL (borderline, 170–199 mg/dL)
—LDL cholesterol: 110 mg/dL (borderline, 110–129 mg/dL)
—Total triglycerides: 100 mg/dL (borderline, 100–140 mg/dL)

- Primary hypercholesterolemia or hypertriglyceridemia (hyperlipidemia): Elevation in serum cholesterol as a result of an inherited disorder of lipid metabolism (i.e., familial hypercholesterolemia)
- Secondary hypercholesterolemia or hypertriglyceridemia: Elevation in serum cholesterol as a result of another disease process (i.e., nephrotic syndrome)

PATHOPHYSIOLOGY

Primary Hypercholesterolemia

- Familial hypercholesterolemia (FH): Defect of LDL receptor, resulting in the body's inability to properly utilize circulating LDL cholesterol
- Familial hypertriglyceridemia (FHTG): A severe elevation in serum triglycerides; can be associated with lipoprotein lipase deficiency or apolipoprotein C-II deficiency

GENETICS

- Familial hypertriglyceridemia (FHTG): Dominantly inherited disorder
- Familial hypercholesterolemia (FH): Dominantly inherited defect of LDL receptor
- Familial combined hyperlipidemia (FCHL): Dominantly inherited lipid disorder

EPIDEMIOLOGY

The incidence of familial hypercholesterolemia homozygotes is 1 in 1,000,000; heterozygotes, 1 in 500, with unknown cause resulting in hypercholesterolemia and/or hypertriglyceridemia occurring in 2% of the population

COMPLICATIONS

Hypercholesterolemia has been linked to:

Premature coronary artery disease and vascular disease.
Severe hypertriglyceridemia can cause pancreatitis.

Autopsy studies demonstrate that early coronary atherosclerosis or precursors of atherosclerosis often begins in childhood and adolescence and are related to high serum total cholesterol levels, LDL-cholesterol plus very low-density lipoprotein-cholesterol levels and low high-density lipoprotein levels. Significant atherosclerotic vessel disease can occur in the first decade of life in children with homozygous familial hypercholesterolemia.

PROGNOSIS

- Familial hypercholesterolemia:

—Homozygotes: Coronary artery disease in first or second decade of life
—Heterozygotes: 50% of males develop premature heart disease by age 50 (females, age 60)

- Familial combined hyperlipidemia: Occurs in 1%–2% of the population and accounts for 10% of all premature heart disease. A reduction of LDL cholesterol by 1% reduces risk by 2%.
- Children and adolescents with high cholesterol levels are more likely than the general population to have high levels as adults.

 Differential Diagnosis

- Hypercholesterolemia

—Primary hypercholesterolemia (see above)
—Hypothyroidism
—Nephrotic syndrome
—Liver disease (cholestatic)
—Renal failure
—Anorexia nervosa
—Acute porphyria
—Myelomatosis
—Medications (antihypertensives, estrogens, steroids, microsomal enzyme inducers, cyclosporine, diuretics)
—Pregnancy
—Dietary: Excessive dietary intake of fat, cholesterol and/or calories

- Hypertriglyceridemia

—Primary hypertriglyceridemia (see above)
—Acute hepatitis
—Nephrotic syndrome
—Chronic renal failure
—Medications (diuretics, retinoids, oral contraceptives)
—Diabetes mellitus
—Alcohol abuse
—Lipodystrophy
—Myelomatosis
—Glycogen storage disease
—Dietary: Excessive dietary intake of fat and/or calories

 Data Gathering

HISTORY

Question: Is there a family history of premature heart disease? Is there occurrence of premature heart disease and hyperlipidemia in parents and grandparents?

Significance: Almost all cases of primary hyperlipidemia are of dominant inheritance.

Question: Does your child smoke?
Significance: Smoking reduces HDL cholesterol levels and increases the risk of vascular disease.

Question: Does your daughter use oral contraceptives?
Significance: Birth control pills have been shown to cause elevations in lipoprotein levels and, when coupled with already elevated lipid levels, can increase the risk of atherosclerosis.

Question: Does your child exercise regularly?
Significance: Lower levels of cholesterol and triglycerides are generally found in children and adolescents who are physically fit.

 Physical Examination

- Eye examination:

—Arcus corneae: Deposits of cholesterol, resulting in a thin, white circular ring located on the outer edge of the iris

- Skin examination:

—Tendon xanthomas: Thickened tissue surrounding the Achilles and extensor tendons
—Xanthelasma: Yellowish deposits of cholesterol surrounding the eye
—Palmar xanthomas: Pale lines in creases of palms
—Eruptive xanthomas: Characteristic of hypertriglyceridemia; papular yellowish lesions with a red base that occur on the buttocks, elbows, and knees.

 Laboratory Aids

TESTS

- Fasting serum lipoprotein levels: Total cholesterol, HDL cholesterol, and triglycerides

—Determine the type of hyperlipidemia

- Calculated LDL cholesterol: LDL cholesterol = total cholesterol − [HDL cholesterol + triglycerides/5]

—Determines the level of LDL cholesterol

- Chemistry panel (ALT, AST, Bili, BUN, creatinine, urinalysis)

—Screening test for liver and kidney disease

- Thyroid evaluation (T4, TSH)

—Determines the presence of hypothyroidism

- Three-day diet history

—Evaluates dietary intake of calories and cholesterol with 3-day diet

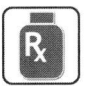 Therapy

GENERAL MEASURES

Outpatient management unless secondary hyperlipidemia caused by liver or renal failure, which would necessitate inpatient management of primary illness. Note: The cause of secondary hyperlipidemia should be treated with disease-specific therapy to reduce elevated lipid levels.

FOR PRIMARY HYPERLIPIDEMIA

It is recommended that once a lipoprotein analysis is obtained, it should be repeated so that an average LDL-cholesterol level can be calculated.

Risk Assessment and Treatment

1. Acceptable LDL-cholesterol level (<110 mg/dL): Provide education on the eating pattern recommended for all children and adolescents and on other risk factors; repeat lipoprotein analysis in 5 years.
2. Borderline LDL-cholesterol (110 to 129 mg/dL): Provide advice about risk factors for cardiovascular disease; initiate the American Heart Association Step-One diet and other risk factor intervention; reevaluate in 1 year.
3. High LDL-cholesterol (130 mg/dL): Examine for secondary causes (thyroid, liver, and renal disorders) and familial disorders, screen all family members, initiate Step-One diet, followed by the Step-Two diet, if necessary.

—Step-One diet: 30% and no less than 20% of calories from total fat; less than 10% of total calories from saturated fat; 10% of calories from polyunsaturated fat; and no more than 300 mg per day of cholesterol.
—If after 3 months does not result in a lower LDL-cholesterol level to the acceptable range, the Step-Two diet should be prescribed.
—Step-Two diet: Requires careful planning and no more than 30% and no less than 20% of calories from total fat; less than 7% of total calories from saturated fat; 10% of
—calories from polyunsaturated fat; and no more than 200 mg per day of cholesterol.

RISK FACTORS

The following are factors that contribute to heart disease:

- Cigarette Smoking
- Severe obesity (95th percentile weight for height)
- Elevated blood pressure
- Diabetes mellitus
- Low HDL cholesterol (<35 mg/dL)
- Physical inactivity
- Family history of premature coronary heart disease, cerebrovascular disease or occlusive peripheral vascular disease (onset before 55 years of age in a parent, grandparent, siblings or siblings of a parent)

DRUG THERAPY

Drug therapy should be considered only for children more than 10 years of age after an adequate trial of diet therapy (for 6 to 12 months) and whose LDL-cholesterol level remains at 190 mg/dL or whose LDL-cholesterol level remains at 160 mg/dL and there is a family history of premature cardiovascular disease (55 years of age) or two or more other risk factors are present in the child or adolescent after vigorous attempts have been made to control these risk factors.
The recommended drugs for the treatment of hypercholesterolemia and high LDL-cholesterol levels in children are: Bile acid sequestrants cholestyramine and colestipol.
Other therapies include:

- Statin group of drugs—Pravachol, lovastatin, Zocor etc. (HMG-CoA reductase inhibitor)—is an effective drug in adults and may prove to be beneficial in children in the future. Side effects include hepatitis and myositis.
- Niacin in megavitamin doses has been effective in the reduction of both serum LDL cholesterol and triglycerides; however, side effects occur in more than 50% of individuals, including flushing, itching, and headache.
- Experimental gene therapy has been shown to be effective in an animal model for familial hypercholesterolemia. Investigational therapy

 Follow-Up

For patients with primary hyperlipidemia who are off medication, follow-up should be performed every 1 to 2 years with lipoprotein profile evaluation. For those patients on medication, follow-up should be conducted every 3 months.

PREVENTION

- General measures:
- Fat intake is unrestricted prior to 2 years of age. After age 2, limit foods high in saturated fats (< 10% of calories per day), cholesterol (<300 mg per day), and trans-fatty acids. Limit salt intake to <6 g per day and intake of sugar.
- Two complementary approaches are recommended:
- The population approach aims to lower the average level of blood cholesterol in all children and adolescents through population-wide changes in nutrient intake and eating patterns. Goals are as follows:

—An overall healthy eating pattern
—Appropriate body weight
—Desirable lipid profile
—Desirable blood pressure
—No new initiation of cigarette smoking
—No exposure to environmental tobacco smoke
—Complete cessation for those who smoke
—Be physically active every day

—Reduce sedentary time (e.g., television watching, computer, video games, or time on the phone)

- The individualized approach aims to lower cholesterol in children and adolescents at high risk of future cardiovascular disease.

—Screen children and adolescents whose parents or grandparents were found to have at or before 55 years of age:
—Coronary atherosclerosis documented myocardial infarction (MI)
—Sudden cardiac death
—Angina pectoris
—Cerebrovascular disease
—Peripheral vascular disease
—Angina pectoris or cholesterol level of 240 mg/dL or higher.

POSSIBLE COMPLICATIONS

- Hypercholesterolemia

—Premature heart disease
—Stroke
—Carotid artery disease

- Hypertriglyceridemia

—Pancreatitis

Clinical Pearls

Serum total cholesterol is inaccurate when serum triglycerides are greater than 400 mg/dL.
Hypertriglyceridemia is associated with falsely lowered serum Na.

ICD-9-CM 272.4

BIBLIOGRAPHY

American Academy of Pediatrics, Committee on Nutrition. Cholesterol in childhood. *Pediatrics* 1998;101(1):141–147.

Kavey RE, et al. American Heart Association guidelines for primary prevention of atherosclerotic cardiovascular disease beginning in childhood. *J Pediatr* 2003;142(4):368–372.

Lauer RM, Sanders SP. Pediatric issues and diseases. *Am Heart J* 2001;142(2):224–228.

Shamir R, Lerner A, Fisher EA. Hypercholesterolemia in children. *Isr Med Assoc J* 2000;2(10):767–771.

Sinaiko AR, et al. End points for cardiovascular drugs trials in pediatric patients. *Am Heart J* 2001;142(2):229–232.

Valente AM, et al. Hyperlipidemia in children and adolescents. *Am Heart J* 2001;142(3):433–439.

Author: Ruben W. Cerri.

Hypertension

Database

DEFINITION

Hypertension is average systolic and/or diastolic blood pressures above the 95th percentile for age and gender as defined by the Second Task Force on Blood Pressure Control in Children. References now include norms based on the patient's age, gender and height percentile. The final determination should be based on at least three measurements obtained on separate occasions. The significance of this definition with regard to morbidity and mortality is unclear.

PATHOPHYSIOLOGY

Hypertension is either primary (essential) or secondary. Secondary causes, with examples, include:

- Renal: Acute glomerulonephritis, chronic renal failure, polycystic kidney disease, reflux nephropathy
- Renovascular: Fibromuscular dysplasia, neurofibromatosis, vasculitis
- Cardiac: Coarctation of the aorta
- Endocrine: Pheochromocytoma, neuroblastoma, glucocorticoid-remediable aldosteronism
- Neurologic: Increased intracranial pressure, Guillain-Barré syndrome
- Drugs: Corticosteroids, oral contraceptives, sympathomimetics, illicit drugs (cocaine, phencyclidine)
- Other: Obesity, burns, traction

GENETICS

Primary hypertension is more likely to develop in individuals when there is a strong family history. The genetics of secondary causes depend on the condition (e.g., polycystic kidney disease: Autosomal dominant, autosomal recessive; neurofibromatosis: Autosomal dominant; glucocorticoid-remediable aldosteronism: Autosomal dominant).

EPIDEMIOLOGY

Primary hypertension is the most common cause of hypertension in adolescents and adults. Various rates of hypertension in children have been reported, from 1.2%–13%, but less than 1% appears to require medication. African American adults have a greater incidence of hypertension. Differences in children, however, are not seen until after age 12. Tracking (i.e., determining the risk of hypertension based on earlier blood pressure measurements) is not reliable in children.

COMPLICATIONS

- Congestive heart failure
- Renal failure
- Encephalopathy
- Retinopathy

PROGNOSIS

The patient's prognosis depends on the underlying cause of the hypertension. It is excellent if the blood pressure is well controlled.

Differential Diagnosis

The initial objective after diagnosing hypertension in children is distinguishing primary from secondary causes. Generally, the younger the child and the more elevated the blood pressure measurements, the more likely the cause of hypertension is secondary.

Data Gathering

HISTORY

Question: Is there a family history of hypertension?
Significance: Several causes of hypertension are familial.

Question: Do you have symptoms of headache or blurry vision?
Significance: These are signs of hypertensive emergency.

Question: Do you have chest pain?
Significance: This may indicate hypertensive heart disease or decreased coronary blood flow.

Question: Do you have epistaxis or unusual weight gain or loss?
Significance: These are other signs of hypertension.

Question: Do you have flushing?
Significance: Flushing may be a sign of pheochromocytoma.

Question: Do you have a history of urinary tract infections?
Significance: Infections can be associated with reflux nephropathy and hypertension.

SPECIAL QUESTIONS

- Medical history: Umbilical artery line, urinary tract infection
- Medications: Corticosteroids, cold preparations, oral contraceptives, illicit drugs
- Family history: Hypertension, phakomatosis, endocrinologic disorders
- Trauma: AV fistula, traction
- Review of symptoms: Other systemic diseases

Physical Examination

- Body habitus: Thin, obese, growth failure, virilized, stigmata of Turner or Williams syndrome
- Skin: Café-au-lait spots, neurofibromas, rashes, acanthosis (suggestive of the metabolic syndrome)
- Head: Moon facies
- Eyes: Funduscopic changes, proptosis
- Lungs: Rales
- Heart: Rub, gallop, murmur
- Abdomen: Mass, hepatosplenomegaly, bruit
- Genitalia: Ambiguous, virilized
- Neurologic: Bell palsy

Laboratory Aids

TESTS

Ambulatory blood pressure monitoring may be helpful in cases where the diagnosis of hypertension is uncertain (white-coat hypertension, labile hypertension).
The laboratory evaluation to determine the etiology of hypertension should proceed in a stepwise fashion.

- All patients should have:

—Urinalysis, urine culture
—Serum electrolytes, BUN, creatinine, calcium, uric acid, cholesterol
—CBC
—Echocardiogram: The most sensitive study to monitor end-organ changes
—Renal ultrasound

- Further evaluation, based on history, physical examination, and/or to prove secondary causes, includes:

—Voiding cystourethrogram
—DMSA renal scan
—Urine or plasma for catecholamines and metanephrines
—Plasma renin activity
—Aldosterone levels

- More invasive studies include:

—Renal angiogram
—Renal vein renin concentrations
—MIBG (metaiodobenzylguanidine) scan
—Renal biopsy
—Genetic studies to identify rare causes of hypertension (Liddle syndrome, glucocorticoid remedial hyperaldosteronism)

Therapy

- Mild primary hypertension may be managed with nonpharmacologic treatment: Weight reduction, exercise, sodium restriction, avoidance of certain medications such as pseudoephedrine.
- Pharmacologic therapy should be directed to the cause of secondary hypertension when this is known or for severe, sustained hypertension. Medications may be needed in children with mild-to-moderate hypertension if nonpharmacologic therapy has failed or if end-organ changes are present.
- Classes of antihypertensive agents include α- and β-blockers, diuretics, vasodilators (direct and calcium-channel blockers), angiotensin converting enzyme (ACE) inhibitors and angiotensin receptor blockers.
- Other specific therapies include surgery (renovascular hypertension, coarctation of the aorta), percutaneous transluminal angioplasty (renovascular hypertension), and dialysis (chronic renal failure).

 Follow-Up

The reduction of blood pressure with medication should be gradual to avoid side-effects. The medications themselves cause adverse effects, such as exercise intolerance (β-blockers), headaches (vasodilators), renal insufficiency (ACE inhibitors), and hypokalemia (diuretics). Certain classes of medication should be avoided in patients with specific conditions, such as asthma and diabetes (β-blockers) and renal artery stenosis (ACE inhibitors).

PITFALLS

- Use the proper cuff size. The inflatable bladder should completely encircle the arm and cover approximately 75% of the upper arm. A cuff that is inappropriately small will artifactually increase the measurement.
- ACE inhibitors and β-blockers alter plasma renin activity levels.
- Several medications, such as labetolol, can affect an MIBG scan.
- Avoid multiple medications with the same mechanism of action.
- Elicit a history of adverse effects and adjust medications accordingly.
- If patients feel the medication is making them feel ill, they will discontinue it themselves.
- Attempt to wean medication intermittently.

 Common Questions and Answers

Q: What is the value of ambulatory blood pressure monitoring?
A: This device is similar to a Holter monitor and measures blood pressures over a 24-hour period while the patient is awake and asleep. By reviewing the blood pressures one can determine if a significant proportion of readings are elevated and whether or not the normal dip in pressures during sleep is seen. Thus conditions such as "white coat" hypertension can be verified or disputed.

Q: What percentage of children have renovascular causes for their hypertension?
A: Studies looking at the etiology of hypertension indicate that 10% to 24% of children may have a renovascular cause. Children under 5 years of age are 4 times more likely to have renal artery stenosis than are adolescents.

Q: What are the indications for invasive studies such as angiography?
A: This decision should be individualized and based on the severity of the hypertension, response to medication, the clinical presentation (e.g., neurofibromatosis), and results of other studies. In general, young children and all children with severe, unexplained hypertension should be completely evaluated.

Q: Can adolescents with elevated blood pressure compete in sports?
A: Adolescents with hypertension should be encouraged to participate in athletics if their blood pressures are well controlled. The use of stress testing in this population is controversial.

Q: Do I need to worry about systolic hypertension?
A: Recent studies in adults have shown that sustained systolic hypertension may be just as dangerous as diastolic hypertension.

ICD-9-CM 401.9 (UNSPECIFIED)

BIBLIOGRAPHY

Bartosh SM, Aronson AJ. Childhood hypertension. An update on etiology, diagnosis, and treatment. *Pediatr Clin North Am* 1999;46:235–252.

Fivush B, Neu A, Firths, et al. Acute hypertensive crises in children: emergencies and urgencies. *Curr Opin Pediatr* 1997;9:233–236.

Lucksted EF. Cardiac risk factors and participation guidelines for youth sports. *Ped Clin North Am* 2002;49:681–707.

Nehal US, Ingelfinger JR. Pediatric hypertension: recent literature. *Curr Opin Pediatr* 2002;14(2):189–196.

Rosner B, Prineas RJ, Loggie JMH, et al. Blood pressure nomograms for child and adolescents by height, sex, and age in the United States. *J Pediatr* 1993;123:871–876.

Roth CG, et al. Evaluation of the hypertensive infant: a rational approach to diagnosis. *Radiol Clin North Am* 2003;41(5):931–944.

Sorof J. Obesity hypertension in children: a problem of epidemic proportions. *Hypertension* 2002;40(4):441–447.

Author: Seth L. Schulman

Hypoparathyroidism

Database

DEFINITION

Hypoparathyroidism is decreased parathyroid hormone (PTH) effect.

PATHOPHYSIOLOGY

• Diminished or absent PTH activity results in:

—Hypocalcemia and hyperphosphatemia
—Reduced vitamin D activation to $1,25(OH)_2$-vitamin D
—Hypocalcemia leads to increased neural excitability.

• Hypoparathyroidism

—Transient
—Fetal parathyroid suppression: Maternal hypercalcemia, diabetic mother
—Hypomagnesemia: Direct effects (suppressed PTH secretion, increased PTH resistance)
—Alcohol intoxication
—Congenital
—Familial: X-linked recessive, autosomal dominant, autosomal recessive
—Sporadic and isolated
—DiGeorge syndrome: Parathyroid gland hypoplasia, thymic hypoplasia/aplasia, facial abnormalities, aortic arch and cardiac defects

• Acquired

—Postsurgical
—Postirradiation
—Following severe burns
—Type 1 polyglandular autoimmune disease (Blizzard syndrome): Hypoparathyroidism associated with chronic mucocutaneous candidiasis and autoimmune adrenal insufficiency; can also have diabetes mellitus, lymphocytic thyroiditis, hypogonadism, pernicious anemia, chronic hepatitis
—Iron deposition: Thalassemia, hemochromatosis
—Copper deposition: Wilson disease
—Metastatic carcinoma
—Miliary tuberculosis

• Pseudohypoparathyroidism: Resistance to PTH

—Albright hereditary osteodystrophy: G protein mutation

GENETICS

• X-linked recessive: Neonatal onset
• Autosomal-dominant and autosomal-recessive forms

—Chromosome 3q13: Mutations in the calcium-sensing receptor gene
—Chromosome 6p23–24: Homozygous loss of function of GCMB gene (transcription factor required for parathyroid gland embryology)
—Chromosome 11p: Mutations in the PTH gene
—Chromosome 22q11: DiGeorge syndrome
—Chromosome 21q22: Type 1 polyglandular autoimmune disease
—Chromosome 20q13: Albright hereditary osteodystrophy

• Mitochondria diseases: Kearns-Sayre syndrome (progressive external ophthalmoplegia before age 20 years and pigmentary retinal degeneration, frequently with other organ system involvement including cardiac, neurologic, and hypoparathyroidism)

EPIDEMIOLOGY

Many normal neonates can have hypocalcemia (serum calcium less than 8 mg/dL) during the first 3 weeks of life due to physiologic transient hypoparathyroidism.

• Parathyroid gland immaturity can lead to deficient PTH release and exaggerated normal fall in serum calcium concentration during the first 3 days of life.
• Relative immaturity of renal phosphorus handling and response to PTH can lead to late neonatal hypocalcemia precipitated by a high phosphate diet (cow's milk–based formulas).

COMPLICATIONS

• Hypocalcemia can cause tetany, arrhythmias, seizures, and respiratory arrest.
• Long-standing untreated hypoparathyroidism and pseudohypoparathyroidism can lead to intracranial calcifications, especially in the basal ganglia. These may cause extrapyramidal signs (e.g., chorioathetosis, dystonic spasms, parkinsonism). Cognitive impairment and psychiatric disturbances can also be seen.
• Untreated hypoparathyroidism can also lead to dilated cardiomyopathy, that improves with restoration of normocalcemia.

PROGNOSIS

Fair; long-term outcome: development of nephrocalcinosis resulting in renal insufficiency

Differential Diagnosis

HYPOCALCEMIA

• Vitamin D deficiency
• Vitamin D-dependent rickets type I and II
• Hyperphosphatemia
• Prematurity
• Acute pancreatitis
• Malignancy: Osteoblastic metastases, tumor lysis syndrome
• Medication: Citrated blood products, phenobarbital, Dilantin, phosphate

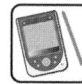
Data Gathering

HISTORY

• In neonates: Maternal calcium and magnesium abnormalities, maternal diabetes
• Family history of calcium disorders
• Medications
• Recurrent infections
• Recurrent muscle cramps
• Paresthesias

Physical Examination

• Chvostek sign: Facial nerve stimulation (tapping anterior of external auditory meatus) causes contraction of orbicularis oris, producing upper lip or mouth twitch.
• Trousseau sign: Inflation of blood pressure cuff reduces the blood flow to peripheral motor nerves and thereby can elicit carpopedal spasm in latent tetany.
• Carpopedal spasm
• Laryngeal stridor
• Mental status changes
• Irritability
• Papilledema
• Cataracts
• Bradycardia, hypotension
• Dry skin, coarse hair, brittle nails
• Albright hereditary osteodystrophy (pseudohypoparathyroidism type Ia): short stature, round face, thick face, barrel chest, obesity, subcutaneous calcifications, brachydactyly (short 4th metacarpal bones)

Laboratory Aids

TESTS

Laboratory Tests

• Total and ionized serum calcium concentrations: Low
• Serum phosphorus concentration: Elevated in hypoparathyroidism; low in rickets
• Serum magnesium concentration: Rule out hypomagnesemia
• Albumin: Assess calcium binding (if cannot get ionized calcium)
• Intact PTH levels
• 25-OH- and $1,25(OH)_2$-vitamin D levels: Distinguish hypoparathyroidism from rickets
• Urinary calcium-to-creatinine ratio: Low in idiopathic hypoparathyroidism, higher (almost equal to normocalcemic controls) in calcium ion-sensing receptor gain-of-function mutations
• Urinary cyclic AMP response to PTH: Diagnostic test if concerned about pseudohypoparathyroidism; otherwise, not routinely done

Imaging

- Chest x-ray: Rachitic rosary (rickets), absence of thymus (DiGeorge syndrome)
- Head CT: Intracranial calcifications are associated with chronic hypoparathyroidism and pseudohypoparathyroidism

False Positives

- Hypomagnesemia

Therapy

DRUGS

Titrate therapy to maintain serum calcium concentrations greater than 8.0 mg/dL. In cases requiring lifelong therapy, compromise for serum calciums in the 8- to 9-mg/dL range to decrease the long-term risk for developing nephrocalcinosis.

- $1,25(OH)_2$-vitamin D: Less than 1 year: 0.04 to 0.08 μg/kg per day; 1 to 5 years: 0.25 to 0.75 μg per day; greater than 6 years and adults: 0.5 to 2 μg per day.
- Calcium: Dose depends on preparation and on patient needs.
- A recent 3-year trial of synthetic human PTH-(1–34) in patients aged 18 to 70 years was promising, but it is dosed as twice daily subcutaneous injections.

DIET

Unrestricted

Follow-Up

Regularly with the endocrinologist

WHEN TO EXPECT IMPROVEMENT

Immediately

SIGNS TO WATCH FOR

- Patients with acute, severe hypocalcemia should be placed on telemetry to monitor for cardiac arrhythmias (especially prolonged QTc).
- Muscle cramps
- Carpopedal spasms
- Seizures

Common Questions and Answers

Q: Is the thyroid also involved?
A: No.

Q: Are seizures common?
A: Yes, seizures are a common presentation of hypoparathyroidism in childhood, and physiologic transient hypoparathyroidism is the most common cause of neonatal seizures.

Q: Can hypoparathyroidism be associated with other abnormalities?
A: Yes. Investigate neonates at the time of diagnosis for cardiac defects and thymic aplasia (DiGeorge syndrome), and monitor patients with hypoparathyroidism for development of other autoimmune endocrinopathies and chronic mucocutaneous candidiasis (type 1 polyglandular autoimmune disease).

Q: When should IV versus oral calcium supplementation be used?
A: IV calcium supplementation provides the quickest correction of hypocalcemia and is therefore useful in severe cases (seizures, stridor, tetany, cardiac arrhythmias) or in the initiation of therapy (as you await establishment of adequate vitamin D levels, which are necessary for enteral calcium absorption). Switch to oral calcium supplementation as soon as possible to reduce the risk of potential IV calcium-mediated venous sclerosis and tissue extravasation.

ICD-9-CM 252.1

BIBLIOGRAPHY

Betterle C, Greggio NA, Volpato M. Clinical review 93: autoimmune polyglandular syndrome type 1. *J Clin Endocrinol Metab* 1998;83:1049–1055.

Cuneo BF, Driscoll DA, Gidding SS, et al. Evolution of latent hypoparathyroidism in familial 22q11 deletion syndrome. *Am J Med Genet* 1997;69:50–55.

Eronocodelu Y, Bober E, Tunnessen W Jr. Picture of the month. Albright hereditary osteodystrophy. *Arch Pediatr Adolesc Med* 1997;151:1263–1264.

Guise TA, Mundy GR. Evaluation of hypocalcemia in children and adults. *J Clin Endocrinol Metab* 1995;5:1473–1478.

Klein GL, Langman CB, Herndon DN. Persistent hypoparathyroidism following magnesium repletion in burn-injured children. *Pediatr Nephrol* 2000;14:301–304.

Kowdley KV, Coull BM, Orwoll ES. Cognitive impairment and intracranial calcification in chronic hypoparathyroidism. *Am J Med Sci* 1999;317:273–277.

Levine MA. Pseudohypoparathyroidism: from bedside to bench and back. *J Bone Miner Res* 1999;14:1255–1260.

Marx SJ. Hyperparathyroid and hypoparathyroid disorders. *N Engl J Med* 2000;343:1863–1875.

Thakker RV. Genetic developments in hypoparathyroidism. *Lancet* 2001;357:974–976.

Thomusch O, et al. The impact of surgical technique on postoperative hypoparathyroidism in bilateral thyroid surgery: a multivariate analysis of 5846 consecutive patients. *Surgery* 2003;133:180–185.

Winer KK, et al. Long-term treatment of hypoparathyroidism: a randomized controlled study comparing parathyroid hormone-(1–34) versus calcitriol and calcium. *J Clin Endocrinol Metab* 2003;88:4214–4220.

Yamamoto M, Akatsu T, Nagase T, et al. Comparison of hypocalcemic hypercalciuria between patients with idiopathic hypoparathyroidism and those with gain-of-function mutations in the calcium-sensing receptor: is it possible to differentiate the two disorders? *J Clin Endocrinol Metab* 2000;85:4583–4591.

Author: Adda Grimberg

Hypoplastic Left Heart Syndrome

 Database

DEFINITION

Hypoplastic left heart syndrome (HLHS) is a continuum of congenital cardiac defects resulting from severe underdevelopment of the structures of the left side of the heart: Left atrium, mitral valve, left ventricle, aortic valve, and ascending aorta.

PATHOPHYSIOLOGY

The etiology of HLHS appears multifactorial, most likely resulting from an in utero reduction of left ventricular inflow or outflow (mechanisms postulated include premature closure of the foramen ovale and fetal cardiomyopathy). As a result, the right ventricle (RV) must supply both the pulmonary and systemic (via the ductus arteriosus) circulations before and after birth. The reduction in pulmonary vascular resistance that occurs with lung expansion at birth reduces the proportion of RV output to the systemic circulation. If the ductus arteriosus closes, shock may occur.

GENETICS

- Familial inheritance:

—Sibling recurrence risk (0.5%), although rare kinships have a frequency approaching autosomal-dominant transmission.
—Other forms of congenital heart disease (CHD) (13.5%)

- Male predominance (67%)
- Definable genetic disorder (10%–28%)

—Turner syndrome, Noonan syndrome, Smith-Lemli-Opitz syndrome, Holt-Oram syndrome
—Trisomy 13, 18, 21, or other microdeletion syndromes
—Major extracardiac anomalies (diaphragmatic hernia, omphalocele)

EPIDEMIOLOGY

- 0.16 to 0.36 per 1,000 live births
- 8% of CHD; third most common cause of critical CHD in the newborn
- 23% of all neonatal mortality from CHD

COMPLICATIONS (NEONATAL PRESENTATION)

—Circulatory collapse with resultant metabolic acidosis
—Multiorgan system failure (i.e., necrotizing enterocolitis, renal failure, liver failure, central nervous system injury)

PROGNOSIS

- Fatal if untreated (95% mortality within the first month of life)
- In the current era, HLHS is often diagnosed prenatally and improved outcomes may result from early diagnosis and prevention of the presentation as neonatal shock.
- 90% early survival after stage I palliation if treated in a timely fashion at experienced institutions
- 5% mortality at stage II hemi-Fontan (bidirectional cavopulmonary) procedure
- Recently, 1% mortality at Fontan operation (with the addition of a fenestration to allow right-to-left shunting)
- Excluding infants that die waiting for a donor organ, the 5-year actuarial survival for either staged palliation (Fontan) or heart transplantation is similar, approximately 75%.

 Differential Diagnosis

- Cardiac: Other causes of circulatory collapse in the neonate include critical aortic stenosis and coarctation of the aorta, cardiomyopathy (infectious, metabolic, or hypoxic), intrauterine supraventricular tachycardia, obstructive cardiac neoplasms, and large arteriovenous fistulae.
- Noncardiac: Neonatal septicemia, respiratory distress syndrome

 Data Gathering

HISTORY

- Respiratory distress (tachypnea, grunting, flaring, retractions)
- Cyanosis
- Cardiovascular collapse and profound metabolic acidosis when the ductus closes

 Physical Examination

- Congestive heart failure (tachycardia, hepatomegaly, gallop)
- Normal S1 and single S2 (A2 absent), a murmur of tricuspid regurgitation may be auscultated
- Varying degrees of cyanosis
- Decreased perfusion and weak peripheral pulses

 Laboratory Aids

- Chest radiograph: Varying degree of cardiomegaly with increased pulmonary vascular markings (if the atrial septum is intact, lungs will appear hazy with a pulmonary venous obstructive pattern)
- Electrocardiogram: Right axis deviation (+90 to +210 degrees), right ventricular hypertrophy with a qR pattern in the right precordial leads, decreased left ventricular forces with an rS pattern in the left precordial leads
- Echocardiogram: Varying degrees of hypoplasia or atresia of the mitral valve, left ventricle, aortic valve, ascending aorta, and aortic arch; patent ductus arteriosus with right-to-left shunt in systole and diastolic flow reversal; atrial septal defect with left-to-right flow
- Cardiac catheterization: No longer routinely performed; similar findings as with echocardiography

 Therapy

MEDICAL

- The preoperative goal is to balance the systemic and pulmonary circulations provided by the right ventricle to a Qp/Qs (ratio of pulmonary to systemic blood flow) of approximately 1:1, usually achieved with a pulse oximetry measurement of 75%.
- Prostaglandin E1 infusion: 0.05 to 0.1 μg/kg per minute
- Aggressive treatment of metabolic acidosis with fluid boluses, bicarbonate, and/or THAM
- .21 FiO_2, goal PaO_2 of 35 to 40 mm Hg
- Careful use of small amounts of inotropic agents (in cases of sepsis or RV failure). Aggressive use of inotropic agents (alpha effect) may worsen systemic perfusion.

SURGICAL

• Palliative surgery is generally performed in three stages:

—Stage I (Norwood) palliation (performed in the first few days of life or soon after presentation): Involves transection of the main pulmonary artery with anastomosis of the augmented aortic arch to the pulmonary valve stump to form a neoaortic valve and arch; placement of an aorta-to-pulmonary artery shunt (modified Blalock-Taussig shunt) and often an atrial septectomy. The RV continues to provide both systemic and pulmonary blood flows. The oxygen saturations after this procedure are usually approximately 75%.

—Hemi-Fontan procedure: Involves anastomosis of the superior vena cava to the pulmonary artery, resulting in volume unloading of the RV. All prior shunts are usually removed. The oxygen saturations after this procedure are usually 85%–90%.

—Modified-Fontan procedure: Baffling the inferior vena cava to the pulmonary artery with placement of a small fenestration in the baffle, permitting a small residual right-to-left shunt. The RV is now supplying only systemic blood flow. The oxygen saturations after this procedure are usually 90%–95%.

• There are many surgical modifications on these three procedures. In addition, these procedures may be performed at different ages based on an institution's experience. Our approach has been to perform the hemi-Fontan operation at 4–6 months of age and the Fontan operation at 18 months to 2 years of age.

• Orthotopic heart transplantation may be performed either as an initial approach or after a stage I palliation.

SUPPORTIVE

While surgical intervention has become the medical standard, supportive measures are sometimes offered especially when multiple noncardiac congenital anomalies exist, or when severe multiorgan system damage is present.

 Follow-Up

Interval pediatric evaluations should include careful consideration of growth parameters, cardiovascular symptoms, and developmental milestones. Examinations should focus on the presence or absence of cyanosis, edema, pleural effusions, diarrhea, ascites and arrhythmias. For Fontan patients, frequent echocardiograms and intermittent cardiac catheterizations may be needed to assess for:

• RV dysfunction
• Aortic arch obstruction
• Branch pulmonary artery narrowing
• Venous collateral formation causing increased cyanosis
• Protein-losing enteropathy
• Sinus node dysfunction
• Atrial arrhythmias

For patients treated alternatively with heart transplantation, other lifelong issues should be addressed as follows:

• Graft rejection and/or coronary vasculopathy
• Infection
• Hypertension
• Lymphoproliferative disease

 Follow-Up

• Lifelong subacute bacterial endocarditis (SBE) prophylaxis (high-risk category).
• Digoxin and furosemide are generally administered until the hemi-Fontan.
• Afterload reduction (i.e., angiotensin converting enzyme inhibitors) may be used to reduce the workload on the heart at any stage.
• Antiplatelet (i.e., aspirin) and anticoagulant (i.e., Coumadin) therapies are used by most physicians after stage 1 and later in the setting of the low-flow state of the cavopulmonary connection.

For transplant patients, immunosuppressive regimens are managed differently according to institution preferences.

PITFALLS

During initial resuscitation and stabilization of a newly diagnosed infant:

• Avoid using oxygen despite low pulse oximetry saturation. Increasing FiO_2 will lower pulmonary vascular resistance and increase blood flow to the lungs, which are already "overcirculated," shunting blood away from the systemic circulation and worsening systemic perfusion.
• Avoid overventilating the infant. Carbon dioxide is a pulmonary vasoconstrictor and may improve systemic perfusion by decreasing pulmonary perfusion. Maintain mildly elevated $PaCO_2$ levels (40–50 mm Hg).

ICD-9-CM 746.7

BIBLIOGRAPHY

Freedom RM, et al. Hypoplastic Left Heart Syndrome. In: Allen HD, Clark EB, Gutgesell HP, Driscoll DJ, eds. *Heart Disease in Infants, Children and Adolescents.* 6th Ed. Philadelphia: Lippincott Williams and Wilkins, 2001: 1011–1025.

Mahle WT, Clancy RR, McGaurn SP, et al. Impact of prenatal diagnosis on survival and early neurologic morbidity in neonates with the hypoplastic left heart syndrome. *Pediatrics* 2001;107(6):1277–1282.

Stamm C, et al. Long-term results of the lateral tunnel Fontan operation. *J Thorac Cardiovasc Surg* 2001;121:28–41.

Tworetzky W, McElhinney DB, Reddy VM, et al. Improved surgical outcome after fetal diagnosis of hypoplastic left heart syndrome. *Circulation* 2001;103(9):1269–1273.

Author: Michael P. Mulreany

Hypospadias

 Database

DEFINITION

Hypospadias is the incomplete development of the anterior urethra due to a failure of the urethral folds to unite over and cover the urethral groove.

GENETICS

- Increased incidence in monozygotic twins (8.5-fold that in singletons).

—Reported mutations include defects in the androgen receptor, 5α-reductase II defects, alterations in homeobox genes, although these are found only in a minority of patients.

ETIOLOGY

- Polygenic/multifactorial
- Higher familial incidence
- Proposed theories include:

—Estrogenic environmental contamination
—Pressure of the fetal limbs on developing penis
—Insufficient HCG in placenta
—Abnormality in androgen metabolism as a local manifestation of a systemic endocrinopathy

EPIDEMIOLOGY

- 1/250 to 1/300 live male births

—Incidence
—With affected father: 8%
—With affected brother: 14%
—With 2 or more affected family members: 21%

- Unexplained increase in incidence since the 1970s
- Higher prevalence in Italian and Jewish populations

 Differential Diagnosis

- Ambiguous genitalia, namely severely masculinized female pseudohermaphroditism

HISTORY

- Important to inquire about

—Other affected family members
—Other congenital anomalies

- Increased incidence of cryptorchidism, inguinal hernia

—May be associated with an enlarged utricle, complicating urethral catheter placement.

 Physical Examination

- Incomplete foreskin
- Distal urethral pit on glans
- Chordee (ventral curvature of penis)

—Localize meatal position by pulling outward on ventral penile shaft skin. Record position as glanular; coronal; distal, middle, or proximal shaft; penoscrotal; or perineal
—Important to document position of testes

 Laboratory Aids

- Karyotype in patients with bilateral undescended testes and hypospadias, may also be obtained in cases of unilateral undescended testis and hypospadias.

IMAGING

- If there is a question of ambiguous genitalia, pelvic ultrasound or cystography may be indicated.
- There is no need for imaging in cases of routine, isolated hypospadias.

Therapy

- If the patient has a very small penis, he may benefit from hormonal stimulation preoperatively.

—Surgical repair is usually performed in the first year of life.
—Mild glandular hypospadias may not need surgery.
—Type of repair depends on position of meatus and degree of chordee.
  —Tubularized incised plate
  —Meatal advancement
  —Onlay island flap
  —Tubularized island flap
—90% success rate for all one-stage repairs
—Potential complications include
  —Urethrocutaneous fistula
  —Urethral diverticulum
  —Urethral stricture
  —Unacceptable cosmetic outcome

 ## Follow-Up

- Compressive dressing for 2 days, removed by parents at home
- Indwelling urethral catheter/stent remains for about 2 weeks
- Postoperative visit at 2 weeks to remove catheter

PITFALLS

Newborn circumcision is absolutely contraindicated

 ## Common Questions and Answers

Q: Does the patient with hypospadias routinely have other anatomic problems?
A: No. The majority of patients with hypospadias have no other problems.

Q: Why is there no need for routine imaging?
A: These studies have been done and show that without symptoms or problems, patients with hypospadias have no other congenital problems.

ICD-9-CM 752.61

BIBLIOGRAPHY

Baskin L. Hypospadias and urethra development. *J Urol* 2000;163:951.

Fisch M. Urethral reconstruction in children. *Curr Opin Urol* 2001;11(3):253–255.

Kelalis P, King K, Belman A, et al, eds. *Clinical Pediatric Urology*. Philadelphia: WB Saunders, 1992:619–652.

Authors: Michele Clement and Douglas Canning

Idiopathic Thrombocytopenic Purpura

Database

DEFINITION
Idiopathic thrombocytopenic purpura (ITP) is a syndrome characterized by:
- Isolated thrombocytopenia (platelet count <100,000/mm^3)
- Shortened platelet survival
- Presence of circulating platelet autoantibodies
- Increased number of megakaryocytes in the bone marrow
- Acute ITP resolves (platelet count >150,000/mm^3) within 6 months after diagnosis, without relapse
- Chronic ITP is defined by persistent thrombocytopenia (<150,000/mm^3) greater than 6 months after initial presentation.
- Recurrent ITP exhibits an intermittent pattern of thrombocytopenia after an initial recovery to normal count.

PATHOLOGY/PATHOPHYSIOLOGY
- Thrombocytopenia results from increased destruction of antibody-coated platelets by phagocytic cells in the reticuloendothelial system, particularly the spleen.
- It is hypothesized that antibodies generated in response to foreign antigen or drug cross-react with platelet membrane glycoproteins (most commonly IIb/IIIa and Ib/IX).
- Compensation for platelet destruction occurs by increased platelet production from megakaryocytes in the bone marrow. Typical bone marrow aspirate shows increased numbers of immature megakaryocytes.

EPIDEMIOLOGY
- ITP is the most common acquired platelet disorder of childhood.
- Incidence is approximately 4 per 100,000 children per year (<15 years of age).
- Greater than 80% of childhood ITP is acute.
- Males and females equally affected in childhood ITP (female:male ratio is 3:1 in adult and chronic ITP).
- Median age at diagnosis is 4 years (range: 2 to 10 years for acute ITP). Children younger than 1 year or older than 10 years are more likely to develop chronic ITP.

COMPLICATIONS
- Intracranial hemorrhage (ICH) is a rare but often fatal event in acute ITP. It occurs in approximately 1 per 1,000 cases.
- Platelet count at time of ICH always below 20,000/mm^3 in published literature (80% of cases below 10,000/mm^3); may be spontaneous without antecedent trauma
- Traditionally thought to occur early in disease course, but more recently shown to occur at any time
- Mucosal bleeding from nose, gums, lower gastrointestinal tract, or kidneys is not uncommon.
- Hematemesis and melena are rare. Menorrhagia may be severe.
- Retinal hemorrhage is rare.

PROGNOSIS
- Acute ITP: 60% of children will have a normal platelet count in 3 months, 90% at 1 year from diagnosis.
- Chronic ITP is more difficult and resistant to treat and therefore has an increased risk of bleeding complications. Platelet count tends to be higher at 40,000–80,000/mm^3. Remissions can continue to occur many years after diagnosis (predicted spontaneous remission rate—61% after 15 years).
- Cannot predict who will resolve acute ITP and who will persist with chronic ITP.
- Patients with chronic ITP must be evaluated for secondary ITP associated with underlying diseases such as systemic lupus erythematosus, HIV infection, or Evans syndrome.

Differential Diagnosis

- Destructive thrombocytopenias (normal or increased megakaryocytes in marrow)
- Immunologic: ITP, infection (HIV, CMV, EBV, VZV, parvovirus B19), drug-induced, post-transfusion purpura, autoimmune hemolytic anemia (Evans syndrome), lymphoproliferative disorders, SLE, hyperthyroidism
- Nonimmunologic: Microangiopathic hemolytic anemia, hemolytic-uremic syndrome, DIC, thrombotic thrombocytopenic purpura, Kasabach-Merritt syndrome (giant hemangioma), cardiac defects (left ventricular outflow obstruction, prosthetic heart valves, repaired intracardiac defects), malignant hypertension
- Impaired or ineffective production (decreased or absent megakaryocytes in marrow)
- Marrow infiltrative processes (leukemias, myelofibrosis, lymphomas, neuroblastoma, other solid tumor metastases, osteopetrosis, storage diseases), drug- or radiation-induced aplastic anemia, nutritional deficiency states (iron, folate, vitamin B12), viral-induced suppression (e.g., hepatitis, EBV, HIV), thrombocytopenia absent radii (TAR) syndrome, Fanconi anemia, trisomy 13 and 18, Bernard-Soulier syndrome, Wiskott-Aldrich syndrome, May-Hegglin anomaly, inherited thrombocytopenias (X-linked or AD), metabolic disorders (e.g., methylmalonic acidemia)
- Clumping of platelets in the laboratory or giant platelets can artificially decrease a machine-generated platelet count. Review the smear to confirm.

Data Gathering

HISTORY
- Onset is acute in an otherwise well child, sometimes with overnight development of bruising, petechiae, and purpura without history of trauma. Not associated with pallor, fatigue, weight loss, or persistent fevers.
- Half of cases are preceded by a viral infection 1 to 3 weeks before onset (particularly varicella; also EBV, CMV)
- Ask about unusual bruising, rashes (petechiae or purpura), blood in urine or stool, epistaxis, gum bleeding with tooth brushing, and any change in neurologic status.
- Recent immunizations, especially MMR vaccine
- Drug history focusing on drugs with antiplatelet effects (e.g., ASA, seizure medications, heparin)
- Evidence of other autoimmune diseases (e.g., rheumatoid or collagen vascular symptoms, thyroid disease, hemolytic anemia)
- Family history is usually negative for bleeding disorders. Inquire about autoimmune disease in the family.

SPECIAL QUESTIONS
Risk factors for HIV should be elicited, because ITP-like thrombocytopenia may be a presentation of HIV in children.

Physical Examination

- Clusters of petechiae or large bruises readily apparent on skin.
- Purpura in the oropharynx and dried blood or clots in the nares.
- The physical examination should otherwise be normal.
- Consider other diagnoses if there is pallor, jaundice, adenopathy, bone pain, arthritis, or organomegaly (mild splenomegaly may occur in 5%–10%)
- A funduscopic examination should be performed on all patients (retinal hemorrhage)

Laboratory Aids

TESTS
Diagnosis based on isolated thrombocytopenia with no other abnormal laboratory values or physical signs (other than bleeding).

- CBC shows thrombocytopenia with a normal WBC count and hemoglobin (mild anemia in proportion to amount of blood loss).
- Mean platelet volume (MPV) is typically increased.
- Peripheral blood smear should always be reviewed to differentiate platelet clumps from true thrombocytopenia. The few platelets present on smear are large. Smear is otherwise normal, with no red-cell fragmentation, no spherocytes, and no blasts.
- Platelet counts are frequently less than 20,000/mm^3 (tend to be >30,000/mm^3 in chronic ITP).
- PT and PTT are normal. Bleeding time would be prolonged, but testing is unnecessary.
- A direct antiglobulin test (DAT) to exclude coexisting autoimmune RBC hemolysis (Evans syndrome).
- ANA in subset of patients for whom causes of thrombocytopenia other than acute childhood ITP must be ruled out: Including older girls, patients with chronic ITP, and with suspicion of autoimmune disease.
- HIV testing if risk factors are identified
- Need for bone marrow aspirate is controversial. It is safe to perform with a low platelet count.

- Bone marrow aspirate is indicated if anemia, abnormal WBC counts, leukemic blasts on peripheral smear, organomegaly, jaundice, or lymphadenopathy is present.
- Most hematologists examine bone marrow before initiating corticosteroids or if child fails to remit within 2 to 3 weeks (with or without treatment).
- Marrow shows normal to increased numbers of megakaryocytes with otherwise normal morphology and cellularity.
- Assays for platelet-associated antibodies (either direct or indirect) are not established as clinically useful.
- Demonstration of platelet-associated IgG may be useful in more complicated patients in whom chronic ITP is a possible diagnosis.

 ## Therapy

Which patients need treatment remains controversial. Though the eventual duration of ITP in children is not affected by therapy, the platelet count can often be increased rapidly to a safer level by treatment. Guidelines put forth by the American Society of Hematology recommend treatment for:

- Any patient with life-threatening bleeding
- Any patient with a platelet count less than 10,000/mm^3 with minor or "wet" purpura should be hospitalized and treated.
- Any patient with a platelet count of 10,000–20,000/mm^3 plus "wet" purpura should be treated.
- Active toddlers or children at risk for trauma are usually treated.
- Medical treatment interferes with the antibody-mediated platelet clearance and raises platelet counts acutely, but does not alter the long-term course.
- Observation alone is acceptable for older children without serious bleeding and in whom adequate supervision and follow-up are assured.
- Avoid medications that affect platelet function, such as aspirin, ibuprofen, and cold medications with antihistamines.
- Precautions to prevent trauma: Limited activity, helmet and pads around bed.
- Parental education should be for signs and symptoms of acute ICH and ICP.

CHOICE OF THERAPY FOR ACUTE ITP
- Corticosteroids: 80% respond with platelet counts over 20,000/mm^3 by 72 hours.
—Oral prednisone at 2 mg/kg per day tapered over 2 to 4 weeks is a typical course.
—Advantages: Ease of dosing (oral, outpatient) and low cost.
—Side effects: Moodiness, increased appetite, weight gain, hypertension.
—Disadvantage: Most pediatric hematologists require a bone marrow aspirate before steroid therapy is begun to exclude leukemia.
—Prolonged steroid treatment has serious side effects.
- Intravenous immunoglobulin G (IVIgG): 94%–97% of children will have a rise in platelet count >20,000/mm^3 by 72 hours with IVIgG.

—The usual dose is 0.8 to 1 g/kg over 6 to 8 hours, and often repeated if slow or no response.
—Advantages: Faster time to platelet count over 20,000/mm^3 (24 hours); marrow aspirate may be deferred.
—Disadvantages: high cost, long infusion time, allergic reactions, 10%–30% have evidence of aseptic meningitis with severe headache and stiff neck, 50%–75% have headache, nausea, vomiting, or fever.
- Premedicate with acetaminophen and diphenhydramine.
- Anti-Rh D immunoglobulin (Win-Rho): Rh D immunoglobulin coats Rh D-positive erythrocytes and causes an immune clearance of the antibody-coated autologous red blood cells (transient hemolysis); blocking Fc receptors of splenic macrophages prolongs the survival of platelets in ITP.
—Platelet count typically rises after 48 hours.
—Patient must be Rh(+) and nonsplenectomized.
—Dose is 50 to 75 μg/kg IV over 3 to 5 minutes.
—Advantages: Anti-D is less expensive than IVIgG but more costly than steroids.
—Lower rate of allergic side effects (10%) than IVIgG and does not cause aseptic meningitis.
—Disadvantages: Mild hemolysis with a transient hemoglobin decrease of 1 to 3 g/dL.

CHOICE OF THERAPY FOR CHRONIC ITP
In general, children with chronic ITP have few bleeding manifestations, and observation alone is often justified.
- Splenectomy: Approximately 60% of patients will respond with complete remission. No presurgical predictors of response have been found.
—Disadvantages: Surgical morbidity and risk of postsplenectomy sepsis with encapsulated organisms (management should include vaccination against *Haemophilus influenzae*, pneumococcus, and meningococcus, and lifelong prophylactic penicillin).
- Medical therapy: IVIG, corticosteroids, anti-D immunoglobulin, immunosuppressives (azathioprine, cyclophosphamide, cyclosporine), vincristine, danazol, and monoclonal anti-Fc receptor have been used.
—Plasmapheresis and staphylococcal protein A column adsorption for antibody removal have been used with limited success in refractory cases.

LIFE-THREATENING HEMORRHAGE
The goal is to stop bleeding. Transfused platelets are destroyed like native platelets but may help with hemostasis. IVIG may be given concomitantly. Multimodality therapy is frequently necessary during life-threatening hemorrhage. Emergent splenectomy is sometimes necessary. Plasmapheresis may also be beneficial.

 ## Follow-Up

- Spontaneous recovery is the norm (60% by 3 months, 80% by 6 months, and 90% by 1 year). The incidence of significant

bleeding-related morbidity and mortality is extremely low (<5%).
- Of patients with chronic ITP, 50%–60% eventually stabilize without need for ongoing therapy or need for splenectomy. Spontaneous resolution of thrombocytopenia can occur as long as 10 to 20 years after diagnosis.

 ## Common Questions and Answers

Q: Why aren't platelet transfusions used to increase the platelet count?
A: Transfused platelets are rapidly consumed and no increase in platelet count is observed.

Q: Will the ITP recur after another viral infection?
A: Only a minority of recovered patients have recurrence in the setting of a viral illness.

Q: How should activities be limited until the platelet count returns to normal?
A: A common sense approach to activities for children with low platelet counts is to avoid any activity in which one foot is not on the ground at all times (e.g., bicycle riding, swinging, jungle gym). Also, avoid all contact sports.

Q: How often should platelet counts be obtained?
A: Initially, quite frequently to follow the response to therapy and until count is >20,000/mm^3 and stable. Thereafter, get counts during times of high risk of relapse (e.g., after steroid taper) and monthly until a normal platelet count is consistently seen. After resolution, platelet counts only for clinical suspicion of recurrent thrombocytopenia.

Q: Can IVIgG or anti-Rh D immunoglobulin be given repeatedly if the platelet count falls as the treatment wears off (4–5 weeks)?
A: Yes. Some patients with chronic ITP have received monthly IVIG for years without problems. Steroids also may be resumed if there is a fall in the platelet count.

ICD-9-CM 287.3

BIBLIOGRAPHY
Blanchette V, Carcao M. Approach to the investigation and management of immune thrombocytopenic purpura in children. *Semin Hematol* 2000;37:299–314.

Bolton-Maggs PHB. Idiopathic thrombocytopenic purpura. *Arch Dis Child* 2000;83:220–222.

Bussel JB. Fetal and neonatal cytopenias: what have we learned? *Am J Perinatol* 2003;20(8):425–431.

Chong BH, Keng TB. Advances in the diagnosis of idiopathic thrombocytopenic purpura. *Semin Hematol* 2000;37:249–260.

De Matta D, et al. Acute childhood idiopathic thrombocytopenic purpura: AIEOP consensus guidelines for diagnosis and treatment. *Haematologica* 2000;85:420–424.

Maslanka K, et al. Long-term outcome of splenectomy for immune thrombocytopenic purpura. *Am J Hematol* 2004;75(2):117–118.

Authors: Don Eslin
Jane E. Minturn, 3rd edition

Immunoglobulin A Deficiency

 Database

DEFINITION

Patients are considered IgA deficient if they have a serum IgA less than 5 mg/dL and a normal serum IgG and IgM, and they are older than 1 year.

PATHOPHYSIOLOGY

Increased incidence of the following:

- Atopy
- Sinopulmonary infections
- Gastrointestinal infections (especially *Giardia lamblia*)
- Crohn disease
- Ulcerative colitis
- Sprue
- Autoimmune illnesses

—Arthritis
—Lupus
—Immune endocrinopathies
—Autoimmune hematologic conditions

- Chronic active hepatitis

GENETICS

Most commonly autosomal-dominant mode of inheritance with variable expressivity, but the following rare associations also occur:

- 18q syndrome
- Partial deletions in the long or short arm, and ring forms of chromosome 18
- Also associated with: HLA-A1, HLA-A2, B8, and Dw3.

EPIDEMIOLOGY

The prevalence is approximately 1 in 500 in the normal population.

COMPLICATIONS

Increased incidence of the following:

- Respiratory tract infections
- Gastrointestinal tract infections
- Atopy

PROGNOSIS

Survival into the seventh decade is common.

 Differential Diagnosis

- Toxic, environmental, drugs

—Penicillamine and anticonvulsants can induce IgA deficiency.

- Genetic/metabolic

—X-linked agammaglobulinemia (Bruton)
—Common variable immune deficiency
—Severe combined immune deficiency
—Ataxia telangiectasia
—DiGeorge syndrome
—Chronic mucocutaneous candidiasis
—Nezelof syndrome
—Selective IgG2 deficiency

- Miscellaneous

—Patients may be completely healthy and IgA deficiency may be an incidental finding.

- Common causes: May be the result of decreased synthesis or impaired differentiation of IgA B lymphocytes into IgA plasma cells

 Data Gathering

HISTORY

Question: Does the patient have frequent sinopulmonary infections?
Significance: Patients with IgA deficiency can have frequent sinopulmonary infections.

Question: Does the patient have frequent gastrointestinal infections?
Significance: Patients with IgA deficiency can have frequent gastrointestinal infections.

Question: Does the patient have allergies?
Significance: Patients with IgA deficiency tend to be allergic.

Question: Does the patient have any autoimmune diseases?
Significance: Patients with IgA deficiency have an increased incidence of autoimmune diseases.

Question: Can healthy patients have IgA deficiency?
Significance: Approximately 30% of patients with IgA deficiency are completely healthy.

 Physical Examination

The physical examination should look for signs of recurrent infection and atopy.

Finding: Cobblestoning of the conjunctiva
Significance: Cobblestoning of the conjunctiva is caused by allergic inflammation in the eyes. Allergies are associated with IgA deficiency.

Finding: Allergic shiners
Significance: Allergic shiners are the result of allergies. Allergies are associated with IgA deficiency.

Finding: Serous otitis media
Significance: Serous otitis may be the result of recurrent ear infections. Increased ear infections can be seen in IgA deficiency. Furthermore, serous otitis media can be secondary to allergies, which is also associated with IgA deficiency.

Finding: Pain on palpation of the sinuses
Significance: Recurrent sinus infections are associated with IgA deficiency.

Finding: Pneumonia
Significance: An increased frequency of pneumonia is associated with IgA deficiency.

Finding: Swollen joints
Significance: An increased frequency of autoimmune diseases are associated with IgA deficiency.

Immunoglobulin A Deficiency

 ## Laboratory Aids

GENERAL GOAL

Decide whether the patient's complaints are consistent with IgA deficiency (frequent upper respiratory and gastrointestinal infections, or allergies).

—Measure serum IgA level.
—If the patient is IgA deficient, exclude other conditions associated with IgA deficiency.

Test: Serum IgA level
Significance: A patient is considered deficient if the serum IgA level is less than 5 mg/dL.

Test: Total immunoglobulins
Significance: If normal, this study would help rule out X-linked agammaglobulinemia (Bruton), common variable immunodeficiency, and severe combined immunodeficiency.

Test: IgG subclasses
Significance: This study would help rule out an associated IgG2 subclass deficiency.

Test: Lymphocyte mitogens
Significance: This is a functional lymphocyte study. If normal, this study would help rule out common variable immunodeficiency, severe combined immunodeficiency, ataxia telangiectasia, DiGeorge syndrome, and Nezelof syndrome.

Test: Lymphocyte *Candida* antigen stimulation
Significance: No response to *Candida* in vivo is consistent with chronic mucocutaneous candidiasis.

Issues for Referral

Factors that may help alert you to make a referral include:

- Suggestion that IgA deficiency may be part of a more complex immune deficiency. An allergist/immunologist can assist with an appropriate immunologic evaluation.
- IgA deficiency associated with autoimmune disease. Evaluation and treatment by a rheumatologist would be indicated.
- Patient likely to need a blood transfusion. There is an increased incidence of anaphylaxis to IgA-containing blood products when administered to IgA-deficient patients. The allergist can help select appropriate blood products for these patients.

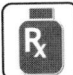 ## Therapy

There is no specific drug therapy.

- Recurrent infections should be treated aggressively with broad-spectrum antibiotics.
- Antibiotic prophylaxis to prevent recurrent sinopulmonary infections is often indicated.
- Intravenous gamma globulin is not indicated.

CONFLICTS WITH OTHER TREATMENTS

Patients with IgA deficiency may develop antibodies against IgA in transfused blood products. These patients are at risk for anaphylactic (or anaphylactoid) transfusion reactions. To avoid these reactions, these patients may receive packed red blood cells (only if these cells have been washed 3 times), or they may receive plasma products from IgA-deficient donors, or they may receive autologous banked blood.

 ## Follow-Up

Patients should be observed for:

—Sinopulmonary infections
—Gastrointestinal infections
—Autoimmune diseases
—Inflammatory bowel disease

Note: It is important to manage infectious complications aggressively, and to intervene promptly when the associated conditions present.

 ## Common Questions and Answers

Q: What is the recurrence risk for a couple with an affected child?
A: It depends on the mode of inheritance. Most commonly, the mode of inheritance is autosomal dominant and the risk would be 50%. However, the expressivity is variable and the patient's phenotype may not be that of an IgA-deficient person.

Q: Does the patient take any medications?
A: IgA deficiency can be induced by some anticonvulsants and by penicillamine.

Q: Should IgA patients wear medical alert bracelets?
A: Yes. These patients can have anaphylaxis if administered blood products containing IgA. In an emergency situation, this is important information for the caregivers to know.

BIBLIOGRAPHY

Burrows PD, Cooper MD. IgA deficiency. *Adv Immunol* 1997;65:245–276.

Rankin EC, Isenberg DA. IgA deficiency and SLE: prevalence in a clinic population and a review of the literature. *Lupus* 1997;6(4):390–394.

Smith CA, Driscoll DA, Emanuel BS, et al. Increased prevalence of immunoglobulin A deficiency in patients with the chromosome 22q11.2 deletion syndrome (DiGeorge syndrome/velocardiofacial syndrome). *Clin Diagn Lab Immunol* 1998;5:415–417.

Authors: Mathew Fogg
Christopher A. Smith, 3rd edition

Imperforate Anus

Database

DEFINITION

Imperforate anus is a congenital abnormality whereby the bowel fails to perforate or only partially perforates the pelvic muscular floor and/or the epidermal covering.

CAUSES

Not determined

PATHOLOGY

• The hindgut comes in contact with the cloacal membrane during the sixth week of fetal development. At this time, the hindgut is divided into a ventral urogenital and dorsal rectal component. By the eighth week, the dorsal half perforates to the exterior. In imperforate anus, the process is arrested during this critical period.
• There are many anatomic variants of imperforate anus. From the prognostic point of view, the most important is classification, distinguishing two main types: supralevator (high) and translevator (low). Separate is a group of cloacal malformations in which the urinary genital and digestive systems drain to a common channel that communicates with the perineum.
• A fistula communicating from the gut to the urogenital system or to the external opening is present in 90% of cases. In females, most commonly the fistula leads to the opening in the posterior fourchette of the vagina (in low lesions) or to the upper vagina (in high lesions). In males, the fistula leads to the raphe of the scrotum (in low lesions) or to the urethra (in high lesions).

GENETICS

• Imperforate anus can be an isolated defect or part of the syndrome or association.
• Syndromic disorders that contain imperforate anus are associated with defects on chromosomes 6, 7, 10, and 16.

EPIDEMIOLOGY

Incidence is estimated between 1 in 3,000 to 1 in 9,000. High lesions are more common in males (2:1). Low lesions occur with equal frequency in both sexes.

COMPLICATIONS

• Other anomalies are present in one-third of patients with an imperforated anus.
• Imperforate anus can be associated with vertebral and cardiac anomalies, tracheoesophageal fistula and, renal and limb anomalies (VACTERL).
• Other anomalies associated with imperforate anus include intestinal atresia, malrotation, omphalocele, annular pancreas, urologic anomalies, spinal anomalies, duplicate uterus, septate vagina, vaginal atresia, and absence of rectal muscles.

PROGNOSIS

Continence can be attained in 90% if patients have low lesions. Less than 50% of patients with high lesions are continent before school age, but most of them continue to improve and achieve continence by adolescence.

Differential Diagnosis

There are no disorders that can mimic imperforate anus. The task is to define the location of the termination of the bowel and the opening of the fistula.

Data Gathering

HISTORY

• A majority of children are diagnosed in the first days of life by abnormal findings on physical examination.
• Failure to pass meconium, a history of constipation, and signs of low intestinal obstruction (abdominal distention and vomiting) should mandate reexamination of the perianal area.

Physical Examination

- Lesion presents as either no opening, an inadequate caliber of anus, or an anterior malposition of the opening.
- Physician should attempt to localize the opening of the fistula and look for associated anomalies.
- Evaluation for lumbosacral neurologic function should be done. Anal wink can usually be elicited, because a vertiginous external anal sphincter is present in a majority of the cases.

Laboratory Aids

TESTS

- Invertogram: After sufficient time for a transit of gas (>12 hours after birth), the child is placed in an upside-down position for 3 minutes, after which a lateral view of the pelvis is obtained.
- Lumbosacral films to evaluate for vertebral anomalies.
- An MRI of the spine should be considered to look for a tethered cord.
- Renal ultrasound, voiding cystoureterogram, and IVP can be used to evaluate for urinary tract anomalies.

Therapy

- Surgery should be performed by an experienced surgeon.
- High lesions require an emergent diverting colostomy and pull-through procedure with a Pena midsagittal anorectoplasty at 3 to 9 months of age. The colostomy is closed after the anoplasty has healed and any necessary secondary dilations have been completed.
- Complications of surgery include stricture of the anocutaneous anastomosis, rectourinary fistula, mucosal prolapse, constipation, and incontinence.

Common Questions and Answers

Q: Is this an isolated defect in my child?
A: Often, imperforate anus can be associated with multiple other anomalies and not necessarily isolated. Renal and vertebral anomalies must be excluded.

Q: What is the genetic basis for this defect?
A: Imperforate anus can be associated with chromosomal anomalies or can be an isolated problem.

BIBLIOGRAPHY

Bill AH, Hatch EI. Neonatal obstruction of the intestinal tract: patterns and management. In: Kelley VC, ed. *Practice of Pediatrics.* Philadelphia: Harper & Row, 1987:27–32.

Chen CJ. The treatment of imperforate anus: experience with 108 patients. *J Pediatr Surg* 1999;34(11):1728–1732.

Javid PJ, Barnhart DC, Hirschl RB, et al. Immediate and long-term results of surgical management of low imperforate anus in girls. *J Pediatr Surg* 1998;33(2):198–203.

Jona JZ. Advances in neonatal surgery. *Pediatr Clin North Am* 1998;45(3):605–617.

Pena A, Hong A. Advances in the management of anorectal malformations. *Am J Surg* 2000;180(5):370–376.

Authors: Andrew E. Mulberg and Gregorz Telega

Impetigo

 Database

DEFINITION

- Impetigo is a bacterial skin infection of the superficial layers of the epidermis characterized by honey-colored, crusted patches or bullae with a central crust.
- It has two clinical varieties: Nonbullous impetigo (impetigo contagiosa), the most prevalent form, and bullous impetigo (staphylococcal impetigo).

CAUSES

- Nonbullous impetigo: Group A beta-hemolytic streptococcus, *Staphylococcus aureus,* or both are the causative agents. Previously, group A streptococcus was the most common bacterium associated with nonbullous impetigo, but now *S. aureus* is the most common.
- Bullous impetigo: *S. aureus* is almost always the causative agent. The formation of bullae is mediated by production of an epidermolytic toxin.

PATHOPHYSIOLOGY

- Bacteria invades areas of the skin that are not intact.
- In early lesions, histology shows vesicopustular formation in the subcorneal region of the epidermis. The blister cavity is larger in the bullous than in the nonbullous form. Neutrophils are present within the cavity.
- A serous crust and neutrophilic debris overlying a superficially eroded epidermis may be seen in later stages on histopathologic evaluation.

EPIDEMIOLOGY

- The most common bacterial skin infection in children.
- Transmitted by direct contact
- Highly contagious and rapidly disseminated through day care centers and school
- Fomites can be a source of infection.
- Associated with crowding, which often is present in socioeconomically disadvantaged populations.
- Incidence is greatest during the summer when there is common close contact between children.

COMPLICATIONS

Nonhematogenous spread may result in:

- Cellulitis
- Lymphangitis
- Scarlet fever
- Acute poststreptococcal glomerulonephritis
- Exacerbation of guttate psoriasis

Hematogenous spread may result in:

- Osteomyelitis
- Septic arthritis
- Pneumonia
- Septicemia

PROGNOSIS

- Without treatment, individual lesions usually resolve spontaneously within 2 weeks.
- Most lesions resolve without scarring.
- Spreading of the infection by fingers or clothing to other areas of the skin is common.
- Rarely, a chronic ulcer may form.

 Differential Diagnosis

NONBULLOUS IMPETIGO

- Atopic dermatitis
- Candidiasis
- Scabies
- Pediculosis
- Childhood discoid lupus erythematosis
- Tinea corporis
- Varicella
- Herpes simplex
- Ecthyma

BULLOUS IMPETIGO

- Thermal burn
- Bullous pemphigoid
- Pemphigus vulgaris
- Stevens-Johnson syndrome
- Bullous erythema multiforme
- Necrotizing fasciitis

 Data Gathering

HISTORY

- Ask about exposure history since lesions are highly contagious.
- Obtain history of other skin conditions that could cause secondary impetigo.

 Physical Examination

Nonbullous impetigo: Starts as a small, tender, erythematous papule. Often, there is evidence of minor interruption of the skin by lesions such as an insect bite, eczema, or a mild abrasion. The papule then becomes "honey-crusted" with a serous discharge.
Bullous impetigo: Appears on exposed and moist skin. It starts as a transparent bulla that ruptures easily, exposing a moist erosion surrounded by a thin rim of scale.
Lesion may itch but produces little or no pain, or surrounding erythema.
Local lymphadenopathy is seen in 90% of cases.
Constitutional symptoms, such as fever, are rare.

 Laboratory Aids

TESTS

- Culture of the lesion: Though not necessary in the majority of cases, can be obtained by swabbing the blister fluid or the skin beneath the lifted edge of a crusted plague; obtain prior to therapy or in cases of treatment failure.
- Biopsy of the lesion: When the cause of the lesion(s) remain(s) in doubt, biopsy should be considered using histopathologic evaluation, and possibly immunofluorescence staining.
- Immunologic tests—can occasionally be used to confirm recent infection with streptococcus.
- Complete blood count (CBC)—will show leukocytosis in approximately 50% of patients.

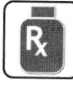 Therapy

- Local wound care, such as cleaning, the removal of crusts, and the application of wet dressing can be helpful.
- For uncomplicated and localized impetigo, a topical preparation is recommended. Mupirocin is as effective as systemic therapy against staphylococcal and streptococcal impetigo, and is associated with fewer side effects. It can be applied 3 times daily for 7 to 10 days.
- Topical fusidic acid cream (not available in the USA), topical hydrogen peroxide cream, lotion and ointment made from tea have been shown to be effective.
- Bacitracin efficacy is questionable since there have been many treatment failures.
- If impetigo is widespread, or is bullous impetigo, oral antimicrobial therapy should be considered for 7 days. Beta-lactamase resistant antimicrobials, such as one of the following: cephalexin, cefadroxil, amoxicillin combined with potassium clavulanate, dicloxicillin or cloxacillin should be used.
- If the staphylococcus is methicillin resistant, vancomycin, trimethoprim/sulfamethoxazide, minocycline, or clindamycin should be considered.

Impetigo

Follow-Up

- If a 7-day course of oral therapy does not eliminate the lesion(s), a culture of the serous fluid from a crusted lesion should be obtained. The antimicrobial susceptibility of the isolate(s) should be performed.
- Consider testing patients with recurrent impetigo for nasopharyngeal carriage. Intranasal application of mupirocin can temporarily eliminate nasal carriage of methicillin-susceptible and resistant strains of *S. aureus* in more than 90% of individuals within 2 to 4 days.

PREVENTION

- Wash hands carefully.
- Cover the lesion with watertight dressing.
- Avoid sharing soiled towels, clothes, or bed sheets, and grooming items, such as nail scissors, tweezers, razors, and toothbrushes.
- Use antibacterial soap to lower the incidence of impetigo.

PITFALLS

- It is impossible clinically to distinguish staphylococcal from streptococcal impetigo; though most cases of bullous impetigo are due to *staphylococcus*.
- Bullous impetigo in neonates must be treated by parenteral antibiotics. First line agents should be beta-lactamase resistant antistaphylococcal penicillins, such as methicillin, oxacillin, or nafcillin.

Common Questions and Answers

Q: Should systemic therapy be started to prevent the development of acute poststreptococcal glomerulonephritis following streptococcal impetigo?
A: There are no data available to show that antimicrobial therapy reduces the incidence of glomerulonephritis. It is postulated that by the time impetigo is diagnosed, there is already extensive antigenic exposure.

Q: My patient is allergic to penicillin. What is the next drug of choice?
A: Erythromycin is often effective but should be avoided in areas where there is known resistance. The two macrolides, azithromycin and clarithromycin, are effective but costly.

Q: When can a child return to school or day care?
A: Children should not return to school until after 24 hours of antibiotic treatment. Lesions should be kept covered when returning to school.

ICD-9-CM: 684

BIBLIOGRAPHY

Brown J, et al. Impetigo: an update. *Int J Dermatol* 2003;42:251–255.

Darmstadt, Gary L. A guide to superficial strep and staph skin infections. *Contemporary Pediatrics* 1997;14:95–116.

Jain A, Daum RS. Staphylococcal infections in children: Part 1. *Pediatr Rev* 1999;20: 183–191.

Koning S, et al. Fusidic acid cream in the treatment of impetigo in general practice: double blind randomized placebo controlled trial. *BMJ* 2002;324:1–5.

Luby S, Agboatwalla M. The effect of antibacterial soap on impetigo incidence. *Am J Trop Med Hyg* 2002;67(4):430–435.

Rubin, GA. A systemic review and meta-analysis of treatments of impetigo. *Br J Gen Pract* 2003;53:480–487.

Sharquie KE, et al. The antibacterial activity of tea in vitro and in vivo (in patients with impetigo contagiosa). *J Dermatol* 2000;27:706–710.

Author: Y. Lily Higgins

Inappropriate Antidiuretic Hormone Secretion

 Database

DEFINITION

Inappropriate antidiuretic hormone (ADH) or ADH-like peptide secretion in the presence of low serum sodium, low serum osmolality, and high urine osmolality, but in the absence of renal or adrenal pathology

CAUSES

- Idiopathic
- CNS pathology, causing increased secretion of ADH or ADH-like peptides: Meningitis, head trauma, neurosurgical procedures, encephalitis, Guillain-Barré syndrome, brain tumor, brain abscess, hydrocephalus, hypoxia, subarachnoid hemorrhage, cerebral venous thrombosis
- Non-CNS tumor with independent secretion of ADH or ADH-like peptides: Bronchogenic carcinoma, pancreatic carcinoma, Hodgkin disease, prostatic cancer
- Pulmonary disease (leading to secondary elevation in ADH secretion or ADH-like peptides): Tuberculosis, pneumonia, asthma, cystic fibrosis, positive-pressure ventilation
- Drugs (which mimic ADH or stimulate its release): Vincristine, cyclophosphamide, carbamazepine, chlorpropamide, phenothiazines, clofibrate, nicotine, fluoxetine, sertraline

PATHOPHYSIOLOGY

- ADH is synthesized within neurons of the hypothalamus, transported in conjunction with neurophysin down the supraopticohypophyseal tract and stored in the posterior pituitary.
- ADH acts on the renal collecting ducts.
- Interaction of ADH with its receptors forms intracellular cyclic AMP (cAMP).
- cAMP increases water permeability through aquaporins (water channels) of the ducts and consequently reabsorption of free water.

The syndrome of inappropriate ADH (SIADH) results when elevated levels of ADH or ADH-like peptides cause free water retention and hypervolemia leading to hyponatremia. Three possible mechanisms include:

- Direct stimulation of the posterior pituitary (e.g., CNS disorders)
- Independent production of ADH or ADH-like substances from ectopic sources (e.g., oat-cell carcinoma, tuberculosis)
- Decreased venous return that stimulates atrial volume receptors and thereby leads to ADH release (e.g., pulmonary and intrathoracic diseases)

EPIDEMIOLOGY

SIADH can occur at any age. Its incidence depends on the various possible etiologies.

COMPLICATIONS

Severe hyponatremia can cause seizures and, rarely, brain damage. Correcting hyponatremia too quickly can lead to central pontine myelinolysis, which impairs vital functions such as breathing.

PROGNOSIS

Based on the primary cause

 Differential Diagnosis

- Hyponatremic dehydration
- Congestive heart failure
- Adrenal insufficiency
- Cirrhosis
- Nephrotic syndrome
- Renal failure
- Severe potassium depletion
- Water intoxication
- Cerebral salt wasting (CSW): Excess production or effects of atrial and/or brain natriuretic peptide hormones
- Hypothyroidism
- Reset hypothalamic osmostat
- Rocky Mountain spotted fever

 Data Gathering

HISTORY

- Unusual water intake (suspicious for psychogenic polydipsia)
- Review of intake and output for inpatients
- Changes in urine output
- Anorexia, lethargy
- Weight gain or weight loss
- Renal disease
- Vomiting
- Diarrhea
- Use of diuretics
- Burns
- Heart disease
- Liver disease
- Brain injury: Trauma, surgery, hypoxia, toxin

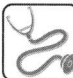 Physical Examination

- No signs of dehydration
- Signs of fluid overload
- Lack of edema
- No hyperpigmentation of skin creases/gums
- Due to hyponatremia, the patient may be lethargic or irritable with muscle cramps. In severe cases, patients may lose deep tendon reflexes, seize, or be comatose.

PITFALL

Failure to distinguish SIADH from various forms of salt wasting such as cerebral salt wasting or adrenal insufficiency

PROCEDURE

A complete neurologic and physical examination must be performed. Classically, patients with SIADH manifest signs of hypervolemia but without increased urine output and without edema.

 Laboratory Aids

TESTS

Specific Tests

- Urinary osmolality and sodium with simultaneous serum osmolality, sodium, and uric acid
- Typically, serum sodium is less than 125 mEq/L, serum osmolality is less than 260 mOsm/L, and serum uric acid is less than 2.4 mg/dL, while simultaneous urinary osmolality is greater than 260 mOsm/L and urine sodium is greater than 30 mmol/L
- Plasma ADH concentration: Diagnostic but not helpful for rapid diagnosis

Nonspecific Tests

- Fractional renal excretion of sodium: Net sodium loss is normal or elevated and is dependent on sodium intake.
- Urinary specific gravity
- Urine output in cc/kg per hour. SIADH usually <1 cc/kg per hour, cerebral salt wasting >2–3 cc/kg per hour)
- Blood glucose
- Triglycerides

Imaging

Head MRI if indicated

Home Testing

Timed urinary volume is helpful.

Therapy

The most important aspects of therapy for SIADH are diagnosis and treatment of the underlying cause.

DIET

• Fluid restriction. Complete until Na >130, insensible losses only until >135 mEq/dL

DRUGS

• For emergency use only: Hypertonic saline (1.5–3% NaCl).
• Diuretics should be avoided because they worsen hyponatremia.
• ADH antagonists: Available only through research trials now but expected to soon become standard of care
• Demeclocycline (for chronic SIADH)

DURATION

• Varies with different etiologies and between patients

POSSIBLE CONFLICTS

• Use of other medications that require a large volume for administration

Follow-Up

WHEN TO EXPECT IMPROVEMENT

Slowly, but usually during the first 48 to 72 hours

SIGNS TO WATCH FOR

Changes in neurologic status

PREVENTION

Clinicians should have a high index of suspicion when administering certain medications, in order to serially monitor serum sodium and fluid status carefully.

Common Questions and Answers

Q: Is the use of diuretics beneficial?
A: No. Although diuretics may relieve the effects of volume overloading, they also worsen hyponatremia. Overall, diuretics usually cause more detriment than benefit.

Q: What distinguishes SIADH from hyponatremic dehydration?
A: The history of dehydrated patients reveals excessive water loss (e.g., vomiting and diarrhea). Dehydrated patients are thirsty and have lost weight. Patients with SIADH have a history of underlying disease and weight gain. On physical examination, patients with dehydration have signs of hypovolemia in contrast to patients with SIADH who do not. Dehydrated patients have elevated blood urea nitrogen (BUN) and serum creatinine, whereas patients with SIADH have low BUN, creatinine, and albumin.

Q: What distinguishes SIADH from cerebral salt wasting (CSW)?
A: Patients with salt wasting appear dehydrated due to decreased plasma volume, but patients with SIADH do not. CSW is associated with very high urine output in contrast to SIADH, which has low urine output. Net sodium loss is very high in CSW, but SIADH has normal to slightly elevated net sodium loss. Distinguishing laboratory features of CSW include suppressed plasma aldosterone concentration and normal serum uric acid concentration. Note that plasma ADH concentration is high in both SIADH and CSW.

Q: Why is it important to distinguish SIADH from CSW (and other causes of hyponatremic dehydration)?
A: Therapies differ dramatically for these conditions. Unlike the water restriction used to treat SIADH, treatment of dehydration, such as that seen in CSW, requires replacement of ongoing salt and water losses.

ICD-9-CM 253.6

BIBLIOGRAPHY

Deen PM, Knoers NV. Physiology and pathophysiology of the aquaphorin-2 water channel. *Curr Opin Nephrol Hypertens* 1998;7(1):37–42.

Gross P, Wehrle R, Bussemaker E. Hyponatremia: pathophysiology, differential diagnosis and new aspects of treatment. *Clin Nephrol* 1996;46(4):273–276.

Kappy MS, Ganong CA. Cerebral salt wasting in children: the role of atrial natriuretic hormone. *Adv Pediatr* 1996;43:271–308.

Olson BR, Gumoski J, Rubino D, et al. Pathophysiology of hyponatremia after transphenoidal pituitary surgery. *J Neurosurg* 1997;87(4):499–507.

Soupart A, Decaux G. Therapeutic recommendations for management of severe hyponatremia: current concepts on pathogenesis and prevention of neurologic complications. *Clin Nephrol* 1996;46(3): 149–169.

Author: Paul S. Thornton

Infantile Spasms

 Database

DEFINITION

Infantile spasms (IS) are myoclonic seizures, usually occurring in clusters, associated with a typical EEG pattern: High voltage slowing, asynchrony, disorganization, multifocal spikes (hypsarrhythmia). Flexor, extensor, mixed flexor/extensor, and arrest/akinetic fits occur. The combination of IS, hypsarrhythmia, and mental retardation is known as West syndrome. Infantile spasms are symptomatic if a specific etiology can be identified and cryptogenic if no underlying cause is found.

CAUSES

• Syndromes: Tuberous sclerosis (TS), Down syndrome, Aicardi syndrome, and recently X-linked infantile spasms syndrome (ISSX: a mutation in the ARX gene)
• Metabolic disorders: Congenital lactic acidosis, PKU
• Malformations of cortical development
• Almost any cause of pre- or perinatal brain injury may lead to infantile spasms, including meningitis, hypoxic-ischemic injury, uremia, and congenital infection.

GENETICS

Families of probands have a higher incidence of epilepsy, suggesting multifactorial inheritance. Tuberous sclerosis may be sporadic or autosomal dominant. ISSX is X linked with variable penetrance.

EPIDEMIOLOGY

Incidence is 0.25 to 0.42 per 1,000 live births. Peak age of onset is 4 to 9 months; onset usually before 1 year of age. Boys more often affected than girls.

ASSOCIATED CONDITIONS

• Intrauterine infection, CNS infections
• Cerebral malformations—malformation of cortical development
• Perinatal asphyxia, prenatal/perinatal stroke
• Lennox-Gastaut syndrome
• Traumatic brain injury
• Intraventricular hemorrhage
• Kernicterus
• Genetic conditions noted above
• 40% of infantile spasms are cryptogenic

PROGNOSIS

Infantile spasms carry a poor developmental prognosis, attributable to the underlying etiology. Approximately 65%–90% of patients are developmentally delayed at diagnosis, and about 10% of these children will achieve normal cognitive, physical, and educational development. About 60% of children with IS go on to develop other seizure types, and 23%–50% develop Lennox-Gastaut syndrome. Prognosis is better in the cryptogenic group, with up to 40% having normal cognitive development and freedom from seizures on long-term follow-up.

 Differential Diagnosis

• Nonepileptic disorders: benign myoclonus, paroxysmal torticollis, posturing related to gastroesophageal reflux (Sandifer Syndrome), shuddering spells, exaggerated startle in children with CP.
• Myoclonic epilepsies of infancy: Benign myoclonic epilepsy of infancy, Severe myoclonic epilepsy (early infantile epileptic encephalopathy)
• Benign sleep myoclonus

 Data Gathering

HISTORY

• Prenatal and perinatal history, including: Maternal age, pregnancy complications, perinatal difficulties
• Family history of TS, seizure, or previous children with infantile spasms should be elicited.
• Detailed developmental history to establish any preexisting developmental delay.
• Description of spells to differentiate spasms from nonepileptic seizures.

 Physical Examination

• Check general growth parameters, especially head circumference—microcephaly suggests preexisting brain abnormality, poorer prognosis.
• Dysmorphisms (Down stigmata, retinal defects as in Aicardi syndrome), suggesting syndromic or genetic basis; hepatomegaly, suggesting inborn errors of metabolism or congenital infection.
• Careful skin examination, including Wood lamp examination, should be performed for evidence of neurocutaneous disorders, especially the hypopigmented macules associated with TS.
• Neurologic examination: Particular attention should be given to level of alertness—visual attentiveness often impaired at presentation; developmental milestones, and motor tone.

 Laboratory Aids

TESTS

• EEG: High voltage, disorganized, multifocal spikes, asynchronous—hypsarrhythmic.
• Routine blood studies: Electrolytes, calcium, and glucose (though generally unrevealing). Chromosomal analysis (should include testing for ARX mutations if family history of lissencephaly, mental retardation, ataxia, or dystonia); test for Tuberous sclerosis if any clinical or radiologic evidence to support diagnosis; metabolic screening, including blood lactate and pyruvate, serum amino acids, urine organic acids; and TORCH titers, depending on level of suspicion for congenital infection or microcephaly.
• If no cause is found, consider lumbar puncture to look for evidence of hypoglycorrhachia, hyperglycinemia, lactic acidosis or abnormalities of neurotransmitter levels.
• MRI is the single most useful laboratory test; intracranial calcifications associated with intrauterine infections and TS are more apparent on CT.
• Infants with cutaneous signs of TS should undergo cardiologic and ophthalmologic evaluation, renal ultrasound, genetic counseling, and evaluation of other family members.
• Infantile spasms is rarely an atypical presentation of pyridoxine-dependent seizures.

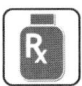 ## Therapy

DRUGS

• Adrenocorticotropic hormone (ACTH) is generally considered the most effective therapy for infantile spasms. Treatment is generally initiated at 150 U/m^2 per day IM (high dose) or 20–30 U per day (low dose) for 1 to 2 weeks, and gradually tapered over 1 to 6 months. No consistent differences established between the high and low dose groups, and the decision on which to treat with is based on the physician's experience.

—ACTH side effects include cushingoid appearance, irritability, sleep disturbance, hyperglycemia, hypertension, electrolyte abnormalities, hypertrophic cardiomyopathy, immunosuppression, gastritis/GI bleeding, osteoporosis, weight gain, and growth failure.
—ACTH therapy has not been proved to affect outcome in infants whose spasms are due to prenatal or perinatal brain abnormalities (symptomatic infantile spasms). Many practitioners use Vigabatrin as first-line agent for infantile spasms in setting of tuberous sclerosis.

• Alternative therapies include:

—Topiramate (at dosages up to 20–60 mg/kg per day)
—Zonisamide (5–15 mg/kg per day)
—Clonazepam (0.1–0.15 mg/kg per day) or Nitrazepam (0.5–3.5 mg/kg per day)
—Tiagabine (0.3–1.3 mg/kg per day)
—Valproate (at dosages up to 100 mg/kg per day) used cautiously due to the increased rate of fatal hepatotoxicity in this age group.
—Phenobarbital (3–6 mg/kg per day)
—Prednisone (2 mg/kg per day).
—A trial of pyridoxine (100 mg IV) should be given to all to rule out pyridoxine-deficiency or dependency. Reports (primarily from Japan) exist of successful treatment of IS with daily high-dose pyridoxine (200–300 mg per day).
—Vigabatrin (100–150 mg/kg per day) is considered the initial treatment of choice in Europe, is not currently available in the United States, concern of visual-field constriction.

 ## Follow-Up

ACTH therapy necessitates weekly follow-up to monitor BP, glucose, electrolytes, BUN/Cr, stool guaiac and signs of infection. Stopping ACTH resolves its side effects.

PITFALLS

• Hypertension and hemorrhagic gastritis may occur during ACTH therapy and must be anticipated by weekly follow-up visits.
• Other seizure disorders may supervene after infantile spasms have remitted and may require alternate anticonvulsant therapy.

 ## Common Questions and Answers

Q: Do infantile spasms ever remit spontaneously?
A: Spontaneous remission of infantile spasms has been reported but appears to be rare.

Q: What predictions can be made about prognosis with idiopathic infantile spasms?
A: Periodic evaluation by a child neurologist or developmental pediatrician helps to detect delays in motor or cognitive development; neither EEG nor any laboratory tests contributes prognostic information in cryptogenic infantile spasms.

ICD-9-CM 345.6

BIBLIOGRAPHY

Baram TZ, Mitchell WG, Tournay A, et al. High-dose corticotrophin (ACTH) versus prednisone or infantile spasms: a prospective, randomized, blinded study. *Pediatrics* 1996;97(3):375–379.

Kramer U. Epilepsy in the first year of life: a review. *J Child Neurol* 1999;14(8):485–489.

Patient information: http://www.epilepsyfoundation.org/

Sherr E. The ARX story (epilepsy, mental retardation, autism, and cerebral malformations): one gene leads to many phenotypes. *Curr Opin Pediatr* 2003;15:567–571.

Wong M, Tevathan E. Infantile spasms. *Pediatr Neurol* 2001;24(2):89–98.

Authors: Amy R. Brooks-Kayal and Eric Marsh

Influenza

Database

DEFINITION
Influenza is an acute febrile illness characterized by fever, respiratory, and gastrointestinal symptoms.

CAUSES
Influenza is caused by the orthomyxoviruses influenza types A, B, and C. Influenza C virus has not been reported as a cause of influenza epidemics.

PATHOLOGY/PATHOPHYSIOLOGY
• The incubation period of influenza virus is approximately 2 to 3 days.
• Persons are considered contagious on the day before symptoms, and remain so until 5 days after illness onset. This period can be longer for children.

EPIDEMIOLOGY
• Although influenza affects persons of all ages, the highest morbidity and mortality occurs in infants and the elderly.
• The attack rate in preschool children is up to 40%.
• Epidemics of influenza occur almost exclusively during winter months, peak approximately 2 weeks after the index case, and last 4 to 8 weeks. Up to 75% of school children in the epidemic region may be affected.
• Transmission of influenza virus occurs by aerosol droplets as well as by direct or indirect contact.

COMPLICATIONS
• Secondary bacterial infections (10% of children): Bacterial pneumonia (pneumococcal or staphylococcal), otitis media (24%), sinusitis
• Primary progressive viral pneumonia: pulmonary hemorrhage, high morbidity, and mortality rates
• Acute myositis during convalescent period is most commonly associated with influenza B infection: Rhabdomyolysis, myoglobinuria, elevated transaminase levels
• Reye syndrome:
• Febrile convulsions
• Drug toxicity: Influenza infection may result in increased serum levels of certain medications that are metabolized by the liver
• Rare sequelae in severe cases of influenza infection include focal and diffuse myocarditis, diffuse cerebral edema, mediastinal lymph node necrosis, sudden death, Guillain-Barré syndrome, and encephalitis.

ASSOCIATED ILLNESSES
• Pharyngitis
• Laryngotracheitis (croup)
• Bronchitis
• Bronchiolitis
• Pneumonia
• Gastroenteritis
• Conjunctivitis

Differential Diagnosis

INFECTION
• Viral infections, including but not limited to respiratory syncytial virus (RSV), parainfluenza, adenovirus
• *Streptococcus pyogenes* infection
• Bacterial sepsis in young infants

Data Gathering

• Infection with the influenza virus causes distinct clinical pictures based on the age of the affected individual.
—Infants and young children may suffer higher fevers and more severe respiratory symptoms.
—Many older children and adults infected with influenza are diagnosed with a "viral respiratory infection," without specific reference to the viral etiologic agent.
—The diagnosis of influenza infection is more commonly made in light of previously identified index cases or specific findings such as myositis.

HISTORY
• Abrupt onset of illness, beginning with dry cough, coryza
• Fever, headache, anorexia, malaise, myalgias, sore throat, irritability
• Respiratory complaints range from mild cough to severe respiratory distress (infants).
• Gastrointestinal complaints in younger children may include vomiting, diarrhea, and severe abdominal pain.

Physical Examination

• Cough is the predominant respiratory sign. Infants and small children may exhibit a "barky" cough (croup).
• Nasal congestion and conjunctival and pharyngeal infections are common.
• Cervical adenopathy is more common in children than in adults.
• Neonates may appear septic: Apnea, circulatory collapse, petechiae.
• A generalized macular or maculopapular rash is sometimes observed.
• The myositis that accompanies the convalescent phase of influenza infection is commonly limited to or most severe in the gastrocnemius and soleus muscles. These patients may present with the inability to walk or toe-walking.

SPECIAL QUESTIONS
• Patients considered to be at high risk for severe disease include those with chronic pulmonary disease or history of an asthma attack, hemodynamically significant cardiac disease, immunosuppressed children including those with HIV infection, those receiving immunosuppressive therapy, with sickle cell anemia, chronic renal disease, diabetes mellitus or other chronic metabolic disease, and those on chronic aspirin therapy.

• Health care professionals, household contacts and caregivers of children under 2 years old, or of any high-risk person listed above, should also receive annual influenza vaccination.
• Persons ≥50 years (formerly 65 years) are recommended for annual vaccination.

Laboratory Aids

TESTS
All specimens should include a throat swab and nasopharyngeal washing.

• Viral culture from nasopharyngeal secretions will be positive within 2 to 6 days.
• Direct immunofluorescent antibody (DFA) and indirect immunofluorescence antibody (IFA) tests have moderate sensitivity (6%–70%) and excellent specificity (>95%), and are completed within 2–4 hours.
• Rapid antigen testing is available for diagnosing influenza A and influenza B. The newer tests are moderately sensitive (70%–80%) and highly specific (94%–97%), and can be completed within 10–15 minutes.
• Serologic evidence of infection involves comparison of acute and convalescent serum antibody titers (6 months). ELISA testing for influenza is also available.

IMAGING
• The chest radiographs in patients with lower airway involvement are indistinguishable from other viral lower respiratory infections.
• Chest radiographs may be normal despite significant respiratory involvement.

FALSE POSITIVES
Culture is the gold standard for diagnosis of influenza. The false-positive rate of DFA, IFA, and rapid antigen testing can be as high as 20% for influenza A and 40% for influenza B. The use of nasopharyngeal aspirates rather than nasopharyngeal swabs can reduce this false-positive rate by 5% to 10%.

PITFALLS
• The leukocyte count in patients with influenza may be high, low, or normal.
• The differential count is too variable to be of help in diagnosis.
• Evaluation of arterial oxygenation by arterial blood gas analysis or, preferably, pulse oximetry may be required in severe cases of influenza infection. Occasional infants without roentgenographic evidence of lower respiratory tract infection have experienced apnea or rapid decrements in pulmonary function.

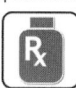

Therapy

• Most patients with influenza infection require supportive oral hydration, antipyresis, and routine decongestant therapy.
• Antitussive medications should be used cautiously, and should be appropriate to the age of the child.
• Neuraminidase inhibitors are most effective if used within the first 2 days of symptom onset.

IMMEDIATE

With the exception of the young infant, previously healthy children with influenza infection rarely require emergency treatment.

- Humidified air, with oxygen as needed, will be helpful to most patients with respiratory symptoms of influenza.
- Supplementary airway maneuvers, including endotracheal intubation, may be required for severe laryngotracheitis or patients with hypoxia that is unresponsive to high-flow oxygen administration.
- Hypovolemic and distributive causes of poor peripheral circulation respond well to intravascular volume repletion.

DRUGS

- Symptom severity and duration may be reduced if antiviral medications are administered within 2 days of symptom onset.
- Antiviral medications have not been proven to reduce serious complications of influenza infection in children, but they may reduce minor complications such as otitis media and shorten the symptom duration by approximately 1 day.
- Amantadine hydrochloride (<9 years of age or <40 kg: 5 mg/kg per day in 1–2 divided doses; ≥40 kg: 200 mg per day in 1–2 divided doses) has in vitro activity against influenza A. Rimantadine (5 mg/kg per day in 2 divided doses, maximum 150 mg per day), a synthetic analog of amantadine, can be used as well. Neither medication is approved for use in infants younger than 1 year of age or for influenza B infection.
- Zanamivir (two 5-mg inhalations twice daily for 5 days), is approved for use in children ≥7 years old.
- Oseltamivir (2 mg/kg orally with maximum 75 mg twice daily for 5 days) is approved for use in children ≥1 year old, and can be used for prophylaxis in children ≥13 years old.

DURATION

Therapy should be given until 1 to 2 days after the disappearance of signs and symptoms. Zanamivir or oseltamivir should be used for 5 days.

POSSIBLE CONFLICTS

- Amantadine dose should be reduced in patients with renal insufficiency, similarly for rimantadine and severe hepatic insufficiency. The side effects of these drugs include insomnia, lightheadedness, and difficulty concentrating.
- Patients with epilepsy have a higher risk of seizure activity when receiving amantadine.
- Inhalation of zanamivir can cause bronchospasm, and it should not be prescribed to asthmatics.
- Oseltamivir may cause nausea or vomiting.

PREVENTION

Vaccination

- American Academy of Pediatrics recommendations for influenza vaccination:
—Children who are between 6 months and 2 years old during influenza season (October through March);

—Children and adolescents who are at high risk for complications due to influenza infection (see Special Questions section).
—Health care professionals and caregivers who have frequent contact with children less than 2 years old or any high-risk persons;
- Household contacts and out of town care givers of high-risk persons.
- Vaccine Types:
—Trivalent inactivated influenza vaccine (TIV): Only one licensed for children younger than 24 months of age.
—Live-attenuated Influenza vaccine (LAIV): Licensed as "FluMist," in the United States; administered as an intranasal spray in two monthly doses. This is not recommended for high-risk persons or those persons' contacts.
- Children who are receiving chronic aspirin therapy should be considered for vaccination because of the associations between aspirin use, influenza infection, and Reye syndrome.
- Children more than 10 years old receiving influenza vaccination for the first time should receive 2 doses of vaccine administered at least 1 month apart.
- Influenza vaccine is recommended for women who will be in the first trimester of pregnancy during the influenza season. Vaccination is safe during any stage of pregnancy and during breast-feeding.
- Persons with a known anaphylactic hypersensitivity to eggs should consult a physician before receiving influenza vaccination.
- Young children are particularly at risk for attenuated flu-like symptoms beginning 6 to 12 hours after vaccination and lasting up to 2 days.

Chemoprophylaxis

- Prophylactic administration of antiviral medications is recommended for certain subgroups of patients:
—High-risk children who are exposed to influenza A infection less than 2 weeks after the final dose influenza vaccination was given (see Special Questions, above)
—Immunocompromised patients (poor response to vaccine)
—High-risk patients who cannot receive the vaccine (anaphylactic reaction to chicken or eggs)
—Control of outbreaks in institutions housing high-risk persons
- The dosages for prophylaxis are the same as those used for treatment.
- Daily therapy should be given during periods of peak influenza activity in a community.
- The neuraminidase inhibitors, zanamivir and oseltamivir, are not yet approved for prophylaxis

 Follow-Up

WHEN TO EXPECT IMPROVEMENT

- Fever associated with influenza infection usually lasts up to 5 days. Recrudescence of fever does not necessarily signify the onset of a secondary bacterial infection.

- Cough may last up to 2 weeks.
- Lethargy or malaise may persist for up to 2 weeks.
- Influenza A infection usually lasts longer than influenza B or influenza C infections.

SIGNS TO WATCH FOR

- Clinical signs of secondary bacterial infection (see Complications, above)
- Deteriorating mental status or respiratory status after initial improvement
- Myoglobinuria in the face of muscle pain

PITFALLS

The patient presenting with benign acute viral myositis might have an elevated creatinine phosphokinase (CPK). However, the presence of myoglobinuria might suggest acute viral rhabdomyolysis, which can be more damaging to the kidney. These patients should be hospitalized and monitored for adequate hydration.

 Common Questions and Answers

Q: When is it safe for a child with influenza to return to daycare or school?
A: Older children with influenza may shed the virus in nasal secretions for up to 7 days from onset of symptoms, and younger children even longer. Therefore, older children with influenza may return to school 1 week after the onset of symptoms, and infants and toddlers should remain home for 10 to 14 days.

Q: Can a child on chronic steroid therapy be immunized against influenza?
A: In general, children who require maintenance steroid therapy for their underlying illness should still receive influenza immunization. If possible, immunize while the child is on the lowest possible dose of steroids and not during a period of high-dose therapy.

Q: What are the chances of acquiring influenza despite annual vaccination?
A: Vaccination against influenza is greater than 70% to 90% effective in preventing disease and greater than 90% effective in preventing death from the infection.

ICD-9-CM 487.1

BIBLIOGRAPHY

American Academy of Pediatrics Committee on Infectious Diseases. Reduction of the influenza burden in children. *Pediatrics* 2002;110:1246–1252.

Cooper NJ, et al. Effectiveness of neuraminidase inhibitors in treatment and prevention of influenza A and B: systematic review and meta-analyses of randomised controlled trials. *BMJ* 2003;326:1235–1241.

Uyeki TM. Influenza diagnosis and treatment in children: a review of studies on clinically useful tests and antiviral treatment for influenza. *Pediatr Infect Dis J* 2003;22:164–177.

Author: Joel A. Fein

Inguinal Hernia

Database

DEFINITION

A hernia is defined as the protrusion of an organ or its portion through the wall normally containing it. Inguinal hernia is a protrusion of abdominal contents (intestine, omentum) through the inguinal canal outside the peritoneal cavity.

PATHOPHYSIOLOGY

Inguinal hernias occur when an outpouching of the peritoneum, called processus vaginalis, fails to become obliterated following the testicular migration.

- During the seventh month of gestation, the testes begin their descent from the peritoneal cavity, where they developed, through the inguinal canal and down into the scrotum.
- Between the seventh and ninth months of gestation, the testes reach the scrotum, at which point the processus vaginalis begins to obliterate spontaneously, leaving a small potential space adjacent to the testes called tunica vaginalis.
- Incomplete obliteration of the processus vaginalis leaves a sac of peritoneum extending all the way from the internal inguinal ring to the scrotum, from which an inguinal hernia may develop.

EPIDEMIOLOGY

- Inguinal hernias are extremely common and represent the most frequent problem requiring surgical intervention in the pediatric age group.
- The incidence of inguinal hernia varies with age and ranges from 3%–5% in full-term babies to 7%–30% in preterm infants.
- Inguinal hernia is much more common in boys (90% of cases) than girls, has a definite familial tendency, and presents more frequently on the right side as a result of later descent of the right testis and delayed obliteration of the right processus vaginalis.
- Clinical presentation is on the right side in 60% of cases, the left side in 30%, and bilateral in 10%.

RISK FACTORS

- Prematurity
- Urologic conditions: Cryptorchidism, hypospadia, epispadia, bladder exstrophy
- Abdominal wall defects: Gastroschisis, omphalocele
- Conditions that increase intraabdominal pressure: Ascites, peritoneal dialysis, ventriculoperitoneal shunt
- Meconium peritonitis
- Cystic fibrosis
- Connective tissue disease (Marfan syndrome, Ehlers-Danlos syndrome)
- Mucopolysaccharidoses
- Family history

Differential Diagnosis

- Lymphadenopathy
- Hydrocele
- Retractile testis
- Undescended testis
- Varicocele
- Testicular tumor

COMPLICATIONS

- Incarceration
- Strangulation
- Intestinal infarction leading to perforation and peritonitis
- Testicular/ovarian ischemia or infarction

Data Gathering

HISTORY

Question: Where is the bulge located?
Significance: Swelling or bulge in the inguinal area is the most common presenting sign of inguinal hernia. Location of the bulge may be helpful in differentiating a complete inguinal hernia (descends into the scrotum) from an incomplete one (does not descend into the scrotum).

Question: Does the bulge change in size, and, if so, what activities bring about these changes?
Significance: The usual history is of an intermittently appearing bulge, especially noted at times of increased intraabdominal pressure, such as crying or straining.

Question: Does the child appear to be bothered by the swelling (extreme fussiness during diaper changes in babies, or complaints of pain/discomfort in older children)?
Significance: Hernias are usually asymptomatic. The parents may perceive the bulge as being painful to the baby since it often is more pronounced when the baby is crying. However, if the parents provide definitive history of a painful bulge in the inguinal region, incarcerated inguinal hernia must be suspected.

Physical Examination

- Examine the child in the supine and standing positions
- If the bulge is apparent in the standing position, but disappears when the child is supine, presence of a hernia is strongly suggested.
- If the bulge is not readily apparent, perform maneuvers that increase intraabdominal pressure (have a patient blow up balloons, or gently press on his/her abdomen, or have him/her cough or strain).
- Transillumination of the scrotum may help in differentiating hernias, which usually do not transluminate, from hydrocele which typically do (unreliable sign).
- Always consider an incarcerated hernia, testicular torsion, epididymitis, orchitis, or trauma when examination reveals a tender scrotal mass.
- Try to reduce the hernia with the child in the supine or head-down position so that gravity assists the maneuver. Use a pacifier to calm the infant. Do not force a difficult incarcerated hernia.

DIAGNOSTIC INVESTIGATIONS

The diagnosis of an inguinal hernia can usually be made on the basis of the clinical history and examination. However, in some cases, use of scrotal or inguinal ultrasonography is indicated:

- Suggestion of torsion (use duplex ultrasound to evaluate blood flow)
- Suggestion of the spermatic cord or testicular tumor
- Scrotal trauma and concern about testicular rupture

TREATMENT

- An inguinal hernia will not resolve spontaneously; herniorrhaphy is accepted universally as the treatment of choice and an outpatient procedure.
- Complication rate after an elective repair is low (1%–2%), but increases dramatically (~20%) if the hernia becomes incarcerated.
- This excessive morbidity, along with a fairly high rate of incarceration in the first year of life, is responsible for the recommendation to repair pediatric inguinal hernias soon after they are diagnosed.
- Approximately 10% of patients will develop a contralateral hernia after a unilateral repair.
- Routine contralateral inguinal exploration in children with unilateral hernia has been a topic of debate for over 50 years.

PITFALLS

- Karyotyping should be considered when a testicle is palpable in the inguinal canal or found at herniorrhaphy in phenotypic females since there is an association between androgen insensitivity and inguinal hernia.
- Sliding hernia occurs when one wall of the hernia is composed of viscera.
- Richter hernia results from the herniation of only a part of the bowel wall, which results in bowel ischemia without bowel obstruction (very rare).
- Hernia of Littre has Meckel diverticulum in the hernia sac

BIBLIOGRAPHY

Geisler DP, et al. Laparoscopic exploration for the clinically undetected hernia in infancy and childhood. *Am J Surg* 2001;182(6):693–696.

Kapur P, et al. Pediatric surgery for the primary care pediatrician, part I. *Pediatr Clin North Am* 1998;45(4):773–789.

Sheldon CA. The pediatric genitourinary examination: inguinal, urethral, and genital diseases. *Pediatr Clin North Am* 2001;48(6):1339–1380.

Tackett LD, Brewer CK, Luks FI, et al. Incidence of contralateral inguinal hernia: a prospective analysis.

Toki A, et al. Ultrasonographic diagnosis for potential contralateral inguinal hernia in children. *J Pediatr Surg* 2003;38(2):224–226.

Erez I, et al. Preoperative ultrasound and intraoperative findings of inguinal hernias in children: A prospective study of 642 children. *J Pediatr Surg* 2002;37(6):865–868.

Author: Eugene Schneider

Intersex

 Database

DEFINITION

Chromosomal sex is established at fertilization, which then directs the undifferentiated gonads to develop into testes or ovaries. Phenotypic sex results from the differentiation of internal ducts and external genitalia under the influence of hormones and transcription factors. If there is any discordance among these three processes (i.e., chromosomal, gonadal, or phenotypic sex determination), then ambiguous genitalia (intersex) develop.

CAUSES

Currently, four main categories of intersex are described:
- Female pseudohermaphroditism (FPH)
- Male pseudohermaphroditism (MPH)
- Gonadal dysgenesis (pure PGD or mixed MGD)
- True hermaphroditism (TH).

FPH is the most common intersex disorder. The ovaries and mullerian derivatives are normal and the sexual ambiguity is limited to masculination of the external genitalia. A female fetus is masculinized only if exposed to androgens and the degree of masculinization is determined by the stage of differentiation at the time of exposure. Masculination may also be secondary to exogenous maternal steroids. Congenital adrenal hyperplasia (CAH) accounts for the majority of FPH patients (most commonly 21a hydroxylase or 11B hydroxylase deficiencies). MPH is a heterogenous disorder in which testes are present but the internal ducts and/or the external genitalia are incompletely masculinized. The phenotype ranges from completely female external genitalia to mild male ambiguity (such as hypospadias or cryptorchidism). MPH can result from eight basic etiologic categories:

- Testicular unresponsiveness to hCG and LH (Leydig cell agenesis/hypoplasia due to hCG/LH receptor defect
- Enzyme defects in testosterone biosynthesis, some of which are common to CAH (StAR, HSD3B2, CYP17, 17-βHSD3)
- Defects in androgen-dependent target tissues (androgen insensitivity syndrome)
- A defect in the enzymatic conversion of testosterone (T) to DHT (5α-Reductase deficiency)
- Defects in the synthesis, secretion, or response to antimullerian hormone (AMH) or mullerian inhibiting substance (MIS) resulting in persistent mullerian duct syndrome
- Aberrations in testicular gonadogenesis (testicular dysgenesis)
- Primary testicular failure (vanishing testes)
- Exogenous insults (maternal ingestion of progesterone/estrogen or environmental hazards).

Gonadal dysgenesis disorders comprise a spectrum of anomalies ranging from complete absence of gonadal development to delayed gonadal failure. Complete or pure GD includes failed gonadal development in genetic males and females due to abnormalities of sex or autosomal chromosomes. Partial gonadal dysgenesis refers to disorders with partial testicular formation at some point in development including MGD, dysgenetic MPH, and some forms of testicular or ovarian regression. TH requires the presence of both ovarian and testicular tissue in the individual. TH can result from sex chromosome mosaicism, chimerism, or Y chromosomal translocation. This uncommon condition may be classified into three groups: Lateral, testis and ovary (usually left); Bilateral, ovotestis and ovotestis; Unilateral (most common), ovotestis and testis or ovary. The genital development is ambiguous with hypospadias, cryptorchidism, and incomplete fusion of labioscrotal folds. Genital duct differentiation generally follows that of the ipsilateral gonad.

PATHOLOGY

- A testis that is poorly formed is called a dysgenetic testis and an ovary that is poorly formed is called a streak gonad.
—A dysgenetic testis usually has discontinuity of the tunica albuginea with hilar disorganization, hypoplastic or disordered tubules, and fibrotic stroma.
—Streak gonads contain ovarian-like stroma with occasional primordial follicles.
—A patient with a Y chromosome is at high risk to develop a tumor in a streak or dysgenetic gonad. Gonadoblastoma is the most common tumor. Although it is a benign growth, it can give rise to a malignant tumor called a dysgerminoma. The risk of tumor formation is about 20% and is age-related (older more at risk).
—An ovotestis has evidence of both seminiferous tubules and ovarian stroma and follicles.

EPIDEMIOLOGY

Low birth weight is a well-established risk factor for cryptorchidism and hypospadias, but associations with low maternal parity and low socioeconomic status are still uncertain. Ambiguous genitalia is also part of the Denys-Drash syndrome (Wilms tumor, hypertension, nephropathy).

GENETICS

- Inactivating or loss of function mutations in five genes involved in steroid biosynthesis can cause CAH: CYP21, CYP11B1, CYP 17, HSD3B2, and StAR. Each of these genetic defects are inherited in an autosomal recessive pattern.
- MPH can result from Leydig cell unresponsiveness to hCG-LH since the production of testosterone by the Leydig cells is critical to male differentiation of the Wolffian ducts and the external genitalia. Familial studies are consistent with autosomal recessive transmission. Multiple cases have been described and conversion and nonsense mutations have been identified in homozygous and compound heterozygous individuals.
- The androgen receptor (AR) gene is located on the long arm of chromosome X. Most of the AR gene mutations affect the steroid-binding domain and result in receptors unable to bind androgens or that bind androgens but exhibit qualitative abnormalities.

- The SRD5A2 gene, which accounts for most fetal 5α-reductase activity, is on chromosome 2. 5α-reductase 2 deficiency is heterogenous and more than 40 mutations have been reported. Consanguinity has also been described in up to 40% of patients' families. Three genetic isolates of this disorder have been described in the Dominican Republic, the New Guinea Samba Tribe, and in Turkey.
- PMDS is inherited in a sex-limited autosomal recessive manner. AMH is encoded by a gene on chromosome 19. AMH mutations are most common in Mediterranean or Arab countries with high rates of consanguinity.
- Mutations or deletions of any of the genes involved in testis determination cascade (SRY, DSS, DAX1, XH2, SOX9, SF1, WT1) have been identified in dysgenetic MPH.
- 47XXY males may develop through nondisjunction of the sex chromosomes during the first or second meiotic divisions in either parent or, less commonly, through mitotic nondisjunction in the zygote at or after fertilization. These abnormalities almost always occur in parents with normal sex chromosomes
- Categories of 46XX sex reversal include classic XX male individuals with apparently normal phenotypes, nonclassic XX males with some degree of sexual ambiguity, and XX true hermaphrodites. 80% to 90% of 46XX males result from an anomalous Y to X translocation involving the SRY gene during meiosis. However, 8% to 20% of XX males have no detectable Y sequences, including SRY.
- XY gonadal dysgenesis (XY sex reversal or Swyer Syndrome) is a heterogenous condition that can result from deletions of the short arm of the Y chromosome. SRY gene mutations, alterations in autosomal genes, or duplications of the DSS locus on the X chromosome.
- A 45X karyotype may be due to nondisjunction or chromosome loss during gametogenesis in either parent resulting in a sperm or ovum without a sex chromosome. 45X/46XX mosaicism may be present in up to 75% of Turner Syndrome patients.
- In TH, the most common karyotype is 46XX followed by 46XX/46XY chimerism, mosaicism, and 46XY. Most 46XX TH are SRY-negative and the genes responsible have not yet been identified. A mutated downstream gene in the sex determination cascade likely allows for testicular determination.

 Differential Diagnosis

The differential diagnosis initially depends on the palpability of gonads on presentation.

- If no gonads are palpable, all four categories are possible (FPH, MPH, GD, TH). Of these, FPH is most commonly seen followed by MGD.
- If one gonad is palpable, FPH and PGD are ruled out because ovaries and streak gonads do not descend. MGD, TH, and MPH remain possibilities.
- If two gonads are palpable, MPH and rarely TH are the most likely diagnoses. In 46XY

boys, hypospadias and cryptorchidism without an underlying intersex etiology would be a diagnosis of exclusion after a full evaluation.

Data Gathering

HISTORY
Prematurity, exogenous maternal hormones (used in infertility treatments), use of oral contraceptives, central nervous system lesions, and family history for urologic abnormalities, neonatal deaths, precocious puberty, infertility, or consanguinity.

Physical Examination

- Any abnormal virilization or cushingoid appearance of the child's mother should be noted.
- The patient should be examined supine in the frogleg position with both legs free.
—Note any dysmorphic features including a short, broad neck or widely spaced nipples. Abnormal phallic size should be documented by width and stretched length measurements.
—Describe the position of the urethral meatus and amount of chordee (ventral curvature).
—Note the number of orifices: three in normal girls (urethra, vagina, and anus) or two in boys (urethra, anus).
—A rectal exam should always be performed for palpation of a uterus.
- Using warmed hands, begin the inguinal examination at the anterior superior iliac spine. Sweep the groin from lateral to medial with the nondominant hand. Once a gonad is palpated, grasp it with the dominant hand, and continue to sweep toward the scrotum with the other hand to attempt to bring the gonad to the scrotum.
—Check the size, location, and texture of both gonads if palpable. Wetting the fingers of the nondominant hand with lubricating jelly or soap can increase the sensitivity of the fingers.
—The undescended testis may be found in the inguinal canal, the superficial inguinal pouch, at the upper scrotum, or rarely in the femoral, perineal, or contralateral scrotal regions.
—For differential diagnosis and treatment purposes, the distinction needs to be made whether or not the testis is palpable. Unless associated with a patent processus vaginalis, ovaries and streak gonads do not descend, while testes, and rarely ovotestes, may be palpable.
- Document development and pigmentation of the labioscrotal folds.

Laboratory Aids

TESTS
All patients require:
- Serum electrolytes
- 17OH progesterone
- T, LH, FSH, karyotype.
- If 17OHP is elevated, 11 deoxycortisol and

DOC will help differentiate 21a from 11B hydroxylase deficiency.
- If 17OHP is normal, T/DHT ratio along with androgen precursors pre/post hCG stimulation (if older than 3 months) will help elucidate the MPH etiology.
- A failure to respond to hCG in combination with elevated LH/FSH levels is consistent with anorchia.

IMAGING
- Ultrasound can detect gonads in the inguinal region, (where they are also most easily palpable) but are only 50% accurate in showing intraabdominal testes. These tests are also helpful in identifying a uterus.
- A genitogram should be performed to evaluate a urogenital sinus including the entry of the urethra and vagina.
- A cervical impression can be identified on the vaginogram.
- Though more expensive, CT and gadolinium-enhanced MRI may also help to delineate the anatomy.

SURGERY
Infants in whom TH, MGD, or MPH are considered will require an open or laparoscopic exploration with bilateral deep longitudinal gonadal biopsies for histologic evaluation.

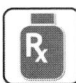

Therapy

Much current research is aimed at understanding the influence of androgens on the fetal/newborn brain and its relationship to gender identity. Diagnosis and management of these children is very individualized and should always involve a "team effort" including the pediatric urologist, endocrinologist, geneticist, and the child's parents immediately after birth.

MEDICAL THERAPY
- Treatment on the newborn with CAH involves correction of dehydration and salt loss by electrolyte and fluid therapy with mineralocorticoid replacement. Glucocorticoid replacement is generally added on confirmation of the diagnosis.
- Estrogen replacement is begun after puberty in girls with complete AIS.
- Testosterone replacement may be needed in some cases of MPH (partial AIS, testicular dysgenesis, primary testicular or Leydig cell failure) to aid in pubertal changes and for maintenance through adulthood.

SURGICAL THERAPY
- Until further data are available, the current recommendation for a girl with CAH is to continue a female sex of rearing and perform a feminizing genitoplasty depending on the degree of masculinization. This surgery has three main aims: reducing the size of the enlarged, masculinized clitoris, reconstructing the female labia, and increasing the opening and possibly length of the vagina. Many surgeons advocate early surgery for technical and psychological reasons, realizing that vaginal revision may be needed after puberty.

- Some gonads need to be removed due to the risk of tumor formation. Controversy exists regarding the best time to perform orchiectomies in a child with complete AIS reared as female (at diagnosis vs. after puberty). Streak gonads in the presence of a Y chromosome and dysgenetic abdominal testes should be removed. All other undescended testes need to be anchored in the scrotum by abdominal or inguinal orchidopexy. Dysgenetic testes in the scrotum need to be followed closely.
- Urethral reconstruction of hypospadias is performed in all children raised as boys at about 6 months of age.

PROGNOSIS
- The overall prognosis for somatic, sexual, and psychosocial growth and development is good with careful management of most of these children. Any thoughts of gender reassignment should only be entertained after thoughtful discussion with the child's parents and all medical staff involved.
- Except for girls with CAH, most of these patients are infertile.

Follow-Up

- Long-term management of mineral and glucocorticoids is done by the pediatric endocrinologist. The vaginal introitus in CAH should be reexamined after puberty to assess adequacy of width and depth.
- Undescended testes, especially dysgenetic testes, have an increased risk of tumor formation even after orchidopexy (seminoma-UDT, gonadoblastoma/dysgerminoma-dysgenetic testis). These boys need to learn testis monthly self-examination after puberty.
- Hypospadias repairs are followed at least through potty training to ensure good voiding habits and absence of meatal stenosis or urethrocutaneous fistulae.

ICD-9-CM 752.7

BIBLIOGRAPHY

Husmann, D. Intersex. In: Gillenwater JY, et al, eds. *Adult and Pediatric Urology*. 4th Ed. St. Louis: Mosby, 2002:2533–2564.

Kolon T, Lamb D. The molecular basis of intersex conditions. AUA Updates, Vol. XX, Lesson 14, 2001.

Mandell J. Sexual differentiation: Normal and abnormal. In: Walsh PC, et al, eds. *Campbell's Urology*. 7th Ed. WB Saunders, Philadelphia: 1998:2145–2154.

Rangecroft L. British association of paediatric surgeons working party on the surgical management of children born with ambiguous genitalia. Surgical management of ambiguous genitalia. *Archives of Disease in Childhood* 2003;88(9):799–801.

Sultan C, et al. Ambiguous genitalia in the newborn. *Seminars in Reproductive Medicine*. 2002;20(3):181–188.

Author: Thomas F. Kolon

Intestinal Obstruction

 Database

DEFINITION

Pathologic blockage of progression of intestinal contents.

Classification

- Partial or complete obstruction

—Mechanical obstruction arising from
—*Intraluminal* causes:
  —Atresia
  —Stenosis
  —Meconium ileus
  —Polyp
  —Bezoar
  —Foreign body or tumor
—*Intramural*:
  —Stricture
  —Tumor
  —Hematoma
—*Extrinsic*:
  —Adhesions
  —Hernia
  —Volvulus
  —Tumor
  —Malrotation, constricting bands or duplications
—*Paralytic* obstruction.

- Simple obstruction (failure of progression of aboral flow of luminal contents) or strangulating obstruction (impaired blood flow to the intestine in addition to intestinal content obstruction).
- Paralytic ileus: Failure of intestinal motor function without mechanical obstruction resulting from:

Infection (pneumonia, gastroenteritis, peritonitis, systemic sepsis)
Drugs (i.e., opiates, loperamide, vincristine)
Associated with surgery
Metabolic abnormalities (hypokalemia, uremia, myxedema, and diabetic ketoacidosis).

Differential diagnosis must include *chronic intestinal pseudoobstruction,* a syndrome of altered intestinal and colonic motility of undefined etiology.

CAUSES

Neonates

- Atresia of the intestine (33% of all neonatal obstructions).
- Anorectal malformation: Anal atresia and stenosis (1:4,000–8,000 of newborns).
- Meconium ileus (30% of all neonatal obstructions, almost all due to cystic fibrosis, CF) and meconium plug.
- NEC (necrotizing enterocolitis).
- Hirschsprung disease

Infants

The most common cause of intestinal obstruction is pyloric stenosis. The second most common is intussusception (the most common cause between 3 months and 6 years

of age with 60% of cases occurring before 1 year of age).

- Other less common causes:
  —Hirschsprung disease
  —Postoperative intestinal obstruction and adhesion
  —Duplications
  —Meckel diverticulum

Older Children

Malrotation
Annular pancreas
Meckel diverticulum
Cancer-related intestinal obstruction
Superior mesenteric artery syndrome (SMA)
Corrosive injury-induced gastric outlet obstruction
Esophageal injury
Postoperative intestinal obstruction and adhesions
Juvenile polyposis and related syndromes, i.e., Peutz-Jeghers
Inflammatory bowel disease (IBD)
Meconium ileus equivalent (occurs only in patients with CF)
Roundworm (*Ascaris lumbricoides*)
Gastric and intestinal bezoars

GENETICS

Familial instances of jeujunoileal and colonic atresias, Hirschsprung disease and pyloric stenosis may have genetic predisposition. Many conditions associated with intestinal obstruction like CF are inherited genetically.

EPIDEMIOLOGY

- Intestinal obstruction occurs in approximately 1 in 1,500 live births.
- The different causes of intestinal obstruction have their own identified epidemiologic patterns:

—Small bowel obstruction secondary to *Ascaris lumbricoides* in tropical and subtropical countries
—Colonic volvulus secondary to aerophagia and constipation in mentally retarded children
—Meconium ileus equivalent in children with CF
—Down syndrome (with a high prevalence, 20%–30%, of duodenal atresia)

PATHOPHYSIOLOGY

In mechanical obstruction, intestinal contents accumulate proximal to the site of obstruction. The bowel distends with swallowed air, ingested food, secretions, and gases from intestinal reactions and bacterial fermentation. Retrograde flow of intestinal contents and reflex gut distension causes vomiting. These internal and external losses result in hypovolemia, oliguria and azotemia. Bacteria proliferate in the small bowel and its contents become feculent.
In addition, in strangulation obstruction there is loss of plasma into the bowel leading more rapidly to shock. When strangulation progresses, gangrene, peritonitis and perforation may ensue. Damage to the normal

gut barrier may enable bacteria, bacterial toxins and inflammatory mediators to enter the circulation.

 Differential Diagnosis

Other causes of abdominal pain and vomiting should be considered:
Appendicitis, torsion of testis or ovary, and lower lobe pneumonia must be ruled out by history and physical examination.

- Other diagnoses include:

—Pancreatitis
—Sickle-cell crises
—Henoch-Schönlein purpura
—Billiary colic
—Lead poisoning
—Acute adrenal insufficiency
—Diabetic ketoacidosis
—Acute intermittent porphyria

 Data Gathering

In most cases, a specific cause can be identified based on patient's age, history and physical examination.

HISTORY

The classic symptoms of intestinal obstruction include nausea and vomiting, abdominal distension, and obstipation.
In neonates, history of maternal polyhydramnios and aspiration of more than 20 mL gastric fluid after birth is suggestive of high intestinal obstruction. All healthy full-term children should pass meconium within 48 hours of birth. Failure to do so raises the suspicion of intestinal obstruction. Neonates, more so than older children, with unrecognized intestinal obstruction, deteriorate rapidly with increased morbidity, mortality, and surgical complications.

CLINICAL PRESENTATION

- Pain is one of the cardinal manifestations of intestinal obstruction. Two types of pain: The distension of the intestine produces visceral pain that is poorly localized, and parietal pain, which is well localized and is associated with rigidity in the presence of peritonitis.
- Nausea and vomiting-high obstruction causes bilious emesis and distal obstruction may lead to abdominal distension and feculent emesis.
- Passage of bloody stool and mucus may suggest strangulation, and is associated with intussusception and volvulus.
- Elicit any family history of CF, polyps, and previous abdominal surgery, as well as recent weight loss or spinal surgery.

Physical Examination

- General assessment and vital signs, as the patient could be dehydrated, septic or malnourished.
- Tenderness and rigidity results from peritonitis.
- Palpation may reveal the presence of a hernia, a mass suggestive of feces or intussusception.
- Anal inspection excludes anal atresia, and stenosis. Rectal examination will reveal, at times, a palpable polyp or intussusceptum, and blood (overt, occult, the currant jelly typical of intussusception).
- Strangulation is suspected when there is fever, tachycardia, signs of peritonitis, and severe pain that persists after nasogastric decompression.

Laboratory Aids

No laboratory studies are diagnostic.

- Electrolyte abnormalities including sodium, chloride, bicarbonate, and potassium, are necessary to identify for the proper assessment of hydration and third-spacing of fluids.
- High obstruction may lead to hypochloremic, hyperkalemic metabolic alkalosis.
- Bowel infarction may lead to marked leukocytosis, thrombocytopenia, and metabolic acidosis.
- Serum amylase and lipase should be determined to rule out pancreatitis, but they might be mildly elevated in intestinal obstruction.

IMAGING

- Plain abdominal radiographs in the supine and erect or decubitus views will identify the classic features of a gasless abdomen, with air-fluid levels and distended loops of intestine.
- However, high small bowel obstruction or strangulation obstruction may present with normal or nearly normal radiographs.
- In small bowel obstruction, dilated bowel, air fluid levels without gas in the colon and multiple dilated loops in distal obstruction.
- Paralytic ileus may present with dilation of the small and large intestines.
- Duodenal obstruction with "double bubble" gas shadow
- Pneumoperitoneum in perforation
- Peritoneal calcifications in meconium peritonitis. Obstruction with intraluminal calcifications in rectourinary fistula, colonic aganglionosis, or intestinal atresia.
- Right lower quadrant ground-glass appearance in meconium ileus.
- Ultrasonography: Identify a mass (i.e., perforated appendix), pyloric stenosis, malrotation, volvulus, or intussusception (where it can replace the contrast

examination in combination with "air" enema).
- Computer tomography: Small and large bowel obstruction, diagnosis of strangulation, and is helpful in postoperative obstruction, Crohn disease, and neoplasms. High cost and radiation exposure makes it a subject of debate in general, and in younger patients particularly.
- Contrast examinations: Barium enema to confirm intussusception or Hirschsprung disease, and upper GI series to exclude malrotation or volvulus). Water-soluble materials should be used when perforation is suspected.
- Evaluation for other associated congenital anomalies (the most frequent are cardiac and renal abnormalities) is mandatory, as some are life-threatening. Associated malformations are frequently associated with duodenal atresia and to a lesser extent with jejunoileal atresia.

COMPLICATIONS

Complications may result from delayed operation.

- Dehydration
- Intestinal ischemia with sepsis and shock
- Bowel perforation and peritonitis
- Short-gut syndrome after extensive necrosis and/or resection, and consequently the prolonged use of parenteral nutrition and its complications

TREATMENT

- Initial stages:

—Hold oral intake.
—Decompress the stomach by nasogastric tube.
—Intravenous hydration, correction of electrolyte imbalance, and ensuring adequate urine output.
—Identify etiology of obstruction and establish definitive repair.
—Cultures and broad-spectrum antibiotics (such as cefoxitin or gentamicin and clindamicin or metronidazole in combination) according to patient's age and status.

- Surgical:

—Definitive treatment requires an urgent operation.
—Exceptions to this rule include: Early postoperative, partial, and recurrent adhesive obstructions, pyloric stenosis, intussusception, meconium ileus, duodenal hematomas, and SMA.
—The surgical procedure is individualized according to the specific type, site, anatomy of the obstruction and associated conditions.
—Nonoperative management

- In intussusception, institution of hydrostatic or air reduction is successful in 90% of cases.
- Nasogastric decompression or antiinflammatory medication for adhesions or inflammatory strictures.
- Contrast material enemas, manipulation and direct enteral irrigation with N-acetylcysteine for uncomplicated meconium ileus

- Colonic volvulus may be treated with endoscopic decompression followed by elective bowel resection.
- Paralytic ileus is usually self-limiting, and resolves with conservative therapy and medication such as prokinetic agents (metoclopramide and erythromycin).

Prevention

Prenatal diagnosis of intestinal atresia has increased with the routine use of fetal ultrasonography, resulting in earlier recognition, prompt surgical intervention and fewer metabolic abnormalities.

Prognosis

Varies with different causes of intestinal obstruction, age of the patient, presence of prematurity and associated anomalies. Associated complications and the institution of prompt treatment influence outcome. Short-bowel syndrome continues to be a major impediment to improved survival rate, permanent parenteral nutrition associated morbidity and mortality.

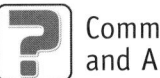

Common Questions and Answers

Q: Will my child need surgery for this problem?
A: Most likely; surgical treatment is necessary to correct the cause of intestinal obstruction except in a few cases, such as intussusception, pseudoobstruction, and paralytic ileus.

Q: What is the most common cause of this problem in my 3-day-old son?
A: In an infant, the most common causes are atresias of the intestine, which are absences of the normal amount of large or small intestine in the abdomen. Other causes are defects in the large intestine, such as Hirschsprung disease. Other notable risk factors include cystic fibrosis and diabetes in the mother.

ICD-9-CM 560.9

BIBLIOGRAPHY

Dalla Vecchia LK, et al. Intestinal atresia and stenosis: a 25-year experience with 277 cases. *Arch Surg* 1998;133:490–496.

Frager D. Intestinal obstruction role of CT. *Gastroenterol Clin North Am* 2002;31:777–799.

Hajivassiliou CA. Intestinal obstruction in neonatal/pediatric surgery. *Semin in Pediatr Surg* 2003;12:241–253.

Sato S, et al. Jejunoileal atresia: A 27-year experience. *J Pediatr Surg* 1998;33:1633–1635.

Wesson DE, Haddock G. The surgical abdomen. In: Walker WA, et al. *Pediatric Gastrointestinal Disease*. Philladelphia: BC Decker, 2000:435–444.

Authors: Vered Yehezkely-Schildkraut and Raanan Shamir

Intoeing—Tibial Torsion

 Database

DEFINITION

- Tibial torsion—twisting (internal or external) of the tibia (can be associated with femoral torsion)
- Medial or internal tibial torsion (MTT) associated with intoeing (most common).
- Lateral or external tibial torsion associated with out-toeing.
- Normal defined as within 2 standard deviations of mean.

CAUSES

- Normal fetal development
- Intrauterine position
- Heredity-familial tendency
- Posturing (sitting position)—cause or effect?
- Associated pathology (e.g., spasticity, fracture malunion, or DDH)

PATHOLOGY

- Tibial torsion—twisting the tibia; usually medial or internal; associated with intoeing.
- If associated with increased femoral anteversion, may be associated with patellofemoral malalignment (knee cap subluxation)

EPIDEMIOLOGY

Common and usually normal (i.e., within 2 standard deviations of the mean)

GENETICS

No strong evidence to suggest that this is an inherited condition (heredity-familial tendency)

COMPLICATIONS

Functional if severe, no long-term complications (osteoarthritis) proven

PROGNOSIS

Good; usually not painful, cosmetically unattractive, or dysfunctional

 Differential Diagnosis

Look for DDH, spasticity (e.g., mild cerebral palsy)

 Data Gathering

HISTORY

Question: Birth history?
Significance: Firstborn common

Question: Pain, limping?
Significance: May indicate other diagnosis

Question: Other "packaging" conditions?
Significance: Metatarsus adductus, torticollis, DDH may be associated

Question: When first noticed? Getting better or worse? Functional limitations (i.e., trips and falls frequently)?
Significance: Functional limitations may suggest other diagnosis such as mild cerebral palsy, especially if abnormal birth history, abnormalities in developmental milestones, and physical findings consistent with cerebral palsy.

 Physical Examination

Finding: If ambulatory, watch gait and assess for foot progression angle.
Significance: The angle formed between the axis of the foot and the axis of forward progression of gait.

Finding: Also assess other aspects of gait.
Significance: Stride, heel-toe gait, cadence, limping, other abnormalities. Unilateral or bilateral torsion.

Finding: Leg length discrepancy, hip abnormalities, contractures, spasticity, thigh foot axis (TFA)
Significance: With the child prone, the knee flexed to 90 degrees, and the ankle at neutral, measure the difference between the axis of the foot and the axis of the femur. If the thigh-foot axis is internal, this suggests internal tibial torsion; if external, external tibial torsion.

Finding: Transmalleolar axis
Significance: With the child seated and the knee flexed to 90 degrees, assess the malleolar axis in reference to the coronal plane (less reliable than TFA).

Finding: Look for abnormalities of the feet.
Significance: Metatarsus adductus or clubfoot may be a primary cause of intoeing. Significant calcaneovalgus may be a component of out-toeing.

Finding: Careful neurologic examination
Significance: To see if intoeing is related to a mild neurologic abnormality, such as mild spastic diplegic cerebral palsy.

SPECIAL QUESTIONS

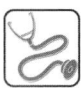 ## Physical Examination

- "Torsional profile" consists of:

—Foot-progression angle
—Medial hip rotation in extension (to assess femoral torsion)
—Lateral hip rotation in extension (to assess femoral torsion)
—Thigh-foot angle (to assess tibial torsion)
—Transmalleolar axis (to assess tibial torsion)
—Configuration of the foot

- "Kissing patellae"

—Occurs when bilateral increased femoral anteversion causes the patellae to face one another, giving the appearance of kissing patellae.

 ## Laboratory Aids

Usually not helpful. (i.e., normal with tibial torsion)

IMAGING STAGES

Usually not needed. Physical examination gives information needed.

Test: Hip x-ray
Significance: If hip pathology (i.e., DDH) is suspected, then may be indicated.

Test: CT
Significance: CT is an accurate way of measuring tibial and femoral torsion but there is radiation exposure. An occasional indication may be a patient who is being evaluated for surgery.

Test: MRI
Significance: Techniques for using MRI to quantify torsion and ultrasound have also been described, but in general are less accurate than CT.

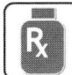 ## Therapy

- Observation and familial and patient reassurance (almost always the treatment of choice).
- Devices such as casts, shoe wedges, twister cables, splints, Denis Brown bars have no proven benefit (i.e., they will not change the natural history). Some of these may in fact cause problems such as ligamentous damage to hip, knee, ankle, and foot.
- Reassurance is usually enough. The condition improves spontaneously. Usually corrects enough by 8 years of age.
- Surgery seldom needed.
- Tibial osteotomy: When done is usually a distal supramaleolar osteotomy.

GENERAL TREATMENT MODALITIES

- Observation
- Physical therapy: Will not change natural history (it may help with associated patellofemoral malalignment pain)
- Devices (casts, shoe wedges, twister cables, splints, Denis Brown bars): No proven benefit
- Tibial osteotomy is seldom, if ever, needed.

 ## Follow-Up

WHEN TO EXPECT IMPROVEMENT

Usually corrects enough by 8 years of age

SIGNS TO WATCH FOR

Should improve with growth and development. There is no substantial evidence that increased femoral anteversion will cause arthritis of the hip or knee.

PROGNOSIS

Overall, good prognosis for the majority of patients

 ## Common Questions and Answers

Q: When are special shoes or braces indicated for tibial torsion?
A: Almost never. The situation will improve without treatment in most. There is no convincing evidence that any of these treatments truly alter the natural history of the condition.

Q: Why do patients with torsional pathology occasionally have knee pain?
A: Children can have increased femoral anteversion with associated external tibial torsion (i.e., an external rotation of the tibia that matches and, in effect, balances the internal rotation of the femur). This can be diagnosed by observing the above rotational profile and by noting increased Q-angle. This situation is sometimes a "setup" for patellofemoral pain.

ICD-9-CM 736.89

BIBLIOGRAPHY

Craig CL, Goldberg MJ. Foot and leg problems. *Pediatrics in Review* 1993;14(10):395–400.

Schoenecker PL, Rich MM. The lower extremity. In: Morrissy RT, Weinstein SL, eds. *Lovell and Winter's Pediatric Orthopaedics*. 5th Ed. Philadelphia: Lippincott Williams & Wilkins, 2001:1059–1104.

Staheli LT. Lower positional deformity in infants and children: a review. *J Pediatr Orthop* 1990;10:559.

Staheli LT. Torsional deformities. *Pediatr Clin North Am* 1977;24:799.

Author: John P. Dormans and Leslie Moroz

Intracranial Hemorrhage

 Database

DEFINITION

Intracranial hemorrhage is extravasation of blood from intracranial vessels to the epidural, subdural, intraparenchymal (intracerebral), or intraventricular space within the cranial vault.

EPIDEMIOLOGY

Stroke in children (birth to 14 years) is 2.5 to 2.7 cases per 100,000 children. 55% are believed to be ischemic, others represent intracranial hemorrhage (ICH). Germinal matrix hemorrhage is the most common ICH in premature infants and trauma is the most common cause of ICH in children. AVMs are the most common cause of nontraumatic ICH in children. Children with change in mental status or seizure at presentation have worse outcome.

CAUSES

Vascular

Congenital vascular anomalies: AVMs, venous angioma, cavernous malformation, hereditary hemorrhagic telangiectasia, aneurysm, coarctation with intracranial aneurysm, vein of Galen malformation (VGAM)
Developmental/acquired vasculopathy: Ehlers-Danlos syndrome type IV, Moyamoya syndrome, pseudoxanthoma elasticum, sickle cell disease, hypertension, mycotic aneurysm, vasculitis (cocaine, inflammatory diseases).

Trauma

Child abuse, angioplasty, trauma (subdural, epidural, subarachnoid).
Other contexts of ICH include prematurity, neonatal asphyxia, sinovenous thromobosis, cerebral infarction—especially due to venous thrombosis.

Hematologic Disorders

Immune thrombocytopenic purpura, thrombotic thrombocytopenic, purpura, congenital autosomal recessive afibrinogenemia, disseminated intravascular coagulation, hemolytic-uremic syndrome, iatrogenic (chemotherapy) thrombocytopenia, congenital serum C2 deficiency, kidney or liver dysfunction with coagulation defect, vitamin K deficiency, factor deficiency (factor V, protein C, or S deficiency), leukemia, lymphoma.

PATHOPHYSIOLOGY

• Epidural hematoma (blood between the dura mater and the skull) is frequently arterial, related to skull fracture, typically middle meningeal artery bleeding following temporal bone fracture. One-fourth of epidural hematomas in children from dural venous laceration.
• Subdural hematoma (blood between the dura mater and the arachnoid membrane) is frequently venous from trauma causing stretching and tearing of bridging cortical veins or coagulopathy.
• Subarachnoid hemorrhage (blood between the arachnoid membrane and brain) ruptured intracranial aneurysm, AVM, or trauma.
• Blood within the brain parenchyma can be the result of trauma, hypertension, infections such as herpes simplex encephalitis, brain tumor, venous sinus thrombosis, or cerebral infarction. Occurs mostly with rupture of medium or smaller branches of major cerebral arteries.
• Subependymal germinal matrix hemorrhage especially premature infants born less than 34 weeks gestational age.
• Intraventricular hemorrhage most commonly occurs when either an intraparenchymal or subependymal germinal matrix (in the subependymal layer of the lateral ventricle) hemorrhage extends into the ventricular system. Germinal matrix hemorrhage is divided into four grades:

—Grade I—isolated to one or both germinal matrices
—Grade II—intraventricular hemorrhage without ventricular dilatation
—Grade III—intraventricular hemorrhage with ventricular dilatation (hydrocephalus)
—Grade IV—intraventricular hemorrhage with ventricular dilatation and extension into the adjacent hemispheric white matter.

GENETICS

Increased frequency with hereditary disorders of coagulation, congenital heart disease, and polycystic kidney disease associated with intracranial aneurysms.

COMPLICATIONS

• Increased intracranial pressure and brain herniation syndromes.
• Hydrocephalus-communicating/noncommunicating.
• Vasospasm secondary to blood and breakdown products of erthrocytes.
• Seizures
• Motor, visual, and cognitive deficits secondary to ischemic infarction.
• Death

 Differential Diagnosis

• Stroke
• Brain tumor
• Migraine headache

Approach to the Patient

Presentations include change or decrease in consciousness, seizure, severe headaches, meningismus (since blood is an irritant), or sudden focal neurologic deficit. With posterior fossa bleed dysconjugate gaze, ataxia and rapid deterioration to coma. Expeditious history, examination, and emergent CT should occur whenever intracranial hemorrhage is suspected. While the bleeding itself may not cause permanent damage to the brain, rapidly increasing intracranial pressure resulting from hemorrhage, edema, or hydrocephalus is life-threatening.

 Data Gathering

HISTORY

• Head trauma
• Circumstances during delivery, especially with prolonged labor and a large infant
• Headache, with attention to severity, quality (worrisome if different from prior headaches)
• Abrupt, severe, headache, and stiff neck may suggest a "warning leak" from aneurysm
• Change in level of consciousness, "lucid interval" with epidural hematoma
• Seizures, especially new-onset
• Visual problems
• Focal neurologic deficits
• Epistaxis (may occur with leakage of CSF if skull fracture is present)
• Meningeal symptoms
• Patient or family history of coagulopathy
• Risk factors for cerebral venous sinus thrombosis: Dehydration, coagulopathy, polycythemia, sepsis, and asphyxia (especially in newborns)
• Risk factors for arterial aneurysms: Polycystic kidney disease, coarctation of the aorta
• Failure to thrive, hydrocephalus with vein of Galen malformation

Physical Examination

- Signs of increased intracranial pressure or herniation, such as Cushing triad (hypertension, bradycardia, abnormal respiratory pattern), papilledema, pupils that do not constrict to light, ophthalmoparesis, decorticate or decerebrate posturing. Intraventricular blood may present with signs of increased intracranial pressure caused by communicating hydrocephalus. Increased ICP may result in a bulging fontanel and splayed sutures.
- Meningeal signs, low-grade fever.
- In setting of trauma:

—Leakage of cerebrospinal fluid from the ear or nose
—Battle sign: Bruising over the mastoid process suggestive of basilar skull fracture
—Raccoon eyes: Periorbital ecchymosis suggestive of basilar skull fracture
—Subhyaline retinal hemorrhages (shaken baby syndrome)

- Herpes simplex type 1 encephalitis: Frequently presents with fever, cognitive impairment, seizures
- Germinal matrix hemorrhages are often clinically silent but may present with apnea in the newborn.
- Intracranial hemorrhage should be suspected in the septic-appearing neonate, especially if there are no obvious risk factors for sepsis.
- Subarachnoid hemorrhage frequently presents as the worst headache ever experienced, subhyaloid hemorrhages, and signs of meningeal irritation.
- Unexplained SDH in infants' particularly bilateral-inflicted trauma until proven otherwise.

Laboratory Aids

TESTS

Hematologic
Complete blood count (platelets), PT/PTT

Imaging

- CT of the head is the most important study to obtain when considering intracranial hemorrhage in the differential diagnosis because of its relative convenience, speed, and low false-negative rate. Fresh intracerebral blood typically appears as an area of increased density on head CT; between 1 and 6 weeks subacute ICHs become isodense with adjacent brain parenchyma on CT scans. Acute ICH can appear isodense if the hematocrit is low i.e., Hb <8–10 g/dL)

—"Biconvex and displacing gray-white interface"—extradural hemorrhage
—"Crescent-shaped"—SDH. Bilateral subdural hemorrhage frequent in intentional injury.

- MRI is also useful for diagnosing acute hemorrhage.
- MRI/MR angiography is the diagnostic study of choice for venous sinus thrombosis, cerebral aneurysms, AVMs, tumors, traumatic brain injury and dissection
- Lumbar puncture will show RBCs, reduced glucose, xanthochromia (best observed in natural light) and bloody CSF. If there is a high suspicion for subarachnoid hemorrhage, and CT does not show hemorrhage, it is important to rule out the condition by spinal fluid evaluation.
- Angiography, either with conventional dye or magnetic resonance angiography, is helpful when looking for vasospasm and arterial venous malformations. It also helps to identify aneurysms that may have ruptured and may require neurosurgical intervention (e.g., insertion of clips or thromboembolic coils).
- Head ultrasound is the most convenient method for diagnosing germinal matrix and intraventricular hemorrhages in infants. Infants born at gestational age of <32 weeks, with birth weight <1,800 g, or infants at high risk due to low hematocrit, low platelets, unstable BP, cardiopulmonary arrest, or pneumothorax. If hemorrhage is identified or until approximately 32 weeks gestational age, serial ultrasound examinations are warranted.

Immediate Stroke Evaluation

- First 24 Hours consider
- head CT
- CXR
- Echocardiogram
- Urine tox screen
- CBC
- Electrolytes
- Ca, Mg, Phos
- BUN/Cr, LFT
- PT/PTT/INR, ESR/ANA
- LP, MRI/MRA/MRV, transcranial and carotid U/S

Therapy

Acyclovir therapy should be instituted if herpes simplex type 1 encephalitis is considered.
Intracranial aneurysms are frequently amenable to neurosurgical/neuroradiologic intervention to decrease the likelihood of rebleeding; in addition, careful control of increased intracranial pressure, decreasing vasospasm with nimodipine or cerebral balloon angioplasty, and prompt attention to hydrocephalus may be necessary.
AVMs definitive treatment consists of surgical resection or interventional neuroradiologic techniques using balloon or coil occlusion of the larger feeding vessels or proton beam irradiation.
Neurosurgical intervention is frequently necessary for subdural and epidural hematomas. Serial neurologic examinations on patients treated for intracranial hemorrhage.

Follow-Up

Long-term observation for signs of hypoxic-ischemic injury—cognitive deficits, focal weakness, and seizures. Often, good neurologic recovery is possible.

PREVENTION

- Automobile seat belts; bicycle, skating, and skateboarding helmets; child abuse prevention; diving safety practices; preventing falls; maintaining safe driving speeds; keeping children away from firearms. Hematologic monitoring for those at risk for hemorrhage due to blood disorders.

PITFALLS

- Epidural hematoma may present in a delayed fashion after head trauma. A "lucid interval" of approximately 24 hours may be followed by change in consciousness, headache, and other neurologic symptoms and signs.
- Early subarachnoid hemorrhage may not be apparent on CT and may require LP (if safe to perform) or serial CT evaluation while a patient is under clinical observation.
- Intracranial hemorrhage, especially in young infants and children without an obvious etiology, should raise the suspicion of nonaccidental trauma.
- Patients with concussion without intracranial hemorrhage may still develop cerebral edema, and these patients should be observed closely for signs of increasing intracranial pressure.

ICD-9-CD 432.9

BIBLIOGRAPHY

Bonnier C, et al. Neuroimaging of intraparenchymal lesions predicts outcome in shaken baby syndrome. *Pediatrics* 2003;112(4):808–814.

deVeber G. Cerebrovascular disease in children. In: Swaima KF, Aswall S, eds. *Pediatric Neurology*. 3rd Ed. St. Louis: Mosby, 1999.

Hemophilia Information: http://www.hemophilia.org

Nelson KB, Lynch JK. Stroke in newborn infants Lancet. *Neurology* 2004;3(3):150–158.

Proust F, Toussaint P, Garnieri J, et al. Pediatric cerebral aneurysms. *J Neurosurg* 2001;94(5):733–739.

Stroke Information: National Stroke Association, http://www.stroke.org

Authors: Q. Bashir
Ann Poduri, 3rd edition

Intussusception

Database

DEFINITION

- Intussusception is the most common abdominal emergency of early childhood and is the telescoping of one part of the bowel into itself or adjacent bowel causing abdominal pain, vomiting and lethargy. Telescoping of the bowel causes diminished venous blood flow due to ischemia, resulting in edema of the bowel, hemorrhage and subsequently to decreased arterial ischemia and infarction of the bowel wall. Peak age of presentation is the first year of life.
- Ileo-colic accounts for 90% of intussusceptions.
- Ileo-ileal and colo-colic types do occur.
- Ischemia of the bowel rarely occurs in the first 24 hours but evolve afterwards.

There are two subtypes of the disease associated with age at diagnosis and underlying lead point:

- In younger patients it is idiopathic type and has been reported secondary to Rotavirus immunization.
- In patients after the 3rd year of life an underlying lead point should be excluded including:

—Anatomical causes (Meckel diverticulum, post surgery)
—Tumors (polyps, lymphoma, sarcoma, lipoma)
—Inflammatory (Henoch-Schönlein purpura, celiac disease)

EPIDEMIOLOGY

- Male to female ratio 3:2
- Peak age from 6 to 12 months

COMPLICATIONS

- Bowel necrosis secondary to local ischemia
- Gastrointestinal bleeding
- Bowel perforation
- Sepsis, shock

PROGNOSIS

- Timely diagnosis results in a highly favorable prognosis.
- Hydrostatic reduction by air or barium enema is therapeutic in 50% to 90%.
- Risk of recurrence is approximately 10% after reduction, 1% after manual reduction, and not reported after intestinal resection.

Differential Diagnosis

- Infection: Parasites (Enterobius)
- Tumors: Known association to intussusception.
- Congenital: Hirschsprung disease
- Immunologic: Henoch-Schönlein purpura, celiac disease
- Miscellaneous:

—Meckel diverticulum: Usually painless rectal bleeding
—Incarcerated hernia
—Incarcerated malrotation (midgut volvulus)
—Obstruction: Adhesions, hernia, volvulus, stricture, bezoar, foreign body, fecal impaction, polyp

Data Gathering

HISTORY

- Intermittent (colicky) abdominal pain with vomiting and blood/mucus in stools is considered the classic presentation, but is only found in 20% of cases.
- Lethargy not explained by the severity of dehydration
- Colicky pain is the major symptom.
- "Currant-jelly" stools appear in about 50% of cases—a sign of longer course

Physical Examination

- Sick lethargic infant with colicky pattern of abdominal pain
- Absent bowel sounds.
- A mass effect in the right upper quadrant may be noted.
- Absence of bowel contents in right lower quadrant (Dance sign)
- Occasionally, the intussusception can be felt on rectal examination.
- "Currant jelly" stool on rectal exam

Laboratory Aids

TESTS

- CBC, electrolytes
- Plain abdominal films: obstruction, air-fluid levels, paucity of distal gas, soft tissue mass; may result in false-negative reading.
- Abdominal ultrasound
- Barium enema: "Cervix-like mass" or "coiled spring" on evacuation film.

PITFALLS

- Some of the classic symptoms may be absent on presentation, and clinical suspicion and good judgment must be sufficient to act upon.
- Clinical status of hypovolemic patients may worsen with high osmotic contrast agents.

Intussusception

 Therapy

- Nasogastric tube placement: Bowel decompression.
- Intravenous line placement: Correction of fluid and electrolyte losses.
- Contraindications to reduction by BE include peritonitis, shock, and perforation.
- Caution should be used when symptoms have been present more than 5 days or if radiologic evidence of obstruction, fever, or leukocytosis are present.
- A barium enema may miss a lead point.
- A surgical consultation should be obtained before the reduction attempt secondary to risk of perforation, and failed reduction requires surgical correction.
- Perforation during reduction occurs in 1% of cases, mostly in the transverse colon.

 Follow-Up

Recurrence after nonoperative reduction has been reported in up to 10% and usually is seen within 24 hours of the reduction

 Common Questions and Answers

Q: Can my child have a recurrent intussusception?
A: Yes, the risk, though, is very low, probably below 10% if the child has had a nonsurgical reduction or removal of the lead point.

Q: Can my child with constipation get this problem?
A: This is doubtful, although in severe cases it might be possible.

Q: What are the common ages for presentation?
A: Six months to 3 years is the age range associated with the greatest risk of intussusception, but it can occur at any age. The prevalence of pathologic conditions rises with the age of a child diagnosed with intussusception.

ICD-9-CM 560.0
BIBLIOGRAPHY

Daneman A, Navarro O. Intussusception. Part 1: a review of diagnostic approaches. *Pediatr Radiol* 2003;33(2):79–85.

Daneman A, Navarro O. Intussusception. Part 2: An update on the evolution of management. *Pediatr Radiol* 2004;34(2):97–108.

Davis CF, et al. The ins and outs of intussusception: history and management over the past fifty years. *J Pediatr Surg* 2003;38(Suppl 7):60–64.

Hyer W. Polyposis syndromes: pediatric implications. *Gastrointest Endosc Clin N Am* 2001;11(4):659–682.

McCollough M, Sharieff GQ. Abdominal surgical emergencies in infants and young children. *Emerg Med Clin North Am* 2003;21(4):909–935.

Peter G, Myers MG. National Vaccine Advisory Committee; National Vaccine Program Office. Intussusception, rotavirus, and oral vaccines: summary of a workshop. *Pediatrics* 2002;110(6):e67.

Author: Dror Wasserman

Iron Deficiency Anemia

 ## Database

DEFINITION

A reduction in hemoglobin production due to an insufficient supply of iron that results in a microcytic, hypochromic anemia.

PATHOPHYSIOLOGY

- Iron is required for oxygen transport by hemoglobin.
- Iron is absorbed primarily in the duodenum
- Iron deficiency develops because of inadequate supply or increased demand for iron, or a combination of these
- Causes of inadequate supply include dietary deficiency and malabsorption

—-Dietary deficiency in infants and young children results from introduction of cow's milk prior to 12 months old, exclusive breastfeeding beyond 6 months old without iron supplementation and excessive cow's milk intake (>24 ounces per day)
—Malabsorption results from surgical resection of intestine—celiac disease
—Certain foods impair iron absorption (tannins in tea and coffee, phytates)

- Causes of increased demand include rapid growth and blood loss

—Periods of rapid growth include infancy (especially low birth weight infants) and adolescence.
—Gastrointestinal blood loss is most common and includes cow's milk enteropathy (seen in infants), inflammatory bowel disease (IBD), and bleeding from Meckel diverticulum
—Other etiologies of blood loss include perinatal loss, menorrhagia, pulmonary hemosiderosis, and hematuria.

- Sequential stages of iron deficiency:

—Depletion of iron stores. Reflected by low serum ferritin and absent bone marrow stores (Prussian blue staining)
—Iron deficient erythropoiesis. Near-normal number of red blood cells produced but have abnormal hemoglobin synthesis with wide distribution in red blood cell size.
—Iron deficiency anemia. Microcytosis evident.

EPIDEMIOLOGY

- Leading cause of anemia among infants and children in the United States. Most commonly seen in children ages 9 months to 3 years and in teenage girls. Prevalence is variable depending on socioeconomic status, availability of iron-fortified formulas, prevalence and duration of breastfeeding, and the way that iron deficiency is defined. Prevalence of iron deficiency anemia is generally between 1% and 5% of children in the United States.

COMPLICATIONS

- Impaired cognitive and motor development in infants and toddlers.
- Impaired immunity
- Short-term memory impairment and poor exercise performance in adolescents

PROGNOSIS

- Anemia readily corrected with iron replacement.
- Developmental delay may be long lasting or irreversible.

 ## Differential Diagnosis

- Recent infection
- Lead poisoning
- Thalassemia trait
- Anemia of chronic inflammation (juvenile rheumatoid arthritis, IBD)
- Sideroblastic anemias

 ## Data Gathering

HISTORY

- Evaluate dietary intake of iron, including breast or formula feeding and type of formula (iron fortified or low iron)
- Age of introduction of cow's milk
- Daily intake of cow's milk
- Birth history for prematurity or blood loss
- Pica
- Lead exposure
- Blood loss from urine, stool, menorrhagia

 ## Physical Examination

- Often normal exam
- Pallor, irritability
- Tachycardia, flow murmur if anemia more severe
- Koilonychia (spoon nails)
- Glossitis or stomatitis
- Test for occult blood in stool and urine

 ## Laboratory Aids

- Hemoglobin level less than 2 standard deviations below the age specific mean—defines anemia.
- Low MCV (red cell volume) and MCH (hemoglobin concentration) for age.
- High RDW (red cell distribution width). Measures the variation in red cell size. Normal is <14.5%. Often increased before anemia is present.
- Low serum ferritin reflects tissue iron stores. Earliest laboratory abnormality. May be normal or increased with concurrent infection.
- Low serum iron
- Increased TIBC (total iron binding capacity)
- Low transferrin saturation; measures the iron available for hemoglobin synthesis
- Increased soluble transferrin receptor. Indicator of increased tissue iron demand. Also increased in thalassemia syndromes but not in anemia of chronic inflammation.
- Decreased reticulocyte hemoglobin content (CHr). This test is an early indicator of iron deficiency because reticulocytes have a short (1–2 day) lifespan.
  Increased free erythrocyte protoporphyrin (FEP), a precursor molecule to hemoglobin synthesis.
- Also increased in lead poisoning and chronic inflammation.
- Thrombocytosis
- Peripheral blood smear with microcytosis, hypochromia, poikilocytosis (varying shapes), pencil forms, and anisocytosis (varying sizes)
- Bone marrow examination shows decreased iron stores by Prussian blue staining. Bone marrow examination is rarely needed to establish diagnosis.

 ## Therapy

- Oral replacement with ferrous iron, 3 to 6 mg/kg per day of elemental iron divided into 2 or 3 doses. Iron should be given on an empty stomach or with a vitamin C-containing juice to increase absorption.
- Family education regarding age-appropriate diet and iron-containing foods
- May require initial inpatient observation in cases of severe anemia
- Red cell transfusion only if evidence of cardiovascular compromise (rarely indicated)
- Parenteral (IM or IV) iron dextran indicated only for severe noncompliance, malabsorption, or if ongoing loss exceeds absorption capacity. Administration may be associated with pain at injection site or anaphylaxis.
- Prevention is preferable. Anticipatory guidance and governmental sponsored programs such as the Special Supplemental Nutrition Program for Women, Infants and Children (WIC).

Follow-Up

- Reticulocyte count begins to increase in 3 to 4 days.
- Hemoglobin concentration should be increased at least 1 g/dL in 2 to 4 weeks.
- Continue iron for 2 months beyond correction of anemia to replete body stores.

PREVENTION

- Maintain breast-feeding for the first 5 to 6 months of life when possible. Although the concentration of iron is lower in breast milk than in formula, iron in breast milk is more bioavailable (50% vs. 10%).
- Iron supplementation (1 mg/kg per day) for infants who are exclusively breast-fed beyond 6 months.
- Iron-fortified formula for the first 12 months of life for infants who are not breast-fed.
- Iron supplementation after 2 months of life for low birth weight and premature infants because of decreased iron stores and increased growth rate.
- Encourage iron-enriched cereal when infants are started on solid food.
- Avoid whole cow's milk during the first year of life to prevent occult GI bleeding.
- Screen hemoglobin level at periodic intervals. (AAP recommends 9 months, 5 years, and 14 years.)

PITFALLS

- Causes of poor response to oral iron supplementation include:

—Noncompliance (most common)
—Ongoing blood loss
—Insufficient duration of therapy
—High gastric pH
—Concurrent lead intoxication
—Incorrect diagnosis (thalassemia trait and anemia of chronic disease are not iron responsive.)

 Common Questions and Answers

Q: What dietary changes can help prevent the reoccurrence of iron deficiency?
A: Limit milk to not more than 24 ounces a day so that the child has a better appetite for iron-containing foods. Heme iron, found in meats, fish, and poultry, is absorbed better than nonheme iron and enhances the absorption of nonheme iron. Other foods that contain iron are raisins, dried fruit, sweet potatoes, lima beans, chili beans, green peas, peanut butter, and enriched foods. Give iron on an empty stomach along with an ascorbic acid-containing juice to increase absorption of iron. Foods that decrease iron absorption include bran, vegetable fiber, tannins found in tea, and phosphates. Antacids may also decrease iron absorption.

Q: What are the side effects of iron therapy?
A: Iron can cause temporary staining of the teeth, which can be decreased by diluting the iron with a small amount of juice. Iron will also change the color of bowel movements to greenish black and may be associated with constipation.

Q: What are the most important tests to do to establish the diagnosis of iron deficiency?
A: For patients with a history of dietary deficiency or known blood loss, a complete blood count that shows a low hemoglobin level and MCV and an elevated RDW is very suggestive of iron deficiency. A therapeutic trial of iron without further laboratory testing is an appropriate next diagnostic step. An increase in the hemoglobin concentration of 1 g/dL or greater after 1 month of therapy confirms the diagnosis. If this does not occur, further laboratory testing is necessary and other diagnoses should be considered.

Q: How does a concurrent infection affect the diagnosis of iron deficiency?
A: Common childhood infections can be associated with a mild microcytic anemia that resembles iron deficiency. Laboratory tests to diagnose iron deficiency can be misleading while a child is acutely ill. Acute infection is associated with a shift of iron from serum to storage sites causing a decrease in serum iron and an increase in ferritin. It is therefore more helpful to screen a child for iron deficiency 3 to 4 weeks after an acute infection.

ICD-9-CM 280

BIBLIOGRAPHY

Anonymous. Iron deficiency—United States, 1999–2000. *MMWR Morbidity & Mortality Weekly Report.* 2002;51(40):897–899.

Booth I, Aukett MA. Iron deficiency anaemia in infancy and early childhood. *Arch Dis Child* 1997;76:549–554.

Griffin IJ, Abrams SA. Iron and breastfeeding. *Pediatr Clin North Am* 2001;48:401–413.

Looker AC. Iron deficiency—United States 1999–2000. *Morbid Mortal Weekly Rev* 2002;51:897–899.

Lozoff B, Jimenez E, Wolf AW. Iron deficiency anemia and infant development: effects of extended oral iron therapy. *J Pediatr* 1996;129:382–389.

Lozoff B, Jimenez E, Wolf AW. Long-term developmental outcome of infants with iron deficiency anemia. *N Engl J Med* 1991;325:687–694.

Nathan DG, et al, eds. *Nathan and Oski's Hematology of Infancy and Childhood, 6th ed.* Philadelphia: WB Saunders, 2003.

Oski FA. Iron deficiency anemia in infancy and childhood. *N Engl J Med* 1993;129:190–193.

Pappas DE. Iron deficiency anemia. *Pediatr Rev* 1998;19:321–322.

Wharton BA. Iron deficiency in children: detection and prevention. *Br J Hematol* 1999;106:270–280.

Wu AC, et al. Screening for iron deficiency. *Pediatr Rev* 2002;23:171–177.

Author: Janet L. Kwiatkowski

Iron Poisoning

 ## Database

DEFINITION

• The nontherapeutic ingestion of an iron-containing preparation, which may be available in a number of iron salts.
• Ingested doses of <20 mg/kg of elemental iron are generally nontoxic; of 20–60 mg/kg lead to moderate toxicity; and of >60 mg/kg lead to severe toxicity, and can be potentially fatal.

PATHOPHYSIOLOGY

• Direct corrosive effects of iron on gastrointestinal mucosa may lead to abdominal pain, vomiting, hematemesis, diarrhea, hematochezia and melena. These effects may cause intestinal ulceration, edema and inflammation.
• Hepatotoxicity from free iron accumulation can lead to periportal necrosis and hepatic failure, as well as coagulopathy.
• Gastrointestinal fluid losses can lead to hypotension and tissue hypoperfusion.
• Decreased cardiac output from decreased venous filling pressures, decreased preload, relative bradycardia, and a possible direct negative inotropic effect of iron on the myocardium can lead to shock.
• Metabolic acidosis results from tissue hypoperfusion with lactate formation, unbuffered hydrogen ion as absorbed ferrous iron is converted to ferric iron, disruption of oxidative phosphorylation, and lipid peroxidation of mitochondrial membranes.
• Adult respiratory distress syndrome (ARDS) may present in severe cases, and may be caused by iron-induced alveolar membrane damage.

Phases of the clinical effects of iron poisoning:

• Phase I (early acute): From 0–6 hours postingestion. Characterized by gastrointestinal (GI), central nervous system (CNS) and cardiovascular (CV) signs and symptoms.
• Phase II (quiescent): From 6–24 hours. Characterized by decrease in GI symptoms and relative improvement in condition.
• Phase III (recurrent): From 12–48 hours. Characterized by cyanosis, profound metabolic acidosis, shock, evidence of hepatic and renal failure, ischemic bowel, myocardial depression, and cerebral dysfunction sometimes causing seizures and coma.
• Phase IV (late): 4–6 weeks postingestion. Characterized by gastric scarring and pyloric stenosis, sometimes leading to obstruction.

EPIDEMIOLOGY

• Most frequent cause of pediatric unintentional ingestion fatalities, accounting for about 30% of fatalities in one series
• Almost all deaths from iron toxicity are in children <3 years of age
• Almost all iron-related injuries are in children <4 years of age, and are usually due to ingestion of adult iron formulations.
• Risk factors for iron poisoning include ready availability of iron preparations in homes with pregnant women and young children, and the similarity in appearance of some pills and vitamins to candy.

COMPLICATIONS

• Small bowel infarction and necrosis
• Gastric or intestinal scarring and strictures, which may present as gastric outlet or intestinal obstruction
• Hepatic failure
• Metabolic acidosis
• Hypovolemic and hemorrhagic shock
• Coagulopathy
• ARDS
• CNS effects including lethargy, seizures and coma
• *Yersinia enterocolitica* infection or sepsis
• Death

PROGNOSIS

• Manifestations of iron ingestion can range from asymptomatic to severe systemic toxicity and death.
• Prognosis can be estimated based on factors such as estimated ingestion dosage, serum iron level, clinical course, and presence of complications.

 ## Differential Diagnosis

INGESTIONS

• Salicylate, theophylline or digoxin ingestions

GASTROINTESTINAL

• GI hemorrhage
• GI trauma with perforation
• Appendicitis with rupture
• Intussusception
• Hemolytic uremic syndrome
• Gastritis
• Esophagitis
• Mallory-Weiss tear
• Vascular malformation

OTHER

• Reye syndrome
• Fulminant sepsis
• Meningitis
• Diabetic ketoacidosis

 ## Data Gathering

HISTORY

Question: Did the parent discover iron-containing pills, pill fragments or other preparations in their young child's mouth or in opened containers in the home?
Significance: Detailed information on iron compound ingested such a iron salt type (determines percent of elemental iron), number of pills ingested and approximate ingestion time can be used to calculate estimated ingested iron dose in mg/kg of elemental iron. As a reference, the percent of elemental iron in ferrous fumarate is 33%; in ferrous chloride is 28%; in ferrous sulfate is 20%; and ferrous gluconate is 12%.

 ## Physical Examination

Finding: A lethargic, hypotensive, vomiting toddler.
Significance: The diagnosis of iron poisoning should be strongly considered for this scenario.

Finding: Decreased blood pressure (hypotension), decreased capillary refill, pallor, increased heart rate (tachycardia) and CNS depression (lethargy or coma).
Significance: Hypovolemic and hemorrhagic shock.

Finding: Abdominal tenderness and evidence of vomiting and diarrhea (test emesis and stool for occult blood)
Significance: Direct corrosive effects of iron on gastric mucosa.

 ## Laboratory Aids

TESTS

Test: Iron level
Significance: The serum iron level at 4–6 hours postingestion is most predictive of the clinical course, and is used in conjunction with the clinical assessment. (TIBC is NOT recommended). Iron levels 300–500 μg/dL are usually associated with GI toxicity and moderate systemic toxicity. Iron levels 500–1,000 μg/dL are usually associated with significant systemic toxicity and shock. Iron levels over 1000 μg/dL are usually associated with significant morbidity and mortality.

Test: Chemistries including hepatic profile
Significance: To assess for hepatic injury and/or metabolic acidosis (positive anion-gap acidosis)

Test: Complete blood count and coagulation studies
Significance: To determine degree of anemia from blood loss as well as monitor for coagulopathy.

Test: Arterial blood gas
Significance: Monitor metabolic acidosis

RADIOGRAPHIC STUDIES

Test: Abdominal radiograph
Significance: May reveal iron pills, which can then guide GI decontamination. Liquid iron preparations and multivitamins with iron are typically not radioopaque. Absence of pills on x-ray does not exclude potential iron ingestion and toxicity.

 Therapy

DISPOSITION

- Asymptomatic patients with minimal or no GI involvement can be observed in the ED for a 6-hour period and discharged home.
- Symptomatic patients with GI or mild symptoms should be admitted for regular inpatient management.
- Symptomatic patients with significant toxicity should be treated in an intensive care setting by specialists skilled in management of this ingestion. Metabolic acidosis and radioopaque material on abdominal radiograph predict significant iron absorption and toxicity.

INITIAL EVALUATION AND SUPPORTIVE CARE

- Evaluation for presence of GI or systemic involvement, including acidosis, shock, or lethargy.
- Supportive care should include assessment of airway, supplemental oxygen, establishing intravenous access and supporting blood pressure with normal saline or Ringer's lactate.
- Orogastric intubation should be considered in a lethargic patient to facilitate GI decontamination.

GI DECONTAMINATION

- Goal is to decrease iron absorption and break up pill concretions, which may directly damage the GI mucosa.
- Syrup of ipecac is not recommended.
- Gastric lavage with normal saline or tap water may be attempted, but iron tablets are often too large to pass through. Iron does not bind well to activated charcoal, so this is not effective.

- Whole bowel irrigation with a polyethylene glycol electrolyte solution until all pill remnants have passed in the stool is recommended for most cases.
- Rarely, endoscopy or gastrotomy may need to be performed to remove embedded pills.

CHELATION WITH DEFEROXAMINE (DFO)

- Given parenterally via continuous IV infusion at 5–15 mg/kg per hour. This is recommended for: Symptomatic or ill patients, patients with a positive abdominal radiograph or significant exposure history, and symptomatic patients with iron levels of 300 μg/dL or higher and all patients with levels of 500 μg/dL or higher.
- Chelation can be discontinued with clinical improvement, resolution of metabolic acidosis, resolution of radiograph radioopacities and urine color normalization.
- If renal failure develops, chelation can be continued and dialysis performed (the iron-deferoxamine complex is dialyzable).

 Follow-Up

- Abdominal x-ray should be followed until complete decontamination is documented.
- Patients should be monitored for possible late complications, such as strictures of the GI tract.

PREVENTION

- Strategies include parental education, package-labeling warning of the potential pediatric ingestion hazard, regulatory change to require prescription status for preparations containing iron, and improved packaging of iron preparations.
- The Consumer Product Safety Commission (CPSC) requires child-resistant packaging for packages containing 250 mg or more of elemental iron, and the Food and Drug Administration (FDA) requires individually-packaged dosage units for products containing 30 mg or higher of elemental iron per dosage unit; however, most children's multivitamin preparations only contain up to 18 mg of elemental iron per tablet.

PITFALLS

- TIBC (total iron-binding capacity) not recommended to assess degree of toxicity.
- Lower iron levels do not necessarily preclude the possibility of serious iron toxicity.
- Abdominal radiograph without radioopaque foreign body does not rule out iron ingestion.

 Common Questions and Answers

Q: Why isn't syrup of ipecac recommended to induce vomiting?
A: Since the major early signs and symptoms involving the GI tract include vomiting, inducing vomiting may interfere with the clinical assessment. There is also the risk of aspiration in the patient with severe poisoning.

Q: What is the recommendation regarding observation of a patient for development of symptoms with iron ingestion of an unknown quantity?
A: Observe for 6 hours. Those asymptomatic 6 hours after ingestion are not likely to exhibit systemic illness.

ICD-9-CM 964.0

BIBLIOGRAPHY

Fine JS. Iron poisoning. *Curr Probl Pediatr* 2000;30(3):71–90.

Henretig FM, et al. Acute iron poisoning. In: Shaw LM, Kwong TC, eds. *The Clinical Toxicology Laboratory: Contemporary Practice of Poisoning Evaluation.* Washington, DC: AACC Press, 2001:401–409.

Howland MA. Antidotes in depth: deferoxamine. In: Goldfrank LR, et al. *Goldfrank's Toxicologic Emergencies.* 7th Ed. New York: McGraw-Hill, 2002:558–562.

Litovitz T, Manoguerra A. Comparison of pediatric poisoning hazards: an analysis of 3.8 million exposure incidents. *Pediatrics* 1992;89(6):999–1006.

Mills KC, Curry SC. Acute iron poisoning. *Emerg Med Clin North Am* 1994;12:397–413.

Morris CC. Pediatric iron poisonings in the United States. *South Med J* 2000;93(4):352–358.

Osterhoudt KC, Shannon M, Henretig FM. Toxicologic emergencies. In: Fleisher GR, Ludwig S, eds. *Textbook of Pediatric Emergency Medicine.* 4th Ed. Philadelphia, PA: Lippincott Williams & Wilkins, 1999:914–917.

Perrone J. Iron. In: Goldfrank LR, et al. *Goldfrank's Toxicologic Emergencies,* 7th ed. New York: The McGraw-Hill Companies, Inc, 2002:548–557.

Tenenbein M. Whole bowel irrigation in iron poisoning. *J Pediatr* 1987;111:142–145.

Watson WA, et al. 2002 annual report of the American Association of Poison Control Centers Toxic Exposure Surveillance System. *Am J Emerg Med* 2003;21(5):353–421.

Author: Carla Campbell

Irritable Bowel Syndrome

 Database

DEFINITION

• A cluster of symptoms that include abdominal discomfort or pain, and at least two of the following three features:

—Improvement in the abdominal pain after a bowel movement
—An increasing number of stools with the start of the pain
—Change in the form and appearance of the stool with the onset of pain.

These symptoms can occur on a recurrent basis and need not be continuous in order for IBS to be considered. The symptoms need to be present for at least 12 weeks in the previous 12-month period. These criteria (Rome II) were developed as a formal symptom-based set of features to make the diagnosis of IBS due to the lack of any specific tests.

• The difficulty in the diagnosis of IBS is the poor understanding of the mechanisms of the disease, lack of completely specific symptoms, lack of specific testing and symptoms that can be associated with a wide variety of other gastrointestinal (GI) organic illnesses.
• Terms such as spastic colon, nervous colon, or spastic colitis have also been used to describe IBS. Spastic colitis, however, is inaccurate because these patients do not have evidence of inflammation of their colon (colitis) at colonoscopy.

PATHOPHYSIOLOGY

• Most commonly, IBS is thought to be a disorder of GI function relating to motility, sensation and/or perception.
• There are no actual histologic, microbiologic, or biochemical abnormalities noted in patients with IBS albeit there is a subset of patients who develop symptoms as a postinfectious complication.
• The pathogenesis of IBS is believed to be multifactorial with a variety of influences on the gut-brain axis at various levels. These factors interact to cause the symptoms of IBS and include: physiologic, social, cultural, behavioral and environmental. The interaction of these factors may be further influenced in the patient with IBS by other triggers such as diet, stress, emotion, physical activity, and hormonal changes.

EPIDEMIOLOGY

• IBS is a highly prevalent disorder and is thought to occur in up to 22% of the general population. It is more prevalent than hypertension, asthma, diabetes and ischemic heart disease.
• In adults, IBS is the seventh most common cause of visits to primary care physicians and the second most common cause of referral to a gastroenterologist. It is responsible for 3.5 million visits per year.
• 50% of patients present with symptoms before age 35, and 33% can trace their symptoms back into childhood.
• Female to male ratio ranges from 1.5 to 2.0:1.
• More common in adolescents in the pediatric population.
• Poses a significant health care burden with a total cost of $30 billion dollars in 1999–2000.
• There is no known genetic predisposition for developing IBS.

COMPLICATIONS

• A large number of the complications that arise from IBS include depression and anxiety causing a decreased QoL.
• Patients with IBS show a significant amount of absenteeism from both school and work.

 Differential Diagnosis

• The diagnosis of IBS is based on a clinical spectrum of formal symptoms (Rome II) but also to some degree still remains a diagnosis of exclusion.
• Common disorders that need to be considered are those that can present with recurrent abdominal pain and altered bowel patterns. These include:

—Chronic inflammatory conditions of the bowel (Crohn disease, ulcerative colitis, in determinate colitis, celiac disease)
—Infectious disorders (parasites, bacterial)
—Lactose intolerance
—Complications of constipation (megacolon, encopresis, intermittent sigmoid volvulus)
—Drug-induced diarrhea or constipation
—Gynecologic disorders
—Neoplasms
—Psychiatric disorders

• Patients fulfilling Rome II criteria for IBS rarely (<1% probability) have an underlying illness. On the other hand, IBS is so prevalent that there can be a cooccurrence with other disorders that can modify and/or amplify the clinical features of IBS. Common disorders include celiac disease and lactose intolerance.

 Data Gathering

HISTORY

• Evaluation of these patients needs to include a careful and detailed history, including a description of the symptoms, with assessment if they recur on a regular basis.

—A detailed diet and travel history
—Inciting and exacerbating factors
—Characteristics of abdominal pain: Sharp, dull, crampy, or burning. It is usually periumbilical or lower abdominal in nature, but not necessarily. The pain starts after a meal and rarely awakens a patient from sleep. Patients, especially children, describe associated symptoms, such as pallor, nausea, anorexia, and fatigue with the abdominal pain.
—Presence or absence of abdominal distension?
—Presence of increased belching and/or flatulence?
—Change in bowel habits: Presence of alternating diarrhea and constipation? Patients tend to have one predominant form. Most patients experience relief of pain after a bowel movement. In patients with constipation, they may go several days to a week without any stool passage.
—In some instances, mucus can be described in this group of patients. However, blood is a rare finding and is usually associated with local/anal irritation or fissure secondary to diarrhea or constipation.
—Presence of fever, anorexia, weight loss, rash and joint complaints? Suggests non-IBS diseases.
—Presence of other "red flags"? Nocturnal symptoms that awaken a patient, family history of GI disorders and a recent major change in the nature or severity of the symptoms.
—Presence of triggers for IBS symptoms? Stress, anxiety, certain foods (wheats, milk, alcohol, caffeine), and cigarette smoking.

Physical Examination

- Findings are usually completely normal including a rectal examination.
- There is usually no evidence of weight loss or growth failure.

 ## Laboratory Aids

TESTS

- There are no laboratory tests that are diagnostic for IBS. Routine CBC, ESR, urinalysis, electrolytes, liver function tests, albumin, amylase, lipase, celiac antibodies and thyroid studies are performed to exclude other diseases.
- Abdominal x-ray, or CAT scan may exclude an intraabdominal Process
- Lactose breath test: Presence of lactose intolerance.
- Stool cultures for routine specimen, clostridium difficile and ova and parasites: Exclude infectious etiologies for symptoms
- Gastric emptying, antralduodenal and anal-rectal manometry are special tests
- Upper endoscopy and/or a colonoscopy. Indications include:

—Bleeding
—Profuse diarrhea
—Weight loss
—Iron deficiency anemia
—Abnormal laboratory or x-ray studies
—Extraintestinal manifestations of inflammatory bowel disease.

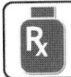 ## Therapy

- The best, but at times the most difficult, treatment for IBS is reassurance of both the parents and the child.
- The symptoms should be addressed, but the patient and/or parents should be made aware that the symptoms are not dangerous to the child.
- Interventions have been attempted to decrease the severity of the symptoms:

—Bulking agents: Fiber supplementation in the diet is a usual first step in therapy which prolongs stool transit time and absorption.
—Laxatives: These have unproven benefits, no real trials and frequent complications.
—Antispasmodics: Dicyclomine (Bentyl) and hyoscyamine (Levsin), can aid in pain relief but overall efficacy in global symptom control is not proven
—Tricyclic antidepressants: Pain relief is somewhat effective, but can have unwanted side effects.

- Newer therapies

—5-HT4 agonist—tegaserod (Zelnorm) activates cholinergic neurons to stimulate GI contractility. Three large studies have shown very good results in controlling global IBS symptoms in patients with constipation predominant features.
—5-HT3 antagonist—alosetron (Lotronex) inhibition of cholinergic neurons and of visceral sensory mechanisms. Presently, it is only available in limited, restricted use in females with severe diarrhea predominant IBS that have failed other therapies. Complications of ischemic colitis (3:1,000) and severe constipation have been reported. A few cases of ischemic colitis resulted in either death or need for surgical resection.

- Future therapies

A variety of new pharmacologic agents are in the development stage that will target specific arms of the gut-brain axis to alleviate the symptoms of IBS. The new agents in the pipeline include 5HT2B antagonists, serotonin and norepinephrine reuptake inhibitors, NK1 modulators (Substance P), NK1 antagonists to block peristalsis, CRF-1 antagonist and alpha-2 adrenergic agonist (clonidine) which can reduce colonic pain sensation in response to distention and relax colonic compliance and tone.

- Psychotherapy: Patients are taught a variety of techniques and exercises to use during the episodes of pain that allow them to focus on other subjects, not on the pain.
- Overall, the most effective intervention may be to combine therapies that will target specific symptoms and arms of the gut-brain axis in order to globally control the symptoms from IBS.

 ## Follow-Up

There is no standard or specific follow-up needed for patients with IBS. They should continue with routine care, and one should ensure effective communication between the patient and physician to review the clinical symptoms and evaluate for any changes in the symptoms that may indicate another underlying problem.

PITFALLS

- Avoid downplaying the clinical symptoms of patients because it will make their acceptance of the treatment plan more difficult.
- Confine testing to basic screening tests so that patients are not left with the impression that there is a significant organic disease present.

 ## Common Questions and Answers

Q: Evidence of microscopic colitis can be consistent with the diagnosis of IBS?
A: There should be no histologic or laboratory abnormalities.

Q: Patients with IBS may have a coexisting GI disorder?
A: Frequently, patients can be diagnosed with lactose intolerance or celiac disease. In these instances both disorders need to be treated in order to alleviate the symptoms.

ICD-9-CM 564.1

BIBLIOGRAPHY

Camilleri M. Management of the irritable bowel syndrome. *Gastroenterology* 2001;120:652–668.

Camilleri M. Treating irritable bowel syndrome: overview, perspective and future therapies. *Br J Pharmacol* 2004;141:1237–1248.

Milla PJ. Irritable bowel syndrome in childhood. *Gastroenterology* 2001;120(1):287–290.

Staiano A, Corazziari E. Irritable bowel syndrome: contrasts and comparisons between children and adults. *J Pediatr Gastroenterol Nutr* 2001;32(suppl 1):S32–S34.

Talley NJ. Irritable bowel syndrome and health care seeking: do we pass our bad habits onto our children? *Am J Gastroenterol* 2000;95(2):340–341.

Author: Edisio Semeao

Kawasaki Disease (Mucocutaneous Lymph Node Syndrome)

 Database

DEFINITION

• An idiopathic, multisystem disease of young children characterized by vasculitis of the small- and medium-sized blood vessels.
• Diagnosis of Kawasaki disease (KD) requires a fever for greater than 5 days and four of the following criteria:
—Nonexudative conjunctival injection
—Polymorphous, nonvesicular rash
—Mucosal involvement of the upper respiratory tract that may include erythema, fissures of the lips, crusting of the lips and mouth, or a strawberry tongue. Exudative pharyngitis and discrete oral lesions (e.g., vesicles, etc.) are rare.
—Edema or erythema of the hands and feet
—Cervical adenopathy of at least 1.5 cm in diameter, which is often unilateral
• Atypical KD
—Patients may present with less than four of the five diagnostic criteria and still develop aneurysms.
—Atypical disease is more common in children younger than 1 year of age.

CAUSES

• Etiology is uncertain. Epidemiologic and clinical features suggest an infectious cause.
• There is some evidence that KD may be associated with infection with superantigen–producing bacteria (either *Staphylococcus aureus* or group A streptococci).
• Association with recent use of rug cleaners or having had rugs shampooed has not been substantiated.

EPIDEMIOLOGY

• Median age of cases is 2 years with 77% of cases in children younger than 5 years of age, 5% of cases in children older than 10 years of age, and almost unheard of in children over age 15. Recurrence is low, approximately 0.8%.
• There has been little change in the incidence in the last several years in the United States. The annual hospitalization rate in the United States for children less than 5 years of age is 17.1 per 100,000 children. Rates were highest among Asian and Pacific Islander children followed by African American children. KD accounted for greater than 4,200 hospitalizations in the United States in the year 2000 with hospital charges of about $35 million. There were no deaths reported among hospitalized patients during the acute phase of illness. KD has surpassed rheumatic fever as the leading cause of acquired heart disease in children in the United States.

COMPLICATIONS

• Aneurysms usually first noted 12–28 days after onset of the disease. Rarely appear more than 28 days after onset.
• Aneurysms may thrombose leading to myocardial infarction and death.
• Rarely, aneurysms may rupture acutely.
• A pancarditis is often present in the first 10 days of the illness. Pericardial effusions may accompany this.

PROGNOSIS

• Without treatment with intravenous immunoglobulin (IVIG) 15% to 25% of patients develop coronary aneurysms.
• Use of IVIG decreased the incidence of coronary artery aneurysms to 4% to 8%.
• Death occurs secondary to cardiac disease in 0.3% to 2% of cases; approximately 10% is related to early myocarditis, and the remainder due to myocardial infarctions.
• Myocardial infarction can occur several years after the initial illness.
• Patients who are younger than 1 year, older than 8 years, male, and whose fevers persist for greater than 14 days are more likely to develop aneurysms.
• Mortality rates are much higher in males and patients who develop giant coronary artery aneurysms (diameter of greater than 8 mm).
• Patients with a history of KD may have a worse cardiovascular risk profile in later life, indicative of an increased risk of atherosclerotic heart disease compared to the general population.

ASSOCIATED ILLNESSES

• Diarrhea and abdominal pain may be seen.
• Patients may develop arthralgias or even frank arthritis.
• Pancarditis may present as myocardial dysfunction early in the course of disease with signs of congestive heart failure.
• Infantile periarteritis nodosa (PAN) is a previously described entity in which the pathologic findings of coronary artery aneurysms are indistinguishable from those seen in KD. Most patients with PAN do not have the other findings of KD.

 Differential Diagnosis

• Infections
—In one series, measles and group A β-hemolytic streptococcal infections most closely resembled KD and accounted for 83% of patients referred who did not have KD.
—Severe staphylococcal infections with toxin release (e.g., toxic shock syndrome) may also resemble KD, although there is usually renal involvement (extremely rare in KD) and low platelets.
—Other infections that must be considered include adenovirus, Epstein-Barr virus, roseola, enterovirus, Rocky Mountain spotted fever, and leptospirosis.
• Immunologic
—Juvenile rheumatoid arthritis and unusual variants of acute rheumatic fever
—Hypersensitivity reactions and Stevens-Johnson syndrome
—In Stevens-Johnson syndrome the conjunctivitis is more likely to be exudative, the rash is more likely to be vesicular with crusting, and there is often a history of drug ingestion.

 Data Gathering

HISTORY

Typical presentation proceeds through three recognizable phases:
• Acute phase (1–2 weeks from onset):
—Highly febrile, irritable, toxic appearing
—Fever usually greater than 40°C and may be as high as 41.6°C
—Oral changes usually quickly follow and also may last 1 to 2 weeks.
—Rash prone to occur in perineal area
—Edema and erythema of the feet are usually painful and limit ambulation.
• Subacute phase (from 2 to 8 weeks after onset)
—Without treatment, gradual improvement occurs; fever decreases and there is desquamation of the perineal area, palms, soles, and/or periungual areas.
—Coronary artery aneurysms often appear during the early portion of this phase and acute myocardial infarction may be seen.
—May have persistent arthritis or arthralgias
• Convalescent phase (from months to years after)
—Resolution of remaining symptoms
—Laboratory values return to normal (see subsequent text).
—Aneurysms may resolve or patients may have persistent aneurysms, persistent cardiac dysfunction, or even myocardial infarction.

 Physical Examination

Finding: High, unremitting fevers that last 1 to 2 weeks
Significance: Fever

Finding: Rash is polymorphous and not vesicular.
Significance: Seen in 99% of cases; predilection for perineum. Often prominent on trunk, usually maculopapular, may coalesce and may be petechial.

Finding: Conjunctivitis
Significance: Bilateral and nonexudative (96% of cases)

Finding: Oral changes may be erythema, fissures, and crusting of lips, diffuse oropharyngeal erythema, or the presence of a strawberry tongue or any combination of these findings.
Significance: Usually not exudative

Finding: Extremity changes may include erythema of the palms and soles and/or induration of the hands and feet (99% of cases).
Significance: Desquamation, especially periungual, usually occurs in subacute phase. Transverse grooves across the fingernails (Beau lines) may be seen 2 to 3 months after onset.

Finding: Adenopathy is usually cervical and often unilateral.
Significance: Least often seen of the major criteria (75%–82% of cases). May be fleeting and easily missed.

Finding: Aseptic meningitis
Significance: Is common and patients are extremely irritable and may show signs of encephalopathy or ataxia.

Kawasaki Disease (Mucocutaneous Lymph Node Syndrome)

Finding: Pancarditis during the acute phase
Significance: May present with tachycardia, gallop rhythms, muffled heart sounds, signs of congestive heart failure, and murmurs consistent with aortic or mitral insufficiency.
Finding: Abdominal exam
Significance: Patients may have a right upper quadrant mass (hydrops of gallbladder), diarrhea, hepatosplenomegaly, or jaundice.
Finding: Meatitis and vulvitis
Significance: May be seen in association with urethritis and sterile pyuria.
Finding: Arthralgias are common; frank arthritis is seen in approximately one-third of patients.
Significance: May involve large and small joints; is nondeforming. Onset may be as late as second or third week. Usually resolves in approximately 1 month.
Finding: Uveitis
Significance: During acute phase, slit lamp examination may reveal anterior uveitis in approximately 80% of KD cases.

 ## Laboratory Aids

Test: Complete blood cell
Significance: WBC usually increased with a left shift; greater than 20,000 in 50% of cases and greater than 30,000 in 15%. Hemoglobin less than 10 mg/dL is an independent predictor of poor response to IVIG.
Test: Increased erythrocyte sedimentation rate; increased CRP
Significance: ESR often greater than 100 mm; CRP greater than 10 predicts a poor response to IVIG.
Test: Platelet count
Significance: Platelets may be low, normal, or high at presentation but increase rapidly after the second week of illness; during subacute phase platelet counts may increase to 1 to 2 × 10⁶.
Test: Lactate dehydrogenase level (LDH)
Significance: LDH greater than 590 IU/L predicts poor response to IVIG.
Test: Other laboratory abnormalities include:
- Sterile pyuria and mild proteinuria on urinalysis
- Mild increases in hepatic transaminases
- A cerebrospinal fluid pleocytosis with a normal protein and glucose
- Mild anemia
- Mild hypoalbuminemia
- Hyponatremia
- Hypophosphatemia
- Severe hemolytic anemias

Test: ECG
Significance: During acute phase may show prolonged PR interval, decreased QRS voltage, flat T waves, and ST changes.
Test: Chest x-ray
Significance: May show dilated heart during acute phase.
Test: Echocardiogram
Significance: During acute phase can show a decreased shortening fraction and effusion. Aneurysms may be detected as early as 6 days into the illness, and peak onset is between 3 to 4 weeks.

Test: Increased BUN or creatinine
Significance: If laboratory indicators of renal involvement are present, then illnesses other than KD should be considered (e.g., toxic shock syndrome).

 ## Emergency Care

- Maintain high suspicion so that cases of KD are not missed in the emergency department.
- If KD is suspected, assess for cardiac dysfunction with an ECG and obtain a cardiology consult.
- Good supportive care should be provided including fluid therapy and possibly inotropes to treat shock when present (rare presentation).
- Admission for definitive treatment and monitoring is imperative.

 ## Therapy

DRUGS

- Intravenous immunoglobulin (IVIG)
—Usual dose is 2 g/kg as a one-time dose over 10 hours.
—Efficacy of IVIG after the 10th day of illness is unclear.
—Patients who fail to respond to an initial dose of IVIG or who have a recrudescence of their symptoms should be retreated (up to two-thirds may have a good response to repeat doses).
—Side effects: Patients may develop signs of fluid overload and congestive heart failure. Aseptic meningitis may also be seen. This may be difficult to differentiate from the aseptic meningitis seen in patients as part of their KD.
- Aspirin
—High-dose aspirin was the mainstay of therapy; still used in conjunction with IVIG, although no data look at IVIG with aspirin versus IVIG alone.
—Usual initial dose is 80 to 100 mg/kg per day in divided doses. High dose required to overcome malabsorption of aspirin seen during acute phase of KD.
- Corticosteroids
—New data suggest IV pulse methylprednisolone may be useful.
—Methylprednisolone has been given in conjunction with early doses of IVIG or as rescue therapy in patients who don't respond to 2 or 3 doses of IVIG. It may need to be tapered to prevent recrudescence of symptoms. There is a need for randomized, controlled trials to study the efficacy of steroids and, if they are found to be useful the most appropriate time for their use.
- Cyclophosphamide has also been reported to be useful in some patients who do not respond to repeated doses of IVIG.

DURATION

- Aspirin is continued at high dose until day 14 of the illness or when the child has been afebrile for 48 hours.
- Aspirin dose is then decreased to 30 mg/kg per day until 4 weeks after onset and additionally decreased to 3 to 10 mg/kg per day for 6 to 8 weeks or until the platelet count returns to normal.

- If there are coronary artery abnormalities dipyridamole at 3 to 5 mg/kg per day should be added to the aspirin for its vasodilatory effect. Aspirin and dipyridamole should be continued for 1 year or until coronary artery aneurysms resolve.

ACTIVITY

- Children with KD should be kept at bed rest until the second or third week of illness or when they have been afebrile for over 72 hours due to the possibility of myocardial involvement during the acute phase.
- Isolation of patients is not indicated.
- Even asymptomatic patients should be restricted from strenuous activities.

 ## Follow-Up

WHEN TO EXPECT IMPROVEMENT

- The natural course is a gradual improvement during the subacute phase.
- With IVIG children usually defervesce and show significant resolution of clinical symptoms within 2 to 3 days of treatment (70% to 80%).
- Two-thirds of patients who receive a repeat dose of IVIG will respond to this dose.

SIGNS TO WATCH FOR

- White blood cell count, platelet count, and ESR should be followed weekly to biweekly until they return to normal.
- Weekly echocardiograms should be done to rule out the development of coronary artery aneurysms from weeks 2 to 6 of the illness.
- If aneurysms are present, cardiology follow-up should include coronary artery catheterization and imaging at some time (usually 8 to 12 weeks after onset of illness).
- Symptoms of cardiac insufficiency (fatigue, chest pain, dyspnea on exertion, etc.) should be respected and an evaluation for myocardial dysfunction undertaken when these are present.

 ## Common Questions and Answers

Q: Do coronary artery aneurysms associated with KD ever resolve?
A: Most coronary artery aneurysms do resolve. Even some giant aneurysms (those greater than 8 mm in diameter) will resolve; there is concern, however, that even if aneurysms resolve, these patients may be at risk for the early development of atherosclerosis.

ICD-9-CD 446.1

BIBLIOGRAPHY

Holman RC, et al. Kawasaki hospitalization in the United States, 1997 and 2000. *Pediatrics* 2003;112:495–501.

Meissner HC, Leung DYM. Kawasaki syndrome: where are the answers? *Pediatrics* 2003;112:672–675.

Silva AA, Maeno Y, Hashmi A, et al. Cardiovascular risk factors after Kawasaki disease: a case-control study. *J Pediatr* 2001;138(3):400–405.

Author: James M. Callahan

Knee Pain, Anterior/Patellofemoral Malalignment Syndrome

 Database

DEFINITION

This condition is characterized by discomfort at the anterior aspect of the knee and is generally associated with activities especially those that involve running, jumping, and climbing stairs.

Also referred to as miserable malalignment syndrome.

PATHOPHYSIOLOGY

Predisposing factors for patellofemoral malalignment syndrome include:

- Femoral anteversion
- Genu valgus
- Pes planus

These three anatomic features have been commonly referred to as a terrible triad contributing to anterior knee pain. Because the entire kinetic chain is linked in function malalignment at one area can lead to secondary stresses at a distant location.

- Excess femoral anteversion as well as marked pes planus can contribute to the increase lateral pull on the patella and subsequent patellofemoral pain.
- Further contributing factors include a wider pelvis and more laterally positioned tibial tubercle both of which also contribute to altered biomechanics at the knee.
- Tight hamstrings, heel cords, and quadriceps as well as diminished quadriceps tone can lead to increased forces across the patellofemoral joint.

 Differential Diagnosis

- Osgood Schlatter disease

Osgood Schlatter disease is tenderness not at the patella but at the anterior tibial tubercle. This is a self-limiting inflammation of the apophysis that tends to occur in growing teenagers. Irregularity and fragmentation of the apophysis is seen on lateral radiographs.

- Meniscus tear

This disruption of the crescent shaped fibrocartilaginous tissue adjacent to the tibial and femoral articular surfaces most commonly presents as posteromedial and posterolateral hemijoint tenderness with knee hyperflexion and rotation.

- Prepatellar bursitis

This is an inflammation of the fluid-filled bursal sac beneath the subcutaneous tissue and immediately anterior to the patella. This is more common in patients that kneel for extended periods of time and has been called carpet layer's knee. This swelling and tenderness is immediately anterior to the patella and does not primarily present with deeper tenderness in the medial and lateral parapatellar regions found in patellofemoral syndrome

 Data Gathering

HISTORY

Question: Pain in under and around the kneecap with activities including squatting, sitting for prolonged periods with the knees bent and going up or down stairs or hills?
Significance: These activities increase patellofemoral contact stress.

Question: Recent history of direct trauma to the kneecap?
Significance: A blunt trauma to the kneecap can cause soft tissue or subchondral contusion which may exacerbate this condition.

 Physical Examination

Finding: Pathologic strength and flexibility including weak quadriceps muscles, tight hamstrings, calf and hip muscles.
Significance: Diminished strength and poor flexibility lead to increased contact pressures within the knee.

Finding: Improper hip, knee and ankle rotation as well as angulation.
Significance: Improper angulation and rotation can lead to lateralized vector forces across the knee.

Finding: Cracking noises from the front of the knee with flexion and extension
Significance: Cracking can be a sign of softening of the undersurface of the patella. Chondromalacia is patellar articular cartilage. These changes range from mild cracking as a result of pathology softening to locking and catching as a result of cartilage disruption.

 Laboratory Aids

Test: Anterior, posterior, lateral, merchant plain radiographs of the knee
Significance: The merchant kneecap view shows the shape of the patella within the trochlea. Patients will frequently be found to have lateral patellar tilt as well as an abnormally shaped patella with excessive elongation of the lateral patellar facet.

Test: MRI
Significance: An MRI is not a first line study for patellofemoral syndrome; however, it may be performed to rule out associated pathology in patients with recalcitrant pain and unusual clinical presentations.

Knee Pain, Anterior/Patellofemoral Malalignment Syndrome

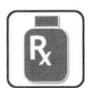 Therapy

- A progressive exercise program is the main focus of treatment.
- Activity restriction in the initial acutely symptomatic stage is instituted to eliminate high impact sports including especially those which involve running and jumping.
- Strength and flexibility exercises are needed to increase the strength and control the quadriceps muscle as well as to stretch the quadriceps, hamstrings and tendoachilles complex.
- Straight leg raising program can help to strengthen the quadriceps.

—This can be performed several times each day as a home exercise program or formally with physical therapy in more recalcitrant cases.
—Quadriceps, hamstrings and tendoachilles stretches can be performed at the same time intervals as the strengthening program

- Patients can be advanced from low resistance exercises such as swimming, stationary bike and elliptical trainers and to higher level running activities.

PITFALLS

Patients with a traumatic effusion, locking, catching, instability to ligamentous stress testing, multiple joint effusions or night waking should be evaluated for other traumatic or medical conditions.

 Common Questions and Answers

Q: Is it acceptable to play sports or is this condition too dangerous?
A: Patients with a history patellofemoral syndrome who have regained their strength and flexibility are permitted to return to sports provided that they do not have pain and limping during their activities. A history of catching, locking, or knee effusions may be a sign of further biomechanical intraarticular pathology that should be addressed.

Q: Is bracing indicated?
A: Some patients with anterior knee pain respond to neoprene sleeves and those with a component of increased lateral translation may benefit from neoprene sleeves with lateral patellar supports. Bracing, however, is not a substitute for a strength and conditioning program.

Q: Is chondromalacia patella the same as patellofemoral syndrome?
A: No. Chondromalacia is a classification of the anatomic pathologic changes of the undersurface of the patella. Patellofemoral syndrome is the clinical condition encompassing the patient's history, physical, and radiographic elements of anterior knee pain.

BIBLIOGRAPHY

Dalton SE. Overuse injures in adolescent athletes. *Sports Med* 1992;13:58–70.

Ganley TJ, et al. Pediatric Sports Medicine. *Curr Opin Orthopaed*, 2001;12:456–461.

Gerrard DF. Overuse injury and growing bones: the young athlete at risk. *Br J Sports Med* 1993;27:14–18.

Lou J, et al. Exercise and Children's Health. *Curr Sports Med Rep* 2002;I:349–353.

Maffulli N, Baxter-Jones ADG. Common skeletal injures in young athletes. *Sports Med* 1995;19:137–149.

Saperstein AL, Nicholas SJ. Pediatric and adolescent sports medicine. *Pediatr Clin North Am* 1996;43:1013–1033.

Smith AD, Tao SS. Knee injures in young athletes. *Clin Sports Med* 1995;14:629–650.

Stanitski CL. Management of sports injures in children and adolescents. *Orthop Clin North Am* 1988;19:689–698.

Author: Ted Ganley

Kwashiorkor

Database

DEFINITION

- Extreme expression of protein-energy malnutrition
- Characterized by edema, growth failure, hypoalbuminemia, fatty infiltration of the liver, and specific dermatosis
- First described in West Africa by Cecily Williams. The word kwashiorkor in Ghanian means "red or yellow boy."

CAUSES

Diet deficient in protein and a low protein-to-energy ratio are important factors in the development of kwashiorkor. Other factors postulated include:

- Carbohydrate overloading of a severely malnourished child
- Aflatoxin poisoning
- Imbalance between the production of toxic-free radical and its disposal
- Essential fatty acid deficiency
- Deficiency of trace minerals (e.g., zinc, copper, manganese, and selenium)
- Oxidative and nitrosative stress

More recent data reveals lower plasma thiols (e.g., G6PDH, glutathione reductase, FAD and glutathione) in children with kwashiorkor and that clinical signs and symptoms disappeared with normalization of the biochemical findings.
Further investigations have shown an association between selenium deficiency and congestive heart failure in kwashiorkor.

PATHOPHYSIOLOGY

- Hypoalbuminemia reduces colloid osmotic pressure, leading to edema.
- Reduction in renal blood flow and glomerular filtration rate due to decreased plasma volume and decreased cardiac output as a consequence of hypoalbuminemia.
- Increase in ferritin stimulates release of antidiuretic hormone and subsequent fluid retention.

EPIDEMIOLOGY

- Most common age group are children younger than 2 years of age.
- Prevalent in Third World countries; occurs in developed countries secondary to nutritional ignorance rather than food deprivation
- Other contributory factors include misconception concerning the use of foods, unstable home environment, high prevalence of alcoholism, poor sanitary conditions, and societal beliefs that prohibit the use of many nutritious foods.

COMPLICATIONS

- Fluid and electrolyte disturbances

—Hypoosmolality with moderate hyponatremia
—Mild-to-moderate metabolic acidosis
—Hypocalcemia
—Decreased body potassium without hypokalemia
—Decreased body magnesium with or without hypomagnesemia

- Infections

—Gram-positive and gram-negative organisms; the latter is more common in severe protein-energy malnutrition

- Cardiac failure

—May occur in the midst of severe anemia, during rehydration, and shortly after the introduction of high-protein and high-energy feedings

- Severe anemia

—Hemoglobin levels usually improve with proper dietary management.
—Blood transfusion should be reserved for patients with hemoglobin less than 4 g/100 mL, hypoxia, or impending cardiac failure.

- Hypothermia and hypoglycemia

—Secondary to either impaired nonregulatory mechanisms, reduced fuel substrate, or severe infection

- Severe vitamin deficiency

—Vitamin A deficiency is common

Differential Diagnosis

Protein energy malnutrition due to the impairment in protein absorption or metabolism

Data Gathering

HISTORY

Question: Dietary history?
Significance: Assess for adequacy of protein and total calories.

Question: Cultural beliefs about feeding?
Significance: May contribute to low protein intake.

Question: Breast-feeding?
Significance: May protect infant but expose older sibling to protein deficiency.

Question: Possible protein loss, diarrhea, renal disease?
Significance: Nondietary cause of decreased serum protein.

Question: Skin rash?
Significance: See Physical Examination.

Question: Growth records?
Significance: Decreased growth velocity commensurate with poor protein intake.

Physical Examination

- Children appear apathetic, irritable, and sad.
- Predominant soft, pitting, painless edema of the soft tissues usually in the feet and legs, perineum, upper extremities, and face.

Finding: Dyspigmentation of the skin
Significance: Hair develops a red-brown color, loses its luster, becomes fragile and easily pluckable. Alternating bands of depigmentation and normal hair known as the "flag sign."

Finding: Characteristic dermatosis of kwashiorkor
Significance: Also known as "flaky" dermatosis. Appears in areas of the body subject to friction or pressure, notably the flexures, groin, buttocks, behind the knees, or at the elbows. It is described as patchy areas of darkly pigmented skin with a clear margin and a slightly raised edge. As the lesions progress, these lesions peel or desquamate. In severe cases, the skin peels away in patches leaving pale, ulcerated lesions lacking pigmentation. The borders of these lesions may have new highly pigmented dark plaques. These severe peeling lesions may resemble second-degree burns, but unlike burns, the dermatosis of kwashiorkor lacks a surrounding of erythema and is accompanied by edema.

Finding: Vesiculations of skin
Significance: Resulting in weeping lesions

Finding: Height
Significance: May be normal or retarded, depending on the chronicity of the illness.

Finding: Pale, cold, and cyanotic extremities
Significance: Decreased vascular volume secondary to decreased protein concentration.

Finding: Abdomen is frequently protuberant secondary to poor peristalsis.
Significance: Leading to distended stomach and intestinal loops.

 Laboratory Aids

Test: Common biochemical findings
Significance:

- Significant reduction in serum concentration of total protein and albumin.
- Hemoglobin and hematocrit are usually low.
- Ratio of nonessential to essential amino acids in plasma is elevated in kwashiorkor and usually normal in marasmus.
- Increased serum elevation of free fatty acids
- Low serum and urine carnitine levels

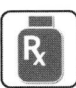 Therapy

Treatment protocol is usually divided into three stages:

- Resolving life-threatening conditions

—Restoration can be achieved by oral rehydration solution. As soon as the patient improves, liquid elemental feeds can be initiated. Intravenous fluids must be used when there is persistent vomiting or abdominal distention. Electrolyte imbalances should be treated.

- Restoring nutritional status

—Nutritional status can be improved by nasogastric feeds with 6 to 12 feedings per day. High-protein, high-energy formulas are used. Initial treatment should provide average energy and protein requirements, followed by a gradual increase to 1.5 times the energy and 3 to 4 times the protein requirements by the seventh day. No change in weight or a decrease caused by loss of edema, accompanied by large diuresis, can occur.

- Ensuring nutritional rehabilitation

—Intravenous alimentation is rarely justified in primary protein-energy malnutrition and can increase mortality rates.
—Introduction of traditional home food and therapy can continue on an outpatient basis. Emotional and physical stimulation must be provided. Emphasizing nutritious use of household foods, personal and environmental hygiene, and dietary management of diarrhea and other diseases is also an aspect of management.

- N-acetylcysteine supplementation has been recently studied with an earlier and faster recovery in clinical signs and symptoms as well as glutathione levels

PROGNOSIS

Early recognition is important in treating kwashiorkor. Treatment corrects the acute signs of the disease, but catch-up growth in height may never be achieved. A higher mortality rate is associated with severe anthropometric deficits. Mortality rate in kwashiorkor can be as high as 40%, but adequate treatment can reduce it to less than 10%. Some of the factors that indicate poor prognosis are:

- Age of less than 6 months
- Infections
- Dehydration and electrolyte abnormalities
- Persistent tachycardia, signs of heart failure
- Total serum protein less than 3 g/100 mL
- Elevated serum bilirubin
- Severe anemia with hypoxia
- Hypoglycemia and/or hypothermia

ICD-9-CM 260

BIBLIOGRAPHY

Badaloo A, et al. Cysteine supplementation improves the erythrocyte glutathione synthesis rate in children with severe edematous malnutrition. *American J Clin Nutr* 2002;76:495–496.

Carvalho NF, Kenney RD, Carrington PH, et al. Severe nutritional deficiencies in toddlers resulting from health food milk alternatives. *Pediatrics* 2001;107(4):E46.

Latham MC. The dermatosis of kwashiorkor in young children Ithaca, NY: Cornell University, 1991.

Liu T, et al. Kwashiorkor in the United States: fad diets, perceived and true milk allergy, and nutritional ignorance. *Arch Dermatol* 2001;137(5):630–636.

Ocal B, Unal S, Zorlu P, et al. Echocardiographic evaluation of cardiac functions and left ventricular mass in children with malnutrition. *J Paediatr Child Health* 2001;37(1):14–17.

Oumeish OY, Oumeish I. Nutritional skin problems in children. [Review] *Clinics in Dermatology* 2003;21(4):260–263.

Rossouw JE. Kwashiorkor is North America. *Am J Clin Nutr* 1989;49:588–592.

Author: Helen Anita John-Kelly

Lacrimal Duct Obstruction

 Database

DEFINITION

Lacrimal duct obstruction is the congenital or acquired blockage of the distal portion of the tear drainage system. The obstruction extends from the lacrimal sac to the opening of the nasolacrimal duct in the inferior meatus in the nose. This results in chronic tearing.

PATHOPHYSIOLOGY

• Congenital obstruction occurs from incomplete canalization of the nasolacrimal duct during embryogenesis
• Acquired obstructions result from scar tissue occluding the duct. This usually results secondarily from infection, inflammation or trauma.

EPIDEMIOLOGY

Approximately 6% of newborns, most of which resolves spontaneously.

COMPLICATIONS

• Acute dacryocystitis (acute infection and inflammation of the lacrimal sac), which rapidly appears as an erythematous nodule and surrounding cellulitis in the inferior medial canthal area and medial lower eyelid
• Chronic low-grade dacryocystitis manifested by subtle mucopurulent discharge from the eye which may be intermittently symptomatic

PROGNOSIS

• Spontaneous resolution in approximately 90% of children by 12 months of age with congenital obstruction. If there is no spontaneous resolution, surgical intervention involving a probing and irrigation is recommended.
• Acquired obstruction requires surgical intervention

 Differential Diagnosis

• Causes of increased tear production: Congenital glaucoma, reflex tearing secondary to dry eye, seventh nerve palsies, trichiasis, entropion, corneal abrasion
• Causes of decreased drainage: Imperforate puncta or canaliculi, ectropion, lateral canthus dystopia, traumatic injury to the nasolacrimal drainage system

 Data Gathering

HISTORY

• Determine when the symptoms began.
• Clarify which eye is more symptomatic and if frank epiphora is present.
• Congenital obstruction usually manifests itself within the first few months of life.
• Patients with acquired obstruction usually have a history of eye infection, dacryocystitis or trauma to the drain system.
• Both present with symptoms including tearing, crusting of eyelashes particularly upon awaking, and discharge from eye.

 Physical Examination

Finding: Increased tear meniscus, maceration of eyelid skin, mucopurulent discharge, crusted debris on the eyelashes, and occasionally conjunctival hyperemia
Significance: Common symptoms

Finding: Palpation of lacrimal sac with expression of sac
Significance: Distal obstruction in lacrimal system allowing accumulation of mucopurulent material from the puncta with pressure on the lacrimal sac

 Laboratory Aids

Test: Dye disappearance test (DDT)
Significance:

• Fluorescein is applied to the conjunctival cul de sac and the patient is observed for 5 minutes.
• In a negative test (normal) the tear meniscus will become relatively unstained as the tears naturally flow down through the drainage system.
• In a positive test (abnormal) the height of the stained tear meniscus will either increase or fail to decrease due to the obstructed lacrimal system.

Lacrimal Duct Obstruction

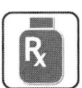 Therapy

- Initially, in congenital obstruction lacrimal sac massage and either ophthalmic antibiotic drops or ointment are applied when ocular discharge increases. Polysporin ophthalmic is typically recommended for coverage of the eyelid normal flora. This conservative approach is applied for the first year of life.
- If symptoms persist after 12 months of age, probing and irrigation of the nasolacrimal system are performed. An inferior turbinate infracture is performed in cases of distal obstruction to increase the space in the inferior meatus and facilitate outflow.
- If the initial probing and irrigation procedure fails, then the procedure is repeated with placement of silastic intubation and/or stretching of the lacrimal duct via balloon dacryoplasty. Silastic intubation can be monocanalicular or bicanalicular and is typically maintained for 3–6 months.
- If all else fails, a dacryocystorhinostomy, a permanent surgical connection between the lacrimal sac and the nose, is created to prevent recurrent infections (dacryocystitis).
- Patients with acquired obstructions typically require surgery. Probing and irrigation are performed to determine the location of the obstruction. These patients may also require silastic intubation, balloon dacryoplasty and/or dacryocystorhinostomy surgery.

 Follow-Up

Children with congenital obstruction should be reevaluated at 9 to 12 months of age and referred for probing and irrigation if still symptomatic. Children with acquired obstruction should be referred to an ophthalmologist for surgical treatment.

PITFALLS

Referral for probing and irrigation is delayed until patient is about 12 months of age; the probing and irrigation should be performed in a timely fashion to ensure a good outcome.

 Common Questions and Answers

Q: Is my child in any danger while the nasolacrimal duct remains obstructed?
A: Not usually. The obstruction presents more of a nuisance. However, occasionally the contents of the sac can become infected and will require oral or parenteral antibiotics.

Q: Why not wait longer to do the probing and irrigation in congenital nasolacrimal duct obstruction?
A: The failure rate of the initial procedure increases with age: if performed before 13 months of age, 96% success rate; between 13 and 18 months of age, 77% success rate; and between 18 and 24 months, 54% success rate.

ICD-9-CM 375.56

BIBLIOGRAPHY

Granet DB, Olitsky S, Burke MJ. Nasolacrimal duct obstruction. *J Pediatr Ophthalmol Strabismus* 2000;37(2):103–106.

Katowitz JA, Welsh MG. Timing of initial probing and irrigation in congenital nasolacrimal duct obstruction. *Ophthalmology* 1987;94:698–705.

Kushner BJ. The management of nasolacrimal duct obstruction in children between 18 months and 4 years old. *J AAPOS* 1998;2:57–60.

Mandeville JT, Woog JJ. Obstruction of the lacrimal drainage system. *Curr Opin Ophthalmol* 2002;13(5):303–309.

Robb RM. Congenital nasolacrimal duct obstruction. *Ophthamoll Clin North Am* 2001;14(3):443–446.

Authors: Femida Kherani
Scott M. Goldstein, 3rd edition

Lactose Intolerance

 ## Database

DEFINITION

- Lactose is a disaccharide built from glucose and galactose and is the major carbohydrate in infant's food (breast milk or milk-based formula).
- Lactose is important as a source of energy and promotes the absorption of calcium, phosphorus, and iron and is a prebiotic effect on the gut flora.
- Inability to digest the disaccharide lactose secondary to deficiency of the enzyme lactase, resulting in clinical symptoms.
- Three types of deficiency have been noted:

Congenital lactase deficiency is extremely rare. It presents during the newborn period, often with the first feeding of lactose-containing formula. Will cause severe diarrhea, failure to thrive and risk the newborns' life.

Acquired lactase deficiency can be divided to two subtypes:

Secondary to an insult /damage to the small bowel mucosa.

Secondary to normal developmental loss of enzyme activity due to genetic predisposition and aging.

PATHOLOGY

- Disaccharide activity can be measured in biopsy specimens of the small bowel and compared to normal values.
- The small bowel intestinal histology will often be normal (unless the reason is insult/damage to the small bowel mucosa).

EPIDEMIOLOGY

- After the lactation period there is gradual reduction of the enzyme activity—with genetic predisposition.
- Deficiency is found in up to 80% of native Australians, Americans, tropical Africans, and East and Southeastern Asians. It is also highly prevalent in African Americans.
- It can be clinically evident in many African Americans by 3–7 years of age.
- In Caucasians the clinical pictures starts in the second decade of life
- Adult lactase production is a dominant trait; lactase deficiency is a recessive trait with single Mendelian locus.

PROGNOSIS

Prognosis of lactase deficiency and clinical intolerance is excellent as elimination and enzyme replacement are possible; with lactose avoidance or with enzyme supplementation, the child can control and eliminate symptoms. However, lactose intolerance may be secondary to disease processes that should be treated promptly.

 ## Differential Diagnosis

Lactose intolerance may be secondary to a generalized small bowel mucosal dysfunction; the presence of other symptoms should prompt an evaluation. The differential diagnosis includes:

- Infection

—Viral and bacterial infections can cause secondary lactose intolerance. Most common pathogen is rotavirus.
—Parasitic infections can mimic lactose intolerance (Giardiasis).

- Inflammatory

—Small intestine Crohn disease can have associated lactose intolerance.

- Congenital

—Other carbohydrate enzyme deficiencies can mimic lactose intolerance. This includes sucrase-isomaltase or glucose-galactose malabsorption.
—Cystic fibrosis
—Shwachman syndrome

- Allergic/immune

—Celiac disease often is associated with lactose intolerance due to small intestinal damage.
—Protein intolerance can cause secondary lactose intolerance.

 ## Data Gathering

HISTORY

Question: Symptoms?
Significance: Classic symptoms include bloating, gaseousness, colicky abdominal pain, and diarrhea after digestion of lactose-containing meal.

Question: Diet history?
Significance: Provides important information.

Question: A detailed history of symptoms.
Significance: Blood or mucus in the stools, failure to thrive, fat malabsorption, or any extraintestinal symptoms strongly suggest different etiologies.

Question: Lactose ingestion?
Significance: Symptoms vary in severity and with dose of lactose.

Question: Milk ingestion?
Significance: Association with milk ingestion may not be evident.

 ## Physical Examination

Finding: Height and weight
Significance: Should be measured and plotted against age-appropriate norms; any deviation should not be evaluated as lactose intolerance alone.

Finding: Abdomen percussion
Significance: Abdomen may be distended.

Finding: Blood in the stool
Significance: Must be evaluated, because lactose intolerance does not cause bleeding.

Laboratory Aids

Test: Stool-reducing substances and fecal acidity
Significance: A positive result indicates malabsorption of carbohydrates. A pH <6.0 or reducing substances greater than 0.5% are interpreted as a positive result.

Test: Lactose hydrogen breath test
Significance:

- Noninvasive and highly sensitive.
- The only source of hydrogen is fermented unabsorbed carbohydrates.
- A rise of breath H_2 concentration of greater than or equal to 20 ppm over baseline appears to correlate with enzyme deficiency.
- However, the frequently poor association between symptoms of lactose intolerance and breath H_2 excretion suggests caution in the interpretation of the clinical significance of the breath hydrogen test.

—False-positive test results occur due to inadequate fasting before the test, rapid intestinal transit, toothpaste, smoking, and bacterial overgrowth.
—False-negative results occur due to diarrhea, hyperventilation, recent antibiotics exposure, and delayed gastric emptying. Up to 10% of the population are colonized with bacteria unable to produce hydrogen and will give a negative result.

Test: Lactase activity measurement of biopsy-invasive and expensive
Significance: saved for patients undergoing upper endoscopy to exclude celiac disease.

 ## Therapy

- Removal of lactose from the diet is effective in eliminating symptoms. However, a milk-free diet may result in calcium deficiency.
- Predigestion of lactose can be done by the addition of commercially available enzyme supplementation. Multiple products are available over the counter. Liquid preparations, capsules, and chewable tablets can be obtained.
- Acquired deficiencies, particularly those associated with infection, may resolve over time. The majority of patients with lactose intolerance will not recover the ability to digest lactose.
- Supplemental probiotics may improve symptoms of lactose intolerance.

PITFALLS

Care must be taken to determine if the lactose intolerance is secondary to a primary pathologic process (i.e., celiac disease, Crohn disease, or giardiasis).

 ## Common Questions and Answers

Q: When is the usual time for presentation of lactose intolerance?
A: In whites, the age of presentation is after 5 years of age. In blacks, 2- to 3-year-old children may present with clinical signs and symptoms. The differential diagnosis must distinguish primary from secondary causes.

Q: Does lactose intolerance prevent the child from ever eating lactose?
A: No, the patient can take smaller amounts of lactose in the diet, or have the enzyme supplemented.

Q: Does this problem ever get better?
A: No, it is a lifelong problem, but seems to become less symptomatic for adults, in light of their individual desire to tolerate symptoms.

ICD-9-CM 271.3

BIBLIOGRAPHY

de Vrese M, Stegelmann A, Richter B, et al. Probiotics—compensation for lactase insufficiency. *Am J Clin Nutr* 2001; 73(Suppl 2):421S–429S.

Kerner JA Jr. Formula allergy and intolerance. *Gastroenterol Clin North Am* 1995;24(1):1–25.

Kokkonen J, Tikkanen S, Savilahti E. Residual intestinal disease after milk allergy in infancy. *J Pediatr Gastroenterol Nutr* 2001; 32(2):156–161.

Murray JA. The widening spectrum of celiac disease. *Am J Clin Nutr* 1999;69(3):354–365.

Rose S. Milk consumption for the lactose intolerant: a clarification. *J Am Diet Assoc* 2000;100(9):1007.

Suarez FL, Saviano DA, Levitt MD. A comparison of milk or lactose hydrolyzed milk by people with self-reported severe lactose intolerance. *N Engl J Med* 1995;333:1–5.

Veligati LN, Treem WR, Sullivan B, et al. Delta 10 ppm versus delta 20 ppm: a reappraisal of diagnostic criteria for breath hydrogen testing in children. *Am J Gastroenterol* 1994;89(5):758–761.

Author: Dror Wasserman

Lead Poisoning

Database

DEFINITION

• One of the most common pediatric environmental health problems, involving a systemic intoxication by the heavy metal lead; most commonly this is with inorganic lead.
• Children in the United States are predominantly exposed to lead through ingestion of contaminated house dust and soil, and paint chips from deterioration of pre-1980 housing containing lead-based paint (LBP).
• The Centers for Disease Control and Prevention (CDC) considers a blood lead level of 10 μg/dL or higher to represent undue lead exposure and absorption, or an elevated blood lead level (EBLL); this term is preferable to lead poisoning, which is less specific.

PATHOPHYSIOLOGY

• Lead adversely affects many organ systems including the neurologic, hematologic, gastrointestinal (GI), renal, and reproductive systems. Many of the toxic effects result from inhibition of enzymes involved in heme biosynthesis, as the electropositive metal binds to the negatively charged sulfhydryl groups on the active sites of δ-aminolevulinic acid dehydratase (ALA-D), ferrochelatase, porphobilinogen synthase, coproporphyrinogen oxidase, and other enzymes. Divalent lead also acts competitively with calcium in various biologic systems.
• Children absorb lead more efficiently from the GI tract and are more likely to ingest lead through hand-to-mouth activity as compared to adults.
• As the developing, immature central nervous system is susceptible to the toxic effects of lead, the neuropsychological effects of lead poisoning on young children have been of particular concern.

EPIDEMIOLOGY

• Prevalence of elevated lead levels and geometric mean blood lead level (BLL) have decreased significantly in the last 20 years.
• Approximately 434,000 American children aged 1 to 5 years (2.2% of a representative national sample) are estimated to have BLLs of 10 μg/dL or higher.
• Higher prevalence occurs among children aged 1 to 3 years, those living in older housing, those from lower income families, and those living in metropolitan areas with populations of 1 million or greater.

CDC CLASSIFICATION

CDC CLASSIFICATION	BLOOD LEAD LEVEL RANGE (μg/dL)
I	0–9
IIa	10–14
IIb	15–19
III	20–44
IV	45–69
V	70+

• Approximately 83% of American pre-1978 privately owned units contain some lead-based paint.
• A recent national survey estimates that 38 million and 24 million housing units have LBP and significant LBP hazards, respectively.

COMPLICATIONS

• Acute encephalopathy
• Seizures
• Coma
• Death (predominantly from cerebral edema)
• Mental retardation
• Cognitive, behavioral, attentional, and neurodevelopmental impairment
• Anemia
• Fanconi syndrome
• Abdominal colic
• Adverse reproductive outcomes

PROGNOSIS

• In general, there is an increased risk for long-term neuropsychological sequelae, which increases with lead exposure and absorption that is more intense, of longer duration, and begins at an early age when the central nervous system is still maturing.
• Recurrent episodes of symptomatic lead poisoning increase the risk for permanent sequelae.
• More subtle effects may not be detected until school entry.

Differential Diagnosis

Most lead poisoning in children is asymptomatic.
• Lead encephalopathy should be considered in the differential diagnosis of a child presenting with seizures, altered mental status, and/or coma.
• Lead poisoning should also be considered in the differential diagnosis of mental retardation, behavioral disorders, and anemia.

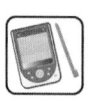

Data Gathering

HISTORY

Question: How do children obtain exposure to a source of lead?
Significance: The most common sources of lead include lead-based paint through residence in or visitation of older, deteriorated housing, a parental occupation or hobby involving lead exposure (construction or battery plant work, stained glass window or pottery making), use of remedies or cosmetics containing lead, and ingestion of contaminated water, food, or beverages.

Question: What are typical symptoms?
Significance: Most children are asymptomatic. Although many of the clinical manifestations of symptomatic lead poisoning are nonspecific, a cluster of complaints including anorexia, intermittent abdominal pain, constipation, sporadic vomiting, change in

mental status (such as irritability or lethargy), decreased play activity, and change in developmental status (particularly with regression of developmental milestones) may herald this condition.

Question: How does lead encephalopathy present?
Significance: Can present with change in consciousness, ataxia, persistent vomiting, seizures, and coma; often this presents after a prodrome of symptoms mentioned above.

Physical Examination

• Not generally helpful at lower lead levels. Symptomatic and/or encephalopathic patients may have acute gastrointestinal, neurologic, hematologic, and systemic manifestations.
• Assess for clinical evidence of developmental delay.
• Burton gum lead line: A blue-gray discoloration at the gum-tooth interface typically along the lower incisors rarely can be seen in the setting of chronic, fairly high lead exposure and poor dental hygiene.

Laboratory Aids

SPECIFIC TESTS

Test: Blood lead test, either venous or capillary.
Significance: Compare result with CDC classification system. Results may be reportable to local health authorities. The test result is a measure only of recent lead exposure and does not indicate total body burden of lead.

NONSPECIFIC TESTS

Test: Complete blood count
Significance: To assess for anemia. Anemia is seen in lead poisoning starting at lead levels of approximately 60 μg/dL from globin and heme synthesis inhibition and hemolysis. Iron deficiency anemia is often seen concomitantly. Anemia related to lead toxicity is typically normocytic and normochromic; a microcytic, hypochromic anemia may be seen with a mixed etiology. Basophilic stippling is sometimes seen on peripheral blood smear.

Test: Free erythrocyte protoporphyrin (FEP)
Significance: Marker of lead-induced inhibition of heme synthesis. FEP can be useful clinically to follow the recovery from heme synthesis inhibition during management.

RADIOGRAPHIC STUDIES

Test: Abdominal radiograph
Significance: Look for radiopaque foreign material suggestive of ingestion of lead paint chips or other lead-containing foreign body, when ingestion of such is suspected in the history.

Test: Long bone x-rays
Significance: Look for "lead lines" or metaphyseal sclerosis, characterized by increased

density along transverse lines in the metaphyses of growing long bones, representing increased mineralization due to interference with the metabolism of the boney matrix. If present, lead lines imply chronic lead exposure. Not recommended for routine use.

Test: X-ray fluorescence for estimation of body lead burden
Significance: Used mainly in experimental settings

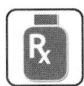 ## Therapy

Environmental management—which includes removing children from the lead source(s), should occur when venous lead levels are recurrently 15 to 19 μg/dL (CDC class IIB) and when levels are greater than or equal to 20 μg/dL (CDC class III).
- Chelation therapy
—should complement environmental management in all children with venous levels of 45 μg/dL (CDC class IV) or higher, using parenteral calcium disodium ethylenediamine tetraacetate (EDTA; also calcium disodium versenate) or oral agents such as meso 2,3-dimercaptosuccinic acid (DMSA, succimer, Chemet).
—Chelation of children with levels in the 25 to 45 μg/dL range may be considered in certain cases, although it is not routinely recommended and evidence suggests it may not be beneficial.
—Outpatient therapy can take place if a lead-safe environment has been identified and compliance is expected.
—Succimer is given at 10 mg/kg/dose (or 350 mg/m² per dose) every 8 hours for 5 days, then every 12 hours for 14 more days.
—Weekly monitoring for neutropenia, platelet abnormality, and increased liver enzymes is recommended.
—Succimer is more lead-specific than other chelators and causes less mineral depletion.
- Children with symptomatic lead poisoning or with levels of 70 μg/dL (CDC class V) or higher should be admitted immediately to a hospital for parenteral chelation with both intramuscular dimercaprol (British antilewisite, BAL) and intravenous or intramuscular calcium disodium EDTA.
—As there are many issues involved with administration of both chelating agents, consultation of appropriate guidelines and pharmacologic information are recommended.
—Children with encephalopathy constitute a medical emergency and should receive the preceding treatment in an intensive care setting with attentive neurosurgical support.
—Consultation with a clinician experienced in lead toxicity treatment is advised for these patients.
- Ingested lead-containing foreign bodies should be evacuated with whole bowel irrigation using a high molecular weight glycol solution.
- Nutritional support—with calcium and iron supplementation should be given if intake is inadequate; deficiencies of these increase lead absorption from the gastrointestinal

tract. Iron supplementation should be withheld during chelation therapy.

 ## Follow-Up

- Prompt environmental follow-up of current lead exposure situations and investigation for additional exposure (e.g., with family moves, visitation of new residences, etc.) should occur.
- Follow-up venous lead levels should be performed for those with levels from 10 to 19 μg/dL (CDC class IIA, IIB) approximately every 3 to 4 months.
- Follow-up venous levels should be performed for those with levels of 20 μg/dL or higher at 1 to 2 month intervals until no additional lead exposure is present and levels have decreased.

PREVENTION

- Primary prevention: Removal of potential environmental lead hazards prior to lead exposure.
- The CDC now recommends that states and cities include primary prevention activities in order to reach the Healthy People 2010 Objective 8–11 of eliminating elevated blood lead levels in children.
- Secondary prevention: Screening for elevated lead levels. Since 1997, the CDC has recommended that state and local health departments make the determination for a universal versus targeted screening approach.
- Minimum screening recommendations are for a blood lead test for children at ages 1 and 2 years, and for those of 36 to 72 months of age without previous screening.
- Universal screening—for communities where the risk for lead exposure is widespread, and where 12% or more of children aged 12 to 36 months have lead levels of 10 μg/dL or higher and/or 27% or greater of the housing stock was built prior to 1950.
- Targeted screening—for communities not meeting above criteria. Screening would be indicated for children meeting local criteria for residence in a specified geographic area, membership in a high-risk group (including children on Medicaid), or a high-risk status as determined by the use of a personal-risk questionnaire.
- Tertiary prevention: Case management and environmental remediation for children with lead poisoning. Closer attention to the first two modes of prevention should obviate the need for this.

CONTROL MEASURES

- Abatement of building-based (residential) lead hazards by removal, encapsulation, or enclosure of lead-containing structures.
- Control of environmental lead dust exposure and ingestion by good housekeeping (wet dusting and mopping of household dust) and personal hygiene (cleaning of child's hands, toys, personal items, etc.).
- Removal of any other known lead source from the child's environment.

PITFALLS

- Delay in checking a blood lead test in the presence of clinical signs, symptoms of lead poisoning, or neuropsychological disorders.
- Failure to inquire about lead exposure possibilities, especially when approaching urban children.

 ## Common Questions and Answers

Q: What is lead abatement?
A: Lead abatement is removal of a lead hazard from the environment either by replacing it (e.g., installing a new window), enclosing the area with the lead source (e.g., installing paneling), removing the lead-based paint from a surface (burning or dry sanding methods should never be used), or encapsulating the area (placement of a specific coating over the lead-containing surface, which prevents access to the lead hazard).

Q: Is lead abatement permanent?
A: Often the lead paint that is chipping or peeling is removed from a home. Any areas with intact lead-based paint may become deteriorated with aging, leading to new lead hazards, although ongoing maintenance and repair may prevent this.

Q: Why didn't my child's brother or sister get lead poisoning at the same age since he/she lived in the same house?
A: Children are different; some do much more hand-to-mouth activity than others, which is the main way that children get lead into their bodies. Also, your home may not have had the same lead dangers (hazards) when the sibling was younger.

ICD-9-CM 984.9

BIBLIOGRAPHY

Centers for Disease Control and Prevention. *Managing Elevated Lead Levels Among Young Children: Recommendations from the Advisory Committee on Childhood Lead Poisoning Prevention.* Atlanta: CDC, 2002.

Jacobs ED, et al. The prevalence of lead-based paint hazards in U.S. housing. *Environ Health Perspect* 2002;110:A599–A606.

Lanphear BP, Matte TD, Rogers J, et al. The contribution of lead-contaminated house dust and residential soil to children's blood lead levels. *Environ Res* 1998;79(section A):51–68.

Meyer P, et al. Surveillance for elevated blood lead levels among children—United States, 1997–2000. *MMWR Surveill Summ* 2003; 52(No. SS-10):1–21.

Piomelli S. Childhood lead poisoning. *Pediatr Clin North Am* 2002;49(6):1285–1304.

Rogan WJ, Dietrich KN, Ware JH, et al. The effect of chelation therapy with succimer on neuropsychological development in children exposed to lead. *N Engl J Med* 2001;344(19): 1421–1426.

Author: Carla Campbell

Lice (Pediculosis)

 Database

DEFINITION

Infestation of the head, body, or anogenital region with one of three species of lice

CAUSES

Three species of ectoparasites (six-legged, wingless, 1- to 4-mm insects that live on humans, feeding on human blood):

- *Pediculus humanus capitis*: Head louse
- *Pediculus humanus corporis*: Body louse
- *Phthirus pubis*: Pubic or crab louse

PATHOPHYSIOLOGY

- Head lice

—Survives for several weeks on scalp
—Typical infestation, 12 to 24 live insects per patient
—Single louse produces up to 120 eggs
—Ova (nits) laid close to the scalp; firmly attached to hair shaft by chitinous ring (usually clustered in the parietal and occipital areas)
—Ova hatch after 8 days, leaving shell of nit on hair (readily visible to examiner).
—Transmitted by personal contact, or fomites (e.g., combs, hats, upholstery, clothing, headsets)
—Prefer to feed on scalp skin; hook onto scalp, pierce skin to feed
—Release poisonous saliva that causes pruritus, dermatitis
—Survive 1 to 2 days off human host

- Body lice

—10%–20% larger than head lice
—Prefer to live on clothing, visiting human only to feed
—Lay eggs along seams of clothing, which hatch when warmed by wear
—Transmitted through contact with infested clothing or bedding
—Viable off of human for 10 to 21 days

- Pubic lice

—Crab-like appearance with predilection for pubic hair
—Transmitted almost exclusively by sexual contact
—Uncommonly spread by fomites (e.g., toilet seats, bedding)
—Occasionally will infest axillary hair, beard, or eyelashes
—May infest eyebrows/lashes (pediculosis palpebrarum) in young children (associated with maternal infestation; but one must consider possible sexual abuse)

EPIDEMIOLOGY

- Head lice

—Common in day-care setting and elementary school children
—Affects all socioeconomic groups
—Not indicative of poor hygiene
—Slightly higher incidence in girls

- Body lice

—Found on persons with poor hygiene
—More common in extreme conditions such as crowding, homelessness, wars, famine, flood, and earthquakes
—Highest incidence in the Sudan and Ethiopia

- Pubic lice

—Most common in adolescents and young adults

COMPLICATIONS

- Head lice

—Secondary dermatitis, impetigo, or furunculosis

- Body lice

—Secondary eczema, impetigo (from scratching)
—Postinflammatory hyperpigmentation
—Known vector for disease; *Rickettsia prowazekii* (epidemic typhus), *Rickettsia quintana* (trench fever), *Borrelia recurrentis* (relapsing fever).

ASSOCIATED ILLNESSES

- These lice are not responsible for the spread of any disease.
- Pubic lice: Up to 50% of patients have another sexually transmitted disease, particularly gonorrhea, or syphilis.

 Differential Diagnosis

- Seborrheic dermatitis
- Contact dermatitis
- Eczema
- Impetigo

 Data Gathering

HISTORY

Question: Pruritus?
Significance: Itching is the most common symptom, however some patients are asymptomatic.

Question: Secondary skin lesion (from scratching)?
Significance: May be chief complaint

SPECIAL QUESTIONS

Question: Contacts?
Significance: Possible infested contacts (home, school, or sexual contact).

Question: Special living circumstances?
Significance: Crowding or institutionalization.

 Physical Examination

Finding: Lice (difficult to find) on the scalp, in the pubic hair or in the seams of clothing.
Significance: Diagnostic.

Finding: Nits clustered in parietal and occipital regions, in the perianal region or in the seams of clothing.
Nits difficult to flick away (unlike dandruff); need to be pulled along entire length of hair shaft to remove.
Significance: Diagnostic.

Finding: Primary skin lesion
Significance: Pinpoint, erythematous macule, papule, or urticarial wheel. These can be obliterated by scratching.

OTHER FINDINGS

- Secondary skin lesions; dermatitis of the neck, shoulder area.
- Examine eyelashes, eyebrows for secondary infestation.
- Posterior occipital lymphadenopathy
- Body lice
- Postinflammatory hyperpigmentation
- Maculae cerulae (bluish/slate macules, 0.5- to 1-mm diameter), from heavy infestation in pubic, trunk, and thigh areas.

 Laboratory Aids

Test: Rarely necessary
Significance: Can examine louse or nit under microscope to confirm characteristic appearance. Dandruff is a false-positive finding.

Test: Home testing
Significance: Parents can be instructed how to examine all family members by using a fine-toothed plastic comb from the scalp to the end of the hair looking for lice and/or nits.

Test: School testing
Significance: Schools can perform examinations during epidemics.

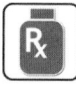 **Therapy**

DRUGS

Head and Pubic Lice

- Permethrin (Nix) 1% creme rinse

—Acts on nerve cell membranes causing paralysis/death of insect
—10-minute application, followed by second application 7 to 10 days later.
—High ovicidal activity; continued activity up to 12 days after application
—High cure rate, prevalence to resistance in the United States is unknown.
—Over-the-counter preparation, low toxicity

- Pyrethrins (Rid, A-200)

—Neurotoxin also, low ovicidal activity
—Some resistance documented in the United States
—10-minute shampoo application, second application in 1 week
—Over-the-counter preparation
—Some develop contact dermatitis to natural chrysanthemum base.

- Malathion (Ovide) 0.5%

—Better ovicidal activity, highly effective
—Probably most effective treatment available, minimal resistance
—Requires 8- to 12-hour application
—Less toxicity than lindane and pyrethrins
—Alcohol base of product causes patient to be flammable while product is on.

- Lindane (Kwell) 1% lotion

—Should no longer be used due to neurotoxicity, lack of efficacy

Other Treatments:
Use of bactrim with topical permethrin has slightly improved cure rate
Ivermectin: Oral or topical may be effective for heavy infestations, but it is not FDA approved for this

- Other considerations:

—Cortisone creams for secondary dermatitis; decreases pruritus
—Antibiotics for impetiginized lesions

GENERAL

Head Lice

- Apply peduculicide cream rinse, and comb the wet hair until no lice are found. Combing should be repeated every few days until no lice have been found for a period of 2 weeks.
- If nit removal desired, soak hair with white vinegar for 30 to 60 minutes, followed by combing with a fine-toothed nit comb.
- Examine household members and treat those who are infested.
- Prophylactically treat bed mates.

Environmental cleaning:
This is controversial and may not be necessary:

- Wash bedding, clothes, and cloth toys in hot water (>128°F).
- Treat combs by washing in hot water, and soaking in pediculicide.
- Seal anything not washable in plastic bags for 10 to 14 days.
- Nit removal not necessary, especially if pediculicide reapplied 1 week later
- Environmental insecticide is not helpful in the control of head lice.

Body Lice

- Pediculicide not necessary (insects live in clothing)
- Improve hygiene.
- Wash clothing and bedding in hot water.
- Dry cleaning is effective, as is hot ironing (particularly along seams of clothing).

Pubic Lice

- Treat sexual contact to prevent reinfestation.
- Removal of nits with fine-toothed comb from pubic hair helpful.

Pediculosis Palpebrarum

- Petrolatum ointment applied to lashes three to four times per day for 8 to 10 days
- Remove nits by hand from the eyelashes.

DURATION

- The pediculicide kills the lice shortly after application; therefore, living lice after treatment is indicative of incorrect use of the pediculicide, very heavy infestation, reinfestation or resistance to therapy. Retreatment with a second pediculicide with reapplication 7 to 10 days later is recommended.

PREVENTION

Head lice is not preventable.

 Follow-Up

WHEN TO EXPECT IMPROVEMENT

Risk of transmission promptly reduced after single application, so child should be allowed to return to school or day care. Removal of nits is not necessary to reduce spread. Pruritus may persist for 2 weeks after therapy.

SIGNS TO WATCH FOR

Recurrence of symptoms represents improper use of the treating agent, reinfestation, resistance, failure to recognize and treat other sites of infestation, such as perianal hair, axillary hair, or sexual contacts: Pediculosis pubis.

PROGNOSIS

Excellent

PITFALLS

Pediculosis palpebrarum: Pediculicides are oculotoxic and must be avoided.

 Common Questions and Answers

Q: Did my child get head lice because my house or my child is not clean enough?
A: No, head lice is unrelated to personal hygiene. Some experts even believe lice prefer a clean scalp.

Q: Should I cut my child's long hair to get the lice out?
A: No, meticulous application of the pediculicide to the entire scalp and pulled through all hair shafts is adequate treatment. Urgently cutting a child's hair to alleviate parental anxiety can be traumatizing to the child.

Q: Can infants become infested with pubic lice (Phthirus pubis)?
A: Yes. Although the primary mode of transmission of the crab louse is via sexual contact, it can be transmitted through close personal contact with an infested individual. Small children become infested on the eyebrows or lashes with crab lice.

Q: If children are infested with the head louse, how can items such as stuffed animals or other cloth toys be decontaminated?
A: Machine washable items can be washed in hot water at temperatures >128°F. An alternative method of decontamination is sealing the items in a plastic bag for 10 to 14 days.

Q: Is removal of nits necessary to prevent spread?
A: No. They can be removed from a cosmetic standpoint by using a fine-toothed comb or by soaking the hair in a solution of white vinegar followed by wrapping the head with a towel soaked in the same solution for 30 to 60 minutes.

Q: What is appropriate treatment of infestation of the eyelashes?
A: A petroleum-based ocular ointment should be applied three to four times daily for a period of 10 days. Nits should be removed mechanically from the lashes.

ICD-9-CM 132.9

BIBLIOGRAPHY

American Academy of Pediatrics. Sexually transmitted diseases. In: Pickering LK, eds. *2003 Red Book: Report of the Committee on Infectious Diseases.* 26th Ed. Elk Grove Village, IL: American Academy of Pediatrics, 2003.

Dirk E. Drug-resistant lice. *Arch Dermatology* 2003;139:1061–1064.

Meinking TL, Burkhart CN. Head lice (correspondence). *NEJM* 2002;347: 1381–1382.

Meinking TL, et al. An observer blinded study of 1% permethrin crème rinse with and without adjunctive combing in patients with head lice. *J Pediatr* 2002;141:665–670.

Roberts, R. Head lice. *NEJM* 2002;345: 1645–1650.

Author: Jane Lavelle

Lupus Erythematosus

 Database

DEFINITION

Multisystem, autoimmune disease characterized by the production of antibodies to various components of the cell nucleus, in conjunction with a variety of clinical manifestations. Four of the following 11 criteria, developed by the American College of Rheumatology, must be met to classify a patient with systemic lupus erythematosus (SLE):

- Malar (butterfly) rash
- Discoid rash
- Photosensitivity
- Oral or nasal ulcers
- Arthritis
- Cytopenia: Anemia, leukopenia, lymphopenia, or thrombocytopenia
- Neurologic disease: seizures or psychosis
- Nephritis: >0.5 g per day proteinuria or cellular casts
- Serositis: Pleuritis or pericarditis
- Immunologic disorder: Antibodies to double-stranded DNA (dsDNA), Smith nuclear antigen, LE cell prep, or false-positive serologic test for syphilis
- Positive ANA

CAUSE

Although the exact etiology is unknown, lupus is an autoimmune disease, with genetic, environmental, and hormonal factors playing a role.

PATHOLOGY

- Immune complex-mediated vasculitis, which can occur in almost any organ system.
- Cutaneous lesions in SLE are very variable. They include the erythematous malar or "butterfly" rash, maculopapular rashes (which can occur anywhere on the body), periungual erythema, and mucosal membrane vasculitis.
- Arthritis in SLE can affect large and small joints and is usually symmetric and nonerosive.
- Hematologic pathology in lupus includes a hemolytic anemia, anemia of chronic disease, leukopenia, lymphopenia, and thrombocytopenia.
- Neurologic impairments in SLE include psychosis, depression, seizures, organic brain syndromes, and peripheral neuropathies.
- Renal pathology includes mesangial changes and glomerulonephritis (focal, diffuse, proliferative, or membranous). The first signs of renal disease in a lupus patient are often proteinuria and active urinary sediment. Hypertension, nephrotic syndrome, and renal failure can also occur.
- Serositis is usually seen as pericarditis or pleuritis, but peritonitis can also occur.

EPIDEMIOLOGY

- Approximately 15% of lupus patients have their onset of symptoms in childhood.
- Peak incidence of SLE is between the ages of 15 and 40.
- It has been estimated that 5,000 to 10,000 children in the United States have SLE.
- Female to male ratio is between 5:1 and 10:1.

GENETICS

- Increased frequency of lupus in first-degree family members of patients with SLE
- Approximately 10% of patients have at least one affected relative.
- Concordance rate of 25%–50% in monozygotic and 5% in dizygotic twins
- Some major histocompatibility antigens are associated with increased incidences of lupus, such as HLA-DR2 and DR-3 in Caucasians and DR2 and DR7 in African Americans.

COMPLICATIONS

- End-stage renal disease
- Infections secondary to the treatments used to control the disease
- Myocardial infarctions at a young age

 Differential Diagnosis

- Systemic onset juvenile rheumatoid arthritis
- Oncologic disease (leukemia, lymphoma)
- Other vasculitic disorders
- Dermatomyositis
- Fibromyalgia
- Drug-induced lupus

 Data Gathering

HISTORY

Question: Photosensitive?
Significance: A history of photosensitivity or a malar rash is common but not necessary in SLE.

Question: Systemic complaints?
Significance: Many patients have systemic complaints, such as fevers, fatigue, and malaise.

Question: Other complaints?
Significance: Many patients complain of joint pain, Raynaud phenomenon, or alopecia.

 Physical Examination

- Rash: May be malar, discoid or vasculitic. Periungual erythema may also be seen.
- Oral or nasal ulcers (usually on the hard or soft palate) that are painless and often go unnoticed by the patients.
- Arthritis of the large and small joints
- Pericardial friction rub if the patient has pericarditis
- Edema may be present secondary to renal disease.
- CNS changes, such as personality changes, psychosis, seizures

Laboratory Aids

Test: Antinuclear antibodies (ANA)
Significance: Found in over 95% patients with SLE, but a positive ANA can occur in many diseases (and in 10%–20% of the normal population).

Test: Anti-dsDNA and anti-Sm.
Significance: Very specific to lupus, but not all patients with lupus have these autoantibodies. In many patients, the anti-DNA levels vary with the activity of disease.

Test: CBC
Significance: Anemia, leukopenia, lymphopenia, and/or thrombocytopenia may be seen.

Test: Urinalysis
Significance: May show proteinuria or an active urinary sediment if there is renal dysfunction.

Test: Complement levels
Significance: Can fall very low during a lupus flare (C3 and C4).

Test: PTT
Significance: Patients may also have a prolonged PTT, as the result of antiphospholipid (APL) antibodies, which are often seen in SLE. Patients with APL antibodies are at an increased risk for thrombotic events, such as deep venous thromboses, strokes, and fetal losses during pregnancies.

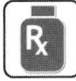 ## Therapy

- Avoid excessive sun exposure and use sunscreen liberally.
- Nonsteroidal antiinflammatory drugs may be used for the musculoskeletal and mild systemic complaints, although ibuprofen has been noted to cause aseptic meningitis in a small number of patients with SLE.
- Hydroxychloroquine is often used to help control the cutaneous manifestations of lupus.
- Steroids are often necessary to control the systemic and renal manifestations.
- Patients with renal disease often need immunosuppressive agents, such as cyclophosphamide (usually given as monthly intravenous boluses). Mycophenolate mofetil, cyclosporin, or azathioprine may also be used.
- Rituximab (anti-CD20 antibody) causes B cell depletion and is now being used in SLE, especially for thrombocytopenia.
- Trials with other biologic agents are also being tested in lupus (antibodies to CD40 ligand, C5, etc.)
- For very severe lupus, bone marrow immunoablation or transplantation is an option.

PITFALLS

Overdiagnosis; a positive ANA in the absence of clinical signs or symptoms of SLE is not lupus.

PROGNOSIS

- Extremely variable. Renal disease and CNS involvement are poor prognostic signs, whereas systemic complaints and joint findings are not.
- The 10-year survival in a child presenting with SLE is over 80%.

 ## Common Questions and Answers

Q: If a patient has a positive ANA but no clinical signs of SLE, how often should the ANA be followed?
A: A positive ANA will usually remain positive indefinitely, but it has no real significance in the absence of clinical or other laboratory disturbances. Up to 20% of the normal population may have a positive ANA, so there is no need to repeat the test.

Q: Can SLE patients with end-stage renal disease obtain renal transplants?
A: Yes, and SLE usually does not recur in the new kidney.

Q: What is neonatal lupus (NLE)?
A: Neonatal lupus is due to maternal autoantibodies (usually SS-A or SS-B antibodies), that cross the placenta and can cause rashes, congenital heart block, cytopenias, and/or hepatitis in the newborn baby. Many mothers of babies with NLE are asymptomatic and unaware that they have these autoantibodies. The rash, erythema annulare, can begin a few days after delivery and usually resolves within 6 to 9 months. Topical steroids can minimize the lesions. Congenital heart block is due to damage of the conducting system of the developing fetal heart. Bradycardia may be noted by 22 weeks' gestation and congestive heart failure with nonimmune hydrops fetalis may ensue.

ICD-9-CM 710.0

BIBLIOGRAPHY

Godfrey T, Hughes GR, et al. Therapeutic advances in systemic lupus erythematosus. *Curr Opin Rheumatol* 1998;10(5):435–441.

Lehman TJA, McCurdy DK, Bernstein BH, et al. Systemic lupus erythematosus in the first decade of life. *Pediatrics* 1989;26:235.

Schumacher HR, eds. *Primer on the Rheumatic Diseases.* 10th Ed. Atlanta: Arthritis Foundation, 1993.

Author: Elizabeth Candell Chalom

Lyme Disease

Database

DEFINITION

Multisystemic illness caused by the spirochete *Borrelia burgdorferi*

CAUSE

The tick-borne spirochete *B. burgdorferi*

PATHOLOGY

• *B. burgdorferi* is injected into the skin with the saliva of the *Ixodes* tick. The spirochetes first migrate within the skin, forming the typical rash, erythema migrans. The rash starts as a red macule or papule and then expands to an annular lesion up to 30 cm in diameter with partial central clearing. The spirochetes then spread hematogenously to other organs, including the heart, joints, and nervous system.
• Joints: Early on, the patient may experience migratory joint pain (often without frank arthritis), myalgias, and painful tendons and bursae. Months later, 60% of untreated patients will develop mono- or pauciarticular arthritis of the large joints, especially the knees. Joint fluid can have a white blood count anywhere from 500–110,000 cells/mm³, and the cells are mostly neutrophils.
• Neurologic: 14% of untreated patients will develop neurologic symptoms of Lyme disease several weeks after the initial rash. These symptoms include aseptic meningitis, cranial nerve palsies (especially facial nerve palsies), mononeuritis, plexitis, and myelitis. Months to years later, chronic neurologic symptoms may occur, including a subtle encephalopathy, memory, mood, and sleep disturbances.
• Cardiac: Approximately 8% of untreated patients develop cardiac disease several weeks after the initial Lyme rash. The most common cardiac lesion is atrioventricular block (primary, secondary, or complete). Pericarditis, myocarditis, or pancarditis can also develop. Most of the cardiac manifestations will disappear with or without treatment in a short time (3–4 weeks), but they may later recur. Severe cardiac involvement rarely may be fatal.

EPIDEMIOLOGY

• Lyme disease can affect people of all ages, but one-third to one-half of all cases occur in children and adolescents.
• Male to female ratio is 1:1 to 2:1.
• Lyme disease has now become the most common tick-borne disease in the United States with approximately 16,000 cases reported each year.
• Onset is most often in the summer months, and the endemic areas are in the northeast, north central, and Pacific Coast states.

GENETICS

Chronic Lyme arthritis seems to be associated with an increased incidence of HLA-DR4 and less so with HLA-DR2.

COMPLICATIONS

• Chronic arthritis occurs in approximately 2% of children with the disease.
• The same ticks that transmit Lyme disease, can also transmit *Ehrichia* and *Babesia*, so infections with those spirochetes can occur simultaneously.
• Other complications arise from the treatment of Lyme disease, such as cholecystitis secondary to treatment with ceftriaxone, and infections from indwelling catheters used for intravenous antibiotics.

Differential Diagnosis

• Viral arthritis/arthralgias
• Septic arthritis
• Juvenile rheumatoid arthritis
• Postinfectious arthritis
• Fibromyalgia syndrome
• Systemic lupus erythematosus

Data Gathering

HISTORY

Question: Tick bite?
Significance: A history of a tick bite can only be elicited in one third of patients with Lyme disease, and most people with tick bites do not develop Lyme disease. Even in endemic areas, the risk of developing Lyme disease after a tick bite is less than 5%.

Question: Rash?
Significance: 50% to 80% will have or will recall the typical rash, which is not painful or pruritic, but does feel warm.

Question: Other symptoms?
Significance: Many patients will complain of fatigue, headaches, fevers, chills, myalgias, and arthralgias early on in the disease.

Question: Joint pain?
Significance: Many patients will complain of painful joints early on, and later will develop joint swelling.

Physical Examination

• The rash of erythema migrans, if seen, is virtually pathognomonic for Lyme disease. If the patient does not have the rash, there is no physical finding that gives a definitive diagnosis of Lyme.
• The physical examination may be completely normal early in the course of the disease.
• The patient may have arthritis, Bell Palsy, a cranial nerve palsy, or an irregular heart beat.

Laboratory Aids

Test: ELISA
Significance: Several weeks after the tick bite, antibodies to *B. burgdorferi* can be detected by ELISA. This test, however, has a relatively high false-positive rate and occasionally false-negative results. It remains positive for years after treatment.

Test: Western blot analysis
Significance: A much more specific test. After 4–8 weeks of the infection, at least five of the following IgG bands must be present for the test to be positive: 18, 21, 28, 30, 34, 39, 41, 45, 58, 66, and 93 kd. During the first 2–4 weeks of the infection, 2 IgM bands may establish the diagnosis.

Test: A positive ELISA with a negative Western blot
Significance: Usually means the patient does not have Lyme disease and the ELISA was a false positive.

Test: Polymerase Chain Reaction
Significance: PCR testing may be done with synovial tissue or fluid, or cerebrospinal fluid. A positive PCR indicates active disease, but a negative result does not rule out Lyme. PCR is not commercially available for serum testing.

Lyme Disease

 Therapy

- Initial therapy for early Lyme disease consists of oral antibiotics. For patients over 8 years old, doxycycline is the drug of choice. For younger children or for people who do not tolerate tetracyclines, amoxicillin plus probenecid is preferred, but penicillin (PCN) V is also acceptable. For PCN-allergic patients, erythromycin may be used, but it is less effective.
- For patients with only the skin rash, 14 days of oral antibiotics is usually sufficient. If other symptoms are present, 30 days are recommended.
- For persistent arthritis unresponsive to oral medications, severe carditis, or neurologic disease (other than an isolated seventh nerve palsy), intravenous antibiotics become necessary.
- Ceftriaxone is the drug of choice, but intravenous PCN V may also be used. Treatment should be given for 14–21 days.
- Some studies suggest that a single dose of doxycycline after a tick bite will prevent Lyme Disease.

PROGNOSIS

In general, the prognosis for children with Lyme disease is much better than that for adults. Only 2% of children have chronic arthritis at 6 months.

PITFALLS

Incorrect diagnosis: Many patients with vague systemic complaints (fatigue, headaches, arthralgias) are incorrectly diagnosed with Lyme disease, even though their Lyme tests are negative (or the ELISA is mildly positive and the Western blot is negative). These patients are then treated with multiple courses of oral antibiotics; if they do not respond, they are often treated with intravenous antibiotics, sometimes for prolonged periods of time. This delays diagnosing the true problem and subjects the patient to the unnecessary risks of long-term antibiotic use and occasionally of central venous lines.

 Common Questions and Answers

Q: What does the deer tick look like?
A: The deer tick is flat, very small (about the size of a pin head), and has eight legs. The adult male is black and the female is red and black. They can grow to three times their normal size when they are engorged with blood.

Q: Do all bites from infected deer ticks cause Lyme disease?
A: No. Even infected ticks will not cause Lyme disease if they are attached to the skin for a short period of time. If the tick is attached for less than 24 hours, the chances of transmitting the disease are very low. The longer the tick is attached, the higher the probability of disease transmission.

Q: Should all patients be retested for Lyme disease after a full course of treatment?
A: No. Lyme titers and the Western Blot will remain positive for years after adequate treatment for Lyme disease. If the patient's symptoms have resolved, there is no point in rechecking the titer. If the patient is still symptomatic, titers and a Western blot may be checked before starting intravenous antibiotic therapy, to look for a rising titer and to be sure the patient truly has Lyme disease. If symptoms remain after intravenous therapy, other diagnoses should be considered.

Q: Should patients with nontraumatic Bell palsy be tested for Lyme disease?
A: Bell palsy is seen in association with Lyme disease infections so testing for Lyme disease is a good idea.

ICD-9-CM 088.81

BIBLIOGRAPHY

Bunikis J, Barbour AG. Laboratory testing for suspected Lyme disease. *Med Clin North Am* 2002;86(2):311–340.

Donta ST. Late and chronic Lyme disease. *Med Clin North Am* 2002;86(2):341–349.

Dressler F, Whalen JA, Reinhardt BN, et al. Western blotting in the serodiagnosis of Lyme disease. *J Infect Dis* 1993;167:392–400.

Hayes E. Lyme disease. *Clinical Evidence* 2002;(7):652–664.

Huppertz HI. Lyme disease in children. *Curr Opin in Rheumatol* 2001;13(5):434–440.

McGinley-Smith DE, Tsao SS. Dermatoses from ticks. *J Am Acad Dermatol* 2003;49(3): 363–392; quiz 393–396.

Nachman SA, Pontrelli L. Central nervous system Lyme disease. *Semin Pediatr Infect Dis* 2003;14(2):123–130.

Shapiro ED, Gerber MA. Lyme disease: fact versus fiction. *Pediatr Ann* 2002;31(3): 170–177.

Shapiro ED. Lyme disease. *Pediatr Rev* 1998;19(5):147–154.

Steere AC. Lyme disease. *N Engl J Med* 2001;345(2):115–125.

Weinstein A, Britchkov M. Lyme arthritis and post-Lyme disease syndrome. *Curr Opin Rheumatol* 2002;14(4):383–387.

Author: Elizabeth Candell Chalom

Lymphadenopathy

Database

DEFINITION

- Lymphadenopathy is the term used to describe one or more enlarged lymph nodes >10 mm in diameter (for inguinal nodes the term is used for nodes >15 mm, and for epitroclear nodes, >5 mm). Any palpable supraclavicular, popliteal and iliac lymph node is considered abnormal.
- Localized lymphadenopathy involves enlarged nodes in any one region secondary to localized process (e.g., inguinal lymphadenopathy secondary to thigh abscess) and generalized lymphadenopathy involves two or more noncontiguous regions secondary to a systemic process (e.g., as with Epstein Barr virus [EBV] infection).
- Lymph nodes drain contiguous areas. The cervical nodes drain the head and neck area; axillary nodes drain the arm, thorax, and breast; epitroclear nodes drain the forearm and hand; and inguinal nodes drain the leg and groin. The supraclavicular nodes drain the thorax and abdomen, and are seen with malignancy. A right-sided supraclavicular node is associated with mediastinal malignancy, and the left-sided node suggests abdominal malignancy.
- Normal lymph nodes are generally <10 mm in size. Lymph nodes are often palpable in normal healthy children. They are present from birth, peak in size between 8–12 years of age, and then regress during adolescence.
- Lymphadenopathy must also be carefully differentiated from lymphadenitis. Lymphadenitis is defined as lymph node enlargement with signs of inflammation (erythema, tenderness, induration, warmth) and is often treated with antibiotics.

PATHOPHYSIOLOGY

Lymphatic flow from adjacent nodes or the inoculation site brings microorganisms to the lymph nodes. Lymph node enlargement may occur via any of the following mechanisms: The nodal cells may replicate in response to antigenic stimulation (e.g., Kawasaki disease) or malignant transformation (e.g., lymphoma); a large number of reactive cells from outside the node (e.g., neutrophils or metastatic cells) may enter the node; foreign material may be deposited into the node by lipid-laden histiocytes (e.g., lipid storage diseases); vascular engorgement and edema may occur secondary to local cytokine release; or suppuration secondary to tissue necrosis (e.g., *Mycobacterium tuberculosis*). Many systemic infections (e.g., Human Immunodeficiency virus [HIV]) cause hepatic or splenic enlargement in addition to generalized lymphadenopathy.

EPIDEMIOLOGY

The incidence of lymphadenopathy is difficult to determine because it is dependent on the underlying pathologic process that causes lymph node enlargement. However, there are palpable nodes present in 5%–25% of newborns (cervical, axillary, inguinal), and in greater than 50% of older children (all areas except epitrochlear, supraclavicular and popliteal).

COMPLICATIONS

- Lymphadenitis
- Local infection (e.g., cellulitis)
- Lymph node abscess
- Sepsis via hematogenous spread of inadequately contained infection
- Fistula (e.g., with atypical mycobacterium)
- Fibrosis secondary to purulence or lymphadenitis
- Stridor secondary to enlarged cervical lymph nodes
- Wheezing secondary to parabronchial mediastinal lymph nodes

PROGNOSIS

- Excellent for reactive lymphadenopathy
- Dependent on underlying diagnosis

Differential Diagnosis

Generalized lymphadenopathy may be seen in many systemic illnesses and the DDx includes:

INFECTIONS

- Viral

—Adenovirus
—Rubella
—Enteroviruses
—Herpes simplex virus
—Measles
—Varicella
—EBV/Cytomegalovirus (CMV)
—HIV
—Hepatitis A or B viruses

- Bacterial

—*Staphylococcus aureus*
—*Bartonella henselae*
—Group A β-hemolytic streptococcus (GAS)
—*Salmonella*
—*Yersenia*
—*Brucellosis*
—Tularemia
—*Mycobacterium tuberculosis*
—*Mycoplasma pneumonia*
—*Rickettsiae*

- Parasitic

—Chagas disease
—Schistosomiasis

Autoimmune Disease

- Systemic lupus erythematosis (SLE)
- Juvenile rheumatoid arthritis (JRA)
- Serum sickness

Malignancy

- Lymphoma (Hodgkin and Non-Hodgkin)
- Histiocytosis
- Neuroblastoma
- Leukemia

MEDICATIONS

- Phenytoin, isoniazid, pyrimethamine, antileprosy drugs, antithyroid drugs, aspirin, barbiturates, penicillin, tetracycline, iodides, sulfonamides, allopurinol, phenybutazone

LYMPHOPROLIFERATIVE DISORDERS

- Wiskott-Aldrich syndrome
- Ataxia-telangiectasia syndrome
- Combined immunodeficiency syndrome
- X-linked lymphoproliferative syndrome

MISCELLANEOUS

- Kawasaki disease
- Castleman disease
- Rosai-Dorfman disease (sinus histiocytosis with massive lymphadenopathy)
- Kikuchi-Fufimoto disease (histiocytic necrotizing lymphadenitis)
- Churg-Strauss syndrome
- Infection-associated hemophagocytic syndrome (IAHS)
- Gianotti-Crosti syndrome (papular acrodermatitis)
- Sarcoidosis
- Lipid storage diseases (Niemann-Pick, Gaucher, Wolman, Faber diseases)
- Hyperthyroidism

Data Gathering

HISTORY

The etiology of lymphadenopathy is usually determined by performing a thorough history and physical examination. The history should focus on the following:

- Preceding symptoms (e.g., upper respiratory symptoms preceding cervical lymphadenopathy)
- Localizing signs or symptoms (e.g., stomatitis for mandibular nodes)
- Duration (e.g., days or weeks)
- Constitutional or associated symptoms (e.g., fever, weight loss, or night sweats)
- Exposures (e.g., cat exposure [cat-scratch disease], uncooked meat [Toxoplasmosis], tick bite [Lyme disease])
- Medications (e.g., Phenytoin or Isoniazid)
- Travel or residence (e.g., travel to or residence in an endemic area [i.e., Tuberculosis, Lyme disease])

Physical Examination

A complete physical exam is imperative to look for signs of systemic disease, such as skin, ocular findings or hepatosplenomegaly. If localized lymphadenopathy is suspected, the area that the lymph node drains must be examined for pathology (e.g., the arm for a papule associated with axillary lymphadenopathy in cat-scratch disease).

- The cervical, axillary, and inguinal nodes, as well as the liver and the spleen, must be palpated to be help determine if there are signs of systemic disease or infection.
- Characterize the nodes. Be sure to note the following characteristics:
—Location—be as exact as possible (see above)
—Size—>10 mm, measure dimensions
—Consistency—soft, firm, solid, cystic, fluctuant, rubbery (e.g., firm, rubbery nodes are associated with lymphomas, soft nodes with reactive lymphadenopathy).
—Fixation—normally freely mobile; infection or malignancy may cause adherence to surrounding tissues or nodes.
—Tenderness—most likely inflammation

Laboratory Aids

Laboratory tests are generally not needed in the workup of lymphadenopathy unless dictated by the history and physical examination. Consider the following tests if one or more nodes are persistently enlarged, have increased in size, have changed in consistently or mobility, or if there are systemic symptoms:

Test: Complete blood count (CBC)
Significance: Consider with generalized lymphadenopathy, or if malignancy is in the DDx.

Test: Purified Protein Derivative (PPD)
Significance: Consider with persistently enlarged node (2–4 weeks), or endemic travel.

Test: Erythrocyte sedimentation rate (ESR)
Significance: Increased with infection or inflammation

Test: Throat culture
Significance: Concern for GAS pharyngitis

Test: EBV/CMV titers
Significance: Consider with persistent generalized adenopathy

Test: *Bartonella henselae* titers
Significance: Persistently enlarged unilateral node and history of cat exposure

Test: HIV
Significance: Consider with persistent generalized lymphadenopathy, failure to thrive, or other concerning history

Test: Rapid Plasma Reagin (RPR)
Significance: Consider with rash and generalized lymphadenopathy, or other suspicion of syphilis.

Test: Anti-nuclear antibody test (ANA)
Significance: Consider if persistent generalized lymphadenopathy and other signs of systemic disease to rule-out SLE.

RADIOGRAPHIC STUDIES

Test: Chest x-ray (CXR)
Significance: Helpful with supraclavicular nodes, systemic symptoms, or a positive PPD

Test: Ultrasound
Significance: May help differentiate cystic from infectious masses (especially cervical)

Test: Computerized axial tomography (CAT) scan
Significance: May help delineate mass or anatomy

OTHER STUDIES

Biopsy should be considered if the nodes are persistent, especially if accompanied by signs of systemic disease such as hepatosplenomegaly, weight loss, and exanthema, or if the nodes are fixed to the underlying skin, there is ulceration, or the node is supraclavicular, nontender or increasing in size or firmness.

Test: Fine needle aspiration
Significance: Cost-effective, but sometimes nondiagnostic; may result in fistulous tract

Test: Open biopsy
Significance: Often diagnostic, but requires general anesthesia

Therapy

- Close observation unless the history and physical examination suggest malignancy or lymphadenitis.
- Acute lymphadenitis should be treated with antibiotics directed against streptococcus and staphylococcus.
—Cephalexin 50 mg/kg per day in 4 doses or cefadroxil 30 mg/kg per day in 2 divided doses
—Penicillin allergic patients: erythromycin 50mg/kd per day in 4 divided doses.
- Treat underlying disease
- Excision for special prolonged cases

Follow-Up

- Children with localized lymphadenopathy may be observed for several weeks, or treated with antibiotics if indicated. Most cases will resolve without intervention.
- Serial observation if the nodes are persistently enlarged. Studies are indicated as outlined above.

PITFALLS

- Need detailed history and thorough physical examination in order to accurately diagnosis most causes of lymphadenopathy.
- Systemic disease or malignancy may occasionally present with localized lymphadenopathy. Close observation and follow-up is important if etiology is unclear.
- May misdiagnose patient if close follow up is not provided.

Common Questions and Answers

Q: When should there be concern about malignancy in a child with lymphadenopathy?

A: Malignancy should be considered in any child who has lymphadenopathy that does not improve in spite of antibiotic therapy, that has a concerning location (e.g., supraclavicular) or concerning physical exam features (hard, large size [>2 cm]), that persistently enlarges, or if the child shows signs of systemic disease.

Q: How much of a workup does a well child with localized lymphadenopathy need?
A: Most children with lymphadenopathy do not require an extensive workup. As long as the lymph nodes are soft, mobile and nontender, the lymphadenopathy is likely to be self-limited. If the etiology is unclear, then children should be observed for a couple of weeks since most cases of lymphadenopathy will self-resolve. Further workup is needed if the nodes persist, enlarge, or there are signs of systemic disease (e.g., hepatomegaly or weight loss).

Q: When should a child with lymphadenopathy be referred to a surgeon?
A: Most cases of lymphadenopathy in children are self-limited and can be observed for a few weeks, and/or treated with antibiotics, if appropriate. Referral to a surgeon should be considered in any child with persistently enlarged lymphadenopathy (>4 weeks), or immediately if there are signs of malignancy.

ICD-9-CM 785.6

BIBLIOGRAPHY

Albright JT, Pransky SM. Nontuberculous mycobacterial infections of the head and neck. *Pediatr Clin North Am* 2003;50(2): 503–514.

Bamji M, et al. Palpable lymph nodes in healthy newborns and infants. *Pediatrics* 1986;78:573–575.

Chesney PJ. Lymphatic system and generalized lymphadenopathy. In: Long SS, Pickering LK, Prober CG, eds. *Principles and Practice of Pediatric Infectious Diseases*. 2nd Ed. New York: Churchill Livingstone, 2003:122–129.

Herzog LW. Prevalence of lymphadenopathy of the head and neck in infants and children. *Clin Pediatr* 1983;22:485–487.

Kelly CS, Kelly RE. Lymphadenopathy in children. *Pediatr Clin North Am* 1998;45(4): 875–888.

Margileth AM. Lymphadenopathy: when to diagnose and treat. *Contemp Pediatr* 1995;12(2):71–91.

Margileth AM. Sorting out the causes of lymphadenopathy. *Contemp Pediatr* 1995;12(1):23–40.

McClain KL, Fletcher RH. Evaluation of peripheral lymphadenopathy in children. In: Rose BD, ed. *UpToDate*. Wellesley, MA: UpToDate, 2003.

Twist CJ, Link MP. Assessment of lymphadenopathy in children. *Pediatr Clin North Am* 2002;49:1009–1025.

Author: Hans B. Kersten

Lymphedema

Database

DEFINITION

• Accumulation of interstitial fluid in part of the body (usually an extremity) secondary to malformation or malfunction of the lymphatic system.
• Divided into primary and secondary forms (although other classification tools exist):

—Primary: Usually an isolated finding, thought to result from abnormal development of the lymphatics. Deep tissues and muscles not affected. Primary lymphedema often divided into:
  —Congenital lymphedema: Presenting in the first few months of life
  —Lymphedema praecox: Presenting from late in first year of life to early adulthood (20–35 years of age)
  —Lymphedema tarda: Presenting in adulthood (after 20–35 years of life)

• Secondary: The etiology of lymphatic damage has been identified, causes include surgery, neoplasm (primary or metastatic), parasitic infestation, infection, irradiation, and trauma.

PATHOPHYSIOLOGY

• Represents state of overproduction or decreased removal of lymph.
• Initially edema is pitting. Chronic edema may result in fibrosis.

GENETICS

• In 1998, a defect in the long arm of chromosome 5 (5q35) was identified to cause dominantly inherited congenital lymphedema.
• Genetic disorders are associated with lymphedema: Fabry disease, Milroy (congenital familial lymphedema with ocular findings), Meige disease (familial lymphedema praecox), and Down, Turner, Noonan, yellow nail, Klippel-Trenaunay-Weber, pes cavus, and other syndromes.
• Inheritance can be autosomal dominant, recessive, or sex-linked.
• No increased rate of congenital anomalies of other organ systems, but may be associated with other vascular malformations.

EPIDEMIOLOGY

• Most lymphedema in childhood is primary lymphedema.
• Congenital lymphedema comprises 10% of primary lymphedema cases; lymphedema praecox, 71%; and lymphedema tarda, 19%.
• Incidence of 1.5 per 100,000 in children less than 20 years.
• Female to male ratio in congenital lymphedema close to 1:1; in praecox and tarda, 2:1 to 9:1 (64%–90% female).
• Case reports of recurrent lymphedema secondary to herpes simplex virus type 2 exist.

COMPLICATIONS

• Cellulitis
• Lymphangitis
• Lymphangiosarcoma
• Psychological problems
• Physical limitations
• Fibrosis

PROGNOSIS

• Edema persists throughout life.
• Natural history: Plateau in severity of edema after an initial few years of progression in 50%, slow constant progression in 50%.
• Edema of contralateral extremity (usually leg) develops in up to 10%.
• Chronic inflammation and edema ultimately lead to fibrosis and induration of the involved area.

Differential Diagnosis

INFECTION

• Cellulitis
• Lymphangitis
• Herpes simplex virus type 2

TUMORS

• Pelvic mass
• Multiple enchondromatosis

METABOLIC

• Cushing disease

ANATOMIC

• Venous stasis
• Deep venous thrombosis
• Hemihypertrophy
• Atrioventricular fistula

MISCELLANEOUS

• Heart failure
• Nephrosis
• Cirrhosis
• Hypoproteinemia
• Reflex sympathetic dystrophy

Data Gathering

HISTORY

Question: Is there a history of cellulitis or trauma?
Significance: Many report prior history of cellulitis or trauma of the limb later affected with lymphedema.

Question: Is the edema unilateral?
Significance: Subacute or chronic painless swelling of one leg in an otherwise healthy pubertal female is classic for lymphedema praecox.

Question: History of surgery?
Significance: Painless swelling in an extremity distal to surgical or trauma site is common for secondary lymphedema.

Physical Examination

• Subcutaneous tissue filled with fluid resulting in pitting edema. Involvement of single limb strongly suggests lymphedema, whereas global involvement suggests other disease states.
• Chronic inflammation leads to fibrosis, which corresponds to a change from pitting to nonpitting edema and induration.
• Hair loss and hyperkeratosis of the affected limb develop over time.
• Pain in affected limb uncommon

Laboratory Aids

Test: Urinalysis for the presence of protein
Significance: The presence of proteinuria should raise the suspicion for glomerulonephrosis

Test: Serum total protein and albumin
Significance: If low, suggests hypoproteinemia, which can result in edema

RADIOGRAPHIC STUDIES

Test: Ultrasound, computed tomography (CT) scan, or magnetic resonance imaging (MRI) of pelvis
Significance: Useful when evaluating lower extremity edema, as obstructive pelvic lesions may be otherwise inapparent.

Test: Doppler ultrasound
Significance: Helpful when deep venous thrombosis is a diagnostic possibility

Test: Radionuclide lymphangioscintigraphy which has largely replaced lymphangiography
Significance: When history and physical examination yield a diagnosis of uncomplicated primary lymphedema in childhood, it is controversial as to whether or not these tests are necessary. Most feel it adds little to diagnosis and treatment in straightforward cases.

Test: Venography and biopsy
Significance: Considered unnecessary for diagnosis.

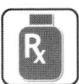 Therapy

- Therapy should be instituted as soon as possible and before fibrosis develops.
- Goals: Maintain or possibly decrease status of swelling, decrease risk of infections, minimize skin changes
- Extremity elevation and compression (e.g., Jobst stocking, Ace wrap) recommended long-term for all patients.
- Meticulous skin care
- Pneumatic machines or manual massage: Short-term recommendation to achieve greatest reduction of edema
- Exercise (walking and/or swimming) thought to enhance lymphatic return
- Cellulitis and lymphangitis treated with hospitalization and intravenous antibiotics
- Complete decongestive physiotherapy is a comprehensive treatment program offered at few selected centers, but seems to be effective in reducing swelling and maintaining reduction in fluid accumulation.
- Diuretics: Not used in children and adolescents; efficacy debated
- Surgery has one of two goals: Removal of excess edematous tissue or attempts to restore lymph drainage; both may decrease the rate of infections but have poor cosmetic results and are recommended only for those with uncontrolled swelling with significant disability. Microsurgical treatment has undergone many advances with excellent outcome in carefully selected patient populations.
- Prophylactic antibiotic use is indicated for patients with recurrent cellulitis or lymphangitis.
- Compression and elevation are lifelong measures.
- In children with chylous reflux syndromes a diet low in long-chain triglycerides may be of benefit.

 Follow-Up

Some edema reduction achieved with pneumatic compression or massage over short term, but persistent use of elevation and compression stockings necessary to maintain benefit.

SIGNS TO WATCH FOR

Fever, chills, red streaks on the extremity, inflamed lymph nodes all point to cellulitis or lymphangitis.

PREVENTION

- Primary disease cannot be prevented, but progression should be minimized with therapies listed here.
- Secondary disease can be prevented by altering surgical approaches to diseases that emphasize sparing of lymphatics and nodes.
- Skin care and properly fitted shoes must be emphasized to avoid skin breakdown, which can lead to cellulitis and/or lymphangitis.

PITFALLS

- Systemic reactions to lymphangiography are not uncommon.
- Compliance with compression stockings is poor because they are often hot and uncomfortable.

 Common Questions and Answers

Q: Is the swelling going to go away?
A: No, this is a lifelong disorder in most cases.

Q: Could this have been prevented?
A: No, primary lymphedema is most likely due to abnormal embryologic development.

Q: If the lymph channels have been abnormal since birth, why does the swelling present during adolescence?
A: No one really knows; hormones may affect lymphedema.

ICD-9-CM 457.1

BIBLIOGRAPHY

Campisi C, et al. Peripheral lymphedema: new advances in microsurgical treatment and long term outcome. *Microsurgery* 2003;23:522–526.

Child AH, Beninson J, Sarfarazi M. Cause of primary congenital lymphedema. *Angiology* 1999;50:325–326.

International Society of Lymphology. The diagnosis and treatment of peripheral lymphedema; Consensus Document of the International Society of Lymphology. *Lymphology* 2003;36:84–91.

Johansson K, Albertsson M, Ingvar C, et al. Effects of compression bandaging with or without manual lymph drainage treatment in patients with postoperative arm lymphedema. *Lymphology* 1999;32:103–110.

Ko DSC, Lerner R, Klose G, et al. Effective treatment of lymphedema of the extremities. *Arch Surg* 1998;133:452–458.

Miller AJ, Bruna J, Beninson J. A universally applicable clinical classification of lymphedema. *Angiology* 1999;50(3):189–192.

Smeltzer DM, Stickler GB, Schirger A. Primary lymphedema in children and adolescents: a follow-up study and review. *Pediatrics* 1985;76:206–218.

Wright NB, Carty HML. The swollen leg and primary lymphedema. *Arch Dis Child* 1994;71:44–49.

Author: Laura N. Sinai

Malaria

 Database

DEFINITION

• Malaria was described by the earliest medical writers in China, Assyria, and India, and by the fifth century BC, Hippocrates was able to describe the characteristic fever patterns and clinical manifestations of the disease.
• Malaria is a febrile illness as a result of the *Plasmodium* species of protozoan parasites. *P. vivax*, *P. malariae*, *P. falciparum*, and *P. ovale* are the species that infect humans.
• Severe malaria is defined as parasitemia > 5% with CNS and other end-organ dysfunction (shock, acidosis, renal failure, and/or hypoglycemia).

PATHOPHYSIOLOGY

• Two discrete stages of the *Plasmodium* life cycle: sexual stage, which develops in the female *Anopheles* mosquito providing the sporozoites to the host; and asexual stage, which occurs in the human, first in the liver producing merozoites and then in the erythrocytes as trophozoites. Trophozoites cause red cell hemolysis, therefore, releasing more merozoites to infect other erythrocytes.
• With the exception of infants with the disease, the cycle is characteristically synchronous and periodic, giving the typical tertian periodicity seen in *P. falciparum*, *P. vivax*, and *P. ovale* and the quartan periodicity seen in *P. malariae*.
• Infection from a contaminated blood transfusion or needle can occur; congenital malaria has also been reported.
• Hemolytic anemia, the most common disease finding, can be severe, especially in *P. falciparum*; the predominant mechanism is a result of intravascular hemolysis from fragile erythrocytes rather than solely rupture from infected cells.
• Cerebral malaria, the most serious consequence of malaria noted in *P. falciparum* infection, is caused by occlusion of the cerebral microvasculature from infected red cells. Prognosis often depends on the management of other complications, e.g., acidosis, renal failure.
• Tropical splenomegaly syndrome seen in chronic infections caused by *P. malariae* produces splenomegaly, hepatomegaly, portal hypertension, and pancytopenia. In *P. vivax* malaria, acute splenomegaly can induce rupture.
• Blackwater fever is a result of acute renal failure caused by accumulation of hemoglobin in the renal tubules resulting in hemoglobinuria with dark urine. This often occurs after repeated attacks of *P. falciparum*.
• Other diseases such as pulmonary edema, distributive shock, dysentery, and nephrotic syndrome have been described.

GENETICS

• Sickle cell disease and trait confers protection against malaria by two postulated mechanisms: release of a toxic form of heme from these erythrocytes that possess antimalarial properties; the hemoglobin S erythrocyte tends to lose potassium required for adenosine triphosphatase (ATPase) activation, thereby depriving the parasites of nutrients.
• Thalassemia and G6PD deficiency may also provide innate resistance to malaria.

EPIDEMIOLOGY

• High-risk areas of the world for malaria include parts of Central and South America, Africa, and Asia under tropical climates.
• Malaria is a major cause of infant death in the tropical regions of the world.
• Infection transmission is acquired through the life of the female *Anopheles* mosquito but can also occur through contaminated blood transfusions or needles as well as be acquired congenitally.
• The most common infecting species are *P. falciparum* and *P. vivax*.
• *P. vivax* and *P. ovale* are associated with relapsing disease because of the persistent hepatic stage of the infection.

COMPLICATIONS

• *P. falciparum* tends to cause more severe disease, and morbidity is significantly increased as a result of the multiorgan system involvement.
• Chronic relapses occur from *P. vivax* and *P. ovale* infections and can occur during periods ranging from every few weeks to a few months.
• In the pregnant patient, increased perinatal mortality has not been reported with malaria in stable, endemic regions. However, for semiimmune or nonimmune mothers, transplacental antibodies may be lacking, and the risk of congenital infection may be higher in this subgroup.

PROGNOSIS

• The prognosis is dependent on the *Plasmodium* species, relapsing nature of the disease, chloroquine resistance, and age of the patient. The infant with *P. falciparum* infection accounts for most of the mortality as a result of malaria.

 Differential Diagnosis

Because there are few clearly distinctive clinical features of malaria, it can be easily overlooked if a good travel history is not obtained in any child with prolonged fever.

 Data Gathering

HISTORY

• Travel
• Dark urine
• Fevers
• Pattern of fevers
• Headaches
• Malaria prophylaxis

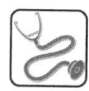 Physical Examination

• High fevers, headache, chills, sweating, and rigors are common presenting findings.
• Other features such as cough, irritability, anorexia, vomiting, abdominal pain, back pain, and arthralgias may also be present.
• Periodicity of fever is less commonly seen in young children and is dependent on the Plasmodium species.
• Hepatosplenomegaly may be present and is more likely observed in chronic infections as a result of *P. falciparum*.
• Cerebral malaria will manifest with signs of increased intracranial pressure with encephalopathy and seizures.

 Laboratory Aids

Test: Hemoglobin
Significance: Hemolytic anemia as a result of intravascular hemolysis as well as direct red cell infection is present initially as mild then more severe, depending on the Plasmodium species.

Test: WBC
Significance: Leukocyte counts are usually normal or low; there is no eosinophilia. Thrombocytopenia as a result of liver and splenic sequestration occurs in the more severe cases.

Test: Peripheral smear
Significance: Thick and thin peripheral blood smears are required for definitive diagnosis (thick smears enable better sensitivity if the parasitemia is low; thin smears provide for species identification). If initial smears are negative, repeat specimens should be obtained every 8 to 12 hours during a 72-hour period to confirm a truly negative result. The percent of red cells involved is an important risk factor for severe disease. A parasitemia greater than 5% of red cells, signs of central nervous system (mental status changes) or other organ involvement are reasons for more intensive therapy.

Test: Quantitative buffy coat (QBC) analysis
Significance: Available as a rapid screening test, but confirmation by blood smears is still necessary.

Test: Serologic tests
Significance: Using indirect immunofluorescent assays may be helpful but have a low sensitivity in the early phases of acute infections.

Test: Polymerase chain reaction (PCR)
Significance: Other tests using PCR techniques are being studied and may be useful in the near future.

 ## Therapy

- For all *Plasmodium* species except chloroquine-resistant *P. falciparum* and chloroquine-resistant *P. vivax*, chloroquine phosphate is recommended at a dose of 10 mg/kg PO (maximum 600 mg), then 5 mg/kg PO in 6 hours (maximum 300 mg), then 5 mg/kg PO in 24 and 48 hours (maximum 300 mg).
- If parenteral therapy is necessary, treatment with quinidine gluconate, 10 mg/kg IV initial dose (maximum 600 mg) over 2 hours followed by 0.02 mg/kg per minute infusion until oral therapy can be started.
- For chloroquine-resistant *P. falciparum* or chloroquine-resistant *P. vivax*; quinine sulfate, 25 mg/kg per day orally in three doses a day for three to 7 days plus doxycycline, 2 mg/kg per day orally twice daily for 7 days (maximum 1 g/d) is recommended. Instead of doxycycline, clindamycin 20 to 40 mg/kg per day orally in three doses for 5 days.
- A safe alternative for children is mefloquine, 15 mg/kg PO followed by 10 mg/kg PO 8 to 12 hours later.
- Other alternatives include pyrimethamine-sulfadoxine (Fansidar), quinine sulfate plus doxycycline, or atovaquone plus proguanil.
- Primaquine phosphate is used for the prevention of *P. vivax* and *P. ovale* relapses but should not be used in patients with G6PD deficiency or in pregnancy.
- Consultation with a pharmacist is recommended to identify other possible contraindications and warnings associated with these medications.

 ## Follow-Up

- Delay in the diagnosis of malaria has been shown to increase the morbidity and mortality up to 20-fold compared with diagnosis and treatment within 24 hours of presentation.
- If treated promptly, even *P. falciparum* malaria will respond well to current treatment options.

PREVENTION

- In the hospital setting, universal precautions should be followed.
- Control measures are targeted toward control of the *Anopheles* mosquito population, and protective measures such as remaining in well-screened areas, and wearing protective clothing should be advised. Use of insect repellents such as DEET is recommended. However, in children younger than 2 years, concentration of less than 10%, and concentrations less than 35% for the older child is recommended.
- Chemoprophylaxis for travelers in endemic areas should begin 1 week before arrival, once weekly during the period of exposure, and then 4 weeks after leaving the endemic region.
- Chloroquine is the drug of choice except in resistant areas (500 mg once a week or 5 mg/kg once a week); in chloroquine-resistant areas, mefloquine is recommended (250 mg once a week; if < 15 kg, 5 mg/kg; if 15 to 19 kg, one-fourth tablet; if 20 to 30 kg, one-half tablet; if 31 to 45 kg, three-fourths tablet). Contraindications to mefloquine use include patients taking beta-blockers or other drugs altering cardiac conduction, patients with seizures or psychosis, and patients requiring fine motor skill performance. Doxycycline or chloroquine plus proguanil are alternatives to mefloquine.
- Travelers should use pyrimethamine-sulfadoxine (Fansidar) if a febrile illness occurs while on chloroquine and access to medical care is not readily available.

PITFALLS

Failure to obtain a thorough travel history to determine exposure risk to developing malaria can delay the diagnosis and appropriate therapy.

 ## Common Questions and Answers

Q: What is the optimal drug regimen for the young infant or child or the lactating or pregnant female?
A: The only drug not contraindicated in any of these patients is chloroquine. In chloroquine-resistant areas, mefloquine has been shown to be safe in the second and third trimesters. Limited data suggest safety in the first trimester also. Mefloquine is excreted in breast milk; however, limited data suggest safety young infants.

Q: Is there a vaccine available to prevent malaria?
A: Although the possibility of vaccination against malaria continues to attract interest, no adequate vaccination is available. Recent advances in the technology for introducing malarial DNA coding into bacteria may lead to an effective vaccine in the future.

Q: How can I determine if the area my patient is traveling to has chloroquine-resistant malaria?
A: The CDC has an automated traveler's hotline accessible from a touch-tone phone 24 hours a day, 7 days a week: (404) 332-4559. Questions can also be faxed to (404) 332-4565. The Internet address for information is www.cdc.gov.

ICD-9-CM 084.6

BIBLIOGRAPHY

Katz M. Treatment of protozoan infections: malaria. *Pediatr Infect Dis J* 1983;2:475–480.

Kramer MH, Lobel HO. Antimalarial chemoprophylaxis in infants and children. *Paediatr Drugs* 2001;3:113–121.

Maitland K, Bejon P, Newton CR. Malaria. *Curr Opin Infect Dis* 2003;16(5):389–395.

Newton CR, Hien TT, White N. Cerebral malaria. *J Neurol Neurosurg Psychiatry* 2000;69:433–441.

Peter G, Halsey NA, Marcuse EK, et al. *Malaria. 2003 Red Book: Report of the Committee on Infectious Diseases*, 26th Ed. Elk Grove Village, IL: American Academy of Pediatrics, 2003:414–419.

Silver HM. Malarial infection during pregnancy. *Infect Dis Clin North Am* 1997;11:99–107.

Steele RW. Malaria in children. *Adv Pediatr Infect Dis* 1997;12:325–349.

White NJ, Miller KD, Churchill FC, et al. Chloroquine treatment of severe malaria in children. *N Engl J Med* 1988;319:1493–1500.

White NJ. Antimalarial drug resistance. *Journal of Clinical Investigation.* 2004;113(8):1084–1092.

Authors: Louis M. Bell
Philip V. Scribano, 3rd edition

Mammalian Bites

 Database

DEFINITION

Injury to the human skin and/or subcutaneous tissues caused by bite, causing usually local, and in some cases systemic, effects.

CAUSES

- Animal bites

—Dogs
—Cats
—Rodents
—Wild animals

- Human bites

PATHOPHYSIOLOGY

- Animal bites

—Crush and tear injuries can result from dog maulings, sometimes even involving bone.
—Cat bites are generally puncture-type wounds, penetrating deeper and carrying a higher risk of infection.

- Human bites generally only violate skin, although penetration into joint and tendon sheath spaces can occur (especially bites overlying the metacarpal-phalangeal areas).
- Reports of rates of infectious complications have yielded varying results.

—Early studies report that infection occurs in 3% to 18% of dog bites, 28% to 80% of cat bites, and 15% to 20% of human bites.
—More recent studies have suggested an incidence of infection after dog and cat bites to be closer to 2% to 3%.
—Bacteriologic analysis of infected animal and human wounds demonstrate polymicrobial cause, most commonly mixed aerobic and anaerobic species.
—*Pasteurella* species are the most frequent isolates from both dog bites (*P. canis*) and cat bites (e.g., *P. multocida* and *P. septica*).
—Common anaerobes include *fusobacterium, bacteroides, porphyromonas,* and *prevotella*.
—For infected human bites, bacterial isolates include *Streptococcus anginosus, Staphylococcus aureus, Eikenella corrodens, fusobacterium* and *prevotella*.

EPIDEMIOLOGY

- Animal bites

—Dogs are responsible for 90% to 95% of cases, although the remainder of cases are divided as follows: cats, 3% to 8%; rodents or rabbits, 1%; and raccoons and other animals, 1%.
—Ninety percent of the offending animals are well known to the victim.
—Children are the most common victims. Boys are twice as likely as girls to be bitten by dogs; girls are more likely to be bitten by cats.

- Human bites

—Incidence is unknown as a result of lack of reporting.
—Most common in children of ages 2 to 5 years.
—In older children may occur accidentally during sports activities or intentionally during altercations or abusive situations.

PROGNOSIS

- Animal bites

—Most injury from animal bites is trivial, but infections, and rarely deaths, do occur.

- Human bites over metacarpals (clenched fist) can penetrate tendon sheaths, become infected, and result in a tenosynovitis.

HISTORY

- Animal bites

—Type of animal?
—Apparent health of the animal?
—Any provocation for the attack?
—Location of the bite or bites?
—Is animal available to undergo observation i.e., it is a known animal as opposed to a stray or wild animal?
—Rabies immunization status of the animal?
—Tetanus immunization status of the child?

 Physical Examination

- Carefully assess neurovascular integrity.
- Location of bite: If bite is located over a joint, assess for violation of joint capsule.
- Examine entire patient to ensure that all wounds are identified and treated.
- Older wounds: assess for signs of infection such as erythema, induration, purulence, regional adenopathy, and elevated temperature.

DIAGNOSTIC AIDS

- No tests routinely done.
- In significant dog bites, consider radiography to evaluate for presence of fracture, foreign body (e.g., tooth), air within joint.
- Blood culture if fever, systemic toxicity

Therapy

- Wound care: Copious irrigation to remove visible debris; cleanse but do not irrigate puncture wounds.
- Human bites over metacarpals (clenched-fist injuries) require orthopaedic evaluation for possible surgical exploration and irrigation.
- Debride devitalized tissue.
- The increased risk of infection associated with suturing a potentially contaminated wound must be weighed against the cosmetic effect as a result of nonclosure. Primary closure of larger wounds or significant facial wounds may be indicated unless wound is old or has evidence of infection. Hand wounds may be an exception as a result of high propensity for infection.
- Antibiotics: Data are often contradictory. In general:

—All cat bites should be treated with prophylactic antibiotics as a result of high risk of infection with *P. multocida*. Amoxicillin-clavulanic acid is drug of choice (50 mg/kg per day divided b.i.d. or t.i.d. for 5 days).
—All human bites should be treated with antibiotic prophylaxis. Amoxicillin-clavulanic acid is drug of choice (50 mg/kg per day divided b.i.d. or t.i.d. for 5 days).
—Alternative antibiotic regimens for penicillin allergic patients is trimethoprim-sulfamethoxazole PLUS clindamycin.
—Bites to the hand, deep puncture wounds, and wounds in immunocompromised hosts may be treated empirically.
—Skin and soft tissue infections requiring hospitalization: ampicillin/sulbactam 150 mg/kg per day in 4 divided doses. For penicillin allergic patients, third-generation cephalosporin. Antibiotics with poor activity against *Pasteurella* include penicillinase-resistant penicillins, clindamycin, and aminoglycosides.

- Tetanus prophylaxis if indicated
- Rabies prophylaxis if indicated:

—Unknown dog or cat; dogs or cats with unknown immunization status that cannot be observed for 10 days
—Bites from wild animals including raccoons, bats, skunks, foxes, coyotes
—Because bat bites may go undetected, especially by a sleeping child, rabies prophylaxis is now recommended after exposure to bats in a confined setting.

- Rabies is unlikely if the child was bitten by an immunized dog or cat, other pet (e.g., hamsters, guinea pigs, gerbils, rabbits), squirrels, mice, or rats.
- The regimen for patients who have not been vaccinated previously should include both human rabies vaccine (a series of 5 doses administered intramuscularly [IM]) and rabies immune globulin (20 IU/kg) administered as much as possible into the wound, the remainder given IM at a site distant from the site used for vaccine administration.

- HIV post-exposure prophylaxis (PEP): There are case reports describing transmission of HIV by human bites; however, the risk of transmission as a result of biting is unknown.

—It is estimated to be extremely small (even if the biter's saliva contains blood), probably less than 0.1%.
—A bite with a break in the skin is considered low risk and a bite with intact skin is felt to pose no risk.
—HIV PEP requires a multi-drug regimen administered over 28 days. It can be associated with significant toxicity.
—No formal recommendations regarding PEP in biting incidents have been made at this time.

- Decisions to initiate PEP might best be made in consultation with local experts.

PREVENTION

- Educate children about the safe handling of animals.
- Ensure children are routinely immunized against tetanus and hepatitis and family pets are immunized against rabies.
- Local regulations dictate the reporting of animal bites to health departments.

BIBLIOGRAPHY

Goldstein EJC. Current concepts on animal bites: bacteriology and therapy. *Curr Clin Top Infect Dis* 1999;19:99–111.

Griego RD, Rosen T, Orengo IF, et al. Dog, cat, and human bites: a review. *J Am Acad Dermatol* 1995;33:1019–1029.

Havens PL and the Committee on Pediatric AIDS. Postexposure prophylaxis in children and adolescents for nonoccupational exposure to human immunodeficiency virus. *Pediatrics* 2003;111:1475–1489.

Moran GJ, Talan DA, Mower W, et al. Appropriateness of rabies postexposure prophylaxis treatment for animal exposures. *JAMA* 2000;284:1001–1007.

Talan DA, Abrahamian FM, Moran GJ, et al. Clinical presentation and bacteriologic analysis of infected human bites in patients presenting to the emergency departments. *Clin Infect Dis* 2003;37:1481–1489.

Talan DA, Citron DM, Abrahamian FM, et al. Bacteriologic analysis of infected dog and cat bites. *N Eng J Med* 1999;340:85–92.

Author: Jill C. Posner

Mastoiditis

Database

DEFINITION

Mastoiditis is an infection of the mastoid air cells that can range from an asymptomatic illness to a severe life-threatening disease.

CAUSES

- Acute mastoiditis is caused by an extension of the inflammation and infection of acute otitis media into the mastoid air cells.
- The bacteria isolated from middle ear drainage or from the mastoid are usually *Streptococcus pneumoniae*, group A β-hemolytic streptococci, and *Staphylococcus aureus*. However, many patients cultures are sterile.
- Chronic mastoiditis is usually caused by *S. aureus*, anaerobic bacteria, enteric bacteria, and *Pseudomonas aeruginosa*. Chronic mastoiditis is often a multiple organism infection.
- Unusual agents of chronic mastoiditis include *Mycobacterium tuberculosis*, atypical mycobacterium, *Nocardia asteroides*, and *Histoplasma capsulatum*.
- Cholesteatomas may contribute to the development of mastoiditis by impeding mastoid drainage or erosion of underlying bone.

PATHOLOGY

- The mastoid process is the posterior portion of the temporal bone and consists of interconnecting air cells that drain superiorly into the middle ear. Because these mastoid air cells connect with the middle ear, all cases of acute otitis media are associated with some mastoid inflammation.
- Acute mastoiditis develops when the accumulation of purulent exudate in the middle ear does not drain through the eustachian tube or through a perforated tympanic membrane but spreads to the mastoid.
- Acute mastoiditis can progress to a coalescent phase when the bony air cells are destroyed and may then progress to subperiosteal abscess or to chronic mastoiditis.

EPIDEMIOLOGY

- At the start of the 20th century, about half the cases of otitis media developed into a coalescent mastoiditis. The routine use of antibiotics for otitis media and aggressive management of treatment failures has decreased this incidence to 0.2% to 0.4%.
- Some recent studies have documented increasing incidence of mastoiditis at their centers. This may be related to regional differences in bacterial resistance, child-care attendance, or practitioners' prescription patterns for otitis media.
- Most patients are between 6 and 24 months old.
- It is unusual to see mastoiditis in the very young because of incomplete pneumatization of the mastoid air cells.

COMPLICATIONS

- The mastoid's proximity to many important structures can result in serious complications from extension of infection or as a response to the inflammatory process.
- Intracranial complications include meningitis and extradural, subdural, or brain parenchymal abscesses.
- Venous sinus thrombophlebitis results from extension of disease to the sigmoid or lateral sinus. Sepsis, increased intracranial pressure, or septic emboli may result.
- Facial nerve palsy is usually unilateral and can be permanent.
- Labyrinthitis or osteomyelitis may result from extension of the infection into adjacent bones.
- Subperiosteal abscess
- Hearing loss can occur from destruction of the ossicles or from labyrinthine damage.
- Bezold abscess is a deep neck abscess along the medial sternocleidomastoid muscle that develops when the infection erodes through the tip of the mastoid bone and dissects down tissue planes.

PROGNOSIS

- Mastoiditis has a good prognosis if treated early. However, intracranial extension of mastoiditis can lead to permanent neurologic deficits and death.
- Chronic mastoiditis can lead to irreversible hearing loss.

Differential Diagnosis

- Parotitis
- Posterior auricular lymphadenopathy or cellulitis
- Otitis externa or an ear canal furuncle
- Neoplastic disease: leukemia, lymphoma, rhabdomyosarcoma, histiocytosis X
- Branchial cleft anomaly

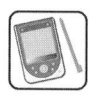

Data Gathering

HISTORY

- Symptoms may include fever, otalgia, otorrhea, and postauricular swelling.
- Children who are already on antibiotics may present with more subtle findings
- Past medical history usually may include a recent or a chronic history of treatment for otitis media.
- Intracranial extension should be suspected if there is lethargy, a stiff neck, headache, focal neurologic symptoms, seizures, visual changes, or persistent fevers despite appropriate antibiotic treatment.
- Labyrinthitis initially presents with tinnitus and nausea, which can progress to vomiting, vertigo, nystagmus, and loss of balance.

Physical Examination

- The ear may protrude away from the scalp. In infants, the ear protrudes out and is displaced down.
- The tympanic membrane often is hyperemic with decreased mobility. The tympanic membranes of children on antibiotics may have a normal appearance.
- The mastoid process is tender with soft tissue swelling. The overlying skin may be warm and erythematous with posterior auricular fluctuance.
- In chronic mastoiditis, the fever and posterior auricular swelling are often not present and the patient presents with ear pain, persistent drainage, or hearing loss.

Laboratory Aids

Test: Middle ear aspirate obtained by myringotomy
Significance: Gram stain and cultures for aerobic and anaerobic bacteria should be done. There is some correlation between middle ear bacterial cultures and mastoid cultures.

Test: Radiographs
Significance: Reveal haziness of the mastoid air cells and can show bony destruction in more advanced disease. However, radiographs are unreliable and can be falsely normal as well as falsely abnormal.

Test: Temporal bone and cranial CT
Significance: Helpful in the confirmation of the diagnosis, identification of coalescence or a subperiosteal abscess, and evaluation for concomitant intracranial complications. However, intracranial complications are best seen with MRI.

Test: Lumbar puncture
Significance: Must be performed in any child with symptoms of meningitis.

Test: CBC with differential
Significance: May show a leukocytosis with a neutrophil predominance.

Test: Erythrocyte sedimentation rate
Significance: May be elevated in acute mastoiditis but is usually normal in the chronic stage.

Test: Purified protein derivative (PPD)
Significance: Should be done if tuberculosis is suspected.

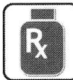 ## Therapy

- Middle ear drainage is essential, and therefore a myringotomy with or without tube placement should be performed early.
- Parenteral antibiotics are chosen on the basis of the most likely organisms and regional bacterial resistance patterns. In acute mastoiditis, oxacillin (150 mg/kg per day in 4 doses) or cefotaxime (150–200 mg/kg per day in 4 doses) can be used. Broad-spectrum coverage such as oxacillin and gentamicin is recommended for chronic mastoiditis. If *M. tuberculosis* is suspected, then antituberculosis therapy should be started.
- Indications for surgical intervention include subperiosteal abscess, coalescence, facial nerve palsy, meningitis, intracranial abscess, venous thrombosis, or persistent symptoms despite adequate antibiotic treatment.

PREVENTION

- Appropriate early treatment of otitis media as well as timely follow-up to identify treatment failures.
- Avoid factors that predispose to otitis media, including smoking and bottle feeding.
- Early recognition of mastoiditis decreases the risk of intracranial complications.
- Streptococcal vaccination may help decrease the occurrence of otitis media.

 ## Follow-Up

- If patients respond quickly to parenteral therapy, they can complete a 3-week course with oral antibiotics and weekly follow-up visits.
- Audiograms should be performed later to screen for hearing loss.

 ## Common Questions and Answers

Q: Do all children with mastoiditis need a CT scan of the head if mastoiditis is suspected?
A: No, in general if the child with mastoiditis has mild swelling, no fluctuance of the mastoid, and responds to therapy, no CT scan is needed. A patient who appears toxic, is not responding to appropriate antibiotic therapy, or one suspects is a surgical candidate should undergo additional imaging studies.

Q: Should all children with mastoiditis be admitted to the hospital?
A: Yes, in general, admission with intravenous antibiotics and ENT evaluation is warranted to assure response to antibiotics and rule out complications.

ICD-9-CM

383.00 (acute)
383.1 (chronic)

BIBLIOGRAPHY

Antonelle PJ, Dhanani CM, et al. Impact of resistant pneumococcus on rates of acute mastoiditis. *Otolaryngol Head Neck Surg* 1999;121:190–194.

Bitar CN, Kluka EA, Steele RW. Mastoiditis in children. *Clin Pediatr* 1996;35:391–395.

Spiegel JH, Lustig LR, Lee KC, et al. Contemporary presentation and management of a spectrum of mastoid abscesses. *Laryngoscope* 1998;108:882–888.

Taylor MF, Berkowitz RG. Indications for mastoidectomy in acute mastoiditis in children. *Ann Otol Rhinol Laryngol* 2004;113(1):69–72.

Vazquez E, Castellote A, et al. Imaging of complications of acute mastoiditis in children. *Radiographics* 2003;23:359–372.

Zapalac JS, Billings KR, et al. Suppurative complications of acute otitis media in the era of antibiotic resistance. *Arch Otolaryngol HNS* 2002;128:660–663.

Author: Frances M. Nadel

Measles (Rubeola-First Disease)

 Database

DEFINITION

Measles is an exanthematous disease that has a relatively predictable course, making diagnosis clinically possible. The disease involves fever, cough, conjunctivitis, or coryza with an erythematous rash, which has a characteristic progression.

CAUSES

Measles is a paramyxovirus, genus *Morbillivirus*. It was first isolated in 1954 in human and monkey kidney tissue cultures.

PATHOPHYSIOLOGY

The infection is probably acquired by inoculation of the nose or conjunctivae.

EPIDEMIOLOGY

- Measles is a highly contagious disease in nonimmune persons.
- Transmission of measles is thought to occur mainly by microaerosolized droplets of respiratory secretions.
- Hospital or clinic waiting rooms (especially pediatric emergency department waiting rooms) have been identified as a major risk accounting for up to 45% of the known exposures in this setting.
- Prior to the 1963 licensure of vaccine, approximately 500,000 cases of measles (330 cases per 100,000) population were reported annually.
- In 1983, there were only 0.7 cases per 100,000 population. However, in 1990, 27,672 cases were reported with 89 deaths.
- The reason for the 1989–1991 outbreak was failure to adequately vaccinate preschool-aged children.
- Patients are contagious from 1 to 2 days before onset of symptoms until 5 days after the appearance of the rash.
- The incubation period is generally 8 to 12 days from exposure to onset of symptoms and about 14 days until the appearance of rash.
- With adequate vaccinations, measles could be eliminated as a disease.
- In 1999 only 86 cases of measles were reported to the CDC.

COMPLICATIONS

- Complication rates in 1989–1990 outbreaks that occurred throughout the country was 23% and included diarrhea (9%), otitis media (7%), pneumonia (6%), and encephalitis (0.1%).
- Encephalitis, which can lead to permanent neurologic sequelae, occurs in 1 of every 1,000 cases reported in the United States.
- In 1990, approximately 18% to 20% of patients required hospitalization, many for either dehydration or pneumonia.
- In patients with poor nutrition, such as found in developing countries, mortality is higher.
- Croup, pneumonia, myocarditis, pericarditis, encephalitis, and disseminated intravascular coagulation (black measles)
- Subacute sclerosis panencephalitis (SSPE) occurs in 1 per 100,000 children with naturally occurring measles. After an incubation period of several years (mean 10.8), a progressive encephalopathy develop among unvaccinated children. Patients with SSPE are not infectious.

PROGNOSIS

- Mortality in the modern outbreak of 1989–1990 occurred in 3 of every 1,000 cases in the United States.
- Case-fatality rates are increased in immunocompromised children.

ASSOCIATED DISEASES

- Typical measles
- Modified measles

—Occurs naturally in infants younger than 9 months of age because of the presence of transplacental antibody or as a result of administration of immunoglobulin to an exposed susceptible child.
—The illness is similar to typical measles but is generally mild. The patient may be afebrile and the rash may last only 1 to 2 days.

- Atypical measles

—Occurs as a result of a hypersensitivity reaction to measles infection in those who received killed virus vaccine between 1963 and 1967 and are subsequently exposed to wild virus.
—This group of young adults (second and third decade of life) become quite ill, with sudden onset of fever from 103°F to 105°F associated with headache. The rash, unlike typical measles, appears first on the distal extremities and progresses in a cephalad direction.
—Virtually all patients with atypical measles have respiratory distress with clinical and radiographic signs of pneumonia often with pleural effusions.
—Diagnosis depends on recognition and on acute and convalescent measles antibody titers.
—The differential diagnoses included meningococcemia, Rocky Mountain spotted fever (RMSF), and toxic shock syndrome.

 Differential Diagnosis

- Steven-Johnson syndrome
- Kawasaki disease
- Viral exanthem
- With a careful history and physical examination it is almost always possible to rule in measles and rule out other possibilities.

 Data Gathering

HISTORY

- Case definition from the CDC includes:

—Generalized rash lasting 3 days or longer
—A temperature of 101°F or higher and cough, coryza, or conjunctivitis

- The mean incubation period is 10 days (range: 8 to 21 days)
- The prodrome of measles lasts 2 to 4 days and begins with symptoms of upper respiratory infection and fever up to 104°F. General malaise, conjunctivitis with photophobia, and cough increasing in severity over this period.
- During the prodrome, Koplik spots (white spots on the buccal mucosa) appear.
- The rash appears on the face (often the nape of the neck, initially) and abdomen 14 days after exposure. The rash is erythematous and maculopapular and spreads from the head to the feet.
- After 3 to 4 days, the rash begins to clear, leaving a brownish discoloration and fine scaling.
- Fever usually resolves by the fourth day of rash.

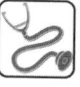 Physical Examination

- The rash appears on the face (often the nape of the neck, initially) and abdomen 14 days after exposure. The rash is erythematous and maculopapular and spreads from the head to the feet.
- Pharyngitis, cervical lymphadenopathy, and splenomegaly may accompany the rash.

Measles (Rubeola-First Disease)

Laboratory Aids

- The course of typical measles follows a predictable pattern and, therefore, laboratory studies to confirm infection are rarely indicated.
- At the beginning of a suspected case, confirmation of the index cases is important.
- Nasopharynx culture: Virus may be cultured from the nasopharynx if inoculated into tissue culture within 24 hours of the onset of rash.
- Monoclonal antibody immunofluorescence cells test: Rapid detection of measles virus from nasal secretions is also possible. Measles infected with epithelial cells will demonstrate fluorescence. However, after the third day of rash, detection of virus by the method becomes increasingly difficult.
- Blood sample: Measles-specific IgM titers will confirm infection but blood samples should be drawn no sooner than 5 days after the rash first appears. Prior to this IgM titers will be negative.
- Blood sample: A comparison of IgG titers obtained during the acute and convalescent stages can be done. Blood samples must be taken at least 7 to 10 days apart.

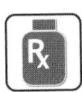

Therapy

SPECIFIC

- There is no specific therapy for this infection other than supportive care. Antipyretics, plenty of oral fluids, and room humidification to help reduce cough are usually all that is needed.
- In April 1993, the American Academy of Pediatrics issued a policy statement concerning vitamin A treatment of measles.

—The use of vitamin A should be considered for children 6 months to 2 years of age who are hospitalized with measles or its complications; and
—Children over 6 months of age who have an immunodeficiency, ophthalmologic evidence of vitamin A deficiency, impaired intestinal absorption, or moderate to severe malnutrition, or who are recent immigrants from areas of high mortality from measles.
—Children 6 months to 1 year should receive 100,000 IU of water-miscible vitamin A.
—The recommended dosage for children over 1 year of age is a single dose of 200,000 IU of water-miscible vitamin A on admission, a second dose the following day.
—The higher dose may be associated with vomiting and headache for a few hours.
—For children with ophthalmologic evidence of vitamin A deficiency, a third dose at 4 weeks is indicated.
—Vitamin A is available in 50,000 IU/mL solution and may be given orally.

PREVENTION

- Vaccine recommendations

—Routine vaccination against measles, mumps, rubella (MMR) for children begins at 12 to 15 months with a second MMR vaccination at entrance to elementary school, age 4 to 6 years or middle school, age 11 to 12 years.
—With the recent resurgence of measles, aggressive employee immunization programs should be pursued for all health care workers.
—Health care workers born in 1957 or after who have no documentation of vaccination or other evidence of measles immunity should be vaccinated at the time of employment and revaccinated no sooner than 1 month later.

- Infection control measures

—Any patient suspected of having measles should be in a negative-pressure isolation room, in respiratory isolation.
—All health care workers involved with the patient must wear masks, gloves, and gowns.
—Isolation is required until 5 days after the first appearance of the rash, except for immunocompromised patients, who require isolation for the course of the illness.
—All suspected cases of measles should be reported immediately to the local health department.

Follow-Up

In uncomplicated measles infection the patient begins feeling better with a fading of rash on the third and fourth day.

PITFALL

Misdiagnosis is the biggest problem with measles infection. Because it is rare and may occur in outbreaks, initially cases are often misdiagnosed as Kawasaki disease or Stevens-Johnson syndrome.

Common Questions and Answers

Q: If a health care worker has had a natural measles infection or measles immunization, should one be concerned about infection following exposure?
A: Those persons born prior to 1957 who had a "wild measles virus" infection are usually immune from reinfection. However, in a report in 1993, four health care workers who were previously vaccinated with positive pre-illness measles antibody levels developed modified measles following exposure to infected patients. Therefore, all health care workers should observe respiratory precautions in caring for patients with measles.

Q: During an outbreak of measles, should children younger than 12 months be vaccinated?
A: In an outbreak of measles, public health officials may recommend vaccination of infants 6 months to 11 months with a single antigen measles vaccine; children initially vaccinated before their first birthday should be revaccinated at 12 to 15 months of age. A second dose should be administered during the early school years.

ICD-9-CM 056.9

BIBLIOGRAPHY

American Academy of Pediatric Measles. In: Peter G, ed. *1994 Red Book: Report on the Committee on Infectious Diseases.* 23rd Ed. Elk Grove Village, IL: American Academy of Pediatrics, 1994:308–323.

Arrieta AC, Zaleska M, Stutman HR, et al. Vitamin A levels in children with measles in Long Beach, California. *J Pediatr* 1992;121:75.

Atkinson W, Wolfe C, Humiston S, Nelson R, eds. *Epidemiology and Prevention of Vaccine Preventable Diseases.* 6th Ed. Washington, DC: Department of Health & Human Services, Public Health Foundation, 2000.

D'Souza RM, D'Souza R. Vitamin A for treating measles in children. *Cochrane Database Syst Rev (1)* 2002:CD001479.

Farizo KM, Stehr-Green PA, Simpsons DM, et al. Pediatric emergency room visits: a risk factor for acquiring measles. *Pediatrics* 1991;98:74.

Hussey GD, Klein M. A randomized controlled trial of vitamin A in children with measles. *N Engl J Med* 1990;323:169.

Rall GF. Measles virus 1998–2002: progress and controversy. *Ann Rev Microbiol* 2003;57:343–367.

Author: Louis M. Bell

Meckel Diverticulum

 Database

DEFINITION

- Meckel diverticulum is a congenital anomaly that is part of the group known as the omphalomesenteric duct remnants.
- A remnant of the embryonic yolk sac found in approximately 2% of all infants; the most common congenital gastrointestinal anomaly.
- This diverticulum originates from the antimesenteric border of the bowel in the region of the terminal ileum and proximal to the ileocecal valve. It can be between 3 and 6 cm in length.
- Other intestinal diverticuli are more common in the jejunum and on the mesenteric border of the bowel.

CAUSES

- Meckel diverticulum results from a partial or complete failure of involution of the omphalomesenteric or vitellointestinal duct.
- The omphalomesenteric duct is the portion of the yolk sac that becomes incorporated into the ventral wall of the primitive gut.

PATHOLOGY

- Meckel diverticulum contains all three layers of the intestinal wall.
- The majority of these diverticuli are lined with ileal mucosa, but ectopic tissue is often present.
- The variety of ectopic tissue that may be present includes gastric (which is the most common), duodenal, colonic, and pancreatic.
- Of the symptomatic cases of Meckel diverticulum, 40% to 80% have some type of ectopic tissue, including gastric or pancreatic type.

EPIDEMIOLOGY

- In asymptomatic and incidentally discovered cases of Meckel diverticuli, there is no sex ratio difference. In cases in which the diverticulum is symptomatic there is a 3:1 male predominance.
- The lifetime risk of developing complications from Meckel diverticulum is approximately 6%.
- The development of symptoms seems to be age related, with the peak incidence being early childhood (2 years of age).
- Eighty percent of all patients requiring surgery were less than 10 years of age and nearly 50% were under 2 years of age.
- There have been reports of a higher incidence of Meckel diverticulum in patients with esophageal atresia (12%), imperforate anus (11%), and minor omphalocele (25%).

 Differential Diagnosis

- The differential diagnosis for Meckel diverticulum is based on its two main clinical symptoms: bleeding and obstruction.
- The causes of a lower gastrointestinal hemorrhage include:

—milk protein colitis
—infectious enteritis—intussusception
—Henoch-Schönlein purpura—polyps
—inflammatory bowel disease (IBD)—volvulus
—lymphonodular hyperplasia—hemolytic uremic syndrome—pseudomembranous colitis
—arteriovenous malformation (AVM)
—duplication cysts.

- The differential for obstruction includes

—malrotation—volvulus—intussusception
—atresias—adhesions—strictures.

 Data Gathering

HISTORY

Question: Bleeding?
Significance: The most common presentation for a Meckel diverticulum is intermittent, painless rectal bleeding secondary to peptic ulceration that arises at the junction of the ectopic gastric mucosa and the normal ileal mucosa. The bleeding can be excessive if the erosion is at the site of the remnant vitelline artery. The bleeding, even in the most severe cases, tends to be self-limiting, because of constriction of the splanchnic vessels secondary to hypovolemia. Bleeding is most commonly seen in children younger than 5 years of age. In diverticuli that bleed, 90% have ectopic gastric mucosa.

Question: Obstruction?
Significance: A second common clinical presentation is partial or complete small bowel obstruction. The mechanism of the obstruction can be secondary to intussusception (most common), intraperitoneal bands, volvulus, or an internal herniation.

Question: Similarity to appendicitis—pain?
Significance: Meckel diverticulum may present with signs and symptoms of appendicitis (inflammatory) with right lower quadrant pain, vomiting, and low-grade fever. This occurs when the diverticulum becomes acutely inflamed secondary to an obstruction or peptic ulceration. Approximately one-third of Meckel diverticulum may progress to perforation before exploration.

 Physical Examination

Finding: Usually normal

 Laboratory Aids

Diagnosis of Meckel diverticulum depends on clinical presentation and suspicion. There are no specific laboratory evaluations that aid in the diagnosis of a Meckel diverticulum. There may be evidence of anemia, which can be significant.

Test: Standard abdominal x-rays
No value in diagnosing a Meckel diverticulum.

Test: Meckel scans
This is an important tool in making the diagnosis. The scan is 80% to 90% sensitive and 95% specific. During the scan, the technetium-99m pertechnetate is taken up by the ectopic gastric tissue (mucous neck secreting cells). Certain substances enhance the detection of the ectopic gastric tissue including cimetidine, glucagon and pentagastrin.
The scan will usually show a focal collection in the mid-abdomen or right lower quadrant. False results can happen in 20% of the scans.

- False + with bleeding

—Intussusception
—Hemangioma
—AVM
—Inflammatory lesion-Crohn disease
—Peptic ulcer

- False + nonbleeding

—Ureteral obstruction
—Sacral meningomyelocele

- False

—Barium
—Bladder overdistension
—No gastric mucosa present

Test: Red cell tagged scans
Not specific for a Meckel diverticulum, but may be useful in localizing the site of bleeding.

Test: Superior mesenteric angiography
Have been used in making the diagnosis but are rarely indicated.

Therapy

- The therapy for a Meckel diverticulum is surgical removal, in cases in which the patient is symptomatic. The important factors in the removal are to remove all ectopic tissue during the surgery and to ensure that the closure of the bowel wall does not cause a narrowing of the lumen.
- In some cases a Meckel diverticulum is found incidentally. Some believe that if found, it should be removed secondary to the potential complications of hemorrhage, perforation, and obstruction. Others feel that the lifetime risk for developing these complications is low, and therefore they would not remove the diverticulum.
- The current favored practice is to examine the diverticulum for evidence of ectopic tissue, which includes either a thickening or a mass within the wall of the diverticulum. If present, then removal is indicated. A second feature that may lead to removal is a narrowing at the base of the diverticulum, therefore increasing the risk for obstruction and perforation.

 Follow-Up

- Once the Meckel diverticulum is removed, standard postoperative care is undertaken. No specific follow-up is indicated.
- In cases in which the diverticulum is found incidentally but not removed, one should be aware of its existence in case symptoms arise later in life that can be attributable to this lesion.
- There have been a few cases in adults in which malignant tumors have developed in the diverticulum.

 Common Questions and Answers

Q: What are the reasons for resection of a Meckel diverticulum?
A: Narrowing at base of diverticulum or presence of ectopic tissue resulting in bleeding.

Q: What is the most common ectopic tissue present in Meckel diverticulum?
A: Gastric

Q: What is the most common presentation of a Meckel diverticulum?
A: Intermittent, painless rectal bleeding

ICD-9-CD 751.0

BIBLIOGRAPHY

Anderson GF, Sfakianakis G, King DR, et al. Hormonal enhancement of technetium-99m pertechnetate uptake in experimental Meckel's diverticulum. *J Pediatr Surg* 1980;15:900–905.

Cullen JJ, Kelly KA. Current management of Meckel's diverticulum. *Adv Surg* 1996;29:207–214.

Emamian SA, Shalaby-Rana E, Majd M. The spectrum of heterotopic gastric mucosa in children detected by Tc-99m pertechnetate scintigraphy. *Clin Nucl Med* 2001;26(6): 529–535.

Soltero MJ, Bill AJ. The natural history of Meckel's diverticulum and its relation to incidental removal. *Am J Surg* 1976;132: 168–173.

Stuvil O, Brandt ML, Panic S, et al. Meckel's diverticulum in children: a 20 year review. *J Pediatr Surg* 1991;26:1289–1292.

Yahchouchy EK, Marano AF, Etienne JC, et al. Meckel's diverticulum. *J Am Coll Surg* 2001;192(5):658–662.

Author: Edisio Semeao

Megaloblastic Anemia

 Database

DEFINITION

Anemia characterized by megaloblastic red blood cells (RBC; large cells with abundant cytoplasm) in the bone marrow and hypersegmented neutrophils on peripheral blood smears.

PATHOPHYSIOLOGY

• Abnormal DNA synthesis in hematopoietic precursors
• Anemia is as a result of ineffective hematopoiesis and hemolysis
• Overall causes are numerous, but the following are the most common general etiologic categories:

—Vitamin B_{12} (cobalamin) deficiency
—Folate (folic acid) deficiency
—Refractory dyserythropoietic anemias—rare in children

• Other disorders may be associated with an increased mean corpuscular volume (MCV) other than megaloblastic anemias, e.g., reticulocytes (young red blood cells), which are increased in hemolytic anemias; liver disease; pregnancy; aplastic anemia; hypothyroidism.

EPIDEMIOLOGY

• Exact incidence and prevalence figures in American children are unknown, but overall the disease is rare.
• In adults, pernicious anemia is a common cause.

COMPLICATIONS

• Mild congestive heart failure may develop as a result of anemia but this is uncommon as a result of the insidious onset of megaloblastic anemia in general.
• Neurologic complications from vitamin B_{12} deficiency.
• Folate deficiency may complicate vitamin B_{12} deficiency.

PROGNOSIS

Prognosis depends on etiology of megaloblastic anemia; usually good if dietary deficiency. Poor prognoses may be associated with inborn errors of metabolism that sometimes present with megaloblastic anemia.

 Differential Diagnosis

Macrocytic anemias must be differentiated from megaloblastic anemias. In macrocytic anemias, the MCV is increased but without megaloblastic bone marrow changes.

 Data Gathering

HISTORY

• Insidious onset of anemia and associated symptoms such as increased pallor, increased fatigue, poor appetite, irritability, and so on.
• Gastrointestinal history may include:

—Malabsorption/diarrhea
—Special diets: particularly strict vegan diets
—Prior gastrointestinal surgery

• Medications such as anticonvulsants and chemotherapeutic agents that interfere with folate metabolism.
• Neurologic symptoms most commonly associated with vitamin B_{12} deficiency; symptoms may include:

—Difficulty walking
—Numbness/tingling in hands and/or feet

 Physical Examination

• Pallor and other associated signs of anemia
• Smooth and sometimes tender tongue
• Neurologic findings: abnormal position and vibratory sensation, ataxia, muscular weakness, peripheral neuropathy, positive Babinski sign

 Laboratory Aids

Test: Complete blood count (CBC)
Significance:

• Decreased hemoglobin
• Increased MCV
• Increased red cell distribution width (RDW)
• Normal to decreased white blood count (WBC) and platelets

Test: Peripheral blood smear
Significance:

• Macro-ovalocytes
• Hypersegmented neutrophils
• Increased anisocytosis (variation in RBC size)
• Increased poikilocytosis (variation in RBC shape)

Test: Reticulocyte count
Significance: Low reticulocyte count

Test: B_{12}
Significance: Low serum vitamin B_{12}

Test: Folate
Significance: Low serum and RBC folate

Test: Bone marrow and biopsy examination
Significance:

• Large RBC, WBC, and platelet precursors with nuclear-to-cytoplasmic dissociation prominent in red cell line.
• Increased iron stores
• Multiple bi- and trinucleate RBC precursors and multiple mitotic figures

Test: Schilling test
Significance: Assesses B_{12} absorption

• Part 1 evaluates vitamin B_{12} absorption by measuring urine radioactivity after oral radioactive vitamin B_{12}. (Note: This test may be performed after the patient has been treated, but the test involves administration of vitamin B_{12} so that all other tests, particularly bone marrow examination, should be performed beforehand or shortly thereafter.)
• If the urinary excretion is lower than expected, then abnormal absorption is present; this may be as a result of malabsorption or intrinsic factor disorders.
• Part 2 should be performed if part 1 is abnormal; this involves oral intrinsic factor. If part 2 is normal and part 1 is abnormal, then pernicious anemia is highly suspected. If part 2 remains abnormal, then a malabsorption syndrome is the most likely diagnosis.

Test: Barium studies
Significance: May be needed to evaluate gastric, small bowel, and large bowel anomalies.

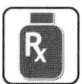 Therapy

- General considerations: the following three categories should be addressed for all patients:

—Replacement of deficient substance, vitamin B$_{12}$, or folate at adequate doses for an adequate duration
—Treatment/management of underlying disorder, such as malabsorption syndromes, chronic hemolytic anemias
—Monitoring response to therapy

- Treating undiagnosed vitamin B$_{12}$ deficiency with high doses of folate may worsen neurologic complications, although a hematologic response may occur.
- Folic acid deficiency: folic acid at 1 to 5 mg oral daily dose for at least 2 to 3 months; parenteral preparation also available if needed.
- Vitamin B$_{12}$ deficiency: acutely, daily doses of 25 to 100 mg IM; long-term, 200 to 1,000 mg monthly IM. Most patients with vitamin B$_{12}$ deficiency require lifelong treatment because most cases are as a result of abnormal absorption.

 Follow-Up

- The reticulocyte count should increase within the first 2 weeks of therapy, whereas the hemoglobin will take longer, in some cases months, to increase.
- If the hemoglobin fails to rise in 2 months, then other causes of anemia including iron deficiency and anemia of chronic disease should be considered.

PITFALLS

- Microcytic anemias such as iron deficiency, thalassemia, and anemia of chronic disease may obscure the diagnosis of megaloblastic anemias by falsely lowering the MCV; however, hypersegmented neutrophils should be present to aid in the correct diagnoses.
- Serum B$_{12}$ and folate rise rapidly after beginning supplements; therefore, diagnostic levels should be drawn prior to administration of supplements or normal diets.

 Common Questions and Answers

Q: What are common dietary sources of vitamin B$_{12}$?
A: Meat, eggs, and milk; liver contains the greatest amount of vitamin B$_{12}$.

Q: What are common dietary sources of folate?
A: Vegetables (primarily green, leafy vegetables), citrus fruits and berries, liver.

Q: Can food preparation destroy vitamin B$_{12}$ and folate?
A: Food preparation cannot destroy vitamin B$_{12}$, but excessive heating can destroy folate.

ICD-9-CM 281.9

BIBLIOGRAPHY

Oh RC, Brown DL. Vitamin B12 deficiency. *Am Fam Physician;* 67:979–986, 993–994.

Rosenblatt DS, Whitehead VM. Cobalamin and folate deficiency: acquired and hereditary disorders in children. *Semin Hematol* 1999;36:19–34.

Snow C. Laboratory diagnosis of vitamin B12 and folate deficiency: a guide for the primary care physician. *Arch Intern Med* 1999;159: 1289–1298.

Author: Kim Smith-Whitley

Meningitis

Database

DEFINITION

Meningitis is inflammation of the membranes of the brain or spinal cord usually caused by bacteria, viruses, fungi, and rarely parasites. It is almost always a result of hematogenous spread.

CAUSES

• Bacterial
—Bacteria causing meningitis differ depending on age:
—Less than 1 month: Group B streptococcus, *Escherichia coli*, other enteric, *Listeria monocytogenes*, *Streptococcus pneumoniae*
—1–3 months: Group B streptococcus, *E. coli*, *S. pneumoniae*, *Haemophilus influenzae* type b (almost disappearing secondary to immunization)
—3 months to 5 years: *S. pneumoniae*, *Neisseria meningitides*, *H. influenzae* type b
—Older than 5 years: *S. pneumoniae*, *N. meningitis*
• Viral
—Enteroviruses (EV): Approximately 70 different strains which include polioviruses, Coxsackie A, Coxsackie B, and echoviruses. Recently discovered EVs are not placed in the above four groups but simply numbered (e.g., enterovirus 68)
—Other less common: Arboviruses (e.g., West Nile virus), mumps, herpes simplex virus
• Fungal
—Fungi most commonly isolated include *Candida* spp, *Coccidioides immitis*, *Cryptococcus neoformans*, Aspergillus
• Aseptic meningitis
—Agents not easily cultured in the viral or microbiology laboratory can cause meningitis and include *Borrelia burgdorferi* (Lyme disease), *Treponema pallidum* (syphilis)
—Tuberculous meningitis

EPIDEMIOLOGY

• Bacterial meningitis
—Most bacterial meningitis (80%) occurs in patients younger than 24 months of age.
—*S. pneumoniae* isolates are becoming more resistant to penicillin. Currently, approximately 20% of isolates causing invasive disease are at least relatively resistant to penicillin.
• Viral meningitis
—85% are as a result of EVs that tend to occur in outbreaks in summer and early fall.
• Fungal meningitis
—*C. neoformans* is a budding encapsulated yeast-like organism found in soil and avian excreta. Although associated with meningitis in immunocompromised adults (especially those with AIDS), this is rare in children with AIDS. Thirty percent of patients with cryptococcal meningitis have no underlying immunodeficiency.
—Meningitis caused by Candida spp. occurs in ill premature infants and other immunocompromised individuals.

• Tuberculous meningitis

—The incidence of disease as a result of *Mycobacteria tuberculosis* (TB) is on the rise throughout the world.
—TB meningitis occurs in 1 of every 300 untreated primary TB infections.
—This is most commonly seen in children ages 6 months to 6 years.
—Meningitis will accompany miliary TB in approximately 50% of cases.
—Increasing number of patients suffer from multidrug resistant TB

COMPLICATIONS

• Bacterial meningitis

Acute Complications

—Syndrome of inappropriate ADH secretion (SIADH)
—Seizures occur in up to one-third of patients
—Focal neurologic signs occur in 10% to 15%.

Long-term Complications

—Mental retardation
—Hearing defects
• Viral meningitis
—SIADH in 10%

LONG-TERM COMPLICATIONS

—Complications from viral meningitis are rare. However, neonates (<1 month of age) may develop severe EV disease and older agammaglobulinemic children may develop chronic EV meningoencephalitis.
• Tuberculous meningitis

Acute Complications

—The most common are cranial nerve findings, especially 6th cranial nerve palsy affecting the eyes.
—Hydrocephalus

Long-term Complications

—Are many and include blindness, deafness, and mental retardation

PROGNOSIS

• Bacterial meningitis
—Approximately 500 to 1,000 deaths each year
—Hearing deficits and neurologic damage may occur in up to 25% of children.
• Viral meningitis
—Prognosis for enteroviral meningitis is quite good.
• Aseptic meningitis
—Lyme disease: prognosis with diagnosis and treatment is quite good (see Lyme Disease).
• Tuberculous meningitis
—The long-term prognosis in children with tuberculous meningitis depends on the stage of disease in which treatment is begun (for staging, see Data Gathering, History, and Physical Examination, below).
—Complete recovery occurs in 94% of those whose treatment was started in stage 1, but only 51% and 18% for those whose treatment began in stage II or stage III, respectively.

Data Gathering

HISTORY

Bacterial Meningitis

• Children older than 12 months of age will often complain of neck pain, headache, or back pain.
• Nausea and vomiting are commonly associated.
• In children younger than 12 months symptoms are often nonspecific. Common chief complaints by the infants' caregivers include:
—Irritable or "sleeping all the time"
—"Won't take to bottle"
—"Not acting right"
—"Cries when moved or picked up"
—"Won't stop crying"
—"Soft spot bulging out"
Other historical information that may affect management:

Question: Is the patient immunocompromised?
Significance: This makes unusual pathogen more likely.

Question: Recurrent meningitis?
Significance: Recurrent meningitis with *S. pneumoniae* or *Enterococcus* may indicate a skull fracture or cribriform plate fracture with contamination of the cerebral spinal fluid (CSF) by nasopharyngeal secretions.

Viral Meningitis

Question: Early symptoms
Significance: Headache and fever may precede signs of meningitis such as stiff neck, vomiting, photophobia.

Question: Duration
Significance: The illness lasts 2 to 6 days.

Fungal Meningitis

Question: Symptoms
Significance: Cryptococcal meningitis is often indolent with complaints of worsening headaches and vomiting for days to weeks.

Question: Exposure
Significance: Exposure to pigeon droppings or other bird droppings can be a valuable clue to etiology if present.

Tuberculous Meningitis

• Symptoms often are nonspecific initially with personality changes, fever, nausea, and vomiting progressing to anorexia, irritability, and lethargy (stage I disease).
• Stage II disease is characterized by focal neurologic signs (most often involving the cranial nerves, III, VI, VII).
• Stage III disease is characterized by coma and papilledema.

Physical Examination

• Stiff neck in older children but not infants with poor neck muscle tone

- Brudzinski and Kernig signs may be present. Brudzinski sign: flexion of the neck elicits involuntary flexion of the hips. Kernig sign: while legs are flexed 90° at the hip, extension of the lower legs are unable to be accomplished beyond 135°.
- Children younger than 12 months may not have nuchal rigidity, Kernig and/or Brudzinski signs.
- Classically, there may be "paradoxical" crying, crying increases when child is picked up.
- Tache cerebri—flaring of skin when stroked.

Laboratory Aids

Test: Lumbar puncture with analysis of the CSF
Significance: Depending on the presentation, age, history, and physical examination, some or all of the following tests should be requested for CSF analysis.
- Opening pressure: normal is less than 200 mm H_2O in lateral recumbent position.
- Cell count and differential
- Glucose: To be compared with the serum glucose; normal is more than 40 mg/dL or one half to two thirds of the serum glucose.
- Protein: Normal 5 to 40 mg/dL except in newborns who may have protein levels of 150 to 200 mg/dL.
- Cultures: For bacteria, fungi, viruses, and mycobacteria. Approximately 80% of blood cultures are positive in children with bacterial meningitis.
Test: PCR
Significance: TB, HSV, EV, *Borrelia burgdorferi*
Test: Antibody studies
Significance: Lyme disease
Test: Other laboratory studies
CBC: platelet count, PT/PTT, electrolytes, BUN, creatinine, glucose, liver function tests, arterial blood gas
- Blood culture

Therapy

- Assure adequate ventilation and cardiac function (ABCs).
- Initiate hemodynamic monitoring and support by achieving venous access and treat shock syndrome, if present.
- Monitor serum sodium concentrations because SIADH is a frequent complication during the first 3 days of treatment.
- Glucose should be given intravenously if <50 mg/dL at a dose of 0.25 to 1 g/kg.
- Acidosis should be corrected if pH is less than 7.2 with 1 to 2 mEq/kg of sodium bicarbonate.
- Coagulopathy should be treated with platelet concentrates (0.2 units per kg) if platelets are less than 50,000/mm³ and fresh frozen plasma (10 mL/kg) if PT/PTT is prolonged.
- Steroids should be used in the initial therapy of TB meningitis along with antituberculosis medication. Use in children with bacterial meningitis is controversial.

Bacterial Meningitis

- Antimicrobial agents
—Less than 1 month: Ampicillin IV 200 mg/kg per day divided q12 hours if < 7 days of age or 300 mg/kg per day divided q8 hours if >7 days of age, and cefotaxime IV 180 mg/kg per day divided q6 hours.
—Greater than 1 month: Vancomycin IV 60 mg/kg per day divided q6 hours; and cefotaxime IV 300 mg/kg per day divided q6 hours or ceftriaxone 100 mg/kg/day divided q12 hours (should not be used in infants less than 2 months of age)
- Note: In children less than 1 month of age, if gram stain or culture reveals gram positive cocci ampicillin should be changed to vancomycin for possible resistant *S. pneumoniae*.

Fungal Meningitis

- Amphotericin B ± 5-flucytosine depending on the type of fungi isolated.

Tuberculous Meningitis

- Treatment is generally with four drugs for 2 months followed by two drugs for 10 months.
- Initially, treatment can start with isoniazid, rifampin, pyrazinamide, and streptomycin.

Viral Meningitis

- Enterovirus: no specific therapy other than supportive
- HSV: Acyclovir 60 mg/kg per day divided q8 hours

PREVENTION

- *H. influenzae* type b (HIB) vaccine has significantly reduced the incidence of meningitis and other invasive HIB infections.
- A seven-valent streptococcus pneumoniae protein conjugate vaccine (PCV 7) has shown greater than 90% efficacy in preventing invasive diagnosis and is recommended for use in all infants given at 2, 4, 6, and 12 to 15 months of age.

Follow-Up

- Most children with bacterial meningitis become afebrile by 7 to 10 days after starting therapy with gradual improvement in activity with less irritability.
- Evaluation for neurologic sequelae, such as hearing and vision testing, is essential.
- Prophylaxis in *H. influenza* type b: Rifampin (20 mg/kg per dose, maximum 600 mg once daily for 4 days) should be given to all household contacts if one member is less than 4 years old and is unvaccinated (for family and for patient before discharge unless received).
- Prophylaxis in *N. meningitidis*: Rifampin (10 mg/kg per dose, maximum 600 mg twice daily for 2 day) should be given to all household contacts, day-care contacts, and other persons with close contact 7 days prior to onset of illness.
- Note: If cefotaxime or ceftriaxone was used for treatment, the patient with *N. meningitidis* or *H. influenza* type b meningitis does not need to receive prophylaxis.

PITFALLS

- If no etiology is discovered after the first lumbar puncture and the child is not responding to therapy, then a repeat lumbar puncture should be performed at 36 to 48 hours.
- Remember that in tuberculous meningitis, up to 50% of children will not react to the five tuberculin unit Mantoux tests. Therapy should be started if suspicious; do not rely on the skin testing.
- Be aware that the isolation of resistant strains of *S. pneumoniae* is increasing; therefore, antibiotics such as vancomycin and cefotaxime or ceftriaxone should be used until antibiotic sensitivity data are available.

Common Questions and Answers

Q: Is a lumbar puncture required before starting antibiotics in the patient with suspected meningitis with unstable vital signs requiring resuscitation?
A: No. In the unstable patient it is contraindicated to perform a lumbar puncture. Appropriate intravenous antibiotic should be started. When resuscitated, a lumbar puncture should be performed.

ICD-9-CM 322.9

BIBLIOGRAPHY

Agarwal R, Emmerson AJ. Should repeat lumbar punctures be routinely done in neonates with bacterial meningitis? Results of a survey into clinical practice. *Arch Dis Child* 2001;84(5):451–452.

Arditi M, Mason EO, Bradley JS, et al. Three-year multicenter surveillance of pneumococcal meningitis in children: clinical characteristics, and outcome related to penicillin susceptibility and dexamethasone use. *Pediatrics* 1998;102(5):1087–1097.

El Bashir H, Laundy M, Booy R. Diagnosis and treatment of bacterial meningitis. *Arch Dis Child* 2003;88(7):615–620.

Hoffman JA, Mason EO, Schutze GE, et al. *Streptococcus pneumoniae* infections in the neonate. *Pediatrics* 2003;112(5):1095–1102.

Lebel MH, Freij BJ, Syrogiannopoulos GA, et al. Dexamethasone therapy for bacterial meningitis: results of two double-blind, placebo-controlled trials. *N Engl J Med* 1988;319(15):964–971.

Saez-Llorens X, McCracken GH. Bacterial meningitis in children. *Lancet* 2003;361: 2139–2148.

Stark JR, Smith KC. Tuberculosis. In: Feigin RD, Cherry JD, Demmler GJ, Kaplan SL, eds. *Textbook of Pediatric Infectious Diseases.* 4th Ed. Philadelphia: WB Saunders, 2004:1337–1370.

van de Beek D, de Gans J, McIntyre P, Prasad K. Corticosteroids in acute bacterial meningitis. *Cochrane Database Syst Rev* 2003;(3):CD004305.

Authors: Jason Newland and Louis M. Bell

Meningococcemia

Database

DEFINITION

• Meningococcemia is a systemic infection with the bacterium *Neisseria meningitidis*, a gram-negative diplococcus that is relatively fastidious. Despite treatment with appropriate antibiotics, this disease may have a fulminant course with a high likelihood of mortality.
• Thirteen serogroups have been described on the basis of capsular polysaccharide antigens; serotypes B, C and Y account for most of the cases in the United States. Serogroup Y accounted for 30% of cases between 1996 to 1998.

PATHOPHYSIOLOGY

• Colonization and infection of the upper respiratory tract occurs after inhalation of, or direct contact with, the organism, usually in oral secretions.
• Disseminated disease occurs when the organism penetrates the nasal mucosa and enters the bloodstream, in which it replicates itself.
• Fulminant disease is signified by diffuse microvascular damage and disseminated intravascular coagulation (see Septic Shock).
• Death results from effects of endotoxic shock including circulatory collapse and myocardial dysfunction.
• Bacteremia without sepsis presents with fever, malaise, myalgias, and headache. Patients may clear the infection spontaneously, or it may invade meninges, joints, lungs, and so on.
• Meningococcemia without meningitis occurs after initial bacteremia with systemic sepsis. A rash erupts, which may be nonspecific maculopapular, morbilliform, or urticarial. Progression to petechiae or purpura signifies evolution of disease.
• Fulminant disease is signified by hypotension, oliguria, disseminated intravascular coagulation (DIC), myocardial dysfunction, and vascular collapse. Death occurs in approximately 20% of these patients.

GENETICS

Inherited deficiency of terminal complement may be found in 5% to 10% of patients during epidemics. The frequency increases to 30% in patients with recurrent disease.

EPIDEMIOLOGY

• The rates of meningococcal disease in the United States have remained stable at 0.9 to 1.5 cases per 100,000 population per year.
• Patients with deficiency of a terminal complement component (C5–9), asplenia, or properdin deficiency are at increased risk for invasive and recurrent disease.
• Children younger than age 5 years are most often affected, with peak incidence between 3 and 5 months.
• During epidemics, more school-aged children may be affected.
• The disease occurs most commonly in winter and spring months.
• Increased disease activity may follow an influenza A outbreak.

COMPLICATIONS

• Complications may result directly from the infection or be classified as allergic immune complex mediated.
• Meningococcemia may be complicated by myocarditis, arthritis, hemorrhage, and pneumonia.
• Meningococcal meningitis is most commonly complicated by deafness in 5% to 10% of survivors.
• Other complications of meningitis include seizures, subdural effusions, and cranial nerve palsies.
• Allergic complications include arthritis, vasculitis, pericarditis, and episcleritis.

PROGNOSIS

• Fatality rate of meningococcemia is 20%, even when recognized and treated.
• Fatality rate of meningococcal meningitis is 5%. The most severe cases often have a rapid progression from onset of symptoms to death over a matter of hours. At the time of hospital admission, the following signs predict poor survival:

—Lack of meningitis
—Shock
—Coma
—Purpura
—Neutropenia
—Thrombocytopenia
—DIC
—Myocarditis

Differential Diagnosis

• Meningitis as a result of *N. meningitidis* is indistinguishable from that of other causes, except for one-third of children who have a petechial rash.
• Sepsis from other microbial causes may appear identically, including the petechiae or purpuric rash.

Data Gathering

HISTORY

Time of onset of fever, malaise, and rash?

Physical Examination

• Recognition of abnormal vital signs and lethargy is necessary.
• Careful examination of the skin for petechiae is important.
• Nuchal rigidity, lethargy, and irritability should be carefully evaluated.

Laboratory Aids

The organism can be cultured from blood, cerebral spinal fluid (CSF), and skin lesions.

Test: Gram stain of CSF or scraped petechia (pressed against a glass slide)
Significance: Revealing gram-negative diplococci will give a presumptive diagnosis.

Test: Rapid test for antigen detection
Significance: Best found in CSF but not sensitive for serogroup B.

 ## Therapy

- Patients with acute onset of petechial rash and fever should receive a prompt initial dose of antibiotics (preferably after blood culture)
- Close monitoring of vital signs and clinical status should follow, preferably in an ICU setting.
- Cefotaxime or ceftriaxone can be initiated as presumptive therapy. Once sensitivity is confirmed, penicillin is preferred.
- After isolate is proven to be sensitive to penicillin, treatment of choice is aqueous penicillin G IV at a dose of 300,000 IU/kg per day every 4 to 6 hours for 5 to 7 days.
- In penicillin-allergic patients, third-generation cephalosporins or chloramphenicol are acceptable alternatives.

 ## Follow-Up

Patients with bacterial meningitis should have hearing test as a follow-up.

PREVENTION

- Isolation of the hospitalized patient.
- Hospitalized patients require respiratory isolation until 24 hours after appropriate antibiotic therapy.

CONTROL MEASURES

- Exposed contacts, including household, day care, and nursery school, should receive rifampin, 10 mg/kg (maximum 600 mg) every 12 hours for four doses. Those contacts less than 1 month should receive 5 mg/kg, orally every 12 hours for four doses.
- Ceftriaxone administered intramuscularly is effective prophylaxis for those contacts less than or equal to 15 years a single dose of 125 mg IM is recommended. For those contacts over 15 years 250 mg IM is recommended. Its safety profile is preferred for pregnant women.
- Medical personnel should receive prophylaxis only if they had close contact with respiratory secretions.
- Vaccines for types A, C, Y, W-135 are available and produce an immune response in 10 to 14 days. The Advisory Committee on Immunization Practices and the American Academy of Pediatrics (AAP) recommend that vaccine be considered for students entering their freshman year of college.

PITFALLS

- Public health officials should be notified of *N. meningitidis* cases.
- Physical examination of a child with fever should include careful evaluation of the skin for petechiae and signs of early shock (tachycardia, delayed capillary refill, abnormal mental status, etc.).

 ## Common Questions and Answers

Q: How long should antibiotic therapy be given in a patient with septic shock?
A: 7 days.

Q: When is meningococcal vaccine indicated?
A: In asplenic, or functionally asplenic patients, in patients with terminal complement deficiency, and in epidemics in conjunction with chemoprophylaxis.

Q: When should one test for complement deficiency?
A: In patients with recurrent disease.

Q: Which hospital personnel should receive prophylaxis?
A: Only those with close contact with secretions.

ICD-9-CM 036.2

BIBLIOGRAPHY

American Academy of Pediatrics. Meningococcal infections. In: Pickering LK, ed. *2003 Red Book: Report of the Committee on Infectious Diseases.* 26th Ed. Elk Grove Village, IL: American Academy of Pediatrics, 2003:396–401.

Apicella MA. *Neisseria meningitidis.* In: Mandell GL, Douglas GR, Bennet JE, eds. *Principles and Practice of Infectious Diseases.* 3rd Ed. New York: Churchill Livingstone, 1990:1600–1613.

Baker CJ, Edwards MS. Meningococcemia. In: Oski FA, ed. *Principles and Practice of Pediatrics.* Philadelphia: JB Lippincott, 1990:1097–1101.

Beaty HN. Meningococcemia. In: Fauci A, Braunwald E, Isselbacher KJ, eds. *Harrison's Principles of Internal Medicine.* New York: McGraw-Hill, 1998:574–576.

Glode MP, Smith AL. Meningococcemia. In: Feigin RD, Cherry JD, eds. *Textbook of Pediatric Infectious Diseases.* Philadelphia: WB Saunders, 1997:1211–1224.

Gupta S, Tuladhar AB. Does early administration of dexamethasone improve neurological outcome in children with meningococcal meningitis? *Arch Dis Child* 2004;89(1):82–83.

Pathan N, Faust SN, Levin M. Pathophysiology of meningococcal meningitis and septicaemia. *Arch Dis Child* 2003;88(7):601–607.

Rosenstein NE, Perkins BA, Stephens DS, Popovic T, Hughes JM. Medical progress: Meningococcal disease. *N Engl J Med* 2001;344:1378–1388.

Welch SB, Nadel S. Treatment of meningococcal infection. *Arch Dis Child* 2003;88(7):608–614.

Author: Louis M. Bell

Mental Retardation

Database

DEFINITION

- Mental retardation essentially means slow rate of learning or slow cognitive processing abilities. By definition there are significant cognitive and adaptive delays first evident in childhood. Significant cognitive delays are defined as two standard deviations below the population mean on a standard cognitive or IQ test.
- This usually indicates an IQ score of less than 70 to 75.
- Adaptive skills are the functional skills of everyday life, including communication, social skills, daily living/self care skills, and the ability to safely move about the home and community.
- Mental retardation is typically subdivided into mild, moderate, severe, and profound categories depending on the severity of the delays. A more recent definition by the American Association on Mental Retardation (AAMR) puts more emphasis on the level of functioning and amount of supports required of an individual.

CAUSES

- The cause of the mental retardation is usually an insult to the brain or abnormal development of the central nervous system. The exact pathophysiology may differ depending on the etiology, which can include:

—Genetic
—Familial
—Metabolic
—Endocrinological
—Infectious
—Environmental toxins
—Traumatic
—Anatomic brain malformation
—The etiology is not evident in many cases of mental retardation.

EPIDEMIOLOGY

- Prevalence of mental retardation is generally listed as 2% to 3% of the population.
- It is found in both sexes and all racial and socioeconomic groups.
- Of the different subcategories of mental retardation, the mild form is the most prevalent at 85% of the mental retardation population.
- Profound mental retardation is least prevalent at about 1% of this group.
- Associated findings are more common in the more sever forms of mental retardation.
- The prognosis for longevity varies with the associated findings and overall health, but individuals with mental retardation can live to adulthood and old age. An individual's level of functioning is variable depending on the level of retardation, special individual skills and family or community supports. In general the following applies:

—Mild mental retardation (IQ 55 to 70): Formerly called educable. May be in school with extra help and may achieve roughly a fourth grade level in reading and math. May be employed in an unskilled to semiskilled job. May live in a group home or independently. Some marry.
—Moderate mental retardation (IQ 40 to 54): May learn to recognize basic words and learn basic skills. May work in a sheltered workshop or with supported employment in an unskilled job. May live with family or in a group home doing much of their own care.
—Severe mental retardation (IQ 25 to 39): May live with family, or in a group home or institution. Some may be in a sheltered workshop. May be able to do some daily self-care or chores with supervision.
—Profound Mental Retardation (IQ <25): Live with family, group home or institution. Usually require full care.

Mental retardation has many associated findings including, seizures, autism, cerebral palsy, communication disorders, failure to thrive, sensory impairments, and psychiatric disorders. Behavioral disorders also can be seen including attention deficit hyperactivity disorder, self-injurious and self-stimulating behaviors. Families often face additional stressors when caring for a child with mental retardation.

Differential Diagnosis

The differential can include several other developmental diagnoses, including:

- Borderline cognitive abilities
- Developmental language disorder
- Autism
- Learning disability
- Cerebral palsy
- Significant visual or hearing impairment
- Degenerative disorders

Specific etiologies are too numerous to list completely but a partial list of the more common causes would include:

- Genetic/familial

—Fragile X syndrome
—Trisomy 21 (Down syndrome)
—Other chromosomal abnormalities
—Tuberous sclerosis
—Neurofibromatosis
—PKU (Phenylketonuria)
—Other inborn errors of metabolism

- Nervous system anomalies

—Hydrocephalus
—Lissencephaly
—Seizures

- Infections

—Prenatal cytomegalovirus, rubella, toxoplasmosis, HIV
—Postnatal bacterial meningitis, neonatal herpes simplex

- Endocrinologic

—Congenital hypothyroidism

- Environmental

—Heavy metal poisoning such as lead
—In utero drug or alcohol exposure, including fetal alcohol syndrome

- Trauma/injury

—Closed head trauma
—Asphyxia

Data Gathering

HISTORY

A complete and detailed history is needed including:

Question: Pregnancy history?
Significance:

- Maternal age and parity
- Maternal complications (including infections and exposures)
- Medications/drugs used
- Tobacco or alcohol used, along with quantities
- Fetal activity

Question: Birth history?
Significance:

- Gestational age
- Birth weight
- Route of delivery
- Maternal or fetal complications/distress
- APGAR scores

Question: General health?
Significance:

- Significant illnesses, hospitalizations, or surgeries
- Accidents or injuries
- Hearing and vision status
- Medications used
- Known exposures to toxins
- Any new or unusual symptoms

Question: Developmental history?
Significance:

- Current developmental achievement in each stream of development
- Age when developmental milestones were achieved
- Any loss of skills
- Where parents think their child is functioning developmentally

Question: Educational history?
Significance:

- Type of schooling and services received, if any
- Any previous educational/developmental testing

Question: Behavioral history?
Significance:

- Any perseverative or stereotypical behaviors
- Interaction skills
- Attention and activity level

Question: Family history?
Significance: Anyone with developmental delays, neurologic disorders, syndromes, inherited disorders, or consanguinity

Physical Examination

A complete physical examination including growth perimeters is needed looking for etiology. Key features to include are:

Finding: Observation of interactions and behavior
Significance: Any atypical behaviors and general impressions

Finding: Head circumference
Significance: Looking for macro or microcephaly

Finding: Skin examination
Significance: Looking for neurocutaneous lesions

Finding: Major or minor dysmorphic features
Significance: Any indication of a syndrome or anatomic malformation

Finding: Neurologic examination
Significance: Looking for cranial nerve deficits, neuromuscular status, reflexes, balance and coordination, and any soft signs

DEVELOPMENTAL TESTING

When developmental delays are present and mental retardation is suspected, more formal developmental screening or testing should be done. Possible testing for the pediatrician would be the Denver Developmental Screening Test or the CAT/CLAMS. The diagnoses needs to be made on standardized tests, usually done by a clinical psychologist. Such standardized testing might involve the Stanford Binet Intelligence Scale, the Wechsler scales, and the Vineland Adaptive Behavior Scales. A referral to a clinical psychologist for the formal diagnosis is indicted.

Laboratory Tests

There is no specific laboratory test battery for mental retardation. The testing needs to be tailored to the individual situation based on the history and physical examination. A high index of suspicion should be maintained for any associated findings and delays in the other streams of development. Listed below are some of the more common studies ordered for mental retardation work up.

Test: Audiologic testing
Significance: Hearing should be checked in any child with speech and language and/or cognitive delays.

Test: Genetic testing
Significance: Warranted for any dysmorphic features, a family history of delays or genetic disorder. A karyotype and Fragile X DNA should be considered particularly for significant cognitive delays.

Test: Metabolic tests
Significance: Tests such as quantitative plasma amino acids, quantitative urine organic acids, lactate, pyruvate or ammonia should be considered if there is any loss of skills or indication of a metabolic disorder. More specific metabolic tests may be indicated depending on symptoms.

Test: Thyroid function tests
Significance: Most infants will have had screening for hypothyroidism shortly after birth. This should be rechecked if symptoms indicate.

Test: Electroencephalogram
Significance: An EEG should be considered if there is any concern about seizures.

Test: Head MRI
Significance: Consider a head MRI for head abnormalities, significant neurological findings, loss of skills, or for work up of a specific disorder such as trauma or leukodystrophy.

Test: Subspecialists
Significance: Referral to other medical specialists may also be indicated. These specialists may include developmental pediatrics, neurology, genetics, or ophthalmology.

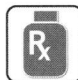

Therapy

There is no specific cure for mental retardation. Therapy should consist of appropriate treatment for any underlying or associated medical condition. Early intervention and special education programs are available for an individualized education program based on the child's needs and abilities. Behavior management programs or selected use of medications is available for patients with severe behavioral problems. The ultimate goal of all therapies is to help the child reach his/her full potential.

Follow-Up

Children with mental retardation will need regular pediatric preventative care in addition to management of any underlying medical conditions. Ongoing monitoring of the educational programs, to ensure that it is still meeting the child's needs, is important. The family will also need ongoing counseling and support in dealing with a child having special needs.

PREVENTION

There is no specific prevention for mental retardation, but prevention of some underlying causes may be possible. Immunization programs and early detection of metabolic disorders as well as education programs for head injury/asphyxia prevention may be useful in some cases. Avoidance of alcohol and some drugs during pregnancy may also decrease some brain insults.

PITFALLS

- Children with behavioral problems may also be masking cognitive delays.
- Hearing impairment may present as a delay in development

- Children with mild mental retardation may not be picked up until they are having difficulties keeping up in elementary school.

Common Questions and Answers

Q: Will my child be "normal" by adulthood?
A: Generally, mental retardation is considered a lifelong condition. Some individuals, usually with the milder form of mental retardation, can function well in the community, especially when given added supports.

Q: Can my child learn?
A: Except for the severest forms of mental retardation, children do learn. This learning may not be as rapid or as extensive as that of a typically developing child.

Q: But my child looks fine and has had appropriate motor development. How can he/she be mentally retarded?
A: Mental retardation is a slowed rate of cognitive development. Many children with mental retardation do not have obvious dysmorphic features. Other streams of development, such as gross motor skills, may be reached on time or nearly so, yet the cognitive developmental streams can be significantly delayed.

ICD-9-CM NUMBER

Mild mental retardation 317
Moderate mental retardation 318.0
Severe mental retardation 318.1
Profound mental retardation 318.2
Unspecified mental retardation 319

BIBLIOGRAPHY

American Psychiatric Association. *Diagnostic and Statistical Manual of Mental Disorders.* 4th Ed. Washington, DC: Author, 1994.

Batshaw ML. Mental retardation. *Pediatr Clin North Am* 1993;40:507–521.

Battaglia A, Carey JC. Diagnostic evaluation of developmental delay/mental retardation: an overview. *Am J Med Genet* 2003;117(1):3–14.

Finucane B, Haas-Givler B, Simon EW. Genetics, mental retardation, and the forging of new alliances. *Am J Med Genet* 2003;117C(1):66–72.

Gilbride KE. Developmental testing. *Pediatr Rev* 1995;16:338–345.

Palmer FB, Capute AJ. Mental retardation. *Pediatr Rev* 1994;15:473–479.

Xu J, Chen Z. Advances in molecular cytogenetics for the evaluation of mental retardation. *Am J Med Genet* 2003;117C(1):15–24.

Author: Rita Panoscha

Mesenteric Adenitis

 Database

DEFINITION

Inflammation of the mesenteric lymph nodes that causes enlargement of the nodes

CAUSES

• Infection

—Viral: echovirus 1 and 14, Coxsackie B1 and B5, mononucleosis (EBV, CMV)
—Bacterial: Tuberculosis, Streptococcus, *Yersinia enterocolitica*
—Inflammation or hypersensitivity reaction to a foreign protein

PATHOPHYSIOLOGY

• Lymph nodes involved are those draining the ileocecal area.
• Absorption of toxic products or bacterial products secondary to stasis
• Nodes are enlarged, discrete, soft, and pink, and with time become firm. Calcification and suppuration are rare.
• Cultures of the nodes are negative.
• Reactive hyperplasia: the adenitis results from a reaction to some material absorbed from the small intestine, reaching the intestine from the blood or lymphatic system.
• Hypersensitivity reaction to a foreign protein

EPIDEMIOLOGY

• Age-related, most common in patients <18 years of age
• Previous history of recent sore throat or upper respiratory tract infection found in 20% to 30% of subjects
• Most common cause of acute abdominal pain in young adults and children
• Self-limiting condition
• Can be diagnosed accurately at laparotomy but imaging is sufficient
• True incidence is not known
• Most common cause of inflammatory adenopathy, more common than tuberculosis.
• Can mimic acute appendicitis.

COMPLICATIONS

• Suppuration
• Rupture of lymph nodes
• Peritonitis
• Abscess formation

 Differential Diagnosis

• Infection:

—Acute appendicitis: 20% of patients treated for possible acute appendicitis had mesenteric adenitis.
—Infectious mononucleosis: Associated lymphadenopathy more generalized. Associated splenomegaly; can screen for positive mono or EBV titers.
—Tuberculosis: Associated intestinal involvement, positive PPD, elevated ESR.
—Pelvic inflammatory disease: A consideration in sexually active adolescents; vaginal examination useful
—Urinary tract infections: Urinalysis is helpful.
—Abscess: Related to missed acute appendicitis, IBD
—*Yersinia enterocolitica* infection: Bloody diarrhea, arthropathy present; stool culture is diagnostic
—Typhlitis: Transmural inflammation of the cecum seen in patients with neutropenia and chemotherapy.

• Tumors: Lymphoma; can get more generalized adenopathy; CT scan of the abdomen and/or laparotomy to confirm the diagnosis
• Trauma: Hematomas of the abdominal wall and intestines; history of trauma will be present.
• Metabolic: Acute intermittent porphyria; cyclical episodes of acute abdominal pain and vomiting; appropriate metabolic workup diagnostic
• Congenital: Duplication cysts; may present with abdominal pain as a result of rupture, bleeding, intussusception, or volvulus
• Miscellaneous:

—Crohn disease: Associated mesenteric adenitis and intestinal involvement
—Intussusception: Acute abdominal pain with currant jelly stools; barium/air enema is diagnostic and therapeutic
—Ovarian cysts: May need abdominal/pelvic ultrasound to differentiate between the two

 Data Gathering

HISTORY

Question: Abdominal pain?
Significance: Ache to severe colic; is the first symptom, as a result of stretch on the mesentery.

Question: Location of pain?
Significance: May initially be in the upper abdomen/right lower quadrant (RLQ) or generalized. If generalized, eventually becomes localized to RLQ. An important point is that the patient cannot localize the exact point of the most intense pain, unlike appendicitis.

Question: Spasms?
Significance: Between spasms the patient feels well and can walk without any difficulty. One-third of patients have nausea and vomiting.

• Anorexia and fatigue are uncommon.

 Physical Examination

• Patient flushed: Early in the attack fever may be 38°C to 38.5°C.
• May have an associated URI symptoms: rhinorrhea or acute pharyngitis.
• Approximately 20% of patients will have cervical adenopathy.
• Abdominal examination shows tenderness of the RLQ: It may be a little higher, more medial, and less severe than acute appendicitis.
• Point of maximal tenderness may vary from one examination to the next.
• Diffuse or periumbilical tenderness without rigidity.
• Voluntary guarding and rebound tenderness occasional

Laboratory Aids

Test: CBC
Significance: One-half of the patients may have WBC counts over 10,000.

IMAGING

Test: Abdominal ultrasound
Significance: Will differentiate between acute appendicitis, pelvic inflammatory disease, ovarian pathology, and mesenteric adenitis.

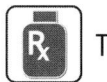 Therapy

Mainly supportive

 Follow-Up

WHEN TO EXPECT IMPROVEMENT

Acute symptoms may take days to resolve and generally last a few days after the associated viral symptoms have resolved.

SIGNS TO WATCH FOR

- Increasing abdominal pain
- Vomiting
- Fevers
- Toxic appearance
- Severe tenderness that is persistent
- Guarding
- Rigidity
- Decreasing bowel sounds

PROGNOSIS

Most patients recover completely without any specific treatment. Death is very unusual and may occur only when secondary specific bacterial infection occurs with suppuration, and rupture of the nodes with resulting abscess and peritonitis.

PITFALLS

Can be difficult to differentiate from acute appendicitis clinically, and many patients may have a laparotomy before the right diagnosis is made.

 Common Questions and Answers

Q: Can one clinically differentiate between acute appendicitis and nonspecific mesenteric adenitis?
A: Patients with nonspecific mesenteric adenitis cannot localize the exact point of the most intense pain, unlike appendicitis. Between spasms patients with nonspecific mesenteric adenitis feel well and can walk without any difficulty. Abdominal examination shows tenderness of the RLQ that is a little higher, more medial, and less severe than in acute appendicitis. Point of maximal tenderness may vary between examinations in patients with nonspecific mesenteric adenitis. There is no rigidity on abdominal examination in patients with nonspecific mesenteric adenitis. However, it is clinically difficult to differentiate the two.

Q: What are the two investigations that can be diagnostic for RLQ pain?
A: An ultrasound of the RLQ can differentiate between acute appendicitis, ovarian pathology, and lymphadenopathy. An upper GI with small bowel follow-through series can be diagnostic for inflammatory bowel disease.

ICD-9-CM 089.2

BIBLIOGRAPHY

Adams JT. Abdominal wall, omentum, mesentery and retroperitoneum. In: Schwartz SI, Shires GT, Spencer FC, eds. *Principles of Surgery.* New York: McGraw-Hill, 1989: 1491–1524.

Bell TM, Steyn JH. Viruses in lymph nodes of children with mesenteric adenitis and intussusception. *Br Med J* 1962;2:700–702.

Black RE, Slome S. *Yersinia enterocolitica. Infect Dis Clin North Am* 1988;2(3):625–641.

Cherry JD. Enteroviruses: poliovirus, Coxsackie virus, echovirus and enterovirus. In: Feigin RD, Cherry JD, eds. *Textbook of Pediatric Infectious Diseases,* vol 2. 3rd Ed. Philadelphia: WB Saunders, 1997;157: 1705–1752.

Macari M, Balthazar EJ. The acute right lower quadrant: CT evaluation. *Radiol Clin North Am* 2003;41(6):1117–1136.

Swischuk LE. Periumbilical pain and fever. *Pediatr Emerg Care* 1998;14(2):159–160.

Zeiter DK, Hyams JS. Recurrent abdominal pain in children. *Pediatr Clin N Am* 2002; 49(1):53–71.

Author: Dror Wasserman

Metabolic Diseases in Acidotic Newborns

 Database

DEFINITION

Inborn errors of metabolism (IEMs) are inherited defects in biochemical pathways affecting fats, amino acids or carbohydrates. In general, they affect the conversion of fuel to energy. Some IEMs present with catastrophic neonatal metabolic acidosis. Because these conditions are life threatening if not treated promptly, a high degree of suspicion is essential. In the newborn period, the immediate goals should be to:

1. Establish a tentative diagnosis
2. Initiate presumptive management
3. Send confirmatory studies
4. Involve a team trained in treating patients with inborn errors of metabolism.

PATHOPHYSIOLOGY

- IEMs presenting with metabolic acidosis usually produce an elevated anion gap as a result of accumulation of an acidic intermediate. Identification of this acid is the first step in establishing the diagnosis.
- Tissue dysfunction results from (a) toxicity of the accumulated byproduct, and/or (b) failure to produce sufficient energy to meet cellular needs.
- CNS toxicity results in increased intracranial pressure, emesis, lethargy, coma, seizures, abnormalities in muscle tone
- Hepatic toxicity causes jaundice, failure to thrive, hypoglycemia, hyperammonemia, coagulopathy
- Other organ systems may be involved, depending on the disease. These include the heart, the proximal renal tubule, the pancreas and the bone marrow.

GENETICS

Generally autosomal recessive. Exceptions include pyruvate dehydrogenase deficiency (a form of lactic acidosis, usually X-linked) and diseases of the mitochondrial genome (maternally inherited).

COMPLICATIONS

- Failure to treat patients promptly can be fatal or result in severe CNS insult and developmental disability. The basal ganglia are particularly susceptible to a variety of metabolic disturbances and damage to these structures can cause "metabolic stroke."
- For many IEMs, recurrent episodes of acidosis, triggered by stress, intercurrent illness or dietary noncompliance, are a major source of morbidity.
- Long-term effects may include progressive tissue dysfunction (e.g., liver or renal failure, cardiomyopathy) or failure to thrive.

 Differential Diagnosis

In neonates, many different IEMs present with similar symptoms, which can easily be confused with other serious diseases.

1. Differential diagnosis in sick, acidotic neonate:

   - Sepsis
   - Congenital heart disease
   - Toxin/drug exposure
   - Perinatal depression
   - IEM

2. Categories of IEM presenting with neonatal acidosis.

- Lactic acidosis

—Pyruvate dehydrogenase deficiency
—Pyruvate carboxylase deficiency
—Phosphoenolpyruvate carboxykinase deficiency
—Defects in tricarboxylic acid cycle enzymes
—Mitochondrial diseases or other conditions affecting oxidative phosphorylation (OXPHOS)
—Severe disorders of gluconeogenesis (e.g., glucose-6-phosphatase deficiency)
—Multiple carboxylase deficiency, biotinidase deficiency
—Disorders of fatty acid oxidation

- Ketoacidosis

—Disorders of ketone utilization (e.g., β-ketothiolase deficiency)
—Ketosis occurs in many disorders that also cause accumulation of lactate (see Lactic Acidosis above) or other organic acids

- Other organic acids

—Maple syrup urine disease
—Branched chain organic acidurias (methylmalonic acidemia, propionic acidemia, isovaleric acidemia) many others. Note that in some cases, other abnormalities (e.g., lethargy, hyperammonemia) may occur prior to severe acidosis.

 Data Gathering

HISTORY

Question: Were there complications with the pregnancy?
Significance: Some IEMs, particularly certain disorders of fatty acid oxidation, are associated with fatty liver of pregnancy or the HELLP (hypertension, elevated liver enzymes, low platelets) syndrome.

Question: What is the current diet and feeding schedule? Does the baby wake spontaneously to feed?
Significance: In many IEMs, acidotic episodes are triggered by specific exposures, or else by prolonged fasting, including relatively short delays "to let the baby sleep longer." In addition, diets low in protein content may delay the onset of symptoms in disorders of amino acid metabolism.

Question: What is the family history?
Significance: Because IEMs are genetic disorders, there may be a family history of poorly explained pediatric death. Diagnoses to inquire about include sepsis (was an organism identified?), sudden infant death syndrome, cardiomyopathy, uncontrollable seizures, coma and liver failure. Unexplained developmental delay or hypoglycemia in older siblings can provide useful clues.

Question: Have the parents noticed any unusual odors?
Significance: Some organic acids are associated with specific odors (see Physical Exam).

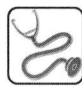 Physical Examination

- ABCs and vital signs. Cushing's triad (apnea, bradycardia, hypertension) should prompt immediate evaluation for elevated intracranial pressure. Are there signs of dehydration?
- Skin: Jaundice as a result of liver toxicity occurs in many neonates with IEMs. Rashes are associated with biotinidase deficiency.
- HEENT: Bulging fontanelle suggests elevated intracranial pressure. Minor dysmorphic features (e.g., frontal bossing, short/upturned nose, long philtrum, low-set ears) are sometimes seen in pyruvate dehydrogenase deficiency and severe disorders of fatty acid oxidation.
- Respiratory: Tachypnea may be a result of respiratory compensation of metabolic acidosis or to hyperammonemia.
- Cardiovascular: Arrhythmias or signs of heart failure may signal a cardiomyopathy.
- GI: Hepatomegaly occurs in many IEMs that also cause acidosis. It can be a result of abnormal accumulation of lipid (e.g., in fatty acid oxidation defects) or glycogen (e.g., glucose-6-phosphatase deficiency). Abdominal pain and emesis can be caused by ketosis.
- Neurologic: IEMs associated with acidosis are often associated with neuronal toxicity. Every neonate with a suspected IEM must have a complete neurologic exam to evaluate level of consciousness, tone, unusual movements, reflexes.
- Assessment for odors:

—"burnt sugar:" maple syrup urine disease
—"fruity:" ketosis
—"sweaty feet:" isovaleric acidemia

- Growth parameters: Normal at birth for most IEMs.

Laboratory Aids

The goal of the lab evaluation is to make a presumptive diagnosis as soon as possible. In most cases, definitive diagnosis requires specialized and time-consuming tests. Two critical management points:

1. Presumptive treatment should not await definitive testing, but should be based on clinical suspicion and initial testing. Delays in treatment can be fatal.
2. Involvement of a biochemical genetics team is invaluable in directing the workup of suspected IEMs.

A rational approach for acidotic neonates is to determine the IEM category using the tests below, then to send metabolic follow-up studies as indicated:
Initial tests:

- Urinalysis for ketones. Obtain urine by catheterization if necessary.
- Dextrose stick
- Basic metabolic profile
- ABG with lactate
- Ammonia
- Liver function tests

Patterns and follow-up testing:
These studies establish a presumptive diagnosis in most IEMs presenting with acidosis.

1. If elevated ketones, consider:
   a. Branched-chain and other organic acidemias (methylmalonic acidemia, propionic acidemia, isovaleric academia, others): ketoacidosis, hyperammonemia, +/− hypoglycemia. Obtain plasma amino acids, urine organic acids, plasma acylcarnitine profile with total/free carnitine.
   b. Primary lactic acidosis syndromes.
2. If elevated lactate, consider:
   a. Primary lactic acidosis syndromes: May be associated with ketosis (OXPHOS deficiency) and/or hypoglycemia (gluconeogenesis defects). Obtain lactate/pyruvate ratio, urine organic acids, CPK and biotinidase quantitation. Consider MRI and MRSpectroscopy if CNS symptoms present.
   b. Fatty acid oxidation defects: hypoketotic hypoglycemia +/− hyperammonemia and lactic acidosis: Obtain CPK, plasma acylcarnitine profile with total/free carnitine, urine organic acids. Perform ECG/ECHO for signs of cardiac failure.
3. If anion is not identified on initial tests, consider branched-chain and other organic acidemias

Other tests:
Consider organic acid, amino acid, and lactate/pyruvate analysis of the CSF in neonates with neurologic dysfunction.

 ## Therapy

GENERAL

In almost all IEMs, the metabolic derangement worsens during times of stress (e.g., perinatal period, infection, fasting, etc.) and accompanying catabolism. A general approach to therapy for patients covered in this section is to provide sufficient calories to reverse the catabolic state. Considerations include:

- Intravenous access.
- Many decompensated patients will have altered mental status and dehydration. Consider intubation if obtunded.
- Bicarbonate boluses and infusions may be necessary, especially if pH <7.22 or bicarb <14. Monitor sodium carefully in patients receiving $NaHCO_3$.
- In most cases, a high glucose infusion rate (e.g., with D10-based fluid) speeds recovery. One important exception is pyruvate dehydrogenase deficiency, a primary lactic acidosis syndrome, in which rapid glucose infusion can worsen the lactic acidosis. These children should receive D5.
- Specific dietary measures require a presumptive diagnosis. For example, long-chain fatty acids are contraindicated in many disorders of fatty acid oxidation, while branched-chain organic acidurias require protein restriction and formulas from which particular amino acids have been eliminated.
- Total parenteral nutrition is a useful option when a presumptive diagnosis has been made. Note that special TPN amino acid mixtures reduced in branched-chain amino acids are available for particular disorders (e.g., MSUD).
- Insulin can help reverse catabolic state but must be used cautiously;
- Nasogastric feeding using appropriate formulas is useful.
- In patients with large acid load and/or concomitant hyperammonemia, hemodialysis may be indicated.

SPECIFIC THERAPEUTIC MEASURES

- Specific therapies are best carried out with the help of a biochemical geneticist or other specialist with experience treating IEMs, and a clinical nutritionist.
- Organic acidemias:

—Protein restriction, protein elimination during times of stress, and avoidance of fasting. High glucose infusion rates during decompensation.

- Primary lactic acidosis syndromes:

—Therapy is supportive and involves avoidance of stresses (fasting, etc.).

- In pyruvate dehydrogenase deficiency, a ketogenic diet may improve chronic acidosis.
- Fatty acid oxidation disorders:

—Low fat, high carbohydrate diets with frequent feeds

 ## Common Questions and Answers

Q: If an infant dies before a diagnosis is made, what can be done to provide information for family members regarding future pregnancies?
A: A postmortem examination and biochemical tests performed on various tissues obtained immediately after death can establish the diagnosis. A skin biopsy (obtained pre- or postmortem) yields fibroblasts for a variety of biochemical assays, including enzyme defects in fatty acid oxidation disorders and organic acidemias. Workup of primary lactic acidosis syndromes requires electron transport chain analysis of muscle, which must be harvested immediately (within 30 minutes) after death.

Q: What determines developmental outcome in children with IEMs?
A: Disease severity depends in part on the specific mutations in each patient. However, prompt initiation of appropriate therapy in the newborn period, as well as compliance with chronic management and avoidance of decompensation periods all contribute to developmental outcome.

BIBLIOGRAPHY

Burton BK. Inborn errors of metabolism in infancy: a guide to diagnosis. *Pediatr* 1998;102:E69–E77.

Ozand PT, Generoso GG. Organic acidurias: a review. Part 2. *J Child Neuro* 1991;6:228–295.

Ozand PT, Generoso GG. Organic acidurias: a review. Part I. *J Child Neuro* 1991;6: 195–219.

Authors: Ralph J DeBerardinis and Sulagna C Saitta

Metabolic Diseases in Hyperammonemic Newborns

 Database

DEFINITION

Inborn errors of metabolism (IEMs) are inherited defects in biochemical pathways affecting metabolism of fats, amino acids or carbohydrates. Some IEMs present with elevated ammonia in newborns (>100 micromolar). Because these conditions are life-threatening if not treated promptly, maintaining a high degree of clinical suspicion in sick neonates is essential. In the newborn period, the immediate goals include:

1. Establish a tentative diagnosis.
2. Initiate presumptive management.
3. Send confirmatory studies.
4. Involve a team trained in treating patients with inborn errors of metabolism.

PATHOPHYSIOLOGY

The urea cycle converts ammonia (NH_3) to water-soluble urea in the liver, and is the major mechanism for ammonia disposal. IEMs causing hyperammonemia interfere with urea cycle function, either directly or indirectly, including the following mechanisms:

- Genetic defects in a urea cycle enzyme per se (see Urea Cycle Defects)
- Decreased production, increased utilization or defective transport of a urea cycle intermediate. Examples:

—Hyperornithinemia, Hyperammonemia, Homocitrullinemia (HHH) syndrome
—Lysinuric protein intolerance
—Fatty acid oxidation defects
—Hyperammonemia/Hyperinsulinemia syndrome
—Organic acidemias
—Pyruvate carboxylase deficiency

- Hepatotoxicity (galactosemia, hereditary fructose intolerance)

GENETICS

Generally autosomal recessive. Ornithine transcarbamylase deficiency (the most common urea cycle defect) is X-linked.

COMPLICATIONS

- Developmental disability.
- Coma
- Elevated intracranial pressure
- Death
- Recurrent episodes of hyperammonemia

 Differential Diagnosis

Neonatal hyperammonemia not caused by IEMs:

- Sepsis or other severe illness
- Liver failure (any cause)
- Transient neonatal hyperammonemia
- Perinatal depression/hypoxia
- Iatrogenic (valproic acid, asparaginase)

IEMs

- Urea cycle defects (N-acetylglutamate synthetase deficiency; carbamoyl phosphate synthase deficiency; ornithine transcarbamylase deficiency (OTCD); argininosuccinate synthetase deficiency (citrullinemia); Argininosuccinate lyase (AL) deficiency)
- Organic acidemias (isovaleric acidemia; propionic acidemia; methylmalonic acidemia; multiple carboxylase deficiency; others.
- Fatty acid oxidation defects (medium chain acyl-CoA dehydrogenase deficiency, multiple acyl-CoA dehydrogenase deficiency; others)
- Hyperornithinemia, Hyperammonemia, Homocitrullinemia (HHH) syndrome
- Pyruvate carboxylase deficiency
- Hyperammonemia/Hyperinsulinemia syndrome
- Galactosemia
- Hereditary fructose intolerance

 Data Gathering

HISTORY

Question: Is there evidence of systemic disease?
Significance: A variety of systemic newborn illnesses, including sepsis, can be complicated by a secondary hyperammonemia.

Question: What is the family history?
Significance: A family history of poorly explained pediatric death or developmental disability raises suspicion for a genetic disorder, such as an IEM. Diagnoses to ask about include sepsis (was an organism identified?), sudden infant death syndrome, cardiomyopathy, uncontrollable seizures, coma and liver failure.

Question: What is the current diet and feeding schedule?
Significance: In urea cycle defects, hyperammonemia is exacerbated by protein intake.

Question: Does the baby wake spontaneously to feed?
Significance: Failure to wake and feed spontaneously, like lethargy, is a sign of CNS dysfunction in neonates.

Question: What is the perinatal history?
Significance: Perinatal hypoxia can cause temporary liver dysfunction and reduced urea cycle capacity. Relative immaturity of the urea cycle can cause hyperammonemia in premature infants.

 Physical Examination

- ABCs and vital signs. Cushing's triad (apnea, bradycardia, hypertension) should prompt immediate evaluation for elevated intracranial pressure, a complication of hyperammonemia.
- Skin: Jaundice as a result of hepatotoxicity is not typical in urea cycle defects but occurs in other IEMs associated with hyperammonemia.
- HEENT: Bulging fontanelle suggests elevated intracranial pressure.
- Respiratory: Hyperammonemia's effects on the brainstem respiratory center may cause tachypnea.
- GI: Hepatomegaly occurs in some of these disorders (fatty acid oxidation disorders, galactosemia).
- Neurologic: Hyperammonemia causes a variety of neurologic abnormalities, including abnormal tone, obtundation, and coma.

 Laboratory Aids

The goal of lab testing is to make a presumptive diagnosis as soon as possible. In most cases, definitive diagnosis requires specialized and time-consuming tests. Two critical management points:

1. Presumptive treatment should not await definitive testing, but should be based on clinical suspicion and initial testing. Delays in treatment can be fatal.
2. Involvement of a biochemical genetics team is invaluable in directing the workup of suspected IEMs.

Initial tests to evaluate neonatal hyperammonemia include:

- Dextrose stick
- Electrolytes, BUN, creatinine
- CBC, blood culture
- Blood gas with lactate
- Liver function tests and PT/PTT
- Urinalysis for ketones, reducing substances
- Frequent ammonia levels

Suspected disorders and follow-up testing:

- Urea cycle defects: plasma amino acids and urine orotic acid
- Organic acidemias: urine organic acids, plasma amino acids and acylcarnitine profile.
- Fatty acid oxidation defects: CPK, urine organic acids, plasma acylcarnitine profile.
- Galactosemia: urine galactitol, GALT activity, and total galactose from blood.
- Definitive diagnosis may require enzyme testing or mutation analysis.

Metabolic Diseases in Hyperammonemic Newborns

 Therapy

GENERAL

• Discontinue protein intake, which exacerbates ammonia production. Protein/amino-acid free formula or parenteral nutrition should be used.
• In many disorders, catabolism and associated breakdown of endogenous protein exacerbates the nitrogen load. This can be treated with calories from high-rate dextrose infusion.
• Obtain intravenous access.
• Many patients will require intensive care transfer. Hyperammonemia interferes with normal CNS and respiratory function, so hyperammonemic neonates often require intubation.
• Nitrogen scavenging agents (e.g., sodium benzoate, sodium phenylacetate, sodium phenylbutyrate) combine with ammonia to form water-soluble compounds that can be excreted. These medications are useful in certain settings (e.g., urea cycle defects).
• In severe hyperammonemia, dialysis may be indicated.

SPECIFIC THERAPEUTIC MEASURES

Specific therapies are best carried out with the help of a specialist experienced in treating IEMs, and a clinical nutritionist. Examples include:

• Urea cycle defects:

—Protein restricted diet, with protein elimination during illness/stress.
—Chronic therapy with nitrogen scavenging agents.
—Amino acid supplements when indicated (e.g., citrulline in OTC deficiency; arginine in Citrullinemia, AL deficiency).

• Fatty acid oxidation disorders:

—Low fat, high carbohydrate diets with frequent feeds

• Organic acidemias:

—Protein restriction, protein elimination during times of stress, and avoidance of fasting.

 Common Questions and Answers

Q: Can females have OTC deficiency?
A: Since OTC is an X-linked gene, females are generally asymptomatic carriers. However, "skewed" X inactivation in which the normal OTC gene is inactive in a large majority of hepatocytes has caused symptomatic disease in a number of females. They are treated similarly to affected males.

Q: Can any of these disorders present outside of the newborn period?
A: Disease severity depends in large part on a patient's "residual" enzyme activity. In some patients, there is enough enzyme activity that hyperammonemia does not occur until later in life, during a period of illness, stress, or high protein intake.

Q: What determines developmental outcome in children with IEMs?
A: In most IEMs, severe mutations cause very low "residual" enzyme activity and a higher disease severity. However, prompt initiation of appropriate therapy in the newborn period, as well as compliance with chronic management and avoidance of decompensation periods all contribute to better developmental outcome.

BIBLIOGRAPHY

Batshaw ML, MacArthur RB, Tuchman M. Alternative pathway therapy for urea cycle disorders: twenty years later. *J Pediatr* 2001;138:S46–S55.

Scriver CR, Baudet AL, Sly WS, Valle D, eds. Urea cycle enzymes. *The Molecular and Metabolic Bases of Inherited Disease.* 8th Ed. New York: McGraw-Hill, 2001.

Burton BK. Inborn errors of metabolism in infancy: a guide to diagnosis. *Pediatr* 1998;102:E69–E77.

Summar M, Tuchman M. Proceedings of a consensus conference for the management of patients with urea cycle disorders. *J Pediatr* 2001;138:S6–S10.

Summar M. Current strategies for the management of neonatal urea cycle disorders. *J Pediatr* 2001;138:S30–S39.

Authors: Ralph J DeBerardinis and Sulagna C Saitta

Metabolic Diseases in Hypoglycemic Newborns

 ## Database

DEFINITION

Inborn errors of metabolism (IEMs) are inherited defects in biochemical pathways affecting metabolism of fats, amino acids or carbohydrates. Some IEMs predispose newborns to hypoglycemia. Because these conditions are life-threatening if not treated promptly, maintaining a high degree of clinical suspicion in sick neonates is essential. In the newborn period, the immediate goals should be to:

1. Establish a tentative diagnosis
2. Initiate presumptive management
3. Send confirmatory studies
4. Involve a team trained in treating patients with inborn errors of metabolism.

PATHOPHYSIOLOGY

- Through glycolysis and oxidative phosphorylation, glucose is a major source of cellular energy (ATP). Failure to produce ATP is probably the main source of hypoglycemia-associated tissue dysfunction.
- The brain preferentially utilizes glucose metabolism to produce energy, and is particularly sensitive to hypoglycemia.
- A long list of metabolic disturbances in a variety of pathways can result in hypoglycemia.
- Neonates are at particular risk for hypoglycemia because they use glucose more rapidly than adults and have immature ability to obtain energy from other sources (glycogen, muscle protein, adipose tissue).

GENETICS

Almost all IEMs causing hypoglycemia are autosomal recessive. One form of hyperinsulinism is autosomal dominant.

COMPLICATIONS

- Hypoglycemic episodes must be recognized and treated promptly, or permanent CNS injury ("hypoglycemic stroke") may occur.
- For many IEMs, recurrent episodes of hypoglycemia may occur. These are avoided by specific dietary measures during times of stress.

 ## Differential Diagnosis

Hypoglycemia is caused by increased glucose utilization or decreased glucose availability. Examples of disorders causing each:

- Increased glucose utilization:

—Sepsis increases metabolic demand and is a leading cause of neonatal hypoglycemia
—Hyperinsulinemia
—Decreased insulin counter-regulatory hormones (glucagon, cortisol, growth hormone)

- Decreased glucose availability/production:

—Infants of diabetic mothers
—From ingested carbohydrate
—Galactosemia
—Hereditary fructose intolerance
—Glycogen storage diseases
—Decreased gluconeogenesis
—Phosphoenolpyruvate carboxykinase deficiency
—Fructose 1,6 diphosphatase deficiency
—Pyruvate carboxylase deficiency
—From decreased efficiency of pathways providing alternate energy sources
—Organic acidemias
—Fatty acid oxidation defects

- A variety of toxins or medications interfere with pathways needed to maintain glucose homeostasis, including salicylates, valproate, β-blockers, ethanol, and exogenous insulin.

 ## Data Gathering

HISTORY

Question: What is the family history?
Significance: Because IEMs are genetic disorders, patients may have a family history of poorly explained pediatric death. Diagnoses to ask about include sepsis (was an organism identified?), sudden infant death syndrome, cardiomyopathy, uncontrollable seizures, coma, and liver failure. Unexplained developmental delay or hypoglycemia in older siblings can provide useful clues.

Question: Were there complications with the pregnancy?
Significance: Maternal diabetes, including gestational diabetes, is a risk factor for perinatal hypoglycemia. Some IEMs, particularly certain disorders of fatty acid oxidation, are associated with fatty liver of pregnancy or the HELLP (hypertension, elevated liver enzymes, low platelets) syndrome.

Question: What are the results of the newborn screen?
Significance: Many children are tested for a variety of IEMs, either through state-mandated or supplemental newborn screens. Some of these disorders predispose to hypoglycemia and have specific therapies.

Question: What is the current diet and feeding schedule?
Significance: The timing of hypoglycemia helps form differential diagnosis.

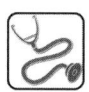 ## Physical Examination

- ABCs and vital signs. Tachycardia and hypotension are commonly seen in hypoglycemia.
- Facies: Decreased interpupillary distance or other midline anomalies occur in association with abnormalities of the pituitary.
- Skin: Diaphoresis is an effect of the catecholamine surge that accompanies hypoglycemia.
- Respiratory: Tachypnea may be a result of respiratory compensation of metabolic acidosis or to hyperammonemia.
- GI: Hepatomegaly occurs in many IEMs causing hypoglycemia and is a key feature in differentiating possible diagnoses. It can be a result of abnormal accumulation of lipid (e.g., in fatty acid oxidation defects) or glycogen (e.g., glycogen storage disease).
- Neurologic: Every neonate with a suspected IEM needs a complete neurologic exam to evaluate level of consciousness, tone, unusual movements, and reflexes. Tremulousness is a common early sign of hypoglycemia. Stupor and coma occur if hypoglycemia is not reversed.
- Growth parameters: Infants of diabetic mothers may be large for gestational age (LGA). Beckwith-Wiedemann syndrome presents with LGA, hyperinsulinism and physical stigmata (hemihypertrophy, macroglossia, abdominal wall defects).

Laboratory Aids

The goal of the lab evaluation is to make a presumptive diagnosis as soon as possible. In many cases, definitive diagnosis requires specialized and time-consuming tests. Two critical management points:

1. Presumptive treatment should not await definitive testing, but should be based on clinical suspicion and initial testing. Delays in treatment can be fatal.
2. Involvement of a biochemical genetics team is invaluable in directing the workup of suspected IEMs.

In a neonate with a hypoglycemic dextrose stick, obtain the following "critical" labs as soon as possible:

- Basic metabolic profile including glucose
- Urinalysis for ketones: Inappropriately low in hyperinsulinism and fatty acid oxidation defects
- ABG with lactate: Lactic acidosis occurs in gluconeogenic defects and in glycogen storage disease type I
- Insulin: Inappropriately high in hyperinsulinemic states
- Cortisol, growth hormone levels: Inappropriately low in deficiency states
- Plasma acylcarnitine profile: Diagnostic for fatty acid oxidation defects, some organic acidemias
- Urine organic acids: Helps quantify accumulation of ketones and intermediates of amino acid and lipid metabolism

 ## Therapy

GENERAL

- A well-appearing neonate with a low dextrose stick should be fed immediately. If feeds are contraindicated or not tolerated, obtain IV access.
- In children with associated physical or laboratory findings consistent with an IEM or other serious illness (e.g., vital sign instability, lethargy, acidosis), IV access should be obtained.
- A dextrose bolus (e.g., 2 cc/kg D10) and infusion rapidly corrects hypoglycemia in most cases. Infants requiring high glucose infusion rates are suspicious for hyperinsulinism.

SPECIFIC THERAPEUTIC MEASURES

Specific therapies vary according to the diagnosis and are best carried out with the help of a specialist familiar with each disease. Examples include:

- Hyperinsulinism:

—May require continuous glucose administration (intravenously or via continuous gastric feeds)
—Medical therapies including diazoxide and octreotide
—Pancreatectomy

- Deficiencies in counter-regulatory hormones:

—Hormone supplementation

- Galactosemia, hereditary fructose intolerance:

—Eliminate offending agent from diet

- Fatty acid oxidation disorders, glycogen storage disease type I, defects in gluconeogenesis:

—Frequent feeds, fasting avoidance, increase caloric intake during stress

 ## Common Questions and Answers

Q: Why is hypoglycemia dangerous?
A: Glucose is a crucial source of rapidly available energy for many tissues, especially the brain. Prolonged hypoglycemia causes CNS damage.

Q: Why are the "critical" labs so important?
A: In some metabolic disorders, the biochemical disturbance is apparent only during hypoglycemic episodes. Collecting this panel of informative labs during an episode greatly increases the chance of making a diagnosis.

Q: If an infant dies before a diagnosis is made, what can be done to provide information for family members regarding future pregnancies?
A: A postmortem examination and biochemical tests performed on various tissues obtained immediately after death can establish the diagnosis. A skin biopsy (obtained pre- or postmortem) yields fibroblasts for a variety of biochemical assays, including enzyme defects in fatty acid oxidation disorders and organic acidemias. Workup of primary lactic acidosis syndromes requires electron transport chain analysis of muscle, which must be harvested immediately (within 30 minutes) after death.

BIBLIOGRAPHY

Hypoglycemia of infancy and childhood. In: Becker KL, ed. *Principles and Practice of Endocrinology and Metabolism*. 2nd Ed. Philadelphia: JB Lippincott Co, 1995.

Saudubray JM, de Lonlay P, Touati G, et al. Genetic hypoglycemia in infancy and childhood: Pathophysiology and diagnosis. *J Inherited Metab Diseases* 2000;23:197.

Authors: Ralph J DeBerardinis and Sulagna C Saitta

Methemoglobinemia

 Database

DEFINITION

• Methemoglobin is a dysfunctional hemoglobin in which the deoxygenated heme moiety has been oxidized from the ferrous (Fe^{2+}) to the ferric (Fe^{3+}) state. Methemoglobinemia is an undue accumulation of methemoglobin within the blood.

PATHOPHYSIOLOGY

• Hemoglobin in the allosteric configuration of methemoglobin cannot carry oxygen.
• Methemoglobin increases the oxygen affinity of normal heme moieties in the blood, and results in impaired oxygen delivery to tissues.
• NADH-dependent cytochrome b5 methemoglobin reductase is the major source of physiologic reduction of methemoglobin.
• A normally dormant NADPH-dependent methemoglobin reductase is the site of action for antidotal methylene blue therapy.

EPIDEMIOLOGY

• Toxic methemoglobinemia, resulting from exposure to oxidant chemicals or drugs, is the most common cause of methemoglobinemia among children older than 6 months.

—Dietary or environmental chemicals: chlorates, chromates, copper sulfate fungicides, naphthalene, nitrates, nitrites.
—Industrial chemicals: aniline and other nitrogenated organic compounds.
—Drugs: amyl nitrite, benzocaine, dapsone, lidocaine, metoclopramide, nitric oxide, nitroprusside, phenazopyridine, prilocaine, and many others.
—Methemoglobinemia is a common iatrogenic complication of drug therapy.

• Enteritis-associated methemoglobinemia is the most common cause among children younger than 6 months.

—As many as two-thirds of infants with severe diarrhea will have methemoglobinemia.
—Intestinal nitrate and nitric oxide promotes methemoglobin formation.
—Innate enzymatic methemoglobin reduction systems may be underdeveloped during infancy.
—Acidemia further inhibits enzymatic methemoglobin reduction systems.
—Methemoglobinemia also reported with nitrite-producing bacterial infections of the intestines or urinary tract.

• Congenital methemoglobinemia is rare.

—Hemoglobin M: heterozygotes for autosomal dominant Hemoglobin M will exhibit lifelong cyanosis.
—NADH-dependent methemoglobin reductase deficiency: homozygotes for this autosomal recessive enzyme will have lifelong cyanosis, heterozygotes may have increased susceptibility to oxidative hemoglobin injury.

COMPLICATIONS

• >10% methemoglobinemia

—Cyanosis

• >30% methemoglobinemia

—Malaise, fatigue, dyspnea, tachycardia

• >50% methemoglobinemia

—Somnolence, tissue ischemia

• >60%

—Potential lethality

PROGNOSIS

• Toxic methemoglobinemia

—Full recovery with recognition, removal of oxidant stress, and appropriate therapy.

• Enteritis-associated methemoglobinemia

—Methemoglobinemia may be prolonged and relapsing until enteritis healed.

• Congenital methemoglobinemia

—Lifelong cyanosis expected.

ASSOCIATED DISEASES

• Heinz body hemolytic anemia: oxidant stress on the globin protein may cause hemolysis. Sulfhemoglobinemia: oxidant stress on the hemoglobin porphyrin ring may cause sulfhemoglobinemia.

 Differential Diagnosis

• Environmental hypoxia
• Cardiovascular disease
• Pulmonary disease
• Sulfhemoglobinemia
• Factitious skin discoloration

 Data Gathering

HISTORY

Question: Age of onset?
Significance: New onset of cyanosis in children older than 6 months is unlikely a result of congenital or enteritis-associated methemoglobinemia.

Question: Source of water?
Significance: Well water may be contaminated with nitrates.

Question: Drug or chemical exposure?
Significance: May suggest a source of toxic methemoglobinemia.

Question: Diarrhea?
Significance: May suggest enteritis-associated methemoglobinemia.

Question: Formula fed?
Significance: Anecdotes suggest an association between enteritis-associated methemoglobinemia and soy formula feeding.

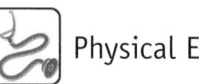 Physical Examination

Finding: Cyanosis
Significance: Cyanosis becomes apparent in the presence of 1.5 g/dL of methemoglobin (in contrast to 5 g/dL of deoxyhemoglobin).

Finding: Heart murmur
Significance: May suggest right-to-left intracardiac shunting, rather than methemoglobinemia.

Finding: Abnormal lung auscultation
Significance: May suggest cyanosis as a result of pulmonary disorder.

Laboratory Aids

TESTS

Test: Oxygen saturation
Significance: Oxygen saturation measured by pulse oximetry is low, but oxygen saturation calculated from arterial blood gas is normal (a "saturation gap").

Test: Co-oximetry
Significance: Multiple-wavelength co-oximetry is the standard for quantifying methemoglobin in the blood.

Test: Hemoglobin quantitation
Significance: The percent methemoglobin concentration must be considered in relation to the total hemoglobin. Anemia may suggest concurrent hemolysis.

Test: Serum bicarbonate
Significance: Metabolic acidosis is relatively mild in cases of <40% toxic methemoglobinemia. Metabolic acidosis is typically profound in cases of enteritis-associated methemoglobinemia.

Test: G-6-PD Assay
Significance: Glucose-6-phosphate dehydrogenase deficiency does not predispose to methemoglobinemia, and should not be routinely ordered.

Test: Hemoglobin electrophoresis
Significance: Hemoglobin M is rare and does not respond to therapy. This test should not be routinely ordered.

PITFALLS

• Pulse oximetry may be inaccurate in the setting of methemoglobinemia or methylene blue therapy.

 ## Therapy

ACQUIRED METHEMOGLOBINEMIA

• Administer 100% oxygen
• Decontaminate or remove from toxic source of oxidative stress
• Alleviate enteritis with IV fluids or elemental formulas
• Treat identified bacterial infections
• Consider administration of 1% methylene blue

—Dose: 1 to 2 mg/kg IV over 5 minutes, repeat as necessary (caution above 4 to 7 mg/kg total)
—Indications: signs of tissue hypoxia, central nervous system depression, >30% methemoglobinemia.
—Contraindications (relative): known, severe, G-6-PD deficiency

• Exchange transfusion is a consideration of last resort

CONGENITAL METHEMOGLOBINEMIA

• No beneficial therapy exists for Hemoglobin M.
• Oral methylene blue or ascorbic acid may provide alternative reduction pathways for patients with NADH dependent reductase deficiencies.

PITFALLS

• Methylene blue therapy may be ineffective if:

—Patient is G-6-PD deficient
—Ongoing drug or chemical absorption, or biotransformation, leads to continuing methemoglobin formation
—Sulfhemoglobin is present
—Hemoglobin M is present
—High doses of methylene blue add to, rather than ameliorate, the oxidant stress

 ## Follow-Up

• Toxic methemoglobinemia

—Consider consultation with a medical toxicologist
—May require environmental investigation

• Enteritis-associated methemoglobinemia

—Careful formula rechallenge is warranted if possibility exists for milk protein allergy or other dietary intolerance

• Congenital methemoglobinemia

—Consider consultation with a hematologist

 ## Common Questions and Answers

Q: Can methemoglobinemia be diagnosed by the color of the blood?
A: The "chocolate-brown" blood of methemoglobinemia is most easily noted when compared to "control" blood on a white filter paper background. In contrast to deoxygenated blood from patients with cardiopulmonary disease, methemoglobin-darkened blood does not redden on exposure to room air.

Q: Is methemoglobin responsible for the profound metabolic acidosis often found in diarrheal infants?
A: Benzocaine-induced methemoglobinemia rarely causes acidosis in infants. In contrast, infants with enteritis-associated methemoglobinemia often have a profound acidemia with a relatively narrow anion gap. Acidosis should be considered a contributing or coexisting factor, rather than a result, of methemoglobinemia among infants with diarrhea.

BIBLIOGRAPHY

Avner JR, Henretig FM, McAnaney CM. Acquired methemoglobinemia: The relationship of cause to course of illness. *Am J Dis Child* 1990;144:1229–1230.

Clifton J 2nd, Leikin JB. Methylene blue. *Am J Ther* 2003;10(4):289–291.

Osterhoudt KC. Methemoglobinemia. In: Ford MD, Delaney KA, Ling LJ, Erickson T, eds. *Clin Toxicol.* Philadelphia: W.B. Saunders, 2001:211–217.

Pollack ES, Pollack CV. Incidence of subclinical methemoglobinemia in infants with diarrhea. *Ann Emerg Med* 1994;24:652–656.

Wright RO, Lewander WJ, Woolf AD. Methemoglobinemia: etiology, pharmacology, and clinical management. *Ann Emerg Med* 1999;34:646–656.

Author: Kevin Osterhoudt

Milia

Database

DEFINITION

White papules that occur commonly and spontaneously on the face, and frequently elsewhere; after healing of blisters when present on mucous membranes; referred to as Epstein pearls

PATHOPHYSIOLOGY

- Retention of keratin and sebaceous material within the pilosebaceous duct, eccrine sweat duct, or sebaceous collar surrounding vellus hair.
- Lamellated keratin deposits are found in the superficial papillary dermis.

EPIDEMIOLOGY

- Common in all age groups
- Up to 40% of newborns have milia on the skin
- In older patients, most often related to trauma, site of irradiation or reepithelializing blister

COMPLICATIONS

- Primarily of cosmetic concern.
- Rare potential for foreign body reaction to occur.
- If persistent milia in an unusual or widespread distribution when seen with other defects: hereditary trichodysplasia (Matie-Unna hypotrichosis) or oral-facial-digital syndrome type I. Often seen in healed areas of dystrophic forms of epidermolysis bullosa.

PROGNOSIS

- Spontaneous regression of milia occur in infants.
- In older individuals the lesions are usually chronic unless treated.
- Lesions uncommonly recur.

Differential Diagnosis

- Infection

—Molluscum contagiosum
—Impetigo (pustules)
—Herpes simplex (clouded vesicles)
—Environmental (poisons)

- Tumors

—Sebaceous gland hyperplasia

- Miscellaneous

—Neonatal acne
—Keratosis pilaris

Data Gathering

HISTORY

- Asymptomatic?
- Recent trauma?
- History of blistering diseases?

Physical Examination

- One- to 2-mm bright white papules with smooth surface: Most often found on cheeks, nose, chin, forehead, but occasionally on dorsal surface of hands and over knees, especially if related to trauma.
- Occasionally, lesions may be seen on upper trunk, extremities, penis, or mucous membranes.
- Distinguish from pustules by palpation

Laboratory Aids

Milia are firm and, when incised, reveal solid keratin rather than liquid contents.

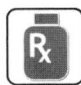 **Therapy**

- No need for treatment in infants because they are benign, asymptomatic, and often resolve on their own. Alternatively, cyst contents may be expressed by squeezing or with a comedone extractor after incision of the overlying epidermis with a needle or no. 11 scalpel blade.

SPECIAL QUESTIONS

If present periocularly, ask about history of atopy/allergic conjunctivitis.

 Follow-Up

Without treatment, most lesions resolve in 1 to 2 weeks in infants.

 Common Questions and Answers

Q: Will the lesions get bigger before they go away?
A: No, there is no tendency to enlarge with time.

ICD-9-CM 706.2

BIBLIOGRAPHY

Hurwitz S. *Clinical Pediatric Dermatology: A Textbook of Skin Disorders of Childhood and Adolescence.* 2nd Ed. Philadelphia: WB Saunders, 1993.

Author: Albert C. Yan

Milk Protein Allergy

 Database

DEFINITION

Symptoms affecting the gastrointestinal tract, skin, and respiratory tract resulting from ingestion of cow's milk protein. Predisposing factors include:

- Age (diagnosis usually before 2 years)
- Immune deficiency (immaturity of the mucosal immune system, immaturity or damage of mucosal barrier function, low IgA)
- History or presence of atopy
- Early milk protein-based formula feeding
- Allergenic formula
- Gastrointestinal infection

PATHOPHYSIOLOGY

- Unprocessed cow's milk protein is 80% casein and 19% whey. The whey fraction contains over 20 types of antigenic proteins, including: β-lactoglobulin, α-lactalbumin, Bovine serum albumin, β2-microglobulin, Transferrin, Lactoferrin
- Infants ingesting cow's milk develop an immune response to the proteins with the formation of circulating IgG antibodies and mucosal IgA antibodies, which is thought to be protective.
- Exclusively breast-fed infants may also develop milk protein allergy through exposure to allergens that appear in breast milk.
- Although β-lactoglobulin is suspected to be an antigen, no single protein fraction has been proven. Most children appear to be allergic to multiple cow's milk proteins; rarely are patients allergic to only one fraction.
- There is 25% to 30% cross-reactivity between milk proteins and soy proteins.

EPIDEMIOLOGY

The prevalence of this entity has been estimated at between 2.0% and 7.5% of otherwise normal infants.

 Differential Diagnosis

Diseases characterized by watery diarrhea, abdominal pain, and blood and mucous in the stool should be considered. Infections etiologies (dysentery, Clostridium) and celiac disease should be excluded.

 Data Gathering

A normal appearing child with blood and mucous in the stool are the most common GI manifestations. No single laboratory test appears to have significant sensitivity for detecting this syndrome. Radioallergosorbent test (RAST) and skin testing may be used with positive predictive value of only 50%.

HISTORY

- Diagnosis is implied if clinical symptoms resolve on removal of cow's milk protein containing products. In some cases no resolution is seen on soy based formula and hydrolyzed formula and even crystalline amino acid-based formulas are needed.
- Patients will present in the first few months of life. Symptoms include:

—Failure to thrive
—Vomiting and diarrhea
—Abdominal distension
—Occult blood loss (without anemia in most cases)
—Hypoproteinemia
—Infants with allergic colitis present with diarrhea associated with blood streaks and mucus.
—Well-appearing
—Rarely, infants may present with hemorrhage or hypovolemic/allergic shock.

 Laboratory Aids

- Occasionally, peripheral blood and stool eosinophilia may be documented.
- Infectious causes of enteropathy may mimic the disorder; therefore, infection should be ruled out with stool cultures and duodenal fluid cultures, if available.
- Recto-sigmoid biopsies are not routinely performed.
- Histologic changes in bowel mucosa tend to be nonspecific.
- Grossly, the mucosa appears friable and inflamed, rarely with erosions or gross ulcerations.
- Pathologic findings may include:

—Partial villous atrophy with reduction in villous height on upper endoscopy
—Moderate increase in intraepithelial lymphocytes
—Prominent eosinophilic infiltrate

 Emergency Care

In the rare situation of severe food allergy with shock-like picture and acidosis, fluids and elimination of food should be given in the hospital.

Milk Protein Allergy

 Therapy

- Removal of cow's milk protein-containing products from the diet is the cornerstone of treatment.
- Approximately 10% to 30% of children allergic to cow's milk will also be allergic to soy, hydrolyzed formulas (Pregestimil, Nutramigen, Alimentum) are the formulas of choice for infants with cow's milk protein intolerance.
- Resolution of bloody stools usually occurs within 24 to 72 hours, but guaiac-positive stools may continue for 2 to 6 weeks.
- Newer therapies have included the Neocate and EleCare formulas, which are amino acid, simple carbohydrate, and fat-based formulas that have been more effective in recalcitrant cases of allergy.

 Follow-Up

- In most cases tolerance to cow's milk protein usually develops at age 1 year, and reintroduction of a normal diet can be safely done.
- Occasionally, symptoms of intolerance may persist past the third year of life, and approximately 10% will have symptoms that persist at 6 years of age.
- Cow's milk protein challenge with RAST, skin testing, and possible gastrointestinal biopsies can help to monitor the degree of allergic response in these older children.
- In cases of severe anaphylactic reactions or acute urticaria, the cow's milk challenge should be performed in a hospital under medical supervision.
- Gastrointestinal intolerance seems to persist in a certain proportion of subjects, with intestinal symptoms and increased prevalence of lactose intolerance.

 Common Questions and Answers

Q: What are the newer formulas for treating milk protein allergy?
A: The newest formulas are Neocate and EleCare. These are amino acid-based formulas that are made with single amino acids and have the least allergic potential. Most patients will do well on soy-based formula or hydrolyzed cows' milk formula

Q: When does this problem usually resolve?
A: In most infants who develop minimal symptoms the problem will resolve by the first year of life, but the range can be several years. Some reports of residual GI disease exist.

ICD-9-CM 995.67

BIBLIOGRAPHY

Host A, Jacobsen HP, Halken S, et al. The natural history of cow's milk protein allergy/intolerance. *Eur J Clin Nutr* 1995;49(Suppl 1):S13–S18.

Host A. Frequency of cow's milk allergy in childhood. *Ann Allergy Asthma Immunol* 2002;89(6 Suppl 1):33–37.

Kokkonen J, Tikkanen S, Savilahti E. Residual intestinal disease after milk allergy in infancy. *J Pediatr Gastroenterol Nutr* 2001;32:156–161.

Sampson HA, Anderson JA. Summary and recommendation: classification of gastrointestinal manifestations due to immunologic reactions to foods in infants and young children. *J Pediatr Gastroenterol Nutr* 2000;30:S87–S94.

Walker-Smith J. Cow's milk allergy: a new understanding from immunology. *Ann Allergy Asthma Immunol* 2003;90(6 Suppl 3):81–83.

Walker-Smith J. Hypoallergenic formulas: are they really hypoallergenic? *Ann Allergy Asthma Immunol* 2003;90(6 Suppl 3):112–114.

Author: Dror Wasserman

Mumps/Parotitis

 Database

DEFINITION

Mumps is an acute viral disease characterized by painful enlargement of the parotids and other salivary glands.

CAUSES

- Parotitis is usually caused by mumps, a Rubulavirus in the paramyxovirus family.
- Other viral causes of parotitis include cytomegaloviruses, influenza, parainfluenza, and enteroviruses.
- Bacterial cases are usually secondary to *Staphylococcus aureus* (suppurative parotitis).
- Recurrent parotitis is an idiopathic, rare, recurrent swelling of the parotids, without suppuration or external inflammatory changes.
- Rare childhood cases may be secondary to an obstructing calculus, foreign body (sesame seed), or various drugs (antihistamines, phenothiazines, iodine-containing drugs/contrast media).

PATHOPHYSIOLOGY

- The mumps virus enters via the respiratory tract, and a viremia ultimately ensues.
- The viremia spreads to many organs, including the salivary glands, gonads, pancreas, and meninges.

EPIDEMIOLOGY

- Humans are the only known host for mumps.
- Spread is via the respiratory route.
- Incidence of this once very common disease has declined dramatically since the advent of universal childhood immunization. Outbreaks, however, continue to occur.
- Period of communicability: 7 days before to 5 days after onset of parotid swelling
- Most communicable period: 1 to 2 days before the parotid swelling
- Incubation period: 12 to 25 days after exposure
- One attack of mumps (clinical or subclinical) confers lifelong immunity.

COMPLICATIONS

- Meningitis: More than 50% of patients have a CSF pleocytosis; this "aseptic meningitis" is usually benign.
- Encephalitis: Rarely causes permanent sequelae
- Cerebellitis
- Facial nerve palsy
- Oophoritis, nephritis, thyroiditis, myocarditis, mastitis, arthritis, transient ocular involvement, deafness, and sterility (all rare)

PROGNOSIS

Complete recovery in 1 to 2 weeks is the rule.

ASSOCIATED ILLNESSES

- Salivary adenitis: This is the most common manifestation of mumps, though one-third of cases occur subclinically.
- Epididymo-orchitis: Up to 35% of adolescent mumps cases are complicated by orchitis. Orchitis develops within 4 to 10 days of the onset of the parotid swelling. Sterility is uncommon.
- Pancreatitis: Mild inflammation is common; serious involvement is rare.

 Differential Diagnosis

- Mumps parotitis can be distinguished from the other viral causes by clinical presentation along with specialized laboratory studies (see below).
- Bacterial parotitis is usually caused by *S. aureus*, but streptococci, gram-negative bacilli, and anaerobic infections are also possible.
- Cases of tuberculous and nontuberculous (atypical) mycobacterial parotitis are rare, but have been reported.
- Parotid enlargement can be an initial sign in HIV-infected children.
- A salivary calculus can be diagnosed by sialogram.
- Recurrent childhood parotitis is a rare disorder in which symptoms initially manifest in children 3 to 6 years of age; it is largely a diagnosis of exclusion.
- Cervical or preauricular adenitis may simulate parotitis; close anatomic localization should be diagnostic.
- Infectious mononucleosis and cat-scratch disease are other considerations.
- Drug-induced parotid enlargement occasionally occurs.
- Malignancies of the parotid are extremely rare.
- Pneumoparotitis is seen in those with a history of playing a wind instrument, glass blowing, scuba diving, and even general anesthesia.

 Data Gathering

HISTORY

- Prodromal symptoms are uncommon in children with mumps, but may include fever, anorexia, myalgia, headache, and malaise.
- Onset of mumps is usually pain and swelling in front of and below the ear.
- Swelling usually starts with one ear and then rapidly progresses to the other ear.
- Mild fever usually accompanies parotid swelling.
- Dysphagia and dysphonia are common.
- Testicular pain and swelling, along with constitutional symptoms, usually begin approximately 1 week after the parotid swelling of mumps.
- Epigastric pain and constitutional symptoms with pancreatic involvement
- Fever, headache, and stiff neck with meningitis
- Behavioral changes, seizures, and other neurologic abnormalities are rare.
- Other symptoms are analogous to the particular organ involved.

 Physical Examination

- Nonerythematous, tender parotid swelling (erythema seen with suppurative parotitis)
- Swelling ultimately obscures the mandibular ramus.
- The ear is often displaced upward and outward.
- Submaxillary and sublingual glands also may be swollen.
- Inflammation may be noted intraorally at the orifice of Stensen duct.
- Presternal edema is occasionally noted.
- Mumps are infrequently associated with truncal rash.
- Tender, edematous testicle in mumps orchitis (usually unilateral)

SPECIAL QUESTIONS

Ask the patient if the pain (at the parotid) intensifies with the tasting of sour liquids.

PROCEDURE

Have the patient suck on a lemon drop or lemon juice, and note any discharge from Stensen duct.

Laboratory Aids

- Uncomplicated parotitis: mild leukopenia with lymphocytosis.
- Suppurative parotitis and mumps orchitis: leukocytosis.
- Pancreatic involvement: hyperamylasemia and elevated serum lipase.
- Salivary adenitis without pancreatic involvement: isolated hyperamylasemia.
- Meningitis: CSF pleocytosis (predominately mononuclear).
- Gram stain and culture of pus expressed from Stensen duct is diagnostic in suppurative parotitis.
- Sialography is useful to evaluate for stones or strictures, but is contraindicated in acute infection.
- Serologic confirmation of mumps parotitis: complement fixation, neutralization, hemagglutination inhibition, or enzyme immunoassays.
- Definitive laboratory diagnosis of mumps parotitis: body fluid isolation of mumps virus in tissue culture.

PITFALLS

Skin tests should not be used for test of immunity; serologic studies are more reliable.

 Therapy

- Supportive therapy is all that is required in mumps parotitis.
- Antibiotics directed against *S. aureus* should be used in cases of suppurative parotitis.

 Follow-Up

- Most children have resolution of glandular swelling by about 1 week.
- Disappearance of testicular pain and swelling can be expected 4 to 6 days after onset.
- Testicular atrophy is common, though infertility is rare.
- Markedly elevated pancreatic enzymes should be monitored until they improve.
- Children should not return to school until at least 9 days after the onset of parotid swelling.

PREVENTION

- A single 0.5-mL subcutaneous injection of live mumps vaccine (usually given together with measles and rubella, the "MMR") at 12 to 15 months usually confers long-lasting immunity.
- Primary vaccine failure and waning vaccine-induced immunity have been reported.
- A second vaccination is recommended between 4 and 6 years of age.
- The first dose of MMR vaccine sometimes causes fever and rash, usually 7 to 10 days after immunization. The measles component is usually the culprit.
- Links of the MMR vaccine to autism have not been substantiated.
- Vaccine should not be administered to children who are immunocompromised by disease or pharmacotherapy, or to pregnant women.
- Children with HIV infection who are not severely immunocompromised should be immunized with the MMR vaccine.

 Common Questions and Answers

Q: Should immunization be deferred in children with intercurrent illness?
A: No, children with minor illnesses, even with fever, should be vaccinated.

Q: Should vaccination be withheld in children living with immunocompromised hosts?
A: No, vaccinated children do not transmit mumps vaccine virus.

BIBLIOGRAPHY

American Academy of Pediatrics. Mumps. In: Pickering LK, ed. *2003 Red Book: Report of the Committee on Infectious Diseases.* 26th Ed. Elk Grove Village, IL: American Academy of Pediatrics, 2003:439–443.

Casella R, Leibundgut B, Lehman K, et al. Mumps orchitis: report of a mini-epidemic. *J Urol* 1997;158(6):2158–2161.

Chitre VV, Premchandra DJ. Recurrent parotitis. *Arch Dis Child* 1997;77(4):359–363.

Elliman D, Bedford H. MMR vaccine: the continuing saga. *BMJ* 2001;332:183–184.

Endo A, Izumi H, Miyashita M, et al. Facial palsy associated with mumps. *Pediatr Infect Dis J* 2001;20(8):815–816.

Galazka AM, Robertson SE, Kraigher A. Mumps and mumps vaccine: a global review. *Bull WHO* 1999;77(1):3–14.

Gold E. Almost extinct diseases: measles, mumps, rubella, and pertussis. *Pediatr Rev* 1996;17(4):120–127.

Majda-Stanislawska E. Mumps cerebellitis. *Eur Neurol* 2000;43(2):117.

Taylor B, Miller E, Farrington CP, et al. Autism and measles, mumps, and rubella vaccine: no epidemiologic evidence for a causal association. *Lancet* 1999;353:2026–2029.

Virtanen M, Peltola H, Paunio M, et al. Day to day reactogenicity and the healthy vaccinee effect of measles-mumps-rubella vaccination. *Pediatrics [serial online]* 2000;106(5):62.

Watson JC, Hadler SC, Dykewicz CA, et al. Measles, mumps, and rubella—vaccine use and strategies for elimination of measles, mumps, rubella, and congenital rubella syndrome and control of mumps. *Morb Mortal Wkly Rep* 1998;47(RR-8):1–57.

Whitelaw CC, Kallis JM. Pediatric facial swelling. *Acad Emerg Med* 1998;5(2):146, 198–202.

Author: Nicholas Tsarouhas

Munchausen Syndrome by Proxy

 Database

DEFINITION

Munchausen syndrome by proxy (MSBP) describes an illness in a child that is fabricated by someone else (usually the parent). This results in repeated interactions with the medical care system, often leading to multiple medical procedures. The perpetrator denies the cause of the child's illnesses. Symptoms decrease when the child is separated from the perpetrator.

CAUSES

It is the parent, commonly the mother, who fabricates the illnesses.
Little is known about the etiology in the parent. The parent may have Munchausen syndrome. They may be seeking secondary gain from the attention of medical staff or financial gain by having the child be disabled.

EPIDEMIOLOGY

- Typical victims are <4 years of age, males = females
- Victims average 21.8 months from onset of symptoms to diagnosis
- Varies with presentation
- Of infants monitored in apnea programs, 0.27% are believed to be secondary to MSBP.
- Five percent of allergy patients in some clinic settings are estimated to be MSBP.
- Mortality is approximately 6% to 9%.

PROGNOSIS

If undiagnosed, mortality has been estimated at 6% to 9%. Some children go on to develop Munchausen syndrome themselves. The long-term consequences to the child are unknown.

 Differential Diagnosis

Diagnosis depends on presentation. MSBP should be considered in unusual presentations of:

- GI bleeding
- Apnea/apparent life-threatening event
- Asthma
- Seizures
- GU bleeding
- Unexplained abnormalities in electrolytes
- Chronic diarrhea or vomiting
- Infections with multiple organisms found in blood or urine culture.

PITFALLS

- Delay in making the diagnosis: The average length of time to diagnosis is 21.8 months.
- Physicians and nursing personnel may be reluctant to suspect the parent because of their own involvement with the family.

 Data Gathering

HISTORY

- Unexplained or unusual illness, symptoms, and signs that are incongruous or present only when the perpetrator is present
- Usual medical treatment is ineffective in treating the presenting symptom.
- The perpetrator may not be concerned about the patient, may be constantly present while the patient is in the hospital, or may form unusually close relationships with the hospital staff.

SPECIAL QUESTIONS

- A history of frequent moves, other siblings who have either died or had unusual medical illnesses may suggest MSBP.
- In the context of divorce, repeated allegations of sexual abuse may represent MSBP.

 Physical Examination

- Examination of the patient with apnea presentation may indicate evidence of intentional suffocation.
- Patients who present with unusual bleeding may have lacerations on other parts of the body.
- The perpetrator also may have lacerations.
- Note the presence of indwelling intravenous, CSF, or bladder catheters.
- The patient may have evidence of old fractures.

 Laboratory Aids

TESTS

Workup is dictated by presentation:

- Pneumogram to rule out apnea
- If bleeding is the major presentation, identify the blood as the patient's (as opposed to that of the perpetrator or an animal).
- A toxicology screen may be helpful for unusual presentations of poisoning.
- Separating the perpetrator from the patient, with resultant decrease in symptoms, may suggest the diagnosis.
- Suspect MSBP when there is blood or urine culture with many organisms.
- If GI bleeding is the presenting symptom, use endoscopy or a Meckel scan to rule out anatomic causes of bleeding.
- Video monitoring of a patient's room may demonstrate the perpetrator harming the child.
- Ensure that the perpetrator cannot tamper with testing.

Munchausen Syndrome by Proxy

 Therapy

- If MSBP is documented, the patient must be separated from the perpetrator. Psychotherapy for the perpetrator is warranted.
- As long as the perpetrator is in need of intensive psychotherapy, the patient should be protected.

 Follow-Up

If the perpetrator agrees to seek help, improvement usually occurs, but long-term follow-up is necessary.

SIGNS TO WATCH FOR

- Recurrence of original presentation, unusual new symptoms

 Common Questions and Answers

Q: Is it legal to use video surveillance or to separate the parent from the patient?
A: If suspicions of MSBP are high and other laboratory tests are negative, it is important to make the diagnosis. Hospital administration and/or risk management should be consulted on how to proceed.

Q: Should this be reported to child abuse authorities?
A: If documented, this should be reported to protect the child.

ICD-9-CM 301.51

BIBLIOGRAPHY

Anderson J, McKane JB. Munchausen syndrome by proxy and apnea. *Br J Hosp Med* 1996;56(1):43–45.

Babcock J, et al. Rodenticide-induced coagulopathy in a young child. A case of Munchausen syndrome by proxy. *Am J Pediatr Hematol Oncol* 1993;15(1):126–130.

Baskin DE, Stein R, Coats DK, Paysse EA. Recurrent conjunctivitis as a presentation of Munchausen syndrome by proxy. *Ophthalmology* 2003;110(8):1582–1584.

Berg B, Jones DP. Outcome of psychiatric intervention in factitious illness by proxy. *Arch Dis Child* 1999;81(6):465–472.

Bryk M, Siegel PT. "My mother caused my illness": the story of a survivor of Munchausen by proxy syndrome. *Pediatrics* 1997;100(1):1–7.

D'Avanzo M, et al. Concealed administration of furosemide simulating Bartter syndrome in a 4.5 year old boy. *Pediatr Nephrol* 1995;9(6):749–750.

Hall DE, et al. Evaluation of covert video surveillance in the diagnosis of Munchausen syndrome by proxy: lessons from 41 cases. *Pediatrics* 2000;105(6):1305–1312.

Kamerling LB, Black XA, Riser RT. Munchausen syndrome by proxy in the pediatric intensive care unit: An unusual mechanism. *Pediatr Crit Care Med* 2002;3(3):305–307.

Lasher LJ, Feldman MD. Celiac disease as a manifestation of Munchausen by proxy. *South Med J* 2004;97(1):67–69.

Light MJ, Sheridan MS. Munchausen syndrome by proxy and apnea. *Clin Pediatr* 1990;29:162–168.

Magen D, Skorecki K. Extreme hyperkalemia in Munchausen-by-proxy syndrome. *N Engl J Med* 1999;340:1293–1294.

Meadow R. False allegations of abuse and Munchausen syndrome by proxy. *Arch Dis Child* 1993;68(4):444–447.

Meadow R. Management of Munchausen syndrome by proxy. *Arch Dis Child* 1985;60:385–393.

Meadow R. Munchausen syndrome by proxy: the hinterland of child abuse. *Lancet* 1977;2:343–345.

Meadow R. Non-accidental salt poisoning. *Arch Dis Child* 1993;68(4):448–452.

Rand DC, Feldman MD. An explanatory model for Munchausen by proxy abuse. *Int J Psychiatry Med* 2001;31(2):113–126.

Schreier H. Munchausen by proxy defined. *Pediatrics* 2002;110(5):985–988.

Sheridan MS. The deceit continues: an updated literature review of Munchausen Syndrome by proxy. *Child Abuse Negl* 2003;27(4):431–451.

Author: Cheryl L. Hausman

Muscular Dystrophies

 ## Database

DEFINITION

Muscular dystrophies (MDs) are hereditary diseases that cause progressive weakness and degeneration of muscle. MDs frequently involve proximal muscles and may also involve cardiac and smooth muscle. These diseases share similar electromyographic (EMG) and muscle pathologic findings and usually show an elevated creatine kinase (CK). The availability of genetic tests for most forms of MDs has changed the diagnostic approach for these disorders. Forms of MDs include:
- Duchenne muscular dystrophy (DMD)
- Becker muscular dystrophy (BMD)
- Myotonic dystrophy (MyD), sometimes presents in neonates as congenital myotonic dystrophy (CMyD)
- Emery-Dreifuss muscular dystrophy (EDMD)
- Facioscapulohumeral muscular dystrophy (FMD)
- Limb-girdle muscular dystrophy (LGMD)
- Congenital muscular dystrophies (CMDs): Fukuyama-type, merosin-deficient type, others

PATHOPHYSIOLOGY

Slowly, progressive weakness involves all muscle groups—some worse than others—in a symmetric fashion.
Common pathologic findings:
- Loss of muscle cells and residual muscle fibers have variability in size.
- Segmental necrosis of the muscle fiber and some regenerative activity
- Accumulation of lipocytes and collagen between muscle fibers
- Smooth muscle and heart are also affected.
- In some types (MyD, EDMD, DMD, BMD, FMD), innervation of the muscle is also affected. The milder clinical course in BMD corresponds to a milder degree of dystrophin deficiency that can be measured in muscle.
- Brain pathology: deficiency of membrane-associated cytoskeletal proteins (e.g., in DMD) also interferes with brain development.

GENETICS

- DMD and BMD are X-linked recessive. One half of cases are sporadic and are a result of new mutations in the dystrophin gene.
- MyD is autosomal dominant.
- EDMD is X-linked recessive (chromosome Xq28), autosomal dominant or autosomal recessive (chromosome 1q21).
- FMD is autosomal dominant, a result of deletions on chromosome 4q35.
- LGMD: Autosomal-recessive types: mutations in α-sarcoglycan gene (17q); β-sarcoglycan gene (4q); γ-sarcoglycan gene (13q); δ-sarcoglycan gene (5q); calpain-3 gene (15q); dysferlin gene (2q); telethonin gene (17q).
- Autosomal-dominant type: mutation in caveolin-3 gene (3q)
- CMDs are autosomal recessive. To date these mutations have been identified:

—Laminin-α-2 gene (6q22): primary merosin deficiency CMD type
—Fukutin gene (9q): Fukuyama CMD type (mostly in Japan)

EPIDEMIOLOGY

- The incidence of DMD is 1 in 3,500 live male births.
- The estimated minimum incidence of MyD is 1 in 8,000, and BMD is 3 to 6 per 100,000 male births.
- Other forms of MD are less common.

COMPLICATIONS

- Patients with DMD usually die in their twenties of heart failure or pneumonia.
- MyD patients frequently die of cardiomyopathy and respiratory failure. Other features include:
- Posterior capsular cataracts, ptosis, and ophthalmoplegia are common in adults.
- Gastrointestinal dysmotility is common in all age groups.
- Hyperinsulinemia with peripheral resistance to insulin, testicular and ovarian atrophy, and hypersomnolence also occur.
- Severe and potentially fatal cardiac arrhythmias are common in EDMD.
- CMDs are often fatal by the end of the first decade because of respiratory failure.
- Cerebro-ocular muscular dystrophy (muscle-eye-brain disease) has ocular anomalies and cerebral malformations (also known as Walker-Warburg syndrome).
- Orthopaedic complications, such as arthrogryposis, contractures, kyphoscoliosis, and lumbar lordosis, frequently occur in CMDs, CMyD, EDMD, DMD, and BMD.
- Retinal telangiectasias are common in FMD.

ASSOCIATED CONDITIONS

- MR or learning difficulty, except in Becker dystrophy, LGMD, FMD, some cases of CMD.
- Seizures: occasional in DMD and CMD
- Sensorineural deafness: some cases of FMD
- A variant of malignant hyperthermia with general anesthesia may occur in MDs.

 ## Differential Diagnosis

- Nonneurologic disorders that may superficially appear to cause muscle weakness include factitious weakness and any disorder causing pain with movement.
- Electrolyte disturbance may acutely produce muscle weakness (hypercalcemia, hypokalemia).
- Weakness as a result of other neurologic disorders that may mimic muscular dystrophy:
—Polyneuropathy: hereditary neuropathy, such as Charcot-Marie-Tooth disease or acquired neuropathy (chronic inflammatory demyelinating polyneuropathy)
—Spinal dysraphism
—Motor neuron disease
—Myasthenia gravis
—Motor degenerative disorders or acquired structural CNS lesions (neoplastic, vascular, or demyelinating)

—Muscle diseases (electromyography usually abnormal) such as inflammatory myopathies, periodic paralyses, and congenital myopathies
—Metabolic myopathies

- Disorders causing creatine kinase isoenzyme elevation: infectious, inflammatory, and metabolic myopathies, hypothyroid myopathy, muscular trauma, and malignant hyperthermia
- Myopathy and medication: steroids, Mevacor (lovastatin), alcohol, penicillamine, antimalarials, and antiparasitic medication

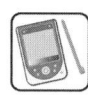 ## Data Gathering

HISTORY

- Age and rapidity of symptom onset
- Symptoms progressive or static
- Disability indicates symmetric, usually proximal, pattern of involvement.
- Pre- and perinatal history is important: paucity of fetal movements, polyhydramnios, neonatal hypotonia, or respiratory failure could be the first sign of MD.
- Pain, fasciculations, rash, or marked fluctuation in weakness are not features of MD.
- Exposure to certain medications (diuretics, steroids, Mevacor) or toxins may suggest alternative causes of muscle weakness (see Differential Diagnosis, above).
- Detailed developmental and family histories are essential.
- DMD is usually apparent by the third year of life, with frequent falls, waddling gait, lumbar lordosis, difficulty climbing stairs, and difficulty arising from the floor. Most boys are wheelchair-bound by 13 years of age and die of cardiac or respiratory failure in their twenties.
- BMD appears usually beyond age 6 years. Progression is slower, and death usually occurs beyond the third decade. Sometimes presents with discolored urine (myoglobinuria).
- CMyD presents with generalized hypotonia, respiratory distress, facial diplegia, distal limb weakness, and skeletal deformities at birth. The long-term prognosis poor: 50% survive into their thirties. Requirement of mechanical ventilation beyond 1 month of age is a poor indicator. Adults with MyD may be diagnosed when CMyD appears in the family, because of weakness during immobilization or during workup for arrhythmias.
- EDMD presents between ages 5 and 15 years with weakness of upper arms and peroneal muscles. Flexion contractures are common in the elbows, neck, and calf muscles. Progression is slow, but some patients have fatal cardiac arrhythmias.
- FMD has onset between ages 5 and 25 years, with weakness of facial, shoulder, and upper arm musculature. There is an inability to close the eyes, whistle, drink through a straw, and raise the arms above the head. Progression is slow, often with periods of nearly complete arrest.

- Autosomal-recessive LGMD has a DMD phenotype in girls and boys and begins between ages 5 and 10 years. In contrast to DMD, the cognitive function is normal.
- Autosomal-dominant LGMD begins in the second or third decade with complaints similar to those of DMD.
- CMDs have neuromuscular symptoms similar to those of CMyD, but may also have brain or ophthalmologic disease as well. Progression is variable, but most die in the first decade.

 ## Physical Examination

- Resting tachycardia may be an early sign of cardiomyopathy in DMD and CMyD. The respiratory pattern may reflect hypoventilation from weakness of respiratory muscles.
- Children with decreased vital capacity may have a rapid, shallow breathing pattern.
- Check for contractures, scoliosis/lordosis, and pseudohypertrophy.
- There is frontal balding and testicular atrophy in MyD.
- Neurologic
—Cognitive developmental milestones, weakness of facial and shoulder girdle muscles. Functional testing may be most helpful in documenting extremity weakness: The ability of the child to raise the arms over the head, write, stand from a seated position, run, squat, sit up from supine position, may be more reproducible, especially when different examiners are involved in follow-up. Myotonia, seen in CMyD and MyD, is a sustained contraction of skeletal muscle in response to voluntary contraction or percussion. It is clinically apparent as an inability to release a hand grip or jaw clench. Deep tendon reflexes are diminished.
—Muscle enlargement also may be seen in motor neuron disease, glycogen storage diseases, hypothyroidism, and amyloidosis. The calf muscles in DMD feel rubbery (pseudohypertrophy).
—Toe walking is also seen in spastic diplegia, spinal tumors, spinal dysraphism, hereditary neuropathies, benign/developmental.
—The Gower sign (propping hands on thighs on rising) and a waddling gait (increased rotational movement of hips) suggest pelvic weakness. The patient stands and walks on a wide base.
—Infants with CMDs and CMyD are hypotonic, with frog-leg posture and head lag: They may be indistinguishable on examination from spinal muscular atrophy, except that MD does not cause tongue fasciculations.

 ## Laboratory Aids

TESTS

- Chemistry: creatine kinase (CK), aspartate aminotransferase (SGOT), alanine aminotransferase (SGOT), lactate dehydrogenase (LDK), and aldolase. Of these,

the CK MM isoenzyme is the most sensitive and specific for primary muscle disease.
—CK measurement should be done before EMG (EMG can raise CK).
—DMD and the Fukuyama-type CMD have the highest CK level. CK level falls with progression of disease as muscle mass decreases. CK level is usually elevated in female carriers of DMD and BMD.
- Molecular genetics: DNA-based mutation studies using polymerase chain reaction (PCR) and Southern blot assay are available for DMD, BMD, EDMD, FMD, LGMD, primary merosin- and Fukuyama-type CMDs.
- The role of traditional diagnostic tests such as electromyography (EMG), nerve conduction studies (NCS), and muscle biopsy has diminished in the era of molecular DNA testing. These tests are now performed in patients with negative genetic analysis, atypical presentation. Immunohistochemistry may be necessary to make a specific diagnosis.
- Immunologic: Muscle biopsy tissue can be immunostained specifically for the presence of dystrophin, emerin, sarcoglycans, dysferlin, calpain-3, telethonin, merosin, and fukutin. These proteins can be quantified by Western blot analysis. Dystrophin is measured in fetal muscle biopsies in difficult cases.
- Electrophysiologic: EMG/NCS helps to differentiate anterior horn cell disease, peripheral neuropathy, and neuromuscular junction disorder from myopathy. In myopathic conditions, nerve conduction velocity is normal, but motor unit action potentials have shortened duration and lower amplitude.
—Spontaneous trains of discharges by inserting the EMG needle are characteristic for myotonia.
- Electrocardiography (ECG) may reveal tall R waves and a deep Q wave in DMD and A-V block in EDMD.
- Prenatal diagnosis possible

 ## Emergency Care

- Respiratory failure: DMD, MyD, CMyD, and CMDs.
- Cardiac or arrhythmias in DMD, MyD, and EDMD.

 ## Therapy

- For DMD, corticosteroids—deflazacort or prednisone, initiated at approximately 6 to 12 years, can prolong walking for 1 to 2 years, but watch for weight gain, other side effects.
- Mainly supportive. Passive muscle stretching and night splinting delay contractures. Maintenance of upright posture delays scoliosis. Major surgery or long bed rest should be avoided while the patient is still walking. Cataract surgery is recommended in MyD. Attention to healthy diet to avoid obesity; exercise as tolerated; swimming is useful; intubation and mechanical ventilation in infantile forms; pacemakers for arrhythmias.

- Vitamin therapies or specific diets have not been proven beneficial, but in many cases effects on disease markers have not been formally tested.
- Dilantin (phenytoin) and Tegretol (carbamazepine) may be helpful for myotonia, but the myotonia of MyD is usually not troublesome. Metoclopramide is useful in gastroparesis.
- Gene therapy is not currently available for any of these disorders.

PITFALLS

- Pain is usually not present in MDs, but polymyositis, dermatomyositis, and infectious myositis may be painful.
- Dermatomyositis has a typical rash not seen in MD.

 ## Follow-Up

- Best done in multidisciplinary neuromuscular clinics.

Common Questions and Answers

Q: What is the recurrence risk in DMD?
A: Because of new mutations, the mothers of probands may not be carriers. Each time a carrier (heterozygous woman) has a child, there is a 25% chance it will be an affected male. Each time a heterozygous mother has a son, the chance that she will transmit the abnormal gene is 50%. Each time a daughter is born, she will have a 50% chance of being a carrier. Affected males transmit the gene to all of their daughters.

ICD-9-CM 359.1

BIBLIOGRAPHY

Basil BT, Jones HR Jr. Diagnosis of pediatric neuromuscular disorders in the era of DNA analysis. *Pediatr Neurol* 2000;23:289–300.

Bushby K. Genetics and the muscular dystrophies. *Dev Med Child Neurol* 2000;42:780–784.

Do T. Orthopedic management of the muscular dystrophies. *Curr Opin Pediatr* 2002;14(1):50–53.

Mathews KD. Muscular dystrophy overview: genetics and diagnosis. *Neurol Clin* 2003;21(4):795–816.

Online information for Parents: Muscular Dystrophy Association: www.mda.org.

Roland EH. Muscular dystrophy. *Pediatr Rev* 2000;21(7):233–237.

Author: Peter M. Bingham and *Olafur Thorarensen, 3rd edition*

Myasthenia Gravis

 Database

DEFINITION

Myasthenia gravis presents as intermittent weakness that worsens with exercise and improves with rest. The majority of patients present with ptosis and diplopia alone or in combination with swallowing difficulties and generalized weakness. It is caused by a disruption in signal transmission from the motor neuron to the muscle. There are no sensory or cognitive symptoms.

PATHOPHYSIOLOGY

• The motor nerve terminal lies in close proximity to the end plate, a region of the muscle cell membrane with a high concentration of acetylcholine receptors. When stimulated, the motor nerve terminal releases vesicles of acetylcholine that traverse the synaptic cleft and bind to the receptors, causing contraction of the muscle. The cleft contains acetylcholinesterase, an enzyme that breaks down acetylcholine and helps terminate the muscle contractions. In the common autoimmune form of myasthenia, an autoantibody binds to the acetylcholine receptor, and blocks its activity. The rate of receptor breakdown also increases and fewer receptors are present, resulting in decreased muscle contraction. Thymic pathology is believed central to the pathogenesis of autoimmune myasthenia; hyperplasia is present in most children who undergo thymectomy.
• In neonatal myasthenia, infants are born with weakness and hypotonia as a result of maternal-fetal transmission of antibodies against the acetylcholine receptor. The severity of maternal symptoms does not predict the likelihood that the infant will be affected. Occasional arthrogryposis (joint contractures) reflects in utero paralysis from transplacental transmission of the antibody. High levels of maternal antibodies against the fetal form of the acetylcholine receptor correspond to an increased risk of disease. A previous pregnancy with an affected infant places future pregnancies at much higher risk. In rare cases, the mother is asymptomatic, despite presence of a placentally transmitted antibody.

EPIDEMIOLOGY

Three types of myasthenia gravis seen in childhood: neonatal transient, congenital myasthenia, and juvenile myasthenia.

• Neonatal transient: 10% to 20% of infants born to mothers with autoimmune myasthenia
• Congenital myasthenia: rare; less than 10% of all childhood myasthenia. Weakness usually starts in the first year of life and is caused by an inherited disorder in neuromuscular transmission. Mutations have been described in the presynaptic nerve terminal, acetylcholinesterase, acetylcholine receptors, and postsynaptic proteins.

• Juvenile myasthenia: an autoimmune disorder similar to adult-onset, autoimmune myasthenia gravis; caused by aberrant production of antibodies against the acetylcholine receptor. It is relatively rare, with one new diagnosis per million patients per year. The average age of onset is 10 to 13 years, with a female predominance of 2:1 or 4:1.

PROGNOSIS

• Neonatal transient: a self-limited disorder that resolves spontaneously over the first few months of life as maternal antibodies disappear. The infant may require ventilatory and nutritional support during the first few months of life. Infants with arthrogryposis multiplex congenita (born to mothers with antibodies against the fetal form of acetylcholine receptors) may gain mobility with time.
• Congenital myasthenia: Prognosis varies, depending on the specific defect. Autosomal-recessive disorders tend to be more severe than the dominant disorders. Weakness shows variable response to cholinesterase inhibitors. Immunosuppressants are not helpful. In general, these are indolent disorders. Ptosis and fatigability resemble the juvenile type, but are more stable over time.
• Juvenile myasthenia: Most patients do extremely well with treatment. Longitudinal studies suggest that the rate of spontaneous remission is approximately 2% per year and can occur throughout the lifetime of the patient. Patients with generalized weakness are slightly less likely to experience remission. The mortality rate from myasthenia is near that of the general population in patients under 50 years of age.

ASSOCIATED ILLNESSES

In juvenile myasthenia, other autoimmune disorders may occur: hyperthyroidism is present in 3% to 9% of patients, and there is a small increase in the incidence of rheumatoid arthritis and diabetes. Some reports suggest an increased incidence of seizures in autoimmune myasthenia. Screening for thymoma at initial diagnosis is appropriate (by chest CT scan)—children appear to have a lower incidence of this tumor than adults in the setting of autoimmune myasthenia.

 Differential Diagnosis

• Generalized botulism

—In specific endemic areas, may cause generalized weakness in infants. It is caused by a Clostridium toxin that blocks the release of acetylcholine from the nerve terminal.
—The infant usually presents with generalized hypotonia and a poor suck for days (or weeks). Prominent symptoms unique to botulism are constipation and pupillary dilation. Nerve conduction studies and stool

tests for the botulism toxin confirm the diagnosis.

• Guillain-Barré syndrome, or acute inflammatory demyelinating polyneuropathy, is a frequent cause of rapidly progressive generalized weakness. Unlike myasthenia, there are often sensory symptoms, and areflexia occurs even with minimal weakness.
• Acute spinal cord compression can present as generalized weakness of the extremities. Look for sparing of facial and extraocular muscles, look for a sensory level, bowel or bladder dysfunction, and hyperactive reflexes.
• Organophosphate ingestion or an overdose of Mestinon (pyridostigmine bromide) can cause profound weakness. Symptoms of parasympathetic hyperactivity, such as hypersalivation, miosis, diarrhea, and bradycardia, will usually be present.
• Penicillamine is used for the treatment of autoimmune disorders and can induce autoantibodies that bind the acetylcholine receptor, causing myasthenia gravis. The weakness usually resolves when the drug is stopped.

 Data Gathering

HISTORY

• Transient neonatal: mother with known autoimmune myasthenia or a history of weakness, ptosis, or dysphagia.
• Congenital myasthenia: usually presents in the first year of life (rarely later) with hypotonia, poor feeding, ptosis, and delayed motor milestones. Possible family history of similar weakness. No response to thymectomy or immunosuppressant medications.
• Juvenile myasthenia: gradual onset of weakness over weeks, months, or even years. The symptoms are worse after prolonged activity or late in the day. Intermittent ptosis, diplopia, dysphagia, and dysphonia are common.

 Physical Examination

• Neonatal: from birth, the infant is hypotonic, with a weak suck, a weak cry, and ptosis.
• Congenital and juvenile myasthenia:

—Weakness of neck flexion
—Ptosis, ophthalmoplegia, variable feeding problems are often the earliest findings.
—Generalized weakness may be asymmetric in the limbs. The weakness is more pronounced with endurance tasks.
—Shallow, rapid respirations suggest impending ventilatory failure. Vital capacity of less than 50% of predicted (in older children) suggests impending respiratory failure.

Laboratory Aids

JUVENILE MYASTHENIA

• Nerve conduction and electromyography studies: Repetitive stimulation of a nerve shows a diagnostic "decremental response" as a result of decreased acetylcholine receptors. Single-fiber electromyography measures the variability in firing rates of two muscle fibers innervated by different branches of the same motor neuron. A large variability, "jitter," suggests a higher threshold for activation because of a limited number of acetylcholine receptors.
• Acetylcholine receptor antibody levels (most specific): elevated in approximately 80% of patients with generalized myasthenia. Only 50% of patients with isolated ocular myasthenia have an elevated level.
• Edrophonium chloride is a fast-acting acetylcholinesterase-blocking agent. Patients with myasthenia often show an immediate, transient improvement in muscle strength after intravenous infusion of this drug. A measurable weakness should be present prior to testing, and a placebo dose of saline should be given initially. Though the risk of a hyperreactive cholinergic response with muscle weakness and bradycardia is low, atropine should always be available, and the patient's vital signs should be closely monitored during the test, which is contraindicated in patients with heart disease. Measurable cranial nerve dysfunction, such as ptosis, is often responsive to edrophonium.
• Children receive 20% of a 0.2-mg/kg dose of Tensilon over 1 minute; if there is no response after 45 seconds, the rest of the dose is then given, up to a maximum of 10 mg. Have atropine and epinephrine readily available.

Emergency Care

Respiratory failure is a rare but serious complication of juvenile myasthenia gravis. Shallow breathing, a vital capacity of less than 50% predicted, or a rapidly worsening vital capacity suggests impending respiratory failure.

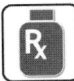 ## Therapy

• Neonatal myasthenia: severity of disability should be used to guide the aggressiveness of therapy. Respiratory or swallowing impairment: pyridostigmine syrup, 60 mg/ 5 mL, 7 mg/kg, 30 minutes before feeds. 1 mg intramuscular = 30 mg oral dose.
• Juvenile myasthenia: most patients benefit from pyridostigmine bromide (Mestinon) given three to four times per day. A long-acting formulation prior to bedtime may alleviate obstructive hypoventilation during sleep. Pyridostigmine improves strength by blocking acetylcholinesterase activity. A normal starting dosage is approximately 7 mg/kg per day. The dosage is slowly titrated upward, following symptoms, at several-day intervals. Common side effects are hypersalivation, blurry vision, and diarrhea. Glycopyrrolate, 1 mg by mouth, may decrease diarrhea.
• Prednisone: considered in patients with disabling symptoms and inadequate response to pyridostigmine. Watch for transient worsening within weeks in up to 50% of patients. Start daily dose at 2 mg/kg, watch for improvement in 3 to 6 weeks, taper toward 1.5 mg/kg per day on alternate-day schedule for 4 months. Taper slowly thereafter by 5 mg/week. Monitor for side effects, including growth stunting. Calcium and every-other-day dosing limit the bone deterioration from chronic steroids.
• Azathioprine induces remission in 30% of patients and results in significant improvement in another 25% to 60%. Azathioprine is a useful adjunctive to steroids and thymectomy; however, it takes 3 to 12 months for its suppressant effects to occur. In one long-term study of juvenile myasthenia, there was no increased risk of cancer or infection with the use of azathioprine.
• Thymectomy generally results in a 20% to 60% remission, and another 15% to 30% of patients show a marked improvement after surgery. As surgical techniques for thymectomy have improved, the complications and recovery times have decreased. Thymectomy earlier in the course of illness appears to produce a higher rate of remission. 80% to 90% of patients undergoing thymectomy have thymic hyperplasia. Effect of thymectomy on risk of infection or autoimmune disorders is uncertain, but apparently not large.
• Juvenile myasthenics with profound weakness and respiratory failure should undergo immediate therapy to decrease the number of circulating receptor antibodies. Plasmapheresis or intravenous immunoglobulin can be effective within a few days by decreasing or diluting, respectively, the acetylcholine receptor antibodies. Steroids diminish antibody production within weeks to months.

Newer immunosuppressants have been reported to be effective in small case series for refractory myasthenia gravis, including Mycophenolate mofetil, and anti-CD20.

 ## Follow-Up

• The following medications can exacerbate myasthenia gravis:

—Corticosteroids may worsen symptoms, but usually only briefly, after increasing the dose.
—Aminoglycosides
—Ciprofloxacin
—β-adrenergic blocking agents, including eyedrops
—Lithium
—Procainamide
—Quinidine
—Phenytoin

• Prolonged recovery of strength after exposure to nondepolarizing neuromuscular blocking agents.
• Always start new medications cautiously.

ICD-9-CM 358.0

Neonatal 775.2

BIBLIOGRAPHY

Gardnerova M, Eymard B, Morel E, et al. The fetal/adult acetylcholine receptor antibody ration in mothers with myasthenia gravis as a marker for transfer of the disease to the newborn. *Neurology* 1997;48:50–54.

Lindner A, Schalke B, Toyka VK. Outcome in juvenile-onset myasthenia gravis: a retrospective study with long-term follow up. *J Neurol* 1997;244:515–520.

Newsom-Davis J. Therapy in myasthenia gravis and Lambert-Eaton myasthenic syndrome. *Semin Neurol* 2003;23:191–198.

Parent Internet Information. Myasthenia Foundation America. Available at http://www.myasthenia.org. Accessed March 10, 2005.

Selcen D, Dabrowski ER, Michon AM, et al. High-dose intravenous immunoglobulin therapy in juvenile myasthenia gravis. *Pediatr Neurol* 2000;22:40–43.

Wittbrodt ET. Drugs and myasthenia gravis: an update. *Arch Intern Med* 1997;157(4):399–408.

Authors: Brenda E. Porter and Grant T. Liu

Myocarditis

Database

DEFINITION

Myocarditis is defined as an inflammation of the myocardium with associated myocellular necrosis.

EPIDEMIOLOGY

- True incidence of acute myocarditis is difficult to estimate because of the wide range in clinical severity. Estimates of the incidence of clinically significant disease in tertiary care facilities have been as high as 0.3% in some case series.
- Cases are more prevalent in the summer months, likely owing to the higher prevalence of enteroviral infections during this season.
- Cardiovascular complications are a rare complication of viral infection, despite their ubiquitous nature.
- May account for more than 15% of cases of sudden infant death syndrome and 60% of cases of peripartum cardiomyopathy.

ETIOLOGY

- Causes of myocarditis may include various infections, drugs, toxins, and systemic diseases. "Idiopathic" myocarditis, however, remains the most common form encountered.
- Among the many infectious agents, viral, bacterial, rickettsial, fungal, and parasitic organisms have been linked to myocarditis.
- In the United States and Europe, viruses are the most frequent infectious cause of myocarditis. Recent studies suggest that adenovirus is the most common viral agent, with enteroviruses (e.g., Coxsackievirus B), also playing a prominent role. Other viruses include Epstein-Barr virus, human herpesvirus, parvovirus B19, human immunodeficiency virus, influenza, and hepatitis C virus.
- Worldwide, *Trypanosoma cruzi* (Chagas disease), and *Corynebacterium diphtheria* (diphtheria) are common causes.
- Recent reinitiation of smallpox vaccination has resulted in recurrence of Vaccinia
- Among the drugs and toxins, cocaine abuse and enterotoxins (occurring during septic shock) have been associated with acute onset of cardiac dysfunction.
- Giant cell myocarditis is a rare, very severe form, associated with various systemic autoimmune diseases, including systemic lupus erythematosis, rheumatic fever, and Kawasaki disease.

PATHOPHYSIOLOGY

- Although many agents, including viruses, may exert direct cytotoxic effects, it is the subsequent autoimmune response that appears to be the major factor leading to cellular injury. This theory is supported by studies linking persistence of viral RNA in the myocardium with induction of autoantibodies and resultant ventricular dysfunction.

- Recent work has identified the coxsackie-adenovirus receptor, offering insight into both the cardiac tropism of these agents and an explanation for the infrequent occurrence of viral myocarditis despite the ubiquitous nature of the agents.
- Regardless of the etiology, symptom severity increases with worsening ventricular function. Fulminant myocarditis may be characterized by both severe systolic and diastolic dysfunction. Progressive left ventricular (LV) systolic dysfunction may lead to hypotension, acidosis and end-organ hypoperfusion. LV diastolic dysfunction may result in elevated LV end-diastolic pressures, leading to pulmonary venous and arterial hypertension, with possible concomitant pulmonary edema.

PROGNOSIS

- Exact statistics are hampered by the lack of complete ascertainment of all cases of acute myocarditis, with many patients likely exhibiting only mild symptoms, which spontaneously resolve.
- Of those patients who present with acute left ventricular failure, approximately one-third will make a full recovery, one-third will develop a stable dilated cardiomyopathy, and one-third will progress to irreversible ventricular failure, necessitating either chronic, mechanical support, or cardiac transplantation.
- A recent report in adults would suggest that those presenting with fulminant myocarditis are far more likely to demonstrate recovery of ventricular function than those presenting with acute myocarditis (without severe initial ventricular impairment) alone.
- Giant cell myocarditis represents a unique subgroup with a particularly poor prognosis—in one series, more than 70% of patients had either died or been transplanted at 1 year from the time of diagnosis.

Differential Diagnosis

- Severe left-sided obstructive heart lesions: mitral stenosis, valvar aortic stenosis, coarctation of the aorta
- Congenital coronary artery anomalies: anomalous left coronary artery from the pulmonary artery and other coronary variants
- Incessant arrhythmias: incessant supraventricular tachycardia, ventricular tachycardia
- Metabolic disorders: selenium and carnitine deficiency
- Mitochondrial disorders
- Genetic syndromes: muscular dystrophies, familial cardiomyopathies

Data Gathering

HISTORY

- Prodromal symptoms: antecedent flu-like illness, gastroenteritis, rheumatologic symptoms, fever
- Duration and presence of symptoms of left heart failure: exercise intolerance, easy fatigability, dyspnea, orthopnea, anorexia, loss of appetite/poor feeding, early satiety, emesis (especially in children)
- Duration and presence of symptoms of right heart failure: abdominal pain/cramping, swelling of abdomen/lower extremities, loose stools
- Travel history
- Family history

Physical Examination

Any of the following may be present:

- Pulmonary

—Rales
—Tachypnea
—Retractions

- Cardiovascular

—Jugular venous distension
—Normal to hyperdynamic precordium +/− right ventricular heave
—Lateral displacement of the point of maximal impulse (PMI)
—Tachycardia
—Arrhythmia (atrial and/or ventricular ectopy may be present)
—Accentuation of second heart sound (secondary to pulmonary artery hypertension)
—Murmur (mitral and/or tricuspid insufficiency)
—Gallop

- Abdomen

—Hepatomegaly

- Extremities

—Weak pulses
—Poor capillary refill
—Cool extremities

Laboratory Aids

Despite limited sensitivity and specificity, endomyocardial biopsy, using the Dallas criteria for histopathologic classification, remains the criterion standard for confirming the diagnosis of acute myocarditis. Recent studies, however, would suggest that isolation of viral genome from tracheal aspirates in the proper clinical setting may have similar diagnostic accuracy to endomyocardial biopsy (which would eliminate the risk of cardiac perforation with the procedure). Other studies supportive of the diagnosis may include:

IMAGING STUDIES

• Chest radiograph: cardiomegaly and varying degrees of pulmonary edema, possible pleural effusions
• Echocardiogram: key findings would include:

—Impaired systolic and/or diastolic ventricular function
—Cardiac chamber enlargement
—Valvar insufficiency (particularly mitral valve insufficiency)

• Autoimmune (Gallium-67) scintigraphy: sensitive, but not specific for acute myocarditis
• Contrast-enhanced magnetic resonance imaging

LABORATORY STUDIES

• Elevated inflammatory markers: erythrocyte sedimentation rate, C-reactive protein
• Elevated markers of myocardial injury: creatine kinase MB fraction, troponin levels
• Cultures (bacterial, viral, fungal) of blood, urine, stool, and nasopharynx may be considered
• Enteroviral PCR of nasopharynx or stool
• Acute and convalescent serologic studies may be considered for selected antibody studies
• Promising markers may include autoimmune serum markers and autoantibodies (anti-adenosine nucleotide translocator, anti-myosin)

OTHER STUDIES

• Electrocardiogram: highly variable findings may include low QRS voltages, ST segment changes, T-wave flattening or inversion, prolongation of the QT interval and arrhythmias (atrial premature beats, atrial fibrillation, or ventricular premature beats)

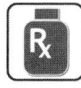 ## Therapy

Major advances in therapy have been realized over the last decade:

• Bed rest and limited activity (during acute phase)
• Standard medical regimens

—Diuretics
—ACE inhibitors
—β-blockers
—+/− Digitalis (animal models suggest increased expression of proinflammatory cytokines and higher mortality rate with higher doses)
—+/− Antiarrhythmics (in cases of hemodynamically significant dysrhythmias)

• Immunosuppression

—High-dose gamma globulin (2 g/kg IVIG over 24 hours) during the acute phase has been associated with improved recovery of LV function and with a tendency to better survival during the first year after presentation

—Steroids, azathioprine, calcineurin-inhibitors, Cytoxan, and OKT3 have all been suggested as effective agents, though insufficient evidence of therapeutic benefit is currently available to recommend routine use

• Mechanical support (in patients with rapidly progressing, severe heart failure; used as a bridge to transplantation)

—Left- or biventricular assist devices
—Extracorporeal membrane oxygenation (ECMO)

• Rescue therapy

—Cardiac transplantation

• Novel therapies (not currently in routine clinical use as a result of a lack of preponderance of evidence of therapeutic benefit)

—Antigenic tolerance, monoclonal antibodies directed at the coxsackie-adenovirus receptor, antiviral agents (including protease inhibitors)

 ## Follow-Up

• Patients with acute myocarditis require close and coordinated follow-up between their pediatric cardiologist and general pediatrician.
• Pediatric cardiology follow-up should be based on the severity of clinical symptoms, the degree of myocardial depression, associated arrhythmias, and longitudinal changes in cardiac function. Additional testing (as described previously) would be expected to monitor for resolution of any inflammatory response and cardiac performance.
• General pediatric follow-up is essential to monitor for interval clinical changes in cardiac function, as well as effects of the illness on other systems: nutritional status, growth, development, and co-morbid illnesses.

 ## Common Questions and Answers

Q: Is acute myocarditis contagious?
A: For some causes of acute myocarditis (drug, toxin, autoimmune, and idiopathic), there is no risk of catching the illness. The degree of contagiousness for infectious causes depends significantly on the particular agent. For most cases of infectious acute myocarditis, viruses are to blame. These viruses are usually ubiquitous in the community, so that the chance an individual has not previously been exposed is usually low. Furthermore, the development of acute myocarditis is rare and usually requires a genetically susceptible person, so that any one individual's chances of contracting the disease are very remote.

Q: Do children with acute myocarditis require subacute bacterial endocarditis (SBE) prophylaxis?
A: The requirement for SBE prophylaxis is solely dependent on the presence of valvular insufficiency and/or intracardiac thrombus. Absence of both of these would imply that SBE prophylaxis is not indicated. However, all elective procedures should be first considered in the context of cardiac function, presence of ongoing inflammation, associated arrhythmias, need for/type of sedation, and necessity of the procedure.

Q: What kinds of activity restrictions should be placed on children with acute myocarditis?
A: During the acute phases of the illness (although active inflammation is present), bed rest and only limited (nonexertional) activity should be encouraged. Activity restrictions after that time depend significantly on the degree of ventricular dysfunction and any associated arrhythmias. Often patients who have had complete recovery of ventricular function may eventually resume all normal activities.

ICD-9-CM

Secondary to rheumatic fever 398.0
Acute myocarditis 422.90

BIBLIOGRAPHY

Batra AS, Lewis AB. Acute myocarditis. *Curr Opin Pediatr* 2001;13:234–239.

Bowles NE, Ni J, Kearney DL, et al. Detection of viruses in myocardial tissues by polymerase chain reaction. Evidence of adenovirus as a common cause of myocarditis in children and adults. *J Am Coll Cardiol* 2003;42(3):473–476.

Drucker NA, Colan SD, Lewis AB, et al. Gamma-globulin treatment of acute myocarditis in the pediatric population. *Circulation* 1994;89:252–257.

Feldman AM, McNamara D. Myocarditis. *N Engl J Med* 2000;343(19):1388–1398.

Halsell JS, Riddle JR, Atwood JE, et al. Myopericarditis following smallpox vaccination among vaccinia-naive US military personnel. *JAMA* 2003;289(24):3283–3289.

Wong ML, O'Kirwan F, Khan N, et al. Identification, characterization, and gene expression profiling of endotoxin-induced myocarditis. *Proc Nat Acad Sci* 2003;100(24):14241–14246.

Authors: David M. Bush
Bradley S. Marino, 3rd edition

Near Drowning

Database

DEFINITION

Near drowning, or submersion injury, is survival, at least temporarily, after suffocation by submersion in water. Near drowning may be described by the water temperature and tonicity—warm water ($\geq 20°C$), cold water ($<20°C$), or very cold water ($<5°C$)—and as "freshwater" versus "saltwater" near drowning.

CAUSES

• "Wet drowning": aspiration of fluid into the trachea and lungs with either denaturation of surfactant by freshwater or washout of surfactant as a result of saltwater, which results in intrapulmonary shunting and hypoxemia.
• "Dry drowning": hypoxemia from prolonged severe laryngospasm as water enters the larynx when the near-drowning victim becomes hypercapnic and takes an involuntary gasp of air. No fluid is aspirated into the lung.

PATHOPHYSIOLOGY

• Grossly, the lungs are edematous, but not filled with aspirated fluid, with focal hemorrhages.
• Microscopically, there is thinning of the alveolar septum with emphysematous changes and frothy fluid in the airways.

EPIDEMIOLOGY

• Second only to motor vehicle accidents as the most common cause of death as a result of injury in childhood
• Children younger than 5 years of age, especially toddlers and boys, who cannot swim and have direct access to swimming pools are at highest risk.
• Bathtub drowning and near drowning are common in babies, and child neglect or abuse should be considered.
• Adolescent near drowning usually involves substance abuse or risk-taking behavior.
• Children with seizure disorders are at higher risk of near drowning.

COMPLICATIONS

• Brain injury secondary to hypoxia
• Pulmonary injury with intrapulmonary shunting secondary to damage of the alveoli
• ARDS
• Metabolic acidosis secondary to hypoxemia
• Ischemic injury to organs such as liver, kidneys, and intestines
• Disseminated intravascular coagulation (DIC) secondary to ischemia
• Electrolyte abnormalities uncommon; may occur if a large volume of freshwater is in the stomach and not removed
• Hypothermia in cold water near drowning

PROGNOSIS

• Most children (60% to 95%) recover with intact neurologic survival.
• Brain injury and death correlate with degree of hypoxia/anoxia.
• Children with warm water submersion time longer than 4 minutes, who do not receive CPR at the scene and who have absent vital signs or a Glasgow Coma Scale (GCS) score less than 5 in the emergency department, usually have a poor prognosis.
• Victims who have prolonged submersions in very cold water may have good prognosis because of "core" cooling with a concomitant decrease in metabolic rate while the brain is still being perfused.
• A good prognostic indicator is continuing improvement in the neurologic examination over the first several hours.

ASSOCIATED CONDITIONS

• C-spine injuries should be considered in older children with diving accidents.
• Signs of child abuse or neglect (burns, whip marks, bruises) should be sought in young children.
• Toxicology screens should be done for adolescents.

Differential Diagnosis

Children with smoke inhalation or hydrocarbon ingestion may have similar presentations. However, the history and physical examination should easily determine the diagnosis.

Data Gathering

HISTORY

• Mechanism: History of diving injury, intoxication, seizure disorder, child abuse
• Prognostic indicators: Length of submersion, vital signs and examination at scene, CPR done at scene, temperature of water

Physical Examination

• Vital signs with temperature
• Neurologic: pupillary response, cranial nerve findings, GCS score
• Respiratory: Lower airway findings (rales, tachypnea, wheezing, retractions)
• Circulation: perfusion, strength of distal pulses, capillary refill, urine output
• GI: abdominal distension from swallowed water or ventilation

Question: Was the child apneic, cyanotic, or pulseless at the scene?
Significance: If so, the child requires admission and close observation even if he or she appears well at presentation to the hospital.

Question: Did the child fall through ice?
Significance: Very cold water near drowning may have a good prognosis despite submersion time longer than 5 minutes.

Question: What was the estimated time of submersion, and when was CPR begun?
Significance: Shorter time periods (<2–5 minutes) for each answer correlate with better prognosis.

• Near-drowning victims may have deteriorating pulmonary involvement, despite an initially normal examination. Watch closely for signs of lower airway involvement, such as tachypnea, retractions, or rales.
• Serial neurologic examinations with pupillary response should be performed to access neurologic outcome. Children with a GCS score less than 5 after resuscitation usually have a poor neurologic outcome.

Glasgow Coma Scale

RESPONSE	POINTS
1. Eye Opening	
Spontaneous	4
To voice	3
To pain	2
None	1
2. Verbal Response	
Oriented	5
Confused	4
Inappropriate words	3
Incomprehensible words	2
None	1
3. Motor Response	
Obeys commands	6
Purposeful movement (pain)	5
Withdraw (pain)	4
Flexion (pain)	3
Extension (pain)	2
None	1
Total GCS points	(1 + 2 + 3)

Laboratory Aids

TESTS

- Pulse oximetry is a critical aid in assessment of pulmonary involvement in the near-drowning victim. Oxygen saturation less than 97% within 4 hours after the near drowning indicates pulmonary involvement and need for admission.
- Arterial blood gases to detect and treat metabolic acidosis and hyperpnea should be done in the child with respiratory distress or apnea.
- An initial chest radiograph is indicated for endotracheal tube placement in the intubated child and as a baseline film for those with pulmonary involvement.
- Cervical spine films are indicated in the diving accident victim.
- Renal electrolytes are not indicated unless a large volume of water has been swallowed and not evacuated from the stomach.
- Anticonvulsant levels for victims with seizure disorders.
- Toxicology screening when suspected.
- ECG to document normal function and evaluate for prolonged QTC if indicated by history

FALSE POSITIVES

Initial pulse oximetry and chest radiographs may be normal in the near-drowning victim. Victims should be monitored with pulse oximetry for 4 to 6 hours for progressive respiratory distress.

Therapy

- Airway: Protect the C-spine if indicated by history. Ensure a patent airway in the arrested or comatose victim.
- Breathing: Supplemental oxygen for oxygen saturations by pulse oximetry less than 95%. The near-drowning victim should be intubated and positive end-expiratory pressure (PEEP) and ventilation given if apneic or unable to maintain a Pao_2 greater than 60 or a pco_2 less than 50 in 50% supplemental oxygen. Prophylactic antibiotics or steroids are not indicated.
- Circulation:

—For the victim with cardiopulmonary arrest, asystole protocol should be followed, using epinephrine via the ET tube or intravenously and chest compressions done.
—Since capillary leak may occur after an ischemic/anoxic episode, isotonic fluids (e.g., normal saline solution or Ringer's lactate) (10-mL/kg aliquots) should be given for signs of intravascular volume depletion (tachycardia, poor perfusion) until normalized.

—ECG monitoring should be provided with appropriate response to dysrhythmias, especially for the hypothermic, cold water near-drowning victim. For core temperature less than 29.5°C, attempts at electrical defibrillation are not likely to be successful, and "chemical defibrillation" with amiodarone or lidocaine and aggressive rewarming are tried.

- Disability: Maintenance of eucapnia and adequate oxygenation to prevent further hypoxemia. There is no indication for measures to reduce ICP (hyperventilation, barbiturates, mannitol, fluid restoration, ICP monitoring, or steroids) because the brain injury and swelling is secondary to hypoxic cell injury as opposed to a traumatic lesion.
- Exposure: The near-drowning victim should be dried and warmed: for core temperatures 32°C to 35°C, active rewarming with heating blankets or radiant warmers; for less than 32°C, active internal rewarming added (heated aerosolized oxygen and intravenous fluids, gastric lavage with warm saline); for severe very cold water drowning cases and where available, peritoneal or hemodialysis, mediastinal irrigation, and cardiac bypass

DURATION

- The cold water near-drowning victim with hypothermia must be rewarmed to greater than 32°C before CPR is terminated. Remember: "The patient is not dead until he is warm and dead."
- Pulmonary treatment is provided as needed (see Breathing, above). Complications may include pneumonia; pneumothorax or pneumomediation in the ventilated patient; and ARDS.

Follow-Up

- Long-term follow-up of apparently neurologically intact survivors has shown mild coordination or gross motor deficiencies.
- The victim may be at increased risk for chronic lung disease, depending on the degree of pulmonary involvement.

PITFALLS

- Failure to observe near-drowning victim for signs of pulmonary involvement, since late deterioration can occur 24 to 48 hours postincident.
- The hypothermic patient who is a warm water near-drowning victim does not have a good prognosis or need vigorous rewarming.

PREVENTION

- Most drownings are preventable.
- Legislation to require adequate fencing and rescue equipment for public and residential pools
- Restriction of sale and consumption of alcohol in boating areas, pools, and beaches
- Parental education regarding adequate supervision during bathing and around swimming pools

Common Questions and Answers

Q: Should the near-drowning victim who arrives at the hospital with cardiopulmonary arrest be resuscitated?
A: Yes, a brief (10 to 15 minutes) attempt at resuscitation is indicated until circumstances of the near drowning and core temperature are known. Warm water near-drowning victims who require CPR in the emergency department may rarely (0% to 25%) have good neurologic recovery but usually respond quickly (<15 minutes) to therapy.

Q: Is artificial surfactant useful in near-drowning victims?
A: Although useful in neonates, surfactant has not been well studied in near-drowning victims. In a dog model and in addicts with ARDS, it has not been beneficial. Further investigation is needed before it can be recommended for clinical use.

ICD-9-CM 994.1

BIBLIOGRAPHY

American Academy of Pediatrics. Policy Statement: prevention of drowning in infants, children and adolescents. *Pediatrics* 2003; 112(2):437–439.

Biggarat MJ, Bohn D. Effect of hypothermia and cardiac arrest on outcome of near-drowning accidents in children. *J Pediatr* 1990;117:179–183.

Bratton SL, Jardine DS, Morra JF. Serial neurologic examination after near drowning and outcome. *Arch Pediatr Adolesc Med* 1994; 148:167–170.

Diekema DS, Quan L, Holt VL. Epilepsy as a risk factor for submersion injury in children. *Pediatrics* 1993;91(3):612–616.

Hwang V, Shofer FS, Durbin DR, Baren JM. Prevalence of traumatic injuries in drowning and near drowning in children and adolescents. *Arch Pediatr Adolesc Med* 2003; 157(1):50–53.

Lavelle JM, Shaw KN. Ten year review of pediatric bathtub near-drownings: evaluation for child abuse and neglect. *Ann Emerg Med* 1995;25:344–348.

Spack L, Rainer G, Gedeit R, et al. Failure of aggressive therapy to alter outcome in pediatric near-drowning. *Pediatr Emerg Care* 1997;13(2):98–102.

Author: Kathy N. Shaw

Neck Masses

Database

To diagnose and appropriately manage neck masses, one must combine the history with a careful examination of the mass. The major task of the differential diagnosis is to distinguish infections from congenital and malignant causes.

Differential Diagnosis

- **Infectious**

—Reactive hyperplasia: self-limited, usually viral enlargement of bilateral minimally tender nodes
—Bacterial lymphadenitis: usually staphylococcal or streptococcal infection of unilateral, tender, swollen, warm, erythematous node. In neonates, a cellulitis-adenitis syndrome is usually caused by group B streptococcus.
—Cat-scratch disease: sometimes protracted illness caused by the gram-negative bacillus *Bartonella henselae*, which starts as a papule at a cat-scratch site, and then progresses to tender, regional adenopathy.
—Tuberculosis (TB): acute or insidious onset of fever and firm, nontender adenopathy in children exposed to adult infected with the acid-fast bacillus *Mycobacterium tuberculosis*.
—Atypical mycobacterial disease: infection usually caused by *M. avium* complex or *M. scrofulaceum* (ubiquitous agents found in the soil). Rapidly enlarging mass of firm, nontender nodes in young children with no known exposure to TB. Nodes often occur with overlying skin discoloration and thinning; some spontaneously drain.
—Infectious mononucleosis: Epstein-Barr viral infection most commonly seen in older children who present with fever, exudative pharyngitis, adenopathy, and hepatosplenomegaly.
—Retropharyngeal abscess: suppurative adenitis of the retropharyngeal nodes that presents in children under 5 years of age. These children often have fever, neck stiffness, dysphagia, respiratory distress, drooling, and stridor.
—Peritonsillar abscess: suppurative sequela of a severe tonsillopharyngitis, usually caused by group A β-hemolytic Streptococcus, which commonly presents in older children and adolescents with trismus, "hot potato" voice, and uvular deviation from a bulging palatal abscess.

- **Congenital**

—Thyroglossal duct cyst: remnant of the embryonic thyroglossal sinus, which presents as a nontender (unless infected) mobile, anterior midline mass near the hyoid bone.
—Branchial cleft cyst: remnant of the second branchial cleft, which presents as a nontender (unless infected) cyst at the anterior border of the sternocleidomastoid.
—Cystic hygroma (lymphangioma): complex, multiloculated mass of lymphatic tissue, which presents in the first year of life as a large, soft, compressible neck structure.
—Dermoid cyst: small, firm, nontender mass, usually high in the midline.
—Hemangioma: bluish purple, blanching mass appearing in first year of life.

- **Malignant**

—Hodgkin lymphoma: slowly enlarging, unilateral, firm, nontender neck malignancy, which usually presents in previously well adolescents.
—Non-Hodgkin lymphoma: presents in young adolescents as a painless, rapidly growing, firm collection of lymph nodes.
—Neuroblastoma: most commonly presents in toddlers as a large, nontender, abdominal mass, often associated with a myriad of signs and symptoms as a result of its propensity for metastasis.
—Rhabdomyosarcoma: head and neck malignancy that usually presents as a rapidly enlarging mass.

- **Thyroid**

—Chronic lymphocytic thyroiditis (Hashimoto thyroiditis): autoimmune childhood goiter that may be euthyroid, hypothyroid, or hyperthyroid.
—Thyrotoxicosis (Grave's disease): clinically hyperfunctioning thyroid caused by circulating thyroid cell-stimulating antibodies.
—Thyroiditis: painful bacterial infection of the thyroid caused by Staphylococcus or Streptococcus.

- **Miscellaneous**

—Kawasaki disease: idiopathic vasculitis distinguished by fever, conjunctivitis, oral involvement, extremity changes, rash, and adenopathy.
—Sinus histiocytosis with massive lymphadenopathy (Rosai-Dorfman disease): benign form of histiocytosis that presents as massive, painless enlargement of cervical nodes.
—Sternocleidomastoid (pseudo) tumor of infancy (congenital muscular torticollis): benign perinatal fibromatosis, often associated with difficult deliveries or abnormal uterine positioning that results in a hard, immobile, fusiform mass in the sternocleidomastoid.
—Cervical wattle: benign pedunculated congenital anomaly on lateral neck with a core of elastic cartilage.
—Hematoma: secondary to trauma.
—Hypersensitivity reaction: secondary to bites, stings, or other allergens.

Data Gathering

HISTORY

Question: Fever?
Significance: Infection, Kawasaki disease, malignancy

Question: Noticed with intercurrent infection?
Significance: Reactive hyperplasia, mononucleosis, adenitis, abscess, congenital cyst

Question: Increasing size?
Significance: Infection, malignancy

Question: Sore throat?
Significance: Mononucleosis, peritonsillar, or retropharyngeal abscess

Question: Swallowing problems?
Significance: Retropharyngeal or peritonsillar abscess, thyroglossal duct cyst

Question: Cats?
Significance: Cat-scratch disease

Question: History of scratch or papule on face?
Significance: Cat-scratch disease

Question: Recurrently infected neck mass?
Significance: Infected congenital cyst (thyroglossal duct, branchial cleft)

Question: Noticed at or shortly after birth?
Significance: Cystic hygroma, hemangioma, sternocleidomastoid tumor of infancy

Question: Weight loss, cough, or other chronic constitutional symptoms?
Significance: Malignancy, tuberculosis

Question: Hypo- or hyperthyroid symptoms?
Significance: Thyroglossal duct cyst, thyroidal diseases

Physical Examination

Finding: Tender, erythematous, indurated mass
Significance: Cervical adenitis, infected congenital lesion, cat-scratch disease

Finding: Nontender, enlarged lymph nodes(s)
Significance: Reactive hyperplasia, malignancy

Finding: Fluctuant
Significance: Adenitis with abscess, cystic hygroma

Finding: Drainage
Significance: Adenitis with abscess, atypical mycobacterial disease, infected thyroglossal duct, or branchial cleft cyst

Finding: Regional adenopathy
Significance: Reactive hyperplasia, cat-scratch disease

Finding: Exudative pharyngitis
Significance: Mononucleosis

Finding: Asymmetric soft palate with uvular deviation
Significance: Peritonsillar abscess

Finding: Pulmonary findings
Significance: Tuberculosis, malignancy

Finding: Midline
Significance: Thyroglossal duct or dermoid cyst, thyroidal disease

Finding: Moves with tongue protrusion
Significance: Thyroglossal duct cyst

Finding: Sinus opening
Significance: Thyroglossal duct, branchial cleft, or dermoid cyst

Finding: Multiloculated
Significance: Cystic hygroma

Finding: Matted down
Significance: Malignancy

Finding: Posterior to sternocleidomastoid muscle
Significance: Malignancy, infectious

Finding: Inferior deep cervical nodes (scalene and supraclavicular)
Significance: Malignancy

Finding: Generalized adenopathy
Significance: Malignancy

Finding: Hepatosplenomegaly
Significance: Malignancy, infectious mononucleosis

Finding: Skin discoloration
Significance: Trauma, abscess, atypical mycobacterial disease

Finding: Conjunctivitis, oral involvement, extremity changes, rash
Significance: Kawasaki disease

 ## Laboratory Aids

Test: CBC
Significance: Leukocytosis in infections; atypical lymphocytosis in mononucleosis; thrombocytosis after first week in Kawasaki disease; most patients with neck malignancies initially have a normal CBC

Test: Epstein-Barr virus titers, mononucleosis spot test
Significance: "Monospot" test less reliable in children younger than 4 years old; therefore, titers more useful

Test: Indirect fluorescent antibody titers for Bartonella
Significance: Reliable test to confirm clinical suspicion of cat-scratch disease

Test: PPD
Significance: Negative or only weakly positive in atypical mycobacterial infections

Test: Chest radiograph
Significance: Cavitary lesions and infiltrates in TB; adenopathy in malignancies and TB

Test: Lateral neck x-ray
Significance: Prevertebral soft tissue space at C2-C3 abnormally wide ($>1/2$ adjacent vertebral body diameter) in cases of retropharyngeal abscess

Test: Ultrasound
Significance: Often the first imaging modality for neck masses; provides immediate, noninvasive information on location, size, and composition of mass (cystic versus solid)

Test: CT or MRI scan
Significance: Useful in evaluating deep neck infections, and complex or extensive neck masses

Test: Thyroid scintigraphy
Significance: Useful in evaluating thyroid lesions, especially when malignancy is a concern

Test: Gram stain and culture of specimen after needle aspiration or incision and drainage
Significance: Diagnostic as well as therapeutic procedure when infection suspected

Test: Histologic evaluation of specimen after fine-needle aspiration or biopsy
Significance: Diagnostic to distinguish malignant causes from congenital and infectious ones

 ## Therapy

• Infectious—antibiotics; drainage for abscesses
• Congenital—antibiotics if infected; ear, nose, and throat (ENT) referral for surgical excision
• Malignancy—oncology referral for chemotherapy/radiation/excision
• Thyroidal—endocrine referral for pharmacotherapy

• Miscellaneous
—Kawasaki disease—IVIG, aspirin; cardiology referral for echocardiography
—Sternocleidomastoid tumor of infancy—massage, range of motion, and stretching exercises

 ## Follow-Up

Close follow-up is essential for all neck masses; consider referral for biopsy in the following cases:

• Failure of antibiotics
• Toxic illness/systemic symptoms
• Clinical signs of malignancy
• Nodes that are firm, nontender, and fixed to skin/deep tissues; nodes located posterior to the sternocleidomastoid or in the lower cervical/supraclavicular regions
• Increasing size after 2 weeks without diagnosis
• No decrease in size after 4 to 6 weeks without diagnosis
• Not back to normal size after 8 to 12 weeks

ICD-9-CM 784.2

BIBLIOGRAPHY

Armstrong WB, Giglio MF. Is this lump in the neck anything to worry about? *Postgrad Med* 1998;104(3):63–78.

Brown RL, Azizkhan RG. Pediatric head and neck lesions. *Pediatr Clin North Am* 1998;45(4):889–905.

Chesney PJ. Cervical adenopathy. *Pediatr Rev* 1994;15:276–285.

Cmejrek RC, Coticchia JM, Arnold JE. Presentation, diagnosis, and management of deep-neck abscesses in infants. *Arch Otolaryngol Head Neck Surg* 2002;128(12):1361–1364.

Kelly CS, Kelly RE. Lymphadenopathy in children. *Pediatr Clin North Am* 1998;45(4):875–888.

McGuirt WF. The neck mass. *Med Clin North Am* 1999;83(1):219–234.

Ponder TB, Smith D, Ibrahim R. Lymphadenopathy in children and adolescents: role of fine-needle aspiration in management. *Cancer Detect Prevent* 2000;24(3):228–233.

Swischuk LE, John SD. Neck masses in infants and children. *Radiol Clin North Am* 1997;35(6):1329–1340.

Weber AL, Siciliano A. CT and MR imaging evaluation of neck infections with clinical correlations. *Radiol Clin North Am* 2000;38(5):941–968.

Wetmore RF, Mahboubi S, Soyupak SK. Computed tomography in the evaluation of pediatric neck infections. *Otolaryngol Head Neck Surg* 1998;119(6):624–627.

Author: Nicholas Tsarouhas

Necrotizing Enterocolitis

 Database

DEFINITION

Necrotizing inflammatory bowel disorder affecting the premature infant; only 10% of cases occur in term infants. Necrotizing enterocolitis (NEC), the most common and most serious acquired gastrointestinal disorder among hospitalized preterm infants, is associated with significant acute and chronic morbidity and mortality. NEC can lead to focal or diffuse ulcerations and necrosis of the gastrointestinal (GI) tract mainly in the distal small bowel and colon.

CAUSES

Unknown etiology but factors causing direct and indirect mucosal disruption, which in turn may lead to an increased permeability in the gut of agents that lead to injuries including:

- Hypoxia/ischemia
- Polycythemia
- Drug exposure
- Cardiac defects
- Exchange transfusions

Enteral alimentation: Since 95% of infants who develop NEC have been enterally fed, the act of initiation of feeds has been implicated as a possible cause of NEC. The composition of the formula (osmolarity), the rate of volume increase, and the immaturity of the mucosa have all been implicated as factors that may increase the risk of NEC.

- Because of the frequent report of epidemic, cluster-type episodes, a variety of microorganisms have been implicated in the development of NEC. In the majority of cases no identifiable organism is recovered, but at times certain microbes, such as *Escherichia coli, Klebsiella, Salmonella,* and *Staphylococcus epidermidis,* have been recovered. Blood cultures may be positive in 20% to 30% of cases.
- As a result of the type of injury that is seen, a cytokine-mediated cascade has also been proposed to play a role in the disease process. In some patients, there have been elevations in serum tumor necrosis factor-α, platelet-activating factor, endothelin-1 and cachectin.
- A variety of host factors may also lead to the development of NEC. These include:

1. Immature gut barrier
2. Low basal acid output
3. Slow intestinal motility
4. Decreased levels of intestinal proteases
5. Low concentrations of immunoglobulins
6. Reduced levels of intestinal T lymphocytes

PATHOLOGY

- Varying degrees of inflammation and early in the course superficial mucosal ulcerations and submucosal edema and hemorrhage leading to transmural coagulation necrosis and perforation.
- NEC can be transmural in nature in the most severe cases.
- The most common sites for NEC include the terminal ileum, ileocecal region, and ascending colon.
- Fifty percent of infants have both colonic and small intestine disease, although the other 50% is divided fairly equally between isolated ileal or colonic involvement.
- In cases that do not progress to perforation, healing occurs by epithelialization and fibroblast proliferation, which can lead to the formation of strictures.
- Changes in neuronal elements within the intestinal wall have been described, which can result in dysfunctional intestinal motility.

GENETICS

There is no known genetic predisposition or component in the development of NEC.

EPIDEMIOLOGY

- The prevalence for NEC is approximately 4%, and the incidence ranges from 1 in 2,000 to 4,000 live births.
- The incidence is highest in infants with birth weights between 500 and 750 g (13% to 20%) and decreases to approximately 2% in infants greater than 750 g.
- NEC usually has an onset within the first 2 weeks of life (3 to 12 days) and after enteral feeds have been initiated. The more premature the infant, the longer the child is at risk for developing NEC, and cases have been reported 3 months after birth.
- There is no association between NEC and sex or race.
- The overall mortality for infants with NEC is between 20% and 40%. Mortality is related to the presence of bacteremia, low birth weight, and low gestational age.
- Mean gestational age is 31 weeks.
- The risk of NEC in full term infants is between 10% and 30% of all cases. Risk factors include:

—Cyanotic heart disease
—Polycythemia
—Exchange transfusions
—Perinatal asphyxia
—Small for gestational age
—Umbilical catheters
—Maternal pre-eclampsia
—Antenatal cocaine abuse.

COMPLICATIONS

- NEC is associated with significant morbidity and mortality.
- A variety of complications may occur in infants with this disease process in the acute setting, including gastrointestinal perforation, DIC, sepsis and shock, fluid and electrolyte imbalance, and respiratory failure.
- Complications related to long term effects on the GI tract occur in 10% to 30%. These include:

—Intestinal strictures
—Acquired short bowel syndrome
—Enterocolic fistulae
—Malabsorption
—Cholestasis
—Anastomotic leaks.

- The most common complication (10% to 35%) are intestinal strictures. These occur mainly in the left colon.

 Differential Diagnosis

The clinical spectrum of signs and symptoms that can be seen in a patient with NEC leads to a variety of other disease processes that must be considered. Some processes can be related to the gastrointestinal tract, although others may be systemic in nature:

- Systemic

—Sepsis with ileus
—Pneumothorax causing a pneumoperitoneum
—Hemorrhagic disease of the newborn
—Swallowed maternal blood
—Postasphyxia bowel necrosis

- Gastrointestinal

—Volvulus
—Malrotation
—Pseudomembranous colitis
—Hirschsprung colitis
—Intussusception
—Spontaneous bowel perforation
—Stress ulcer
—Meconium ileus
—Milk protein allergy
—Umbilical arterial thromboembolism

Data Gathering

HISTORY

- The clinical presentation is variable in this group of patients, but the triad of abdominal distension, bloody stools, and bilious emesis is frequently seen shortly after initiating enteral feeds.
- A number of more subtle, nonspecific findings may be the initial sign of NEC and include apnea and/or bradycardia, lethargy, diarrhea, acidosis, and temperature instability, ileus, and feeding intolerance.
- Patients who have more advanced disease may present with more serious problems: coagulopathy (DIC), increased fluid requirements, and shock.

 Physical Examination

- Clinical symptoms that are helpful in raising suspicion include:

—abdominal distension
—Increased stool output
—Heme positive stools
—Clinitest positive stools
—Emesis
—Increased gastric residuals
—Decreased bowel sounds
—Mottling of the extremities.

- Patients who have more advanced disease may present with more serious problems: vital sign instability (shock), ascites, and peritonitis.

PITFALLS

The major pitfall occurs when there is a delay in making the correct diagnosis and in the institution of appropriate therapy. This leads to a rapid progression of symptoms and usually a worse outcome.

 Laboratory Aids

TESTS

- Presence of pneumatosis intestinalis or hepatic venous gas on x-ray. Perforation in the setting of other clinical symptoms is also indicative of NEC.
- Laboratory abnormalities may include:

—Thrombocytopenia
—Disseminated intravascular coagulopathy
—Metabolic acidosis
—Anemia
—Neutropenia
—Peripheral eosinophilia.

- Other radiologic findings may include ileus, isolated dilated intestinal loop, ascites, and free air.

 Therapy

- For patients who develop NEC, therapy is based on the severity and progression of the symptoms.
- Initial management of all patients with suspected or proven NEC needs to include NPO status, intravenous fluids, nasogastric (NG) tube placement for decompression, and intravenous antibiotics.
- Patients need to have blood and stool cultures sent and need to have frequent evaluation of CBC, fluid status, and abdominal x-ray. These should be evaluated every 6 hours to once a day, depending on the severity of the episode.
- Length of therapy and reinstitution of feeds tend to be based on the severity of the episode and on clinical, laboratory, and radiologic abnormalities.
- If the infant responds immediately to therapy and there are no laboratory or radiographic abnormalities, feeds may be started as early as 72 hours after the episode.
- If mild abnormalities arise and the patient remains only mildly ill, a 10-day course of therapy is considered.
- In cases in which laboratory and radiologic abnormalities include pneumatosis intestinalis, acidosis, and/or thrombocytopenia, a 14-day course is indicated.
- Surgical intervention is required in 25% to 50% of all cases. Indications include pneumoperitoneum, cellulitis of the anterior abdominal wall, metabolic acidosis unresponsive to medical therapy, and progressive respiratory failure.
- Overall, the best therapy for NEC is prevention. Modifying the feeding regimen especially using a low osmolar, protein hydrolysate, high medium chain triglyceride (MCT) fat, or breast milk has been reported to reduce the risk of developing NEC. Interventions to prevent bacterial proliferation (formula supplemented with IgA-IgG preparation, use of probiotics) and enhance the intestinal maturity of the neonate (corticosteroids) have been used in animal models with some success. Human studies are yet to be completed.

 Follow-Up

- Despite early recognition and intervention, NEC is associated with a significantly high morbidity and mortality.
- Mortality results from perforation, sepsis, shock, and DIC.
- Morbidity may be related to anemia, intravenous access difficulties, and the risk for infection.
- The other most common, long-term sequelae seen in 15% to 35% of infants with NEC are intestinal strictures and short gut syndrome if the patient undergoes surgical resection of bowel.
- However, the overall prognosis for infants surviving the acute stage of NEC is very good. 80% to 95% of infants who are discharged from their first hospitalization have a good long-term survival.

 Common Questions and Answers

Q: What is the most common complication of NEC?
A: Not recognizing the problem and the development of intestinal strictures.

Q: Is this preventable?
A: The development of NEC is not clearly preventable, but clinicians should be careful to start feeds in extremely premature infants and use low osmolar, protein hydrolysate, MCT formulas, and/or breast milk.

ICD-9-CM 557.0

BIBLIOGRAPHY

Bell MJ, Ternberg JL, Feigin RD. Neonatal necrotizing enterocolitis: therapeutic decisions based upon clinical staging. *Ann Surg* 1978;187:1B7.

Isreal EJ, Morera C. Necrotizing enterocolitis. In: Walker W, Watkins J, et al, eds. *Pediatric Gastrointestinal Disease*. 3rd Ed. Ontario: BC. Decker, 2000:665–676.

Ladd AP, Rescorla FJ, West KW, et al. Long-term follow-up after bowel resection for necrotizing enterocolitis: factors affecting outcome. *J Pediatr Surg* 1998;33(7):967–972.

Lee JS, Polin RA. Treatment and prevention of necrotizing enterocolitis. *Sem Neonatol* 2003;8(6):449–459.

Pierro A, Hall N. Surgical treatments of infants with necrotizing enterocolitis. *Sem Neonatol* 2003;8(3):223–232.

Udall JN. Gastrointestinal host defense and necrotizing enterocolitis. *J Pediatr* 1990; 117:533–543.

Author: Edisio Semeao

Neonatal Alloimmune Thrombocytopenia

 Database

DEFINITION

Neonatal alloimmune thrombocytopenia (NAIT) is analogous to hemolytic disease of the newborn.

PATHOPHYSIOLOGY

• Caused by maternal antibodies directed against fetal platelet antigens, inherited from the father, which cross the placenta and enter the fetal circulation
• Antibody-coated platelets in the fetus or newborn are destroyed at an increased rate.

EPIDEMIOLOGY

• Occurs in 1 in every 1,000 to 5,000 live births, including first-born offspring.
• The most common antigens responsible are human platelet antigen-1a (HPA-1a, formerly PL^{A1}), responsible antigen in over 75% of cases, HPA-5b (formerly Br^a), and HPA-3 (formerly Bak); however, many other antigens can be responsible and vary in frequency according to ethnic group.
• Severe thrombocytopenia (platelet counts >50,000/μL) as a result of HPA-1a antibodies occurs in 1 in 1,100 births.
• Mothers who are HPA-1a negative and HLA-DR3, -B8, or -DR52a positive form platelet antibodies at increased rates and are more likely to have severely affected neonates.
• Less commonly, maternal antibodies directed against fetal histocompatibility antigens may cause thrombocytopenia or neutropenia.

COMPLICATIONS

• Abnormal bleeding: primarily skin and mucous membrane bleeding, including but not limited to:

—Petechiae and ecchymoses: These lesions are progressive and not confined to areas of birth trauma, such as the head and shoulders.
—Prolonged bleeding from the umbilical stump, phlebotomy sites, and/or at circumcision sites
—Cephalohematomas
—Hematuria
—Gastrointestinal bleeding
—Intracranial hemorrhages: Reported in 2% to 20% of cases; 50% of these occur in utero.

PROGNOSIS

• The overall prognosis is fair, as the majority of patients will experience little morbidity or mortality associated with bleeding; however, the risk of bleeding is higher than in infants of mothers with idiopathic thrombocytopenic purpura (ITP), and reported mortality is 10% in some series.
• The majority of future pregnancies are equally or more severely affected, but this is controversial.

 Differential Diagnosis

• Infection: primarily related to disseminated intravascular coagulation (DIC)

—Bacterial: sepsis
—Viral: congenital rubella or cytomegalovirus
—Spirochetal: syphilis
—Protozoal: toxoplasmosis

• Tumor/malignancy

—Bone marrow disease: congenital leukemia, neuroblastoma

• Metabolic

—Methylmalonic or isovaleric acidemia

• Congenital

—Thrombocytopenia with absent radii (TAR) syndrome
—Wiskott-Aldrich syndrome
—May-Hegglin anomaly
—Hemangiomata with Kasabach-Merritt syndrome

• Immunologic

—Autoimmune neonatal thrombocytopenia: primarily seen in infants of mothers with a history of ITP
—Infants of mothers with systemic lupus erythematosus (SLE)

• Miscellaneous

—Catheter-associated thrombosis with increased platelet consumption
—Renal vein and other large-vessel thromboses
—DIC
—Necrotizing enterocolitis

 Data Gathering

HISTORY

• Family history of bleeding disorders, particularly a history of thrombocytopenia or ITP in the mother
• Medications used during pregnancy or in the newborn
• Infectious diseases in mother and/or newborn

SPECIAL QUESTIONS

Affirmative answers to the following questions increase the likelihood of NAIT in the thrombocytopenic newborn:

• Is there no history of maternal ITP or SLE?
• Is the mother's platelet count presently normal?
• Has the mother had prior newborns with thrombocytopenia, NAIT, or in utero intracranial hemorrhage?
• Has the mother ever been told that she was HPA-1a- or PL^{A1}-negative?

 Physical Examination

• Most neonates with NAIT are well appearing unless they have already experienced an intracranial hemorrhage.
• Skin and mucous membrane bleeding, petechiae, and ecchymoses are common findings.
• Less commonly, if significant hemorrhaging occurs, the following signs may be noted: irritability, pallor, and signs of intracranial hemorrhage, including those related to increased intracranial pressure.
• If congenital anomalies, hepatosplenomegaly, or masses are present, causes of thrombocytopenia, other than immune-mediated, should be investigated.

PITFALLS

NAIT is a difficult diagnosis to confirm and often requires expensive tests, the results of which are often not available to guide the acute management of the newborn; however, a complete workup is necessary for management of future pregnancies in the affected neonate's mother.

Neonatal Alloimmune Thrombocytopenia

 Laboratory Aids

TESTS

• Complete blood count (CBC) in newborn

—Low platelet count: less than 150,000 often below 50,000
—Hemoglobin and hematocrit should be normal: Infants with low values may have experienced perinatal blood loss or could have active bleeding.
—White blood cell (WBC) should be normal in uncomplicated NAIT.

• Consider a PT/PTT to evaluate for DIC, particularly if the infant is ill-appearing or has a complicated pre- and/or perinatal history.
• Maternal platelet count: This is usually normal in NAIT, but a normal maternal platelet count does not rule out autoimmune thrombocytopenia.
• Maternal serum for antiplatelet antibody analysis: To confirm the diagnosis of NAIT, the antibody detected should be specific for a known platelet antigen.
• Maternal and paternal platelet antigen typing: This is crucial for counseling regarding future pregnancies.
• Newborn platelet antigen typing: Use only when absolutely necessary to make the diagnosis, as large amounts of blood are required for this test.
• Consider urine and stool for detection of occult blood.
• Head ultrasound to rule out intracranial hemorrhages

 Therapy

• Therapy primarily involves close monitoring for severe bleeding, including intracranial hemorrhage
• Daily platelet counts at minimum during the first several days of life
• If significant bleeding occurs, the neonate should receive a platelet transfusion with the first available product, in order of preference:

—Washed, irradiated maternal platelets
—Platelets cross-matched with maternal serum
—Irradiated PL^{A1}-negative platelets
—Irradiated random donor platelets: often very limited success in increasing platelet count, as 98% of the U.S. population is PL^{A1}-positive

• Platelet transfusions, when needed, are usually required only once.
• The treatment of severely thrombocytopenic neonates without evidence of significant bleeding is controversial, because of the small but real risk of intracranial hemorrhages.
• Often transfusions are performed at platelet counts of 20,000 to 30,000.
• Other therapies have been reported with limited success, such as steroids, intravenous gamma globulin, and exchange transfusions.

 Follow-Up

• The thrombocytopenia of NAIT usually resolves within 3 to 4 weeks but can be present for up to 12 weeks.
• Family counseling regarding management of future pregnancies after a thorough diagnostic evaluation is strongly recommended.

SIGNS TO WATCH FOR

If the thrombocytopenia persists after 3 months, other etiologies of thrombocytopenia should be investigated.

PREVENTION

Although the disease cannot be prevented, mothers of infants with NAIT can be monitored and possibly treated during subsequent pregnancies.

ISOLATION OF HOSPITALIZED PATIENTS

Isolation of hospitalized patients is not required.

 Common Questions and Answers

Q: What is the HPA-1a- or PL^{A1}-negative mother's risk of having other affected newborns?
A: This depends on the genotype of the father:

• If the father is homozygous for HPA-1a or PL^{A1}, all offspring will be heterozygous PL^{A1}-positive and at great risk for developing NAIT.
• If the father is heterozygous for HPA-1a or PL^{A1}, 50% of offspring will be at risk for developing NAIT.

Q: What is the management of future pregnancies in mothers known to be HPA-1a- or PL^{A1}-negative?
A: This depends on the risk of having an affected child and the clinical course of past affected children. Some perinatal monitoring and therapeutic techniques have shown limited success but not without risks. However, if the risk of having an affected child is 100% and the clinical course of prior affected newborns was associated with significant morbidity and/or mortality, consider the following perinatal management:

• Percutaneous umbilical blood sampling for a platelet count
• Maternal intravenous gamma globulin therapy
• Maternal low-dose prednisone
• Weekly intrauterine platelet transfusions
• Early elective cesarean section to avoid birth trauma

Q: Will the affected neonate be at increased risk for other bleeding problems later in life?
A: If the neonate has confirmed NAIT, there is no increased risk for bleeding problems later in life relative to the general population.

BIBLIOGRAPHY

Bussel J, Kaplan C, MacFarland J, et al. Recommendations for the evaluation and treatment of neonatal autoimmune and alloimmune thrombocytopenia. *Thromb Haemost* 1991;65:631–634.

Bussel JB, Zabusky MR, Berkowitz RL, et al. Fetal alloimmune thrombocytopenia. *N Engl J Med* 1997;337:22–26.

Lanzkowsky P. *Manual of Pediatric Hematology and Oncology.* New York: Churchill Livingstone, 1995.

Ouwehand WH, Smith G, Ranasinghe E. Management of severe alloimmune thrombocytopenia in the newborn. *Arch Dis Child Fetal Neonat Edit* 2000;82:F173–F175.

Roberts I, Murray NA. Neonatal thrombocytopenia: causes and management. *Arch Dis Child Neonatal Edition* 2003;88: F359–F364.

Author: Kim Smith-Whitley

Neonatal Apnea

 ## Database

DEFINITION

• The American Academy of Pediatrics (AAP) defines apnea of infancy as "an unexplained cessation of breathing for 20 seconds or longer, or shorter respiratory pause if accompanied by bradycardia, cyanosis, pallor, and/or marked hypotonia."
• Apnea may be central, characterized by decreased central nervous system (CNS) phrenic nerve efferent activity with resultant absence of respiratory effort; obstructive, in which obstruction of the upper airways results in no flow of air despite respiratory effort; or mixed, which shares features of both.
• Apnea of prematurity (AOP)—also called idiopathic or simple—is a diagnosis of exclusion, and may be central, obstructive, or mixed.
• It is defined as apnea occurring in the infant of less than 37 weeks gestational age without any identifiable pathologic condition.
• Apnea of infancy (AOI) is apnea occurring without identified cause in the term infant, i.e., greater than 37 weeks gestational age.
—Periodic breathing: a form of central apnea characterized by at least three cycles of brief pauses in respiratory effort lasting <10 seconds, followed by normal respiratory patterns for >20 seconds.
—Periodic breathing after the first 2 days of life is extremely common in infants—even in term infants, and is not considered pathologic if these periods are fairly brief and account for a small proportion of the patient's respirations.

EPIDEMIOLOGY

Incidence of apnea of prematurity is inversely proportional to birth weight and gestational age. Incidence is approximately 65% at 34 to 35 weeks postconceptional age.
• More than 50% of infants weighing less than 1,500 g and 90% of infants less than 1,000 g exhibit apnea. Periodic breathing is very common in premature infants (∼ 30%), and decreases to ∼ 10% by term. Term neonates exhibit periodic breathing for 2% to 6% of their respiratory time.

PROGNOSIS

• Apnea as a result of a secondary cause will have the prognosis of the underlying condition.
• Prognosis for AOP depends in large part on the degree of prematurity.
—For those born at 35 to 36 weeks gestational age, apneic spells are managed easily and resolve quickly.
—Infants >28 weeks gestational age at birth typically experience resolution of clinical AOP by 35 to 36 weeks.
—Extremely small preterm infants (24 to 28 weeks gestational age at birth), may have apneic episodes that persist beyond 40 weeks gestational age. Average time to resolution of symptoms is prolonged in patients with significant lung disease and associated with duration of supplemental oxygen.

—As the infant grows, severe apneic events requiring caregiver intervention resolve first, followed by the eventual disappearance of spontaneously resolving episodes.
—Ex-premature infants may be expected to have subtle, generally subclinical, respiratory control abnormalities up to 43 weeks postmenstrual age, thus, the maturity of their respiratory system lags behind their corrected gestational age.
—Unrecognized and untreated apnea can be deadly or cause significant morbidity.
—However, currently, there are no data showing conclusively that appropriately managed recurrent neonatal apneic spells, in themselves, result in significant developmental or neurologic problems.

 ## Differential Diagnosis

While apnea spells occur frequently in the neonate, apnea of prematurity is a diagnosis of exclusion, and these episodes are frequently a sign of a concomitant serious illness.

INFECTIONS

• Sepsis, including line-associated sepsis
• Pneumonia
• Meningitis
• Encephalitis
• Urinary tract infection
• Viral infections, particularly respiratory syncytial virus (RSV)
• Fungal infections

ENVIRONMENTAL

• Hyper- or hypothermia

TUMORS

Congenital central nervous system tumors (rare)

NEUROLOGIC

• Apnea of prematurity (most common, but diagnosis of exclusion)
• Seizures
• Intraventricular hemorrhage
• Encephalopathies
• Hydrocephalus
• Congenital hypoventilation syndrome (rare)
• CNS anomalies (rare)

PULMONARY/AIRWAYS

• Choanal atresia or stenosis
• Laryngeal web
• Laryngomalacia
• Congenital or acquired subglottic stenosis
• Vocal cord dysfunction
• Increased airway secretions or edema of the airways from suctioning or other manipulation
• Inappropriate neck positioning, especially excessive flexion, can also obstruct the flow of air through the trachea.
• Respiratory distress syndrome (RDS)
• Pulmonary edema
• Hypoplastic lungs

METABOLIC

• Hypoglycemia
• Inborn errors of metabolism.

HEMATOLOGIC

• Anemia (controversial whether mild anemia can be cause of apnea)

CARDIOVASCULAR

• Unrepaired patent ductus arteriosus (PDA)
• Congestive heart failure (CHF)
• Hypotension/shock
• Prostaglandin-E1 therapy
• Arrhythmia

TOXIN/DRUGS

• Exposure to narcotics or other respiratory depressants—either directly or via treatment of mother during labor and delivery
• Maternal magnesium therapy and general anesthesia

GASTROINTESTINAL

• Gastroesophageal reflux
• Nasopharyngeal reflux
• Necrotizing enterocolitis (probably via systemic inflammation and its depressive effects on the CNS respiratory centers)

 ## Data Gathering

HISTORY

• Did apnea present during the first 24 hours of life?
—Early onset of apnea increases the likelihood that the apnea is as a result of a complication of labor and delivery (birth trauma, intracranial hemorrhage, neonatal infection, birth asphyxia, or medications administered to the mother) or a separate complicating condition of the infant.
• Are there risk factors present for neonatal sepsis, such as maternal fever, prolonged rupture of membranes, or group B streptococcal (GBS) colonization?
• Did the episode occur during feeds? Does milk or formula regurgitate through the nose?
—Common in premature infants to have dyscoordination of suck, swallow, and breathing reflexes. This generally resolves by the time the infant has reached term by corrected gestational age.
• Does the baby spit up frequently or have other signs of gastroesophageal reflux?
• Are there signs of sepsis or infection,
• Is the infant sleeping when the apneic spells occur?
—Apnea of prematurity events are more likely to occur during sleep. Episodes occurring while awake may indicate another cause.
• Has there been a formal sleep study or multichannel recording to elucidate central and obstructive components of the apneic episodes?

 ## Physical Examination

• General: level of alertness; signs of birth trauma; temperature instability

—If apneic episodes are observed—are there chest or abdominal movements? Is there cyanosis? Is there posturing?
—Adicales respiratory effort.
• HEENT: patency of nasal passageways; nasal septum—examine for dislocation; obstructive nasal secretions. How well does airflow through each nares? Is there stridor or wheezing? Is the facial anatomy normal with signs of normal musculature, innervation, and movements? Is the cry loud and nonhoarse?
• Pulmonary—chest excursions; evaluation of air movement; signs of respiratory distress (accessory muscle use, retractions, grunting, flaring), adventitious breath sounds such as crackles, stridor, or wheezing.
• Cardiovascular
—Focus on signs of shock, congenital anomalies, heart failure: pulses, capillary refill time, pulse rate, blood pressure, color, heart tones, murmurs, liver span.
• Abdominal: (signs of necrotizing enterocolitis) is the abdomen distended? Tender? Discolored? Is the stool bloody? Is there (bilious) emesis?
• Neurologic: cranial nerve anomalies (could point to poor airway tone, aspiration risk, or vocal cord dysfunction); mental status and tone (signs of systemic or CNS illness).

 ## Laboratory Aids

Test: CBC with differential

Test: Blood gas

Test: Electrolytes, serum minerals and glucose

Test: Ammonia and other studies for metabolic disorders

Test: Chest radiograph

Test: Head ultrasound; Head CT or MRI
Significance: Useful to look for signs of possible intracranial hemorrhage or congenital abnormalities.

OTHER STUDIES

Test: Multichannel study, sleep study (pneumogram, polysomnogram)
Significance: These studies are used to distinguish among central, obstructive, and mixed apneas; sequence events occurring during apneic spells to point to specific causes; and detect subtle apnea.

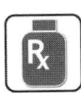 ## Therapy

• Management has two aims: treating the individual episodes to prevent hypoxic injury, and reducing the frequency and severity of further apneic spells.
• Treatment depends on proper classification of apneas as central, obstructive, or mixed and identification of any complicating condition.
• Periodic breathing without accompanying oxygen desaturations does not require therapy; otherwise it is treated similarly to apnea.
• When apneic spells are not alleviated by therapy, babies should be placed under cardiorespiratory monitoring to help caregivers recognize when episodic interventions are needed.
• Treatment for apneic spells
—Tactile stimulation
—Positive pressure ventilation
—Oxygen therapy, if hypoxia does not resolve with other therapy
—Intubation and mechanical ventilation, if severe
—Treatment of underlying concomitant illness, if present
• Nonpharmacologic therapy
—Prone positioning CPAP (continuous positive airway pressure)—a second-line therapy as a result of its invasiveness.
—High-flow nasal cannulae alone appear to have similar efficacy as nasal CPAP for reducing central apnea as well as splinting open upper airways to reduce obstructive airway. It may be better tolerated than CPAP, is less expensive, and can be delivered in lower acuity settings.
• Pharmacologic therapy
• Methyxanthine
—Caffeine citrate is generally preferred over theophylline because of possible improved efficacy, once-per-day dosing, oral route of administration, and a larger therapeutic window with a lower incidence of adverse effects.
—Oral caffeine citrate is typically given as a 20 mg/kg loading dose, followed by 5 to 10 mg/kg per day maintenance therapy. Criteria for discontinuing caffeine therapy vary, but typically includes 5 to 7 apnea-free days, and the infant weight exceeding 1,500 to 2,000 g.
—The therapeutic range of caffeine is between 5 and 20 mg/mL, but there is not agreement on the need to check these levels. Higher levels are generally tolerated without significant toxicities.
—In neonates, the half-life of caffeine can be 75 to 144 hours, so levels do not fluctuate rapidly, and caffeine therapy can be stopped abruptly as there is a natural wean. With increasing hepatic maturation and p450 cytochrome activity, the half-life of caffeine decreases to adult levels by 3 to 5 months postconceptual age.
—Adverse effects include irritability, jitteriness, restlessness, possibly increased vomiting, reflux, and regurgitation, possibly hypoglycemia, and reduced growth as a result of increased metabolic consumption of oxygen. At very high serum levels, seizures may occur.
—Oxygen: may be utilized when apnea is accompanied by desaturation.
—Doxapram: a respiratory stimulant that increases sensitivity to carbon dioxide and may be efficacious when methylxanthines fail.
—There is concern regarding long term effects of exposure to the preservative used in this solution, benzyl alcohol.

 ## Follow-Up

• Many recommend follow-up apnea testing following termination of methylxanthine therapy.

• There is some controversy regarding discharge plans for babies with different types and severity of neonatal apnea. Babies who have been on methylxanthines without apneic events for 1 week are discharged on medications without monitors from some nurseries. At other hospitals, all babies on caffeine are prescribed home monitors on discharge.
• Prior to discharge, premature babies should be evaluated in car seat by apnea study (e.g., pneumogram), and moved to a car bed if they are unable to tolerate the neck flexion inherent to car seat use.

PITFALLS

• Reliance on reports of apnea can underestimate episode frequency because alarms are frequently ignored as a result of high prevalence of false positives, and often the events have resolved by the time the alarms are investigated. Monitoring equipment with memory features or polysomnograms may address these issues.
• Failure to look for underlying causes of apnea in the premature infant—apnea of prematurity is a diagnosis of exclusion.
• Keeping babies who are not to receive home monitors, on cardiorespiratory monitors up until day of discharge can give parents a false sense of insecurity. Monitoring should be stopped once no longer indicated rather than at the time of discharge.

 ## Common Questions and Answers

Q: My baby had apnea of prematurity. Should I be prescribed a home monitor, and if so, what kind?
A: The AAP recommends against the use of home cardiorespiratory monitors to try to prevent SIDS. However, there are some babies for whom home monitors may be indicated. These include premature infants, less than 43 weeks corrected gestational age, or who are still having extreme episodes of apnea. Additionally, monitors may be appropriate for infants with significant respiratory disease, including those with significant chronic lung disease, congenital airway abnormalities, tracheotomy, neuromuscular disease, disorders affecting respiratory, or history of an acute life-threatening event (ALTE). Home monitoring should be limited to a specified course, and withdrawn when no longer needed.

ICD-9-CM 770.8 (APNEA NEONATORUM)

BIBLIOGRAPHY

American Academy of Pediatrics Committee on Fetus and Newborn. Policy statement: apnea, sudden infant death syndrome, and home monitoring. *Pediatrics* 2003;111(4):914–917.

Peter CS, Sprodowski N, Bohnhorst B, Silny J, Poets CF. Gastroesophageal reflux and apnea of prematurity: no temporal relationship. *Pediatrics* 2002;109(1):8–11.

Author: David L. Robinowitz

Nephrotic Syndrome

 Database

DEFINITION

Nephrotic syndrome (NS) applies to any glomerular disorder associated with heavy proteinuria, hypoproteinemia, edema, and hypercholesterolemia. Nephrotic-range proteinuria is found when there is 4+ protein on the urine dipstick, which correlates with proteinuria of more than 40 mg/kg per day.

PATHOPHYSIOLOGY

Causes

- Most pediatric cases are primary; 10% are secondary to other diseases.
- The most common primary cause of NS in childhood is minimal change nephrotic syndrome (MCNS). It is characterized by minimal histologic changes on light microscopy, usually responds to steroid therapy, and follows a relapsing course.
- Other causes of primary nephrotic syndrome include focal segmental glomerulosclerosis and membranous and membranoproliferative glomerulonephritis (GN).
- Secondary causes of NS include infections, vasculitis, diabetes, drugs, and hereditary disorders.

Immunologic Abnormalities

A number of immunologic abnormalities are seen with NS that predispose to infection. These include defective opsonization, decreased serum levels of complement factors D and B, abnormal humoral immunity, decreased delayed hypersensitivity and proliferative responses, and increased suppressor-cell activity and suppressor lymphokine levels.

Pathology (in MCNS)

- The glomerular tuft and size are normal. Mesangial expansion is absent or minimal.
- Immunofluorescence is usually negative, although scanty staining for C3, IgM, and IgA may occasionally be found; these patients are usually steroid dependent.
- Electron microscopy reveals widening and effacement of the visceral epithelial foot processes, which are reversible, occur in association with proteinuria, and are not specific for MCNS.

EPIDEMIOLOGY

- The peak age of onset is 3 years.
- The incidence of new cases is 2 to 7 per 100,000 in children less than 16 years of age.
- The prevalence is 16 per 100,000 in children less than 16 years of age.
- Boys are more commonly affected than girls (3:2).
- A positive family history is present in 3.5% of patients.
- Atopy and MCNS have an association.
- The most common MHC haplotype associated with MCNS is HLA-DR7.
- African American children have a higher incidence of focal glomerulosclerosis (FSGS) than do Caucasian and Asian children.
- Examples of congenital NS are Finnish, mesangiosclerotic, and syphilitic nephrosis.

COMPLICATIONS

- Most complications are secondary to steroid therapy and include growth retardation, glaucoma, posterior lens cataracts, obesity, mood changes, hirsutism, osteoporosis, and infection.
- Primary peritonitis and cellulitis may occur de novo or with steroid therapy.
- Diarrhea and vomiting may result in rapid severe hypovolemia.
- Vascular thromboses are found with NS in relapse, especially if hypovolemia is present.
- Acute reversible renal failure is an uncommon complication of NS of childhood.
- MCNS does not result in chronic renal failure.

PROGNOSIS

The prognosis for MCNS is excellent, with a mortality rate of less than 1%.

 Differential Diagnosis

- Edema

—Congestive cardiac failure
—Liver failure
—Protein-losing enteropathy
—Protein energy malnutrition (Kwashiorkor)

- Nephrotic syndrome

—Focal glomerulosclerosis (FSGS)
—Membranous GN
—Membranoproliferative GN
—Diffuse mesangial proliferation

 Data Gathering

HISTORY

- Fatigue and general malaise
- Reduced appetite
- Weight gain and facial swelling
- Abdominal swelling or pain
- Urine that is foamy
- Atopy

 Physical Examination

- Pitting-dependent edema
- Fluid accumulation in body spaces (ascites, pleural effusions, scrotal swelling)
- White nails, lusterless hair, soft ear cartilage
- Hepatomegaly
- Mild hypertension

SPECIAL QUESTIONS

- Inquire about known atopy or food intolerance.
- Inquire about drug exposure (especially nonsteroidal antiinflammatory agents).
- Inquire about any infections or hernias.

PROCEDURE

Look for edema in the most dependent area of the child.

Laboratory Aids

TESTS

- The urine dipstick usually shows 2,000 mg/dL (4+) of protein.
- Timed or spot urine protein collection: The 24-hour urine shows more than 40 mg/kg per day, and the spot urine protein/creatinine ratio is above 1.

IMAGING

In complicated cases, renal ultrasound to look at the kidney size and parenchymal architecture

PITFALLS

- In small children with NS, the urine dipstick may be less than 4+.
- Failure to monitor complications of glucocorticoid therapy. Growth failure, especially, must be monitored for.

HOME TESTING

The first morning urine is tested for protein.

REQUIREMENTS

Educate the family about urine testing, complications, diet, and therapy.

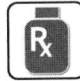 ## Therapy

DRUGS

- Corticosteroids used as first-line agents
- Alkylating agents (cyclophosphamide, chlorambucil)
- Mycophenolate mofetil (MMF)
- Cyclosporine, Tacrolimus
- Diuretics
- Albumin

DURATION

There are a number of similar regimens.

- On presentation: daily corticosteroids for 4 weeks, followed by alternate-day therapy for 4 weeks
- On relapse: daily corticosteroids until in remission, followed by alternate-day therapy for 8 to 12 weeks

DIET

Restrict salt intake while in relapse or on daily corticosteroids.

POSSIBLE CONFLICTS

- Live vaccines are contraindicated while daily corticosteroids or alkylating agents are being given. Children in relapse, on corticosteroids, or on alkylating agents and who are nonimmune and exposed to varicella should receive VZIG.
- Albumin and/or Lasix must be used cautiously to prevent fluid overload or intravascular dehydration.

 ## Follow-Up

WHEN TO EXPECT IMPROVEMENT

Remission occurs 2 to 4 weeks after starting corticosteroids in MCNS.

SIGNS TO WATCH FOR

Fever, abdominal pain, oliguria

PITFALLS

Recognize situations in which hypovolemia may occur.

 ## Common Questions and Answers

Q: Will the MCNS recur?
A: The clinical course tends to be one of multiple remissions and relapses. Relapses usually stop about the time of puberty.

Q: Can the NS return in adult life?
A: Although uncommon, this does occur.

Q: Is macroscopic hematuria ever found with MCNS?
A: Gross hematuria suggests a renovascular event or a diagnosis other than MCNS. Microscopic hematuria occurs in approximately 25% of cases.

Q: What other agents are used to treat NS?
A: Cyclosporin A, Tacrolimus, MMF, and angiotensin converting enzyme inhibitors/angiotensin receptor blockers are used in children with steroid-dependent or -resistant NS.

ICD-9-CM 581.9

BIBLIOGRAPHY

Barratt TM, Clark G. Minimal change nephrotic syndrome and focal segmental glomerulosclerosis. In: Holliday M, Barratt TM, Avner ED, eds. *Pediatric Nephrology*. 3rd Ed. Baltimore: Williams & Wilkins, 1994:767–787.

Chesney RW. The idiopathic nephrotic syndrome. *Curr Opin Pediatr* 1999;11(2):158–161.

Eddy AA. Symons JM. Nephrotic syndrome in childhood. *Lancet* 2003;362(9384):629–639.

Hodson EM, Knight JF, Willis NS, et al. Corticosteroid therapy for nephrotic syndrome in children. *Cochrane Database Syst Rev* 2000;4:CD001533.

Hodson EM, Knight JF, Willis NS, Craig JC. Corticosteroid therapy for nephrotic syndrome in children [update of Cochrane Database Syst Rev 2001;(2):CD001533;PMID:11405997]. *Cochrane Database Syst Rev* 2003;(1):CD001533.

Meyers KEC, Kaplan BS. Minimal-change nephrotic syndrome. In: Neilson EG, Couser WG, eds. *Immunologic Renal Diseases*. Philadelphia: Lippincott-Raven, 2001:969–985.

Vande Walle JG, Donckerwolcke RA. Pathogenesis of edema formation in the nephrotic syndrome. *Pediatr Nephrol* 2001;16(3):283–293.

Author: Kevin E. C. Meyers

Neural Tube Defects

 Database

DEFINITION

Neural tube defects (NTDs) include clinical and subclinical defects, resulting from failure of neural tube closure between the third and fourth week of gestation. NTDs include anencephaly, encephalocele, myelomeningocele, and occult spinal dysraphism.

PATHOPHYSIOLOGY

- Neural tube closure begins midway along the neural axis, spreads like a zipper in both rostral and caudal directions, and is completed in a few days. Failure of neural tube closure most often occurs in the lumbosacral region.
- The defect itself may be only the tip of the iceberg, since the total extent of the malformation may involve the entire central nervous system. This includes disorganized brainstem nuclei or brainstem herniation (Chiari II malformation).

GENETICS

Most cases are as a result of a combination of genetic, environmental, and dietary factors. However, a chromosomal or gene abnormality can be identified in about 10% of children with NTDs, and this number increases if there are multiple congenital anomalies. Five percent of patients are born to a couple with a family history of NTD. After one NTD, the recurrence rate is 2% to 4% for subsequent pregnancies.

EPIDEMIOLOGY

- One per 1,000 live births in the United States (not including occult defects, for which no accurate epidemiologic data are available)
- Anencephaly: 0.2 per 1,000
- Encephalocele: 1 per 5,000
- Myelomeningocele: 0.2 to 0.4 per 1,000

COMPLICATIONS

- Encephalocele: hydrocephalus (50%), intellectual deficits (40%), motor and cognitive deficits, seizures likely as a result of dysplastic cortex surrounding the encephalocele
- Myelomeningocele: hydrocephalus (80%); Chiari II malformation (80%), with some exhibiting feeding difficulties, stridor, and apnea as a result of lower cranial nerve dysfunction; neurogenic bladder (80%) with risk of renal damage; orthopaedic deformities; seizures (25%); below average intelligence (15% to 20%); and tethered spinal cord later in childhood
- Occult dysraphism: progressive lower extremity motor or sensory deficit, gait dysfunction, sphincter dysfunction, foot deformities, scoliosis

PROGNOSIS

- Anencephaly is uniformly fatal.
- Encephalocele: Prognosis is largely dependent on the size of the defect, the amount of brain tissue contained within the sac, and any associated brain malformations.
- Myelomeningocele: Prognosis for ambulation depends on the location of the lesion. The lower the lesion, the more likely the patient will ambulate. Cognitive outcome depends in part on associated brain malformations and treatment of hydrocephalus.

 Differential Diagnosis

Diagnosis reflects the embryogenesis and anatomy of each defect.

- Anencephaly results from failure of anterior neural tube closure. The diagnosis is obvious at birth. The cerebral hemispheres, basal ganglia, and variable amounts of the upper brainstem are absent; 75% are stillborn and the remainder die in the neonatal period.
- Encephalocele results from limited failure of anterior neural tube closure. Abnormal brain tissue protrudes through a skull defect usually covered by skin. Seventy percent to 80% are occipital, 20% are frontal. Ten percent to 20% of occipital defects are meningoceles and contain no brain tissue. Frontal encephaloceles, unless accompanied by craniofacial abnormalities, may not be identified unless a neuroimaging study is performed for an associated symptom (such as developmental delay or seizures).
- Myelomeningocele is a failure of posterior neural tube closure. Abnormal neural tissue protrudes through a vertebral column defect. Eighty percent are thoracolumbar, lumbar, or lumbosacral. By definition, this is an open defect, and the diagnosis is obvious at birth.
- Occult spinal dysraphism has intact skin over the defect. Wide spectrum of defects includes dermal sinus tracts, cysts, lipomas, other tumors, diastematomyelia (bifid spinal cord), and tethered spinal cord.
- A syndromic basis for dysraphism should be considered when non-neural congenital defects are present (e.g., telecanthus-Waardenburg syndrome; conotruncal defect [chromosome 22q11 deletion]).

 Data Gathering

HISTORY

- NTDs are associated with maternal folic acid deficiency, gestational diabetes, maternal hyperthermia during days 20 to 28 of gestation, and use of valproic acid, carbamazepine, and alcohol during pregnancy.
- Occult frontal encephaloceles may come to attention because of a history of developmental delay, seizures, or focal neurologic signs.

- Occult spinal dysraphism presents with lower extremity weakness or sensory loss, gait abnormalities, bowel and bladder dysfunction, foot deformities, and, rarely, recurrent meningitis.

 Physical Examination

- Plot head circumference as a marker of developing hydrocephalus.
- Are there dysmorphic features pointing to a syndrome?
- Integrity of the skin covering the defect, because this affects the timing of surgical intervention. A bony defect or sinus may be palpable in occult cases.
- Neurologic exam of the lower extremities in a myelomeningocele outlines the functional level of the lesion and provides an estimate of future ambulatory potential. Intact hip flexion (L1–L2) and knee extension (L3–L4) are favorable signs for future ambulation.
- Flaccid paralysis is present below the level of the lesion, and ultimate limb growth may be asymmetric. Sensory level may not correspond to motor level. Cranial neuropathies, such as strabismus, laryngeal paresis, and stridor, may be present at birth or may develop in the first months of life.
- Local signs of occult spinal dysraphism include a dimple, sinus, lipoma, skin pigment change, or tuft of hair in the lumbosacral area. Examination may show foot deformities, tight heel cords, unequal leg or foot length, decreased sphincter tone, lower extremity weakness, or sensory changes.

 Laboratory Aids

TESTS

- Maternal serum alpha-fetoprotein (MSAFP) testing, done at 16 to 18 weeks' gestation, can identify 88% of cases of anencephaly and 79% of cases of myelomeningocele.
- Ultrasonography—diagnoses more than 99% of cases of anencephaly and 90% of cases of myelomeningocele. Encephaloceles are more likely to be diagnosed by ultrasound than by MSAFP testing.
- Serial cranial ultrasounds or CT scans can evaluate hydrocephalus, which can occur without rapid head growth in patients with NTDs.
- MRI for other brain anomalies, including areas of cortical dysplasia, found in 92% of patients in one neuropathologic study.
- EEG for suspected seizures.
- Urodynamic evaluation should be performed in all children with myelomeningocele to anticipate/prevent renal damage as a result of reflux.
- Suspected occult spinal dysraphism—evaluate with spine x-rays and ultrasound (in the newborn period). CT scan provides more detail of bony anatomy, and MRI more detail of spinal cord anatomy.

Emergency Care

Urgent stabilization in the newborn period, followed by prompt neurosurgical closure. Acute hydrocephalus from shunt failure or tethered spinal cord from occult spinal dysraphism may arise later in life.

 Therapy

- Route of delivery: For most patients with NTDs and vertex presentation, no clear benefit of cesarean section. One study demonstrated improved neurologic outcome in patients delivered via cesarean section.
- Neurosurgical closure of a myelomeningocele within the first few days of life to prevent infection and for cosmetic reasons. Prophylactic antibiotics given while awaiting surgery decrease the incidence of meningitis and ventriculitis. Closure of the defect in the first hours of life is not necessary, keep defect clean and moist.
- An encephalocele with adequate skin covering can be repaired less urgently.
- V-P shunts should be placed in infants with hydrocephalus, because early treatment of hydrocephalus may improve cognitive outcome.
- Infants with high bladder pressure typically are treated initially with anticholinergics and clean intermittent catheterization.
- Occult spinal dysraphism with possible neurologic signs or symptoms should be referred to neurosurgery for evaluation.
- Promising results are reported for fetal surgery closures.

 Follow-Up

- Multidisciplinary approach includes a primary pediatrician, neurosurgeon, urologist, orthopaedist, neurologist, physiatrist, and others.
- Prognosis for ambulation depends on the location of the myelomeningocele. Virtually all children with sacral lesions are able to ambulate; 95% of adolescents and 40% of younger children with low lumbar lesions will ambulate; 30% of adolescents with high lumbar or thoracic lesions will ambulate.
- Approximately 80% of children with myelomeningocele will have a neurogenic bladder (urodynamic testing). The goal of therapy is urinary continence and control of high bladder pressure.
- Many children can ultimately achieve bowel control with bowel programs involving high-fiber, low-fat foods; enemas; stool softeners; and biofeedback.
- Approximately 60% of children with encephalocele and 80% to 85% with myelomeningocele are of normal intelligence.
- Risk of epilepsy corresponds to degree of mental retardation, high with frontal encephaloceles.

- Anticipation of skin breakdown, decubitus ulcers, and leg injuries are important.
- In an older child with a myelomeningocele, loss of motor function in the legs, increased spasticity, gait difficulties, pain, bladder dysfunction, and scoliosis may be signs of a tethered cord.

PREVENTION

- Folic acid supplementation in early pregnancy can reduce the incidence of NTDs by 50% in the general population, and by 70% in women with a history of NTD in a previous pregnancy.
- Since many pregnancies are not discovered until after the fourth week of gestation, when neural tube closure occurs, the CDC recommends that all women of childbearing age receive a minimum of 0.4 mg of folic acid daily.
- The American Academy of Pediatrics recommends women with a history of NTD in a previous pregnancy receive 4 mg of folic acid daily, starting 1 month before and through the first 3 months of pregnancy.
- Women on anticonvulsants and other medications linked to NTDs may benefit from receiving 4 mg of folic acid daily.

PITFALLS

- The neurologic status of a patient with a repaired neural tube defect should remain stable overall. Have a high index of suspicion for worsening hydrocephalus, syringomyelia, and tethered spinal cord—all treatable conditions, which may develop over time.
- Tethered cord may accompany occult dysraphism and is a surgically treatable cause of acquired neurogenic bladder/cauda equina syndrome in young children.
- Vocal cord paralysis may appear episodically, resembling croup, in children with myelomeningocele.
- Shunt blockage or infection must be diagnosed early and may be heralded by subtle symptoms of irritability, increased sleep, or low-grade fever.
- Latex allergy is common in children with myelomeningocele and may be prevented by avoiding latex-containing products.

 Common Questions and Answers

Q: Will my child have learning problems?
A: At least 50% of those with myelomeningocele have normal intelligence. Cognitive outcome appears improved with the advent of early shunting of hydrocephalus.

Q: Could my baby have other problems besides neurologic problems?
A: Infants with NTDs need to be checked periodically for signs of bladder problems. Some develop problems with control of eye movements (strabismus), but this is often correctable.

Q: Do the child's uncles or aunts have an increased risk of having a child with a birth defect?
A: Though some families do seem to carry an increased risk for NTDs, the increase is small and seems to affect the immediate, not the extended, family.

Q: Should I stop taking anticonvulsants during pregnancy to reduce my risk of NTDs?
A: Not unless your doctor recommends doing so. In general, continuing the lowest dose of the medicine that best controls your seizures is recommended during pregnancy. There are risks to the fetus from poorly controlled seizures during pregnancy. The overall risks and benefits of medications must be weighed. Any woman of childbearing age who is taking anticonvulsants should receive folic acid supplementation.

ICD-9-CM

Myelomenigocele 741.9
Anencephaly 740.0

BIBLIOGRAPHY

Adzick NS, Walsh DS. Myelomeningocele: prenatal diagnosis, pathophysiology and management. *Semin Pediatr Surg* 2003;12(3):168–174.

Blum RW, Pfaffinger K. Myelodysplasia in childhood and adolescence. *Pediatr Rev* 1994;15:480–484.

Botto LD, Moore CA, Khoury MJ, Erickson JD. Neural-tube defects. *N Engl J Med* 1999; 341(20):1509–1519.

Bruner JP, Tulipan N, Paschall RL, et al. Fetal surgery for myelomeningocele and the incidence of shunt-dependent hydrocephalus. *JAMA* 1999;282(19):1819–1825.

Drolet B. Birthmarks to worry about. Cutaneous markers of dysraphism. *Dermatol Clin* 1998;16:447–453.

Hunt JA, Hobar PC. Common craniofacial anomalies: facial clefts and encephaloceles. *Plast Reconstr Surg* 2003;112(2):606–615.

Johnson MP, Sutton LN, Rintoul N, et al. Fetal myelomeningocele repair: short-term clinical outcomes. *Am J Obstet Gynecol* 2003;189(2): 482–487.

Patient Information. Spina Bifida Association of America Web site. Available at http://www.sbaa.org, accessed May 13, 2005.

Authors: Dennis J. Dlugos and Sabrina E. Smith

Neuroblastoma

 ## Database

DEFINITION

Neuroblastoma is a tumor derived from neural crest cells that form the sympathetic ganglia and adrenal medulla.

PATHOPHYSIOLOGY

- Etiology unknown
- Neuroblastoma should be distinguished from ganglioneuroma and ganglioneuroblastoma, which, in general, show features of differentiation or maturation.
- Included in the category of small, round blue-cell tumors of childhood
- Metastatic spread by lymphatic and hematogenous routes

GENETICS

- Familial neuroblastoma has been reported but is rare (autosomal dominant with variable penetrance, 1% of patients)
- Neuroblastoma cells may acquire specific genetic alterations, which are of prognostic importance, i.e., amplification of the N-myc gene.

EPIDEMIOLOGY

- Most common extracranial solid tumor of children; 7% to 10% of all childhood cancers
- Prevalence: 1 in 7,000 live births in the United States; 600 new cases a year
- Majority of children are younger than 4 years of age and have disseminated disease at diagnosis
- Fifty percent of tumors arise from the adrenal gland.
- Eighty percent of tumors occur below the diaphragm; 20% occur in cervical and thoracic sites.

COMPLICATIONS

Common sites of metastases include:

- Liver
- Bone marrow
- Skin: nontender subcutaneous nodules with a bluish hue
- Lymph nodes
- Bone, particularly the skull and facial bones as well as long bones
- Mass effect at the site of the primary lesion (e.g., spinal cord compression, Horner syndrome)
- Paraneoplastic syndromes
- Vasoactive intestinal peptide (VIP) syndrome: as a result of VIP production by tumor; watery diarrhea, abdominal distention, and electrolyte imbalances usually resolve with treatment.
- Opsoclonus-myoclonus: etiology unknown but thought to be on an autoimmune process; associated with chaotic eye movements ("dancing eyes") and myoclonic jerks ("dancing feet") with or without cerebellar ataxia; may not resolve with treatment of

tumor. Specific therapy includes high-dose steroids and IVIG.
- Catecholamine excess: flushing, sweating, tachycardia, headache, hypertension (hypertension more commonly of renal origin than catecholamine excess)

PROGNOSIS

- Most important adverse prognostic factors are N-myc amplification, metastatic disease, and age over 1 year
- The following biologic properties have prognostic significance:

—Histology: "Favorable" vs. "unfavorable"
—N-myc amplification: Amplification is associated with more aggressive, higher stage tumors (22% of patients).
—Serum ferritin: High levels are associated with more aggressive tumor.
—DNA index (ploidy): Hyperdiploid tumors are associated with less aggressive tumors than diploid tumors (in infants).
—Chromosome analysis: Chromosome 1 deletions associated with more advanced stage tumors.
—Lactate dehydrogenase (LDH): High levels associated with more aggressive tumors.
—Neuron-specific enolase (NSE): May be elevated in pediatric tumors other than neuroblastoma.
—Children with low-risk disease, such as those younger than 1 year with low-stage tumors, have an overall cure rate of greater than 90%.
—Older children with advanced-stage tumors have historically significantly lower cure rates of 15% to 30%. With intensive multimodal therapies, including high-dose therapy with stem cell rescue and cis-retinoic acid, long-term survival may approach 50% to 60%.

 ## Differential Diagnosis

- Depends on the presentation of the patient and the site of the primary tumor
- Included in the differential diagnosis of abdominal or thoracic mass:

—Abdominal primaries include Wilms tumor, Burkitt lymphoma, and germ-cell tumor.
—Thoracic primaries include lymphoma (usually non-Hodgkin), leukemia with bulky disease, and germ-cell tumors.

- The differential diagnosis of a "small, round, blue-cell tumor" should include neuroblastoma, lymphoma, Ewing sarcoma, and rhabdomyosarcoma.

 ## Data Gathering

HISTORY

- Presenting signs and symptoms of neuroblastoma depend on the primary site of the tumor and the degree of dissemination.

- General well-being: Ask about activity level, change in appetite, irritability, specific areas of discomfort, and so forth. This may give some indication of the extent of disease. Patients with neuroblastoma may present appearing either well or sick, though those with disseminated disease generally appear both chronically and acutely ill.

 ## Physical Examination

ABDOMINAL MASS

- Abdominal mass is usually firm, fixed, irregular, and frequently crosses the midline.
- Abdominal distension with or without tenderness
- Mass effect
- Signs of bowel obstruction: anorexia, vomiting, low stool output
- Hypertension
- Genital and lower extremity edema from obstruction of venous and lymphatic drainage

CERVICAL/THORACIC MASS (POSTERIOR MEDIASTINAL)

- Respiratory distress or stridor with thoracic masses
- Horner syndrome with cervical or high thoracic masses: ptosis, myosis, and anhydrosis
- Anisocoria
- Superior vena cava syndrome with large mediastinal tumors

PARASPINAL MASS

- Vertebral body involvement and nerve root compression
- Bladder and bowel dysfunction, paraplegia, and back pain as a result of spinal cord compression

METASTATIC DISEASE

- Liver: hepatomegaly
- Bone: with or without bony pain, periorbital ecchymoses and/or proptosis
- Bone marrow: cytopenias, pain from marrow expansion
- Lymph nodes: adenopathy
- General: fever, irritability, failure to thrive
- Periocular ecchymosis

 ## Laboratory Aids

TESTS

- Office evaluation should include CBC, a basic chemistry panel to assess electrolyte imbalance, and a radiographic study of the suspected primary tumor site (generally an ultrasound or CT scan; MRI may be necessary for paraspinal tumors).
- Further studies should be obtained at the referral center where the patient will receive treatment; this will avoid repeating expensive tests.

Laboratory Aids

- CBC: decreased hemoglobin, platelets, and/or white blood cell counts may indicate bone marrow involvement.
- Urine catecholamines: homovanillic acid (HVA); vanillylmandelic acid (VMA); secreted by some neuroblastomas
- Liver function tests: may indicate liver involvement when elevated
- Lactate dehydrogenase (LDH): may have prognostic value
- Serum ferritin: may have prognostic value
- Bone marrow aspirate and biopsy: to evaluate bone marrow involvement

IMAGING

- Plain films of the primary site (calcification suggests neuroblastoma)
- US, CT, and/or MRI of the primary site and possible metastatic sites
- Skeletal survey or bone scan to rule out bone lesions
- MIBG scan: can detect both bone and soft tissues that are involved

STAGING

- The International Neuroblastoma Staging System (INSS) is the commonly used, current staging system.
- Low-risk groups usually have localized disease.
- High-risk groups have disseminated disease often involving the bones, bone marrow, liver, and/or skin. Biologic characteristics of the tumor can also help stratify risk (e.g., N-myc amplification).
- Stage 4S (IVS or D) are patients younger than 12 months of age who have a localized primary mass (stage 1 or 2) with disseminated disease involving the liver, skin, or (minimal) bone marrow but sparing the bones.

PITFALLS

Do not use the spot VMA or HVA to screen for neuroblastoma. False positives (excretion on other sources) and false negatives (nonsecreting tumors) are both possible.

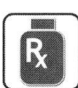

Therapy

Treatment protocols are based on prognostic categories:

- Patients with low-risk disease, such as stage 4S or stage 1, may only require surgery alone, particularly if surgical resection is complete and the biologic characteristics of the tumor are favorable.
- Patients with advanced-stage disease, such as stage 4 (extensive metastases), usually require a combination of surgery, chemotherapy, and radiation therapy with or without high-dose therapy and stem-cell rescue (HDT/SCR).

SURGERY

- Total surgical resection at the time of diagnosis is attempted but not aggressively; if gross total resection is risky, partial resection or biopsy alone is indicated.
- After a histologic diagnosis has been established, chemotherapy and radiation therapy can be instituted to obtain tumor shrinkage for a later attempt at total gross resection.

CHEMOTHERAPY

- Multiagent chemotherapy is often used for patients with intermediate- and high-risk disease.
- Common chemotherapeutic agents for neuroblastoma include cyclophosphamide (Cytoxan), doxorubicin (Adriamycin), etoposide (VP-16), vincristine, ifosfamide, cisplatin, and carboplatin.

RADIATION

- Radiation therapy is used for control of local disease and/or for palliation.
- Total body radiation may be a component of preparative regimens for bone marrow transplantation (BMT).

BIOLOGIC THERAPY

- 13-Cis-retinoic acid: cellular differentiating agent that has shown improved survival when used posttransplant

BONE MARROW TRANSPLANTATION

- Autologous bone marrow transplantation (ABMT) or peripheral SCR after intensive chemotherapy is used in high-risk protocols. Tandem transplants, using high-dose chemotherapy with or without total body irradiation, are currently being explored.

DURATION

- Depends on stage of disease, response, and complications: generally under 12 months. Prolonged maintenance chemotherapy does not play a role in therapy, although biologic response modification therapy may be given in the second year after diagnosis.

SIGNS TO WATCH FOR

- Patients are often followed by radiographic studies of the primary site and sites of metastases as well as laboratory tests and bone marrow studies, depending on the presentation and staging of the patient—for example, urine catecholamines, serum ferritin, and abdominal CT for a patient with an adrenal primary without metastases.
- Complications depend on the primary site of the tumor and the therapy received; acute and late effects of chemotherapy and radiation therapy require close monitoring.

ISOLATION OF HOSPITALIZED PATIENTS

- Patients with neuroblastoma should take measures to avoid contact with persons known to have active varicella.

- Neutropenic patients do not require special isolation precautions except in the transplant setting.

Common Questions and Answers

Q: Are siblings of children with neuroblastoma at increased risk for neuroblastoma compared with the general population?
A: No, except in rare families with a known history of neuroblastoma (<1%).

Q: Can neuroblastoma spontaneously regress?
A: Yes; however, this is usually seen only in children under 1 year of age with lower stage disease.

Q: What are the biggest risks during therapy?
A: The risk of infection is quite high as a result of the presence of an indwelling catheter and severe neutropenia secondary to aggressive chemotherapy. Platinum-containing regimens can cause significant hearing loss that may worsen the higher the cumulative dose.

Q: What therapy is available to patients who either fail to go into remission or relapse following aggressive therapy?
A: There is no standard approach to a refractory or relapsed patient with neuroblastoma. Generally, phase I or II therapies may be offered, although the outcome for these patients is generally very poor.

ICD-9-CM 194.0

BIBLIOGRAPHY

Brodeur AE, Brodeur GM. Abdominal masses in children: neuroblastoma, Wilms tumor, and other considerations. *Pediatr Rev* 1991;12(7): 196–206.

Castleberry RP. Biology and treatment of neuroblastoma. *Pediatr Clin North Am* 1997; 44:919–937.

Caty MG, Shamberger RC. Abdominal tumors in infancy and childhood. *Pediatr Surg* 1993; 40(6):1253–1271.

Finklestein JZ. Neuroblastoma: the challenge and the frustration. *Hematol Oncol Clin North Am* 1987;1(4):675–694.

Grupp SA, Stern JW, Ross AA, et al. Tandem high dose therapy in rapid sequence for children with high-risk neuroblastoma. *J Clin Oncol* 2000;18(13):2567–2575.

Lee KL, Ma JF, Shortliffe LD. Neuroblastoma: management, recurrence, and follow-up. *Urol Clin North Am* 2003;30(4):881–890.

Author: Julie W. Stern

Neurofibromatosis

Database

DEFINITION

Neurofibromatosis Type 1 (NF1) is a neurocutaneous syndrome in which tumors grow along various types of nerves, both internal and external. Neurologic features include cognitive disability, intra- and extracranial tumors of the nervous system, and stroke (rare). The diagnosis is based on the presence of any two of the following physical/familial criteria:

• Two or more cutaneous neurofibroma(ta) or one plexiform neurofibroma
• Two or more Lisch nodules
• Inguinal or axillary freckling
• Six or more (smooth-edged) café-au-lait spots, at least 1.5 cm in diameter in postpubertal individuals or 0.5 cm in diameter in prepubertal individuals
• Optic nerve glioma
• Osseous lesions, including sphenoid wing dysplasia, pseudarthrosis
• A first-degree relative (parent, sibling or offspring) with NF

Tumors may be cosmetically disfiguring and physically limiting; they rarely undergo sarcomatous transformation.

GENETICS

• Neurofibromatosis type 1 (NF1) is an autosomal dominant disorder; 50% of the cases are inherited, although the other half occur as a sporadic mutation.
• NF1 is one of the most commonly inherited autosomal dominant disorder (approximately 1 in 4,000), with no known gender or ethnic predisposition.
• The NF1 gene is located on chromosome 17.
• Expression of NF1 varies widely within and among families, from mildly affected to severely impaired.
• The course of NF1 is impossible to predict; even a relative's disease will not be an indication of progression.

EPIDEMIOLOGY

• The frequency is 1 in every 3,000 to 4,000 live births.
• NF1 affects 100,000 Americans.
• Occurrence appears to be independent of sex, race, or environmental factors.

COMPLICATIONS

• Oncologic

—Neurofibromas are benign tumors of Schwann cells, nerve fibers, and fibroblasts that arise along the nerves.
—Plexiform neurofibromas occur in approximately 15% of patients with NF1; these are extensive tumors that grow along the nerve root and may invade adjacent structures, threatening vital structures (especially in the neck and throat) or cause gross disfigurement. Approximately 10% of

these tumors undergo sarcomatous degeneration.
—CNS tumors include optic nerve/pathway gliomas or gliomas elsewhere in the brain.

• Neurologic: learning disability, language disorders, autism, seizures, retardation, and attention deficit occur with higher than background frequency in NF.
• Renal: hypertension
• Circulatory: moya-moya, stroke
• Endocrine: pheochromocytoma
• Hematologic: leukemia

ASSOCIATED CONDITIONS

• Head circumference greater than the 98% percentile
• Developmental speech delay, motor incoordination, learning disorders, attention deficit disorder
• Hypertension
• Brain tumor, moya-moya disease
• Sarcoma, leukemia, Wilms tumor, pheochromocytoma
• Headaches, scoliosis
• Abnormalities in growth, hemihypertrophy

Differential Diagnosis

• Café-au-lait spots are most often benign findings unrelated to NF.
• NF2 may resemble NF1.

—NF1 versus NF2: NF2 is also known as central bilateral acoustic NF, a rare disorder characterized by multiple tumors on the cranial and spinal nerves, and by other lesions of the brain and spinal cord.
—NF2 is genetically and clinically distinct from NF1. The NF2 gene is located on chromosome 22.
—The diagnosis of NF2 is made if the individual has the following:
  —Bilateral acoustic neuromas
OR
  —A first-degree relative with NF2 and either
    —a unilateral acoustic neuroma
OR
  —Two of the following:
    —meningioma
    —glioma
    —schwannoma
    —juvenile posterior subcapsular lenticular opacity

• Sotos syndrome features macrosomia, hypertelorism, ventriculomegaly, and cognitive difficulties.
• McCune-Albright syndrome has large café-au-lait spots with irregular margins and polyostotic fibrous dysplasia
• Tuberous sclerosis (TS) may share autosomal dominant transmission, CAL, and hypopigmented lesions in common with NF; features distinctive for TS include adenoma sebaceum, cardiac and renal tumors, and prominent epilepsy. Genetic testing for TS may soon be available.

Approach to the Patient

N/A

Data Gathering

HISTORY

• A family history is from a first-degree relative, mother, or father of the proband. The disorder shows 100% penetrance.
• Vision: Optic path tumors generally occur between the ages of 2 and 6 years.
• Development: Learning problems and ADHD are common.
• Seizures: Also more common in NF
• Joint/extremity pain: Neuropathic pain or abrasion as a result of neurofibroma
• Back pain: Could signal potentially serious cord or root compression
• Headache: (Hydrocephalus); migraine also common in NF
• Respiratory problems: Neurofibromas may encroach on the airway; sexual development; abnormalities as a result of hypothalamic disease; psychiatric concerns; and depression are common.

Physical Examination

• Café-au-lait spots are noted at birth or within the first year of life; the macules are generally flush and circular, although they may have jagged edges or areas of hypertrichosis. Café-au-lait spots result from collection of heavily pigmented melanocytes of neural crest origin in the epidermis. The macules will appear for the first 5 years of life and then slow or stop, although they will grow with the child.
• Axillary and inguinal freckling are generally seen by puberty. The freckling is a cluster often seen in the skin folds.
• Lisch nodules are best assessed by slit-lamp examination. The Lisch nodules are small bumps on the iris that do not interfere with vision. They are uncommon during infancy, but by age 20, 99% of NF1 patients will have Lisch nodules.
• Optic pathway tumors (OPT) are present in 20% of patients with NF1, though only approximately 20% of those will require intervention. Treatment should be limited to those patients who have uncorrectable visual acuity, a change in visual fields, and/or endocrine abnormalities, or to those lesions that extend to the hypothalamus.
• Bony dysplasias occur in approximately 3% of patients with NF1. Dysplasias frequently occur in the tibia or the sphenoid wing. A pseudarthrosis will occur as a result of thinning of the long bone and its inability to heal after it breaks.

GENERAL

- Blood pressure
- Review of palpable tumors for extension or "stoney" feel that could signal cancerous change
- Abdominal examination for masses
- Funduscopy and acuity check for evidence of optic pathway tumor
- Neck and spine palpation/mobility
- Reflexes for evidence of nerve root tumor
- Growth parameters (including head circumference) for evidence of hydrocephalus, hypothalamic disturbance
- Scoliosis screen

 ## Laboratory Aids

TESTS

Laboratory Tests

- In most cases, the diagnosis of NF1 remains a clinical diagnosis. However, DNA testing has become more available and therefore may be useful in atypical cases or in making reproductive choices. DNA-based testing of the NF1 gene is undertaken in a step-wise approach using a cascade of complementary tests that are able to detect a mutation in the NF1 gene in 95% of patients who meet the NIH diagnostic criteria.
- Renal studies may be indicated for persistent hypertension or difficulty with urine flow.

Imaging

- Bright areas in cerebral white matter on T2-weighted MR images are common in NF1 and their clinical significance is uncertain. Indications for neuroimaging depend on findings that may warrant it, such as progressive macrocrania, sensory deficits (especially visual), new-onset seizure, and chronic headaches. Some clinicians obtain a scan as a baseline on all new cases, but this is controversial.

 ## Therapy

- Presently, there is no treatment for tumor growth, except surgical interventions; tumors cannot be predicted based on their occurrence in another member of the family with NF. Interventions are palliative and supportive.
- Surgical intervention is performed on those tumors that are medically compromising, painful, or cosmetically disfiguring. Subcutaneous nodules are flesh-colored, raised, "pealike" nodules that may be present during childhood; these commonly appear and grow during puberty or pregnancy and do not grow into plexiform tumors.
- Family counseling regarding genetic implications, possible genetic testing using linkage, or, in some cases, mutation testing of the gene neurofibromin.
- Vigilance/anticipatory care regarding common psychological and developmental issues, such as speech delay, incoordination, hyperactivity/attention deficit, and learning disabilities. Early educational assessment and interventions may improve developmental outcome.

 ## Follow-Up

- Anticipatory care issues (see Data Gathering) are all pertinent to follow-up: monitoring for the development of tumors, hypertension, and psychological and developmental disabilities.
- Continuous yearly ophthalmologic examinations: Goldman visual field perimetry is suggested in those with any question of an optic nerve tumor. Some practitioners use yearly visual field testing (by an ophthalmologist) in lieu of MRI scanning.
- Orthopaedic, oncologic, endocrine, surgery, and plastic surgery consultants may be helpful, depending on individual issues.
- Blood pressure checks are increasingly important in adolescents and adults with NF.
- Deaths have been associated with cancer, heart disease, and strokes, similar to the general population.
- Optimism: Natural history studies indicate that people with NF1 can live long, full lives.

PITFALLS

- Macrocrania is a common feature of NF, but growth curve for the head is necessary to determine whether it signifies a concern.
- Regrowth of plexiform neurofibromas: Even after apparent total resection, regrowth is common, and should be discussed before surgery.
- The possibility of nerve injury after surgery on plexiform neurofibromas should also be considered with the family/individual before surgery.

 ## Common Questions and Answers

Q: Can neurofibromatosis develop into cancer?
A: Most tumors caused by NF are benign and remain benign (even large tumors). In rare cases, they may become malignant.

Q: My child has NF1. What specialists must he see?
A: Your child should have yearly checkups with a physician familiar with the issues of NF (could be a family physician, pediatrician, child neurologist, or geneticist) who will know when to refer to other specialists. Otherwise, periodic visits to an ophthalmologist with experience in NF is the only routine recommendation.

ICD-9-CM 237.70

BIBLIOGRAPHY

American Academy of Pediatrics Committee on Genetics. Health supervision for children with neurofibromatosis. *Pediatrics* 1995;96: 368–372.

Gabriel KR. Neurofibromatosis. *Curr Opin Pediatr* 1997;9(1):89–93.

Gutman DH, Aylsworth A, Carey JC, et al. The diagnostic evaluation and multidisciplinary management of neurofibromatosis 1 and neurofibromatosis 2. *JAMA* 1997;278:51–57.

Lynch TM, Gutmann DH. Neurofibromatosis 1. *Neurol Clin* 2002;20(3):841–865.

North KN, Riccardi V, Samango-Sprouse C, et al. Cognitive function and academic performance in neurofibromatosis 1: consensus statement from the NF1 Cognitive Disorders Task Force. *Neurology* 1997;48: 1121–1127.

Rosser T, Packer RJ. Intracranial neoplasms in children with neurofibromatosis 1. *J Child Neurol* 2002;17(8):630–637; discussion 646–651.

Author: Leah Burke

Neutropenia

 Database

DEFINITION

A decrease in the number of circulating neutrophils (both segmented and band forms), strictly defined as an absolute total neutrophil count (ANC) of less than 1,500/mm^3. To calculate ANC, multiply the total WBC count by the percentage of segmented neutrophils and band forms. For example: WBC count 5,200 with 15% segs/polys, 4% bands, 76% lymphocytes, 5% monocytes: ANC = 5,200 × [0.15 + 0.04] = 988).

PATHOPHYSIOLOGY

Causes include:

- Decreased production in the bone marrow (congenital and acquired)
- Immune-mediated destruction
- Increased utilization (usually with overwhelming infection)
- Sequestration in the spleen

GENETICS

Some neutropenia syndromes can be inherited (e.g., Kostmann syndrome: autosomal recessive).

EPIDEMIOLOGY

- Normal values for total WBC counts and ANCs vary with age and race.
- African American children have lower total WBC counts and lower ANCs than do Caucasian children.
- Infants have a higher total WBC count and a higher percentage of lymphocytes in their differential counts.

COMPLICATIONS

- Systemic bacterial infection or localized infections such as cellulitis, labial abscesses, perirectal abscesses, oral mucosal ulceration, thrush

PROGNOSIS

- Varies
- Death from overwhelming infection does occur.
- Neutropenia resulting from infection or drug related marrow suppression is usually short-lived, but the congenital neutropenia syndromes may result in chronic lifelong neutropenia.
- Immune-mediated neutropenia frequently improves with age.

 Differential Diagnosis

- Neutropenia associated with infection

—Bacterial: Group B streptococcal disease, tuberculosis, brucellosis, tularemia, typhoid, paratyphoid
—Viral: hepatitis A and B, parvovirus B19, respiratory syncytial virus (RSV), influenza A and B, rubeola, rubella, varicella, cytomegalovirus (CMV), Epstein-Barr virus (EBV), human immunodeficiency virus (HIV)
—Other: malaria, visceral leishmaniasis, scrub typhus, sandfly fever

- Drug-induced

—Antibiotics: sulfonamides (trimethoprim-sulfamethoxazole is a common offender), penicillin, chloramphenicol (may be irreversible)
—Chemotherapy agents: alkylating agents, antimetabolites, anthracyclines
—Antipyretics: aspirin, acetaminophen (uncommon)
—Sedatives: barbiturates, benzodiazepines
—Phenothiazines: chlorpromazine, promethazine
—Antirheumatic agents: gold, penicillamine, phenylbutazone

- Tumors

—Leukemia
—Solid tumors that invade bone marrow

- Metabolic

—Nutritional: malnutrition, copper deficiency, megaloblastic anemia secondary to folate or vitamin B12 deficiency
—Inborn errors of metabolism: hyperglycinemia, isovaleric acidemia, propionic acidemia, methylmalonic acidemia

- Congenital

—Kostmann syndrome (severe congenital neutropenia)
—Cyclic neutropenia (regular oscillations in the number of circulating neutrophils: periodicity every 7 to 36 days; duration of neutropenia, 3 to 10 days)
—Chronic benign neutropenia of childhood (diagnosis of exclusion)
—Schwachman-Diamond syndrome (neutropenia and exocrine pancreatic insufficiency)
—Cartilage—hair hypoplasia (neutropenia, dwarfism, abnormal cellular immunity)
—Reticular dysgenesis

- Immunologic

—Neutropenia associated with primary immunodeficiencies (abnormalities in T and B lymphocytes)
—Autoimmune neutropenia: idiopathic (common in childhood; onset usually before age 2 years; diagnosis established by demonstrating antineutrophil antibodies; typically a benign course with resolution within several years; steroids may help in severe cases); Felty syndrome (neutropenia, splenomegaly, and rheumatoid arthritis); secondary to drugs, infection, or rheumatologic process
—Isoimmune neonatal neutropenia

- Miscellaneous

—Hypersplenism
—As part of evolving aplastic anemia (idiopathic, Fanconi anemia, familial aplastic anemia, dyskeratosis congenita)
—Bone marrow infiltration (tumor, osteopetrosis, Gaucher disease)
—Radiation injury

 Data Gathering

HISTORY

- Current or recurrent history of fever, skin abscesses, infection, or oral ulceration (helps establish duration of neutropenia)
- Medication use (many medications can cause neutropenia)
- Results of prior CBC with differential (a prior normal WBC count and ANC essentially rule out Kostmann syndrome)
- Symptoms of systemic infection: fever, rash, upper respiratory symptoms, jaundice
- Diet (looking for evidence of nutritional deficiency)
- Family history of neutropenia, recurrent infection, or early death (points to an inherited condition)

 Physical Examination

- Fever (temperature should not be taken rectally), tachycardia, and hypotension may indicate systemic infection.
- Oral ulceration, gingival irritation, pharyngitis, thrush
- Cellulitis, perirectal, or labial abscesses
- Hepatomegaly or splenomegaly
- Bruises, petechiae, pallor (other cell lines may be involved)
- Phenotypic abnormalities (thumb anomalies, dwarfism, joint findings)

Laboratory Aids

TESTS

- CBC with differential count (serial testing two to three times a week for 3 to 4 weeks may be necessary to evaluate for cyclic neutropenia)
- Bone marrow aspirate and biopsy (may be normal or may reveal a decrease in the number of myeloid precursors or a maturational arrest of the myeloid line [usually in the later stages], depending on the cause of neutropenia)
- Antineutrophil antibodies (present in autoimmune and isoimmune neutropenia) both on the neutrophils (direct) and in the serum (indirect)
- Cultures

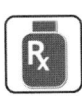
Therapy

GENERAL

- Correction of underlying cause of neutropenia (discontinue drug, treat infection, correct nutritional deficiency)
- Treatment of fever and suspected infection when neutropenic. Initially, broad-spectrum antibiotics are indicated; once the diagnosis has been established, this may not be necessary.
- Prophylactic antibiotics are not usually beneficial and may predispose to systemic fungal infection.
- Stool softeners may be helpful in the profoundly neutropenic patient at risk for constipation to prevent development of a perirectal abscess.

SPECIFIC

- Hematopoietic growth factors

—Granulocyte colony-stimulating factor (G-CSF): drug of choice for Kostmann syndrome
—Granulocyte-macrophage colony-stimulating factor (GM-CSF)

- Granulocyte transfusions (rarely indicated)
- Corticosteroids and/or plasmapheresis (most helpful in immune-mediated neutropenia)
- No therapy may be required if neutropenia is not severe and there are no serious or recurrent infections (often the case in autoimmune neutropenia and chronic benign neutropenia).

Follow-Up

- CBCs and physical examinations at regular intervals while the patient is neutropenic
- Management of febrile episodes: prompt evaluation by a physician, obtain blood culture, hospitalize, and treat with intravenous antibiotics

PREVENTION

Neutropenia syndromes are not predictable and thus are not preventable.

ISOLATION OF HOSPITALIZED PATIENT

Isolation would be prudent until the etiology of the neutropenia is identified.

PITFALLS

Factitious causes of a low WBC count:

- Long time period between when blood sample is drawn and when it is tested
- Excessive leukocyte clumping (in presence of certain paraproteins)
- Leukocyte fragility secondary to leukemia or medication use

Common Questions and Answers

Q: Do all episodes of fever and neutropenia require antibiotics?
A: In severe neutropenia syndromes or when the etiology of the neutropenia is unclear, it is prudent to evaluate the child promptly, draw a blood culture, and administer intravenous broad-spectrum antibiotics. Certain neutropenia syndromes are not associated with an increased risk of infection; children with these syndromes should be evaluated when they have fever but probably do not require intravenous antibiotics if they look well.

Q: Should a child with neutropenia be allowed to go to school?
A: Yes.

Q: Do such children need to wear a mask?
A: No.

Q: When should a hematologist be consulted?
A: With any of the following:

- Chronic or profound neutropenia
- History of recurrent skin infections
- When bone marrow examination is indicated
- When hematopoietic growth factors, plasmapheresis, or granulocyte transfusion are being considered

ICD-9-CM 288.0

BIBLIOGRAPHY

Alexander SW, Pizzo PA. Current considerations in the management of fever and neutropenia. *Curr Clin Topics Infect Dis* 1999;19:160–180.

Boxer L, Dale DC. Neutropenia: causes and consequences. *Semin Hematol* 2002;39:75–81.

Boxer LA. Neutrophil abnormalities. *Pediatr Rev* 2003;24:52–62.

Christensen RD, Calhoun DA, Rimsza LM. A practical approach to evaluating and treating neutropenia in the neonatal intensive care unit. *Clin Perinatol* 2000;27(3):577–601.

Dale DC. Immune and idiopathic neutropenia. *Curr Opin Hematol* 1998;5(1):33–36.

Kyono W, Coates TD. A practical approach to neutrophil disorders. *Pediatr Clin N Am* 2002;49:929–971.

Rolston KV. New trends in patient management: risk-based therapy for febrile patients with neutropenia. *Clin Infect Dis* 1999;29(3):515–521.

Author: Cynthia F. Norris

Non-Hodgkin Lymphoma

Database

DEFINITION

Non-Hodgkin lymphoma (NHL) is a malignant proliferation of cells of lymphocytic or histiocytic lineage that spread in a pattern similar to the migration of normal lymphoid cells.

PATHOPHYSIOLOGY

The exact cause is unknown. In contrast to adult lymphomas, childhood NHL is almost never nodular alone and rarely occurs in peripheral nodal areas.

Pediatric NHL can be divided into three major categories according to the NCI Formulation:

• Small noncleaved-cell lymphomas
—40% to 50% of childhood NHL
—Subdivided into Burkitt and Burkitt-like based on the degree of pleomorphism
—A variety of B-cell markers are usually present (e.g., CALLA, CD20).
—Express surface immunoglobulins, majority bearing IgM of either kappa or lambda light-chain subtype
—Terminal deoxyribonucleotidyl transferase (TdT) is negative.
—Characteristic chromosomal translocation, usually t(8;14), rarely t(8;22) or t(2;8); all translocations involve the c-myc proto-oncogene.

• Lymphoblastic lymphomas
—Comprise 30% of childhood NHL
—Predominantly of thymocyte (T-cell) origin: Morphologically identical to acute leukemia T lymphoblasts. Bone marrow involvement of >25% blasts is considered leukemia.
—T-cell lymphomas are positive for TdT and have a T-cell immunophenotype (e.g., CD7).
—Majority lack chromosomal translocations; seldom involve T-cell receptor genes on chromosomes 7 and 14q.

• Large-cell lymphomas
—20% of childhood NHL
—The large noncleaved or cleaved type is of B-cell origin.
—Immunoblastic types are primarily of B-cell origin except for the Ki-1 antigen-positive type (anaplastic), which is of T-cell origin.

EPIDEMIOLOGY

• Third most common childhood malignancy (approximately 12% cancers in children <20 years of age in developed countries)
• Incidence is approximately 1.0 to 1.5 per 100,000 children.
—Higher frequency of endemic Burkitt type in equatorial African countries (10 to 15 per 100,000 children under 5 to 10 years of age)
—Incidence increases steadily with age; in children, usually occurs in first two decades of life (unusual <3 years of age)
• Sex: male to female ratio is 3:1
• Genetic predisposition: increased risk in patients with immunologic defects (e.g., Bruton agammaglobulinemia, ataxia-telangiectasia, Wiskott-Aldrich, severe combined immunodeficiency)
• Environmental factors

—Drugs: immunosuppressive therapy and diphenylhydantoin
—Radiation: atomic-bomb survivors and ionizing radiation
—Viruses: Epstein-Barr virus (EBV), human immunodeficiency virus (HIV); EBV present in greater than 95% of cases of endemic Burkitt's versus fewer than 20% cases of sporadic

COMPLICATIONS

• Tumor lysis syndrome
—Combination of hyperuricemia, hyperkalemia, and hyperphosphatemia with hypocalcemia, resulting in uric acid nephropathy that leads to renal failure
—Correct before starting chemotherapy.
• Gastrointestinal obstruction, perforation, bleeding, intussusception
• Inferior vena cava obstruction and venous thromboembolism
• Neurologic (e.g., paraplegia, increased intracranial pressure)
• Superior vena cava (SVC) and superior mediastinum syndrome (SMS)
—Associated with lymphoblastic lymphomas that invade the thymus and nodes surrounding the vena cava and airways
• Massive pleural effusion
• Cardiac tamponade or arrhythmia

PROGNOSIS

Important prognostic factors for outcome include tumor burden at presentation.
• Favorable: stages I and II with primary site being head and neck (nonparameningeal), peripheral nodes, or abdominal site (80% or greater 2-year survival).
• Unfavorable: stage III or IV, parameningeal stage II, stage IV with CNS involvement (worst); incomplete initial remission within 2 months (60% to 80% 2-year survival)

Differential Diagnosis

• Abdominal masses
—Newborns: hydronephrosis, renal cysts, Wilms' tumor, or neuroblastoma.
—Older children: constipation, full bladder, hamartoma, hemangioma, cysts, leukemic or lymphomatous involvement of the liver and/or spleen, Wilms' tumor, or neuroblastoma
• Mediastinal masses
—Anterior: masses of thymic origin, teratomas, angiomas, lipomas, or thyroid tumors
—Middle: metastatic or infection-related lesions involving the lymph nodes, pericardial or bronchogenic cysts, esophageal lesions, or hernias
—Posterior: neurogenic tumors (e.g., neuroblastoma, ganglioneuroma, neurofibroma), enterogenous cysts, thoracic meningocele, or hernias

Data Gathering

A diagnosis needs to be made expeditiously, as pediatric lymphomas generally have a rapid growth rate.

HISTORY

• B-cell lymphomas
—Systemic manifestation (e.g., fever, weight loss, anorexia, fatigue) if disseminated; less likely if tumor localized
—Lump in neck that does not respond to antibiotics
—Abdominal mass with pain, swelling, change in bowel habits, nausea, or vomiting
• T-cell lymphomas
—Mediastinal tumor symptoms include cough, hoarseness, dyspnea, orthopnea and chest pain, anxiety, confusion, lethargy, headache, distorted vision, syncope, and a sense of fullness in the ears.
—Marrow involvement
—Bleeding and/or bruising, bone pain, pallor, fatigue

Physical Examination

• Small non–cleaved-cell lymphomas
—Intraabdominal mass (up to 90%): involving ileocecal region, appendix, ascending colon, or some combination of these sites. Lymphadenopathy may be present in inguinal or iliac region; hepatosplenomegaly. Acute abdomen with intussusception, peritonitis, ascites, and acute GI bleeding. Lymphoma is the most frequent cause of intussusception in children over age 6 years.
—In endemic Burkitt lymphoma, jaw tumors are the most frequent; orbital involvement in infants; abdominal masses in 50%.
—Other sites: testis, unilateral tonsil hypertrophy, peripheral lymph nodes, parotid gland, skin, bone, CNS, and marrow.
• Lymphoblastic lymphoma
—Mediastinal mass (50% to 70%) with pleural effusion present with decreased breath sounds, rales, and cough with or without SVC or SMS syndrome. Signs include swelling, plethora, and cyanosis of the face, neck, and upper extremities; diaphoresis; and stridor and wheezing.
—Lymphadenopathy (50% to 80%) is primarily above the diaphragm.
—Abdominal involvement is uncommon, likely to involve only liver and spleen.
—Cranial nerve involvement is rarely seen.
• Large cell lymphomas
—Sites involved include mediastinum, bone, inguinal nodes, and skin.
—Bone marrow and CNS involvement are rarely found at diagnosis.

Laboratory Aids

TESTS

The diagnosis should be established with the least invasive method possible. A bone marrow aspirate and biopsy may establish the diagnosis without further testing. Fluid from ascites in patients with abdominal disease, or pleural fluid should be obtained for cytology, immunophenotyping and cytogenetics. Biopsy of an enlarged lymph node may be performed.

Laboratory Tests

- CBC
- Liver and renal function studies
- Serum LDH and uric acid
- Adequate surgical biopsy

Imaging

- Abdominal ultrasound
- Chest PA and lateral
- CT scan of chest, abdomen, and pelvis
- Gallium scan
- Bone scan (optional or if gallium scan suggests bone involvement)
- MRI (especially for bone involvement)

Special Tests

- CSF examination
- Peritoneal or pleural fluid examination
- Bone marrow aspiration and biopsy
- Cytogenetics and immunophenotyping of tumor

STAGING

No uniform staging system exists for childhood NHL. The St. Jude Children's Research Hospital staging system is as follows:

Stage I: single-tumor (extranodal) or single-nodal area, excluding mediastinum or abdomen
Stage II: single tumor with regional nodal involvement, two or more tumors or nodal areas on one side of the diaphragm, or a primary GI tract tumor (resected) with or without regional node involvement
Stage III: tumors or lymph node areas on both sides of the diaphragm, any primary intrathoracic or extensive intraabdominal disease (unresectable), or any primary paraspinal or epidural tumors
Stage IV: bone marrow or CNS disease regardless of other sites; marrow involvement defined as 0.5% to 25% of malignant cells.

Therapy

A multidisciplinary approach is imperative to ensure the best therapy.

RADIOTHERAPY (XRT)

- Radiation adds no therapeutic benefit in children with limited disease.
- Increases both short- and long-term toxicity
- XRT used as emergent treatment for SVC obstruction, CNS, or testicular involvement.

SURGERY

- Performed if total resection can be achieved
- Additional indications: intussusception, intestinal perforation, suspected appendicitis, or serious GI bleeding
- It is important to avoid extensive surgery in patients with NHL.

PRECHEMOTHERAPY MANAGEMENT

Allopurinol, hydration, and urinary alkalinization to prevent tumor lysis syndrome. Monitor uric acid, BUN, creatinine, K+, Ca2+, and PO4−.

CHEMOTHERAPY

- Histology and stage determine choice of a particular protocol.
- Because of a high-conversion rate of lymphomas to leukemias, prophylactic CNS treatment is given (except in patients with totally excised intraabdominal tumor).
- Duration: 6 to 18 months
- Drugs: cyclophosphamide, vincristine, methotrexate (IV + IT), prednisone, daunorubicin, asparaginase, cytarabine, thioguanine, carmustine, hydroxyurea, hydrocortisone, doxorubicin, mercaptopurine, etoposide
- Common side effects: hair loss, myelosuppression with transfusions required, nausea/vomiting

IMMUNOTHERAPY

- Rituximab is a chimeric monoclonal antibody directed against the CD20 antigen, which is almost universally expressed on tumor cells in pediatric B-cell NHL.
- This is a new active agent for patients with lymphoma. It has been used successfully in patients with relapsed/refractory B-cell NHL.
- There are few overlapping side effects with the combination of rituximab and conventional chemotherapeutic agents.

MANAGEMENT OF RELAPSE

- Relapse indicates extremely poor prognosis.
- No uniform approach to rescue therapy
- In patients refractory to or relapsing after initial therapy, different chemotherapy combinations may induce a new response, but long-term survival is rarely seen.
- Allogeneic or autologous bone marrow transplant should be considered.
- For patients with chemosensitive relapse, salvage therapy followed by high-dose therapy with stem cell support is recommended, since this may result in prolonged survival.

Follow-Up

- Patient monitoring weekly to monthly with CBC and examination.
- Radiologic imaging at intervals during and off therapy.
- Monitor for toxicity-related complications (cardiac, gonadal function, second malignancies)

PITFALLS

Late effects from therapy:
- Cardiomyopathy from anthracyclines
- Impaired reproductive function or infertility from alkylating agents or radiation
- Second malignant neoplasms from etoposide and alkylators
- Psychological consequences of life-threatening illness

Common Questions and Answers

Q: Did I do something to cause this?
A: No. The majority of cases are sporadic and not associated with diet, underlying immune dysfunction, or viral illness.

Q: When will my child be "cured"?
A: For patients with small- or large-cell lymphomas, relapse most commonly occurs in the first 10 months. Therefore, a child may be considered cured if he or she remains in remission after the first year off therapy. A patient with lymphoblastic lymphoma is considered cured if he or she remains in remission after about 3 years from onset of therapy.

Q: Is this contagious?
A: No. Siblings may have slightly higher inherent risk than the general population, but they are not at risk from the affected child.

ICD-9-CM 200

BIBLIOGRAPHY

Coiffier B, Haioun C, Ketterer N, et al. Rituximab (anti-CD20 monoclonal antibody) for the treatment of patients with relapsing or refractory aggressive lymphoma: a multicenter Phase II study. *Blood* 1998;92:1927–1932.

Pinkerton CR. The continuing challenge of treatment for non-Hodgkin's lymphoma in children. *Br J Haematol* 1999;107(2): 220–234.

Rheingold SR, Lange BJ. Oncologic emergencies. In: Pizzo PA, Poplack DG, eds. *Principles and Practice of Pediatric Oncology*. 4th Ed. Philadelphia: JB Lippincott, 2002:1177–1203.

Shad A, Magrath I. Diagnosis and treatment of non-Hodgkin's lymphoma in childhood. In: Wernik P, Canellos G, Putcher J, eds. *Neoplastic Diseases of the Blood*. 3rd Ed. New York: Churchill Livingstone, 1996:925.

Author: Jill P. Ginsberg

Nosebleeds (Epistaxis)

 Database

DEFINITION

Epistaxis is bleeding from the nose. Bleeding may be evident anteriorly through the nares or posteriorly through the nasopharynx.

CAUSES

- Inflammation of, or trauma to, the nasal passages accounts for most nosebleeds:

—Viral upper respiratory infections, allergic rhinitis, bacterial rhinitis
—Nose picking, external trauma, foreign bodies, postsurgical bleeding, chemical, or caustic agents/inhalants

- Local structural abnormalities may predispose to epistaxis:

—Rhinitis sicca, or environmental drying of the nasal mucosa, commonly promotes epistaxis
—Nasal polyps, telangiectasias, meningoceles, angiofibromas, vascular malformations, septal deviations or spurs

- Less commonly, nosebleeds may herald, or accompany, systemic illnesses:

—Hematologic diseases such as leukemias, thrombocytopenias, hemophilias (and von Willebrand disease), and hemoglobinopathies
—Clotting disorders as a result of infection, hepatic failure, or poisoning/envenomation
—Hypertension (usually not the cause but can make hemostasis difficult)

- Pseudoepistaxes from pulmonary hemoptysis, bleeding esophageal varices or pharyngeal/laryngeal tumors that bleed can be mistaken for epistaxis

PATHOPHYSIOLOGY

- The nasal mucosa has a rich blood supply originating from both the internal and external carotid arteries.
- Blood vessels of the nasal septum and lateral nasal walls have little anatomic support or protection. The thin mucosal surface is prone to drying.
- Blood vessels of the nose form many plexiform networks. Especially important is Kiesselbach plexus in the anterior nasal septum, the most common site of nosebleeds in children.
- The nose is subject, by position, to traumatic injury.

EPIDEMIOLOGY

- Nosebleeds occur in all ages throughout the year.
- Children aged 2 to 10 years are most commonly affected.
- Nosebleeds are more common in the winter.

COMPLICATIONS

- Nosebleeds are most commonly uncomplicated.
- Rare complications include significant blood loss, airway obstruction, aspiration, and vomiting.

PROGNOSIS

- Uncomplicated epistaxis is most often self-limited or resolves with simple first-aid techniques.
- Refractory or recurrent epistaxis may require more specialized techniques, surgical intervention, and/or otorhinolaryngologic intervention.

ASSOCIATED ILLNESSES

Hemoptysis, hematemesis, or melena may be the presenting concerns in individuals with bleeding from the nasopharynx.

 Differential Diagnosis

Epistaxis is a common event in normal children. A careful history and physical examination should identify those children with unusual predisposing causes for nosebleeds.

 Data Gathering

HISTORY

- Frequency of occurrence
- Persistence of bleeding
- Nose-picking behavior/traumatic injury
- Nasal congestion, discharge, obstruction
- Allergies
- Medications or drugs of abuse (especially cocaine)
- Previous or concurrent bruising or bleeding
- Menstrual history
- Family history of systemic disease or hemorrhagic disorder

 Physical Examination

- Vital signs with blood pressure determination
- Inspection of nose, nasopharynx, and oropharynx
- General examination with attention to lymph nodes, liver and spleen size, rashes, icterus, pallor

PROCEDURE

- Examination of the nose may be facilitated by application of a topical vasoconstricting agent and/or anesthetic agent.
- Anxiety may interfere with examination and treatment of children. Sedation and analgesia may be beneficial in some circumstances.

Laboratory Aids

TESTS

• Laboratory evaluation is not indicated in healthy children with readily controlled epistaxis from an anterior site.
• Recurrent or refractory nosebleeds, or suspicious findings from the history and physical examination, may warrant a directed laboratory evaluation (such as platelet count, prothrombin and partial thromboplastin times, complete blood count, and/or bleeding time) and/or consultation.

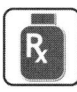 ## Therapy

• Elevate the head of the bed.
• Direct pressure, applied by gently squeezing the nostrils, is usually sufficient to stop most nosebleeds.
• Ice or cold packs to the neck or nasal dorsum appear not to have a significant benefit, but may be combined with application of pressure.
• A cotton pledget beneath the upper lip may aid hemostasis by compressing the labial artery.
• Vasoconstricting agents (0.25% phenylephrine, 0.05% oxymetazoline, 1:1,000 epinephrine, or 1% to 5% cocaine) will help reduce bleeding as well as improve visualization.
• Application of topical thrombin or fibrin glue may be used when direct visualization of the bleeding site is achieved.
• Once identified, an offending vessel may be cauterized with a silver nitrate stick or a swab dipped in trichloroacetic acid.
• Antiseptic creams combining chlorhexidine and neomycin applied topically are more effective than no treatment and just as effective as cautery with silver nitrate.
• An anterior nasal packing with oxycellulose or petroleum jelly gauze may be required to control refractory epistaxis when the site of bleeding cannot be precisely identified.
• Otorhinolaryngologic consultation may be needed for severe nosebleeds or when posterior nasal packing, fracture reduction, surgery, or embolization are required. Nasal endoscopy is now routinely used.
• Parental reassurance is an important, but often neglected, aspect of therapy.

PREVENTION

• Vaporizers, humidifiers, or saline sprays prevent desiccation of the nasal mucosa.
• Petroleum jelly applied to the anterior nasal septum aids healing of inflamed nasal mucosa.
• Antigen avoidance and medical therapy should be used to reduce allergic symptoms.
• Fingernails should be cut short, and nose-picking behavior should be discouraged.
• Protective athletic equipment should be worn.

 ## Follow-Up

• Nosebleeds are easily controlled and self-limited in most instances.
• Families should be given instructions in basic first aid for nosebleeds, because minor insults, such as sneezing or excessive manipulation, may cause nosebleeds to recur.
• Referral to an otorhinolaryngologist is indicated for patients with specific local abnormalities, such as polyps, tumors, or vascular malformations.
• Severe nosebleeds, recurrent nosebleeds, and/or posteriorly located nosebleeds may warrant evaluation by an otorhinolaryngologist.
• Identification of systemic illness may require referral to the appropriate specialist.
• Postsurgical nosebleeds can be particularly problematic.

PITFALLS

• Blood clots in the nasopharynx should be removed because they may obscure engorged, bleeding vessels.
• Failure to detect a posterior location within the nasal cavity as the source of bleeding may interfere with measures to control bleeding.
• After nasal packing, it is essential to examine the oropharynx to confirm adequate hemostasis.
• Absorbable-type packings should be used, if required, in patients with bleeding disorders. Standard packings are prone to rebleeding on removal.
• Impregnation of nasal packings with antibiotic ointment reduces the risk of toxic shock syndrome.

 ## Common Questions and Answers

Q: How should the patient with nosebleeds be positioned?
A: When possible, patients with nosebleeds should be kept erect. The upright position decreases vascular congestion. Recumbent patients may appear to have less bleeding, but this is as a result of redirection of blood flow through the posterior pharynx.

Q: How does rhinitis sicca contribute to epistaxis, and why does it occur?
A: The nose warms, humidifies, and filters inspired air. Many modern heating systems and air-conditioning units reduce household humidity to unnaturally low levels. Rhinitis sicca is the direct result of inhaling dry air and results in friable nasal mucosa. Turbulent airflow from a septal deformity also promotes drying.

ICD-9-CM 784.7

BIBLIOGRAPHY

Kubba H, MacAndie C. A prospective, single-blind, randomized controlled trial of antiseptic cream for recurrent epistaxis in childhood. *Clin Otolaryngol* 2001;26(6): 465–468.

Mahmood S, Lowe T. Management of epistaxis in the oral and maxillofacial surgery setting: An update on current practice. *Oral Surg Oral Med Oral Pathol Oral Radiol Endod* 2003;95(1):23–29.

Tan LS, Calhoun KH. Epistaxis. *Med Clin North Am* 1999;83:43–56.

Authors: Suzanne Beno
Kevin C. Osterhoudt, 3rd edition

Obesity

 Database

DEFINITION

Obesity is a complex, multifactorial, chronic disease that develop from an interaction of genotype and the environment. Obesity is defined as excess body fat. The body mass index (BMI) is the ratio of weight in kilograms to the height in meters, squared and is a widely accepted proxy measure of adiposity. Children with a BMI >25 are overweight and a >30 are obese.

CAUSES

- Obesity is caused by chronic intake of calories in excess of energy utilization as a result of modifiable causes such as a sedentary lifestyle, social pressure such as advertising, absence of healthy choices, and the increased availability of inexpensive high caloric foods at all times.
- Factors that may be difficult to modify without intensive medical intervention include corticosteroid treatment, hypothyroidism, Prader-Willi syndrome, Down syndrome, and other disorders.

EPIDEMIOLOGY AND RISK FACTORS

- Data from the Centers for Disease Control and Prevention indicate that >10% of children ages 2 to 5 years old, 15.3% of children ages 6 to 11 years, 15.5% of children aged 12 to 19 years are overweight.
- There has been a dramatic increase from 1971–1974, when 4% of children aged 6 to 11 years, and 6% of children aged 12 to 19 years were overweight.
- Prevalence of overweight children varies by racial/ethnic group, with the highest rates for Mexican-American children, followed by non-Hispanic blacks.
- Risk factors:

—Interactions between genetic, biological, psychological, sociocultural, and environmental factors clearly are clearly important.
—Children with an overweight parent are more likely to be overweight.
—Extent and duration of breast feeding seem inversely related to obesity.
—Low-income families may face lack of consistent access to healthful food choices, particularly fruits and vegetables.
—The earlier a child becomes obese, the more likely obesity develops later.
—Less active children are more likely to be overweight.

COMPLICATIONS

Immediate

- Pulmonary: asthma, sleep apnea, and sudden death.
- Endocrine: insulin resistance and type 2 diabetes, hypercholesterolemia, early menarche, polycystic ovarian syndrome, and irregular menses.
- Hypertension.
- Gastroenterologic: gallstones, liver steatosis/liver fibrosis secondary to nonalcoholic steatohepatitis (NASH).
- Orthopaedic: slipped epiphyses, tibia vara (Blount's disease).
- Neurologic: pseudotumor cerebri.
- Psychosocial: decreased self-esteem, discrimination, and depression

Long-Term, All of the Above Including

- Persistence of obesity
- Ischemic heart disease
- Cerebrovascular disease
- Osteoarthritis, gout
- Some cancers
- Increased mortality from all causes in adulthood

PROGNOSIS

- Long-term maintenance of weight loss is poorer in adults than in children.
- Better prognosis is seen when the children adhere to self-monitoring (see Behavior Modification, below).
- Significant health benefits are seen from an even modest decrease in BMI
- Setting realistic targets with gradual weight loss achieve better results in the long term.

 Differential Diagnosis

- Vast majority of obese patients do not have a disease process as we understand it today. Genetic predisposition may be a factor.
- Some medical conditions associated with obesity include:

—Down Syndrome
—Prader-Willi syndrome
—Lawrence Moon Biedl syndrome
—Hypothalamic dysfunction
—Brain tumor
—Excessive tube feeding in children with mental retardation and cerebral palsy
—Cushing syndrome: iatrogenic and spontaneous
—Hypothyroidism
—Hyperinsulinism
—Growth hormone deficiency

HISTORY

A full medical history is important but one would need to focus on the following aspects:

- Level of concern, readiness to change, weight loss expectation
- Psychosocial history: school, family support, counseling, depression, eating disorders
- Dietary history: 3-day diet record, portion size
- Dietary pattern: number of meals and snacks, eating in front of the television, family meals.
- Physical activity: type and duration of physical activity
- Duration of inactivity: television, computer and video games, Internet, telephone
- Duration of obesity—lifelong or recent onset.

Physical Examination

While a full examination is required, the focus may include:

- Anthropometric measurements: height, weight, BMI, possibly waist circumference, skinfold thickness
- Pediatric growth charts for the U.S. population now include BMI for age and gender: (http://www.cdc.gov/growthcharts) allowing longitudinal tracking of BMI
- Blood pressure
- Dysmorphic signs, xanthoma, acanthosis nigricans

TESTS

Case Specific

- Lipid profile
- Fasting glucose or a glucose tolerance test
- Thyroid function
- AST, ALT, GGT
- Insulin level
- Genetic studies—Prader Willi gene

In addition these tests may be helpful

- Ultrasound or MRI to look for fatty liver.
- Resting energy expenditure (REE): guidance on the caloric requirement of a child and guide the dietary manipulation.

Obesity

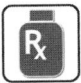 Therapy

As in other chronic conditions, the objective of the treatment should be to control obesity, and to prevent complications.

When possible, a multidisciplinary team approach is recommended.

Family and school involvement especially gym teachers, as well as recognition of the difficulty of weight management, is critical for success.

DRUGS

I. Appetite suppressants—affects serotonin or catecholamine levels

Generic names	Trade names
• Dexfenfluramine	• Redux—recalled by FDA
• Diethylpropion	• Tenuate
• Fenfluramine	• Podimin—recalled by FDA
• Mazindol	• Sanorex, Mazanor
• Phendimetrazine	• Bontul, Plagine, Prelu-2, X-Trozine Ionamin, Adipex-2
• Sibutramine	• Meridia (approved for >16 years old)
• Phentermine	• Fastin, Oby-trim

II. Lipase inhibitor—fat malabsorption.

• Orlistat	• Xenacal

REFERRALS

Referral to other subspecialist for apnea, hypertension, diabetes, dysmorphic features, elevated liver enzymes, psychological, and orthopaedic problems that are more common in obese patients.

SURGERY

Gastric bypass surgery may have a role in the morbidly obese patient (BMI >40) with other comorbid conditions:

- Advanced steatohepatitis with fibrosis
- Severe apnea with cor pulmonale
- Diabetes mellitus
- Hypertension
- In children, further studies are needed before this can be recommended.

BEHAVIOR MODIFICATION

- Goal-setting, contracting, reward system
- Self-monitoring of time of inactivity, time of physical activity, sometimes food intake and body weight
- Environmental control to reduce cues and opportunities for energy intake and inactivity and to increase cues and opportunities for physical activity
- Management of high-risk situations, such as parties, dining out, holidays, dining out, emotional fluctuations, and feelings of deprivation
- Improvement of parenting skills

DIETARY CHANGES

- Encourage structured family meal
- Encourage eating slowly
- Eliminate eating or snacking in front of the television
- Eliminate sugar-containing drinks
- Decrease portion size
- Replace high-energy density foods with an increased variety of fruits and vegetables
- The "Atkins diet" may be effective in achieving weight loss but the long-term effects of the high-fat diet is unknown. There are no pediatric data regarding this dietary intervention.

PHYSICAL ACTIVITY AND INACTIVITY

- Monitor and limit time of physical inactivity: television, computer and video games, Internet, and telephone.
- Establish and monitor regular physical activities.
- Establish healthy lifestyles: using stairs, walking to the store, visiting friends rather than talking on the phone.
- Help parents, teachers, coaches, and others discuss health habitus, not body habitus, as part of their efforts to control overweight and obesity.
- Different types of exercise may have a different fat burning index, in particular, quick walking is thought to be more useful than aggressive weight lifting. Excellent exercise for obese patients includes swimming, which protects the weight bearing joints and rapid walking.

 Follow-Up

Initially frequent, every 4 to 6 weeks
After healthy habits have been established, less frequent follow-up

 Common Questions and Answers

Q: Is childhood obesity a result of a slow metabolism or hormonal problem?
A: Hormonal and metabolic causes of obesity are unusual. Most often, obesity is a result of exogenous causes, such as physical inactivity and excessive food intake.

Q: Can childhood obesity be treated despite parental obesity?
A: Familial obesity results from a genetic predisposition, but also from a shared environment that can be modified.

Q: How can obesity be prevented in high-risk children?
A: By limiting television watching, establishing healthy lifestyles, regular physical activities, and a healthy balanced diet.

Q: Is child obesity a risk for adult chronic diseases?
A: Obese children are at much higher risk for hypertension, dyslipidemia, insulin resistance and type 2 diabetes, ischemic heart disease, cerebrovascular disease, sleep apnea and increased mortality for all causes when they become adults.

ICD-9-CM

Obesity 278.0
Morbid obesity 278.01

BIBLIOGRAPHY

Berkowitz RI, Wadden TA, Tershakovec AM, Cronquist JL. Behavior therapy and sibutramine for the treatment of adolescent obesity: a randomized controlled trial. *JAMA* 2003;289(14):1805–1812.

BMI. 2000 CDC Growth Charts: United States. Atlanta: Centers for Disease Control and Prevention, 2002. Available at: htpp://www.cdc.gov/growthcharts. Accessed February 10, 2004.

Krebs NF, Jacobson MS. Prevention of pediatric overweight and obesity. American Academy of Pediatrics, Committee on Nutrition 2002–2003. *Pediatrics* 2003; 112(2):424–430.

Ogden CL, Flegal KM, Carroll MD, Johnson CL. Prevalence and trends in overweight amongst US children and adolescents 1999–2000. *JAMA* 2002;288(14):1728–1732.

Robinson TN. Reducing children's television viewing to prevent obesity: a randomized controlled trial. *JAMA* 1999;282:1561–1567.

Strauss RS. Childhood obesity. *Pediatr Clin North Am* 2002;49(1):175–201.

Styne DM. Childhood and adolescent obesity. *Pediatr Clin North Am* 2001;48(4):823–854, vii.

Sugerman HJ. Bariatric surgery for severely obese adolescents. *J Gastrointest Surg* 2003;7(1):102–107.

Authors: Ruben W. Cerri and John Tung

Omphalitis

 ## Database

DEFINITION

Omphalitis, an infection of the umbilical stump, begins in the neonatal period as a superficial cellulitis but may progress to necrotizing fasciitis, myonecrosis, or systemic disease.

CAUSES

• Most (85%) cases of omphalitis are polymicrobial.
• The most common organisms include gram-positive cocci (*Staphylococcus aureus*, group A *Streptococcus*) and gram-negative enteric bacilli (*Escherichia coli*, *Klebsiella pneumoniae*, and *Proteus mirabilis*).
• Gram-positive organisms predominated in the past; however, the introduction of antistaphylococcal cord care (triple dye) has led to an increase in colonization and infection with gram-negative organisms.
• Anaerobic bacteria, including *Bacteroides fragilis* and *Clostridium perfringens*, are isolated in one-third of infections.
• Anaerobic organisms are more likely in cases complicated by necrotizing fasciitis or myonecrosis than in cases of superficial abdominal wall cellulitis.
• *C. tetani* and *C. sordellii* have been reported when deliveries have occurred outside a medical facility and when the cultural practice of placing cow dung on the umbilical stump after delivery was observed.

PATHOPHYSIOLOGY

• Potential bacterial pathogens normally colonize the umbilical stump after birth.
• These bacteria invade the umbilical stump, leading to omphalitis.
• Established aerobic bacterial infection, necrotic tissue, and poor blood supply facilitate the growth of anaerobic organisms.
• Infection may also extend beyond the subcutaneous tissues to involve fascial planes (fasciitis), abdominal wall musculature (myonecrosis), and the umbilical and portal veins (phlebitis).

EPIDEMIOLOGY

• Incidence varies from 0.2% to 0.7% in industrialized countries.
• Incidence is higher in hospitalized preterm infants compared to term infants.
• Episodes of omphalitis are usually sporadic, but rare epidemics occur.
• Mean age of onset is 5 to 9 days in term infants and 3 to 5 days in preterm infants.
• Risk factors for the development of omphalitis include low birth weight, prior umbilical catheterization, septic delivery, and prolonged rupture of membranes.

COMPLICATIONS

• Necrotizing fasciitis, a bacterial infection of the subcutaneous fat, and superficial and deep fascia, complicates 8% to 16% of cases of omphalitis. It is characterized by rapidly spreading infection, often with systemic toxicity.
• Myonecrosis refers to infectious involvement of the muscle. The rapid development of edema may constrict the muscle within its fascia and cause a superimposed ischemic myonecrosis.
• Extensive areas of necrotic tissue facilitate the growth of anaerobic organisms.
• Portal vein thrombosis and septic embolization follow infection of the umbilical vessels.
• Sepsis complicates omphalitis in 13% of cases.

PROGNOSIS

• The outcome of infants with uncomplicated omphalitis is generally good. The mortality rate among all infants with omphalitis, including those who develop complications, is 7% to 15%. The mortality rate is significantly higher (38% to 87%) with necrotizing fasciitis or myonecrosis.
• Risk factors for poor prognosis include male gender, prematurity, low birth weight, and septic delivery, including delivery outside a medical facility.

ASSOCIATED DISEASES

• Omphalitis may be the initial manifestation of an underlying disorder of neutrophil migration such as leukocyte adhesion deficiency, a rare immunologic disorder with an autosomal-recessive pattern of inheritance. These infants present with leukocytosis, delayed separation of the umbilical cord, and recurrent infections.
• Omphalitis may also be a manifestation of neutropenia in the neonate.

—In neonatal alloimmune neutropenia, maternal IgG antibodies cross the placenta and result in an immune-mediated destruction of fetal neutrophils bearing antigens that differ from the mother's. The resultant neutropenia can last for several weeks to as long as 6 months. Antineutrophil antibodies are found in the serum of the mother and the infant. Affected infants may also present with other cutaneous bacterial infections, pneumonia, sepsis, and meningitis.
—Causes of neutropenia associated with immune dysfunction include autoimmune neutropenias, X-linked agammaglobulinemia, hyper-IgM immunodeficiency syndromes, and HIV.
—Other causes of neutropenia include metabolic disorders such as hyperglycinemia, isovaleric acidemia, propionic acidemia, methylmalonic acidemia, tyrosinemia, and glycogen storage disease type IB.

• Omphalitis complicated by sepsis can also be associated with neutropenia. Therefore, the underlying disease process producing neutropenia may not be immediately appreciated in affected newborns.
• Rarely, an anatomic abnormality such as a patent urachus or patent omphalomesenteric duct may be present.

 ## Differential Diagnosis

• The characteristic clinical picture of omphalitis allows diagnosis on clinical grounds. Determine the presence of associated complications, such as necrotizing fasciitis, myonecrosis, or systemic infection. Consider an underlying immunologic or metabolic disorder.

 ## Data Gathering

HISTORY

• Review the pregnancy, labor, delivery, and neonatal course in detail.
• A history of change in mental status such as irritability, lethargy, somnolence, or decreased level of activity may indicate systemic dissemination of the infection.
• A history of urine or stool discharge from the umbilicus suggests an underlying anatomic abnormality.
• Family history may reveal individuals with metabolic disorders or recurrent infections.

 ## Physical Examination

Physical signs vary with the extent of disease. Signs of localized infection include the following:

• Abdominal tenderness
• Periumbilical edema and erythema
• Purulent or malodorous discharge from the umbilical stump

The following indicate more extensive local disease such as necrotizing fasciitis or myonecrosis:

• Periumbilical ecchymoses or gangrene
• Abdominal wall crepitus
• Progression of cellulitis despite antimicrobial therapy
• Signs of systemic disease are nonspecific and include thermodysregulation and evidence of multiorgan dysfunction:

—Fever or temperature instability
—Tachycardia, hypotension, delayed capillary refill
—Apnea, tachypnea, flaring of the alae nasi, grunting, intercostal/subcostal retractions, hypoxemia
—Abdominal distension, diminished bowel sounds
—Cyanosis, petechiae, jaundice
—Lethargy, hypotonia

Laboratory Aids

LABORATORY STUDIES

Test: Umbilical stump Gram stain and culture for aerobic and anaerobic organisms
Significance: Identify potential organisms and antimicrobial susceptibility patterns. While suggestive, cultures of umbilical discharge may reflect only colonization of the stump and are not proof of an etiologic role in the underlying process. Therefore, if myonecrosis is suspected, specimens of muscle should be sent for culture.

Test: Blood culture
Significance: There is a risk of systemic dissemination of infection in the neonate.

Test: Complete blood count
Significance: Neutropenia or neutrophilia may be present. An immature-to-total neutrophils ratio >0.2 is suggestive of systemic infection. Thrombocytopenia may be present.

Test: Prothrombin time, partial thromboplastin time, fibrinogen, fibrinogen split products
Significance: Indicated for sepsis or disseminated intravascular coagulation.

Test: Lumbar puncture
Significance: Indicated in any neonate with a focal bacterial infection.

RADIOLOGIC IMAGING (CASE DEPENDENT)

Test: Abdominal radiographs
Significance: Portal venous or intramural air requires immediate surgical consultation.

Test: Abdominal CT
Significance: Confirms involvement of fascia and muscle and delineates the extent of infection.

Test: Voiding cystourethrogram
Significance: Diagnoses a patent urachus.

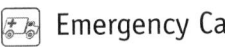 ## Emergency Care

Immediate evaluation, antimicrobial therapy, and supportive care are essential to survival.

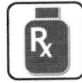 ## Therapy

• Empiric coverage: An antistaphylococcal agent (e.g., oxacillin, vancomycin) plus an aminoglycoside (e.g., gentamicin, amikacin, tobramycin) or 3rd generation cephalosporin (e.g., cefotaxime).
• Add anaerobic coverage (e.g., metronidazole) in cases complicated by necrotizing fasciitis or myonecrosis. Clindamycin also provides anaerobic coverage and may be substituted for the antistaphylococcal penicillin.
• As with antimicrobial therapy for other infections, consider local antibiotic susceptibility patterns.
• Early and complete surgical debridement of affected tissue and muscle is important. Delay in diagnosis or surgical intervention allows local progression of infection and worsening systemic toxicity.
• The use of hyperbaric oxygen to treat anaerobic necrotizing fasciitis and myonecrosis is controversial. No prospective data are available. The delivery of high concentrations of oxygen to marginally perfused tissues may have a detrimental effect on the growth of anaerobic organisms and improve phagocyte function. However, surgical therapy remains the highest priority.

PREVENTION

• Antimicrobial agents applied to the umbilicus decrease bacterial colonization and prevent omphalitis.
• Effective methods of umbilical cord care include:

—Triple dye daily until cord separation
—Triple dye once and then alcohol daily until cord separation
—Triple dye once and no further treatment
—Povidone-iodine daily until cord separation
—Silver sulfadiazine daily until cord separation
—Bacitracin daily until cord separation

There are no significant differences in the incidence of omphalitis with these regimens. However, the duration of umbilical cord attachment is significantly longer with triple dye daily compared to the other regimens (17 days vs. 6 to 12 days).

• Dry cord care—spot cleaning of soiled skin in periumbilical area without application of any antibacterial agents—is acceptable but requires extreme vigilance for signs of infection. Infants treated with dry cord care as opposed to any of the above regimens are more likely to experience foul-smelling umbilical exudates (7% vs. <1%), bacterial colonization of umbilical stump, and omphalitis.

 ## Follow-Up

• Infants developing associated portal vein thrombosis require follow-up for complications as a result of portal hypertension.

 ## Common Questions and Answers

Q: Do all infants who develop omphalitis require evaluation for immunologic disorders?
A: No, particularly if predisposing factors such as an umbilical catheter are present. Infants requiring further evaluation include those with persistent neutropenia, recurrent infections, delayed separation of the umbilical cord, or a family history of immunologic disorders.

Q: Is surgical consultation required for all infants with omphalitis?
A: No, surgical consultation is not required for uncomplicated omphalitis. However, a high degree of suspicion should exist for associated complications. The presence of necrotizing fasciitis or myonecrosis requires immediate surgical consultation.

ICD-9-CM 771.4

BIBLIOGRAPHY

Bradley JS. Wound and deep-tissue infections. In: Jenson HB, Baltimore RS, eds. *Pediatric Infectious Diseases: Principles and Practice.* Norwalk: Appleton and Lange, 1995:723–732.

Cushing AH. Omphalitis: a review. *Pediatr Infect Dis J* 1985;4:282–285.

Gladstone IM, Clapper L, Thorpe JW. Randomized study of six umbilical cord regimens. *Clin Pediatr* 1988;27:127–129.

Mason WH, Andrews R, Ross LA. Omphalitis in the newborn infant. *Pediatr Infect Dis J* 1989;8:521–525.

Samuel M, Freeman N, Vaishnav A, et al. Necrotizing fasciitis: a serious complication of omphalitis in neonates. 1994;29:1414–1416.

Author: Samir S. Shah and Leslie Moroz

Osteogenesis Imperfecta

 Database

DEFINITION

Osteogenesis imperfecta (OI) is a group of genetically and clinically heterogeneous connective tissue disorders affecting bone and soft tissue, causing abnormal fragility of bone, resulting in recurring fractures and deformity.

CAUSES

Abnormality of collagen production and organization; failure of maturation of procollagen to type 1 collagen and failure of normal collagen cross-linking

PATHOLOGY

- In general, both enchondral and intramembranous bone formation are disturbed.

—Osteoid seams are wide and crowded by osteoblasts (woven bone).
—Osteoclasts are normal. Collagen fibrils are disorganized (by EM).

- Physis broad and irregular

—Osteopenia
—Long bones are slender and smaller.
—Fractures (recent or healed)
—Deformities
—Spine: scoliosis, compression fractures, kyphosis, upper cervical spine instability
—Skull: multiple centers of ossification, wormian bones, basilar invagination/ platybasia

GENETICS

- Sillence classification:

—Type 1: autosomal dominant, blue sclera, onset preschool
—A: teeth involved
—B: teeth not involved
—Type II: autosomal recessive, lethal, blue sclera
—Type III: autosomal recessive, severe, normal sclera
—Type IV: autosomal dominant, normal sclera, mild form
—A: teeth involved
—B: teeth not involved

- Some cases of OI occur as spontaneous mutations.

EPIDEMIOLOGY

Approximately 1 in 20,000

PROGNOSIS

- In general, the earlier the fractures occur, the more severe the disease.
- For moderate and mild types, there is a gradual tendency to improvement, with the incidence of fractures decreasing after puberty.

 Differential Diagnosis

- Severe: congenital hypophosphatasia, achondroplasia, camptomelic dwarfism
- Mild: cystinosis, pyknodysostosis, child abuse, leukemia, idiopathic juvenile osteoporosis, steroid treatment, rickets in very-low-weight infants, Menkes' kinky-hair syndrome (newborn male [X-linked recessive] with failure to thrive, metaphyseal corner fractures, and abnormal hair)

 Data Gathering

HISTORY

Variable; family history

 Physical Examination

- Severe congenital forms: multiple fractures, limbs deformed and short, skull soft
- Mild and moderate forms

—General: short stature, hernias
—Extremities: bowing, coxa vara deformity, cubitus varus, hypermobility of joints: subluxations and dislocations
—Pelvis: trefoil pelvis, protrusio acetabuli
—Spine (cause: osteoporosis, compression fractures, and ligamentous laxity): kyphoscoliosis (30% to 40%), platybasia
—Skin: thin skin, subcutaneous hemorrhages, wide surgical scars
—Eyes: blue sclera caused by thin collagen layer, Saturn's ring (white sclera immediately) hyperopia, embryotoxon or arcus juvenilis occasionally, retinal detachment occasionally
—Teeth: dentinogenesis imperfecta, enamel normal, both deciduous and permanent teeth affected, teeth easily broken, discoloration
—Deafness: either conduction or nerve type

Laboratory Aids

TESTS

Blood Tests

- Serum calcium and phosphorus is normal.
- Alkaline phosphatase may be elevated.
- There is no widely available specific laboratory test that is diagnostic of this abnormality.
- Collagen testing is becoming more available.

Radiographs

- Osteopenia
- Fractures: new, healing, or healed; malunions
- Deformity
- Metaphyseal ends of long bones: honeycomb appearance of ends of long bones, popcorn calcifications, Erlenmeyer flask appearance, acetabular protrusio
- Spine: atlantoaxial subluxation, spondylolisthesis, scoliosis, compression fractures

 ## Emergency Care

- For unstable fractures, such as femur fractures, spine instability
- Depends on location of fracture and details of individual situation

Therapy

DRUGS

Bisphosphonates are being used currently in clinical trials for children with severe involvement (gene therapy possibly in future). Sex hormones, fluoride, magnesium oxide, calcitonin, and special diets have all been tried.

ORTHOPAEDIC

- Fracture treatment: Fractures heal at a normal rate; splinting, orthoses, casting, operations (intramedullary rod).
- Education: Fracture prevention is key.
- Scoliosis: Seen in approximately 50%; orthoses usually ineffective; spinal fusion for curves greater than 50 degrees.
- Correction of deformities (e.g., realignment osteotomies with intramedullary fixation most common for long bone deformity)

 ## Follow-Up

PROGNOSIS

- Depends on severity of OI
- Spranger scoring system
- Moderate and mild types: gradual tendency to improvement, with incidence of fractures decreasing after puberty

PITFALLS

- Hyperplastic callus formation may be confused with osteogenic sarcoma.
- Education and injury prevention are key.

ICD-9-CM 756.51

BIBLIOGRAPHY

Gertner JM, Root L. Osteogenesis imperfecta. *Orthop Clin North Am* 1990;21(1):151–162.

Minch CM, Kruse RW. Osteogenesis imperfecta: a review of basic science and diagnosis. *Orthopedics* 1998;21(5):558–567, 568–569 (quiz).

Sillence DO. Osteogenesis imperfecta: an expanded panorama of variants. *Clin Orthop* 1981;159:11.

Spanger JW, Cremin B, Beighton P. Osteogenesis imperfecta congenita. *Pediatr Radiol* 1982;12:21.

Tosi LL. Osteogenesis imperfecta. *Curr Opin Pediatr* 1997;9(1):94–99.

Zaleske DJ. Metabolic and endocrine abnormalities. In: Morrissy RT, Weinstein SL, eds. *Lovell and Winter's Pediatric Orthopaedics.* 5th Ed. Philadelphia: Lippincott Williams & Wilkins, 2001:177–242.

Authors: John P. Dormans and Leslie Moroz

Osteomyelitis

 ## Database

DEFINITION

Osteomyelitis is infection of the bone.

CAUSE

- *Staphylococcus aureus*: causes 90% of osteomyelitis in otherwise healthy children of all ages
- *Streptococcus pyogenes* or *Haemophilus influenzae* can also be the etiologic agent.
- Group B streptococci and *Escherichia coli* are often isolated in children under 1 month of age.
- *Salmonella* can be the cause in children with sickle cell anemia.
- *Pseudomonas aeruginosa* can be found in puncture wounds to the foot.

PATHOLOGY

- Usually, osteomyelitis begins as bacteremia with hematogenous spread to the bone, but direct inoculation of bacteria into the bone by trauma is also possible.
- Most bacteria that enter the bone are phagocytized, so that no infection develops. When bacteria enter areas of the bone with low blood flow, however, such as the metaphysis directly beneath the physeal plate, they may not be phagocytized, and an infection may develop.
- The first changes noted in osteomyelitis are the death of the osteoblasts in the infected area and resorption of trabeculae. Inflammation develops, which further compromises blood flow, and microabscesses are formed within the bone. Pus can spread through the bone and between the bone and the periosteum. This pus can lift the periosteum, causing point tenderness.

GENETICS

- Increased incidence in patients with sickle cell disease and other immunodeficiencies

EPIDEMIOLOGY

Incidence of 0.016% per year. The femur and tibia are most often affected.

COMPLICATIONS

- Permanent damage to the growth plate, septic arthritis, fracture in a weakened bone

 ## Differential Diagnosis

- Cellulitis
- Septic arthritis
- Inflammatory arthritis or JRA
- Malignancy
- Trauma
- Sickle cell crisis
- Toxic synovitis

 ## Data Gathering

HISTORY

A child with osteomyelitis usually complains of sudden onset of bone or joint pain and fever. A younger child may refuse to bear weight on or move the extremity that is involved.

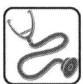 ## Physical Examination

- Physical examination usually reveals a febrile child with point tenderness over the area of infected bone. The child is often unwilling to move the involved extremity.
- As the infection progresses, swelling, warmth, and erythema of the skin overlying the infection may be noted.
- An infant with osteomyelitis may appear septic.

 ## Laboratory Aids

TESTS

- Patients usually have an elevated white blood cell count and a high sedimentation rate.
- C-reactive protein levels are usually elevated and are useful for monitoring response to therapy.
- Blood cultures are positive in over 50% of patients.
- Aspiration of the infected bone, even in the absence of debridement, is useful to determine the etiologic organism.

IMAGING

- Plain films begin to show the changes of osteomyelitis 10 to 14 days into the infection, with periosteal elevation and bone destruction.
- 99Tc bone scans are 80% accurate, and gallium scans are thought to be 91% accurate in diagnosing osteomyelitis.
- MRI can be useful in defining abscesses and extent and anatomy of bone sequestra; it is also the most useful imaging study to delineate chronic osteomyelitis.

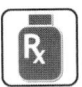 ## Therapy

- Antibiotic therapy for 4 to 6 weeks is usually required for osteomyelitis. Intravenous oxacillin is usually the empiric drug of choice until an organism can be isolated. Gram-negative coverage should be added for neonates, and Salmonella coverage is needed in sickle cell patients.
- If a recent foot puncture wound was experienced, coverage for Pseudomonas is recommended.
- Once the organism is known and sensitivities are established, the patient may be switched to oral antibiotics, as long as the serum bactericidal titer can be maintained.
- If an abscess is present in the bone, surgical débridement may also be necessary.

 ## Follow-Up

Patients should be followed to ensure adequate treatment of infection and continued growth of the extremity involved.

PITFALLS

- Delayed diagnosis, difficulty distinguishing osteomyelitis from a sickle cell crisis

 ## Common Questions and Answers

Q: Do you need to surgically debride osteomyelitis?
A: This is a very controversial topic. Many physicians feel that all osteomyelitis should be surgically débrided, although others believe that in the absence of an abscess, antibiotic therapy alone is adequate. Most agree, however, that if an abscess is present, it should be drained.

Q: Will osteomyelitis cause permanent damage in the bone?
A: If the growth plate is not damaged and the infection is adequately treated, there should be no permanent sequelae of osteomyelitis. If the growth plate is damaged, however, the affected limb may not grow evenly, or at all, even after the infection is treated.

Q: Is CRP a more useful laboratory study than ESR for osteomyelitis?
A: The CRP level is known to respond more quickly to changes in the inflammatory state than the ESR, reflecting changes in as short a period as 6 to 8 hours. Studies have shown that the CRP normalizes sooner in osteomyelitis than does the ESR, and studies have also shown that a persistently high CRP is a better indicator than ESR of inadequate therapy, the need for repeated drainage procedures, worsened radiographic appearance, and symptoms of greater duration.

ICD-9-CM 730.2

BIBLIOGRAPHY

Barron SA. Index of suspicion. Case I. Diagnosis: osteomyeltis. *Pediatr Rev* 1998;19(2):51–52.

Dirschl DR. Acute pyogenic osteomyelitis in children. *Orthop Rev* 1994;(May):305–312.

Fink CW, Nelson JD. Septic arthritis and osteomyeletis in children. *Clin Rheum Dis* 1986;12:423.

Mandell GA. Imaging in the diagnosis of musculoskeletal infections in children. *Curr Prob Pediatr* 1996;26(7):218–237.

Roine IR, Faingezicht I, Arguedts A, et al. Serial serum C-reactive protein to monitor recovery from acute hematogenous osteomyelitis in children. *Ped Infect Dis J* 1995;14:40–44.

Roy DR. Osteomyelitis. *Pediatr Rev* 1995;16(10):380–384, 385 (quiz).

Sonnen GM, Henry NK. Pediatric bone and joint infections. Diagnosis and antimicrobial management. *Pediatr Clin N Am* 1996;43(4):933–947.

Wall EJ. Childhood osteomyelitis and septic arthritis. *Curr Opin Pediatr* 1998;10(1):73–76.

Author: Aaron Donoghue

Osteosarcoma

 Database

DEFINITION

Osteosarcoma is a tumor of the bone composed of spindle cells that produce malignant osteoid.

CAUSES

- The etiology of most cases is unknown.
- There is an association of osteosarcoma with exposure to ionizing radiation.
- Secondary osteosarcoma is seen in up to 5% of patients who received radiation therapy for an initial malignancy.
- Children with hereditary retinoblastoma are at increased risk of developing osteosarcoma with and without prior exposure to radiation.
- Osteosarcoma can arise in patients with Paget disease of the bone, Rothman-Thompson syndrome, enchondromatosis, hereditary multiple exostoses, and fibrous dysplasia.

PATHOLOGY/PATHOPHYSIOLOGY

- Osteosarcoma most often involves the medullary region of bone.
- Rarely, osteosarcoma occurs in soft tissue separate from underlying bone.
- Classic or conventional osteosarcoma, the largest group of osteosarcomas, is composed of connective tissue stroma containing highly malignant spindle-shaped cells as well as areas of osteoid production and calcification.
- Four microscopic subtypes are osteoblastic, chondroblastic, fibroblastic, and telangiectatic.
- These variants are rare in the pediatric population, and lack prognostic significance at present.
- Two rare clinical subtypes, periosteal and parosteal osteosarcoma, rarely metastasize and carry a better prognosis.

EPIDEMIOLOGY

- Osteosarcoma is the most common malignant bone tumor of childhood, representing 60% of all bone tumors in the pediatric age group.
- Overall, it accounts for less than 1% of all malignant neoplasms.
- Peak incidence is in adolescence and early adulthood, with a median age of 18 at diagnosis.
- Osteosarcoma is thought to begin during the adolescent growth spurt.
- Approximately 90% of tumors occur at the metaphyseal ends of long tubular bones, but any portion of the skeleton may be involved.
- The most frequent site is the distal femur, followed by the proximal tibia and the proximal humerus.

COMPLICATIONS

Ten percent to 20% of patients have pulmonary metastases at the time of diagnosis; a smaller proportion have metastases to other bones.

PROGNOSIS

The majority of patients with osteosarcoma involving an extremity without pulmonary metastases can be cured. Five-year survival for nonmetastatic disease ranges from 60% to 70%. The following have been associated with a poorer prognosis:

- Pulmonary metastases
- Disseminated bone metastases
- Poor response of the tumor to preoperative chemotherapy
- Inability to achieve a total surgical excision of the tumor

 Differential Diagnosis

- Infection: osteomyelitis, septic arthritis
- Trauma: stress fracture
- Benign Tumors: unicameral bone cyst, osteoblastoma, eosinophilic granuloma, giant-cell tumor, aneurysmal bone cyst, osteochondroma, fibrous dysplasia
- Malignant Tumors: Ewing sarcoma, chondrosarcoma, fibrosarcoma, leukemia, metastatic lesions of other primary tumors

 Data Gathering

HISTORY

- Pain at the site of the tumor is the most common presentation.
- Swelling over the involved area is also reported.
- The duration of symptoms varies.
- A history of recent trauma is common, but unrelated. Trauma often brings the affected area to the patients' or parents' attention, but does not actually cause osteosarcoma.
- Weight loss is rare but may occur in advanced disease.
- If fever is present, it may indicate an infectious etiology (osteomyelitis) rather than osteosarcoma.

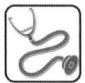 Physical Examination

- A tender, soft tissue mass and increased warmth may be present in the involved area.
- Localized erythema is uncommon.
- Unless there exists an underlying fracture range of motion of the limb is normal and there is no difficulty weight bearing.
- Regional lymphadenopathy is rare.

 Laboratory Aids

TESTS

- Laboratory tests are not generally helpful in osteosarcoma. Serum lactate dehydrogenase (LDH) and alkaline phosphatase may be elevated.
- The prognostic significance of alkaline phosphatase is controversial.
- An elevated WBC, C-reactive protein, or sedimentation rate may suggest osteomyelitis.

IMAGING

- A plain radiograph of the involved area always reveals some abnormality. Most commonly, one sees a lytic or blastic region of the bone with ill-defined borders. Other findings may include periosteal elevation adjacent to the primary lesion, a sunburst appearance of the primary lesion caused by neoplastic spicules adjacent to the bony cortex, or a pathologic fracture.
- Radiographic examination should include the primary tumor site as well as areas of potential metastases. A chest CT and bone scan should be done to assess for pulmonary and bone metastases.
- An MRI should be done to better evaluate the extent of the tumor. It should include the joint above and below the involved bony area. MRI can delineate the intra- and extraosseous extent of the tumor as well as evaluate the neurovascular structures involved.

REFERRAL AND STAGING

- When a malignant bone tumor is suspected, the patient should be referred immediately to a pediatric cancer center. Children's cancer centers can provide the multidisciplinary team needed to diagnose, biopsy, treat, and rehabilitate children with bone tumors.
- A staging workup should include a bone scan to look for bone metastases and local skip lesions, as well as a chest radiograph and chest CT to detect macroscopic pulmonary metastases.
- The diagnosis of osteosarcoma can be confirmed only by a biopsy, which should be done by an experienced pediatric orthopaedic surgeon in conjunction with a pediatric oncologist and pediatric pathologist.
- Certain surgical incisions at the time of biopsy may make patients ineligible for limb-sparing procedures.

Osteosarcoma

Therapy

DRUGS

- At present, therapy incorporates preoperative chemotherapy followed by surgical resection.
- The goals of adjuvant chemotherapy are treatment of pulmonary micrometastases and shrinkage of the primary tumor mass, particularly when limb-salvage procedures are surgical options.
- Response to adjuvant chemotherapy (degree of necrosis at the time of complete resection) is a very important prognostic factor.
- Groups such as the Children's Oncology Group (COG) have developed chemotherapy protocols for osteosarcoma. The majority of children with osteosarcoma are treated on these chemotherapy protocols.
- The mainstays of treatment are cisplatin and doxorubicin, with many protocols also using high-dose methotrexate and ifosfamide.

—The duration of chemotherapy varies from 8 to 12 months according to the extent of the tumor at diagnosis, tumor response to therapy, and the individual protocol.

SURGERY

In the past, when osteosarcoma was managed by surgery alone, the majority of patients subsequently developed pulmonary metastases and died of progressive disease. Surgical options depend on the primary site of the tumor and the extent of tumor involvement. Complete surgical resection with wide margins is necessary for cure. Surgical options for osteosarcomas of the extremities include:

- Amputation
- Limb salvage with allograft or prosthetic reconstruction
- Rotationplasty

Macroscopic pulmonary metastases should be resected at the time of surgery if still visible by radiographic examination. Localized pulmonary recurrences that develop after treatment also should be resected, as this can result in long-term cure or a prolonged symptom-free period.

RADIATION

Osteosarcoma is a radiation-insensitive tumor, but radiation has been used in individual cases.

PHYSICAL THERAPY/REHABILITATION

All patients need to work with specialists to learn how to adapt to their surgically induced disability. The duration of physical therapy and rehabilitation is dependent on the disability and the individual patient's needs.

Follow-Up

SIGNS TO WATCH FOR

- Wound infections may develop in surgical sites in the initial postoperative period.
- Significant pain, fever, swelling, discharge, and foul odor from the surgical site should be evaluated, preferably by the surgeon. Poor healing of the surgical site may be a problem, particularly in patients receiving chemotherapy or in those with poor nutrition. Patients may require intravenous antibiotics, supplemental feeding or surgical revision of the wound.
- If prostheses are required, skin breakdown and fitting difficulties with prosthetic devices, such as adjustments for changes in height and weight, should be diagnosed and corrected. Scoliosis and back pain may develop in patients using improperly adjusted crutches and/or prosthetic devices after lower extremity or pelvic procedures. This requires expertise in prosthetic devices for children.
- "Phantom" pain is a normal phenomenon after amputation. Patients and their families should be reassured if this occurs. Sometimes medication can reduce the pain.
- All children need to be followed by an oncologist regularly after treatment is completed to monitor for recurrence as well as long-term side effects of the chemotherapy, such as cardiac toxicity, infertility, or secondary malignancy.

Common Questions and Answers

Q: How does one differentiate osteosarcoma from Ewing sarcoma, the second most common bone tumor of childhood?
A: Ultimately, only a biopsy can differentiate the two. In general, Ewing sarcoma is seen in younger children and tends to affect the axial bones, such as the pelvis. When found in the long bones, it is usually in the diaphyseal regions. Symptomatology does not differ, but Ewing sarcoma is metastatic to the bone marrow, as well as the bone and lung.

Q: How does one differentiate osteosarcoma from a benign bone lesion?
A: Ultimately, only a biopsy can differentiate the two. Benign lesions tend to be very well circumscribed with smooth edges on radiograph. They are generally not associated with soft tissue masses, swelling, or fever. Fractures are just as likely through benign bone lesions as malignant ones. Only in very rare situations should bony lesions be presumed to be benign observed and without biopsy.

Q: Is there an increased risk of osteosarcoma in the contralateral limb?
A: No.

Q: Does limb salvage incur a greater risk of recurrence than does amputation?
A: Recent studies have shown that there is no increase in recurrence if wide margins are achieved at the time of surgery.

ICD-9-CM 170.9

BIBLIOGRAPHY

Arndt CAS, Crist WM. Medical progress: common musculoskeletal tumors of childhood and adolescence. *N Engl J Med* 1999;341(5): 342–352.

Ferguson WS, Goorin AM. Current treatment of osteosarcoma. *Cancer Invest* 2001;19(3): 292–315.

Himelstein BP, Dormans JP. Malignant bone tumors of childhood. *Pediatr Clin North Am* 1996;43(4):967–984.

Marec-Berard P, Philip T. Ewing sarcoma: the pediatrician's point of view. *Pediatric Blood Cancer* 2004;42(5):477–480.

Miller SL, Hoffer FA. Malignant and benign bone lesions. *Radiol Clin North Am* 2001;39(4):673–699.

Rodriguez-Galindo C, Spunt SL, Pappo AS. Treatment of Ewing sarcoma family of tumors: current status and outlook for the future [erratum appears in *Med Pediatr Oncol.* 2003 Dec;41(6):594] 2 *Med Pediatr Oncol* 2003; 40(5):276–287.

Rougraff BT, Simon MA, Kneisl JS, et al. Limb salvage compared with amputation for osteosarcoma of the distal end of the femur. A long-term oncologic, functional, and quality-of-life study. *J Bone Joint Surg* 1994;76(5):649–656.

Author: Susan R. Rheingold

Otitis Externa

 Database

DEFINITION

Otitis externa is inflammation or infection of the external auditory canal and/or the auricle. May be categorized as follows:

- Acute: also known as swimmer's ear; usually an acute bacterial infection of the external auditory canal.
- Chronic: persistent, low-grade infection and inflammation of the external ear.
- Atopic: encompasses otitis externa as a result of atopic dermatitis, seborrheic dermatitis, psoriasis, and other inflammatory conditions.
- Fungal: occurs more commonly in patients with diabetes mellitus or an immunodeficiency.
- Malignant or Necrotizing: severe otitis externa with invasive disease into the surrounding soft tissue, cartilage and bone; seen more commonly in patients with diabetes mellitus or immunodeficiency; may progress to invasive disease of the surrounding structures.

ETIOLOGY

- Bacteria: *Pseudomonas aeruginosa* (particularly in malignant otitis externa), *Staphylococcus aureus*, *S. epidermidis*, other staphylococcal species, *Microbacterium* species, *Streptococcus pyogenes*, *S. pneumoniae*, *Escherichia coli*, *Haemophilus influenzae*, Klebsiella, and other gram-negative species
- Fungal: *Candida albicans*, *Aspergillus niger*, *A. versicolor*
- Viral: herpes simplex virus (acute infection and herpes zoster) and varicella

PATHOPHYSIOLOGY

- Cerumen provides an acidic layer, which prevents infection of the external auditory canal. Warm, humid air can disrupt the integrity of cerumen.
- Trauma to the squamous epithelium of the external auditory canal or an increase in the pH of the external auditory canal increases the risk of inflammation and infection.
- Cleaning or removal of cerumen, or introduction of water into the canal from swimming, playing water sports can lead to maceration of the canal and the onset of infection.

EPIDEMIOLOGY

- Occurs more commonly in summer months
- Ten percent of the population is diagnosed with acute otitis externa at some point in their lives.
- Ninety percent of cases are unilateral.
- Risk factors include increased environmental temperature, high humidity, local trauma, and exposure to water with high bacterial counts.

COMPLICATIONS

- Cellulitis of adjacent tissues (facial or auricular)
- Lymphadenitis of upper neck or parotid lymph nodes
- Otitis media and rarely mastoiditis
- Facial nerve neuritis
- Canal stenosis (usually in chronic otitis externa that results in hypertrophy of the canal walls)
- Hearing loss, if there is significant edema of the canal walls

PROGNOSIS

Very good, with rapid response to treatment

 Differential Diagnosis

INFECTIOUS

- Otitis media
- Mastoiditis
- Furunculosis

TUMORS

- Squamous cell carcinoma
- Basal cell carcinoma
- Acoustic neuroma
- Other metastatic tumors

MISCELLANEOUS

- Foreign body
- Cerumen impaction
- Cholesteatoma

 Data Gathering

HISTORY

- Ask about known risk factors, including swimming, ear cleaning, history of atopic or seborrheic dermatitis.
- Has there been any hearing loss (associated with involvement of the tympanic membrane), pain that is worse with chewing or activities that result in motion of the ear, pruritus (associated with inflammation of the external auditory canal), and/or ear discharge?
- The presence of fever may suggest a more severe infection.
- Ask about use of earrings or other ear jewelry, which is associated with atopic dermatitis as the etiology of the otitis externa.
- Ask about use of topical treatments for the ear or canal (including tattooing permanent or nonpermanent), which is also associated with atopic dermatitis as the cause of the otitis externa.

 Physical Examination

- Pain with traction of pinna or with applied pressure to the tragus
- Canal appears macerated with erythema, purulent discharge, and/or edema
- Look for the presence of foreign bodies, including pieces of cotton from cleaning with cotton swabs
- Tympanic membrane should appear intact with normal landmarks. If not, there may be a concurrent otitis media.
- In cases of fungal infection, "mold" or black or white fungal hyphae with spores may be seen.
- In viral infections, vesicles may be present.
- In eczematous otitis externa, the skin is dry and flaky with crust. Excoriation may be visible as well.
- A somewhat fruity smell suggests infection as a result of *Pseudomonas*.

 Laboratory Aids

- In simple, uncomplicated otitis externa, testing is generally not indicated.
- In more severe infections, recalcitrant infections or immunocompromised patients, bacterial culture with gram stain and fungal cultures should be obtained.
- Herpes has been described as an etiologic agent; therefore, direct fluorescence antibody (DFA) testing for herpes may be helpful. Viral cultures should be considered when there is a vesicular component to the otitis externa.

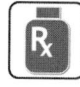 Therapy

GENERAL MANAGEMENT

- Hydrogen peroxide or 3% hypertonic saline may be used to clean the ear. Be sure to use a cotton swab to dry the canal after cleansing.
- Pain can usually be managed with mild analgesics, such as acetaminophen or ibuprofen.
- If there is significant edema of the canal, using ophthalmic drops (which tend to be less viscous than otic drops) in combination with a wick to facilitate introduction of medication into the ear canal may be useful. However, if there is concern about a concomitant otitis media with perforation, caution must be used with the introduction of any topical treatment to the external auditory canal.

SPECIFIC THERAPIES, DEPENDING ON THE PRESENTATION

- Remove foreign body if present
- For acute localized otitis externa with abscess, incision and drainage of the abscess in combination with antistaphylococcal penicillins or first-generation cephalosporins.
- For fungal otitis externa, antifungal drops such as clotrimazole 1% solution are used.
- For atopic otitis externa, appropriate management of the underlying dermatologic condition is appropriate along with the topical application of corticosteroid to the affected parts of the ear.
- Skin testing for specific allergies should be considered if atopic otitis externa is severe or recalcitrant.
- For cellulitis, lymphadenitis, or otitis media, oral antimicrobials are used.
- For malignant otitis media and/or mastoiditis, intravenous antimicrobials and consultation with an otolaryngologist (ear, nose and throat specialist; ENT) are indicated.
- In the case of chronic otitis externa, surgical intervention is rare, and occurs only when there is failure of long-term medical therapy. Such cases should be referred to ENT for debridement and further evaluation.
- When pseudomonal infection is suspected, an antipseudomonal agent, such as a third-generation cephalosporin (e.g., ceftriaxone sodium) or a fluoroquinolone (ofloxacin) should be used.

TOPICAL ANTIBIOTICS/ ANTIINFLAMMATORY AGENTS

- Polymyxin B, neomycin, and hydrocortisone combination otic solution or suspension can be used to treat a simple infection. In some cases, the neomycin component may cause allergy leading to exacerbation of the otitis externa. Fluoroquinolones, such as ofloxacin and ciprofloxacin (available only as a combination with hydrocortisone), have also shown high cure rates.
- Topical benzocaine with antipyrine can serve as a topical analgesic, but should not be used if tympanic membrane perforation is suspected
- Topical ophthalmic antimicrobial/steroid drops, such as Cortisporin ophthalmic solution, may be tolerated better if there is severe maceration of the canal since they are less acidic.

 Follow-Up

- Reevaluation if there is no symptomatic improvement 24 to 48 hours after starting treatment.
- Fever or progression of symptoms in spite of treatment warrants more aggressive or broader therapy.
- Immunocompromised, including those with diabetes mellitus, should be followed closely depending on severity, to ensure improvement.

PREVENTION

- Earplugs that prevent water from entering the ear canal should be used prior to swimming or participation in other water sports.
- Acetic acid drops (which can be made at home with one part vinegar to two parts rubbing alcohol) followed by wicking away moisture with cotton can be used to restore the acidic pH of the ear canal and decrease moisture to prevent otitis externa after swimming.
- Discourage removal of cerumen with vigorous ear cleaning, especially by using cotton swabs in the ear.
- If there is a known allergen avoid usage.

 Common Questions and Answers

Q: How should I clean my child's ear?
A: Only the external tragus, pinna, and visible parts of the ear should be cleaned with a cotton ball or washcloth. No foreign object should be placed in the canal. Ear cerumen is a normal protective substance to maintain protection of the fragile tympanic membrane. If impaction is suspected use a cerumen loosening agent such as carbamide peroxide. Although there is still common use of ear candles, small narrow candles that are placed at the opening of the external auditory canal and then lit with the goal of the heat causing the cerumen to loosen and exit the ear. This method has not been shown to remove significant impacted cerumen and can leave candle wax in the ear canal

Q: When can my child return to swimming after an episode of otitis externa?
A: After completion of the prescribed therapy, your child may resume water sports. He/she should use waterproof earplugs and acetic acid drops to prevent another infection.

Q: When should otitis externa be referred to an otolaryngologist?
A: In refractory cases, chronic otitis externa, or persistent hearing loss after treatment, and when there are severe complications (e.g., malignant otitis externa, mastoiditis).

ICD-9-CM 380.10

BIBLIOGRAPHY

Bojrab DI, Bruderly T, Abdulrazzak Y. Diseases of the external auditory canal: otitis externa. *Otolaryngol Clin North Am* 1996;29(5): 761–782.

Cantor RM. Pediatric emergencies: otitis externa and otitis media. A new look at old problems. *Emerg Med Clin North Am* 1995;13(2):445–455.

Dohar JE. Evolution of management approaches for otitis externa. *Pediatr Infect Dis J* 2003;22:299–308.

Hughes E, Lee JH. Otitis externa. *Pediatr Rev* 2001;22(6):191–197.

Mirza N. Otitis externa: management in the primary care office. *Postgrad Med* 1996;99(5):153–158.

Roland PS, Stoman DW. Microbiology of acute otitis externa. *Laryngoscope* 2002;112(7 Pt.1): 1166–1177.

Sood S, Strachan DR, Tsikoudas A, Stables GI. Allergic otitis externa. *Clin Otolaryngol* 2002;27:233–236.

Author: Lee R. Atkinson-McEvoy

Otitis Media

 Database

DEFINITION

Otitis media refers to inflammation of the middle ear. A distinction is usually made between otitis media with effusion (OME) and acute otitis media (AOM). AOM implies that infection is present.

ETIOLOGY

- *Streptococcus pneumoniae*: up to 40%
- Nontypeable *Haemophilus influenzae*: 25% to 30%
- *Moraxella catarrhalis*: 10% to 20%
- Other organisms include group A streptococcus, *Staphylococcus aureus*, and gram-negative organisms, such as *Pseudomonas*. Respiratory viruses are often noted as part of acute otitis media, but are the sole pathogen in <10% of cases.

PATHOPHYSIOLOGY

- Dysfunction of the eustachian tube is the most important factor.
—The eustachian tube in younger children is shorter, and more compliant and horizontal than in older children and adults.
—Children with craniofacial anomalies have an increased risk of eustachian tube dysfunction and subsequent otitis media.
- Viral upper respiratory infection often precedes or coincides with AOM. Viral infections may lead to development of AOM by several mechanisms:
—Inducing inflammation in the nasopharynx and eustachian tube
—Enhancing nasopharyngeal bacterial colonization
—Impairing host immune system and increasing susceptibility to secondary bacterial infection
- Interaction of viruses and bacteria may lead to increased inflammation and delay in clearance of bacteria from the middle ear fluid.

EPIDEMIOLOGY

- Reported frequency of otitis media has increased over the past two decades. The reported incidence is likely to decrease with the current focus on improving diagnostic accuracy and use of pneumococcal conjugate vaccine.
- Increased incidence in those younger than 2 years of age, with the peak incidence between 6 to 12 months of age
- More common in fall and winter, and less common in spring and summer
- Risk increased with exposure to large numbers of children (e.g., day care). Additive factors include number of hours spent in childcare, number of children, younger age at entry, and type of childcare setting (center vs. family day care).
- Inverse relationship with breast-feeding duration
- More common in males

- Exposure to environmental tobacco smoke is an independent risk factor.

COMPLICATIONS

Suppurative complications of AOM are much less common with current antibiotic therapy. The recent increase in resistant organisms could lead to a resurgence of suppurative complications.
- Hearing loss—acute conductive hearing loss is common and usually resolves as the effusion resolves. Fluid of long-standing duration may lead to permanent conductive hearing loss. Sensorineural hearing loss may result from spread of infection into the labyrinth.
- Tympanic membrane perforation
- Chronic suppurative otitis media
- Tympanosclerosis
- Cholesteatoma
- Acute mastoiditis
- Petrositis
- Labyrinthitis
- Facial nerve paralysis
- Bacterial meningitis
- Epidural abscess
- Subdural empyema
- Brain abscess
- Lateral sinus thrombosis

PROGNOSIS

- Symptoms of acute infection (fever and otalgia) relieved within 24 hours in most patients.
- Treatment failures more likely with increased severity of disease and younger age.
- Development of another infection within 30 days usually represents a recurrence caused by a different organism, rather than a relapse.
- Recurrences are frequent, and more common in younger children and if initial episode is severe.
- Thirty percent to 70% of treated children will have an effusion at 2 weeks. Middle ear effusion may persist for weeks to months.

 Differential Diagnosis

- OME—the tympanic membrane may appear dull with a diffuse light reflex, fluid bubbles may be visible and mobility may be decreased.
- Otitis externa
- Other causes of fever—including viral upper respiratory infections, pharyngitis, pneumonia, meningitis, urinary tract infections, and bone and joint infections.
- Pharyngitis and dental pain may be mistaken for otalgia.

 Data Gathering

HISTORY

- History of current episode with presence of ear pain, fever, and associated symptoms

- Past medical history, including underlying disorders (e.g., cleft palate, Down syndrome), immune deficiency, and previous history of otitis media
- Recent treatment with antibiotics
- Exposure to large numbers of children (school, day care, large family)

 Physical Examination

- Physical exam of the patient should look for other causes of fever and irritability in children: upper respiratory infections, pharyngitis, lymphadenitis, meningitis, urinary tract infection, and bone and joint infections.
- Physical examination of the ear is best done with pneumatic otoscopy.
—The patient should be adequately restrained if uncooperative.
—Cerumen in the canal should be removed if view of the tympanic membrane is inadequate.
—The tympanic membrane is visualized at rest, and with gentle positive and negative pressure via pneumatic otoscopy.
- The presence of a middle ear effusion is determined by the characteristics of the tympanic membrane:
—Contour: normal, retracted, full, or bulging
—Color: gray, pink, yellow, white, or red
—Translucency: translucent or opaque
—Mobility: normal, decreased, or absent
- The presence of a middle ear effusion is suggested by abnormal color, opacification, decreased mobility, or visible fluid bubbles. A diagnosis of acute otitis media is suggested if a middle ear effusion is present along with ear pain, erythema, fullness, or bulging.
- The concomitant presence of conjunctivitis (otitis media-conjunctivitis syndrome) suggests the presence of *H. influenzae* as a causative organism.

 Laboratory Aids

TESTS

Tympanometry

- A tympanogram is easily performed by office personnel.
- Provides information on middle ear pressure and tympanic membrane compliance
- Sensitive in detecting middle ear effusion, but poor positive predictive value
- May be a useful as an objective tool to follow up middle ear effusions

Tympanocentesis

- For episodes of AOM that are resistant to antibiotic therapy, tympanocentesis and culture and sensitivity of the middle ear fluid may help guide antibiotic therapy.
- Tympanocentesis or myringotomy may also be required as part of the treatment of suppurative complications.

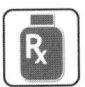 ## Therapy

DRUGS

Note: since many patients who have physical findings consistent with diagnosis of AOM may recover without treatment, some experts recommend withholding treatment for 48 to 72 hours before starting antibiotics, especially in older patients.

First-Line Therapy

- Amoxicillin (45 mg/kg per day divided b.i.d.) is still the drug of choice for most episodes of AOM. Reasons for this include cost, safety profile, and its activity against the common organisms causing otitis media. The recommended duration of therapy is 10 days, but a 5- to 7-day course may be considered for uncomplicated and isolated cases of AOM in children over the age of 2 years.
- Using higher doses of amoxicillin (80 to 90 mg/kg per day) will cover many of the moderately resistant strains of *S. pneumoniae*. Increasing the dose of amoxicillin should be considered when the risk of resistant *S. pneumoniae* is increased:
—Children less than 2 years of age
—Recent β-lactam use
—Exposure to day care
—Communities with a high incidence of resistant organisms. Routine use of higher dose amoxicillin is recommended when the rate of nonsusceptible pneumococcus exceeds 40%.

- Azithromycin may be used in patients who are allergic to penicillin.

Second-Line Therapy

- Failure of antibiotic therapy may be related to bacterial resistance or a viral etiology. The choice of a second-line antibiotic depends on suspected mechanism of resistance. *H. influenzae* and *M. catarrhalis* produce β-lactamase. *S. pneumoniae* alters penicillin binding proteins. Failure caused by a resistant pathogen is more likely for *S. pneumoniae* than for *H. influenzae* or *M. catarrhalis*.
- In cases in which resistant *S. pneumoniae* is likely, treatment with higher doses of amoxicillin (80 to 90 mg/kg per day) is recommended if not done initially.
—Amoxicillin-clavulanate, cefuroxime axetil, and intramuscular ceftriaxone are also effective against resistant strains.
—The macrolides and trimethoprim-sulfa do not provide reliable coverage for resistant *S. pneumoniae*.
- Amoxicillin-clavulanate or a second-generation cephalosporin may be used if *H. influenzae* or *M. catarrhalis* is suspected.

- Intramuscular ceftriaxone is not recommended for routine treatment of AOM. It may be considered when oral therapy is impossible or when appropriate first- and second-line therapy for *S. pneumoniae* has already failed. When used for treatment of resistant organisms, ceftriaxone 50 mg/kg IM should be given every 1 to 3 days for 3 doses.

Adjunctive Therapy

- Fever relief may be provided with acetaminophen or other antipyretic.
- Pain may be treated with acetaminophen, ibuprofen, or topical anesthetic drops.

 ## Follow-Up

- Expect symptomatic improvement within 48 to 72 hours of treatment. May need to switch antibiotic therapy and/or reevaluate for complications.
- Tympanic membrane may appear abnormal for some time after treatment. In infants or young children, initial follow-up exam should be scheduled 3 to 4 weeks after completion of antibiotic therapy. If effusion is present, follow monthly. For persistent effusions of more than 3 months duration, a hearing evaluation is recommended.
- Consider otolaryngology referral:
—Persistent otitis media not responding to antibiotic therapy. Tympanocentesis may be helpful.
—Recurrent otitis media with more than four episodes during a respiratory season, especially if earlier in the season. Prior to ENT referral some clinicians recommend prophylactic antibiotic therapy with once-daily amoxicillin (20 mg/kg daily).
—Persistent and/or recurrent otitis with abnormal hearing and/or speech

SIGNS TO WATCH FOR

- Watch for signs of persistent infection including persistent fever, persistent or severe otalgia, or ear discharge.
- Signs of complications include posterior auricular swelling or erythema, headache, and meningismus

PREVENTION

- Breast-feeding protects against otitis media in the first year of life.
- Preventing exposure to environmental tobacco smoke can decrease the risk of otitis media.
- Decreasing exposure to multiple respiratory pathogens by delaying entrance to group childcare or choosing settings with fewer numbers of children may be helpful.
- Vaccines
—Influenza vaccine can decrease the incidence of otitis media by preventing the preceding viral illness.
—In addition to preventing invasive disease, conjugated pneumococcal vaccine significantly reduces the risk of AOM.

—Other vaccines being developed against both viruses and bacteria (*Moraxella*, nontypeable *H. influenzae*, respiratory syncytial virus [RSV]) may help to prevent episodes of AOM.

 ## Common Questions and Answers

Q: When should children with otitis media be treated?
A: The presence of a middle ear effusion may occur commonly with an upper respiratory infection. The presence of an effusion is suggested by fluid bubbles or a dull tympanic membrane with decreased mobility. An effusion that is likely to be complicated by infection, and therefore represents AOM, shows significant pressure with a bulging and immobile tympanic membrane. This may be accompanied by fever and ear pain. The presence of infection usually warrants treatment with antibiotics, especially in children less than 2 years of age, those who are prone to infection, and those with AOM during the winter season.

Q: What is the current strategy for dealing with resistant *S. pneumoniae*?
A: *S. pneumoniae* develops resistance by alteration of penicillin binding proteins. *H. influenzae* and *M. catarrhalis* produce β-lactamase. A previous strategy to deal with these resistant organisms was to use antibiotics resistant to β-lactamase, such as second-generation cephalosporins. This strategy is not effective for resistant strains of pneumococcus. The most effective strategy is to increase the dose of amoxicillin, bringing the concentration of antibiotic in the middle ear fluid above the MIC. These higher doses of amoxicillin, 80 to 90 mg/kg per day, are recommended when initial treatment has failed and resistant organisms are suspected. It is also recommended as initial therapy if resistant strains are likely in the community or in younger children, those in day care, and those treated with β-lactam antibiotics recently.

ICD-9-CM 382.9

BIBLIOGRAPHY

Bluestone CD. Clinical course, complications and sequelae of acute otitis media. *Pediatr Infect Dis J* 2000;19:S37–S46.

Harrison CJ. Changes in treatment strategies for acute otitis media after full implementation of the pneumococcal seven valent conjugate vaccine. *Pediatr Infect Dis J* 2003;22(8 Suppl):S120–S130.

Rothman R. Does this child have acute otitis media? *JAMA* 2003;290:1633–1640.

Weber SM, Grundfast KM. Modern management of acute otitis media. *Pediatr Clin N Am* 2003;50(2):399–411.

Author: William R. Graessle

Pancreatic Pseudocyst

 ## Database

DEFINITION

Localized intrapancreatic or peripancreatic fluid collection, which is rich in pancreatic enzymes but devoid of significant solid debris, enclosed by a wall of nonepithelialized granulation tissue. Arises as a complication of acute or chronic pancreatitis.

PATHOPHYSIOLOGY

• Pancreatic pseudocysts develop shortly after an attack of acute pancreatitis or insidiously in chronic pancreatitis.
• Disruption in the pancreatic ductular system resulting in the extravasation of pancreatic enzymes evoking an inflammatory response.
• The inflammatory reaction leads to a fluid collection that is rich in pancreatic enzymes and is termed as acute Pancreatic Fluid Collection (PFC).
• If the duration of the pancreatic fluid collection is more than 4 weeks, gets localized (intrapancreatic or extrapancreatic) and a fibrin capsule develops over time, it is called as a pseudopancreatic cyst.
• The pseudocyst does not have a true epithelial lining.
• If there is communication between the pseudocyst and the pancreatic duct, the enzyme level in the fluid remain elevated and if there is no communication, the enzyme level falls with time.

PROGNOSIS

More than 50% of pseudocysts resolve without intervention.

DIFFERENTIAL DIAGNOSIS OF PANCREATIC CYSTS

• Congenital/genetic

—Congenital cysts
—Polycystic disease
—Von Hippel Lindau disease
—Cystic fibrosis

• Infections

—Pancreatic abscess
—Echinococcal (hydatid) cyst
—Taenia solium cyst

• Tumor

—Serous cystadenoma
—Mucinous cystadenoma
—Cystic islet cell tumors
—Teratoma
—Pancreatoblastoma
—Cystadenocarcinoma
—Frantz tumor
—Angiomatous cystic neoplasms
—Lymphangiomas
—Hemangioendothelioma

• Miscellaneous

—Splenic cyst
—Adrenal cyst
—Enterogenous cyst
—Duplication cyst
—Endometriosis

 ## Data Gathering

HISTORY

Question: When is pancreatic pseudocyst suspected?
Significance: Pancreatic pseudocyst should be suspected in patients recovering from acute pancreatitis or patients with chronic pancreatitis who have recurrent/persistent abdominal pain, a palpable abdominal mass or persistently elevated pancreatic enzymes in blood.

Question: What are the usual presenting symptoms?
Significance:

• Abdominal pain
• Nausea and vomiting
• Weight loss
• Jaundice
• Abdominal distension (mass/ascites)

 ## Physical Examination

• In many situations there are no clinical signs that are seen.
• Abdominal mass.
• Abdominal tenderness.
• Sometimes clinical signs secondary to complications:

—Jaundice in hepatobiliary obstruction
—Lower limb edema in compression of inferior vena cava
—Ascites in peritonitis
—Pleural effusion

 ## Laboratory Aids

• Persistently elevated pancreatic enzymes in blood could be a clue but is not an absolute indicator.
• CT scan to diagnose presence of pseudopancreatic cyst and to gauge size and relationship to adjacent organs.
• Ultrasonography: to diagnose pancreatic pseudocysts and for follow-up of the cyst size.
• Endoscopic ultrasonography is evolving in the adult settings and will probably be used in the pediatric population soon.
• Endoscopic retrograde cholangiopancreatography (ERCP) is used in some cases to delineate the pancreatic ductular system before drainage to distinguish ductal stenosis, stones and other causes of obstructions.

Therapy

- Medical management

—Majority of the cases resolve by supportive care.
—Follow up with ultrasound or CT scan to make sure there are no complications.
—More than 60% have complete resolution by the end of 1 year.

- Indications for drainage

—Indications of urgent drainage include infection, rupture with cardiopulmonary compromise, biliary and gastric outlet obstruction.
—Indications for drainage in a chronic setting include persistent symptoms, rapid enlargement, failure of large pseudocysts (>6 cm) to shrink after 6 weeks and obstruction of other structures (biliary, bowel etc.).

- Different modalities for drainage include percutaneous, endoscopic and surgical procedures.

—Percutaneous drainage (aspiration or catheter drainage) is done in cases in which the pseudocyst has a less mature wall. Percutaneous aspiration has a high recurrence rate of 63% and failure rate of 54%. Continuous drainage has a recurrence rate of 8% and a failure rate of 19%.
—A mature cyst wall is required for surgical and endoscopic cystoenterostomies.
—Endoscopic procedures are becoming the first-line drainage modality, as they are less invasive than surgery. Endoscopic procedures include transmural cystoenterostomies and transpapillary route procedures like stent placement for pseudocysts that communicate with the main pancreatic duct.
—Surgical procedures now a days are getting more reserved for failed endoscopic procedures, complicated pseudocysts and for multiple pseudocysts. Surgical procedures include internal drainage (cystogastrostomy, cystoduodenostomy and Roux-Y cystojejunostomy), resection and external drainage. As reported in two surgical reviews, the recurrence rate was between 0% and 17% and mortality rate between 5% and 6% following surgical procedures.

COMPLICATIONS

- Perforation/Rupture

—Cardiopulmonary compromise secondary to pleural effusion and ascites.
—Peritonitis and ascites; can be fatal.

- Hemorrhage

—Erosions of vessels lining the cyst cause intracystic bleeding and rapid increase in the cyst size.
—Bleeding may occur directly into stomach, duodenum (clinically manifesting as GI bleeding) or peritoneal cavity.

- Obstruction

—Biliary obstruction: jaundice.
—Portal obstruction: portal hypertension.
—Gastric outlet obstruction.
—Inferior vena caval obstruction: peripheral edema.
—Urinary obstruction.
—Colonic obstruction.

- Infection is rare in children compared to adults

—Has a high mortality rate as stated in adult literature.
—Management usually requires surgical drainage.

Common Questions and Answers

Q: What is the incidence of pancreatic pseudocysts?
A: Some series suggest a 30% to 50% incidence of pseudocyst after severe pancreatitis.

Q: Can a pancreatic pseudocyst go unnoticed?
A: Yes, as the natural history of the disease process is healing by itself.

Q: What mode of therapy has least recurrence rate?
A: Surgical excision.

ICD-9-CM 577.2

BIBLIOGRAPHY

Law NM, Freeman ML. Emergency complications of acute and chronic pancreatitis. *Gastroenterol Clin North Am* 2003;32(4):1169–1194, IX

Reber HA. Surgery for acute and chronic pancreatitis. *Gastrointest Endoscop* 2002;56(6):(Suppl):246–248.

Robertson MA. Acute and chronic pancreatitis. In: Walker WA, ed. *Pediatric Gastrointestinal Disease*. 4th Ed. Hamilton, Ont.: BD Decker, 2004.

Vidyarthi G, Steinberg SE. Endoscopic management of pancreatic pseudocysts. *Surg Clin North Am* 2001;81(2):405–410, XII

Authors: Raman Sreedharan, MD, DCH, MRCPCH and Dev Mehta

Pancreatitis

 Database

DEFINITION

Pancreatitis is inflammation of the pancreas characterized by variable local and systemic inflammatory responses. Pancreatitis can be classified into acute and chronic.

- Acute pancreatitis is characterized by abdominal pain, nausea and vomiting with elevation of pancreatic enzymes and is usually self-limiting. Recurrent episodes of pancreatitis may occur, but the pancreatic function and morphology is restored between episodes. Severe acute pancreatitis is rare in children, and has a high mortality.
- Chronic pancreatitis is characterized by recurrent or persistent abdominal pain with morphological changes in the pancreas leading to pancreatic exocrine or endocrine insufficiency in some patients.

CAUSES OF ACUTE PANCREATITIS

- Idiopathic 22%
- Trauma 20%
—Bicycle handle injuries
—Motor vehicle accidents
—Child abuse
—Postoperative
  —ERCP
  —Scoliosis surgery
  —Posttransplant
- Infections 15%
—Bacterial (typhoid, mycoplasma)
—Viral (measles, mumps, Epstein-Barr virus, Coxsackie B, rubella, influenza, echovirus, hepatitis A and B)
—Parasites (*Ascaris lumbricoides, Echinococcus granulosus, Cryptosporidium parvum, Plasmodium falciparum*)
- Biliary tract disease 14%
—Gallstones
—Sclerosing cholangitis
—Congenital anomalies
  —Pancreatic divisum
  —Annular pancreas
  —Anomalous choledochopancreaticoduodenal junction
  —Biliary tract malformations
  —Duplication cyst of the duodenum/gastropancreatic/common bile duct
—Metabolic
  —Hyperlipidemia
  —Hypercalcemia
  —Uremia
  —Inborn errors of metabolism
—Systemic disease
  —Shock/hypoxemia
  —Hemolytic uremic syndrome
  —Crohn disease
  —Celiac disease
  —Malnutrition (anorexia nervosa, bulimia and refeeding syndrome)
  —Diabetes mellitus
  —Mitochondropathy
  —Hemochromatosis
  —Vasculitis (SLE, Henoch-Schönlein purpura, Kawasaki disease)
—Drug (L-asparaginase, azathioprine/ 6-MP, mesalamine, sulfonamides, thiazides, furosemide, tetracyclines, valproic acid,

corticosteroids, estrogens, procainamide, ethacrynic acid etc.)
—Toxins
  —Alcohol, organophosphates, Yellow scorpion sting
—Hereditary
  —Cystic fibrosis
  —Hereditary pancreatitis gene
  —SPINK 1 gene
  —Protease Serine 1 (PRSS 1)

PATHOPHYSIOLOGY

- Mechanisms of acute pancreatitis are still obscure, but many mechanisms lead to stasis in the pancreatic duct.
- This leads to activation of pancreatic proenzymes by cathepsin, as well as cytokine release.
- Premature activation of trypsin sets of a cascade of zymogen activation of proteolytic enzymes leading to autodigestion of pancreas, necrosis, and hemorrhage.
- Autodigestion leads to local and systemic inflammatory response, which are characterized by cytokine release (TNF, IL1, IL2, IL6, platelet activating factor, etc.), neutrophil activation, and leucocyte recruitment.
- Systemic inflammatory response can lead to multi-organ failure and death.

COMPLICATIONS

- Pancreatitis can lead to local and systemic complications.

LOCAL COMPLICATIONS

- Ascites
- Pancreatic phlegmon
- Pancreatic abscess
- Pancreatic pseudocyst
- Hemorrhagic pancreatitis
- Necrotizing pancreatitis
- Pancreatic calculi
- Exocrine insufficiency
- Diabetes mellitus
- Pancreatic fistula
- Pancreatic fibrosis
- Pancreatic carcinoma

SYSTEMIC COMPLICATIONS

- Gastrointestinal and Hepatobiliary
—Paralytic ileus
—Gastritis
—Stress ulcer
—Upper gastrointestinal bleeding
—Portal vein thrombosis/splenic vein thrombosis/obstruction
—Liver disease
—Bile duct obstruction
- Pulmonary
—Atelectasis
—Pleural effusion
—Pneumonitis
—ARDS
- Cardiovascular
—Hypotension/circulatory collapse
—Pericarditis/pericardial effusion
—ECG changes
—Sudden death
- Hematologic
—Hemoconcentration
—Disseminated intravascular coagulation
- Renal
—Oliguria

—Azotemia and renal failure
—Hepatorenal syndrome
- Neurologic
—Psychosis
—Coma
- Metabolic
—Acidosis
—Hyperkalemia
—Hyperglycemia
—Hypertriglyceridemia
—Hypocalcemia

PROGNOSIS

- The prognosis in children is mostly related to the associated medical condition, though inflammatory complications in other organs may be caused or exacerbated by the inflammatory response from acute pancreatitis.
- The adult criteria to predict outcome of acute pancreatitis (Ranson's criteria) and APACHE-11 are not very useful in children. CT scan changes in severe cases guide management.
- In children, acute pancreatitis may progress to recurrent pancreatitis, and eventually, chronic pancreatitis. These tend to occur in those with structural anomalies of the pancreatic or biliary tree, or hereditary. Many are idiopathic.

 Data Gathering

HISTORY

Question: Describe the abdominal pain in pancreatitis.
Significance: Upper abdominal pain, usually epigastric with radiation to the back. There could be some relief of pain on stooping forward. Pain is aggravated by food intake.

Question: What are the other symptoms?
Significance: Low-grade fever could be part of the disease process and high-grade fever is usually as a result of infection. Nausea and vomiting are very common. Vomiting could be bilious.

Question: Any history of trauma?
Significance: Even trivial abdominal trauma should be a red flag for pancreatitis and evidence for child abuse should also be looked for.

Question: Family history?
Significance: Hereditary pancreatitis runs in the family.

 Physical Examination

- General examination
—Growth parameters (weight and height), vitals, capillary refill, pulse-oximetry, pallor, jaundice, edema, clubbing. Low-grade fever could be a manifestation of pancreatitis and high-grade fever could indicate infections.
—Shock is a complication of pancreatitis.
—Pallor could be the result of chronic systemic disease or a result of hemorrhage.
—Clubbing could be an indicator of Cystic fibrosis.

- GI examination
—Mouth: presence of aphthous ulcers: possibility of Crohn disease.
—Inspection:
  —Abdominal distension or flank fullness (ascites or mass-like pseudopancreatitis cyst)
  —Bluish discoloration (Grey Turner's sign in the flanks and Cullen's sign around the umbilicus in hemorrhagic pancreatitis).
—Palpation:
  —Tenderness with guarding and rebound tenderness, especially in the epigastric or upper abdomen.
  —Palpable mass could be a pancreatic pseudocyst.
  —Palpate for liver, gall bladder, spleen and for other masses.
—Percussion:
  —Ascites.
—Auscultation:
  —Bowel sounds decreased or absent in paralytic ileus.
  —Perianal region:
—Skin tags, fistulas, abscesses and healed scars, which could be indicative of IBD
—Per-rectal examination for mass and for melena/occult blood.
—Respiratory system
  —Pleural effusion and ARDS
  —Diffuse respiratory findings could be indicative of CF.
—CNS
  —Stupor or coma

Laboratory Aids

Test: CBC
- Hemoglobin may be decreased in hemorrhagic pancreatitis or in intestinal hemorrhage.
- Hemoconcentration occur in shock states.
- WBC count is elevated.

Test: Basic metabolic panel
- Electrolyte imbalance as a result of fluid shift and renal complications.
- Calcium is decreased.
- Glucose may be transiently elevated.

Test: Liver function tests
- Elevated transaminases.
- Elevated bilirubin.

Test: Amylase level
- 3- to 6-fold increase in the level increases the specificity for the diagnosis of pancreatitis.
- Starts rising 2 to 12 hours after the insult and remain elevated for 3 to 5 days.
- Persistent elevation could be a result of complication like pseudocyst.
- Degree of elevation does not have any correlation to the severity or the course of the illness.
- Necrotizing and hemorrhagic pancreatitis may develop with normal amylase levels.
- Other causes of elevated amylase levels:
Bowel obstruction
Acute appendicitis
Biliary obstruction
Salivary duct obstruction
Diabetic ketoacidosis

Cystic fibrosis
Cerebral trauma
Burns
Macroamylasemia

LIPASE
- Start rising 4 to 8 hours after the insult and remain elevated for 8 to 14 days.
- Three-fold increase in the level is very sensitive and specific for pancreatitis.
- Levels do not correlate with severity or the clinical outcome.

IMAGING

Abdominal Radiographs
- Sentinel loop: distended small intestinal loop near the pancreas.
- Colon cut-off sign: absence of gas shadow in the colon distal to transverse colon.
- Multiple fluid levels in paralytic ileus.
- Calcification or stones in pancreas or gall bladder.
- Diffuse haziness: ascites.

Contrast Studies
- UGI: "Reverse 3 sign"/Frostberg sign: the curves of the 3 indicate swelling of the pancreas and the middle apex of the 3 suggests the origin of the duct. Anterior displacement of the stomach is seen in pseudopancreatic cyst or retroperitoneal swelling. Barium enema: may show displacement of the transverse colon and extrinsic compression.

Chest Radiograph
- Pleural effusion
- Diaphragmatic involvement
- ARDS

Ultrasound Abdomen
- Pancreatic size, echogenicity, calcification or stones, abscess and pseudocysts.
- Endoscopic ultrasound is more useful than the trans-abdominal ultrasound study.

CT Scan
- In acute cases as in trauma, to look at extent of injury to pancreas and other intraabdominal structures.
- Can identify complications like abscess, hemorrhage, pseudocyst etc.
- Identify pathology in the hepatobiliary system.

Magnetic Resonance Cholangiopancreatography (MRCP)
- Useful for delineation of the ductal pattern of the pancreas and also to identify pathology in the hepatobiliary system leading to pancreatitis in the older child. Note, still of limited use in small children and infants.

Endoscopic Retrograde Cholangiopancreatography (ERCP)
- Persistent/ chronic pancreatitis. Limited to therapeutic use in older children.

Therapy

Supportive care and pancreatic rest is still the main stay of therapy.

- Close monitoring of vitals and intake/output.
- Fluid management—Need 1.5 × maintenance initially as there is extreme third spacing.
- In moderate to severe cases, or vomiting, nasogastric decompression by placement of NG tube and NPO helps to decrease the pancreatic stimulation during the acute phase of the illness. Mild cases may be started on feeds after a few days.
- Pain management—narcotics may be used and Meperidine is preferable to Morphine as Meperidine has less effect on the sphincter of Oddi.
- H_2 blockade—prevents pancreatic stimulation in severe cases.
- Nutrition—NJ feeds worth considering first if oral feeding is not possible. An alternative is TPN.
- Antibiotics—prophylaxes in severe cases in which necrotizing pancreatitis is suspected; note, few antimicrobials, such as imipenem-cilastatin, get adequate penetration.
- Therapeutic ERCP
—For decompression of pancreatic or common bile duct obstruction/ removal of ductal stones, and drainage of certain pseudocysts.
- Interventional radiology/surgery
—For abscess and pseudocysts drainage.
- Surgery
—Peritoneal lavage, and rarely for salvage in necrotizing/ hemorrhagic pancreatitis.

Common Questions and Answers

Q: What is hereditary pancreatitis?
A: Hereditary pancreatitis presents as recurrent inflammation of the pancreas and runs in families over two or more generations and is inherited as an autosomal dominant trait with variable penetrance.

Q: Can pancreatitis be a presenting symptom for cystic fibrosis?
A: Yes.

Q: Normal ultrasound or CT scan of pancreas excludes acute pancreatitis?
A: No. Normal US and CT common in mild cases.

BIBLIOGRAPHY

Jackson WD. Pancreatitis: etiology, diagnosis and management. *Curr Opin Pediatr* 2001;13:447–451.

Lerner A, Branski D, Lebenthal E. Pancreatic diseases in children. *Pediatr Clin North Am* 1996;43(1):125–156.

Pietzak MM, Thomas DW. Pancreatitis in childhood. *Pediatr Rev* 2000;21(12):406–412.

Somogyi L, Martin SP, Venkatesan T, et al. Recurrent acute pancreatitis: an algorithmic approach to identification and elimination of inciting factors. *Gastroenterology* 2001;120:708–717.

Authors: Raman Sreedharan, MD, DCH, MRCPCH and Dev Mehta

Panhypopituitarism

 Database

DEFINITION

Deficiency of multiple pituitary hormones

CAUSES

- Idiopathic
- Congenital
—Absence of the pituitary (empty sella syndrome)
—Pituitary malformations (ectopic posterior pituitary, hypoplastic infundibular stalk)
—Familial panhypopituitarism
- Acquired
—Birth trauma or perinatal insult
—Surgical resection of the gland or damage to the stalk
—Child abuse
- Infection
—Viral encephalitis
—Bacterial or fungal infection
—Tuberculosis
- Vascular
—Pituitary infarction
—Pituitary aneurysm
- Cranial irradiation
- Chemotherapy
- Tumors
—Craniopharyngioma
—Germinoma
—Glioma
—Pinealoma
—Primitive neuroectodermal tumor (medulloblastoma)
—Histiocytosis
—Sarcoidosis

PATHOPHYSIOLOGY

Pathology is based on specific deficiency:
- Growth hormone: hypoglycemia in newborns and poor growth in other patients
- ACTH: hypocortisolism
- TSH: hypothyroidism
- LH/FSH: hypogonadism
- ADH: diabetes insipidus
- Prolactin: hyperprolactinemia

GENETICS

There are rare cases of autosomal-recessive, autosomal-dominant, and X-linked forms.

EPIDEMIOLOGY

Congenital forms affect both sexes equally and are diagnosed at a young age.
The incidence of secondary forms depends on the underlying cause.

COMPLICATIONS

- Hypoglycemia in the newborn period
- Short stature
- Adrenal crisis
- Dehydration

PROGNOSIS

- Prognosis for congenital forms is excellent.
- Prognosis for secondary forms depends on the primary disease.

 Differential Diagnosis

- Hyperinsulinism in newborns
- Isolated growth hormone deficiency in newborns

 Data Gathering

HISTORY

Question: Birth history?
Significance: Hyperinsulinemic infants are typically large for gestational age, which can be associated with shoulder dystocia; hypopituitary babies are not large. Midline defects are associated with hypopituitarism and not hyperinsulinism.

Question: Complications during pregnancy or delivery?
Significance: Birth trauma may be associated with pituitary injury. Breech delivery or vacuum extraction has been associated.

Question: Birth weight?
Significance: Hypopituitary infants are usually normal or small for gestational age in contrast to hyperinsulinemic infants who are typically large.

Question: History of hypoglycemia during the neonatal period?
Significance: Ask about symptoms of lethargy, poor feeding, irritability, or seizures, which could suggest hypoglycemia.

Question: History of surgeries and previous diseases?
Significance: Congenital hypopituitarism is often associated with midline facial defects (such as bifid uvula or cleft palate), which require repair.

Question: Growth pattern?
Significance: Plot previous heights and look for growth pattern. GH deficiency usually manifests as poor linear growth by the end of the first year of life.

Question: Delayed puberty?
Significance: Children with delayed puberty show further growth failure in adolescence. Sense of smell should be assessed to rule out Kallmann syndrome (isolated central hypogonadism and anosmia).

Question: Increased thirst and urination?
Significance: Children with hypothalamic disorders may present with symptoms of diabetes insipidus.

SPECIAL QUESTIONS

Question: Any complaints of headache?
Significance: Headache can be a symptom of a brain tumor.

Question: Any neurologic signs or symptoms?
Significance: Focal neurologic symptoms are highly suggestive of CNS pathology.

 Physical Examination

Finding: Actual height and weight
Significance: Patients with panhypopituitarism have normal size in the newborn period. Patients with hyperinsulinism are typically large for gestational age.

Finding: Prolonged hyperbilirubinemia
Significance: May be first sign of hypothyroidism with or without hypopituitarism. Some state newborn screens will not detect central hypothyroidism. Hypopituitarism can lead to neonatal cholestasis.

Finding: Micropenis in males
Significance: Neonatal penis should be at least 2.5 cm in length; micropenis suggests gonadotropin deficiency.

PHYSICAL EXAMINATION TRICKS

Finding: Penile and testicular size
Significance: Measure stretched phallic length (from pubic ramus to glans) with patient lying supine and phallus at 90° to the body; use Prader beads to assess testicular volume.

Finding: Midline defects
Significance: Palpate for submucosal cleft palate.

Finding: Visual field testing
Significance: Visual field defects suggest a brain tumor.

ASSOCIATIONS

- Midline defects (e.g., cleft lip/palate, hypotelorism, single central maxillary incisor)
- Septo-optic dysplasia (de Morsier syndrome)
- Holoprosencephaly

 Laboratory Aids

SPECIFIC TESTS

Test: Liver function tests
Significance: Typically elevated liver enzymes in the newborn period.

Test: Thyroid function tests including free thyroxine (T4)
Significance: Total T4 and TSH may be normal, but free T4 will be low.

Test: TRH stimulation test
Significance: Delayed, normal, or exaggerated TSH response is consistent with a hypothalamic lesion.

Test: Serum IGF-I and IGFBP-3
Significance: May be low but normal growth factors do not exclude GH deficiency in children with brain tumors.

Test: Free thyroxine by equilibrium dialysis
Significance: Must measure, not calculate, the free T4 concentration in serum.

Test: Growth hormone stimulation tests
Significance: Should be performed by a pediatric endocrinologist.

Test: Cortrosyn stimulation test
Significance: More helpful in the diagnosis of primary adrenal insufficiency than secondary (ACTH) or tertiary (CRH) deficiency.

Test: Metyrapone or CRH stimulation test
Significance: The definitive tests for ACTH or CRH deficiency but must be performed by a pediatric endocrinologist.

Test: Water deprivation test
Significance: The definitive test for ADH deficiency but must be performed by a pediatric endocrinologist.

IMAGING

Test: Bone age
Significance: Typically delayed in GH deficiency or hypothyroidism.

Test: MRI with contrast of brain with fine cuts through the pituitary hypothalamus
Significance: Look for tumors and presence of normal "bright spot" in posterior pituitary. Absence of the bright spot is highly associated with central diabetes insipidus.

COMMENTS ON TESTING

Test: Measurement of water intake and urine output over 24 hours at home.
Significance: Can help diagnosis diabetes insipidus.

- Baseline serum tests
- Can all be done in a nonfasting state.
- Stimulation tests
- Need to be performed by a pediatric endocrinologist.

Emergency Care

If ACTH deficient, stress dosing of glucocorticoids is necessary

Therapy

DRUGS

- Recombinant human growth hormone (rhGH) by subcutaneous injection daily: 0.3 mg/kg per week
- Levo-thyroxine orally: 25 to 150 μg daily, based on weight, age, and free thyroxine levels
- Hydrocortisone
—Replacement doses if needed: 8 to 15 mg/m^2 per day orally, divided q8h (or three times daily)
—In stress circumstances such as fever, illness, dose increased to 25 to 100 mg/m^2 per day PO
—For surgery, major illness, vomiting, etc.: 50 to 100 mg/m^2 per day IV or PO
—Intravenous doses should be divided q4h; oral stress doses should be divided q8h
—To calculate hydrocortisone dose, estimate body surface area (BSA) using a nomogram or the following formula: BSA (m^2) = Square root of (height (cm) × weight (kg)/3600)

—DDAVP: available in oral and intranasal formulations

DURATION

- Long-term therapy: monitored by a pediatric endocrinologist
- Recombinant human growth hormone (rhGH)
—In children and adolescents:
 —Until growth velocity drops to 2.5 cm/year
 —Once puberty is complete
—In adulthood:
 —GH-deficient adults may benefit from lifelong rhGH therapy as a result of the impact of GH on body composition, lipid profile, and cardiac function
 —Patient should again undergo GH provocative testing (off rhGH therapy, of course)
- Levo-thyroxine: for life
- Hydrocortisone
—Replacement dose based on individual's need
—Stress dose coverage for life
- DDAVP: for life as needed to control symptoms of polyuria/polydipsia

DIET

There are no restrictions; it is important to know if patient has intact thirst mechanism.

POSSIBLE CONFLICTS WITH OTHER TREATMENTS

There is a theoretical risk that growth hormone might stimulate tumor growth as a result of its mitogenic effect. Current data generally argue against growth hormone as a tumor stimulant.

Follow-Up

Initially, every 3 months by a pediatric endocrinologist

WHEN TO EXPECT IMPROVEMENT

- Immediately, if hypoglycemic
- Growth velocity should increase within 3 to 6 months
- The growth response to thyroid hormone replacement is slow, but free T4 levels should normalize within 4 to 6 weeks.

SIGNS TO WATCH FOR

- Headache
- Vision problems
- Seizures
- Changes in activity level
- Limp, knee, or hip pain

PITFALLS

- rhGH therapy is associated with idiopathic intracranial hypertension (pseudotumor cerebri), which typically improves whether or not medication is stopped.
- rhGH deficiency/therapy is associated with slipped capital femoral epiphysis (SCFE).

Carefully evaluate any limp or knee or hip pain in patients on rhGH therapy. SCFE mandates orthopaedic consultation.
- Growth hormone is a mitogenic factor so there has been a theoretical potential for increasing the incidence of leukemia. Clinical studies have not confirmed this hypothesis.
- The family and the patient must understand the importance of taking stress doses of steroid appropriately (e.g., with surgery, vomiting, or febrile illnesses).
- You must consider the diagnosis of panhypopituitarism in patients with hypoglycemic seizures.
- Normal children can fail to respond to growth hormone provocative testing.
- Ordering a TSH level is generally not helpful when evaluating pituitary/hypothalamic causes of hypothyroidism. The unbound thyroxine level (free T4 by equilibrium dialysis) is the most useful test in these cases both to establish the diagnosis and to monitor L-thyroxine replacement therapy.

Common Questions and Answers

Q: When do I give the stress dose of steroid and for how long?
A: Whenever the patient has fever, vomiting, serious illness, or surgery. Continue until 24 hours after stress resolves (e.g., the day after fever breaks or vomiting stops).

Q: What are the chances of cretinism if hypopituitarism is congenital?
A: Minimal, if medication is taken properly.

ICD-9-CD 253.2

BIBLIOGRAPHY

Cohen LE, Radovick S. Other transcription factors and hypopituitarism. *Rev Endocr Metab Disord* 2002;3(4):301–311.

De Vries L, Lazar L, Phillip M. Craniopharyngioma: presentation and endocrine sequelae in 36 children. *J Endocrin Metab* 2003;16(5):703–710.

Maghnie M. Diabetes Insipidus. *Horm Res* 2003;59(Suppl 1):42–54.

McGauley G, Cuneo R, Salomon F, et al. Growth hormone deficiency and quality of life. *Horm Res* 1996;45(1–2):34–37.

Parks JS, Brown MR, Hurley DL, et al. Heritable disorders of pituitary development. *J Clin Endocrinol Metab* 1999;84:4362–4370.

Romeo JH. Hyperfunction and hypofunction in the anterior pituitary. *Nurs Clin North Am* 1996;31(4):769–778.

Sklar CA, Constine LS. Chronic neuroendocrinological sequelae of radiation therapy. *Int J Radiat Oncol Biol Phys* 1995;31(5):1113–1121.

Soule SG, Jacobs HS. The evaluation and management of subclinical pituitary disease. *Postgrad Med J* 1996;72(847):258–262.

Authors: Craig A. Alter
Robert Ferry, 3rd edition

Parvovirus B19 (Erythema Infectiosum, Fifth Disease)

 Database

DEFINITION

Parvovirus B19 (B19) is a common viral infection of school-aged children that is most commonly associated with an erythematous macular rash in a patient whose appearance remains well.

CAUSES

• B19 is a single-stranded DNA virus, one of the smallest of the human viruses.
• It was first isolated from asymptomatic blood donors in 1975.

PATHOPHYSIOLOGY

• Parvovirus B19 replicates in the red blood cell (RBC) precursors in the bone marrow and is associated with a number of different diseases ranging from benign to severe.
• There is no practical in vitro system for isolation or culture of the virus.

ASSOCIATED DISEASES

• Aplastic crisis secondary to B19 in patients with hereditary hemolytic anemias or any condition that shortens the RBC lifespan, such as sickle cell disease or spherocytosis, may cause severe anemia.
• Fifth disease or erythema infectiosum caused by B19 occurs in up to 35% of school-aged children.
• Human parvovirus arthropathy, symmetrical joint pain, and swelling, especially of the hands, knees, and feet is seen in adults much more frequently than children; among women with B19 infection, 80% to 100% develop polyarthritis.
• Hydrops fetalis may develop following maternal B19 infection and intrauterine involvement.
• Chronic bone marrow failure as a result of persistent B19 infection in immunocompromised patients has been reported.
• Extremity numbness and tingling, hemophagocytic syndrome, and Henoch-Schönlein purpura has recently been sporadically reported as being associated with B19 infection.
• Papular–purpuric gloves and socks syndrome is a rash localized to the hands and feet. It is associated with edema, erythema, and paresthesia.

EPIDEMIOLOGY

• Most B19 infections occur in school-aged children.
• Seroprevalence of B19 IgG antibodies:

—>5 years, 2% to 9%
—Five to 18 years, 15% to 35%
—Adults, 30% to 60%

• Route of spread includes exposure to:

—Nasal secretions
—Aerosolized large-droplet respiratory secretions
—Blood (1,011 virions per mL or serum in patients with hereditary hemolytic anemias)

• Attack rates range from 15% to 60% of susceptibles, i.e., seronegative, will become infected on exposure.
• Forty percent of susceptible health care workers were infected in a Philadelphia outbreak in 1989.

COMPLICATIONS

• Parvovirus B19 during pregnancy

—Fetal loss or hydrops fetalis may occur if infected with B19 during pregnancy.
—50% of women are susceptible to B19 infection.
—The infection is not a teratogen to the fetus.
—Fetal death occurs in 3% to 9%.
—The greatest risk for B19 infection to affect the fetus exists in the first 20 weeks of gestation.
—There is no indication for elective abortion in cases of maternal infection.
—The risk of fetal death after exposure, if antibody status is unknown, is from 0.05% to 1%.

• Aplastic crisis

—Transfusions may be necessary to treat symptoms of severe anemia.

• Arthritis/arthropathy

—Although most cases of polyarthritis resolve within 2 weeks, persistent symptoms for months to even years (rarely) have been reported.

PROGNOSIS

The prognosis is quite good for all manifestations of B19 infections; in general, they require supportive care only until spontaneous recovery.

 Differential Diagnosis

B19 infection should be considered in all patients with arthritis or viral exanthems with a history and examination that is consistent.

 Data Gathering

HISTORY

Question: Asymptomatic infection?
Significance: May occur in approximately 20% of children and adults.

Question: Erythema infectiosum?
Significance: The most common form of parvovirus infection recognized. The incubation period is 4 to 14 days; prodromal symptoms are mild and include headache, sore throat, lethargy, and low-grade fevers lasting 1 to 4 days. A facial rash that is erythematous (slapped cheeks) is noticed next, which spreads to the body and extremities. The body rash is macular erythematous and lacy appearing. It may become more intense with exercise and may be pruritic. Occasionally, it involves the palms and soles and rarely can be papular, vesicular, or purpuric. It may last for approximately 7 days but can persist more than 20 days. The child is usually unaffected and remains active and playful. Symptoms in adults are similar although often more severe. During the illness, 80% of adults have arthralgias or arthritis.

Question: Aplastic crisis?
Significance: Prodromal symptoms in B19-infected children with sickle cell disease or other hereditary hemolytic anemias are nonspecific and consist of fever, malaise, and headache. Laboratory testing confirms the diagnosis.

Question: Chronic marrow suppression?
Significance: In immunocompromised patients, B19 infection may persist for months, leading to chronic anemia with B19 viremia. Low-grade fever and neutropenia may accompany anemia.

Parvovirus B19 (Erythema Infectiosum, Fifth Disease)

 Physical Examination

- Fifth disease

—A facial rash that is erythematous (slapped cheeks) is noticed next, which spreads to the body and extremities.
—The body rash is macular erythematous and lacy appearing. It may become more intense with exercise and may be pruritic.
—Occasionally, it involves the palms and soles and rarely can be papular, vesicular, or purpuric.

 Laboratory Aids

The diagnosis of B19 infection depends on recognition of typical symptoms and the following tests:

Test: Antibodies
Significance: Presence of specific IgM or IgG antibodies as determined by EIA and/or detection of virus. In patients with symptoms of erythema infectiosum or aplastic crisis, the presence of B19-specific IgM antibodies is diagnostic. IgM- and IgG-specific antibodies are detected in 90% of such patients by 3 to 7 days of illness. B19-specific IgG antibodies persists for years, although specific IgM antibodies begin to fall 30 to 60 days after onset of illness.

Test: Polymerase chain reaction (PCR) techniques
Significance: Immunocompromised patients with chronic marrow may be unable to produce B19-specific IgG or IgM antibodies. In such cases, B19 viral DNA can be detected using nuclear and hybridization or PCR techniques. Such techniques are also useful for detecting infection in fetuses.

Test: Hematocrit and reticulocyte count in patients with aplastic crisis
Significance: Laboratory studies reveal reticulocytopenia, usually with counts of >1%. During the illness, the patient's hematocrit may fall as low as 15%.

 Therapy

- There is no specific therapy for this infection other than supportive care.
- Intravenous immunoglobulin therapy has been given with some success to a few patients with chronic marrow suppression secondary to B19 infection.

PREVENTION INFECTION CONTROL

In the hospital environment, secondary attack rates approaching 40% were reported in susceptive health care workers exposed to two children with sickle cell disease and unsuspected B19 infections. In response, all patients with suspected aplastic crisis secondary to B19 should be placed in contact isolation. No measures are needed for normal hosts with rash. In addition, pregnant teachers who are at risk for infections should consider a leave of absence during community outbreaks of B19.

 Follow-Up

EXPECTED COURSE OF ILLNESS

- During aplastic crisis secondary to B19 the reticulocytopenia usually remains low (often >1%) for approximately 8 days before spontaneous recovery.
- The rash of erythema infectiosum in the child or adult may last up to 20 days. It may, at times, fade and/or intensify depending on sunlight exposure, exercise, or body surface temperature changes (bathing).

 Common Questions and Answers

Q: When may children with B19 infection return to school?
A: Children are not infectious when the rash appears. Therefore, they may return to school or day care. The infectious period is only during the prodromal phase of illness, which is often unrecognized.

Q: What can be done to reduce risk of fetal infection?
A: Because B19 infections during pregnancy may result in fetal death, and B19 infections often occur in community outbreaks, fetal risks following maternal exposure to persons with recognized B19 infection are a frequent concern. Among pregnant women of unknown antibody status, the risk of fetal death after exposure to B19 is estimated to be <1.5%. Risk to the fetus appears to be greatest if the infection occurs prior to the 20th week of gestation. Pregnant teachers who are at risk for infection should consider a leave of absence during community outbreaks of B19.

ICD-9-CM 057.0

BIBLIOGRAPHY

Anderson LJ, Tsou C, Parker RA, et al. Detection of antibodies and antigens of human parvovirus B19 by ELISA. *J Clin Microbiol* 1986;24:522–526.

Bell LM, Naides SJ, Stoffman P, et al. Human parvovirus B19 infection among hospital staff members after contact with infected patients. *N Engl J Med* 1989;321:485–491.

Bell LM. Parvovirus B19 infection: a decade of discovery. In: Long SS, Starr SE, eds. *The report on pediat infect dis* 1992;2:6.

Cherry JD. Parvovirus infections in children and adults. *Adv Pediatr* 1999;46:245–269.

Kerr JR. Pathogenesis of human parvovirus B19 in rheumatic disease. *Ann Rheum Dis* 2000;59(9):672–683.

Török TJ. Parvovirus B19 and human disease. *Adv Intern Med* 1992;37:431–455.

Ware R. Human parvovirus infection. *J Pediatr* 1989;114:343–348.

Young NS, Brown KE. Parvovirus B19. *N Engl J Med* 2004;350:586–597.

Author: Louis M. Bell

Patent Ductus Arteriosus

 Database

DEFINITION

• Patent ductus arteriosus (PDA) is the persistence into postnatal life of the normal fetal vascular conduit between the central pulmonary and systemic arterial systems. Normally, the ductus arteriosus (DA) functionally closes within the first 1 to 3 days of life. Structural closure is usually completed by the third week of life. If the DA remains patent beyond 3 months of life, it is considered abnormal and is unlikely to close spontaneously (spontaneous closure rate 0.6% per year).
• In the infant with a normal left aortic arch, the DA connects the main pulmonary artery at the origin of the left pulmonary artery to the descending aorta, distal to the origin of the left subclavian artery.
• Many variations can occur although they are less common. The main, proximal right or proximal left pulmonary artery may be connected to virtually any location on the aortic arch or proximal portions of the brachiocephalic vessels.
• There are five distinct clinical conditions associated with PDA:

—Isolated cardiovascular lesion in premature infants.
—Isolated cardiovascular lesion in otherwise healthy term infants and children.
—Incidental finding associated with more significant structural cardiovascular defects.
—Compensatory structure in cases of neonatal persistent pulmonary hypertension (PPHN) without congenital heart disease (CHD).
—Critical compensatory structure in some cyanotic or left-sided obstructed lesions.

In this chapter, the PDA as an isolated cardiovascular lesion is discussed.

CAUSES

• Prematurity
• Rubella infection in the first trimester
• Genetic or familial factors
• High altitude
• Idiopathic

EPIDEMIOLOGY

• As an isolated defect, PDA is the sixth most common congenital cardiovascular lesion.
• Incidence 1/2,000 (5% of all types of CHD).
• Female:male ratio 2:1
• The incidence increases with the degree of prematurity (50% to 80% in preterm infants <26 weeks' gestation). The incidence varies significantly depending on management style (e.g., amount of maintenance fluid prescribed, surfactant administration), coexisting diseases (e.g., respiratory distress syndrome, hypoxemia, fluid overload, necrotizing enterocolitis, sepsis, hypocalcemia), and environmental factors (altitude).

PATHOLOGY

In premature infants and term infants with PPHN, delayed closure represents an impaired developmental process, although in the full-term infant a PDA probably reflects an anatomic abnormality of the ductal tissue.

PHYSIOLOGY

Fetal blood flows from the main pulmonary artery (MPA) to the DA to the aorta, thus bypassing the pulmonary vascular bed and supplying systemic blood flow. With the first postnatal breaths, the pulmonary vascular resistance falls abruptly, the DA constricts, and pulmonary blood flow is directed into the lungs. With a PDA, excessive blood flow will continue from the aorta into the pulmonary artery causing increased pulmonary blood flow and volume overloading of the left side of the heart.

COMPLICATIONS

• Pulmonary edema and congestive heart failure
• Pulmonary hemorrhage
• Pulmonary vascular obstructive disease
• Increased chronic lung disease
• Failure to thrive
• Recurrent respiratory infections
• Lobar emphysema or collapse
• Infective endarteritis
• Thromboembolism of cerebral arteries
• Aneurysm of the ductus
• Intracranial hemorrhage
• Necrotizing enterocolitis
• Renal dysfunction

 Differential Diagnosis

• Aortopulmonary window
• Systemic or pulmonary arteriovenous communications
• Ruptured sinus of Valsalva
• Coronary artery fistula
• Truncus arteriosus
• Innocent venous hum in older children
• Pulmonary atresia with collaterals
• Ventricular septal defect with aortic regurgitation
• Ventricular septal defect in infancy

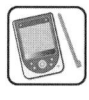 Data Gathering

HISTORY

Premature Infants

• Variable, ranging from asymptomatic to complete cardiovascular collapse.
• Increased ventilatory support, pulmonary hemorrhage, respiratory or metabolic acidosis from low cardiac output and excessive pulmonary blood flow.
• Tachypnea, feeding intolerance, apnea, bradycardia, necrotizing enterocolitis, and decreased urine output.

Infants and Older Children

• Small PDA: usually asymptomatic with incidental heart murmur found on routine exam.
• Moderate PDA: Possible congestive heart failure, poor feeding, and poor weight gain.
• Large PDA: Symptoms as above and also recurrent respiratory infections.

 Physical Examination

PREMATURE INFANTS

Findings:

• Tachypnea, rales, tachycardia (± S3 gallop)
• Hyperdynamic precordium and bounding pulses with wide pulse pressure (as a result of diastolic "run off" from the aorta to the pulmonary artery).
• The typical PDA murmur in a premature infant is a pansystolic murmur audible at the left upper or midsternal border.
• With a large PDA and equalization of pressure between the MPA and the aorta, no murmur may be heard.
• Hepatomegaly may exist with heart failure (late sign).

INFANTS AND OLDER CHILDREN

Findings: Varies with size of shunt.

- Small PDA

—A pansystolic murmur may be heard at the second left intercostal space. Murmur becomes continuous i.e., extends into diastole as the pulmonary vascular resistance decreases over the first months of life.

- Moderate or large PDA

—The murmur is louder, has a harsh quality, and acquires a machine-like quality often being heard posteriorly. In that case, a systolic thrill may be felt at the left upper sternal border.
—Tachycardia, bounding pulses with a wide pulse pressure, and a mid-diastolic low-frequency rumbling murmur may be audible at the apex with a large PDA.
—With severe left ventricular failure the classic PDA signs may disappear, but there will be findings consistent with congestive heart failure (CHF) (tachycardia, S3 gallop at the apex, hepatomegaly, tachypnea, rales).
—In extreme cases, pulmonary hypertension may occur with the murmur shortening, the diastolic component disappearing, and S2 becoming accentuated. At advanced stages of irreversible pulmonary vascular disease cyanosis begins to appear, often more pronounced in the lower limbs, with reversal of shunting.

 ## Laboratory Aids

1. Electrocardiogram—usually normal with a small PDA; left atrial enlargement and left ventricular hypertrophy with moderate and large PDA; biventricular hypertrophy in later stages
2. Chest radiograph—usually normal with a small PDA, although prominence of main and peripheral pulmonary arteries may be seen. In moderate and large PDA these findings become more pronounced along with an enlarged heart. Increased pulmonary vascular markings are proportionate to the left-to-right shunt. Pulmonary edema can be seen if CHF develops. In premature infants with respiratory distress syndrome there is evidence of deteriorating lung disease with unclear cardiac borders.
3. Echocardiogram—delineates the PDA and assesses the size of the left atrium and the left ventricle. Doppler techniques assess the ductal flow pattern and may be useful for estimating the pulmonary artery pressure.
4. Cardiac catheterization—most often not essential for diagnosis; indicated for suspected pulmonary hypertension; also can be performed for treatment via transcatheter closure techniques

 ## Therapy

PREMATURE INFANT

- Supportive treatment (careful use of O_2, respiratory assistance, correction of metabolic acidosis)
- Management of CHF with fluid restriction and diuretics
- If PDA persists despite above management or patient is symptomatic, closure of PDA is indicated.
- Medical closure: Indomethacin most often used.
- Contraindications to medical management include: renal failure (creatinine >1.8 mg/dL), thrombocytopenia (platelets <100,000), associated conditions (necrotizing enterocolitis, intraventricular hemorrhage grade IV)
- Surgical closure indicated if medical treatment fails or use of indomethacin is contraindicated

INFANTS AND OLDER CHILDREN

- Medical management of CHF with digoxin and diuretics.
- SBE prophylaxis for any at-risk procedures.
- Spontaneous closure rate low and closure with indomethacin not usually effective in this group of patients.
- Closure is indicated whenever a symptomatic PDA exists.
- For asymptomatic audible PDA, closure can be performed electively after the first year of age and is mainly performed to reduce the risk of endocarditis. Recommendations for closure of an asymptomatic, incidentally found ("silent" ductus) vary by cardiologist.
- Closure of ductus can be achieved by one of three means:

—Open surgical ligation or division—mostly in premature infants
—Videoscopically assisted ligation—used at few institutions
—Transcatheter occlusion with coils or devices—most common

Most infants and children can have a PDA safely and effectively closed via cardiac catheterization, obviating the need for a surgical procedure.

 ## Follow-Up

PROGNOSIS

- Outcome in treated premature infants is generally good but mostly depends on the degree of prematurity and the presence of associated conditions.
- Outcome in term infants and older children is excellent if no complications have occurred.
- PDA among adults may be associated with significant mortality with or without surgery.
- Postclosure of PDA no endocarditis prophylaxis is needed if complete obliteration of flow is achieved. Most cardiologists continue prophylaxis for 6 months after the procedure that closed the DA.

ICD-9-CM 747.0

BIBLIOGRAPHY

Cowley CG, Lloyd TR. Interventional cardiac catheterization advances in nonsurgical approaches to congenital heart disease. *Curr Opin Pediatr* 1999;11(5):425–432.

Knight DB. The treatment of patent ductus arteriosus in preterm infants. A review and overview of randomized trials. *Semin Neonatol* 2001;6(1):63–73.

Moore JW, et al. The duct-occlud device: design, clinical results, and future directions. *J Interv Cardiol* 2001;14(2):231–237.

Moore P, et al. Patent ductus arteriosus. In: Allen HD, Clark EB, Gutgesell HP, Driscoll DJ, eds. *Heart Disease in Infants, Children and Adolescents.* 6th Ed. Philadelphia: Lippincott Williams & Wilkins, 2001:652–669.

Sullivan ID. Patent arterial duct: when should it be closed? *Arch Dis Child* 1998;78(3): 285–287.

Author: Michael P. Mulreany

Pelvic Inflammatory Disease (PID)

 Database

DEFINITION

An ascending, polymicrobial, genital tract infection of sexually active females. It includes an array of inflammatory disorders, including endometritis, parametritis, salpingitis, oophoritis, tubo-ovarian abscess (TOA), peritonitis, and perihepatitis. PID is a clinical diagnosis. The Centers for Disease Control and Prevention (CDC) has established the following clinical criteria. If the following minimum criteria are present, and no other cause can be identified, empiric therapy for PID should be initiated in sexually active young women:

- Uterine adnexal tenderness or
- Cervical motion tenderness.

The additional criteria can be used to enhance the specificity of the diagnosis of PID in women with more severe clinical signs:
—Oral temperature higher than 101°F (38.3°C)
—Abnormal cervical or vaginal mucopurulent discharge
—Presence of white blood cells (WBCs) on saline microscopy of vaginal secretions
—Elevated erythrocyte sedimentation rate (ESR)
—Elevated C-reactive protein (CRP)
—Laboratory documented evidence of infection with *Neisseria gonorrhoeae* or
—*Chlamydia trachomatis*
- Definitive criteria
—Histopathologic evidence of endometritis on endometrial biopsy
—Transvaginal sonography or other imaging techniques showing thickened fluid-filled tubes with or without free pelvic fluid or TOA
—Laparoscopic abnormalities consistent with PID

ETIOLOGY

Although a polymicrobial infection, cervical infection or vaginal bacterial overgrowth with the following organisms can lead to acute PID:
- *N. gonorrhoeae* cervicitis
- *C. trachomatis* cervicitis: tends to be associated with less fever, pain, and systemic symptoms than PID as a result of gonococcus
- Bacterial vaginosis: bacteroides, mobiluncus, and peptostreptococcus species

EPIDEMIOLOGY

- Affects more than 1 million American women per year
- Estimated total cost over $4.2 billion per year
- Adolescent cases account for 20% to 30% of all cases, with adolescents having a 10-fold risk when compared to adults.
- Risk increases with failure to use condoms, number of lifetime partners, having new partners in the last 3 months, past history of sexually transmitted infections (STIs), and the presence of an IUD.
- Oral contraceptive pill (OCP) use decreases the risk of PID, but does not reduce the risk of vaginal or cervical infection.

COMPLICATIONS

- Chronic pelvic pain or dyspareunia (up to 18%)
- Ectopic pregnancy
- Infertility
- Tubo-ovarian abscess (TOA)
- Fitz-Hugh-Curtis syndrome (perihepatitis resulting from tracking of pus along the paracolic gutters)

PROGNOSIS

- Excellent if adequate treatment obtained early and acute complications absent
- One episode is associated with a 13% to 21% risk of infertility, two episodes with a 35% risk, and three or more episodes with a 55% to 75% risk.
- One episode of PID increases the risk of future ectopic pregnancy 10-fold.
- Long-term sequelae are present in 25% of affected women, with a higher likelihood in adolescents as a result of later presentation, delay in diagnosis, and inadequate treatment.

 Differential Diagnosis

INFECTION

- Cervicitis
- Vulvovaginal candidiasis
- Trichomoniasis
- Bacterial vaginosis
- Tubo-ovarian abscess
- Pyelonephritis or cystitis
- Appendicitis, appendiceal abscess
- Tuberculosis
- Viral or bacterial enteritis
- Acute cholecystitis
- Mesenteric lymphadenitis
- Pelvic thrombophlebitis

GYNECOLOGIC

- Dysmenorrhea
- Pregnancy, intrauterine or ectopic
- Ovarian cyst or torsion
- Chronic pelvic pain
- Endometriosis
- Teratoma or other mass

MISCELLANEOUS

- Foreign body or pelvic trauma
- Functional pain

 Data Gathering

HISTORY

Assessment begins with sensitive, private interview with a practitioner who can assure confidentiality.

Question: Review of systems.
Significance: Presentation may be "silent," with relatively few or mild symptoms.

Question: Ask about pain, fever, and gynecologic symptoms.

Significance: Classic presentation of PID includes:
- Lower abdominal pain
- Abnormal vaginal discharge or bleeding
- Fever

Question: Take complete menstrual, sexual, gastrointestinal, and urinary histories.
Significance: Associated symptoms may include:
- Dysmenorrhea
- Dyspareunia
- Vomiting, diarrhea, or constipation

Question: Past medical history, including gynecologic history, should be obtained.
Significance: Supportive historical data for PID include:
- Recent menstruation
- Use of IUD or douche
- Inconsistent condom use
- Multiple or new sexual partners
- Prior history of PID

 Physical Examination

- Perform a thorough abdominal exam, noting tenderness, rebound or guarding, and signs of perihepatic involvement.

Finding: Pelvic examination
Significance: Document the following:
- Presence of external or vaginal lesions
- Origin, quality, and quantity of discharge (e.g., "copious, mucopurulent cervical discharge," or "scant, thin vaginal discharge")
- Signs of cervical inflammation (e.g., erythema, friability)
- Cervical motion tenderness
- Adnexal tenderness and/or fullness
- Blot away discharge to better assess the source of new fluid accumulation

 Laboratory Aids

TESTS

- Urine β-Human Chorionic Gonadotropin (β-HCG)—is essential to know if the patient is pregnant, regardless of sexual history
- Complete blood count with differential
- ESR or CRP
- Wet prep of discharge for trichomonads, hyphae, or clue cells
- Gram stain of cervical discharge
- Testing for *N. gonorrhoeae* and *C. trachomatis*
- Culture is technique dependent, yielding an 80% sensitivity.
- Antigen detection tests (e.g., direct fluorescent antibody [DFA], enzyme-linked immunosorbent assay [ELISA]) have lower sensitivities.
- Genetic amplification (LCR) requires a single specimen for both organisms, has a 24-hour turnaround time, and has 90% to 95% sensitivity.
- Syphilis serology (e.g., rapid plasma reagin [RPR] testing) and human immunodeficiency virus (HIV) testing with appropriate counseling and follow-up.

RADIOGRAPHIC STUDIES

Test: Pelvic ultrasound
Significance: To rule out TOA or other pelvic pathology

Test: Laparoscopy
Significance: Not routinely used, but considered the criterion standard for diagnosis.

 Emergency Care

- TOA rupture—requires immediate surgical or gynecologic consultation, can present as acute peritonitis.
- If an IUD is in place, it must be removed immediately.

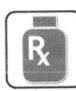 Therapy

Inpatient treatment has been the standard of care, and should be done if:

- Suspected TOA
- Patient has failed outpatient treatment
- Patient is clinically ill or is at high risk for sequelae
- Patient is immunocompromised or suppressed

When choosing outpatient treatment:

- Repeat bimanual exam must be done within 72 hours of initiating therapy.
- Patient must be compliant with medications and follow-up.
- The patient should be given a full course of doxycycline (or other oral medications) and tolerate the first dose under supervision.
- All patients with PID should receive intensive education about STI prevention.

DRUGS

Inpatient Management

- CDC regimen A:

—Cefotetan 2 g IV every 12 hours or cefoxitin 2 g IV every 6 hours
—Plus, doxycycline 100 mg PO twice a day for 14 days.

- Regimen B:

—Clindamycin 900 mg IV every 8 hours
—Plus, gentamicin loading dose 2 mg/kg IV or IM, followed by maintenance dose 1.5 mg/kg every 8 hours

- Alternative parenteral regimens include:

—Ofloxacin 400 mg IV every 12 hours or Levofloxacin 500 mg IV once daily
—With or without metronidazole 500 mg IV every 8 hours, or ampicillin/sulbactam 3 g IV every 6 hours
—Plus doxycycline 100 mg IV or PO every 12 hours, or
—The choice between parenteral regimens A or B is based on availability and the drug allergy history of the patient. Data to support the use of alternative regimens are limited.

- Regimen A should be continued for at least 48 hours after clinical improvement, and is followed by the completion of a 14-day course of doxycycline 100 mg PO twice a day.
- Regimen B should be continued for at least 24 hours after clinical improvement, and is followed by completion of a 14-day course of either doxycycline or clindamycin 450 mg PO twice a day.

Outpatient Management

- Regimen A

—Ofloxacin 400 mg PO twice a day for 14 days or Levofloxacin 500 mg orally once daily for 14 days; approved for ages >16 years
—With or without metronidazole 500 mg PO twice a day for 14 days

- Regimen B

—Ceftriaxone 250 mg IM once or cefoxitin 2 g IM with probenecid 1 g PO once or other parenteral third-generation cephalosporin
—Plus doxycycline 100 mg PO twice a day for 14 days
—With or without metronidazole 500 mg PO twice a day for 14 days

- The choice between oral regimens is based on availability, cost, and patient history of drug allergy.

 Follow-Up

- For inpatients, substantial clinical improvement should occur within 3 to 5 days if the patient has been properly diagnosed and treated.
- Outpatients should have significant improvement after 48 to 72 hours of treatment.
- Test of cure examination and laboratory testing should be done for all patients 6 to 8 weeks after diagnosis.

PREVENTION

- Primary prevention involves early education and aggressive screening for STIs.
- Abstinence and barrier contraceptive use should be advocated and facilitated.
- Screening and treatment of sexual partners should be encouraged and facilitated.

PITFALLS

- Doxycycline lowers the efficacy of oral contraceptives.
- Most bacteriologic studies are technique-dependent, and require trained clinicians.
- All home pregnancy tests should be repeated.
- Pelvic ultrasound requires a full urinary bladder, unlike transvaginal ultrasound.
- Overzealous education concerning possible sequelae or future infertility may lead to the patient "testing" fertility in the future.

Common Questions and Answers

Q: A patient states she is not sexually active. Should I continue to consider PID?
A: Yes. Because of the risk and severity of sequelae, PID should always be considered. Continue considering alternative diagnoses.

Q: A patient does not meet the criteria for PID; however, it is still the most likely diagnosis. Should I start therapy even though other studies are pending?
A: Yes, appropriate therapy for PID may be initiated even though other workups are in progress. Delay in therapy results in increased risk of sequelae from PID. When considering other diagnoses, the most life-threatening processes, including ectopic pregnancy, septic abortion, and appendicitis, should be considered first. Always consider ovarian torsion high among the differential diagnoses because it must be corrected in a timely fashion to maintain ovarian function.

Q: An adolescent patient with PID has inquired about fertility. What should I tell her?
A: Many clinicians would argue that an episode of PID could serve as a "wake-up" call to teenagers, inspiring them to abstain or comply with barrier contraception. However, a young woman who is told that she may have impaired fertility might try testing it through unprotected sex.

Q: Does the absence of cervical motion tenderness exclude the diagnosis of PID?
A: No, cervical motion tenderness is one of three major diagnostic criteria that are recommended by the CDC. The presence of all three major, or two major and two minor, criteria is needed to make the clinical diagnosis of PID. If adnexal and abdominal tenderness are present along with two of the minor criteria described above, then the absence of cervical motion tenderness does not exclude the diagnosis of PID.

ICD-9-CM 614.9

BIBLIOGRAPHY

Centers for Disease Control and Prevention. 2002 sexually transmitted disease treatment guidelines [serial online]. MMWR 2002; 51(RR-6). Available from http://www.cdc.gov/std/treatment. Accessed March 15, 2005.

Hollier LM, Workowski K. Treatment of sexually transmitted diseases in women. *Obstet Gynecol Clin North Am* 2003;30(4):751–775, vii–viii.

Pletcher JR, Slap GB. Pelvic inflammatory disease. In: Neinstein LS, ed. *Adolescent Health Care: A Practical Guide*. 4th Ed. Baltimore: Lippincott Williams & Wilkins, 2002.

Author: Jonathan R. Pletcher

Penile and Foreskin Problems

 Database

DEFINITION

Complaints relating to problems with retracting the foreskin, discharge from the foreskin, and problems relating to circumcision. These are common causes for concern in male infants. The most common diagnoses are listed below.

- Phimosis—two types:

—Physiologic attachment of the prepuce to the glans, which it protects and gradually separates from as desquamated cells (smegma) accumulate and separate the two layers.
—Ring of fibrotic scar tissue that prevents the foreskin, which has already separated from the glans, from being retracted.

- This probably results from recurrent bouts of irritation of the foreskin from improper hygiene habits such as voiding through the foreskin.
- It is important that all parents of uncircumcised boys teach them proper hygiene habits during potty training.
- Penile adhesions—Attachments of the foreskin back to the glans after circumcision.

—Physiologic adhesions, in which the prepuce has stuck back down onto the glans after it was separated during the circumcision
—Surgical adhesions, between the raw surface in which the foreskin was removed (the junction between the inner preputial skin and the skin of the penis) and the glans.
  —Sometimes referred to as skin bridges

- Meatal stenosis—narrowing of the urethral meatus as a result of recurrent irritation of the meatus, likely from rubbing against moist diapers. Occurs almost exclusively in circumcised boys. Significant narrowing will produce an upwardly deflected stream, which is tiny and strong. In severe cases straining and prolonged voiding.
- Epidermal inclusion cysts—small, enlarging white bumps occurring at the scar from circumcision. These are caused by small islands of epithelium buried beneath the skin surface that progressively accumulate desquamated skin cells. These may also occur from congenital rests of skin cells buried during development but these are rare and occur along the median raphae of the penis.
- Balanitis—infection of the glans. May also involve the prepuce (balanoposthitis).

—Probably overdiagnosed as a result of physiologic drainage of smegma or urea dermatitis from failure to retract foreskin during voiding in potty trained boys.
—When infections do present, there can be significant cellulitis of the penis and fever.
—Most common causative organisms are gram-positive. Yeast is another causative organism.

 Data Gathering

HISTORY

- Problems associated with newborn circumcision, when the changes occurred, character of urinary stream, presence of fever, or discharge in cases of balanitis. Retraction of foreskin in uncircumcised males during voiding. Ballooning of the foreskin with voiding.
- In older boys inquire about sexual activity or masturbation.

 Physical Examination

- Circumcised males—size and position of meatus, redundancy of inner preputial skin, presence of adhesions to the glans, and whether or not they involve the scar line between the shaft skin and the inner preputial skin. Lesions or erythema of glans or shaft. Watch patient void if meatal stenosis is suspected.
- Uncircumcised males—ability to retract foreskin with gentle retraction, presence of phimotic ring. Lesions or erythema of prepuce. Do not try to forcefully retract the foreskin. It can take 8 to 10 years before the foreskin is able to be retracted.

 Laboratory Aids

In cases of balanitis with drainage, cultures may be taken. If urethral discharge is present, culture for gonorrhea and chlamydia.

 Therapy

- Phimosis

—Physiologic—no need for intervention. Good hygiene practices should be encouraged such as pulling the foreskin back to expose the meatus when voiding and not voiding through the foreskin. Pamphlets that explain the care of the penis for uncircumcised males are helpful to give to the parents.
—Fibrotic ring—If there is a fibrotic ring of scar tissue preventing the retraction of the foreskin, a trial of betamethasone cream 0.05% applied to the foreskin b.i.d. for 4 weeks with daily gentle retraction may soften the scar tissue enough to resolve the phimosis. In cases in which conservative measures fail, a circumcision is indicated.

- Penile adhesions:

—Physiologic—Practices in the past have included separation using eutectic mixture of local anesthetics (EMLA) cream.
  —If there is redundancy of the foreskin or a prominent suprapubic fat pad that can tend to hide the penis in infants, adhesions often recur or require constant application of barrier creams or ointments to the penis and manual retraction of the redundant foreskin by the parents to prevent recurrence.
  —In many cases no treatment is necessary, as the adhesions will break down with time over a period of years.
  —If there are extensive adhesions with significant redundancy of foreskin, then consideration should be given to revision of the circumcision if the adhesions are to be treated.
—Surgical—These adhesions or skin bridges are a result of scar tissue formation between the raw cut edges in which the foreskin was removed to the raw surface of the glans.
  —As this represents true scarring and not two epithelial surfaces stuck together, the surfaces cannot be simply pulled apart like physiologic adhesions.
  —They will not resolve with time, and if left in place, with growth, penile skin will be transferred to the glans, resulting in discoloration, especially in patients with darker skin tones.
  —These adhesions need sharp division either in the office with EMLA cream anesthesia or under general anesthesia if they are extensive.

- Meatal stenosis—When the narrowing at the meatus is producing an upwardly deflected, narrow stream (which can make aiming into the toilet tricky) or is causing straining and prolonged voiding, treatment is indicated.
  —A meatotomy can be done in the office using EMLA anesthesia or as an outpatient surgical procedure.

- Epidermal inclusion cysts—These subcutaneous islands of skin cells will progressively enlarge over time. Complete excision under general anesthesia is nearly always curative.
- Balanitis—When the inflammation and irritation seem to be from chronic dampness and exposure to urine, treat with barrier creams or ointments.

—Keeping the area clean and dry will help prevent future episodes.

—If there are small whitish plaques (not smegma), associate with redness, yeast may be present and an antifungal cream such a 1% clotrimazole can be used to help speed the healing.

—In cases in which there is purulent drainage and cellulitis of the penis, which can often be rapidly spreading over 24 hours, treatment with antibiotics is recommended.

—If the child is afebrile, oral antibiotics such as a first-generation cephalosporin would be the first line of treatment.

—If the child develops fever or there is progression of cellulitis despite 24 to 48 hours of antibiotics, then admission and treatment with intravenous antibiotics (ampicillin/sulbactam is a good choice) should be considered.

—Genital infections of this nature should be taken quite seriously, and if treatment as an outpatient is attempted, close follow-up (return visit in 24 to 48 hours) is prudent.

 ## Common Questions and Answers

Q: The foreskin stuck back down to my son's penis. Does that mean he needs another circumcision?
A: Not necessarily. If there is minor redundancy and a small physiologic adhesion, then no treatment at all may be needed.

Q: My uncircumcised son had some thick white drainage from his foreskin. Is that from an infection?
A: Probably not. The thick white material is probably shed skin cells, which have been slowly separating the foreskin from the glans.

BIBLIOGRAPHY

Bartholomew TH, McIver B. Other disorders of the penis and scrotum. In: Gonzales ET, Bauer SB, eds. *Pediatric Urology Practice*. Baltimore: Lippincott Williams & Wilkins, 1999:533–546.

Elder JS. Congenital anomalies of the genitalia. In: Walsh PC, Retik AB, Vaughan ED, et al., eds. *Campbell's Urology*. Philadelphia: WB Saunders, 1998:2120–2143.

Orsola A, Caffaratti J, Garat JM. Conservative treatment of phimosis in children using a topical steroid. *Urology* 2000;56:307–310.

Authors: J. Christopher Austin and Stephen A. Zderic

Pericarditis

 Database

DEFINITION

Inflammation of the pericardium, usually resulting in the accumulation of fluid in the pericardial space between the visceral (intimately related to the myocardium) and parietal (several layers of elastic fibers and collagen) pericardium; may be serous, fibrinous, purulent, hemorrhagic, or chylous.

CAUSES

- Infectious: viral (coxsackie, echo, mumps, varicella, Epstein-Barr, adenovirus, influenza, human immunodeficiency virus), bacterial (streptococcus, pneumococcus, staphylococcus, meningococcus, mycoplasma, tularemia, *Haemophilus influenzae* type B, *Pseudomonas aeruginosa*, *Listeria monocytogenes*, *Pasteurella multocida*, *Escherichia coli*), tuberculosis, fungal (candidiasis, histoplasmosis, actinomycosis), parasitic (toxoplasmosis, echinococcus, *Entamoeba histolytica*, rickettsia)
- Rheumatologic/inflammatory: acute rheumatic fever, rheumatoid arthritis, systemic lupus erythematosus, systemic sclerosis, sarcoidosis, Kawasaki disease and familial Mediterranean fever
- Metabolic/endocrine: hypothyroidism, uremia (chemical irritation)
- Neoplastic disease: lymphoma, lymphosarcoma, leukemia, metastatic disease to the pericardium, radiation therapy induced
- Postoperative: postpericardiotomy syndrome (after cardiac surgery), chylopericardium
- Other: trauma, drug-induced (hydralazine, isoniazid, procainamide), aortic dissection, idiopathic

PATHOPHYSIOLOGY

Fine deposits of fibrin develop next to the great vessels and this leads to altered function of the membranes of the pericardium, including changes in oncotic and hydrostatic pressure with subsequent accumulation of fluid in the pericardial space. In postpericardiotomy syndrome, there appears to be a nonspecific hypersensitivity reaction to the direct entrance into the pericardial space.

EPIDEMIOLOGY

- Infectious pericarditis is more frequently seen in children younger than 13 years, with predominance in children younger than 2 years.
- Can occur in any age group.
- Overall incidence is slightly higher in males. Postpericardiotomy syndrome occurs in approximately 5% to 10% of children after uncomplicated cardiac surgery, particularly when the atrium has been entered.

COMPLICATIONS

- Cardiac tamponade: Intrapericardial pressure rises at a rapid rate secondary to decreased compliance of the pericardial membranes, resulting in restriction of ventricular filling and eventual decrease in stroke volume and cardiac output.

—The compliance of the pericardium is influenced by the disease process itself, i.e., the pericardium is thickened and stiff in bacterial and tuberculous pericarditis.
—During cardiac tamponade, ventricular end-diastolic, atrial, and venous pressures are all equal.
—In acute pericarditis, tamponade may occur with small amounts of fluid because of a rapid increase in the intrapericardial pressure.
—In contrast, large amounts of fluid may be tolerated if the accumulation is a chronic, slow process.

- Constrictive pericarditis: Thick, fibrotic and often calcified pericardium is seen, usually a late result of purulent or tuberculous pericarditis; it can occur months to years after the initial infection.

—It can also be seen in oncology patients with direct invasion of tumor into the pericardium or after significant radiation to the chest.
—Poor compliance of the pericardium leads to diminished diastolic filling of the ventricle.
—Patients may complain of exercise intolerance and fatigue.
—Additionally they may have signs of right heart failure. This entity may be difficult to distinguish from restrictive cardiomyopathy.

PROGNOSIS

Most children recover fully from pericarditis, even if it is bacterial in etiology. However, there is significant morbidity and mortality associated, especially in young infants, when the diagnosis is delayed and/or when *S. aureus* is the etiologic agent. Pericarditis can also recur in as many as 15% of patients. The prognosis varies with the other causes of pericarditis, but generally is directly related to the primary disease.

 Differential Diagnosis

- Acute myocarditis
- Restrictive cardiomyopathy
- Other nonspecific causes of chest pain

 Data Gathering

HISTORY

Question: Fever, cough, precordial chest pain, and shoulder pain (which is aggravated by changes in position)?
Significance: Most common symptoms.

Question: Respiratory distress?
Significance: Seen if there is rapid accumulation of fluid.

Question: Pain?
Significance: Often relieved if the child sits leaning forward.

Question: No symptoms?
Significance: Slow, chronic accumulation may be associated with no symptoms at all. Other symptoms are dependent on the etiology of the pericarditis.

Question: Recent upper respiratory infection or gastroenteritis?
Significance: With viral pericarditis, there may be a preceding history of a recent upper respiratory infection or gastroenteritis.

 Physical Examination

Finding: Pericardial friction rub is the pathognomonic finding
Significance: It may be heard if only a small amount of fluid is in the pericardial space.

Finding: Quiet precordium, tachycardia, and muffled heart sounds
Significance: May be heard when there is a large amount of fluid and/or tamponade

Finding: Right-sided heart failure
Significance: Tamponade, including peripheral edema, jugular venous distension, and hepatomegaly

Finding: Pulmonary edema
Significance: Rare because the heart is underfilled, and left atrial pressure, though elevated, does not exceed right atrial pressure

Finding: Pulsus paradoxus
Significance: An exaggerated decrease in systolic blood pressure with inspiration

Finding: Kussmaul sign
Significance: Paradoxical rise in jugular venous pressure during inspiration, often considered diagnostic of tamponade

Pericarditis

Laboratory Aids

Test: Chest roentgenogram
Significance: Often shows enlargement of the cardiac silhouette ("water bottle"), usually in association with normal pulmonary vascular markings. However, heart size may appear normal in acute pericarditis. Calcification may be seen in constrictive pericarditis.

Test: Echocardiography
Significance: Most sensitive and specific test for pericardial thickening and fluid in the pericardial space. In the presence of a large effusion, the heart may appear to swing within the pericardial cavity. In tamponade, diastolic collapse of the right atrium and right ventricle may be seen as well.

Test: Electrocardiogram
Significance: Nonspecific, but generally demonstrates low-voltage QRS complexes secondary to dampening of the signal transmitted through the pericardial fluid. One can also see diffuse ST segment elevation with or without T wave inversion. These findings may be secondary to inflammation of the myocardium. Electrical alternans can be seen with large effusions.

Test: Pericardiocentesis
Significance: Fluid obtained should be sent to the lab for cell count, cytology, and culture (including bacteria, viruses, *Mycobacterium tuberculosis*, and fungi).

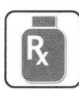

Therapy

• Treatment should be directed toward the etiology of the disease.
• However, no matter the cause, pericardiocentesis is required if there is an effusion that causes hemodynamic compromise. It may be lifesaving in patients with bacterial pericarditis.
• Pericardiocentesis may also be indicated for diagnostic purposes when the etiology of the effusion is in question.
• Complications of pericardiocentesis include myocardial puncture, coronary artery/vein laceration, hemopericardium, and pneumothorax.
• Echocardiographic or fluoroscopic guidance is useful for this procedure, but is not required if there is impending cardiovascular collapse.

THERAPY BY DIAGNOSIS

• Viral pericarditis usually resolves spontaneously in 3 to 4 weeks with bed rest and analgesics.
• Bacterial pericarditis is potentially life-threatening and requires immediate decompression of the pericardial space (often with open drainage and pericardial window creation), intravenous antibiotic therapy for at least 4 weeks, and supportive therapy i.e., volume expansion, inotropes. *S. aureus* is the

most common organism responsible for bacterial pericarditis.
• Rheumatologic causes of pericardial inflammation usually respond to corticosteroids and/or salicylates and rarely require pericardiocentesis.
• Uremic pericarditis usually responds to dialysis but pericardiotomy (surgical removal of the pericardium) may be necessary in chronic situations.
• Neoplastic pericarditis is addressed by treating the primary disease and performing pericardiocentesis if indicated for diagnostic and/or hemodynamic reasons.
• Hemorrhagic pericarditis with effusion accumulation secondary to trauma should be drained because of the risk for developing constrictive pericarditis.
• Constrictive pericarditis is treated with complete stripping of the pericardium (pericardiectomy). Often, immediate clinical improvement is not seen because there has been myocardial damage. However, eventual full recovery is the norm.
• Postpericardiotomy syndrome occurs 1 to 4 weeks after cardiac surgery and is usually treated with antiinflammatory drugs, bed rest, and occasionally steroids. Pericardiocentesis is indicated if tamponade develops.

Follow-Up

WHEN TO EXPECT IMPROVEMENT

Most forms of pericarditis resolve on their own, or with antiinflammatory medication, over the course of several weeks. Follow-up is necessary to be sure that effusions have resolved and to assess for recurrence (up to 15% relapse). Patients with bacterial pericarditis require long-term therapy and close follow-up to assess for the development of constrictive pericarditis.

SIGNS TO WATCH FOR

All cardiac surgical patients need an evaluation 2 to 4 weeks after surgery to assess for postpericardiotomy syndrome, with treatment and follow-up as necessary. Signs of low cardiac output and right heart failure indicate impending cardiac tamponade. Constrictive pericarditis may present with a rapidly decreasing cardiac silhouette, calcifications on chest roentgenogram, and signs or symptoms of right heart failure.

PREVENTION

Viral and rheumatologic pericarditis cannot be prevented. The incidence of bacterial pericarditis has decreased with immunization for bacterial infections, such as *H. influenzae* type B.

PITFALLS

The history, physical examination, and laboratory findings of acute pericarditis can be quite similar to those found in acute myocarditis. In addition, myocarditis can be

associated with pericardial disease and vice versa. Echocardiography is an excellent tool to help differentiate between these two entities.

Common Questions and Answers

Q: How does cardiac tamponade present?
A: Patients with impending tamponade appear quite ill with tachycardia, chest pain, and signs of right heart failure including jugular venous distension, hepatomegaly, ascites, and peripheral edema. They may also have signs of poor systemic perfusion secondary to low cardiac output. The chest radiograph may or may not show an enlarged cardiac silhouette, depending on how acutely the process occurs. It takes much less fluid to cause tamponade in an acute process than in a chronic process. Echocardiography is the standard diagnostic tool and pericardiocentesis is the treatment.

Q: What is pulsus paradoxus and how does one measure it?
A: Pulsus paradoxus is an exaggerated response of the systolic blood pressure to the normal respiratory cycle. Normally with inspiration, the systolic blood pressure drops approximately 5 mmHg secondary to the increased capacitance of the pulmonary veins from the increased systemic venous return. In tamponade, this response becomes more profound (>10 mmHg), most likely secondary to diminished filling of the left heart. Pulsus paradoxus can also be seen in patients with severe respiratory distress, such as in asthma and emphysema.

To assess for pulsus paradoxus, measure the systolic blood pressure first in expiration; then allow it to fall to the place in which it is heard equally well in inspiration and expiration. A difference of greater than 10 mmHg is considered abnormal.

ICD-9-CM 420.91, 420.90, 423.20

BIBLIOGRAPHY

Dupuis C, Gonnier P, Kachaner J, et al. Bacterial pericarditis in infancy and childhood. *Am J Cardiol* 1994;74:807–809.

Fyler DC. Pericardial disease. In: Fyler DC, eds. *Nadas' Pediatric Cardiology*. Philadelphia: Hanley and Belfus, 1992:S1590–S1599.

Golinko RJ, Kaplan N, Rudolph AM. The mechanism of pulsus paradoxus during acute pericardial tamponade. *J Clin Invest* 1963;42:249–257.

Goyle KK, Walling AD. Diagnosing pericarditis. *Am Fam Physician* 2002;66(9):1695–1702.

Rheuban KS. Pericardial diseases. In: Allen HD, Gutgesell HP, Clark EB, Driscoll DJ, eds. *Heart Disease in Infants, Children, and Adolescents: Including the Fetus and Young Adult*. 6th Ed. Baltimore: Lippincott, Williams & Wilkins, 2001.

Author: Meryl S. Cohen

Periodic Breathing

 Database

DEFINITION

Periodic breathing is a respiratory pattern in which three or more apneas lasting 3 or more seconds in duration occur separated by less than 20 seconds of respiration

CAUSES

• Periodic breathing can be seen in healthy infants, children, and adults.
• Periodic breathing in infants is associated with:

—Apnea of prematurity or infancy
—Familial history of sudden infant death syndrome (SIDS)
—Anemia of prematurity
—Hypoxemia
—Hypochloremic alkalosis

• Periodic breathing with adults is associated with:

—Cardiac abnormalities (congestive heart failure)
—Neurologic dysfunction (meningitis, encephalitis, brainstem dysfunction)
—Also referred to as Cheyne-Stokes respiration

• Abnormalities in any component of the breathing control system may result in an increased amount of periodic breathing
• Possible etiologies for periodic breathing include:

—A delay in detecting changes in blood gas values by the chemoreceptors
—Increased chemoreceptor gain

PATHOLOGY

• There is no common pathologic finding
• Abnormalities, when they exist, are related to the underlying disorder causing the periodic breathing

EPIDEMIOLOGY

• Usually absent in the first 48 hours of life
• More frequent during REM (active) sleep versus non-REM (quiet) sleep
• Less common in prone versus supine position
• In full-term infants:

—Amount of periodic breathing usually, <4% of their sleep time
—Amount gradually decreasing through the first year of life
—By 1 year of age, the mean amount of periodic breathing is <1% of total sleep time.

• In premature infants:

—Amount of periodic breathing higher than in full-term infants
—Amount correlates inversely with the gestational age

• Incidence among healthy children and adults is unknown.

COMPLICATIONS

Relationship between periodic breathing and SIDS is controversial.

PROGNOSIS

• In otherwise normal premature or term infants: excellent
• With an underlying cardiac or neurological disorder, the prognosis is governed by this primary process

 Differential Diagnosis

• Other forms of apnea:

—Central apnea
—Obstructive apnea

• Other forms of periodic breathing:

—Cheyne-Stokes respiration
—Biot breathing
—Kussmaul respiration

• Normal irregular respiration seen in infants

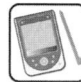 Data Gathering

HISTORY

• In most cases, parents notice periodicity in the respiration of the child.
• An apparent life-threatening episode (ALTE) might precipitate an evaluation on which periodic breathing is thereafter documented.
• In otherwise healthy premature or term infants, there are no other symptoms.

 Physical Examination

In otherwise healthy premature or term infants, the physical examination is normal.

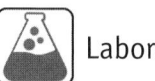 Laboratory Aids

TESTS

Polysomnography

• Assesses the extent of periodic breathing episodes
• Determines if there is accompanying hypoxemia, hypercarbia, or bradycardia with events
• Distinguishes between periodic breathing and obstructive and/or central apnea
• Useful for following response to treatment (normalization of polysomnogram)
• Variables to be monitored include:

—EEG, EOG, and EMG (for sleep state determination)
—O_2 saturation
—End-tidal CO_2 tension
—Respiratory movements (abdomen, chest)
—Airflow

• pH probe (if gastroesophageal reflux is suspected) record for a minimum of 6 hours

• Two-Channel Pneumogram

—Gives less information than polysomnography
—Can document periodic breathing, but may miss episodes of obstructive apnea
—Variables to be monitored include:

—Heart rate
—Respiratory effort
—O_2 saturation

IMAGING

• Chest radiograph

—Usually normal

Periodic Breathing

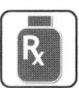 Therapy

- Therapy should be directed to treating any underlying primary disease.
- If periodic breathing is associated with apnea, hypoxemia, and/or other sleep disturbances, appropriate treatment should be instituted.

DRUGS

Stimulants

- Caffeine

—Loading dose: 10 mg/kg
—Maintenance dose: 2.5 mg/kg daily
—Therapeutic level: 5 to 20 mg/L

- Theophylline

—Loading dose: 4 to 5 mg/kg
—Maintenance dose: 3 to 5 mg/kg per day divided t.i.d.
—Therapeutic level: 6 to 10 mg/L

- Supplemental oxygen

—Useful if periodic breathing is secondary to hypoxemia

- Nasal CPAP

—Very effective in eliminating periodic breathing

- Home monitoring

—Indicated when:
    —The amount of periodic breathing is significant.
    —There is accompanying apnea.
    —There is associated hypoxia and/or bradycardia.

DURATION

- Dependent on the underlying cause of the periodic breathing
- Treatment does not change the natural course of periodic breathing in otherwise healthy infants.
- Therapy should continue until the periodic breathing resolves or is no longer clinically significant.

 Follow-Up

WHEN TO EXPECT IMPROVEMENT

- Dependent on the underlying cause of the periodic breathing
- Improvement is anticipated as the infant ages.
- When treatment is started, a decrease in the amount of periodic breathing should be seen almost immediately.

PITFALLS

Confusing periodic breathing with obstructive or central apnea

 Common Question and Answer

Q: What is the risk of the patient dying of SIDS?
A: The relationship between periodic breathing and SIDS is not clear, although most studies have not found a higher frequency of SIDS among patients with periodic breathing.

ICD-9-CM 786-09

BIBLIOGRAPHY

Glotzbach SF, Ariagno RL. *Respiratory Control Disorders in Infants and Children* Baltimore: Williams & Wilkins, 1992:142–160.

Horemuzova E, Katz-Salamon M, Milerad J. Breathing patterns, oxygen and carbon dioxide levels in sleeping healthy infants during the first nine months after birth. *Acta Paediatr* 2000;89:1284–1289.

Hunt CE, Corwin MJ, Lister G, et al. Longitudinal assessment of hemoglobin oxygen saturation in healthy infants during the first six months of age. *J Pediatr* 1999;134:580–586.

Schechter MS, and the Section on Pediatric Pulmonology, Subcommittee on Obstructive Sleep Apnea Syndrome. Technical report: diagnosis and management of childhood obstructive sleep apnea syndrome. *Pediatrics* 2002;109(4):e69.

Shannon DC, Carley DW, Kelly DH. Periodic breathing: quantitative analyses and clinical description. *Pediatr Pulmonol* 1986;4:98–102.

Sterni LM. Tunkel DE. Obstructive sleep apnea in children: an update. *Pediatr Clin N Am* 2003;50(2):427–443.

Author: Richard M. Kravitz

Periorbital Cellulitis

 Database

DEFINITION

Periorbital cellulitis is an acute infection of the superficial skin and subcutaneous tissues of the eyelids. It is also known as preseptal cellulitis because the inflammation is localized in the tissues anterior to the orbital septum. Thus the eyeball and orbital structures are not involved.

PATHOPHYSIOLOGY

• Preseptal cellulitis is an infection caused by a variety of bacteria. The most common pathogens are *Staphylococcus aureus*, *Streptococcus pneumoniae*, *S. epidermis*, and *Haemophilus influenzae*.
• Predisposing factors that may lead to infection include skin trauma, insect bites, and upper respiratory infections with paranasal sinusitis.

EPIDEMIOLOGY

This infection usually occurs in young children, commonly under the age of 5.

COMPLICATIONS

Orbital extension (2.5% to 17%), skin abscess (8%), eyelid necrosis (1% to 2%), sepsis, intracranial extension (2% to 3%)

PROGNOSIS

Excellent with minimal incidence of long-term sequelae unless a complication is encountered

 Differential Diagnosis

• Infectious

—Early orbital cellulitis
—Dacryocystitis
—Stye
—Severe viral conjunctivitis

• Allergic

—Periocular allergic reaction
—Insect bite
—Angioneurotic edema

• Other

—Periocular trauma
—Rhabdomyosarcoma
—Idiopathic orbital inflammatory syndrome (IOIS)

 Data Gathering

• It is important to inquire about the history of onset, time course of symptom progression, and any predisposing factors.
• Any history of trauma or underlying respiratory infection may be helpful, although these types of questions have a low yield.
• The presence of pain would support cellulitis, although complaints of itching are more suggestive of an allergy.
• Quantify systemic symptoms such as fever and lethargy as these indicate a more severe, disseminated infection.

 Physical Examination

• The lids will be edematous, erythematous, warm to the touch, and typically tender on palpation. The findings can start in one eyelid but both the upper and lower eyelids are usually swollen.
• The globe should be carefully examined. In preseptal cellulitis, the ocular exam is normal. The eye is almost always white, although patients can have some conjunctival edema. Any change in vision or pupillary function, or limitations in eye motility suggest orbital involvement. Pediatric orbital cellulitis is an ophthalmologic emergency and requires prompt therapy.
• Many patients with preseptal cellulitis appear to have proptosis but actually do not. The presence of proptosis suggests deep orbital involvement.
• Finally, signs of fever, respiratory infection, and sepsis should be identified.

PHYSICAL EXAM TRICKS

Occasionally the eyelids are so swollen it is difficult to examine the globe. To do so, place anesthetic eyedrops on the eye and fashion a paperclip into a lid retractor to lift the eyelid.

 Laboratory Aids

• Lab tests are usually not helpful or indicated.
• CBC is warranted only if bacteremia is suspected.
• Skin cultures and blood cultures have a low yield. Blood cultures are only obtained when the child is febrile or appears septic.

IMAGING

• CT scanning is a helpful modality to appreciate sinus and orbital disease. It is important to obtain imaging studies if orbital cellulitis is suspected and especially, in cases that do not respond to medical treatment.
• Of note, imaging findings will lag behind clinical findings by several days. Thus serial CT scanning should only be done if the child is not improving with treatment.

Periorbital Cellulitis

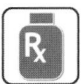 Therapy

GENERAL MANAGEMENT

• New antibiotics are constantly being introduced to replace older medications. Antibiotics that cover Staphylococcus, Streptococcus, and Haemophilus, such as second-generation cephalosporins or β-lactamase-resistant penicillins, should be started as soon as possible.
• Children under the age of 2 years should be hospitalized for intravenous therapy and very close observation.
• Children between the age of 2 and 5 should be watched closely. Mild cases may be managed on an outpatient visit.
• Children over the age of 5 years can usually be treated with an oral regimen as long as they do not appear toxic.

DRUGS

• In nontoxic children, oral antibiotics (Augmentin, cefaclor, Pediazole, etc.) are started on an outpatient basis and the child should be seen again in within 24 hours.
• Children who do not improve or deteriorate, and children who present with fever or septic symptoms, should be admitted for intravenous antibiotic (Unasyn, ceftriaxone, etc.). These children should be watched closely.

SURGERY

• Surgical intervention is usually required when an abscess or a foreign body is present.

 Follow-Up

WHEN TO EXPECT IMPROVEMENT

• Patients usually take 24 to 48 hours to respond to therapy.
• Patients should be seen daily until a definite improvement is noted.

SIGNS TO WATCH FOR

Watch patients closely for signs of orbital extension, bacteremia, or other forms of disseminated infection.

PITFALLS

• Neonates and infants can become septic very quickly, so they need to be closely monitored.
• Periorbital cellulitis may be a secondary extension of another process like sinusitis
• CT scans will lag behind clinical findings once treatment is started. In fact, a repeat scan 24 to 48 hours after starting antibiotics will usually look worse than the preantibiotic scan.

ICD-9-CM 376.01

BIBLIOGRAPHY

Donahue SP, Schwartz G. Preseptal and orbital cellulitis in childhood. A changing microbiologic spectrum. *Ophthalmology* 1998;105:1902–1905.

Foster JA, Katowitz JA. Pediatric orbital and periocular infections. In: Katowitz JA, eds. *Pediatric oculoplastic surgery*. Springer-Verlag, 2001.

Lessner A, Stern GA. Preseptal and orbital cellulitis. *Infect Dis Clin North Am* 1992;6:933–952.

Powell KR. Orbital and periorbital cellulitis. *Pediatr Rev* 1995;16:163–167.

Authors: Femida Kherani
Scott M. Goldstein, 3rd edition

Perirectal Abscess

Database

DEFINITION

Abscess in the perirectal area, which may extend into surrounding soft tissues

- Most common cause of anorectal suppuration
- May or may not be associated with a fistula
- Infection usually starts in one of the small anal glands leading to pus in the intersphincteric space.

CAUSES

- Nonspecific anal gland infection
- Crohn disease
- Perforation by a foreign body
- External trauma
- Tuberculosis
- Carcinoma
- Immune deficiency (e.g., AIDS, neutropenia, diabetes mellitus)

PATHOPHYSIOLOGY

- Majority of anal abscesses and fistulas originate from infected anal glands.
- Infection from the anal glands penetrate through the internal sphincter and end in the intersphincteric space.
- Abscess formation is the acute phase; fistula is the chronic phase.

EPIDEMIOLOGY

- Can occur in any age group but more common between the ages of 20 and 45 years.
- No racial predilection

COMPLICATIONS

- Fulminant sepsis
- Fistulas can occur if abscesses are not drained as soon as possible.

PROGNOSIS

Prognosis is good if there is early detection and drainage of abscesses.

Differential Diagnosis

- Pilonidal infection
- Hidradenitis suppurativa
- Crohn disease
- Gangrenous hemorrhoids
- Foreign body
- Tuberculosis

Data Gathering

HISTORY

- History of constipation?
- Fevers?
- Painful defecation?
- Refusing to walk?
- Rectal pain?
- Weight loss, diarrhea, abdominal pain, and poor growth are symptoms associated with Crohn disease.
- Foreign body?
- Trauma?

Physical Examination

The classic triad in patients with abscess are rubor, tumor and calor.
The various types of anorectal abscesses give rise to the following presentations:

Finding: Intersphincteric abscess
Significance: Is limited to the primary site in the intersphincteric space between the internal and external sphincters associated with throbbing pain on defecation and continues for hours thereafter; severe enough to prevent sleep. It often does not cause perianal skin changes.

Finding: Perianal abscess
Significance: Result of distal vertical spread of the infection to the anal margin. Presents as tender, red swelling; often misdiagnosed as an external anal thrombosis.

Finding: Intermuscular abscess/supralevator abscess
Significance: Results from two different sources. One source is a proximal vertical spread of infection from the gland through the intersphincteric space to the supralevator space. The other source is an abscess resulting from a pelvic pathology such as Crohn disease. Patients usually complain of vague pelvic discomfort, fever, and urinary retention; rectal exam usually reveals an indurated swelling above the anorectal ring.

Finding: Ischiorectal abscess
Significance: As a result of horizontal spread of infection across the external anal sphincter into the ischiorectal fossa. Sometimes infection may track across the internal anal sphincter into the anal canal. Patients may complain of pain and fever before a swelling is visible. Induration then occurs under the skin over the ischiorectal fossa and eventually a typical red fluctuant abscess is seen.

Finding: Circumferential spread
Significance: May occur from one side to the other in the intersphincteric space and can present with pain

Laboratory Aids

- CBC
- Culture
- CT scan

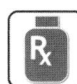 Therapy

- Abscesses should all be drained as soon as diagnosed. Lack of fluctuation should not delay treatment. Whether a fistulotomy or fistulectomy should be performed for an accompanying fistula is still a matter of debate.
- Pus should be sent for culture, and use of antibiotics is usually reserved for an infection that does not respond to drainage or if gut organisms are present. The most common organism is *Escherichia coli*.
- At times, a repeat exploration of the abscess/fistula under general anesthesia may be performed to drain residual abscess.
- Sitz baths may be helpful postprocedure.

 Follow-Up

EXPECTED COURSE OF ILLNESS

- Patients usually recover well after surgical drainage of abscess.
- Fistulae may occur after aspiration of abscess.
- Additional follow-up to determine the cause of the abscess formation is crucial in attempting to prevent recurrence.

 Common Questions and Answers

Q: What are complications of this problem?
A: Fistula formation is seen in up to 25% of patients with a predilection for males.

Q: What are the most common organisms of the abscess?
A: *Staphylococcus* species.

Q: What other disease may my child have if he has perirectal abscess?
A: Crohn disease must be excluded. If there is exposure to tuberculosis, this also must be excluded.

Q: Will the abscess recur after surgery?
A: Yes, if the disease process is secondary to a chronic disease-like inflammatory bowel disease.

Q: What treatments can be done other than surgery?
A: Antibiotics, sitz baths, and warm compresses can give symptomatic improvement.

ICD-9-CM 566

BIBLIOGRAPHY

al-Salem AH, Qaisaruddin S, Qureshi SS. Perianal abscess and fistula in ano in infancy and childhood: a clinicopathological study. *Pediatr Pathol Lab Med* 1996;16(5):755–764.

Festen C, van Harten H. Perianal abscess and fistula-in-ano in infants. *J Pediatr Surg* 1998; 33(5):711–713.

Rosen NG, Gibbs DL, Soffer SZ, et al. The nonoperative treatment of fistula in ano. *J Pediatr Surg* 2000;35:938–939.

Authors: Helen Anita John-Kelly and Andrew E. Mulberg

Peritonitis

Database

DEFINITION

Peritonitis is defined as inflammation of the peritoneal cavity. This inflammation may be categorized as spontaneous bacterial peritonitis (no intraabdominal source of infection) or secondary bacterial peritonitis (intraabdominal source of infection present).

PATHOPHYSIOLOGY

Spontaneous bacterial peritonitis (SBP) occurs when pathogenic bacteria are cultured from peritoneal fluid but no intraabdominal surgical treatable source of infection is identified. Recognized as a complication in patients with ascites as a result of cirrhosis of any etiology.
There have also been isolated patients reported with noncirrhotic diseases associated with ascites:

- Budd-Chiari syndrome
- Congestive heart failure
- Nephrotic syndrome
- Systemic lupus erythematosus
- Rheumatoid arthritis

Secondary bacterial peritonitis results from any process leading to perforation of the gastrointestinal tract including:

- Necrotizing enterocolitis
- Volvulus with ischemia
- Intussusception with ischemia
- Trauma
- Perforation from duodenal/gastric ulcers and postoperative

Generalized bacteremia and translocation of organisms from the gut into the portal veins or lymphatics or, less likely, directly into the ascitic fluid may account for the source of the infection. Clearance of bacteria from the bloodstream may be impaired in patients with cirrhosis and ascites because of diminished phagocytic activity of the hepatic reticuloendothelial system (RES) secondary to cellular functional defects or shunting of blood away from the liver.
Complement, necessary for the opsonization of bacteria and ultimately clearance by phagocytes, is decreased in the ascitic fluid of patients with ascites.

EPIDEMIOLOGY

Infectious organisms include:

- Aerobic-gram negative organisms:
Escherichia coli (approximately 50%)
- Klebsiella (approximately 13%)
- Aerobic gram-positive organisms:

—Streptococcus (approximately 19%)
—Enterococcus (5%).
    —Anaerobes rarely cause SBP and polymicrobial infections occur in relatively few patients (approximately 8%).
    —Urine cultures have been found to be positive for the same organism in approximately 44% of patients.
    —Pneumonia and soft tissue infections have also been suggested as sources.

- In secondary bacterial peritonitis, the underlying bacterial infection tends to be a complex polymicrobial infection with an average of 2.9 to 3.9 different isolates, the most common isolates are combination of organisms is *E. coli* and *Bacteroides fragilis* and the most common gram-positive organism is nonenterococcal streptococci and enterococci.

Predisposing Factors to SBP

- Advanced liver disease or nephritic syndrome causing ascites
- Decreased RES activity
- Decreased serum complement levels
- Decreased ascitic protein and complement levels
- Presence of gastrointestinal hemorrhage

PROGNOSIS

- SBP is associated with a high mortality, with about 50% fatality rate during hospitalization. The combination of underlying disease and the infection causes acute decompensation in a marginally compensated host.
- Retrospective studies have indicated that SBP appears to be recurrent with 51% of patients who survive the first episode going on to develop one or more recurrences.

Data Gathering

HISTORY

Clinical features depend on the stage at which peritonitis is diagnosed.

- Fever, chills?
- Generalized abdominal pain with rebound tenderness?
- Decreased bowel sounds? In SBP, approximately 10% of cases are entirely asymptomatic.

Other less common findings include:

- Hypothermia
- Hypotension
- Diarrhea
- Increased ascites despite diuretics
- Worsening encephalopathy
- Unexplained decrease in renal function.

Physical Examination

- Painful palpation of abdomen
- Decreased bowel sounds
- Evidence of chronic liver disease
- Evidence of ascites

Laboratory Aids

- Diagnosis may be confirmed with paracentesis. To improve culture yield, culture bottles should be inoculated immediately at the bedside in large volume blood culture bottles. Elevated PMN count in ascitic fluid is important in the early diagnosis of SBP and is considered the most important laboratory indicator of SBP.
- Diagnostic criteria for SBP include:

—Polymorphonuclear leukocyte counts of greater than 250/mm^3
—Ascitic fluid culture usually for a single organism

- Diagnostic criteria for secondary bacterial peritonitis include:

—Ascitic fluid culture positive for polymicrobial infection
—Total protein greater than 1 g/dL
—Glucose less than 50 mg/dL
—LDH greater than 225 mU/mL

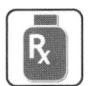

Therapy

- Support the patient's cardiovascular and respiratory systems.
- Control the underlying infection with antibiotics or surgery (in secondary bacterial peritonitis). Empirical antibiotic coverage should be directed primarily toward enteric gram-negative aerobes and gram-positive cocci.
- In SBP, cefotaxime, has been shown to have higher resolution of infection and lower hospital mortality than the traditional ampicillin and an aminoglycoside as empiric coverage.
- Once the organism is identified, the antibiotic coverage may be optimized.
- Patients at significant risk for SBP will benefit from selective intestinal decontamination as an effective preventive measure. Antibiotics that have been studied for this use in adults include: Norfloxacin, Ciprofloxacin and Trimethoprim-sulfamethoxazole

In SBP, surgery is the primary management tool with control of the source of the intraabdominal infection. No particular antibiotic regimen has been shown to be superior in controlled clinical trials. Both single agents and combination regimens have been used.

COMPLICATIONS

- Hypovolemia results from extravascular extravasation and sequestration from the inflamed peritoneal membrane. Intravascular volume must be supported with crystalloids and blood products.
- Respiration may be impaired via mechanical mechanisms through diaphragmatic spasm and reflex abdominal rigidity and through increased permeability of the pulmonary vasculature in response to systemic inflammation.
- Control of the underlying source of the abdominal infection by repairing the affected bowel through laparotomy/laparoscopy should be considered.

—The degree of contamination may be decreased through intra operative peritoneal lavage, and débridement of loculations and abscesses.
—Adding antibiotics to lavage fluid has lost favor after the discovery that this procedure appears to impair neutrophil chemotaxis, inhibit neutrophil bacteriocidal activity, and increases the formation of adhesions.
—Catheters may be placed to drain well-defined abscess cavity, form a controlled fistula, or provide access for continuous postoperative peritoneal lavage.

Common Questions and Answers

Q: Is peritonitis common in children with ascites?
A: Despite the frequency of ascites from many different causes, peritonitis occurs rarely. In the setting of children with chronic liver disease and ascites, spontaneous bacterial peritonitis may occur rarely.

Q: What are the most useful laboratory aids for this diagnosis?
A: Paracentesis and analysis of the fluid for pH, glucose content, and amount of inflammatory cells provides the most useful information regarding the diagnosis of peritonitis.

ICD-9-CM 567.9

BIBLIOGRAPHY

Farber MS, Abrams JH. Antibiotics for the acute abdomen. *Surg Clin North Am* 1997;77(6):1395–1417.

Gilbert J, Kamath P. Spontaneous bacterial peritonitis: an update. *Mayo Clin Proc* 1995;70:365–370.

Guarner C, Soriano G. Spontaneous bacterial peritonitis. *Semin Liver Dis* 1997;17(3): 203–217.

Nathans AB, Rotstein OD. Therapeutic options in peritonitis. *Surg Clin North Am* 1994;74(3):6577–6592.

Sabri M, Saps M, Peters JM. Pathophysiology and management of pediatric ascites. *Curr Gastroenterol Rep* 2003;5(3):240–246.

Schaefer F. Management of peritonitis in children receiving chronic peritoneal dialysis. *Paediatr Drugs* 2003;5(5):315–325.

Author: Dror Wasserman

Peritonsillar Abscess

 Database

DEFINITION

Infectious complication of tonsillitis or pharyngitis resulting in an accumulation of purulence in the tonsillar fossa. Also referred to as "quinsy."

CAUSE

- Group A β-hemolytic *Streptococcus* (GABHS)
- α-Hemolytic streptococci
- Miscellaneous anaerobic bacteria
- *Staphylococcus aureus*

PATHOPHYSIOLOGY

- Infectious tonsillopharyngitis progresses from cellulitis to abscess.
- Purulence collects within one, and sometimes both, tonsillar fossae.
- Tonsillar and peritonsillar edema may lead to compromise of the upper airway.

EPIDEMIOLOGY

Seen most commonly in adolescents, but occasionally in younger children.

ASSOCIATED ILLNESS

- Tonsillitis or pharyngitis usually precedes its development.
- Peritonsillar cellulitis is often associated with infectious mononucleosis.

COMPLICATIONS

- Upper airway obstruction is the most feared complication.
- Dehydration, from decreased oral intake, is the most common complication.

PROGNOSIS

- Complete swift recovery can be expected with appropriate therapy.
- Recurrence of peritonsillar abscesses are not uncommon.

 Differential Diagnosis

- Peritonsillar cellulitis: the most common diagnostic consideration; can be distinguished by its lack of peritonsillar space "fullness," uvular deviation, dysphonia, and trismus
- Retropharyngeal abscess: Minimal peritonsillar findings, along with a widened prevertebral space on lateral neck x-ray is diagnostic of this airway-compromising disease, which almost always occurs in preschool children.
- Epiglottitis: This life-threatening airway emergency presents abruptly with fever, stridor, increased work of breathing, and drooling; usually occurs in toxic-appearing children 3 to 7 years of age, but becoming a rare entity since the advent of the *Haemophilus influenzae* type B vaccine.
- Other infectious etiologies of severe tonsillopharyngitis: Epstein-Barr virus (infectious mononucleosis), coxsackievirus (herpangina), *Corynebacterium diphtheriae*, *Neisseria gonorrhoeae*

 Data Gathering

HISTORY

Question: Fever and sore throat?
Significance: Most common initial complaints

Question: Trouble swallowing, pain with opening the mouth (trismus), muffled ("hot-potato") voice?
Significance: Classic presenting symptoms

Question: Unilateral neck or ear pain?
Significance: Other common presenting symptoms

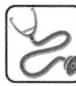 Physical Examination

Finding: Unilateral peritonsillar fullness, or bulging of the posterior, superior, soft palate
Significance: Diagnostic physical exam finding

Finding: Uvular deviation
Significance: Another classic physical exam finding

Finding: Palpable fluctuance of palatal swelling
Significance: Calls for urgent aspiration

Finding: Erythematous, edematous pharynx, with enlarged and exudative tonsils
Significance: Coexisting tonsillopharyngitis is common.

Finding: Cervical adenopathy
Significance: Common

Finding: Drooling
Significance: Often present

Finding: Torticollis
Significance: Sometimes seen

 Laboratory Aids

Test: White blood cell count
Significance: Usually elevated with prominent "left shift"

Test: Rapid streptococcal throat antigen studies
Significance: Helpful to diagnose GABHS infection

Test: Gram stain and culture of aspirate specimen
Significance: Confirms causative microorganism

Test: CT scan or ultrasound
Significance: Differentiation of peritonsillar cellulitis from peritonsillar abscess; radiographic studies, however, are rarely necessary.

Therapy

- True abscesses should be urgently/emergently drained via either needle aspiration or surgical incision and drainage.
- Antibiotic therapy can be initiated with high-dose intravenous penicillin.
- Clindamycin, nafcillin, oxacillin, cefazolin, and ampicillin/sulbactam, are acceptable, broader-spectrum alternatives.
- Surgical drainage with tonsillectomy should be considered in children not responding to parenteral antibiotics within 24 to 48 hours.
- Appropriate analgesia and adequate hydration should be ensured.

 ## Follow-Up

- Patients may be discharged on oral antibiotics to complete a 10- to 14-day course when afebrile and peritonsillar swelling has subsided.
- Tonsillectomy should be considered after severe or recurrent peritonsillar abscesses.

PREVENTION

Abscess formation can often be prevented if appropriate antimicrobial therapy is initiated when the infection is still at the cellulitis stage.

PITFALLS

Treating a true abscess without incision and drainage is inadequate, and can have airway-threatening implications.

 ## Common Questions and Answers

Q: Are radiographs necessary to make the diagnosis of peritonsillar abscess?
A: No. The physical examination is diagnostic; a lateral neck radiograph is useful only if retropharyngeal abscess or epiglottitis are diagnostic concerns.

Q: Is surgical consultation necessary in cases of peritonsillar abscess?
A: Yes. Otorhinolaryngology consultation is indicated for both acute as well as chronic management.

ICD-9-CM 475

BIBLIOGRAPHY

Blotter JW, Yin L, Glynn M, et al. Otolaryngology consultation for peritonsillar abscess in the pediatric population. *Laryngoscope* 2000;110:1698–1701.

Cherukuri S, Benninger MS. Use of bacteriologic studies in the outpatient management of peritonsillar abscess. *Laryngoscope* 2002;112(1):18–20.

Friedman NR, Mitchell RB, Pereira KD, et al. Peritonsillar abscess in early childhood. Presentation and management. *Arch Otolaryngol Head Neck Surg* 1997;123(6):630–632.

Herzon FS, Nicklaus P. Pediatric peritonsillar abscess: management guidelines. *Curr Probl Pediatr* 1996;26(8):270–278.

Johnson RF, Stewart MG, Wright CC. An evidence-based review of the treatment of peritonsillar abscess. *Otolaryngol Head Neck Surg* 2003;128(3):332–343.

Scott PMJ, Loftus WK, Kew J, et al. Diagnosis of peritonsillar infections: a prospective study of ultrasound, computerized tomography, and clinical diagnosis. *J Laryngol Otol* 1999;113:229–232.

Author: Nicholas Tsarouhas

Persistent Pulmonary Hypertension of the Newborn (PPHN)

Database

DEFINITION

• Clinical syndrome of severe respiratory failure and hypoxia in a neonate characterized by high systemic pulmonary arterial pressures, tricuspid regurgitation and intracardiac shunting from right to left through persistent fetal pathways, including a patent foramen ovale and ductus arteriosus.

CAUSES

• Idiopathic
• Secondary to underlying disease—infection, pneumonia, meconium aspiration, chronic intrauterine asphyxia, perinatal asphyxia, polycythemia
• Secondary to an anatomic abnormality—Congenital Diaphragmatic Hernia (CDH), pulmonary hypoplasia, alveolar capillary dysplasia

PATHOPHYSIOLOGY

• When a neonate takes his/her first breath after delivery, the pulmonary vascular resistance (PVR) normally decreases in order to redirect approximately half of the cardiac output to the pulmonary circulation. This normal decline in PVR does not occur in PPHN, hence its previous name of "persistent fetal circulation" or PFC.
• Increased PVR increases right ventricular afterload, causing a backflow of blood to the right heart (and subsequent tricuspid regurgitation) and increased right heart pressures, which can lead to right ventricular failure.
• Increased pulmonary arterial pressures also cause intracardiac shunting across any patent foramen ovale, ductus arteriosus, or atrioseptal or ventriculoseptal defect that may be present. Blood shunts from right to left as a result of the supranormal systemic pulmonary arterial pressures. This causes more deoxygenated blood to go to the left heart and then to the body, which manifests as lower oxygen saturation in the lower extremities (postductally) and hypoxia.
• Deoxygenated blood in the left heart can lead to ischemic damage to the heart and right or left ventricular failure.
• The cardiac and/or respiratory failure is occasionally severe enough to require extracorporeal membrane oxygenation (ECMO).
• If there is no shunting of blood, or the blood cannot get from the right to left heart because of a lack of persistent fetal pathways, a neonate may develop poor systemic perfusion, severe acidosis, shock, right ventricular failure, or even death.
• Any hypoxia, acidosis or stress that occurs after birth, further increases pulmonary vascular resistance.
• In most cases, the pulmonary vasculature begins to relax within 3 to 5 days of life and the process reverses. There is continued vascular remodeling over the first 2 weeks of life. In some instances, the pulmonary vascular resistance remains elevated as a result of an underlying disease process or anatomic abnormality.

GENETICS

• Sporadic in occurrence
• Alveolar capillary dysplasia has been documented in one set of siblings; however, it is also primarily sporadic.

EPIDEMIOLOGY

• Mostly occurs in full-term newborns as a result of the presence of the muscular layer of arterioles.
• Incidence of approximately 1 in 1,000 term newborns. There has been no noted decline in the incidence even with the decrease in the incidence of group B streptococcal (GBS) sepsis, a cause of PPHN.
• More common in postdate newborns as a result of the risk of uteroplacental insufficiency leading to hypoxic stress and the passage of meconium.

COMPLICATIONS

• Myocardial dysfunction
• Congestive heart failure
• Hypoxic ischemic insult

ASSOCIATED ILLNESSES

Related to the underlying disease or as a complication of treatment:

• Pneumothorax or air leak syndrome
• Chronic lung damage
• Long term developmental delays
• Cerebral palsy
• Seizure disorder
• Neurosensory hearing loss

PROGNOSIS

• PPHN usually either resolves spontaneously or as the underlying parenchymal lung disease improves.
• The survival rate is good even for those neonates who receive ECMO. The survival rate and incidence of long term sequelae depend on the underlying disease and severity of illness.
• The survival rate for all causes of PPHN in those not needing ECMO is about 90%. Approximately 10% to 20% of these babies have sensorineural hearing loss or an abnormal neurological exam at follow-up.
• For those with PPHN requiring ECMO, the survival rate is approximately 80% for idiopathic PPHN, 90% for meconium aspiration syndrome, 80% for PPHN secondary to sepsis, and only 50% to 60% for those babies with CDH. Roughly 20% of these survivors have sensorineural hearing loss or abnormal neurological examinations at follow up.
• Even with the advances in technology and the availability of ECMO, the prognosis is poor for those babies with severe underlying lung pathology (CDH).

Differential Diagnosis

CONGENITAL

• Cyanotic congenital heart disease
• Total anomalous pulmonary venous return
• Congenital diaphragmatic hernia (CDH)
• Congenital cystic adenomatoid malformation (CCAM)
• Alveolar capillary dysplasia

INFECTIOUS

• Pneumonia
• Sepsis

PULMONARY

• Surfactant deficiency (respiratory distress syndrome)
• Meconium aspiration syndrome
• Blood or amniotic fluid aspiration
• Pneumothorax or air leak syndrome

Data Gathering

HISTORY

Question: Were any abnormalities seen on prenatal ultrasound?
Significance: A normal prenatal ultrasound would make the diagnosis of CDH, CCAM, and congenital heart disease less likely. A history of oligohydramnios is associated with pulmonary hypoplasia.

Question: Were there any problems during labor and delivery?
Significance: Fetal distress and/or hypoxia during labor and delivery can lead to PPHN; therefore, it is important to ask about events that can cause fetal distress—maternal chorioamnionitis, GBS infection, difficult delivery, or meconium aspiration. It is also important to ask about these events and any evidence of fetal distress in order to generate a differential diagnosis for a neonate with respiratory failure and hypoxia.

Question: What was the infant's initial clinical course?
Significance: Infants with PPHN usually present with mild respiratory distress that worsens in the first minutes to hours of life, progressing to respiratory failure, hypoxia, and poor perfusion. This is in contrast to infants with cardiac disease, CCAM or CDH which are usually cyanotic and in significant distress from birth.

Physical Examination

The following physical exam findings suggest a diagnosis of PPHN:
• Significant respiratory distress with nasal flaring, grunting and retractions
• Clear breath sounds (if idiopathic pphn)
• Pale, grey color with poor perfusion

- Tricuspid regurgitation murmur heard at the left lower sternal border

The following physical exam findings suggest diagnoses other than idiopathic PPHN:

- Any murmur other than tricuspid regurgitation would suggest congenital heart disease
- A barrel chest suggests a pneumothorax or meconium aspiration
- A scaphoid abdomen suggests CDH

 Laboratory Aids

TESTS

Test: Complete blood count with differential
Significance: Leukocytosis, leukopenia, bandemia or neutropenia suggest bacterial infection

Test: Blood culture
Significance: Should be performed in all cases of PPHN to rule out infection.

Test: Frequent arterial blood gases
Significance: Help to determine the degree of hypoxia, hypercapnia, and acidosis, and the degree of illness; to help manage ventilator support; and to determine the need for ECMO by calculating the oxygenation index (see below).

Test: Oxygenation index (OI)
Significance: Used to express the severity of the respiratory distress and to determine if a neonate is a candidate for ECMO. OIs should be calculated with every blood gas. Three OIs >40 suggest the need for ECMO. OI = (Mean Airway Pressure x FiO_2/PaO_2) x 100.

Test: Hyperoxia test
Significance: While on 100% oxygen, a paO_2 >250 mmHg almost completely rules out cyanotic heart disease.

RADIOGRAPHIC STUDIES

Test: Chest radiography
Significance: In idiopathic PPHN, the chest radiograph usually shows clear lungs. The chest x-ray will help to rule out pneumothorax, hyperinflation, meconium aspiration, and atelectasis. Assessing the cardiac silhouette and the pulmonary vascular markings may help rule out some congenital heart disease.

Test: Echocardiogram
Significance: Very important to make the diagnosis of PPHN and to rule out congenital heart disease; to follow cardiac output and function; to assess cardiac function if deciding to start ECMO.

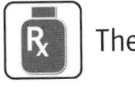 Therapy

All infants should be transferred to a Level III Neonatal Intensive Care Unit where High Frequency Ventilation (HFV) and inhaled nitric oxide (iNO) are available. If the neonate

meets criteria for starting ECMO or is close to it (OI >40 on 3 different blood gases), then ECMO should also be available at the receiving institution.

SUPPORT RESPIRATORY STATUS

- Conventional ventilation or high frequency ventilation to improve oxygenation and control ventilation although minimizing lung damage. There are no set guidelines for the ventilator management of PPHN, but most institutions feel that high frequency ventilation minimizes lung damage when high mean airway pressures (MAP) are needed, i.e., MAPs approximately greater than 15.
- Frequent monitoring to keep PaO_2 between 80 and 100, pCO_2 >35 to 45, and OI below ECMO criteria (OI >40 times 3).
- Avoid hyperventilation as this has been associated with poor neurodevelopmental outcome.

LOWER THE PVR AND THUS PROMOTE PULMONARY BLOOD FLOW

- Give 100% oxygen.
- Keep blood gas pH alkalotic (>7.40) while keeping pCO_2 >35 to 45 by ventilator manipulation or bicarbonate infusion.
- Keep systemic blood pressures high (mean BP >45 to 50) with volume, transfusions, or pressors.
- Treat acidosis with fluid, blood, or bicarbonate infusion.

IMPROVE OXYGEN SATURATION AND THUS OXYGEN DELIVERY TO THE TISSUES

- Initially 100% oxygen should be used to keep the PaO_2 >80 to 100 and the oxygen saturation 99% to 100%. The oxygen can be weaned very slowly (about 2% per hour if saturation remains >98%).
- iNO, a pulmonary vasodilator, should be used if the infant is on 100% oxygen and significant ventilator support (MAP >15), and the above noted PaO_2 goal is not achieved. iNO has been shown to decrease the need for ECMO in term neonates with hypoxic respiratory failure secondary to PPHN except for those babies with CDH. iNO should only be used as a bridge to ECMO in babies with CDH.
- WEAN SLOWLY! If the oxygen and /or the iNO is weaned too quickly, the baby can become critically ill since PPHN is a very labile condition.
- ECMO if the OI is >40 on three blood gases. With the current therapeutic alternatives (iNO and HFV), ECMO can usually be avoided.

REDUCE OXYGEN DEMAND

- Sedatives and paralytics may be given to prevent fluctuations in oxygenation during care.
- Minimize stimulation.

TREATMENT OF ANY UNDERLYING LUNG DISEASE

- Antibiotics
- Surfactant
- Chest tube
- Surgery

 Follow-Up

- All newborns with PPHN and those who go on ECMO need to be followed after discharge for the development of long-term sequelae including: neurosensory hearing loss, developmental delay, and growth failure.

PITFALLS

- It can be difficult to differentiate cyanotic congenital heart disease from PPHN. Before starting ECMO, be sure to repeat an echocardiogram to rule out any heart disease that may be amenable to repair and/or a different therapy.
- Those infants who fail to improve after one week of therapy should be reevaluated for any evidence of an underlying disease process.
- PPHN is a very labile condition. Neonates can change from being stable to being very sick and emergently needing ECMO.
- ECMO, though life saving and with a good survival rate, is not without problems. Side effects include: being repeatedly exposed to blood products, risk of intraabdominal or intracardiac bleed, potential for long-term neurological sequelae, and long-term risk of having only one patent carotid artery.

 Common Questions and Answers

Q: Does iNO improve outcome in newborns with severe PPHN?
A: Yes. iNO, used at a dose of 20 ppm, has been shown to decrease the need for ECMO and the incidence of death in term infants with PPHN without CDH. Follow up studies done at one year of age have shown no difference in long-term disabilities between those babies treated and not treated with iNO. Long-term outcome is mainly determined by the underlying disease and the severity of illness.

BIBLIOGRAPHY

Lipkin PH, Davidson D, Spivak L, Straube R, Rhines J, Chang CT. Neurodevelopmental and medical outcomes of persistent pulmonary hypertension in term newborns treated with nitric oxide. *J Pediatr* 2002;140:306–310.

Sadiq HF, Mantych G, Benawra RS, Devaskar UP, Hocker JR. Inhaled nitric oxide in the treatment of moderate persistent pulmonary hypertension of the newborn: a randomized controlled trial. *J Perinatol* 2003;23:98–103.

Walsh MC, Stork EK. Persistent pulmonary hypertension of the newborn. Rational therapy based on pathophysiology. *Clin Perinatol* 2001;28:609–627.

Author: Wendy J. Kowalski

Perthes Disease

 Database

DEFINITION

Self-limited osteonecrosis of the proximal femoral epiphysis of unknown etiology.

CAUSES

Unknown; related to a combination of trauma and vascular insult (recent evidence suggests thrombophilia).

PATHOLOGY

- Four stages

—Initial: bone necrosis
—Fragmentation: fragmentation of necrotic bone with early revascularization
—Reossification: revascularization, resorption, and repair via creeping substitution
—Healing: remodeling

EPIDEMIOLOGY

- Seen most commonly between ages 4 and 8 years of age
- Boys affected more than girls, with ratio of 4.5:1
- Ten percent bilateral
- Majority have delayed bone age
- More common in lower socioeconomic groups

GENETICS

No strong evidence to suggest that Perthes is an inherited condition.

COMPLICATIONS

- Mild limb length discrepancy
- Restriction of hip range of motion
- Pain, limping
- Osteoarthritis (late)

PROGNOSIS

- Based on the following factors:

—Age of the patient at onset of the disease (earlier onset gives better prognosis); if onset older than 8 years of age, poorer prognosis than if onset at younger age
—Extent of femoral head involvement; if more than one-half of epiphysis involved, poorer prognosis
—Subluxation of femoral head, poorer prognosis
—Growth disturbance of the physis, poorer prognosis

 Differential Diagnosis

- Toxic synovitis
- Chondrolysis (idiopathic and secondary)
- Infection (Brodie abscess—subacute osteomyelitis of proximal femoral epiphysis)
- Tuberculosis of the hip
- Juvenile rheumatoid arthritis
- Rheumatic fever
- Tumors (chondroblastoma of proximal femoral epiphysis)
- Meyer dysplasia
- Bone dysplasias

—Multiple epiphyseal dysplasia
—Trichorhinophalangeal syndrome
—Spondyloepiphyseal dysplasia

- Hypothyroidism, juvenile cretinism
- Sickle cell disease, hemophilia
- Gaucher disease

 Data Gathering

HISTORY

Question: Age at onset of symptoms/signs?
Significance: Older age at onset implies worse prognosis.

Question: Limping?
Significance: Weeks to months duration

Question: Hip, thigh, or knee pain?
Significance: Hip pathology may cause referred pain at thigh or knee.

 Physical Examination

Finding: Limitation of range of motion
Significance: Especially internal rotation and abduction

Finding: Irritability and tenderness of hip joint area
Significance: Usually early—related to synovitis from early repair

Finding: True hip joint irritability
Significance: Early finding indicating intraarticular synovitis

Finding: Atrophy of thigh
Significance: Late finding

Finding: Slight shortening of affected limb
Significance: As a result of collapse (real) or contracture (apparent)

Finding: Trendelenburg gait
Significance: Leaning over affected leg during stance phase of gait cycle, as a result of mechanical disadvantage from collapse and pain/synovitis

SPECIAL QUESTIONS

Finding: Distribution of pain may follow the sensory distribution of the obturator nerve.
Significance: Referred pain from hip pathology may cause symptoms in medial thigh and knee.

PHYSICAL EXAMINATION TRICKS

The Trendelenburg test is positive when a patient stands on the affected side and the pelvis drops on the opposite side.

Laboratory Aids

Test: Laboratory tests
Significance: Generally are not helpful, but may be necessary to rule out other conditions such as infection and JRA

IMAGING STAGES

- Incipient (or initial) stage (first)
- Aseptic or avascular stage (second)
- Fragmentation stage (third)
- Residual or remodeling stage (fourth)
- The first radiographic sign of Perthes is smaller size of the femoral head epiphysis and a widened articular cartilage space compared with the other side; the second sign is the subchondral fracture.

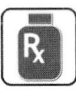 ## Therapy

- Most do not need surgery
- Treatment needed generally for those with more severe involvement (one-half of head involved or late onset).
- Two basic treatment principles:

—Maintenance and/or restoration of range of motion
—Containment of the femoral head epiphysis in the acetabulum

- General treatment modalities

—Bed rest early during collapse
—Weight relief early during collapse (usually crutches)
—Physical therapy to maintain range of motion
—Traction—less popular now
—Bracing
—Surgery

DRUGS

NSAIDs for pain and inflammation

DURATION

Generally continues until patient enters the reossification phase

 ## Follow-Up

WHEN TO EXPECT IMPROVEMENT

- The magnitude and duration of symptoms depend on the age of the patient at onset of the disease and the degree of involvement of the disease process. Most patients show improvement in symptoms by 6 months after the onset of disease.
- Patients with Perthes disease preferably should be seen and followed by a pediatric orthopaedic surgeon.

SIGNS TO WATCH FOR

- Stiffness—loss of range of motion
- Limping
- Pain
- Subluxation of the hip joint

PROGNOSIS

Overall, good prognosis for the majority of patients

PITFALLS

The majority of patients with Perthes disease do not need surgery. For those who do, early recognition and appropriate early referral are key.

 ## Common Questions and Answers

Q: How long do you observe a patient with hip pain before ordering an x-ray?
A: It depends on the presence or absence of abnormalities on the physical examination. If any of the signs mentioned above are seen in conjunction with significant hip pain, an x-ray is indicated. An x-ray should be done early to establish the diagnosis and rule out other abnormalities.

Q: Why do patients with hip pathology have knee pain?
A: This is because the nerves that innervate the hip joint also have cutaneous sensory distributions. Both the obturator and femoral nerves innervate the hip joint and both also have cutaneous sensory distribution in the region of the thigh and knee joint.

ICD-9-CM 732.1

BIBLIOGRAPHY

Kaniklides C, Lonnerholm T, Moberg A, et al. Legg-Calve-Perthes disease. Comparison of conventional radiography, MR imaging, bone scintigraphy and arthrography. *Acta Radiol* 1995;36(4):434–439.

Salter RB. The present status of surgical treatment of Legg-Perthes disease: current concept review. *J Bone Joint Surg* 1984; 66A:961.

Weinstein SL. Legg-Calve-Perthes Syndrome. In: Morrissy RT, Weinstein SL, eds. *Lovell and Winter's Pediatric Orthopaedics.* 5th Ed. Philadelphia: Lippincott, Williams & Wilkins, 2001:957–998.

Authors: John P. Dormans and Leslie Moroz

Pertussis

Database

DEFINITION

- *Bordetella pertussis* is a small, nonmotile, fastidious, gram-negative rod.
- The first description of the disease appeared in 1578 during an epidemic in Paris, France.

PATHOPHYSIOLOGY

- Replicates only in association with ciliated epithelium, causing congestion and inflammation of the bronchi; peribronchial lymphoid hyperplasia followed by a necrotizing process occurs and results in a bronchopneumonia; atelectasis can occur as a result of bronchiolar obstruction from accumulated secretions.
- Filamentous hemagglutinin (FHA), lymphocytosis promoting factor (LPF), and adenylate cyclase play a role in the organism's attachment and adversely affect immune cell function.
- The long incubation period (7 to 21 days) reflects the time necessary for *B. pertussis* to increase in numbers needed for progressive spread of infection in the respiratory tract and produce enough toxins for eliciting damage and dysfunction of the respiratory epithelium.
- Respiratory illness characterized as a bronchopneumonia.
- Apnea is a common manifestation in the young infant, <6 months of age. The characteristic "whoop" is typically absent.

EPIDEMIOLOGY

- One of the most highly communicable diseases with attack rates close to 100% in susceptible individuals.
- A disease of young children; the infant either nonimmunized or partially immunized is at greatest risk.
- Approximately one-third of cases reported to the CDC are in infants, <6 months of age.
- Disease in adolescents and adults is not usually recognized as pertussis despite a cough that is paroxysmal and may last for weeks. In a recent Canadian study, the prevalence of pertussis in 422 adolescents and adults with prolonged cough illness was 20%. Despite improved vaccination rates in the United States, pertussis infection rates have steadily risen since the early 1980s. This is thought to be attributed to the growth of a susceptible adult population, and these patients are the major source of pertussis infection in children.
- Route of spread includes aerosolized respiratory droplets, direct contact with nasal secretions, and indirect contact with secretions through hand contact.

COMPLICATIONS

- Pneumonia, the most frequent complication, is responsible for more than 90% of deaths in young children with pertussis, and is usually owing to secondary bacterial disease rather than *B. pertussis* itself.
- Superinfections as a result of viruses (adenovirus, respiratory syncytial virus, cytomegalovirus) or bacteria (*Streptococcus pneumoniae*, *Staphylococcus aureus*) and gram-negative iatrogenic infections can complicate pneumonias.
- Other pulmonary complications include atelectasis, pneumothorax, pneumomediastinum, and subcutaneous emphysema.
- Seizures (3%) and encephalopathy (0.9%) have been observed in infants with pertussis, although these findings may be related to fever causing febrile convulsions and cerebral hypoxia as a result of the pulmonary complications.

PROGNOSIS

The prognosis is directly related to patient age; the highest mortality is observed in infants, <6 months of age. Infants have a 0.5% to 1% risk of death, whereas, in the older child, prognosis is good.

Differential Diagnosis

- *B. parapertussis* and adenoviruses
- *B. pertussis*
- Bronchiolitis
- Bacterial pneumonia
- Cystic fibrosis
- Tuberculosis
- Foreign body aspiration should also be considered.

Data Gathering

HISTORY

Question: What are clinical stages of pertussis infection?
Significance:

- Three stages:

—Catarrhal stage (1 to 2 weeks) with symptoms of an upper respiratory infection
—Paroxysmal stage (2 to 4 weeks or longer) characterized by paroxysmal cough with increased severity and frequency producing the characteristic whoop during the sudden forceful inspiratory phase; posttussive vomiting is also observed during this stage.
—The convalescent stage begins and lasts 1 to 2 weeks but cough can persist for several months. In the adolescent or adult, long-standing cough of 2 to 3 weeks is the hallmark symptom. Most patients report a paroxysmal or staccato quality to the cough.

Physical Examination

- Rhinorrhea, lacrimation, conjunctival hyperemia, and fever seen in the early stage of disease
- Cyanosis observed during the paroxysmal stage
- Lung auscultatory examination is usually normal unless significant atelectasis or pneumonia has occurred.

Laboratory Aids

Test: CBC
Significance: Leukocytosis with predominant lymphocytosis (77%) is commonly observed at the end of the catarrhal stage and throughout the paroxysmal stage of illness, although this phenomenon is not frequently observed in infants.

Test: Chest radiographs
Significance: May reveal perihilar infiltrates or a "shaggy right heart border," although these findings can be seen with other respiratory infections.

Test: Culture of *B. pertussis*
Significance: Achieved using calcium alginate or Dacron swabs of the nasopharynx and plated onto selective media such as Regan-Lowe or Bordet-Gengou and incubated for 7 days.

Test: Culture isolation of *B. pertussis*
Significance: Most frequently successful during the catarrhal or early paroxysmal stages and is rarely found beyond the fourth week of illness. The overall sensitivity is 60% to 70%.

Test: Direct immunofluorescent assays of nasopharyngeal specimens
Significance: Can provide a rapid and specific diagnosis but is limited by the experience of the laboratory personnel for interpretation

Test: Polymerase chain reaction (PCR) techniques
Significance: Available in most centers, and have been shown to have a higher sensitivity than culture in the detection of *B. pertussis* from nasopharyngeal specimens

Test: Recently developed monoclonal immunofluorescent antibody (BL-5)
Significance: Has been shown to be at least as sensitive and specific as culture but needs additional investigation

Test: Serology
Significance: Has excellent sensitivity and specificity when the acute serum is collected early in the course of illness and compared to the convalescent serum specimen

Therapy

- Patients with more severe disease manifestations (apnea, cyanosis, feeding difficulties) or other complications require hospitalization for supportive care.
- If antibiotic treatment is initiated during the catarrhal stage, it can prevent disease from progressing. Antibiotics have not been shown to shorten the course of illness if begun during the paroxysmal stage, although it will eliminate the organism from the nasopharynx within 3 to 4 days, thus shortening the potential for contagion.
- Erythromycin (50 mg/kg per day) in four doses for 14 days is recommended; an alternative dose with 40 mg/kg of erythromycin estolate twice a day for 14 days has shown equal efficacy. Note, an association between oral erythromycin use and hypertrophic pyloric stenosis has been reported in infants younger than 6 weeks of age. Given the limited study of this causal relationship, the American Academy of Pediatrics continues to recommend erythromycin for treatment and prophylaxis against *B. pertussis*.
- Newer macrolides, azithromycin and clarithromycin, may be effective in shorter courses of 5 to 7 days, however, their efficacy has not been fully studied.
- Trimethoprim-sulfamethoxazole is another alternative to erythromycin, although its efficacy is unproved.
- Infants under 6 months may develop apnea from fatigue secondary to excessive coughing. They need close observation, preferably in the hospital.

Follow-Up

- The paroxysmal stage can last up to 4 weeks and the convalescent stage up to several months and can be quite problematic for patient and family.
- The complications of pertussis are more likely to occur in the younger infant and therefore tend to have a more serious, protracted course.

PITFALLS

The most likely source of pertussis in young infants is from the adolescent or adult with mild symptoms of pertussis. Therefore, a high index of suspicion must exist in this population before adequate control of exposure to the partially or unimmunized infant can be successful.

PREVENTION

Infection Control

- Isolation of hospitalized patient: respiratory isolation for 5 days after starting erythromycin therapy or until at least 3 weeks after the onset of the paroxysmal stage, if antibiotics were not given, is recommended.

- Control measures: exposed individuals (all household contacts, other close contacts, other children in child care) should receive erythromycin chemoprophylaxis to limit secondary transmission, regardless of immunization status.

Immunizations

- Vaccinations available in the United States include acellular vaccines in combination with diphtheria and tetanus toxoids as the preferred vaccination product over previous whole cell products. Universal immunization of the preschool child is paramount to control the rate of infection.
- Combination DTaP and HiB vaccine is available with the benefit of fewer injections and immunization visits; however, lower antibody responses have been reported.
- The DTaP licensed vaccines in the United States have variable efficacy, and further study of the immunity data is necessary to determine the optimal pertussis vaccine.
- It seems prudent to vaccinate adults with periodic booster vaccinations given the risk they create for young infants.

Common Questions and Answers

Q: Why is the transmission of pertussis difficult to control in the young infant?
A: Unfortunately, many physicians do not consider pertussis in an adolescent or adult because they assume that childhood immunization will protect adults against pertussis. In addition, delays in antimicrobial treatment are common in adults as a result of the lack of index of suspicion of pertussis by their providers. The immunity protection by pertussis vaccination is limited and, as a result of the poor tolerability of booster immunizations in adults, this has not been a universal recommendation.

Q: Are there any risks associated with the pertussis vaccine?
A: The rates of local reactions, fever, and other common systemic symptoms of somnolence, fussiness, and loss of appetite, are significantly lower with the acellular pertussis vaccine than with whole-cell pertussis vaccine. Moderate to severe systemic reactions, including high temperature, persistent, inconsolable crying for more than 3 hours, seizures, and collapse, have rarely been reported with DTaP, and the frequency is much lower than DTP immunization. Because of the temporal relation between administration of pertussis vaccine and severe adverse events such as death, encephalopathy, developmental delay with learning, and behavioral problems or onset of seizures, much publicity has been given to this vaccine, yet causation has not been established.

Q: What are the contraindications to pertussis vaccination?
A: Contraindications to avoid initial or subsequent doses of pertussis vaccine (DTP and DTaP) include the following: an immediate anaphylactic reaction, encephalopathy within

7 days of a prior injection or a seizure within 3 days or persistent crying, a shock-like state or fever greater than 104.9°F within 48 hours of a prior injection. A progressive neurologic disorder or history of seizure disorder is a contraindication also.

ICD-9-CM 033.9

BIBLIOGRAPHY

Bass JW, Wittler RR. Return of epidemic pertussis in the United States. *Pediatr Infect Dis J* 1994;13:343.

Black S. Epidemiology of pertussis. *Pediatr Infect Dis J* 1997;16:S85–S89.

Cherry JD, Olin P. The science and fiction of pertussis vaccines. *Pediatrics* 1999;104:1381–1384.

Edwards KM. Pertussis in older children and adolescents. *Adv Pediatr Infect Dis* 1998;13:49–77.

Eskola J, Ward J, Dagan R, et al. Combined vaccination of Haemophilus influenzae type B conjugate and diphtheria-tetanus-pertussis containing acellular pertussis. *Lancet* 1999;354:2063–2068.

Feigin RD. Pertussis. In: Feigin RD, Cherry JD, eds. *Textbook of Pediatric Infectious Diseases* 3rd Ed. Philadelphia: WB Saunders. 1990:1208.

Gordon M, Davies HD, Gold R. Clinical and microbiologic features of children presenting with pertussis to a Canadian pediatric hospital during an eleven year period. *Pediatr Infect Dis J* 1994;13:617–622.

He Q, Mertsola J, Soini H, et al. Sensitive and specific polymerase chain reaction assays for detection of *Bordetella pertussis* in nasopharyngeal specimens. *J Pediatr* 1994;124:421–426.

Hewlett EL. Pertussis: current concepts of pathogenesis and prevention. *Pediatr Infect Dis* 1997;16:S78–S84.

Hoppe JE. Comparison of erythromycin estolate and erythromycin ethylsuccinate for treatment of pertussis. *Pediatr Infect Dis J* 1992;11:189–193.

Hoppe JE. Neonatal pertussis. *Pediatr Infect Dis J* 2000;19:244–247.

Muller FMC, Hoppe JE, Wirsing Von Konig CH. Laboratory diagnosis of pertussis: state of the art in 1997. *J Clin Microbiol* 1997;35:2435–2443.

Peter G, Halsey NA, Marcuse EK, et al. Pertussis. *2000 Red Book: Report of the Committee on Infectious Diseases.* 25th Ed. Elk Grove Village, IL: American Academy of Pediatrics, 2000:435–448.

Senzilet LD, Halperin SA, Spka JS, Alagaratnam M, Morris A, et al. Pertussis is a frequent cause of prolonged cough illness in adults and adolescents. *Clin Infect Dis* 2001;32(12):1691–1697.

Authors: Louis M. Bell
Philip V. Scribano, 3rd edition

Pharyngitis

 Database

DEFINITION

Pharyngitis (sore throat) is inflammation of the mucous membranes and underlying structures of the pharynx and tonsils, usually secondary to viral or bacterial infection.

CAUSES

Viral

- Adenovirus types 1 through 7, 7a, 9, 14, 15, and 16
- Epstein-Barr virus (EBV)
- Influenza A, B: usually associated with more severe systemic complaints
- Parainfluenza 1, 2, and 3.
- Enteroviruses—coxsackie A, B, and echoviruses
- Measles and rubella and coronavirus, cytomegalovirus
- Herpes simplex virus (HSV)
- Rhinovirus and RSV: not usually associated with pharyngeal inflammation.
- Human immunodeficiency virus (HIV)

Bacterial

- *Streptococcus pyogenes* (group A β-hemolytic *streptococcus*)
- Group C or G streptococci
- *Arcanobacterium hemolyticum*
- *Corynebacterium diphtheriae* (Diphtheria)
- *C. hemolyticum*
- *Neisseria gonorrhoeae* and *N. meningitidis*
- *Mycoplasma pneumoniae*
- *M. hominis*
- *Chlamydia pneumoniae, C. psittaci*
- *Yersinia enterocolitica*
- *Francisella tularensis* (tularemia)
- *Treponema pallidum* (syphilis)
- Oral anaerobes (Vincent angina)

Fungi

- *Candida species* (oral thrush)

COMPLICATIONS

- *S. pharyngitis*—suppurative complications include peritonsillar abscess, cervical lymphadenitis, and mastoiditis. The most significant nonsuppurative complication is acute rheumatic fever.
- Lemierre syndrome—postanginal sepsis or necrobacillosis originates as pharyngitis or tonsillitis then progresses to sepsis and suppurative thrombophlebitis of the internal jugular vein. Septic thromboemboli seed various organs especially the liver, lungs, and joints.

PROGNOSIS

- *S. pharyngitis*: usually excellent. Morbidity associated with acute rheumatic fever (ARF) and acute poststreptococcal glomerulonephritis (APGN).
- Viral pharyngitis is usually self-limited.

 Differential Diagnosis

INFECTIOUS

- Herpangina (enterovirus)
- Hand-foot-and-mouth disease (enterovirus)

- Peritonsillar abscess or cellulitis
- Retropharyngeal abscess or cellulitis
- Laryngitis
- Epiglottitis

INGESTIONS

- Caustic or irritant ingestions
- Inhaled irritant

TRAUMA

- Vocal abuse from shouting

INFLAMMATORY

- Allergy

MISCELLANEOUS

- PFAPA syndrome (Periodic Fever, Aphthous ulcers, Pharyngitis and cervical Adenitis)
- Psychogenic pain (globus hystericus)
- Vitamin deficiency (A, B complex, C)
- Dehydration

 Data Gathering

HISTORY

Question: Is the pharyngitis associated with the sudden onset of fever with headache, nausea and vomiting?
Significance: Frequent in streptococcal pharyngitis, which is usually exudative but with cough or rhinorrhea in only about 10% of cases.

Question: Is the pharyngitis associated with rhinorrhea, cough, hoarseness, conjunctivitis and ulcerative pharyngeal lesions?
Significance: More likely to be a viral etiology.

Question: Are there significant systemic complaints (e.g., fever, malaise)?
Significance: Characteristic of EBV or HIV (acute retroviral syndrome).

Question: Has the patient been swimming in an inadequately chlorinated pool?
Significance: Consider adenoviral pharyngoconjunctival fever.

 Physical Examination

Finding: Moderate to severe pharyngeal erythema and tonsillar enlargement.
Significance: Erythema may be associated with petechiae, exudate or ulceration.

Finding: Follicular, exudative pharyngotonsillitis that may occur in association with conjunctivitis.
Significance: Common with adenovirus infections (e.g., pharyngoconjunctival fever).

Finding: Ulcerative lesions or characteristic enanthem consisting of 2 to 14 ulcers and vesicles (1 to 2 mm in size) in the posterior pharynx.
Significance: Common with enteroviral infections (e.g., Coxsackie A, B, echovirus).

Finding: Ulcerative lesions on anterior oropharynx (gingivostomatitis).
Significance: Characteristic of HSV infection which can also cause an exudative pharyngitis in adolescents that may be difficult to differentiate from streptococcal or EBV pharyngitis.

Finding: Scarletiniform rash
Significance: Strongly suggests diagnosis of GAS but also reported with *Arcanobacterium hemolyticum*.

Finding: Presence of an adherent membrane that may extend from the tonsils, uvula and pharyngeal walls to the larynx and trachea with foul or sweet odor to breath and/or severe lymphadenitis creating "bull neck" appearance.
Significance: Suggests diphtheria.

Finding: Splenomegaly and/or generalized adenopathy
Significance: Suggests EBV.

Finding: Presence of more than six palatal petechiae
Significance: Strongly associated with streptococcal pharyngitis.

 Laboratory Aids

Because of the importance of its complications, streptococcal disease should be confirmed or excluded by laboratory testing, except in presentations suggestive of viral or other etiology of pharyngitis (e.g., a toddler with conjunctivitis and rhinorrhea, presence of gingivostomatitis, findings consistent with IM, etc.).

SPECIFIC TESTS

Test: Rapid streptococcal antigen detection tests (RADTs)
Significance: Are effective as initial tests with greater than 95% specificity and 50% to 80% sensitivity. Cultures should be performed when rapid test is negative. (Hint: culture throat using two swabs initially, keeping one for culture if the rapid test is negative.) Positive rapid tests do not require culture confirmation. The best technique is to swab both tonsillar pillars and the retropharynx.

Test: Throat culture
Significance: The criterion standard with best sensitivity (>90%) for group A β-hemolytic streptococci.

Test: Monospot (heterophile antibody) test or Epstein-Barr virus serology

 Therapy

- Usually no therapy indicated, except for streptococcal pharyngitis (and other rare cases of bacterial or fungal pharyngitis).
- May withhold treatment for GAS pharyngitis until throat culture result is available.
- Steroids have not been found to significantly alter the course or symptoms of acute pharyngitis and are not recommended.
- Tonsillectomy for recurrent pharyngitis is still controversial with only modest reductions in the number of subsequent episodes weighed against the morbidity of the procedure.

DRUGS

- Oral penicillin V: is the drug of choice for GAS pharyngitis except in penicillin-allergic individuals. Resistant strains have not been documented in vitro.
—Children: use 400,000 units (250 mg) b.i.d. or t.i.d. for 10 days.
—Adolescents/Adults: use 800,000 Units (500 mg) b.i.d. for 10 days or 400,000 units (250 mg) t.i.d. or q.i.d. for 10 days.
- Intramuscular benzathine penicillin G: assures compliance, useful in outbreaks.
—Children (<60 lbs.): 600,000 Units IM (1 dose). Children (>60 lbs.) and adults: 1,200,000 Units IM (one dose). Bringing to room temperature reduces discomfort, also procaine penicillin combinations are less painful.
- Amoxicillin, clindamycin, and first generation oral cephalosporins (up to 15% of penicillin-allergic persons are also allergic to cephalosporins): are reasonable alternatives to penicillin in GAS pharyngitis. Amoxicillin suspension is reported to be more palatable than penicillin VK in young children where palatability may affect compliance.
- Clarithromycin and azithromycin have also been shown to eradicate streptococci; however, because of the broad spectra of these antibiotics and the increasing incidence of antibiotic-resistant bacteria, penicillin is still recommended by most experts except in cases of penicillin hypersensitivity, when patient nonadherence to a 10-day penicillin regimen is suspected or for patients who fail therapy with a β-lactamase.
- Oral erythromycin: is indicated in penicillin-allergic individuals. Erythromycin ethyl succinate (40 to 50 mg/kg per day in two to four divided doses). Resistance is rare in the United States (<5% of isolates).
- Cefdinir and cefpodoxime proxetil are approved for use in a more convenient 5-day dosing schedule.
- Tetracyclines and sulfonamides should not be used as a result of resistance of group A streptococci.

DURATION OF THERAPY

Recent trials comparing 10-day courses of penicillin with newer oral cephalosporins or macrolides used for 3 or 5 days have shown similar bacteriologic and clinical cure rates; but efficacy in prevention of nonsuppurative sequelae (e.g., acute rheumatic fever) is unknown, and these agents have broad spectra and greater expense.

 Follow-Up

PATIENTS WITH STREPTOCOCCAL PHARYNGITIS

- Clinical improvement is usually rapid.
- Cure rate is excellent except in noncompliant patients, rare coinfection with pathogens that elaborate β-lactamase (consider therapy with clindamycin) or in cases of a new infection acquired from family or classroom contact (also rare).

- No need to perform posttreatment cultures for GAS in asymptomatic patients in areas in which incidence of ARF is low (e.g., United States, Canada, Western Europe).
- Watch for suppurative complications (e.g., peritonsillar abscess, cervical adenitis, mastoiditis).

PREVENTION

- Long-term penicillin prophylaxis for patients with a history of rheumatic fever.

ISOLATION OF HOSPITALIZED PATIENT

- Isolation of hospitalized patients with respiratory viruses and pharyngitis.
- Droplet precautions for hospitalized children with streptococcal pharyngitis until 24 hours after initiation of therapy.

CONTROL MEASURES

- Children with GAS pharyngitis can return to school or day care 24 hours after starting antimicrobial therapy.
- Cultures of asymptomatic contacts of patients with streptococcal pharyngitis are not indicated except in outbreak situations in school or day care (in which treatment of patients with positive RADT or culture is indicated) or in contacts with a history of nonsuppurative complications.

PITFALLS

- Swabbing the throat from anywhere other than the tonsils and posterior pharyngeal wall.
- Even experienced clinicians may overestimate the diagnosis of GAS pharyngitis by up to 80%, using clinical grounds alone.
- About 20% of children with GAS pharyngitis who have mild symptoms may go unrecognized if cultures are not performed.
- Failure to use throat culture to rule out streptococcal pharyngitis when rapid test is negative.
- Failure to request identification of other organisms in the appropriate clinical setting. (e.g., N. gonorrhoeae or A. hemolyticum)
- Reliance on Monospot test in young children (<5 years) because of a high incidence of false negatives (consider EBV serology instead).
- Positive throat culture or RADT in patients with viral pharyngitis may represent streptococcal carrier state. Diagnostic tests for GAS should be utilized in patients suspected to have streptococcal disease on clinical and epidemiologic grounds, not on all patients who complain of a "sore throat."
- Overtreatment of patients who are streptococcal carriers—asymptomatic patients (or patients with intercurrent viral infections) who have a positive test for GAS are at low, or no risk of developing suppurative or nonsuppurative complications and unlikely to spread the organism to close contacts.

 Common Questions and Answers

Q: Are rapid antigen detection tests (RADT) alone adequate for the diagnosis of GAS pharyngitis?
A: No, only if they are positive. A negative RADT result should be confirmed by the more sensitive culture.

Q: Is there any benefit to starting therapy while waiting for culture results?
A: Immediate therapy probably shortens the symptomatic period, but waiting for a positive test result avoids overuse of antibiotics.

Q: Does an asymptomatic patient with a positive test for GAS from the pharynx (e.g., chronic carriers) require therapy?
A: Usually not. Between 8% and 20% of children in school or day care will have asymptomatic carriage of GAS and generally do not require therapy. Exceptions are those with a history of ARF, outbreak situations, or to achieve eradication in families with recurrent episodes of GAS pharyngitis.

Q: Is there any evidence of GAS resistance to penicillin and other beta lactam antibiotics?
A: No, GAS has never been found to be resistant to penicillin but some studies suggest tolerance to penicillin in which penicillin is bacteriostatic rather than bactericidal. However, 2% to 8% of GAS strains will be resistant to macrolides.

Q: Is tonsillectomy indicated for recurrent GAS pharyngitis?
A: Rare patients in whom multiple symptomatic episodes of laboratory-confirmed GAS pharyngitis occur despite appropriate therapy, may be considered for tonsillectomy.

Q: Is continuous antimicrobial prophylaxis for recurrent GAS pharyngitis recommended?
A: No, there is insufficient evidence to show that it is effective, except for preventing recurrences of acute rheumatic fever.

Q: What is the association of pharyngitis and recurrent fever?
A: There is an increasingly recognized syndrome of periodic fever, aphthous stomatitis, pharyngitis and cervical adenitis, also known as PFAPA. The fever is usually high, recurs at fixed intervals of 2 to 8 weeks and resolves spontaneously within 4 days. It does not appear to be familial, begins before the age of 5 years, the patient is well between episodes, and there are no known sequelae or etiology.

ICD-9-CM

Pharyngitis (streptococcal) 034.0
Pharyngitis (acute, viral, infective) 462.0
Pharyngitis (influenza) 487.1
Pharyngitis (coxsackie) 074.0, and others

BIBLIOGRAPHY

American Academy of Pediatrics. Group A streptococcal infections. In: Pickering LK, ed. *2003 Red Book: Report of the Committee on Infectious Diseases.* 26th Ed. Elk Grove Village. IL: American Academy of Pediatrics, 2003.

Author: Mark L. Bagarazzi

Photosensitivity

 Database

DEFINITION

Adverse or abnormal reaction of the skin to sunlight

CAUSES

- Combination of sunlight with some abnormality in the skin such as loss of pigment, a chemical agent, a metabolic product, another skin disorder, a genetic disease, or an unknown factor, produces a cutaneous abnormality.
- Specific wavelengths of the radiant energy emitted by the sun and reaching the earth are usually responsible for each photosensitivity disorder, most commonly ultraviolet B (UVB, 290 to 320 nm), ultraviolet A (UVA, 320 to 400 nm), and visible light (400 to 800 nm).

PATHOLOGY

Findings are diverse for the different disorders and rarely diagnostic.

EPIDEMIOLOGY

- Variable for each disorder
- Photosensitivities with onset in childhood include albinism, hydroa aestivale, hydroa vacciniforme, the porphyrias (e.g., erythropoietic, erythropoietic protoporphyria, hepatoerythropoietic), and genetic disorders (e.g., xeroderma pigmentosa, Hartnup disease, poikiloderma congenitale, Bloom syndrome, and Cockayne syndrome).
- Photosensitivities that occur frequently in adults but can occur in childhood are vitiligo, chemically induced photosensitivities, polymorphous light eruption, and connective tissue disease.

GENETICS

- The genetic disorders include the porphyrias and others as previously listed.
- The various porphyrias have variable inheritance patterns, although most of the other genetic disorders are inherited in an autosomal-recessive pattern.
- There is a positive familial history in many cases of polymorphous light eruption.

 Differential Diagnosis

- Photosensitivity resulting from pigment loss:

—Albinism
—Vitiligo

- Idiopathic photosensitivity:

—Polymorphous light eruption
—Solar urticaria

- Chemically induced reactions

—Topical agents: perfumes, plant-associated phytophotodermatitis (e.g., lemons, limes, celery, parsnips, carrots, dill, parsley, figs, meadow grass, giant hogweed, mangos, wheat, clover, cocklebur, buttercups, Shepherd's purse, and pigweed), blankophores (e.g., optical brighteners in detergents), sunscreens, topical retinoids (e.g., tretinoin, adapalene)
—Systemic agents: tetracyclines, sulfonamides, nalidixic acid, griseofulvin, phenothiazines, oral hypoglycemic agents, amiodarone, quinine, isoniazid, and thiazide diuretics

- Metabolic disorders:

—Porphyrias: disorders of hemoglobin synthesis producing various porphyrins that are photosensitizers

- Genetic disorders:

—(see Epidemiology, above)

- Cutaneous diseases aggravated by sunlight:

—Connective tissue diseases

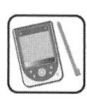 Data Gathering

HISTORY

- Age of onset of rash?
- Occurrence in spring and summer?
- Occurrence after sun exposure?
- How long after sun exposure?
- Occurrence after exposure to sun through glass?
- Any oral medications? May be related to oral contraceptives, sulfa drugs, iodines/bromides, or phenytoin.
- Any new topical agents (e.g., perfumes, lemons, limes, sunscreens, etc.)? Photosensitivity may occur on neck or places in which agents were placed on skin.

 Physical Examination

Finding: Distributed lesions
Significance: The distribution of lesions is the main sign of photosensitivity reactions. Lesions are prominent on sun-exposed skin such as the face, pinnae of the ears, the V of the neck, the nuchal area, and the dorsa of the hands. Often, sparing of the philtrum, the area below the chin, the eyelids, and other covered areas is seen. In phytophotodermatitis, linear or bizarre shapes can occur, including, as an example, hand prints if a caregiver has been squeezing limes and then picks up a child and the child is then exposed to sunlight.

Finding: Lesion characteristics
Significance: The characteristics of individual lesions vary with the particular disease and can include papules, vesicles, and plaques (polymorphous light eruption), sunburn (chemical reaction to a systemic agent), linear areas of hyperpigmentation (chemical reaction to a topical agent), skin cancers (xeroderma pigmentosum), vesicles (porphyria). In some cases, scarring can also be seen related to severe burns (porphyria).

PHYSICAL EXAMINATION TRICKS

Careful examination reveals accentuation of the rash on the nose, cheeks, and forehead with sparing of the eyelids and the submental portion of the chin. There is often a sharp cutoff in the nuchal area at the collar line.

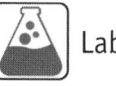 Laboratory Aids

Test: Phototesting
Significance: Using an artificial source of light, can confirm the presence of certain photosensitivities. Procedures are of two types. The first is exposure of skin to increasing doses of ultraviolet A and ultraviolet B to determine the erythema response (present at lower exposures than usual) and possibly reproduce lesions in certain diseases.
The second is photopatch testing in which photoallergic chemicals are applied under patches in duplicate, and one set is subsequently exposed to UVA. Patients who have photoallergic contact dermatitis develop a reaction under only the exposed patch of the agent causing the problem.

Test: Biochemical tests
Significance: Helpful for the diagnosis of the porphyrias with elevated levels of various porphyrins specific to each type in the urine, blood, or stool

- Measurement of antinuclear antibodies are helpful in connective tissue diseases.

SPECIALIZED TESTS FOR GENETIC DISEASES

- Cell culture: to evaluate DNA repair for xeroderma pigmentosum, or demonstrate chromosomal breaks in Bloom disease
- Measurement of specific amino acid and indole excretion patterns in Hartnup disease

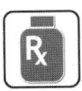

Therapy

- Protection against sun exposure is necessary.

—Avoiding the sun, particularly between 10 A.M. and 3 P.M., and wearing protective clothing is important.
—Sunscreens are helpful for those sensitive to UVB. Sunscreens should be waterproof and reapplied every 2 hours.
—The higher the sun protection factor (SPF—ratio of minimal erythema dose of sunscreened skin to minimal erythema dose of unprotected skin), the better.
—Sunscreens are less effective for blocking UVA and therefore less effective in helping patients with sensitivities to longer wavelengths.
—Sunscreens that contain both UVA and UVB blocking capabilities offer better protection than most. These include sunscreens containing avobenzone (Parsol 1789), titanium dioxide, and zinc oxide.
—Opaque formulations such as zinc oxide and titanium dioxide block ultraviolet and visible light but may be less cosmetically appealing.
—Patients with severe photosensitivities may have to avoid any significant light exposure.

- Removal of the offending agent is necessary in chemically induced photosensitivities.

—Any severe and acute eruptions may require a short course of oral prednisone.
—Antimalarial agents have been used for polymorphous light eruption, lupus erythematosus, solar urticaria, and porphyria cutanea tarda and require the experience of a specialist.

DURATION

Most patients require chronic protection against sun exposure. However, the problem is generally more acute in spring and summer months.

Follow-Up

WHEN TO EXPECT IMPROVEMENT

Variable, depending on the specific condition

PROGNOSIS

With the exception of chemically induced photosensitivities, most of the conditions are chronic.

PITFALLS

If possible, it is important to accurately document the specific wavelength of light and the degree of photosensitivity in order to accurately advise the patient. This requires phototesting by a specialist.

Common Questions and Answers

Q: What is the best sunscreen to use?
A: It depends on your particular problem. If you are sensitive to UVB, use a sunscreen with the highest SPF. If you are sensitive to UVA, sunscreens containing avobenzone, titanium dioxide, or zinc oxide are best.

Q: I have heard that sunscreens with an SPF above 15 are not necessary?
A: This is definitely not true for patients with photosensitivities, who have abnormal responses to light and require excessive protection. Even for the normal person, it is often not true. An SPF of 15 suggests that someone may receive 15 times more sun exposure with the sunscreen applied than without and not become sunburned. Some physicians have suggested that this is more than anyone should need. However, this number is calculated by testing in a controlled laboratory. Normal outdoor conditions, such as wind, reflection from water and sand, perspiration, and water exposure, can significantly decrease the effectiveness of the sunscreen.

Q: What is "sun allergy"?
A: This is a lay term for polymorphous light eruption, one of the most common photosensitivities presenting with papules, vesicles, and plaques 1 to 2 days after sun exposure. It usually recurs every spring and most patients learn to avoid sun exposure. However, ironically, it can improve with slow gradual sun exposure.

Q: Can I become allergic to sunscreens?
A: Certain active agents in sunscreens can produce an allergic response in rare individuals. If the rash recurs with each use, switch to another sunscreen with different ingredients. If the problem continues, it is necessary to consult a specialist for evaluation.

ICD-9-CM 692.72

BIBLIOGRAPHY

Harber LC, Bickers DR. *Photosensitivity Diseases: Principles of Diagnosis and Treatment.* 2nd Ed. Toronto: BC Decker, 1989.

Hurwitz S. Photosensitivity and photoreactions. *In Clinical Pediatric Dermatology: A Textbook of Skin Disorder of Childhood and Adolescence.* 2nd Ed. Philadelphia: WB Saunders, 1993:83.

Morison WL. Clinical practice. Photosensitivity. *N Engl J Med* 2004;350(11): 1111–1117.

Roelandts R. The diagnosis of photosensitivity. *Arch Dermatol* 2000;136(9): 1152–1157.

Author: Albert C. Yan

Pinworms

Database

DEFINITION

- Infection by a small white nematode (roundworm), typically *Enterobius vermicularis*, measuring 8 to 13 mm for females and 2 to 5 mm for males. Pinworms may also be caused by *Enterobius gregorii* in Europe, Africa, and Asia.
- Infection is characterized by perianal pruritus that occurs at night or just prior to waking. Difficulty sleeping, decreased appetite and/or abdominal pain may occur.

PATHOPHYSIOLOGY

- *E. vermicularis* eggs are ingested and hatch in the human's stomach and duodenum. Then the larvae migrate to the ileum and cecum. Adult worms copulate in the cecum.
- The pregnant female pinworm migrates from the cecum to the anus approximately 5 weeks later and deposits eggs on the perianal skin (at which point the female pinworm usually dies).
- Thousands of eggs are laid which may result in hundreds of worms.
- Pruritus is caused by the perianal deposition of eggs and a mucosal mastocytosis response. Other gastrointestinal symptoms, such as anorexia or abdominal pain, may occur as a result of the mucosal inflammatory response.
- Granulomas may form if dead worms and eggs invoke an inflammatory response in ectopic locations such as the peritoneal cavity, vulva, cervix, uterus, and fallopian tubes.

EPIDEMIOLOGY

- Considered the most common helminthic infection of humans (the only known natural host) and the most common worm infection in the United States.
- Occurs in school-aged children (5 to 10 years) and preschool children predominantly. Does occur in adults, usually in those caring for infected children. Some individuals may be predisposed to having either heavy or light worm burdens.
- Infection rates in the United States are 5% to 15%.
- Occurs worldwide, but is more prevalent in temperate climates.
- Not associated with poverty or personal hygiene
- Transmitted fecal-orally. Can be spread directly, hand to mouth, or via fomites, such as toys, bedding, clothing, toilet seats, and baths.

COMPLICATIONS

- Urethritis
- Vulvo-vaginitis
- Granuloma formation
- Pelvic inflammatory disease
- Bacterial superinfection of perianal excoriations

PROGNOSIS

- Reinfection is common.
- With appropriate treatment, symptoms resolve within a few days.
- Any chronic symptoms are likely to be as a result of recurrence rather than "chronic infection," because the life cycle of the adult worm is short with eggs being laid by the adult worm within 5 weeks.

Differential Diagnosis

INFECTION

- Other parasites (e.g., *Strongyloides stercoralis*)
- Nonparasitic vulvo-vaginitis (as a result of bacterial or fungal causes)

DERMATOLOGIC

- Contact or irritative diaper dermatitis
- Irritative vulvo-vaginitis secondary to soaps, bubble baths, or lotions
- Anal fissures (usually cause pain rather than itching)

MISCELLANEOUS

- Behavioral: self-touching (normal)
- Sleep disorders not as a result of nocturnal pruritus
- Hemorrhoids

Data Gathering

HISTORY

Question: Has this child or a sibling had pinworms before or recently?
Significance: Eggs can survive for several days in the environment, and the incubation period can be 1 to 2 months. Spread can occur between family members. Treat all those who are symptomatic, and consider treating close household contacts, especially if repeat infections have occurred.

Question: Does the child itch during the day?
Significance: Pinworm infections usually cause perianal itching during the night or just prior to waking in the morning. Daytime perianal or perivulvar itching or irritation is likely a result of other causes.

Question: Has the child had fevers, diarrhea, or vomiting?
Significance: Pinworms are highly unlikely to cause systemic symptoms (except in rare cases in which they migrate aberrantly).

Question: Can you see worms around the anus at night?
Significance: Pinworms may be seen 2 to 3 hours after the child has gone to sleep. Female worms are 8 to 13 mm, and males are 2 to 5 mm. They may be visible as small, white worms in the perianal area at night.

Physical Examination

- Exam may be normal. Well-appearing child.
- Self-inflicted, perianal excoriation
- Pinworms visible perianally

Laboratory Aids

Test: Transparent tape, "Scotch-tape" test. In the morning, prior to the child awakening and before defecation or washing, the adhesive side of transparent tape is applied to the perianal area.
Significance: After removal, the tape is applied to a glass slide and examined under light microscopy for pinworm ova. Several samples may be necessary to see the pinworms.

Test: Stool or urine samples for ova or parasites.
Significance: Generally not helpful or recommended. Very few ova present in stool (even rarer in the urine).

Test: Blood count for eosinophilia.
Significance: Generally not helpful or recommended. Eosinophilia is not observed because usually there is no tissue invasion.

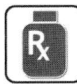

Therapy

Drugs of choice—single drug and dose therapy with one of the following agents:

- Mebendazole, 100 mg (available as a chewable tablet) PO once, may repeat in 2 weeks if symptoms still present.
- Pyrantel Pamoate, 11 mg/kg (maximum 1 g) once, may repeat in 2 weeks.
- Albendazole, 400 mg once, may repeat in 2 weeks.

Experience is limited in children less than 2 years. Consider risks and benefits before use.

PREVENTION

- Decontaminate the environment by washing underclothes, bedclothes, bed sheets, and towels.
- Maintain good hand hygiene, including hand washing and proper toileting.
- Keep fingernails short and avoid nail biting.
- Treat family members and close contacts.

PITFALLS

- Reinfection is common especially if all close contacts are not treated.
- Infection may be asymptomatic but transmitted to others.
- Auto-reinfection can occur if eggs remain under the nails.
- Caution in treating pregnant individuals with antihelminthic medications, because Mebendazole, Pyrantel pamoate, and Albendazole are all Category C and not recommended in pregnancy.

Common Questions and Answers

Q: When can an infected child return to daycare?
A: After receiving the first treatment dose, the child can return to school or daycare. It is prudent to bathe the child and to trim and scrub his/her nails prior to school reentry.

Q: Is it necessary to reevaluate and retest a child once treated?
A: No. However, reinfection is common.

Q: Can pinworm eggs survive on bedding, toilet seats, or clothing?
A: Yes, eggs can remain infectious in an indoor environment for up to 3 weeks.

Q: How do the antihelminthic medications work?
A: They inhibit microtubule function and cause glycogen depletion in the adult worms.

ICD-9-CM 127.4

BIBLIOGRAPHY

Drugs for parasitic infections. *Med Lett Drugs Ther* 2002:1–12. In Abramowicz M Ed. Available from: http://www.medletter.com/freedocs/parasitic.pdf. Accessed. February 26, 2004.

American Academy of Pediatrics. Pinworm Infection (*Enterobius vermicularis*). In: Pickering LK, ed. *2003 Red Book: Report of the Committee on Infectious Diseases.* 26th Ed. Elk Grove Village, IL: American Academy of Pediatrics, 2003:486–487.

Elston DM. What's eating you? Enterobius vermicularis (pinworms, threadworms). *Cutis* 2003;71:268–270.

Grencis RK, Cooper ES. Enterobius, trichuris, capillaria and hookworm including ancylostoma caninum. *Gastroenterol Clin North Am* 1996;25:579–597.

Author: Terry Kind

Plague

Database

DEFINITION

Plague is an enzootic infection that (usually) results in lymphadenitis and fever. Severe constitutional, gastrointestinal, neurologic, and respiratory symptoms (pneumonic plague) can also occur. "The black death" has a secure place in history as a devastating epidemic that affected one-third of the population of Europe during the 14th century.

CAUSES

The illness commonly known as the plague is caused by *Yersinia pestis*, a gram-negative pleomorphic bacillus that is part of the Enterobacteriaceae family.

PATHOLOGY/PATHOPHYSIOLOGY

Dermatologic Portal of Entry

• *Y. pestis* is most commonly transmitted from fleas to humans via the regurgitation of the organism into the bite during the flea's blood meal into a foregut already obstructed with plague organisms. Rodents, as well as dogs, cats, and rabbits, can thereby act as reservoirs of infection by harboring infected fleas. Alternatively, direct skin inoculation of organisms from infected animal tissue or blood can occur through breaks in the skin.
• Lymphatic spread of infection to the regional lymph nodes creates a localized inflammatory response.
• Subsequent hematogenous spread of the organism to other organs results in the production of greater levels of bacterial endotoxin. This endotoxin is responsible for the systemic manifestations, as well as the high mortality rate, of the untreated illness.

Respiratory Portal of Entry

Pneumonic Plague

• Acquired via contact with the saliva or respiratory droplets (either from a human or more commonly in the United States, from a cat with plague pneumonia)
• Replication of the organism within the alveolar spaces results in a fulminant localized infection and endotoxemia.

Other Organ Systems Involved

• Liver
• Spleen
• Kidney
• Meninges

EPIDEMIOLOGY (AGE-RELATED)

• More than half of the contemporary cases of plague occur in persons under 20 years of age, possibly because of an increased tendency for children to come into contact with small animals and rodents.
• An outbreak of the pneumonic plague has been reported recently in India; however, the identification of the specific causative organism has been called into question.
• A large proportion of the cases in the United States have occurred in the Southwest.
• No cases of person-to-person transmissions of plague pneumonia have been reported in the United States since 1925.

CLINICAL PRESENTATIONS

• Bubonic plague: lymphadenitis (usually inguinal); systemic manifestations; 75% of plague cases worldwide
• Septicemic plague: tachycardia, hypotension, other organ involvement; either bubonic or pneumonic (septicemic) plague may progress to pneumonic plague.
• Pneumonic plague: pneumonia; systemic manifestations; rapidly progressive, often fatal

Differential Diagnosis

• Diagnosis of plague follows a high index of suspicion and a thorough review of the patient's lifestyle, travel history, and recent activities.
• The appearance of septicemia and endotoxin-mediated shock includes a large differential diagnosis that includes sepsis as a result of other bacteria or viruses, as well as distributive shock resulting from toxic ingestion or anaphylaxis.

INFECTION

• Recent reports of plague-like illnesses have been associated with infections by other organisms such as *Pseudomonas pseudomallei* (melioidosis) and *Francisella tularensis* (tularemia).
• Streptococcal infections especially between the toes can result in tender inguinal lymph nodes.

Data Gathering

HISTORY

Question: What is the incubation period for this disease?
Significance: There is usually 2 to 6 days between exposure and first presentation of symptoms, but this period can be shorter for pneumonic plague.

Question: In the context of exposure to *Y. pestis*, what are the initial symptoms of exposure?
Significance: Initial symptoms include abrupt onset of fever, weakness, malaise.

Question: What are the initial symptoms of bubonic plague?
Significance: The patient may complain of pain in the groin or axillae prior to lymph node swelling.

Physical Examination

• Patients may present initially with suppurative lymphadenitis in the groin, axillae, or neck regions.
• Patients with rapidly progressive illness are tachycardic, hypotensive, and toxic in appearance. Rashes and fever are more likely to be the initial presentation of patients with an initial pneumonic focus of infection. Other organ system involvement is common.

—Gastrointestinal: Abdominal pain, nausea, and diarrhea are usually as a result of the presence of inflammatory mediators. Hepatosplenomegaly is a common finding.
—Neurologic: Weakness, delirium, and coma are a result of the effects of the endotoxin of *Y. pestis*.

• Patients with septicemia can experience renal (glomerular and parenchymal damage), hematologic (disseminated intravascular coagulation), and hepatic necrosis.

SPECIAL QUESTIONS

• A thorough travel history, especially to the Southwest United States is imperative in order to raise the index of suspicion for diagnosing plague.
• Environmental history should include die offs of rats, ground squirrels, or prairie dogs in the patient's locale.

Laboratory Aids

Test: Total white blood count
Significance: Usually 10,000 to 20,000, but may be as high as 100,000

Test: *Y. pestis* culture
Significance: Can be cultured on blood agar plates from lymph node aspirate, blood, cerebrospinal fluid, or sputum from patients with pneumonic plague.

Test: Gram stain, Wayson stain, Giemsa stain, or fluorescent antibody staining of the specimen.
Significance: May reveal the bipolar organisms.

Test: Comparison of acute and convalescent sera
Significance: Taken 3 to 4 weeks apart, show at least a four-fold increase in antibody titers by passive hemagglutination

Test: ELISA or direct fluorescent antibody (DFA) for *Y. Pestis*
Significance: Detects F1 antigen in blood or bubo during the acute phase of illness

Test: PCR assay for *Y. Pestis* (not available in commercial laboratories)
Significance: Detects, through amplification methods, dead bacteria from bubo aspirate

Emergency Care

For septicemic patients, initial attention should be given to airway management and fluid resuscitation.

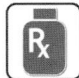 Therapy

DRUGS

- In the acutely ill patient suspected of *Y. pestis* infection, streptomycin (30 mg/kg per day) can be administered by the intravenous or intramuscular route. (Strep must be obtained from CDC, which takes too long. Use gentamicin in full doses.)
- Tetracycline (20 to 30 mg/kg IV per day), or chloramphenicol (75 to 100 mg/kg per day IV), should be added in severe cases or if meningitis is present.
- For the patient who does not require hospitalization, streptomycin (30 mg/kg per day), tetracycline (20 to 30 mg/kg per day) or chloramphenicol (75 to 100 mg/kg per day) may be administered enterally after cultures are obtained.
- Drainage of affected lymph nodes or abscesses, if necessary, should wait until there is persisting fever and a fluctuant node.

DURATION

Therapy continued for at least 10 days. Severely ill patients may require a substantially longer course of therapy. Patients treated with streptomycin can be switched to other medications a few days after improvement is noted.

POSSIBLE CONFLICTS WITH OTHER TREATMENTS

To avoid permanent dental staining, patients younger than 8 years of age should not receive tetracycline unless absolutely necessary.

PREVENTION

- General prevention: Suppression (or flea deinfestation) of the rodent population in endemic areas, as well as deinfestation of cats and dogs, may reduce the prevalence of disease considerably.
- Hospital isolation (negative pressure) should be continued for 3 days after initiation of therapy.

—Pneumonic plague patients require strict respiratory and secretion isolation precautions.
—Bubonic plague patients with no evidence of pneumonia require drainage and secretion precautions (after 24 hours of respiratory isolation and a persistently clear chest radiograph).

- Exposed persons: All contacts of patients thought to suffer from plague should undergo:

—Deinfestation of all clothing, pets, bedding, and homes
—Observation for fever or symptoms of disease for 7 to 10 days (inpatient or outpatient)

- Persons who have had contact with a patient with pneumonic plague require antimicrobial prophylaxis with tetracycline (15 mg/kg per day). For children under 8 years old, use trimethoprim-sulfamethoxazole (40 mg/kg per day), or IM streptomycin (20 mg/kg per day) for a total of 7 days.
- State public health authorities should be notified in cases of suspected plague.
- Vaccination with a five-vaccine regimen (three primary and two boosters) of inactivated whole-cell product is indicated for:

—Persons who intend to travel to or reside in endemic regions in which the domestic rats are infested.
—Laboratory workers or other professional who will be in contact with potentially infected rodents or their fleas
—Booster doses should continue every 1 to 2 years as long as the exposure exists.

 Follow-Up

WHEN TO EXPECT IMPROVEMENT

Resolution of symptoms should begin in the first 3 days after initiation of therapy; however, the rate of clinical improvement depends on the initial severity of illness.

SIGNS TO WATCH FOR

Neurologic sequelae of the plague often manifest during the course of treatment for the illness.

PITFALLS

- Failing to consider septicemic plague in the appropriate epidemiologic setting and withholding appropriate antibiotics or using an empiric betalactam
- Certain strains of *Y. pestis* are resistant to streptomycin. In general, these organisms are sensitive to chloramphenicol.
- A high index of suspicion is needed to diagnose plague. Patients who present with fever, tachycardia, or tachypnea, rather than lymphadenitis, are at higher risk for delayed diagnosis and serious sequelae, i.e., septicemic plague.

 Common Questions and Answers

Q: Can one determine the risks of being exposed to plague during international travel?
A: Yes. The CDC provides a service that contains updated information for international travel. This automated traveler's hotline is accessible from a touch-tone telephone at all hours. The telephone number is (404) 332–4559. Similar information is available by facsimile at (404) 332–4565.

Q: Does persistent fever during treatment for plague warrant altering the antibiotic regimen?
A: No, fever can persist for up to 2 weeks after appropriate antibiotic therapy for plague.

ICD-9-CM 020.9

BIBLIOGRAPHY

American Academy of Pediatrics. Plague. *2003 Red Book: Report of the Committee on Infectious Diseases.* 25th Ed. Elk Grove IL: American Academy of Pediatrics, 2003.

Centers for Disease Control and Prevention. Fatal human plague—Arizona and Colorado, 1996. *MMWR Morb Mortal Wkly Rep* 1997;46: 617–620.

Centers for Disease Control and Prevention. Human plague—United States, 1993–1994. *MMWR Recomm Rep* 1994;43:242–246.

Centers for Disease Control and Prevention. Update: human plague—India, 1994. *MMWR Morb Mortal Wkly Rep* 1994;43:722–723.

Cleri DJ, Vernaleo Jr, Lombardi LJ, et al. Plague pneumonia disease caused by *Yersinia pestis. Semin Respir Infect* 1997;12:12–23.

Crook LD, Tempest B. Plague: a clinical review of 27 cases. *Arch Intern Med* 1992;152:1253.

Darling RG, Catlett CL, Huebner KD, Jarrett DG. Threats in bioterrorism. I: CDC category A agents. *Emerg Med Clin North Am* 2002;20(2): 273–309.

Gage KL, Dennis DT, Orloski KA, et al. Cases of cat-associated human plague in the western US, 1977–1998. *Clin Infect Dis* 2000;30: 893–900.

Gomez NF, Cleary TG. *Yersinia* species. In: Long SS, Pickering LK, eds. *Principles and Practice of Pediatric Infectious Diseases.* New York: Churchill Livingstone, 1997:935–939.

Krishna G, Chitkara RK. Pneumonic plague. *Semin Respir Infect* 2003;18(3):159–167.

Perry RD, Featherston JD. *Yersinia pestis*—etiologic agent of plague. *Clin Microbiol Rev* 1997;10:35–66.

Rahalson L, Vololonirina M, Ratsitornahina M, et al. Diagnosis of bubonic plague by PCR in Madagascar under field conditions. *J Clin Microbiol* 2000;38:260–263.

Authors: Bruce Tempest
Joel A. Fein, 3rd edition

Pleural Effusion

Database

DEFINITION

Accumulation of fluid in the pleural cavity

CAUSES

- There is normally 1 to 15 mL of fluid in the pleural space.
- Alterations in the flow and/or absorption of this fluid leads to its accumulation.
- Mechanisms influence this flow of fluid:
—Increased capillary hydrostatic pressure (e.g., congestive heart failure, overhydration)
—Decreased pleural space hydrostatic pressure (e.g., postthoracentesis, atelectasis)
—Decreased plasma oncotic pressure (e.g., hypoalbuminemia, nephrosis)
—Increased capillary permeability (e.g., infection, toxins, connective tissue diseases, malignancy)
—Impaired lymphatic drainage from the pleural space (e.g., disruption of the thoracic duct)
—Passage of fluid from the peritoneal cavity through the diaphragm to the pleural space (e.g., hepatic cirrhosis with ascites)

PATHOPHYSIOLOGY

- Dependent on the underlying disease
- Two types of pleural effusion:
—Transudate: Mechanical forces of hydrostatic and oncotic pressures are altered, favoring liquid filtration.
—Exudate: Damage to the pleural surface occurs that alters its ability to filter pleural fluid; lymphatic drainage is diminished
- Stages associated with parapneumonic effusions (infectious exudates):
—Exudative stage: free flowing fluid; pleural fluid glucose, protein, LDH, and pH are normal
—Fibrinolytic stage: loculations are forming; increase in fibrin, polymorphonuclear leukocytes, and bacterial invasion of pleural cavity are occurring; pleural fluid glucose and pH falls although protein and LDH increase
—Organizing stage (empyema): fibroblasts grow; pleural peal forms; pleural fluid parameters worsen

EPIDEMIOLOGY

- Dependent on underlying cause
—Pneumonia (most common cause effusion)
—For parapneumonic effusion, the most common organisms include:
—*Staphylococcus aureus* (increasing incidence of methicillin-resistant species)
—*Streptococcus pneumoniae* (increasing incidence of penicillin–resistant species)
—*Haemophilus influenzae* (decreasing incidence since introduction of HiB vaccine)
—No identified organisms (all cultures sterile)
—Congenital heart disease
—Malignancy

COMPLICATIONS

- Hypoxia
- Respiratory distress
- Persistent fevers
- Decreased cardiac function
- Malnutrition (seen in chylothorax)
- Shock (secondary to blood loss in cases of hemothorax)
- Trapped lung

PROGNOSIS

- Dependent on underlying disease process:
—Properly treated infectious etiology: excellent prognosis
—Malignancy: poor prognosis

Differential Diagnosis

TRANSUDATE

- Cardiovascular
—Congestive heart failure
—Constrictive pericarditis
- Nephrotic syndrome with hypoalbuminemia
- Cirrhosis
- Atelectasis

EXUDATE

- Infection
—Bacterial effusions (*S. aureus* is most common organism)
—Tuberculous effusion
—Viral effusions: adenovirus; influenza

—Fungal effusions: most not associated with effusions; Nocardia and Actinomyces are most common
—Parasitic effusions
- Neoplasm
—Seen mostly in leukemia and lymphoma
—Uncommon in children
- Connective tissue disease
—Rheumatoid arthritis
—Systemic lupus erythematosus
—Wegener granulomatosis
- Pulmonary embolus
- Intraabdominal disease
—Subdiaphragmatic abscess
—Pancreatitis
- Others
—Sarcoidosis
—Esophageal rupture
—Hemothorax
—Chylothorax
—Drugs
—Chemical injury
—Postirradiation effusion

Data Gathering

HISTORY

- Underlying disease determines most of systemic symptoms
- The patient may be asymptomatic until the amount of fluid is large enough to cause cardiorespiratory distress
- Dyspnea and cough are associated with large effusions
- Fever
- Pleuritic pain (pneumonia may cause irritation of the parietal pleura causing pleural pain; as the effusion increases and separates the pleural membrane, the pain may disappear)

Physical Examination

- Decreased thoracic wall excursion on the ipsilateral side
- Fullness of intercostal spaces on the ipsilateral side
- Trachea and cardiac apex displaced toward the contralateral side (may produce a mediastinal shift that can reduce venous return and compromise the cardiac output)
- Dull or flat percussion on the ipsilateral side (suggesting the presence of consolidation of pleural effusion)
- Decreased tactile and vocal fremitus
- Decreased whispering pectoriloquy
- Pleural rub during early phase (may resolve as fluid accumulates in the pleural space)
- Decreased breath sounds

Laboratory Aids

- Tests

—Thoracentesis: indicated whenever etiology is unclear or effusion is symptomatic

Pleural Fluid Analysis

TEST	TRANSUDATE	EXUDATE
pH	7.4	<7.3
Protein (g/100 mL)	<3.0	≥3.0
Pleural/serum protein	<0.5	≥0.5
LDH (IU)	<200	≥200
Pleural/serum LDH	<0.6	≥0.6
Pleural/serum amylase	<1	≥1
Glucose (mg/dL)	>40	≤40
RBC	<5,000	≥5,000
WBC	<1,000 (mostly mononuclear cells)	<1,000 (mostly PMNs)

—Pleural biopsy: if thoracentesis is nondiagnostic; most useful for diseases that cause extensive involvement of the pleura (e.g., tuberculosis, malignancies); confirms neoplastic involvement in 40% to 70% of cases
—Serology values (to follow the degree of inflammation and the response to therapy):
   —Erythrocyte sedimentation rate (ESR); C reactive protein (CRP)
• Imaging
—Chest radiograph (upright film): anteroposterior projection can see pleural fluid when there is >400 mL; lateral projection can see pleural fluid when there is <200 mL
—Chest radiograph (lateral decubitus film); can evaluate for free-flowing pleural fluid; can identify as little as 50 mL of pleural fluid
—Ultrasound: can diagnose small (3 to 5 mL) loculated collections of pleural fluid; useful as a guide for thoracentesis; can distinguish between pleural thickening and pleural effusion
—CT scan: can clearly identify effusions/empyemas, abscess, or pulmonary consolidations; useful for defining the extent of loculated effusions

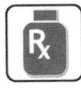 ## Therapy

OVERVIEW

• Supportive measures
—Maintain adequate oxygenation, fluid status, and nutritional balance
—Antipyretic agents when febrile
—Pain control
—Note: pleural fluid glucose of less than 40 mg/dL suggests a parapneumonic, tuberculosis, malignant, or rheumatic etiology to the effusion.
• Treat the underlying disease
—Antibiotics for infections
—Cardiac medications for congestive heart failure
—Chemotherapeutic agents for malignancies
—Antiinflammatory agents (e.g., steroids) for connective tissue diseases
—Medium-chain triglycerides and low-fat diet for chylothorax
• Effective drainage of pleural fluid
—Thoracentesis
—Chest tube drainage
—Surgical drainage

DRAINAGE METHODS

• Thoracentesis
—For diagnosis (to distinguish between a transudate and an exudate; for culture material if infection is suspected)
—For relief of dyspnea or cardiorespiratory distress
• Chest tube thoracostomy
—Reduce reaccumulation of fluid
—Drain parapneumonic effusion (before loculations prevent drainage)
• Intrapleural fibrinolytics
—Adjunct to complete drainage in complicated (e.g., multiloculated empyema) pleural effusions
—Streptokinase and urokinase are agents of choice

SURGICAL MANAGEMENT

• Video-assisted thoracic surgery (VATS)
—Alternative to more invasive procedures (e.g., open thoracotomy/decortication)
—Débridement through pleural visualization and lysis of adhesions/loculations
—Useful when initial drainage is delayed, when loculations prevent adequate drainage, or patient is failing more conservative therapy
• Open thoracotomy with rib resection
—Encapsulated empyema
• Decortication
—Symptomatic chronic empyema
—Relief of thick fibrous peal
• Pleurectomy
—Chylothorax
—Malignant effusions
• Pleurodesis
—For recurrent effusions
—Chemical agents frequently used: tetracycline, doxycycline, talc, quinacrine
—Surgical methods include mechanical abrasion, pleurectomy via VATS, or open thoracotomy route

ANTIBIOTICS

• Used when effusion is caused by an infection
• Specific antibiotics dictated by organism identified
• If effusion is sterile, broad-spectrum antibiotics are indicated to cover for the usual organisms.

DURATION OF THERAPY

• Drainage
—Stopped when patient is asymptomatic (afebrile, no distress) and drainage <50 mL/hour
—Thick, loculated empyema requires prolonged drainage (and possibly a VATS procedure if not improving).
• Antibiotics
—Clinical improvement usually occurs in 48 to 72 hours
—Dependent on organism and degree of illness (total duration is controversial; usually at least 3 to 4 weeks minimum of total IV + PO)
—Should remain on IV antibiotics until afebrile
—Complete remainder of therapy on oral antibiotics

DIET

• Chylothorax
—Medium-chain triglycerides
—Nutritional replacement
—(At least) 4 to 5 weeks on this regimen

 ## Follow-Up

WHEN TO EXPECT IMPROVEMENT

• Clinical improvement usually within 1 to 2 weeks
• With empyemas, may have fever spikes for up to 2 to 3 weeks after improvement noted

PITFALLS

• Cytologic examination
—Fresh and heparinized specimen should be refrigerated at 4°C until it can be processed.
—Fixatives should not be added.
• Malignant effusions
—Sclerosing procedures usually ineffective
—Chest tube drainage can create a pneumothorax because the lung is incarcerated by the tumor.

 ## Common Questions and Answers

Q: How long of a treatment course of antibiotics is required for empyemas?
A: Dependent on the underlying organism; usually between 2 to 4 weeks total of IV/PO.

Q: When will the chest radiograph normalize?
A: May take up to 6 months (or longer) to normalize.

Q: When will the pulmonary function tests normalize?
A: Dependent on extent of effusion, it may take up to 6 to 12 months.

ICD-9-CM 511.9

BIBLIOGRAPHY

Buckingham SC, King MD, Miller ML. Incidence and etiologies of complicated parapneumonic effusions in children. *Pediatr Infect Dis* 2003;22:499–504.

de Benedictis FM, De Giorgi G, Niccoli A, et al. Treatment of complicated pleural effusion with intracavitary urokinase in children. *Pediatr Pulmonol* 2000;29(6):438–442.

Doski JJ, Lou D, Hicks BA, et al. Management of parapneumonic collections in infants and children. *J Pediatr Surg* 2000;35:265–268; discussion 269–270.

Givan DC, Eigen H. Common pleural effusions in children. *Clin Chest Med* 1998;19:363–371.

Heffner JE. Infection of the pleural space. *Clin Chest Med* 1999;20:607–622.

Merino JM, Carpintero I, Alvarez T, et al. Tuberculous pleural effusion in children. *Chest* 1999;115(1):26–30.

Montgomery M. Air and liquid in the pleural space. In: Chernick V, eds. *Kendig's Disorders of the Respiratory Tract in Children.* Philadelphia: WB Saunders, 1998:389–411.

Ramnath RR, Heller RM, Ben-Ami T, et al. Implications of early sonographic evaluation of parapneumonic effusions in children with pneumonia. *Pediatrics* 1998;101(1 Pt 1): 68–71.

Author: Richard M. Kravitz

Pneumocystis Jiroveci (Previously Known as *P. Carinii*) Pneumonia

Database

DEFINITION

Opportunistic lung infection caused by *P. jiroveci* (PJ). This organism is currently considered a primitive fungus based on DNA sequence analysis. It has two developmental forms: a cyst containing sporozoites and an extracystic one named trophozoite.

• The acronym PCP is still in use and refers to Pneumocystis pneumonia. PCP occurs almost exclusively in the immunocompromised host. Children with congenital or acquired immune deficiency syndrome (AIDS), and recipients of suppressive therapy in the treatment of malignancies or after organ transplantation are at high risk.
• PCP is an AIDS-defining illness. It is the most common opportunistic life-threatening lung infection in infants with perinatally acquired HIV disease.
• PJ causes a diffuse pneumonitis characterized by fever, dyspnea at rest, tachypnea, hypoxemia, nonproductive cough and bilateral diffuse infiltrates in the roentgenogram. It is a severe condition frequently leading to respiratory failure necessitating intubation and mechanical ventilation.
• Chemoprophylaxis against this microorganism has proven successful. Therefore, early identification of the HIV-infected mother becomes essential.
• Despite advances in therapy, infection continues to carry severe morbidity and mortality.

PATHOPHYSIOLOGY

• In the immunodeficient child the pathologic changes occur predominantly in the alveoli. Cysts and trophozoites are seen adhering to the alveolar lining cells or in the cytoplasm of macrophages.
• As infection progresses, the alveolar spaces are filled with a pink, foamy exudate containing fibrin, abundant desquamative cells, and large number of organisms. Alveolar septal thickening with mononuclear cell infiltration is also seen.

EPIDEMIOLOGY

• Ubiquitous in mammals worldwide.
• Growth in respiratory tract surfaces.
• Mode of transmission is unknown.

—Airborne person-to-person transmission is possible, but case contacts are rarely identified.
—Environmentally acquired.

• Asymptomatic infection appears early in life; more than 70% of healthy individuals have antibodies by age 4.
• Primary infection is likely to be the prominent mechanism in infants, whereas reactivation of latent disease may play a significant role later in life.

• PCP in the HIV patient can occur at any time, but usually presents during the first year of life. The greatest incidence is between 3 and 6 months of age.
• In patients with leukemia, the incidence of PCP has been directly related to the degree of immunodeficiency resulting from chemotherapy.
• Epidemics of PCP were reported in premature and malnourished infants during wartime. This type has been termed the infantile form.

COMPLICATIONS

High rate of respiratory failure necessitating intubation and mechanical ventilation (about 60%)

PROGNOSIS

• Five percent to 40% mortality in treated patients
• Near 100% mortality if patient is untreated
• About 35% of patients will have reoccurrence unless lifetime prophylaxis is instituted.

Differential Diagnosis

VIRAL INFECTIONS

• Common viral respiratory pathogens
• Cytomegalovirus
• Epstein-Barr virus

BACTERIAL INFECTIONS

• *Mycobacterium tuberculosis*
• *Mycobacterium avium-intracellulare*

OTHER

Lymphocytic interstitial pneumonitis

Data Gathering

HISTORY

Question: Malnourished?
Significance: Infantile form has a subacute onset with nonspecific manifestations:

• Poor feeding, weight loss, and restlessness
• Chronic diarrhea
• Usually without fever
• After 1 to 2 weeks, the patient develops progressive tachypnea, respiratory distress, and cough.

Question: Sporadic or immunocompromised host?
Significance: This form has a more abrupt onset, even a fulminant one:

• Fever (>38.5°C)
• Nonproductive cough
• Dyspnea at rest

These forms are general clinical guidelines. Symptoms may be superimposed and can be seen in infants, children, and adolescents.

Physical Examination

Finding: Fever and significant tachypnea
Significance: Are characteristic

Finding: Hypoxemia
Significance: Early in the course of disease that seems disproportionate with the auscultatory findings

Finding: Rapidly progressive respiratory distress with cyanosis
Significance: Respiratory failure early in course

Finding: Absence of crackles
Significance: A common initial finding

Finding: Chest auscultation
Significance: Can reveal decreased breath sounds, crackles, and rhonchi

Finding: Coryza and wheezing
Significance: Have infrequently been reported

Laboratory Aids

Test: Arterial blood gas
Significance:

• pH is usually increased
• Reduced PaO_2 in room air (<70 mmHg)
• Alveolar-arterial oxygen gradient (>30 mmHg)
• Decreased $PaCO_2$

Test: Chest radiograph
Significance:

• Most common radiologic presentation is diffuse bilateral alveolar infiltrates:

—Initially of perihilar distribution with spread to the periphery
—Apices are the least affected
—Interstitial infiltrates and air bronchograms can be seen
—Rapid progression to whole lung consolidation

• Presence of hilar or mediastinal adenopathy may indicate another process such as *M. tuberculosis*, *M. avium-intracellulare*, fungal infections, cytomegalovirus, or lymphoma.

Test: Lactate dehydrogenase (LDH)
Significance: Can be elevated in patients with AIDS and PCP, but this finding is nonspecific.

Test: White blood count
Significance: Is usually normal

Pneumocystis Jiroveci (Previously Known as *P. Carinii*) Pneumonia

PATHOLOGY

• Definitive diagnosis can be obtained by demonstration of PJ in pulmonary specimens:

—Induced sputum
—Bronchoalveolar lavage (BAL) (90% sensitivity), usually through flexible bronchoscopy
—Open lung or transbronchial biopsy

Test: Staining
Significance:

• Cysts stain with Gomori methenamine-silver nitrate or toluidine blue-O stains
• Sporozoite and trophozoites are identified with polychrome stains (Giemsa, Wright, polychrome methylene blue)
• Immunofluorescent monoclonal antibodies (high sensitivity)

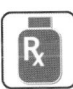 Therapy

ANTIBIOTICS

• Trimethoprim-sulfamethoxazole (TMP-SMX) is the drug of choice.

—TMP (15 to 20 mg/kg per day) and SMX (75 to 100 mg/kg per day) IV or PO divided every 6 hours.
—Oral therapy is reserved for patients with mild illness who do not have malabsorption or diarrhea.
—Minimum 2 weeks; 3 weeks of therapy recommended in patients with AIDS.

ALTERNATIVE THERAPY

• Pentamidine isethionate

—4 mg/kg per day IV (or IM) given in a single daily dose for minimum 2 weeks.
—Total daily dose should not exceed 300 mg.
—Used in patients who cannot tolerate TMP-SMX or unresponsive after 5 to 7 days of therapy.
—Same efficacy as TMP-SMX, but with higher incidence of side effects.
—Concomitant use with didanosine increases the risk of pancreatitis.

• Atovaquone is approved for adults who cannot tolerate TMP-SMX.

—Limited pediatric experience. Suggested dose is 40 mg/kg daily divided b.i.d.

SUPPORTIVE THERAPY

• Supply oxygen as necessary to keep PaO_2 above 70 mmHg
• Mechanical ventilation must be considered if PaO_2 is less than 60 mmHg on FiO_2 of 0.5
• Corticosteroids

—May be beneficial in HIV patients with moderate to severe PCP
—Not systematically evaluated in children
—Consider when PaO_2 is less than 70 mmHg or the alveolar-arterial gradient is greater than 35 mmHg

—In patients over 13 years of age: prednisone 40 mg PO b.i.d. for days 1 to 5, 40 mg PO q.d. for days 6 to 10, 20 mg PO q.d. for days 11 to 21. Younger patients may receive 2 mg/kg per day of prednisone for 7 to 10 days followed by a tapering dose over the next 10 to 14 days.

PROPHYLAXIS

• During high-risk periods, PCP can be effectively prevented in the immunodeficient host by chemoprophylaxis in the following groups:

—HIV-exposed: 4 weeks to 4 months of age
—HIV-infected or indeterminate: 4 to 12 months of age
—HIV-infected: 1 to 5 years of age if CD4+ T-lymphocyte count is <500 cells/μL or percentage is <15%
—HIV-infected: >5 years of age if CD4+ T-lymphocyte count is <200 cells/μL or percentage is <15%
—Severely symptomatic HIV patient or with rapidly declining CD4+ count
—HIV patients who had previous episode of PCP
—HIV-exposed: birth to 4 to 6 weeks require no prophylaxis
—Children who have received hematopoietic stem cell transplants (HSCT)
—All HSCT recipients with hematologic malignancies (e.g., leukemia, lymphoma)
—All HSCT recipients receiving intense conditioning regimens or graft manipulation
—Prophylaxis is initiated at engraftment and administered for 6 months, and longer than 6 months in children receiving immunosuppressive therapy or with chronic graft vs. host disease

RECOMMENDED STRATEGY

• TMP (150 mg/m^2 per day) with SMX (750 mg/m^2 per day) PO divided b.i.d. daily on 3 consecutive days per week, or
• TMP (5 mg/kg per day) and SMX (25 mg/kg per day) PO divided b.i.d. daily on 3 consecutive days per week.

ALTERNATIVE REGIMEN

• Dapsone (>1 month of age) 2 mg/kg (100 mg maximum) PO once daily
• Aerosolized pentamidine (<5 years old)

—300 mg via Respirgard II inhaler once monthly

• Atovaquone

—1 to 3 months and >24 months: 30 mg/kg orally once daily
—4 to 24 months: 45 mg/kg orally once daily

• If neither dapsone nor pentamidine is tolerated, IV pentamidine 4 mg/kg administered every 2 to 4 weeks is recommended.

 Follow-Up

WHEN TO EXPECT IMPROVEMENT

• After 5 to 7 days of treatment
• If no improvement, TMP-SMX should be replaced with pentamidine.

ISOLATION OF HOSPITALIZED PATIENT

Standard precautions required. Isolation from other immunodeficient patients is recommended.

PITFALLS

• HIV-infected patients have a higher rate (15%) of adverse reactions (rash, fever, neutropenia, anemia, renal dysfunction, nausea, vomiting and diarrhea) to TMP-SMX than the general population
• Prophylaxis is protective as long as the drug is administered, but does not eradicate PJ.
• Aerosolized pentamidine prophylaxis failure is usually associated with organisms in the upper lobes. BAL of this area becomes the procedure of choice.

 Common Questions and Answers

Q: What are the most common side effects of pentamidine?
A: Side effects include hypoglycemia, impaired renal or liver function, anemia, thrombocytopenia, neutropenia, hypotension, and skin rashes, and can be expected in 50% of patients.

Q: How frequently is prophylaxis failure seen?
A: Appropriate TMP-SMX treatment has only a 3% failure rate.

Q: What is the recommended course of action if adverse reactions to TMP-SMX are seen during PCP therapy?
A: Continuation of treatment, if the reactions are not severe, is recommended.

ICD-9-CM 136.3

BIBLIOGRAPHY

Abrams EJ. Opportunistic infections and other clinical manifestations of HIV disease in children. *Pediatr Clin North Am* 2000;47:79–103.

American Academy of Pediatrics. *2003 Red Book: Report of the Committee on Infectious Diseases.* 26th Ed. Elk Grove Village, IL: American Academy of Pediatrics. 2003:500–505.

Hughes WT. Pneumocystis carinii pneumonitis. In: Chernick V, ed. *Kendig's Disorders of the Respiratory Tract in Children.* 46th Ed. Philadelphia: WB Saunders, 1998:503–511.

Authors: Danna Tauber
Roberto V. Nachajon, 3rd edition

Pneumonia—Bacterial

 Database

DEFINITION

- Inflammation of lung tissue secondary to bacterial infection. Can be recognized by clinical signs and symptoms and/or pulmonary infiltrate(s) on chest radiograph

CAUSES

- Group B streptococci (newborns)
- *Listeria monocytogenes* (newborns)
- *Enterococcus* (newborns)
- *Escherichia coli* (newborns)
- *Chlamydia trachomatis* (young infants)
- *Streptococcus pneumoniae* (25–30% of all cases)
- *Staphylococcus aureus*
- *Moraxella catarrhalis*
- Group A streptococci
- *Haemophilus influenzae*; type b and nontypable
- *Mycoplasma pneumoniae* (generally seen in school-aged children)
- *Bordetella pertussis*
- *Chlamydia pneumonia* (school-aged children)
- *Legionella pneumophila*
- *Mycobacterium tuberculosis*

EPIDEMIOLOGY

- Four percent of children per year in the United States are diagnosed with pneumonia from any cause.
- Highest incidence in children less than one year of age

PREDISPOSING FACTORS

- Cystic fibrosis, sickle cell anemia, cerebral palsy, immunodeficiency (e.g., HIV disease or AIDS), malignancy, tracheoesophageal fistula, congenital pulmonary malformations, bronchopulmonary dysplasia), seizure disorder, altered mental status

COMPLICATIONS

- Pleural effusion, empyema, lung abscess, pneumatoceles, pneumothorax, bacteremia/sepsis

PROGNOSIS

- Otherwise healthy children with uncomplicated pneumonia typically have rapid improvement with treatment (3 to 5 days).

 Differential Diagnosis

INFECTIOUS

- Viral pneumonia, bronchiolitis, upper respiratory tract infection (URI), croup (laryngotracheobronchitis), sepsis, fungal infection, parasitic infection

PULMONARY

- Asthma, atelectasis, pneumonitis (e.g., chemical), Pulmonary hemorrhage
- Pulmonary embolism

CONGENITAL

- Pulmonary sequestration

GENETIC

- Cystic fibrosis

TUMORS

- Lymphoma, primary lung tumor, metastatic tumor

MISCELLANEOUS

- Foreign body aspiration, congestive heart failure, sarcoidosis, gastroesophageal reflux disease

 Data Gathering

HISTORY

Question: Has the patient had fever and/or chills (hypothermia in neonates)?
Significance: May indicate bacterial infection

Question: Is the patient experiencing difficulty breathing, or rapidly breathing?
Significance: Often seen in bacterial pneumonia. Also seen in other lower respiratory tract diseases

Question: Has the patient had chest pain?
Significance: Can indicate pleuritis. In children, can rarely be a sign of cardiac disease.

Question: Has the patient been coughing? Describe the cough.
Significance: Cough is often seen in bacterial pneumonia. The character and duration of the cough can help you identify an etiology. For example, *B. pertussis* pneumonia often presents with a paroxysmal cough and post-tussive vomiting.

Question: Does the patient have abdominal pain and/or vomiting?
Significance: Lower lobe pneumonia can present with abdominal pain.

Question: Does the patient have irritability, lethargy and/or malaise?
Significance: These can all be signs of significant bacterial infection.

Question: In young infants, has the patient had poor feeding or apnea?
Significance: Poor feeding may be a sign of more significant infection. It may also be a symptom of congestive heart failure. Apnea can be seen in infants who have *B. pertussis* infection.

Question: For infants less than 3 months of age, what was the birth history, including maternal infections?
Significance: C. trachomatis can be transmitted to an infant through a mother's genital tract at delivery.

Question: What is the child's immunization status?

Significance: In a fully immunized child, *H. influenzae* type b and *B. pertussis* infections are less common.

Question: Is there a recent history of upper respiratory tract infection (URI)?
Significance: Children with URIs can go on to develop both viral and bacterial pneumonia. Physical exam and chest radiograph findings help to distinguish one from the other.

Question: Is there a family history of significant chronic medical illnesses, such as cystic fibrosis or sickle cell anemia?
Significance: Certain illnesses (i.e., cystic fibrosis) are risk factors for bacterial pneumonia.

Question: Is there exposure to sick contacts, including day care exposure?
Significance: This can increase a patient's risk of infection, particularly for highly contagious organisms, such as *B. pertussis*.

Question: Does the patient have any risk factors for tuberculosis, or recent travel?
Significance: Travelers, health care workers, and those working in prisons or institutional settings are at greater risk for tuberculosis.

Question: Is there exposure to pets or tobacco smoke?
Significance: Cigarette smoke and contact with pets may precipitate an allergic or asthma exacerbation.

 Physical Examination

Finding: Ill appearance
Significance: Most children with bacterial pneumonia appear ill. General examination can range from mildly ill appearing to toxic in appearance. Patients can be dehydrated or in shock.

Finding: Fever
Significance: Most children with bacterial pneumonia have fever. Patients with atypical bacterial pneumonia are sometimes afebrile.

Finding: Tachypnea or increased work of breathing (flaring, grunting and/or retracting)
Significance: These are very useful clinical predictors of pneumonia.

Finding: Decreased oxygen saturation
Significance: Should raise the suspicion for pneumonia.

Finding: Localized rales, rhonchi, decreased breath sounds or wheezing
Significance: These are all significant clinical findings of pneumonia. Crackles and rhonchi are essentially diagnostic of pneumonia.

 Laboratory Aids

TESTS

Not indicated for patients with uncomplicated pneumonia

Test: Blood culture
Significance: Not usually indicated in healthy children with uncomplicated pneumonia. Should be obtained in severely ill patients,

patients with abnormal immunity and infants <3 months of age. Unlikely to lead to identification of pathogen causing pneumonia.

Test: Cold agglutinin test
Significance: A positive test suggests *M. pneumoniae*. This test is usually not indicated since empiric treatment of this pathogen is typically safe and effective

Test: Purified protein derivative (PPD) test
Significance: Should be obtained in all patients in whom *M. tuberculosis* is suspected

RADIOLOGIC STUDIES

Test: Chest radiograph, upright
Significance: Alveolar or lobar infiltrate with air bronchograms are typically seen in bacterial pneumonia. "Round" infiltrates may be seen with *S. pneumococcus*. Diffuse interstitial infiltrates and hyperinflation may be seen with atypical pneumonia such as *M. pneumoniae* or *Chlamydia pneumonias*. It is important to realize that an infiltrate may not be seen if it is early in the disease course, or if the patient is dehydrated. A chest radiograph is not required for diagnosis if clinical symptoms clearly suggest uncomplicated pneumonia. However, a chest x-ray should typically be obtained if pneumonia is suspected but clinical findings are unclear, if a pleural effusion or other complication is suspected, if the patient has evidence of respiratory distress, if the patient requires admission to the hospital or if the patient is not responding to treatment. Consider obtaining a chest radiograph in patients less than 5 years old who have a high fever (>39 degrees) and leukocytosis (>20,000/mm³) but no known source of infection as these patients have a higher likelihood of having bacterial pneumonia.

Test: Chest radiograph, lateral decubitus
Significance: More sensitive than an upright radiograph in detecting pleural effusions or foreign body aspiration.

Test: Computed tomography
Significance: Not recommended as first line imaging for patient with suspected pneumonia. Can help distinguish between empyema and effusion and is useful in helping to interpret ambiguous radiograph findings. It is mainly used as adjunct imaging for patients who are worsening or not improving despite treatment.

ADDITIONAL STUDIES

For severely ill patients who are not responding to treatment or in whom diagnosis is unclear, consider

- Flexible fiberoptic bronchoscopy with bronchoalveolar lavage or lung biopsy
- Transthoracic-needle aspiration
- Thoracentesis if clinically indicated

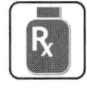

Therapy

OUTPATIENT

Empiric Treatment

- Less than 5 years of age (unless atypical pneumonia suspected based on exposure to sick contacts greater than 5 years old with cough, clinical symptoms or, in infants 4 to 12 weeks of age, perinatal exposure to *C. trachomatis*). Treatment is for 7 to 10 days
—Amoxicillin: 45 to 90 mg/kg per day divided BID or TID
- Consider for additional coverage of *H. influenzae,* nontype b:
- Amoxicillin/clavulanate: 25 to 45 mg/kg per day divided b.i.d. or t.i.d.
- Cefuroxime 30 mg/kg per day divided b.i.d., Cefprozil 30 mg/kg per day divided b.i.d., Cefdinir 14 mg/kg per day divided QD or b.i.d., or Cefpodoxime 10 mg/kg per day divided b.i.d.
- May consider use of Ceftriaxone 50 mg/kg IM to initiate therapy
- For penicillin allergic may use macrolide or cephalosporin
- 5 years of age or greater (unless organism other than atypical pathogen suspected; atypical pathogens are much more common in this age group)
- Erythromycin 30 to 50 mg/kg per day divided every 6 to 8 hours or other macrolide
- May consider tetracycline 25 to 50 mg/kg per day divided q.i.d. in patients 9 years of age and over
- May consider fluoroquinolones in patients 16 years of age and over
- If specific pathogen is known or suspected, use appropriate antibiotic therapy
- For patients with more severe disease may consider combining β-lactamase antibiotic and macrolide.

INPATIENT

- Oxygen as needed to keep oxygen saturations greater than 94% to 95%
- Intubation and positive pressure ventilation if clinically indicated
- Empiric antibiotic treatment
—Less than two months of age
—Ampicillin 200 mg/kg per day divided every 6 to 8 hours plus Cefotaxime 100 to 200 mg/kg per day divided every 6 hours or Gentamicin 6 mg/kg per day divided every 8 hours
—2 months to 5 years of age (if atypical pathogens are not suspected)
—Cefuroxime 75 to 150 mg/kg per day divided every 8 hours, Ceftriaxone 50 to 75 mg/kg per day divided every 12 to 24 hours, or Cefotaxime 100 to 200 mg/kg per day divided every 6 to 8 hours
—For seriously ill patients add Vancomycin 60 mg/kg per day divided every 6 hours
—For antistaphylococcal coverage add nafcillin 50 to 100 mg/kg per day divided every 6 hours, oxacillin 100 to 200 mg/kg per day divided every 4 to 6 hours, cefazolin 50 to 100 mg/kg per day divided every 8 hours or clindamycin 25 to 40 mg/kg per day divided every 6 to 8 hours
—If atypical pneumonia also suspected, may add macrolide
—May also consider macrolides or clindamycin IV as alternative for cephalosporin allergic patients
—Five years of age and older
—Add macrolide to above therapy (however patients with lobar pneumonia are less likely to have atypical pneumonia)

Follow-Up

- If treated as outpatient, follow up within 1 to 3 days (may follow up by phone if patient only appeared mildly ill)
- If worsening or not responding to treatment may need repeat or additional diagnostic studies
- Consider follow up chest radiograph if indicated for severe disease or other complications (e.g., effusion). Note that radiographs may be abnormal for up to 6 weeks after successful treatment.

Common Questions and Answers

Q: What are the indications for admission and inpatient treatment of pneumonia in children?
A: Severe respiratory distress, oxygen requirement, severely ill appearance, dehydration or inability to feed or take oral medications, infants less than 2 months of age, patients with effusion or other complication, history or risk of apnea, patients with abnormal immunity (e.g., neutropenia or HIV disease), or patients with chronic medical conditions which predispose them to more severe disease. Strongly consider in infants <6 months of age or if noncompliance is a major concern.

Q: Why does the recommended treatment for bacterial pneumonia vary by age?
A: The causes of bacterial pneumonia vary significantly by age. The most common pathogens are as follows:
—Age 0 to 4 weeks: (a) Group B *Streptococcus* (b) Gram-negative enteric bacteria (c) *L. monocytogenes*
—Age 4 to 12 weeks: (a) *C. trachomatis* (b) *S. pneumoniae* (c) *B. pertussis*
—Age 12 weeks to 4 years: (a) *S. pneumoniae* (b) *H. influenza* (non-type b) (c) *M. catarrhalis*
—Age 5 years to adolescence: (a) *M. pneumoniae* (b) *C. pneumoniae* (c) *S. pneumoniae*

ICD-9-CM 482.9

BIBLIOGRAPHY

Bradley JS. Management of community-acquired pediatric pneumonia in an era of increasing antibiotic resistance and conjugate vaccines. *Pediatr Infect Dis J* 2002;21: 592–598.

Lerou PH. Lower respiratory tract infections in children. *Curr Opin Pediatr* 2001;13: 200–206.

Lichenstein R, Suggs AH, Campbell J. Pediatric pneumonia. *Emerg Med Clin North Am* 2003;21:437–451.

Tan TQ, Mason EO Jr, Wald ER, et al. Clinical characteristics of children with complicated pneumonia caused by *Streptococcus pneumoniae*. *Pediatrics* 2002;110:1–6.

Author: Lee Ann Savio Beers

Pneumothorax

 Database

DEFINITION

Air in the pleural space

PATHOPHYSIOLOGY

- Air can enter the pleural space via:

—Chest wall (e.g., penetrating trauma)
—Intrapulmonary (e.g., ruptured alveoli)

- Usually collapse of the lung on the affected side seals the leak.
- If a ball valve mechanism ensues, however, air can accumulate in the thoracic cavity, causing a tension pneumothorax (a medical emergency).

CAUSES

- Spontaneous (secondary to rupture of apical blebs)
- Mechanical trauma

—Penetrating injury (e.g., knife or bullet wound)
—Blunt trauma

- Barotrauma

—Mechanical ventilation
—Cough (if severe enough)

- Iatrogenic

—Central venous catheter placement
—Bronchoscopy (especially with biopsy)

- Infection: most common organisms:

—*Staphylococcus aureus*
—*Streptococcus pneumoniae*
—*Mycobacterium tuberculosis*
—*Bordetella pertussis*
—*Pneumocystis carinii*

- Airway occlusion

—Mucus plugging (asthma)
—Foreign body
—Meconium aspiration

- Bleb formation (e.g., idiopathic, secondary to cystic fibrosis)
- Malignancy

EPIDEMIOLOGY

- Dependent on the underlying lung disease
- Spontaneous pneumothorax:

—Incidence: 7.4 to 18/100,000
—Male/female ratio 6:1
—Peak incidence: 10 to 30 years old

- Cystic fibrosis

—Incidence:
  —overall CF population: 5% to 8%
  —CF patients >18 years old: 16% to 20%
    —Risk increases as pulmonary function deteriorates

COMPLICATIONS

- Pain
- Hypoxia
- Respiratory distress
- Tension pneumothorax

—Hypoxia
—Hypercarbia with acidosis
—Respiratory failure

- Pneumomediastinum with subcutaneous emphysema
- Bronchopulmonary fistula

PROGNOSIS

- Dependent on the underlying etiology of the pneumothorax
- If simple, spontaneous pneumothorax recovery is excellent

 Differential Diagnosis

PULMONARY

- Congenital lung malformations

—Cysts (e.g., bronchogenic cysts)
—Cystic adenomatoid malformation
—Congenital lobar emphysema

- Acquired emphysema
- Hyperinflation of the lung
- Postinfectious pneumatocele
- Bullae formation

MISCELLANEOUS

- Diaphragmatic hernia
- Infections (e.g., pulmonary abscess)
- Muscle strain
- Pleurisy
- Rib fracture

 Data Gathering

HISTORY

- Patient may be asymptomatic (pneumothorax discovered on chest film obtained for other reasons)

- Cough
- Shortness of breath
- Dyspnea
- Pleuritic chest pain that is usually sudden in onset and localized to apices (referred pain to shoulders)
- Respiratory distress

SPECIAL QUESTIONS

Question: Does the patient have any underlying medical problems that are associated with an increased risk for pneumothoraces?
Significance: Patients with asthma, cystic fibrosis, pneumonia, or collagen vascular diseases have an increased risk for developing a pneumothorax.

Question: Did the patient do anything prior to developing symptoms that might have caused the pneumothorax?
Significance: Heavy lifting or increased coughing

 Physical Examination

- May be normal
- Decreased breath sounds on the affected side
- Decreased vocal fremitus
- Hyperresonance to percussion on the affected side
- Tachypnea
- Tachycardia
- Shortness of breath
- Respiratory distress
- Shifting of the cardiac point of maximal impulse away from the affected side
- Shifting of the trachea away from the affected side
- Subcutaneous emphysema
- Cyanosis
- Scratch sign: listening through the stethoscope, a loud scratching sound is heard when a finger is gently stroked over the area of the pneumothorax

 Laboratory Aids

Tests:

- Arterial blood gas

—Po$_2$ can frequently be decreased
—Pco$_2$: elevated with respiratory compromise; decreased from hyperventilation

- Pulse oximetry

—Useful for assessing oxygenation

- Electrocardiogram (ECG)

—Diminished amplitude of the QRS voltage
—Rightward shift of the QRS axis (if left-sided pneumothorax)

IMAGING

- Chest radiograph

—Radiolucency of the affected lung
—Lack of lung markings in the periphery of the affected lung
—Collapsed lung on the affected side
—Possible pneumomediastinum with subcutaneous emphysema

- Chest CT

—Useful for finding small pneumothoraces
—Can help distinguish a pneumothorax from a bleb or cyst
—Helpful for locating small apical blebs associated with spontaneous pneumothoraces

Therapy

OVERVIEW

- Stabilization of the patient
- Evacuation of the pleural air

—Should be done urgently if tension pneumothorax is suspected
—In small asymptomatic pneumothoraces, observation of the patient indicated

- Treat the underlying condition predisposing for the pneumothorax:

—Antibiotics for infection
—Bronchodilators and anti-inflammatory agents for asthma attacks

DRUGS

- Oxygen

—Used to keep $SaO_2 \geq 95\%$

Breathing 100% O_2 can speed the intrapleural air's reabsorption into the bloodstream (useful for treating smaller pneumothoraces, especially in neonates) hastening lung reexpansion

SURGERY

- Needle thoracentesis

—Useful for evacuation of the pleural air in simple, uncomplicated spontaneous pneumothorax

- Chest tube drainage

—Used for evacuation of the pleural air in recurrent pneumothoraces, complicated pneumothoraces, and cases with significant underlying lung disease
—Thoracotomy vs. video-assisted thoracoscopic surgery (VATS)

- Surgical removal of pulmonary blebs

—Blebs have a high rate of rupturing with resultant pneumothorax.
—In patients with established pneumothoraces, the blebs should be removed or oversewn to prevent reoccurrence of the pneumothorax (blebs have a high rate of reoccurrence if not repaired).

- Pleurodesis

—Used to attach the lung to the intrathoracic chest wall to prevent reoccurrence of a pneumothorax
—Useful in cases of recurrent pneumothorax or if the pneumothorax is unresponsive to chest tube drainage (e.g., cystic fibrosis, malignancy)
—Mechanism of action: the surface of the lung becomes inflamed and adheres to the chest wall via the formation of scar tissue.
—Two commonly used methods:
—Surgical pleurodesis
—Mechanical abrasion of part of the lung or pleurectomy
—Advantages: very effective: low reoccurrence rate; site specific (limits affected area)

—Disadvantages: requires surgery and general anesthesia; contraindicated if unstable

- Chemical pleurodesis

—Chemicals are used to cause inflammation
—Chemicals commonly used: tetracycline, minocycline, doxycycline, quinacrine
—Advantages: requires no surgery or general anesthesia
—Disadvantages: less effective than surgery; generalized inflammation (rather than site-specific; makes future thoracic surgery more difficult; painful)

DURATION

- Chest tube should be left in until:

—Majority of the air is reabsorbed
—No reaccumulation of air is seen on sealing of the chest tube
—Usually 2 to 4 days

Follow-Up

WHEN TO EXPECT IMPROVEMENT

Symptomatic relief within seconds of the air being evacuated

SIGNS TO WATCH FOR

Unable to remove the chest tube without reaccumulation of air (suggestive of a bronchopulmonary fistula; requires surgical exploration if no improvement in 7 to 10 days)

PITFALLS

- Not considering the diagnosis in otherwise healthy patients
- Confusing the symptoms with those of an underlying lung disease
- Inserting a needle into a cyst or bleb (can cause a tension pneumothorax with rapid respiratory compromise)

Common Question and Answer

Q: Can a pneumothorax reoccur?
A: Reoccurrence is dependent on the underlying cause of the pneumothorax.

- Spontaneous pneumothorax (reoccurrence rates):

—Observation alone: 20% to 50%
—If thoracentesis performed: 25% to 50%
—If chest tube drainage performed: 32% to 38%
—Overall reoccurrence rate: 16% to 52%

- Chemical pleurodesis:

—Twenty-five percent for tetracycline
—Eight percent to 10% for talc

- Surgical pleurodesis:

—Thirteen percent for VATS
—Three percent for thoracotomy
—Zero percent to 4% for thoracotomy with pleurectomy

- Cystic fibrosis (reoccurrence rates):

—If no drainage attempted: 68%
—Thoracentesis alone: 90%
—Chest tube drainage alone: 72%
—Chemical pleurodesis:
—Forty-two percent to 86% for tetracycline
—Twelve and one-half percent for quinacrine
—Eight percent for talc
—Surgical pleurodesis:
—Zero percent to 4% for thoracotomy with pleurectomy

ICD-9-CM 512.8

BIBLIOGRAPHY

Perron AD. Chest pain in athletes. *Clin Sports Med* 2003;22(1):37–50.

Briassoulis GC, Venkataraman ST, Vasilopoulos AG, et al. Air leaks from the respiratory tract in mechanically ventilated children with severe respiratory disease. *Pediatr Pulmonol* 2000;29(2):127–134.

Cook CH, Melvin WS, Groner JI, et al. A cost-effective thoracoscopic treatment strategy for pediatric spontaneous pneumothorax. *Surg Endosc* 1999;13(12):1208–1210.

Flume PA. Pneumothorax in cystic fibrosis. *Chest* 2003;123:217–221.

Jantz MA, Pierson DJ. Pneumothorax and barotrauma. *Clin Chest Med* 1994;15:75–91.

Montgomery M. Air and liquid in the pleural space. *Kendig's Disorders of the Respiratory Tract in Children*. Philadelphia: WB Saunders, 1998:389–411.

Noppen M. Management of primary spontaneous pneumothorax. *Curr Opin Pulm Med* 2003;9(4):272–275.

Sahn SA, Heffner JE. Primary care: spontaneous pneumothorax. *N Engl J Med* 2000;342:868–874.

Ullman EA, Donley LP, Brady WJ. Pulmonary trauma emergency department evaluation and management. *Emerg Med Clin N Am* 2003; 21(2):291–313.

Author: Richard M. Kravitz

Polyarteritis Nodosa

 Database

DEFINITION

An inflammatory process of small and medium-sized muscular arteries resulting in dysfunction of affected organs.

CAUSES

- Idiopathic
- Postinfectious (streptococcal, hepatitis B)

PATHOLOGY

Necrotizing arteritis of small- and medium-sized arteries resulting in segmental fibrinoid necrosis

EPIDEMIOLOGY

- Extremely rare in childhood
- Prevalence equal in boys and girls

GENETICS

No specific HLA types known to be at increased risk

COMPLICATIONS

- Hypertension
- Renal failure
- Digital necrosis
- Intestinal infarction
- Stroke

 Differential Diagnosis

INFECTION

- Bacterial endocarditis
- Brucellosis
- Influenza B (calf pain)

TUMORS

- Left atrial myxoma
- Burkett lymphoma

METABOLIC

- Homocystinuria

CONGENITAL

- Immunologic

—Systemic necrotizing vasculitis
—Systemic lupus erythematosus
—Kawasaki disease
—Systemic juvenile rheumatoid arthritis
—Wegener granulomatosis
—Takayasu arteritis
—Cryoglobulinemia
—Antiphospholipid antibody syndrome

PSYCHOLOGICAL

- Münchhausen syndrome

MISCELLANEOUS

- Degos disease (malignant atrophic papulosis)

 Data Gathering

HISTORY

- Persistent constitutional symptoms?
- Bilateral calf pain?
- Abdominal pain?
- Weight loss?
- Unexplained fever?
- Headache?
- Arthralgia/myalgia?
- Rashes?
- Seizures?
- Weakness?

 Physical Examination

- Assess BP and pulses
- Check skin for livedo reticularis, splinter hemorrhages, erythema nodosum, and necrotic digits
- Neurologic examination for findings consistent with neuropathy (mononeuritis multiplex)
- Ophthalmologic examination for cotton wool spots
- Check testes for tenderness or swelling
- Check muscles for tenderness, especially calves

PHYSICAL EXAMINATION TRICKS

Finding: The lacy network of superficial vessels of livedo reticularis
Significance: Does not blanch and is somewhat tender. Mottling of the skin seen in fair-skinned individuals will blanch and is not tender, and disappears with warming.

 Laboratory Aids

Test: ESR
Significance: Usually extremely elevated; leukocytosis and thrombocytosis are seen.

Test: Urine analysis
Significance: Proteinuria and hematuria can be present.

Test: Cr and BUN
Significance: May be elevated

Test: ANA and RF
Significance: Usually negative

Test: Muscle enzymes (CK, LDH, AST, Aldolase)
Significance: muscle involvement is common, especially in those with calf pain.

Test: Antineutrophil cytoplasmic antibody (ANCA)
Significance: Detectable in some; usually perinuclear (p) type, rarely cytoplasmic (c) type

Test: Hepatitis B serologies
Significance: Hepatitis B has been associated in some series of PAN patients.

Test: Biopsy of affected tissue/organ
Significance: As indicated, usually skin, kidney, nerve, testicle

Test: Streptococcal titers
Significance: Polyarteritis nodosa may develop following streptococcal infections in children.

Test: MRI of tender muscles
Significance: STIR images can show edema so a directed biopsy can be done to avoid false-negative muscle biopsy, which used to be common.

Test: MRA (magnetic resonance angiography) or angiography
Significance: Can demonstrate vessel wall stenoses and aneurysm.

FALSE POSITIVES

Elevated ESR is seldom as a result of PAN. Consequently, a vigorous search for alternate explanations should be sought prior to making this diagnosis.

PITFALLS

The detection of ANCA, previously thought to be highly specific for vasculitis, now appears to be less so. Hence, it remains important to confirm the diagnosis of PAN with biopsy or angiography.

HOME TESTING

May wish to have patients monitor blood pressure periodically if renal involvement suspected

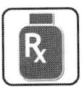 Therapy

DRUGS

- Corticosteroids are mainstay; usually start at dose of 1 to 2 mg/kg per day and adjusting based on response.
- Immunosuppressives such as methotrexate, azathioprine, and cyclophosphamide may be necessary.
- Hypertension should be managed aggressively, especially with calcium channel blockers.

DURATION

May require long-term therapy

DIET

- If renal system involved, low in sodium and potassium
- Possible conflicts with medications

 Follow-Up

WHEN TO EXPECT IMPROVEMENT

Initiation of steroid therapy may bring response in 1 to 2 weeks; however, management of specific organs affected during acute stage is essential.

SIGNS TO WATCH FOR

- Rising creatinine and BUN
- Abdominal pain
- Uncontrolled hypertension

PROGNOSIS

- May be extremely poor over the long term
- Risk high for renal failure, hypertension, stroke, myocardial infarction, bowel infarction, and death
- As a result of low incidence/prevalence, precise data not available

PITFALLS

Initiation of therapy prior to efforts to establish the diagnosis

 Common Questions and Answers

Q: What is the difference between PAN and systemic necrotizing vasculitis?
A: PAN has a fairly strict definition. There are many children who clearly have vasculitis of the small and medium-sized arteries who do not fit precisely into the description of PAN. In most ways the search for organ involvement and therapy is the same.

Q: Who should manage the patient with PAN?
A: Usually one discipline provides comprehensive management plan (either the pediatrician or rheumatologist). Subspecialist(s) of the affected organ systems provide management guidelines for specific organ issues.

ICD-9-CM 446.0

BIBLIOGRAPHY

Cassidy JT, Petty RE. *Textbook of Pediatric Rheumatology.* 4th Ed. Philadelphia: WB Saunders, 2001.

Cuttica RJ. Vasculitis in children: a diagnostic challenge. *Curr Probl Pediatr* 1997;27(8): 309–318.

Fink CW. The role of the streptococcus in poststreptococcal reactive arthritis and childhood polyarteritis nodosa. *J Rheumatol Suppl* 1991;29:14–20.

Hughes LB, Bridges SL Jr. Polyarteritis nodosa and microscopic polyangiitis: etiologic and diagnostic considerations. *Curr Rheumatol Rep* 2002;4(1):75–82.

Ozen S, Besbas N, Saatci U, et al. Diagnostic criteria for polyarteritis nodosa in childhood. *J Pediatr* 1992;120:206–209.

Ozen S. The spectrum of vasculitis in children. *Best Pract Res Clin Rheumatol* 2002;16(3):411–425.

Authors: David D. Sherry and Randy Q. Cron, 3rd edition

Polycystic Kidney Disease

 Database

DEFINITION

Polycystic kidney disease (PKD) is a heritable disorder with diffuse cystic involvement of both kidneys without other dysplastic elements.
There are two forms with considerable overlap in the pediatric population:

• Autosomal-dominant polycystic kidney disease (ADPKD):

—Characterized by the presence of cysts at any point along the nephron or collecting duct
—Occasionally associated with characteristic cardiovascular and GI manifestations
—Referred to as adult polycystic kidney disease because it usually presents with clinical symptoms in the third to fifth decade
—May present in early childhood

• Autosomal-recessive polycystic kidney disease (ARPKD):

—Cystic dilation of renal collecting ducts
—All cases accompanied by hepatic abnormalities such as biliary dysgenesis and periportal fibrosis (congenital hepatic fibrosis)
—Was called infantile polycystic kidney disease but can present at any time from the prenatal period through adolescence

• Diffuse cystic disease occurs in several other conditions in children and adults. Examples include tuberous sclerosis, multicystic dysplastic kidney, and a variety of malformation syndromes. Nephronophthisis and medullary cystic diseases are also germ-line mutations in single genes.

PATHOPHYSIOLOGY

• ARPKD

—In the infant and young child the kidneys are enlarged, spongy, and reniform. The cystic cortical collecting ducts are grossly visible as pinpoint dots on the capsular surface. The dilated ducts are 1 to 2 mm in diameter.
—Microscopic examination reveals medullary ductal ectasia, which is the characteristic feature of ARPKD. The glomeruli and remaining tubular structures are decreased in number.
—In older patients larger renal cysts and fibrosis develop.
—Hepatic involvement is invariably present.

• ADPKD

—Kidneys are enlarged with numerous round protuberances on their surfaces, and cysts are irregularly dispersed through the parenchyma. The cysts may measure from a few millimeters to many centimeters.

GENETICS

• ARPKD

—Mutations in the PKHD1 gene (chromosome 6) result in a loss of functional fibrocystin. Fibrocystin is a receptor-like membrane protein with intracellular signaling sites and extracellular-matrix-interaction domains on the .

• ADPKD

—Type I ADPKD accounts for 85% to 90% of cases of ADPKD, and is caused by mutations in the PKD1 gene (chromosome 16) resulting in decreased functional polycystin-1, with defects in polarity on renal tubular epithelia.
—Type II ADPKD is caused by mutations in the PKD2 gene (chromosome 4) with decreases in functional polycystin-2. Polycystin-2 is a calcium-permeable channel on renal tubular epithelia. Type II ADPKD has a later onset of symptoms and slower rate of progression.

EPIDEMIOLOGY

• Estimated incidence of ARPKD is 1:10,000 to 1:40,000 live births.
• ADPKD is one of the most common hereditary disorders and accounts for 8% to 10% of cases of end-stage renal disease. Prevalence rates range from 1:200 to 1:1,000.

COMPLICATIONS

• ARPKD

—Most patients present in infancy.
—Severely affected infants may have the oligohydramnios sequence at birth, with pulmonary hypoplasia and Potter phenotype.
—As renal function diminishes, the child may develop growth failure, anemia, and renal osteodystrophy.
—In the older child, complications of hepatic fibrosis and portal hypertension predominate. Hepatosplenomegaly, bleeding esophageal varices, and hypersplenism causing thrombocytopenia, anemia, and leukopenia may occur.

• ADPKD

—Patients may present with hypertension, urinary tract infection, abdominal pain, hematuria, or a palpable abdominal mass.
—The extrarenal complications seen in adults with ADPKD such as hepatic cysts, pancreatic cysts, colonic diverticula, cardiac valvular abnormalities, and intracranial aneurysms are very rarely seen in pediatric patients.

PROGNOSIS

• ADPKD

—Patients who are symptomatic at birth may die from pulmonary insufficiency.
—In ARPKD, those who survive to 1 year have a much better prognosis.
—Renal insufficiency begins in early childhood and the progression is extremely variable.

—Causes of death outside of the neonatal period include renal failure, sepsis, hypertension, and complications of bacterial cholangitis and portal hypertension.
—Treatment with renal transplantation and liver transplantation may increase longevity.

• ADPKD

—Patients who present during infancy with symptomatic renal involvement may have an ominous prognosis and up to 50% die in the neonatal period.
—Presentation of ADPKD in the older child has a better prognosis.
—Control of hypertension and urinary tract infection improves the prognosis.

 Differential Diagnosis

• Multicystic dysplastic kidney (MDK)

—Congenital condition with multiple large cysts of various sizes with no overall structural pattern to the kidney and no functional tissue, rarely bilateral renal involvement; often associated with cardiac, gastrointestinal, and CNS abnormalities

• Glomerular cystic kidney disease (GCKD)

—Consists of bilateral cystic dilations of Bowman space with lack of significant tubular involvement and may have clinical and radiologic features consistent with ARPKD or ADPKD.

• Malformation syndromes
• Renal cysts occur in many hereditary syndromes in the form of peripheral cortical microcysts:

—Examples include trisomy 9, trisomy 13, Meckel syndrome, Jeune syndrome, Ivemark syndrome, Zellweger syndrome, and Bardet-Biedl syndrome.
—Acquired cystic disease may occur in patients with end-stage renal disease.

 Data Gathering

HISTORY

ARPKD

• Patients usually present in infancy.
• Prenatal ultrasound may reveal oligohydramnios, large renal masses, or absence of urine in the bladder.
• Patients may present during the neonatal period with flank masses or respiratory distress.
• May present in older children with symptoms of enlarged kidneys or hepatosplenomegaly.
• A concentrating defect may result in polydipsia and polyuria.
• Hypertension is common and may result in cardiac hypertrophy and congestive heart failure.

ADPKD

- The most common presenting complaint in adults is pain.
- Older children may present with hypertension, abdominal pain, abdominal mass, hematuria, or urinary tract infection.
- Cerebral vessel aneurysms are rarely detected before age 20.

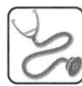 ## Physical Examination

ARPKD

- Flank mass most common.
- May also reveal evidence of portal hypertension (hematemesis, hepatosplenomegaly) or hypersplenism (pallor, petechiae).

ADPKD

- The clinical spectrum of disease is highly variable.
- Most common presentation in neonates is flank masses or palpable kidneys
- Older children may present with hypertension, abdominal pain, abdominal mass, hematuria, urinary tract infection, or renal insufficiency.

 ## Laboratory Aids

Patients should undergo evaluation for renal insufficiency including BUN, creatinine, electrolytes, calcium, phosphorus, and CBC.

IMAGING

ARPKD

Test: Ultrasound
Significance:

- Will reveal, in patients with ARPKD, bilateral, enlarged kidneys with increased echogenicity of the parenchyma, and loss of corticomedullary differentiation
- Occasional macrocysts may be present, >2 cm in diameter.
- The liver is enlarged and hyperechoic but usually less echogenic than the kidney. Dilated intrahepatic biliary ducts or decreased visualization of peripheral portal veins as a result of fibrous tissue may be seen.
- The disease may be diagnosed after 24 to 30 weeks' gestation by ultrasonographic evidence of hyperechogenic enlarged kidneys, oligohydramnios, and no evidence of bladder filling.

Test: Intravenous pyelogram (IVP)
Significance:

- Usually shows the classic finding of medullary streaking (radial striations) corresponding to accumulation of contrast in dilated collecting ducts.

- In older children with ARPKD the kidneys may be less enlarged, with evidence of macrocysts and loss of radial striations.

ADPKD

Test: Ultrasound
Significance:

- The kidneys of ADPKD may be enlarged with macrocysts of varying size. In children, renal involvement is frequently asymmetric and occasionally unilateral. However, the renal enlargement and macrocysts may not develop until adulthood. In children at risk, even single cysts in normal-sized kidneys are highly predictive of future ADPKD.
- Extrarenal cysts may also be seen in the liver, pancreas, ovary, or spleen, although rarely in children.
- May not always distinguish ADPKD and ARPKD

Test: IVP
Significance:

- Will reveal enlarged, lobular kidneys
- The calyces are stretched and distorted.
- Numerous cysts of various sizes are seen in the parenchyma.

FALSE POSITIVES/NEGATIVES

- The sonographic features of ADPKD and ARPKD may be present in the second trimester but usually are not manifested until after 30 weeks. Both false positives and false negatives have been reported.
- Although the combination of renal collecting tubule ectasia and biliary ectasia with periportal fibrosis is unique to ARPKD, portal duct fibrosis and bile duct proliferation may be seen in a variety of renal diseases such as Jeune and Zellweger syndromes and trisomy 9 and 13.

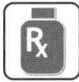 ## Therapy

- Medical management of PKD is supportive.

—Hypertension is common in ADPKD and ARPKD. Patients may require antihypertensive therapy such as calcium-channel blockers.

- Supplemental bicarbonate may be indicated for metabolic acidosis.

—Urinary tract infections or bacterial cholangitis require aggressive antibiotic therapy.
—Infection of hepatic cysts may require drainage.

- Overall, renal replacement therapy with maintenance dialysis and renal transplantation is at least as successful in PKD as in non-PKD patients.

DIET

The degree of renal insufficiency will dictate the need for a low potassium or low phosphorus diet.

 ## Follow-Up

SIGNS TO WATCH FOR

- Asymptomatic children in families with ADPKD are at risk and should be followed closely for hypertension, hematuria, and the development of an abdominal mass and the extrarenal manifestations.
- Routine screening with cerebral arteriography for evidence of possible intracranial aneurysms in pediatric ADPKD patients is not recommended.

 ## Common Questions and Answers

Q: What can be done to slow the progression of renal insufficiency in ADPKD?
A: Well-controlled blood pressure and rapid treatment of urinary tract infections may decrease the progression of renal failure.

Q: Should asymptomatic, older siblings of an infant with ARPKD be evaluated?
A: Yes. An older child may have congenital hepatic fibrosis with minimal renal involvement.

Q: Should one screen ADPKD-affected family members for the presence of cerebral vessel aneurysms if other family members have berry aneurysms?
A: Although routine screening is not recommended, intrafamilial clustering of aneurysms has been reported and it may be advisable to screen children with MRI or cranial CT in a family with aneurysms.

ICD-9-CM 753.1

BIBLIOGRAPHY

Gabow PA. Polycystic kidney disease. *N Engl J Med* 2004;350:151–164.

Kaplan BS, Kaplan P, Rosenberg HK, et al. Polycystic kidney disease in childhood. *J Pediatr* 1989;115(6):867.

Rizk D, Chapman AB. Cystic and inherited kidney diseases. *Am J Kidney Dis* 2003;42:1305–1317.

Author: Mary B. Leonard

Polycystic Ovary Syndrome

 Database

DEFINITION

Polycystic ovary syndrome (PCOS) is an endocrinologic disorder characterized by chronic anovulation, excessive androgen production, and noncyclical gonadotropin secretion. It begins perimenarcheally, and its clinical manifestations include hirsutism, amenorrhea or oligomenorrhea, and obesity.

CAUSES

- The characteristic polycystic ovary emerges when a state of anovulation persists for any length of time.
- Although the ovaries of these women produce excessive amounts of androgens, there is no inherent endocrinologic abnormality in the ovaries.
- The tonically elevated levels of luteinizing hormone (LH) cause the ovarian stromal tissue to produce more androgens, which in turn produce premature follicular atresia.
- Because there are many causes of anovulation, there are many causes of polycystic ovaries.
- It has been suggested that heredity, central catecholamine abnormalities, psychological stress, insulin resistance, and obesity may be involved.
- At least one group of patients with this condition inherits the disorder, possibly by means of an X-linked dominant transmission.

PATHOPHYSIOLOGY

- The ovaries of most women with PCOS are enlarged as much as 5 cm in diameter, and the ovarian capsule is smooth, white, and thickened.
- Beneath the capsule are numerous small follicular cysts.
- For years it was erroneously believed that the thick sclerotic capsule acted as a mechanical barrier to ovulation.
- Instead of the characteristic picture of fluctuating hormone levels in the normal menstrual cycle, a steady state of gonadotropin and sex steroids is produced in association with persistent anovulation.
- There is increased pulse amplitude of gonadotropin-releasing hormone (GnRH) and tonically elevated levels of LH.
- The polycystic ovary is a sign of these underlying endocrinologic abnormalities, not a disease intrinsic to the ovary.

EPIDEMIOLOGY

PCOS is relatively common and usually begins soon after menarche.

COMPLICATIONS

- The elevated levels of androgens that are produced are associated with hirsutism.
- The lack of a normal menstrual cycle leads to irregular bleeding, amenorrhea, and infertility.
- Because of the increased levels of unopposed estrogens, there is a threefold increased risk of endometrial cancer, and a 34-fold greater risk of breast cancer appearing in the postmenopausal years.

 Differential Diagnosis

- Congenital adrenal hyperplasia
- Cushing syndrome
- Adrenal androgen-producing tumors
- Ovarian androgen-producing tumors
- Extragonadal sources of androgens

 Data Gathering

HISTORY

- Complete menstrual history
- Amenorrhea or irregular vaginal bleeding
- Infertility

 Physical Examination

HIRSUTISM

- Most patients with this syndrome are obese.
- Obesity probably enhances the syndrome because of the decrease in sex hormone—binding globulin, but is probably not important in its pathogenesis, because the syndrome occurs in some thin women and because many obese women do not have PCOS.

 Laboratory Aids

- Because FSH levels are normal or low, an LH/FSH ratio greater than 3 (provided the LH level is not lower than 8 mIU/mL) may be used to suggest the diagnosis in women with clinical features of PCOS.
- Androgen levels are elevated. Serum testosterone levels are usually between 70 and 120 ng/dL, and androstenedione levels are usually between 3 and 5 ng/mL.

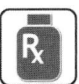 Therapy

- The best treatment for PCOS is oral contraceptives, unless pregnancy is desired, because these agents inhibit LH, decrease circulating testosterone levels, and increase levels of sex hormone–binding globulin, which binds and inactivates more of the testosterone in the circulation.
- Use oral contraceptives that contain less than 50 μg estrogen and a progestin other than norgestrel, which is the most androgenic progestin in current use.
- Patients who desire fertility should be treated with ovulation-inducing agents, starting with clomiphene citrate and proceeding to human menopausal gonadotropin or GnRH agonists if unresponsive.
- If adrenal androgens (DHEAs) are elevated, dexamethasone (0.25 to 0.5 mg at bedtime) should be given along with the oral contraceptive to reduce adrenal androgens to normal.
- Patients with amenorrhea or irregular bleeding should be treated with monthly progestins, such as oral medroxyprogesterone acetate 10 mg daily for the first 10 days of the month, to prevent the effects of unopposed estrogens.
- Spironolactone 50 to 100 mg twice daily causes regression of the hirsutism in women with PCOS by decreasing androgenic action in the target organs.
- Ovarian wedge resection was advocated in the past for treatment of androgen excess, but the decrease in circulating androgens occurred for only a short time, and this therapy should no longer be used.

 Follow-Up

In the patient who has long-standing anovulation, an endometrial biopsy, with extensive sampling, should be done because of the link between unopposed estrogen and endometrial cancer.

 Common Questions and Answers

Q: Can I still get pregnant if I have this syndrome?
A: Yes. Although the best treatment for this syndrome is oral contraceptives, those patients who desire to become pregnant can be treated with ovulation-inducing agents.

Q: I've noticed increased facial hair recently. Is there anything I can do about this?
A: Yes. In most cases, the oral contraceptives will decrease circulating androgen levels sufficiently so that this will regress, but if increased body hair (hirsutism) persists, another drug, spironolactone, blocks the action of androgens, can be added to more effectively treat this.

ICD-9-CM 256.4

BIBLIOGRAPHY

DeVane GW, Czckala NM, Judd HL, et al. Circulating gonadotrophins, estrogens, and androgens in polycystic ovarian disease. *Am J Obstet Gynecol* 1975;121:496.

Dramusic V, Rajan U, Chan P, Ratnam SS, Wong YC. Adolescent polycystic ovary syndrome. *Ann N Y Acad Sci* 1997;816:194–208.

Givens JR, Andersen RN, Wiser WI, et al. The effectiveness of two oral contraceptives in suppressing plasma androstanedione, testosterone, LH and FSH and stimulating plasma testosterone binding capacity in hirsute women. *Am J Obstet Gynecol* 1976;124:333.

Goldzicher JW. Polycystic ovarian syndrome. *Fertil Steril* 1981;35:371.

Goudas VT, Dumesic DA. Polycystic ovary syndrome. *Endocrinol Metab Clin North Am* 1997;26(4):893–8912.

Kazar AR, Kessel B, Yen SSC. Circulating luteinizing hormone pulse frequency in women with polycystic ovary syndrome. *J Clin Endocrinol Metab* 1987;65:233.

Lobo RA, Goebelsmann U. Effect of androgen excess on inappropriate gonadotropin secretion as found in polycystic ovary syndrome. *Am J Obstet Gynecol* 1982;142:394.

Author: Ernest M. Graham

Polycythemia

 Database

DEFINITION

- Polycythemia is elevated hemoglobin and hematocrit owing to an absolute increase in red-cell mass. Polycythemia can be divided into subcategories, as follows:

—Primary polycythemia: primary defect of bone marrow erythropoiesis, resulting in overproduction of red cells
—Secondary polycythemia: stimulation of red-cell production by increased levels of erythropoietin (EPO), which may be appropriately secreted in response to tissue hypoxia, or may be inappropriately secreted because of renal disease or from a tumor.
—Apparent or relative polycythemia: increased hematocrit without true increase in red-cell mass
—Erythrocytosis is another term describing increased red cell mass, which some authors prefer because it avoids confusion with the diagnosis of polycythemia vera.

PATHOPHYSIOLOGY

Primary Polycythemias

- Polycythemia vera (PCV): myeloproliferative disease with abnormal multipotent progenitor cells with abnormally high sensitivity to erythropoietin (EPO); EPO levels are normal.
- Primary familial and congenital polycythemia (PFCP): red-cell precursors highly sensitive to EPO. Usually autosomal dominant; some families have truncation mutations in the EPO receptor (EPOR), leading to a loss of downregulation of EPO signaling.

Secondary Polycythemias

Relative tissue hypoxia resulting from deficiency of oxygen delivery, as a result of:

- Chronic lung disease and inadequate oxygenation as a result of a defect in gas exchange
- Cyanotic heart disease: desaturation of arterial blood because of admixture of oxygen-poor venous blood as a result of right-to-left shunt
- Circulatory: right-to-left shunting outside the heart
- Hemoglobinopathy: abnormal oxygen transport to tissues because of a mutant hemoglobin with higher than normal oxygen affinity.
- At the partial pressure of oxygen of the tissues, high oxygen-affinity hemoglobins release less oxygen than normal, resulting in hypoxia.
- Tissue hypoxia leads to supernormal secretion of EPO by the kidney, and increased production of red cells from the marrow.
- 2,3-bisphosphoglycerate (2,3-BPG) deficiency: increased oxygen affinity of hemoglobin because of reduced level of red-cell 2,3-BPG
- A genetic defect von Hippel-Lindau gene (VHL) that causes a defect in the hypoxia

sensing mechanism and leads to familial polycythemia has been described.
- Inappropriate EPO secretion associated with kidney disease (not end stage, in which EPO is usually deficient)
- Malignant tumor, which secretes EPO

GENETICS

- High oxygen-affinity hemoglobins: autosomal dominant
- Primary familial and congenital polycythemia: usually autosomal dominant; Finnish clusters described
- VHL gene mutation with defect of hypoxia sensing: autosomal recessive; Chuvash polycythemia
- 2,3-BPG mutase deficiency: autosomal recessive

EPIDEMIOLOGY

- Uncorrected cyanotic congenital heart disease: most common cause of polycythemia
- PCV: Fewer than 50 reported childhood cases; 0.1% of cases of PCV are in children.
- High oxygen-affinity hemoglobins; 2,3-BPG dismutase deficiency; EPOR mutations, VHL mutations, primary familial and congenital polycythemia: all rare

COMPLICATIONS

- Hyperviscosity: Blood viscosity increases dramatically when hematocrit >65%.
- Decreased exercise tolerance, dyspnea, and mental status changes are as a result of slowed microcirculation in the CNS.
- Thrombosis: Budd-Chiari syndrome from hepatic vein thrombosis, deep vein thrombosis, pulmonary embolus; seen especially in PCV
- Stroke: Cerebral thrombosis as a result of hyperviscosity
- Malignant transformation of PCV; not seen in PFCP

PROGNOSIS

Depends on underlying condition:

- High oxygen-affinity hemoglobinopathies: very good for normal life
- PCV: guarded, as may progress to myelodysplastic syndrome
- Eisenmenger syndrome (see below): poor; progressive pulmonary hypertension and cor pulmonale

 Differential Diagnosis

PRIMARY POLYCYTHEMIA

- PCV
- Myeloproliferative disease
- May have thrombocytosis or leukocytosis
- Primary familial and congenital polycythemia

SECONDARY POLYCYTHEMIA

- Cyanotic congenital heart disease

- Eisenmenger syndrome
—Pulmonary hypertension from long-standing uncorrected congenital heart disease with left-to-right shunting (acyanotic) leads to elevated right-sided pressures and reversal of shunt to flow right to left, leading to cyanosis
- Extreme high altitude
—Compensation for low O_2 pressure includes an increase in red-cell mass.
- Alveolar hypoventilation: neuromuscular
—Muscular dystrophy
—Poliomyelitis
—Pickwickian syndrome
—Central hypoventilation
- End-stage lung disease
- Abnormal hemoglobins with high O_2 affinity
- 2,3-BPG mutase deficiency
- Inappropriate EPO secretion may occur in:
—Renal disease, including posttransplant erythrocytosis after renal allografting
—Iatrogenic
—Excessive red-cell transfusion, possible in trauma, resuscitations, neonatal blood exchange
—Excessive exogenous dosing of EPO
- Neonatal polycythemia
- Twin-to-twin or placental transfusion
- Cobalt poisoning

RELATIVE POLYCYTHEMIA

- May be seen in smokers
- Dehydration or diuretic use

 Data Gathering

HISTORY

- Diagnosis of congenital heart disease, uncorrected or partially corrected
- History of cyanosis
- Delivery history
- Baby held below placenta
- Delayed clamping of cord
- Twins of disparate size
- Transfusion history
- Headache, paresthesias, dizziness, syncope
- Transient blindness
- Decreased exercise tolerance, respiratory distress, dyspnea on exertion, oxygen requirement
- Pruritus
- Lethargy
- Cigarette smoking
- Prolonged time spent at extremely high altitude
- Family history of cyanosis, high hematocrit, need for phlebotomy
- Cobalt poisoning: Homemade beer and magnets may contain cobalt.

 Physical Examination

- Central and acral cyanosis
- Signs of dehydration: dry mucous membranes, no tears, poor skin turgor
- Heart murmur

- Clubbing
- Plethora: conjunctival, mucous membranes, nail beds
- Splenomegaly: present in 75% of PCV

 ## Laboratory Aids

TESTS

Initial

- CBC
- Serum EPO: Distinguish 1° from 2° polycythemia, but much overlap in EPO levels
- Pulse oximetry: to determine percent saturation of hemoglobin
- Arterial blood gas with co-oximetry: Po_2 low in lung disease or right-to-left shunt

To Investigate High Oxygen-Affinity Hemoglobin

- Hemoglobin electrophoresis
- Whole-blood P50 and red-cell 2,3-BPG level
- Met-hemoglobin level: apparent cyanosis

To Investigate PCV

- Total red-cell mass measurement by chromium 51–tagged red cells: top normal range (adults) is less than 36 mL/kg in men, less than 32 mL/kg in women, or less than 25% above the predicted normal range normalized by body surface area; gold standard test for true polycythemia
- Bone marrow aspirate with chromosomes: morphologic evidence of myelodysplastic syndrome; abnormal clone by karyotype or X chromosome inactivation studies
- Serum B12, unsaturated B12-binding capacity (UB12BC): markedly elevated in PCV
- Erythroid progenitor culture studies for BFU-E that grow independent of EPO

Other Testing

- Total blood viscosity: rarely measured
- Iron studies: serum Fe, TIBC, ferritin
- BUN, creatinine, urinalysis: underlying renal disease

IMAGING

- Echocardiography: to evaluate shunting
- Chest radiograph: to evaluate chronic lung disease, lung malignancies
- Abdominal ultrasound: to evaluate renal disease, spleen size, abdominal tumors
- Sleep study: looking for nighttime airway obstruction and desaturation

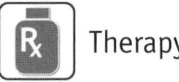 ## Therapy

OBSERVATION ONLY

Many patients require no therapy.

THERAPEUTIC PHLEBOTOMY

- Removal of red cells every 3 to 4 weeks to maintain hematocrit below threshold for symptoms; usually below 50% to 55%
- Patients with Eisenmenger syndrome and symptoms of hyperviscosity may not tolerate intravascular volume reduction if a large volume of blood is removed at one time.
- Patients on a chronic phlebotomy program may require iron supplementation.

DRUGS

- Hydroxyurea, alkylating agents, ^{32}P (in adults) to suppress red-cell production in PCV
- Interferon-α for PCV

SUPPLEMENTAL OXYGEN

Helpful for secondary polycythemia as a result of underlying lung disease; may not help in right-to-left shunt

SURGERY

Correction of underlying cardiac disease

DIET

- No specific recommendation
- Dietary restriction of water and salt intake may be required for underlying renal disease.

 ## Follow-Up

SIGNS TO WATCH FOR

- Insufficient phlebotomy
- Headache
- Dizziness
- Syncope
- Decreased exercise tolerance between phlebotomies
- Progression of myelodysplastic disease
- Thrombocytopenia
- Bleeding
- Thrombosis
- Stroke
- Severe headache
- Jaundice
- Ascites

PREVENTION

- There are no preventive measures for primary conditions such as PCV, hemoglobinopathies, or PFCP
- Treatment of the underlying condition, such as correction of a cyanotic heart lesion, will prevent the development of secondary polycythemia.

PITFALLS

- Fingerstick CBC: Squeezing the finger to collect a specimen may give a falsely elevated hematocrit.
- Arterial blood gas: cannot interpret low Po_2 if specimen is mixture of venous and arterial blood
- Relative polycythemia: red-cell mass normal

- Decreased plasma volume with normal red-cell mass; seen in adult cigarette smokers
- Dehydration; elevated hematocrit as a result of hemoconcentration
- Hemoglobin electrophoresis does not identify all high-affinity hemoglobins.

—Many comigrate with normal hemoglobins
—Hemoglobin electrophoresis cannot be interpreted if the patient has been transfused within the past 3 months.

- Whole blood P50

—Fresh specimen required; normals different from red cell lysates, purified hemoglobin

 ## Common Questions and Answers

Q: Can a child with uncorrected cyanotic congenital heart disease be supported indefinitely with phlebotomy?
A: No. Phlebotomy relieves the symptoms of hyperviscosity, but does not stop the progression of pulmonary hypertension.

Q: When should a child with polycythemia be referred to a pediatric hematologist?
A: If the high hematocrit is persistent and not clearly related to dehydration or neonatal causes (e.g., placental transfusion), then the child should be referred to a pediatric hematologist. Unexplained cyanosis is also a reason for referral. In the case of congenital heart disease, the pediatric cardiologist may be comfortable managing polycythemia without consultation with a hematologist.

ICD-9-CM 238.4

BIBLIOGRAPHY

Danish EH, Rasch CA, Harris JW. Polycythemia vera in childhood: case report and review of the literature. *Am J Hematol* 1980;9:421.

Kralovics R, Prchal JT. Congenital and inherited polycythemia. *Curr Opin Pediatr* 2000;12:29.

Messinezy M, Pearson TC. The classification and diagnostic criteria of the erythrocytoses (polycythaemias). *Clin Lab Haem* 1999;21:309–316.

Pearson TC, Messinezy M. Investigation of patients with polycythemia. *Postgrad Med J* 1996;519–524.

Prchal JF, Prchal JT. Molecular basis for polycythemia. *Curr Opin Hematol* 1999;6:100.

Prchal JT, Sokol L. "Benign erythrocytosis" and other familial and congenital polycythemias. *Eur J Haematol* 1996;57:263–268.

Prchal JT. Classification and molecular biology of polycythemias (erythrocytoses) and thrombocytoses. *Hematol/Oncol Clin of North Am* 2003;17:

Vlahakos DV, Marathias KP, Agroyannis B, Madias NE. Posttransplant erythrocytosis. *Kidney Int* 2003;63:1187–1194.

Author: David F. Friedman

Porencephaly Cortical Dysplasia/Neuronal Migration Disorders—Malformations of Cortical Development

 Database

DEFINITION

Malformations of cortical development (MCD) are a heterogeneous group of development brain malformations that are highly associated with epilepsy, developmental delay, and mental retardation. Associated features may include autism, learning difficulties, hypotonia, and spasticity. In some cases, there is global neurodevastation and failure to thrive. The key histological feature of MCD is that the structural organization of the cerebral cortex is abnormal. MCD may affect focal regions of the brain as in focal cortical dysplasia, tuberous sclerosis complex, or porencephaly or may affect more widespread regions of the brains such as in lissencephaly or hemimegalencephaly. As a general rule, the more extensive the malformation, the greater the degree of neurological impairment.

MCD AFFECTING WIDE REGIONS OF CORTEX

• Etiologic agent likely before 20 weeks' gestation
• Lissencephaly (smooth brain): loss of cerebral cortical convolutions (sulci) and cortical laminations; may occur in combination with agyria-pachygyria (see below).
• Agyria-pachygyria: a more heterogeneous pathologic classification in which there are broad regions of cortex without gyri (similar to lissencephaly), but, in addition, focal areas of thickened cortical gyri also may be present.
• Hemimegalencephaly: a rare condition in which one cerebral hemisphere is enlarged and may exhibit concomitant agyric-pachygyric features. The normal-sized hemisphere may also contain subtle, focal abnormalities.

MCD AFFECTING FOCAL REGIONS OF CORTEX

• Etiologic agent likely after 20 weeks' gestation
• Dysplastic cortical architecture: focal regions of disorganized cortical architecture and abnormally shaped neurons
• Heterotopia: clusters of neurons found within the white matter (in which neurons are not typically found); may be nodular and confined to small region in cortex or adjacent to the ependyma (nodular forms); may extend across portions of a hemisphere (laminar heterotopia)
• Schizencephaly: nonloculated cavities or clefts (uni-or bilateral) in the brain that communicate with the system and/or subarachnoid space

RECENT CLASSIFICATION SCHEME FOR MCD (BARKOVICH ET AL., 2001)

Disorders of Cell Proliferation

• Tuberous Sclerosis Complex
• Focal Cortical Dysplasia
• Hemimegalencephaly
• Microcephaly syndromes
• DNET (Dysembryoplastic neuroepithelial tumors)
• Ganglioglioma
• Gangliocytoma

Disorders of Neural Migration

• Lissencephaly Type I (Classical)
—Miller-Dieker syndrome
—X-linked lissencephaly (XLIS)
• Lissencephaly Type II (Cobblestone)
—Walker-Warburg syndrome
—Muscle-eye-brain disease
—Fukuyama Congenital Muscular Dystrophy
• Subcortical Band Heteropsia ("Double cortex syndrome")
• Periventricular Nodular Heterotopia

Disorders of Brain Organization

• Polymicrogyria
• Schizencephaly
• Taylor Type I dysplasia
—Microdysgenesias

Malformations, Not Otherwise Classified

• Mitochondrial disorders
• Peroxisomal disorders (e.g., Zellweger syndrome)

CAUSES

CD/NMDs result from a variety of in utero causes, including infectious, toxic-metabolic, ischemic insults. Several MCDs result from single gene mutations.
• Genetic
—Lissencephaly may occur as a sporadic syndrome but has been associated with mutations in select genes
　　—Miller-Dieker lissencephaly syndrome
　　—Chromosome 17p13.3
—Lissencephaly with cerebellar hypoplasia
　　—Chromosome 7q22
　　—XLIS
　　—Chromosome Xq22
—Periventricular nodular heterotopia
　　—Chromosome Xq28
—Subcortical band heterotopia
　　—Chromosome Xq22
—Tuberous Sclerosis Complex
　　—Chromosome 9q34
　　—Chromosome 16p13
—Fukuyama Congenital Muscular Dystrophy
　　—Chromosome 9q31
• Other lissencephaly-associated syndromes, including the Norman-Roberts, Neu-Laxova, and Walker-Warburg syndromes, are believed to have an autosomal-recessive pattern of inheritance.
• The HARD syndrome (hydrocephalus, agyria, retinal dysplasia and encephalocele is autosomal recessive.
• Cortical cytoarchitectural abnormalities may also occur in trisomy 13,18 and 21.
• Infectious
—Polymicrogyria, pachygyria-agyria, and heterotopias may occur in the setting of toxoplasmosis, other agents, rubella, cytomegalovirus, and herpes virus (TORCH) infections of the central nervous system during early development. They may also occur as a consequence of intrauterine hypoxic-ischemic injury.
• Ischemic
—Polymicrogyria and heterotopia may occur in the setting of in utero hypoxic-ischemic injury.
—Schizencephaly may reflect intrauterine infarction and is characterized by a large cleft in one or both hemispheres. Whether schizencephaly is truly an MCD remains to be shown.
—Porencephaly (porencephalic cysts) are intraparenchymal cavities that communicate with the ventricular system, which also result from intrauterine hypoxic-ischemic injury.
• Toxins
—Ethanol
—Ionizing radiation
—Carbon monoxide
—Isotretinoin
—Methyl mercury
• Metabolic
—CD/NMDs have been reported in association with Zellweger syndrome, neonatal adrenoleukodystrophy, Menkes disease, and GM2 gangliosidoses.
• Miscellaneous
—MCDs may occur in syndromes characterized by numerous other congenital anomalies, such as the Smith-Lemli-Opitz, Potter, and Meckel syndromes.

PATHOLOGY

The most characteristic feature is disruption of normal cerebral cortical architecture. In lissencephaly, there are few cerebral convolutions (sulci and gyri) in the entire brain, and the normal layering of cortex is abnormal. Neurons are often abnormally shaped and are oriented incorrectly within the cortex. In heterotopias, clusters of neurons are located inappropriately in the subcortical white matter. A large bilateral subcortical heterotopia is found in patients with "double cortex syndrome" and clusters of heterotopic neurons line the ventricles in periventricular nodular heterotopia. Disruption of the synaptic connections between various brain regions likely accounts for epilepsy and other neurologic problems such as mental retardation or autism associated with MCDs.

GENETICS

See Causes, above.

EPIDEMIOLOGY

• Incidence varies according to syndrome.
• Some children die at birth or in early childhood, owing to global devastation.
• Epilepsy may be associated with MCD in as many as 70% to 90% of cases. MCD are also a common cause of infantile spasms (especially tuberous sclerosis complex and lissencephaly).

• Approximate estimates are that from 20% to 40% of specimens resected during epilepsy surgery contain MCD.

PROGNOSIS

Most patients with CD/NMDs will continue to suffer from seizures and cognitive impairment as well as other neurological and behavioral abnormalities.

Differential Diagnosis

In patients presenting with either overt or subtle neurologic symptoms or signs, consider a developmental central nervous system abnormality. Seizures and/or developmental delay are especially common manifestations of MCDs. Epilepsy in pediatric patients may be a manifestation of a neurocutaneous disorder such as TSC. Tumors, vascular malformations, and in utero ischemic insults also should be considered.

Data Gathering

HISTORY

• Important questions include family history of genetic or chromosomal syndromes, family members with mental retardation, neurologic dysfunction or seizures, and infant deaths associated with profound neurologic impairment.
• Ask about parental consanguinity.
• Subtle manifestations of neurocutaneous syndromes may be identified in family members with skin lesions or, in more overt cases, as individuals with CNS or other cancers, as in TSC. Inquire about head or truncal flexion movements suggestive of infantile spasms.

Physical Examination

• Many children with MCDs have no overt signs of dysfunction, although others have global neurologic impairment.
• Developmental delay, seizures (especially infantile spasms), and focal neurologic signs may be observed.
• Microcephaly or macrocephaly also may be identified.
• Some children will have dysmorphic facies characterized by hypotelorism, malformed skull, and midline deformities.
• Characteristic facies of the Miller-Dieker lissencephaly syndrome include a thin upper lip and microcephaly.
• Cutaneous manifestations such as hypomelanotic lesions ("ash leaf spots"), facial angiofibromas, a shagreen patch, or other regions of hyper/hypo pigmentation may identify patient with neurocutaneous disorders such as tuberous sclerosis.
• Funduscopic examination may reveal retinal hamartomas in TSC.
• A linear sebaceous nevus on the forehead is associated with hemimegalencephaly.
• Hypomelanosis of Ito is also associated with MCDs.

PHYSICAL EXAMINATION TRICKS

• Cutaneous examination with a Wood's lamp may be useful in identifying ash leaf or café-au-lait spots.
• Tooth enamel pits may be identified in TSC.

Laboratory Aids

TESTS

• Most routine blood tests and cerebrospinal fluid will be normal.
• Metabolic derangements characteristic of disorders such as gangliosidoses may be identified with specific blood tests.
• Chromosomal karyotyping analysis (genetic screening) for Miller-Dieker syndrome, and various trisomies can be performed to aid in both diagnosis and further genetic counseling.
• Screening for select gene mutations is available through several research labs and will become commercially available.
• EEG is critical in diagnosing seizures and assessing the degree of underlying brain dysfunction. Characteristic findings may be sharp waves, spikes, hypsarrhythmia (in infantile spasms), and slow spike-wave discharges (Lennox-Gastaut syndrome). In children with developmental delay, formal neuropsychiatric assessment may be useful.

IMAGING

• Brain MRI with and without gadolinium contrast is essential in identifying and classifying MCDs. Brain CT may be useful but has lower resolution that does MRI.
• Functional brain imaging with single-photon emission computed tomography (SPECT) and positron-emission tomography (PET) is gaining popularity in assessing regional changes in glucose or oxygen metabolisms within regions of dysplasia.

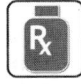

Therapy

DRUGS

In general, neurologic consultation is recommended to help manage children with MCD and epilepsy. Virtually all children with MCD and seizures will require anticonvulsant drugs for adequate seizure control. These regimens must be tailored to account for drug interactions, potential side effects, and long-term efficacy in seizure control. Children with infantile spasms may respond to ACTH or vigabatrin therapy.

EPILEPSY SURGERY

A significant proportion of children with MCD and seizures will not respond to medications and will require epilepsy surgery to remove the seizure focus within the MCD. In some cases, the surgery is a small focal resection although in others, removal of a brain hemisphere is indicated. Some cases are not amenable to epilepsy surgery and other treatment modalities include the vagal nerve stimulator or the ketogenic diet.

Follow-Up

WHEN TO EXPECT IMPROVEMENT

Adequate seizure control may be difficult in MCD patients. Cognitive and other neurologic deficits may benefit somewhat from neuropsychological intervention, education, and physical therapy. In children with a documented MCD and refractory seizures, resective epilepsy surgery provides a safe and often successful alternative to conventional anticonvulsant medications.

SIGNS TO WATCH FOR

Most worrisome would be a persistent change in mental status, which could indicate status epilepticus. Other worrisome signs include development of new neurologic symptoms in patients with TSC, suggesting hydrocephalus.

ICD-9-CM LISSENCEPHALY 742.2

BIBLIOGRAPHY

Barkovich AJ, Kuzniecky RI, Jackson GD, Guerrini R, Dobyns WB. Classification system for malformations of cortical development: update 2001. *Neurology* 2001;57:2168–78.

Barkovich AJ, Kuzniecky RI. Gray matter heterotopia. *Neurology* 2000;55:1603–1608.

Crino PB, Chou K. Epilepsy and cortical dysplasias. *Curr Treat Options Neurol* 2000;2:543–552.

Crino PB, Henske EP. New developments in the neurobiology of the tuberous sclerosis complex. *Neurology* 1999;53:1384–1390.

Eller KM, Kuller JA. Fetal porencephaly: a review of etiology, diagnosis and prognosis. *Obstet Gynecol Surv* 1995;50:684–687.

Ho SS, Kuzniecky RI, Gilliam F, et al. Congenital porencephaly: MR features and relationship to hippocampal sclerosis. *AJNR* 1998;19(1):135–141.

Author: Peter B. Crino

Portal Hypertension

 ## Database

DEFINITION

An elevation of portal blood pressure above 5 to 10 mmHg.

PATHOPHYSIOLOGY

- The portal vein receives nutrient-rich blood from the stomach, spleen, pancreas, gallbladder, and intestine.
- Normally, the portal system, which has no valves, has very low resistance and the direction of flow reflects the pressure gradient and vessel patency.
- An increase in portal resistance is the main pathogenetic factor that initiates the process of portal HTN.
- Other factors include hyperdynamic circulation, expanded intravascular volume, systemic arteriolar vasodilatation, and other, yet unidentified, humorally mediated factors (probably nitric oxide) contributing to increased portal blood flow and pressure.
- Decompression of the high venous pressure through porto-systemic collaterals leads to all the major sequelae of portal HTN:

—Splenomegaly
—Varices
—Hemorrhoids
—Caput medusa (periumbilical varices)
—Hepatic encephalopathy
—Hepato-pulmonary syndrome

COMPLICATIONS

- The clinical complications of portal hypertension:

—Hemorrhage from varices (hematemesis, hematochezia, melena)—most common presenting symptom (70%)
—Hypersplenism (resulting in pancytopenia) from splenic engorgement
—Malabsorption as a result of congestion of the intestinal mucosa
—Abnormal sodium retention by the kidney
—Ascites as a result of increased mesenteric venous congestion, and impaired lymphatic drainage; presence of ascites increases risk of spontaneous bacterial peritonitis.
—Hepatorenal syndrome occurs in patients with severe liver disease and leads to rapidly progressive renal failure; although its cause is unknown, its pathophysiology involves renal cortical vasoconstriction and decreased renal blood flow.
—Hepatopulmonary syndrome (intrapulmonary right-to-left shunting) leads to shortness of breath, exercise intolerance, and digital clubbing.
—Pulmonary hypertension can be a life-threatening complication of portal HTN.

 ## Differential Diagnosis

Portal HTN can be seen in many different diseases. Conceptually, it is easiest to divide the causes of increased portal pressure by location of the underlying lesion.

- Prehepatic causes

—Portal vein thrombosis (umbilical vein catheterization, sepsis, dehydration, hypercoagulable state)
—Splenic vein thrombosis

- Intrahepatic causes

—Hepatocellular disorders:
  —Congenital hepatic fibrosis
  —A1-antitrypsin deficiency
  —Chronic hepatitis
  —Autoimmune hepatitis
  —Hepatoportal sclerosis
  —Wilson disease
  —Glycogen storage disease
  —Tyrosinemia
  —Schistosomiasis
  —Peliosis hepatitis
  —Vitamin A toxicity

- Biliary tract disorders

—Extrahepatic biliary atresia
—Intrahepatic cholestasis syndromes
—Sclerosing cholangitis
—Choledochal cyst
—Cystic fibrosis

- Posthepatic causes

—Budd-Chiari syndrome–occlusion of suprahepatic IVC or hepatic veins by congenital web, tumor, or thrombus
—Congestive heart failure
—Veno-occlusive disease of hepatic venule

 ## Data Gathering

HISTORY

- History of umbilical catheterization
- History of hepatitis, abdominal trauma, clotting disorder, contraceptive pills, underlying medical problem such as cystic fibrosis, tyrosinemia, Wilson disease
- Ingestion of excessive amounts of vitamin A
- Hematemesis

—Upper GI bleed from varices may be the first sign of long-standing silent liver disease or previously undiagnosed portal vein thrombosis.
—Patients with a stoma and portal HTN can develop life-threatening stomal variceal bleeds

 ## Physical Examination

- Splenomegaly (size of spleen does not correlate with pressure)
- Hepatomegaly may or may not be present. (Budd-Chiari is associated with a large, tender liver although chronic hepatitis and cirrhosis eventually leads to a shrunken liver)
- Hemorrhoids
- Prominent vascular pattern on the abdomen (caput medusa)
- Digital clubbing
- Telangiectasia
- Palmar erythema
- Growth failure

 ## Laboratory Aids

TESTS

- CBC and smear: detect hypersplenism, GI blood loss, and chronic liver disease)
- PT, PTT: detect coagulation defects
- Liver function tests (ALT, AST, albumin, alkaline phosphatase, GGT)
- Ultrasound with Doppler
- To investigate liver size and echogenicity
- Biliary anatomy
- Spleen size
- Renal abnormalities associated with cystic liver disease
- Presence of ascites
- Vessel diameter
- Direction of blood flow
- Presence of esophageal varices
- Esophagogastroduodenoscopy (EGD): definitively identifies the presence of esophageal varices and determines if variceal rupture is the cause of a GI bleed
- Barium swallow: an insensitive detector of varices so rarely useful in this setting (only 70% detection in adults)
- Liver biopsy and other specific serologic tests: identify the underlying cause of the portal hypertension
- In adult patients, hepatic venous wedge pressure gradient correlates well with the risk of variceal bleeding and has been used to document response to therapy. Selective angiography has been used to delineate extrahepatic vascular anatomy. These invasive studies are not used in pediatrics because of a lack of well-documented pediatric measurements and lack of a favorable risk-benefit ratio. Hopefully, in the future, noninvasive studies will become useful for measuring portal pressures in pediatric patients.

Portal Hypertension

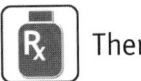 Therapy

ACUTE MANAGEMENT OF VARICEAL BLEED

- Vital signs

—Remember that hemodynamic instability can be masked by β-blockers

- Fluid resuscitation

—Crystalloid initially, then red blood cell transfusion with goal hemoglobin 10 g/dL

- Nasogastric tube placement

—Lavage with room temperature saline until clear

- Correction of coagulopathy

—Platelet transfusion if <50,000/μL
—Parenteral vitamin K
—Fresh frozen plasma

- Intravenous antibiotics

—Acute variceal hemorrhage increases the risk of spontaneous bacterial peritonitis in the setting of ascites

- Pharmacotherapy

—Octreotide (somatostatin analog) decreases splanchnic blood flow via its inhibition of intestinal vasoactive peptide secretion
—Vasopressin decreases splanchnic blood flow via its vasoconstriction effects but its use is limited as a result of a poor side effect profile (nitroglycerin, a venodilator, has been used in conjunction to decrease the side effects)

- Endoscopy (after stabilization)

—Document source of hemorrhage (variceal rupture or other, such as gastric ulcer)
—Sclerotherapy
—Ligation therapy (band or clip)

- Direct tamponade

—Sengstaken-Blakemore tube: severe uncontrollable hemorrhage but high rate of complications

- Surgical intervention

—Portosystemic shunt
—Esophageal devascularization and/or transection
—TIPS (transjugular intrahepatic portosystemic shunt)
—Liver transplantation

CHRONIC MANAGEMENT OF VARICES

- Surveillance endoscopy and primary prophylaxis in pediatric patients with portal HTN who have not had a first variceal bleed is controversial and not yet recommended.
- Long-term management of patients with portal HTN who have had a variceal bleed depends on the underlying cause of the portal HTN and may include β-blockers, endoscopic sclerotherapy or ligation, portosystemic shunts, and liver transplantation.

- B-blockade: Nonselective β-blockers, such as propranolol, have been shown to be effective in preventing both initial and recurrent variceal bleeds and may improve long-term survival in patients with esophageal varices. They function to lower portal blood flow and thus portal pressure by both β2-blockade, which increases splanchnic tone and β1-blockade which decreases cardiac output. Propranolol, specifically, may also decrease collateral circulation. However β-blockers are rarely used in patients younger than adolescence for fear of a lack of adaptive cardiovascular response in the event of a hemorrhage and they cannot be used in patients with asthma or diabetes.
- Endoscopic sclerotherapy: Reduces rebleeding episodes and long-term mortality when initiated after the first bleeding episode; it is unclear whether it will prevent occurrence of a first bleed.
- Endoscopic ligation therapy with bands or clips: Alternative methods that may be as effective as and carry fewer complications than sclerotherapy; limited pediatric data available is favorable.
- Portosystemic shunt: this is not commonly used in pediatric patients; May be helpful in the setting of prehepatic causes of portal HTN, does not improve long-term survival in patients with intrahepatic disease, and its complications may include thrombosis and worsening of hepatic encephalopathy; TIPS procedure may be a more effective bridge to liver transplantation in pediatric patients with progressive liver disease and recurrent variceal bleeds.
- Liver transplantation: A number of studies have established that long-term survival is better for transplanted patients than for patients treated with any other mode of therapy for bleeding.
- Therefore, the current approach at most institutions is liver transplantation for those patients with life-threatening bleeds not amenable to β-blockade or endoscopic therapies.

OTHER MANAGEMENT ISSUES

- When ascites is present, sodium restriction and diuretic therapy are helpful.
- Hepatorenal syndrome requires intensive care, intravascular volume expansion, splanchnic vasoconstrictors, and imminent liver transplantation.

 Follow-Up

- Depends on the etiology of the disease
- Most patients are followed closely for hepatic decompensation
- Growth failure, recurrent life-threatening bleeds not controllable with prophylactic intervention, and poor quality of life are indications for liver transplantation

PITFALLS

- The site of bleeding needs to be identified and managed appropriately

- Not all GI bleeding in a patient with portal HTN is an upper GI source, i.e., hemorrhoids; NG lavage will help determine if the problem is from the upper tract.
- The second most common pitfall is to overestimate the hemoglobin, because equilibration may not have taken place at the time of presentation with an acute bleed.

 Common Questions and Answers

Q: What is my child's long-term prognosis?
A: The disease course and prognosis depend on the underlying etiology. Variceal bleeding associated with prehepatic causes of portal HTN such as portal vein thrombosis typically becomes less problematic as the child ages. Therefore, these patients will most likely not require a shunt and may be easily managed with endoscopic therapy. Similarly, patients with congenital hepatic fibrosis also do very well, because the underlying disease is not progressive and bleeding may be easily managed with endoscopic therapy. In contrast, progressive liver disease has a worse prognosis and often requires liver transplantation.

Q: Should I restrict my child's activities?
A: Limit contact sports and use a spleen guard if splenomegaly is present.

Q: Are there any medications I should avoid?
A: Avoid aspirin and NSAID-containing products.

ICD-9-CM 306.2

BIBLIOGRAPHY

Gitnick G, LaBrecque DR, Moody FG. *Diseases of the Liver and Biliary Tract.* St. Louis: Mosby-Year Book, 1992.

Molleston JP. Variceal bleeding in children. *J Pediatr Gastroenterol Nutr* 2003;37(5):538–545.

Reif S, Blendis L. Portal hypertension and ascites. In: Walker WA, Durie PR, Hamilton JR, et al., eds. *Pediatric Gastrointestinal Disease: Pathophysiology, Diagnosis, Management.* 3rd Ed. Philadelphia: BC Decker, 2000:233–247.

Ryckman FC, Alonso MH. Causes and management of portal hypertension in the pediatric population. *Clin Liver Dis* 2001;5(3):789–818.

Shashidhar H. et al. Propranolol in prevention of portal hypertensive hemorrhage in children: a pilot study. *J Pediatr Gastroenterol Nutr* 1999;29(1):12–17.

Shneider BL. Portal Hypertension. In: Suchy FJ, et al, eds. *Liver disease in children*, 2nd ed. Philadelphia: Lippincott, Williams & Wilkins, 2001:129–151.

Authors: Rose C. Graham-Maar
Barbara Haber, 3rd edition

Posterior Urethral Valves

Database

DEFINITION

Valvular obstruction of the posterior urethra that results in variable dysfunction of all segments of the urinary tract, including the bladder, ureters, and renal parenchyma

PATHOPHYSIOLOGY

- The embryogenesis of posterior urethral valves (PUVs) is unclear.
- PUVs may arise from abnormal insertion and persistence of the distal end of the mesonephric duct.
- The valve is a fold of mucosa and fibrous tissue that usually forms a diaphragm with a slit-like orifice.
- Children with PUVs commonly have renal parenchymal dysplasia.
- With flow of urine from the bladder in patients with PUVs, the valves balloon into the urethra, causing obstruction. As a result of the increased work of voiding, the bladder hypertrophies, with trabeculation and diverticulum formation. The bladder develops poor compliance, decreased capacity, increased pressure, and spastic hyperreflexia.
- The segment of the urethra proximal to the obstruction dilates and elongates.
- Obstructive uropathy produced by PUVs is the result of transmission of high bladder pressures to the ureters and kidneys.
- Hydroureteronephrosis, vesicoureteral reflux, perirenal urinoma, or urinary ascites may occur.
- Renal parenchymal damage may result.

GENETICS

- The genetic basis of PUVs remains unclear.
- The majority of cases are sporadic, although rare cases in siblings have been reported.

EPIDEMIOLOGY

- PUVs is the most common cause of lower urinary tract obstruction in male infants.
- There are rare reports of obstructive valves in the female urethra; however, they differ embryologically from PUVs seen in males.
- The majority of boys with PUVs present in the first year of life.

COMPLICATIONS

- Severe cases may suffer the effects of intrauterine oligohydramnios, including Potter syndrome and pulmonary hypoplasia.
- The renal parenchymal damage results in the sequelae of progressive renal failure, such as anemia, acidosis, fluid and electrolyte abnormalities, and failure to thrive.
- Urinary tract infections and vesicoureteral reflux are common complications.
- Urinary incontinence may result from uninhibited bladder contractions, bladder noncompliance, and polyuria.

PROGNOSIS

- The prognosis for infants with severe PUVs has improved as a result of earlier recognition and improved management of pulmonary hypoplasia and fluid and metabolic derangements.
- Pulmonary hypoplasia and renal dysplasia account for most causes of death in infants with PUVs.
- Measures of renal function at the time of presentation may not correlate with ultimate outcome.
- Rather, the rate of improvement following relief of obstruction is more indicative of prognosis.
- An early nadir creatinine below 1.0 mg/dL does not preclude renal failure, as the child attains greater body mass.
- During the course of many years, many children who seem to do well initially will suffer progressive renal failure and require renal transplantation.
- Patients with an abnormal serum creatinine at 2 years of age often develop end-stage renal disease by adolescence or young adulthood.
- Children with significant bilateral reflux, renal dysplasia, and/or bladder dysfunction are more likely to eventually develop renal insufficiency and hypertension.

Differential Diagnosis

- Nonobstructive urinary tract dilation may occur secondary to:

—Vesicoureteral reflux
—Prune-belly syndrome
—Detrusor-sphincter dyssynergia
—Polyuria
—Urinary tract infection

- Other entities that may mimic PUVs include:

—Urethral strictures
—Primary vesical neck contractures
—Anterior urethral valves

Data Gathering

HISTORY

- The clinical presentation depends on the age of presentation and the severity of the obstruction.
- Many severe cases are diagnosed postnatally as the result of evaluation of hydronephrosis detected antenatally on maternal ultrasound.
- Severely affected infants may present with respiratory distress and other sequelae of oligohydramnios, azotemia, sepsis, dehydration, acidosis, and electrolyte disorders.
- Patients may present with palpable bladder, urinary tract infection, abnormal urinary stream, or failure to thrive as a result of renal failure.
- Toddlers may present with urinary tract infection or voiding symptoms such as dysuria and a weak urinary stream.
- Older boys may present with daytime incontinence, nocturnal enuresis, or urinary frequency as a result of bladder hypertrophy coupled with polyuria secondary to a renal concentrating defect.
- A strong urinary stream does not exclude the diagnosis of PUVs because an adequate flow may be generated by the hypertrophied bladder.

Physical Examination

Palpably enlarged bladder and kidneys are the most common physical finding.

 ## Laboratory Aids

Infants with severe PUVs may have urinary tract infections and/or azotemia and fluid and electrolyte abnormalities such as dehydration, acidosis, hyperkalemia, and hyponatremia.

IMAGING

- The voiding cystourethrogram (VCUG) is the most important study in the diagnosis of PUVs. VCUG will reveal a sharply defined lucency in the posterior urethra and bladder hypertrophy. Bladder trabeculation, diverticula, and vesicoureteral reflux may also be demonstrated.
- Abdominal ultrasound may demonstrate hydroureteronephrosis, evidence of renal dysplasia, and dilation of the posterior urethra, a thickened bladder, and urinary ascites.
- Hydronephrosis is present in 90% of infants with PUVs.
- Definitive diagnosis requires endoscopic examination.

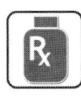 ## Therapy

SUPPORTIVE

- Initial management in the neonate consists of inserting a fine urethral catheter into the bladder and treating any fluid and electrolyte disturbances and/or urinary tract infection.
- A large postobstructive diuresis may occur, requiring ongoing management of fluids and electrolytes.

SPECIFIC

- Valve ablation (destruction of the obstructive valve leaflet) is the definitive treatment of the primary lesion. The most common approach is to incise the valves transurethrally through an endoscope.
- In utero drainage of the fetal bladder, with unclear benefits, has been attempted at a few medical centers.
- Unless the patient has renal insufficiency that does not improve after fluid resuscitation and catheter drainage, the next step is endoscopic ablation of the valves.
- If the infant's urethra is too small for the endoscope, cutaneous vesicostomy may be necessary.
- If rapid recovery does not occur following placement of the catheter or after valve ablation, vesicostomy or supravesical urinary diversion (such as ureterostomy or nephrostomy) may be required. The optimal anatomic level of urinary diversion remains controversial.
- Following valve ablation, the posterior urethra will appear less dilated on VCUG. However, improvement in hydroureteronephrosis and vesicoureteral reflux occurs more slowly, over years.

 ## Follow-Up

- Growth problems, renal insufficiency, and end-stage renal disease can occur at any time during childhood, puberty, or beyond.
- Patients who require extensive urinary diversion, such as vesicostomy, pyelostomy, or ureterostomy, will require long-term reconstruction, including possible bladder reconstruction.
- Delayed obstruction may occur owing to urethral stricture.
- Patients with persistent incontinence require urodynamic evaluation to determine the case and individualized therapy.
- All children with PUVs should have careful follow-up through childhood and puberty. Each visit should include imaging for renal function and upper tract dilation and drainage, urodynamic studies of bladder function, assessment of growth, blood pressure, urinary protein, and serum creatinine.

PITFALLS

When a catheter is passed into the bladder, the valves flatten and are nonobstructive. This may give the misleading impression that there is no obstruction.

 ## Common Questions and Answers

Q: What can be done for children with long-term bladder dysfunction and incontinence?
A: Voiding dysfunction may occur as the result of myogenic failure, detrusor hyperreflexia, and bladder hypertonia. Patients may require a combination of clean intermittent catheterization (CIC), pharmacologic therapy, and bladder augmentation. Approximately 20% of patients with PUVs have secondary bladder pathology that is not reversible by primary therapy of the valves.

Q: Are patients with PUVs good candidates for renal transplantation?
A: Patients with valves have a 5-year graft survival rate of only 50%, compared with 75% for patients with other diagnoses. The main adverse factor is poor bladder function. Better results may follow more aggressive correction of the bladder anomalies. Transplantation has been successful in patients with bladder augmentation and in patients using clean intermittent catheterization.

Q: Do patients with PUVs have impaired sexual and reproductive function?
A: In a small study, patients had good sexual function and some were fertile. Ninety-five percent had normal erections and were able to achieve penetration. Thirty-four percent and 50% had normal and slow ejaculation, respectively. Approximately one-half had normal semen.

ICD-9-CM 753.6

BIBLIOGRAPHY

Chertin B, Cozzi D, Puri P. Long-term results of primary avulsion of posterior urethral valves using a Fogarty balloon catheter. *J Urol* 2002;168(4 Pt 2):1841–1843; discussion 1843.

Churchill BM, McLorie GA, Khoury AE, et al. Pediatric renal transplantation into the abnormal urinary tract. *Urol Clin North Am* 1990;17:343.

Holmes N, Harrison MR, Baskin LS. Fetal surgery for posterior urethral valves: long-term postnatal outcomes. *Pediatr* 2001;108(1):E7.

Parkhouse HF, Woodhouse CRL. Long-term status of patients with posterior urethral valves. *Urol Clin North Am* 1990;17:373.

Radhakrishnan J. Obstructive uropathy in the newborn. *Clin Perinatol* 1990;17:215–239.

Roth KS, Carter WH Jr, Chan JC. Obstructive nephropathy in children: long-term progression after relief of posterior urethral valve. *Pediatrics* 2001;107(5):1004–1010.

Author: Mary B. Leonard

Premature Adrenarche

 ## Database

DEFINITION

Premature adrenarche is characterized by the appearance of small amounts of pubic hair before age 8 in girls and age 9 in boys. Recent data suggest that the onset of normal sexual development in girls is younger than previously recognized, but lowering of the traditionally accepted limits is subject to debate. With premature adrenarche, axillary hair, acne, and apocrine sweat gland secretion are not always present. No other signs of sexual development are exhibited. The presence of breast development suggests precocious puberty and not premature adrenarche.

PATHOPHYSIOLOGY

• Dehydroepiandrosterone (DHEA) and dehydroepiandrosterone sulfate (DHEAS) from the adrenal glands rise earlier than typically seen in normal puberty.
• Zona reticularis of the adrenals normally begins to increase androgen secretion at age 7 to 8 years.

GENETICS

A familial pattern suggesting either recessive or dominant inheritance has been described.

COMPLICATIONS

Can be the first sign of true precocious puberty when followed by the development of breast tissue and advancement of bone age, and thus warrants careful observation. Boys with premature adrenarche and precocious puberty are more likely than girls to have an underlying CNS disorder.

PROGNOSIS

• Undergo puberty appropriately with normal fertility
• Development of ovarian or adrenal hyperandrogenism during adolescence (also known as polycystic ovarian syndrome) is more common in some girls with premature adrenarche. Insulin resistance, a common finding in ovarian hyperandrogenism, has been reported in some children and adolescents with a history of premature adrenarche.
• Final adult height is normal.

 ## Differential Diagnosis

• Tumors
—Androgen-secreting tumors can arise in the gonads or adrenal glands.
• Congenital
—Nonclassic congenital adrenal hyperplasia (CAH)
• Miscellaneous
—Central precocious puberty
—Familial male precocious puberty (testotoxicosis)
—Exogenous male hormone ingestion

 ## Data Gathering

HISTORY

• Careful attention to presence of any other signs of sexual precocity as well as rate of progression
• Family history of pubertal development, infertility, irregular menses, hirsutism, premature male pattern balding

 ## Physical Examination

• The presence of pigmented, curly hairs in the pubic area is consistent with the androgen effect.
• In girls, clitoromegaly suggests CAH or androgen-secreting tumors.
• The finding of acanthosis nigricans suggests that insulin resistance and the risk of developing ovarian hyperandrogenism are present.

PITFALLS

Failure to differentiate between true pubic hair (curly and short) and dark lanugo hair (straight and long)

 ## Laboratory Aids

TESTS

• Adrenal steroids: DHEA and DHEAS are often elevated in the early pubertal range, but testosterone and 17α-hydroxyprogesterone (17-OHP) should be in the prepubertal range.
• GnRH stimulation test: not routinely recommended but would show a normal prepubertal response
• Children with systemic signs of virilization (such as a significantly advanced bone age) or elevated adrenal steroids (17-OHP or DHEA) should have ACTH stimulation testing to exclude CAH and other hyperandrogen syndromes.

IMAGING

• Bone age usually is normal (not significantly advanced).
• Abdominal US, CT scan, or MRI should be considered if signs of significant virilization are present or if rapid progression has occurred; look for intracranial or intraabdominal masses, especially if androgens are markedly elevated.

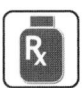 ## Therapy

- No treatment
- Reassure parents and children that this is a benign process.
- Reassess every 6 months to look for signs of virilization and pubertal progression.

 ## Follow-Up

WHEN TO EXPECT IMPROVEMENT

Regression does not occur.

SIGNS TO WATCH FOR

- Watch for other signs of puberty, such as breast development, testicular enlargement (= 4 mL) or growth acceleration, that suggest onset of true precocious puberty.
- Increasing virilization suggests nonclassic CAH or early polycystic ovarian syndrome.
- Acanthosis nigricans or signs of insulin resistance as these have been reported in girls with a history of premature adrenarche.

 ## Common Questions and Answers

Q: Is there a dietary cause of excess adrenal hormones?
A: No.

Q: Does premature adrenarche mean puberty will be early?
A: The onset of puberty in these children is within the normal range and should follow the familial pattern.

Q: Can anything be done to reverse the changes?
A: This is a benign process that does not have long-term sequelae. Antiandrogen drugs are available but are not recommended.

ICD-9-CM 255.3

BIBLIOGRAPHY

Herman-Giddens ME, Slora EJ, Wasserman RC, et al. Secondary sexual characteristics and menses in young girls seen in office practice: a study from the pediatric research office in settings network. *Pediatrics* 1997;99:505–512.

Ibanez L, Potau N, Virdis R, et al. Postpubertal outcome in girls diagnosed of premature pubarche during childhood: increased frequency of functional ovarian hyperandrogenism. *J Clin Endocrinol Metab* 1993;76:1599–1603.

Kaplowitz P, Oberfield SE, and the Drug and Therapeutics and Executive Committees of the Lawson Wilkins Pediatric Endocrine Society. Reexamination of the age limit for defining when puberty is precocious in girls in the United States: implications for evaluation and treatment. *Pediatrics* 1999;104:936–941.

Kornreich L, Horev G, Blaser S, et al. Central precocious puberty: evaluation by neuroimaging. *Pediatr Radiol* 1995;25(1): 7–11.

Midyett LK, Moore WV, Jacobson JD. Are pubertal changes in girls before age 8 benign? *Pediatrics* 2003;111:47–51.

Morris AH, Reiter EO, Geffner ME, et al. Absence of non-classical congenital adrenal hyperplasia in patients with precocious adrenarche. *J Clin Endocrinol Metab* 1989; 69:709.

Oppenheimer E, Linder B, DiMartino-Nardi J. Decreased insulin sensitivity in prepubertal girls with premature adrenarche and acanthosis nigricans. *J Clin Endocrinol Metab* 1995;80:614–618.

Pere A, Perheentupa J, Peter M, et al. Follow up of growth and steroids in premature adrenarche. *Eur J Pediatr* 1995;154(5): 346–352.

Styne DM. New aspects in diagnosis and treatment of pubertal disorders. *Pediatr Clin North Am* 1997;44(2):505–529.

Author: Andrea Kelly and J. Nina Ham

Premature Thelarche

 Database

DEFINITION

• Premature thelarche is breast development before age 8 years in girls with no other signs of pubertal development.
• A recent study suggested that African American girls are developing pubertal characteristics as early as age 6 and Caucasian girls as early as age 7. However, physicians should be cautious about lowering these normal limits and should evaluate children on an individual basis because signs of puberty at these younger ages may not be normal.

CAUSE

Intermittent estrogen secretion by ovarian cysts

PATHOPHYSIOLOGY

• Low levels of estrogen secretion by normal follicular cysts
• Increased sensitivity of breast tissue to low levels of estrogen (surmised to be environmental)
• Ovarian response to transient increases in FSH levels and possibly to variations in ovarian sensitivity to FSH

EPIDEMIOLOGY

Sixty percent noted between 6 months to 2 years of age

COMPLICATIONS

May be the first sign of precocious puberty

PROGNOSIS

• No known effects on growth or fertility
• Onset after age 2 years may be associated with increased risk of progression to precocious puberty.

 Differential Diagnosis

• Environmental

—Exposure to exogenous estrogens in form of creams or birth control pills
—Intake of food with high estrogen levels (e.g., chicken liver)

• Tumors

—Benign lipomas

• Congenital

—Neonatal breast hyperplasia (ICD-9-CM 778.7) is benign breast enlargement in newborn boys or girls that is apparent shortly after birth and is a result of gestational hormones. This form of breast development usually regresses.

• Severe acquired hypothyroidism: High levels of TSH may cross-stimulate gonadal FSH and/or LH receptors.
• McCune-Albright syndrome: triad of precocious puberty, café-au-lait spots, and polyostotic fibrous dysplasia as a result of gain of function mutations of G proteins
• True precocious puberty

 Data Gathering

HISTORY

• Careful assessment of onset and progression of breast tissue
• Family history of early puberty
• Exposure to estrogens

SPECIAL QUESTIONS

Ingestion of foods with high estrogen levels?

 Physical Examination

• Areolar enlargement is usually not present.
• Galactorrhea is not present.
• Look carefully for other signs of puberty:

—Menstrual blood
—Dull, gray-pink, or rugose vaginal mucosa (vs. prepubertal appearance: shiny, bright red, and smooth)
—Pubic or axillary hair

• Inspect skin for birthmarks suggestive of McCune-Albright syndrome (café-au-lait spots in a "coast of Maine" pattern)
• Evaluate for signs of hypothyroidism: goiter, short stature.

PROCEDURE

Palpate carefully to distinguish fat from true breast tissue.

 Laboratory Aids

TESTS

No test is specific. Serum FSH and estradiol may be slightly higher than age-matched controls but are not consistently elevated. In isolated premature thelarche serum ultrasensitive LH is pre-pubertal.

IMAGING

• Bone age is not significantly or very mildly advanced (<1 year ahead of chronologic age). Useful in guiding the need for more intensive evaluation of true precocious puberty
• Pelvic ultrasonography may demonstrate presence and regression of small ovarian cysts (1 to 15 mm) and a prepubertal uterus.

Premature Thelarche

 Therapy

- Observation
- Reassurance that this is a benign process

 Follow-Up

WHEN TO EXPECT IMPROVEMENT

Regression may occur up to 6 years after onset.

SIGNS TO WATCH FOR

Evidence of pubertal progression should prompt additional evaluation by an endocrinologist:

- Rapid increase in size of breast tissue
- Vaginal bleeding
- Growth spurt
- Development of pubic and axillary hair

PITFALLS

- Must distinguish fat from breast tissue in obese girls
- Removal of a breast bud will result in failure of that breast to develop during adolescence.

 Common Questions and Answers

Q: Does premature thelarche predispose the child to abnormalities in pubertal development?
A: If onset occurs after age 2 years, the girl may be more likely to enter puberty earlier. However, the majority of girls with premature thelarche will have normal pubertal development and fertility.

Q: Is my child susceptible to breast cancer?
A: There are no data to suggest that premature thelarche increases the risk of breast neoplasia.

Q: Can it happen in boys?
A: Many newborn male and female infants have breast buds as a result of exposure to maternal estrogen in utero. This neonatal gynecomastia usually resolves quickly.

Q: My daughter has breast development on only one side. Is this a tumor?
A: Asymmetric breast development is quite common in the early stages of normal pubertal development. Malignant tumors of the breast during childhood are extremely rare. As mentioned earlier, any removal of breast tissue prior to or during puberty must be avoided if possible.

ICD-9-CM 259.1

BIBLIOGRAPHY

Haber HP, Wollmann HA, Ranke MB. Pelvic ultrasonography: early differentiation between isolated premature thelarche and central precocious puberty [see comment in *Eur J Pediatr* 1997;156(1):78–79]. *Eur J Pediatr* 1997;154(3):182–186.

Herman-Giddens ME, Slora EJ, Wassermn RC, et al. Secondary sexual characteristics and menses in young girls seen in office practice: a study from the pediatric research office in settings network. *Pediatrics* 1997;99:505–512.

Kaplowitz P, Oberfield SE, and the Drug and Therapeutics and Executive Committees of the Lawson Wilkins Pediatric Endocrine Society. Reexamination of the age limit for defining when puberty is precocious in girls in the United States: implications for evaluation and treatment. *Pediatrics* 1999;104:936–941.

Klein Ko, Mericq V, Brown-Dawson JM, et al. Estrogen levels in girls with premature thelarche compared with normal prepubertal girls as determined by an ultrasensitive recombinant cell bioassay. *J Pediatr* 1999; 134(2):190–192.

Lebrethon MC, Bourguignon JP. Management of central isosexual precocity: diagnosis, treatment, outcome. *Curr Opin Pediatr* 2000; 12(4):394–399.

Midyett LK, Moore WV, Jacobson JD. Are pubertal changes in girls before age 8 benign? *Pediatrics* 2003;111(1):47–51.

Pasquino AM, Pucarelli I, Passeri F, et al. Progression of premature thelarche to central precocious puberty [see comment in *J Pediatr* 1995;127(2):336–337]. *J Pediatr* 1995; 126(1):11–14.

Salardi S, Cacciari E, Mainetti B, et al. Outcome of premature thelarche: relation to puberty and final height. *Arch Dis Child* 1998;79(2):173–174.

Stanhope R. Premature thelarche: clinical follow-up and indication for treatment. *J Pediatr Endocrinol Metab* 2000;13(Suppl 1): 827–830.

Styne DM. New aspects in the diagnosis and treatment of pubertal disorders. *Pediatr Clin North Am* 1997;44(2):505–529.

Traggiai C, Stanhope R. Disorders of pubertal development. *Best Practice & Research in Clinical Obstetrics & Gynaecology* 2003;17(1): 41–56.

Author: Olga T. Hardy and Andrea Kelly

Premenstrual Syndrome (PMS)

 Database

DEFINITION

Premenstrual syndrome (PMS), also called luteal phase disorder, is a disorder characterized by psychological and physical symptoms (such as irritability, moodiness, tearfulness, anxiety, headaches, mastalgia, bloating/weight gain, and fatigue) that occur cyclically and consistently during the second half (luteal phase) of the menstrual cycle and negatively impact a woman's usual activities of daily living.

Premenstrual dysphoric disorder (PMDD) most extreme variant of PMS; defined in DSM-IV-TR as (a) severe psychologic symptoms (see below) causing (b) significant dysfunctions which (c) are not an exacerbation of symptoms of a chronic condition and (d) are confirmed through prospective daily ratings of three consecutive cycles. The criteria for PMDD are:

- At least five symptoms must be present during most of the luteal phase, with at least one of the symptoms being among the first four: (a) feeling sad, hopeless, or self-deprecating; (b) feeling tense, anxious or "on edge"; (c) marked lability of mood interspersed with frequent tearfulness; (d) persistent irritability, anger, and increased interpersonal conflicts; (e) decreased interest in usual activities, which may be associated with withdrawal from social relationships; (f) difficulty concentrating; (g) feeling fatigued, lethargic, or lacking in energy; (h) marked changes in appetite, which may be associated with binge eating or craving certain foods; (i) hypersomnia or insomnia; (j) a subjective feeling of being overwhelmed or out of control; and (k) physical symptoms such as breast tenderness/swelling, headaches, bloating or weight gain, arthralgias, or myalgias.

PATHOPHYSIOLOGY

- Etiology unknown, but presumed to be multifactorial
- Occurrence of symptoms seems related to ovarian function/ovulation; PMS does not occur before menarche, during pregnancy, or after menopause; PMS can occur after hysterectomy, but not after bilateral oophorectomy.
- Research suggests altered cyclic interactions between sex hormones and neurotransmitters (in particular relationships between sex hormones, prostaglandins, and serotonin); β-aminobutyric acid (GABA) and opioid neurotransmitter systems have also been studied, along with trace elements, vitamins, and minerals.
- Women with PMS do not have abnormal serum concentrations of estrogen or progesterone; research suggests women with PMS have abnormal responses to variations in sex hormones.

EPIDEMIOLOGY

- Forty percent to 75% of women experience some PMS symptoms at some time.
- Fifteen percent to 30% of women report recurrent symptoms suggestive of PMS.
- Two percent to 5% of women have symptoms which interfere with their usual activities (PMDD).

COMPLICATIONS

- Psychological morbidity includes difficulty with interpersonal relationships (family and friends) and school absence/failure.

 Differential Diagnosis

PSYCHIATRIC

- Mood disorder, including major depression, dysthymia, bipolar illness,
- Postpartum depression, anxiety disorder
- Substance abuse
- Physical, sexual, or emotional abuse
- Somatization disorder
- Eating disorder

ENDOCRINOLOGIC

- Thyroid disease
- Cushing disease
- Diabetes mellitus

GYNECOLOGIC

- Dysmenorrhea (primary or secondary)
- Pregnancy
- Endometriosis
- Hormonal contraceptive use
- Perimenopause

IMMUNOLOGIC/HEMATOLOGIC

- Anemia
- Fibromyalgia
- Systemic Lupus Erythematosis (SLE)
- Chronic fatigue syndrome
- Neurally mediated hypotension

NEUROLOGIC

- Migraine headache

 Data Gathering

HISTORY

- Complete medical history (including use of medications or illicit substances, cigarettes, dietary evaluation)
- Gynecologic history (age at onset of pubertal development, menstrual pattern, sexual activity, contraceptive use, dysmenorrhea)
- Psychiatric history (history of mental health disorders, medications)
- Family history (including mental health and substance use/abuse history)
- Psychosocial history (living situation, school/vocational activities and goals, hobbies, peers)
- Complete review of systems including both physical symptoms (fatigue, breast tenderness/swelling, bloating, edema, weight gain, headache, arthralgias, myalgias, pelvic discomfort, changes in bowel habit, reduced coordination) and emotional/psychological symptoms (depression, mood lability, irritability, tension, anxiety, tearfulness, restlessness, reduced concentration, fatigue, altered libido, altered appetite/eating habits, altered sleep)
- Chronologic review to determine if symptoms are recurrent with majority of menstrual cycles, isolated to luteal phase of cycle, and remit with onset of menses.

 Physical Examination

There are no specific physical findings of PMS

Finding: Enlarged thyroid gland
Significance: May suggest hypothyroidism and need to evaluate for thyroid disease.

Finding: Virilization (hirsutism, clitoromegaly)
Significance: May suggest hyperandrogenism and need to evaluate for adrenal disease (including Cushing syndrome) or other hormonal disorders, such as polycystic ovarian syndrome.

Finding: Pallor
Significance: May suggest anemia.

Finding: Orthostatic hypotension
Significance: May suggest neurally mediated hypotension.

Laboratory Aids

TESTS

Test: CBC
Significance: To rule out anemia

Test: Thyroid Stimulating Hormone Assay (TSH)
Significance: To rule out thyroid disease

Test: PAF (Premenstrual Assessment Form), PRISM (Prospective Record of Severity of Menstruation), or COPE (Calendar of Premenstrual Experiences)
Significance: Prospective symptom calendars can help establish diagnosis and provide information about symptom patterns (recurrence and relation to menses)

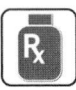

Therapy

• Treatment goals include reducing both symptom frequencies and severities and the impact of symptoms on patients' activities.
• Patient education, counseling, and reassurance may be all that is needed for women with milder symptoms.
• Many pharmacologic and nonpharmacologic modalities have not been formally evaluated.

NONPHARMACOLOGIC

Lifestyle/Diet

• Increasing physical activity, ensuring adequate and regular sleep, and maintaining a healthy diet are important first steps.
• Research supports reducing caffeine intake, and suggests that reductions in salt and refined sugars may also be beneficial.
• Meta-analyses of research to date has shown that some supplements are beneficial in reducing symptom frequencies and severities, including calcium carbonate (1,200 mg/day), pyridoxine/Vitamin B6 (50 mg/day), and possibly magnesium (400 mg/day).
• A wide range of herbal therapies are used by patients, including evening primrose oil, chasteberry, black cohosh, ginkgo, and St. John's wort; to date there is no strong evidence to support their use in PMS.
• Mind/Body therapies are frequently used including individual psychotherapy, relaxation techniques, guided imagery, yoga, massage, biofeedback, and group therapy; to date there is no strong evidence to support their use in PMS.

Pharmacologic

1. Initial intervention: Many menstrually associated symptoms can be managed through the use of nonsteroidal anti-inflammatories, i.e., (NSAIDs).

• NSAIDs (e.g., naproxen sodium 275 to 550 mg b.i.d.) relieve premenstrual/menstrual cramping, headaches, myalgias/arthralgias.

Side effects include gastrointestinal upset and renal dysfunction.

2. Secondary intervention: Selective serotonin reuptake inhibitors (SSRIs) are first-line therapy for women, especially those with predominantly psychological symptoms. Both continuous and intermittent (during luteal phase) dosing can be used, and symptom amelioration can occur during the first cycle treatment. Intermittent use includes administration during the last 14 days of the menstrual cycle or treatment begun at expected date of symptom onset.

• Fluoxetine (10 to 20 mg/day), sertraline (50 mg/day) and citalopram (20 to 40 mg/day) are three of the most commonly used SSRIs for PMS/PMDD; side effects include gastrointestinal upset, insomnia, tremor/agitation, fatigue, dry mouth, and sexual dysfunction.
• Hormonal contraceptives that suppress ovulation may ameliorate hormonally mediated symptoms such as breast swelling/tenderness, bloating but may exacerbate mood symptoms.

Referral

• A gynecologist/reproductive endocrinologist can assist in the management of severe PMS/PMDD. Other pharmacologic agents which are used include gonadotropin releasing hormone (GnRH) analogs, danazol, estrogen implants, androgens.

Follow-Up

• Frequent follow-up and the use of prospective menstrual/symptom calendars are important. Patient education and counseling are crucial to successful treatment. Once the diagnosis of PMS is established, and after recommending appropriate lifestyle changes (and possibly NSAIDs), the patient should be reevaluated after 3 months. If there has not been substantial improvement, secondary pharmacologic therapies (SSRIs) may need to be considered.

PITFALLS

• Many women report that their PMS symptoms are not taken seriously

Common Questions and Answers

Q: Can adolescent girls have PMS and PMDD?
A: The incidence of PMS and PMDD in adolescents is not well established. Although up to 50% of cycles are anovulatory during the first 1 to 2 years postmenarche, younger patients do experience many PMS symptoms, and menstrual problems are some of the most common reasons for school absence. Most experts believe that PMS/PMDD will not

develop until a regular ovulatory pattern is established, 2 to 3 years after menarche.

Q: Is family history important?
A: Genetic factors may play a role in the development of PMS/PMDD; twin studies show a 93% concordance rate in monozygotic twins, with only a 44% rate in dizygotic twins.

Q: Are there any common comorbidities?
A: The symptoms of PMS/PMDD are also seen with depression, anxiety, and other mood disorders. Psychiatric symptomatology can fluctuate, and symptoms may change in relation to the menstrual cycle. Careful and thorough history taking and prospective symptom diaries can help differentiate PMS/PMDD from another mental health disorder.

ICD-9-CM 625.4

BIBLIOGRAPHY

American Psychiatric Association. *Diagnostic and Statistical Manual of Mental Disorders.* 4th Ed, Text Revision. Washington, DC: Author, 2000.

Bhatia SC. Diagnosis and treatment of premenstrual dysphoric disorder. *Am Fam Physician* 2002;66:1239–1248, 1253–1254.

Cronje WH, Studd JWW. Premenstrual syndrome and premenstrual dysphoric disorder. *Prim Care* 2002;29(1):1–12.

Dickerson LM, Mazyck PJ, Hunter MH. Premenstrual syndrome. *Am Fam Physician* 2003;67:1743–1752.

Girman A, Lee R, Kligler B. An integrative approach to premenstrual syndrome. *Am J Obstet Gynecol* 2003 May;188(5 Suppl): 556–65.

Gundersen DC. Premenstrual syndrome and premenstrual dysphoric disorder. In: Jacobson JL, Jacobson AM, eds. *Psychiatric secrets,* 2nd ed. Philadelphia, PA: Hanley & Belfus, 2001:348–351.

Halbreich U. The etiology, biology, and evolving pathology of premenstrual syndromes. *Psychoneuroendocrinology* 2003; 28(Suppl 3):55–99.

Halbreich U, Bornstein J, Pearlstein T, Kahn LS. The prevalence, impairment, impact, and burden of premenstrual dysphoric disorder (PMS/PMDD). *Psychoneuroendocrinology* 2003;28(Suppl 3):1–23.

Murray PM. Medical and other noncontraceptive uses of combined oral contraceptives. *J Pediatr Adolesc Gynecol* 2003;16:243–252.

Author: Ann B. Bruner

Primary Adrenal Insufficiency

 Database

DEFINITION

Primary adrenal insufficiency is a deficiency in the secretion of cortisol by the adrenal glands. This may be associated with deficiencies of other hormones, including aldosterone and adrenal androgens.

PATHOPHYSIOLOGY

- Addison disease: primary hypoadrenalism is a result of bilateral destruction of the adrenal cortices; this can be as a result of autoimmune destruction (isolated or as part of polyendocrine autoimmune syndromes), tuberculosis, hemorrhage, fungus, neoplastic infiltration, or AIDS
- Adrenoleukodystrophy: inherited disorders of impaired peroxisomal degradation of very long chain fatty acids, resulting in adrenal insufficiency and progressive neurologic deterioration
- ACTH unresponsiveness: an inherited defect in the ACTH receptor, resulting in isolated glucocorticoid deficiency with hypoglycemia in infancy and hyperpigmentation
- Adrenal hypoplasia congenita: a defect in adrenal organogenesis
- Congenital adrenal hyperplasia: a group of enzymatic disorders of steroid metabolism, of which 21-hydroxylase deficiency is the most common.

GENETICS

- Addison disease: autoimmune adrenal insufficiency may be isolated or part of autoimmune polyglandular syndromes type 1 and 2. Familial and sporadic cases have been reported.
- Mutations in the AIRE-1 gene have been identified as the cause of autoimmune polyglandular syndrome type 1. An association exists between idiopathic Addison disease and HLA-138 and -Dw3.
- Adrenoleukodystrophy: X-linked recessive disorder of very long chain fatty acid metabolism. An autosomal-recessive form of the disease exists, with presentation during infancy.
- ACTH unresponsiveness: autosomal recessive ACTH receptor defect
- Adrenal hypoplasia congenital: X-linked mutation in DAX-1 gene
- Congenital adrenal hyperplasia: autosomal-recessive inheritance

EPIDEMIOLOGY

Age

- Addison disease is uncommon in children and usually presents between ages 20 and 50 years. In the pediatric population, it is most often seen in late childhood and adolescence.
- Adrenoleukodystrophy typically presents late in the first decade of life with neurologic symptoms. Signs and symptoms of adrenal insufficiency may present at any age.
- ACTH unresponsiveness presents in late infancy or the toddler period.
- Adrenal hypoplasia congenita presents in infancy or early childhood.
- Adrenal insufficiency associated with CAH presents in the newborn period.

Sex

- Addison disease is more common in females.
- Adrenoleukodystrophy, an X-linked disorder, predominantly affects males.
- ACTH unresponsiveness affects both sexes equally.
- Congenital adrenal hypoplasia, an X-linked disorder, predominantly affects males.

COMPLICATIONS

- If not diagnosed and/or treated properly, a significant physical stress such as surgery or illness may result in a life-threatening adrenal crisis.
- Adrenoleukodystrophy results in severe neurologic impairment and death.
- Unrecognized ACTH unresponsiveness is associated with recurrent hypoglycemia, seizures, mental retardation, and death.
- Pubertal delay or hypogonadotropic hypogonadism is seen with congenital adrenal hypoplasia as a result of DAX-1 mutations.
- CAH can cause virilization/ambiguous genitalia in female infants with the disease and can cause salt-wasting crises in infants of both sexes.

PROGNOSIS

- The long-term prognosis of isolated adrenal insufficiency is good, provided adequate hydrocortisone is provided, particularly in times of illness.
- The diagnosis of adrenoleukodystrophy carries a poor prognosis.

 Differential Diagnosis

- Autoimmune adrenal cortical destruction
- Infectious adrenal cortical destruction

—Tuberculous
—Fungal
—AIDS

- Adrenal hemorrhage
- Neoplastic adrenal infiltration
- Adrenoleukodystrophy
- ACTH unresponsiveness
- Adrenal hypoplasia congenita
- CAH

 Data Gathering

HISTORY

- Weakness and fatigue
- Anorexia, weight loss
- Headache
- Nausea, vomiting, diarrhea, abdominal pain
- Orthostatic symptoms
- Muscle or joint pains
- Emotional lability
- Salt craving
- Hyperpigmentation,
- Decreased axillary or pubic hair in females as a result of lack of adrenal androgens
- Amenorrhea in females

 Physical Examination

- Hyperpigmentation, especially on lip borders, buccal mucosa, nipples, and over skin creases
- Weight loss
- Hypotension
- Evaluate for other signs of autoimmune disease (e.g., thyromegaly, vitiligo).
- Pubertal staging
- Signs of virilization in females

Primary Adrenal Insufficiency

 Laboratory Aids

TESTS

Specific

- Cortrosyn stimulation test: administer cosyntropin (synthetic ACTH) 250 μg IV and measure cortisol at 30 and 60 minutes. A normal response is a final cortisol exceeding 18 μg/dL. An insufficient cortisol response is diagnostic of adrenal insufficiency.
- A baseline ACTH greater than 200 pg/mL with inadequate cortisol is seen in primary adrenal insufficiency
- Serum adrenal antibodies may be positive in autoimmune Addison disease.
- Very long chain fatty acids are elevated in adrenoleukodystrophy.
- Low gonadotropin and sex steroid levels suggesting hypogonadotropic hypogonadism may be seen with adrenal hypoplasia congenita
- Adrenal steroid precursors will be elevated in CAH.

Nonspecific

Electrolytes

- Hyponatremia: result of the mineralocorticoid deficiency and glucocorticoid deficiency; combination sodium loss from kidneys and the inability to excrete a water load
- Hyperkalemia and acidosis: chronic mineralocorticoid deficiency with the inability to excrete potassium and acid
- Hypercalcemia: most likely a result of increased calcium absorption as a result of the lack of glucocorticoid effect on the gut
- Hypoglycemia: glucocorticoids have permissive effects on gluconeogenesis.
- Renin levels are elevated when a mineralocorticoid deficiency is present.

 Emergency Care

ACUTE ADRENAL CRISIS

An intercurrent illness or surgical procedure may provoke an episode of hypotension, tachycardia, and shock. Electrolytes reveal decreased serum sodium, elevated potassium, metabolic acidosis, and a decreased or normal glucose. Serum should be drawn and saved to aid in diagnosis, but treatment should not be delayed for a diagnostic Cortrosyn stimulation test.

Treatment

- D5NS for volume repletion and treatment of salt-wasting
- Stress dosage of hydrocortisone: 100 mg/m² followed by 100 mg/m² per 24 hours of hydrocortisone divided q4h. Taper steroids over the next 1 to 2 days to a physiologic replacement dosage.
- Mineralocorticoid replacement: Florinef 0.1 mg daily when able to take PO.

Therapy

CHRONIC ADRENAL INSUFFICIENCY

Treatment

- Hydrocortisone 10 to 12 mg/m² per day PO divided as t.i.d. This oral dose should be tripled for minor stress such as fever, illness, or vomiting. For major stress (surgery, significant illness), give hydrocortisone 50 to 100 mg/m² followed by 50 to 100 mg/m² per 24 hours IV divided q4h. Intramuscular hydrocortisone is recommended for emergency home use.

- Florinef 0.1 mg PO per day
- Patient education

—Stress dosing
—Seek medical attention for significant illness, persistent vomiting, or the inability to take fluids by mouth.
—Medic-Alert bracelet

 Follow-Up

An acute adrenal crisis usually improves rapidly with the administration of fluids and glucocorticoids. Steroids can usually be tapered over 12 days.

LONG-TERM MONITORING

- Clinical: reduction in hyperpigmentation
- Electrolytes, ACTH, renin
- Screen for polyautoimmune disorders.
- Growth
- Very long chain fatty acid levels and neurologic function in adrenoleukodystrophy
- Pubertal development

PITFALLS

- The symptoms of primary adrenal insufficiency are nonspecific and are similar to those found in many disease processes. The electrolyte picture of adrenal insufficiency can be seen in renal disorders, obstructive uropathy, and isolated aldosterone deficiency.
- Cosyntropin testing should definitively separate out those with true adrenal insufficiency.

Common Questions and Answers

Q: What are the indications for stress dosing and how rapidly can the stress hydrocortisone dose be tapered?
A: Patients will require stress dosing of hydrocortisone for surgical procedures, fever (>100°F), vomiting, diarrhea, and particularly vigorous exercise. The stress dose is typically given for 24 hours, after which the usual dose is resumed. Should it be necessary to administer the stress dosage for a more prolonged period, the dosage can usually be tapered to a physiologic dosage over 12 days, once the patient's clinical condition has improved.

ICD-9-CM 255.4

BIBLIOGRAPHY

Anderson MS, Venanzi ES, Klein J, et al. Projection of an immunological self shadow within the thymus by the aire protein. *Science* 2002;298(5597):1395–1401.

Baker JR. Autoimmune endocrine disease. *JAMA* 1997;278(22):1931–1937.

Dorin RI, Qualls CR, Crapo LM. Diagnosis of adrenal insufficiency. *Ann Intern Med* 2003;139:194–204.

Listenberg MJL, Kemp S, Sarde CO. Spectrum of mutations in the gene encoding the adrenoleukodystrophy protein. *Am J Hum Genet* 1995;56:44–50.

Peter M, Viemann M, Partsch CJ, et al. Congenital adrenal hypoplasia: clinical spectrum, experience with hormonal diagnosis, and report on new point mutations of the DAX-1 gene. *J Clin Endocrinol Metab* 1998;83(8):2666–2674.

Speiser PW, White PC. Congenital adrenal hyperplasia. *N Engl J Med* 2003;349:776–788.

Tsigos C. Isolated glucocorticoid deficiency and ACTH receptor mutations. *Arch Med Res* 1999;30(6):475–480.

Vaidya B, Pearce S, Kendall-Taylor P. Recent advances in the molecular genetics of congenital and acquired primary adrenocortical failure. *Clin Endocrinol* 2000; 53(4):403–418.

Author: Lorraine Katz and J. Nina Ham

Prion Diseases (Transmissible Spongiform Encephalopathies, TSE)

 Database

DEFINITION

• The transmissible spongiform encephalopathies (TSEs) or prion diseases are a family of slowly progressive neurodegenerative diseases of humans and animals that are uniformly fatal, causing irreversible cumulative brain damage.
• The human TSEs include Creutzfeldt-Jakob disease (CJD), the recently identified new variant CJD (vCJD), kuru, Gerstmann-Sträussler-Scheinker syndrome, and fatal familial insomnia syndrome.
• Six TSEs in animals have been described: bovine spongiform encephalopathy (BSE, also known as mad cow disease) scrapie in sheep and goats, feline spongiform encephalopathy, transmissible mink encephalopathy, exotic ungulate encephalopathy, and chronic wasting disease of mule deer and elk.

CAUSES

• Prions are infectious proteins lacking nucleic acids that are believed to cause TSE. Infection arises when normal protease-sensitive host proteins, involved in neuronal function, undergo spontaneous misfolding to yield the abnormal protease-resistant form associated with infectivity.
• Prions reproduce by recruiting neighboring normal cellular prion protein and stimulating its conversion to the infectious form. Not all scientists believe the prion hypothesis and some have argued that the causative agent is virus-like and possesses nucleic acids.

PATHOLOGY/PATHOPHYSIOLOGY

• Progressive accumulation of abnormal prion protein in the CNS disrupts function leading to vacuolization and cell death. There is no host immune response or inflammation involved in the pathologic process.
• Neuropathologic findings include neuronal loss, atrophy, vacuolization or spongiform change, reactive astrogliosis, and cell death.

ASSOCIATED DISEASES AND EPIDEMIOLOGY CJD

• CJD is the most prevalent form of TSE in humans and occurs as both a sporadic and familial disease.
• Approximately 90% of cases are sporadic because there is no family history, and no known source of transmission, and occurs throughout the world at a rate 1/1,000,000 people.
• Familial cases are associated with a gene mutation in the gene encoding normal prion protein and account for approximately 10% of cases.
• Less than 5% of CJD cases are iatrogenic resulting from accidental transmission of the causative agent via contaminated surgical equipment, as a result of cornea or dura mater transplants, or administration of human-derived pituitary growth hormones.
• There is no evidence of person-to-person transmission among family members via direct contact, by droplet or by airborne spread.
• Disease is characterized by progressive dementia, myoclonus, visual or cerebellar disturbance, pyramidal/extrapyramidal dysfunction, and/or akinetic mutism.
• Classic sporadic CJD most often occurs between the ages of 50 and 70 and affects both sexes equally.
• Death usually occurs within 1 year of onset of symptoms.

Variant CJD (vCJD)

• vCJD is a new form of CJD, first reported in 1994, which has unique clinical features.
• vCJD, in contrast to CJD, affects younger patients including adolescents (average age, 29 years) and has a longer duration of illness with median of 14 months as opposed to 4.5 months with CJD.
• There is strong epidemiologic evidence that links vCJD to BSE. BSE is a TSE affecting cattle and was first reported in the United Kingdom. The most likely route of exposure is through bovine-based foods derived from BSE-infected cattle. The highest incidence of vCJD is seen in the U.K., the country with the largest potential exposure to BSE. There are no confirmed cases of vCJD in North America.
• Clinical features, early in the illness, include prominent psychiatric symptoms such as depression and schizophrenia-like psychosis, and ataxia. Other neurologic signs such paresthesia/dysesthesia, chorea, dystonia, myoclonus, and akinetic mutism develop as the disease progresses.

Fatal-Familial Insomnia

• An autosomal-dominant disorder, caused by genetic mutation in normal prion protein gene.
• Clinical features include insomnia, dysautonomia, ataxia, myoclonus, and late dementia.
• Pathology reveals minimal vacuolization and no plaques.

Gerstmann-Sträussler-Scheinker Syndrome

• A disorder with autosomal-dominant inheritance
• Clinical features include ataxia and dementia
• Pathology reveals amyloid plaques.

 Differential Diagnosis

• Neurodegenerative disorders—mostly seen in older adults with the exception of Alpers disease

—Alzheimer disease
—Parkinson disease
—Frontotemporal dementia
—Pick disease
—Alper disease (progressive cerebral hemiatrophy)
—Amyotrophic lateral sclerosis
—Huntington disease
—Spinocerebellar ataxia

• Psychiatric disorders—especially when considering vCJD as a diagnosis

—Depression
—Schizophrenia
—Drug-induced psychosis

• Encephalitis—infectious
• Sydenham chorea
• Subacute sclerosing panencephalitis
• Progressive multifocal leukoencephalopathy
• Toxic encephalopathy
• Inborn errors of metabolism
• Hashimoto thyroiditis
• CNS vasculitis
• CNS tumors

Prion Diseases (Transmissible Spongiform Encephalopathies, TSE)

Data Gathering

HISTORY

- Evidence of a familial form of TSE
- Potential iatrogenic exposures such as administration of human-derived pituitary growth hormones, implantation of dura mater or corneal grafts from humans, epilepsy surgery or other CNS surgery involving stereotactic electrodes.
- Duration of symptoms greater than 6 months.
- Afebrile illness
- In vCJD, progressive neuropsychiatric symptoms including:

—Depression, anxiety, apathy, withdrawal, or delusions
—Painful sensory symptoms including pain and/or dysesthesia.
—Ataxia
—Myoclonus, chorea, or dystonia
—Dementia

Physical Examination

- Afebrile
- Abnormal mental status examination with defects in memory, personality, and other higher cortical functions, or psychosis
- Neurologic signs include unsteady gait and the presence of involuntary movements.
- Late findings include mutism and complete immobility.

Laboratory Aids

The diagnosis of TSE in humans can only be confirmed following pathologic examination of the brain. Microscopic examination of patients with all types of human TSEs reveals spongiform change accompanied by neuronal loss and gliosis. Amyloid plaques or immunohistochemical demonstration of abnormal prion protein in the brain may also be seen. "Florid" plaques (amyloid plaques encircled by holes or vacuoles resulting in a daisy-like appearance) are consistently present in patients with vCJD. Tonsil biopsy may be helpful in suspected cases of vCJD; the biopsy may reveal accumulation of abnormal prion protein.

LABORATORY TESTS

Most laboratory tests are of little value in the diagnosis of TSE. Examination of the CSF may reveal a mild elevation of protein, but otherwise the CSF is normal.

ELECTROENCEPHALOGRAM (EEG)

- In CJD, generalized slowing is seen early in the disease with progression to periodic burst of biphasic or triphasic sharp-wave complexes.
- In vCJD, the EEG does not show the wave forms characteristic of sporadic CJD. Although EEG abnormalities are seen in the majority of patients, these findings are not specific.

IMAGING

- In patients with vCJD, MRI reveals abnormal bilateral pulvinar high signal.
- In CJD, MRI often demonstrates hyperintense signals in the basal ganglia.
- In later stages of CJD and vCJD, imaging studies such as MRI or CT scan reveal generalized atrophy with large ventricles.

Therapy

No treatment is effective in slowing or stopping the progression of disease. Appropriate supportive care should be provided. The prognosis for human TSEs is uniformly poor.

INFECTION CONTROL

Standard universal precautions are indicated for infection control. Strict isolation is not necessary. Caution should be used in obtaining CSF and handling tissues obtained at autopsy. Equipment contaminated by high-risk tissue should be soaked in ≥ 1 N sodium hydroxide solution for at least 1 hour and then autoclaved at 134°C for at least 1 hour.

Common Questions and Answers

Q: Is transmission of TSEs from human blood possible?
A: There are no known cases of TSEs attributed to transfusion of blood products or reuse of devices contaminated with blood products.

Q: Is our food supply safe?
A: No cases of vCJD or BSE have been recognized in North America. The incidence in the U.K. has been low and is not increasing rapidly. Measures have been taken by the World Health Organization and the FDA to reduce the risk of TSE, including a ban on the use of ruminant tissues in animal feed, and surveillance systems to detect TSE in animals and to prevent any part or product of an animal with suspected TSE to enter the human or animal food chain. The FDA has banned biologic agents of bovine origin produced in countries at risk of BSE.

ICD-9-CM

Creutzfeldt-Jakob 046.1
Kuru 046.0
Sträussler-Scheinker syndrome 784.69

BIBLIOGRAPHY

American Academy of Pediatrics. Prion diseases. In: Pickering LK, ed. *2000 Red Book: Report of the Committee on Infectious Diseases*. 25th Ed. Elk Grove Village, IL: American Academy of Pediatrics, 2000: 471–473.

Kretzschmar HA. Diagnosis of prion diseases. *Clin Lab Med* 2003;23(1):109–128, viii.

MacKnight C. Clinical implications of bovine spongiform encephalopathy. *Clin Infect Dis* 2000;32:1726–1731.

Prusiner SB. Shattuck Lecture— neurodegenerative diseases and prions. *N Engl J Med* 2001;344:1516–1526.

Weissmann C, Enari M, Klohn PC, Rossi D, Flechsig E. Transmission of prions. *J Infect Dis* 2002;186(Suppl 2):S157–S165.

Whitley RJ, MacDonald N, et al. Technical report: transmissible spongiform encephalopathies: a review for pediatricians. *Pediatrics* 2000;106:1160–1165.

Author: Jason Kim and Theoklis Zaoutis

Prolonged QT Interval Syndrome

 Database

DEFINITION

Prolonged QT interval syndrome, also known as congenital long QT syndrome (LQTS), is characterized by prolongation of the surface ECG QT interval, syncope, and sudden death as a result of malignant ventricular tachyarrhythmias. This electrical instability is a result of an abnormality in ventricular repolarization.

PATHOPHYSIOLOGY

There are two hypotheses to explain the pathogenesis of congenital LQTS:

- An abnormality or imbalance in the sympathetic innervation to the heart, which would explain the sinus bradycardia, abnormal repolarization, adrenergic dependence of arrhythmias, and response to antiadrenergic medications associated with the syndrome
- An intrinsic abnormality in the mechanisms responsible for cardiac repolarization. Because some of the identified gene mutations resulting in congenital LQTS occur at loci that also encode a cardiac ion protein, ion channels have been proposed as the intrinsic abnormality that is responsible for abnormal repolarization.

GENETICS

- Autosomal dominant (Romano-Ward syndrome)
- Autosomal recessive (associated congenital nerve deafness [Jervell and Lange-Nielsen syndrome])
- Genetic linkage analysis studies have demonstrated an association between several gene mutations encoding specific ion channel subunits and LQTS. (see table.)

EPIDEMIOLOGY

- Exact prevalence of LQTS is not known, but it may be a common cause of syncope and sudden unexplained death in children and young adults.
- Extrapolation from sudden death data suggests that the frequency may be as high as 1 in 5,000.

COMPLICATIONS

- Complications, especially in untreated patients, include:

—Ventricular tachyarrhythmias, specifically torsades de pointes
—Syncope
—Sudden death

- In patients with the congenital, inherited form of the condition, asymptomatic family members may be affected.

PROGNOSIS

- Children have a higher incidence of sudden death than do adults, which may reflect a bias that adult patients have already survived childhood. The risk of cardiac events is higher in males before puberty and in females during adulthood.
- Pediatric patients with greatest risk for sudden death are believed to be those with QTc greater than 600 msec. Gender, environmental factors, genotype, and therapy are other factors that influence the clinical course.
- β-blocker therapy has been shown to reduce the incidence of sudden death.

 Differential Diagnosis

Congenital LQTS is most commonly misdiagnosed as vasovagal syncope or a seizure disorder. All patients who have a syncopal event or who are diagnosed with epilepsy should have a baseline screening ECG. Sudden infant death syndrome (SIDS) may be related to congenital LQTS, but this relationship remains controversial. QT interval prolongation may be subtle, such that up to 10% of affected individuals may have a normal screening ECG and up to 40% may have borderline prolongation of the QT interval. Acquired forms of LQTS should be differentiated from the congenital, inherited form. Acquired LQTS may be a result of the following:

- Electrolyte abnormalities: hypokalemia, hypocalcemia, hypomagnesemia, and metabolic acidosis
- Toxins: organophosphates
- CNS trauma
- Malnutrition: anorexia
- Primary myocardial disease: myocarditis, ischemia
- Medications

—Cardiac medications: quinidine, procainamide, disopyramide, sotalol, amiodarone
—Antibiotics/antifungals: erythromycin, trimethoprim/sulfa, pentamidine, ketoconazole, fluconazole
—Psychotropic medications: tricyclic antidepressants, phenothiazines, haloperidol
—Antihistamines: Seldane, Hismanal, Benadryl
—Gastrointestinal: cisapride.

 Data Gathering

HISTORY

- The history may be notable for:

—Palpitations
—Symptoms of presyncope
—Syncope

- These symptoms may be related to provocative stimuli, especially emotional or physical stress. Any use of medications known to prolong the QTc interval should be noted
- Most importantly, a thorough family history for arrhythmia, syncope, epilepsy, or sudden unexplained death should be obtained.

 Physical Examination

Usually normal, but there may be bradycardia

 Laboratory Aids

- Bazett's formula: $QTc = QT/$(square root of RR interval). Generally, a QTc greater than 500 msec is considered abnormal, although some clinicians allow a slightly longer QTc for infants younger than 6 months of age.
- Some clinicians believe that the QTc should not be corrected at heart rates less than 60 bpm. The measurement should be taken in lead II without significant sinus arrhythmia.
- Children frequently have a prominent U wave. It should generally be included in the measurement of the QTc if it is greater than half the amplitude of the T wave.
- A single measured prolonged QTc interval does not make the diagnosis of LQTS,
- There is currently no single diagnostic test to confirm the diagnosis.

—Scoring systems may help stratify patients into high, moderate, and low probability of having the syndrome. (See table, Diagnostic Criteria for Long QT Syndrome.)

- Atrioventricular block can be seen in infants with relatively rapid heart rates and P waves that occur during the prolonged repolarization period and ventricular refractoriness.
- Other tests that may help confirm the diagnosis include 24-hour ambulatory Holter monitoring.

—This recording may disclose asymptomatic ventricular ectopy or arrhythmias, T-wave alternans, or variability in the QTc interval during different periods of the day.

- Exercise stress testing may also be helpful in identifying ventricular arrhythmias or prolongation of the QTc interval, particularly during the early recovery phase.
- The echocardiogram should demonstrate normal cardiac structure and function.

Genetic Linkage Analysis Results

	LQT1	LQT2	LQT3	LQT4	LQT5	LQT6	LQT7
Gene	KVLQT1	HERG	SCN5A	ANKB	minK	MiRP1	KCNJ2

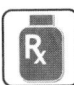 ## Therapy

- Most clinicians treat asymptomatic children with medications because of a high incidence of sudden death occurring as the first symptom.
- The primary method of therapy is β-blockade, most commonly with propranolol, atenolol, or nadolol.
- The class Ib antiarrhythmic medications, such as mexiletine, are also used in patients with congenital LQTS, especially in those with documented ventricular arrhythmia.
- Medications do not generally help treat patients with acquired LQTS.
- Occasionally, implantation of a permanent pacemaker is indicated based on the theory that long pauses may help to promote the induction of tachyarrhythmias, such as torsades de pointes.
- Left stellate ganglionectomy is a controversial therapy performed to eliminate the hyperactive left sympathetic ganglion output.
- Automatic implantable cardioverter-defibrillators (AICD) are usually reserved for older children and adolescents who have significant symptoms and/or documented ventricular arrhythmias.
- Current research may lead to the development of therapy specific to the precise ion channel defect.

Diagnostic Criteria for Long QT Syndrome

Family history	
Family members with definite LQTS	1
Unexplained sudden cardiac death before age 30 among immediate family members	0.5
Symptoms	
Syncope[a]	
With stress	2
Without stress	1
Congenital deafness	0.5
Electrocardiographic findings	
QTc > 480 msec	3
QTc 460 to 470 msec	2
QTc 450 msec (in males)	1
Torsades de pointes	2
T-wave alternans	1
Notched T wave in 3 leads	1
Low heart rate for age	0.5
Prominent U waves	1
Miscellaneous	1

[a]Mutually exclusive

Total score: 0 to 2 = unaffected; 2.5 to 4.0 = intermediate; ≥4.5 = affected.

 ## Follow-Up

- Follow-up outpatient appointments should include the review of new or recurrent symptoms, including palpitations, near-syncope or syncope, and the efficacy and adverse effects of medical therapy.
- The ECG may demonstrate a normal or prolonged QTc.
- Follow-up 24-hour ambulatory Holter monitor recordings and exercise stress tests may help in the assessment of adequate β-blocker therapy and the identification of ventricular arrhythmias.

PREVENTION

Preventive measures should focus on the avoidance of exposure to medications or situations that may provoke prolongation of the QTc interval or the induction of torsades de pointes, such as certain antihistamines and antibiotics, sympathomimetics, caffeine, electrolyte abnormalities, and highly stressful environments.

PITFALLS

- The primary pitfall is missed recognition of the syndrome. This may occur when an affected patient has a normal screening ECG (up to 10% of patients) or when a wrong diagnosis is made.
- Once the diagnosis is made, family members should be screened.

 ## Common Questions and Answers

Q: Should activity be restricted in patients with congenital LQTS?
A: Because sudden rises in serum catecholamine levels may precipitate symptoms, it is appropriate to restrict competitive and vigorous athletics. Symptomatic patients may require greater restrictions. Documentation of appropriate β-blockade, by a lower maximal heart rate at peak exercise, on follow-up exercise stress test may be helpful.

Q: If someone is identified as having LQTS, should family members be evaluated?
A: Yes, with a high degree of suspicion. Most cases of congenital LQTS are inherited in an autosomal-dominant pattern, so that each child of an affected parent has a 50% chance of having the gene. This does not predict the severity of symptoms, but parents, all siblings, and children of patients should have ECGs. Holter monitoring and exercise stress testing may be helpful in provoking an abnormal QTc interval in suspected family members.

ICD-9-CM 426.8

BIBLIOGRAPHY

Ackerman MJ. The long QT syndrome. *Pediatr Rev* 1998;19(7):232–238.

Garson A Jr, Dick M II, Fournier A, et al. The long QT syndrome in children: an international study of 287 patients. *Circulation* 1993;87:1866–1872.

Hoffman JI. The prolonged QT syndrome. *Adv Pediatr* 2001;48:115–156.

Roden DM, Lazzara R, Rosen M, et al. Multiple mechanisms in the long QT syndrome: current knowledge, gaps, and future directions. *Circulation* 1996;94:1996–2012.

Schwartz PJ, Moss AJ, Vincent GM, et al. Diagnostic criteria for the long QT syndrome: an update. *Circulation* 1993;88:782.

Zupancic JA, Triedman JK, Alexander M, et al. Cost-effectiveness and implications of newborn screening for prolongation of QT interval for the prevention of sudden infant death syndrome. *J Pediatr* 2000;136(4):481–489.

Author: Ronn E. Tanel

Prune-Belly Syndrome

 Database

DEFINITION

The prune-belly syndrome is a rare congenital disorder characterized by the triad of:

- Deficiency of the abdominal musculature
- Bilateral cryptorchidism
- Dilated, anomalous development of the bladder and upper urinary tract
- It presents in a broad spectrum of severity, from severe renal dysplasia and pulmonary hypoplasia to mild uropathy with stable renal function.

CAUSES

The etiology of the prune-belly syndrome remains unclear. Two theories have been proposed:

- The triad of congenital defects may be the result of a primary mesodermal defect in development with congenital deficiency of smooth muscle in the bladders, ureters, and renal pelvis.
- Outflow obstruction of the bladder in utero may result in dilation of the bladder and upper urinary tract with subsequent renal injury. The expanded bladder may block the route of the descending testicles and may cause abdominal distension and abdominal wall muscle atrophy.

PATHOPHYSIOLOGY

- Prune-belly bladder is large, irregular in shape, and thick walled. Many patients have poor urinary flow and high residual volumes.
- Ureters are usually markedly dilated, tortuous, and elongated. Peristalsis is ineffective and the distal ureters are most severely affected.
- Renal involvement is variable; the most severe dysplasia occurs in patients with worse dilation of the urinary tract. The dysplastic changes are usually symmetric.
- Usually, the bladder neck is wide and the prosthetic urethra is dilated and triangular. Most patients do not have anatomic obstruction at this point.

GENETICS

- The genetic basis of prune-belly syndrome remains unclear. A majority of patients have normal karyotypes.
- A majority of cases are sporadic, although rare cases in siblings have been reported.

EPIDEMIOLOGY

- Most patients are detected during the neonatal period or prenatally during maternal ultrasound.
- Prune-belly syndrome is much more common in males.

COMPLICATIONS

Many patients have other associated anomalies:

- Gastrointestinal anomalies include imperforate anus and increased risk of volvulus.
- Lower extremity musculoskeletal anomalies include talipes equinovarus and congenital hip dislocation.

Complications of the syndrome include:

- Pulmonary hypoplasia
- Vulnerability to recurrent pulmonary infections and postoperative atelectasis secondary to chest wall instability and ineffective cough because of abdominal wall deficiency
- Frequent urinary tract infections (UTIs) secondary to upper urinary stasis, vesicoureteral reflux, and bacteriuria
- Sequelae of progressive renal insufficiency

PROGNOSIS

- Patients with the most severe renal dysplasia die in the neonatal period.
- Those with a mild form do not require surgical treatment of the urinary tract; renal function is usually stable and the prognosis is excellent.
- For patients with moderate involvement, the degree of renal dysplasia and insufficiency determines outcome. In addition, upper urinary tract stasis, poor bladder emptying, vesicoureteral reflux, and bacteriuria are factors that may combine to result in a worse long-term prognosis.

 Differential Diagnosis

- The distinctly abnormal physical examination of the affected infant results in an early, accurate diagnosis in most cases.
- Pseudo–prune-belly syndrome (prune-belly syndrome uropathy, normal abdominal wall examination, and incomplete or absent cryptorchidism)

 Data Gathering

HISTORY

In patients with mild involvement of the abdominal wall that are not detected in the neonatal period, evaluation of UTIs may reveal the dilated urinary tract.

 Physical Examination

- In most cases, the abdominal wall is characterized by multiple wrinkles and redundant skin.
- A large, distended bladder creates a suprapubic mass.
- Ureters and kidneys are readily palpable.
- Intestinal loops and peristalsis may be observed.
- Testes are undescended.
- Myopathy results in difficulty in sitting up from a supine position.

 Laboratory Aids

TESTS

- The initial evaluation should include assessment of renal function.
- May see elevated serum levels of creatinine and BUN
- Renal failure may result in anemia and elevated levels of potassium, phosphorus, hydrogen ion, and uric acid, and decreased concentrations of sodium, calcium, and bicarbonate.

IMAGING

- An ultrasound will demonstrate the dilatation and redundancy of the upper urinary tract.
- When considering a voiding cystourethrogram, consider the risk of introducing infection into the dilated, poorly draining urinary tract.
- Renal function and drainage of the dilated tract can be assessed by radioisotope renal scan or an excretory urogram.

Prune-Belly Syndrome

 Therapy

SUPPORTIVE

- The basic principles of supportive care and management of renal failure apply.
- Antibiotics in the neonatal period and antibiotic prophylactic of indefinite duration are indicated to prevent infection.

SPECIFIC

- The dilated, tortuous urinary tract is managed by urologists. The optimal approach to patients with severe uropathy who survive the newborn period is very controversial.
- Some advocate minimal surgical intervention, based on the observation that there is no functional obstruction and the dilated system has a low pressure owing to the deficient smooth musculature. If renal function deteriorates, the urinary tract dilation progresses or the patient develops a urinary tract infection despite antibiotic prophylaxis; cutaneous vesicostomy is recommended to facilitate drainage.
- Others advocate extensive surgical remodeling. Possible procedures include, as indicated:

—Internal urethrotomy, reduction cystoplasty
—Excision of the redundant ureter with reimplantation of the remaining segment
—Cutaneous ureterostomy
—Pyelostomy

- Reconstruction of the abdominal wall has yielded good cosmetic results with questionable improvements in function.
- Bilateral orchiopexy is indicated.

 Follow-Up

Regardless of how patients might be managed, they require long-term follow-up, with meticulous attention to renal function, pulmonary function, and urine bacteriology.

 Common Questions and Answers

Q: Are patients with prune-belly syndrome candidates for renal transplantation?
A: Yes. However, special pretransplant consideration should be given to the dilated urinary tract in order to optimize function.

Q: How does the urinary tract function in older children?
A: A tendency for bladder tone and ureteral peristalsis to improve with age has been noted.

Q: Are these patients infertile?
A: Normal sexual activity has been described. However, there are no reports of fertility, and the patients usually have azoospermia.

Q: What is the usual cause of morbidity in the newborn period?
A: Respiratory failure.

ICD-9-CM 756.7

BIBLIOGRAPHY

Coplen DE, Snow BW, Duchett JW. Prune-belly syndrome. In: Gilwater JY, Grayhack JT, Howards SS, et al., eds. *Adult and Pediatric Urology.* 3rd Ed. St. Louis: Mosby, 1996:2297–2310.

Greskovich FJ III, Nyberg LM Jr. The prune belly syndrome: a review of its etiology, defects treatment and prognosis. *J Urol* 1988;140:707–712.

Jennings RW. Prune belly syndrome. *Semin Pediatr Surg* 2000;9(3):115–120.

Noh PH, Cooper CS, Winkler AC, et al. Prognostic factors for long-term renal function in boys with the prune-belly syndrome. *J Urol* 1999;162(4):1399–1401.

Sutherland RS, Mevorach RA, Kogan BA. The prune-belly syndrome: current insights. *Pediatr Nephrol* 1995;9(6):770–778.

Wheatley JM, Stephens FD, Hutson JM. Prune-belly syndrome: ongoing controversies regarding pathogenesis and management. *Semin Pediatr Surg* 1996;5(2):95–106.

Woodard JR, Zucker I. Lessons learned in 3 decades of managing the prune-belly syndrome. *Urol Clin North Am* 1990;17:407.

Author: Mary B. Leonard

Pseudotumor Cerebri—Idiopathic Intracranial Hypertension

Database

DEFINITION

Diagnostic criteria of idiopathic intracranial hypertension (IIH) include:

- Signs and symptoms of increased intracranial pressure, such as headache, vomiting, visual changes and papilledema
- Elevated CSF pressure with otherwise normal CSF
- Normal neurologic examination except for papilledema (and occasional abducens or other motor cranial neuropathy)
- Normal neuroimaging study

CAUSES

- Pathogenesis may involve decreased CSF absorption as a result of arachnoid villi dysfunction or elevated intracranial venous pressure. For example, obesity may lead to increased intraabdominal, intrathoracic and cardiac filling pressure, eventually leading to elevated intracranial venous pressure.
- Numerous precipitants of pseudotumor have been reported. In adolescents, it is clearly associated with obesity and weight gain, but is not clearly linked to obesity in children below age 11 years. Many weaker associations may be as a result of chance. Pseudotumor is often linked to minocycline, tetracycline, sulfonamides, and withdrawal from corticosteroids, isotretinoin, and thyroid replacements; it is also linked to vitamin A deficiency or intoxication, chronic anemia, and hypothyroidism.

GENETICS

Sporadic, no clear genetic predisposition, unless related to an underlying hormonal, toxic, or inflammatory condition; no data are available in children.

EPIDEMIOLOGY

- Incidence in children is unknown.
- Males and females are affected equally, unlike adults.
- Pseudotumor has been reported as early as 4 months of age, with a median age of 9 years.

ASSOCIATED CONDITIONS

- Visual loss as a result of optic nerve pressure
- Endocrinopathies, exogenous steroids, lead exposure, tetracycline, and several other antibiotics may be associated with pseudotumor.

DIFFERENTIAL DIAGNOSIS

The following may all be confused with IIH, but the clinical picture and CSF analysis usually permit their distinction.

- Chronic meningitis (such as CNS Lyme disease), encephalitis, or cerebral edema (may show minimal changes on neuroimaging with elevated CSF protein and little pleocytosis)
- Cerebral venous sinus thrombosis

APPROACH TO THE PATIENT

IIH should be considered in any child with chronic headache or unexplained visual changes. Examination of the fundi is essential.

Data Gathering

HISTORY

- Headache is the most common presenting complaint.
- Blurred vision, diplopia, transient visual obscurations, neck stiffness, pulsatile tinnitus and dizziness may be present.
- Infants and young children may present with irritability, somnolence, or ataxia.
- Directed history for signs of associated endocrinopathy, antibiotic or steroid exposure, sleep disturbance, sinus infection, connective tissue disease, abnormal clotting, familial tendency to thrombosis

PHYSICAL EXAMINATION

- Papilledema is almost always present in older children with IIH.
- Most infants have some degree of papilledema, even with open fontanelles and split sutures.
- Sixth cranial nerve palsies are common in children with IIH; they were found in 29 of 68 patients in one series.
- Other cranial nerve deficits are rarely seen.
- Recording baseline visual acuity and visual fields in older children is essential.

Laboratory Aids

TESTS

- Cranial CT or MRI should be normal. MRI is recommended because of superior imaging of brainstem, posterior fossa, and sinuses. MRA/MRV is strongly suggested to evaluate for venous sinus thrombosis which can be difficult to distinguish from idiopathic intracranial hypertension.
- Lumbar puncture manometry, performed while the patient is relaxed and placed in the left lateral decubitus position, should show an opening pressure of greater than 250 mm H_2O, but otherwise normal CSF composition.
- Goldmann perimeter visual field testing or computerized visual fields are useful in children over 5 years of age to document field deficits and monitor response to therapy.
- CBC and TFTs should be obtained because anemia, hypothyroidism, and hyperthyroidism have rarely been associated with pseudotumor.

The following may be useful in selected cases:

- ANA
- ESR
- Urine cortisol
- Serum lead level
- Serologic testing for Lyme disease

Emergency Care

The urgency of diagnosis and treatment depends on the severity of visual loss. Most patients present with mild-to-moderate visual loss, rather than severe or progressive visual loss.

Pseudotumor Cerebri—Idiopathic Intracranial Hypertension

 Therapy

- Treatment depends on the degree of visual loss.
- For patients with no visual loss, removal of possible causative agents may be the only intervention needed, along with treatment of associated conditions (obesity, anemia, thyroid disease). Consider treatment with acetazolamide (Diamox). Headache can be treated symptomatically if needed.
- For patients with mild-to-moderate visual loss, acetazolamide, a carbonic anhydrase inhibitor that decreases CSF production, is the drug of choice.

—The pediatric dosage is 60 mg/kg per day divided q.i.d. for the standard form and b.i.d. for the long-acting form (Diamox sequels).
—The initial adult dose is 250 mg q.i.d. or 500 mg b.i.d., increased to 750 mg qid or 1,500 mg b.i.d. if tolerated.

- Furosemide can be used if acetazolamide is ineffective or has intolerable side effects.
- Serial lumbar punctures are not recommended as standard therapy, although the initial LP can be useful to relieve symptoms acutely.
- Surgical therapy (optic nerve sheath fenestration or lumboperitoneal shunt) is indicated for progressive visual loss despite medical therapy and may also be considered at presentation depending on degree of visual loss. Optic nerve sheath fenestration may be the preferred surgical treatment, especially in children, because of the high-failure rates of lumboperitoneal shunting. High-dose IV steroids and acetazolamide are indicated while awaiting surgical therapy.

 Follow-Up

- Initially, patients should have visual acuity, visual fields, and fundi evaluated weekly or biweekly.
- If vision is stable, then monthly visits may be adequate for 3 to 6 months.
- More frequent follow-up is required for any signs of progressive visual loss.
- Follow-up and tapering of acetazolamide should be done in conjunction with a neurologist or neuro-ophthalmologist.
- If visual loss, papilledema, and symptoms of pressure resolve, acetazolamide can be tapered after 2 months of therapy.

PITFALLS

- Children are not exempt from permanent visual loss as a consequence of IIH.
- Ophthalmologic follow-up is important.
- Occasional patients, especially adolescents, may experience headache weeks or months after resolution of objective signs of IIH, even though intracranial pressure has returned to normal.
- IIH may be diagnosed erroneously if:

—Pseudopapilledema is mistaken for papilledema
—CSF abnormalities, such as isolated increase in protein, are overlooked
—Neuroimaging fails to identify a cerebral venous sinus thrombosis

 Common Questions and Answers

Q: What are the side effects of acetazolamide?
A: Side effects of acetazolamide include GI upset, paresthesias, loss of appetite, drowsiness, metabolic acidosis, and renal stones. An alternative is furosemide.

Q: If IIH occurs on tetracycline, can the child take penicillin?
A: Penicillins/cephalosporins have not been reported as a significant cause of IIH.

Q: Are there any limitations on physical activity?
A: Activity can be graded entirely according to the child's symptoms

ICD-9-CM 348.2

BIBLIOGRAPHY

Friedman, DI, Jacobson, DM. Diagnostic criteria for idiopathic intracranial hypertension. *Neurology* 2002;59(10): 1492–1495.

Jones JS, Nevai J, Freeman MP, McNinch DE. Emergency department presentation of idiopathic intracranial hypertension. *Am J Emerg Med* 1999;17:517–521.

Scott IU, Siatkowski RM, Eneyni M, Brodsky MC, Lam BL. Idiopathic intracranial hypertension in children and adolescents. *Am J of Opthalmol* 1997;124:253–255.

Shin, RK, Balcer, LJ. Idiopathic intracranial hypertension. *Curr Treat Options Neurol* 2002;4:297–305.

Soler D, Cox T, Bullock P, Calver DM, Robinson RO. Diagnosis and management of benign intracranial hypertension. *Arch Dis Child* 1998;78:89–94.

Authors: Dennis J. Dlugos and Sabrina E. Smith

Psittacosis

Database

DEFINITION

Psittacosis is an acute febrile disease characterized by pneumonitis and other systemic symptoms. The name is derived from the Greek word for parrot, *psittakos*.

CAUSE

Chlamydia psittaci, an obligate intracellular parasitic bacterium; proposed new name: *Chlamydophila psittaci*.

PATHOPHYSIOLOGY

- Inhalation of aerosolized organisms into the respiratory tract
- Incubation period of 5 to 21 days
- Spreads via bloodstream to lungs, liver, and spleen
- Lymphocytic inflammatory alveolar response

EPIDEMIOLOGY

- Birds are the major reservoir (pigeons, parrots, parakeets, turkeys, chickens, and ducks).
- Infecting agent present in bird nasal secretions, urine, feces, feathers, viscera, carcasses.
- Although inhalation is the most common route of infection, bird bites and mouth-to-beak contact also spread infection.
- Birds may be healthy or sick.
- Most reported cases (70%) are the result of exposure to pet caged birds (especially parrots, parakeets).
- Most common mammalian source of infection is sheep.
- Occupational hazard of workers in poultry plants, pet shops, zoos, farms.
- Rarely transmitted person to person.
- Only 100 to 200 total cases reported in United States each year.
- Very rare disease in young children.

COMPLICATIONS

- Hepatitis, anemia
- Thrombophlebitis, pulmonary embolus
- Arthritis, keratoconjunctivitis
- Endocarditis, myocarditis, pericarditis
- Encephalitis: agitation, delirium, confusion, stupor

PROGNOSIS

Complete recovery is expected in all but a few rare cases (even without antibiotic use).

ASSOCIATED ILLNESS

Pneumonitis, along with severe headache, is the most common presentation.

Differential Diagnosis

- Psittacosis should be considered in all fevers of unknown origin or atypical pneumonitis.
- *Mycoplasma* and *Chlamydia pneumoniae*, Legionella spp., *Coxiella burnetii* (Q fever), tuberculosis, viral and fungal pneumonitis, as well as pneumococcal pneumonia.

Data Gathering

HISTORY

- Abrupt onset of symptoms is usual.
- Fever, headache, cough, weakness, chills, muscle aches, and joint pain are common.
- A nonproductive cough is usual.
- Vomiting, confusion, and photophobia are less common.

PITFALLS

Failure to question parents as to the exposure of the patient to any type of bird—wild or domestic.

Physical Examination

- Ill appearance, tachypnea, rales, and splenomegaly are common.
- A relative bradycardia is a unique finding in some cases.
- Rash, meningismus, pharyngeal injection, cervical adenopathy, hepatomegaly, and mental status changes are less common.

Laboratory Aids

TESTS

- Chest radiograph demonstrates diffuse interstitial infiltrates.
- Routine laboratory studies are not helpful.
- Complement fixation titers (see Common Questions and Answers)
- Microimmunofluorescence studies and PCR assays are more specific than complement fixation studies, but are not yet widely available.
- Isolation of the organism is diagnostic.

PITFALLS

Note that complement fixation titers do not distinguish between the various chlamydial infections (*C. psittaci*, *C. pneumoniae*, and *C. trachomatis*).

Therapy

- Tetracycline (40 mg/kg per day) or doxycycline (100 mg b.i.d.) in children older than 8 years.
- Erythromycin (40 mg/kg per day) in children younger than 8 years.
- Azithromycin, clarithromycin, and chloramphenicol are additional options.
- Antibiotics should be continued for at least 10 to 14 days after defervescence.

Follow-Up

- Resolution of fever and most other systemic symptoms can be expected within 48 hours of antibiotic therapy.
- Untreated patients may have severe pulmonary symptoms for 1 to 3 weeks.

PREVENTION

- Epidemiologic investigation is indicated in all possible cases.
- Birds suspected to be infected should be sacrificed, transported, and analyzed by appropriate experts.
- Potentially contaminated bird areas should be disinfected and aired.

Common Questions and Answers

Q: In children with pneumonia who have a pet bird, how is the diagnosis confirmed?
A: A fourfold rise in antibody titers by complement fixation or microimmuno-fluorescence (acute and convalescent specimens; 2 to 3 weeks apart); a single titer of 1:32 or higher (highly suggestive); culture (done through the CDC).

Q: Does the source bird usually exhibit signs of disease?
A: No. Although the bird may show signs like anorexia, ruffled feathers, depression, or watery green droppings, often the bird is totally asymptomatic.

ICD-9-CM 073.9

BIBLIOGRAPHY

American Academy of Pediatrics. Chlamydia (Chlamydophila) psittaci. In: Pickering LK, ed. *2003 Red Book: Report of the Committee on Infectious Diseases.* 26th Ed. Elk Grove Village, IL: American Academy of Pediatrics, 2003:237–238.

Butler JC, Whitney CG. Compendium of measures to control Chlamydia psittaci infection among humans (psittacosis) and pet birds (avian chlamydiosis), 1998. *MMWR Morb Mortal Wkly Rep* 1998;47(RR-10):1–14.

Cotton MM, Partridge MR. Infection with feline Chlamydia psittaci. *Thorax* 1998; 53:75–76.

Gregory DW, Schaffner W. Psittacosis. *Semin Respir Infect* 1997;12(1):7–11.

Heddema ER, Kraan MC, Buys-Bergen HE, et al. A woman with a lobar infiltrate due to Psittacosis detected by polymerase chain reaction. *Scand Infect Dis J* 2003; 35(6–7):422–424.

Scully RE. Weekly clinicopathological exercises: psittacosis causing acute respiratory distress syndrome. *N Engl J Med* 1998;338(21):1527–1535.

Author: Nicholas Tsarouhas

Psoriasis

 ## Database

DEFINITION

Psoriasis is a skin disease characterized by a chronic relapsing nature and, most commonly, clinical features of scaly, erythematous papules and plaques with thick white scale usually involving elbows, knees, and scalp (psoriasis vulgaris). Other variants include guttate, inverse erythrodermic, and pustular psoriasis (see Physical Examination).

CAUSES

The pathogenesis is unknown. Trigger factors are well defined and include:

- Trauma to normal skin, producing psoriasis in the area (Koebner phenomenon)
- Infections (upper respiratory infections, *Streptococcus pyogenes,* human immunodeficiency virus)
- Stress
- Winter
- Certain drugs (systemic corticosteroids, lithium, β-adrenergic blockers, nonsteroidal antiinflammatory drugs, and antimalarials)

PATHOPHYSIOLOGY

- Plaque-type psoriasis is characterized by a thickened, parakeratotic epidermis with an absent granular layer above dermal papillae containing dilated tortuous capillaries.
- Collections of polymorphonuclear leukocytes extend from the dermal papillae into the epidermis (Munro microabscesses).
- A mixed perivascular infiltrate is confined to the papillary dermis.

GENETICS

- Psoriasis has a strong genetic influence.
- The mode of genetic transmission is not defined. It is likely multifactorial with more than one gene involved and modified by environmental influence.

—One-third of patients with psoriasis report a relative with the disease.
—8.1% of offspring develop psoriasis in family studies, when one parent is affected.
—When both parents have psoriasis, the percentage increases to 41%.
—In twin studies, 65% of monozygotic twins are concordant for the disease, although only 30% of dizygotic twins are concordant.

EPIDEMIOLOGY

- Psoriasis is universal in occurrence, but the prevalence varies in different populations. The average prevalence in the United States is estimated at 1% to 3%.
- Males and females are equally affected.
- Onset of psoriasis is bimodal, commonly presenting in the third decade with a smaller second peak of onset in the sixth decade; however, it can present at any age, with a mean age of onset in children of 8.1 years.

- Earlier onset is associated with more severe disease.

PROGNOSIS

- Once psoriasis appears, it generally persists throughout life.
- Spontaneous remissions of variable length and frequency occur but are unpredictable.

 ## Differential Diagnosis

Classic plaque psoriasis is easily diagnosed. Variants of psoriasis, including guttate, erythrodermic, and pustular disease, are more difficult to recognize. The differential varies with the type of psoriasis and includes:

- Nummular eczema
- Cutaneous T-cell lymphoma
- Tinea corporis
- *Pityriasis rosea*
- *Pityriasis lichenoides et varioliformis acuta*
- Secondary syphilis
- Atopic dermatitis
- Drug eruption
- Candidiasis
- Seborrheic dermatitis

 ## Data Gathering

HISTORY

- When the eruption first appeared
- Area involved
- Recent illness, particularly sore throat
- Recent medications, particularly systemic steroids
- Any appearance of lesions with trauma to skin
- Joint pain
- Previous treatments and response
- Improvement with sun exposure
- Family history of psoriasis

 ## Physical Examination

- A complete cutaneous examination is necessary.
- In psoriasis vulgaris, sharply demarcated erythematous plaques with white scale are located most commonly on the elbows, knees, scalp, lumbar area, and umbilicus, but they can cover any surface and large areas of the body. Intertriginous regions are often involved, but scale is absent.
- Guttate psoriasis presents often in children and young adults as small papules (0.5 to 1.5 cm), with limited scale over the trunk and proximal extremities, and is frequently associated with streptococcal infection.
- Erythema with variable scale involving the majority of the body accompanied by chills is characteristic of erythrodermic psoriasis.
- Generalized pustular psoriasis is the most serious variant, with 23-mm sterile pustules arising on erythematous skin over large areas of the body and accompanied by high fevers.
- A chronic and localized variant of pustular disease involves only the palms and soles.

PHYSICAL EXAMINATION TRICKS

Classic plaque psoriasis is easily diagnosed, but variants and mild cases require careful examination for physical clues.

- Nails are frequently involved, with pinpoint pits, hyperkeratosis, and oil spots.
- Areas of hidden disease are the retroauricular portion of the scalp and the perianal region.
- Removal of scale on plaques results in bleeding points, a feature known as the Auspitz sign.
- The Koebner phenomenon may produce linear or geometric lesions corresponding to areas of trauma.
- Swollen or deformed joints suggest associated psoriatic arthritis.
- Infants may present with a chronic diaper dermatitis that is well-demarcated and often shows limited response to topical therapy

 ## Laboratory Aids

TESTS

- An elevated uric acid level is a common finding.
- *Streptococcus pyogenes* infection is frequent in guttate disease, and throat culture is appropriate.
- Other laboratory values are generally within normal limits. However, in more severe variants, anemia, elevated erythrocyte sedimentation rate, and decreased albumin levels can be seen.
- In pustular psoriasis, leukocytosis and hypocalcemia are associated.

Therapy

- Therapy is delivered by topical medications, phototherapy, or systemic medications.
- Localized disease is treated with topical therapy and more diffuse disease with phototherapy.
- Systemic medications are reserved for resistant cases.
- Except in the most severe cases, therapy for children should be limited to topical medication and ultraviolet B (UVB) phototherapy.
- General skin care should include gentle washing, soaking to remove scale, and application of emollients, preferably ointments and creams.

DRUGS

Topical

- Topical corticosteroids

—Mid- to high-potency topical corticosteroid ointments are applied twice daily.
—Midpotency preparations (0.025% fluocinolone ointment, 0.1% triamcinolone acetonide) are preferred in children.
—Low-potency corticosteroids (1.0% and 2.5% hydrocortisone) are used on the face and intertriginous regions to prevent atrophy.
—Can also be found in shampoo preparations (Dermasmoothe FS and Capex)

- Anthralin

—Anthralin is applied to plaques for a 30-minute application, and is washed off carefully.
—Lower concentrations are used initially (0.1%, 0.25%) and are increased gradually as tolerated (0.5%, 1.0%).
—Irritation and staining are common, and the face and intertriginous regions cannot be treated with this approach.

- Calcipotriene

—Calcipotriene ointment is a vitamin D3 derivative often used for treatment of adults.
—It is applied twice daily, with avoidance of the face and intertriginous regions.
—Maximum use in adults is 100 g/week.
—Rare cases of hypercalcemia have been reported.
—Although effective in children, safety guidelines have not been established.

- Tazarotene gel

—A topical retinoid (0.05% and 0.1%)
—Can be mildly to moderately irritating when used as monotherapy.
—Often combined with topical steroids as adjunctive therapy applied once or twice daily.
—Coal tar

—A weak therapeutic agent when employed as monotherapy
—More effective when combined with UVB phototherapy
—Used in multiple shampoo preparations

PHOTOTHERAPY

UVB

- Administered between three and seven times weekly in a booth with bulbs that emit the appropriate wavelength of ultraviolet radiation
- Very effective for guttate and plaque psoriasis
- Average treatment time: 3 months and gradually increasing the time. Sunscreen should be used on the face.
- Narrowband UVB represents a form of monochromatic UVB using wavelengths of 311 nm and appears to be a somewhat more effective form of delivering UVB phototherapy.
- PUVA (psoralen and UVB)

—PUVA and oral medications (methotrexate and etretinate) should be reserved for severe cases and carefully monitored by a dermatologist.

Possible Conflicts with Other Drugs

Photosensitizing medication (tetracyclines, sulfa derivatives, phenothiazines, and others) should be avoided with phototherapy.

Duration

- Topical therapy is administered chronically with breaks to minimize side effects.
- Remissions occur in summer with sun exposure, and medications may often be discontinued.
- The average treatment course with UVB therapy is 3 months; if the patient clears, treatment may be followed by an average remission period of 5 months.

 Follow-Up

WHEN TO EXPECT IMPROVEMENT

- Response will depend on the potency of medication and frequency of treatment.
- Improvement with topical medication is obvious at 2 weeks and usually maximum at 2 months.
- One month of UVB therapy produces a decrease in disease.

SIGNS TO WATCH FOR

Pustules, a significant increase in degree or extent of erythema, or fever suggest progression of the disease to more serious variants and may require hospitalization and systemic therapy.

PITFALLS

- If therapy is too aggressive, disease may become irritated and worsen.
- Scrubbing by the patient to remove scale also irritates the disease.
- Psychological aspects of the disease, particularly in children, should be addressed.

 Common Questions and Answers

Q: Will my disease get worse?
A: It is impossible to predict the course of an individual's disease, since it is influenced by both heredity and everyday factors in the environment. Although there is no cure, with treatment the disease can be kept under control. Remissions do occur and maybe for prolonged periods of time.

Q: When my disease is in remission, what can I do to prevent it from returning?
A: Avoidance of trauma and frequent moisturization of the skin is important. In the summer, controlled sun exposure is helpful. You may have to continue other treatments at less frequent intervals. Any sore throats should be cultured and treated if streptococcal disease is present. However, frequently it is impossible to prevent recurrence of the disease.

Q: Will my other children get psoriasis?
A: If neither parent has psoriasis, the chances are <10% that another child will develop the disease; if one parent is affected, the chances increase to 15%; if both parents are affected, the chances are 50%. Therefore, unless both parents are affected, it is more likely that other children will not have psoriasis.

Q: Does stress make psoriasis worse?
A: Some studies have suggested that flare-ups of psoriasis are associated with increased stress. It is difficult to evaluate whether stress is the cause or the result of the disease. Do all you can to reasonably relieve stress, but do not focus on this as the cause of your psoriasis.

ICD-9-CM 696.1

BIBLIOGRAPHY

Capella GL, Finzi AF. Psoriasis and other papulosquamous diseases in infants and children. *Clin Dermatol* 2000;18(6):701–709.

Christophers E, Sterry W. Psoriasis. In: Fitzpatrick TB, Eisen AZ, Wolff K, et al., eds. *Dermatology in General Medicine*. 4th Ed. New York: McGraw-Hill, 1993:489.

de Jong EM. The course of psoriasis. *Clin Dermatol* 1997;15(5):687–692.

Farber EM. Early intervention can reduce risks for problems later. *Postgrad Med* 1998;103(4):89–92, 95–96, 99–100 passim.

Leman J, Burden D. Psoriasis in children: a guide to its diagnosis and management. *Paediatr Drugs* 2001;3(9):673–680.

Stern RS. Epidemiology of psoriasis. *Dermatol Clin* 1995;13(4):717–722.

Author: Albert C. Yan

Pubertal Delay

 Database

DEFINITION

Pubertal delay is delay in age at onset of puberty. It is also delay in the rate of progression of pubertal development greater than 2 standard deviations from the mean, thus 2.5% of the population can be viewed as having delayed puberty.

Constitutional or Physiologic Delay of Puberty

- Late onset of puberty is usually a normal variant
- Patients grow slowly through childhood, enter puberty late and then progress through puberty at a normal rate.

Male pubertal development is considered delayed if:

- Genital stage 1 persists beyond 13.7 years.
- Pubic hair stage 1 persists beyond 15.1 years.
- More than 5 years pass before completion of genital growth.
- Pubertal development begins but progression stalls, such that the duration of a given sexual maturity rating is longer than expected:

—Genital 2: 2.2 years
—Genital 3: 1.6 years
—Genital 4: 1.9 years
—Pubic hair 2: 1.0 year
—Pubic hair 3: 0.5 year
—Pubic hair 4: 1.5 years

Female pubertal development is considered delayed if:

- Breast stage 1 persists beyond 13.4 years.
- Pubic hair stage 1 persists beyond 14.1 years.
- No menarche beyond age 16 years
- More than 5 years pass between initiation of breast stage 2 and menarche
- Pubertal development begins but progression stalls, such that the duration of a given sexual maturity rating is longer than expected:

—Breast 2: 1.0 year
—Breast 3: 2.2 years
—Breast 4: 6.8 years
—Pubic hair 2: 1.3 years
—Pubic hair 3: 0.9 year
—Pubic hair 4: 2.4 years

PATHOPHYSIOLOGY

- Constitutional delay is a normal variant that is believed to result from persistence of the prepubertal (childhood) hypogonadotropic state.
- Delayed puberty and short stature associated with chronic disease is not well explained from a pathophysiologic perspective. New insights indicate that endogenous opiates may play a crucial role in the pathways connecting the cerebral cortex to the hypothalamus, which is key to hypothalamic activation before the onset of puberty.

GENETICS

- Patients with constitutional delay will often have a family history of late pubertal onset with subsequently normal stature and development.
- The genetic transmission of delayed puberty otherwise depends on the underlying disorder.

EPIDEMIOLOGY

- Constitutional delay of puberty explains 90% to 95% of pubertal delay.
- Constitutional delay occurs in approximately 2.5% of adolescents of both sexes.
- More than 60% of patients with constitutional delay of puberty have a positive family history.

 Differential Diagnosis

INFECTION

- Viral or tuberculosis infection, resulting in acquired panhypopituitarism

TUMORS (MAY RESULT IN PANHYPOPITUITARISM)

- Craniopharyngioma
- Hypothalamic glioma
- Astrocytoma
- Pituitary adenoma

TRAUMA

- Panhypopituitarism resulting from severe head trauma

CONGENITAL

- Congenital panhypopituitarism
- Mixed gonadal dysgenesis
- Turner syndrome, Noonan syndrome
- Prader-Willi syndrome

IMMUNOLOGIC

- Juvenile rheumatoid arthritis
- Systemic lupus erythematosus
- Autoimmune oophoritis

ENDOCRINOLOGIC

Hypothyroidism

PSYCHOSOCIAL

- Anorexia nervosa
- Athleticism
- Substance abuse
- Chronic psychosocial stress

ENVIRONMENTAL

- Postradiation
- Chemotherapy

MISCELLANEOUS

- Constitutional delay of puberty (majority of cases)
- Unrecognized chronic disease

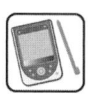 Data Gathering

HISTORY

- Obtain long-term growth record. Patients with gonadotropin or gonadal disorders usually have had normal growth during childhood but no increase in growth during the expected pubertal spurt where growth retardation is a new event. Most children with constitutional delay have slow growth throughout childhood.
- Obtain history of progression of secondary sex characteristics. Adolescents with complete gonadal or gonadotropin deficiencies will not enter puberty, unless initiated by exogenous or adrenal hormones, whereas those with constitutional delay will progress at a normal rate after initiation of puberty. Adolescents with partial deficiencies may reach pubarche at a normal time, but will fail to progress.
- Obtain family history of pubertal development.
- Assess nutrition and socioeconomic history to rule out chronic malnutrition or eating disorder.
- Elicit history of drug use (e.g., glucocorticoids or cytotoxins).

 Physical Examination

Examine all patients with pubertal delay thoroughly, with particular attention to:

- Thyroid examination
- Neurologic and funduscopic examinations to check for intracranial pathology
- Genital and gynecologic examination: external examination for all patients; internal gynecologic examination for females with amenorrhea may be indicated; breast, pubic hair, and genital examination to assess sexual maturity ratings
- The first sign of puberty in males is when testicular size is greater than 2.5 cm. Find which one of your finger segments approximates 2.5 cm, and use it as a gross measure. As a means of screening size, using a finger is more subtle than using an orchidometer. However, when a clinician needs to follow pubertal progression closely, an orchidometer is necessary to accurately establish testicular size.

Pubertal Delay

Laboratory Aids

TESTS

Initial Workup

Routine screening tests for chronic or systemic disease:

- Complete blood count
- Urinalysis
- Erythrocyte sedimentation rate
- Chemistry profile
- Thyroid stimulating hormone

If screening studies abnormal

- Gonadotropin levels (low levels suggest prepuberty or hypothalamic-pituitary failure; high levels suggest gonadal failure or absence)
- If hypergonadotropic, obtain karyotype (XX is suggestive of ovarian failure, XO or abnormal X could be indicative of Turner Syndrome or gonadal dysgenesis)
- If all of the above studies are normal, and there is no evidence to support constitutional delay, reevaluation for cryptic chronic illness, substance abuse, eating disorder, or ongoing psychosocial stress should occur until puberty progresses or the underlying cause of delay becomes clear.

RADIOGRAPHIC STUDIES

- Bone age: plain film of the epiphyseal growth centers in the hand. Epiphyses change in response to growth hormone, thyroxine, and steroids of adrenal or gonadal origin. Comparison to chronologic age can help to differentiate constitutional delay from organic disorders. A bone age that is more than 2 years delayed from chronologic age is consistent with constitutional delay, but not specific, and can be found with any hypogonadotropic cause of delayed puberty.
- Pelvic ultrasound: can be useful in locating intraabdominal testicular structures, or in determination of the presence or absence of müllerian structures. Pelvic ultrasound is indicated when testes cannot be detected in patients with a male phenotype or when müllerian structures cannot be confirmed on physical examination in patients with a female phenotype.
- Computed tomography (CT) or magnetic resonance imaging (MRI) of the head: useful in assessing pituitary or hypothalamic structures, mass lesions, pathologic calcifications, or increased intracranial pressure if a central cause of delayed puberty is suspected.

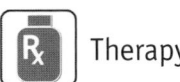

Therapy

PSYCHOSOCIAL INTERVENTIONS

Most patients with pubertal delay do not require drugs, but all need psychological and social support.

DRUGS

- In cases of presumed constitutional delay, hormones can be used to affect hypothalamic maturation, thereby initiating endogenous puberty.
- Referral to an endocrinologist or adolescent specialist is usually recommended prior to the initiation of hormonal therapy to aid in diagnosis and management.

Follow-Up

In cases of permanent hypogonadism, because of gonadal absence, failure, or gonadotropin deficiency, long-term hormonal therapy is necessary.

PREVENTION

- Undue stress and unnecessary tests can be avoided by discussing pubertal changes with patients and their families at the outset, in late childhood.
- Even though they will not ask health care providers, teens with chronic disease may be actively worrying about slow growth and pubertal development. Open discussion with a caring provider can help allay fears and stress.

PITFALLS

- No test can make a definitive diagnosis of constitutional delay.
- Levels of sex steroids and gonadotropins vary significantly in a single patient because of pulsatile or rhythmic secretions, and are generally not necessary in the work-up of pubertal delay.
- Sex steroid therapy in a patient with hypopituitarism can affect adult height if given before growth hormone therapy is optimized.
- Consultation with a specialist or experienced laboratory personnel is recommended before obtaining pituitary stimulation tests, as they may require special conditions.

Common Questions and Answers

Q: Since approximately 95% of pubertal delay is constitutional or physiologic in nature, when can I avoid an expensive workup and just observe the patient?
A: Unfortunately, only the spontaneous onset of puberty confirms the diagnosis of constitutional delay. Anxiety from delayed puberty may preclude waiting. To make a presumptive diagnosis of constitutional delay, pathology must be ruled out. Physical examination, including genital anatomy and smell sense, must be normal. There should be no signs or symptoms consistent with chronic disease. The history, including nutritional history and review of systems, must be negative. The screening blood work must be negative. Growth must progress at least

3.7 cm per year, and bone age must be delayed no more than 4.0 years compared with chronologic age. Although not always indicated, the next level of tests can be ordered. Normal prepubertal levels of lutenizing hormone (LH) and follicle stimulating hormone (FSH) must be present. Presumptive diagnosis is strongly supported, but not proven, by a positive family history and a height between the 3rd and 25th percentiles.

Q: When should patients with pubertal delay be seen by an endocrinologist or adolescent specialist?
A: Often, the initial workup of pubertal delay can be completed by the primary care provider. For complex stimulation tests, or if help is needed in interpreting test results, referral to an experienced specialist is warranted. If a specific chronic disease is suspected as the underlying etiology, then referral should be made to the appropriate subspecialist.

Q: Do racial differences exist concerning pubertal onset and development?
A: Several recent studies indicate that the mean ages for onset of breast development and menarche are younger for African American females than for Caucasian females. One such study reported the mean age of onset for breast development as 8.87 years for African American girls and 9.96 years for Caucasian girls. Mean age at menarche was found to be 12.16 and 12.88 years for African American and Caucasian girls, respectively. These differences are rarely, if ever, clinically relevant.

ICD-9-CM 255.0

BIBLIOGRAPHY

Argente J. Diagnosis of late puberty. *Horm Res* 1999;51(Suppl 3):95–100.

Brook CG. Treatment of late puberty. *Horm Res* 1999;51(Suppl 3):101–103.

Gordon C, Mansbach J. Demystifying delayed puberty. *Contemp Pediatr* 2001;4:43.

Pletcher JR, Slap GB. Menstrual disorders: amenorrhea. *Pediatr Clin of North Am* 1999; 46:505–518.

Reiter EO, Lee PA. Delayed puberty. *Adolescent Medicine State of the Art Reviews* 2002;13(1): 101–118, vii.

Rosen DS, Foster C. Delayed puberty. *Pediatr Rev* 2001;22(9):309–315.

Styne DM. New aspects in the diagnosis and treatment of pubertal disorders. *Pediatr Clin North Am* 1997;44:505–529.

Traggiai C, Stanhope R. Delayed puberty. *Best Practice & Research Clinical Endocrinology & Metabolism* 2002;16(1):139:151.

Authors: Jonathan R. Pletcher and Kenneth R. Ginsburg

Pulmonary Embolism

 ## Database

DEFINITION

Pulmonary embolism (PE) is the occlusion of a pulmonary vessel by a thrombus.

PATHOPHYSIOLOGY

- Thromboemboli may develop anywhere in the systemic venous system.
- PE is characterized by the triad of hypoxemia, pulmonary hypertension, and right ventricular failure.
- Diminished pulmonary perfusion causes a ventilation/perfusion (V/Q) mismatch, resulting in hypoxemia. Hyperventilation occurs secondary to stimulation of proprioceptors in the lung.
- Hypercapnia is seen with severe occlusion of the pulmonary artery (often not seen with smaller emboli).
- Pulmonary infarction is uncommon owing to the presence of collateral pulmonary and bronchial arteries along with the airways providing additional sources of oxygen to the tissues.

EPIDEMIOLOGY

- PEs are seen more frequently in adults and tend to occur in postsurgical situations, especially when patients have been bedridden.
- PE is rarely recognized in children; the incidence in children is 3.7%.
- Increasing incidence is secondary to increased central catheter utilization.
- Approximately 10% of adults who present with an acute pulmonary embolus die within 1 hour of onset.
- The mortality rate can be as high as 30% if delays in diagnosis are made.
- Death occurs with 85% obstruction of the pulmonary artery.
- Risk factors vary according to age groups and gender.
- In children, risk factors include:

—Presence of a central venous catheter
—Lack of mobility
—Congenital heart disease
—Ventriculoatrial shunt
—Trauma
—Solid tumors or leukemia
—Postsurgical procedures (especially scoliosis repair)
—Hypercoagulable states

- In adults, the most common risk factor is the presence of a deep vein thrombosis, usually in the legs or pelvis.

PROGNOSIS

- If treated promptly, prognosis is good.
- If treatment is delayed, especially if the patient is hemodynamically compromised prior to the event, prognosis is poor.

 ## Differential Diagnosis

- Cardiac

—Cardiac tamponade
—Constrictive pericarditis
—Restrictive cardiomyopathy

- Pulmonary

—Chronic cough
—Status asthmaticus
—Pneumonia with empyema
—Pneumothorax

 ## Data Gathering

HISTORY

- Are there any chest symptoms?
- PE should be suspected in children who present with:

—Pleuritic chest pain
—Shortness of breath
—Hemoptysis
—Cough
—Acute respiratory distress
—Apprehension or anxiety
—Syncope
—Cardiovascular shock

- Symptoms may be nonspecific and indicative of other disorders.
- The clinician must have a high index of suspicion and recognize risk factors in order to establish the correct diagnosis.

 ## Physical Examination

Findings on physical examination are nonspecific.

- General

—Fever
—Diaphoresis
—Nervousness or apprehension (altered mental status is uncommon)

- Cardiovascular

—Increased intensity of the pulmonic component of S_2
—Tachycardia
—Gallop rhythm
—New murmur

- Pulmonary

—Tachypnea
—Rales
—Cyanosis (present with 65% obstruction of the pulmonary artery)
—Pleuritic chest pain
—Dyspnea
—Cough
—Hemoptysis
—Wheezing (uncommon)

- Extremities

—Deep venous thrombosis is frequently found in the adult population.
—Phlebitis
—Edema

PITFALLS

Failure to make the diagnosis is the most common mistake. PE must be suspected in critically ill children who have a central venous catheter and develop sudden respiratory failure. Since the symptoms for severe lung disease and PE are similar, the diagnosis might be missed if the index of suspicion is low.

 ## Laboratory Aids

TESTS

Blood Tests

- In general, blood tests are nonspecific and of no significant value in making the diagnosis of a pulmonary embolus.
- Arterial blood gas:

—Decreased PaO_2 and $PaCO_2$
—Increased alveolar-arterial (A-a) gradient

Cardiac Studies

- ECG

—Useful in ruling out other conditions
—May show sinus tachycardia or nonspecific ST-T wave changes

- Echocardiogram

—Useful for identifying:
  —Abnormalities of cardiac anatomy
  —Thrombi on catheter tips
—If there are emboli seen by echocardiogram, there is a 40% to 50% mortality rate. Also, if signs of right ventricular dysfunction are noted, such as right ventricular dilatation, abnormal right ventricular wall motion, or increased tricuspid regurgitation jet velocity, there is an associated risk of poor outcome.

Pulmonary function testing

—Results are nonspecific.

Evaluation of the lower extremities

—Finding deep vein thrombosis via:
  —Impedance plethysmography
  —Doppler technology
  —Venography

Imaging

- Spiral CT

—New modality for the diagnosis of PE
—Greater sensitivity than V/Q scan in the diagnosis of PE as a result of the ability to image abnormal pulmonary pathology.

- Chest radiograph

—May be abnormal in 70% of patients with pulmonary embolus
—Most frequent findings:
—Parenchymal infiltrates
—Atelectasis
—Pleural effusions: seen in 33% of cases, mostly unilateral
—Hampton hump (pyramid-shaped wedge pointing toward the hilum)

- Ventilation/perfusion (V/Q) scan

—Results of a V/Q scan performed to rule out a pulmonary embolus are reported in one of five categories, ranging from high probability to normal.
—An abnormal V/Q scan with normal ventilation and decreased perfusion in the appropriate clinical setting is 90% specific for a pulmonary embolus.
—A normal V/Q scan does not completely rule out pulmonary embolus, although if the patient is at low risk, a pulmonary embolus is highly unlikely.

- Pulmonary angiography

—Most sensitive and specific test
—Not done as frequently in children as in adults because of complications of the procedure
—With the introduction of newer, improved catheters and safer contrast solutions, this test is now safely performed in the pediatric population.
—Indicated for cases:
—Intermediate-probability V/Q scans
—High-probability scans in patients who are:
—Poor candidates for anticoagulation
—Hemodynamically unstable or require an embolectomy

 Therapy

DRUGS

- Stabilize the patient before anticoagulation or thrombolytic therapy is begun:

—Improve oxygenation
—Correct acidosis
—Stabilize blood pressure
—Analgesia for severe pleuritic chest pain. Avoid the use of opiates in cases of cardiovascular collapse.

- The goal of therapy is anticoagulation and/or thrombolysis
- In patients with an intermediate or high suspicion of PE, begin anticoagulation prior to investigations

ANTICOAGULATION THERAPY

To prevent further thrombus formation

Heparin

- Bolus dose: 100 to 200 U/kg
- Maintenance dose: 10 to 25 U/kg per hour
- Keep partial thromboplastin time (PTT) in the range of 55 to 60 seconds
- Should be given for 7 to 10 days

Coumadin

- Coumadin should be started 24 to 48 hours after heparin therapy is begun.
- Maintenance dose: 2.5 to 10.0 mg/d
- Keep prothrombin time (PT) twice normal and maintain the International Normalized Ratio (INR) between 2.0 and 3.0
- Should be continued for 3 to 6 months

Thrombolytic Therapy

Agents Available

- Streptokinase: No difference in outcome has been found using streptokinase over urokinase.
- Urokinase
- rtPA (tissue plasminogen activator): Same efficacy as streptokinase and lower incidence of allergic reactions

Indications

- Hemodynamically unstable
- Large embolus
- Low-molecular-weight heparins have been used as prophylaxis or as treatment for preexisting conditions in both adults and children.
- A synthetic, nonthrombocytopenic heparin pentasaccharide with pure antifactor Xa activity is currently being tested.
- Ticlopidine and clopidogrel have been used successfully for the prevention of thrombotic strokes and arterial thrombotic syndromes.

Contraindications to Anticoagulation Therapy

- Active internal bleeding
- Recent cerebrovascular accident
- Major surgery
- Recent gastrointestinal bleed

EMBOLECTOMY

- Indicated when hemodynamic instability persists; reserved for patients who have failed thrombolytic therapy or in whom medical treatment is contraindicated.
- Late results are excellent if the patient has not suffered from a perioperative cardiac arrest, which is associated with early mortality.

Percutaneous Caval Filtration

- Indicated if commencement or continuation of anticoagulation is strongly contraindicated, or if full anticoagulation has failed to prevent recurrent emboli.

- This should be considered in patients undergoing venous thrombolysis since up to 20% may have embolization during treatment.

 Follow-Up

Patients on Coumadin therapy should have the usual follow-up for those receiving an anticoagulant.

 Common Questions and Answers

Q: Is it safe for children on Coumadin to play contact sports?
A: The general recommendation is that no contact sports should be allowed while children are on Coumadin therapy because of the increased risk of bleeding.

ICD-9-CM 415.1

BIBLIOGRAPHY

Arcasoy SM, Kreit JW. Thrombolytic therapy of pulmonary embolism: a comprehensive review of current evidence. *Chest* 1999;115(6):1695–1707.

Evans DA, Wilmott RW. Pulmonary embolism in children. *Pediatr Clin North Am* 1994;41:569.

Fedullo PF, Tapson VF. Clinical practice. The evaluation of suspected pulmonary embolism. *N Engl J Med* 2003;349(13):1247–1256.

Goldhaber SZ, Elliott CG. Acute pulmonary embolism: part I: epidemiology, pathophysiology, and diagnosis. *Circulation* 2003;108(22):2726–2729.

Kruip MJ, Leclercq MG, van der Heul C, Prins MH, Buller HR. Diagnostic strategies for excluding pulmonary embolism in clinical outcome studies: a systematic review. *Ann Intern Med* 2003;138(12):941–951.

Velmahos GC, Vassiliu P, Wilcox A. Spiral computed tomography for the diagnosis of pulmonary embolism in critically ill surgical patients: a comparison with pulmonary angiography. *Arch Surg* 2001;136(5):505–511.

Zierler BK. Ultrasonography and diagnosis of venous thromboembolism. *Circulation* 2004;109(12 Suppl 1):I9–I14.

Author: Akinyemi O. Ajayi

Pulmonary Hypertension

 Database

DEFINITION

Pulmonary hypertension is increased pulmonary vascular resistance.

CAUSES

- Hypoxemia-induced pulmonary hypertension:
- Chronic lung disease

—Cystic fibrosis
—Bronchopulmonary dysplasia
—Interstitial lung disease

- Upper airway obstruction

—Tonsillar and/or adenoid hypertrophy
—Obesity

- Hypoventilation

—Neurologically mediated process
—Secondary to muscle weakness

- High pulmonary blood flow secondary to left-to-right shunting (seen in congenital heart disease):

—Patent ductus arteriosus
—Atrial septal defect
—Ventricular septal defect

- Left-sided cardiac disorders that increase pulmonary venous pressure:

—Left ventricular failure
—Mitral valve stenosis
—Obstructed anomalous pulmonary veins

- Occlusion of pulmonary vessels:

—Sickle cell disease
—Veno-occlusive disease
—Thromboembolism

- Pulmonary vasculitis

—Systemic lupus erythematosus
—Rheumatoid arthritis
—Scleroderma

- Persistent pulmonary hypertension of the newborn
- Idiopathic cases (primary pulmonary hypertension)

PATHOPHYSIOLOGY

Structural alternations in pulmonary vessel architecture (remodeling):

- Smooth muscle hypertrophy
- Extension of blood vessel's smooth muscle into smaller vessels
- Inflammation

EPIDEMIOLOGY

Incidence in children is unknown.

COMPLICATIONS

- Chronic hypoxia
- Exercise intolerance
- Right-sided heart failure (cor pulmonale)
- Death

PROGNOSIS

- Dependent on the underlying disease, but in general, poor
- In cases of primary pulmonary hypertension, improvement of pulmonary hypertension with administration of vasodilators during initial catheterization is associated with a better survival rate than if there is no response.
- Ten percent to 40% mortality in treated patients
- Near 100% mortality if patient is untreated

 Differential Diagnosis

- Pulmonary

—Asthma
—Cystic fibrosis
—Chronic obstructive pulmonary disease (COPD)
—Emphysema
—Pulmonary arteriovenous malformations (AVM)

- Miscellaneous

—Congestive heart failure
—Noncardiogenic pulmonary edema
—Fatigue

 Data Gathering

HISTORY

- Dyspnea (earliest complaint usually reported)
- Fatigue:

—Early on with exercise or exertion
—At rest in later stages or if severe

- Exercise intolerance
- Feeding intolerance
- Failure to thrive
- Excessive sleeping
- Diaphoresis
- Chest pain
- Syncope
- Palpitations (late finding)

 Physical Examination

Typically governed by the signs of the underlying lung or heart disease

COMMON FINDINGS

- Tachypnea
- Arrhythmias
- Narrowed splitting of S_2 heart sound
- Increased P_2 heart sound
- Presence of S_3 and/or S_4 heart sounds
- Murmur of pulmonary or tricuspid insufficiency (tricuspid insufficiency more common)
- Jugular venous distention
- Peripheral edema
- Hepatomegaly

SPECIAL QUESTIONS

Consider obstructive sleep apnea as cause of pulmonary hypertension. Ask about snoring if suspecting pulmonary hypertension in the absence of overt cardiac or pulmonary disease.

 Laboratory Aids

TESTS

- Arterial blood gas

—Measurement of PO_2 assesses degree of hypoxia
—Evaluation of PCO_2 determines presence or absence of hypoventilation

- Electrocardiogram (ECG)

—Can be normal if cor pulmonale has not yet developed
—If cor pulmonale present, ECG can demonstrate:
　　—Right QRS axis deviation
　　—Right ventricular hypertrophy
　　—Right atrial hypertrophy

IMAGING

- Chest radiograph

—Will vary according to the underlying disorder and extent of pulmonary hypertension
—Pulmonary hypertension correlates poorly with chest radiograph findings
—In primary pulmonary hypertension:
   —Cardiomegaly
   —Enlarged pulmonary artery
   —Peripheral lung appears underperfused ("pruning" of pulmonary vessels)

- Echocardiogram with Doppler flow

—Increased pulmonary artery pressure
—Right ventricular hypertrophy
—Paradoxical movement of the intraventricular septum
—Pulmonic and tricuspid valve regurgitation
—Right-to-left shunting via an open foramen ovale

- Cardiac catheterization

—The most accurate measurement of pulmonary artery pressure is done by right heart catheterization.
—Criteria for pulmonary hypertension in children:
   —Mean pulmonary arterial pressure >25 mmHg (at rest)
   —Mean pulmonary arterial pressure >30 mmHg (with exercise)
   —Pulmonary vascular resistance >3 U/m^2
—Pressures should be measured before and after vasodilator to assess reversibility of pulmonary hypertension

Therapy

- Therapy is directed toward:

—Treating the underlying disease
—Vasodilators to decrease the pulmonary hypertension and improve right heart function

DRUGS

- Oxygen

—Keep Sao_2 ≥95%

- Anticoagulation therapy (Coumadin)

—Prevents clot formation in the narrowed pulmonary vessels
—Helpful even in the absence of thromboembolic disease

- Vasodilators

—Calcium-channel blockers—PO (e.g., nifedipine)
—Nitric oxide—inhaled
—Prostacyclin—IV (e.g., epoprostenol)
—Endothelin receptor antagonist—PO (e.g., bosentan)

MECHANICAL VENTILATION

Useful for correcting hypoxia and hypercarbia secondary to hypoventilation

SURGERY

- Tonsillectomy and/or adenoidectomy if obstructive sleep apnea is present
- Transplantation (lung or heart-lung transplantation): reserved for patients with refractory, severe pulmonary hypertension

DURATION

Treatment can be lifelong unless the primary cause of the pulmonary hypertension can be corrected.

Follow-Up

WHEN TO EXPECT IMPROVEMENT

- In acute pulmonary hypertension, response to most treatment modalities will be almost immediate.
- Oxygen has been shown to reverse hypoxia-related remodeling of the airways after a month of therapy.

PITFALLS

- Signs and symptoms of pulmonary hypertension are not specific and can easily be missed.
- In patients with severe disease, catheterization is associated with increased risk of complications.
- Supplemental oxygen can sometimes cause hypercapnia by blunting the hypoxia-driven respiratory drive.
- Vasodilators should be used under close supervision because of their effect on systemic blood pressure (systemic hypotension can be a significant problem).

Common Questions and Answers

Q: How many hours per day should supplemental oxygen be used?
A: Studies have shown decreased mortality in patients using oxygen 24 hours per day compared with patients using supplemental oxygen for only part of the day.

Q: Should the dosage of oxygen be adjusted during the day as per the patient's activity?
A: Increasing the supplemental oxygen should be considered for activities that require increased oxygen consumption (e.g., exercise, eating, sleeping).

ICD-9-CM 416.0

BIBLIOGRAPHY

Barst RJ. Recent advances in the treatment of pediatric pulmonary hypertension. *Pediatr Clin North Am* 1999;46:331–345.

Chatterjee K, De Marco T, Alpert JS. Pulmonary hypertension: hemodynamic diagnosis and management. *Arch Intern Med* 2002;162(17):1925–1933.

Klings ES, Farber HW. Current management of primary pulmonary hypertension. *Drugs* 2001;61:1945–1956.

Ravishankar C, Tabbutt S, Wernovsky G. Critical care in cardiovascular medicine. *Curr Opin Pediatr* 2003;15(5):443–453.

Widlitz A, Barst RJ. Pulmonary arterial hypertension in children. *Eur Respir J* 2003;21:155–176.

Yeh TF. Persistent pulmonary hypertension in preterm infants with respiratory distress syndrome. *Pediatr Pulmonol* 2001;Suppl 23:103–106.

Author: Richard M. Kravitz

Purpura Fulminans

 Database

DEFINITION

Purpura fulminans is a congenital, acquired, or idiopathic condition of rapidly progressive microvascular hemorrhage into the skin. It is associated with an underlying acquired or congenital disorder of coagulation, and may lead to skin necrosis.

PATHOPHYSIOLOGY

- Common features of purpura fulminans

—Inflammation: endothelial injury from bacterial endotoxin or other trigger may initiate secretion of inflammatory cytokines or activation of coagulation and complement proteins.
—Purpura: extravasation of formed elements of the blood from injured capillaries into the skin
—Dermal vascular thrombosis: formation of microthromboses in blood vessels of the skin, leading to hemorrhage in the skin (purpura), necrosis of skin, and gangrene

- Infection-associated purpura fulminans

—Overwhelming sepsis, usually bacterial; *Neisseria meningitidis* most common
—May be a complication of varicella infection.
—Disseminated intravascular coagulation (DIC): state of sustained activation of coagulation cascade and fibrinolytic mechanisms, leading to consumption of platelets, fibrinogen, and often formation of microthromboses

- Inherited defect of coagulation presenting as neonatal purpura fulminans

—Deficiency of protein C: leads to a loss of important inhibitory regulation of coagulation and uncontrolled clotting
—Protein C slows ("brakes") the coagulation cascade at two steps: by degrading activated coagulation factor Va in the common part of the coagulation pathway, and by degrading factor VIIIa in the intrinsic pathway.
—Protein S is a cofactor for protein C.

- Idiopathic

—Postinfectious complication—formation of antibodies to protein S causing protein S deficiency has been described as a postinfectious autoimmune phenomenon.
—Complication of Coumadin therapy
—Other unknown mechanisms

GENETICS

- Deficiencies of protein C and protein S are autosomally inherited with variable penetrance.
- Many different genetic mutations, leading to both qualitative and quantitative defects of the proteins, have been described.
- Heterozygous protein C and S deficiency states usually cause a hypercoagulable condition, with increased risk of venous or arterial thrombosis throughout life.
- Homozygous protein C or S deficiency states lead to severe deficiency (less than 5% of normal factor activity) and neonatal purpura fulminans and are usually fatal.
- Factor V Leiden, a known risk factor for thrombosis, may also predispose to infection-associated purpura fulminans. May also predispose to purpura fulminans in patients who are heterozygotes for protein C or S deficiency.
- Other genetic predispositions to thrombosis, such as prothrombin mutations, may also contribute to risk for purpura fulminans.

EPIDEMIOLOGY

Depends on underlying cause:

- Neonatal purpura fulminans related to homozygous protein C deficiency: 1 in 250,000 to 1 in 500,000 births. Homozygous protein S deficiency is rarer.
- Purpura frequently seen in bacterial sepsis with meningococcus and other pathogens

COMPLICATIONS

- Skin necrosis and gangrene
- Scarring
- Acral amputations, from tips of digits to whole limbs
- Thrombosis in internal organs
- Death

PROGNOSIS

- Related to underlying cause of purpura fulminans
- Overall, poor for homozygous deficiencies of proteins C and S

 Differential Diagnosis

- Infection

—*N. meningitidis*, most common infectious cause of purpura fulminans
—Streptococci
—Haemophilus species
—Staphylococci
—Gram-negative bacteremia: *Escherichia coli*, Klebsiella, Proteus, Enterobacter
—Rickettsia: Rocky Mountain spotted fever
—Varicella

- Environmental

—Coumadin-induced skin necrosis: 1 in 500 to 1 in 1,000 individuals starting Coumadin therapy develop necrosis in subcutaneous fat, thought to be as a result of relative depletion of anticoagulant protein C (a vitamin K-dependent factor) during the initial phase of Coumadin effect.

- Tumor

—Myeloid leukemia

- Congenital

—Inherited deficiencies of protein C and protein S. Only severe, homozygous (less than 5% activity) deficiencies of proteins C and S are associated with purpura fulminans.
—Milder, heterozygous deficiencies of protein C and protein S, as well as deficiency of antithrombin III, dysfibrinogenemias, the carrier state for factor V Leiden, and other prothrombotic defects all give rise to hypercoagulable states, but not neonatal purpura fulminans. Patients with one or more risk factors for thrombosis may be more likely to develop purpura fulminans with an environmental stimulus.

- Immune
- Heparin-induced thrombocytopenia: Antibody to heparin-platelet complex causes platelet activation, thrombocytopenia, and microthrombosis, including dermal vessels.
- Antiphospholipid antibody syndrome: Predisposition to thrombosis can include skin necrosis.
- Miscellaneous

—Thrombotic thrombocytopenic purpura
—Paroxysmal nocturnal hemoglobinuria
—Henoch-Schönlein purpura

 Data Gathering

HISTORY

- Current bacterial sepsis: fever, weakness, dizziness, nausea, vomiting, onset of petechial rash
- Family history suggestive of hypercoagulable state: blood clots or thromboses at an early age, such as stroke, deep vein thrombosis, pulmonary embolism; family members taking Coumadin or heparin
- Previous affected child with purpura fulminans or hypercoagulable state
- Prior exposure to heparin, therapeutically or via intravenous "heplock"
- Medications, including anticoagulation

 Physical Examination

- Signs of sepsis: fever, hypotension, tachycardia, poor perfusion, cool extremities, decreased pulses, shock
- Nonblanching purpura
- Acral purpura and necrosis: check fingers, nose, toes, and penis for black areas.
- An erythematous border may surround purpuric areas.
- Bullae may form over purpuric skin.
- Oozing at sites of venipuncture
- Pain, ischemia, and edema of extremities, or internal organ dysfunction may result from deep vein thrombosis or arterial thrombosis, depending on location and severity.

PHYSICAL EXAMINATION TRICKS

Depress the purpuric area with a glass slide to determine whether it blanches.

Laboratory Aids

TESTS

Screening

- CBC: Platelet count may be low; hemoglobin may be low.
- Prothrombin time (PT): prolonged as in DIC
- Partial thromboplastin time (PTT): prolonged as in DIC
- Fibrinogen: decreased with consumption and fibrinolysis
- Fibrin split products or D-dimer increased fibrinolysis as in DIC

Etiologic

- Protein C activity in patient and parents
- Protein S antigen (total and free) in patient and parents
- Test for antiphospholipid antibodies: usually lupus anticoagulant or anticardiolipin antibody
- Factor V Leiden mutation assay

Imaging

To document presence and extent of suspected large vessel thrombosis:

- Ultrasound with Doppler flow study
- CT
- MRI: better for visualization of vessels
- Angiography: most invasive, requires vascular injury for access

Imaging is potentially useful to:

- Distinguish thrombosis from other pathology
- Judge age of thrombus (based on collateralization)
- Assess clot size prior to anticoagulant or thrombolytic therapy
- Distinguish baseline old clot from new thrombosis

The most useful imaging strategy depends on location and clinical situation.

FALSE POSITIVES

- Protein C and S levels may decrease during a thrombotic episode that is not related to an underlying deficiency. Low measurements often need to be repeated at baseline after recovery.
- Protein C and S levels may be below adult normal ranges for the first 3 to 6 months of life in healthy infants.

PITFALLS

- Proteins C and S are vitamin K-dependent. Level may be affected if vitamin K is not administered at birth.
- Protein C determination is affected by Coumadin therapy. It is difficult to confirm a deficiency state, especially mild deficiency, by repeat testing if Coumadin is started empirically.

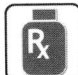 ## Therapy

DRUGS

- Antiinfective agents depending on underlying cause
- Fresh frozen plasma (FFP) every 12 hours to replace proteins C and S in acute DIC of purpura fulminans
- Periodic FFP infusions for chronic replacement
- Prothrombin complex concentrates
- Protein C concentrate—shown to be of benefit in meningococcemia in adults
- Oral Coumadin
- Low molecular weight heparin

DURATION

- Protein C has half-life of 10 hours in circulation.
- Protein C replacement by periodic infusion of protein C concentrate
- Anticoagulation indefinitely usually recommended for documented protein C or S deficiency

DIET

Patients on Coumadin therapy may need to avoid foods with high vitamin K content, especially if there is variation in the dose of Coumadin required to maintain adequate anticoagulation.

POSSIBLE CONFLICTS

- Many drugs can affect Coumadin metabolism.
- Chronic infusion therapy for neonates may run into access problems.

 ## Follow-Up

WHEN TO EXPECT IMPROVEMENT

Related to underlying cause of purpura fulminans

SIGNS TO WATCH FOR

Spread of purpura, hypotension, gangrene

PITFALLS

- Individuals with protein C and protein S deficiency may have increased risk of Coumadin-induced skin necrosis when starting Coumadin. Patients should be heparinized for several days prior to the start of oral anticoagulation.
- Management of an infant on oral anticoagulation is difficult because of the practical problem of obtaining reliable measurements of PT, the increased risk associated with deep venipunctures for blood samples, and difficulty in establishing a stable Coumadin dose.
- Low molecular weight heparin is often preferable.

 ## Common Questions and Answers

Q: What is the risk of a second affected child with protein C or S deficiency?
A: If the diagnosis is confirmed by family studies that show both parents to be carriers of the deficiency and the affected child to be homozygous, then there is a 25% chance that each subsequent infant would have purpura fulminans, and 50% chance that each child would be a carrier. However, other hypercoagulable states have been described that may be risk factors for purpura fulminans.

Q: Should a child with purpura fulminans be followed by a specialist?
A: Generally yes, with a pediatric hematologist, to assist in acute management of purpura, establishment of diagnosis, and management of anticoagulation.

ICD-9-CM 286.6

BIBLIOGRAPHY

Adcock DM, Brozna J, Marlar RA. Proposed classification and pathologic mechanisms of purpura fulminans and skin necrosis. *Semin Thromb Hemost* 1990;16:333.

Francis RB. Acquired purpura fulminans. *Semin Thromb Hemost* 1990;16:310.

Gerson WT, Dickerman JD, Boville G, et al. Severe acquired protein C deficiency in purpura fulminans associated with disseminated intravascular coagulation: treatment with protein C concentrate. *Pediatrics* 1993;91:418.

Kleijn ED, deGroot, R, et al. Activation of protein C following infusion of protein C concentrates in children with severe meningococcal sepsis and purpura fulminans: a randomized, double-blinded, placebo-controlled dose-finding study. *Crit Care Med* 2003;31:1839–1847.

Leclerc F, Leteurtre S, Cremer R, et al. Do new strategies in meningococcemia produce better outcomes? *Crit Care Med* 2000;28:S60.

Marlar RA, Neumann A. Neonatal purpura fulminans due to homozygous protein C or protein S deficiencies. *Semin Thromb Hemost* 1990;16:299.

Rivard GE, David M, Farrell C, Schwarz HP. Treatment of purpura fulminans in meningococcemia with protein C concentrate. *J Pediatr* 1995;126:646.

Smith OP, White B. Infectious purpura fulminans: diagnosis and treatment. *Br J Haematol* 1999;104:202.

Pathan N, Faust, SN, Levin M. Pathophysiology of meningogoccal meningitis and septicaemia. *Arch Dis Child* 2003;88:601–607.

Author: David F. Friedman

Pyelonephritis

 Database

DEFINITION

Acute pyelonephritis (upper urinary tract infection) is defined clinically by fever and flank pain, and histologically by acute renal parenchymal (interstitial) inflammation secondary to bacterial invasion.

PATHOPHYSIOLOGY

Specific factors relating to the development of pyelonephritis:

- Host related

—Anatomic abnormalities (e.g., obstruction, fistula)
—Functional abnormalities (e.g., dysfunctional voiding)

- Pathogen related

—Adherence factors (P-fimbriae)
—Virulence factors (lipopolysaccharide, capsular antigen)

CAUSES

- Enterobacteriaceae: (*Escherichia coli*, most frequent cause [80%]; *Proteus*; *Klebsiella*; *Enterobacter*)
- Gram-positive organisms (cause 10% to 15%): *Staphylococcus aureus, epidermidis, saprophyticus*, and enterococci
- Other organisms: *Pseudomonas, Haemophilus influenzae, Streptococcus* group B

PATHOLOGY

- Patchy infiltration of the medullary parenchyma by polymorphonuclear leukocytes and lymphocytes, tubular disruption and interstitial edema occurs
- Parenchymal scarring may result as a consequence of the infection.

EPIDEMIOLOGY

- 5% of girls develop urinary tract infection (UTI) during childhood.
- Urinary infections are more likely to involve the upper renal tracts in children younger than 3 years of age.
- UTIs are more common in females, except in uncircumcised males under 6 months of age.

COMPLICATIONS

- Acute: reduced concentrating ability, hyperkalemic RTA, bacteremia
- Chronic: focal renal scarring, hypertension, proteinuria, azotemia, xanthogranulomatous pyelonephritis

 Differential Diagnosis

- Cystitis
- Sterile pyuria

—Vulva-vaginitis
—Balanitis
—Systemic viral illness
—Postvaccination
—Pregnancy
—Appendicitis
—Cystic renal disease
—Tuberculosis

- Lower lobe pneumonia
- Acute appendicitis

HISTORY

- A fever of 38.5°C may represent the only complaint.
- In the neonate inquire about vomiting, lethargy, irritability, fever, hypothermia, and jaundice.
- Older children will be able to tell the examiner about flank pain, dysuria, frequency, urgency, and incontinence.

The following are important factors that predispose to the development of UTIs and should be specifically inquired after:

- Constipation
- Bubble baths
- Incorrect toilet training
- Perineal skin irritation
- Antibiotic exposure
- Uncircumcised males

 Physical Examination

- Findings may be nonspecific.
- Fever, irritability, rigors, lethargy
- Flank tenderness

—May be related to the underlying renal tract abnormality such as flank mass as a result of obstruction with hydronephrosis or cystic kidney disease, spina bifida apparent or occult as evidenced by a dimple, pilonidal sinus, or hemangioma.

SPECIAL QUESTIONS

- Previous UTIs
- Investigations already performed
- A family history of UTIs or reflux nephropathy
- Symptoms suggestive of dysfunctional voiding such as the bladder always feels full, infrequent use of the bathroom, and urgency incontinence
- Previous surgery or trauma to the lower back, lower motor milestones, and gait to assess the lower limb neuromuscular status and stool continence.

PHYSICAL EXAMINATION TRICKS

- Gentle posterior punch test will reveal tenderness at the costovertebral angle.
- Bimanual palpation of the kidneys for tenderness and size
- Careful neuromuscular exam of the lower limbs and of the back to evaluate for a neurogenic bladder
- Assess the rectal tone

Laboratory Aids

TESTS

- Collect urine via one of the sterile methods (midstream, catheter, or suprapubic).
- Urine dip for WBC and nitrites as a rapid screen for infection
- As a screening test, an unspun clean-catch urine specimen with bacteria on stained microscopic examination correlates (80% to 90%) with culture results of greater than 100,000 colonies per milliliter of urine.
- Urine for culture and sensitivity: A positive culture is defined by the growth of a single pathogenic organism of clean-catch 100,000 colonies/mL, catheter 1,000 colonies/mL, and by any growth from a suprapubic specimen.

IMAGING

- Renal ultrasound to rule out obstruction and to assess the renal size and parenchyma
- Voiding cystourethrogram (VCUG) to rule out anatomic anomalies including obstruction (e.g., posterior urethral valves) and vesicoureteric reflux
- ^{99m}Tc-dimercaptosuccinic acid (DMSA) can be done to confirm the presence of acute pyelonephritis and to look for renal scarring. This is a sensitive and specific test that some clinicians believe to be the imaging study of choice for diagnosing acute pyelonephritis and renal scarring.

FALSE POSITIVES

May be owing to nonsterile collection techniques, allowing the urine to stand unrefrigerated, or owing to prior antibiotic exposure.

FALSE NEGATIVES

The rapid test for nitrites requires the urine to stay in the bladder for several hours and is therefore not good for infants who do not store urine in the bladder.

PITFALLS

- Imaging evaluation of the urinary tract following a UTI should be individualized based on the child's clinical presentation and on clinical judgment.
- All children 5 years or younger should have an ultrasound and VCUG; over 5 years of age an ultrasound is recommended.
- Once the urine is sterile, a VCUG can be performed; there is no need to wait 4 weeks.
- Administer antibiotic prophylaxis prior to the VCUG.

REQUIREMENTS FOR TESTING

Educate the caregivers in the use and interpretation of the dipstick, and about the symptoms and signs of urinary tract infection.

 ## Therapy

DRUGS

- Antibiotics such as co-trimoxazole, Augmentin, and the second-generation cephalosporins
- Familiarity with local antibiotic patterns of resistance is particularly important in treating hospital-acquired infections.
- Antipyretics such as acetaminophen

DURATION

- Give intravenous antibiotics until afebrile for at least 24 hours, then change to an oral formulation.
- In total, 10 to 14 days of antibiotic therapy are required.
- Patients with first-time urinary infections should receive low-dose antibiotic prophylaxis until their workup is completed.
- Children with frequent symptomatic recurrences of UTI and those with vesicoureteric reflux (VUR) require long-term antibiotic prophylaxis.

DIET

Ensure adequate hydration.

 ## Follow-Up

- The fever usually defervesces in 3 to 5 days.
- Ongoing fever or persistent flank pain requires further evaluation to exclude a resistant organism and or an unrecognized urinary tract obstruction.
- The diagnosis and treatment of any underlying voiding dysfunction and constipation is required for the successful management of UTIs in children.
- The outcome of acute pyelonephritis (APN) is usually good, but may result in parenchymal scarring.
- Risk factors for renal damage include obstruction, reflux with dilation, young age, delay in treatment, number of episodes of pyelonephritis, and bacterial virulence factors.

 ## Common Questions and Answers

Q: Should a DMSA scan be used to help diagnose APN?
A: Routine use of the DMSA scan to diagnose APN is controversial as there is disagreement about the therapeutic implications of a positive test and routine testing will be costly. Children with hypertension and previous UTIs require a DMSA scan to look for renal cortical scarring.

Q: Does renal parenchymal scarring occur in the absence of reflux?
A: Yes. The causal relationship between reflux, acute pyelonephritis, and renal parenchymal scarring is complex.

ICD-9-CM 590.10

BIBLIOGRAPHY

Agarwal S. Vesicoureteral reflux and urinary tract infections. *Curr Opin Urol* 2000;10(6):587–592.

Bartkowski DP. Recognizing UTIs in infants and children. Early treatment prevents permanent damage. *J Postgrad Med* 2001;109(1):171–172, 177–181.

Bloomfield P, Hodson EM, Craig JC. Antibiotics for acute pyelonephritis in children. *Cochrane Database System Rev* 2003;(3):CD003772.

Jodal U, Hansson S. Urinary tract infection. In: Holliday M, Barratt TM, Avner ED, eds. *Pediatric Nephrology*. 3rd Ed. Baltimore: Williams & Wilkins, 1994:950.

Martinell J, Hansson S, Claesson I, et al. Detection of urographic scars in girls with pyelonephritis followed for 13–38 years. *Pediatr Nephrol* 2000;14(10–11):1006–1010.

Rushton HG. Urinary tract infections in children. Epidemiology, evaluation and management. *Pediatr Clin North Am* 1997;44(5):1133–1169.

Weir M. Brien J. Adolescent urinary tract infections. *Adolescent Medicine State of the Art Reviews* 2000;11(2):293–313.

Author: Kevin E. C. Meyers

Pyloric Stenosis

 Database

DEFINITION

Hypertrophy of the muscular layers of the pylorus with elongation and thickening, leading to obstruction of the gastric outlet.

ETIOLOGY

- Unknown
- No specific pattern of inheritance established
- Multifactorial inheritance likely
- Neonatal hypergastrinemia and gastric hyperacidity have a role.
- An association between infantile hypertrophic pyloric stenosis and the administration of oral erythromycin given for postexposure prophylaxis for pertussis has been described.

PATHOPHYSIOLOGY

- There is diffuse hypertrophy and hyperplasia of the pylorus, leading to narrowing of the gastric antrum.
- The antrum becomes thickened, elongated, and firm in consistency.
- Hypergastrinemia associated with hyperactivity, elevations of prostaglandins and deficiency of nitric oxide as a smooth muscle neurotransmitter have been suggested as etiologic factors.

INCIDENCE AND EPIDEMIOLOGY

- Exceedingly rare in newborns as well as in patients older than 6 months of age
- Occurs in approximately 1 in 950 live births.
- More frequent among Caucasians

COMPLICATIONS

- Dehydration
- Electrolyte abnormalities, primarily hypochloremic metabolic alkalosis from loss of hydrochloric acid caused by persistent vomiting

PROGNOSIS

Morbidity and mortality are very low, and surgery is curative.

ASSOCIATED ANOMALIES

Increased occurrence of esophageal atresia and malrotation was noted in 5% of infants with pyloric stenosis.

 Differential Diagnosis

- Gastroesophageal reflux
- Gastroenteritis
- Pyloric atresia
- Antral web

 Data Gathering

HISTORY

- Nonbilious vomiting, classically projectile in an otherwise well and hungry child between 2 and 8 weeks of age
- The infant is typically a "hungry vomiter," refeeding immediately, only to vomit again.
- Possible weight loss
- Varying degrees of dehydration and lethargy

 Physical Examination

- Visible peristalsis may be appreciated just after the infant feeds, which is seen as a waveform proceeding from the left upper quadrant toward the pylorus in the right upper quadrant.
- A palpable, hard, mobile, and nontender mass in the epigastrium to the right of the midline, referred to as an olive
- Best palpated after the infant has vomited

 Laboratory Aids

TESTS

- Hypochloremia and alkalosis
- Hyponatremia
- Hypokalemia
- One percent to 2% of infants have indirect hyperbilirubinemia associated with jaundice.

RADIOLOGIC FEATURES

GASTROINTESTINAL STUDIES

- An upper gastrointestinal study can differentiate between antral webs and pylorospasm and other obstructive lesions.
- Vigorous gastric peristalsis with little or no gastric emptying is seen in pyloric stenosis.
- An elongated narrow pyloric anal canal can be seen as a single or sometimes a double tract of barium, commonly known as the "string sign."
- A pyloric bulge into the distal antrum, producing an umbrella appearance, also may be seen.

Ultrasound

- Ultrasonography identifies the hypertrophic pyloric musculature as a broad ring with low-echo density and an inner layer of high-echo density corresponding to the mucosa.
- To confirm the diagnosis, the muscle thickness should be greater than 4 mm or the pyloric length greater than 16 mm.

 ## Emergency Care

Early identification of electrolyte abnormalities and correction with appropriate IV fluids.

 ## Therapy

- Correction of the metabolic abnormalities by replacing sodium, chloride, and potassium
- Pyloromyotomy (Ramstedt procedure): longitudinal incision of the antropyloric muscle.
- Laparoscopic pyloromyotomy is a minimally invasive version of the Ramstedt procedure.
- Pyloric stenosis is a medical emergency, not a surgical emergency.
- Postoperative vomiting is well recognized and is most likely caused by persistent local edema.
- Initiate feedings very slowly; most patients can be advanced to maintenance oral feedings 48 hours after surgery.

 ## Follow-Up

Vomiting may persist for several days after surgery.

PITFALLS

- Failure to appreciate that chloride loss is the most significant electrolyte disorder when replacing fluids and electrolytes
- Failure to appreciate that this disorder does occur in girls as well as boys

 ## Common Questions and Answers

Q: Can ultrasound help make the diagnosis?
A: Yes. Many will order this test first to avoid the possible aspiration of contrast material.

Q: Why is there so much chloride loss?
A: The chloride loss occurs with the loss of gastric acid, which contains HCl.

Q: What plan should I follow when replacing electrolytes?
A: Correct the deficiency of fluids with twice maintenance fluid volumes. Correct the chloride loss with normal saline, and correct the potassium loss with KCl.

ICD-9-CM 537.0

BIBLIOGRAPHY

D'Agostino J. Common abdominal emergencies in children. *Emerg Med Clin North Am* 2002;20(1):139–153.

Hernanz-Schulman M. Infantile hypertrophic pyloric stenosis. *Radiology* 2003;227(2):319–331.

Letton RW Jr. Pyloric stenosis. *Pediatr Ann* 2001;30(12):745–750.

Mitchell LE, Risch N. The genetics of infantile hypertrophic pyloric stenosis: a reanalysis. *Am J Dis Child* 1993;147(11):1203.

Authors: Andrew E. Mulberg and Helen John-Kelly

Rabies

Database

DEFINITION

Rabies is a viral infection of the central nervous system (CNS) that is transmitted from animals to people.

CAUSES

Transmission of the virus, a rhabdovirus containing single-stranded RNA, occurs through animal bites and, rarely, via corneal transplants (from donors with unexplained encephalitis) or inhalation among laboratory workers.

PATHOPHYSIOLOGY

Except for rare cases, the rabies virus enters the body through a bite that causes a break in the skin and introduces infected saliva. From there, the virus gains access to muscle, in which it is sequestered. The virus then enters the peripheral nerves, in which it moves centripetally to the CNS at a rate of approximately 3 mm/hour. Once in the CNS, infection spreads rapidly to involve nearly all neurons. This, if untreated, leads to cardiopulmonary arrest and death shortly thereafter by poorly understood mechanisms.

EPIDEMIOLOGY

- Although the current annual incidence of reported human rabies in the United States is about one to two cases per year, incidence rates elsewhere in the world are much higher. In addition, thousands of infected animals are identified each year in the United States.
- Endemic regions of the United States include the mid-Atlantic, southeast, south central, and north central areas, and California.
- Common vectors: Seven species of animals account for 98% of all reported U.S. animal rabies cases: skunks (38% to 43%), raccoons (28% to 31%), bats (14%), cats (4%), foxes (4%), cattle (4%), dogs (3%), and other (2%).
- Of the 30 human rabies cases since 1990 believed to be contracted in the United States, only two cases reported a suspicious bite.
- Uncommon vectors: As noted, transmission rarely occurs via corneal transplants or inhalation among laboratory workers.

CLINICAL MANIFESTATIONS

- The incubation period can range between 10 days and 2 years! Most cases, however, present within 20 to 90 days postexposure.
- Prodrome: 2 to 10 days with vague and insidious symptoms such as sore throat, malaise, anxiety, depression, and, at times, fever or nausea. A fairly specific prodromal symptom is itching, pain, or tingling at the site of the bite.
- Acute neurologic phase: furious (80%) vs. paralytic (20%) rabies

—Furious rabies: Agitation, hyperactivity, bizarre behavior—nuchal rigidity, sore throat, and hoarseness. The pathognomonic sign is hydrophobia and, at times, aerophobia.
—Paralytic rabies: Starts with flaccid paralysis in the limb that was bitten; subsequently spreads to other limbs. Cranial nerve involvement can give an expressionless face.
—Coma: Follows the acute neurologic phase; may persist up to 2 weeks and is followed by death almost universally.

PROGNOSIS

- Once the patient is infected with the rabies virus, the prognosis is grim.
- Without postexposure rabies immunization, the disease is uniformly fatal.
- There are three documented cases of rabies in humans in which the patient survived after receiving postexposure immunization and intensive medical management.

Differential Diagnosis

- Other causes of encephalitis (e.g., HSV, enterovirus) can mimic rabies.
- Paralytic rabies can present much like Guillain-Barré syndrome or poliomyelitis.
- Pseudorabies is hysteria in an individual who thinks he or she has rabies, but does not. Here, though, normal blood gases and lack of variation in bizarre behavior are distinguishing.

Data Gathering

HISTORY

- Rabid animals: Although signs of rabies in animals vary greatly, atypical behavior for the animal is the norm (e.g., passive animals become aggressive, nocturnal animals roam in daylight). Foaming at the mouth and lack of coordination may be present.
- A small minority of humans with rabies have no identifiable preceding animal exposure.

Physical Examination

- Although the neurologic findings can vary, cranial nerve paralysis (palate, vocal cords) is common. Therefore, hoarseness and stridor can be seen.
- Meningismus is also fairly common, along with involuntary movements. Beyond this, findings depend on type of presentation (furious vs. paralytic) (see Clinical Manifestations, above).

SPECIAL QUESTIONS

- Type of animal inflicting the bite (domestic vs. wild)?
- Location of the animal and availability for observation?
- History of previous rabies vaccination of the animal and patient?

Laboratory Aids

- There are no known methods for identification of rabies virus infection prior to the onset of clinical signs. However, once signs appear, laboratory diagnosis is now possible as early as day 5 of illness by several techniques:

—Enzyme linked antibodies stain of brain tissue from apprehended animal.
—Fluorescent antibodies (FA) stain of corneal epithelial cell smears or a section of skin from the neck at the hairline of affected individual.
—Serologic diagnosis is possible if the patient survives beyond the acute period. A rise in virus-neutralizing antibody will be seen.
—Viral isolation from saliva, CSF, urine sedimentation, and brain is, at times, possible between days 4 and 24.

- Postmortem diagnosis is made by the presence of pathognomonic cytoplasmic inclusions (Negri bodies) in brain tissue (sensitivity, 80%).

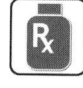

Therapy

LOCAL WOUND CARE

- The first step in preventing infection is washing out the virus mechanically or inactivating it before it has a chance to attach to and enter a neuron.
- The wound should be flushed with copious amounts of soap and water or saline.
- For puncture wounds, insertion of a catheter (e.g., angiocatheter) and irrigation with fluid by means of an attached syringe should be performed. If irrigation is too painful, infiltration of the area with local anesthesia can help.

IMMUNIZATION

Passive

• Human rabies immune globulin (HRIG) derived from the plasma of volunteers hyperimmunized with rabies vaccine should be given to those who are bitten by any variety of wild animal known to be at high risk for rabies infection (skunk, raccoon, fox, coyote, bat) and any domestic dog or cat not in good health and in the custody of someone able to observe the animal for a 10-day period. Local health departments can advise about the risk of specific animal exposures.

• The present recommendation for HRIG vaccination is 20 IU/kg instilled locally into the tissue at the site of the bite. Remaining vaccine can be given IM. In cases of multiple wounds, to ensure that all wounds receive an injection of HRIG, dilution in saline (twofold to threefold) is acceptable. Using more than the recommended dosage is contraindicated because it may interfere with the immune response to the active vaccine.

Active

• Three forms of rabies vaccine are commercially available. These include human diploid cell rabies vaccine (HDCV), rabies vaccine absorbed (RVA), and purified chicken embryo cell vaccine (PCEC). These should be administered by the same criteria given above for passive immunization. In addition, vaccination is recommended for those at high risk for exposure (veterinarians, animal handlers, etc.).

• Dosing: 1 mL IM in the deltoid region on days 0, 3, 7, 14, and 28 postexposure. The anterolateral thigh can be used in infants or young children. Discontinue the vaccine series if fluorescent antibody testing of the animal is conducted and is negative.

PREVENTION

Immunoprophylaxis: Preexposure vaccines are offered to persons at high risk, such as veterinarians and animal handlers. Because wild animals are the largest source of rabies in the United States today, avoiding unnecessary contact is helpful. More importantly, attempts are being made to orally vaccinate wild animals by using vaccine-laden food in several areas of the United States. Last, it is essential that pet owners vaccinate their pets.

 Common Questions and Answers

Q: Does a wild squirrel or rabbit bite necessitate rabies prophylaxis?
A: In general, rodents (squirrels, rats, mice, hamsters, gerbils), lagomorphs (rabbits and hares), and opossums are not known to serve as natural rabies reservoirs. They should not be considered rabid unless they exhibit unusual behavior.

Q: Is there any evidence of human-to-human spread?
A: No, however health care workers or others exposed to a patient with known or suspected rabies should receive vaccination if they have suffered a bite wound or if mucosal surfaces or open wounds have been exposed to the patient's body fluids.

Q: Are there any countries that require routine rabies vaccination?
A: Yes, Nepal.

Q: What if a severe allergic reaction occurs during postexposure rabies prophylaxis?
A: The reaction should be treated at the time, as you would any systemic anaphylactic reaction. Subsequently, the rabies vaccine adsorbed (RVA), produced in rhesus diploid cells, can be given on the same schedule as HDCV.

Q: If a bat is found in the house, should the family members receive immunoprophylaxis?
A: If a bat is found in the room of a sleeping person, previously unattended child, or mentally disabled person, prophylaxis should be considered. The injury inflicted by a bat bite or scratch may not be noticed in the above situations.

ICD-9-CM 071

BIBLIOGRAPHY

American Academy of Pediatrics. Rabies. In: Pickering LK, ed. *2003 Red Book: Report of the Committee on Infectious Diseases.* 26th Ed. Elk Grove Village, IL: American Academy of Pediatrics, 2003.

Centers for Disease Control and Prevention. First human death associated with raccoon rabies—Virginia 2003. *MMWR Morbid Mortal Wkly Rep* 2003;52(45):1102–1103.

Centers for Disease Control and Prevention. Rabies surveillance, United States, 1987. *MMWR Morbid Mortal Wkly Rep* 1988;37:1.

Gomez-Alonso J. Rabies: a possible explanation for the vampire legend. *Neurology* 1998;51(3):856–859.

NASPHV Compendium Committee. Compendium of animal rabies control. *MMWR Morbid Mortal Wkly Rep* 1987;35:815.

Nicholson KG. Modern vaccines. *Lancet* 1990;335:1201.

Plotkin SA. Rabies. *Clin Infect Dis* 2000;30(1):4–12.

Authors: Suzanne Dawid and Louis M. Bell

Rectal Prolapse

 Database

DEFINITION

There are three types of rectal prolapse:

- Complete: The full thickness of the rectum prolapses through the anus (two layers of rectum with an intervening peritoneal sac, which may contain small bowel).
- Incomplete: The prolapse is limited to the two layers of mucosa only.
- Concealed: An internal intussusception of the upper rectum into the lower rectum, which does not emerge through the anus

CAUSES

The exact etiology is uncertain, but is related to the following:

- Constipation
- Excessive straining with bowel movements
- Diarrhea; may be more of a cause in tropical countries
- Cystic fibrosis (CF)
- Malnutrition; can cause loss of the ischiorectal fat pad
- Complete prolapse more rare in children, but when occurs may be related to poor fixation of rectum to sacrum and weak pelvic and anal musculature
- Complication of past surgery, such as imperforate anus repair
- Infections: hookworms

GENETICS

- No known inheritance pattern aside from the association with CF
- An autosomally recessive inherited disease

EPIDEMIOLOGY

- Occurs in more than 19% of children with CF
- It usually presents between 1 and $2\frac{1}{2}$ years of age in patients with CF. Presentation in these children after age 5 is rare.
- In older children and adults, it is six times more common in women than in men.
- It is seen more in underdeveloped countries, perhaps secondary to poor nutrition.

COMPLICATIONS

- In certain older patients who may also have an overactive external sphincter, the need to generate high rectal pressures in order to defecate, together with the rectal prolapse, may cause venous congestion; it may lead to the solitary rectal ulcer syndrome.
- The repetitive trauma to the mucosa can lead to a proctitis.

PROGNOSIS

With proper medical management, excellent prognosis; surgery not usually required

 Differential Diagnosis

- Tumors
- Prolapsing rectal tumor: very rare
- Trauma
- Sexual abuse (e.g., anal penetration)
- Metabolic
- CF: Of significance is the fact that many (anywhere from 10% to 50%) of the patients who are diagnosed with CF after age 4 have experienced rectal prolapse (either at the time of the diagnosis or as a past event).
- Anatomic

—Solitary rectal ulcer syndrome: an uncommon benign condition usually affecting older children (teenagers). Rectal bleeding on defecation common. Some studies report an association between this entity and rectal prolapse.
—Prolapsing polyp
—Large hemorrhoids

- Surgical

—Colonic intussusception

 Data Gathering

HISTORY

- It is usually first noted by a parent after the child has defecated, and may be associated with painless rectal bleeding.
- It often reduces spontaneously. If not, it is usually easily reduced manually by the parent.
- Rectal prolapse may cause some discomfort during bowel movements.
- Trauma to the recurrently prolapsed mucosa may lead to ulceration and mucus discharge.

 Physical Examination

- Usually, prolapse is not seen on examination while the patient is at rest, unless it is irreducible.
- May see poor anal tone and/or large anal orifice, especially within hours after the prolapse
- In complete rectal prolapse, concentric mucosal rings can be seen, whereas incomplete prolapse reveals radial folds. If one sees more than 5 cm of rectum emerging, it is most likely a complete prolapse.

SPECIAL QUESTIONS

- Has the patient had history of wheezing, pneumonia, or failure to thrive?
- Does this patient have CF?

PHYSICAL EXAMINATION TRICKS

- Asking the patient to strain may allow the mucosa to prolapse. However, this is obviously not very helpful in the very young patient.
- A polyp is differentiated in that it is plum-colored and does not involve the entire anal circumference.
- In an intussusception, it is possible to insert the finger around the prolapsing apex of the intussusception, between it and the lining of the anal canal.

 Laboratory Aids

TESTS

- Sweat test: All children with prolapse should have a sweat test to rule out CF. This is a simple, noninvasive, inexpensive test with good specificity and sensitivity when performed by an experienced laboratory.
- Stool cultures: For bacterial and parasitic infestations, if diarrhea is present as a possible causative factor

IMAGING

Evacuation proctography: A barium enema is given, and the movement of barium is observed under fluoroscopy during defecation. This may reveal an internal prolapse not easily recognizable on examination alone. This is not commonly used in children, as good cooperation is necessary.

PITFALLS

Although the history of rectal prolapse may be evident, it is often difficult to elicit on examination, and by the time the patient is seen after a prolapse at home, it may already be spontaneously reduced. Thus, the assumption of the diagnosis may have to rest primarily on the parental history for some time.

Therapy

- Rectal prolapse has a tendency to spontaneously resolve over time.
- The prolapse will more successfully and quickly resolve if the patient is treated for constipation. This should include both dietary manipulations (increased fiber, water) and improved toilet regimen. It also will usually necessitate the use of supplemental aids such as mineral oil and, occasionally, laxatives. A small child should try to defecate on a regular toilet and not a potty. In this way, the feet are off the floor, relieving pressure on the abdomen.
- In the rare case of stool infection with diarrhea as the underlying etiology, the appropriate therapy for that infection should be instituted.

DRUGS

In a patient with CF, the addition of pancreatic enzyme supplementation, if not already a part of the regime, has been shown to cause dramatic improvement in rectal prolapse.

DURATION

The treatment of constipation should continue indefinitely, or until the child has demonstrated regular bowel habits on a high-fiber diet on his or her own without evidence of prolapse for at least several months.

SURGICAL

Numerous approaches have been attempted and advocated with varying degrees of enthusiasm, suggesting that none is perfect. These include:

- Perianal sutures: Has poor results and high complication rate
- Delorme procedure: The rectal mucosa is excised and underlying rectal muscle is plicated with sutures.
- Abdominal rectopexy: The rectum is mobilized and attached to the sacrum by prosthetic material. Although this procedure provides good results, it has a high complication rate of constipation (greater than 50%).
- Anterior resection rectopexy: Includes resection of the sigmoid loop and upper rectum; good results, but again, high complication rate because of the anastomosis
- Perineal resection: Perineal rectosigmoidectomy with a coloanal anastomosis; good results

 Follow-Up

WHEN TO EXPECT IMPROVEMENT

Over a period of months to years on a good dietary and behavioral regimen.

SIGNS TO WATCH FOR

The child is beginning to strain in order to defecate.

PITFALLS

- Although usually a benign event, rectal prolapse is a very distressing condition to both the parents and the child.
- Although surgery seems to be a quicker and more definite solution, in most cases it is more prudent to allow time and medical management to solve the problem. The results from surgical procedures are not foolproof and may lead to further complications.

 Common Questions and Answers

Q: What should I do if my child has a rectal prolapse but I cannot reduce it?
A: You should wrap the prolapse in moist towels and bring your child to the emergency room. There, the physicians will try to reduce it. Rarely, if a prolapse is irreducible and left for a period of time, it can cause bowel ischemia and may require surgery.

Q: My child has rectal prolapse and now he is supposed to have a sweat test to determine whether or not he has cystic fibrosis. Is this very likely?
A: No. Although it is important to rule out this disease, the majority of patients with rectal prolapse do not have CF. On the other hand, many children with CF suffer from rectal prolapse.

Q: My child, who has rectal prolapse, is in day care. How will I know if he is having the prolapse?
A: You should inform someone in the school (a teacher or guardian) of his condition and he or she should check the child for prolapse after a movement. Although, if present, it usually spontaneously resolves, the teacher should inform you so you can do a manual reduction, if necessary.

ICD-9-CM 569.1

BIBLIOGRAPHY

Andrews NJ, Jones DJ. Rectal prolapse and associated conditions. *BMJ* 1992;305:242.

Bartolo DC, Kamm MA, et al. Working party report: defecation disorders. *Am J Gastroenterol* 1994;89(8):S154.

Du Boulay DF, Fairbrother J, et al. Mucosal prolapse syndrome: a unifying concept for solitary ulcer syndrome and related disorders. *J Clin Pathol* 1983;36:1264.

Siafakas C, Vottler TP, Andersen JM. Rectal prolapse in pediatrics. *Clin Pediatr* 1999;38(2):63–72.

Author: Andrew E. Mulberg

Refractive Error

 Database

DEFINITION

For eyes to be able to see, light coming into the eye must be focused on the retina. Refractive errors are aberrations in the optical components of the eyes that cause the eye to be out of focus. Uncorrected refractive error result in blurred vision in one or both eyes, and in children may cause strabismus and amblyopia.

PATHOPHYSIOLOGY

The most important optical components of the eye are the cornea and the lens, which refract light coming into the pupil to focus an image on the retina. The cornea and lens determine the focal length of the eye, which must match the actual eye length (distance from cornea to retina). A sharply focused image on the retina is necessary for recognition of small objects and normal visual acuity; refractive errors cause blurring. Refractive errors can be classified in three groups based on the optical effects:

• Myopia,
also called "near-sightedness," correctable with concave lenses with negative diopteric power. Myopic eyes may be in focus for closer targets, but blurred for more distant targets.
• Hyperopia, correctable with convex lenses with positive diopteric power. Although hyperopia is sometimes called "far-sightedness," this is a misnomer in children. Small hyperopic refractive errors are easily overcome by focusing the eye, or accommodation, and many hyperopic children have no difficulty seeing near or distant targets. Larger amounts of hyperopia may blur both near and distant targets, or cause eye strain or esotropia because of the focusing effort required for focusing (see Strabismus).
• Astigmatism, correctable with toric lenses, is caused by aspheric aberration. Uncorrected astigmatism creates images that are not focusable for near or distant targets. Astigmatism may occur simultaneously with myopia and hyperopia.

Other terms referring to refractive error are:

• Emmetropia, or neutral refraction (no refractive error)
• Anisometropia, or unequal refractive error between the two eyes
• Accommodation, the ability to change the focus the eyes for near targets, and to overcome hyperopia

In children under 8 years of age, because of visual development and plasticity, uncorrected refractive errors may have a significant effect on life-long vision. Amblyopia, which may cause permanent, uncorrectable vision loss, and strabismus are among the risks of untreated refractive errors in young children (see Strabismus, Amblyopia).

PATHOLOGY

The refractive components of the eye (cornea, lens, eye length) normally develop simultaneously to allow focused images during early childhood. Factors determining the relative growth and development of these ocular features are not completely understood, and abnormal growth of any component may result in refractive error. Normally, infants and young children are mildly hyperopic (+ 1.5 to + 3.00 diopters), and growth of the eye (primarily increase in eye length) causes a progressive loss of hyperopia, becoming emmetropic during late childhood. Because of this refractive growth, hyperopic refractive errors are much more common in early childhood, and myopic errors in older children and adults. Except for patients with other ocular and systemic abnormalities, the retina, sclera, cornea and lens is normal in patients with moderate refractive errors. High myopia (generally >−5.00 diopters) may lead to retinal thinning, retinal holes, and retinal detachment.

GENETICS

Both genetic and environmental factors are important determinates of refractive status. It has been estimated that 60% of myopia can be predicted by parental refraction, although inheritance seems to be polygenic in most cases. Some genetic syndromes associated with refractive errors include

• Myopia

—Stickler syndrome
—Albinism
—Marfan syndrome
—Down syndrome
—Ehlers-Danlos syndrome

• Hyperopia

—Senior-Loken syndrome
—WAGR syndrome

• Astigmatism

—Down syndrome
—Cruzon syndrome
—Albinism

EPIDEMIOLOGY

Because of the age-related growth of the optical components of the eye, the prevalence of refractive errors varies during childhood. At birth the median refractive error is low hyperopia, approximately + 2.00 diopters. In adults, the median is emmetropia. The distribution of refractive errors in large populations is a bell-curve around these averages, skewed toward myopia.
In school-aged children in the United States, 7% to 25% have refractive error significant enough to affect visual acuity. About 25% of the United States adult population has myopia, with about 5% with hyperopia. Certain populations have increased prevalence of myopia, including individuals with native American, Chinese, and Japanese descent. Refractive errors are frequently associated with other ocular conditions. These include:

• Myopia

—Childhood glaucoma
—Retinitis pigmentosa
—Coloboma
—Microphthalmia
—Retinopathy of prematurity
—Congenital cataract
—Achromatopsia

• Hyperopia

—Esotropia
—Leber congenital amaurosis
—Surgically treated cataracts (aphakia)

• Astigmatism

—Congenital ptosis
—Coloboma
—Forceps birth injury
—Glaucoma
—Retinopathy of prematurity

COMPLICATIONS

In children, the most significant complications of uncorrected refractive errors are strabismus and amblyopia.

• Accommodative esotropia: uncorrected hyperopia in young children can be overcome by focusing, or accommodation. This involuntary change in the lens of the eye to focus (increase the positive diopteric power of the lens) is controlled reflexively, and is integrated with convergence (crossing the eyes inward). Usually, accommodation is used to focus on near targets, and convergence keeps both eyes pointed at the near target. If there is excessive hyperopia, or if there is an abnormal ratio of accommodative convergence to accommodation (AC/A ratio), the eyes may cross with accommodation. This is esotropia (see Strabismus).
• Amblyopia: amblyopia, or poor visual development, results from a poorly focused image. Anisometropia (unequal refractive error), which blurs vision in one eye, is the most frequent cause of unilateral amblyopia, and occurs in about 3% to 5% of children. Less frequently, bilateral high refractive errors (>4 diopters of hyperopia, >6 diopters of myopia, or >2 diopters of astigmatism) may cause bilateral amblyopia (see Amblyopia).

 Differential Diagnosis

Any cause of monocular or binocular vision loss can simulate refractive error. Since refraction is not easily measured without eye drops and special equipment, the possibility of refractive error must be considered in all children with reduced visual acuity, and should also be considered in children with strabismus and normal vision. Cycloplegic refraction (measuring refraction after the use of eye drops to relax accommodation), and in younger children, a trial of correction with glasses is necessary to eliminate the possibility of residual amblyopia or other causes of poor vision.

Data Gathering

HISTORY

- Age of onset of vision loss
- Associated ocular abnormalities, trauma, injury or surgery
- History of strabismus, amblyopia
- History of prematurity, genetic disorders, collagen disorders (Ehler-Danlos, Marfan syndromes)
- History of headaches, squinting, or subjective vision problems
- Family history of glasses or refractive error, amblyopia, strabismus

Physical Examination

Visual acuity is the most effective diagnostic tool for detecting refractive errors. Vision must be tested with each eye separately, using a patch, opaque card, or plastic occluder. Testing charts are available with letters as well as pictures and illiterate figures (Es). In children who are too young to test with charts, the Bruchner simultaneous red reflex examination can detect high refractive errors and anisometropia, which appear as asymmetrical or distorted red pupillary reflex using the direct ophthalmoscope. Strabismus is frequently a secondary sign of refractive error in children, and can be detected by cover test, Hirschberg corneal light reflex test, or Bruchner test. Photoscreening, which uses the principle of red reflex testing, is also effective in detecting high or asymmetrical refractive errors.

Laboratory Aids

TESTS

There are no effective laboratory tests for refractive errors.

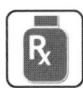

Therapy

Refractive errors are treated by corrective lenses. In young children, this is usually glasses although contact lenses are frequently used in teenagers.

Unlike adults, children with neglected refractive error are at great risk for significant long-term complications, including amblyopia and strabismus. Hyperopia and anisometropic hyperopia pose the greatest risk for amblyopia. Therefore, smaller amounts of hyperopia and anisometropia are generally corrected with glasses. Glasses are prescribed to improve vision and treat or prevent amblyopia in children for:

- Myopia, −3.00 diopters or more in infants and young children, −1.00 diopter or more in school-age children, or −3.00 diopters or more anisometropia
- Hyperopia, +4.00 diopters or more in infants, +3.00 diopters or more in school-age children, or +1.50 diopters or more anisometropia.
- Any hyperopia in accomodative esotropia. Bifocals may also be prescribed to treat residual esotropia for near targets (high AC/A ratio)
- Astigmatism of >3.00 diopters in infants and young children, or >1.50 diopters in school-age children

In general, children accept full correction of all refractive error although undercorrection of hyperopia by 0.50 to 1.00 diopter may enhance the acceptance of new glasses. Occasionally, if hyperopic correction is not well accepted, a brief period of cycloplegia with topical atropine can reinforce use of the glasses.

When there is suspicion of amblyopia, vision should be retested after glasses have been worn for several weeks to measure visual improvement. Children wearing glasses must be remeasured regularly, usually at least annually, until they have reached visual maturity and the risk of amblyopia has passed (8 to 10 years old).

Hyperopic patients may develop accommodative esotropia when their glasses are off, after wearing the glasses for some time. Full correction of hyperopia and continuous correction is the best approach to this unusual complication.

Follow-Up

Refractive errors will change over time as a result of growth of the eye and its optical components. In general, the younger children will need re-refraction and new glasses more frequently. All children wearing glasses should have acuity tested and be re-refracted at least annually.

PITFALLS

- Early detection and correction of refractive errors is important to prevent amblyopia and strabismus. Recognition visual acuity testing using charts should start by age 4 years.
- Children with significant refractive errors will not necessarily be symptomatic. All children should be screened for visual acuity in each eye.
- Glasses may not reverse amblyopia, even if the refractive error is appropriately corrected. Patients with suspected amblyopia (anisometropia, unilateral poor vision, and strabismus) should be followed closely even after wearing the glasses.

Common Questions and Answers

Q. Will my child always need glasses?
A. Not necessarily. Many children who wear glasses are able to see well without correction as adults. Contact lenses and refractive surgery are also possible in older children or adults, if correction remains necessary.

Q. Will wearing glasses weaken my child's eyes?
A. No, wearing correction for refractive errors will not weaken the eyes or vision, and is important to prevent amblyopia and permanent vision loss. Occasionally, children with hyperopia will develop esotropia when the glasses are off, after wearing correction for some time. This is rarely a problem as long as the glasses are worn continuously.

Q. Is my child too young for glasses?
A. Glasses can be worn in children as young as a few months old, with appropriate frames. Usually, children get used to glasses quickly and accept correction easily.

Q. My child could see well, why does he need glasses?
A. Some children with hyperopia can see charts well, but the accommodation (focusing) necessary to overcome the refractive error may cause eye strain, fatigue, and esotropia. Others may need glasses for unilateral refractive error, and seem to see well with both eyes open. In these children, wearing correction may treat or prevent problems even though they may seem to see well without correction.

Q. Everyone in my family has needed glasses for myopia in childhood. Is there anything we can do for my child that will prevent the development of myopia?
A. Unfortunately very few environmental factors have been clearly identified to affect the development of myopia. Reading, particularly at an early age; excessively close visual targets (holding books or toys too close to the face); and light exposure during nighttime have been suggested as factors in myopia development. Avoiding long periods of reading, avoiding intensive near work, using a reasonable reading distance (16 to 18 inches), and avoiding nightlights may reduce some of the environmental stimuli.

ICD-9-CM 367.9

BIBLIOGRAPHY

Drack AV. Inheritance of refractive errors. In: Traboulsi EI, ed. *Genetic Diseases of the Eye*. New York: Oxford University Press, 1998.

Kuo A, Sinatra RB, Donahue SP. Distribution of refractive error in healthy infants. *J Am Assoc Pediatr Ophthalmol* 2003;7:174–177.

Mills, MD. The eye in childhood. *Am Fam Physician* 1999;60:907–918.

Paysse EA, Williams GC, Coats DK, Williams EA. Detection of red reflex asymmetry by pediatric residents using the Bruchner reflex versus the MTI photoscreener. *Pediatrics* 2001;108:E74.

Thorn F. Development of refraction and strabismus. *Curr Opin in Ophthalmol* 2000;11(5):301–305.

Author: Monte D. Mills

Renal Artery Stenosis

 Database

DEFINITION

Renal artery stenosis is narrowing of one or both renal arteries or their more distal branches, resulting in decreased perfusion, increased renin release, increased vascular resistance, and systemic hypertension.

PATHOPHYSIOLOGY

• The most common cause is fibromuscular dysplasia (FMD).
• Other causes include hypoplasia of the renal artery, partial obstruction from a thromboembolism, severe dehydration, extrinsic compression of the artery, vasculitis, neurofibromatosis type 1 (NF), and following renal artery surgery (e.g., renal transplantation or trauma).
• Arterial narrowing by atheroma is very common in adults but rarely is seen in childhood.

PATHOLOGY

• FMD is a segmental sclerotic process involving smooth muscle hyperplasia of the media layer of the artery. In 75% of patients it is unilateral. Stenosis is usually distal in the renal artery and sometimes involves intrarenal branches. FMD frequently gives a beaded appearance on angiography.
• In NF, the arterial narrowing is proximal, often at the vessel ostium and usually involves the intimal layer.

GENETICS

• FMD is sporadic.
• NF is autosomal dominant.
• Williams syndrome involves a heterozygous deletion on chromosome 7.

EPIDEMIOLOGY

The majority of older children and adolescents with elevated blood pressure (readings consistently greater than 95th percentile for height and weight) have primary or idiopathic hypertension. Hypertension in infants and young children is most often secondary to an identifiable cause. Of those with secondary hypertension, the majority have intrinsic renal disease (e.g., glomerulonephritis or renal scarring). Approximately 10% have renal artery stenosis. Its importance, therefore, is not its frequency but the fact it is potentially curable.

COMPLICATIONS

• Renal artery stenosis often causes severe blood pressure elevation which may be asymptomatic or may be associated with headache, encephalopathy, seizures, or stroke.
• Chronic hypertension may cause damage to end-organs, including the heart and kidney.
• Angiography may be associated with acute renal failure induced by radiocontrast. There may be injury to the renal artery or embolism to the kidney.

PROGNOSIS

• Long-term outcome of percutaneous transluminal angioplasty (PTA) in FMD is excellent, and most children require no chronic antihypertensive medications.
• Restenosis of the vessel is very infrequent.

ASSOCIATED ILLNESSES

• FMD is not associated with other conditions.
• Renal artery stenosis may occur in many other conditions, including NF Type 1, vasculitis including polyarteritis nodosa, Kawasaki disease, Takayasu arteritis, moyamoya syndrome, Williams syndrome, Marfan syndrome, tuberous sclerosis, congenital rubella, and following trauma.
• In neonates, renal artery occlusion/stenosis is usually the result of a thromboembolus, which is a complication of an umbilical artery catheter.
• Some tumors including Wilms tumor, neuroblastoma, pheochromocytoma and lymphoma may compress the renal artery and compromise its blood flow.
• Renal artery stenosis has been associated with multicystic dysplastic kidney.

 Differential Diagnosis

• Renal artery stenosis should be suspected and investigated in children with severe, progressive, and/or difficult-to-manage hypertension.
• The differential diagnosis consists of other causes of significant hypertension, including coarctation of the aorta, the midaortic syndrome, rapidly progressive glomerulonephritis, and renal failure and pheochromocytoma.

 Data Gathering

HISTORY

• Symptoms in infants may include irritability, vomiting, and poor feeding.
• In children, symptoms may include headaches, vomiting, dizziness, and seizures.
• Many children are asymptomatic.

SPECIAL QUESTION

Has the child ingested any medication that can increase blood pressure, such as sympathomimetic drugs, steroids, amphetamines, oral contraceptives, or illicit drugs such as cocaine or phencyclidine?

 Physical Examination

• Accurate determination of blood pressure with appropriate-size cuff; done in the upper and lower extremities
• Blood pressure should be repeated until the patient is judged to be relaxed.
• Pulses should be checked in all four extremities.
• The skin must be examined for signs of neurofibromatosis (e.g., café-au-lait spots and neurofibromas) and vasculitis.
• The optic fundi must be checked for hypertensive vascular changes. Often, an ophthalmologist's examination is necessary.
• Auscultation of the lower back and abdomen should be checked for the presence of bruits.
• In infancy, signs of congestive heart failure may be present.

PHYSICAL EXAMINATION TRICKS

• The resting, relaxed blood pressure is likely to be obtained when the pulse rate has reached a basal resting level.
• Listen for an abdominal bruit just to the left of and superior to the umbilicus.
• Listen over the flanks with a bell stethoscope for a bruit.

Renal Artery Stenosis

Laboratory Aids

TESTS

- BUN and creatinine to exclude intrinsic renal disease
- Electrolytes: a hyperrenin state leads to hyperaldosteronism and may produce hypokalemia and mild metabolic alkalosis.
- Selective renal vein renin determinations are suggestive of unilateral stenosis if the affected side is one and a half times the contralateral normal side. However, the test is invasive and requires catheterization of the femoral vein. Random venous renin concentrations have little value and may be misleading.
- Electrocardiogram and/or echocardiogram to investigate the presence of ventricular strain or hypertrophy

IMAGING

- Although a variety of imaging studies are available that may suggest renal artery stenosis, the only definitive test is selective renal arteriography, and, if indicated, transluminal angioplasty.
- Renal ultrasonography may demonstrate a smaller kidney on the suspected side, but this study cannot make or exclude the diagnosis. Doppler ultrasonography and color-coded duplex sonography have some usefulness and may detect increased blood velocity at the origin of the renal artery. Doppler ultrasound may be particularly helpful in the postoperative transplant period when immediate information regarding the renal artery is essential.
- MR Angiography with gadolinium may be useful when radiocontrast is contraindicated because of renal failure.
- Other studies, such as captopril-enhanced nuclear medicine scans using DMSA or MAG-3, digital subtraction angiography and CT angiography have not proved to be confirmatory for all patients, but they may be helpful when used in selective children with a high likelihood of renal artery stenosis.

Therapy

DRUGS

- Hypertension that accompanies renal artery stenosis is often difficult to control with antihypertensive medications. In small infants, however, long-term medical therapy may be necessary until the child is large enough for definitive correction. Multiple medications are often required.
- Because renal artery stenosis results in a high renin state, the angiotensin-converting enzyme (ACE) inhibitors, including captopril and enalapril, are most effective. When used in conjunction with renal scintigraphy or selective renin measurements, ACE inhibitors

may improve diagnosis of renal artery stenosis.
- ACE inhibitors may significantly decrease renal perfusion and function and should not be used in cases of known or suspected bilateral renal artery stenosis.
- Thrombolytic therapy with urokinase should be considered in rare instances of bilateral renal artery thrombosis.

DEFINITIVE CORRECTION

- PTA dilatation of the stenosis, using an intravascular balloon catheter during arteriography, is the treatment of choice. This therapy is very effective in FMD but less effective in the proximal stenosis associated with NF. Stent implantation is occasionally used as an adjunct to angioplasty.
- Surgery is indicated in cases in which PTA is not possible or successful. Autotransplantation and patch grafting may be effective, especially in children with bilateral renal artery and aortic narrowing.

DURATION

- Effective medical therapy should be monitored closely and continued until the renal artery stenosis can be corrected. The need for progressively higher doses and/or additional medications is common.
- Medication is generally discontinued prior to the angioplasty and used postprocedure only if the blood pressure remains elevated.

Follow-Up

- If effective, response to antihypertensive therapy with ACE inhibitors should occur within 1 to 2 weeks. The dose should be titrated upward until a favorable blood pressure change is achieved, side-effects occur or until a maximum recommended dose is reached. At that point, a second drug should be begun.
- Response to dilation of the renal artery stenosis is often immediate, although transient vessel spasm may occur postprocedure and temporarily be associated with hypertension significant enough to require treatment.

PITFALLS

- Excessive investigation for renal artery stenosis or other secondary causes of hypertension in the majority of children identified with elevated blood pressure
- Failure to proceed rapidly to an arteriogram in a child appropriately suspected of having renal artery stenosis

ICD-9-CM 440.1

BIBLIOGRAPHY

Airoldi F, Palatresi S, Marana I, et al. Angioplasty of atherosclerotic and fibromuscular renal artery stenosis: time course and predicting factors of the effects on renal function. *Am J Hypertens* 2000;13(11):1210–1217.

Baxter BM. Ultrasound of renal transplantation. *Clin Radiol* 2001;56:802–818.

Deal JE, Snell ME, Barratt TM, et al. Renovascular disease in childhood. *J Pediatr* 1992;121:378–384.

Ellis D, Shapiro R, Scantlebury VP, et al. Evaluation and management of bilateral renal artery stenosis in children: a case series and review. *Pediatr Nephrol* 1995;9:259.

Fossali E, Signorini E, Intermite RC, et al. Renovascular disease and hypertension in children with neurofibromatosis. *Pediatr Nephrol* 2000;14(8–9):806–810.

Guzzetta PC, Davis CF, Ruley EJ. Experience with bilateral renal artery stenosis as a cause of hypertension in childhood. *J Pediatr Surg* 1991;26:532.

Leung DA, Hagspiel KD, Angle JF, et al. MR angiography of the renal arteries. *Radiol Clin North Am* 2002;40:847–865.

Lillehei CW, Shamberger RC. Staged reconstruction for middle aortic syndrome. *J Pediatr Surg* 2001;36(8):1252–1254.

Ng CS, de Bruyn R, Gordon I. The investigation of renovascular hypertension in children: the accuracy of radio-isotopes in detecting renovascular disease. *Nucl Med Commun* 1997;18:1017–1028.

Shahdadpuri J, Frank R, Gauthier BG, et al. Yield of renal arteriography in the evaluation of pediatric hypertension. *Pediatr Nephrol* 2000;14:816–819.

Tyagi S, Kaul UA, Satsangi DK, et al. Percutaneous transluminal angioplasty for renovascular hypertension in children: initial and long-term results. *Pediatrics* 1997;99:44–49.

Vade A, Agrawal R, Lim-Dunham J, et al. Utility of computer tomographic renal angiogram in the management of childhood hypertension. *Pediatr Nephrol* 2002;17:741–747.

Author: Thomas L. Kennedy III

Renal Failure—Acute

 Database

DEFINITION

Acute renal failure is a rapidly progressive, and potentially reversible, cessation of renal function that results in the inability of the kidney to control body homeostasis. It manifests in retention of nitrogenous waste products and fluid and electrolyte imbalances.

- Oliguria: urine output less than 0.5 mL/kg per hour in infants or less than 500 mL/1.73 m^2 per day in older children
- Anuria: total cessation of urinary output

PATHOPHYSIOLOGY

Acute renal failure has many causes, which can be categorized into three subgroups.

- Prerenal

—Decreased perfusion of the kidney secondary either to decreased extracellular volume or diminished cardiac output
—It is the most common form of acute renal failure in children.

- Postrenal

—An obstructive process (either structural or functional)
—The obstruction can reside in the lower tract or bilaterally in the upper tracts unless the patient has a single kidney.
—This form of renal failure is more common in newborns.

- Intrinsic disorders that directly affect the kidney. This form can be subcategorized:

—Acute tubular necrosis is the most common form of intrinsic renal failure and usually follows hypoxic or nephrotoxic injury.
—Glomerular disorders include the various forms of acute glomerulonephritis (AGN) such as postinfectious AGN and rapidly progressive (crescentic) AGN.
—Vascular lesions compromise glomerular blood flow. Hemolytic-uremic syndrome is the most common disease that causes intrinsic acute renal failure in children.
—Interstitial nephritis can be idiopathic or caused by reactions to drugs or infections.
—Acute renal failure is commonly precipitated by an ischemic or nephrotoxic event. Initial vasodilatation is followed by intense vasoconstriction, with blood redistributed from the cortex to the juxtamedullary nephrons. The delivery of oxygen to the kidney is impaired, leading to acute tubular necrosis. Intratubular debris and cast formation develop. Tubular fluid leaks backward across the injured tubular membrane, which, in addition to tubular obstruction, causes further hemodynamic changes.

EPIDEMIOLOGY

Acute renal failure secondary to acute tubular necrosis is commonly seen in the hospitalized patient. The combination of ischemia plus nephrotoxic agents such as aminoglycosides, amphotericin B, contrast, or chemotherapeutic agents place these individuals at increased risk.

COMPLICATIONS

- Fluid overload, resulting in congestive heart failure and hypertension
- Hyperkalemia, affecting cardiac function by causing arrhythmias
- Uremia, manifest by mental status changes, increased risk of bleeding, and infection
- Metabolic acidosis
- Hypocalcemia, causing tetany

PROGNOSIS

- Generally, patients with nonoliguric renal failure have a lower mortality rate than patients with oliguria or anuria.
- The mortality rate increases in patients with multisystem organ failure, despite good supportive care

 Differential Diagnosis

- Chronic renal failure: insidious, associated with poor growth, polyuria, and anemia
- Azotemia: caused by corticosteroid therapy, upper gastrointestinal bleeding, hypercatabolic state
- Elevated creatinine: caused by rhabdomyolysis, drugs (trimethoprim-sulfa, cimetidine)

 Data Gathering

Key: POST, obstruction; PRE, prerenal; ATN, acute tubular necrosis; AIN, acute interstitial nephritis; AGN, acute glomerulonephritis; HUS, hemolytic-uremic syndrome

HISTORY

- Symptoms: fever, rash (AIN, AGN), bloody diarrhea, pallor (HUS), severe vomiting or diarrhea (PRE), abdominal pain (POST), hemorrhage, shock (ATN), anuria (AGN, POST), polyuria (ATN, AIN)
- Medical history: previous infection (AGN), neurogenic bladder, single kidney (POST)
- Medications: exposure to various medications such as nonsteroidal antiinflammatory agents, beta lactam antibiotics, acyclovir (AIN), nephrotoxic drugs such as aminoglycosides, amphotericin B, cisplatinum (ATN)
- Toxins: exposure to heavy metals, organic solvents (ATN)
- Family: history of HUS
- Trauma: crush injury (ATN)
- Review of symptoms: various systemic symptoms (AGN)

 Physical Examination

- General: dehydration, shock (PRE, ATN), edema (AGN), jaundice (HUS, ATN)
- Eyes: uveitis (AIN)
- Lungs: rales (AGN)
- Heart: gallop (AGN)
- Abdomen/pelvis: mass (POST)
- Skin: rash (AIN, AGN), petechia (HUS)
- Joints: arthritis (AGN)

Laboratory Aids

TESTS

• Urinalysis: normal sediment or eumorphic RBCs, crystalluria (POST), eosinophiluria, pyuria (AIN), granular casts (PRE, ATN), pigmenturia (ATN), RBC casts, proteinuria (HUS, AGN), U_{osm} less than 350 mOsm (POST, AIN, ATN), U_{osm} greater than 500 mOsm (PRE, AGN, HUS)
• Serum chemistries: hyponatremia, hyperchloremic acidosis (POST), hyperkalemia (POST, AGN, HUS), BUN: Cr greater than 20 (PRE)
• CBC: microangiopathic hemolytic anemia, thrombocytopenia (HUS), eosinophilia (AIN)
• Serologies: hypocomplementemia (AGN), antineutrophil cytoplasmic antibodies (AGN), antinuclear antibodies (AGN)
• Renal ultrasound: hydronephrosis, trabeculated bladder (POST), increased echogenicity (ATN, AIN, AGN, HUS)
• Renal biopsy: indicated in patients with prolonged, unexplained acute renal failure

SPECIAL LABORATORY TRICKS

The fractional excretion of sodium (FENa) is a useful urinary index that determines tubular function.

• $FE_{Na} = ([U_{Na}/P_{Na}]/[U_{creat}/P_{creat}]) \times 100$
• The FE_{Na} should not be obtained after diuretics are administered.
• FE_{Na} greater than 2 (AIN, ATN), FE_{Na} less than 1 (HUS, AGN, PRE)

Emergency Care

• If severe hyperkalemia is present, consider

—Calcium gluconate (0.5 to 1.0 mL/kg IV) over 5 to 10 minutes if severe
—Glucose (0.5 g/kg) and insulin (0.1 U/kg) IV over 30 minutes
—Sodium bicarbonate (1 to 2 mEq/kg) IV over 10 to 30 minutes if acidotic
—Kayexolate (1 g/kg) PO or PR in sorbitol
—Furosemide (1 to 2 mg/kg) if renal function is adequate.
—Hemodialysis or peritoneal dialysis

Therapy

Therapy is preventive, supportive, or specific.

PREVENTIVE

The use of mannitol or furosemide to prevent acute renal failure is controversial. They may be used prophylactically (amphotericin B, cisplatinum, contrast) or in cases of hemoglobinuria or myoglobinuria to augment urine flow. Some feel this may convert oliguric renal failure to nonoliguric renal failure.

SUPPORTIVE

• Establish an effective circulatory volume. If the patient is in shock, administer fluids (normal saline, lactated Ringer's) liberally, even if there is no urine output.
• Maintain a normal intravascular volume. Carefully monitor urine output and provide appropriate fluids accordingly. Consider fluid restriction and diuretics if the patient is volume overloaded.
• Monitor serum potassium levels frequently. Avoid potassium-containing drugs, fluids, or foods in patients with oligo/anuria.
• Hyponatremia is usually secondary to free water excess and should be managed with fluid restriction. Hypertonic saline should be used if only CNS symptoms are present.
• Hypocalcemia, if mild, may be treated by phosphate restriction. Severe hypocalcemia requires treatment with calcium gluconate (100 mg/kg) given slowly. Severe acidosis (pH <7.2) requires supplementation with bicarbonate. However, this may cause hypernatremia, fluid overload, and symptomatic hypocalcemia.
• The effect of aggressive nutritional support is controversial, with the exception of use for a significantly malnourished or hypercatabolic child.
• Hypertension should be treated aggressively if encephalopathy is present.
• Dialysis or hemofiltration are indicated for refractory acidosis, severe hyperkalemia, volume overload, and uremic symptoms (pericarditis, lethargy), or for the removal of toxins (uric acid, salicylate).

SPECIFIC

Each cause of renal failure may have a specific treatment, such as fluid resuscitation (PRE), urologic intervention (POST), and corticosteroids (AIN, some forms of AGN).

Follow-Up

Patients usually remain hospitalized until their renal function improves. Long-term follow-up to monitor sequelae is indicated in patients with prolonged anuria.

PITFALLS

The excretion of many medications is influenced by acute renal failure. Careful attention to drug dosing and levels can minimize toxicity.
A significant postobstructive diuresis can be seen after treatment for obstructive acute renal failure.

Common Questions and Answers

Q: What is the expected recovery time in patients with acute renal failure who present with anuria?
A: Recovery time depends on the etiology of the acute renal failure. Children with HUS may recover in days to weeks. Others with ATN recover days after treatment of the inciting cause. Finally, children with an obstructive etiology usually recover as soon as the obstruction is relieved.

Q: When should renal function return to normal values?
A: Renal function may not return to normal in patients with prolonged periods of anuria. In other cases, once recovery starts, a normal serum creatinine is seen within weeks.

Q: What indices should be followed after a patient recovers from acute renal failure?
A: Patients recovering from acute renal failure should have blood pressures and urinalysis for proteinuria monitored regularly. Serum creatinine should be checked if the course of acute renal failure was prolonged.

ICD-9-CM 584.0

BIBLIOGRAPHY

Andreoli, SP. Acute renal failure. *Curr Opin Pediatr* 2002;14:183–188.

Flynn, JT. Causes, management approaches, and outcome of acute renal failure in children. *Curr Opin Pediatr* 1998;10:184–189.

Malinoski DJ, Slater MS, Mullins RJ. Crush injury and rhabdomyolysis. *Crit Care Clin* 2004;20(1):171–192.

Sehic A, Chesney RW. Acute renal failure: diagnosis. *Pediatr Rev* 1995;16:101–106.

Sehic A, Chesney RW. Acute renal failure: therapy. *Pediatr Rev* 1995;16:137–141.

Singri N, Ahya SN, Levin ML. Acute renal failure. *JAMA* 2003;289(6):747–51.

Thadhani R, Pascual M, Bonventre JV. Acute renal failure. *N Engl J Med* 1996;334: 1448–1460.

Author: Seth L. Schulman

Renal Failure—Chronic

 Database

DEFINITION

- Chronic renal failure is a reduction in the glomerular filtration rate to <25% of normal for at least 3 months' duration.
- Chronic renal insufficiency describes a reduction in the glomerular filtration rate between 25% to 50%.

PATHOPHYSIOLOGY

- Infants younger than 2 years of age usually develop chronic renal failure secondary to either obstructive uropathy or renal hypodysplasia.
- Children 2 to 5 years of age develop chronic renal failure secondary to neonatal vascular accidents and hemolytic uremic syndrome, obstructive uropathy, or renal hypodysplasia.
- More common etiologies of chronic renal failure in older children and adolescents include glomerulonephritis (focal segmental glomeruli-sclerosis, crescentic glomerulonephritis, lupus nephritis), reflux nephropathy, or hereditary causes such as Alport syndrome.

GENETICS

Several hereditary diseases can cause chronic renal failure, including:

- Alport disease (partially X-linked dominant)
- Polycystic kidney disease (autosomal recessive or dominant)
- Familial juvenile nephronophthisis (autosomal recessive)
- Cystinosis (autosomal recessive)
- Hyperoxaluria (autosomal recessive)
- Congenital nephrotic syndrome (autosomal recessive)
- Nail patella syndrome (autosomal dominant)
- Sickle cell disease (autosomal recessive)

EPIDEMIOLOGY

- The incidence of chronic renal failure is not known.
- Approximately three to eight new cases of end-stage renal failure are reported per 1 million children per year
- Prevalence of chronic renal failure has been reported to be 32.4 per 1 million children in Western Europe, with 6% younger than 3 years of age, 30% between 3 and 9 years of age, and 64% between 9 and 15 years of age.
- Among children in the United States with chronic renal insufficiency entered into the North American Pediatric Renal Transplant Cooperative Study, 65.9% are male and 63.9% are white.

COMPLICATIONS

- Growth retardation is particularly severe when chronic renal failure develops in the first year of life. The etiology of growth failure may be secondary to poor nutrition, bone disease, acidosis, or a direct effect on the growth hormone-IGF-1 axis.
- Renal osteodystrophy may be seen early in chronic renal insufficiency and manifest as growth failure, bowing of the lower extremities, and slipped epiphysis. Vitamin D deficiency and secondary hyperparathyroidism are the major factors leading to bone disease.
- Anemia develops secondary to decreased erythropoietin secretion and decreased red cell survival. The anemia is normocytic associated with a low reticulocyte count.
- Neurodevelopmental delay is increased in children with chronic renal failure. This is probably secondary to uremic effects on the developing brain.
- Hypertension may be seen in some patients with chronic renal failure secondary either to hyperreninemia or hypervolemia.
- Platelet abnormalities, protein-calorie malnutrition, and immunologic disturbances are also seen in uremic patients.

PROGNOSIS

- Depends on underlying cause, child's age, degree of renal insufficiency, and need for dialysis or transplantation

 Differential Diagnosis

- Differentiate acute from chronic renal failure.
- Usually chronic renal failure is insidious and associated with poor growth, polyuria, and anemia. The kidneys may be small on renal ultrasound. A renal biopsy may be indicated to determine the cause of renal failure if genetic causes are suspected (for counseling) or if treatment is being considered.

 Data Gathering

HISTORY

Question: Symptoms?
Significance:

- Malaise
- Poor appetite
- Vomiting
- Bone pain
- Headache (if hypertensive)
- Polyuria

Question: Past history?
Significance:

- Perinatal complications
- Oligohydramnios
- Recurrent urinary tract infections
- Enuresis

Question: Familial history?
Significance:

- Renal disease
- Hearing impairment

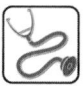 Physical Examination

Finding: General
Significance:

- Short stature
- Poor weight gain
- Pale
- Fetid breath

Finding: HEENT
Significance:

- Retinal changes
- Preauricular pits
- Hearing deficit

Finding: Chest
Significance: Rales

Finding: Heart
Significance:

- Flow murmur
- Gallop
- Rub

Finding: Abdomen
Significance:

- Palpable kidneys
- Suprapubic mass

Finding: Extremities
Significance:

- Rachitic changes
- Edema
- Absent patella

Finding: Neurological
Significance:

- Developmental delay
- Altered mental status
- Hypotonia
- Irritability

Laboratory Aids

Test: Serum chemistries
Significance: Azotemia, hyperkalemia (if advanced), acidemia, hypocalcemia, hyperphosphatemia, elevated alkaline phosphatase

Test: CBC
Significance: Normocytic anemia with low reticulocyte count

Test: Urinalysis
Significance: Isosthenuria, mild proteinuria

Test: Intact parathyroid hormone
Significance: Elevated

Test: Chest radiograph
Significance: Pulmonary edema, cardiomegaly

Test: Bone films
Significance: Delayed bone age, rickets, osteomalacia, osteitis fibrosa

Test: Renal ultrasound
Significance: Small echogenic kidneys, cystic kidneys, hydronephrosis

Test: ECG (if hyperkalemic)
Significance: Peaked T waves

SPECIAL LABORATORY TRICKS

Test: 24-hour urine collection (= 1440 minutes)
Significance: The glomerular filtration rate can be estimated with concomitant blood sampling by calculating the creatinine clearance:

- Ucreat $\times$ (volume voided/1440)/Pcreat $\times$ 1.73/B.S.A.
- The resultant value is expressed as mL/min per 1.73 m^2. Normal range is 80 to 120 mL/min per 1.73 m^2.
- B.S.A. = body surface area.
- A simpler calculation that is already corrected for surface area and does not require a urine collection:
- Height (cm) $\times$ 0.55/Pcreat

The correction factor (0.55) is applicable to most children 1 year of age. A lower factor (0.45) is suggested for infants $<$ 1 year of age and a higher one (0.7) for adolescent males. Plotting the reciprocal of the serum creatinine versus time can approximate the rate of decline of renal function.
This may be useful in determining when renal replacement therapy will be necessary.

 Therapy

MEDICATIONS

- Phosphate binders (calcium carbonate, calcium acetate, sevelamer; avoid aluminum if possible).
- 1,25 dihydroxy vitamin D
- Alkali therapy (sodium bicarbonate/citrate)
- Diuretic therapy
- Recombinant erythropoietin
- Recombinant human growth hormone

DIETARY RESTRICTIONS

- Protein
- Phosphate
- Potassium
- Sodium (indicated if edematous)
- Fluid (indicated in oliguric conditions)

RENAL REPLACEMENT THERAPY

- Dialysis: Indications similar to those for acute renal failure or when glomerular filtration rate $<$ 10 mL/min per 1.73 m^2 and patient is experiencing fatigue, poor school performance, or weight loss secondary to severe dietary restrictions.
- Transplantation: In some cases a preemptive transplant may be offered in lieu of dialysis.

 Follow-Up

General pediatricians should follow patients with chronic renal failure with assistance from a pediatric nephrologist.

PITFALLS

During episodes of gastroenteritis, infants with chronic renal failure may be prone to dehydration because they have obligatory polyuria secondary to a concentrating defect. Do not use urine output or specific gravity as indices for hydration. If hospitalized, "maintenance" fluids may be insufficient as a result of the polyuria.

 Common Questions and Answers

Q: What over-the-counter medications should be avoided in children with chronic renal failure?
A: Nonsteroidal anti-inflammatory drugs, pseudoephedrine (if hypertensive), phosphate containing enemas and magnesium or aluminum-containing antacids should not be taken.

Q: Can children with chronic renal failure receive immunizations?
A: Children with chronic renal failure should receive all necessary immunizations especially since after transplantation some vaccines are contraindicated. In some cases booster immunizations are necessary because of an inadequate response to the initial series (e.g., hepatitis B, MMR, varicella).

Q: When is recombinant human erythropoietin indicated?
A: Generally this medication should be considered when the hematocrit is $<$33%.

ICD-9-CM 585.0

BIBLIOGRAPHY

Benfield MR, McDonald R, Sullivan EK, Stablein DM, Tejani A. The 1997 annual renal transplantation in children report of the North American Pediatric Renal Transplant Cooperative Study (NAPRTCS). *Pediatric Transplant* 1999;3:152–167.

Dabbagh S. Renal osteodystrophy. *Curr Opin Pediatr* 1998;10:190–196.

Friedman AL. Etiology, pathophysiology, diagnosis, and management of chronic renal failure in children. *Curr Opin Pediatr* 1996;8: 148–151.

Seidman A, Freidman A, Boineau F. Nutritional management of the child with mild to moderate chronic renal failure. *J Pediatr* 1996;129:13–18.

Author: Seth L. Schulman

Renal Tubular Acidosis

 Database

DEFINITION

• Renal tubular acidosis (RTA) is a clinical syndrome of disordered renal acidification in which the kidney fails to maintain a normal plasma concentration of bicarbonate in the setting of a normal rate of acid production from diet and metabolism.
• This syndrome is characterized by a hyperchloremic metabolic acidosis, bicarbonaturia, decreased production of titratable acids and ammonium with, usually, an elevated urinary pH.

TYPES

• Distal (Type I)

—Distal RTA is a primary renal acidification defect secondary either to an inability to secrete hydrogen ions or a backleak in the collecting tubule. In some cases there may be bicarbonate wasting as well.
—These infants and children present with failure to thrive, hypokalemia, nephrolithiasis, nephrocalcinosis, or rickets. The nephrolithiasis is secondary to the persistent alkaline urine, hypercalciuria, and hypocitraturia.
—Patients with complete distal RTA can never acidify their urine and, therefore, always have a urine pH higher than 6.0.

• Proximal (Type II)

—This form of RTA is caused by a defect in the sodium-hydrogen ion exchange mechanism. These infants and children spill bicarbonate into their urine because the renal threshold for reabsorption is reduced. Because the distal mechanism is intact, acidification of the urine is possible once the serum bicarbonate falls below the threshold.
—Isolated proximal RTA is rare; most children present with this abnormality as part of the Fanconi syndrome (bicarbonaturia, amino aciduria, glycosuria, and phosphaturia).
—Hypokalemia is usually present but hypercalciuria and hypocitraturia are not. Therefore, nephrocalcinosis, nephrolithiasis, and rickets are not the presenting features of this form of RTA.

• Distal Hyperkalemic (Type IV)

—Type IV RTA is the most common form of RTA in adults and children.
—Hyperkalemia distinguishes this form from types I and II.
—There are five subtypes of type IV RTA but the predominant feature is aldosterone deficiency or unresponsiveness.
—One form in children occurs with obstructive uropathy and renal insufficiency. This causes a defect in the juxtaglomerular apparatus leading to hyporeninemia with secondary hypoaldosteronism. Children with this form of RTA may present with failure to thrive.

GENETICS

• In infants and children type I RTA is usually inherited as an autosomal dominant trait. It may occur in association with other diseases such as elliptocytosis, sickle-cell disease, and the Ehlers-Danlos syndrome.
• Type II RTA with Fanconi syndrome occurs with several disorders that are autosomal recessive, including cystinosis, Löwe's syndrome, Wilson disease, tyrosinemia, hereditary fructose intolerance, and galactosemia.
• Certain subtypes of type IV RTA have been reported to be familial.

EPIDEMIOLOGY

Renal tubular acidosis is an extremely rare condition.

COMPLICATIONS

• Children with RTA may develop severe growth failure, rickets, nephrocalcinosis, and nephrolithiasis.

—During episodes of vomiting or diarrhea they may be at risk of developing profound acidosis and hypokalemia.

PROGNOSIS

• Prognosis depends on the underlying etiology.
• Growth velocity increases following treatment with alkali for isolated type I and II RTA and normal stature can be achieved.
• Isolated type I RTA is a chronic condition that requires constant monitoring to avoid nephrocalcinosis.

 Differential Diagnosis

• Renal tubular acidosis is associated with a normal anion gap ($Na^+ - [Cl^- + HCO_3^-] =$ 8 to 16 mEq/L).
• Other causes of metabolic acidosis with a normal anion gap include diarrhea, acetazolamide, ileal conduits, and fistulas draining the small bowel, pancreas, or biliary tree.

 Data Gathering

HISTORY

Question: Symptoms?
Significance: Failure to thrive, renal colic, bone pain, photophobia (cystinosis)

Question: Past medical history?
Significance: Prior admissions for dehydration and acidosis not associated with significant diarrhea.

Question: Medications/drugs
Significance: Amphotericin B, lithium, tetracycline (outdated), toluene.

Question: Familial history
Significance: See Genetics.

Question: Review of symptoms
Significance: Other systemic diseases

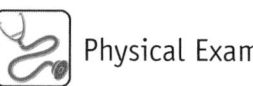 Physical Examination

Finding: General
Significance: Failure to thrive

Finding: Head
Significance: Frontal bossing

Finding: Eyes
Significance:

• Cystine deposition
• Kayser-Fleischer ring
• Cataracts

Finding: Chest
Significance: Rachitic rosary

Finding: Abdomen
Significance:

• Hepatosplenomegaly
• Enlarged kidneys

Finding: Extremities
Significance:

• Bowing
• Widening of the epiphysis of wrists

Laboratory Aids

Test: Serum electrolytes
Significance: Identify the presence of a normal anion gap metabolic acidosis, hyperkaluria/hypokalemia.

Test: Urinalysis
Significance: Exclude features of the Fanconi syndrome.

Test: Urine pH
Significance: Can exclude type I RTA if, <6.0; best if performed in the face of acidosis. Best if determined with a pH probe as quickly as possible after collection

Test: Serum creatinine
Significance: To exclude renal insufficiency

Test: Urine anion gap
Significance:

- Negative ($Cl^- > Na^+ + K^+$) seen in gastrointestinal losses, proximal RTA
- Positive ($Cl^- < Na^+ + K^+$) seen in distal RTA

Test: Urine
Significance: Should be measured by pH meter from a fresh specimen. If this is not possible oil should be added to cover urine and protect dissipation of CO_2.

IMAGING

Test: Abdominal flat plate
Significance: Nephrocalcinosis, nephrolithiasis

Test: Bone films
Significance: Rachitic changes, delayed bone age

 ## Therapy

- Alkali administration is the primary therapy for children with RTA.
- Sodium/potassium citrate (Polycitra 2 mEq HCO_3-/mL) is preferable for children with types I or II RTA.
- Sodium citrate (Bicitra 1 mEq HCO_3-/mL) is used in infants with type IV RTA.
- Older children can take sodium bicarbonate tablets (7.7 mEq HCO_3-)
- Patients with type I RTA require 1 to 4 mEq/kg of alkali therapy per day in 3 to 4 divided doses. This usually decreases the chances of complications such as nephrolithiasis, nephrocalcinosis, and rickets.
- Patients with type II RTA require considerably more alkali therapy (5 to 20 mEq/kg per day in 4 to 6 divided doses).
- The dosage of alkali in children with type IV RTA ranges from 1 to 5 mEq/kg per day, which is usually sufficient to correct the hyperkalemia.

 ## Follow-Up

- Patients with RTA should be closely monitored with frequent serum potassium and plasma bicarbonate levels until a steady state is reached.
- Normal growth may be attained once the metabolic acidosis is corrected.

PITFALLS AND PREVENTION

- Avoid hemolyzed specimens that may artificially increase the serum potassium and reduce the plasma bicarbonate levels.
- Administer alkali over several divided doses.
- Closely monitor patients during episodes of gastroenteritis to avoid dehydration and severe metabolic acidosis.

 ## Common Questions and Answers

Q: Do children outgrow renal tubular acidosis?
A: Types I and II RTA are chronic disorders that require life-long treatment. Some children outgrow certain subtypes of type IV RTA.

Q: Can children with renal tubular acidosis develop renal failure?
A: Untreated type I RTA can lead to renal failure by causing progressive nephrocalcinosis. Children with inherited disorders associated with Fanconi syndrome such as cystinosis can also develop renal insufficiency.

ICD-9-CM 588.8

BIBLIOGRAPHY

Battle DC, Hizon M, Cohen E, et al. The use of the urinary anion gap in the diagnosis of hyperchloremic metabolic acidosis. *N Engl J Med* 1988;318:594.

Gregory MJ, Schwartz GJ. Diagnosis and treatment of renal tubular disorders. *Semin Nephrol.* 1998;18:317–329.

McSherry E. Renal tubular acidosis in children (nephrology forum). *Kidney Int* 1981;20:799.

Rodriguez Soriano J. Renal tubular acidosis: the clinical entity. *J Am Soc Nephrol* 2002;13(8):2160–2170.

Rodriguez-Soriano J. New insights into the pathogenesis of renal tubular acidosis—from functional to molecular studies. *Pediatr Nephrol* 2000;14:1121–1136.

Roth KS, Chan JC. Renal tubular acidosis: a new look at an old problem. *Clin Pediatr (Phila)* 2001;40:533–543.

Author: Seth L. Schulman

Renal Venous Thrombosis

 Database

DEFINITION

• Renal venous thrombosis (RVT) is the thrombotic process that begins in the intrarenal venous radicals and usually progresses forward toward the main renal vein.
• Rarely, the thrombosis progresses in the opposite direction.

PATHOPHYSIOLOGY

• RVT in newborns and infants is commonly associated with asphyxia, dehydration (as with diarrhea), shock, sepsis, hypertonicity, and hemoconcentration.
• Additional predisposing factors in the newborn include congenital renal anomalies and maternal diabetes.
• In older children it is associated with the nephrotic syndrome, cyanotic heart disease, and hyperosmolar states such as with the use of angiography contrast agents.
• In many children, no underlying cause is apparent.
• The slow double circulation of the kidney is especially vulnerable to thrombosis.
• Thrombus formation may be initiated by vascular endothelial cell injury in conjunction with diminished vascular flow.
• RVT usually starts in the small venous radicals with progression through the arcuate and interlobular veins toward the main renal vein.
• RVT causes renal congestion and occasionally infarction.

GENETICS

• Familial occurrence is rare.
• No hereditary factors have been described.

EPIDEMIOLOGY

• RVT is predominantly a disease of the newborn.
• The incidence and prevalence are poorly defined.
• There is a small male preponderance.
• The disease is more frequently unilateral than bilateral.

COMPLICATIONS

• Bilateral RVT may lead to chronic renal failure.
• Scarring may result in hypertension.

 Differential Diagnosis

• The differential diagnosis includes other causes of renal enlargement such as hydronephrosis, cystic renal disease, renal tumors, abscess, and hematoma.
• Hemolytic uremic syndrome should also be considered because RVT may also result in fragmented red blood cells and thrombocytopenia.

PROGNOSIS

• The degree of irreversible renal damage depends on the degree of involvement and associated conditions.
• Recovery of function in affected kidneys may occur.
• Hypertension is seen in 20%.
• The majority have residual renal structural abnormalities, such as atrophy and coarse renal scarring.

 Data Gathering

HISTORY

• The majority present in the newborn period.
• Most of the symptoms are as a result of an underlying disorder.
• RVT is usually heralded by the sudden onset of hematuria and unilateral or bilateral flank masses.

 Physical Examination

• Sixty percent will have a palpably enlarged kidney.
• Associated signs and symptoms include pallor, tachypnea, abdominal distention, shock, flank pain, fever, oliguria, or anuria.
• If in the thrombosis, the lower limbs may become edematous, cyanotic, and hypothermic the inferior vena cava (IVC) is involved.

 Laboratory Aids

• Proteinuria is common.
• The majority have macroscopic hematuria.
• Ninety percent have progressive thrombocytopenia, and the majority also has microangiopathic hemolytic anemia.
• Fibrin split products may be elevated with low-plasma fibrinogen levels.
• Azotemia and other biochemical evidence of acute renal failure may be present.
• Variations in plasma electrolytes depend on the presence of diarrhea or renal failure.

IMAGING

Test: Intravenous urograms
Significance: Almost always contraindicated because of the osmolar load of intravenous contrast material.

Test: Ultrasonography
Significance: The most useful study; it will differentiate between renal enlargement and extrarenal masses. It will also identify obstruction, cystic changes, and many congenital anomalies, and show renal enlargement, increased echogenicity, and loss of corticomedullary differentiation.

Test: Doppler evaluation
Significance: Of renal arterial and renal venous flow, and radioisotopic reperfusion and excretion studies may be helpful.

Therapy

GENERAL

- Treatment is supportive and includes correction of fluid and electrolyte disturbances and treatment of infection.
- Correction of underlying pathophysiologic abnormalities should be attempted.
- Management of the complications of azotemia and uremia, including metabolic acidosis, hyperphosphatemia, fluid overload, and hyperosmolality, may require dialysis, particularly in infants.

ANTICOAGULANT

- The effect of anticoagulant therapy has not been documented in controlled studies and remains controversial.
- Heparin should be considered if there is laboratory evidence of continuing disseminated intravascular coagulation.
- Because the lesions are often asynchronous and asymmetrical, prophylactic heparin has been proposed for cases of RVT that are identified early and do not appear to have bilateral involvement.

SURGERY

- A surgical approach in the acute phase is rarely indicated. Surgery, complicated by disturbed fluid balance and acid-base status and altered coagulation, is risky.
- Because the thrombosis begins deep within the kidney and spreads to the larger veins, thrombectomy should be considered only in the event of bilateral involvement with IVC involvement.
- Ultimately, if the kidney has negligible function and contributes to hypertension or recurrent infections, nephrectomy may be indicated.

 Follow-Up

PROGNOSIS

- Depends on the degree of involvement and associated conditions
- Mortality in infants is approximately 30%.
- Recovery of function in affected kidneys may occur. Varying degrees of renal impairment is seen in 30%.
- Hypertension is seen in 20%.
- The majority have residual renal structural abnormalities, such as atrophy and coarse renal scarring.

SIGNS TO WATCH FOR

All patients should be followed closely for evidence of hypertension.

PREVENTION

Infants at increased risk should be recognized. The infant of a diabetic mother should be followed for evidence of RVT. Patients with nephrotic syndrome are at increased risk of thrombosis in general when treated with diuretics. If cyanotic congenital heart disease is present, contrast agents should be used judiciously. Parents and caregivers should be educated about the importance of adequate intake and good hydration in the newborn and infant. Finally, there should be an increased index of suspicion among medical staff when faced with an infant with diarrhea or a hyperosmolar state.

 Common Questions and Answers

Q: Can RVT occur in the absence of gross hematuria?
A: Most patients have hematuria that may be gross. However, the hematuria is often microscopic or absent.

Q: Do patients with RVT usually have hypertension during the acute phase?
A: Hypertension is uncommon at presentation.

ICD-9-CM 453.3

BIBLIOGRAPHY

Adelman RD. Long-term follow-up of neonatal renovascular hypertension. *Pediatr Nephrol* 1987;1:35.

Arneil GC, MacDonald AM, Murphy AV, et al. Renal venous thrombosis. *Clin Nephrol* 1973;1:119.

Duncan RE, Evans TA, Martin LW. Natural history and treatment of renal vein thrombosis in children. *J Pediatr Surg* 1977;12:639.

Jobin J, O'Regan S, Demay G, et al. Neonatal renal vein thrombosis—long-term follow-up after conservative management. *Clin Nephrol* 1982;17:36.

Kaplan BS, Chesney RW, Drummond KN. The nephrotic syndrome and renal vein thrombosis. *Am J Dis Child* 1978;132:367.

Markowitz GS, Brignol F, Burns ER, et al. Renal vein thrombosis treated with thrombolytic therapy: case report and brief review. *Am J Kidney Dis* 1995;25:801–806.

Mocan H, Beattie TJ, Murphy AV. Renal venous thrombosis in infancy: long term follow-up. *Pediatr Nephrol* 1991;5:45.

Oliver WJ, Kelsch RC. Renal venous thrombosis in infancy. *Pediatr Rev* 1982;4:61.

Schmidt B, Andrew M. Neonatal thrombosis: report of a prospective Canadian and international registry. *Pediatrics* 1995;96:939–943.

Author: Mary B. Leonard

Respiratory Syncytial Virus (RSV)

 Database

DEFINITION

- RSV is a pleomorphic, enveloped RNA virus of the family Paramyxoviridae. There are two major groups, A and B, which differ in the largest surface glycoprotein, the G protein. The fusion protein, F protein, is approximately 95% homologous between the two subgroups.
- It is the most common cause of bronchiolitis, a viral lower respiratory disease of infants and young children.

PATHOPHYSIOLOGY

- The F protein is responsible for fusing infected cells to adjacent cells, generating a syncytium.
- Infection is initiated in the upper respiratory tract with inoculation of the nose or eyes, and may spread to the lower respiratory tract.
- Obstruction of smaller airways occurs secondary to onset of edema, necrotic tissue, and inflammatory cells.
- Virus-induced epithelial damage may expose certain receptors for environmental irritants. Receptor-irritant complexes may contribute to the signs and symptoms of reactive airway disease.

EPIDEMIOLOGY

- Incubation period for RSV is 2 to 4 days.
- Virus is detected in secretions 4 days prior to clinical symptoms and 7 days following the resolution of symptoms (viral shedding demonstrated for as long as 20 days).
- Most effective mode of transmission is via person-to-person spread: by droplet or hand-to-nose contact.
- Nosocomial spread occurs from infected hospital personnel-to-patient spread.
- Peak incidence is the first 2 years of life.
- Fifty percent of children are infected by their first birthday with similar attack rate for the uninfected child during the second year of life.
- Forty percent to 70% of preschool children and 20% of school-age children are reinfected with exposure.
- There is a worldwide distribution. Temperate climates experience an annual, midwinter epidemic, although epidemics are less predictable in the tropics.
- U.S. epidemics may begin in November (or as late as May) and last as long as 12 weeks in urban areas.
- One antigenic strain predominates during any given epidemic.

COMPLICATIONS

- Apneic episodes in very young and premature patients
- Pneumonia, rarely bacterial
- Pneumonitis
- Croup
- Respiratory failure
- Hypoxemia
- Hypercarbia
- Asthma
- Acute otitis media
- Dehydration

Those at greatest risk for severe infection include:

- Age less than 1 year, especially those between the ages of 6 weeks and 6 months
- Children with compromised cardiorespiratory status (e.g., bronchopulmonary dysplasia, congenital heart disease)
- Prematurity
- Immune deficits

PROGNOSIS

- The majority of patients have a mild-to-moderate disease course with symptomatic support. Some infected children proceed to more serious illness, necessitating hospitalization. An average hospital stay for previously healthy children is 5 to 7 days; full recovery is 2 weeks.
- Infants with underlying cardiac or pulmonary disease are at increased risk for more severe and longer duration of disease; mortality as high as 30%.
- Reinfections occur throughout life.

 Differential Diagnosis

INFECTION

- Influenza virus
- Parainfluenza virus type 3
- Adenovirus
- Chlamydia

ENVIRONMENTAL

- Foreign body in airway

TUMORS

- Mass compressing upper airway

CONGENITAL

- Tracheomalacia

 Data Gathering

HISTORY

Question: Initial symptoms?
Significance: Nasal discharge, cough, and fever

Question: Cough?
Significance: Typically progresses over 1 to 2 days, with tachypnea developing

Question: Duration of symptoms?
Significance: This will help in the assessment of the typical clinical progression of illness and the anticipated time course for the child.

Other significant points within the history:

- Lethargy, apnea, and possible cyanotic episodes
- Dehydration is secondary to decreased oral intake as well as increased insensible losses. Assess oral intake and urine output to rule out dehydration.
- Increasing respiratory distress?
- Did the child stop breathing/have apnea?

 Physical Examination

- Nasal discharge
- Otitis media
- Pharyngeal injection
- Conjunctivitis
- Respiratory distress with nasal flaring and retractions, grunting, rales, rhonchi, and expiratory wheezing noted on auscultation.
- Risk for hypoxemia increases as the respiratory rate approaches and surpasses 60 breaths per minute.
- Chest may become barrel-shaped in appearance as respiratory distress increases.
- Hyperinflation of the lungs will push liver and spleen into palpable positions within the abdomen.

 Laboratory Aids

- A definitive diagnosis of RSV can be made by viral isolation
- Three basic techniques are used for RSV detection

—Immunochromatographic assay
—Enzyme immunoassay
—Immunofluorescent assay

- Nasopharyngeal aspirate/washings are specimens of choice for testing
- Pulse oximetry to rule out hypoxemia

RADIOGRAPHIC STUDIES

Test: Chest radiographs are performed with clinical concerns of pneumonia.
Significance: Reveals hyperexpansion, increased bronchial markings, and areas of atelectasis/infiltrate. Note: the pulmonary densities, referred to as "RSV pneumonia," are frequently areas of atelectasis but may represent bacterial infection, especially in the seriously ill patient.

 Emergency Care

Life-threatening apnea may require emergent ventilatory support with mechanical ventilation.

Therapy

- Supportive care: hydration therapy and supplemental oxygen as needed to maintain oxygen saturation greater than 94%.
- Cardiorespiratory monitoring and pulse oximetry are necessary for infants at risk for apnea and hypoxemia. Duration of hospitalization monitoring is dependent on the clinical course.
- Mechanical ventilation as clinically indicated

DRUGS

- Ribavirin: an antiviral agent, has in vitro antiviral activity against RSV but ribavirin aerosol treatment for RSV infections is controversial. The controversy centers on the teratogenicity of ribavirin in humans, its high cost, as well as efficacy trials with conflicting results.
- Studies are ongoing to determine the possible benefit of corticosteroid use.
- β-adrenergic agents have not been proven to be effective, but some studies have shown that 25% to 50% of patients with bronchiolitis respond to this therapy. A trial of a bronchodilator is frequently recommended.
- Mist use is considered controversial because it may irritate the airways.
- Antibiotics are rarely indicated since bacterial disease (lung or blood) is uncommon in hospitalized infants with RSV bronchiolitis.

Follow-Up

- Bronchiolitis will peak in severity over 48 to 72 hours; therefore, reassess the patient if seen early in the disease course.
- Symptoms usually last 7 days but may last up to 2 to 3 weeks with the evidence of reactive airway disease persisting for months to years.
- Periodic breathing may occur 48 to 72 hours postextubation, but recurrent apneic episodes are rare, and home monitoring is usually not indicated.
- Fever commonly resolves over 48 hours.
- Respiratory symptoms commonly improve between days 2 and 5 of illness.
- Evidence of airway hyperactivity may continue for months to years in patients who have had bronchiolitis.

SIGNS TO WATCH FOR

- Increased respiratory rate and increased work of breathing as seen in use of accessory muscles
- Lethargy, altered mental status
- Prolonged high fever

PREVENTION

- Nosocomial and household spread can be minimized by strict hand washing and avoidance of contact with infected individuals.
- Routine use of gowns and gloves has been shown to decrease RSV nosocomial spread.
- Patients with RSV infection should be isolated in private or RSV-cohorted rooms.
- Nursing care should be cohorted so that nurses are not caring for both RSV infected and noninfected patients.
- Two products are available for the prevention of RSV infection: Respiratory Syncytial Virus Immune Globulin Intravenous (RSV-IGIV), made from RSV antibody positive donor serum and Palivizumab, a humanized monoclonal antibody produced by recombinant DNA technology. Both products are approved for the prevention of RSV disease in select children younger than 2 years of age with bronchopulmonary dysplasia or with a history of prematurity (birth at less than 35 weeks' gestation). Specific recommendations are available from the American Academy of Pediatrics Committee on Infectious Diseases and Committee on Fetus and Newborn for the use of Palivizumab and RSV-IGIV and these criteria should guide the use of these products. RSV-IGIV is given 1 month prior to and monthly throughout RSV season, although Palivizumab is given intramuscularly monthly throughout RSV season.

PITFALLS

- RSV is labile at room temperature. Samples should be placed in viral transport media at the bedside and transported to the lab for immediate inoculation to cell culture.
- Instillation and aspiration of 5 mL of isotonic saline is the preferred method of viral collection as opposed to nasal swabs.

Common Questions and Answers

Q: How did my child get this illness?
A: RSV bronchiolitis is caused by respiratory syncytial virus, which is passed from one person to another by contact with nasal secretions and through airborne transmission of droplets.

Q: For how long is my child contagious?
A: Viral shedding occurs for 24 hours prior to the onset of clinical symptoms and for up to 21 days from the onset of symptoms.

Q: Will my child develop asthma because of the wheezing that is occurring now?
A: Evidence of airway hyperactivity following RSV bronchiolitis may continue for months or even years in some children. It is impossible to predict future episodes of reactive airway disease, but the child should be monitored clinically over time.

Q: If a patient has severe chronic lung disease with a supplemental oxygen requirement and is less than 2 years of age at the onset of the RSV season, should RSV-IGIV or Palivizumab be recommended for this patient?
A: The risks and benefits of each therapy must be evaluated on a patient-by-patient basis. RSV-IGIV provides additional protection against other respiratory viral illnesses and may be considered for some selected high-risk infants. However, Palivizumab is preferred for most high-risk children secondary to its ease of administration, safety and effectiveness.

ICD-9-CM 466.1

BIBLIOGRAPHY

American Academy of Pediatrics. Respiratory syncytial virus. In: Pickering LK, ed. *2003 Red Book: Report of the Committee on Infectious Diseases.* 26th Ed. Elk Grove Village, IL: American Academy of Pediatrics; 2003:523–528.

AAP Committee on Infectious Diseases and Committee on Fetus and Newborn. Revised indications for the use of palivizumab and respiratory syncytial virus immune globulin intravenous for the prevention of respiratory syncytial virus infections. *Pediatrics* 2003;112:1442–1446.

Barton LL, Grant KL, Lemen RJ. Respiratory syncytial virus immune globulin: decisions and costs. *Pediatr Pulmon* 2001;32:20–28.

Darville T, Yamauchi T. Respiratory syncytial virus. *Pediatr Rev* 1998;19:55–61.

DeVincenzo JP, Aitken J, Harrison L. Respiratory syncytial virus (RSV) loads in premature infants with and without prophylactic RSV fusion protein monoclonal antibody. *J Pediatr* 2003;143:123–126.

Jacoby DB. Virus-induced asthma attacks. *JAMA* 2002;287:755–761.

McBride JT. Dexamethasone and bronchiolitis: A new look at an old therapy? *J Pediatr* 2002;140:8–9.

Midulla F, Villani A, Panuska Jr, et al. Respiratory syncytial virus lung infection in infants: immunoregulatory role of infected alveolar macrophages. *J Infect Dis* 1993;168:1515–1519.

Purcell K, Fergie J. Concurrent serious bacterial infections in 2396 infants and children hospitalized with respiratory syncytial virus lower respiratory tract infections. *Arch Pediatr Adolesc Med* 2002;156:322–324.

Schuh S, Coates AL, Binnie R, et al. Efficacy of oral dexamethasone in outpatients with acute bronchiolitis. *J Pediatrics* 2002;140:27–32.

Author: Kathleen Wholey Zsolway

Retinoblastoma

 Database

DEFINITION

- The most common primary intraocular tumor of childhood
- Malignant tumor of the embryonic neural retina

PATHOPHYSIOLOGY

- Originates in retinal cell precursor (retinoblast)
- Histology: small round blue cells with large hyperchromatic nuclei and scant cytoplasm
- Growth of tumor may be endophytic (from inner surface of retina to vitreous) or exophytic (from outer layer of retina into subretinal space); may cause retinal detachment.
- Spread is via optic nerve (common) with potential to invade CNS, direct extension beyond the eye, and lymphatic or hematogenous spread (uncommon).
- Tumor cells may break off from primary mass and grow independently within the eye (called vitreous seeding); single tumor with seeding may be confused with multifocal disease.

GENETICS

- Tumor development depends on loss of function of both copies of the RB1 gene (located on chromosome 13) in a retinoblast.
- Hereditary and nonhereditary (sporadic) forms exist.

HEREDITARY RB

- Forty-five percent of all retinoblastoma.
- One RB1 gene is dysfunctional in all cells (germline mutation); mutation in remaining RB1 gene in any retinal cell will lead to development of a tumor.
- Ninety percent probability of second mutation occurring in at least one (but usually more) retinal cells leading to tumor development (high penetrance)
- Therefore, multiple tumors are common (bilateral and/or multifocal).
- Mean age at diagnosis: 12 months
- Only 8% have positive familial history; remainder are new germline mutations.
- Approximately 40% to 45% of offspring will develop RB (autosomal-dominant transmission, 90% penetrance).
- RB1 gene mutation in all cells predisposes to second (nonretinoblastoma) malignancies as well.

NONHEREDITARY RB

- Fifty-five percent of all retinoblastoma
- No germline RB1 mutation; two acquired (somatic) RB1 mutations must occur in a single retinal cell (a rare event).
- Always unilateral
- Rarely diagnosed before 6 months (mean, 24 months)
- No increased risk of RB in offspring
- No increased risk of second malignancy

EPIDEMIOLOGY

- 1:16,000 to 1:25,000 live births
- The most common primary intraocular tumor of childhood (ocular leukemia most common overall)
- Represents 3% of all pediatric malignancies
- No sex, race, geographic, or socioeconomic predilection
- Ninety percent diagnosed before age 4 years
- Median age at diagnosis for unilateral disease is 24 months and 12 months for bilateral disease (see Genetics, above)

COMPLICATIONS

- Metastatic spread: local spread within orbit, through the optic nerve to brain, or to distant sites (uncommon)
- Loss of eye: surgical enucleation in advanced cases
- Blindness: in advanced, bilateral disease; bilateral enucleation rarely required
- Cosmetic deformity: from enucleation, ocular prosthesis lacks normal eye movements; potential orbital bone hypoplasia secondary to external beam radiation therapy
- Second malignancy: patients with hereditary RB have a predisposition to cancer; this risk is greatly increased by exposure to radiotherapy.

PROGNOSIS

- Mortality from retinoblastoma is 8% (United States)
- Survival depends on extent (stage) of disease
- Metastatic disease is uncommon in the United States but can occur up to 5 years after diagnosis and has a poor outcome (same for hereditary and nonhereditary).
- Prognosis for vision depends on size and location of tumor(s)
- Second malignancy is most common cause of death in hereditary RB

—These include osteosarcoma (most frequent), pineal blastoma, melanoma, fibrosarcoma, and others.
—Rates of second malignancy in hereditary RB are 10% at 10 years and as high as 40% at 30 years in patients who received XRT (70% of second tumors occur in the field of radiation, 30% elsewhere).

 Differential Diagnosis

- Coats disease: acquired anomaly, males, retinal telangiectasias
- Persistent hyperplastic primary vitreous (PHPV)
- Inflammatory conditions: hypopyon, uveitis, iritis, endophthalmitis
- Toxoplasmosis, *Toxocara canis*, other ocular infections
- Retinopathy of prematurity (ROP)

 Data Gathering

HISTORY

Question: Familial history of retinoblastoma or any eye tumors?
Significance: Hereditary retinoblastoma; siblings may require eye exam

Question: Leukocoria (white pupil, "cat's eye reflex")?
Significance: Often noted in photographs of children with advanced intraocular RB (60%)

Question: Strabismus, either esotropic or exotropic (20%)?
Significance: Esotropia is more common in the general population, so exotropia is more suspicious.

Question: Eye complaints?
Significance: RB is rarely painful (unless secondary glaucoma or inflammation is present); vision problems are rare complaints because tumor is usually unilateral.

Question: Inflammation, heterochromia, and glaucoma?
Significance: Rare presentations (<10%)

Question: Neurologic signs, orbital/periorbital masses, bone pain, anorexia, signs of cytopenias?
Significance: May represent metastatic disease

Question: Associated conditions?
Significance: 13q deletion syndrome has RB, dysmorphism, mental retardation, and GU or other anomalies.

 Physical Examination

- Only 3% diagnosed with routine funduscopic examination. Leukocoria more common as presenting sign.

Finding: Proptosis and orbital/periorbital masses
Significance: Late sequelae of mass effect

Finding: Check for red reflex in darkened room.
Significance: Screen for RB in office.

- Evaluate for anisocoria.
- Cover test to assess for strabismus (20%)
- Test vision of each eye independently to identify unilateral RB.

Laboratory Aids

Test: Ophthalmologic examination
Significance: Confirmation of diagnosis based on ophthalmologic examination by a specialist in pediatric ocular tumors via direct and indirect ophthalmoscopy (and examination under anesthesia, EUA) and by imaging modalities (MRI or CT). Parents and siblings should also undergo ophthalmologic screening in many cases.

Test: Biopsy
Significance: Biopsy confirmation is rarely necessary.

Test: CBC
Significance: Assess for bone marrow involvement

Test: CSF cytology
Significance: Evaluate for leptomeningeal spread (only necessary if tumor has spread beyond the globe).

Test: Chromosome analysis
Significance: Should be performed, but even in hereditary cases only 5% have mutations detectable by this means.

IMAGING

Test: CT or MRI
Significance: Evaluate primary tumor (80% have calcification) and optic nerve extension, leptomeningeal spread, pineal blastoma (in 4% of patients with hereditary RB = "trilateral RB").

STAGING

- Intraocular and extraocular staging systems exist.
- Most RB in the United States is intraocular without metastatic disease.
- Patients with tumor extension outside the globe should have an LP and bone marrow evaluation for complete staging.

 Therapy

- Primary goals

—Eradicate tumor.
—Prevent metastasis.

- Secondary goals

—Salvage the eye and retain useful vision.
—Cosmetic considerations

Treatment must be individualized, depending on bilateral or unilateral disease, potential for salvageable vision, and evidence of local extension or metastatic disease. Referral to a center with oncologic and ophthalmologic specialists is essential.

—Minimal (nonbulky) intraocular disease
—Plaque radiotherapy (sewn to episcleral surface above RB lesion): local XRT to tumor in selected solitary RBs, up to 16 mm in diameter with or without vitreous seeds
—Photocoagulation (laser): for selected small RBs, usually less than 3 mm
—Cryotherapy (topical freeze technique): for selected RBs less than 3 to 4 mm in diameter without vitreous seeding, which are located anteriorly in the eye

- Bulky intraocular disease

—Current trend is toward eye salvage therapy: initial chemotherapy for tumor reduction followed by local definitive therapy (as for nonbulky disease).

—Tumor resection without enucleation is not possible because of risk of tumor spillage; enucleation of involved eye (with long segment of optic nerve removal to ensure tumor-free margins) may be required for large tumors refractory to chemoreduction or when vision is not salvageable.
—External beam radiation therapy (EBRT): RB is extremely radiosensitive; however, increases risk of second malignancy (especially in hereditary RB). Other effects: dry eye, cataract, retinopathy, and cosmetic deformity from bone maldevelopment. EBRT is still an important modality but is avoided whenever effective alternative therapies are available.

- Metastatic disease

—Multiagent chemotherapy with or without autologous bone marrow transplantation; poor results to date
—Effective treatment requires multidisciplinary collaboration between ophthalmologists, oncologists, and radiation oncologists.

 Follow-Up

- Frequent ophthalmologic examinations (including EUA) are mandatory to evaluate response to therapy and to screen for disease progression, particularly in hereditary RB.
- Therapy must include genetic counseling regarding the risk of second malignancies (with or without adjuvant XRT), risk to siblings, as well as the risk to future children of affected patients with hereditary RB.
- Primary care physicians must be aware of the risks of second malignancies (see Prognosis, above) and maintain an appropriately high index of suspicion for their development.
- Primary care physicians should be aware of the genetics of RB and screen siblings appropriately.

PREVENTION

Siblings and children of patients with RB should undergo ophthalmologic examinations under anesthesia to detect the presence of RB early.

PITFALLS

- Missed or delayed diagnosis: ophthalmologic examination by a specialist in pediatric ocular tumors required to establish diagnosis and follow regression or recurrence in treated eyes, follow for development of new tumors in hereditary cases
- Failure to recognize the possibility that a child with RB has a genetic predisposition, especially in the frequent setting in which there is no familial history of RB
- Failure to refer for appropriate genetic counseling

 Common Questions and Answers

Q: What is the risk that a child with RB will become blind?
A: Vision is salvageable in 100% of eyes with low-stage involvement, and in 81% overall. In less than 10% of patients are both eyes affected severely enough to threaten vision (bilateral disease only occurs in hereditary RB).

Q: What is the chance that a child with RB in one eye will get it in the other?
A: Bilateral disease is seen with hereditary RB. A child with unilateral disease has a 15% chance of having hereditary RB, which would put the contralateral eye at risk; this risk is much higher if the child has multifocal involvement or is less than 1 year of age.

Q: What happens to the eye socket after an enucleation?
A: Prostheses can be made to fit the socket of the enucleated eye to give excellent cosmetic results.

Q: Is there a test to identify hereditary cases?
A: Routine chromosome analysis does not reveal the defective RB gene in the majority (95%) of hereditary cases. Specialized molecular tests may be used in research labs, but since there are many possible mutations, this is costly and time-consuming. In general, hereditary cases are determined clinically because of young presentation, family history, and/or bilateral or multifocal unilateral disease.

ICD-9-CM 190.5

BIBLIOGRAPHY

Abramson DH, Frank CM, Susman M, et al. Presenting signs of retinoblastoma. *J Pediatr* 1998;132(3 Pt 1):505–508.

Castillo BV Jr, Kaufman L. Pediatric tumors of the eye and orbit. *Pediatr Clin North Am* 2003;50(1):149–172.

Deegan WF. Emerging strategies for the treatment of retinoblastoma. *Curr Opin Ophthalmol* 2003;14(5):291–295.

Gallie BL, Dunn JM, Chan HS, et al. The genetics of retinoblastoma: relevance to the patient. *Pediatr Clin North Am* 1991;38:299–315.

Hurwitz RL, Shields CL, Shields JA, et al. Retinoblastoma. In: Pizzo PA, Poplack DG, eds. *Principles and Practice of Pediatric Oncology.* 4th Ed. Philadelphia/New York: Lippincott-Raven, 2001:825–864.

Nahum MP, Gdal-On M, Kuten A, et al. Long-term follow-up of children with retinoblastoma. *Pediatr Hematol Oncol* 2001;18(3):173–179.

Author: Kelly C. Goldsmith

Retropharyngeal Abscess

 Database

DEFINITION

A relatively rare but potentially life-threatening infection occurring in the potential space bounded by the layers of cervical fascia posterior to the esophagus and anterior to the deep cervical fascia.

CAUSES

• Infectious: Cultures frequently reveal multiple organisms. The predominant organisms isolated include:

—*Streptococcus* (group A and others)
—*Staphylococcus aureus*
—Various anaerobic species (*Bacteroides*, *Peptostreptococcus*, and *Fusobacterium*)
—One pediatric study cultured *Haemophilus influenzae* type b in 20% of cases; however, the study took place before the routine use of *H. influenzae* type b conjugate vaccines.
—Many of the isolates are β-lactamase producers.

PATHOPHYSIOLOGY

The majority of infections follows a pharyngitis or supraglottitis and occurs secondary to suppuration of the retropharyngeal lymph nodes, which lie in two paramedial chains and drain various nasopharyngeal structures. Other sources of infection in this space include penetrating trauma, such as from foreign object aspiration, dental procedures, or attempts at intubation. Extension of infection into this space can arise from vertebral body osteomyelitis or petrositis.

EPIDEMIOLOGY

Most large children's hospital centers report one to three cases per year. Children younger than 6 years of age are most at risk, with half of the cases occurring in infants younger than 36 months of age.

COMPLICATIONS

• Spontaneous rupture with aspiration of infected material, with subsequent asphyxia or overwhelming pulmonary infection
• Hemorrhage from extension into local arteries, and/or venous thrombosis from involvement of major neck vessels
• Extension of the infection inferiorly can occur, leading to a subdiaphragmatic or psoas abscess.

PROGNOSIS

Excellent with appropriate antibiotics, expectant care, and surgery, if needed, at optimal time.

 Differential Diagnosis

• Pharyngitis
• Peritonsillar or lateral wall abscess
• Epiglottitis/supraglottitis

 Data Gathering

HISTORY

• Symptoms may be present from hours to days before correct diagnosis. Many patients will have been on oral antibiotics for presumed pharyngitis/sinusitis.
• Most frequent symptoms include sore throat, decreased oral intake, muffled voice, drooling, stiff or painful neck, fever, dysphagia, and stridor.
• Preceding neck trauma? Especially penetrating injuries, recent surgery (especially dental), and history consistent with aspiration of a foreign object.

Retropharyngeal Abscess

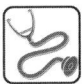 Physical Examination

Most frequent signs are:

- Fever
- Stridor (seen in up to 50% of children in one study, but only 5% in a recent series)
- Drooling
- A tender cervical neck region/mass and restricted range of motion
- Classic diagnostic finding of a bulging posterior pharyngeal wall. May be absent or difficult to appreciate in an ill, apprehensive child.

 Laboratory Aids

Test: CBC
Significance: Frequently reveals an elevated total WBC, with a significant left shift

Test: Lateral neck x-ray
Significance: Reveals widening of retropharyngeal space and at times an air fluid level. Negative plain neck film does NOT rule out retropharyngeal abscess.

Test: CT scan or MRI of the neck
Significance: The most definitive test, which can usually differentiate abscess from local cellulitis/adenitis

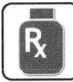 Therapy

- Emergent therapy requires maintaining patent airway; be wary of sudden spontaneous drainage of the abscess, with catastrophic aspiration.
- Careful in-hospital monitoring of airway and fluid intake.
- Start broad-spectrum parental antibiotics, active against *Streptococcus pneumoniae*, *S. aureus*, and oral anaerobic organisms. If patient does not improve, broaden coverage to include drugs active against β-lactamase producing organisms and anaerobic organisms. Clindamycin or ampicillin/sulbactam are good initial choices.
- Immediate consultation with otolaryngology surgical team. Schedule of incision/aspiration of abscess at optimal time, with team experienced in airway management of small children. CT-guided aspiration of the abscess has aided the surgical approach at many sites.
- In selected mild, early cases (especially if the CT scan is consistent with cellulitis rather than true abscess), parenteral antibiotics may be sufficient for therapy. Recent data suggest that up to 50% of patients can be successfully managed without surgical intervention. Patients treated with antibiotics alone must be followed closely for signs of worsening clinical status.

PITFALLS

- Physicians must maintain a high index of suspicion. The presentation of a retropharyngeal abscess can be subtle, with the most frequent initial diagnostic impression usually epiglottitis or severe pharyngitis.
- Both plain films and CT scan have false positives and false negatives.
- Once diagnosis is made, urgent consultation with experienced surgical staff is mandatory.

ICD-9-CM 478.24

BIBLIOGRAPHY

Brook I. Microbiology of retropharyngeal abscess in children. *Am J Dis Child* 1987;141:202–204.

Craig FW, Schunk JE. Retropharygeal abscess in children: clinical presentation, utility of imaging, and current management. *Pediatrics* 2003;111:1394–1398.

Hammerschlag PE, Hammerschlag MR. Retropharyngeal abscess. In: Feigin R, Cherry JD, eds. *Textbook of Pediatric Infectious Diseases*. 3rd Ed. Philadelphia: WB Saunders, 1992:168–171.

Lee SS, Schwartz RH, Bahadori RS. Retropharyngeal abscess: epiglottitis of the new millennium. *J Pediatr* 2001;138(3): 435–437.

Nagy M, Pizzuto M, Backstrom J, et al. Deep neck infections in children: a new approach to diagnosis and treatment. *Laryngoscope* 1997;107:1627–1634.

Wang LF, Kuo WR, Tsai SM, Huang KJ. Characterizations of life-threatening deep cervical space infections: a review of one hundred ninety-six cases. *Am J Otolaryngol* 2003;24(2):111–117.

Weber AL, Siciliano A. CT and MR imaging evaluation of neck infections with clinical correlations. *Radiol Clin North Am* 2000;38(5): 941–968, ix.

Author: Richard M. Rutstein

Reye Syndrome

 Database

DEFINITION

Acute encephalopathy and fatty degeneration of the liver

CDC CASE DEFINITION

An illness that meets all of the following criteria:

- Acute, noninflammatory encephalopathy that is documented clinically by (a) an alteration in consciousness and, if available, (b) a record of the CSF containing less than or equal to 8 leukocytes/cu per mm or a histologic specimen demonstrating cerebral edema without perivascular or meningeal inflammation
- Hepatopathy documented by either (a) a liver biopsy or an autopsy considered to be diagnostic of Reye syndrome or (b) a threefold or greater increase in the levels of the serum glutamic-oxaloacetic transaminase (SGOT), serum glutamic-pyruvic transaminase (SGPT), or serum ammonia
- No more reasonable explanation for the cerebral and hepatic abnormalities

PATHOPHYSIOLOGY

- Mitochondrial injury of unknown etiology in a viral-infected host results in dysfunction of oxidative phosphorylation and fatty-acid oxidation
- Mitochondrial toxins, usually salicylates, exacerbate condition when ingested after mitochondrial injury

EPIDEMIOLOGY

- Peak incidence age 6
- Most children range from 4 to 12 years
- More common amongst Caucasians in rural and suburban communities
- Association with ingestion of aspirin-containing medicines by children with varicella or influenza B
- Peak incidence of 555 cases in U.S. children in 1980.
- In 1982 the Surgeon General issued an advisory on the salicylates and Reye syndrome.
- From 1994 to 1997 there were no more than two cases of Reye syndrome a year.

COMPLICATIONS

- Elevated intracranial pressure secondary to cerebral edema
- Cardiovascular collapse
- Overall mortality of 31%

 Differential Diagnosis

It is important to distinguish between "classic" Reye syndrome, associated with aspirin, and "Reye-like" syndromes, often as a result of metabolic disorders and other causes, as below.

- Metabolic diseases: In a report by Hou and colleagues, Reye-like syndrome was secondary to hereditary organic acidemias ($n = 13$), urea cycle defects ($n = 4$), mitochondrial disorders ($n = 3$), fulminant hepatitis ($n = 2$), tyrosinemia ($n = 1$), and valproate-associated hepatotoxicity ($n = 1$). In the United Kingdom, 12% of Reye syndrome cases between 1981 and 1996 were subsequently reclassified as metabolic disorders.
- CNS infections (e.g., meningitis, encephalitis)
- Toxins
- Drug ingestion (e.g., salicylates, valproate)

 Data Gathering

HISTORY

Question: Prodromal illness?
Significance: URI (73%)—influenza B, influenza A, and varicella

Question: Abrupt onset of vomiting?
Significance: Onset within 4 to 7 days of initial illness.

Question: What is the natural history?
Significance: Followed by neurologic deterioration in which delirium may progress to seizures, coma, or death

 Physical Examination

- Slight liver enlargement without jaundice
- Absence of focal neurologic signs

Neurologic examination varies with stage of disease:

- Stage 0: Alert, wakeful
- Stage 1: Difficult to arouse, lethargic, sleepy
- Stage 2: Delirious, combative, with purposeful or semipurposeful motor responses
- Stage 3: Unarousable, with predominantly flexor motor responses, decorticate
- Stage 4: Unarousable, with predominantly extensor motor responses, decerebrate
- Stage 5: Unarousable, with flaccid paralysis, areflexia, and pupils unresponsive
- Stage 6: Treated with curare or equivalent drug, and therefore unclassifiable

Reye Syndrome

 Laboratory Aids

Test: Ammonia
Significance: May be normal at the onset of vomiting. Serum level greater than 45 mg/dL predicts higher mortality.

Test: Liver and muscle function testing
Significance: Elevated transaminases, creatinine kinase, lactate dehydrogenase, ammonia, and prothrombin time (PT)

Test: CSF
Significance: Normal except for elevated intracranial pressure (ICP)

Test: EEG
Significance: Characteristic of metabolic encephalopathy with generalized slow wave abnormalities

Test: Metabolic workup
Significance: Abnormalities of organic and amino acids may be present if symptoms caused by a metabolic disorder

PATHOLOGY (POSTMORTEM)

Test: Liver
Significance: Grossly yellowish white in appearance secondary to increased triglycerides; foamy cytoplasm with increased microvesicular fat, decreased glycogen.

Test: Brain
Significance: Marked edema with increased intracellular fluid, and loss of neurons

Abnormally appearing mitochondria can be detected in many tissues

 Therapy

- Should be tailored based on severity of presentation
- IV glucose to counteract effects of glycogen depletion
- Fluid restriction in patients with cerebral edema (1,500 mL/m^2 per day), along with mannitol to increase serum osmolality and induce cerebral dehydration
- Vitamin K, fresh frozen plasma, and platelets as needed for treatment of secondary coagulopathy

 Follow-Up

- Cerebral function at presentation is the best predictor of outcome.
- Majority have mild illness without progression
- Patients with milder disease (stage 0, 1, 2) tend to recover completely
- Patients with stage 3 disease are equally likely to recover completely or die
- Patients with stage 4 to 5 disease usually do not survive.

PITFALLS

Failure to recognize early and control or prevent cerebral edema—the immediate cause of death

 Common Questions and Answers

Q: Is Reye syndrome fatal?
A: Around 30% of children will die, usually secondary to cerebral edema. Mortality rates are best predicted by neurologic state at the onset of presentation.

Q: How can the neurologic findings of Reye syndrome be differentiated from meningitis?
A: Aside from an elevated ICP, the lumbar taps of patients with Reye syndrome are at best unremarkable. Elevated white count is not seen in these cases.

ICD-9-CM 331.81

BIBLIOGRAPHY

Belay ED, Bresee JS, Holman RC, et al. Reye's syndrome in the United States from 1981 through 1997. *N Engl J Med* 1999;340(18): 1377–1382.

DeVivo DC. Acute encephalopathies of childhood. In: Rudolph AM, eds. *Rudolph's pediatrics*, 19th ed. Norwalk, CT: Appleton & Lange, 1991:1713–1720.

Duerksen DR, Jewell LD, Mason AL, et al. Co-existence of hepatitis A and adult Reye's syndrome. *Gut* 1997;41(1):121–124.

Glasgow JF, Middleton B, Moore R, Gray A, Hill J. The mechanism of inhibition of beta-oxidation by aspirin metabolites in skin fibroblasts from Reye's syndrome patients and controls. *Biochim Biophys Acta* 1999;1454(1): 115–125.

Glasgow JF, Middleton B. Reye syndrome—insights on causation and prognosis. *Arch Dis Child* 2001;85(5): 351–353.

Green CL, Blitzer MG, Shapiro E. Inborn errors of metabolism and Reye's syndrome: differential diagnosis. *J Pediatr* 1988;113:156.

Hou JW, Chou SP, Wang TR. Metabolic function and liver histopathology in Reye-like illnesses. *Acta Paediatr* 1996;85(9): 1053–1057.

Lichtenstein PK, Heubi JE, Dougherty CC, et al. Grade I Reye's syndrome: a frequent cause of vomiting and liver dysfunction after varicella and upper respiratory tract infection. *N Engl J Med* 1983;309:133.

Reye RDK, Morgan G, Baral J. Encephalopathy and fatty degeneration of the viscera: a disease entity in childhood. *Lancet* 1963;2:749.

Authors: Andrew E. Mulberg and Seth L. Ness

Rhabdomyolysis

 ## Database

DEFINITION

• Skeletal muscle injury resulting from trauma, infection, or inadequate delivery, production, or consumption of energy or oxygen relative to demands. The release of intracellular contents may cause severe electrolyte disturbances including life-threatening hyperkalemia, myoglobinuria, and acute renal failure.

PATHOPHYSIOLOGY

• Rhabdomyolysis is uncommon in childhood
• The most common causes include muscle trauma from crush or compression injury, burns, or electric shock. Others include viral illnesses such as influenza and Epstein-Barr virus infection, heat stroke, severe exertion, status epilepticus, and vasculitis with myositis.
• Uncommon causes in childhood include congenital metabolic myopathies, acute dystonic reactions, the malignant hyperthermia syndrome, other infections, exposure to some medications, toxins or illicit drugs and severe electrolyte disturbances.
• Myopathies involving muscle enzyme or energy substrate deficiencies include Carnitine Palmityl Transferase (CPT) deficiency, McArdle disease (glycogenosis Type V), mitochondrial deficiency disorders and phosphofructokinase deficiency.
• Rhabdomyolysis is more likely to occur following exertion in the dystrophinopathies, which include all forms of muscular dystrophy.
• Infections, in addition to the viral illnesses listed above include coxsackie, HIV, malaria, legionella and toxic shock syndrome.
• Medications include the lipid lowering "statin" drugs (HMG-CoA reductase inhibitors), inhalation anesthetics, propofol, cyclosporine, Amphotericin B, Itraconazole and Isotretinoin.
• Toxins and illicit drugs include snake, spider and vespid venoms, fish toxins, some mushrooms, hydrocarbons, ethanol, cocaine, heroin and phencyclidine (PCP). Rhabdomyolysis has almost been reported, possibly as a result of copper toxicity, in Wilson disease.
• Electrolyte disturbances include hypokalemia, severe hypophosphatemia, hypernatremia and hyponatremia, hypocalcemia and hyperosmolar states.
• The insult may lead to muscle cell destruction or failure of membrane function with release of intracellular contents including proteins and electrolytes and uptake of large amounts of extracellular water leading to severe hypovolemia and decreased renal perfusion.
• The above list of causes is not exhaustive. Any child with sudden onset of muscle pain, tenderness or weakness should be suspected of having rhabdomyolysis and any child with dark urine suspected of myoglobinuria.

GENETICS

Many of the unusual causes of rhabdomyolysis, including muscle enzyme deficiencies, muscular dystrophy, and disorders of mitochondrial metabolism, are heritable disorders, and a familial history should be sought.

EPIDEMIOLOGY

Rhabdomyolysis is more common in adults, in which it is seen most frequently in comatose patients resulting from heroin or cocaine abuse and long periods of being motionless.

COMPLICATIONS

• Electrolyte release from muscle can lead to hyperkalemia, hyperphosphatemia, and secondarily to hypocalcemia.
• Acute renal failure may occur secondary to myoglobinuria and occurs in approximately 40% of patients. Myoglobin may exert direct renal cytotoxicity, tubular obstruction with myoglobin casts and decreased renal blood flow and GFR as a result of hypovolemia.
• Compartment syndrome may occur secondary to muscle swelling.

ASSOCIATED ILLNESSES

In addition to the previously mentioned causes, rhabdomyolysis has also been reported associated with diverse conditions, including asthma, hemolytic uremic syndrome, and diabetes mellitus.

PROGNOSIS

The prognosis depends on the extent of preexisting irreversible renal disease, prompt recognition and institution of appropriate therapy, and the diuretic response to fluid replacement. In general, however, the outlook for recovery is very good.

 ## Differential Diagnosis

• Includes any condition associated with muscle pain, tenderness, and/or weakness. Many of the causes of rhabdomyolysis may be associated with these signs and symptoms but demonstrate no elevation in Creatine Phosphokinase (CK).
• Examples include many viral illnesses, Lyme disease, suppurative myositis, Guillain-Barré syndrome, and collagen vascular diseases.

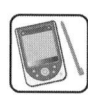 ## Data Gathering

HISTORY

Question: Has there been increased exertion, viral illness, muscle injury, or electrical shock?
Significance: These conditions are associated with muscle breakdown and rhabdomyolysis.

Question: Is there familial history of muscle disease or reaction to anesthesia?
Significance: Rhabdomyolysis is associated with muscular dystrophy and reaction to drugs such as anesthetics.

SPECIAL QUESTIONS

• Antecedent history of illness or insult associated with rhabdomyolysis? Rhabdomyolysis may follow certain illnesses (e.g., influenza) and insults (e.g., crush injury) and thus a history of these should be sought.
• Muscle pain or weakness? These may result from rhabdomyolysis and may help suggest the diagnosis if present.
• Brownish discoloration of the urine?

 ## Physical Examination

• Palpation of muscle for tenderness and uncommonly, swelling or fullness
• Testing for motor strength
• Eliciting reflexes to exclude neuropathy
• Examination of skin and mucous membranes for signs of vasculitis

Laboratory Aids

- Serum electrolytes, calcium, and phosphorus looking for hyperkalemia, hyperphosphatemia, and/or hypocalcemia. There may be metabolic acidosis with a wide anion gap in those conditions associated with lactate production.
- BUN and creatinine: creatinine may be elevated out of proportion to BUN.
- Creatine phosphokinase (CK) will be elevated greater than 100 times normal in rhabdomyolysis.
- Serum carnitine
- Serum lactate
- Serum uric acid
- Urinalysis: urine may appear brown and test positive for blood on dipstick without erythrocytes on microscopy. Granular pigmented casts are common.
- CBC may show anemia with or without microangiopathic changes in cases of hemolytic processes and hemoglobinuria.

Finding: Definitive tests for myoglobinuria
Significance: Urine immunoelectrophoresis and radioimmunoassay are not generally available in clinical laboratories. Ammonium sulfate solubility testing is a reasonable screening test to help differentiate myoglobin from hemoglobin. The two proteins are best distinguished by the clinical setting in which they occur, the CK level, and the presence or absence of hemolytic anemia.

Finding: Muscle biopsy
Significance: Necessary to diagnose the metabolic myopathies. A biopsy will demonstrate immunohistochemical features of a myopathy. Immunoblotting is helpful in evaluating the dystrophinopathies.

Finding: False positives
Significance: The dipstick for blood is positive, but examination of a freshly voided urinary sediment reveals few or no erythrocytes. In this instance, the possibilities are myoglobinuria or hemoglobinuria.

Finding: Very rapid rise in serum creatinine
Significance: May occur as a result of release from muscle

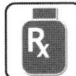 ## Therapy

GENERAL

- Treatment is supportive. If an underlying cause is identified, it should be corrected or removed.
- Adequate hydration (e.g., 2 to 3 times maintenance fluids) should be sufficient to provide brisk urine flow (e.g., greater than 4 mL/kg per hour). Myoglobinuric nephrotoxicity is the only clinical situation in which acute renal failure can be averted by maintaining good urine flow. Alkalinization of the urine is probably beneficial. Furosemide and/or mannitol may be helpful to maintain urine output.
- Dialysis is indicated if oliguric acute renal failure occurs and/or if severe electrolyte disturbances are present.

DRUGS

- With myoglobinuria, bicarbonate therapy should be given intravenously to maintain the urine pH above 7.0.
- If urine output falls in the face of adequate hydration, furosemide (1 to 4 mg/kg per dose IV) should be given to attempt to prevent oliguric renal failure.
- If severe hyperkalemia occurs, measures should be taken to prevent cardiac dysrhythmias (B-agonists, calcium, bicarbonate, glucose, and insulin) and to maximize elimination of potassium by the kidneys (furosemide) and/or gastrointestinal tract (Kayexalate).
- With hypocalcemia, give calcium only if symptoms are present.

POSSIBLE CONFLICTS

- Furosemide may interfere with alkalinization of the urine.
- Use of bicarbonate may precipitate symptomatic hypocalcemia.
- Calcium therapy for severe hyperkalemia is necessary, but its use with hyperphosphatemia increases risk of vascular calcification.
- Risk factors for acute renal failure include preexisting renal disease, delay in recognition and treatment, concurrent use of potential nephrotoxic agents (e.g., NSAIDS), volume depletion, and either hypotension or hypertension.
- Failure to discontinue intravenous fluids if oligoanuric renal failure develops could result in iatrogenic fluid overload.

 ## Follow-Up

WHEN TO EXPECT IMPROVEMENT

- Prompt cessation of rhabdomyolysis may be expected when the inciting cause is corrected or resolves.
- With resolution of the myoglobinuria, return to normal renal function is the rule.

PITFALLS

- Failure to check for muscle breakdown in cases of child abuse
- Use of radiocontrast in imaging studies as part of diagnostic evaluation can worsen acute renal failure.
- Occasionally hypercalcemia may develop during the recovery from myoglobin induced renal failure.

ICD-9-CM 728.89

BIBLIOGRAPHY

Brumback RA, Feeback DL, Leech RW. Rhabdomyolysis in childhood. *Pediatr Clin North Am* 1992;39:821–858.

DiGiacomo JC, Frankel H, Haskell RM, et al. Unsuspected child abuse revealed by delayed presentation of periportal tracking and myoglobinuria. *J Trauma* 2000;49(2):348–350.

Eberhard Ritz. Rhabdomyolysis. *J Am Soc Nephr* 2000;II:1553–1561.

Malinoski DJ, Slater MS, Mullins RJ. Crush injury and rhabdomyolysis. *Crit Care Clin* 2004;20(1):171–192.

Vanholder R, Sever MS, Erek E, Lameire N. Rhabdomyolysis. *J Am Soc of Nephrol.* 2000;11(8):1553–1561.

Zager RA, Brurkhart K. *Kidney Int* 1997;51:728–738.

Author: Thomas L. Kennedy III

Rhabdomyosarcoma

 ## Database

DEFINITION

Malignant tumor of mesenchymal cells committed to skeletal muscle lineage. Etiology is unknown.

PATHOLOGY

- One of the "small round blue" cell tumors of childhood.
- Two major subtypes:

—Alveolar (19% of cases): small round cells with dense appearance, line up along spaces resembling pulmonary alveoli, associated with translocation between chromosomes 2 and 13, or less commonly 1 and 13.
—Embryonal (60% of cases): spindle-shaped cells, less densely cellular with stroma-rich appearance, associated with a chromosomal abnormality on the short arm of chromosome 11 (chromosome 11p15).

- Undifferentiated and pleomorphic types comprise the remaining cases.

GENETICS

- Majority of cases occur sporadically
- Several predisposing factors include:

—Li-Fraumeni syndrome (family cancer syndrome associated with germline mutations of the p53 gene on chromosome 17 and an autosomal-dominant inheritance) includes rhabdomyosarcoma and other soft tissue sarcomas, leukemia, brain tumors, adrenocortical carcinoma, and early-onset breast carcinoma in female relatives.
—Patients with Beckwith-Wiedemann syndrome (fetal overgrowth syndrome characterized by an abnormality at chromosome 11p15) have an increased incidence of primarily Wilms tumor, but also hepatoblastoma, rhabdomyosarcoma, and other tumors of embryonal origin.
—Neurofibromatosis type I (autosomal-dominant genetic disorder characterized by mutation of the NF1 gene on chromosome 17q11.2) is associated with an increased risk of rhabdomyosarcoma, other soft tissue sarcomas (malignant nerve sheath tumors, neurofibrosarcomas), leukemia, Wilms tumor, and brain tumors.
—Previous radiation exposure, especially in patients with Li-Fraumeni, neurofibromatosis type I or hereditary retinoblastoma (RB1 germline mutation)

Prognosis Primary Site

Orbit	95%
Other head and neck	78%
Parameningeal	74%
Paratesticular/vagina	89%
Bladder/prostate	81%
Extremities	74%
Other sites	67%

—Congenital anomalies of the genitourinary system and central nervous system are more frequent than expected in children with rhabdomyosarcoma.

EPIDEMIOLOGY

- Slightly more than 200 new cases are diagnosed each year in the United States.
- Third most common extracranial solid tumor of childhood after neuroblastoma and Wilms tumor
- Fifty percent of cases are diagnosed in children younger than 6 years of age with smaller incidence peak in midadolescence.
- 1.3 times more common in males than females.

COMPLICATIONS

- Rhabdomyosarcoma can compromise function of surrounding organs.
- Metastatic spread may occur to lymph nodes, lung, bone, bone marrow, liver, or brain.

PROGNOSIS

- Overall, 70% of patients can be cured.
- Tumor anatomic site and initial complete surgical resectability have prognostic significance, such that both are used together to direct therapy.
- Prognosis by primary site (5-year survival): (See table, Prognosis by Primary Site.)
- Although 50% of patients with distant metastatic disease can be placed into remission, only 20% can be cured.
- Tumors with alveolar histology (typically extremity lesions) tend to metastasize early.
- The presence of the PAX3-FKHR gene rearrangement (seen in tumors with alveolar histology) is an adverse prognostic factor, associated with older patients and more advanced stage disease.
- Recurrence can occur many years after completion of therapy but is rare after 3 years.

 ## Differential Diagnosis

- Malignant

—Ewing sarcoma
—Neuroblastoma
—Non-Hodgkin lymphoma
—Leukemic chloroma
—Germ cell tumor
—Rare soft tissue sarcomas

- Nonmalignant

—Trauma
—Benign tumors: lipoma, rhabdomyoma, neurofibroma
—Langerhans cell histiocytosis
—Abscess

 ## Data Gathering

HISTORY

- A painless, firm swelling or mass is the most common presentation.
- Other symptoms depend on site of origin:

—Head/neck: nasal congestion or discharge, epistaxis, snoring, sinusitis, dysphagia, otorrhea, chronic otitis media, cranial nerve palsies, proptosis, headache, vomiting or systemic hypertension (with intracranial growth of tumor)
—Genitourinary/pelvic: urinary frequency or retention, hematuria, constipation, vaginal discharge or bleeding
—Extremity: painful or painless lumps or erythema
—Trunk: usually few symptoms until tumor widespread

 ## Physical Examination

- Can occur in any location, even in sites in which skeletal muscle is not normally found
- Distribution of primary tumor sites include the following:

—Head and neck (38%): parameningeal (middle ear, nasal cavity, paranasal sinuses, nasopharynx, infratemporal fossa, pterygopalatine fossa, parapharyngeal area); orbit (orbit, eyelid); nonparameningeal (scalp, parotid, oral cavity, larynx, oropharynx, cheek, hypopharynx, thyroid, parathyroid, neck)
—Genitourinary tract (21%): bladder and prostate; uterus, vagina, vulva, and paratesticular region
—Extremity (18%)
—Trunk (7%)
—Retroperitoneum (7%)

- Special attention should be given to physical examination of lymphatic structures and surrounding tissues as this may identify local invasion and/or lymphatogenous spread.

 ## Laboratory Aids

TESTS

Laboratory Tests

- CBC
- Electrolytes, liver and renal function tests, serum calcium, phosphorus in anticipation of starting chemotherapy

Imaging and Other Tests

To evaluate primary site and confirm diagnosis:

- CT scan or, preferably, MRI scan

- Biopsy: Biopsy should be performed by an experienced physician so as to avoid contamination of the tumor site or removal of insufficient tissue to make the diagnosis. In addition to routine morphologic and immunohistochemical stain assessments, analysis of tumor chromosomes by traditional cytogenetics, fluorescent in situ hybridization or reverse-transcriptase PCR is helpful in making the diagnosis and may provide information regarding prognosis. Because of the importance of these studies, consultation with a pediatric oncologist before the biopsy is strongly encouraged.

To evaluate for evidence of distant metastases (present in 20% of patients at diagnosis):

- Chest radiograph and CT scan
- ^{99m}Tc-diphosphonate bone scan
- Bilateral aspiration and biopsy of iliac bone marrow
- Lumbar puncture for CSF cytology (parameningeal tumors only; to determine if CNS invasion has occurred)

 ## Therapy

- Therapy is a multimodal approach based on location and extent of disease.

—Surgery
—Chemotherapy: common agents used include vincristine, dactinomycin, cyclophosphamide, doxorubicin, etoposide, and ifosfamide. Other agents including topotecan and irinotecan are being investigated.
—Radiation therapy: used in all patients except those with completely resected, embryonal tumors.

 ## Follow-Up

WHEN TO EXPECT IMPROVEMENT

All patients with rhabdomyosarcoma require 1 to 2 years of chemotherapy to prevent recurrence in the original site of tumor or distant spread. However, some improvement in signs and symptoms is usually seen within the first several weeks of therapy.

ACUTE EFFECTS OF THERAPY

Therapy for rhabdomyosarcoma is intensive. Patients can expect many of the following side effects:

- Frequent admissions to the hospital for chemotherapy or complications of the therapy.
- Complications from bone marrow suppressive effects of chemotherapy or radiotherapy:

—Anemia: Blood transfusions are usually necessary; erythropoietin (a stimulator of erythropoiesis) may be given to reduce the number of transfusions required.

—Thrombocytopenia: Platelet transfusions are often necessary to reduce the risk of serious bleeding.
—Neutropenia: Increased risk of bacterial and fungal infections; G-CSF (granulocyte-colony stimulating factor) is usually administered daily following chemotherapy to shorten the duration of neutropenia.

- Complications from the gastrointestinal side effects of chemotherapy or radiotherapy:

—Nausea and vomiting; Relieved with ondansetron and other antiemetic agents.
—Malnutrition secondary to reduced appetite and mucosal ulcerations; nutritional supplements (oral, nasogastric, gastrostomy tube or parenteral) may be necessary.

- Complication from radiotherapy:

—Skin erythema or breakdown.

LATE EFFECTS OF THERAPY

Therapy for rhabdomyosarcoma is intensive, and is associated with significant long-term adverse effects. Regular follow-up with a pediatric oncologist is strongly recommended.

- Cardiomyopathy

—Anthracyclines (doxorubicin) weaken cardiac muscle leading to reduced left ventricular function many years after therapy.
—Approximately 5% of patients receiving cumulative doses of doxorubicin greater than 500 mg/m^2 will develop congestive heart failure.
—Radiation to the heart can lower the cumulative dose threshold to 300 mg/m^2.
—Any patient who has received an anthracycline should be cautioned against initiating strenuous physical activity without adequate preparation.
—Pregnant women who have received anthracyclines in the past should inform their obstetrician so that appropriate cardiac assessment can be completed prior to vaginal delivery.

- Kidney and bladder damage

—Urinalysis should be performed to detect hemorrhagic cystitis or tubular damage.
—Blood pressure should be monitored in patients who received irradiation to the kidneys; vascular damage and hypertension may develop many years after therapy.

- Infertility and delayed puberty

—Reduced or absent gonadal function is related to high doses of alkylating agents (cyclophosphamide, ifosfamide): males are at high risk of azoospermia; females may be fertile, but are at risk for premature menopause.
—Low-dose estrogen therapy with oral contraceptive medications may be necessary for amenorrheic women.
—Retrograde ejaculation may be seen following surgery for paratesticular tumors.

- Second malignant neoplasms

—Sarcomas may occur within the radiation field.

—Myelodysplastic syndromes and acute myeloid leukemia may occur secondary to radiation or chemotherapy (cyclophosphamide, ifosfamide, etoposide)

- Bowel obstruction and enteritis (abdominal-pelvic tumors)

—Adhesions as a consequence of surgery or radiation
—A history of failure to gain weight or symptoms of malabsorption suggests a need for additional evaluation.

- Growth abnormalities/functional defects at the primary site

—Radiation doses greater than 20 Gy will cause growth retardation in growing children.
—Scoliosis can occur if the vertebrae are involved in the radiation field.
—Cataracts can occur after irradiation involving the head.

- Learning difficulties

—Radiotherapy directed to the central nervous system in children <3 years old with head/neck primaries may result in significant cognitive deficits.

 ## Common Questions and Answers

Q: Is aggressive surgical resection indicated?
A: For all but a small minority of patients, aggressive surgical resection with wide negative margins is not indicated. With improvements in medical therapy, survival rates have improved despite the use of more conservative surgical approaches.

Q: Can a child with rhabdomyosarcoma attend school?
A: As the chemotherapy for rhabdomyosarcoma is intensive, most children are unable to continue with school during this time, but will benefit from home-bound instruction.

ICD-9-CM 171.9

BIBLIOGRAPHY

Herzog CE, Stewart JMM, Blakely ML. Pediatric soft tissue sarcomas. *Surg Oncol Clin North Am* 2003;12:419–447.

McCarville MB, Spunt SL, Pappo AS. Rhabdomyosarcoma in pediatric patients: the good, the bad, and the unusual. *AJR Am J Roentgenol* 2001;176(6):1563–1569.

McDowell HP. Update on childhood rhabdomyosarcoma. *Arch Dis Child* 2003;88:354–357.

Ruymann FB, Grovas AC. Progress in the diagnosis and treatment of rhabdomyo-sarcoma and related soft tissue sarcomas. *Cancer Invest* 2000;3:223–224.

Author: Kara M. Kelly

Rheumatic Fever (RF)

 Database

DEFINITION

Postinfectious immune response to group A streptococcus that results in a diffuse inflammatory disease involving multiple organ systems

PATHOPHYSIOLOGY

• Immune-mediated inflammatory reaction to specific rheumatogenic strains of group A β-hemolytic streptococci (GABHS) that affects the heart, joints, brain, blood vessels, and subcutaneous tissue. Streptococcal pharyngitis precedes the onset of acute rheumatic fever (ARF) by approximately 3 weeks.
• "Antigenic mimicry" occurs in which antigen similarities between epitopes of specific rheumatogenic streptococci and host tissue cause an autoimmune cross-reaction in which produced antibodies damage the host.
• Aschoff nodules are proliferative lesions noted in the myocardium that may persist for months to years after the initiation of disease.

GENETICS

There is an increased familial incidence reported, and patients with a previous episode of ARF have an approximate 50% chance of recurrence following untreated pharyngitis, suggesting a genetic predisposition.

EPIDEMIOLOGY

• Estimated 2% to 3% of patients with untreated or inadequately treated streptococcal pharyngitis develop ARF.
• Initial episode primarily seen between 5 and 15 years of age.
• Incidence (United States) is 0.5 to 3.1/100,000 with outbreaks in the mid-1980s among school children and military recruits.
• There are no racial or ethnic differences in susceptibility.
• No longer a disease mainly found in socially and economically disadvantaged groups in the United States, yet the incidence is higher in underdeveloped countries.
• Rheumatogenic strains of group A streptococci with specific M proteins have been associated with outbreaks of ARF.
• Strains of GABHS that cause impetigo do not cause ARF.

COMPLICATIONS

Cardiac

• Pancarditis (always a component of valvulitis)
—Pericarditis (including pericardial effusion) and/or myocarditis (these entities are almost always associated with valvulitis).
—Transient arrhythmias occur infrequently.
—Carditis accounts for the greatest mortality in the acute phase and significant morbidity/mortality chronically.
• Valvulitis
—Mitral valve is most commonly affected followed by aortic (usually associated with mitral involvement). Tricuspid and pulmonary valvar involvement is rare.

—Valve inflammation leads to insufficiency.
—Prolonged immune response causes fibrosis, calcification, and valve stenosis.

Arthritis

• Two or more large joints (knees, ankles, wrists, and elbows)
• Involvement is asymmetric and migratory.
• Limitation of motion may occur.
• Symptoms improve rapidly with aspirin. If symptoms persist beyond the acute illness, many authors suggest investigation into another cause (e.g., systemic lupus erythematosus [SLE]).
• Sydenham Chorea (St. Vitus Dance)
• Involuntary, purposeless, and uncoordinated movements associated with muscle weakness and/or abnormal behavior
• As a result of inflammation of the basal ganglia/cerebellum
• Symptoms occur late, 2 to 6 months after the onset of ARF, and usually resolve within weeks but may last months to years.

PROGNOSIS

• Patients with a previous episode of ARF are at high risk for a recurrence following streptococcal pharyngitis unless secondary prophylaxis is instituted. The highest risk is in the 5 years following the initial occurrence.
• Carditis can abate spontaneously or progress. The severity of the initial carditis is a major determinant of progression to rheumatic heart disease.
• Rheumatic carditis resolves in approximately 70% to 80% of patients who adhere to prophylaxis guidelines.

 Differential Diagnosis

• Carditis: viral, bacterial, rickettsial, parasitic, or mycoplasma myocarditis; Kawasaki disease
• Arthritis: poststreptococcal arthritis, serum sickness, septic arthritis (e.g., gonococcal), Lyme disease
• Collagen vascular disease: juvenile rheumatoid arthritis (small joints, not migratory, and not relieved promptly with aspirin), systemic lupus erythematosus, bacterial endocarditis
• Chorea: congenital choreoathetosis, brain tumors, Huntington chorea, Wilson disease, pediatric autoimmune neuropsychiatric disorders associated with streptococcus (PANDAS)
• Hematologic disorders with joint involvement: sickle cell anemia, leukemia
• Congenital heart defects: previously undiagnosed valvar heart disease, mitral valve prolapse with regurgitation

 Data Gathering

HISTORY

Q: How do you use the Jones criteria to make the diagnosis of ARF?

A: The modified Jones criteria are used to aid in the diagnosis (and avoid the misdiagnosis) of ARF. The diagnosis of ARF is suggested by the presence of either two major criteria or one major and two minor criteria, with evidence of a recent streptococcal infection.
• Major criteria
—Polyarthritis: 70% of patients with ARF (more common in adults) and manifest by a migratory arthritis of major joints.
—Carditis: 50% of patients and always associated with a murmur of valvulitis. It is more common and more severe in children.
—Sydenham chorea: 15% of patients and manifest by abnormal behavior and/or involuntary, purposeless movements.
—Erythema marginatum: 10% of patients and is an evanescent, pink rash with serpiginous borders.
—Subcutaneous nodules: 2% to 10% of patients and manifest by painless nodules over extensor surfaces of large joints, the occiput, and/or vertebral processes.
• Minor criteria
—Fever
—Arthralgia (mild pain without objective findings): can only be considered in the absence of arthritis
—Elevated acute phase reactants (erythrocyte sedimentation rate [ESR], C-reactive protein)
—Prolongation of the PR interval on electrocardiogram

Exceptions to the Jones criteria include:

• Sydenham chorea alone or indolent carditis alone. Each of these may appear late, and therefore, may not be associated with supporting evidence of a recent streptococcal pharyngitis.
• Patients with a previous diagnosis of ARF who have a recurrence may not fulfill the Jones criteria as a result of the subtle presentation.

 Physical Examination

CARDIAC

Finding: Murmur of valvulitis
Significance: Holosystolic mitral regurgitant murmur, Carey-Coombs apical mid-diastolic murmur, or a basal diastolic murmur of aortic insufficiency (major criterion).

Finding: Pericardial friction rub (in association with a murmur)
Significance: Pericardial effusion.

MUSCULOSKELETAL

Finding: Pain, limited motion, erythema, warmth of two or more large joints
Significance: Arthritis (major criterion).

NEUROLOGIC

Finding: Choreiform movements (must be differentiated from tics, athetosis, and hyperkinesis)
Significance: Sydenham chorea (major criterion).

SKIN

Finding: Evanescent, pink rash with pale centers and serpiginous borders on the trunk and proximal extremities
Significance: Erythema marginatum (major criterion).

Finding: Firm, painless nodules over the extensor surface of large joints, occiput and/or spinous processes
Significance: Subcutaneous nodules (major criterion).

Laboratory Aids

SPECIFIC TESTS

Test: No diagnostic test is available.

NONSPECIFIC TESTS

Test: Throat culture
Significance: May be negative in two-thirds of patients, or the patient may be a chronic carrier.

Test: Rapid streptococcal antigen test
Significance: Evidence for infection with GABHS.

Test: Elevated or rising streptococcal antibody titers (antistreptolysin O [ASO], anti-DNase B, antihyaluronidase)
Significance: Evidence for recent infection with GABHS.

Test: ESR and C-reactive protein
Significance: Minor criteria if elevated.

Test: Additional hematologic evaluation
Significance: Leukocytosis on complete blood count (may be normal).

Test: ECG
Significance: Prolonged PR interval (minor criterion), junctional rhythm, transient arrhythmias, ST-T wave changes.

Test: CXR
Significance: Cardiomegaly may indicate carditis or pericardial effusion.

Test: Echocardiogram
Significance: Assess valve involvement, ventricular dilatation, function, and pericardial effusion.

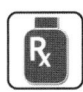

Therapy

• Primary prevention
—Full treatment of streptococcal pharyngitis infection
—Penicillin V 250 mg PO t.i.d. for 10 days; or
—Benzathine penicillin G IM (600,000 U ≥27 kg or 1,200,000 U >27 kg); or
—Erythromycin estolate, cefpodoxime proxetil, or azithromycin.
• Secondary prevention
—Benzathine penicillin G (1,200,000 U IM every 3 weeks); or
—Penicillin V 250 mg PO b.i.d.; or
—Sulfadiazine or erythromycin PO daily.
—Duration depends on clinical presentation and cardiac extent of ARF.
—Patients without rheumatic carditis require

prophylaxis for 5 years or until age 21, whichever comes later.
—Patients with a history of rheumatic carditis but with no residual cardiac disease (clinical or echocardiographic) require prophylaxis for at least 10 years and well into adulthood, whichever is longer.
—Patients with rheumatic heart disease should have prophylaxis for at least 10 years and at least until 40 years of age.
• Treatment of inflammation
—Aspirin: 90 to 100 mg/kg per day for 6 to 8 weeks
—Prednisone: 1 to 2 mg/kg per day for 2 weeks (with a taper over the following 2 to 3 weeks) is recommended only for patients with severe carditis.
—Treatment length is controversial, but often anti-inflammatories are used until the erythrocyte sedimentation rate or C-reactive protein normalizes
• Cardiac support
—Digoxin or other inotropic agents
—Afterload reducing agents such as captopril, intravenous nitroprusside, or milrinone
—Bed rest indicated during episode of acute carditis
—Surgical valvuloplasty or valve replacement if indicated
• Treatment of chorea
—Usually supportive
—Phenobarbital, haloperidol are most commonly used; also chlorpromazine, diazepam, or valproic acid

Follow-Up

• Patients without carditis
—Close follow-up is needed for 2 to 3 weeks to assess for development of acute carditis.
—Long-term pediatric follow-up is needed to diagnose patients with indolent carditis.
—Patients with new murmurs or clinical evidence of heart failure should be referred to a cardiologist.
—Long-term follow-up is needed to evaluate those who develop chorea.
—Prophylaxis should be stressed even in individuals without carditis.
• Patients with carditis
—Cardiology follow-up is needed to assess the development or evolution of rheumatic heart disease.
—Symptoms of worsening heart failure suggest progression of valvar or myocardial disease, recurrent ARF, or endocarditis.
—Secondary prophylaxis and bacterial endocarditis prophylaxis should be stressed.

PITFALLS

No definitive diagnostic test exists and certain clinical criteria must be present and excluded from other disease states to assure the proper diagnosis.

Common Questions and Answers

Q: Does a negative throat culture rule out ARF?

A: No. Throat cultures may be negative in two-thirds of patients.

Q: Is there a vaccine available to prevent ARF?
A: Not presently; however, research efforts to develop a recombinant multivalent vaccine have been promising. Note that over 90 antigenic strains of group A streptococcus have been identified; any vaccines developed will focus on those with the greatest virulence.

Q: What genetic factors predispose to ARF?
A: Several studies done worldwide have reported a high incidence of certain HLA-DR antigens in patients with rheumatic fever. The specific antigen/allele involved varies with the ethnic group studied.

Q: Can echocardiographic evidence of carditis alone be used to diagnose rheumatic fever?
A: This is currently under debate, however most authorities assert that carditis in ARF can only be diagnosed with a murmur consistent with valvulitis. An echocardiographic finding of valvar insufficiency without the appropriate auscultation findings cannot be used to fulfill the Jones criterion of carditis.

Q: Can intravenous gamma globulin (IVIG) be used as a treatment for ARF?
A: A recent study revealed that IVIG did not alter the natural history of ARF with no detectable difference in the cardiac outcome, laboratory findings, or echocardiographic parameters when compared to placebo.

ICD-9-CM 398.99

BIBLIOGRAPHY

Aron AM, Freeman JM, Caters S. The natural history of Sydenham's chorea. *Am J Med* 1965;38:83–95.

Ayoub E. Acute rheumatic fever. In: Allen HD, eds. *Moss and Adams Heart Disease in Infants, Children, and Adolescents Including the Fetus and Young Adult.* 6th Ed. Baltimore: Williams & Wilkins, 2001:1226–1241.

Dajani A, Taubert K, Ferrieri P, et al. Treatment of acute streptococcal pharyngitis and prevention of rheumatic fever. *Pediatrics* 1995;96(4):758–764.

Jones TD. Diagnosis of rheumatic fever. *JAMA* 1944;126:481–484.

Special Writing Group of the Committee on Rheumatic Fever, Endocarditis, and Kawasaki's Disease of the Council on Cardiovascular Disease in the Young of the American Heart Association. Guidelines for the diagnosis of rheumatic fever, Jones criteria update. *JAMA* 1992;268(15):2069–2073.

Stollerman GH. Rheumatic fever in the 21st century. *Clin Infect Dis* 2001;33:806–814.

Voss LM, Wilson NJ, Neutze JM, et al. Intravenous immunoglobulin in acute rheumatic fever: a randomized controlled trial. *Circulation* 2001;103(3):401–406.

Author: Sepehr Sekhavat

Rhinitis—Allergic

Database

DEFINITION

- Inflammation of the nasal and sinus mucosa, associated with sneezing, swelling, increased mucus production, and nasal obstruction
- May be classified as seasonal, perennial, or both
- Seasonal: periodic symptoms, involving the same season for at least 2 consecutive years; most often as a result of pollens (tree, grass, weed) and outdoor spores
- Perennial: occurring at least 9 months of the year; may be more difficult to detect because of overlap with other infections; may be as a result of multiple seasonal allergies or continual exposure to allergens (such as dust mites, cockroaches, molds, and animal dander)
- Perennial with seasonal exacerbations

CAUSES

- Indoor allergens: house dust mite, cockroaches, animal dander, cigarette smoke, hair spray, paint, molds
- Pollens: tree pollens in early spring, grass in late spring and early summer, ragweed in late summer and autumn
- Multiple environmental factors
- Changes in air temperature

ASSOCIATED PROBLEMS

- Asthma
- Allergic conjunctivitis
- Atopic dermatitis (eczema)
- Urticaria
- Otitis media
- Sleep, taste, and/or smell disturbance
- Nasal polyps
- Mouth breathing
- Snoring
- Adenoidal hypertrophy and sleep apnea
- Decreased appetite

EPIDEMIOLOGY

- Most common allergic disease, affecting more than 20 million Americans; affects 8% to 20% of children and 15% to 30% of adolescents.
- Estimated that up to 75% of children with asthma also have allergic rhinitis.
- Most commonly begins during childhood and young adulthood, with the peak incidence being in midadolescence; symptoms of allergic rhinitis develop in 80% of cases before age 20.
- Perennial allergic rhinitis can occur at any age; seasonal allergic rhinitis is rare before age 3 years.

GENETICS

- Increased incidence in families with atopic disease
- If one parent has allergies, each child has a 30% chance of having an allergy; if both parents have allergies, each child has a 70% chance of having an allergy.

COMPLICATIONS

- Chronic sinusitis
- Recurrent otitis media
- Hoarseness
- Loss of smell
- Loss of hearing
- High-arched palate and dental malocclusion from chronic mouth breathing

Differential Diagnosis

INFECTION

- Viral upper respiratory tract infection
- Bacterial sinusitis

ENVIRONMENTAL

- Foreign body

TUMORS

- Nasal polyps
- Dermoid cyst
- Nasal glioma

CONGENITAL

- Cystic fibrosis
- Choanal atresia
- Immotile cilia syndrome
- Septal deviation
- Primary atrophic rhinitis

IMMUNOLOGIC

- Sarcoidosis
- Wegener granulomatosis
- Systemic lupus erythematosus
- Sjögren syndrome

MISCELLANEOUS

- Idiopathic (vasomotor) rhinitis
- Nonallergic perennial rhinitis
- Rhinitis medicamentosa
- Rhinitis associated with pregnancy/other hormonal rhinitis
- Hypothyroidism
- Idiopathic neonatal rhinitis
- Drug-induced rhinitis
- Food-induced rhinitis

Data Gathering

HISTORY

Question: What are typical symptoms?
Significance: Patient often reports stuffy nose, sneezing, itching, runny nose, noisy breathing, snoring, cough, halitosis, and repeated throat clearing. Sensation of plugged ears and wheezing may occur.

Question: Are eyes red and itchy?
Significance: Suggestive of allergic conjunctivitis

Question: Are symptoms seasonal, perennial, or episodic?
Significance: May help to identify potential allergens

Question: Any exacerbating factors including pollen, animals, cigarette smoke, dust, molds?
Significance: Useful information to prevent symptoms from occurring

Question: Is there a family history of atopic disease, such as asthma or atopic dermatitis?
Significance: Supports the diagnosis

Question: Any related illnesses?
Significance: Asthma, urticaria, eczema, ear infections, and delayed speech are commonly associated conditions.

Physical Examination

- Allergic shiners: dark discoloration beneath the eyes as a result of obstruction of lymphatic and venous drainage, chronic nasal obstruction, and suborbital edema
- Dennie-Morgan lines: creases in the lower eyelid radiating outward from the inner canthus; caused by spasm in the muscles of Müller around the eye as a result of chronic congestion and stasis of blood
- Allergic salute: a gesture characterized by rubbing the nose with the palm of the hand upward to decrease itching and temporarily open the nasal passages
- Allergic crease: transverse crease near the tip of the nose, secondary to rubbing
- Nasal mucosa may appear pale and/or edematous; mucoid or watery material may be seen in the nasal cavity; check for nasal polyps, septal deviation.

Laboratory Aids

- Nasal cytology: specimen of nasal discharge to check for the presence of eosinophils. Have the patient blow his/her nose into a piece of nonporous paper or collect discharge with a cotton swab and transfer the discharge to a glass slide. Greater than 10% eosinophils are considered positive for nasal eosinophilia. Note: use of intranasal steroids may reduce the number of eosinophils found in nasal discharge.
- RAST (radioallergosorbent tests): in vitro test to measure allergen-specific IgE; expensive; useful in patients who have diffuse atopic dermatitis. The ImmunoCAP system, (Pharmacia Diagnostics): preferred method for specific IgE testing; uses a single blood sample to identify levels of specific IgE to a number of common respiratory (available as a profile specific to the region of the country in which the patient resides) and food antigens (food allergy profile), or both (childhood allergy profile).
- Total IgE: elevated in allergic rhinitis; not routinely indicated, but may come as part of specific IgE testing; >100 ku/L is considered elevated.
- Sweat test if cystic fibrosis is suspected or if nasal polyps are present.
- Audiometry and tympanometry when indicated
- CBC: may show eosinophilia; not routinely indicated

SKIN TESTING

- Prick test: percutaneous, qualitative test in which antigen concentrate is placed on the skin of the volar surface of the arm or upper back, and a needle is inserted; the skin reaction is subjectively graded from zero to four.
- Intradermal test: qualitative test in which antigen is introduced intradermally (0.02 mL with a 26- to 30-gauge needle); more sensitive than the prick test and often used if prick test is negative or equivocal; the degree of swelling and erythema is graded from zero to four.

PROCEDURES

Rhinoscopy to assess the nasal turbinates and to look for nasal polyps

 Therapy

AVOIDANCE THERAPY

Identify and eliminate known/suspected allergens.

DRUGS

- Mucolytics: act to thin the mucus and thereby improve mucociliary flow
  —Steam inhalation
  —Normal saline drops
  —Bicarbonate spray
  —N-acetylcysteine (orally or inhaled)
  —Oral guaifenesin
- Antihistamines: competitively blocking H1 receptors; suppress itching, ocular symptoms, sneezing, and rhinorrhea; not very effective against nasal congestion
- Second-generation antihistamines: tend to not cross the blood–brain barrier and therefore do not have central nervous system (CNS) side effects such as drowsiness.
  —Loratadine (Claritin, Schering): FDA-approved for children as young as 2 years. Dose: ages 2 to 5 years—5 mg PO daily; ages 6 years or older—10 mg PO daily.
  —Cetirizine HCl (Zyrtec, Pfizer): FDA-approved for children as young as 6 months. Dose: age 6 months to 5 years: 2.5 mg = 1/2 tsp (1 mg/mL banana-grape flavored syrup) PO daily with maximum dose of 5 mg per day (must be divided into 2.5 mg twice a day for children under 2 years of age).
  —Fexofenadine (Allegra, Aventis): 6 to 11 years: 30 mg tab b.i.d.; ≥12 years: 60 mg b.i.d. or 180 mg daily.
- First-generation antihistamine side effects include drowsiness, performance impairment, paradoxical excitement; anticholinergic side effects (e.g., dry mouth, tachycardia, urinary retention, and constipation)
  —Diphenhydramine (Benadryl) 5 mg/kg per day divided q.i.d.
- Intranasal steroids: Blunt early phase reactions and block late phase reactions; may not be fully effective until several days to 2 weeks after initiation of therapy. Must be used regularly and best when administered lying down with the head back.

—Beclomethasone (Vancenase, Beconase): for use in children ≥6 years
—Flunisolide (AeroBid): for use in children ≥6 years
—Fluticasone propionate (Flonase 0.05%): for use in children ≥4 years
—Budesonide (Rhinocort): for use in children ≥6 years
—Triamcinolone acetonide (Nasacort): ≥6 years
—Mometasone furoate monohydrate (Nasonex): for use in children ≥2 years
- Topical cromolyn (NasalCrom): mast-cell stabilizer; minimal side effects; does not provide immediate relief (may take 2 to 4 weeks to see clinical effect): for use in children ≥2 years
- Oral decongestants: α1- and α2-adrenergic agonists (e.g., ephedrine, pseudoephedrine and phenylephrine) act to cause vasoconstriction, decreased blood supply to the nasal mucosa, and decreased mucosal edema. Cardiovascular and CNS side effects include tremors, agitation, hypertension, insomnia, and headaches.
- Topical decongestants: Sympathomimetics such as short-acting phenylephrine (Neo-Synephrine) and long-acting oxymetazoline (Afrin) may be useful for a few days to open nasal passages to allow for delivery of topical steroids; side effects include drying of the mucosa and burning. Use for more than a few (3 to 5) days may result in rebound vasodilatation and congestion (rhinitis medicamentosa).
- Combined oral decongestants and antihistamines: numerous preparations on the market.

IMMUNOTHERAPY

- Also referred to as hyposensitization or desensitization. Consists of a series of injections with specific allergens, with increasing concentrations of allergens, once or twice weekly
- Recommended for patients who have not responded to pharmacologic therapy
- Extremely effective and long-lasting. After several months to years of treatment, total serum IgE levels decrease, and the intensity of the early-phase response is reduced.
- Side effects include urticaria, bronchospasm, hypotension, and anaphylaxis

SURGERY

- Removal of allergic polyps
- Inferior turbinate surgery to reduce the size of the turbinate and relieve obstruction
- Endoscopic sinus surgery to relieve obstruction

PREVENTION

- Minimize exposure to dust mites: consider removing carpets, upholstered furniture, and curtains; washing bedding in hot water frequently, at least every 1 to 2 weeks; using pillow and mattress covers.
- Minimize exposure to animal danders: minimize exposure to all animals, consider using solutions containing tannic acid, which will denature animal allergens; shampoo pets

frequently if pets cannot be removed from the household; use air vent filters.
- Minimize exposure to pollens: keep windows closed, use air conditioning, and avoid leaf-raking or lawn-mowing.
- Minimize exposure to molds: keep houseplants out of the bedroom; avoid spending time in the basement, keep humidity at 35% to 50%.

 Follow-Up

Two to 4 weeks after initial evaluation; then every 3 to 6 months

SIGNS TO WATCH FOR

Fever, prolonged or severe headache, dizziness, pain, or purulent discharge should suggest a diagnosis other than allergic rhinitis alone.

PROGNOSIS

Generally good. Complete recovery occurs in 5% to 10% of patients.

PITFALLS

- Skin tests may be difficult to interpret in patients with diffuse eczema and dermatographism.
- Cardiac arrhythmias have been seen with patients taking terfenadine and astemizole.

 Common Questions and Answers

Q: How does one minimize exposure to dust mites?
A: Keep household temperature low; maintain humidity at approximately 40% to 50%; wash linens weekly at hot temperatures; use a microfilter when vacuuming; place mattress and box spring in tightly woven casing; use air conditioning; use high-efficiency particulate air filter units.

Q: When used on a daily basis, are intranasal steroids safe?
A: Yes. It is generally accepted that inhaled steroids are safe. However, there is increasing evidence that inhaled and intranasal steroids are associated with a decrease in linear growth velocity.

ICD-9-CM 477.9

BIBLIOGRAPHY

Meltzer EO. Treatment options for the child with allergic rhinitis. *Clin Pediatr* 1998;37:1–10.

Skoner DS. New perspectives on pediatric allergic rhinitis: allergic rhinitis: definition, epidemiology, pathophysiology, detection, and diagnosis. *J Allergy Clin Immunol* 2001;108(1):S2–S8.

Lasley MV, Shapiro GG. Testing for allergy. *Pediatr Rev* 2000;21:39–43.

Authors: Esther K. Chung and Karen P. Zimmer

Rickets

 Database

DEFINITION

Failure or delay in the mineralization of growing bone primarily caused by a deficiency of vitamin D, calcium or phosphate

CAUSES

• See table, Causes and Management of Rickets.
• Children at risk for rickets:

—Low birth weight and/or premature infants
—Breast-fed infants who do not receive supplemental vitamin D
—Chronic renal insufficiency
—Cholestatic liver disease
—Inflammatory bowel disease
—Vegan diet

 Data Gathering

HISTORY

• Symptoms of hepatic, renal, or gastrointestinal disease?
• Prolonged breast-feeding without vitamin D supplementation?
• Little or no sunlight exposure (or being covered when exposed to sunlight)
• Adequate calcium intake? Lactose intolerance? Vegetarian diet?
• Factors influencing calcium absorption?

—Vitamin D intake
—Steatorrhea
—Antacids
—Anticonvulsants
—Diet high in foods containing oxalic acid

• Vitamin D fortified milk in children over 1 year of age.
• Prolonged use of cholestyramine?

Question: Factors influencing calcium excretion?
Significance:

• Diuretics, polyuria, or glycosuria suggestive of renal tubular dysfunction.
• Bone pain?
• Delayed standing or walking?
• Anorexia?
• Seizures?
• Pathologic fractures?
• Tetany?
• Familial history of rickets?

 Physical Examination

• Failure to thrive
• Long bone deformities (varus deformity or valgus deformity)
• Fractures following minimal trauma
• Skull abnormalities (delay in closure of anterior fontanelle, craniotabes and frontal bossing)
• Chest deformities (enlargement of costochondral junctions leading to rachitic rosary)
• Muscular hypotonia
• Waddling gait

 Laboratory Aids

See table, Classification of Rickets and Vitamin D Metabolite Levels.

• Circulating vitamin D metabolites (25-hydroxyvitamin D, 1,25-dihydroxyvitamin D)
• Circulating levels of parathyroid hormone (PTH)
• Serum Ca, P, Mg, alkaline phosphatase, and total CO_2
• Urinary Ca, P, Mg, pH, creatinine, and amino acids, exclude Fanconi syndrome and proximal renal tubular acidosis.

IMAGING

• Knee or wrist films (the earliest sign at the wrist is a loss of clear demarcation between the growth plate and the metaphysis with loss of the provisional zone of calcification)
• Radiographic findings: irregular cortices and bony margins, widened metaphyses, widened growth plates, osteopenia

Causes and Management of Rickets

CAUSE	MANAGEMENT
Calcium deficiency	
Low intake	<6 months of age 400 mg/d 6–12 months of age 600 mg/d 1–10 years of age 800 mg/d
Extreme prematurity (birth weight <1,500 g)	Adjust intake to 200 mg/kg per day
Steatorrhea	25-OH-D_3 (5–7 μg/kg per day) if serum levels are low and supplement dietary calcium between 25–100 mg/kg per day
Anticonvulsant (Phenobarbital or phenytoin)	Calcium <6 months of age 400 mg/d 6–12 months of age 600 mg/d 1–10 years of age 800 mg/d Vitamin D 200 IU/d of ergocalciferol
Renal tubular acidosis	Base supplement: 3–10 mM/kg per day as $NaHCO_3$ or citrate
Vitamin D deficiency	
Insufficient UV light exposure	200 IU/d of vitamin D of ergocalciferol
Breast-fed infants who are not supplemented with vitamin D	200 IU/d of vitamin D of ergocalciferol
Liver disease	4,000–8,000 IU/d ergocalciferol
Renal disorders	4,000–40,000 IU/d of Calcitriol
Nutritional rickets and osteomalacia	1,000–5,000 IU/d of ergocalciferol 3,000–5,000 IU/d of Calcitriol
Vitamin D-dependent rickets Vitamin D-resistant rickets	40,000–80,000 IU/d of ergocalciferol with phosphate supplements, daily dosage is increased at 3–4 month intervals in 10,000–20,000 IU increments
Phosphorus deficiency	
Diet (limited to premature infants)	Adjust formula or parenteral source to give 10 mg/kg per day
Antacid excess	Alternative gastric acid control
Excessive phosphaturia from tubular dysfunction	Supplemental P and calcitriol if low

Therapy

See table, Causes and Management of Rickets.

Follow-Up

- Monitor serum calcium, alkaline phosphatase, and phosphorus every 2 to 4 weeks; x-ray bones monthly until stabilized. An early radiographic sign of healing in the appearance of the provisional zone of calcification at the boundary between the physis and metaphysis

Common Questions and Answers

Q: What is the best way to diagnose rickets?
A: Laboratory investigation and radiographs are the best ways to diagnose rickets. The most common biochemical findings of children with vitamin D deficient rickets are hypocalcemia, hypophosphatemia, low 25-(OH)D concentrations, elevated PTH, and elevated alkaline phosphatase. The classic radiographic findings occur at the growth plate of long bones and are best seen at the distal end of the radius and ulna or at the tibial and femoral growth plates around the knee. Widening of the physis with fraying, cupping, and splaying of the metaphyses and underdevelopment of the epiphysis are common findings.

Q: What are the recommendations for vitamin D supplementation in infants and children?
A: To prevent rickets and vitamin D deficiency in healthy infants and children and acknowledging that adequate sunlight exposure is difficult to determine, the American Academy of Pediatrics recommends a supplement of 200 IU per day for the following:

All breast-fed infants unless they are weaned to at least 500 mL per day of vitamin D-fortified formula or milk.
All nonbreast-fed infants who are ingesting less than 500 mL per day of vitamin D-fortified formula or milk.
Children and adolescents who do not get regular sunlight exposure, do not ingest at least 500 mL per day of vitamin D-fortified milk, or do not take a daily multivitamin supplement containing at least 200 IU of vitamin D.

Q: What are the distinguishing features of vitamin D deficient and calcium deficient rickets?
A: The biochemical features (hypocalcemia, high alkaline phosphatase and high PTH) and radiographic (growth plate changes) are very similar. The distinguishing feature is the difference in vitamin D status. In vitamin D deficient rickets, 25(OH)D levels are low. Typically in calcium deficient rickets 25(OH)D levels are normal (>10 ng/mL) and $1,25(OH)_2D$ are high.

ICD-9-CM

Rickets 268.0
Renal rickets 588.0
Vitamin D-resistant rickets 275.3

BIBLIOGRAPHY

Abrams SA. Nutritional rickets: an old disease returns. *Nutr Rev* 2002;60(4):111–115.

Lawrence M, Gartner F, Greer R, and Section on Breastfeeding and Committee on Nutrition. Prevention of rickets and Vitamin D deficiency: new guidelines for Vitamin D intake. *Pediatrics* 2003;111(4):908–910.

Wharton B, Bishop N. Rickets. *Lancet* 2003;362(9393):1389–400.

Authors: Alisha J. Rovner and Maria Mascarenhas

Classification of Rickets and Vitamin D Metabolite Levels

	CALCIUM	PHOSPHORUS	ALKALINE PHOSPHATE	25 (OH)D
Deficient synthesis and supply	N or ↓	↓	↑	↓
No sunlight				
Poor diet				
Immaturity				
Malabsorption	N or ↓	↓	↑	↓
Liver disease	N or ↓	↓	↑	↓
Chronic renal failure	N or ↓	↑	↑	N
Vitamin D-dependent rickets (recessively inherited)	↓	↓	↑	N
Vitamin D-resistant rickets (sex-linked dominant)	N	↓	↑	N
Renal tubular disorders (defect of phosphate reabsorption)	N	↓	↑	N

N, normal; ↓, decreased; ↑, increased.

Rickettsial Disease

Database

DEFINITION

• The rickettsial diseases are a group of illnesses caused by the Rickettsiaceae family of organisms. Despite some minor differences in epidemiologic, clinical, and laboratory characteristics, the illnesses caused by these organisms have similar manifestations and treatment.
• The rickettsial diseases can be divided into subgroups based on clinical presentation: the spotted fever group, the typhus group, Q fever, and ehrlichiosis.
• Because these illnesses are organized primarily by clinical similarities, the spotted fever group includes the tick-borne typhus classification.

CAUSES

• The rickettsial illnesses with the exception of Q fever are transmitted to humans via insect vectors such as ticks, fleas, lice, or mites. Q-fever is acquired via inhalation of the body fluids of infected mammals.
• Rickettsial diseases occur in patients of all ages. Rocky Mountain spotted fever (RMSF) has a predilection for children.
• The rickettsial diseases that occur in the United States are RMSF (see Rocky Mountain Spotted Fever), murine typhus, rickettsialpox, epidemic typhus, Q fever, and ehrlichiosis.

PATHOLOGY/PATHOPHYSIOLOGY

• For the spotted fever, typhus, and ehrlichiosis groups: vasculitis caused by proliferation of organisms in the endothelial lining of small blood vessels
• Q fever: pneumonitis

COMPLICATIONS

• Venous thrombosis
• Pneumonitis
• Pericarditis, myocarditis, heart failure
• Severe disease occurs more commonly in patients with G6PD deficiency, cardiac insufficiency, or immunocompromise.

Differential Diagnosis

INFECTION

• Before the appearance of the rash, the constitutional symptoms associated with the spotted fevers result in a very wide differential diagnosis. After the appearance of the rash, the diagnoses are more limited: measles, meningococcemia, secondary syphilis, viral infections, coxsackievirus (hand-foot-and-mouth disease), infectious mononucleosis, enteroviral infection.
• Environmental (poisons): drug hypersensitivity reaction (toxicodermatosis)
• Tumors: leukemia with thrombocytopenia
• Immunologic: idiopathic thrombocytopenia purpura (ITP)
• Miscellaneous: leukocytoclastic angiitis, erythema multiforme/Stevens-Johnson syndrome

Data Gathering

Differentiating the illnesses listed depends on the travel history, history of exposure to certain mammals or insects, and the initial clinical presentation of the patient. This clinical presentation is categorized by the grouping: spotted fever group, typhus group, Q fever, and ehrlichiosis.

HISTORY

Question: Fever, headache, and rash?
Significance: In general, rickettsial disease should be considered in a patient with these complaints. The progression of the rash can be particularly helpful in considering the diagnosis.

Physical Examination

Differentiating clinical findings of each group are described subsequently, and the rashes associated with each illness are described in the table, Characteristics of the Generalized Rashes of the Rickettsial Diseases.

• Constitutional symptoms
• Hepatosplenomegaly
• "Tache noir" (black spot): the earliest finding in the spotted fever group originates at the site of the infecting bite; becomes necrotic, forming eschar; regional lymphadenopathy related to eschar; lesion usually found on the head in children and on the legs in adults; is present in between 30% and 90% of cases.

Significance: These symptoms suggest illness caused by the spotted fever group. Tache noir is present in 30% to 90% of cases.

• Impaired level of consciousness
• Myocardial and renal involvement
• Brill-Zinsser disease (BZD) is actually a recrudescence of a previous infection with epidemic (louse-borne) typhus caused by *Rickettsiaceae prowazekii*; BZD can occur years after the initial infection and is usually less severe than the initial episode of louse-borne typhus.

Significance: These symptoms suggest illness caused by the typhus group.

• A self-limited febrile illness characterized by headache, myalgias, and chest pain
• Pulmonary symptoms occur in some form in over 50% of cases: mild pneumonitis/cough usually an incidental finding; radiographically confirmed pneumonia in moderately ill patients; rapidly progressive pneumonia
• Endocarditis may occur.
• Hepatitis may range in severity.
• Nervous system findings range from headache to meningitis and encephalitis.

Significance: These symptoms suggest illness caused by *Coxiella burnetii*, the organism responsible for Q fever.

Characteristics of the Generalized Rashes of the Rickettsial Diseases

	APPEARANCE	DISTRIBUTION	ASSOCIATED FINDINGS
Spotted fever group			Tache noir in 30% to 90% of patients
Tick typhus	Macular → papular	Extremities → palms/soles → trunk	
Rickettsialpox	Macular → papular → Vesicles	Extremities → palms/soles → trunk	
Scrub typhus	Macular	Limited to trunk	Rash of shorter duration lymphadenopathy is a prominent symptom
Typhus group			No tache noir
Epidemic (louse-borne) typhus	Macules → maculopapules → petechiae → hemorrhage	Trunk → extremities	
Murine typhus		Trunk → extremities	Less extensive rash of shorter duration
Miscellaneous			
Q fever	Macular or maculopapular or petechial	Trunk and extremities	No rash
Ehrlichiosis			Rash common in children; rare in adults

- Acute febrile illness characterized by headache, anorexia, and vomiting
- A relative bradycardia is often noted.
- Hyponatremia, leukopenia, and thrombocytopenia

Significance: These symptoms and signs suggest illness caused by *Ehrlichia chaffeensis*, the organism primarily responsible for human ehrlichiosis.

PHYSICAL EXAM TRICKS

Rashes that involve the palms and soles present a limited differential diagnosis. This list includes rickettsial diseases, certain viral infections such as coxsackievirus (hand-foot-and-mouth), syphilis, erythema multiforme, and urticarial rash.

 ## Laboratory Aids

Test: Polymerase chain reaction (PCR) from blood or tissue
Significance:

- Allows the identification of rickettsial-specific DNA sequences
- *R. rickettsii*, *R. typhi*, and *R. prowazekii*

Test: Immunofluorescent (IgM) tests
Significance:

- Sensitive, specific, and simple
- Can differentiate acute from past infection
- This technique is only useful early in the course of *R. tsutsugamushi* (scrub typhus) infection.
- Biopsy of the tache noir may reveal rickettsial organisms of the spotted fever group by direct immunofluorescent staining. Similar testing of the generalized rash is not useful for rickettsial illnesses other than RMSF.

Test: Serologic tests

- Complement fixation tests
- Enzyme-linked immunosorbent assay (ELISA)
- Latex agglutination test
- The Weil-Felix reaction assays the patients' serologic response to rickettsiae; the highest titers occur during the second and third weeks of illness; this test will be negative in patients with rickettsialpox and Q fever.
- PCR tests in blood and tissue are available for many rickettsial diseases.

FALSE POSITIVES

The Weil-Felix reaction may be falsely positive in testing for any of the above organisms.

PITFALLS

The headache associated with rickettsial infections can be severe. However, radiographic imaging is not necessary if there are no signs or symptoms of increased intracranial pressure.

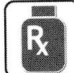 ## Therapy

EMERGENCY

- Fluid resuscitation for patients who appear moderately to severely ill.
- Antimicrobial therapy should be instituted as soon as the diagnosis is suspected and should not be delayed while awaiting serological confirmation.
- Therapy is most effective if instituted within the first week of illness.

DRUGS

- All of the rickettsial diseases respond rapidly to treatment doxycycline. Recommended dosage is dependant on the specific rickettsial infection being treated.
- Studies have shown that there is little risk of tooth staining in children under 8 years old who receive less than 14 days of doxycycline.
- Erythromycin, trimethoprim-sulfamethoxazole and fluoroquinolones have been used with variable success against rickettsial infections.

DURATION

The optimum duration of treatment for rickettsial infections has not been determined. In general, the more severe infections warrant 7 to 14 days of antimicrobial therapy.

POSSIBLE CONFLICTS

Prevention

- Except for *R. tsutsugamushi* (scrub typhus) and *Ehrlichia*, all of the rickettsial diseases produce long-term immunity to the etiologic organisms within the same group.
- Fleas, ticks, and mites should be controlled in endemic areas with the appropriate insecticides.
- Clothing to cover the entire body should be worn in tick-infested areas.
- In areas in which louse-borne typhus is epidemic, periodic delousing and dusting of insecticide into clothes is recommended.
- No vaccines are currently available in the United States.

 ## Follow-Up

WHEN TO EXPECT IMPROVEMENT

Improvement in the patient's clinical status usually takes place within 1 to 2 days of initiation of therapy. This improvement is delayed in severe cases, particularly if there is endocardial involvement (Q fever) or treatment is begun after the first week of illness.

PITFALLS

- Paradoxical effect of rodenticides: fleas, mites will seek alternate hosts such as humans when mice or rats are "unavailable." Therefore, rodenticides should not be the only prevention measure taken in endemic areas.
- In children younger than 8, failure to treat rickettsial infections promptly with doxycycline can result in the development of severe disease. The benefits of a single, short course of doxycycline outweighs the very small risk of dental staining in these children

 ## Common Questions and Answers

Q: What do I do if I or my child receives a tick bite in an endemic area to rickettsial disease?
A: There is no role for prophylaxis against rickettsial diseases for patients who have suffered tick bites.

Q: Are there differences between typhoid and typhus?
A: Typhoid, or typhoid fever, is a separate entity from typhus. Typhoid is an enteric infection caused by *Salmonella typhi* and is unrelated to the rickettsial diseases.

Q: If I contract a rickettsial illness, can I get that illness or a similar illness again?
A: With the exception of scrub typhus and *Ehrlichia*, infection with a rickettsial organism confers immunity to other rickettsia within the same group.

ICD-9-CM 083.9

BIBLIOGRAPHY

American Academy of Pediatrics. *2003 Red Book: Report of the Committee on Infectious Diseases.* 26th Ed. Elk Grove Village, IL: American Academy of Pediatrics, 2003.

Boyd AS. Rickettsialpox. *Dermatol Clin* 1997;15:313–318.

Dumler JS, Dey C, Meier F. Human monocytic ehrlichiosis: a potentially severe disease in children. *Arch Pediatr Adolesc Med* 2000;154: 847–849.

Edwards MS, Feigin RD. Rickettsial diseases. In: Feigin RD, Cherry JD, Demmler GJ, Kaplan SL eds. *Textbook of Pediatric Infectious Diseases.* 5th Ed. Philadelphia: WB Saunders, 2004.

Purvis JJ, Edward MS. Doxycycline use for rickettsial disease in pediatric patients. *Pediatr Infect Dis J* 2000;19:871–874.

Authors: Suzanne Dawid Joel A. Fein, 3rd Edition

Rocky Mountain Spotted Fever (RMSF)

Database

DEFINITION

Systemic illness (small vessel vasculitis) caused by infection with obligate intracellular gram-negative bacterium, *Rickettsia rickettsii*, carried by tick vectors: wood tick (*Dermacentor andersoni*) in east and far west United States; dog tick (*D. variabilis*) in East; Lone star tick (*Amblyomma americanum*) in Southwest; Rocky Mountain Wood tick (*D. andersoni*) in western United States; *Rhipicephalus sanguineus* in Mexico; *A. cajennense* in Central and South America

PATHOPHYSIOLOGY

• Transmission usually from tick (reservoir) bite; can be by transfusion and aerosol route
—Usually takes more than 6 to 10 hours (often 24 hours) to be transmitted with tick bite
• Incubation period 2 to 14 days, average approximately 7 days
• After exposure, *Rickettsia* multiply in small-vessel endothelium and disseminate via bloodstream, with focal areas of endothelial proliferation, thrombus, blood, and protein leakage
• Local vascular lesions account for signs and symptoms

EPIDEMIOLOGY

• Most prevalent rickettsial disease in United States (600 to 1,200 cases/year), most by *D. variabilis* ticks. Rickettsial disease reported worldwide.
• Seasonal (April to September most common) and geographic (0% to 20% prevalence in tick population reported)
—Endemic to south Atlantic and west south central regions. Reported from all states except Alaska, Hawaii, Maine, and Vermont
—Less often seen in Rocky Mountain states
—Also seen in Mexico, Central, and South America
—Has been reported in family (4% to 8%) and local clusters; pets (dogs) as well
• Up to two-thirds of patients younger than 15 years of age (usually 5 to 9 years of age)
• Usually requires >6 to 10 hours of tick exposure/feeding

COMPLICATIONS

• Complications uncommon with early and appropriate treatment
• Neurologic sequelae
—More common in children with severely impaired states of consciousness
—Behavioral disturbances and learning disabilities common
—Emotional lability, hyperactivity, memory loss, seizures
• Skin
—Gangrene of extremities, end-organs, skin necrosis
—Skin rash usually heals without sequelae
• Hematologic
—Can progress to DIC
• Gastrointestinal
—Hepatic dysfunction

—Hypoalbuminemia from protein loss, hepatic dysfunction, protein leak from damaged vessels
• Cardiac
—Can have persistent cardiac findings, congestive heart failure, cardiovascular collapse
• Metabolic
—Hyponatremia from water shift to intracellular spaces, sodium loss in urine
• Renal
—Acute tubular necrosis

PROGNOSIS

• No known asymptomatic infection (prognosis related to recognition and timing of appropriate therapy)
—May be mild if treated early
• Recovery the rule if treated in 5 to 7 days
• Case fatality approximately 3% to 7% if treated, 25% if untreated (23% before antibiotics in 1939 to 1945)
—Death usually between eighth and 15th day (fulminant cases with death in 5 to 6 days)

Differential Diagnosis

• Infection
—Sepsis, meningitis, encephalitis, rubeola, atypical measles, meningococcemia, typhoid fever, leptospirosis, toxic shock, rubella, scarlet fever, disseminated gonococcal disease, *Haemophilus influenzae*, secondary syphilis, rheumatic fever, bacterial pneumonitis, poliomyelitis, pharyngitis, mumps, hepatitis, mononucleosis, enterovirus and other virus infections, fever of unknown origin, ehrlichiosis (has been reported to occur concurrently), other rickettsial disease, Kawasaki disease, gastroenteritis, meningitis, URI, pneumonitis
• Other
—Immune thrombocytopenic purpura (ITP), thrombotic thrombocytopenic purpura (TTP), immune complex vasculitis, drug reaction, ischemic heart disease, rheumatoid arthritis, erythema multiforme, intra-abdominal process, acute surgical abdomen

Data Gathering

HISTORY

Question: Abrupt or gradual onset of fever
Significance: Often unresponsive to antipyretics or antibiotics, headache (retrobulbar, frontal), rash, confusion, myalgia, nausea, vomiting, abdominal pain
• Classic triad of fever, headache, and rash only in approximately 50%
• Headache: characteristic; intense, persistent night and day, intractable; young child may not complain of headache
• Fever to more than 40°C (104°F) with oscillations of approximately 2°C (two-thirds with fever >38.9°C [>102°F] in first 3 days)
• Onset usually 2 to 8 days post-tick bite
• Tick bite history obtained in only 50% to 70% of cases

Physical Examination

Finding: Rash
Significance: Usually appears by second or third day of illness; may be delayed until sixth day or later; small percentage (10% to 15%) never develop rash; absence of rash should not delay presumptive diagnosis or appropriate therapy if disease suspected.
• Usually small, irregular, erythematous macules that blanch, become maculopapular and petechial (mixed rash), and confluently hemorrhagic
• Appears first (usually) on wrists and ankles, spreads centrally within hours to extremities to trunk, neck, and face; regularly occurs on palms and soles (may be spared) and scrotum; may initially appear on trunk or diffusely in some patients; can progress to necrosis of toes, ears, nose, scrotum, fingers
• May be more difficult to detect in African Americans

Finding: CNS
Significance: Meningismus, restless, irritable, apprehensive, confusion, delirium, lethargy, stupor, coma, ataxia, opisthotonos, aphasia, papilledema, seizures, cortical blindness, central deafness, ataxia, spastic paralysis, cranial nerve palsy

Finding: Cardiac
Significance: CHF, myocarditis, arrhythmias, vascular collapse (often volume related)

Finding: Pulmonary
Significance: Pneumonitis, cough, dyspnea, pulmonary edema, hypoxemia, pleural effusions, alveolar infiltrates

Finding: Gastrointestinal
Significance: Nausea, vomiting, abdominal pain, diarrhea, hepatomegaly, splenomegaly, anorexia, jaundice, mild pancreatitis

Finding: Myalgias
Significance: Especially calf or thigh

Finding: Ocular involvement
Significance: Conjunctivitis, venous engorgement, papilledema, cotton wool spots, retinal hemorrhages, retinal artery occlusion, uveitis

Finding: Other
Significance: Edema of extremities or face; parotitis, orchitis, pharyngitis

Laboratory Aids

Make presumptive diagnosis on signs, symptoms, history, exposures and epidemiologic considerations rather than on laboratory aids.

• No quick or early specific laboratory test; serologic data reliable by days 10 to 12; negative test does not exclude diagnosis.
• Culture impractical and potentially dangerous

SPECIFIC TESTS

Test: Serology
Significance: Not usually useful in acute management as a result of time required for

serology to become positive (6 to 10 days after clinical onset of disease)

Test: Probable confirmation
Significance: Fourfold increase in antibody titer by complement fixation (CF), indirect hemagglutination (IHA), indirect fluorescent antibody (IFA), latex agglutination (LA), microagglutination (MA), or single titer of at least 1:320 by Proteus OX-19 or OX-2 (Weil-Felix); 1:128 by LA, IHA, MA, 1:64 by IFA, or at least 1:16 by CF

Test: Enzyme-linked immunosorbent assay (ELISA)
Significance: Sensitive and accurate, but not useful until seroconversion at approximately day 6

Test: Direct immunofluorescence
Significance: Most sensitive and specific, but observer bias; can see immunofluorescent Rickettsia from skin rash biopsy between days 4 and 8

Test: IFA
Significance: Sensitivity 94% to 100%; specificity 100%

Test: IHA
Significance: Sensitivity 91% to 100%; specificity 99%

Test: LA
Significance: Sensitivity 71% to 94%; specificity 96% to 99%; false positive noted during pregnancy

Test: DNA polymerase chain reaction (PCR)
Significance: Takes 48 hours but can detect the organism from lesion or blood (depends on organism load; therefore, lesion usually better than blood), specific, low sensitivity.

Test: Weil-Felix
Significance: Nonspecific and insensitive, but readily available and rapid (3 to 5 minutes); sensitivity 47% to 70%, specificity 78% to 96%; positive early in course; titer greater than 1:160 suspicious. False positive with *Proteus* infections (UTI), leptospirosis, brucellosis, typhoid fever, liver disease, pregnancy. Not recommended for RMSF evaluation.

Test: CF
Significance: Sensitivity 0% to 63%, specificity 100%

Test: MA
Significance: Specific, not sensitive

NONSPECIFIC TESTS

Test: CBC, electrolytes, BUN, CR, LFT, DIC screen, CXR, ABG, ECG, echocardiogram
Significance: Nonspecific, not especially helpful in diagnosis. WBC normal or low for first 4 to 5 days; after that, leukocytosis (11,000 to 30,000/mm^3) associated with secondary bacterial disease; elevated band count; anemia (30%); thrombocytopenia (consumptive coagulopathy); hyponatremia; hypoalbuminemia, prolonged prothrombin time, decreased fibrinogen (consumption), increased transaminases, and creatine kinase.

Test: CSF
Significance: Usually clear (WBC <10), but may see pleocytosis in one third and increased protein one-half of patients.

 ## Therapy

- Supportive care very important
—Volume, electrolyte support as indicated
- Platelets as indicated for thrombocytopenia
- Vitamin K (IM) for prolonged clotting time
- Hyponatremia management with fluid restriction as able (avoid sodium supplements)
- Albumin if indicated

MEDICATIONS

- All rickettsiostatic, not rickettsicidal
—Hinder replication so host can eradicate disease
—Duration: 5 to 10 days of therapy or until afebrile 2 to 5 days
- Doxycycline (usual medication of choice in all patients, except those who are pregnant)
—Dosage: child: 2.2 mg/kg PO b.i.d. for 1 day, then 2.2 mg/kg per day PO in single dose; adult: 100 mg PO b.i.d. (IV route if indicated)
—Also treats ehrlichiosis (similar presentation) if diagnosis uncertain
—Side effects: less likely to stain teeth than tetracycline, contraindicated during pregnancy
- Chloramphenicol
—Dosage: child: 75 to 100 mg/kg per day IV (initially) (modify if age <1 month), follow by 50 mg/kg per day divided q.i.d.; adult: 500 to 1,000 mg q.i.d.
—Side effects: peripheral neuropathy, aplastic anemia, "gray baby syndrome" with high levels, possible association with leukemia, hemolytic anemia with G6PD
—May not be as effective as tetracyclines or against ehrlichiosis
- Tetracycline
—Dosage: child: 25 to 50 mg/kg per day PO divided q.i.d. or 20 to 30 mg/kg per day IV; adult: 500 mg q.i.d. PO or IV
—Side effects: tooth discoloration if child younger than 8 years of age (dose and duration related); pseudotumor cerebri, photosensitivity reaction, contraindicated during pregnancy
- Other antibiotics
- Corticosteroids
—May be helpful in severe cases, though no controlled studies
—Not recommended for mild or moderately ill patients

 ## Follow-Up

- Expect improvement in 24 to 36 hours and defervescence in 2 to 3 days.
- Majority improve if treated early (<1 week)

CONTROL MEASURES

- Avoidance of tick-infested areas and tick contact; wear long clothing, pants tucked in socks or boots, limit skin access to ticks, frequent inspection (buddy checks)
- Tick repellants
- Early removal; ticks must attach and feed for 4 to 6 hours or longer to transmit disease; avoid direct contact with tick during removal; remove tick with tweezers (or gloved fingers

if tweezers not available) at point of attachment (as close to skin as possible), apply steady upward traction until tick's grip released and clean wound. Don't crush tick as this may increase disease transmission. Matches, petroleum jelly, fingernail polish, and rubbing alcohol do not appear to be effective for removal.
- Vaccine not available in United States; may not prevent disease but does prevent deaths
- Immunity conferred after disease

PITFALLS

- Not considering diagnosis until rash present; fatal disease often without rash at initial presentation
- Not treating empirically (with tetracyclines) if clinical suspicion of diagnosis
- Do not exclude diagnosis even if without history or evidence of tick bite and/or negative serologic test(s).
- Disease may occur outside endemic or reported areas and the usual summer months.
- Classic descriptions of RMSF occur in second week. Initial presentations often are not classic.

 ## Common Questions and Answers

Q: For whom should RMSF as a differential diagnosis be entertained?
A: Anyone with a fever during the spring and summer who has been in an RMSF endemic area, regardless of presence of rash or history of known tick bite. Nonspecific symptoms or signs (GI, respiratory, rashes) may lead to misdiagnosis and delay in therapy.

Q: Should a child with a tick bite receive antibiotic prophylaxis when a tick is discovered?
A: To contract disease, one must be bitten by a tick that actually carries the disease (low risk), the tick must transmit the Rickettsia before it is removed (low risk-requires >6 to 10 hours of feeding), and the Rickettsia must be pathogenic if inoculated (low risk). There is no evidence that prophylaxis is necessary or efficacious in preventing disease. If considered, one must weigh risks and benefits of the therapy to be used.

ICD-9-CM 082.0

BIBLIOGRAPHY

Bleck TP. Central nervous system involvement in rickettsial diseases. *Neurol Clin* 1999;17(4):801–812.

Holman RC, Paddock CD, Curns AT, et al. Analysis of risk factors for fatal Rocky Mountain spotted fever: evidence for superiority of tetracyclines for therapy. *J Infect Dis* 2001;184(11):1437–1444.

Masters EJ, Olson GS, Weiner SJ, Paddock CD. Rocky Mountain spotted fever: a clinician's dilemma. *Arch Intern Med* 2003;163(7):769–774.

Author: George Anthony Woodward

Roseola—Herpes 6,7—*Exanthema subitum*

 Database

DEFINITION

Roseola infantum is a common illness in preschool-aged children characterized by fever lasting 3 to 7 days followed by rapid defervescence and the appearance of a blanching maculopapular rash (usually on the fourth day of illness) lasting only 1 to 2 days.

CAUSES

- Roseola-like illnesses have been associated with a number of different viruses including enteroviruses (Coxsackie virus A and B, echoviruses); adenoviruses (types 1, 2, 3); parainfluenza virus; measles vaccine virus.
- A major cause of roseola appears to be human herpesvirus 6 and 7 (HHV-6). HHV-6 is a herpes virus similar to Epstein-Barr virus and cytomegalovirus.
- HHV-6 was first associated with roseola infantum by Yamanishi and associates in 1988.
- HHV-6 and -7 account for 20% to 40% of unexplained febrile illness in emergency department visits by febrile infants 6 months to 2 years of age.

PATHOPHYSIOLOGY

- Unknown
- The typical pattern of rash appearing as the fever disappears may represent virus neutralization in the skin.

EPIDEMIOLOGY

- Roseola can occur throughout the year; outbreaks have occurred in all seasons of the year.
- Roseola affects children from 3 months to 4 years. The peak age is 7 to 13 months.
- Ninety percent of cases occur in the first 2 years of life.
- Cases occur in males and females equally.
- Incubation period is 5 to 15 days.

COMPLICATIONS

- Seizures are the most common complication of roseola. Between 5% and 10% of children will have a generalized tonic-clonic seizure associated with fever.
- Aseptic meningitis with less than 200 cells with primarily mononuclear cells has been reported.
- Encephalitis
- Thrombocytopenic purpura

PROGNOSIS

The vast majority of children with roseola infantum recover without sequelae.

 Differential Diagnosis

- Roseola has a distinctive presentation but resembles other viral exanthems.
- Antibiotic-associated rash in a child taking oral antibiotics when rash develops after defervescence.
- Rubella and enteroviral infections.

 Data Gathering

HISTORY

Question: Febrile?
Significance: Period of 3 to 5 days; commonly in the 38.9°C to 40.6°C range (102°F to105°F)

Question: Rash?
Significance: Appears as the fever disappears and lasts for 1 to 2 days

Question: Mild cough and coryza?
Significance: Common symptoms

Question: Appearance?
Significance: Usually children remain alert and are not ill appearing.

Question: Lymphadenopathy?
Significance: Common in the suboccipital, posterior cervical, and postauricular regions

Question: Eyelid edema and a bulging fontanelle?
Significance: Has also been noted

Laboratory Aids

Laboratory tests are not helpful in diagnosis. Commercial assays for antibody and/or antigen detection for HHV-6 are being developed.

Test: CBC
Significance: Occasionally, leukopenia with lymphocytosis is noted.

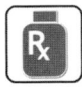 ## Therapy

SUPPORTIVE CARE

Prevention

• The virus associated with roseola infantum is usually transmitted via respiratory secretions or the fecal/oral spread.
• Outbreaks in hospitals have been reported, and infection control measures, such as bedside secretion precaution, should be instituted.

PITFALLS

Calling viral exanthems in preschool-aged children roseola even when fever is concomitant with rash

 ## Common Questions and Answers

Q: When can the child with roseola return to day care?
A: As soon as the child is afebrile; then there is no infectious risk of spread. The child may return to day care even with the rash visible.

Q: Will there be long-term sequelae in the child who has a seizure associated with roseola?
A: In general, these seizures are typical febrile seizures that hold no risk for long-term neurologic sequelae, e.g., epilepsy.

ICD-9-CM 056.9

BIBLIOGRAPHY

American Academy of Pediatrics. Human herpes virus 6. In: Peter G, ed. *1994 Red Book: Report of the Committee on Infectious Diseases.* 23rd Ed. Elk Grove Village, IL. American Academy of Pediatrics, 1994:272–273.

Cherry JD. Roseola infantum. In: Feigin RD, Cherry JD, eds. *Textbook of Pediatric Infectious Diseases.* 3rd Ed. Philadelphia: WB Saunders, 1992:1789–1791.

Jackson MA, Sommeraver JF. Human herpes virus 6 and 7. *Pediatr Infect Dis J* 2002;21:565–566.

Leach CT, Sumaya CV, Brown NA. Human herpes virus-6: clinical implication of a recently discovered, ubiquitous agent. *J Pediatr* 1991;121:173–181.

Stoeckle MY. The spectrum of human herpes virus 6 infection: from roseola infantum to adult disease. *Annu Rev Med* 2000;51: 423–430.

Author: Louis M. Bell

Rotavirus

 Database

DEFINITION

Infection with rotavirus causes high fever, profuse nonbloody diarrhea and vomiting lasting 4 to 8 days. It is the most common cause of severe gastroenteritis in children in both the developed and developing worlds. All children have serologic evidence of infection by 4 years of age.

PATHOPHYSIOLOGY

• The cause of diarrhea is unknown but is believed to be a result of multiple disruptions in the normal mechanisms of water reabsorption in the gut:

—Peptides encoded in the viral genome disrupt the transport of glucose and salt resulting in increased water within the gut.
—Decreased levels of intestinal disaccharidases including lactase result in malabsorption of sugars.
—Viral replication within enterocytes results in atrophy and ischemia of small intestinal villi.
—Infection with rotavirus results in activation of the enteric nervous system resulting in abnormal stimulation of water secretion into the GI tract.

EPIDEMIOLOGY

• Rotavirus is the most common cause of severe gastroenteritis throughout the world.
• Infection accounts for 20% to 50% of pediatric hospitalizations for gastroenteritis.
• Causes more than 500,000 deaths/year in developing countries
• In the United States, rotavirus infection causes at least 50,000 hospitalizations/year and 20 to 40 deaths/year.
• Rotavirus has a predictable seasonality depending on location. In North America, peaks occur in the late summer in the south, moving northward and eastward. In the northeast United States and Canada the highest incidence of disease occurs in late winter. In tropical regions, disease occurs throughout the year.
• Majority of disease occurs in children 6 to 24 months old.
• All children have serologic evidence of disease by the age of 4.
• Incubation period is 12 hours to 4 days.
• Exposure to as few as 200 viral particles can result in disease. The virus can persist on surfaces for prolonged periods of time.
• Virus can be shed asymptomatically but shedding can precede disease by 2 days and typically persists for 10 days.

COMPLICATIONS

• Disease is typically self-resolving, however, 20% if first time infections are moderate to severe and require medical attention. Severe dehydration can occur resulting in acidosis and electrolyte disruptions.
• Diarrhea may be more severe and protracted in immunocompromised hosts.

 Differential Diagnosis

• Viral—Adenovirus, astrovirus and calicivirus (Norwalk virus)
• Bacterial—*Salmonella*, *Shigella*, Campylobacter, *Eschericha. coli*, *Yersina*, *Vibrio*, *Plesiomonas*, *Aeromonas*, *Clostridium difficile*
• Parasitic—*Giardia*, *Cyclospora*, *Isospora*, *Cryptosporidium*

 Data Gathering

HISTORY

• Presents with high fever and vomiting with as many as 20 watery stools a day.
• Diarrhea can test heme positive but is not grossly bloody.
• Up to 10% of children present with vomiting and/or fever without diarrhea.
• Fifty percent of parents of infected infants are also infected, however, only one-third of these are symptomatic.

 Physical Examination

• Consistent with dehydration.

Laboratory Aids

- Rotavirus ELISA testing for the presence of viral protein in the stool is highly sensitive and specific.
- Stool tends to be negative for leukocytes, however this testing is rarely useful.
- Testing for malabsorption via stool assays for reducing substances or by D-xylose absorption assays are often positive.
- Sixty-seven percent of hospitalized children have mild elevations in their transaminases.

Therapy

- Supportive care with either oral or intravenous rehydration depending on disease severity.
- Limited studies have suggested that the addition of lactobacillus early in infection may decrease the duration of symptoms.

CONTROL MEASURES

- Reduction of person-to-person transmission by proper hygiene especially in childcare settings.
- A tetravalent simian/human rotavirus reassortant vaccine was licensed in 1998 and recommended as part of the routine infant immunization schedule. Vaccination was associated with a 60% reduction in rotavirus related diarrhea and an 85% reduction in severe illness associated with infection. The vaccine was withdrawn from the market in 1999 after administration of the vaccine was linked to a small but significant increase in the incidence of intussusception.
- Two new vaccines using a bovine/human reassortant virus and an attenuated human strain are currently undergoing testing in large clinical trails.
- Small studies on hospitalized patients have suggested that the prophylactic use of probiotics may decrease the incidence of nosocomially acquired rotavirus infection.

Common Questions and Answers

Q: When should children with rotavirus infection resume feeding?
A: Feeding early in the course of disease promotes intestinal healing and should be instituted within 24 hours of illness. Infants should be given breast milk, diluted or regular strength formula. Children should be given lactose-free carbohydrate-rich foods. Juices and sodas should be avoided because of their high sugar content.

Q: Are antiemetics or antidiarrheal agents useful in the treatment of children with rotavirus infection?
A: No. There have been no studies demonstrating efficacy of these medications in children.

Q: Is natural infection protective against subsequent infections?
A: Somewhat. The first episode of rotavirus infection tends to be the most severe, however, reinfection can occur although it is often asymptomatic.

BIBLIOGRAPHY

Offit PA, Clark HF. Rotavirus. In: Mandell GM, Bennett JE, Dolin R, eds. *Mandell: Principles and Practice of Infectious Diseases.* 5th Ed. Philadelphia: Churchill Livingstone, Inc., 2000:1696–1700.

Rosenfeldt V, Michaelsen KF, Jakobsen M, et al. Effect of probiotic Lactobacillus strains in young children hospitalized with acute diarrhea. *Pediatr Infect Dis J* 2002;21(5):411–416.

Szajewska H, Kotowska M, Mrukowicz JZ, Armanska M, Mikolajczyk W. Efficacy of Lactobacillus GG in prevention of nosocomial diarrhea in infants. *J Pediatr* 2001;138(3): 361–365.

Author: Suzanne Dawid

Salicylate Poisoning (Aspirin)

 Database

DEFINITION

- Salicylate poisoning may occur with acute or chronic overdosage of:

—Acetylsalicylic acid (aspirin)
—Methyl salicylate (oil of wintergreen)
—Bismuth subsalicylate (PeptoBismol)
—Salicylic acid (a keratolytic)

- The potentially toxic acute oral dose of acetylsalicylic acid is >150 mg/kg.

PATHOPHYSIOLOGY

- Ingested drug is absorbed in stomach and proximal intestine.
- With therapeutic aspirin dosing, serum levels peak in 1 to 2 hours (standard preparations) or 4 to 6 hours (enteric coated).
- After oral overdose, absorption may be prolonged and erratic.
- Acetyl salicylate ingestion may produce gastritis, and may trigger centrally mediated vomiting.
- After overdose, the elimination half-life of salicylate becomes prolonged.
- As blood pH falls, the proportion of nonionized salicylate rises, and more salicylate shifts into tissues including brain.
- Toxic salicylate exposures uncouple mitochondrial oxidative phosphorylation and increase oxygen consumption.
- Direct stimulation of the medullary respiratory center leads to hyperventilation and respiratory alkalosis.
- Multiple metabolic derangements produce a wide anion gap metabolic acidosis.
- Dehydration and electrolyte shifts are common.
- Pulmonary and/or cerebral edema may occur.

EPIDEMIOLOGY

- Analgesics are the most common drugs implicated in poisoning exposures among children less than 6 months of age.
- Salicylate preparations comprise approximately 12% of all analgesic poisoning exposures reported to poison control centers.

COMPLICATIONS

- Nausea and vomiting
- Dehydration
- Metabolic acidosis
- Electrolyte abnormalities
- Disorientation, coma, seizures
- Noncardiogenic pulmonary edema
- Renal failure
- Cerebral edema and death

PROGNOSIS

- Chronic therapeutic misuse often leads to delayed diagnosis, and has the most serious prognosis.
- Single acute ingestion of >300 mg/kg acetyl salicylic acid should be considered life-threatening.

ASSOCIATED DISEASES

- Aspirin is often marketed in combination with other pharmaceuticals, which may complicate drug overdose situation.
- Adolescents frequently overdose on more than one drug preparation.
- Therapeutic use of acetyl salicylic acid among children with influenza has been associated with the occurrence of Reye Syndrome.

 Differential Diagnosis

- Gastroenteritis
- Pneumonia
- Metabolic disease
- Ketoacidosis
- Sepsis
- Meningitis/encephalitis

 Data Gathering

HISTORY

Question: Taking aspirin?
Significance: Aspirin poisoning mimics many illnesses, and chronic overdosage often results in delayed diagnosis.

Question: Enteric coated?
Significance: Enteric coating may lead to significantly delayed drug absorption.

Question: Timing of ingestion?
Significance: Allows for proper consideration of the risks versus benefits of gastrointestinal (GI) decontamination.

Question: Tinnitus?
Significance: Frequently associated with serum salicylate levels >25 mg/dL.

 Physical Examination

Finding: Hyperpnea
Significance: Indicates primary central hyperventilation and compensation for metabolic acidosis.

Finding: Hyperpyrexia
Significance: Presence of "fever" may confuse salicylism with infection.

Finding: Hypoxia
Significance: Pulmonary edema complicates therapy of aspirin overdose.

Finding: Hypotension
Significance: Indicates severe dehydration, likely complicated by metabolic acidosis and salicylate-mediated cardiotoxicity.

Finding: Encephalopathy
Significance: CNS depression or seizures represent grave toxicity.

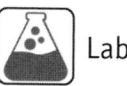 Laboratory Aids

TESTS

Test: Serum electrolytes
Significance: A wide anion gap metabolic acidosis is common, and hypoglycemia or hyperglycemia may occur.

Test: Arterial blood gas
Significance: May show mixed respiratory alkalosis/metabolic acidosis.

Test: Salicylate level
Significance: Serum salicylate levels greater than 60 to 100 mg/dL (acute) or 30 to 40 mg/dL (chronic) portend serious toxicity.

Test: Urine pH
Significance: Allows monitoring of adequacy of urinary alkalinization.

Test: Acetaminophen level
Significance: Acetaminophen may be a coingestant.

Test: Ferric chloride test
Significance: A few drops of 10% ferric chloride will turn brown or purple in 1 mL of urine that contains salicylate.

PITFALLS

- Respiratory acidosis suggests CNS depression and is an ominous sign.
- Salicylate levels after chronic, or acute-on-chronic, overdose correlate poorly to clinical condition.
- Serial salicylate levels may be necessary to rule-out ongoing drug absorption.

Salicylate Poisoning (Aspirin)

 Therapy

GI DECONTAMINATION

• Activated charcoal, 1 g/kg (max ~75 g), may be administered if aspirin is judged to be present in the stomach or proximal intestine.
• Many authorities suggest a second charcoal dose 2 to 4 hours after the first, or if salicylate levels continue to rise.
• Whole-bowel irrigation may reduce drug absorption after large overdoses.

FLUIDS/ALKALINIZATION

• Intravascular volume should be repleted with intermittent boluses of 10 to 20 mL/kg of normal saline.
• Altered mentation may imply CNS hypoglycemia, and should be treated with dextrose.
• Acidemia should be treated with sodium bicarbonate to limit salicylate distribution to the brain.
• With significant poisoning, an intravenous infusion of 5% dextrose with 100 to 150 mEq/L of sodium bicarbonate and up to 20 to 40 mEq/L of potassium chloride should be initiated at 1.5 to 2 times maintenance requirements.

—Titrate fluid volume to produce urine output of 1 to 2 mL/kg per hour
—Titrate alkalinization to produce urine pH between 7.5 and 8
—Greatly increases the urinary elimination of salicylate via "ion-trapping" effect

HEMODIALYSIS INDICATIONS

• Acute serum salicylate level >100 mg/dL
• Chronic serum salicylate level >60 mg/dL
• Severe acidosis or severe electrolyte disturbance
• Renal failure
• Persistent neurologic dysfunction
• Progressive clinical deterioration

PITFALLS

• Endotracheal intubation, if performed, must be accompanied by hyperventilation to prevent worsening acidemia and salicylate distribution to the brain.
• Hypokalemia may interfere with the ability to achieve urinary alkalinization.
• Pulmonary edema and/or cerebral edema may complicate fluid management.
• Hemodialysis equipment must be carefully primed to prevent worsening hypovolemia and cardiovascular collapse.

 Follow-Up

• Drug administration education should be offered to victims of chronic overdose.
• Mental health services should be provided to victims of intentional overdose.

 Common Questions and Answers

Q: What amount of the candy-scented oil of wintergreen is toxic to a toddler?
A: Oil of wintergreen may contain as much as 98% methyl salicylate. One milliliter of methyl salicylate is the equivalent of 1,400 mg of aspirin. Therefore, one teaspoon full of oil of wintergreen represents a very serious "aspirin" overdose.

Q: Is there a prognostic nomogram for aspirin poisoning similar to that used for acetaminophen overdose?
A: The Done nomogram was only applicable to ingestion of nonenteric coated aspirin by children with normal mentation and normal blood pH, and the validity of its prognostication is suspect. Its use is not widely recommended.

BIBLIOGRAPHY

Baxter AJ, Mrvos R, Krenzelok EP. Salicylism and herbal medicine. *Am J Emerg Med* 2003;21(5):448–449.

Bell AJ, Duggin G. Acute methyl salicylate toxicity complicating herbal skin treatment for psoriasis. *Emerg Med* 2002;14(2): 188–190.

Flomenbaum NE. Salicylates. In: Goldfrank LR, Flomenbaum NE, Lewin NA, et al, eds. *Goldfrank's Toxicologic Emergencies*. New York: McGraw-Hill, 2002:507–527.

Hahn IH, Chu J, Hoffman RS, Nelson LS. Errors in reporting salicylate levels. *Acad Emerg Med* 2000;7(11):1336–1337.

Wolowich WR, Hadley CM, Kelley MT, Walson PD, Casavant MJ. Plasma salicylate from methyl salicylate cream compared to oil of wintergreen. *J Toxicol Clin Toxicol* 2003;41(4):355–358.

Yip L, Dart RC, Gabow PA. Concepts and controversies in salicylate toxicity. *Emerg Med Clin North Am* 1994;12:351–364.

Author: Kevin C. Osterhoudt

Salmonella Infections

 Database

DEFINITION

Salmonella is responsible for a broad spectrum of pathologic states ranging from asymptomatic infection to acute gastroenteritis to enteric fever.

EPIDEMIOLOGY

• Three species are responsible for most human salmonellosis: *S. enteritidis* (over 2,000 serotypes exist), *S. choleraesuis*, and *S. typhi*.
• Reservoirs

—*Salmonella* species other than *S. typhi*: animals and animal products (mammals, birds, reptiles, and insects); contaminated food and water; infected humans (fecal excretion may persist several months).
—Humans are the only natural reservoir for *S. typhi*: most commonly transmitted via fecally contaminated food and water; may be transmitted congenitally; chronic carriers may excrete *S. typhi* in stool for years.

• Incubation period

—*Salmonella* species other than *S. typhi*: 6 to 72 hours; symptoms typically begin within 24 hours.
—Incubation period of invasive *Salmonella* strains and *S. typhi* is 1 to 3 weeks.

• Age distribution: children under 5 and the elderly most commonly infected with nontyphoidal *Salmonella*; *S. typhi* most common in 5- to 25-year-olds.

COMPLICATIONS

• Dehydration and/or electrolyte imbalance is the most common complication arising from acute gastroenteritis.
• Invasive *Salmonella* may lead to complications of bacteremia:

—Sepsis: most common in neonates and immunosuppressed individuals
—Meningitis: vast majority of cases occur in first month of life
—Osteomyelitis: most common in patients with sickle cell anemia
—Other local infections: pneumonia, pericarditis

• Complications of enteric fever include intestinal or splenic rupture (at areas of lymphoid hypertrophy), hepatitis, pancreatitis, parotitis, orchitis, arthritis, myocarditis.
• A postinfectious form of hemolytic uremic syndrome may occur following *Salmonella* infection.

PROGNOSIS

• Most normal hosts with *Salmonella* gastroenteritis will recover spontaneously.
• Some individuals will develop a chronic carrier state, persistently shedding bacteria in the stool.

• The relapse rate of enteric fever may approach 20% of patients even when adequately treated.

ASSOCIATED ILLNESSES

• Acute asymptomatic infection

—No clinical signs or symptoms become apparent.
—Probably most common *Salmonella* syndrome
—Patients can be identified only by recovery of organisms in stool.

• Acute gastroenteritis

—*Salmonella* is the most common type of infectious "food poisoning" in the United States.
—Symptoms begin 6 to 48 hours after *Salmonella* ingestion.
—Predominant manifestations are nausea, vomiting, crampy (often severe) abdominal pain, diarrhea (rarely, gross blood can be found).
—Other common features are malaise, myalgia, headache, and fever.
—Symptoms usually resolve spontaneously in 2 to 7 days.

• Bacteremia

—*Salmonella* organisms may produce acute or intermittent bacteremia.
—Symptoms: fever/chills, diaphoresis, myalgia, anorexia
—Bacteremia may occur before clinical gastroenteritis or, in infants, present as a persistent bacteremic state with failure to thrive.
—Up to 1 in 20 patients with *Salmonella* gastroenteritis may develop bacteremia (perhaps as high as 1 in 4 in infants).

• Enteric fever (typhoid fever, paratyphoid fever)

—Caused by *S. typhi* and several other *Salmonella* serotypes
—Incubation period 1 to 3 weeks
—Insidious onset of symptoms over 2 to 7 days: fever as high as 41°C, malaise, anorexia, abdominal pain, constipation.
—Additional symptoms and signs: lethargy, myalgia, headache, cough, either diarrhea or constipation, rigors, delirium, lymphadenopathy, organomegaly, "rose spots"
—Progression of illness: when untreated, illness with high fevers may last weeks; severe morbidity or death can result from especially virulent *Salmonella* strains.

• Asymptomatic chronic carriage

—Approximately 1% of patients infected with *Salmonella* gastroenteritis or enteric fever will continue to shed *Salmonella* in the stool for more than 1 year.

 Differential Diagnosis

The following illnesses may mimic *Salmonella* gastroenteritis and/or enterocolitis:

• Shigellosis: severe abdominal pains often are present, associated with high fevers, ulcers of the gastrointestinal lining are common, stools are often grossly bloody with "sheets" of fecal leukocytes.
• Staphylococcal food poisoning
• Other bacterial infections of the gastrointestinal tract
• Viral enteritis: rotavirus, Norwalk virus, and other viruses
• Parasitic infections
• Toxic ingestion
• Noninfectious systemic illnesses marked by inflammatory colitis

Enteric fever from *Salmonella* infection may be confused with:

• Invasive bacterial disease
• Spirochetal infection

 Data Gathering

HISTORY

• Exposure.

—History of eating raw or undercooked meat or eggs
—Exposure to pet lizards, turtles or snakes.

• Common historical features of *Salmonella* gastroenteritis:

—Nausea and vomiting begin 6 to 48 hours after ingestion.
—Diarrhea and abdominal pain with tenesmus follow; pain is typically periumbilical and in the right lower quadrant.
—Diarrhea lasts 2 to 4 days.
—Fever occurs in half of affected patients and seldom exceeds 39°C.

• Common historical features of enteric fever

—Symptoms begin 3 to 60 days after exposure.
—Commonly acquired during foreign travel
—Diarrhea uncommon early in course
—Fever ensues, which gradually increases in magnitude.
—Malaise, anorexia, myalgia, headache, abdominal pain, and vomiting may occur.

 Physical Examination

Salmonella gastrointestinal disease may display certain features:

• Dehydration may be evident.
• Abdominal pain may closely mimic appendicitis and/or cholecystitis.
• Stools may be bloody, watery, or mucousy.
• Enlarged liver and spleen
• Relative bradycardia for height of fever is a frequently distinguishing finding.
• Rose spots: 2 to 4 mm in diameter; blanching pink papules; most commonly found on anterior thorax; 5 to 20 are generally apparent at a time; fade in 3 to 4 days after appearance; characteristic of enteric fever, but not specific.

Salmonella Infections

 Laboratory Aids

There are several nonspecific laboratory aids to diagnosis:

Test: Stool and blood culture and identification of *Salmonella* organisms
Significance: The gold standard method for laboratory confirmation of infection

Test: Bone marrow aspirate
Significance: The most sensitive source for isolation of *Salmonella* in patients with enteric fever; early in the course of invasive illness bone marrow culture may be positive even when stool samples fail to grow the bacteria; may provide positive cultures even after initial antibiotic pretreatment.

Test: Urine culture
Significance: May be a source of *Salmonella* organisms in the young or elderly and in those with enteric fever

Test: Biopsy
Significance: Needle aspiration of purulent material may yield positive cultures; punch biopsy and culture of rose spots may confirm diagnosis of *S. typhi*.

FALSE POSITIVES

Leukocytes in the stool are suggestive of colitis but are more typical of *Campylobacter, Shigella,* or milk allergy.

PITFALLS

Enteric fever may precede enteritis symptoms and fecal shedding of bacteria.

Therapy

- Acute asymptomatic infection

—Should not be treated with antibiotics: antibiotics do not have impact on duration of diarrhea and may lengthen duration of carrier state.

- Acute gastroenteritis (see Common Questions and Answers)

—Supportive care: maintain intravascular volume; correct electrolyte abnormalities
—Do not administer antidiarrheal agents; they prolong gastrointestinal transit time.
—Consider antibiotics in individuals at high risk of subsequent systemic invasive illness: children younger than 3 months of age; immunocompromised hosts; patients with hemoglobinopathies; patients with chronic gastrointestinal tract disease.

- Bacteremia, enteric fever, and/or chronic carrier state:

—Supportive care
—Antibiotics are indicated; initial therapy usually to be administered intravenously
—Surgical drainage of local suppuration is indicated as in most other infections.
—Corticosteroids (3 mg/kg load, 1 mg/kg every 6 hours) may be beneficial to critically ill patients with enteric fever exhibiting neurologic complications.

—Antipyretics are controversial in enteric fever syndromes because they may cause precipitous declines in temperature and shock.

- Various antibiotics may be used to treat *Salmonella* infection:
- *Salmonella* gastroenteritis at high risk of invasive disease:

—Increasing resistance to amoxicillin, ampicillin, and trimethoprim-sulfa
—Parenteral third-generation cephalosporins or fluoroquinolones preferred.

- Invasive *Salmonella* disease

—Intravenous ampicillin for 2 weeks has been first-line therapy
—Chloramphenicol, a third-generation cephalosporin, or a quinolone may be used for resistant organisms
—Cefotaxime for treatment of meningitis; meningitis or osteomyelitis may require 4 to 6 weeks of parenteral antibiotic therapy.

- Some authorities treat chronic carriers of *Salmonella* who shed more than 1 year:

—High-dose parenteral ampicillin; high-dose oral amoxicillin (with or without probenecid),
—ciprofloxacin
—Consider cholecystectomy for recalcitrant cases.

PREVENTION

Personal hygiene and sanitation measures are the primary means by which to prevent *Salmonella* infections:

- Carriers of *Salmonella* are a public health concern:

—Hospitalized patients: enteric precautions for length of illness
—Outpatients: should be restricted from food preparation for others

- Two vaccines against *Salmonella typhi* are licensed for use in those living in high risk environments including those residing with a chronic carrier or living in an endemic area.

—The Ty21a vaccine is a live attenuated strain is given orally in four doses on alternating days. It is only approved for children older than 6 years old.
—The Vi capsular polysaccharide vaccine is a parenteral vaccine that is licensed for children over 2 years old.
—Both vaccines require frequent booster doses.

 Follow-Up

- Acute gastrointestinal illness

—Symptoms usually resolve spontaneously within 7 days.
—Supportive care to prevent or treat dehydration may be required.
—Young children and those with underlying disease processes may be at higher risk of complications.

- Enteric fever

—Untreated, this illness will have a prolonged course over weeks.
—Life-threatening complications are most common during the second or third week of illness, often after a period of apparent clinical improvement.
—Even with appropriate treatment up to 20% of patients may suffer relapse.

- Chronic carriage

—One percent to 3% of patients with *Salmonella* infection will shed bacteria in the stool for longer than 1 year.
—Chronic carriers should be identified because they represent a public health threat.

PITFALLS

- More people with *Salmonella* infestation are asymptomatic than are symptomatic.
- Antibiotic resistance is a growing problem.
- Even with appropriate therapy, patients may shed bacteria on a persistent basis or may suffer relapse.

 Common Questions and Answers

Q: Should all infants with *Salmonella* gastroenteritis be treated with antibiotics?
A: Clinicians caring for children younger than 1 year of life with proven, or suspected, *Salmonella* infection face many treatment dilemmas. Any toxic-appearing infant and any infant with proven *Salmonella* bacteremia should be admitted to the hospital for parenteral antibiotics. High-risk infants (those under 3 months of age) with positive stool cultures should be treated with antibiotics after obtaining blood cultures. Well-appearing infants above the age of 3 months with *Salmonella* enterocolitis and fever can be observed off antibiotics once surveillance blood cultures are obtained.

ICD-9-CM 003.9

BIBLIOGRAPHY

American Academy of Pediatrics. Salmonella. In: Pickering LK, ed. *2003 Red Book: Report of the Committee on Infectious Diseases.* 26th Ed. Elk Grove Village, IL: American Academy of Pediatrics, 2003.

Fierer J, Swancutt M. Non-typhoid salmonella: a review. *Curr Clin Top Infect Dis* 2000;20:134–157.

Goldberg MB, Rubin RH. The spectrum of Salmonella infection. *Infect Dis Clin North Am* 1988;2:571–598.

Sirinavin S, Garner P. Antibiotics for treating salmonella gut infections. *Cochrane Database of Systematic Reviews* 2000;(2):CD001167.

Stephens I, Levine MM. Management of typhoid fever in children. *Pediatr Infect Dis J* 2002;21(2):157–158.

Authors: Suzanne Dawid
Kevin C. Osterhoudt, 3rd edition

Sarcoidosis

Database

DEFINITION

A multisystem chronic granulomatous disease that has two distinct variations often differentiated by age of onset

CAUSES

Unknown

PATHOLOGY

- A T-cell–mediated disease, resulting in noncaseating granulomas in affected organs

EPIDEMIOLOGY

- Disease occurs before age 4 as arthritis, uveitis, fever, and rash, and in adolescence as Löfgren syndrome of erythema nodosum, polyarthritis, and hilar adenopathy. Adult-type disease with marked pulmonary involvement may also occur in older adolescents. CNS involvement (rare): seizures, cranial neuropathy, hypothalamic dysfunction.

GENETICS

Blacks are more commonly affected than Whites; specific genetic tendencies not identified.

COMPLICATIONS

In children, usually related to uveitis, or from hypercalciuria resulting in renal injury; in older adolescents, pulmonary problems such as restrictive lung disease can occur, and severe growth delay.

Differential Diagnosis

- Infection: tuberculosis, bacterial sepsis, mumps, HIV, gonorrhea, Lyme disease, pulmonary mycoses
- Tumors: leukemia, neuroblastoma, lymphoma
- Immunologic: pauciarticular JRA (for early onset type), systemic JRA, SLE, dermatomyositis, Behçet disease
- Genetic: Blau syndrome (hereditary granulomatous syndrome of synovitis, uveitis, and cranial neuropathy, as a result of defective CARD15/NOD2 gene)

Data Gathering

HISTORY

Question: Malaise, fever, rash, evanescent painful arthritis, swollen lymph nodes, chronic cough, and hematuria?
Significance: May be initial complaints.

Physical Examination

- Peripheral lymphadenopathy is most common manifestation.
- Eyes may be injected.
- Bilateral parotid gland enlargement and hepatosplenomegaly can be present.
- The arthritis, usually in the ankles, is extremely tender.
- Rash is diffuse, erythematous, macular, popular or plaque-like. Eythema nodosum occurs also.

SPECIAL QUESTIONS

Finding: History of papule?
Significance: Forming after needlestick (pathergy)

Laboratory Aids

- CBC
- ESR
- Synovial effusions are typically noninflammatory.
- Biopsy of peripheral lymph gland, skin, conjunctivae, or minor salivary gland demonstrating noncaseating granuloma is helpful.

Test: Angiotensin-converting enzyme (ACE) level
Significance: Produced in most granulomatous diseases, but is useful where index of suspicion is high

Test: Lysozyme level
Significance: May be more sensitive than ACE level for detecting sarcoidosis

Test: Serum calcium and creatinine levels
Significance: Are important for baseline

Test: Urine for blood
Significance: Seen in patients with hypercalciuria

IMAGING

Test: Chest radiograph
Significance: May demonstrate hilar adenopathy

Test: Gallium scan
Significance: Will demonstrate uptake diffusely in lungs (extremely sensitive test)

FALSE POSITIVES

Test: ACE level
Significance: May be elevated in patients with miliary TB and biliary cirrhosis. Not a good screening test; however, can follow levels in response to treatment

Test: Lysozyme level
Significance: also elevated in lymphoma

PITFALLS

Uveitis may be occult; ophthalmology evaluation is important.

Sarcoidosis

 Therapy

DRUGS

Nonsteroidal antiinflammatory drugs, analgesics, and steroids all have a role. In cases of chronic disease, immunosuppressive drugs, such as corticosteroids (oral and/or inhaled) and methotrexate, can be used. Tumor necrosis factor-α inhibitors (infliximab, etanercept) show promising preliminary results. In cases of hypercalciuria/hypercalcemia, hydration and furosemide should be considered.

DURATION

During times of disease activity causing clinical symptoms

DIET

Hydration is important in patients with hypercalcemia

 Follow-Up

WHEN TO EXPECT IMPROVEMENT

Early childhood sarcoid and Löfgren syndrome may resolve over several months. Rarely, older children with pulmonary manifestations may develop chronic interstitial lung disease or bony infiltrates over years of disease.

SIGNS TO WATCH FOR

Climbing creatinine, shortness of breath, or persistent uveal tract inflammation

PROGNOSIS

Generally good for most children. Löfgren syndrome resolves. Over 40% of older children with adult-type disease have persistent pulmonary changes, but only a few will have pulmonary symptoms.

PITFALLS

Overtreatment of asymptomatic lymphadenopathy and not detecting hypercalciuria

 Common Questions and Answers

Q: Why is the outcome better in childhood sarcoid compared with adults with sarcoid?
A: These may be two distinct granulomatous diseases. The two clearly have different patterns of organ involvement.

ICD-9-CM 135.0

BIBLIOGRAPHY

Baughmann RP, Iannuzzi M. Tumor necrosis factor in sarcoidosis and its potential for targeted therapy. *BioDrugs* 2003;17:425–431.

Baumann RJ, Robertson WC Jr. Neurosarcoid presents differently in children than in adults. *Pediatrics* 2003;112:e480–e486.

Cron RQ, Wallace CA, Sherry DD. Childhood sarcoidosis—does age of onset predict clinical manifestations? *J Rheumatol* 1997;24:1654–1656.

Fink CW, Cimaz R. Early onset sarcoidosis: not a benign disease. *J Rheumatol* 1997;24:174–177.

Gedalia A, Molina JF, Ellis GS Jr, et al. Low-dose methotrexate therapy for childhood sarcoidosis. *J Pediatr* 1997;130:3–4.

Hafner R, Vogel P. Sarcoidosis of early onset. A challenge for the pediatric rheumatologist. *Clin Exp Rheumatol* 1993;11:685–691.

Lindsley CB, Petty RE. Overview and report on international registry of sarcoid arthritis in childhood. *Curr Rheumatol Rep* 2000;2:343–348.

Pattishall EN Kendig EL Jr. Sarcoidosis in children. *Pediatr Pulmonol* 1996;22(3):195–203.

Shetty AK, Gedalia A. Sarcoidosis: a pediatric perspective. *Clin Pediatr* 1998;37:707–717.

Tomita H, Sato S, Matsuda R, et al. Serum lysozyme levels and clinical features of sarcoidosis. *Lung* 1999;177:161–167.

Authors: Frank Pessler and Randy Q. Cron

Scabies

Database

DEFINITION

• Scabies results from the infestation of the stratum corneum by the human mite, *Sarcoptes scabiei* (subspecies hominis, phylum Arthropoda, class Arachnida, and order Acarina). Etiologic agent is the gravid female mite, 0.2 to 0.4 mm in size.
• Animal scabies, sarcoptic mange, occurs from contact with an infested canine and produces only a transient rash in humans.
• Norwegian scabies, a variant of human scabies, occurs in institutional settings and is highly contagious, requiring isolation measures and diligent use of medications for elimination.
• Postscabetic syndrome consists of persistent pruritus, caused by hypersensitivity to the mite antigen and may persist for several days after the live mite has been eliminated.

PATHOPHYSIOLOGY

• The female mite burrows into the stratum corneum, rarely penetrating the epidermis, for 15 to 30 days, traveling 2 to 4 mm per day and laying one to three eggs per day.
• Egg laying is completed in 4 to 5 weeks when the female dies within the burrow. Eggs, hatching within the burrow, will undergo several molts and emerge on the skin surface as nymphs. After a 2- to 3-week maturation period, mating will occur; the male will die, and the gravid female will restart the cycle with burrowing.
• Signs and symptoms will develop ten to 30 days after scabies infestation, perhaps the time lag necessary for the body to develop humoral or cellular hypersensitivity to the mite and/or its byproducts or the time necessary for an adequate mass of mites to exist.

EPIDEMIOLOGY

• Affects all age groups.
• Approximately 300 million cases of scabies in the world annually.
• Epidemics are reported to occur in 15-year cycles.
• Sole reservoir of *S. scabiei* is the human.
• Close personal contact with an infested human (with or without clinical symptoms) is required for transmission.
• Mites can live isolated from a human body for 2 to 3 days; however, the extent of fomite transmission is unclear.

COMPLICATIONS

• Secondary infections, including impetigo and folliculitis
• Id eruption or autosensitization
• Pruritus

PROGNOSIS

Excellent outcome with therapy. Resistant cases, necessitating referral to a dermatologist and consideration for oral therapy, have been reported.

Differential Diagnosis

INFECTION

• Impetigo
• Papular viral exanthem

ENVIRONMENTAL

• Contact dermatitis

IMMUNOLOGIC

• Atopic dermatitis
• Papular urticaria

MISCELLANEOUS

• Drug eruption
• Psoriasis
• Infantile acropustulosis

Data Gathering

HISTORY

Question: Pruritus?
Significance: Intensity worse at night when mite activity increases secondary to a rise in body temperature.

Question: Evolution of the rash?
Significance: Characteristically changes over time both in appearance and distribution. The rash may consist of burrows, papules and vesicular lesions. Recurrent clusters of vesicles and pustules can occur over time. The rash may be seen in older children involving the webs of fingers, axillae, arms, wrists, waist line, and genitalia. In young children, the rash may include palms, soles, head, neck and face.

Question: Symptoms in other family members or close contacts?
Significance: Close contact is required for transmission.

Physical Examination

• Examine the entire body surface area with particular attention to the web spaces in the hands.
• Distribution of the rash is usually from the neck down in infants, although in children the neck and face also may be involved.
• Lesions are typically more numerous on the hands, especially the web spaces, and the thenar and hypothenar eminences in older children and adults. The palms and proximal half of the foot and heel are sites of numerous lesions in infants.
• Lesions are also seen on the wrists, in the axillae, around the waistline, on the gluteal cleft, and surrounding the nipples and genitalia.
• A burrow, the characteristic lesion of scabies, is present in 90% to 95% of all symptomatic patients, and forms a "lazy S" shape with a broad base and a punctate brown-black dot at the leading edge of the mite's path. If burrows are not easily identified, washable felt tip marker can be rubbed across the web space, and after the superficial ink is removed with alcohol or water, the ink will have penetrated through the stratum corneum outlining the burrow.
• Secondary lesions are more numerous and obvious than the burrows and may consist of crusted papules, small vesicles, pustules, excoriated broad areas of dermatitis, and areas of secondary infection from impetigo and folliculitis.

Laboratory Aids

• Skin scrapings may be done to secure a definitive diagnosis. The burrows most commonly found on the hands and feet should be moistened with alcohol or mineral oil.
• A no. 15 round-bellied blade attached to a scalpel handle should be briskly scraped across the burrows.
• Scraped material is placed on a slide with a drop of KOH or mineral oil with a coverslip.

—Under a scanning microscope, the presence of the gravid female, eggs, larvae, and/or feces are diagnostic.

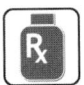

Therapy

DRUGS

• Five percent permethrin cream (Elimite) is used for infants older than 2 months and children. Apply to the entire body surface and leave on for 8 to 14 hours, then wash off. One application is usually effective, although some recommend a second application 10 to 14 days later.
• One percent lindane is effective for older children and nonpregnant adults; should remain on the body for 8 to 12 hours. Lindane use in young children is considered to be potentially toxic and hence lindane use in young children is generally not recommended.
• Ten percent crotamiton cream may be used for infants older than 6 months and is applied for 2 days followed by a cleansing bath 48 hours after the last application. There have been reported treatment failures with crotamiton.
• Six percent sulfur in a petrolatum base may be used; it is applied for 3 consecutive days in older children and adults.
• Mild-to-moderate topical steroids (e.g., 1% hydrocortisone, 0.025% to 0.1% triamcinolone) may be beneficial in the postscabetic syndrome.
• Oral agents, such as ivermectin, are sometimes used in adult patients for resistant scabies, particularly in crusted scabies and in institutional setting outbreaks. Ivermectin, in a solution of propylene glycol, has been used as a topical agent in some trials. Referral to a dermatologist is recommended prior to the consideration of oral therapy or topical use of ivermectin to verify the diagnosis and to assess treatment alternatives.

Follow-Up

• Pruritus may take up to 4 weeks to resolve after effective treatment. Use of a mild-to-moderate topical steroid may improve these symptoms.
• Continued appearance of new burrows may indicate ineffective treatment (most commonly misapplication) and warrants repeat physician evaluation.

PREVENTION

• Bedding, clothing, and items of close contact should be washed and dried in hot temperatures at the time of treatment.
• All family members and close contacts should be treated concurrently regardless of clinical symptoms. Contacts may be infested without symptoms.

PITFALLS

There is a need to treat close contacts, symptomatic and asymptomatic, to eliminate the mite and prevent immediate reinfestation.

Common Questions and Answers

Q: How did my child get scabies?
A: From close contact with an infected person.

Q: How long will my child continue to itch?
A: Pruritus may continue for weeks; the use of topical hydrocortisone may be helpful.

Q: Do I need to wash my child's bedding in a special detergent?
A: Simply wash all bedding in hot soapy water after your child has been treated.

ICD-9-CM 133.0

BIBLIOGRAPHY

American Academy of Pediatrics. Scabies. In: Pickering LK, ed. *Red Book: 2003 Report of the Committee on Infectious Diseases.* 26th Ed. Elk Grove Village, IL: American Academy of Pediatrics; 2003:547–549.

Buffet M, Dupin N. Current treatments for scabies. *Fundament Clin Pharmacol* 2003;17:217–225.

Cestari SC, Petri V, Rotta O, et al. Oral treatment of crusted scabies with ivermectin: report of two cases. *Pediatr Dermatol* 2000;17:410–414.

Chosidow O. Scabies and pediculosis. *Lancet* 2000;355:819–826.

Chouela E, Abeldano A, Pellerano G, Hernandez MI. Diagnosis and treatment of scabies: a practical guide. *Am J Clin Dermatol* 2002;3(1):9–18.

Dourmishev AL, Serafimova DK, Dourmishev LA, et al. Crusted scabies of the scalp in dermatomyositis patients: three cases treated with oral ivermectin. *Int J Dermatol* 1998;37:231–234.

Elston DM. Controversies concerning the treatment of lice and scabies. *J Am Acad Dermatol* 2002;46(5):794–796.

Hurwitz S. Insect Bites and Parasitic Infestations: Scabies. In: *Clinical Pediatric Dermatology.* 2nd Ed. Philadelphia, PA: W.B. Saunders, 1993:405–412.

Orion E, Matz H, Ruocco V, Wolf R. Parasitic skin infestations II, scabies, pediculosis, spider bites: unapproved treatments. *Clin Dermatol* 2002;20(6):618–625.

Victoria J, Trujillo R. Topical ivermectin: a new successful treatment for scabies. *Pediatr Dermatol* 2001;18:63–65.

Author: Kathleen Wholey Zsolway

Scarlet Fever

 Database

DEFINITION

- A clinical syndrome consisting of fever, pharyngitis, cervical lymphadenitis, and the characteristic "sandpaper rash," which results from infection with a strain of *Streptococcus pyogenes* (group A β-hemolytic streptococcus) that elaborates streptococcal pyrogenic toxin.
- Toxins include: A, B, or C. Toxin A is associated with more virulent disease.
- Similar syndrome may also be seen after infection with certain toxin-producing (enterotoxin G, I) strains of *Staphylococcus aureus*, known as, "staphylococcal scarlet fever."
- Some investigators feel that both streptococcal and staphylococcal forms of Scarlet Fever and Toxic Shock Syndrome (TSS) are on a continuum of disease. Bacteria may produce multiple toxins and the severity of disease is determined by the relative amounts of pyrogenic and TSS-producing toxins produced by the offending strain.

PATHOPHYSIOLOGY

- Susceptible individuals thought to lack toxin-specific immunity. Supported by results of "Dick test" in which a small amount of toxin introduced intradermally produces local erythema in susceptible individuals, but no reaction in those with toxin-specific immunity.
- Rash and other toxic manifestations of scarlet fever have been attributed to the development of hypersensitivity to the toxin, which therefore would require prior exposure to the toxin.
- Toxin production is dependent on lysogeny of the infecting streptococcus by a temperate bacteriophage.
- Pharyngitis is characterized by mucosal erythema and frequently by small crypt abscesses with punctate exudate in enlarged tonsils.
- Edematous papillae protrude from coated mucosa to produce a "strawberry tongue."
- Histologic examination of affected skin shows dilated blood and lymphatic vessels and engorged capillaries, most prominently around hair follicles.
- Acute, edematous polymorphonuclear inflammatory reaction is seen microscopically within affected tissues.
- Epidermal inflammatory reaction is usually followed by hyperkeratosis, which accounts for scaling during defervescence.

EPIDEMIOLOGY

- Peak incidence during the first few school years.
- Occurs uncommonly before the age of 3 years or after the age of 15 years, possibly related to the requirement for prior sensitization and toxin-specific immunity.
- By age 10, 80% of children have developed toxin-specific antibodies.
- No sex predilection.

- All forms of streptococcal pharyngitis (i.e., with or without pyrogenic toxin) are more common in temperate and cold climates, and winter and spring months, with some areas reporting an increased incidence in the fall.
- Incubation period is usually 24 to 48 hours.

COMPLICATIONS

- Acute otitis media
- Sinusitis
- Suppurative cervical lymphadenitis
- Pneumonia with or without effusion/empyema
- Peritonsillar cellulitis/abscess
- Retropharyngeal abscess
- Meningitis
- Brain abscess
- Thrombosis of intracranial venous sinuses
- Osteomyelitis
- Hepatitis
- Arthritis
- Acute rheumatic fever (ARF)
- Acute postinfectious glomerulonephritis (APGN)
- Erythema nodosum, possibly

PROGNOSIS

- Overall prognosis is excellent.
- Few patients suffer suppurative complications.
- Risk of developing ARF in untreated streptococcal infections is about 3% under epidemic conditions (0.3% in endemic situations).
- Risk of developing APGN depends on nephritogenicity of infecting strain. Attack rate is 10% to 15% with nephritogenic strains.

 Differential Diagnosis

- Nonscarletinal streptococcal pharyngitis/tonsillitis
- Viral exanthems (measles, rubella, erythema infectiosum)
- Drug eruptions
- Staphylococcal scalded skin syndrome (SSSS)
- Toxic epidermal necrolysis (TEN)
- Toxic shock syndrome (streptococcal or staphylococcal)
- Kawasaki disease

UNCOMMON ENTITIES

- Infection with *Corynebacterium hemolyticum*
- Mercury poisoning (acrodynia)
- Atropine intoxication
- Boric acid poisoning
- Rifampin overdose

 Data Gathering

HISTORY

Question: Was there sudden onset of fever up to 40.5°C, sore throat, headache, nausea, vomiting and toxicity?
Significance: Classic symptoms for group A streptococcal disease.

Question: Does the rash feel like sandpaper?
Significance: Texture is more important than appearance.

Question: When did the rash start?
Significance: Characteristic rash typically occurs 12 to 48 hours after onset of fever.

Question: Any abdominal pain or muscle aches prior to rash?
Significance: May complain of abdominal pain before onset of rash, and aching in extremities or back.

Question: Any close contacts with streptococcal infection?
Significance: Helps in identification.

 Physical Examination

Finding: Fine maculopapular (sandpaper texture) rash on erythematous background.
Significance: Usually begins on the trunk and spreads to involve almost the entire body within hours to days. Although the rash seen with scarlet fever is generally fine and sandpaper-like, larger papules and petechiae may be seen.

Finding: Deep, red, nonblanching lesions in the antecubital and popliteal areas.
Significance: "Pastia lines," develop in the skin folds of joints.

Finding: Circumoral pallor present.
Significance: Classic finding.

Finding: Rash blanches with pressure and ultimately desquamates.
Significance: Desquamation occurs within 7 to 21 days from onset of illness.

Finding: Characteristic toxin-induced scarlet fever exanthem.
Significance: Can rarely be seen without pharyngitis in the setting of pyoderma or an infected wound (known as "surgical scarlet fever").

Finding: Systemic toxicity.
Significance: May indicate incorrect diagnosis.

Finding: Dorsum of tongue.
Significance: Has white coat early in illness with edematous red papillae. White covering desquamates and reveals swollen, red and mottled "strawberry tongue."

OTHER FINDINGS

- Pharynx and tonsils are beefy red and may contain exudate.
- Hemorrhagic spots on interior pillar of tonsils and soft palate.
- Large, tender anterior cervical nodes.

Laboratory Aids

Test: Rapid streptococcal antigen tests
Significance: Effective as screening tests; 50% to 80% sensitivity and greater than 95% specificity. Positive rapid tests do not require culture confirmation.

Test: Throat culture
Significance: The "gold standard" with best sensitivity (>90%) for group A β-hemolytic streptococci. A culture should be performed when rapid test is negative.

Test: White blood cell count
Significance: Usually elevated, although may be elevated in viral pharyngitis as well. Low count would be rare with streptococcal infection.

Test: Eosinophilia (up to 30%)
Significance: Is common in the recovery phase.

Test: Dick test
Significance: Of historic interest, no longer used clinically.

Therapy

- Identical to therapy for streptococcal pharyngitis.
- Therapy started as late as 9 days after illness onset should be effective in preventing ARF.
- May withhold treatment until throat culture result is available.
- Immediate therapy probably shortens symptomatic period.

DRUGS

- Oral penicillin VK: drug of choice except in penicillin-allergic individuals. Resistant strains have not been documented in the United States. Dose: 25,000 to 50,000 Units/kg (1,600 units = 1 mg) divided into 3 to 4 doses for 10 days. 400,000 Units (250 mg) twice daily for 10 days has also been shown to have comparable efficacy and is endorsed by the American Academy of Pediatrics.
- Intramuscular benzathine penicillin G: equally effective as oral penicillin. Dose: 600,000 Units for children less than 60 pounds. 1,200,000 Units in larger children and adults. Assures compliance. Bringing to room temperature reduces discomfort. Benzathine/Procaine penicillin combinations are less painful.
- Clarithromycin and azithromycin have also been shown to eradicate streptococci; however, because of the broad spectra of these antibiotics and the increasing incidence of antibiotic-resistant bacteria, penicillin is still recommended by most experts except in cases of penicillin hypersensitivity, when patient nonadherence to a 10-day penicillin

regimen is suspected or for patients who fail therapy with a beta-lactam.
- Azithromycin, total dose of 60 mg/kg, given either as 12 mg/kg once daily for 5 days or 20 mg/kg once daily for 3 days
- Clarithromycin, 15 mg/kg per day, given every 12 hours for 10 days or 500 mg extended release tablets given once a day for 5 days (studied in adolescents 12 and above)
- There are reports of acute rheumatic fever after the 3-day course of azithromycin.
- Oral erythromycin: is indicated in penicillin-allergic individuals. Erythromycin ethyl succinate (40 to 50 mg/kg per day in 2 to 4 divided doses). Resistance is rare in the United States (<5% of isolates).
- Amoxicillin, clindamycin, and first-generation oral cephalosporins (up to 15% of penicillin-allergic persons are also allergic to cephalosporins) are reasonable alternatives to penicillin.
- Recent trials comparing 10 day course of penicillin with shorter duration of therapy with newer oral cephalosporins have shown similar bacteriologic and clinical cure rates, but efficacy in prevention of nonsuppurative sequelae is unknown.
- Cefdinir and cefpodoxime proxetil are approved for use in a more convenient 5-day dosing schedule.
- Tetracyclines and sulfonamides should not be used as a result of resistance of group A streptococci.
- Positive posttreatment cultures in asymptomatic patients: retreatment is not recommended.

Follow-Up

- Fever and symptoms usually resolve within 24 to 48 hours of antibiotic treatment.
- Nonsuppurative complications occur after unrecognized disease and when treatment is delayed for more than 9 days. ARF occurs an average of 18 days after untreated infection. APGN occurs an average of 10 days after untreated infection.

PREVENTION

- Prompt treatment leads to fewer secondary cases of streptococcal disease.
- Chemoprophylaxis with penicillin recommended by some experts in children with repeated documented episodes occurring at short intervals.

PITFALLS

- A positive throat culture may only be evidence of carriage in some cases of acute pharyngitis that are actually viral (e.g., Epstein Barr virus).
- Milder disease is becoming more common, and is easier to miss. Rash may only involve the bridge of the nose, face, shoulders, and upper chest. Circumoral pallor and severe exudative pharyngitis are being seen less frequently.

Common Questions and Answers

Q: Should household contacts have throat cultures performed?
A: Only obtain cultures from symptomatic household contacts. Cultures should not routinely be obtained in asymptomatic contacts.

Q: Should posttreatment throat cultures be performed?
A: Only in symptomatic individuals and patients at risk for ARF and APGN.

Q: Can scarlet fever recur?
A: Yes, there have been documented reports of recurrent scarlet fever.

Q: Have there been documented day care outbreaks of scarlet fever?
A: Yes, outbreaks have been traced back to a single strain.

Q: How soon can children return to school or day care?
A: When they are afebrile, and after at least 24 hours of antibiotic therapy.

ICD-9-CM 034.1

BIBLIOGRAPHY

Altemeier WA. A pediatrician's view. A brief history of group A beta hemolytic strep. *Pediatr Ann* 1998;27:264–267.

American Academy of Pediatrics. Group A streptococcal infections. In: Pickering LK, ed. *Red Book 2003: Report of the Committee on Infectious Diseases.* 26th Ed. Elk Grove Village, IL: American Academy of Pediatrics, 2003:573–591.

Barnett BO, Frieden IJ. Streptococcal skin diseases in children. *Semin Dermatol* 1992;11:3–10.

Breese BB. Streptococcal pharyngitis and scarlet fever. *Am J Dis Child* 1978;132: 612–616.

Duncan SR, Scott S, Duncan CJ. Modeling the dynamics of scarlet fever epidemics in the 19th century. *Eur J Epidemiol* 2000;16: 619–626.

Jarraud S, Cozon G, Vandenesch F, Bes M, Etienne J, Lina G. Involvement of enterotoxins G and I in staphylococcal toxic shock syndrome and staphylococcal scarlet fever. *J Clin Microbiol* 1999;37:2446–2449.

Richardson M, Elliman D, Maguire H, Simpson J, Nicoll A. Evidence base of incubation periods, periods of infectiousness and exclusion policies for the control of communicable diseases in schools and preschools. *Pediatr Infect Dis J* 2001;20: 380–391.

Shiseki M, Miwa K, Nemoto Y, et al. Comparison of pathogenic factors expressed by group A streptococci isolated from patients with streptococcal toxic shock syndrome and scarlet fever. *Microb Pathog* 1999;27:243–252.

Author: Mark L. Bagarazzi

Scleroderma

Database

DEFINITION

Scleroderma means hard skin.

• Systemic sclerosis (SSc) or progressive systemic sclerosis (PSS)

—Diagnostic criteria: one major or two minor
—Major: sclerodermatous changes (tightness, thickening, induration) proximal to the MCP or MTP
—Minor: sclerodactyly sclerodermatous changes limited to the digits; digital pitting; bibasilar pulmonary fibrosis not as a result of primary lung disease

• CREST (a variant form of SSc)

—Calcinosis
—Raynaud phenomenon
—Esophageal dysmotility
—Sclerodactyly
—Telangiectases
—Affects approximately one-half of patients with SSc
—Females more than males
—Earlier age of onset than SSc
—Same characteristics as SSc, but calcinosis is more severe
—Distal symptoms are more severe
—Associated with anticentromere antibody

• Localized: fibrosis limited to the skin, subcutaneous tissue, and muscle

—Systemic features

—Rare: visceral involvement later in the disease
—Occasional: evolution into another connective tissue disease such as MCTD or SLE
—Very rarely: Raynaud Phenomenon
—Forms

—Morphea: one or more oval or round indurations that become hard and whitish early on, have active inflammatory border with violaceous color; forms: plaque or guttate; limited number of lesions; generalized: extensive; nodular: subcutaneous
—Linear: one or more linear areas affecting subcutaneous tissue, muscle, and bone
—Coup de sabre: involving face or scalp may be associated with seizures
—Parry-Romberg syndrome: form of linear scleroderma; congenital dysplasia of the subcutaneous tissue, neurologic changes such as TIAs.

PATHOPHYSIOLOGY

The following theories have been proposed:

• Alteration of normal glycosylation and hydroxylation of collagen
• Serum factors: endothelin
• Vasculopathy: based on high association with Raynaud
• Immune dysfunction: autoimmunity directed against connective tissue antigen such as laminin or type IV collagen
• May represent distinct early and late processes:

—Early: increase of hydrophilic glycosaminoglycan; increased T cells, macrophages, and plasma cells; mast cell hyperplasia
—Late: increase collagen content; collagen is embryonic with narrow fibrils and immature cross banding; atrophy of rete pegs

EPIDEMIOLOGY

• Systemic

—Incidence: annually 4.5 to 12 per million
—Age of onset: 30 to 50 years; very rare in children
—Sex ratio: younger than 7 years, no difference; older than 7 years, F/M 3:1; 15 to 44 years, F/M 15:1
—Genetics: unknown

• Localized

—More common than SSc
—Exact incidence is unclear

COMPLICATIONS

• Systemic

—see Physical Examination

• Localized

—Skin thickening
—Joint contractures
—Leg length discrepancies

PROGNOSIS

• Natural course includes several phases: initial: inflammation; late: sclerotic, occasional regression over 3 to 5 years
• Ultimate prognosis depends on severity of skin tightness, joint contracture, and visceral involvement
• Mortality: males more than females and non-Whites more than Whites
• Most common cause of death in children is secondary to cardiac, renal, and pulmonary complications

Differential Diagnosis

• Graft-versus-host disease
• Phenylketonuria
• Borrelia infection: acrodermatitis chronica atrophicans
• Porphyria cutanea tarda
• Scleredema

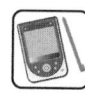

Data Gathering

HISTORY

• Thickening of skin
• Tightness of joints
• Discoloration of skin
• Often insidious onset
• Morning stiffness
• Heartburn, dysphagia, reflux, cough with swallowing

Physical Examination

Finding: Skin
Significance:

• **Stage 1:** Edema: tense, nonpitting, perhaps warm or tender, but often asymptomatic
• **Stage 2:** Sclerosis: waxy hard texture, bound to subcutaneous structures, back of digits, face (loss of forehead wrinkles, reduced mouth orifice)
• **Stage 3:** Atrophy: shiny appearance, hypo- or hyper-pigmented, calcium deposits in subcutaneous tissue. Telangiectases: macular dilatations that fill slowly, unlike spider telangiectasias.

Finding: Raynaud phenomenon associated with underlying disease
Significance:

• Subtypes:

—Phenomenon: associated with underlying disease
—Disease: isolated
—Triple phase: blanching, cyanosis, erythema
—Present in approximately 90% of patients with systemic sclerosis
—Usually fingers, also toes, nose, ears, and tongue, often spares the thumb
—Pathophysiology: arterial vasoconstriction: to blanching venous stasis to cyanosis, reflex vasodilatation to erythema

• Calcinosis, especially over extensor joint surfaces
• Musculoskeletal:

—"Creaking" of thickened tendons
—Contractures, especially PIP and elbows
—No intraarticular inflammation
—Muscle inflammation in approximately 30% of cases

• Gastrointestinal

—Mucosal telangiectasias of mouth

- Decreased incisor distance secondary to skin thickening
- Sicca syndrome with parotitis
- Loosening of teeth secondary to periodontal membrane disease
- Esophageal disease: esophagitis, occasional ulceration or stricture
- Large bowel disease less common
- Cardiac
—Primary cause of morbidity
—Possibly as a result of Raynaud of coronary arteries
- Pulmonary forms
—Interstitial fibrosis with gradual obliteration of vascular bed and resulting cor pulmonale
—Parenchymal disease is almost universal, frequently asymmetric, may have hacking cough, dyspnea on exertion, pleural rub
—Combined pulmonary vascular and pulmonary parenchymal
—Primary pulmonary vascular disease with right ventricular failure
- Renal, as a result of decreased renal plasma flow, ominous, proteinuria, hypertension
- CNS: cranial nerve involvement, especially sensory branch of trigeminal nerve
- Sicca syndrome
—Xerostomia (dry mouth)
—Keratoconjunctivitis sicca (dry eyes)
—Diagnosis: lip biopsy; rose bengal staining of cornea

PROCEDURES

- Schirmer test for dry eyes
- Capilloroscopy Periungual nailfold changes: capillary dropout and dilated loops; occasional redundant cuticular growth and digital pitting

Laboratory Aids

There are no specific diagnostic tests.

NONSPECIFIC TESTS

Systemic Form

- ANA often positive

Test: Hb
Significance: 25% have anemia as a result of chronic disease or vitamin B12 and folate deficiencies as a result of chronic malabsorption in sclerodermatous gut.

Test: Eosinophilia
Significance: 15%

Test: Sclero-70 (Scl-70 or Topoisomerase 1)
Significance: 26% of adults; more common with diffuse disease than peripheral vascular disease

Test: Anticentromere antibody
Significance: 22%; almost exclusively with CREST

Histologic Findings

Test: Muscle
Significance: Increased collagen and fat; negative immunofluorescence

Test: Esophageal
Significance: Atrophic muscle replaced by fibrous tissue more commonly affects smooth muscle of lower two-thirds of esophagus

ECG Findings

- ECG: first-degree block
- Right and left bundle-branch block (BBB)
- PACs and PVCs: Nonspecific T-wave changes, ventricular hypertrophy

PFTs

Test: Restrictive lung disease
Significance: 34% of SSc

Test: Decreased DLCO
Significance: 18% SSc

Test: Acro-osteolysis
Significance: Resorption of tufts of distal phalanges, especially with severe Raynaud

- Earliest changes are decreased FVC and small airway disease
- Bone x-ray
- Periarticular or subcutaneous calcification (15% to 25% of patients)
- Bony erosions

CXR

- Bibasilar pulmonary fibrosis
- Rib notching
- Calcifications (in CREST)

High-Resolution Chest CT

- Ground glass attenuation
- Honeycombing

Esophageal Studies

Test: Manometry and pH probe
Significance: Decreased or absent peristalsis of distal esophagus: distal dilatation, hiatus hernia, stricture

- Dilatation of second and third part of duodenum and proximal jejunum

LOCALIZED FORMS

- 25% to 50% eosinophilia during active disease
- 37% to 67% have positive ANA

Therapy

- Disease modification: Many agents have been tried; however, there are few controlled trials and no proven treatment. Medications include D-penicillamine: breaks down collagen cross-linkages; colchicine: inhibits fibroproliferative process; immunosuppressives: steroids, chlorambucil, MTX, cyclosporine, cyclophosphamide
- Supportive care: avoid cold, trauma, and excessive cold.
- Management of Raynaud: avoid cold, beta-blockers, biofeedback.

Follow-Up

- Localized forms
—Physical examination for joint mobility, muscle bulk, and growth
- Systemic forms
—Physical examination for joint mobility, muscle bulk, and growth
—Yearly PFTs
—Yearly barium swallow

PITFALLS

- Difficulty following slow disease progression, thus recommend photography of lesions every 3 to 6 months
- Failure to appreciate limited mouth opening
- Insufficient physical therapy resulting in permanent joint contractures
- Excessive use of immunosuppressive therapy late in disease when inflammatory component has resolved.

Common Questions and Answers

Q: Is a biopsy necessary?
A: Biopsy is often useful to confirm diagnosis and assess degree of inflammation.

Q: Is the sclero-70 antibody useful?
A: Not for diagnosis; it is only positive in a subset of individuals with the systemic form and, therefore, useful for predicting more severe disease.

ICD-9-CM 710.1

BIBLIOGRAPHY

Athreya B. Juvenile scleroderma. *Curr Opin Rheumatol* 2002;14:553–561.

Cron RQ, Swetter SM. Scleredema revisited. A poststreptococcal complication. *Clin Pediatr* 1994;33:606–610.

Foeldvari I. Scleroderma in children. *Curr Opin Rheumatol* 2002;14:699–703.

Murray KJ, Laxer RM. Scleroderma in children and adolescents. *Rheum Dis Clin North Am* 2002;28:603–624.

Rosenkranz ME, Lehman TJ. Clinical trials for pediatric scleroderma. *Curr Rheumatol Rep* 2002;4:449–451.

Seely JM, Jones LT, Wallace C, et al. Systemic sclerosis: using high-resolution CT to detect lung disease in children. *AJR* 1998;170:691–697.

Uziel Y, Feldman BM, Krafchik BR, et al. Methotrexate and corticosteroid therapy for pediatric localized scleroderma. *J Pediatr* 2000;136:91–95.

Author: Randy Q. Cron

Scoliosis (Idiopathic)

 Database

DEFINITION

Scoliosis: Lateral curvature of the spine exceeding 10° (with rotation of the spine); considered idiopathic only after other causes have been excluded
Kyphosis: Anteriorly concave curvature of the vertebral column

POSSIBLE CAUSES

Idiopathic Scoliosis

- By definition, unknown; listed are some theories, none proven in isolation
- Genetic

—Positive familial history for scoliosis in 30% (not predictive for severity)

- Connective tissue disorder

—Associated with several connective tissue disorders

- Neurologic (equilibrium system)

—Most widely supported theory
—Abnormalities noted in vestibular, ocular, proprioceptive, and vibratory functions

- Hormonal

—Lower levels of melatonin secreted from pineal body in those with adolescent idiopathic scoliosis
—Growth stimulating hormone: more of an influential factor than etiologic factor studies

PATHOLOGY

Lateral curvature of the spine with rotation

EPIDEMIOLOGY

- Prevalence

—Generally considered 1% for curves exceeding 10°
—0.3% for curves exceeding 20°

- Female/male ratios

—1.4:1 for curves 11° to 20°
—5:1 for curves more than 20°

GENETICS

Positive familial history for idiopathic scoliosis in 30% (not predictive for severity)

COMPLICATIONS (NATURAL HISTORY)

- Reduced pulmonary function for patients with thoracic curves over 60°
- Progression of lumbar curves over 50° in adult life with degenerative disc disease and pain in some
- Cosmetic and emotional factors

PROGNOSIS

- Risk of curve progression is related to patient's maturity (Risser sign, menarcheal status) and to the size of the curve.
- Curves less than 20° to 25° have a low risk of progression, even if patient is immature.
- Curves 25° to 45° have higher risk of progression, particularly in the immature.
- Curves >45° to 50° have much higher risk of progression, regardless of maturity.

 Differential Diagnosis

- Adolescent idiopathic scoliosis: onset after 10 years of age
- Juvenile idiopathic scoliosis: onset between 3 and 10 years of age
- Infantile idiopathic scoliosis: onset younger than 3 years of age
- Congenital scoliosis (malformation of spine)
- Scoliosis associated with neurofibromatosis
- Scoliosis associated with tumors (osteoid osteoma, other)
- Neuromuscular scoliosis (e.g., cerebral palsy, spina bifida, muscle disorders)
- Postural scoliosis (from leg length discrepancy for example)

—No rib hump or rotation
—Disappears with forward bending
—Long curve
—No progression

 Data Gathering

HISTORY

Question: Onset?
Significance: Consider when first noted, by whom, rate of worsening, previous treatment, associated signs or symptoms, familial history, etc.

Question: Pain?
Significance: Patients with idiopathic scoliosis usually should not have pain.

Question: Night pain?
Significance: If night pain, consider tumor such as osteoid osteoma or other tumor.

Question: Other signs or symptoms?
Significance: Review of systems (especially neurologic)

 Physical Examination

Finding: General inspection to look for skin changes such as:

- Café-au-lait spots, pigmentation, or other signs of neurofibromatosis; also dysraphic signs (hairy patches, etc.)
- Assess for maturity, hyperelasticity, contracture, congenital anomalies
- Assess for deformity; symmetry of spine, shoulders, and trunk, including decompensation; abnormalities of thoracic kyphosis, or cervical or lumbar lordosis
- The Adam forward bending test is used to look for rib or paraspinous elevations.
- Assess for leg length discrepancy, congenital anomalies, and neurologic abnormalities (including abnormal abdominal reflex).

SPECIAL QUESTIONS

Finding: Crankshaft phenomenon
Significance: Progression of curve size and rotation following posterior spinal fusion in a young child, a result of continued anterior spinal growth. Patient is Risser 0, open triradiate cartilages, younger than 10 years old, and is prior to the occurrence of peak height velocity (the time of maximum spinal growth). Consider anterior fusion in addition to posterior fusion.

PHYSICAL EXAMINATION TRICKS

Finding: Scoliometer test
Significance: To measure rib rotation

Finding: Abnormal abdominal reflex
Significance: May suggest intraspinal pathology including syrinx

Laboratory Aids

• Usually not helpful unless to rule out associated metabolic conditions
• Pulmonary function testing is useful preoperatively for more severe curves.

IMAGING STAGES

• Plain standing PA and lateral scoliosis films on a long 3-foot x-ray cassette
• Risser classification of iliac apophysis ossification is an indicator of maturity.
• MRI is not routinely necessary.
• Seven percent prevalence of intraspinal abnormalities found in left thoracic curves
• Curve patterns are classified according to the King or Lenke classifications.
• Renal ultrasound or IVP is used for evaluation of patient with congenital scoliosis (look for associated renal abnormalities).

Therapy

• Treatment

—Concepts for treatment are based on the severity of the deformity and on the likelihood of progression.

• Observation

—Curves less than 25°
—Immature patients (Risser 0, 1, 2) should be reevaluated in 4 to 6 months.
—Skeletally mature patients (Risser 4 or 5) usually do not require ongoing follow up unless there are special circumstances.
—Curves 25° to 45° in skeletally mature patients
—Risser 4 or 5 patients usually reevaluated in 6 months to 1 year
—Mature patients usually yearly

BRACE TREATMENT

• Curves 25° to 45° (Risser 0, 1): brace on initial evaluation; 30 to 45 degrees (Risser 2 or 3): brace on initial evaluation.
• Curves 25° or greater (in Risser 0 to 3 patient) that have demonstrated more than 10° progression during the period of observation
• Continue brace treatment until maturity (2 years postmenarchal and Risser 4 in females, Risser 5 in males).

OPERATIVE MANAGEMENT

• Recommended when curves exceed 45° to 50°

—Exception: Balanced thoracic and lumbar curves less than 55° may be observed for progression.

• Thoracic curves and double major curves

—Posterior segmental fixation instrumentation remains current state-of-the-art
—Anterior spinal instrumentation for selected curves
—The role of thoracoscopic technique being defined

• Isolated thoracolumbar and lumbar curves

—Anterior spinal fusion using solid rod segmental constructs

GENERAL TREATMENT MODALITIES

• Brace types

—Thoracolumbosacral orthosis (TLSO): success reported with use more than 16 to 18 hours daily; significantly improved outcome when compared to natural history.
—Milwaukee: seldom needed except higher thoracic or cervical curves

DRUGS

Postoperative continuous epidural infusion helpful for pain control

SIGNS TO WATCH FOR

• Back pain associated with idiopathic scoliosis (may indicate other diagnosis)

—Present in 23% at time of initial evaluation (additional 9% during follow-up)
—Of those with back pain, only 9% found to have identifiable cause such as spondylolysis, Scheuermann, syrinx, disc herniation, tumor, tether cord

PROGNOSIS

Overall, good prognosis for the majority of patients

Common Questions and Answers

Q: How long do you observe a patient with spinal asymmetry before ordering an x-ray?
A: It depends on the presence or absence of abnormalities on the physical examination. If any of the signs mentioned here are seen or significant back pain, an x-ray or referral is indicated. The scoliometer is also a useful tool in screening patients.

Q: If a child presents with scoliosis and back pain which occurs especially at night and is relieved with aspirin, what diagnosis is suggested?
A: Scoliosis associated with osteoid osteoma

ICD-9-CM

Scoliosis idiopathic 737.30
Scoliosis infantile progressive 737.32

BIBLIOGRAPHY

Kim HW, Weinstein SL. Spine update. The management of scoliosis in neurofibromatosis. *Spine* 1997;22(23):2770–2776.

Lonstein JE, Carlson JM. The prediction of curve progression in untreated idiopathic scoliosis during growth. *J Bone Joint Surg* 1984;66A:1061–1071.

Newton PO, Wenger DR. Idiopathic and Congenital Scoliosis. In: Morrissy RT, Weinstein SL, eds. *Lovell and Winter's Pediatric Orthopaedics.* 5th Ed. Philadelphia: Lippincott, Williams & Wilkins, 2001:677–740.

Redla S, Sikdar T, Saifuddin A. Magnetic resonance imaging of scoliosis. *Clin Radiol* 2001;56(5):360–371.

Author: John P. Dormans

Seborrheic Dermatitis

 Database

DEFINITION

• Seborrheic dermatitis is a yellow to erythematous, scaly, greasy lesion located in areas of high concentrations of sebaceous glands (the scalp, face, postauricular, and intertriginous areas).
• The pattern of seborrheic dermatitis varies with different age groups. In infants, it is commonly referred to as "cradle cap" and located on the vertex of the scalp.
• The term seborrhea refers to excessively oily skin.

PATHOPHYSIOLOGY

• Specific etiology is controversial, both genetic and environmental factors seem to influence the course of the illness
• Infections: Does not appear to be bacterial, although there is increasing acceptance that the yeast *Pityrosporum ovale*/Malassezia is a causative factor. Further evidence for this is that ketoconazole, an antifungal agent, significantly decreases the number of Malassezia yeasts in seborrheic dermatitis patients, and improves the clinical appearance of the disease. Seborrheic dermatitis is one of the most common cutaneous manifestations of AIDS in adults and may present before other symptoms.
• May be hormonally driven because it first appears in infancy and disappears until puberty.
• Histopathologic findings are nonspecific and include evidence of low-grade inflammation, parakeratosis, acanthosis, elongation of the rete ridges, and slight intracellular edema and spongiosis.

GENETICS

• Controversial whether there is a constitutional predisposition. There is evidence that it is more common in families, but not spouses of affected patients.

EPIDEMIOLOGY

This skin disorder is first seen in infancy, and usually spontaneously resolves by the end of the first year of life. It is not usually seen again until adolescence.

COMPLICATIONS

• Usually none

PROGNOSIS

The infantile form will self-resolve by the end of the first year of life. The adolescent forms may persist through middle age as a chronic skin dermatitis.

 Differential Diagnosis

• Infection: Fungal infections such as *Trichophyton tonsurans* and *Candida* may complicate these lesions, and are commonly confused with seborrhea. Tinea capitis results in a diffuse or patchy, fine, white, adherent scale on the scalp with tiny, perifollicular pustules and/or hair stubs that have broken off at the level of the scalp. Less commonly, there is patchy or diffuse hair loss. Adenopathy is often present. These can be differentiated by microscopic examination of hairs using a potassium hydroxide wet mount preparation and by fungal culture.
• Tumors: Letterer-Siwe (or Langerhans cell histiocytosis) is an uncommon disease that may present with a rash that begins with a scaly erythematous eruption on the scalp, behind the ears, in the intertriginous regions; differentiated by the presence of small reddish-brown papules or vesicles, purpuric lesions, hepatosplenomegaly, and adenopathy.
• Immunologic: Atopic dermatitis (usually affects infants at a later onset, is very pruritic, and often accompanied by a familial history of atopy). Recurrence after treatment is more indicative of atopic dermatitis. Psoriasis lacks the reddish color of seborrhea and is characterized by a micaceous scale and a tendency to locate on the flexural aspects of the extremities; it is less likely to be confined to the scalp.
• Miscellaneous: Leiner disease results in a severe generalized erythematous, exfoliative seborrheic dermatitis, and is accompanied by severe diarrhea, recurrent infections, and failure to thrive. It is the phenotypic appearance of a number of nutritional and immunologic disorders, such as acrodermatitis enteropathica, and complement deficiencies.

 Data Gathering

HISTORY

These infants usually lack a personal or familial history of atopy. The lesions are typically not pruritic and may begin early in the first few months of life. As with other dermatologic disorders, it is important to learn what treatments (especially topical steroids) have previously been tried.

 Physical Examination

• Characteristic lesions are yellow to erythematous, scaly, and greasy.
• In infants, the disorder may be confined to the scalp or may spread downward to the face and back of head.
• Thickened lesions of the scalp in infants are commonly referred to as cradle cap.
• Blepharitis is red eyelid margins with fine white scales.
• After adolescence, this disorder frequently manifests as dandruff, an increase over the normal desquamation of the scalp.
• Axillary involvement, the absence of pruritus, oozing, and weeping help distinguish seborrhea from atopic dermatitis.

 Laboratory Aids

SPECIFIC TESTS

There are no specific tests for seborrhea.

Test: Microscopic examination of hairs and fungal culture
Significance: Fungal infections can be differentiated by using a potassium hydroxide wet mount preparation, and by fungal culture. Culture is often necessary to make the diagnosis because only 29% of affected patients have a positive potassium hydroxide examination.

NONSPECIFIC TESTS

Test: Skin biopsy
Significance: May help in situations that are confusing; however, findings are not necessarily diagnostic for seborrhea.

Seborrheic Dermatitis

 Therapy

- Infantile seborrhea commonly affects the scalp and may respond to a mild shampoo. A sulfur or salicylic acid shampoo (leave on 5 minutes before rinsing off, use 2 to 3 times in the first week, then weekly afterwards) may be used if no improvement. If particularly thick, the scales can be loosened first with warm mineral oil or petrolatum, and then gently scrubbed.
- Lesions resistant to treatment may respond to a short course of topical steroid lotion rubbed into the scalp with the fingertips.
- Adolescents should use shampoos with zinc pyrithione (e.g., Head and Shoulders), selenium sulfide (e.g., Selsun), or tar. Those with erythema and severe pruritus can consider treatment with topical corticosteroid lotions. Dense, diffuse scalp involvement can be treated overnight with Derma-smoothe FS lotion (peanut oil, mineral oil, fluocinolone acetonide 0.01%) under a shower cap, and then shampoo off in the morning. This should be done nightly for no longer than 1 to 3 weeks.
- Ketoconazole cream or shampoo applied once a day for several weeks may be tried with resistant and widespread cases. Other alternative treatments are fluconazole and metronidazole.
- If the seborrheic dermatitis is particularly widespread or is refractory to topical treatment, oral ketoconazole, has been shown to be effective against seborrheic dermatitis of the scalp and body.
- Additionally, a new class of medications, topical tacrolimus ointment and pimecrolimus cream, are being recommended for treating seborrheic dermatitis and other skin disorders. Topical tacrolimus and pimecrolimus not only lack side effects associated with corticosteroids but also have been shown to have potent antifungal activity against *Malassezia furfur* and *Pityrosporum ovale* in vitro.
- Blepharitis should be treated with warm compresses, cleansing with a baby shampoo, and if necessary, sodium sulfacetamide ophthalmic ointment. Topical steroids can suppress this lesion, but the side effects of its use around the eye (such as glaucoma) make this a poor choice for chronic therapy.

 Follow-Up

Some improvement should be seen with therapy by 10 to 14 days. Although this dermatitis is usually self-limited in infancy, it often takes months to resolve completely. Seborrhea may rarely be complicated by secondary bacterial or candidal infections, with erythema, tenderness, and ulceration. Long term therapy may be required in the adolescent in which it may become chronic. Seborrhea may be caused or complicated by associated underlying disorders, such as immune defects such as acquired immunodeficiency syndrome. This should be considered with seborrhea resistant to treatment.

PREVENTION

Frequent washing with selenium lotions (such as Exsel or Selsun) can suppress activity and maintain a remission. There are no other preventative measures.

PITFALLS

Treatments to infant scalp should be left on long enough to allow the scales to loosen, and then can be scrubbed off. Parents may need to be reassured that for stubborn and persistent seborrhea, scrubbing the scalp is safe (even over the fontanelles) and may be necessary to keep the lesions under control.

 Common Questions and Answers

Q: Does therapy speed resolution of the disorder?
A: Treatment does not appear to influence the underlying cause of this disorder (presumably hormonal influence on the sebaceous glands) although some suggest use of an antifungal therapy to presumptively treat *Pityrosporum ovale*/Malassezia may resolve the lesion.

Q: Shouldn't the use of high potency steroids worsen the dermatitis if caused by a fungal infection?
A: Topical corticosteroids are commonly used to treat seborrheic dermatitis. These agents seem to work because of their anti-inflammatory effect. Although in the past high-potency steroids were used for this indication; there are adverse effects associated with their prolonged use. Currently, low-potency corticosteroids are preferred.

Q: Does seborrheic dermatitis cause permanent hair loss?
A: Patients can be reassured that it does not cause permanent hair loss.

ICM-9-CM 690

BIBLIOGRAPHY

Habif T. *Clinical Dermatology*. 3rd Ed. St Louis: CV Mosby, 1996.

Hay RJ, Graham-Brown RAC. Dandruff and seborrheic dermatitis. *Clin Exp Dermatol* 1997;22:3–6.

Gupta AK, Bluhm R, Cooper EA, Summerbell RC, Batra R. Seborrheic dermatitis. *Dermatol Clin* 2003;21:3.

Janniger C, Schwartz R. Seborrheic dermatitis. *Am Fam Physician* 1995;52(1):149–155.

Mimouni K, Mukamel M, Zeharia A, Mimouni M. Prognosis of infantile seborrheic dermatitis. *J Pediatr* 1995;127(5):744–746.

Author: Robert Kamei

Seizures—Febrile

 Database

DEFINITION

• Simple febrile seizures: Single, brief (less than 15 minutes), generalized seizures during fever (rise or fall) in developmentally and neurologically normal children between 6 months and 5 years of age without intracranial infection or other cause.
• Complex febrile seizures: A febrile seizure that either lasts longer than 15 minutes, is focal, or recurs within 24 hours.

GENETICS

• Inheritance: Multifactorial in the majority of cases. A small subgroup of patients, the trait is dominantly inherited with about a 60% penetrance rate. To date, at least five different genetic loci have been identified.
• Febrile seizure syndrome: Generalized epilepsy with febrile seizures plus (GEFS+)— Febrile seizures with generalized tonic clonic seizures, complex partial seizures and absence spells, after (or before) the age of six. Multiple genes identified including SCN1A, SCN1B, and GABA(A) γ^2 subunit genes.

EPIDEMIOLOGY

Two percent to 5% of children experience a febrile seizure. It is strongly age dependent: 4% occur before 6 months, 90% in the first 3 years, and 6% after age 3.

ASSOCIATED CONDITIONS

Associated with rapid rise in fever; familial history of febrile seizures

 Differential Diagnosis

Nonepileptic causes of seizures. Also, fever may be the precipitant of seizure as a result of any other cause of an epileptic spell. History, physical exam, and (especially if patient is under 18 months) lumbar puncture are usually sufficient to exclude:

• CNS infection
• Anoxia/stroke/hemorrhage
• Trauma
• Intoxication
• Metabolic encephalopathy
• Neurodegenerative disorder
• Brain tumor
• Neurocutaneous syndromes (tuberous sclerosis, Sturge-Weber, neurofibromatosis)
• Previous brain injury (history of stroke, hemorrhage, birth asphyxia, CP, meningitis)

 Data Gathering

HISTORY

• Previous history of seizures, febrile or afebrile, or neurologic abnormality: One-third of children with one simple febrile seizure will have another. Neurologic abnormality or prior afebrile seizure increases risk of subsequent epilepsy.
• Precipitating factors (height and duration of fever, length and symptoms of preceding illness, recent history of head trauma, possibility of ingestion): low fever, prolonged illness before seizure, ingestion, or head trauma suggests cause other than fever alone.
• Past medical history: gestation, birth, general health, growth and development, and current medications. Birth complications and developmental delay may increase risk of epilepsy, but not febrile seizures.
• Family history: Both febrile and afebrile seizures can be hereditary.
• Neurological findings: Recent onset of headaches, vomiting, lethargy, weakness, sensory deficits, or change in vision, behavior, balance, or gait. Suggests underlying brain pathology and need for neuro-imaging.

 Physical Examination

• Vital signs: Degree of fever, tachycardia or hypotension (suggests sepsis) tachypnea (suggests respiratory infection), head circumference
• Signs of head trauma or possible child abuse: Retinal hemorrhages and evidence of intracranial hypertension such as bulging fontanelle should be noted on HEENT exam.
• Possible meningitis: Kernig and Brudzinski signs, nucal rigidity.
• Careful neurological examination: Specific attention to mental status and any focal abnormalities of motor strength, tone, or sensation should be performed.
• Routine testing: Not necessary—After a simple febrile seizure if the child appears well. Otherwise consider complete blood count, electrolytes, calcium, glucose, toxicology screen.
• Lumbar puncture: Should be performed in any child who is thought to have a possible CNS infection, including any new onset febrile seizure in a child under 18 months of age as clinical signs of meningitis may be difficult to accurately assess. Any older child who appears toxic or has clinical signs suggesting CNS infection should undergo a spinal tap.
• EEG: Not routinely indicated after a simple febrile seizure. EEG should be performed on children who are neurologically abnormal or experience a complex febrile seizure. This can/should be done after the acute illness has resolved.
• MRI: Reserved for children with complex (focal or prolonged) febrile seizures; focal neurologic deficits, even transitory, after a seizure; and children with focal abnormality on EEG. Should be done after the febrile illness has resolved.

Therapy

- Because only one-third of children with an initial febrile seizure have a second seizure, treatment of a single febrile seizure is not indicated.
- Anticonvulsant prophylaxis may be considered in children with an underlying neurologic abnormality and in children who have had two prolonged or more than three brief febrile seizures.
- When the initial febrile seizure is multiple, prolonged, or focal but the child recovers rapidly and completely, further investigations including EEG and possibly MRI are indicated. Decisions regarding anticonvulsant prophylaxis in these children must be individualized.

DRUGS

- Oral administration of diazepam, 0.3 mg/kg every 8 hours, during all febrile illnesses reduces the risk of recurrent febrile seizures. However, has disadvantage of significant sedation during each febrile illness and if seizure is at the onset of fever therapy is not initiated early enough.
- Alternatively, rectal diazepam, 0.3 to 0.5 mg/kg, can be administered at the time of a febrile seizure if it persists for greater than 5 minutes.
- Phenobarbital prophylaxis (3 to 6 mg/kg daily) should be avoided because of possible behavioral and cognitive side effects. Daily valproate and primidone are considered as effective as phenobarbital but also have limiting side effects.
- Phenytoin and carbamazepine are ineffective as prophylaxis.

 ## Follow-Up

PROGNOSIS

- One-third of children who have a first simple febrile seizure will have a second during a subsequent febrile illness, and half of these will have a third febrile seizure.
- One-half of recurrences occur within 6 months of the first febrile seizure, three fourths within a year, and 90% within 2 years.
- Less than 9% of children with febrile seizures have more than three.
- Risk of recurrence is increased by: familial history of febrile seizures, first febrile seizure before 1 year, and body temperature less than 40°C.
- Only 2% of neurologically normal children who experience a simple febrile seizure will have a nonfebrile seizures by age 7. In children with a prolonged or focal febrile seizures, a prior neurologic deficit, or a family history of epilepsy there is an increased, but still small (6%) probability of subsequent epilepsy.
- There is no evidence that occasional febrile seizures or even febrile status epilepticus causes neurologic damage, mental retardation, a decrease in IQ, cerebral palsy, or learning problems.

PITFALLS

- Diagnosis of febrile seizure in a child less than 18 months old usually entails spinal fluid examination with normal cell count, chemistry, Gram stain, and culture.
- Continued seizures with fever beyond age 6 are not compatible with diagnosis of febrile seizure.
- Infants with febrile seizures may have serious bacterial infections (bacteremia, meningitis or sepsis) causing fever of primary clinical significance.

 ## Common Questions and Answers

Q: What should be done if the child has another febrile seizure?
A: Emergency measures include placement of the child recumbent or supine with head turned to avoid aspiration. Place nothing in the mouth. Antipyretic medications that can be administered PR should be kept in the home. For children who have had prolonged seizures, arrangements and instructions to administer rectal diazepam can be considered.

Q: What restrictions should be placed on general activity of a child with recurrent febrile seizures?
A: No specific activity restrictions are recommended. Children at risk for recurrent seizures should not be left unattended when bathing or swimming.

ICD-9-CM 780.3

BIBLIOGRAPHY

Baumann RJ, Duffner PK. Treatment of children with simple febrile seizures: the AAP practice parameter. American Academy of Pediatrics. *Pediatr Neurol* 2000;23(1):11–17.

Knudsen FU. Febrile seizures: treatment and prognosis. *Epilepsia* 2000;41(1):2–9.

Offringa M, Moyer VA. Evidence based paediatrics: Evidence based management of seizures associated with fever. *BMJ* 2001;323(7321):1111–1114.

Shinnar S, Glauser TA. Febrile seizures. *J Child Neurol* 2002;17 (Suppl 1):S44–S52.

Verity CM, Greenwood R, Golding J. Long-term intellectual and behavioral outcomes of children with febrile convulsions. *N Engl J Med* 1998;338(24):1723–1728.

Vining EP. Gaining a perspective on childhood seizures. *N Engl J Med* 1998;338(26):1916–1918.

Authors: Eric Marsh and Amy R. Brooks-Kayal

Seizures—Partial and Generalized

Database

DEFINITION

Transient involuntary alteration of consciousness, behavior, motor activity, sensation, or autonomic function as a result of abnormal electrical neuronal discharges. Seizures are classified by location of their onset: partial (begins in local area of cerebral cortex), primary generalized (begins simultaneously in both hemispheres). Partial seizures types: simple partial (consciousness not impaired), complex partial (consciousness impaired), and partial seizures evolving to generalized tonic-clonic convulsions. Primary generalized seizure types: absence, atypical absence, myoclonic, clonic, tonic, atonic, and tonic-clonic, seizures.

GENETICS

• Idiopathic seizures may have a multi-factorial genetic pattern. Several epilepsy syndromes have recently been associated with defined genetic loci (e.g., generalized epilepsy with febrile seizures plus; autosomal-dominant nocturnal frontal lobe epilepsy; benign familial neonatal convulsions, severe myoclonic epilepsy of infancy).
• Other common epilepsy syndromes (including benign rolandic, childhood and juvenile absence, and juvenile myoclonic epilepsy) are genetically heterogeneous and have an AD inheritance pattern with variable penetrance.

EPIDEMIOLOGY

Four percent to 6% of children will have at least one seizure in the first 16 years of life; the highest incidence is in childhood, with 30% of first seizures occurring before age 4 years and nearly 80% occurring before age 20 years.

RISK FACTORS

• History of previous seizure (afebrile or febrile)
• Recent withdrawal of anticonvulsant medication
• Brain tumor
• Neurodegenerative disorder
• History of remote neurologic insult (stroke, intracranial hemorrhage, cerebral palsy, head trauma, meningitis)
• Family history of seizures

Differential Diagnosis

OF SUSPECTED SEIZURES

• Seizure (generalized T/C, complex partial, absence, myoclonic, tonic, atonic, etc.)
• Syncope, Breath-holding syncope
• Hyperventilation
• Psychogenic
• Movements related to gastro-esophageal reflux (Sandifer syndrome)
• Narcolepsy-cataplexy

• Night terrors
• Startle disease
• Migraine
• Shuddering spells, paroxysmal dyskinesias, tics, drug-induced dystonia
• Benign sleep myoclonus (in neonates/infants), segmental myoclonus

OF DEFINITE SEIZURE OR EPILEPSY

• Idiopathic (presumed genetic)
• Remote symptomatic (previous history of stroke, intracranial hemorrhage, birth asphyxia, head trauma, meningitis)
• Febrile
• Acute symptomatic: CNS infection, anoxia, trauma, stroke/hemorrhage, intoxication, metabolic encephalopathy, anticonvulsant withdrawal
• Neurodegenerative disorder
• Brain tumor
• Malformations of cortical development (lissencephaly, agenesis of corpus callosum, holoprosencephaly)
• Neurocutaneous syndromes (tuberous sclerosis, Sturge-Weber, neurofibromatosis)

Data Gathering

HISTORY

• Previous history of seizures or neurologic abnormality: suggests child at risk of epilepsy
• Precipitating factors: Fever, preceding illness, recent head trauma, ingestion, change in antiepileptic medication
• Risk factors (see Database)
• Gestation, birth, general health, growth and development, and current medications, recent onset of headaches, weakness, sensory deficits, change in vision, behavior, balance, or gait

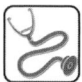

Physical Examination

• Vital signs: fever, respiratory failure (such as adequacy of air exchange, abnormal breathing pattern), tachy/bradycardia, or hypertension (suggesting intracranial hypertension),
• Signs of head trauma and child abuse: retinal hemorrhages, evidence of intracranial hypertension (bulging fontanelle)
• Head circumference: microcephaly suggests underlying neurologic abnormality.
• Signs of systemic infection: meningismus suggests CNS infection
• Skin exam: café-au-lait or ash leaf spots, facial hemangioma suggesting neurocutaneous disorder
• Neurological exam: pupillary asymmetries, altered mental status, fixed eye deviations, and focal motor weakness (Todd's paralysis) suggest focal onset of seizures and possibility of an underlying structural lesions.
• Convulsions: if actively convulsing, neurologic examination is often limited and should be directed toward determining possibility of intracranial hypertension and

any focal abnormalities (see Status Epilepticus chapter).

Laboratory Aids

• Initial: Glucose, electrolytes, BUN, antiepileptic drug levels, CBC, LFTs, toxicology screen, urinalysis. Oximetry or ABG indicated if child is actively seizing.
• Secondary: Lumbar puncture (LP) is indicated in nearly all children under 2 years of age and any older child in whom CNS infection is suspected (unless contraindicated: intracranial hypertension, cerebral mass lesion, or obstructive hydrocephalus). If these conditions are suspected, LP should be deferred until after head CT.

—EEG: indicated immediately if convulsions continue, or the patient fails to awaken within hours after convulsions cease (children with neurological deficits may have longer recovery).
   —Nonurgent EEGs are indicated in all children with first afebrile seizure, complicated febrile seizure, and known epilepsy with recent significant clinical change.
—Neuroimaging: CT or MRI. Urgent imaging, usually CT, is indicated in children with new onset partial seizures, focal neurologic signs, history of head trauma, or difficult-to-control seizures.
—Repeat imaging may be indicated in known epileptics with a significant change in clinical status.
—Focally abnormal EEG following a generalized seizure should prompt (nonurgent) MRI.

For nonurgent imaging, MRI is preferred as it provides more detailed images.

Emergency Care

See Status Epilepticus.

Therapy

PREVENTION

• Need for long-term antiepileptic drug (AED) therapy after a first seizure depends on the etiology, patient's age, and circumstances in which seizure occurred.
• Chronic AED therapy is not indicated after acute symptomatic seizures (transient metabolic disturbances [hyponatremia, intoxication]) or after a single unprovoked seizure in a child with normal neurologic examination and EEG.
• Chronic AED therapy is usually indicated after first seizure symptomatic of a structural brain lesion; after two or more unprovoked seizures; and in patients with a history of epilepsy who have had recurrent seizures.

MEDICATIONS

- The choice of AED for long-term management depends on the specific seizure type. Therapy should be started with a single drug, because approximately 75% of children with epilepsy will be fully controlled with monotherapy, and polytherapy increases the risk of toxicity and decreases compliance.
- Partial-onset seizures (with or without secondary generalization): Carbamazepine is frequently the initial therapy and begun at 5 to 10 mg/kg per day and slowly advanced to 20 to 30 mg/kg per day divided b.i.d. (sustained release preparations only) or t.i.d. Therapeutic blood concentrations range from 8 to 12 mg/mL. LFTs and CBC must be monitored because of potential risk of thrombocytopenia, aplastic anemia, and hepatotoxicity. Newer agents (see below) may have lower toxicity.
- Partial-onset alternatives for whom carbamazepine is ineffective or poorly tolerated: (a) oxcarbazepine (20 to 30 mg/kg per day), (b) lamotrigine (5 to 15 mg/kg per day in patients not taking valproate; 1 to 5 mg/kg per day in patients on VPA), (c) topiramate (4 to 10 mg/kg per day; build up dose slowly to minimize cognitive side effects), (d) Valproate (10 to 15 mg/kg per day increased to 20 to 60 mg/kg per day for blood levels of 50 to 100 mg/dL, (e) gabapentin (20 to 30 mg/kg per day). These medications also all have pediatric labeling and formulations.
- Other options: Levetiracetam (initial dosing of 10 to 40 mg/kg per day and increase to a max dose of 60 mg/kg per day in twice daily dosing) and Zonisamide (initial dosing 1 to 2 mg/kg per day and increase to max dose of 10 mg/kg per day in daily or twice daily dosing). Both demonstrated to be effective for partial seizures in children but do not yet have FDA indication for use under 16 years of age.
- Phenytoin (5 to 7 mg/kg per day) and phenobarbital (3 to 7 mg/kg per day) are older AEDs that are frequently used acutely to rapidly control seizures but used less for chronic maintenance therapy because of cognitive, behavioral, and cosmetic side effects. In young infants (less than 1 year), phenobarbital continues to be used as a first-line agent.
- Primary generalized epilepsies (including myoclonic, tonic, or clonic seizures or for refractory absence): Ethosuximide (20 mg/kg per day in two to three divided doses, increased as needed for blood levels of 40 to 100 mg/mL) is initial AED of choice for childhood absence seizures.
- Generalized seizures alternatives: Valproate, Lamotrigine, Topiramate, and Zonisamide. Adverse effects of Valproate include thrombocytopenia, pancreatitis, hyperammonemia, and fatal hepatotoxicity. CBC and LFTs should be routinely monitored. Be aware that children under 5 years have an increased risk of hepatotoxicity from valproate, and children under 10 years have an increased risk of serious rash from lamotrigine.
- Prolonged seizures (greater than 5 minutes) or acute repetitive seizures: rectal diazepam (0.3 to 0.5 mg/kg per dose) can be administered. Very effective at stopping the seizure with minimal risk of respiratory depression, but families should be CPR-trained.
- Refractory patients to medical therapy: other therapeutic options include the ketogenic diet, vagal nerve stimulator, and surgical resection.

 Follow-Up

PROGNOSIS

- The reported risk of recurrence after a single unprovoked seizure in children varies from 27% to >70%.
- The risk is lowest (27% to 40%) in children with normal neurologic examinations, day time spells, and normal EEGs. The risk is increased (up to 80%) in children with abnormal examinations, focally abnormal EEGs, onset of seizures in sleep, positive familial history of seizures, partial seizure, or postictal (Todd) paralysis.

COMPLICATIONS

- Brain damage: From brief seizures—No convincing evidence exists. From prolonged seizures (>30 minutes)—brain injury can occur secondary to hypoxia (respiratory compromise) and loss of cellular energy stores (see Status Epilepticus).
- Injuries: Rarely, serious injury occurs with brief seizures from loss of consciousness and resultant falls.
- Daily precautions: Few restrictions are needed: Exceptions of driving, operating heavy machinery, or particularly dangerous sports, such as scuba diving, parachuting, and rock climbing. All children with epilepsy should be closely supervised when in, or around, water (swimming or bathing).
- Very frequent seizures, even if brief, may impair learning.

PITFALLS

- Hyponatremic seizures: serum sodium below 120 mEq/dL in infants with gastroenteritis. Judicious Na correction may prevent neurologic effects of rapid shifts in osmolarity: many clinicians administer normal saline to bring the sodium up to 120 mEq/dL, with slower correction thereafter.
- Apnea and hypoventilation may result from excessive administration of benzodiazepines or Phenobarbital. In general, patients treated with these drugs IV should have their ventilation and oxygenation closely monitored. Excessively large or rapidly administered doses should be avoided when possible.
- Febrile seizure is a diagnosis of exclusion in a child with first seizure associated with fever. History may suggest other possibilities; those under 18 months should undergo lumbar puncture (see Seizures—Febrile chapter).

 Common Questions and Answers

Q: How do you know my child has epilepsy?
A: The term epilepsy is applied to children with recurrent seizures (more than one) not as a result of fever or other transient toxic/metabolic disturbance.

Q: Will my child always be an epileptic?
A: Depending on the circumstances, children may grow out of their seizure disorder. In many cases, anticonvulsants can be discontinued if the child has been seizure-free for 2 years.

Q: Why take an anticonvulsant(s)?
A: The purpose of anticonvulsant medication is to prevent interference with normal behavior associated with brief seizures, accidents, and status epilepticus. .

ICD-9-CM 345.1

BIBLIOGRAPHY

Bourgeois BF. Differential cognitive effects of antiepileptic drugs. *J Child Neurol* 2002;17 Suppl 2:2S28–2S33.

Bourgeois BF. New antiepileptic drugs in children: which ones for which seizures? *Clin Neuropharmacol* 2000;23(3):119–132.

Camfield P, Camfield C. Childhood epilepsy: what is the evidence for what we think and what we do. *J Child Neurol* 2003;18(4): 272–287.

Cowan LD. The epidemiology of the epilepsies in children. *Ment Retard Dev Disab Res Rev* 2002;8(3):171–181.

Crumrine PK. Antiepileptic drug selection in pediatric epilepsy. *J Child Neurol* 2002;17 Suppl 2:2S2–2S8.

Glauser TA. Expanding first-line therapy options for children with partial seizures. *Neurology* 2000;55(11 suppl 3):S30—S37.

Pellock JM. Managing pediatric epilepsy syndromes with new antiepileptic drugs. *Pediatrics* 1999;104(5):1106–1116.

Smith R, Ball R. Discontinuing anticonvulsant medication in children. *Arch Dis Child* 2002;87(3):259–260.

Authors: Eric Marsh and Amy R. Brooks-Kayal

Sepsis

Database

DEFINITION

The terms sepsis, bacteremia, sepsis syndrome, and septic shock have been used interchangeably in the medical literature, leading to confusion regarding the correct definition of each:

- Sepsis: the presence of pathogenic organisms or their toxins in the blood or tissues, and the systemic response to them.
- Bacteremia: the presence of viable bacteria in the bloodstream.
- Sepsis syndrome: sepsis accompanied by evidence of altered end-organ perfusion (e.g., changes in mental status, oliguria, elevated plasma lactate levels). This term has recently been used interchangeably with the systemic inflammatory response syndrome, which can be related to infection, trauma, burns, and other etiologies.
- Septic shock: sepsis syndrome with hypotension (systolic blood pressure <5% for age).

CAUSES

The etiology of sepsis varies with age in otherwise healthy children.

- Most common pathogens in the first 4 weeks of life: group B Streptococcus, gram-negative enterics (particularly *Escherichia coli*); *Listeria monocytogenes*.
- When there is a history of hospitalization, instrumentation, or mechanical ventilation: *Staphylococcus aureus, Staphylococcus epidermidis, Pseudomonas aeruginosa*.
- In older infants and children: *Streptococcus pneumoniae, Neisseria meningitidis*, group A Streptococcus, Salmonella spp.

EPIDEMIOLOGY

- Sepsis is among the most common (10% to 25%) medical diagnoses on admission to pediatric intensive care units.
- Mortality rates from sepsis vary with age from 5.6 deaths per 100,000 in infants less than 1 year to 0.5 per 100,000 age 1 to 4, and 0.1 per 100,000 age 5 to 14 years.
- Although sepsis may occur in previously healthy children, it is a particular concern for children with a number of chronic underlying conditions that may render them either immunosuppressed or vulnerable to invasive infections.

—Hyposplenism, either surgical or functional (e.g., sickle cell anemia), highly prone to sepsis from encapsulated organisms—
S. pneumoniae and *H. influenzae* type b
—Neutropenia (<1,000 neutrophils/mm³ of blood), whether resulting from disease (e.g., leukemia) or from chemotherapy
—Congenital or acquired syndromes of immunodeficiency (AIDS, SCID)
—Organ transplant recipients
—Chronic use of high doses of steroids
—Patients with indwelling central venous catheters

COMPLICATIONS

The most common complications of sepsis are those resulting primarily from either acute hypoperfusion of vital organs, or to organ injury incurred by the uncontrolled systemic inflammatory response:

- Acute lung injury
- Acute renal failure
- Disseminated intravascular coagulation (DIC)
- Hypoglycemia
- Adult respiratory distress syndrome (ARDS)
- Refractory shock
- Multiple organ dysfunction syndrome (MODS)

PROGNOSIS

- Case fatality rates have improved from nearly 50% to approximately 10%.
- Mortality higher if shock exists on initial presentation
- Development of ARDS or MODS associated with increased mortality
- Survival improved in patients receiving greater than 60 mL/kg of volume resuscitation in the first hour of management
- Presence of coagulopathy (elevated PT and PTT) associated with elevated mortality from meningococcal sepsis

ASSOCIATED ILLNESSES

See Epidemiology, for identification of subgroups of children at high risk of sepsis.

Differential Diagnosis

The differential diagnosis of the "septic-appearing" child varies somewhat with age:

- For children, <2 months:
—Viral infections (e.g., enterovirus, respiratory syncytial virus)
—Congenital heart disease (e.g., congenital heart failure as a result of hypoplastic left heart syndrome, coarctation of the aorta, ventricular septal defect [VSD], valvular insufficiency)
—Myocarditis, pericarditis
—Cardiac arrhythmia (e.g., supraventricular tachycardia)
—Myocardial infarction secondary to anomalous coronary artery insertion
—Congenital adrenal hyperplasia
—Inborn errors of metabolism (e.g., maple syrup urine disease, methylmalonic or propionic acidemia, urea cycle disorders)
—Hypoglycemia
—Severe anemia
—Methemoglobinemia
—Gastroenteritis with dehydration
—Pyloric stenosis
—Volvulus
—Infant botulism
—Occult trauma: child abuse
- For older infants and children:
—Viral infections
—Myocarditis, pericarditis

—Cardiac arrhythmia (e.g., supraventricular tachycardia, ventricular tachycardia)
—Intussusception
—Toxic ingestion/poisoning (e.g., iron, salicylates, tricyclic antidepressants, oral hypoglycemic agents, ethanol, calcium channel blockers, beta-blockers, clonidine, opioids)
—(Occult) trauma
—Infant botulism
—Diabetic ketoacidosis

Data Gathering

HISTORY

Identify children at risk of sepsis (see Epidemiology).

Question: Duration of illness before presentation?
Significance: Abrupt onset of symptoms more typical of invasive bacterial infection

Question: Presence of chronic underlying illness?
Significance: Identifies children at higher risk of sepsis

Question: Change in behavior?
Significance: May be initial sign of systemic infection

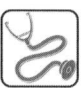
Physical Examination

All patients with suspected sepsis should have a full set of vital signs (e.g., temperature, pulse, respiratory rate, blood pressure).

Finding: Temperature
Significance: Fever is the hallmark of an infection; however, infants in particular may demonstrate hypothermia.

Finding: Stertor, stridor
Significance: Assess for signs of airway obstruction.

Finding: Auscultation of the chest
Significance: Assess adequacy of breathing (tachypnea, rales)

Finding: Tachycardia, hypotension, poor skin perfusion, delayed capillary refill, presence of mottling
Significance: Evidence of inadequate circulatory function

Finding: Altered mental status (somnolence, confusion, disorientation, agitation)
Significance: Evidence of severe systemic disease, possible poor cerebral perfusion

Finding: Presence of petechiae and purpura
Significance: Meningococcemia or DIC

Finding: Thorough physical examination
Significance: Looking for focus of infection

Laboratory Aids

All patients with suspected sepsis should have a thorough laboratory evaluation including:

Test: CBC with WBC differential, platelet count
Significance: Elevated WBC count with increased band count suggestive of invasive infection

Test: Electrolytes, glucose
Significance: Metabolic, acidosis, hypoglycemia

Test: Blood culture
Significance: Identification of causative organism

Test: Arterial blood gas
Significance: Monitoring acid-base status

Test: Urinalysis and urine culture
Significance: Potential source of infection

Test: Lumbar puncture (when hemodynamically stable)
Significance: Required for diagnosis of meningitis

Test: Chest radiograph
Significance: Potential source of infection

Test: Prothrombin time, partial thromboplastin time
Significance: Monitor development of DIC

Test: Fibrinogen, fibrin degradation products
Significance: Monitor development of DIC

Test: Gram stain and culture of petechiae or abscess contents
Significance: May yield causative organism

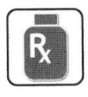

Therapy

- Ensure a patent airway (consider endotracheal intubation).
- Provide supplemental oxygen.
- Assist ventilation (e.g., bag-valve-mask device) as needed.
- Obtain intravenous access (consider placement of a femoral venous line or intraosseous line if difficulty securing peripheral IV).
- Volume resuscitation: bolus 20 mL/kg of normal saline solution, repeat as needed; consider colloid solutions (5% albumin, plasma) after initial 60 to 80 mL/kg of crystalloid)

—Giving 60 mL/kg in first hour improves outcome

- Inotropic agents: dopamine (begin at 5 mg/kg per minute, titrate up to 20 mg/kg per minute as needed), dobutamine (begin at 5 mg/kg per minute), epinephrine (begin at 1 to 2 mcg/kg per minute); to be used for persistent hemodynamic instability after 60 mL/kg isotonic crystalloid resuscitation.

—Consider stress-dose hydrocortisone for catecholamine-resistant hypotension
—Correct hypoglycemia (0.5 to 1 g/kg of dextrose)

- Antibiotics (depends on age, presence of meningitis, central venous catheter, immune function of patient); generally given IV for at least 10 days

—Neonates, <6 weeks, no meningitis: ampicillin and gentamicin; meningitis: vancomycin and cefotaxime

—Infants and children, ≥6 weeks: cefotaxime or ceftriaxone
—Suspected meningitis with penicillin-resistant *S. pneumoniae*: vancomycin and cefotaxime or ceftriaxone
—Suspected Salmonella sepsis: third-generation cephalosporin or trimethoprim-sulfamethoxazole
—Nosocomially acquired infections or patients with immunosuppression and/or central venous catheters: antistaphylococcal penicillin or vancomycin, plus aminoglycoside, and third-generation cephalosporin
—Patients with an intraabdominal focus of infection: ampicillin/sulbactam or ampicillin, gentamicin, and clindamycin

- Drainage and/or eradication of focus of infection

PREVENTION

- Routine vaccination for *Haemophilus influenzae* type b and *S. pneumoniae*, particularly in high-risk patients (e.g., sickle cell anemia, asplenia)
- Rifampin prophylaxis for household or day-care exposure to *H. influenzae* type b or *N. meningitidis*
- Prompt evaluation for fever in immunosuppressed patients

Follow-Up

- Admit all patients with suspected sepsis to the hospital; consider intensive care unit admission.
- Continuous blood pressure monitoring for the development of refractory shock
- Serial vital signs and physical examinations to monitor response to therapy
- Monitor for complications of sepsis and the development of MODS.
- Chest radiograph and serial arterial blood gases for evidence of acute lung injury/ARDS
- Urine output, BUN, creatinine for acute renal failure
- Serial coagulation studies (PT/PTT) for development of DIC
- Serial blood glucose levels for hypoglycemia
- Serial liver function tests (glucose, albumin, ALT, AST, GGT, bilirubin) for evidence of hepatic dysfunction
- Serial neurologic examinations for evidence of central nervous system dysfunction

PITFALLS

- Recognize the patient at risk for sepsis (see Epidemiology).
- Initial priorities in management are the proper assessment of airway, breathing, and circulation.
- Provide adequate initial volume resuscitation; improved outcome is associated with giving greater than 60 mL/kg isotonic saline in the first hour of resuscitation.
- Eradicate the focus of infection (abscess) if present.

- Continuous monitoring and reassessment of the patient is essential.

Common Questions and Answers

Q: What are the earliest signs and symptoms of compensated shock?
A: Unexplained tachycardia and widened pulse pressure are among the earliest signs of septic shock and warrant additional observation and laboratory investigation.

Q: Are colloid solutions (e.g., 5% albumin, fresh frozen plasma) better than isotonic crystalloid (e.g., Ringer's lactate, normal saline) for volume resuscitation?
A: Both are effective for intravascular volume expansion, although less (approximately 25%) of the crystalloid volume initially given ultimately remains in the intravascular compartment. Generally, because of their ready availability and lower cost, crystalloid solutions are given for the first 60 to 80 mL/kg of resuscitation, and consideration is then given to the addition of colloid solutions for additional volume resuscitation.

ICD-9-CM 638.9

BIBLIOGRAPHY

Angus DC, Wax RS. Epidemiology of sepsis: an update. *Crit Care Med* 2001;29(7):S109–S116.

Butt W. Septic shock. *Pediatr Clin North Am* 2001;48(3):601–625, viii.

Buttery JP. Blood cultures in newborns and children: optimising an everyday test. *Arch Dis Child Fetal Neonatal Ed* 2002;87(1):F25–F28.

Carcillo JA. Pediatric septic shock and multiple organ failure. *Crit Care Clin* 2003;19(3):413–340, viii.

Carcillo JA, Fields AI. Clinical practice parameters for pediatric and neonatal patients in septic shock. *Crit Care Med* 2002;30(6):1365–1378.

Han YY, Carcillo JA, Dragotta, MA et al. Early reversal of pediatric-neonatal septic shock by community physicians is associated with improved outcomes. *Pediatrics* 2003;112:793–799.

Marshall JC. Inflammation, coagulopathy, and the pathogenesis of multiple organ dysfunction syndrome. *Crit Care Med* 2001;29(7):S99–S106.

Rivers E, Nguyen B, Havstad S, et al. Early goal-directed therapy in the treatment of sepsis and septic shock. *New Engl J Med* 2001;345:1368–1377.

Watson RS, Carcillo JA, Linde-Zwirble WT et al. The epidemiology of severe sepsis in children in the United States. *Am J Resp Care Med* 2003;167:695–701.

Author: Dennis R. Durbin

Septic Arthritis

Database

DEFINITION
Septic arthritis is an inflammatory response to the presence of infectious organisms within the joint space. See table, Types of Organisms.

CAUSES

Bacterial
- *Staphylococcus aureus*
- Streptococci
- *Haemophilus influenzae*
- *Salmonella*
- *Neisseria gonorrhoeae*
- *Neisseria meningitidis*

Aseptic Arthritis
- Rubella
- Parvovirus
- Hepatitis B or C
- Mumps
- Herpesviruses (EBV, CMV, HSV, VZV)
- Epstein-Barr virus
- Varicella
- *Candida albicans* (neonatal)

PATHOLOGY/PATHOPHYSIOLOGY
- Entry of bacteria into joint space
—Hematogenous spread
—Direct inoculation (penetrating trauma) or extension from bone infection
—Influx of inflammatory cells within the joint capsule
—Destruction of cartilaginous structures within the joint by bacterial and lysosomal enzymes
—If left untreated, can progress to necrosis of the intraarticular epiphysis

EPIDEMIOLOGY
- Predominant age: 2 to 6 years, adolescent (*N. gonorrhea*)
- Sex predominance: male/female 2:1
- Predominantly affected joints: knee, hip, elbow, ankle

COMPLICATIONS
- Permanent limitation of range of motion as a result of tissue destruction and scarring
- Growth disturbance if the epiphysis is involved

PROGNOSIS
Depends on duration of illness prior to institution of appropriate therapy

ASSOCIATED ILLNESSES
- Neonatal septic arthritis can be associated with *S. aureus*, group B streptococcus, *Escherichia coli*, and Candida.
- Sickle cell disease is associated with Salmonella infection, although *S. aureus* is still the most common.
- Immunocompromise associated with Myco-plasma, Ureaplasma, Aspergillus infection

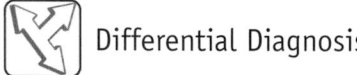

Differential Diagnosis

INFECTION
- Osteomyelitis with contiguous spread of infection
- Lyme arthritis
- Tuberculous arthritis
- Psoas abscess or retroperitoneal abscess with associated hip pain
- Cellulitis causing decreased range of motion of joint secondary to pain

TUMORS
- Osteogenic sarcoma (long-bone pain spreading to joint space)
- Leukemia/lymphoma

TRAUMA
- Occult fracture in proximity to growth plate
- Ligamentous injury (sprain)
- Foreign-body synovitis
- Traumatic knee effusion/hemarthrosis

IMMUNOLOGIC
- Toxic synovitis/Reactive arthritis
- Acute rheumatic fever
- Reactive arthritis
- *Campylobacter, Shigella*
- Reiter syndrome (after gastrointestinal or chlamydial infection) arthritis, uveitis, urethritis
- Henoch-Schönlein purpura
- Behçet syndrome (iridocyclitis, genital and oral ulcerations)
- Inflammatory bowel disease (Crohn disease, ulcerative colitis)
- Serum sickness
- Erythema multiforme/Stevens-Johnson syndrome

COLLAGEN VASCULAR
—Systemic lupus erythematosus
—Juvenile rheumatoid arthritis

MISCELLANEOUS
- Knee
—Apophysitis (e.g., Osgood-Schlatter disease)
—Patellofemoral pain syndrome (chondromalacia patella)
—Osteochondritis desiccans
- Hip
—Slipped capital femoral epiphysis

Data Gathering

HISTORY
Question: Was there trauma?
Significance: History of recent trauma does not rule out septic arthritis.

Question: Can you describe the pain?
Significance: Pain of bacterial arthritis worsens over 1 to 3 days and does not wax and wane.

Question: How many joints are involved?
Significance: Septic arthritis is rarely polyarticular.

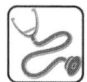

Physical Examination

- Fever occurs within the first few days of illness in 75% of patients, but less commonly in infants. Only 50% of children with gonococcal arthritis will have fever.
- Children with septic arthritis usually appear ill.
- The joint appears warm and swollen.
- Pseudoparalysis: decreased range of motion
- Hip effusion causes the leg to be held flexed and externally rotated.
- The child with septic arthritis will usually have pain through any range of motion. In contrast, most traumatic injuries will allow some painless range of motion of that joint.
- There are usually no external findings when the hip or shoulder joints are infected.
- Consider hip involvement when the patient complains of knee or thigh pain.
- In the frightened or uncooperative child, it is possible to have the parent perform an examination for tenderness and range of motion while the physician observes from a distance.

Laboratory Aids

TESTS

Joint Fluid in Septic Arthritis
- The WBC is often greater than 100,000/mm^3, but can be as low as 50,000/mm^3 in early infections.
- The glucose level in the synovial fluid is less than 50% that of the serum.
- Culture of the joint reveals an organism in 70% to 80% of cases (except for gonorrhea).
- A Gram stain of synovial fluid reveals pathogens in 50% of cases.

Other Supportive Tests
- The ESR is elevated (>30 mm/hr) in 95% of cases. Retain suspicion if >20 mm/hr.
- The C-reactive protein is increased. In one study, a CRP less than 1.0 mg/dL had a negative predictive value of 87% in a population in which the prevalence of septic arthritis in tested patients was 29%.
- Blood cultures are positive in 30% to 40% of cases.
- A high peripheral WBC count is neither sensitive nor specific for septic arthritis.
—A immunofluorescent antibody assay (EIA) for Borrelia burgdorferi, when available, may be helpful in the rapid differentiation between bacterial arthritis and Lyme disease.

IMAGING
- Radiography is rarely helpful in diagnosis, can show widening of joint space and/or displacement of the normal fat pads in the knee or elbow, and is less often positive in the shoulder or hip.
- A technetium-99 bone scan reveals increased uptake in the perimeter of the joint during the "blood pool" phase of the study.
- Ultrasound of the affected joint usually delineates the amount of fluid within the joint capsule. However, this test cannot differentiate between an infectious and a purely inflammatory disease.

FALSE POSITIVES
- Bone scan cannot easily differentiate septic arthritis from epiphyseal osteomyelitis.

- Evaluation of synovial fluid from patients with rheumatologic disease can mimic that of infectious arthritis; however, the clinical picture should allow differentiation of these entities.
—An algorithm using four or more of the following factors has been used to successfully differentiate septic arthritis and transient synovitis of the hip: fever, ESR >20 mm/hr, CRP >1.0 mg/dL, WBC >11,000 cells/mL, and joint space fluid apparent on plain radiograph.

 ## Emergency Care

- Drainage of infection: should occur as soon as possible if bacterial cause is suspected
- Indications for open surgical drainage/irrigation:

—Hip involvement
—Shoulder involvement (controversial)
—Thick, purulent, or fibrinous exudate unable to pass through 18-gauge needle
—All other joints not undergoing open drainage should undergo needle aspiration.
- Antibiotic administration as soon as possible after joint aspiration is performed
- Immobilization of extremity
- Pain management

DRUGS
Choice of antibiotics depends on age of child as outlined in the tables. In communities in which the prevalence of methicillin-resistant S. aureus is high, vancomycin should be considered.

DURATION OF THERAPY (IV AND PO) FOR VARIOUS ORGANISMS
- Treat for at least 2 weeks after resolution of fever and joint effusion.

- ≥28 days: S. aureus, gram-negative organisms, group B streptococcus
- ≥14 days: H. influenzae, N. meningitidis, streptococci
- ≥7 days: N. gonorrhoeae

 ## Therapy

See table, Empiric Therapy Prior to Identification of Organism.

 ## Follow-Up

- Involve orthopaedic surgery and physical therapy services in follow-up.
- Once the patient is receiving oral therapy, serum bactericidal titers (SBTs) must be monitored on a weekly basis if possible. Oral antibiotic titers should be kept at eight times the SBT.

WHEN TO EXPECT IMPROVEMENT
With appropriate antibacterial therapy, one should see improvement of symptoms with 2 days of initial administration.

SIGNS TO WATCH FOR
- Continued pain, fever, or lack of improvement of range of motion after 3 to 4 days of appropriate antibiotic treatment.
- Rising ESR or CRP in the face of antibiotic treatment.

PITFALLS
- Clinical examination in conjunction with the history of acute onset should raise the suspicion of septic arthritis even in the face

of "negative" laboratory screening tests. The most accurate determinations can be inferred from analysis of the synovial fluid.
- Realize that some children, especially neonates and young infants, will not manifest signs of systemic disease early in the course of the illness.
- Observe failure or success of therapy, especially when the extremity is immobilized.

 ## Common Questions and Answers

Q: How can one differentiate toxic synovitis from septic arthritis on the initial visit?
A: Although this is sometimes a difficult diagnosis to make with certainty, patients with toxic synovitis usually exhibit certain characteristics that patients with septic arthritis do not:
- Almost always involves the hip joint
- History of previous viral infection
- Some painless range of motion of the involved joint is possible.
- The ESR is lower than 20 mm/hr.
- Fever is low grade.

BIBLIOGRAPHY

Do TT. Transient synovitis as a cause of painful limps in children. *Curr Opin Pediatr* 2000;12:48–51.

Jung ST, Rowe SM, Moon ES, Song EK, Yoon TR, Seo HY. Significance of laboratory and radiologic findings for differentiating between septic arthritis and transient synovitis of the hip. *J Pediatr Orthop* 2003;23:368–372.

Khachatourians AG, Patzakis MJ, Roidis N, Holtom PD. Laboratory monitoring in pediatric acute osteomyelitis and septic arthritis. *Clin Orthop and Related Research* 2003;(409):186–194.

Kocher MS, Mandiga R, Murphy JM, et al. A clinical practice guideline for treatment of septic arthritis in children. *J Bone Joint Surg* 2003;85-A(6):994–999.

Maraqa NF, Gomez MM, Rathore MH. Outpatient parenteral antimicrobial therapy in osteoarticular infections in children. *J Pediatr Orthop* 2002;22(4):506–510.

Vinod MB, Matussek J, Curtis N, Graham HK, Carapetis JR. Duration of antibiotics in children with osteomyelitis and septic arthritis. *Journal of Pediatr Chil Health* 2002;38(4):363–367.

Wall EJ. Childhood osteomyelitis and septic arthritis. *Curr Opin Pediatr* 1998;10:73–76.

Wang CL, Wang SM, Yang YJ, Tsai CH, Liu CC. Septic arthritis in children: relationship of causative pathogens, complications, and outcome. *J Microbiol, Immunol Infect* 2003;36(1):41–46.

Willis AA, Widmann RF, Flynn JM, Green DW, Onel KB. Lyme arthritis presenting as acute septic arthritis in children. *J Pediatr Orthop* 2003;23(1):114–118.

Author: Joel A. Fein

Types of Organisms

AGE	MOST COMMON ORGANISM	OTHER ORGANISMS
Newborn	S. aureus	Candida albicans Group B streptococcus Gram-negative organisms
	(Klebsiella, Salmonella)	
Infants and children ≤5 years	S. aureus	Haemophilus influenzae* Streptococcus pneumoniae
Children >5 years	S. aureus	S. pneumoniae, Neisseria meningitidis
Adolescents	N. gonorrhoeae	S. aureus, S. pneumoniae, N. meningitidis

*Less likely in fully immunized children.

Empiric Therapy Prior to Identification of Organism

AGE	FIRST CHOICE*	SECOND CHOICE	DURATION
Neonatal	Cefotaxime	Ampicillin and Gentamicin	IV for ≥14 days PO for ≥14 days
≤5 years	Cefuroxime	O/N/M	IV + PO = 28 days
>5 years Adolescent	O/N/M, Cefazolin	Clindamycin	IV + PO = 28 days
Gonococcal	Ceftriaxone	Penicillin	IV + PO = 7–10 days
Nongonococcal	O/N/M	Cefazolin	IV + PO = 28 days

O/N/M = oxacillin or nafcillin or methicillin.
*In communities in which the prevalence of methicillin-resistant S. aureus is high, vancomycin should be considered.

Serum Sickness

Database

DEFINITION

- Serum sickness: type III hypersensitivity reaction that occurs 7 to 21 days after injection of foreign protein or serum (usually in the form of antiserums). The clinical syndrome consists of skin rash, itching, fever, malaise, proteinuria, vasculitis, and joint pain.
- Serum sickness–like reactions are characterized by fever, rash, lymphadenopathy, and arthralgia, and occur 1 to 3 weeks after drug exposure. Immune complexes, vasculitis, and hypocomplementemia are absent. This is the type of reaction, associated with cefaclor, is commonly referred to as serum sickness also.

—Serum sickness–like reactions are more common than true serum sickness because equine serum antitoxins have been replaced with human antitoxin sera. Clinically, they present identically and are treated the same.
—Common causative agents: horse anti-thymocyte globulins, human diploid-cell rabies vaccine, streptokinase, hymenoptera venom, penicillins, cephalosporins, sulfonamides, hydralazine, thiouracils, metronidazole, naproxen, and dextrans.

PATHOPHYSIOLOGY

- Type III immune complex, antigen-antibody complement reaction.
- Antibodies form 6 to 10 days after the introduction of foreign material. Antibodies interact with antigens forming immune complexes that diffuse across the vascular walls. They become fixated in tissue and activate the complement cascade. C3a and C5a are produced, resulting in increased vascular permeability and activated inflammatory cells. Polymorphonuclear cells and monocytes cause diffuse vasculitis.

GENETICS

People with a genetic predisposition to produce IgE are more susceptible.

EPIDEMIOLOGY

- Limited information is available regarding the incidence of adverse drug reactions in children; generally believed to occur less frequently in children than in adults.
- More than 90% of serum sickness cases are drug-induced.
- Less than 5% of serum sickness cases are fatal.

COMPLICATIONS

- Shock
- Digital necrosis
- Guillain-Barré syndrome (rare)
- Generalized vasculitis (rare)
- Peripheral neuropathy (rare)
- Glomerulonephritis (rare)

—Acute flaccid paralysis (case report)

- Increased risk of anaphylaxis with repeat exposure to substance
- Fatality (rare, usually as a result of continued administration of antigen)

PROGNOSIS

- Excellent. Most cases are mild and transient with no sequelae.
- Symptoms resolve in a few days to weeks.

Differential Diagnosis

- Erythema multiforme
- Mononucleosis
- Systemic lupus erythematosus
- Rocky Mountain spotted fever
- Henoch Schönlein purpura
- Hypersensitivity syndrome reaction
- Drug-induced pseudoporphyria
- Acute generalized exanthematous pustulosis
- Wegener granulomatosis

Data Gathering

HISTORY

- Suspect in any patient with an unexplained vasculitic rash who has been taking any new drug during the last 2 months.
- Ask about presentation and evolution of rash. Typically, the rash first appears on the sides of the fingers, hands, and feet before becoming widespread.
- Is there associated pruritus? Often present.
- Fever? Often present, usually mild.
- Ask about the presence of arthritis or arthralgia. Present over half the time; usually involves the metacarpophalangeal and knee joints.
- Is there associated abdominal pain? Some cases may have visceral involvement.
- Is there a history of hematuria? There can be modest renal involvement usually presenting as proteinuria and microscopic hematuria.
- Does the patient report any neurologic symptoms? Peripheral neuropathy, brachial plexus involvement and Guillain-Barré syndrome have been reported associations.
- Is there a previous history of a similar rash? Was it associated with any medications in the past? The rash and symptoms of serum sickness will occur sooner on repeat exposure.
- Try to differentiate from simple drug rash, timing of rash after exposure is important in differentiating the two.
- Has the patient had any drug or antitoxin exposure in the last month, especially to penicillins, cephalosporins, sulfonamides, hydralazine, thiouracils, streptokinase, metronidazole, naproxen, dextrans, bupropion?

Physical Examination

- Erythematous purpuric rash starts at the sides of the feet, toes, hands, and fingers and then becomes more widespread.
- Erythema multiforme, maculopapular, purpuric, or urticarial type rash
- Mild to severe fever
- Generalized lymphadenopathy; may be localized to lymph nodes that drain the injection site.
- Splenomegaly, occasionally
- Edema of the face and neck
- Joint pain

Laboratory Aids

Not extremely helpful in establishing diagnosis because no abnormality is universally present. Diagnosis usually apparent by classic findings and history of foreign protein or drug exposure.

- Urinalysis: may show proteinuria and/or hematuria.
- Complements levels variably reduced before returning to normal.
- Leukocytosis or leukopenia with or without eosinophilia.
- Erythrocyte sedimentation rate may be slightly elevated.
- Direct immunofluorescent staining of rash biopsy (not routinely recommended as part of workup) shows deposits of IgM and C3 complement in capillary walls.

Therapy

- Stop suspected medication/antigen immediately and avoid its future use.
- Topical steroids to relieve itching.
- Antihistamines to inhibit the action of vasoactive mediators.
- NSAIDs to relieve joint pain.
- Oral corticosteroids for severe cases. Recommended to administer and taper over 10- to 14-day period. Shorter course may result in relapse and recurrent symptoms are more difficult to alleviate.
- Admit if symptoms are severe or diagnosis is unclear.

Serum Sickness

 Follow-Up

WHEN TO EXPECT IMPROVEMENT

- Usually self-limited illness that resolves in a few days to weeks.
- If symptoms persist for more than 1 month, reconsider the diagnosis.

PREVENTION

- No known way to prevent first occurrence.
- Take careful history of previous allergic reactions.
- Skin testing prior to antiserum administration will prevent anaphylaxis but not serum sickness.
- When the need for antiserum arises, consider prophylactic antihistamines.

PITFALLS

- A history of fever, rash, and arthralgias is commonly seen with many childhood illnesses. One must always consider differential diagnoses.
- Symptoms may be so minimal that patient does not seek medical attention.
- Often misdiagnosed as simple drug allergy

 Common Questions and Answers

Q: What is the difference between serum sickness and drug allergies?
A: Drug allergies are type I IgE-mediated hypersensitivity reactions that occur very soon after drug exposure in a previously sensitized individual. Serum sickness is a type III antibody-antigen immune complex and complement amplified hypersensitivity reaction that occurs 1 to 3 weeks after an initial exposure.

Q: If my child has had serum sickness, is she at risk for getting it again?
A: Yes, if she receives the same medication or related medications again. The symptoms will occur more quickly, usually in 2 to 4 days and may be more severe.

Q: Will my child have long-term effects from this illness?
A: No, this is a self-limited disease and as long as the offending agent is stopped your child will completely recover.

Q: Is there any way to prevent my child from getting serum sickness?
A: Unfortunately, there is no way to predict if your child will have a serum sickness–like reaction to a particular medication. It is extremely important to be aware of your child's exact allergies to medications and to inform all health care providers caring for your child.

Q: My child has had serum sickness while taking an antibiotic. Can he take other antibiotics?
A: Yes, but your child should never receive that particular antibiotic or any closely related antibiotic again. Repeat exposure will likely result in serum sickness occurring more quickly than after the first exposure. Your child can safely take antibiotics from other drug classes.

Q: If one of my children has had serum sickness from an antibiotic, are my other children at risk?
A: No, there is no known genetic predisposition for serum sickness. Your other children do not need to avoid the medication that caused serum sickness.

Q: How is the Arthus reaction different from serum sickness?
A: The Arthus reaction is also a type III hypersensitivity reaction but only causes a local reaction. It is a local vasculitis caused by formation of antigen-antibody complexes in local vessel walls, which then activate the inflammation process. The reaction occurs within hours after an individual is injected intradermally with an antigen against which he or she has been actively immunized.

ICD-9-CM 999.5

BIBLIOGRAPHY

Erffmeyer JE. Serum sickness. *Ann Allergy* 1986;56:105–109.

Evans R, Kim K, Mahr TA. Current concepts in allergy: drug reactions. *Curr Probl Pediatr* 1991;21:185–192.

Heckbert SR, Stryker WS, Coltin KL, Manson JE, Platt R. Serum sickness in children after antibiotic exposure: estimates of occurrence and morbidity in a health maintenance organization population. *Am J Epidemiol* 1990;132:336–342.

Jain S, Swami G, Arya A, Chowdhry B. A case of acute flaccid paralysis as an unusual presentation of serum sickness. *Neurology India* 2003;51:293.

Knowles S, Shapiro L, Shear NH. Serious dermatologic reactions in children. *Curr Opin Pediatr* 1997;9:388–395.

Lawley TJ, Frank MM. Immune complexes and allergic disease. In: Middleton E, ed. *Allergy Principles and Practice*. 5th Ed. St. Louis: Mosby-Year Book, 2003;702–712.

McCollum R, Elbe DH, Ritchie AA. Bupropion indirect serum sickness-like reaction. *Ann Pharmacother* 2000;34:471–473.

Roujeau J, Stern RS. Severe adverse cutaneous reactions to drugs. *N Engl J Med* 1994;331:1272–1285.

Author: Denise A. Salerno

Severe Acute Respiratory Syndrome (SARS)

 Database

DEFINITIONS

• "Clinical criteria for severe acute respiratory syndrome (SARS) must be interpreted in the context of the prevailing epidemiologic laboratory criteria as published by the Centers for Disease Control and Prevention (CDC) and the World Health Organization (WHO).

WHO Clinical Criteria (5/1/03):
Suspect SARS case:

• A person presenting after November 1, 2002, with high fever (>38°C), and
• Cough or difficulty breathing, and
• "Close contact" with SARS patient or "travel criteria" to SARS area (see History).

Probable SARS case:

• A "suspect" case with radiographic pneumonia or respiratory distress syndrome, or
• A "suspect" case with confirmatory laboratory studies (see Laboratory Aids), or
• A "suspect" case with autopsy findings.

CDC Clinical Criteria (12/12/03):
Early illness:

• Two or more constitutional symptoms: fever, chills, rigors, myalgia, headache, diarrhea, sore throat, or rhinorrhea.

Mild to Moderate illness:

• Temperature of >100.4°F (>38°C), and
• One or more lower respiratory findings: cough, shortness of breath, or difficulty breathing.

Severe illness:

• Clinical criteria of mild to moderate illness, and
• One or more: radiographic evidence, acute respiratory distress syndrome, or autopsy findings.

CAUSE

• A previously unrecognized Coronavirus (a single-stranded RNA virus).
• Coronaviruses are a common cause of mild to moderate URIs in humans, and have occasionally been linked to pneumonia.
• Many believe that the virus originated in an animal species in China, then mutated itself in such a way that it was able to attach itself to human receptor cells.

PATHOPHYSIOLOGY

• The virus attaches itself to human receptor cells and initiates a nonspecific acute lung injury response leading to diffuse, severe alveolar damage.

EPIDEMIOLOGY

SARS Timeline

• November 2002: a series of severe, idiopathic, respiratory illnesses begin occurring in Southeast Asian countries (China, Hong Kong, Vietnam, and Singapore.)
• February 11, 2003: The Chinese Ministry of Health notifies the WHO that 305 cases of acute respiratory syndrome of unknown etiology have occurred in Guangdong province in southern China from November 16, 2002, to February 9, 2003.
• Late February: SARS outbreak in Toronto.
• March 12: WHO issues global SARS alert as number of reported cases steadily increases.
• March 14: CDC activates emergency operations center with first confirmed death of SARS patient.
• March 15: WHO issues travel advisories and warnings.
• March 17: 167 cases reported, 4 deaths, 7 countries.
• March 24: CDC implicates a Coronavirus AS a causative SARS agent.
• April 10: *New England Journal of Medicine* (NEJM) e-publishes "A Novel Coronavirus Associated with SARS."
• April 13: Vancouver team sequences the Coronavirus.
• April 16: WHO confirms Coronavirus as the cause of SARS as a Netherlands team infects monkeys with the virus. The monkeys go on to develop SARS, and then have the Coronavirus recovered from them.
• April 18: World-wide cases rapidly multiplying: 3461 cases, 170 deaths, 27 countries.
• May 17: Deaths dramatically rise: 7,761 cases, 623 deaths, 31 countries.
• June 9: Reported cases slow: 8,421 cases, 784 deaths, 32 countries.
• Early July: WHO declares the SARS epidemic over.
• July 31—final "probable" world cases: 8,096 cases, 774 deaths, 29 countries.
• July 31—final U.S. cases: 134 suspected, 19 probable, 8 confirmed, no deaths, 17 states.
• Since July 2003: Less than 12 confirmed new cases.

TRANSMISSION

• Direct or indirect contact of mucous membranes with infectious respiratory droplets or fomites.
• Period of infectivity: Most likely during period with active symptoms (fever, cough).
• Incubation period: 2 to 10 days; mean 6 days.
• All cases can be traced to contact with individuals from Asian countries or community spread from an individual whose illness could be traced to Asia.
• There have been no suspected SARS cases among casual contacts of the U.S. cases.

• Many health care workers infected after providing care to SARS patients.
• No evidence that SARS is transmitted from asymptomatic individuals.
• However, health care workers who developed SARS may have been a source of transmission within health care facilities during the early phases of illness when symptoms were mild and not recognized as SARS.
• Children pose a lower risk of transmission than adults.

COMPLICATIONS

• In 10% to 20% of cases, the respiratory illness is severe enough to require mechanical ventilation.

PROGNOSIS

• Fatality rate: 9.6%.

 Differential Diagnosis

• Bacterial: *Pneumococcus, Staphylococcus, Legionella, Mycoplasma* and *Chlamydia* pneumoniae.
• Viral: RSV, Influenza A and B.

 Data Gathering

HISTORY

Question: Has there been any recent travel?
Significance: Travel (including transit in an airport) within 10 days of onset of symptoms to an area with recently documented or suspected transmission of SARS is important an epidemiologic criterion for the diagnosis of a SARS case. At the height of the SARS epidemic, these areas included China, Hong Kong, Singapore, Taiwan, Toronto, and Hanoi.

Question: Has there been any recent contact with a SARS patient?
Significance: Close contact within 10 days of onset of symptoms with a person known or suspected to have SARS infection is another important epidemiologic criterion.

Question: Constitutional symptoms, such as fever, chills, rigors, headache, malaise, and myalgias?
Significance: Common in older patients.

Question: Respiratory symptoms?
Significance: At the onset of illness, most cases have mild respiratory symptoms. After 3 to 7 days, the onset of a dry, nonproductive cough begins, often with dyspnea that may be accompanied by, or progress to, hypoxemia.

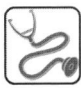 ## Physical Examination

Finding: Fever.
Significance: The illness generally begins with fever.

Finding: Tachypnea, increased work of breathing, or rales.
Significance: Adult patients generally present with evidence of respiratory distress. Importantly, however, although some children present with cough or difficulty breathing, many have remarkably normal examinations. Thus, the case definitions above may not be sufficiently sensitive for young children.

 ## Laboratory Aids

Tests: Detection of SARS-Coronavirus: (a) antibody by enzyme-linked immunosorbent assay (ELISA) or indirect fluorescent-antibody assay (IFA), (b) RNA by reverse transcriptase polymerase chain reaction (PCR) assays, (c) by viral culture.
Significance: Confirmatory laboratory criteria for the diagnosis of SARS.

Test: Nasopharyngeal aspirate.
Significance: The common specimen of choice for detection of respiratory viruses.

Test: Chest radiograph
Significance: The respiratory phase is often characterized by early focal infiltrates progressing to more generalized, patchy, interstitial infiltrates. Focal consolidation is also common. Many patients, however, have normal chest radiographs.

Test: Complete blood count.
Significance: Many patients have leukopenia (especially lymphopenia) and thrombocytopenia.

Test: Liver enzymes.
Significance: Some patients have elevated transaminases.

 ## Therapy

• There is no proven effective treatment.
• CDC currently recommends that patients with SARS receive the same treatment and supportive care that would be used for any patient with serious community-acquired atypical pneumonia of unknown cause.
• Steroids, ribavirin, oseltamivir, and other antivirals have been used without consistent success.

 ## Follow-Up

PREVENTION

Vaccine

• Experiments on mice have shown promise.
• Human trials began in China in May 2004.

Hospital Infection Control Precautions

• Hospitalized patients meeting SARS case definition should be placed in a negative pressure, single examination room.
• Protective equipment appropriate for standard, contact, and airborne precautions (e.g., hand hygiene, gown, gloves, and N95 respirator) in addition to eye protection, are recommended for health care workers to prevent transmission of SARS in health care settings.

Pediatric Patients with Potential SARS Exposure

• Children who have been exposed to an ill individual who is suspected of having SARS, or children who have traveled to an area in which SARS is occurring, should be evaluated based on the following:

—If well, parents should self-monitor the child's condition for fever or respiratory tract illness. Attendance at child care or school is not restricted.
—If the child is not well, parents should contact their physician and the child should be isolated at home.
—If a child is not well and experiencing breathing difficulty, he or she should be hospitalized. Health care workers should be informed before the admission, so SARS precautions can be initiated.

• Children who have been exposed to individuals who are not ill, but have traveled to areas in which SARS is occurring, do not require isolation.

PITFALLS

• Not searching for alternative diagnoses; even during an epidemic of SARS, other microbiologic studies should still be performed to confirm or rule out other infectious diseases.
• Not performing convalescent antibody testing in equivocal cases; undetectable antibody >28 days after onset of illness excludes the diagnosis.

 ## Common Questions and Answers

Q: Is the clinical presentation and course different in children?
A: Fortunately, younger children tend to have a shorter and milder course, consisting mainly of low grade fever, cough, and rhinorrhea. Adolescents, conversely, follow a more severe course, similar to adults.

Q: What constitutes "close contact" with a SARS patient?
A: Close contact includes having cared for or lived with a person known to have SARS, or having a high likelihood of direct contact with respiratory secretions and/or body fluids of a patient known to have SARS.

BIBLIOGRAPHY

Bitnun A, Allen U, Heurter H, et al. Children hospitalized with SARS-related illness in Toronto. *Pediatrics* 2003;112(4):e261–e268.

Booth CM, Matukas LM, Tomlinson GA, et al. Clinical features and short-term outcomes of 144 patients with SARS in the greater Toronto area. *JAMA* 2003;289(21):2801–2809.

Fong NC, Kwan YW, Hui YW, et al. Adolescent twin sisters with SARS. *Pediatrics* 2004;113(2):e146–e149.

Hon KLE, Leung CW, Cheng PKS, et al. Clinical presentations and outcome of SARS in children. *Lancet* 2003;361:1701–1703.

Ksiazek TG, Erdman D, Goldsmith C, et al. A Novel Coronavirus Associated with Severe Acute Respiratory Syndrome. *N Engl J Med* 2003;348(20):1953–1966.

Peiris SM, Phil D, Yuen KY, et al. The Severe Acute Respiratory Syndrome. *N Engl J Med* 2003;349(25):2431–2441.

Author: Nicholas Tsarouhas

Severe Combined Immunodeficiency

 ## Database

DEFINITION

Severe combined immunodeficiency (SCID) is primary immunodeficiency characterized by onset of severe, life-threatening infections in infancy as a result of defective or absent T- and/or B-lymphocyte-mediated immunity.

CAUSES

- A variety of defects lead to a similar clinical presentation.
- The X-linked subset is caused by a defect of the common gamma chain of the IL-2, IL-4, IL-7, IL-9, IL-15, and IL-21 receptor.
- The autosomal-recessive (AR) subset is as a result of various defects. The most common:

—Adenosine deaminase deficiency
—Purine nucleoside phosphorylase deficiency
—JAK3 deficiency
—Absent expression of MHC class I or II molecules

GENETICS

X-linked and autosomal-recessive inheritance (see table, Disorders and Diagnostic Tests)

EPIDEMIOLOGY

- Incidence: estimated to be 1 in 66,000 to 100,000 live births
- Most patients present by 6 months of age.
- The X-linked form accounts for 45% of SCID cases.
- ADA deficiency accounts for 15% of SCID cases.
- IL-7R deficiency accounts for 10% of SCID cases.
- JAK3 deficiency accounts for 6% of SCID cases.

COMPLICATIONS

- Untreated, most patients succumb to overwhelming infection.
- Graft-versus-host disease (GVHD) may result from maternal T cells that cross into fetal circulation or from transfusion of nonirradiated blood products.
- Clinical disease can be caused by live vaccines in previous undiagnosed SCID patients.
- Increased incidence of malignancy:

—Overall risk of malignancy is approximately 5%
—Thirty-fold increased incidence of lymphoma

 ## Differential Diagnosis

- Reticular dysgenesis
- Letterer-Siwe syndrome (histiocytosis)
- Omenn syndrome
- HIV infection
- Failure to thrive is the most common presenting problem.
- Recurrent and or life-threatening infections in infancy with a variety of pathogens (both common and atypical organisms)
- Chronic diarrhea
- Persistent thrush
- Skin rashes are commonly in unusual patterns or locations. They may be the presenting symptom of GVHD.

 ## Data Gathering

HISTORY

- Description of infections, severity, duration, response to treatment
- Family history of unexplained deaths or unusual infections

 ## Physical Examination

- Evaluation should focus on the presence of infection.
- Often an emaciated-appearing infant
- Marked absence of lymphoid and tonsillar tissue
- Dermatologic evaluation may reveal atypical rashes.

 ## Laboratory Aids

TESTS

- CBC with differential to assess for degree of lymphopenia absolute lymphocyte count in the neonatal period normally greater than 2800/mm^3
- T- and B-lymphocyte enumeration:

—T lymphocytes are markedly decreased or absent.
—B lymphocytes are variable but can be normal.

- Mitogen and antigen stimulation tests are markedly decreased or absent.
- Immunoglobulin levels are usually low or absent.

—Patients can have normal IgG levels in the first few months of life as a result of trans-placentally derived maternal IgG.

- Appropriate cultures to identify pathogens

 ## Therapy

- Bone marrow transplant (BMT) is the definitive treatment in most cases. Because of the impairment of recipient immune function, conditioning for BMT may be less rigorous than in other situations requiring BMT.
- Aggressive and early specific antibiotic/antifungal/antiviral therapy for infections
- Pneumocystis carinii prophylaxis
- If required, patients should receive only irradiated blood products. There is a risk of GVHD as a result of viable donor leukocytes that may survive in nonirradiated products.
- Intravenous immunoglobulin replacement: This may be required even after BMT because of variable B-lymphocyte reconstitution.
- Enzyme replacement therapy has been used in ADA-deficient patients.

Follow-Up

• Close monitoring of clinical status should be done before BMT. This may be every 2 to 4 weeks, depending on the patient's status.
• The posttransplant course is variable.

—The overall success rate for matched BMT in SCID is approximately 65%. Success is also being seen in partially matched BMT.
—Patients should still be followed closely for signs of infection, graft failure, and GVHD.

Common Questions and Answers

Q: How should children with SCID be managed before BMT?
A: Children suspected to have SCID should be isolated from potential sources of infection. They should not attend public places such as school because of the risk of obtaining an infection. They should be kept away from ill siblings or relatives. This is especially true if there has been an exposure to chickenpox or other viral illnesses.

Q: Should patients with SCID receive live viral vaccines?
A: Live viral vaccines are contraindicated in SCID. Patients suspected of severe immunodeficiency should not receive live viral vaccines until their immunodeficiency is defined. If the patient is receiving IVIG therapy, vaccinations are not required. Additionally, siblings of patients with SCID who live in the same household should not receive live viral vaccines. This is as a result of the risk of viral shedding in the siblings.

Q: What is the chance of another child being affected with SCID?
A: The risk of another child being born with SCID in a family with a previously affected child will depend on the type of SCID. X-linked: 50% chance of an affected male or carrier female. Autosomal-recessive causes: 25% chance of an affected child. Genetic counseling should be offered to female carriers of X-linked SCID.

Q: Can SCID be diagnosed prenatally?
A: Prenatal testing is available. Amniocentesis can be performed, and fetal cells can be tested for known genetic cause of SCID.

ICD-9-CM 279.2

BIBLIOGRAPHY

Buckley RH. Primary cellular immunodeficiencies. *J Allergy Clin Immunol* 2002;109:747–757.

Gaspar HB, Gilmour KC, Jones AM. Severe combined immunodeficiency-molecular pathogenesis and diagnosis. *Arch Dis Child* 2001;84(2):169–173.

Gelfand EW, Dosch HM. Diagnosis and classification of severe combined immunodeficiency. *Birth Defects* 1983;19:65–72.

Stephan JL, Vlekova V, Le Deist F. Severe combined immunodeficiency: a retrospective single center study of clinical presentation and outcome in 177 patients. *J Pediatr* 1990;123:564–572.

Stites DP, Terr AI. *Basic and Clinical Immunology*. 7th Ed. Norwalk, CT: Appleton & Lange 1991:341–344.

Winkelstein JA, et al., eds. Immune Deficiency Foundation. *Patient and Family Handbook: for the Primary Immune Deficiency Diseases*. 3rd Ed. Towson, MD: Immune deficiency foundation, 1999–2000.

Author: Timothy Andrews

Disorders and Diagnostic Tests

DISORDER (YEAR OF DEFINITION OF MOLECULAR BASIS)	CHROMOSOMAL LOCATION	GENE	DIAGNOSTIC TESTS OTHER THAN DIRECT MUTATION ANALYSIS
X-linked severe combined immunodeficiency	Xq13	Common γ chain (γc)	γc expression by FACS analysis
Adenosine deaminase (ADA) deficiency (1983)	20q12–13	Adenosine deaminase	Red cell ADA levels and metabolites
Purine nucleoside phosphorylase (PNP) deficiency (1987)	14q11	Purine nucleoside phosphorylase	Red cell PNP levels and metabolites
Recombinase activating gene (RAG 1&2) deficiency (1996), Omenn's syndrome (1998)	11p13	RAG 1 and RAG 2	
T-cell receptor deficiency (1987)	11q23	CD3γ/CD3ε	
Zap 70 deficiency (1994)	2q12	ZAP 70	ZAP 70 expression
JAK3 deficiency (1995)	19p13	JAK3	JAK3 expression/signaling
IL-7 receptor deficiency (1998)	5p13	IL-7 receptor α	IL-7 receptor α expression
MHC class II deficiency			
(1993)	16p13	CIITA	HLA-DR expression
(1998)	19p12	RFX-B	
(1995)	1q21	RFX5	
(1997)	13q13	RFXAP	

From Gaspar HB, Gilmour KC, Jones AM. *Arch Dis Child* 2001;84(2):169–173.

Sexual Abuse

Database

DEFINITION

Sexual abuse is the involvement of children in sexual activities that they cannot understand, for which they are not developmentally prepared, to which they cannot give informed consent, and/or that violate societal norms. It is a result of a complex interaction of societal, familial, and individual factors. Associated problems are:

- Physical abuse
- Domestic violence
- Neglect
- Emotional abuse

EPIDEMIOLOGY

- Approximately 150,000 substantiated cases are identified each year in the United States.
- This is likely to be a significant underestimation of the actual numbers.
- Girls are victimized more than boys, although abuse of boys is believed to be underreported.
- Boys represent approximately 20% of cases reported to child protection agencies each year.
- Children of all ages are victimized, with a peak age of vulnerability between 7 to 13 years.
- Race and socioeconomic status are not believed to play a role in the epidemiology of sexual abuse.

COMPLICATIONS

- Sexually transmitted infections, such as gonorrhea, genital warts, *Chlamydia trachomatis*, syphilis, and herpes simplex virus, are identified in only a small percentage of sexually abused children.
- Emotional problems such as posttraumatic stress disorder (PTSD), feelings of helplessness, impaired trust, low self-esteem, depression, adolescent substance abuse, and suicide attempts are seen in some victims of sexual abuse.
- Aggressive, hypersexual, withdrawn behavioral problems may be consequences of having been abused.

PROGNOSIS

- Varies greatly depending on specifics of abuse sustained, available support systems
- More extensive injuries (e.g., deep lacerations, tears) may take weeks to months to heal.
- The emotional impact of sexual abuse is very slow to resolve, and may take years to resolve.

Differential Diagnosis

INFECTION

With genital discharge:

- *Neisseria gonorrhoeae*
- *C. trachomatis*
- *Trichomonas vaginalis*
- Group A streptococcus
- *Haemophilus influenzae*
- *Staphylococcus aureus*
- *Corynebacterium diphtheriae*
- *Mycoplasma hominis*
- *Gardnerella vaginalis*
- *Shigella flexneri* (discharge may be bloody)

With genital bleeding:
- Urinary tract infection
- Vulvovaginitis

With genital inflammation/pruritus:
- Sexually transmitted diseases or infections (STDs or STIs)
- Pinworms
- Scabies
- *Candida albicans* (in pubertal girls)
- Group A streptococcal vulvovaginitis or perianal cellulitis

TUMORS

- Sarcoma botryoid (highly malignant sarcoma, typically of the urogenital tract)

TRAUMA

- Accidental trauma, including straddle and impaling injuries
- Mechanical friction from tight clothing or obesity
- Accidental tourniquet of genitals by hair

CONGENITAL

- Variations in hymenal configuration (septated, cribriform, microperforate, imperforate hymens)
- Urethral caruncles; vestibular bands
- Ectopic ureterocele; hemangiomas
- Syndromes associated with anogenital anomalies

PSYCHOSOCIAL

- Normal behaviors (masturbation, playing doctor)
- Exposure to sexual activity (e.g., in which the child witnesses others or sees adult videos/movies)
- False allegations of sexual abuse

DERMATOLOGIC

- Contact dermatitis
- Seborrhea
- Diaper dermatitis
- Lichen sclerosis et atrophica
- Balanitis xerotica
- Nevi

ENDOCRINE

- Pseudomenses (neonatal withdrawal bleeding)
- Physiologic leukorrhea

MISCELLANEOUS

- Nonspecific vulvovaginitis
- Rectovaginal fistula
- Labial adhesion (agglutination)
- Urethral prolapse
- Phimosis, paraphimosis
- Foreign body

Data Gathering

HISTORY

- The physician interview should be detailed especially if it is the first professional interview of the child. Prior to the examination, however, the child may have been interviewed by the police, social service workers, or a forensic interviewer. In this case, the history does not need to include all of the following details, but should include information needed to perform an appropriate medical assessment of the child.
- The interview should be conducted with the child separate from family members; diagnosis often depends on the history obtained from the child.
- Ask nonleading questions.
- Use developmentally appropriate language.

SPECIAL QUESTIONS

Ask about:

- Identity of alleged perpetrator/relationship to child
- Time of last possible contact
- Method of disclosure
- Frequency of abuse (one time versus multiple)
- Specific types of sexual contact included in the abuse
- Whether the perpetrator ejaculated, if a male
- Threats made to child by alleged perpetrator
- Previous official reports of the abuse
- Review of systems including genital pain, bleeding, dysuria, constipation, painful bowel movements, and behavioral changes

Physical Examination

- Varies depending on age of child
- Prepubertal children require detailed genital inspection only. Genital examination can be done with child in supine frog-leg position.
- A few physical findings are diagnostic of abuse. These include the presence of semen or sperm, acute genital/anal injuries without an adequate accidental explanation, syphilis (excluding perinatal infection), and culture-proven *N. gonorrhoeae*.
- Look for acute genital injuries in the absence of an appropriate history, and marked disruptions in hymenal tissue.
- Many genital findings are unlikely to be related to abuse. These include small labial adhesions in girls who are not yet toilet trained, *Candida albicans* dermatitis, erythema of the vestibule, and small mounds or projections on an otherwise normal hymen.

PROCEDURE

- The labial traction technique (gently grasping labia majora and pulling laterally, down and toward the examiner) allows for the best visualization of the hymenal edges.

Laboratory Aids

TESTS

- Universal STD screening is not necessary.
- Vaginal cultures are obtained from within the vaginal canal. The unestrogenized hymen is very sensitive so great care should be taken in inserting a swab through the hymen opening. Allow 10 to 15 seconds for swabs to absorb secretions.
- Cultures for *N. gonorrhoeae* from rectum, vagina (prepubertal), cervix (adolescent), penile urethra, and/or throat. Misidentification of *N. gonorrhoeae* can be a problem if confirmatory tests (e.g., sugar fermentation, latex agglutination) are not properly done. Be familiar with the laboratory's methods of identification and confirmation. Cultures are the gold standard and are the only acceptable method for diagnosing STDs in prepubertal children.
- *Chlamydia* cultures from rectum, vagina (prepubertal), cervix (adolescent), and/or penile urethra. Obtain cells for *Chlamydia* culture by gently scraping the vaginal wall with a swab (in young children). Because of the low prevalence of *Chlamydia* in the prepubertal population and normal flora that can produce false-positive results, culture remains the gold standard for *Chlamydia* testing. Rapid urine tests are not recommended for young children. Nucleic acid amplification tests can be used for adolescent screening, but have not been approved for young children.
- Routine genital culture
- Rapid plasma reagin (RPR), hepatitis serology, HIV if indicated
- Forensic evidence collection (for an acute assault)

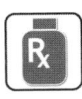

Therapy

- Ensure the safety of the child.
- Report suspected abuse to the local child welfare agency.
- Report suspected sexual abuse to law enforcement.
- Consult a social worker.
- Inform the parents of the report.

DRUGS

- Prophylactic antibiotics that are effective against common STDs, such as gonorrhea, chlamydia, and syphilis, are generally not used for prepubertal children, because these infections are uncommon. Prophylaxis against STDs may be considered for stranger assaults.
- Identified STDs should be treated with the appropriate regimen.

- Consider pregnancy prevention (e.g., emergency hormonal contraceptive) for adolescents.
- Tetanus booster for patients with acute, serious genital, or other injuries.
- Sitz baths for comfort

Follow-Up

- Cases will be investigated by child welfare and/or the police.
- Need for foster care placement and/or ongoing supervision is decided by child welfare investigators.
- Most children are referred for short-term or long-term counseling.
- Persistent physical/genital complaints, which may indicate ongoing abuse, an STD, or psychological problems
- Patient victimizing younger child: young perpetrators are often victims of previous abuse.
- It is important to get help for the child perpetrator so that the pattern of abuse does not continue.

PREVENTION

The efficacy of sexual abuse prevention programs is difficult to measure. Although children who are taught about personal safety learn from the experience, it is unknown whether their behavior is changed by such education.

PITFALLS

- Failing to consider sexual abuse in the differential diagnosis of nonspecific behavioral and physical complaints.
- If cultures are not properly performed, the results may be uninterpretable or misleading.

Common Questions and Answers

Q: What does an "intact hymen" mean?
A: "Intact hymen" is not a medical term and should be avoided in describing the medical examination of the genitals. The hymen is a membranous structure at the entrance to the vaginal canal. It should have an opening that varies in size depending on the child, the child's age, the position in which the child was examined, and so on. The hymen should be inspected for signs of trauma. There is a wide variation of normal hymenal appearances, and caution should be used in interpreting findings.

Q: Can there be penetration without physical findings?
A: Yes. Although full penetration of an erect penis into the prepubertal vaginal canal (through the hymen) will leave injury, the healing properties of the hymenal tissue are great, so that past injuries are sometimes difficult or impossible to identify. Furthermore, penetration may be partial (as in vulvar coitus) and may not leave any injuries to the tissue. For these reasons, physical injuries may not be identified despite a history of penetration.

Q: Are STDs always transmitted sexually?
A: No. All STDs may be transmitted vertically (from mother to infant). The incubation periods of different infections vary, so they are expressed at different ages accordingly. Casual transmission of STDs is postulated for some organisms, but not for others. Gonorrhea and syphilis are considered diagnostic of sexual abuse outside of congenital infection. Chlamydia, herpes simplex virus 2, and trichomonas are probably a result of sexual abuse and should be reported for evaluation. Condyloma acuminata is quite controversial at this time, is probably related to sexual abuse in school-aged and older children, and should be referred for evaluation. Herpes simplex virus type 1 and bacterial vaginosis are nonspecific infections that are not usually related to sexual abuse. Candida is unlikely to be related to sexual abuse.

Q: How often do sexually abused children have physical evidence of the abuse?
A: In the majority of cases, there are no specific physical indicators of abuse. Only a small minority of patients (4% to 14%) have physical evidence considered diagnostic of abuse. Many children have nonspecific abnormalities of the physical examination, and many have normal examinations.

ICD-9-CM 995.5

BIBLIOGRAPHY

American Academy of Pediatrics, Committee on Child Abuse and Neglect. Guidelines for the evaluation of sexual abuse of children. *Pediatrics* 1999;103:186–191.

Bays J, Jenny C. Genital and anal conditions confused with child sexual abuse trauma. *Am J Dis Child* 1990;144:1319–1322.

Berenson AB, Chacko MR, Wiemann CM, et al. A case-control study of anatomic changes resulting from sexual abuse. *Am J Obstet Gynecol* 2000;182:820–834.

Christian CW, Lavelle JM, De Jong AR, et al. Forensic evidence findings in prepubertal victims of sexual assault. *Pediatrics* 2000;106:100–104.

Girardet RG, Lahoti S, Parks D, McNeese M. Issues in pediatric sexual abuse—what we think we know and where we need to go. *Curr Probl in Pediatr Adolesc Health Care* 2002;32(7):216–246.

Gushurst CA. Child abuse: behavioral aspects and other associated problems. *Pediatr Clin North Am* 2003;50(4):919–938.

Heger AH, Ticson L, Guerra L, et al. Appearance of the genitalia in girls selected for non-abuse: review of hymenal morphology and non-specific findings. *J Pediatr Adolesc Gynecol* 2002;15:27–35.

Heger A, Ticson L, Velasquez O, Bernier R. Children referred for possible sexual abuse: medical findings in 2384 children. *Child Abuse Negl* 2002;26:645–659.

Authors: Cindy W. Christian and Matthew J. Cox

Sexual Ambiguity

Database

DEFINITION

Genitalia can be defined as ambiguous when it is not possible to categorize the gender of the child based on outward appearances.

PATHOPHYSIOLOGY

Gonadal Dysgenesis

- Partial dysgenesis of the gonads following differentiation into testes will result in a spectrum of abnormalities ranging from phenotypically female external genitalia with the absence of müllerian structures to micropenis or cryptorchidism.
- Mixed gonadal dysgenesis: Individuals with the mosaic genotypes XO/XY and XX/XY have gonads containing both ovarian and testicular elements and external genitalia ranging from normal female, intersex, to normal male.
- Hermaphroditism: True hermaphrodites have gonads possessing both ovarian and testicular elements. This condition includes the patients with mixed gonadal dysgenesis discussed above, in addition to those with the karyotype 46XX, and less commonly 46XY.

Disorders of Sexual Phenotype

- Female pseudohermaphroditism: Masculinization of the female fetus is usually caused by androgens produced by the fetus or transferred across the placenta from the mother. The most common cause is congenital adrenal hyperplasia (CAH) in which the fetal adrenal glands overproduce androgens in an attempt to correct cortisol deficiency.
- Male pseudohermaphroditism: Incomplete masculinization of the male fetus can be caused by enzyme disorders of testosterone synthesis (e.g., CAH and 5α-reductase deficiency) or unresponsiveness to testosterone action (androgen resistance syndromes).

GENETICS

- Gonadal dysgenesis is associated with chromosomal aberrations.
- Syndromes of gonadal dysgenesis can also arise from mutations in the Wilms tumor-suppressor gene (WT-1), steroidogenic factor 1 (SF-1), SRY, and the SRY homeobox gene SOX9.
- CAH is caused by defects in the genes encoding adrenal steroidogenic enzymes. Thus, it follows an autosomal recessive inheritance pattern. The most common form is 21-hydroxylase deficiency (encoded by the gene CYP21), but sexual ambiguity can also be seen in defects in 17-hydroxylase (CYP17), 3β-hydroxysteroid dehydrogenase (HSD3B2), 17-ketosteroid reductase (HSD17B3), and 11β-hydroxylase (CYP11B1). Congenital lipoid adrenal hyperplasia has been associated with defects in steroidogenic acute regulatory protein (StAR), and less commonly, cholesterol desmolase.

- 5α-Reductase deficiency is an autosomal-recessive disorder that manifests only in genetic males.
- Androgen resistance syndromes are a result of defects in the androgen receptor, whose gene is located on the X chromosome. Thus, they follow an X-linked recessive pattern.

EPIDEMIOLOGY

Incidence

Inherited adrenal enzymatic defects of adrenal biosynthesis are the most common cause of virilization of the newborn female. Ninety percent of these females have 21-hydroxylase deficiency.

Age

Disorders causing sexual ambiguity occur congenitally, and the time of presentation is the newborn period. Children with 5α-reductase deficiency demonstrate virilization with puberty.

COMPLICATIONS

- 21-hydroxylase, 3β-hydroxysteroid dehydrogenase, and StAR protein deficient forms of CAH are associated with mineralocorticoid deficiency and consequent life-threatening salt-losing adrenal crises presenting in the first 2 weeks of life.
- CAH is also associated with cortisol deficiency, requiring emergent and chronic cortisol replacement.
- Dysgenetic testes and ovotestes have an increased risk of malignant degeneration and should be removed.
- An incorrect or hastily made sexual assignment can cause family members undue emotional stress.

PROGNOSIS

The cosmetic outcome from surgery is usually good. The potential for gender-appropriate sexual function is usually good with therapy. The potential for reproductive function depends on the diagnosis. Long-term studies of psychological adjustment are underway.

Differential Diagnosis

- Gonadal dysgenesis

—Partial dysgenesis of the gonads
—Mixed gonadal dysgenesis
—Hermaphroditism

- Female pseudohermaphroditism

—Congenital adrenal hyperplasia: Inherited adrenal enzymatic defects, including 21-hydroxylase, 11-hydroxylase, and 3β-hydroxysteroid dehydrogenase (3β-HSD) deficiencies can cause virilization of females.
—Maternal androgen exposure
—Exogenous androgens or endogenous production (e.g., maternal virilizing tumor)
—Multiple congenital anomalies

—Ambiguous genitalia can be a part of a spectrum of congenital anomalies, especially those of the urologic system and rectum.
—Idiopathic

- Male pseudohermaphroditism

—Congenital adrenal hyperplasia (CAH): Deficiencies in 3β-HSD, 17α-hydroxylase, StAR protein, and cholesterol desmolase result in insufficient androgen synthesis potentially causing undervirilization of males.

- 5α-Reductase deficiency prevents the conversion of testosterone to dihydrotestosterone (DHT), which is necessary for the development of the male external genitalia.
- Syndromes of androgen resistance are a result of abnormalities in androgen receptor or postreceptor defects. Patients with incomplete forms of androgen resistance may present with sexual ambiguity.
- Multiple congenital anomalies
- Idiopathic

Data Gathering

Ambiguous genitalia in the neonate should be treated as an emergency, and the diagnostic evaluation undertaken as soon as possible.

HISTORY

Obtain a careful pregnancy and family history addressing:

- Drug ingestion
- Exposure to teratogens
- Infections during the pregnancy
- Androgenic changes in the mother
- Family history suggestive of CAH

Physical Examination

Notable features include:

- Palpable gonads: imply the presence of Y-chromosome material
- Fusion of the labia
- Existence of a vagina
- Position of the urethra
- Length and diameter of the penis or clitoris
- Development of the scrotum
- Other dysmorphic features
- Hypertension is seen with 17α-hydroxylase and 11-hydroxylase deficiencies.
- See table, Features of the Classic Disorders of Adrenal Steroidogenesis.

Laboratory Aids

TESTS

Specific Tests

- Karyotype
- Steroid levels

—17-Hydroxyprogesterone
—17-Hydroxypregnenolone
—DHEA
—Testosterone
—Dihydrotestosterone
—11-Deoxycortisol
—Androstenedione

IMAGING

- Pelvic ultrasound
- Urethrogram

Nonspecific Tests

Electrolytes: Hyponatremia, hyperkalemia, and metabolic acidosis are associated with several adrenal enzyme deficiencies.

 Emergency Care

- Gender assignment

—The results of the diagnostic evaluation should be available within 48 to 72 hours, and gender assignment made by this time. A team approach with consultations from endocrinology, urology, and psychiatry is useful.

- Treatment of CAH

—Acute salt-wasting adrenal crisis
—Volume resuscitation with D5NS
—Stress hydrocortisone 25 to 50 mg IV immediately after the serum studies are drawn. This should be followed by 100 mg/m^2 per 24 h of hydrocortisone IV divided q4h.
—Hydrocortisone is gradually tapered over the next few days.
—Fludrocortisone 0.05 to 0.3 mg/day when able to take PO

 Therapy

- Surgery

—Surgery may be necessary so that the sexual phenotype and gonads are consistent with the gender assignment. Dysgenetic testes and ovotestes should be removed.

- Treatment of CAH

—Acute salt-wasting adrenal crisis
—Volume resuscitation with D5NS
—Stress hydrocortisone 25 to 50 mg IV immediately after the serum studies are drawn. This should be followed by 100 mg/m2 per 24 h of hydrocortisone IV divided q4h.
—Hydrocortisone is gradually tapered over the next few days.
—Fludrocortisone 0.05 to 0.3 mg/day when able to take PO
—Chronic management of CAH consists of cortisol replacement 12 to 25 mg/m^2 per 24 h divided as q8h and fludrocortisone 0.05 to 0.3 mg/day.

- Counseling of families

 Follow-Up

- Hormone replacement therapy at puberty may be necessary.
- Long-term follow-up may involve monitoring hormone levels, linear growth, and sexual development.

PREVENTION

- Avoid the use of androgenic steroids during pregnancy.
- Prenatal diagnosis of CAH and maternal steroid treatment to prevent virilization of female fetuses is available.

PITFALLS

Girls with CAH may appear quite virilized at birth and be mistaken for boys. Nevertheless, they have good female reproductive potential with adequate control of their disease, and should be assigned a female sex.

Common Questions and Answers

Q: Should a child's sex assignment be consistent with the karyotype?
A: Karyotype should not be the major factor in gender determination because gonadal and future sexual function are more important.

Q: What clues can the physical examination give to the timing of in utero events causing sexual ambiguity?
A: In the virilized female, labioscrotal fusion results from androgen exposure prior to 12 weeks' gestation. Thereafter, androgen exposure can only cause clitoromegaly.

ICD-9-CM 752.7

BIBLIOGRAPHY

Anhalt H, Neely EK, Hintz RK. Ambiguous genitalia. *Pediatr Rev* 1996;(6):213–220.

Carlson AD, Obeid JS, Kanellopoulou N, et al. Congential adrenal hyperplasia: update on prenatal diagnosis and treatment. *J Steroid Biochem Mol Biol* 1999;69(1–6):19–29.

MacLaughlin DT, Donahoe PK. Sex determination and differentiation. *N Engl J Med* 2004;350:367–378.

Mercado AB, Wilson RC, Cheng WK, et al. Prenatal treatment and diagnosis of congenital adrenal hyperplasia owing to steroid 21-hydroxylase deficiency. *J Clin Endocrinol Metab* 1995;80:2014–2020.

Moshang T, Thornton PS. Endocrine disorders. In: Avery GS, eds. *Neonatology: Pathophysiology and Management.* Philadelphia: JB Lippincott, 1993.

New MI. Inborn errors of adrenal steroidogenesis. *Mol Cell Endocrinol.* 2003;211:75–83.

Speiser PW, White PC. Congenital adrenal hyperplasia. *N Engl J Med* 2003;349:776–788.

White PC, Curnow KM, Pascoe L. Disorders of steroid 11 beta-hydroxylase isoenzymes. *Endocr Rev* 1994;15:421–438.

Yong EL, Lim J, Qi W, et al. Molecular basis of androgen receptor diseases. *Ann Med* 2000;32(1):15–22.

Authors: Lorraine Katz and J. Nina Ham

Features of the Classic Disorders of Adrenal Steroidogenesis

ENZYME	CLINICAL MANIFESTATIONS	SEXUAL AMBIGUITY		PREDOMINANT STEROIDS
		FEMALE	MALE	
Desmolase StAR protein	Salt losing	No	Yes	Low levels (all steroids)
3β-HSD	Salt losing	Yes	Yes	17-OH pregnenolone, DHEA
21-Hydroxylase	Salt losing	Yes	No	17-OH progesterone, androstenedione
11-Hydroxylase	Hypertension	Yes	No	11-Deoxycortisol
17-Hydroxylase	Hypertension	No	Yes	DOC, corticosterone

Sexual Precocity

Database

DEFINITION

Sexual precocity has traditionally been defined as physical signs of sexual development before age 8 years in girls and age 9 years in boys. Recently, new guidelines were proposed for lowering the age considered to be normal for sexual development in girls. Signs of puberty as young as age 7 years in White girls and age 6 in Black girls may be normal. These new guidelines have not been adopted universally. The entire clinical picture, including rate of progression and the presence of neurologic symptoms, must be taken into account.

CAUSES

• Central precocious puberty (GnRH-dependent): associated with gonadotropin (LH and/or FSH) levels that are elevated beyond the normal prepubertal range
• Peripheral precocious puberty (GnRH-independent): gonadotropin-independent elevation of sex steroids arising from gonads/adrenals

PATHOPHYSIOLOGY

• Central precocious puberty is associated with CNS disorders.
• Peripheral precocious puberty is associated with gonadal and adrenal disorders.
• Peripheral precocious puberty can progress to central precocious puberty, as a result of maturation of the hypothalamic-pituitary axis by sex steroids.

GENETICS

• Familial male precocious puberty (testotoxicosis): sex-limited, autosomal-dominant inheritance of activating mutation in the LH receptor
• McCune-Albright syndrome: sporadic, postzygotic, somatic mutation in the stimulatory subunit of G-protein receptor; more common in females

EPIDEMIOLOGY

• Precocious puberty occurs in approximately 1 in 5,000 children.

—Precocious puberty is 5 to 6 times more common in girls.
—Eighty percent to 90% of affected girls have central precocious puberty.

• Precocious puberty in boys is more likely to be associated with underlying pathology.

—Approximately 50% of boys have central precocious puberty.

COMPLICATIONS

• Short stature
• Psychosocial stresses of early puberty

PROGNOSIS

• With treatment, improvement in predicted height is achieved, but most do not reach target height predicted by mid-parental height measurements. Early treatment improves final height.
• Effect of GnRH agonists on fertility has not been fully elucidated.

Differential Diagnosis

• Tumors

—CNS tumors
—Hypothalamic hamartoma: The CNS mass most commonly causing precocious puberty, it is a nonprogressive (benign), congenital malformation of neurons that secrete GnRH.
—Hypothalamic-chiasmatic glioma: often associated with neurofibromatosis
—Astrocytoma
—Ependymoma
—hCG-secreting tumors: may arise from pineal gland or liver
—Gonadal tumors
—Adrenal tumors

• Post-CNS trauma or damage

—Surgery
—Radiation: may occur after 18-Gy exposure

• Hydrocephalus
• Infection: Brain abscess, meningitis, encephalitis, granuloma. These CNS lesions may result in abnormal stimulation or lack of inhibition of the GnRH-secreting area of the hypothalamus, resulting in early activation of the pituitary gland.
• Environmental: Exogenous estrogen exposure (such as creams and oral contraceptives) and/or exogenous androgen exposure (such as anabolic steroid injections)
• Congenital adrenal hyperplasia (CAH): Poorly controlled CAH can activate the hypothalamic-pituitary-gonadal axis in either gender.
• Severe acquired hypothyroidism: High levels of TSH may cross-stimulate gonadal FSH and/or LH receptors.
• McCune-Albright syndrome: Triad of precocious puberty, café-au-lait spots, and polyostotic fibrous dysplasia
• Familial male precocious puberty (familial testotoxicosis)
• Refeeding after severe undernutrition during early development (such as adopted children who had kwashiorkor)
• Premature thelarche
• Premature adrenarche
• Obesity

Data Gathering

HISTORY

• Careful chronology of physical changes, growth spurt, onset of menses
• Presence of neurologic, visual, or behavioral changes may suggest a CNS lesion.
• Family history of early puberty

SPECIAL QUESTIONS

• Family history suggestive of familial male precocious puberty

Physical Examination

• Plot accurate height (using wall-mounted stadiometer), weight, and growth velocity.
• Carefully stage breasts, color of vaginal mucosa, and pubic hair in girls.
• Carefully stage testicular volume, penile size, and pubic hair in boys.
• Carefully evaluate for abdominal masses.
• Examine skin for acne (comedones) and café-au-lait spots.
• Perform comprehensive neurologic evaluation to assess for possible CNS pathology.

PROCEDURE

Use standard beads (Prader gonadometer) to assess testicular volumes accurately.

Laboratory Aids

TESTS

Nonspecific Tests

Bone age: If advanced, further studies are warranted, guided by history and physical examination. If not advanced, or if the patient has only mild breast or pubic hair development (but not both), premature thelarche or premature adrenarche, respectively, is the most likely diagnosis.

Specific Tests

- Sex steroids: estradiol, testosterone
- Adrenal steroids: dehydroepiandrosterone sulfate (DHEA-S)
- Gonadotropins: FSH, LH (ultrasensitive or ICMA-LH if possible)
- Prolactin: often elevated with CNS tumors
- TSH and T4
- In males, hCG levels
- Provocative tests should be done in cases in which the aforementioned tests are abnormal or equivocal:

—GnRH test for central precocious puberty; prepubertal GnRH response is predominately FSH, whereas pubertal response is predominately LH.
—ACTH stimulation test for adrenal abnormalities. Exogenous corticosteroid therapy will interfere with ACTH test but does not interfere with GnRH test of pituitary-gonadal axis.

IMAGING

- MRI of head: As indicated by history, physical examination, and laboratory tests; almost always done in males because boys are much less likely than are girls to have idiopathic sexual precocity.
- Ultrasound of gonads/adrenals: as indicated by examination and studies

 Therapy

As indicated by cause of the precocious puberty, for example, removal of CNS lesions or cessation of exogenous sex steroids

DRUGS

- Central precocious puberty: GnRH agonists such as Lupron are the treatment of choice. Adjunctive therapy with recombinant human growth hormone may improve final adult height; calcium supplementation may preserve bone mass accretion in girls during GnRH agonist therapy.
- Peripheral precocious puberty: Aromatase inhibitors (testolactone) and antiandrogens (spironolactone or ketoconazole). Glucocorticoids for CAH.

—Tamoxifen therapy may be beneficial in McCune-Albright Syndrome.

DURATION

Until endocrinologist and family agree that pubertal progression is appropriate, guided by bone age and predicted final adult height

DIET

No restrictions

 Follow-Up

WHEN TO EXPECT IMPROVEMENT

- Depends on cause. For example, sexual changes of McCune-Albright syndrome are a result of autonomously functioning ovarian cysts, which regress variably over time.
- Treatment of central precocious puberty with a GnRH agonist usually results in cessation of menses within 2 months, slowing or nonprogression of pubertal changes over 4 to 6 months, and decreased acceleration of bone age within 12 months.

SIGNS TO WATCH FOR

Typically, GnRH agonists are given in a depot form every 28 days, but some children require shortening of this time interval. Such dosing is often prompted by parental reports of moodiness, development of acne near the time of injection, or breakthrough menses (failure to suppress).

PITFALLS

- Obese children often have advanced bone age.
- Palpation of breast tissue (buds) can be difficult as a result of adiposity.

—Adiposity can be mistaken for breast tissue.

 Common Questions and Answers

Q: If my child is treated with GnRH agonists, will he or she go through puberty when we stop the medication?
A: Yes, children on GnRH agonist treatment do proceed through normal puberty when the medication is stopped. Effects on fertility have not been fully elucidated.

Q: If a child already has some pubertal changes, can they be reversed?
A: If GnRH agonists are used, menses will cease, and breast tissue and pubic hair often regress.

ICD-9-CM 259.1

BIBLIOGRAPHY

Antoniazzi F, Bertoldo F, Lauriola S, et al. Prevention of bone demineralization by calcium supplementation in precocious puberty during gonadotropin-releasing hormone agonist treatment. *J Clin Endocrinol Metab* 1999;84(6):1992–1996.

Egli CA, Rosenthal SM, Grumbach MM, et al. Pituitary gonadotropin-independent male limited autosomal dominant sexual precocity in nine generations: familial testitoxicosis. *J Pediatr* 1985;106:33–40.

Eugster EA, Rubin SD, Reiter EO, et al. Tamoxifen treatment for precocious puberty in McCune-Albright syndrome: a multicenter trial. *J Pediatr* 2003;143:60–66.

Herman-Giddens ME, Slora EJ, Wasserman RC, et al. Secondary sexual characteristics and menses in young girls seen in office practice: a study from the pediatric research office in settings network. *Pediatrics* 1997;99:505–512.

Kaplowitz P, Oberfield SE, and the Drug and Therapeutics and Executive Committees of the Lawson Wilkins Pediatric Endocrine Society. Reexamination of the age limit for defining when puberty is precocious in girls in the United States: implications for evaluation and treatment. *Pediatrics* 1999;104:936–941.

Oostdijk W, Rikken B, Schreuder S, et al. Final height in central precocious puberty after long term treatment with a slow release GnRH agonist. *Arch Dis Child* 1996;75(4):292–297.

Pasquino AM, Pucarelli I, Segni M, et al. Adult height in girls with central precocious puberty treated with gonadrotropin-releasing hormone analogues and growth hormone. *J Clin Endocrinol Metab* 1999;84(2):449–452.

Saenger P, Rincon M. Precocious puberty: McCune-Albright syndrome and beyond. *J Pediatr* 2003;143:9–10.

Shankar RR, Pescovitz OH. Precocious puberty. *Adv Endocrinol Metab* 1995;6:55–89.

Styne DM. New aspects in diagnosis and treatment of pubertal disorders. *Pediatr Clin North Am* 1997;44(2):505–529.

Authors: Malaka B. Jackson and Andrea Kelly

Short-Bowel Syndrome

 Database

DEFINITION

Malnutrition, malabsorption, fluid, and electrolyte loss after extensive small-bowel resection.

ETIOLOGY

- Intestinal resection for necrotizing enterocolitis.
- Congenital anomalies including intestinal atresias and gastroschisis
- Malrotation may result in volvulus with bowel resection secondary to ischemic injury
- Neoplasms and radiation enteritis
- Intestinal resection secondary to Crohn disease

PATHOPHYSIOLOGY

- Markedly decreased mucosal surface area as a result of resection
- Abnormal transit
- Malabsorption of protein, fat, carbohydrate, vitamins, electrolytes, and trace elements, depending on site of resected intestine (see table, Site of Absorption of Various Nutrients in the Intestine). The patient can lose as much as half of the intestine if the duodenum, distal ileum, and ileocecal valve (ICV) are present. If the ICV is gone, patients may not be able to tolerate even a 25% loss of intestine without the help of total parenteral nutrition (TPN).
- Normal bowel length: at 26 weeks' gestation: 150 to 200 cm; at birth in full-term infant: 200 to 300 cm; adult: 600 to 800 cm
- Infants have no intestinal reserve and do not tolerate small-bowel resection and adults. Long-term prognosis may be better because of hypertrophy and hyperplasia of the intestine.
- Gastric acid hypersecretion occurs soon after intestinal resection, but is transient.
- Complications include:

—Bacterial overgrowth and D-lactic acidosis as a result of stasis causing encephalopathy, ataxia and other neurological symptoms.
—Renal stones as a result of fat malabsorption and increased oxalate absorption
—Gallstones as a result of disturbed entero-hepatic circulation of bile salts and lithogenic bile formation

- Bowel adaptation can occur over time. Increased surface area as a result of bowel dilatation and villus hypertrophy and bowel lengthening can occur. Need stimulation of luminal contents for bowel growth, and factors such as glutamine, short-chain fatty acids, tropic hormones, and growth factors may be important for bowel growth.

COMPLICATIONS

- Fluid and electrolyte loss, resulting in diarrhea and dehydration and metabolic acidosis
- Calcium and magnesium deficiency, resulting in bone disease and osteoporosis

- Carbohydrate malabsorption
- Fat malabsorption
- Vitamin A deficiency: increased susceptibility to infections
- Vitamin D deficiency: bone disease (e.g., rickets)
- Vitamin E deficiency: peripheral neuropathy, hemolysis
- Vitamin K deficiency: prolonged clotting time, bruising
- Vitamin B12: macrocytic anemia and thrombosis
- Folic acid: macrocytic anemia
- Gallstones
- Renal stones
- Failure to thrive
- TPN-dependent liver disease: cholestasis, end stage is cirrhosis and portal hypertension
- Zinc deficiency: poor growth, infections
- Carnitine deficiency: contributes to development of steatosis

PROGNOSIS

- Depends on site and amount of bowel resected
- The greater the amount of bowel resected, the worse is the prognosis
- Loss of ICV portends a worse prognosis
- Loss of jejunum and ileum creates a poorer clinical condition than loss of colon
- The longer it takes to tolerate full enteral feeds in a patient, the worse is the prognosis. Most progress is made in the first year after bowel resection.
- Development of severe TPN liver disease: poor prognosis

 Differential Diagnosis

- Infants: necrotizing enterocolitis, volvulus, atresia (jejunal and ileal), gastroschisis, meconium peritonitis, congenital short-bowel syndrome
- Older children: midgut volvulus (as a result of malrotation), Crohn disease, adhesions causing intestinal obstruction, strictures, trauma, aganglionosis of the intestine

 Data Gathering

HISTORY

- Stooling pattern: number, size, nature (watery, bulky, foul smelling), presence of blood and mucus
- Weight loss or gain; gaining length/height
- Abdominal distention and flatulence
- Intense perianal rashes related to stool acidity and malabsorption of carbohydrates
- Appetite
- Abdominal pain and characteristics
- Vomiting and characteristics
- Diet history: oral intake, tube feeds, parenteral nutrition
- Medication history
- Surgical history

 Physical Examination

- Weight, length, and head circumference measurements (if applicable); try to get previous growth chart if available
- Look for signs of vitamin deficiencies in examination of mouth, lips, and skin.
- Abdominal examination: surgical scars, ostomies, distention, hepatosplenomegaly, bowel sounds
- Rectal examination: consistency of stool, heme positivity, perianal rash

 Laboratory Aids

TESTS

Blood Tests

- CBC: Check for anemia and MCV.
- Electrolytes: Sodium, potassium, chloride and bicarbonate; check for losses and adequacy of replacement.
- Minerals: Calcium, phosphorus magnesium, iron; check for losses and adequacy of replacement therapy.
- Albumin and prealbumin: Check for protein stores and nutritional status.
- PT/PTT and PIVKA: Assess vitamin K status. A new test known as the PIVKA-II assay is a more sensitive measure of Vitamin K status; however it is more useful in adolescents.
- Liver function tests: ALT, GGT, bilirubin, if on parenteral nutrition (PN) to check for TPN-associated liver disease
- Vitamin levels: Vitamin A, 25-hydroxy vitamin D, vitamin E, folic acid, B12; check for adequacy
- Zinc level: Check status and adequacy of supplementation.
- Carnitine: Check status if on long-term parenteral nutrition and have liver disease.
- Breath tests: Lactose and lactulose breath test to check for lactase deficiency and bacterial overgrowth, respectively

Stool Tests

- Stool for pH and reducing substances: Check for carbohydrate malabsorption.
- Stool smear for fat (Sudan stain-qualitative): Check for excessive fat loss.
- Stool for blood: Check for mucosal damage.

—Stool elastase: A measure of pancreatic insufficiency.

Tests of Absorption

- Xylose absorption test and lactose breath test to check for carbohydrate malabsorption
- Seventy-two-hour quantitative fecal fat collection along with concomitant diet record
- Carotene levels to check for fat absorption
- Twenty-four-hour stool collection for α1-antitrypsin clearance to check for protein absorption

IMAGING

Upper GI series with small-bowel follow-through and barium enema to evaluate length, caliber, and location of remaining bowel

ENDOSCOPY

- Upper endoscopy: Look for presence of inflammation that may be contributing to malabsorption; get cultures for bacterial overgrowth.
- Lower endoscopy: Look for presence of colitis, especially eosinophilic colitis, and caliber of anastomotic site if in colon.

 Therapy

DRUGS

- Supplementation of vitamin (E, D, K, B12, folic acid) deficiency, calcium, magnesium, iron, and zinc
- H2-receptor antagonists and proton pump inhibitors decrease gastric acid hypersecretion and reduce gastric secretory volume.
- Antidiarrheal drugs: Codeine, diphenoxylate, and anticholinergic drugs (e.g., loperamide) to decrease motility
- Ion-exchange resins: Cholestyramine binds intraluminal dihydroxy bile acids to prevent bile acid–induced diarrhea.
- Octreotide: Decreases gastric, pancreatic, and intestinal secretions; slows gastro-intestinal motility and splanchnic blood flow
- Bacterial overgrowth: Commonly used oral antibiotics are metronidazole, trimethoprim-sulfamethoxazole, vancomycin, and gentamicin.
- Prokinetic agents: Reglan to treat delayed gastric emptying
- Miscellaneous: sucralfate to treat bile reflux, probiotics to treat bacterial overgrowth

Site of Absorption of Various Nutrients in the Intestine

SITE	NUTRIENT
Stomach	Fat
Duodenum	Calcium
	Magnesium
	Iron
	Folate
	Zinc
Jejunum	Monosaccharides
	Disaccharides
	Fat-soluble vitamins A and D
	Water-soluble vitamins: thiamin, riboflavin, pyridoxine, folic acid, ascorbic acid
	Protein
Ileum	Fat
	Vitamin B12
	Bile salts
Colon	Fluid
	Electrolytes
	Short-chain fatty acids

DURATION

Depends on amount and site of bowel resected and degree of intestinal adaptation that occurs. The more the resection, the longer is the therapy. Successful enteral feeds decrease the duration of parenteral nutrition. Macronutrient losses decrease with intestinal adaptation. Micronutrient supplementation may be lifelong (e.g., vitamin B12).

SURGICAL/TRANSPLANT

Surgery is useful in patients who develop strictures and partial obstruction, or in those who have very short intestine length. Intestinal interpositions (isoperistaltic or antiperistaltic) can be used to delay gastric emptying, slow intestinal transit, and increase absorption. Intestinal lengthening and tapering procedures, including the Bianchi and step enteroplasty procedures, increase absorptive surface area. In patients with extremely short intestines and PN dependency, small-bowel transplantation is considered.

DIET

- Oral diet: In those patients who are able to avoid PN or tube feeds, a low-lactose diet may be well tolerated. Low-oxalate diets are helpful in preventing oxalate stones. In general, a high-calorie diet irrespective of carbohydrate and fat composition should be the mainstay of treatment.
- Fluid and electrolyte therapy: Extremely important in the acute phase immediately after bowel resection. In the chronic phase, it is important to keep up with ongoing losses, especially when enteral feeds are started.
- Enteral feeds: More successful in the patient with less extensive resection, intact ICV, and colon in continuity; no advantage of elemental formulas over intact formulas, with respect to tolerance, unless small-bowel damage is present.
- Parenteral nutrition: Important in the acute phase postoperatively when nutrition must be maintained in the face of paralytic ileus; indispensable in the chronic phase when full enteral feeds cannot be instituted and nutrition needs to be maintained. Balanced solutions of protein, glucose, and fat should be administered. Prophylactic measures to prevent parenteral nutrition-induced liver damage should be instituted (e.g., prevention of overfeeding, early introduction of enteral feeds, cycling of parenteral nutrition when patient is stable). Need permanent central access to deliver concentrated PN solutions.

 Follow-Up

WHEN TO EXPECT IMPROVEMENT

Depends on site and extent of bowel resection

SIGNS TO WATCH FOR

Vomiting, diarrhea, weight loss, severe fluid and electrolyte abnormalities, sepsis, bowel dilatation, intestinal obstruction

 Common Questions and Answers

Q: What are the favorable prognostic factors in short-bowel syndrome?
A: Poor prognosis is related to the greater length of the bowel resected, loss of the ICV, loss of jejunum and ileum, longer time to tolerate full enteral feeds, and development of severe TPN-liver disease. Neonates have greater chances of bowel adaptation than do adults.

Q: Are elemental formulas better than intact formulas in the management of patients with short-bowel syndrome?
A: Recent studies have shown similar rates of absorption, stomal output, and electrolyte losses between elemental and intact formulas. The disadvantages of elemental formulas include high osmolality and cost.

ICD-9-CM 579.3

BIBLIOGRAPHY

Buchman AL, Scolapio J, Fryer J. AGA technical review on short bowel syndrome and intestinal transplantation. *Gastroenterology*. 2003;124(4):1111–34.

Sigalet DL. Short bowel syndrome in infants and children: an overview. *Semin Pediatr Surg* 2001;10(2):49–55.

Vanderhoof JA. Short-bowel syndrome including adaptation. In: Walker WA, Watkins JB, eds. *Nutrition in Pediatrics*. Philadelphia: BC Decker, 2000:771–789.

Vanderhoof JA, Young RJ. Enteral and parenteral nutrition in the care of patients with short-bowel syndrome. *Best Prac Res Clin Gastro* 2003;17(6):997–1015.

Warner BW, Vanderhoof JA, Reyes JD. What's new in the management of short Gut syndrome in children. *J Am Coll Surg* 2000;190(6):725–736.

Westergaard H. Short bowel syndrome. *Sem Gastrointest Dis* 2002;13(4):210–220.

Authors: Maria R. Mascarenhas and Meena Thayu

Sickle Cell Disease

 Database

DEFINITION

Sickle cell disease (SCD) is a group of hemoglobin disorders in which sickle hemoglobin (HbS) predominates. SCD is characterized by hemolysis, vascular occlusion, and an increased risk of bacterial infection. Common genotypes include SCD-SS, SCD-SC, SCD-Sβ^+ thalassemia, and SCD-Sβ^0 thalassemia.

GENETICS

SCD has an autosomal-recessive pattern of inheritance.

PATHOPHYSIOLOGY

- The production of HbS is caused by a genetic mutation leading to a valine for glutamic acid substitution at the sixth position of the β-globin chain.
- HbS polymerizes within red cells, particularly under deoxygenated conditions, which leads to (a) changes in red blood cell shape, (b) vascular occlusion, and (c) subsequent ischemic tissue/organ injury.

EPIDEMIOLOGY

- One in 375 Black newborns has SCD.
- One in 12 Black has sickle cell trait.
- The frequencies of SCD genotypes from highest to lowest are SCD-SS (60%), SCD-SC (25% to 30%), SCD-Sβ^+ thalassemia, SCD-Sβ^0 thalassemia, and other relatively infrequent variants.
- Although population data indicate that patients with SCD-SS and SCD-Sβ^0 thalassemia experience more complications than patients with other variants, disease severity varies widely among all individuals with SCD regardless of disease genotypes.

COMPLICATIONS

Acute

- Painful episodes: Sudden, unpredictable pain that develops anywhere in the body
- Dactylitis: Painful swelling of hands and feet
- Bacterial infection: Younger children are at greatest risk for sepsis/meningitis as a result of *Streptococcus pneumoniae*, whereas older children and adults are at greatest risk for sepsis with gram-negative organisms. Salmonella infections are problematic for patients of all ages.
- Acute chest syndrome: A pneumonia-like illness defined as a new infiltrate on chest radiograph
- Neurologic: Including stroke (infarctive and hemorrhagic) and transient ischemic attack (TIA)
- Acute splenic sequestration: Acute enlargement of the spleen, with a decreased hemoglobin and increased reticulocyte count
- Aplastic episode: Transient decrease in RBC production characterized by a decrease in hemoglobin and reticulocyte count; human parvovirus B19 is most common cause
- Cholecystitis: Risk is greatest after age 10 years
- Priapism: A prolonged penile erection, which can be seen in males of all ages

Chronic

- Delayed linear growth and puberty
- Cholelithiasis
- Retinopathy: particularly in children with SCD-SC
- Neurologic: neurologic sequelae of stroke, silent infarction, cerebral vasculopathy and/or abnormal cerebral blood flow velocity (flow rates $\geq$200 cm/second by transcranial Doppler [TCD] ultrasonography), arterial-venous malformations, moyamoya, neuropsychological abnormalities
- Hypersplenism: particularly in young children or patients with SCD-SC or SCD-S$\beta+$ thalassemia
- Avascular necrosis: particularly of the hips
- Renal: nephrotic syndrome, acute glomerulonephritis
- Pulmonary function abnormalities
- Primary nocturnal enuresis

PROGNOSIS

Population estimates of life expectancy from 1978 to 1988 data range from 42 to 48 years for SCD-SS and 60 to 68 years for SCD-SC. However, many believe that early SCD diagnosis (newborn screening), penicillin prophylaxis, comprehensive medical care, and hydroxyurea therapy may increase life expectancy. Children ages 2 to 16 years with SCD-SS or SCD-Sβ^0 thalassemia are at increased risk for developing stroke if they have repeatedly abnormal TCDs. This risk is reduced with chronic transfusion therapy (see Measures for Specific Complications).

 Data Gathering

HISTORY

- SCD-genotype
- Baseline hemoglobin and reticulocyte count
- Baseline pulse oximetry values (Spo^2)
- History of SCD complications
- Prior blood transfusions and complications

 Physical Examination

- Fever
- Pallor (may be accentuated at time of splenic sequestration or transient aplastic episode)
- Scleral icterus
- Signs of respiratory distress (as a result of acute chest syndrome)
- A flow murmur may be present (as a result of anemia).
- Splenomegaly
- Warmth, tenderness, decreased range of motion at site of pain
- Abnormal neurologic findings suggestive of CNS infarction or hemorrhage

 Laboratory Aids

TESTS

Diagnostic

- Hemoglobin electrophoresis: Definitive test along with DNA analysis
- Screening test: "Sickledex" or "shake" tests are not recommended to establish a diagnosis or carrier status; do not use for screening in children less than 12 months of age as a result of false-negative results.
- CBCs: Hemoglobin values vary depending on age and SCD genotype; peripheral blood smear-sickled forms, targets, nucleated RBCs, and increased polychromasia are common RBC findings (sickle forms may be absent in transfused patients or in patients with phenotypes other than SCD-SS).
- Reticulocyte count: Increased
- Quantitative hemoglobin electrophoresis
- Chemistry panel: Elevated LDH, unconjugated bilirubin, AST
- Prior to the first transfusion in any sickle cell patient, draw blood for a red-cell antigen profile for future reference. (This is because of the high risk of alloimmunization in repeatedly transfused patients.)
- Neuropsychological testing: Strongly recommended for children with a history of stroke, silent infarction, abnormal TCD, or learning difficulties

IMAGING

- Bone scan and bone marrow scan (to help differentiate osteomyelitis from bony infarction)
- Chest radiograph study (at the time of pulmonary complications): cardiomegaly
- Abdominal ultrasound (if considering cholecystitis)
- TCD examinations at least yearly in children with SCD-SS or SCD-Sβ^0 thalassemia ages 2 to 16 years; these studies should be performed by trained examiners, experienced with the procedural modifications used for children with SCD
- CT/MRI/MR angiography (MRA) (if considering stroke)

 Therapy

GENERAL MEASURES (GENERAL WELL-PATIENT CARE)

- Children should be seen by a pediatric hematologist at least twice a year for: (a) an interim history, physical examination, and laboratory tests; (b) other ancillary studies, including TCD when appropriate; (c) patient and parent education; (d) psychosocial evaluation; and (e) referrals to other specialists, such as ophthalmology, urology, and general surgery when needed.

- Infection prophylaxis with penicillin starting by 2 months of age
- Pneumococcal vaccines (7-valent as per AAP recommendations and 23-valent at 2 and 5 years)
- Routine immunizations, including hepatitis B series; consider yearly influenza vaccine
- Consider folic acid supplementation.
- Parental monitoring for fever, splenomegaly, pain (including dactylitis), increased jaundice
- Encourage good oral hydration and supply family with medications to treat uncomplicated painful episodes at home.
- Transfusion therapy can prevent the development of SCD complications and decrease associated morbidity or recurrence of complications when used appropriately. When children with SCD-SS receive erythrocyte transfusions, avoid posttransfusion hemoglobin levels above 12 g/dL. Erythrocyte antigen matching for ABO and C, D, E, and Kell is recommended. Monitor children carefully for erythrocyte antibodies and/or delayed transfusion reactions.

MEASURES FOR SPECIFIC COMPLICATIONS

- Fever (rule out sepsis)
—History, physical examination, CBC, reticulocyte count, blood culture (urine, CSF culture, throat culture as indicated by examination)
—Parenteral antibiotics to provide 24- to 48-hour coverage until blood cultures are negative
—Close monitoring for other SCD complications
- Pain (vaso-occlusive episode)
—History, physical examination; consider CBC, reticulocyte count
—Hydration
—Analgesics: Therapy should be directed toward the level of pain the child is experiencing, the medications that have been used prior to presentation, and the past experience of the child with certain interventions. Patients and their families can often tell physicians what therapies have been helpful in the past. In general, for mild pain, start with mild nonnarcotic medications (acetaminophen, ibuprofen) and mild oral narcotic analgesics (codeine, oxycodone). Consider stronger agents such as oral ketorolac, hydromorphone, and morphine for initial management of moderate pain. For severe pain, use parenteral medications such as morphine, hydromorphone, and ketorolac.
—Comfort measures (massage, heating pad, warm soaks)
—Frequent reassessment for pain control and side effects of medications is mandatory.
- Acute chest syndrome
—History, physical examination, CBC, reticulocyte count, chest radiograph film (blood culture as indicated), pulse oximetry
—Initial findings: Chest tenderness, cough, hypoxia, fever, infiltrate on chest radiograph
—Management
—Parenteral antibiotics
—Pain management
—Supplemental oxygen for hypoxia
—Incentive spirometry or chest physiotherapy

—Red blood cell transfusion for moderate to severe disease
- Splenic sequestration
—History, physical examination, CBC, reticulocyte count blood culture as indicated, type and crossmatch
—Initial findings: Increased spleen size, acute pallor, shock (if episode severe), anemia, and thrombocytopenia
—A sequestration episode may have a more insidious onset or be chronic in nature.
—Management
—Fever management (if indicated)
—Close, frequent observation of hemoglobin level, reticulocyte count, spleen size, and cardiovascular (CV) status
—Fluid bolus and maintenance hydration
—Red blood cell transfusion: Avoid transfusing to hemoglobin values above 10 g/dL as hemoglobin may increase as the episode resolves and red cells are released from the spleen.
—Repeated sequestration episodes may be an indication for splenectomy.
- Transient aplastic episode
—History, physical examination, CBC, reticulocyte count (blood culture as indicated), type and crossmatch, human parvovirus B19 serology
—Initial findings: Pallor, tachycardia, absent or low reticulocytes unless recovery phase
—Management
—Fever management (if indicated)
—Close observation of hemoglobin level, reticulocyte count, and CV status
—Respiratory isolation (95% of cases are a result of infection with human parvovirus B19)
—Red-cell transfusion for evidence of CV compromise
- Stroke: acute care
—History, physical examination, CBC, reticulocyte count blood culture as indicated, type and crossmatch
—Initial findings: Syncope, weakness, numbness, limp, hemiparesis, seizure, slurred speech, aphasia, somnolence, coma
—Imaging: Head CT, brain MRI and MRA; consider arteriogram if aneurysm suspected
—Management
—Intravenous fluid bolus and maintenance hydration
—Red blood cell transfusion (given as simple or exchange transfusion)
—Supportive (anticonvulsives, etc.)
- Stroke (primary and secondary stroke prevention): Chronic care
—Monthly red-cell transfusions to keep HbS level below 30%

 Common Questions and Answers

Q: How long will my baby with SCD live?
A: No one can predict how long a child with SCD will live. When studies were done on a large number of individuals with SCD almost two decades ago, these individuals were living, on average, into their 40s if they had the SS type of SCD and into their 60s with the SC type of SCD. Most likely, new treatments

such as daily penicillin, comprehensive medical care, and hydroxyurea therapy have prolonged the life expectancy of children with SCD.

Q: Is there any "cure" for sickle cell disease?
A: Bone marrow transplantation (BMT) is the only known cure for sickle cell disease in children. BMT requires destroying all the bone marrow of the child with SCD with strong drugs and/or radiation and replacing it with the bone marrow of a person without SCD. This marrow donor should be a relative, preferably a full sibling, whose bone marrow matches that of the child with SCD. Only those children with SCD who have experienced severe illness complications should be exposed to the morbidity and mortality risks of BMT at this time.

Q: What is hydroxyurea therapy?
A: Hydroxyurea is a medication that has been shown to reduce the number of painful episodes and acute chest syndrome events in adults with sickle cell disease. Individuals who receive this medication must be monitored closely for serious side effects, such as a decreased white blood count, hemoglobin, or platelets. Once these problems are detected and the drug is stopped, these problems usually resolve. Hydroxyurea therapy in children over five years of age has a similar safety profile to that of adults.

Q: What triggers or starts off a pain episode?
A: Some children say that changes in the weather (e.g., hot to cold or vice versa) will bring on painful episodes. Others say that jumping into a cold swimming pool will bring on pain. Trauma (e.g., being tackled in football), fatigue, stress, infection, and menses can also exacerbate painful episodes. However, in the majority of painful episodes, the triggers are unknown.

ICD-9-CM 282.6

BIBLIOGRAPHY

Adams RJ. Lessons from the stroke prevention trial in sickle cell anemia (STOP) study. *J Child Neurol* 2000;15:344–349.

National Institutes of Health, National Heart, Lung and Blood Institute. The Management of Sickle Cell Disease. 4th Ed. NIH publication No. 02-2117, 2002.

Vinchinsky E, Lubin BH. Suggested guidelines for the treatment of children with sickle cell disease. *Hematol Oncol Clin North Am* 1987;1:483–501.

White DA, DeBaun M. Cognitive and behavioral function in children with sickle cell disease: a review and discussion of methodological issues. *J Pediatr Hematol Oncol* 1998;20(5):458–462.

Author: Kim Smith-Whitley

Sinusitis

Database

DEFINITION

Sinusitis is inflammation of the mucous membranes lining the paranasal sinuses, but most commonly is used to describe bacterial rhinosinusitis, which is a clinical diagnosis made by the presence of upper respiratory tract symptoms that have not improved in 10 days or have worsened after 5 to 7 days. Diagnosis of sinusitis should be considered based on persistence and/or severity of symptoms. Severity of disease, independent of duration, may be used for diagnosis in older children and adolescents.

Classification based on duration of symptoms:

- Acute: persistent nasal and sinus symptoms for 10 to 30 days
- Subacute: clinical symptoms for 4 to 12 weeks
- Chronic: symptoms lasting at least 12 weeks
- Recurrent: acute sinusitis with complete resolution between episodes; three episodes in 6 months or ≥4 episodes in 1 year

Classification by severity of illness:

- Mild: otherwise healthy, but with ≥10 days of persistent anterior and posterior rhinorrhea and fatigue
- Moderate to severe: temperature of >39°C (102.2°F) for 3 days with concurrent purulent nasal discharge and facial pain, periorbital edema and/or headache

CAUSES

- Viral pathogens (e.g., rhinovirus, parainfluenza virus) have been recovered in respiratory isolates, but their significance is unknown.
- Most illnesses of short duration (<7 days) are thought to be from viral infections and should not be treated with antibiotics.
- Bacterial pathogens: increasing prevalence of penicillin-resistance
—*Streptococcus pneumoniae* (30% to 40%)
—*Haemophilus influenzae,* nontypeable (approximately 20% to 28%)
—*Moraxella catarrhalis* (approximately 20% to 28% in children)
—Group A streptococci
—Group C streptococci
—Peptostreptococci
—Other *Moraxella* species
—*S. viridans*
—*Eikenella corrodens*
—*Staphylococcus aureus*
—*Pseudomonas aeruginosa* (in patients with cystic fibrosis)
—Anaerobic organisms
—Fungal pathogen: *Aspergillus*

COMPLICATIONS

- Periorbital cellulitis
- Orbital cellulitis
- Orbital abscess
- Meningitis
- Intracranial abscess
- Optic neuritis
- Cavernous or sagittal sinus thrombosis
- Epidural, subdural, and brain abscesses
- Osteomyelitis of the maxilla

- Osteomyelitis of the frontal bone (Pott puffy tumor)

PROGNOSIS

- Spontaneous resolution in 40% to 50% of patients
- Usually improves within 72 hours of initiation of antibiotics
- Excellent for those who are otherwise healthy

Differential Diagnosis

INFECTION

- Viral URI with or without mucopurulent rhinitis

ENVIRONMENTAL

- Allergic rhinitis

DRUG-INDUCED

- Rhinitis medicamentosa

TUMORS

- Nasal polyps
- Hypertrophied adenoids
- Neoplasms

TRAUMA

- Foreign body (e.g., bead, cotton, tissue)

CONGENITAL

- Septal deviation
- Unilateral choanal atresia
- Immotile cilia

OTHER

- Vasomotor rhinitis

Data Gathering

HISTORY

Some or all of the following may be present:

- Nasal discharge: consistency, color. In older patients, nasal discharge may not be the primary complaint, but concurrent rhinitis is a common feature.
- Postnasal drainage
- Nasal congestion
- Fever
- Recent history of a URI
- Sore throat from mouth-breathing as a result of nasal obstruction
- Cough present during the day; may be worse at night
- Malodorous breath
- Hyposmia/anosmia
- Maxillary dental pain
- Ear pressure or fullness
- Headache and facial pain are rare in children
- Fatigue
- Irritability
- Snoring
- Hyponasal speech

Physical Examination

- Fever may be present.

- Nasal-sounding voice may be present.
- Malodorous breath may be noted.
- Purulent drainage in the nose and/or oropharynx may be appreciated.
- Nasal mucosa may be erythematous, pale, boggy.
- Frontal, maxillary, and ethmoid areas may be tender to palpation/percussion.
- Headache and/or facial pain may change with position, increasing in intensity as the patient leans forward.
- Transillumination is not a reliable aid in diagnosis.
- Proptosis, eye swelling, and impaired extraocular movements suggest orbital infection.

Laboratory Aids

Keep in mind that the overall clinical impression is thought to be more accurate than any single test.
For chronic or recurrent sinusitis, consider:

- Sweat chloride test to rule out cystic fibrosis
- Immunoglobulin levels, IgG subclass levels, complement levels, and testing for human immunodeficiency virus
- Mucosal biopsy to assess ciliary function

RADIOGRAPHIC STUDIES

Imaging is not recommended in uncomplicated cases of sinusitis in children ≤6 years of age.
Imaging controversial in children >6 years of age

—Sinus radiographs
- Plain radiographs do not adequately identify ethmoid sinusitis
- Findings suggestive of sinusitis include complete sinus opacification, mucosal thickening ≥4 mm and air-fluid levels
- CT scans of the paranasal sinuses: useful in complicated, recurrent and chronic sinusitis; poor response to medical therapy; and/or history of polyposis
- MRI of the sinuses: reserve for complicated cases; will show mucosal thickening and fluid; imaging modality of choice for fungal sinusitis

PITFALLS

- Sinus radiographs may be abnormal in asymptomatic children.
- Studies have shown a relatively high incidence of sinus abnormalities on CT scan in asymptomatic children, especially in infants less than 12 months. The significance of opacified sinuses in asymptomatic children is not well understood.
- Up to one-third of patients with symptoms of chronic sinusitis may have normal CT scans.

Therapy

If orbital or central nervous system infection is suspected by history and examination, antibiotics should be started immediately, and emergent CT studies should be performed.

ANTIBIOTICS

- Mild disease (no antibiotics in the previous 4 to 6 weeks): treat for 10 days if symptoms markedly improve in the first 3 to 4 days; treat for 10 to 14 days if no dramatic improvement in the first 3 to 4 days; or treat until symptom free plus 7 days
—Amoxicillin (45 to 90 mg/kg per day divided in two doses): first-line agent for uncomplicated cases of acute sinusitis. Side effects include hypersensitivity, diarrhea.
—Macrolides (including azithromycin, clarithromycin, and erythromycin) or trimethoprim/sulfamethoxazole: if patient allergic to penicillin.
- Moderate disease (no antibiotics in the previous 4 to 6 weeks); mild disease (treated with antibiotics in the previous 4 to 6 weeks); patients not responsive to first-line agents; consider for patients less than 2 years of age, patients living where there is well-described antibiotic resistance or living with smokers, patients attending day care:
—Amoxicillin, high-dose (80 to 90 mg/kg per day divided in two doses)
—Amoxicillin/clavulanic acid (45 mg/kg per day divided in two doses alone or in combination with amoxicillin (45 mg/kg per day divided in two doses): expensive; side effects include vomiting and diarrhea
—Cefpodoxime proxetil (10 mg/kg per day divided in two doses): second-generation cephalosporin; side effects include nausea, vomiting, diarrhea
—Cefuroxime axetil (30 mg/kg per day divided in two doses): second-generation cephalosporin
- Moderate disease (treated with antibiotics in the previous 4 to 6 weeks) and patients not responsive to second-line agents:
—Amoxicillin/clavulanic acid (45 mg/kg per day divided in two doses alone or in combination with amoxicillin (45 mg/kg per day divided in two doses): second-line therapy
—Amoxicillin or clindamycin plus a third-generation cephalosporin
- Complicated sinusitis—central nervous system or orbital involvement
—Intravenous antibiotics and hospitalization
—Cefotaxime (300 mg/kg per day divided into four doses)
—Vancomycin (60 mg/kg per day divided into four doses) is added to cefotaxime if source of infection is known or highly likely to be caused by penicillin-resistant *Streptococcus pneumoniae*.
- Chronic sinusitis
—Use a broad-spectrum antibiotic for 4 weeks.
—Amoxicillin/clavulanic acid (45 mg/kg per day divided in two doses)
—Erythromycin/sulfisoxazole (50 mg/kg per day erythromycin divided qid), cefuroxime axetil (250 to 500 mg in two divided doses), or trimethoprim-sulfamethoxazole (8 mg/kg per day of the trimethoprim component divided in two doses)

OTHER PHARMACEUTICALS

- Decongestants: these decrease nasal airway resistance and increase ostia patency in some studies, but the overall effect on acute sinusitis is unknown.

- Topical decongestants should be used only for short-term therapy (5 to 7 days) because rebound mucosal congestion may occur.
- Systemic decongestants (e.g., pseudoephedrine) have side effects that include tachycardia, hypertension, jitteriness, and insomnia.
- Mucolytics, such as guaifenesin: may improve mucous clearance
- Topical nasal steroids: reduce and prevent mucosal swelling, which can lead to ostial occlusion; particularly useful for patients with allergic rhinitis; used empirically by some experts, although there are no controlled studies for nasal steroids and sinusitis.

OTHER

- Humidifier: improves mucociliary clearance.
- Normal saline: squirt into each nostril daily or twice per day; removes sensitizing agents, increases humidity, and enhances mucociliary transport; vasoconstrictors and improves drainage and ventilation.

SURGERY

- Maxillary sinus aspiration: if unresponsive to multiple antibiotics, severe facial pain, and orbital or intracranial complications; should be performed by a trained otolaryngologist
- Surgery: performed as a last resort after medical therapy attempted and in patients with orbital or CNS complications.

Follow-Up

- Immediate referral is indicated if there are CNS symptoms, periorbital edema, visual changes, facial swelling, extraocular muscle involvement or proptosis.
- Radiographic soft tissue changes may last for up to 8 weeks; therefore, reimaging is of limited value.
- Referral to an ear, nose, and throat (ENT) specialist when the sinusitis is chronic and not responsive to medical therapy; recurrent; complicated; or when there is polyposis

PITFALLS

- Diagnosis of sinusitis is being made with increasing frequency and may result in overtreatment, given that up to 45% will have spontaneous resolution.
- With widespread antibiotic use, there are increasing numbers of resistant organisms.

PREVENTION

- Use prophylactic amoxicillin or sulfisoxazole for refractory sinusitis.
- Avoid allergen exposure and treat allergies if present.
- Practice daily nasal hygiene through the use of normal saline drops/spray.
- Improve mucociliary clearance by increasing ambient humidity with a humidifier.

Common Questions and Answers

Q: Are all of the sinuses present at birth?
A: No, the maxillary and ethmoid sinuses form

during the third and fourth gestational month, and are present at birth. They continue to enlarge until the preteen years. The sphenoid sinuses develop between 3 and 7 years; isolated sphenoid sinusitis is rare. The frontal sinuses are present at age 5 to 6 years and are not completely developed until late adolescence.

Q: Does the nasal discharge seen with sinusitis have to be purulent and thick?
A: No. Although the nasal discharge is often described as purulent and thick, it may also be clear or mucoid, or thick or thin. Multiple studies have shown that a change in color or consistency is not a specific sign of a bacterial infection.

Q: Are radiographs useful in the diagnosis of sinusitis?
A: There is evidence to suggest that x-rays have limited value in the diagnosis of sinusitis, and are not recommended in cases of uncomplicated sinusitis. Mucosal thickening may be seen with viral upper respiratory tract infections and allergic rhinitis. Studies have shown that x-rays do not correlate well with CT scans in the diagnosis of chronic sinusitis.

Q: Can one make the diagnosis of sinusitis based on CT scan results alone?
A: No. Up to 50% of patients who had CTs performed for other reasons had soft tissue changes in their sinuses. Mucosal thickening and opacification on CT imaging have been seen in large numbers of asymptomatic patients. These findings seem to occur more frequently in infants younger than 12 months. Given the poor specificity of CT imaging of the paranasal sinuses, results must be used in the context of the patient's clinical presentation.

ICD-9-CM

Chronic 473.9; Frontal 461.1; Maxillary 461.0; Ethmoid 461.2

BIBLIOGRAPHY

Aitken M, Taylor JA. Prevalence of clinical sinusitis in young children followed up by primary are pediatricians. *Arch Pediatr Adolesc Med* 1998;152:244–248.

Brooks I, Gooch WM, Jenkins SG, et al. Medical management of acute bacterial sinusitis. *Ann Otol Rhinol Laryngol Suppl* 2000;182(9):2–20.

Dyskewicz M. Rhinits and sinusitis. *J Allergy Clin Immunol* 2003;111:S520–S9.

Ioannidis, JPA, Lau JL. American Academy of Pediatrics: Technical report: evidence for the diagnosis and treatment of acute uncomplicated sinusitis in children: a systematic overview. *Pediatrics* 2001;108(3):e57.

Sinus and Allergy Health Partnership. Antimicrobial treatment guidelines for acute bacterial rhinosinusitis. *Otolaryngol Head Neck Surg* 2000;123(1 pt 2):S1–S32.

Authors: Esther K. Chung and Karen P. Zimmer

Sleep Apnea-Obstructive Sleep Apnea Syndrome

 Database

DEFINITION

Obstructive sleep apnea syndrome (OSAS) refers to a spectrum of disorders associated with upper airway obstruction during sleep.

- Obstructive apnea is defined as the cessation of airflow at the nose and mouth despite respiratory effort, associated with some gas exchange abnormality and/or loss of regular sleep patterns.
- Distinct from central apnea—cessation of airflow that is not accompanied by respiratory effort—which indicates brain immaturity or dysfunction.
- Many children with OSAS exhibit partial airway obstruction. This is known as obstructive hypoventilation or hypopnea
- OSAS may be subdivided into: mild, moderate, and severe forms according to degree of severity
- Upper airway resistance syndrome is a respiratory disorder characterized by partial airway obstruction and arousals leading to sleep fragmentation and not associated by gas-exchange abnormalities
- Primary snoring or habitual snoring implies snoring that does not lead to abnormalities in gas-exchange or sleep fragmentation
- Central apneas up to 20 seconds may be a normal finding in premature or newborn infants during the first months of life
- Periodic breathing: three or more central apneas at least 3 seconds each, separated by less than 20 seconds. Periodic breathing may be found in the newborn, however, it should not exceed more than 4% of sleep time (from a sleep study) and is not associated with bradycardia or hypoxemia
- Pediatric incidence estimated between 1% and 2%.

COMPLICATIONS

Complications are as a result of chronic hypoxemia, hypercarbia, acidosis, and impaired sleep and include:

- Pulmonary hypertension, later cor pulmonale (rare)
- Systemic hypertension has been reported in adults and a few pediatric cases
- Congestive heart failure; arrhythmias are common in adults with an underlying coronary heart disease
- Neurodevelopmental complications: daytime somnolence, poor school performance, hyperactivity, and social withdrawal
- Poor growth and failure to thrive
- Respiratory failure and death have also been reported in children with OSAS postanesthesia

ASSOCIATED CONDITIONS

- Adenotonsillar hypertrophy
- Craniofacial anomalies including midfacial hypoplasia and mandibular hypoplasia
- Laryngomalacia

- Neurologic and neuromuscular disorders causing hypotonia may underlie poor ventilation during sleep
- Gastroesophageal reflux
- Obesity
- Metabolic disorders
- Allergic rhinitis, nasal septal deviation, nasal polyps
- Sedatives, seizure medications, and anesthesia

 Differential Diagnosis

- Primary snoring or habitual snoring: By definition not associated with sleep-disordered breathing, may progress to OSAS. Up to 50% of children with habitual snoring may have OSAS
- Upper airway resistance syndrome: This condition is associated with sleep fragmentation and day time sleepiness
- Obesity-hypoventilation syndrome—a variant of OSAS
- Central apnea and periodic breathing
- Congenital central hypoventilation syndrome

Other causes of excessive daytime sleepiness include:

- Disorganized home environment, emotional stress
- Substance abuse/drug intoxication: Psychotropic medications, antihistamines, anticonvulsants, narcotics
- Narcolepsy: Onset rare before adolescence; associated cataplexy, sleep paralysis
- Epilepsy: Absence spells of unresponsiveness; EEG changes
- Causes of obstructive apnea include any cause of lymphoidal hypertrophy in the upper airway (allergies viral/bacterial tonsillitis, neoplasm, epiglottitis, retropharyngeal abscess); chronic phenytoin exposure; excessive storage material in upper airway submucosa
- Causes of abnormal laxity of upper airway soft tissues: Down syndrome, acute polyneuropathy (Guillain Barré syndrome), chronic neuromuscular disease, Prader-Willi syndrome, myasthenia gravis
- Causes of abnormal control/coordination of upper airway musculature: Almost any cause of diffuse CNS dysfunction including cerebral palsy, and acquired lesions of the CNS such as stroke and head trauma
- Causes of central apnea: Beyond infancy, most commonly as a result of drugs suppressing ventilatory drive; in premature infants may be as a result of nonspecific immaturity of neural ventilatory control mechanism, sepsis, and, rarely, seizures, brainstem compression, brain tumors, Arnold Chiari type 2
- Reflux may potentiate central apnea and should be investigated.
- Androgen steroids may cause central apnea in adults

 Data Gathering

HISTORY

- Nocturnal symptoms include difficulty breathing when asleep, snoring, apneas, and restless sleep with frequent arousals.
- Daytime symptoms: excessive sleepiness, frequent upper respiratory/ear infections, conductive hearing loss, mouth breathing, poor appetite, and a hyponasal voice.
- Other concerns: attention deficit hyperactivity, gastroesophageal reflux, poor school performance, and headaches (especially morning time and on awakening)

—Obstructive sleep apnea syndrome rarely produces these symptoms acutely, but tends to occur over weeks to months.
—Parents may notice that symptoms worsen with upper respiratory infections.

- The possibility of sleep disordered breathing or a primary sleep disorder should be considered in children evaluated for attention deficit hyperactivity

 Physical Examination

- Assessment of the child's growth should be made. In severe cases of OSAS, failure to thrive has been reported
- Obesity remains a risk factor especially in older children
- Assessment of tonsils size
- Presence of mouth breathing, hyponasal speech, adenoidal facies, midfacial hypoplasia, retrognathia, micrognathia, or other craniofacial anomalies may be present at times and may suggest the diagnosis
- Observation for nasal obstruction as a result of polyps, nasal septal deviation, turbinate hypertrophy or congestion
- Tongue size
- Mobility and elevation of the soft palate; hard palate integrity
- In extreme cases cardiac involvement may lead to cor-pulmonale and heart failure. Examination may suggest signs of pulmonary hypertension or congestive heart failure, such as an increased second heart sound
- A neurologic examination to evaluate general muscle strength, tone, and developmental status, especially in infants and in children who do not improve after adenotonsillectomy

Sleep Apnea-Obstructive Sleep Apnea Syndrome

 Laboratory Aids

TESTS

Polysomnography

The gold standard for the diagnosis of OSAS is nocturnal polysomnography, to differentiate the type of sleep apnea, and to assess severity.

- Eight- to 10-hour-long multichannel study performed in a controlled setting that can assess respiratory or sleep abnormalities.
- Indices such as oxygenation, ventilation, apnea hypopnea index (AHI) are determined along with sleep parameters as sleep efficiency, sleep stages, number of arousals, and movements throughout the night.
- Monitoring includes electroencephalogram, electrooculogram, electromyogram, arterial oxygen saturation, end tidal CO_2 tension, airflow, respiratory effort, and electrocardiogram.
- Scoring for pediatric polysomnography differs from that of adults (e.g., no minimum time requirement for apnea). Lower AHI values are considered significant in children, compared to adults

Other Studies

- Lateral neck x-ray is easy to perform to assess adenoid and tonsillar size and patency of the nasopharyngeal airway
- Validated questionnaires are helpful to screen for OSAS in the office
- Nocturnal audiotaping and videotaping, and abbreviated nap polysomnography, are useful studies if the results are positive, but generally have a poor negative predictive value
- Upper airway endoscopy and bronchoscopy may be performed to evaluate anatomical or dynamic causes for airway obstruction (pharyngeal hypotonia, pharyngeal stenosis, laryngotracheomalacia, vocal cord polyps, papilloma)
- In severe cases of OSAS, a cardiac evaluation, including ECG, chest radiograph, and Doppler echocardiogram, may be indicated
- Routine blood work generally noncontributory; in severe forms, polycythemia, hypercarbia, and elevated bicarbonate may be noted
- Evaluation for gastroesophageal reflux may include pH monitoring during sleep, barium swallow, or radionuclide studies (milk scan).

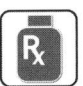 Emergency Care

Obstructive sleep apnea syndrome is usually an insidious disorder.
Mild and moderate cases may be treated on an elective or even on an urgent basis. However, severe cases may require urgent intervention.

- Severe cases of upper airway obstruction are usually diagnosed during polysomnography or during procedures involving sedation or anesthesia.

—Ensure adequate ventilation and oxygenation with quick assessment of the cause
—Temporary relief of the obstruction should be undertaken by an experienced team.
—Transfer to an intensive care unit in which the airway can be monitored carefully
—Following relief of airway obstruction, pulmonary and airway edema, and copious production of secretions may develop.
—Modalities of care should include at this time: placement of a nasopharyngeal airway, noninvasive ventilation (CPAP/BiPAP), or placement of an endotracheal tube and mechanical ventilation.

- Risk factors for postoperative complications in children with OSAS include age less than 3 years, severe OSAS, pulmonary hypertension, obesity, prematurity, failure to thrive, craniofacial or neuromuscular disorder, upper respiratory tract infection

 Therapy

- In most cases, adenotonsillectomy is first line therapy. However, some patients continue to have significant OSAS after surgery that require further evaluation.
- Noninvasive ventilatory support as CPAP or BiPAP may be helpful
- In complicated cases when craniofacial malformations are involved; surgical procedures such as: tongue reduction, uvulopalatopharyngoplasty, mandibular, or maxillary advancement may be indicated.
- When there is evidence of gastroesophageal reflux, treatment with acid suppression agents, and chalasia precautions are indicated
- Weight loss may be useful in obese children

 Follow-Up

Clinical improvement is expected soon after adenotonsillectomy. In children <1 year of age, in severe forms of OSAS, or if there is an underlying craniofacial anomaly or a neurological disorder, repeat overnight polysomnogram is indicated 6 to 8 weeks after surgery.

- Regrowth of adenoid tissue may occur months to years after adenoidectomy. Therefore, if clinical symptoms such as: snoring, difficulty breathing while asleep, or decline in school performance recur—a reevaluation is indicated
- Follow-up sleep studies may help to monitor therapy

PITFALLS

- Habitual snoring may be confused with snoring of a clinical severity causing clinical degree of upper airway obstruction. The need for polysomnography depends on the patient's symptoms.
- Normal size tonsils does not exclude OSAS
- Tonsillar size does not predict the presence of OSAS
- Treatment of reflux in infants with obstructive apnea may be helpful even in the absence of obvious symptoms of reflux

Common Questions and Answers

Q: Can my child still have OSAS after adenotonsillectomy?
A: Yes, at times the adenoid tissue can grow back again. Additionally, some cases of OSAS are related to a small upper airway that is restricted by anatomical or neurological conditions, in these cases adenotonsillectomy will not always resolve OSAS

Q: Does OSAS cause neurological problems?
A: Few studies suggest neurocognitive deficits in children with OSAS. The most common findings include reduced school performance and attention deficit and hyperactivity. However, more studies are indicated to establish this association.

ICD-9-CM 780.57

BIBLIOGRAPHY

American Academy of Pediatrics. Clinical practice guidelines: diagnosis and management of childhood obstructive sleep apnea syndrome. *Pediatrics* 2002;109(4):704–712.

D'Andrea LA. Diagnostic studies in the assessment of pediatric sleep-disordered breathing: techniques and indications. *Pediatr Clin North Am* 2004;51(1):169–286.

Marcus CL. Sleep-disordered breathing in children. *Am J Respir Crit Care Med* 2001;164:16–30.

Rosen CL. Obstructive sleep apnea syndrome in children: controversies in diagnosis and treatment. *Pediatr Clin North Am* 2004;51(1):153–167, vii.

Authors: Thomas Lahiri
Ranaan Arens, 3rd edition

Slipped Capital Femoral Epiphysis

 Database

DEFINITION

Slipped capital femoral epiphysis (SCFE) is displacement of the epiphysis of the head of the femur.

PATHOPHYSIOLOGY

- Unclear: Abnormal stress on normal physeal plate versus a process that weakens the plate.
- The femoral head slips posteriorly and inferiorly, exposing the anterior and superior aspects of the metaphysis of the femoral neck.
- Associations: Obesity, endocrine dysfunction, primary hypothyroidism, pituitary dysfunction, hypogonadism, cryptorchidism, chemotherapy, pelvic radiotherapy, renal rickets

GENETICS

Five percent of children have a parent with SCFE.

EPIDEMIOLOGY

- Incidence: 1 to 5 per 100,000
- Race: Blacks than Whites
- Sex: Males more than females (3:2)
- Left hip twice as often at the right, 25% bilateral
- Age of onset: Boys, 14 to 16 years; girls, 11 to 13 years (essentially premenarche)
- Associated with obesity, increased height, genital underdevelopment, pituitary tumors

COMPLICATIONS

- Ischemic necrosis of epiphysis: Usually as a result of manipulative reduction of the slippage; more common in males; radiographs reveal increased density, irregularity, and ultimately collapse of epiphysis.
- Chondrolysis (acute cartilage necrosis): 1% to 40%, more common in females and Blacks; etiology unclear; radiographs reveal narrowed joint space, sclerosis of acetabular rim, and osteoporosis of femoral head.

 Differential Diagnosis

- Septic arthritis of the hip
- Ischemic necrosis
- Tuberculosis of the hip; however, pain is associated with movement in all directions, and there should be other evidence of disease.
- Renal rickets
- Achondroplasia
- Shwachman syndrome: metaphyseal chondrodysplasia with pancreatic insufficiency

 Data Gathering

HISTORY

- Pain in hip or knee
- Occasional history of trauma; however, usually not sufficient to explain the findings
- Three patterns:

—Chronic: Most common, onset of symptoms greater than 3 weeks, lack of full internal rotation of hip
—Acute: Sudden onset with inability to walk or severe pain and difficulty walking
—Acute-on-chronic: Sudden exacerbation of symptoms that have been present for a while

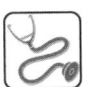

Physical Examination

- Limp if unilateral, or waddling gait if bilateral
- Tenderness and occasional palpable thickening over hip
- Thigh atrophy
- Lack of full internal rotation of hip and decreased motion in all planes secondary to mechanical limitation as a result of the slip.

PROCEDURE

When the hip is flexed, the thigh is forced into external rotation.

Laboratory Aids

TESTS

Radiographs

- AP and lateral view (frog leg or Löwenstein).
- Measure degree of displacement:

—Minimal: alteration in plane of epiphysis relative to femoral neck; significant if angle less than 82%
—Mild: displacement less than 1 cm
—Moderate: displacement greater than 1 cm, less than two-thirds diameter of femoral neck

- Epiphyseal plate widened and irregular
- Decreased height of physis
- "Blanch sign" dense area in femoral neck
- A "Klein line" drawn along the superior femoral neck on the AP view should transect the epiphysis but not on the slipped side.
- Hormonal evaluation if suspected

Pathology

Histologic findings include widening of the epiphyseal plate, large clefts, and necrotic debris in the cartilage and synovitis.

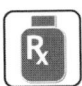

Therapy

- Designed to prevent complications and further slipping, urgent orthopaedic consultation mandatory.
- Conservative: bed rest with traction; probably does not reduce slipping; temporizing until surgery can be scheduled
- Manipulative reduction: risk of damage to epiphyseal vessels or breakdown of callus; probably only to be considered if within 24 hours of acute slip
- Epiphyseal fixation: risk of damage to articular surface or growth plate
- Intertrochanteric osteotomy
- Salvage: hip fusion

PITFALLS

- Diagnosis is most often missed when slipped capital femoral epiphysis is not considered.
- Hip pain may be absent; there may be no pain, or only thigh or knee pain as a result of referred pain.

Follow-Up

Chondrolysis and avascular necrosis are uncommon side effects of slipped capital femoral epiphysis.

Common Questions and Answers

Q: What type of radiographs should be obtained?
A: AP and frog lateral of hips.

Q: Is there a role for CT or MRI?
A: CT can be useful to demonstrate degree of slip. MRI may demonstrate early changes not detectable by radiograph and CT.

ICD-9-CM 732.9

BIBLIOGRAPHY

Loder RT. Slipped capital femoral epiphysis. *Am Fam Physician* 1998;57:2135–2142.

Lubicky JP. Chondrolysis and avascular necrosis: complications of slipped capital femoral epiphysis. *J Pediatr Orthop B* 1996;5:162–167.

Rattey T, Piehl F, Wright JG. Acute slipped capital femoral epiphysis. Review of outcomes and rates of avascular necrosis. *J Bone Joint Surg* 1996;78A:398–402.

Reynolds RA. Diagnosis and treatment of slipped capital femoral epiphysis. *Curr Opin Pediatr* 1999;11:80–83.

Umans H, Liebling MS, Moy L, et al. Slipped capital femoral epiphysis: a physeal lesion diagnosed by MRI, with radiographic and CT correlation. *Skeletal Radiol* 1998;27:139–144.

Weiner D. Pathogenesis of slipped capital femoral epiphysis: current concepts. *J Pediatr Orthop B* 1996;5:67–73.

Authors: David D. Sherry
Randy Q. Cron, 3rd edition

Smallpox (Variola Virus)

 Database

 Differential Diagnosis

 Data Gathering

DEFINITION

Smallpox is an acute eruptive contagious disease caused by the Poxvirus family. The disease has the characteristics of fever, chill, backache and headache that progresses to papular rash to a vesicular rash then to a pustular rash. The vesicles in time fall off leaving scars that are known as pockmarks.

• The two most fatal forms of smallpox are the hemorrhagic and malignant. Hemorrhagic are uniformly fatal to all age and sexes, but especially to pregnant women. There is a shorter incubation time with hemorrhagic with leads to the skin becoming dusky and bleeding occurs in the skin and mucous membranes. Death occurs 5 days after the onset of the rash. Malignant smallpox has an abrupt onset of the prodromal phase with lesions present never progressing to pustules. The skin lesions remain flatten and appear red fine grained. If the patient survives there is minimal scarring, but in severe cases there can be large losses of the epidermis.

CAUSES

Smallpox are particles that contain double stranded DNA, disc shape core and a lipoprotein envelope. It is a member of the Poxvirus family, Orthopoxvirus.

TRANSMISSION

• Transmitted via respiratory aerosol or by direct contact with the virus with the skin lesions.
• The virus infects the upper respiratory tract and local lymph nodes.
• The virus enters the blood stream, which is primary viremia.
• The internal organs are infected an the virus enter the blood stream for a second time which is the secondary viremia (this occurs around day 8 of the disease).
• After secondary viremia the virus spreads to the skin. These events occur during the incubation period when the infected individual is well.
• Humans are the only vectors that— transmit the disease.
• There are no known animal or insect vectors. Infected clothes or bedding can spread smallpox virus.

COMPLICATIONS

The risk of secondary infection is common when the pustules are present. The risk of mortality is estimated at 30%.

• Varicella
• Viral Exanthem
• Meningococcemia (If hemorrhagic form of small pox)

HISTORY

• After the incubation period, which usually lasts 7 to 14 days, there is a abrupt onset of the fever and malaise.
• Followed by the rash, which usually starts in the face and spreads over the body to the extremities.
• The rash starts with macules to papules to vesicles to pustules and then crusting lesions, which occurs around 2 to 3 weeks.
• The patient is infectious during the entire illness until the scabs fall off. The patient is most infectious during 7 to 10 days of the rash.

Laboratory Aids

- In the past the diagnosis was made by growing virus in cell culture or by detecting viral antigens in the vesicular fluid by immunofluorescence.
- Electron microscopy pustular fluid can assist in the diagnosis. Active skin lesions under the microscope have the appearance of altered epithelial cells that contain Guarnieri bodies, which are eosinophilic intracytoplasmic bodies.

PREVENTION

Prior to 1972 all children in the United States were vaccinated at age 1. The smallpox vaccine is also known as Vaccinia. The vaccine immunity is lasts 10 years. There is lifelong immunity after the smallpox illness. Vaccinia is effective for as a result of five factors.

1. There is one serotype of the virus.
2. Humans are sole reservoir of the virus.
3. There is no subclinical or carrier state.
4. There is a rapid antibody response that help protects those people exposed to small pox.
5. The illness is easily recognized to help vaccinate postexposure persons.

- Vaccination is inoculated intradermally on arm or hip.

—The formation of a vesicle is an indication of successful vaccination.

- With possible threats of bioterrorism after the September 11, 2001, terrorist attacks, the U.S. government has increased the production of vaccine.

—Currently, health and emergency services workers are being vaccinated on a volunteer basis.
—There is no current plan to reintroduce routine mandatory smallpox vaccination.
—There has not been a case in the United States since the late 1940s and the last documented case was in Somalia in 1977.

- The major concern with restarting routine smallpox vaccination is vaccine associated side effects.

—These side effects can include encephalitis, generalized Vaccinia and Vaccinia gangrenosa.
—The incidence of complications of vaccination has been estimated to be 1 and 4,000.
—With the presence of human immuno-deficiency virus (HIV), immunosuppression as a result of organ/ bone marrow transplants and other types of immunocompromised illness, the incidence of vaccine side effects could be much higher in these groups of people.

- Vaccinia immune globulin could be administered with the vaccine to help reduce complications in those who are at higher risk of side effect from the vaccine.

- The availability of Vaccinia immune globulin is limited. In the event of a outbreak of smallpox.

—Rapid inoculation of vaccine would be given to those people exposed to the small pox within 4 days.
—The vaccination can help prevent or ameliorate the illness.
—It would be imperative to immunize all health care officials, police, firefighters, morticians, transit workers and emergency management workers if an outbreak occurred.

INFECTION CONTROL

- Home care for those infected with smallpox should be tried initially because there is medical antiviral treatment for smallpox. This would also prevent infecting other patients in the hospital who do not have small pox. Supportive care is most helpful in maintaining fever and pain control and fluid management.
- Any patient admitted to the hospital suspected of having smallpox should be placed in a negative pressure isolation room with high efficiency particulate air filtration. Gowns and mask should be worn. Used gowns and laundry should be placed in biohazard bags and be autoclaved prior to laundering or incinerated.
- Persons who die of smallpox should be cremated if possible.
- Any suspected case should be reported immediately to local/state health departments.

PITFALL

In those cases of hemorrhagic or malignant smallpox, diagnosis can be prolonged as a result of absence of classic symptoms. Laboratory tests can assist in making the diagnosis. The major obstacle is that most physicians and health care workers have not seen this disease in person, only in textbooks. The lack of familiarity with the diseases initial symptoms could delay the diagnosis and delay vaccination of close contact individuals.

Common Questions and Answers

Q. Can I go to my doctor and request the smallpox vaccine?
A. The last case of smallpox was in 1977. The vaccine has not been recommended since 1972. The CDC has an emergency supply of vaccine for small outbreaks. The U.S. government has ordered a larger supply of vaccine.

Q. Is smallpox fatal?
A. Death may occur in up to 30% of cases, but the majority of people survive.

Q. How many people have not had the vaccination?
A. About half of the population has not been vaccinated. Those people were immunized are not protected from smallpox because the vaccine immune efficacy wanes after ten years.

BIBLIOGRAPHY

Besser JM, Crouch NA, Sullivan M. Laboratory diagnosis to differentiate smallpox, vaccinia, and other vesicular/pustular illnesses. *J Lab Clin Med* 2003;142(4):246–251.

Henerson DA, et al. Small pox as a biological weapon. Medical and public health management. *JAMA* 1999;281(22):2127–2137.

Levinson WE, Jawetz E. *Medical Microbiology and Immunology.* East Norwalk: Appleton & Lange, 1992:174–175.

Author: Charles I. Schwartz

Snake and Insect Bites

 ## Database

DEFINITION

Injury to the human skin and/or subcutaneous tissues caused by bite, envenomation, or sting, causing usually local, but in some cases systemic effects

- Snake bites

—Crotalinae (pit vipers: cotton mouths, copperheads, and rattlesnakes)
—Elapidae (coral snakes)

- Spider bites

—Black widow (*Lactrodectus mactans*)
—Brown recluse (*Loxosceles reclusa*)

- Insect stings

—Hymenoptera: fire ants (Solenopsis), yellow jackets, wasps, bees

EPIDEMIOLOGY

- Snake bites

—Only 15% of all snake bites are from poisonous snakes, and only about two-thirds of those involve true envenomation. Coral snake bites constitute less than 1% of all snake bites.
—About 8,000 people sustain a poisonous snake bite annually in the United States, and 12 to 15 fatalities occur.

- Spider bites

—The incidences of black widow and brown recluse spider bites are unknown mainly as a result of the inability to identify the species of spider involved in the majority of cases.
—The black widow is found in most areas of North America but especially in southern New England. The brown recluse is found mainly in southern and midwestern states.

- Insect bites

—One percent to 4% of American population is at risk for anaphylaxis from Hymenoptera stings; 50 to 150 people die each year from sting anaphylaxis.

PROGNOSIS

- Snake bites

—Because the majority of snake bites are from nonvenomous snakes, and about one-third of bites from venomous snakes do not involve envenomation, the majority of bites cause only local injury.
—Significant envenomation can result in considerable tissue destruction, and severe envenomation can cause death.
—Aggressive supportive care and early consideration of antivenom may improve outcome.

- Spider bites

—Most bites do not produce serious effects; some bites can cause severe local and systemic reactions, including death.

—The most severe reactions and the rare fatalities occur with greater frequency in children.

- Insect bites

—Most bites and stings cause minimal local effects, although some cause series systemic reactions and, rarely, death.

 ## Differential Diagnosis

- Black widow spider bites: acute abdomen, renal colic, opioid withdrawal, and tetanus
- Poisonous snake bites: nonpoisonous snake bite (leaves scratches, not punctures), rodent bites, thorn wounds
- Brown recluse spider bite: other spider bites, insect bites and stings (including Lyme), cellulitis, poison ivy/oak, Stevens-Johnson syndrome, toxic epidermal necrolysis, erythema nodosum, chronic herpes simplex, purpura fulminans, diabetic ulcer, gonococcal hemorrhagic lesion

HISTORY

- Snake bites

—A description of the snake can be used to differentiate poisonous from nonpoisonous snakes. Poisonous snakes have triangular-shaped heads, a pit (heat sensor in front of each eye), fangs, slit-like pupils, a single row of subcaudal plates, and may have a rattle. Nonpoisonous snakes have oval heads, no pits, rows of small teeth, round pupils, a double row of subcaudal plates, and no rattles. The corals have oval heads, yet are still poisonous.
—In the Elapidae family, the coral snake can be differentiated from the benign king snake by the pattern of the colored bands: "Red on yellow, kill a fellow; red on black, venom lack."
—If the snake is brought in for identification, use caution! The head of the dead snake can deliver a venomous bite for up to 1 hour after death/decapitation.
—Onset of symptoms in relation to time of bite

- Spider bites

—Identification of spider (rare). The black widow is about the size of a quarter, glossy black, gray or brown, with a red, orange, or yellow hourglass-shaped marking on the ventral surface. The brown recluse is small (1 to 1.5 cm), gray or reddish/brown, with a brown fiddle-shaped mark on the dorsum of the cephalothorax.
—Onset of symptoms in relation to time of bite (history of bite is uncommon)

 ## Physical Examination

- Crotalinae (pit viper) bites

—Intense local pain and burning occur in first few minutes, followed by edema and perioral numbness that may extend to the scalp and periphery. Paresthesias may be accompanied by a metallic taste in the mouth.
—Local ecchymosis and vesicles appear within the first few hours, and by 24 hours hemorrhagic blebs are present. Lymphadenitis may result.
—Necrosis extending throughout the bitten extremity generally ensues without treatment.
—Nausea, vomiting, weakness, chills, and sweating can also occur with systemic absorption of venom.
—Within several hours neuromuscular involvement can develop (diplopia, dysphagia, lethargy, etc.).
—Sign of hypovolemic shock, hemorrhagic diathesis, and neuromuscular dysfunction may occur in life-threatening envenomations.

- Elapidae (coral snake) bites

—Mild, often unimpressive local signs and symptoms (pain, swelling), but significant neurologic effects that include extremity paresthesias, weakness, fasciculations, and bulbar dysfunction that can progress to flaccid paralysis.
—Inspect bite wound for fang punctures.
—Carefully assess neurovascular integrity, consider compartment pressures if severe edema

- Black widow spider bites

—No local symptoms associated with bite
—One to 8 hours after bite, generalized pain and muscle rigidity, cramping abdominal pain
—Children often have nausea and vomiting.
—Respiratory difficulty may occur.
—Hypertension, tachycardia, and cholinergic effects (diaphoresis, salivation, lacrimation, and bronchorrhea)

- Brown recluse spider bites

—Spectrum from minor local reaction to severe necrosis
—Local reaction: pain, erythema, swelling, and pruritus
—Ischemia and skin necrosis: A bright red papule appears within a few hours of the bite and can evolve within 48 to 72 hours into a hemorrhagic vesicle surrounded by purple discoloration (necrosis) or blanching (vasospasm). Shortly after, a firm, purple necrotic lesion appears, and within 7 to 14 days black eschar is visible. Ulcer healing can take weeks to months.

- Insect bites

—Small local reactions: painful, pruritic, urticarial lesion at the sting site
—Large local reaction: swelling and erythema, may become several centimeters in diameter. Anaphylaxis is rare with fire ants but occurs more frequently with bee stings.

DIAGNOSTIC AIDS

- Snake bites

—CBC, platelet count, PT/PTT, fibrinogen, fibrin split products, serum electrolytes, CPK, creatinine, urinalysis

- Spider bites

—CBC, serum electrolytes, creatinine, CPK, urinalysis

- Insect bites

—No tests routinely done

 Therapy

- Crotalinae (pit vipers) bites:

—Prehospital: Remove constrictive items (jewelry or clothing) and immobilize extremity at or below level of heart. Cryotherapy, arterial tourniquets, excision and incision are not recommended. Oral suctioning is never recommended!
—Rapid transport to medical facility
—Address airway, breathing, and circulation
—The use of a constrictive band to decrease systemic absorption of venom is controversial. Its main indication is for cases of prolonged transport time to a medical facility or rapid progression of systemic symptoms. A flat band is placed 5 to 10 cm proximal to the bite, with enough pressure to impede lymphatic and superficial venous flow but not arterial flow. One to two fingers should fit easily between the band and the patient's extremity.
—Wound care: irrigation and dressing.
—Determine if envenomation has occurred via serial examinations (every 30 minutes) and laboratory studies (every 4 hours).
—Antivenom is the mainstay of therapy. Administration of antivenom should be made in consultation with a toxicologist and/or herpetologist. General indications include progressive local swelling, pain or ecchymosis, and any systemic signs or symptoms.
—Two Crotalinae antivenoms are available: Antivenin (Crotalidae Polyvalent [ACP][Wyeth Laboratories]) and Crotalidae Polyvalent Immune Fab (Ovine)(Altana, Inc.) approved by the FDA in October 2000. Some hospitals (in endemic areas) and many zoos may stock antivenoms. Additionally, the regional poison control center may have access to The Antivenom Index and will be able to help locate the nearest supply.
—Administration of ACP antivenom commonly is associated with the development of serum sickness and may be complicated by anaphylaxis. Skin testing prior to administration is recommended.

—Early data suggest that the use of Fab preparations is safe and effective and is associated with fewer immediate and delayed hypersensitivity reactions than ACP.
—Supportive care: volume replacement, packed red blood cells, platelets, fresh-frozen plasma, cryoprecipitate as indicated for hypovolemia and bleeding diathesis. Observe closely for respiratory and renal failures.
—Fasciotomy only for elevated compartment pressures
—Empiric antibiotics are controversial but may be indicated in cases of extensive tissue involvement.
—Analgesia and tetanus prophylaxis

- Elapidae (coral snakes)

—Constriction bands, suction, and drainage do not prevent coral snake venom absorption.
—Crotalinae antivenom is ineffective in treating Elapidae envenomation. Antivenom is available from Wyeth Laboratories to treat envenomation by Micrurus (Eastern and Texas coral snakes) but no antivenom is available for the Arizona coral snake (Micruroides)
—Local wound care, supportive care, analgesia, and tetanus vaccination as above.

- Black widow spider bites

—To alleviate muscle pain and cramping, parenteral opioids and benzodiazepines can be administered.
—Ten percent calcium gluconate has been used anecdotally, but is not of proven benefit.
—Lactrodectus-specific antivenom is available for more severe envenomations. Specific indications include young age, pregnancy, life-threatening hypertension and tachycardia, or severe symptoms refractory to other treatment measures. Administration of an equine serum preparation has been associated with hypersensitivity reactions and occasionally death. One vial is generally all that is needed.

- Brown recluse spider bites

—Most bites can be treated on an outpatient basis with local wound care and symptomatic treatment for pain and pruritus.
—Patients with systemic symptoms, serious infection, or extensive necrosis warrant hospitalization for aggressive supportive care.
—Large, necrotic areas may require surgical excision and skin grafting. Early surgical excision is contraindicated as it may lead to further necrosis. The area of necrosis may not be fully demarcated until 4 to 8 weeks after the bite.

—There have been several anecdotal reports of treatment of some severe brown recluse spider bites with dapsone and others with hyperbaric oxygen therapy. Neither of these treatment modalities has proved efficacy. The administration of dapsone to children has been associated with the development of methemoglobinemia.

- Insect bites or stings

—Rarely require more than local wound care and symptomatic treatment (antihistamine) for pruritus.
—If stinger remains in skin, remove by pinching or scraping. Emphasis should be on quick removal (to decrease exposure to venom) rather than method of removal.
—Life-threatening anaphylaxis should be treated with subcutaneous epinephrine (0.01 mL/kg 1:1,000 max of 0.5 mL), methylprednisolone (2 mg/kg), diphenhydramine (1.25 mg/kg).
—Bacterial superinfection is rare, but if present can usually be treated with oral and/or topical antibiotics with activity against common skin flora.

ICD-9-CM

Chigger 133.8
Snake and Spider 989.5

BIBLIOGRAPHY

Clark RF, Wethern-Kestner S, Vance MV, et al. Clinical presentation and treatment of black widow spider envenomation: a review of 163 cases. *Ann Emerg Med* 1992;21:782–787.

Dart RC, McNally J. Efficacy, safety, and use of snake antivenoms in the United States. *Ann Emerg Med* 2001;37:181–188.

Offerman SR, Bush SP, Moynihan JA, Clark RF. Crotaline Fab antivenom for the treatment of children with rattlesnake envenomation. *Pediatrics* 2002;110:968–971.

Walter FG, Bilden EF, Gibly RL. Envenomations. *Crit Care Clin* 1999;15:353–386.

Author: Jill C. Posner

Speech Problems

 ## Database

DEFINITION

- Speech problems may occur in children with difficulties in speech, language, or both.
- Speech problems can be broken down into the following categories:

—Articulation problems:
  —Articulation disorder: substituting sounds ("w" for "r"), leaving sounds out, or adding sounds to words
  —Apraxia: impairment of voluntary control of the muscles necessary to generate speech sounds.
  —Dysarthria: inability to produce the sounds of speech but not as a result of inability to control the muscles.
  —Phonologic disorder: phonologic errors inappropriate for age as a result of inaccurate production of a specific sound.
—Voice problems:
  —Hoarseness.
  —Resonance: problems in resonance result in hyponasal or hypernasal quality to sound production.
—Fluency problems like stuttering

EPIDEMIOLOGY

- At 5 years old, 19% have speech and language disorders (6.4% speech, 8% language, and 4.6% both speech and language).
- Articulation problems occur in 5% of school-aged children and 10% of preschool-aged children.

 ## Differential Diagnosis

INFECTIOUS

- Chronic/recurrent otitis media

ENVIRONMENTAL

- Lack of stimulation
- Lead poisoning

CONGENITAL

- Hearing impairment
- Fragile X syndrome
- Down syndrome
- Fetal alcohol syndrome/effects
- Cleft lip/palate

NUTRITIONAL

- Malnutrition
- Iron deficiency

TUMORS

- Tuberous sclerosis
- Neurofibromatosis

DEVELOPMENTAL

- Mental retardation
- Autistic spectrum disorders
- Dysarthria
- Apraxia

NEUROMUSCULAR

- Muscular dystrophy
- Acquired hearing loss
- Intracranial hearing loss
- Cerebral palsy
- Hydrocephalus

Approach to Patient

- Determine if there is an underlying cause for the delays (hearing impairment, oromotor tone).
- Determine if there are delays in other areas of development.
- Determine if the speech problems are new, or if there is a regression in skills.
- Refer to the appropriate provider for additional evaluations as needed.

 ## Data Gathering

The parent spends the most time with the child and is more likely to hear errors in speech than anyone else. Some parents may not be as aware of what is appropriate at various ages and may be overly or under concerned. Misarticulations or stuttering can be appropriate at some ages, but should resolve by a certain age.

Question: How much of the child's speech is intelligible?
Significance: The rule of four applies here. The amount of speech that should be understandable by a visiting family member is the child's age in years divided by 4. So a 2 year-old should have speech that is at least one-half understandable.

Question: Does you child have a problem with eating or drooling?
Significance: Problems beyond what is normal for age could suggest problems with apraxia or dysarthria.

Question: Does your child have trouble hearing?
Significance: Chronic hearing loss can lead to trouble in sound production. If the child is having distortions in sounds, she or he may have trouble in production.

Question: Does your child stutter? If so, is your child bothered by the stutter?
Significance: One of the major indicators for referral for stuttering is when a child is starting to have emotional reaction to either the stuttering or the teasing by others because of the stuttering.

Question: Did your child ever have skills that he or she lost?
Significance: Regressions can be seen in undetected chronic diseases (such as HIV, acquired hearing loss) but also in Landau Kleffner syndrome.

Past medical history, including birth history, is important.

 ## Physical Examination

The goal of the physical examination in a child with speech problems is to rule out anatomic abnormalities or syndromes that may explain why a child is having difficulties with speech.

Finding: hypernasal or hyponasal speech.
Significance: Hyponasal speech could suggest an obstruction of the upper airway, such as adenoid hypertrophy, although hypernasal suggests velopharyngeal insufficiency, such as cleft palate.

Finding: Dysmorphic features.
Significance: Signs of syndromes such as fetal alcohol syndrome, Williams syndrome, Down syndrome, Angelman syndrome.

Finding: Abnormal tympanic membrane
Significance: Signs of chronic ear infections or congenital abnormalities of TMs may lead to hearing impairments.

Finding: Pooling of food in mouth or excessive drooling.
Significance: Signs of poor oromotor control, which can be helpful in assessing a child for apraxia and dysarthria.

Finding: Poor social skills
Significance: Speech problems and social communication problems are suggestive of autistic spectrum disorders.

Finding: Skin abnormalities
Significance: Findings consistent with neurofibromatosis or tuberous sclerosis. Also look for scars from tracheostomy.

- Watching a child eat or drink can be valuable in starting to think about why a child is having speech problems.
- A thorough neurologic examination and developmental screening will help determine the need for additional testing.

Laboratory Aids

Test: Hearing evaluation.
Significance: Hearing impairment can alter speech development.

- Pure tone audiometry: high false-negative rate, only useful in older children and those capable of cooperating.
- Otoacoustic emissions: useful for children of all ages as a screening tool for hearing impairment.
- Bilateral audio-evoked response testing: gold standard for hearing evaluations.

Test: Speech and language evaluation.
Significance: Comprehensive assessment of receptive and expressive language and extent of articulation difficulties.

Test: Modified barium swallow.
Significance: This is a good tool to assess a child with excessive drooling or pocketing of food in their mouth. It will help in assessing for oromotor dysfunction.

Test: Genetic testing
Significance: Useful in children with physical or historical features suggestive of genetic syndromes.

Test: Electroencephalogram (EEG)
Significance: May help rule out seizure disorder or Landau Kleffner syndrome. Used when the history or physical indicate need.

Therapy

Speech and language therapy should have the following goals:

- Progression in the normal developmental order
- Fixing errors in child's speech
- Encourage understanding of patterns and meanings of language
- Encourage flexibility in language
- Fine tuning of skills

SPEECH AND LANGUAGE PATHOLOGISTS

- All children with significant speech problems should be referred to speech and language pathologists.
- Stuttering should be referred when it is distressing to the child, or if the child is experiencing excessive repetitions (greater than 5 per 100 words), physical struggle with words (grimacing), trouble getting the word started, or behaviors to avoid speaking or saying particular words

Otolaryngologists: All children with hearing loss; and children with speech problems and history of chronic ear infections.
Developmental pediatrician: Children with speech problems and delays in other developmental areas including social skills. Also children with behavioral problems related to their delays (selective mutism, tantrums, aggressive behaviors)
Neurologist: Children with signs or symptoms of a seizure disorder, children with hypotonia or hypertonia, or children with regressions.
Geneticist: Children with dysmorphic features of unclear etiology; or for genetic counseling for parents if etiology clear.
Occupational therapist: Children with poor oromotor tone can benefit from therapy. This is sometimes done by speech pathologists.

Follow-Up

Children with speech problems should be followed on the regular well-child periodicity schedule.

Common Questions and Answers

Q: How do I assess a bilingual child?
A: Bilingual children should be assessed by the same criteria as any other child. The only difference is both languages should be taken into consideration when determining the extent of the vocabulary or syntax used.

Q: Are children with speech problems more likely to be mentally retarded?
A: Children with mental retardation all have speech delays. Children with isolated speech delays are not mentally retarded.

Q: How can parents help a child with speech problems?
A: Using multiple means of communication can be very valuable. Parents can use pictures of their child's favorite things or activities to help the child communicate and reduce his or her frustration level. Additionally, saying the word when the child points at objects can reinforce the use of language for requests.

BIBLIOGRAPHY

Coplan J. Normal speech and language development: An overview. *Pediatr Rev* 1995; Vol 16, No 3:91–100.

Guitar B, Belin-Frost G. Stuttering. In: Parker S, Zuckerman B, eds. *Behavioral and Developmental Pediatrics: A Handbook for Primary Care.* Boston, MA: Little, Brown and Company, 1995:294–296.

Kelly DP, Sally JI. Disorders of speech and language. In: Levine MD, Carey WB, Crocker AC, eds. *Developmental-Behavioral Pediatrics.* 3rd Ed. Philadelphia, PA: WB Saunders Company, 1999:621–631.

McCauley R. Articulation disorders. In: Parker S, Zuckerman B, eds. *Behavioral and Developmental Pediatrics: A Handbook for Primary Care.* Boston, MA: Little, Brown and Company, 1995:70–72.

Simms MD, Schum RL. Preschool children who have atypical patterns of development. *Pediatr Rev* 2000;21(5):147–158.

Toppelberg CO, Shapiro T. Language disorders: A 10-year research upate review. *J Am Acad Child Adolesc Psychiatry* 2000;39:143–152.

Author: Nathaniel S. Beers

Spinal Muscular Atrophy

 ## Database

DEFINITION

A progressive disorder of motor neurons in the spinal cord. Major symptom is weakness. Most common and severe form, type I, also known as Werdnig-Hoffman disease, begins before 6 months. Onset in type II between 6 and 18 months. Onset in type III (Kugelberg-Welander disease) is after 18 months.

CAUSES

• The classic form (types I, II, and III) follows an autosomal recessive inheritance and is caused by mutations in the survival motor neuron (SMN) gene on 5q11.2 to 13.3.
• Two copies of SMN on each chromosome. SMN1 (SMNt), the telomeric copy, produces stable SMN protein. Homozygous deletion is the most common cause of SMA type I. SMN2 (SMNc), the centromeric copy, produces unstable, truncated protein products. SMA types II and III often result from a conversion of SMN1 to SMN2.
• The SMN protein plays a role in RNA processing, unclear why motor neurons (anterior horn cells) are selectively vulnerable to this defect.

EPIDEMIOLOGY

• One of the most common inherited causes of death in humans.
• Incidence estimated at 1 in 6,000 to 1 in 24,000 live births, carrier frequency 1 in 40.

COMPLICATIONS

• Respiratory complications, including recurrent pneumonias, are common.
• Swallowing difficulties may be severe enough in SMA I to require tube feeding.
• Scoliosis frequently occurs in SMA types II and III, may require surgery.

OTHER ANTERIOR HORN CELL DISEASES

• SMA variants are associated with arthrogryposis, pontocerebellar hypoplasia, congenital fractures, and congenital heart disease. Few such cases have been shown to have SMN mutations.
• Fazio-Londe disease. Rare degeneration of anterior horn cells in the brainstem. Childhood onset.
• Kennedy disease. X-linked recessive anterior horn cell disease with adult onset. Affected males have gynecomastia, testicular atrophy, and reduced fertility.

 ## Differential Diagnosis

• Other genetic neuromuscular disorders include congenital muscular dystrophy, congenital myopathy, glycogen storage disorders, myotonic dystrophy, mitochondrial disease, and congenital myasthenia gravis. Prader-Willi syndrome may mimic SMA I.
• More acute course may suggest infant botulism, Guillain-Barré syndrome, although the latter is rare in this age group. More generalized disorders that may cause acute hypotonia include sepsis and meningitis.
• SMA II differential: congenital muscular dystrophy, congenital myopathy, and congenital myasthenia gravis.
• SMA III differential includes Duchenne, Becker, and the limb girdle muscular dystrophies.
• Spinal cord mass lesion may rarely resemble SMA.

 ## Data Gathering

HISTORY

• Hypotonia and weakness are the primary features. Infants with SMA I will be floppy, less active, and have delayed motor milestones.
• The mother's perceived vigor of prenatal movements may be helpful.

 ## Physical Examination

• Weakness suggests a neuromuscular cause, while normal strength is more consistent with a central etiology. Absent or reduced reflexes also suggest a neuromuscular disorder. A proximal pattern of weakness is consistent with SMA, myopathies, and muscular dystrophies; a distal pattern suggests polyneuropathies.
• Extraocular movements remain intact in SMA.
• Dysmorphic features, or involvement of other organs may point to a diagnosis other than SMA. Occasionally, SMA presents with contractures.
• Tongue fasciculations strongly suggest SMA, but their absence does not exclude the diagnosis.

 ## Laboratory Aids

GENETIC TESTING

• Genetic testing of DNA extracted from blood (SMN deletions) is now the gold standard in diagnosis; may be done prenatally; >95% sensitive.
• Genetic testing for Prader-Willi syndrome (FISH and methylation) may be indicated if there is no SMN gene deletion and EMG is normal in an infant who appears to have SMA.

OTHER TESTING

• Serum creatinine kinase (CK) measurements are often normal in SMA, but may be mildly elevated.
• Electromyography (EMG) may be helpful if the clinical presentation is atypical for SMA or if genetic testing is negative. EMG shows high-amplitude, long-duration motor units.
• With the advent of molecular testing, muscle biopsy is rarely performed. Biopsy is sometimes helpful in atypical presentations or when genetic testing is unrevealing. The characteristic findings are fiber type grouping with generalized atrophy of muscle fibers.
• If the entire evaluation is negative, MRI of the spine may reveal a mass lesion.

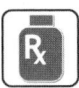 ## Therapy

- Physical therapy is appropriate, although it may not affect the course of SMA I. Most helpful in SMA types II and III.
- A wheelchair will maintain mobility in SMA type II. Adults with SMA III may require the use of a wheelchair later in their course.
- Spinal fusion surgery may preserve respiratory function.
- Low threshold for empiric antibiotics for respiratory infection is appropriate. Chest physiotherapy can help prevent pneumonia and atelectasis.
- Noninvasive positive pressure ventilation (BiPAP) may improve quality of life in patients with decreased respiratory function.
- Avoiding catabolic state with proactive nutritional support, including tube feeding in some cases, is important.

 ## Follow-Up

PROGNOSIS

- Most children with SMA type I die by 2 years; a few live as long as a decade.
- Children with SMA type II typically survive into late adolescence or early adulthood.
- Individuals with SMA type III survive well into adulthood. In SMA type IIIa, approximately two-thirds of affected individuals cannot walk independently by age 40. In SMA type IIIb, only one-third of patients lose the ability to walk by age 40.
- Intelligence is generally preserved.
- Death typically ensues from respiratory complications. Discuss resuscitation status early in SMA I and in the advanced stages of SMA II and III.

PITFALLS

- Genetic testing should be performed in all cases, even when the diagnosis appears clear.
- An apparently minor respiratory infection may carry a higher risk of respiratory failure in SMA I and later stages of SMA II and III. Depending on resuscitation status, there should be no hesitation in admitting such a patient to the hospital for observation.
- Genetic counseling is critical for all families with children affected by SMA, as the chances of recurrence are 25%.

 ## Common Questions and Answers

Q: Can routine vaccinations be given to children with SMA?
A: Yes. In addition to routine vaccinations, yearly influenza vaccinations are recommended for older children.

Q: Are more effective therapies for SMA being developed?
A: There are ongoing studies in animal models and proposed studies on humans, involving both pharmacologic and gene-based therapies. The Muscular Dystrophy Association and other groups are the best sources of information on such research.

ICD-9-CM 335.10

BIBLIOGRAPHY

Birnkrant DJ, Pope JF, Eiben RM. Management of the respiratory complications of neuromuscular diseases in the pediatric intensive care unit. *J Child Neurol* 1999;14(3):139–143.

Dubowitz V. *Muscle Disorders in Childhood.* 2nd Ed. London: W.B. Saunders Company Ltd., 1995.

Iannaccone ST, Burghes A. Spinal muscular atrophies. *Adv Neurol* 2002;88:83–98.

Lefebvre S, Burglen L, Reboullet S, et al. Identification and characterization of a spinal muscular atrophy-determining gene. *Cell* 1995;80(1):155–165.

Nicole S, Diaz CC, Frugier T, Melki J. Spinal muscular atrophy: recent advances and future prospects. *Muscle Nerve* 2002;26(1):4–13.

Zerres K, Rudnik-Schoneborn S. Natural history in proximal spinal muscular atrophy. Clinical analysis of 445 patients and suggestions for a modification of existing classifications. *Arch Neurol* 1995;52(5):518–523.

Author: Peter B. Kang

Staphylococcal Scalded Skin Syndrome (SSSS)

Database

DEFINITION

- A spectrum of generalized exfoliative skin eruptions, which resemble scalding injuries but are caused by an epidermolytic toxin produced by certain strains of *Staphylococcus aureus*.
- Known as Ritter disease or pemphigus neonatorum in neonates.

Spectrum of disease ranges from:

- Bullous impetigo: characterized by discrete, flaccid bullae containing clear or cloudy yellow fluid.
- Staphylococcal scarlet fever: a mild generalized scarletiniform eruption with exfoliation, but without the strawberry tongue and palatal enanthem of streptococcal scarlet fever.
- Evidence based on toxin production now suggests that staphylococcal scarlet fever often represents an abortive form of toxic shock syndrome.
- Classic SSSS: characterized by abrupt onset of fever, irritability and diffuse, blanchable erythema in association with marked skin tenderness.

PATHOPHYSIOLOGY

- The soluble exotoxin, referred to as exfoliative (epidermolytic) toxin A or B (ETA or ETB), produced by certain strains of *S. aureus* and usually belonging to phage group II in the United States are responsible for SSSS.
- The exotoxins are glutamate-specific trypsin-like serine proteases. The active site of the exfoliative toxins appears to be conformationally blocked in its native state. The target for the toxins has recently been identified as desmoglein-1, a desmosomal glycoprotein that plays an important role in maintaining cell-to-cell adhesion in the superficial epidermis. It is speculated that binding of the exfoliative toxin's active site to desmoglein-1 results in a conformational change that opens the active site of the toxin to cleave the extracellular domain of desmoglein-1 resulting in disruption of intercellular adhesion and formation of superficial blisters.
- Generalized desquamation with early intraepidermal bullae demonstrating a cleavage plane just beneath the granular cell layer.
- Nikolsky sign develops within 12 hours to 3 days accompanied by flaccid thin-walled bullae. Bullae spontaneously rupture within hours separating the superficial epidermis into large sheets revealing moist red surfaces resembling burns. One to three days later the denuded areas dry and the entire body surface undergoes a secondary flaky desquamation. Entire skin heals within a total of 10 to 14 days.

EPIDEMIOLOGY

- Most cases are caused by type 71 (75% of cases) or type 70, with occasional cases as a result of types 3A, 3B, 3C, and 55.
- The vast majority of cases occur in neonates or even in the intrauterine environment (as in Ritter disease) and young children <5 years of age.
- Large screening experiments reveal toxin-producing strains in 5% to 6% of individuals.
- Antibodies to ETA have been found in 88% of cord blood samples and are absent in acute sera of patients with SSSS.
- Rarely occurs in adults as a result of increased circulating antibodies and adult kidney excretion of the toxin.
- Most frequently occurs in association with immunosuppression or renal impairment in adults.
- No differences in incidence based on gender or socioeconomic status.

COMPLICATIONS

- Occasional shedding of hair and nails.
- Fungal or bacterial superinfection following desquamation.
- Serious fluid and electrolyte disturbances in cases involving large surface areas that may lead to poor temperature control, hypovolemia, sepsis syndrome, and death. Neonates are particularly susceptible.

PROGNOSIS

- Exfoliated areas eventually dry with a flaky desquamation in 3 to 5 days of initiating appropriate antibiotic therapy.
- Usually complete recovery within 10 to 14 days without scarring.
- More guarded in infants and those with underlying illness.
- Mortality reported as 1% to 10% in neonates and 3% in children.

Differential Diagnosis

- Toxic epidermal necrolysis (TEN)
- Kawasaki disease
- Erythema multiforme bullosum
- Erythema multiforme major (Stevens-Johnson syndrome)
- Streptococcal or staphylococcal toxic shock syndrome (TSS)
- Bullous varicella
- Burns
- Primary bullous disorders (e.g., Bullous mastocytosis)
- Chronic bullous disease of childhood
- Pemphigus vulgaris or foliaceus
- Epidermolysis bullosa

Data Gathering

HISTORY

Question: Was there a nonspecific virus-like prodrome with irritability?
Significance: This is the typical presentation of SSSS.

Question: Where did the rash begin?
Significance: It typically begins periorally then extends to the trunk and extremities and finally desquamates.

Question: Was there any recent, seemingly trivial, localized extracutaneous infection?
Significance: Infections involving the nasopharynx, middle ear, conjunctiva, pharynx, tonsils, umbilicus or urinary tract are frequently recalled.

Question: Was there any recent medication use?
Significance: A history of recent drug use suggests TEN.

Physical Examination

Finding: Erythroderma
Significance: Usually extremely painful.

Finding: Fever
Significance: Usually abrupt onset after prodrome.

Finding: Large flaccid bullae that leave behind denuded skin resembling a burn after rupturing.
Significance: Bullae often appear in areas of trauma, or in areas that are rubbed or touched, including intertriginous zones.

Finding: Distribution of lesions
Significance: Usually involve perineal, periumbilical, and intertriginous areas of the neonate; although the extremities are usually involved in older children.

Finding: Crusting seen in a radial pattern (sunburst) around the mouth, nose and eyes
Significance: Occurs without mucous membrane involvement.

Finding: Sandpaper texture of rash and increased erythema or petechiae in skin creases
Significance: Pastia lines are seen in the Scarletiniform variant.

Finding: Nikolsky sign
Significance: Gentle friction applied obliquely to apparently healthy skin will cause wrinkling then sloughing.

Staphylococcal Scalded Skin Syndrome (SSSS)

 ## Laboratory Aids

TESTS

Test: Skin biopsy
Significance: Used to differentiate SSSS from TEN; the cornified skin layer is recovered in SSSS, whereas the entire necrotic epidermis should be recognized in TEN.

Test: Excision of some exfoliated skin for frozen or permanent histologic section
Significance: Easier to obtain than a biopsy is often useful in arriving at the diagnosis.

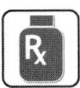 ## Therapy

- Apply principles of good burn care in severe cases including:
- Fluid and electrolyte management should include daily maintenance requirements and replacement of "third-space" fluid loss based on the percentage of affected body surface area (BSA). Fluid should be replaced as an isotonic solution calculated at 3 mL/kg of affected BSA. Most experts recommend replacement of one-half of losses over the first 8 hours and the other half over the next 16 hours.
- Children should be allowed to rest unclothed on sterilized linens, and handling of the child should be kept to a minimum. Wound care should focus on maintenance of developing eschars. This is usually followed by debridement, and affected areas are eventually dressed with silver sulfadiazine or a similar agent.

DRUGS

- Antistaphylococcal agents: parenteral antibiotic therapy (e.g., nafcillin, oxacillin, cephalosporins, clindamycin) should be used for extensive skin involvement or serious systemic disease. Oral therapy (e.g., dicloxacillin, cloxacillin, amoxicillin/clavulanate, cephalexin, clindamycin) is generally sufficient for bullous impetigo. Duration of therapy is typically 7 to 10 days. Topical preparations are of no benefit.
- Corticosteroids have been shown to be detrimental both in experimental animal models and clinical trials.

 ## Follow-Up

- Patients may be followed via telephone as long as lesions are healing well and parents do not report significant complications.

PREVENTION

- Eradication of staphylococci to prevent recurrences after first attack.
- Preventing skin from becoming overly moist or macerated.

ISOLATION OF HOSPITALIZED PATIENT

- Suspected or documented cases should be placed in contact isolation.

PITFALLS

- Confusion with TEN may lead to possible use of corticosteroids or simple discontinuation of antibiotics, resulting in enhanced infection from prolonged toxin production.
- Differentiation from streptococcal disease with need for penicillinase-resistant antibiotic therapy (e.g., nafcillin).
- A methicillin-resistant strain of Staphylococcal aureus has been reported to cause SSSS.
- Adhesive occlusive dressings used to apply topical local anesthetic prior to venipuncture have been shown to cause injury and discomfort in areas previously free of blistering in patients with SSSS.
- Diagnosis should be made clinically and should not be delayed several days while waiting for the results of cultures or other diagnostic tests which are largely confirmatory.

 ## Common Questions and Answers

Q: Can SSSS recur?
A: Yes.

Q: Is SSSS contagious?
A: Yes, the staphylococci are primarily spread from person-to-person (familial clusters have been reported), even mother-to-fetus, most efficiently by someone with lesions, but asymptomatic carriers may also spread infection. Spread of organisms does not necessarily lead to signs of toxin production in those acquiring infection.

Q: How can one distinguish TEN from SSSS?
A: TEN is frequently confused with SSSS and may be differentiated by skin biopsy showing cleavage plane at the dermal-epidermal junction. TEN or Lyell disease is more common in adults and is usually secondary to drug hypersensitivity (e.g., sulfonamides, barbiturates, pyrazolone derivatives).

Q: Can staphylococcus be isolated from the bullae?
A: SSSS bullae are sterile although organisms may be found in a distant focus, such as the nares or conjunctivae. In bullous impetigo, staphylococci may be isolated from the bullae.

ICD-9-CM 695.1

BIBLIOGRAPHY

Anbu AT, Williams S. Miliaria crystallina complicating Staphylococcal scalded skin syndrome. *Arch Dis Child* 2004;89:94.

Eichenfield LF, Honig PJ. Blistering disorders in childhood. *Pediatr Clin North Am* 1991;38:959–976.

Farrell AM. Staphylococcal scalded skin syndrome. *Lancet* 1999;354:880–881.

Ladhani S. Understanding the mechanism of action of the exfoliative toxins of Staphylococcus aureus. *FEMS Immunol Med Microbiol* 2003;39:181–189.

Ladhani S, Evans RW. Staphylococcal scalded skin syndrome. *Arch Dis Child* 1998;78:85–88.

Lina G, Gillet Y, Vandenesch F, Jones ME, Floret D, Etienne J. Toxin involvement in Staphylococcal scalded skin syndrome. *Clin Infect Dis* 1997;25:1369–1373.

Resnick SD. Staphylococcal toxin-mediated syndromes in childhood. *Semin Dermatol* 1992;11:11–18.

Schenfeld, LA. Images in clinical medicine. Staphylococcal scalded skin syndrome. *N Engl J Med.* 2000;342:1178.

Author: Mark L. Bagarazzi

Status Epilepticus

Database

DEFINITION

Status epilepticus (SE) is defined as more than 30 minutes of continuous seizure activity or two or more sequential seizures in 30 minutes without full recovery of consciousness between seizures. As the convulsive phase of nearly all generalized tonic-clonic seizures terminates within 5 minutes, convulsive seizures continuing >5 minutes should be treated as presumptive SE. SE presents in several forms:

- Either a single or repeated generalized convulsion(s) with symmetric or asymmetric movements, with persistent loss of consciousness (may be a result of postictal depression) and neurologic function during and/or between seizures.
- Nonconvulsive seizures manifesting as alteration in consciousness, variable subtle motor signs such as twitching and nystagmus.
- Repeated partial seizures manifested as focal motor convulsions or sensory symptoms not associated with altered consciousness (epilepsia partialis continua)
- Absence status epilepticus in which the individual may be in a persistent staring spell (with or without simple motor automatisms) or in a stuporous state, not fully responsive.

GENETICS

Some inherited conditions increase risk of SE, including neurocutaneous syndromes (tuberous sclerosis, Sturge-Weber) and familial epilepsy syndromes.

EPIDEMIOLOGY

126,000 to 195,000 cases/year with an increased risk in young children and the elderly. The incidence of SE in the pediatric population is 38 per 100,000 and in children <1 year, >150 per 100,000.

PATHOLOGY

SE can be a result of either acute or chronic factors. Most common inciting acute factors are high fever, metabolic derangements (electrolyte imbalances, renal failure, etc.), intoxications, trauma, neoplasm, anoxia, stroke/hemorrhage. Chronic causes include preexisting epilepsy, discontinuation of seizure medications, neurodegenerative disorders, brain tumors, and neurocutaneous syndromes (tuberous sclerosis, Sturge-Weber). Idiopathic cases may be a result of an abnormality of brain development which is beyond MRI resolution.

RISK FACTORS

History of seizure disorder, recent withdrawal of anticonvulsant medication, brain tumor, neurodegenerative disorder, history of remote neurologic insult (stroke, intracranial hemorrhage, birth asphyxia, cerebral palsy, head trauma, meningitis)

PROGNOSIS

The morbidity and mortality of SE reflect etiology and are lower in children than in adults. Recent mortality estimates in children range from 1% to 3%, with risk of new neurologic sequelae estimated between 9% and 29%.

Differential Diagnosis

- Nonepileptic seizures (including psychogenic seizures or pseudoseizures) may mimic status epilepticus. Pseudoseizures may be characterized by asynchronous limb movements, and purposeful resistance to passive movement, and normal concurrent EEG. Induction of a seizure by suggestion further supports this diagnosis.
- Movement disorders (including dystonia, chorea and very frequent tics) can be mistaken for persistent seizure activity.
- Post anoxic myoclonus: status post prolonged cardiopulmonary arrest. These movements are usually nonrhythmic and segmental but can appear rhythmic at times.

Data Gathering

HISTORY

- Ask about prior seizures or neurologic abnormality.
- Ask specifically about precipitating factors: fever; preceding illness; head trauma; change in antiepileptic medication; family history of seizures

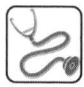

Physical Examination

- Vital signs: fever, Respiratory rate/O_2 sats (adequacy of air exchange and abnormal breathing patterns), heart rate, BP (hypertension suggests intracranial hypertension)
- Signs of head trauma: Retinal hemorrhages; Evidence of intracranial hypertension such as bulging fontanelle

—Meningismus may be absent in CNS infection, or may signal intracranial hemorrhage or spine trauma

- Signs of systemic infection: Especially meningismus suggesting CNS infection.
- Skin examination: Wood's lamp should be used to look for neurocutaneous disorders.
- During convulsions: neurologic, look for a movement asymmetry
- Postictal examination: Transient neurologic abnormalities (pupillary asymmetries, eye deviation, and focal motor weakness (Todd paresis)—may not correlate with the underlying structural lesion). After seizure has stopped a neurologic examination should be performed with attention to mental status, focal weakness, tone, or sensation.

Laboratory Aids

TESTS

Initial

- STAT glucose, electrolytes, calcium, magnesium, and arterial blood gas
- Antiepileptic drug levels
- CBC, liver function tests
- Toxicology screen, urinalysis

Other Tests

- Lumbar puncture: indicated to rule out CNS infection. Contraindications include intracranial hypertension known or suspected from examination or CT scan, cerebral mass lesion, or obstructive hydrocephalus. LP may be deferred until after head CT if suspicion of CNS infection is low.
- Brain imaging with CT or MRI: is indicated for SE, especially with partial-onset seizures (including aura), focally abnormal EEG, focal neurologic signs, or history of head trauma. MRI gives more detailed images; however, CT (more appropriate if urgent imaging or the patient is medically unstable).
- EEG: indicated if convulsions continue; if the patient remains comatose for 1 hour or longer after convulsions cease, or if pharmacologic interventions such as pentobarbital-induced coma, sedation, and neuromuscular blockade for intubation are considered. If a child has been in SE >30 minutes the likelihood of prolonged unresponsiveness possibly as a result of ongoing nonconvulsive SE is a significant possibility that is best addressed by an urgent EEG.

Therapy

- Initial management: ABCs—stabilization of airway, supporting respiration, maintaining blood pressure, and gaining intravascular access. BP, ECG, and respiratory function should be monitored.
- Airway control may be maintained by head positioning, and oral airway placement and oxygen supplementation provided via nasal cannula, mask, or bag-valve-mask ventilation. If the need for respiratory assistance persists, endotracheal intubation may be required.
- 2 to 4 mL/kg of D25 (25% dextrose) for hypoglycemia.
- Rectal acetaminophen and a cooling blanket for fever.
- Antiepileptic drug administration should be initiated whenever seizure activity persists for longer than 5 minutes. Benzodiazepines are initial management of patients with active convulsions. Most commonly, Lorazepam (0.05 to 0.1 mg/kg per dose at 2 mg/min maximum, up to a total dose of 0.3–0.5 mg/kg) and Diazepam (0.1 to 0.2 mg/kg per dose at 5 mg/min, up to a total dose of 1.0 mg/kg, not to exceed a total dose of 10 mg). Be aware that hypotension and respiratory depression can occur with benzodiazepines.
- SE persists: administer an IV loading dose of 20 mg/kg phenytoin or fosphenytoin (preferred; 20 mg/kg as phenytoin-equivalents). Additional 5 mg/kg doses may be given if needed to stop convulsions (to maximum total dose of 30 mg/kg). Monitor BP and ECG during phenytoin infusion and rate reduced if hypotension or arrhythmias occur.
- Intravenous phenobarbital at a loading dose of 20 mg/kg (maximum rate, 100 mg/min) is generally a third-line drug for older children and adults but is usually given before phenytoin in infants younger than 1 year of age. Additional 5- to 10-mg/kg increments (to total maximum dose of 30 to 40 mg/kg) may be given as necessary to stop convulsions. Sedation, respiratory depression, and hypotension are potential side effects.
- Intravenous valproate a loading dose of 10 to 20 mg/kg (maximum rate of 3mg/kg per minute [manufacturer recommends no faster than 20 mg/min but studies have reported successful trials of faster rates of administration]) followed by maintenance doses of up to 60 mg/kg per bid to qid. Monitoring to keep total VPA levels between 50 to 100 is recommended. Thrombocytopenia, pancreatitis, hepatitis, and skin rashes are potential side effects. IV VPA should be changed to a PO formulation before 14 days.

- If intravenous access is difficult to obtain, diazepam (0.5 mg/kg to a maximum of 20 mg), paraldehyde (0.3 to 0.5 mL/kg diluted 1:1 in vegetable oil), or valproic acid (20 mg/kg of liquid formulation diluted 1:1 in water) can be administered rectally.
- Refractory SE exists if the above medications fail and the patient continues to clinically have convulsions or is in nonconvulsive SE. Alternate agents for this situation include Propofol, Midazolam, iterative 5 mg/kg boluses of phenobarbital (in anesthetic doses; EEG monitoring is required with the goal of inducing a suppression-burst pattern for a minimum of 12 hours), pentobarbital, and inhalational anesthetics (isoflurane) may be administered with the patient in an intensive care unit and with neurological consultation.

Follow-Up

PREVENTION

Need for long-term antiepileptic drug (AED) therapy after SE depends on the etiology, patient's age, and circumstances in which SE occurred. Chronic AED therapy is indicated when SE is caused by structural brain lesions or in patients with known epilepsy. Chronic AED therapy generally not needed in children who have SE from transient metabolic disturbances (hyponatremia, intoxication, fever), or in idiopathic SE as a first seizure. Educate family members regarding first aid of seizures. Discussion of potential risks of seizure recurrence even if the child is taking an AED, emphasizing exposures dangers of climbing and swimming. Consider providing caregivers with rectal diazepam with detailed instructions that it is for seizure >5 minutes in duration. Neurology consultation is recommended.

PITFALLS

- Anticonvulsant intoxication may occasionally cause SE (phenytoin, carbamazepine); check levels on any patient known to take anticonvulsants.
- Neuromuscular blockers used in intubation may obscure ongoing electrical seizures. EEG monitoring is mandatory for all patients who have had pharmacologic paralysis for airway control during SE.
- Psychogenic status is often mistaken for status epilepticus. If the diagnosis is in doubt get an EEG to differentiate these possibilities.

—Rhabdomyolysis may complicate SE. Check serial CK levels and keep patient well hydrated.

Common Questions and Answers

Q: Does SE cause brain injury?
A: Research suggests that neuronal loss may occur at 30 to 60 minutes of SE. This illness represents a neurologic emergency. Other determinants of outcome are hypoxic brain injury as a result of hypoventilation during a seizure and brain injury because of an identifiable underlying cause of SE, such as encephalitis. Outcome in children with idiopathic SE without hypoxia is usually very good. Outcome of SE as a result of other brain injury (hypoxia, encephalitis, trauma) depends on severity of the inciting process.

Q: What is the value of PET or other functional imaging in refractory epilepsy?
A: Functional imaging studies may help localize "hot spots" for staging of surgical therapy of refractory epilepsy. Functional imaging generally is not useful in status epilepticus.

Q: How safe is administration of rectal diazepam for children with cluster seizures?
A: Studies suggest that when dosing guidelines are closely followed, this agent is safe and effective in terminating clusters of seizures, obviating a trip to the emergency room. Toxicity of other agents used to control SE includes hypotension (phenytoin), hypoventilation/respiratory arrest (barbiturates, benzodiazepines), and sedation.

ICD-9-CM 345.3

BIBLIOGRAPHY

Appleton R, Martland T, Phillips B. Drug management for acute tonic-clonic convulsions including convulsive status epilepticus in children. *Cochrane Database of Systematic Reviews.* 2002;(4):CD001905.

Crawford TO, et al. Very-high-dose Phenobarbital for refractory status epilepticus in children. *Neurol* 1988;38:1035–1040.

Fountain NB. Status epilepticus: risk factors and complications. *Epilepsia* 2000;41(S2): S23–S30.

Hanhan UA, Fiallos MR, Orlowski JP. Status Epilepticus. *Ped Clin North Am* 2001;48(3): 683–694.

Lowenstein DH. Treatment options for status epilepticus. *Curr Opin Pharmacol* 2003;3(1): 6–11.

Mitchell WG, Conry JA, Crumrine PK, et al. An open-label study of repeated use of diazepam rectal gel (Diastat) for episodes of acute breakthrough seizures and clusters: safety, efficacy, and tolerance. North American Diastat Group. *Epilepsia* 1999;40:1610–1617.

Authors: Eric Marsh, Keith Nagle, and Amy R. Brooks-Kayal

Stevens-Johnson Syndrome

 Database

DEFINITION

Stevens-Johnson Syndrome (SJS) is a severe hypersensitivity reaction, characterized by diffuse bullous lesions, mucocutaneous involvement, and marked constitutional symptoms.

SJS is often considered to lie on a spectrum, between erythema multiforme minor (EM minor) on one extreme, and toxic epidermal necrolysis (TEN) on the other, but this classification is controversial. In this schema, SJS is defined as involving >2 mucous membranes and <10% of total body surface area, and TEN as involving >30%, with overlap in between.

ETIOLOGY

SJS is an acute hypersensitivity reaction to the following:

- Medications—classically anticonvulsants, antibiotics (penicillins, sulfonamides, and erythromycin), nonsteroidal anti-inflammatory medications, and allopurinol.
- Infections—specifically herpes simplex virus (HSV) or Mycoplasma, but any viruses, bacteria or fungi can be involved.
- Environmental factors—foods, immunizations, and other chemical exposures.
- Reexposure to a causative agent can lead to more severe recurrences.

PATHOPHYSIOLOGY

- SJS is an acute hypersensitivity reaction, characterized by a cell-mediated immunologic reaction.
- A prodrome of 1 to 14 days is often seen, consisting of constitutional symptoms, including high fever, myalgias, and arthralgias.
- A rash often starts on the torso, face, and neck, but spreads to the entire body within a few days.
- The rash generally starts as macular lesions, which may resemble the "target lesions" seen in EM minor. The target lesions progress to raised, purpuric lesions and bullae. As these bullae coalesce, the epidermis may slough.
- Ulcers and bullae may form on all mucous membranes (oropharynx and nasopharynx, eyes, genitals; and the respiratory, urinary, and gastrointestinal tracts).
- Ophthalmic involvement includes severe keratitis and conjunctivitis, which can lead to ulcerations, perforations, and scarring.
- The pathologic findings of SJS are an inflammatory infiltration of the epidermis progressing to full-thickness necrosis of the epidermis, which leads to sloughing.

EPIDEMIOLOGY

- Incidence is 2 to 3 cases per million people each year.
- Affects all ages, ethnicities, and both genders equally.

COMPLICATIONS

- Dehydration as a result of fluid loss from damaged skin
- Sepsis
- Bacterial superinfection
- Pneumonia, pneumonitis, pleural effusion, and respiratory failure (as a result of infection or sloughing of respiratory mucosa)
- Gastrointestinal bleeding, ulcers, diarrhea, or constipation (as a result of painful anal ulcerations
- Hepatitis
- Urinary retention, nephritis and renal failure
- Chronic eye dryness and scarring; rarely blindness

PROGNOSIS

- Average length of hospital stay is 3 weeks.
- Mortality is approximately 5% with most children recovering with only minimal sequelae
- Skin lesions generally heal without scarring, but pigment changes may occur.
- Loss of hair and nails is rare.
- Eyes are the major source of long-term morbidity, with chronic dryness, scarring, and rarely blindness.

 Differential Diagnosis

INFECTIONS

- Varicella
- Staphylococcal Scalded Skin Syndrome
- Measles (and other macular rashes)

RHEUMATOLOGIC

- Kawasaki disease
- Henoch-Schönlein purpura

TRAUMA

- Thermal or chemical burns

DERMATOLOGIC

- Erythema multiforme minor
- Fixed drug eruption
- Pemphigus

OTHER

- Graft versus host disease

 Data Gathering

HISTORY

Question: Has the child been on any new medications in the last several weeks, specifically anticonvulsants or antibiotics?
Significance: These medications are known to cause SJS, with the highest incidence in the first 8 weeks after initiation of therapy.

Question: Has the child had recent infections or chemical exposures?
Significance: HSV, Mycoplasma, foods, and immunizations have all been associated with SJS.

Question: Has this child had SJS previously?
Significance: Recurrences of SJS may occur and may be a result of recurrent HSV infection.

 Physical Examination

- Examine entire skin surface and all mucous membranes to determine extent of involvement. Also, look for signs of secondary infection.
- Nikolsky sign (sliding a finger across the affected skin causing sloughing of the epidermis) may be present.
- Evaluate hydration status.
- Evaluate respiratory, nutritional, gastrointestinal, and urologic status.

Laboratory Aids

- There is no specific test for SJS. Laboratory tests should be used to support the diagnosis and to evaluate the extent of the illness.
- Complete blood count—to screen for evidence of superinfection
- Electrolytes—to assess hydration status and renal function
- Liver function tests—to determine the presence of hepatitis
- Acute phase reactants, including erythrocyte sedimentation rate (ESR), are often elevated
- Bacterial cultures, both blood and surface, may be used to assess for secondary infection
- Specific microbiologic tests may be used to evaluate for HSV, Mycoplasma, or other causes of infection.
- Chest radiograph and pulse oximetry may be used to evaluate pulmonary status

Emergency Care

- Evaluate and address respiratory and circulatory problems (ABCs), if present.
- Evaluate and treat sepsis, if present.
- Children with significant pulmonary complications may require mechanical ventilation and should be managed in an intensive care unit.
- Widespread skin involvement is an indication for burn unit admission, as these children will require intensive wound management by pediatric burn specialists.

 ## Therapy

- Therapy is supportive for most patients.
- If an offending drug is identified, it must be discontinued immediately, because this may reduce mortality.
- Fluid resuscitation and ongoing, aggressive fluid management are crucial.
- Many patients are unable to tolerate oral feedings because of ulcerations of the gastrointestinal tract. Nasogastric or parenteral nutrition must be considered to provide supraphysiologic calorie requirements.
- Meticulous skin care, including topical care, debridement, and skin grafting.
- Any eye involvement warrants urgent ophthalmologic evaluation. Ocular lubrication may be required.
- Close monitoring for bacterial superinfection, both superficial infections and sepsis.
- Close monitoring of respiratory, renal, hepatic, or gastrointestinal complications. Mechanical ventilation may be warranted in severe cases.
- Underlying medical conditions, e.g., epilepsy, may become exacerbated if chronic medications are discontinued.

DRUGS

- Open skin lesions should be covered with an antibiotic ointment, such as bacitracin or chlorhexidine, and gauze (with or without petrolatum). Sulfa containing antibiotics such as sulfadiazine may exacerbate SJS and should be avoided
- Prophylactic antibiotics are not indicated. Treat only with antibiotics if diagnosed with secondary bacterial infections.
- Acyclovir may be used to treat HSV, if present. Consider using acyclovir empirically in cases of recurrent SJS.
- Systemic corticosteroids—their use has been controversial for some time. Corticosteroids are of questionable efficacy for SJS and can increase the risk of infection. Some authors have found benefit when used in high doses early in the course of disease. Generally, corticosteroids should NOT be used for the majority of cases of SJS. They may be considered in cases of recurrent SJS, in which the disease is quickly identified, but for no longer than 3 days, as their use raises the risk of superinfections.

- Intravenous immunoglobulin (IVIG)—some small studies have reported that doses of 0.5 mg/kg per day over 4 days may be effective at slowing the progression of SJS. IVIG is proposed to work by blocking apoptosis induced by the inciting agent.
- Plasmapheresis, cyclosporine, and cyclophosphamide have been investigated but have not clearly shown a benefit.

 ## Follow-Up

- Hydration and nutrition must be managed until the lesions are healed and the patient tolerates oral feedings.
- Meticulous skin care until all lesions are healed.
- Long-term ophthalmologic follow-up is necessary if there has been any eye involvement.
- If a preceding exposure is identified, it must be avoided.
- Prophylactic acyclovir may be used in patients with recurrent SJS as a result of HSV.

PITFALLS

- Failure to recognize significant complications, especially infection and dehydration.

Common Questions and Answers

Q: When should corticosteroids be considered?
A: In patients with recurrent SJS in which the disease is quickly identified, corticosteroids may be of benefit if started early. This is the only instance in which corticosteroids should be strongly considered. Corticosteroids started later in the illness are not helpful. They may also exacerbate underlying HSV infection.

Q: Do all patients with SJS require an ophthalmologic evaluation?
A: The presence of any ocular manifestation of SJS mandates ophthalmologic consultation, as eye involvement can progress and be quite severe. Children with no signs of eye involvement (redness, dryness, pain) can be managed without ophthalmology.

Q: How should seizures be managed in patients with epilepsy who develop SJS from their antiepileptic medication?
A: It is vital that the causative medication be discontinued immediately. Seizures should be managed with benzodiazepines until the SJS begins to resolve. At that point, neurologic consultation should be obtained to assist in choosing an antiepileptic medication as the initial, causative medication can not be used again.

ICD-9-CM 695.1

BIBLIOGRAPHY

Forman R, Koren G, Shear NH. Erythema multiforme, Stevens-Johnson, and toxic epidermal necrolysis in children: a review of 10 years' experience. *Drug Saf* 2002;25:965–972.

Fritsch PO, Sidoroff A. Drug-induced Stevens-Johnson syndrome/toxic epidermal necrolysis. *Am J Clin Dermatol* 2000;1:349–360.

Leaute-Labreze C, Lamireau T, Chawki D, Maleville J, Taieb A. Diagnosis, classification, and management of erythema multiforme and Stevens-Johnson syndrome. *Arch Dis Child* 2000;83:347–352.

Martinez AE, Atherton DJ. High-dose systemic corticosteroids can arrest recurrences of severe mucocutaneous erythema multiforme. *Pediatr Dermatol* 2000;17:87–90.

Metry DW, Jung P, Levy ML. Use of intravenous immunoglobulin in children with Stevens-Johnson syndrome and toxic epidermal necrolysis: seven cases and review of the literature. *Pediatrics* 2003;112:1430–1436.

Prendiville J. Stevens-Johnson syndrome and toxic epidermal necrolysis. *Adv Dermatol* 2002;16:151–173.

Roujeau JC, Kelly JP, Naldi L, et al. Medication use and the risk of Stevens-Johnson syndrome or toxic epidermal necrolysis. *N Engl J Med* 1995;333(24):1600–1607.

Roujeau JC, Stern RS. Medical progress: severe adverse cutaneous reactions to drugs. *N Engl J Med* 1994;331(19):1272–1285.

Rzany B, Correia O, Kelly JP, Naldi L, Auquier A, Stern R. Risk of Stevens-Johnson syndrome and toxic epidermal necrolysis during the first weeks of antiepileptic therapy: a case-control study. *Lancet* 1999;353:2190–1294.

Author: Paul S. Matz

Stomatitis

 Database

DEFINITION

- Stomatitis is inflammation of the mucous membranes of the mouth. There are multiple etiologies, with viral infections (e.g., herpes simplex virus, HSV, type 1) and recurrent aphthous stomatitis being the most common in children.
- Recurrent aphthous stomatitis, known more commonly as canker sores, does not have an identified infectious agent. These lesions are believed to be mediated by immunologic response to a variety of insults, including trauma, stress, hormonal fluctuations, infections, vitamin or nutritional deficiencies, and food allergies.
- Herpangina is a disease caused by coxsackievirus group A and marked by stomatitis consisting of 1- to 2-mm oral vesicles and ulcers, and systemic symptoms, most notably fever.

PATHOPHYSIOLOGY

- Infection, inflammation, or trauma leads to interruption of the integrity of the mucosal epithelium.
- Ongoing inflammation leads to further denudation of the epithelium.
- Inflammatory cells and mediators can produce exudates and erythema of the ulceration. The most common causes of this process are enteroviruses (such as coxsackievirus), HSV (particularly type 1), and recurrent aphthous ulcers (usually caused by microtrauma, stress, vitamin deficiencies and food allergies).

EPIDEMIOLOGY

- HSV type 1: up to 90% of the adult population has serologic evidence of previous infection.
- Enteroviral infections occur commonly in summer and fall months.

COMPLICATIONS

Infectious

- Cellulitis
- Lymphadenitis

Miscellaneous

- Dehydration
- Pain

PROGNOSIS

- Most cases of stomatitis are mild and resolve within 1 to 2 weeks.
- HSV stomatitis is most severe during the initial infection; however, it tends to recur in response to stress or trauma as the virus has a long latent period within the nerves of the face, particularly the trigeminal nerve.
- Recurrent aphthous stomatitis also recurs in response to stress or trauma.

 Differential Diagnosis

- Coxsackie viruses
- Herpes Simplex Virus (HSV)
- Varicella

—Smallpox (Variola)

- Trauma
- Medications (e.g., chemotherapeutic agents)
- Stevens-Johnson syndrome
- Candidal infections
- Lichen planus
- Reiter syndrome or disease (reactive arthritis, rash, conjunctivitis, urethritis, diarrhea, and stomatitis with painless erosive ulcers)
- Behçet syndrome (associated with ulcerations of the oral and genital mucous membranes)
- Crohn disease
- HIV-associated aphthous ulcers
- Cyclic neutropenia
- PFAPA syndrome: periodic fever, aphthous stomatitis, pharyngitis, and adenitis

 Data Gathering

HISTORY

Question: How old is the child?
Significance: Herpangina and herpetic gingivostomatitis occur in infants, toddlers, and preschool-aged children. Coxsackievirus (hand-foot-and-mouth disease) occurs most frequently in toddlers and young school-aged children. Aphthous stomatitis occurs in older children and adults.

Question: Are there any associated symptoms?
Significance: Fever, malaise, diarrhea, or other constitutional symptoms occur with coxsackievirus, herpangina, and primary herpetic gingivostomatitis.

Question: Does the child have chronic medical problems?
Significance: Immunodeficiency states (e.g., HIV and neutropenia), poor nutritional status, and inflammatory bowel disease are associated with development of mucosal ulceration.

Question: Does the child take any medications or have any possible exposures to medications?
Significance: Medications, particularly penicillins, sulfa-containing drugs, and antiepileptics, have been associated with Stevens-Johnson syndrome, which has oral mucositis as part of its constellation of symptoms.

Question: Does the child have other lesions on the body?
Significance: Varicella consists of lesions mainly on the trunk and extremities. Coxsackievirus when part of hand-foot-and-mouth disease consists of lesions in the mouth and the palms and soles. HSV can cause lesions on the lips.

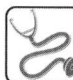 Physical Examination

- Enteroviral infections are associated with small shallow ulcerations with smooth borders on the posterior oral cavity structures such as the tonsils, soft palate, and pharynx. Also vesicular lesions may be present on the palms and soles.
- Herpes simplex infections are shallow ulcers with irregular, erythematous borders that coalesce; they are found on the lips, tongue, and gingiva.
- Varicella infections are shallow ulcers with erythematous borders that usually do not coalesce. Additionally, diffuse vesicles in varying stages of healing can be found on the skin, particularly the trunk and extremities. In severe cases there may be lesions in the oral cavity particularly on the soft palate.

—Smallpox may also present with small red spots on the tongue and in the oral mucosa following a prodromal period with fever. These then can become ulcerated. This is followed by the development of a diffuse erythematous rash that becomes papular over the entire body including the palms and soles. The rash becomes pustular then crusted.

- Stevens-Johnson syndrome presents with large irregular ulcers, which may occasionally be deep. There is occasionally a hemorrhagic component to these ulcers. Ulcers are also sometimes present on other mucosal surfaces. Target lesions, bullae, and urticarial lesions may also be present.
- Behçet syndrome and Reiter syndrome may have painless ulceration of the oral mucous membranes.
- Gingivitis in association with stomatitis is usually present in drug-induced causes of stomatitis, and with HSV.
- Herpetic whitlow is the transmission of herpes virus and development of lesions on the extremities, notably the fingers as a result of direct contact with lesions in the mouth.
- Herpangina consists of oral vesicles and ulcers typically around the fauces, near the tonsillar pillars.

Laboratory Aids

- Usually there is no need for laboratory testing for simple stomatitis. If there are other systemic signs of illness (e.g., diarrhea or arthritis), a more thorough workup for more severe illnesses such as Crohn disease, Reiter syndrome, or cyclic neutropenia should be done.
- HSV can be diagnosed with direct fluorescent antibody staining, rapid enzyme immunoassay, or viral culture of the lesion.
- Enteroviruses can be cultured from stool, nasopharyngeal, throat, CSF, and blood specimens. PCR of CSF fluid also can diagnose an enteroviral infection

Therapy

RINSES

- Salt water rinses (normal saline or 1 tsp of table salt mixed with 16 oz of tepid water or 1 tsp of baking soda with 32 oz of water) every 1 to 2 hours while ulcers are present may aid in reducing pain and shortening the duration of the ulceration.
- Magic mouthwash equal parts of diphenhydramine and Maalox or Kaopectate. In severe cases, 2% viscous lidocaine can be added in an equal amount, but care must be taken to limit the application of lidocaine on ulcerated mucosa, as it may be absorbed and possibly result in arrhythmias. Also, when applied to the posterior pharynx lidocaine can decrease the gag reflex, increasing the risk of aspiration.

ANALGESICS

- Viscous lidocaine 2% (see caution above)
- Acetaminophen or ibuprofen
- Acetaminophen with codeine may be used in severe cases, when intake of fluids is greatly affected by pain. Codeine should be used cautiously as it may cause constipation and central nervous system depression.
- Acyclovir can be given orally for herpes simplex infections to decrease the length of the infection, but to be effective needs to be given within the first 48 hours of development of oral lesions. Acyclovir usually is more beneficial when used for household contacts who begin to exhibit symptoms, and when treatment can be initiated early. Topical acyclovir has not been shown to be effective.

Follow-Up

In young children, the greatest risk is their inability to take in liquids adequately, leading to dehydration. They should be followed closely. If dehydration occurs as a result of poor oral intake, intravenous rehydration should be considered.

PREVENTION

- Hand washing can prevent spread of viral infections.
- As a result of the long life of enteroviruses on surfaces, toys and other objects used by affected children should be sterilized before being used by other children.
- Contact isolation should be observed for children with viral stomatitis in the hospital setting.

Common Questions and Answers

Q: Is stomatitis contagious?
A: Yes, this is a contagious infection. To avoid spreading the illness, careful hand washing should be done. In cases of suspected enteroviral infections, careful sterilization of toys and surfaces with which the affected child has contact should be done before use by unaffected children.

Q: How can I get my child to take food and liquids if stomatitis is painful?
A: The inability to stay hydrated is one of the complications of stomatitis. Children will not have their regular intake of solids as a result of mechanical effects of these on painful ulcers. Using regular analgesics, such as acetaminophen or ibuprofen, can help decrease pain. Topical administration of magic mouthwash (see above) before offering fluids may be helpful. Offering small amounts of nonacidic, cool liquids (and popsicles) frequently may be better tolerated than large amounts given all at once. If your child has decreased urine output or altered mental status, seek medical attention.

Q: When can my child return to school/day care?
A: Young children with herpes or enteroviral stomatitis can transmit these from oral secretions. In cases of young children who drool frequently, or place toys in their mouths, this is a high risk for transmitting the illness. Children become less contagious when the lesions heal. In the case of varicella, children are contagious until all vesicles are crusted over.

ICD-9-CM 528.0

BIBLIOGRAPHY

American Academy of Pediatrics. Summaries of infectious diseases. In: Pickering LK, ed. *2003 Red Book: Report of the Committee on Infectious Diseases.* 26th Ed. Elk Grove Village, IL American Academy of Pediatrics 2003:269–270, 344–353, 554–558, 672–686.

Feder HM. Periodic fever, aphthous stomatitis, pharyngitis, adenitis: a clinical review of a new syndrome. *Clin Opin Pediatr* 2000;12:233–236.

Pichichero ME, McLinn S, Rotbart HA, et al. Clinical and economic impact of enterovirus illness in private pediatric practice. *Pediatrics* 1998;102(5):1126–1134.

Scott DA, Coulter WA, Lamey P-J. Oral shedding of herpes simplex virus type 1: a review. *J Oral Pathol Med* 1997;26:441–447.

Scully C, Gorsky M, Lozada-Nur F. The diagnosis and management of recurrent aphthous stomatitis: a consensus approach. *J Am Dent Assoc* 2003;134(2):200–207.

Siegel MA. Strategies for management of commonly encountered oral mucosal disorders. *J Calif Dent Assoc* 1999;27(3):210–227.

Woo S-B, Sonis ST. Recurrent aphthous ulcers: a review of diagnosis and treatment. *J Am Dent Assoc* 1996;127:1202–1213.

Author: Lee R. Atkinson-McEvoy

Strabismus

Database

DEFINITION

From the Greek strabismus (to squint), strabismus is abnormal misalignment of the eyes. The misalignment can be constant or intermittent, and the eyes can be misaligned in any direction.

- When the deviation between the eyes is constant in all gaze positions, the deviation is comitant. Most childhood strabismus is comitant.
- Incomitant strabismus, with a variable angle depending on the direction of gaze, is seen with palsy of cranial nerves III, IV, or VI, and in some strabismus syndromes such as Duane and Brown syndromes and Graves' ophthalmopathy.
- The strabismus is identified by the relative direction of the eyes. Esotropia is an inward deviation or crossing; exotropia is an outward deviation; hypertropia and hypotropia are deviations up and down.

PATHOPHYSIOLOGY

- The pathophysiology of the most common forms of childhood strabismus is poorly understood.
- Infants with strabismus demonstrate subtle abnormalities in both motor function (asymmetrical smooth pursuit movements) and binocular sensory function (suppression, anomalous retinal correspondence).
- No neuroanatomic abnormalities have been consistently demonstrated in infants with idiopathic strabismus.
- Accommodative esotropia, a common strabismus syndrome, is caused by abnormalities in the reflexive convergence that is necessary for looking at near objects. If the ratio of accommodation (focusing for near) to convergence (rotating eyes inward to keep each eye on the target) is abnormally high, focusing on near targets leads to excessive convergence and esotropia.
- Less often, strabismus syndromes are caused by anatomic restriction to extraocular rotation (Graves disease, Brown syndrome), congenital or acquired paresis or palsy of extraocular muscles (III, IV, or VI palsy, Duane syndrome, Moebius syndrome) or abnormalities of vision (sensory strabismus).

PATHOLOGY

No specific pathological abnormality of the motor nerves, extraocular muscles or orbits is seen in most patients with idiopathic, comitant strabismus. Patients with paretic strabismus demonstrate atrophy of cranial nerves and extraocular muscles. Graves' disease, myasthenia, and other neuromotor diseases causing strabismus have specific pathological features in the extraocular muscles.

GENETICS

Genetic factors are clearly important in the development of many childhood strabismus patterns, with about 30% of strabismus patients having affected family members. The inheritance appears to be multigenic. No specific genes have been associated with idiopathic childhood strabismus syndromes, but genetic causes have been identified for some more rare strabismus syndromes including congenital fibrosis syndromes (chromosome 12p) and Kearn Sayer syndrome (mitochondrial deletion).

EPIDEMIOLOGY

- Strabismus of all types has an overall prevalence of 4% to 5%.
- Frequent coincident ophthalmic diagnoses are amblyopia (30% to 60%), nystagmus (8% to 10%) and refractive error (30% to 50%).
- Premature birth, cerebral palsy, seizure disorders, and developmental delays are frequently associated with strabismus, but most patients with idiopathic comitant strabismus are otherwise developmentally and neurologically normal.

COMPLICATIONS

- Amblyopia occurs in 30% to 60% of children with strabismus, and may require additional treatment. Amblyopia must be recognized and treated early in childhood, during the sensitive period of visual development, to restore normal vision
- Loss of binocularity (ability to use both eyes together, for example, depth perception) frequently occurs with strabismus in early childhood. Restoration of normal alignment is necessary for binocularity, and the best binocularity is associated with correction of strabismus in early childhood (before 2 years of age). In older children and adults, diplopia (double vision) may occur.
- The disfigurement of strabismus, with secondary psychological and social effects, may be a significant problem for children and adults with strabismus.

Differential Diagnosis

- The most common reason for mistaken referral of infants for esotropia is "pseudoesotropia," caused by wide epicanthal folds giving the false appearance of esotropia. This can be easily recognized by the normal corneal light reflex (Hirschberg test) and normal cover test.
- Sensory strabismus, as a result of reduced vision in one or both eyes, can be comitant or incomitant and can be caused by any ocular, optic nerve, or central cause of vision loss. Sensory deviations are most frequently exotropic, but may be in any direction.

- The differential diagnosis of abnormal eye movement in childhood includes palsy of cranial nerves III, IV, or VI, orbital fracture or craniofacial anomaly, systemic or localized motor abnormalities like myasthenia gravis, orbital fibrosis syndrome, infantile botulism, and idiopathic orbital pseudotumor.
- Special strabismus syndromes include Duane syndrome (congenital aberrant innervation of cranial nerve III), Moebius syndrome (congenital absence of cranial nerve VI and VII), Brown syndrome (congenital or acquired monocular elevation defect as a result of abnormality of the trochlea-superior oblique tendon complex), and thyroid ophthalmopathy (Graves' disease).

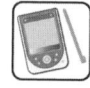

Data Gathering

HISTORY

- Age of onset of deviation
- Frequency, duration, and direction of deviation
- Subjective vision problems or complaints
- History of eye or head trauma, premature birth, seizure disorder, neurologic abnormality, or other motor problems
- Previous use of glasses, patching, or other therapy
- Family history of strabismus, amblyopia, refractive error, or childhood vision problems

Physical Examination

- Vision: patients capable of recognition are tested with charts (letters, pictures, Es), younger patients are tested by the ability to fixate and hold visual fixation on targets (toys, lights) in each eye. It is very important to test each eye separately, to detect possible amblyopia and other causes of monocular vision loss (see Amblyopia). Patients capable of reading charts should have complete ophthalmic examination if they cannot recognize at least the 20/40-size target with each eye, or if there is a difference of >1 chart line between eyes.
- Ocular alignment:
- Hirschberg test: with patient looking at a flashlight, observe the location of the reflection of the light on the corneal surface. Normally, the reflection should be centered in the pupil and symmetrical. In strabismus, the reflection will be displaced laterally (esotropia) or medially (exotropia) in one eye.
- Bruchner test: with a direct ophthalmoscope using the largest light, and the patient looking directly at the light, the light is shone into the patient's eyes. Normally, the pupils should be orange or red and the pupils should symmetrically fill with light. Asymmetrical brightness or color between the two eyes or shadows in the pupil of either eye is abnormal, and may indicate strabismus or other eye problems.

• Cover test (alternate cover test): with the patient holding the visual attention on a single target, the eyes are alternately occluded to force the patient to switch fixation between eyes. Normally, switching fixation should not cause the eyes to move. Movement of the eyes with alternate occlusion signifies strabismus, and merits complete evaluation.

• Ocular rotations: Comitant strabismus will demonstrate a consistent angle of deviation in all gaze directions. Incomitant strabismus, including cranial nerve palsies, thyroid ophthalmopathy, and Duane and Brown syndromes, will be greater in one direction and smaller or absent in others. Ductions (movements of each eye) may be restricted in certain directions with incomitant strabismus.

• Complete ophthalmic examination, including evaluation of vision, alignment, ocular anatomy, and cycloplegic refraction, is indicated whenever there is suggestion or suspicion of strabismus or abnormal vision based on history, screening tests, or examination.

 ## Laboratory Aids

TESTS

The diagnosis of strabismus is based on clinical examination, and no laboratory or radiological tests are routinely necessary. Depending on the clinical situation, imaging studies of the orbits and brain may be helpful in evaluating cranial nerve palsies, suspected traumatic strabismus, and strabismus associated with neurologic disease. Serologic testing for antiacetylcholine receptor antibodies is a specific test for myasthenia gravis, but may be negative in some cases.

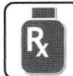 ## Therapy

• Prompt diagnosis and treatment are important for successful outcome from childhood strabismus. Depending on the diagnosis, treatment may include glasses, patching, orthoptic exercises, surgery, or a combination of these therapies.

• Glasses are useful, and may be curative, in certain forms of strabismus, especially accommodative esotropia. With accommodative esotropia, glasses reduce or eliminate esotropia by reducing the need to focus the eyes to overcome hyperopia.

• Occlusive therapeutic patching is used to treat amblyopia. In addition to the improved prognosis for long-term stability of surgical correction after amblyopia is treated, patching may sometimes improve alignment even without surgery. However, patching and other amblyopia treatments are usually only an adjunct to strabismus treatment.

• Surgery is frequently necessary to realign the eyes to treat strabismus. The ocular insertions of the extraocular muscles are shifted, either weakening or strengthening the muscle's effectiveness relative to the other muscles. In most patients, strabismus surgery can be performed in an ambulatory setting with minimal operative risk and postoperative morbidity. In large case series, approximately 20% of patients require more than one surgery for satisfactory alignment.

 ## Follow-Up

Recurrences of strabismus and amblyopia are common. Close monitoring of treatment, and frequent follow-up until visual maturity is achieved at 8 to 10 years of age is important as a result of the frequently unstable outcome of strabismus and amblyopia treatment. Most patients will benefit from reassessment each 6 to 12 months after treatment is complete, until age 10 years.

PITFALLS

• Strabismus is frequently recognized by parents and primary care practitioners, but amblyopia may be asymptomatic. Visual acuity testing with each eye separately, and long-term follow-up until patients reach the age of visual maturity (about 10 years) is important even after successful treatment.

• Patients rarely "grow out of" strabismus. Infants as young as 3 months can have careful eye movement and alignment examinations. Delayed diagnosis may worsen prognosis.

• Patients with intermittent strabismus may benefit from treatment, even if the deviation is not present constantly.

• Strabismus can be a sign of more significant ocular or neurologic abnormality. Retinoblastoma, retinal detachment, brain tumor, and other treatable conditions may initially present with ocular misalignment.

 ## Common Questions and Answers

Q. Does strabismus interfere with learning?
A. No. Patients with normal vision and childhood strabismus should not necessarily have difficulty learning. Learning problems should not be blamed solely on strabismus.

Q. Is "vision training therapy" an effective treatment for strabismus?
A. Eye exercises are rarely helpful in treating childhood strabismus. There is very little practical or scientific evidence that vision training therapy as commonly practiced has value in patients with comitant childhood strabismus, except for treatment of amblyopia with patching or penalization (see Amblyopia).

Q. Does early surgical correction of strabismus improve the long-term outcome?
A. Correction of esotropia prior to 2 years of age has been demonstrated to improve the chance of developing normal binocularity. However, not all patients develop binocularity even after early treatment. Many other factors influence the visual outcome in strabismus patients.

Q. Is correction of strabismus in older children and adults just cosmetic?
A. No. Older children and adults may have measurable visual improvement after treatment of strabismus, including expansion of visual fields and restoration of binocularity. Additionally, the psychological and social effects of disfiguring strabismus may justify corrective surgery even if no visual improvement is expected.

Q. In patients with accommodative esotropia treated with glasses, will the glasses be necessary for the rest of the patient's life?
A. Many patients wearing glasses for accommodative esotropia are able to stop wearing glasses later in childhood (12 to 14 years) without recurrence of esotropia.

BIBLIOGRAPHY

Engle EC. The genetics of strabismus: Duane, Moebius, and fibrosis syndromes. In Traboulsi EI, ed. *Genetic Diseases of the Eye.* New York: Oxford University Press, 1998.

Mills MD. Fundamental principles of strabismus surgery. In Albert DM, ed. *Ophthalmic Surgery: Principles and Techniques.* Malden, MA: Blackwell Science, Inc., 1999.

Mills MD. The eye in childhood. *Am Fam Phys* 1999;60:907–918.

Von Noorden GK. *Binocular Vision and Ocular Motility; Theory and Management of Strabismus.* 5th Ed. St. Louis: Mosby-Year Book, 1996.

Wright KW, ed. *Pediatric Ophthalmology and Strabismus.* St. Louis: Mosby-Year Book, 1995.

Author: Monte D. Mills

Strep Infection—Invasive Group A β-Hemolytic Streptococcus

 Database

DEFINITION

Infection associated with isolation of group A β-hemolytic streptococci (GABHS) from a normally sterile body site.

Syndromes

• Deep and systemic infections (e.g., bacteremia, meningitis, pneumonia, osteomyelitis, septic arthritis, surgical wound infection)
• Necrotizing fasciitis (NF)
• Streptococcal toxic shock syndrome (STSS)

Case Definition for STSS

• I. Isolation of GABHS

—A. From a normally sterile site (e.g., blood, CSF, tissue, peritoneal fluid)
—B. From a nonsterile site (e.g., throat, vagina, sputum)

• II. Clinical signs of severity

—A. Hypotension
—B. ≥2 of the following signs:

—Renal impairment
—Coagulopathy
—Hepatic involvement
—Adult respiratory distress syndrome
—A generalized erythematous macular rash that may desquamate
—Soft tissue necrosis, including NF or myositis, or gangrene

• Definite case: an illness fulfilling criteria IA and II (A and B)
• Probable case: an illness fulfilling criteria IB and II (A and B) and no other identifiable cause

CAUSES

Streptococcus pyogenes is the only species within this group of β-hemolytic streptococci. The M1 and M3 strains predominate in cases of severe GABHS infections.

PATHOPHYSIOLOGY

• The pathogenic mechanism has not been fully elucidated; however, an association with streptococcal pyrogenic exotoxin (SPE) has been suggested. These toxins, especially SPE A, B, and C, and mitogens and superantigens stimulate large numbers of T cells to release a variety of cytokines.
• Portal of entry may be inapparent or unimpressive.
• Shock and multiorgan system failure may ensue.
• In NF, an area of cellulitis develops initially followed by bullous skin changes and the rapid progression of subcutaneous tissue necrosis involving fat and fascia. Skeletal muscle is rarely involved.

EPIDEMIOLOGY

• In children, the most common antecedent is varicella.
• Since the mid-1980s there has been a notable increase in the incidence, morbidity, and mortality.
• The CDC has estimated that the annual incidence in the United States is 3.5 cases per 100,000 persons, approximately 8,500 cases per year.
• Several reports have suggested an association between the use of nonsteroidal antiinflammatory drugs and invasive GABHS infection. There are no data to support a causal link.
• Other high-risk groups include patients with diabetes mellitus, chronic cardiac or pulmonary disease, HIV infection or AIDS, and intravenous drug use.
• The rate of STSS and fatal cases of invasive GABHS appears to be lower in children as compared with adults.

COMPLICATIONS

FROM DEEP AND SYSTEMIC INFECTIONS

• Sepsis syndrome
• Hematologic seeding and development of focal infection
• Complications associated with specific site of involvement (e.g., meningitis—neurologic impairment, septic arthritis—joint destruction)

From NF

• Severe tissue necrosis usually requires extensive surgical débridement and often results in amputation of involved extremities.
• Compartment syndrome
• Functional disabilities
• Cosmetic sequelae

From STSS

• Multiorgan system failure from systemic hypotension and direct effects of inflammatory mediators:
• Adult respiratory distress syndrome
• Disseminated intravascular coagulopathy (DIC)
• Acute tubular necrosis resulting in renal failure
• Hepatic failure
• Cardiac insufficiency
• Cerebral ischemia and edema
• Metabolic derangements

PROGNOSIS

• Fulminant course with rapid deterioration is characteristic of invasive GABHS infections.
• Improved prognosis with early recognition and aggressive management.
• Case-fatality rate in pediatric series approximately 5% to 10%.

 Differential Diagnosis

INFECTION

• Bacterial sepsis
• Staphylococcal toxic shock syndrome
• Other soft tissue infections: cellulitis, erysipelas, clostridial or mixed anaerobic and aerobic fasciitis/gangrene

 Data Gathering

HISTORY

Historical features vary depending on the GABHS syndrome

• Consider GABHS infection in any child with varicella who has any of the following:

—Return of fever after defervescence
—A temperature of ≥39°C beyond the third day of illness
—A fever persisting beyond the fourth day of illness

• In children without varicella, presentation can be nonspecific with fever, chills, myalgias, malaise, pain, macular erythematous rash.
• Severe pain and hyperesthesia out of proportion to the clinical findings
• Portal of entry is unknown in 25% to 50% of cases.
• A preceding clinical pharyngitis is not common.

 Physical Examination

• Vital signs: elevated temperature, tachycardia early, hypotension is a later sign
• Toxic appearance is common but not the rule, especially early in the disease course.
• Skin exam varies. In many instances there are no cutaneous findings or, in cases of varicella, the lesions may not appear superinfected. Alternatively, there may be an initial erythematous cellulitic area that rapidly progresses to a violaceous color with bullous formation.
• A generalized macular erythematous rash is sometimes observed with STSS.
• Deep infections will have physical examination findings consistent with the specific focus (e.g., joint pain and limitation of mobility in septic arthritis, respiratory symptoms in GABHS pneumonia)

Strep Infection—Invasive Group A β-Hemolytic Streptococcus

Laboratory Aids

TESTS

- CBC, electrolytes, BUN, CR, glucose, LFTs, DIC screen

—CK may be helpful in differentiating NF from cellulitis.

- WBC not elevated in all pediatric case series
- Blood culture positive for *S. pyogenes* in >50%
- Culture of wound and tissue aspirates
- Throat culture positive in 50%

IMAGING

MRI to define the extent of involvement in NF

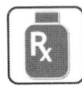

Therapy

SUPPORTIVE CARE

- Volume resuscitation
- Replete electrolytes as indicated
- Blood products as indicated for anemia or thrombocytopenia
- Airway support for severe depression of level of consciousness or respiratory insufficiency

DRUGS

- Intravenous antibiotic therapy covering for both GABHS and *Staphylococcus aureus* should be instituted promptly. Oxacillin (150 mg/kg per day divided q6) or nafcillin (200 mg/kg per day divided q4 to 6h, max 12 g daily) plus clindamycin (25 to 40 mg/kg per day divided q6 or q8). In penicillin allergic patients, consider vancomycin (40 mg/kg per day divided q6) plus clindamycin.
- Following the identification of GABHS from blood, body fluid, or tissue specimens, the drugs of choice are high-dose penicillin G (200,000 to 400,000 U/kg per day in four to six divided doses) plus clindamycin.
- There have been no penicillin G-resistant isolates of GABHS reported. There are strains resistant to clindamycin, so this drug should not be used alone until it is shown to be sensitive.
- Large numbers of GABHS organisms can overcome the efficacy of penicillin. The synergistic use of clindamycin should be considered in cases of NF and STTS.
- Inotropes should be administered as indicated.
- There are a few case reports suggesting that the use of intravenous immunoglobulin may be beneficial in patients with STSS. Various regimens have been used: 150 to 400 mg/kg per day for 5 days; 1 to 2 g/kg as single dose

At this time, the optimal regimen is unknown

SURGICAL TREATMENT IN NF

- Consider surgical consult early in management of NF
- Fasciotomy to relieve compartment syndrome
- Extensive débridement of necrotic tissue is often indicated.

PREVENTION

Routine immunization against varicella

ISOLATION OF HOSPITALIZED PATIENTS

In addition to standard precautions, droplet precautions are recommended for children with pneumonia, and contact precautions should be used for children with extensive or draining cutaneous infections for at least 24 hours after the start of antimicrobial therapy.

PITFALLS

- Not considering the diagnosis until hemodynamic instability is apparent
- Do not exclude diagnosis even in the absence of rash, cellulitis, or superinfected varicella lesions. Rash is only one of six clinical signs of severity in the criteria for STSS.
- Recognize that the involvement of subcutaneous structures in NF may be much more extensive than what might be suggested on physical examination.
- Failing to search for a localized infection as a source of toxin in STTS

Common Questions and Answers

Q: For whom should the diagnosis of invasive GABHS be entertained?
A: Consider GABHS in any child with varicella who experiences recrudescence of fever, fever $\geq 39°C$ beyond the third day of illness, or any fever beyond the fourth day of illness. A high index of suspicion should be maintained in patients with septicemia, and in febrile patients with pain and hyperesthesia out of proportion to the clinical findings.

Q: Should the use of nonsteroidal antiinflammatory drugs (NSAIDs) be restricted in patients with varicella?
A: There are several reports suggesting an association between the use of NSAIDs and the development of invasive GAS diseases, however, there has been no study to establish a causal relationship. It has been demonstrated that NSAIDs inhibit immune-mediated defense mechanisms, enhance the production of cytokines, and suppress the pain and fever that might encourage a patient with invasive GABHS infection to seek medical attention sooner. No formal recommendations for restricting the use of NSAIDs are being made at this time.

Q: Should close contacts of patients with invasive GABHS infections receive chemoprophylaxis?

A: Chemoprophylaxis of household contacts of people with invasive GAS remains controversial. Although the risk of developing disease for household contacts is elevated in comparison to the risk of sporadic disease development, the overall frequency of invasive GAS disease remains small. Testing for GAS colonization and chemoprophylaxis of household contacts of people with invasive GAS is not routinely recommended. However, in high risk populations (people over 65 years old, HIV infection, chickenpox, diabetes mellitus), targeted chemoprophylaxis may be considered. Chemoprophylaxis is not recommended in schools or child care facilities.

ICD-9-CM

Streptococcal infection 034.0
Necrotising fasciitis 728.86

BIBLIOGRAPHY

American Academy of Pediatrics. Group A streptococcal infections. *Red Book: Report of the Committee on Infectious Diseases.* 26th Ed. Washington, DC: American Academy of Pediatrics, 2003.

Aronoff DM, Bloch KC. Assessing the relationship between the use of nonsteroidal anti-inflammatory drugs and necrotizing fasciitis caused by group a streptococcus. *Medicine* 2003;82:225–235.

Herbst R. Perineal streptococcal dermatitis/disease: recognition and management. *Am J Clin Dermatol* 2003;4(8):555–560.

Hoffman JA, Mason EO, Schutze GE, et al. Streptococcus pneumoniae infections in the neonate. *Pediatrics* 2003;112(5):1095–1102.

Ibia EO, Imoisili M, Pikis A. Group A beta-hemolytic streptococcal osteomyelitis in children. *Pediatrics* 2003;112(1 Pt 1):e22–e6.

Kaul R, McGeer A, Norrby-Teglund A, et al. Intravenous immunoglobulin therapy for streptococcal toxic shock syndrome—a comparative observational study. The Canadian Streptococcal Study Group. *Clin Infect Dis* 1999;28(4):800–807.

Laupland KB, Davies HD, Low DE, et al. Invasive group A streptococcal disease in children and association with varicella-zoster virus infection. *Pediatrics* 2000;105(5):E60.

Lesko SM, O'Brien KL, Schwartz B, Vezina R, Mitchell AA. Invasive group a streptococcal infection and nonsteriodal anti-inflammatory drug use among children with primary varicella. *Pediatrics* 2001;107:1108–1115.

Reich HL, Crawford GH, Pelle MT, James WD. Group B streptococcal toxic shock-like syndrome. *Arch Dermatol* 2004;140(2):163–166.

Robinson KA, Rothrock G, Phan Q, et al. Risk for severe group A streptococcal disease among patients' household contacts. *Emerg Infect Dis* 2003;9:443–447.

Author: Jill C. Posner

Stroke

 Database

DEFINITION

Stroke is a neurologic deficit progressing over minutes to hours as a result of insufficient perfusion of the brain or spinal cord.

PATHOPHYSIOLOGY

Abnormalities of the blood, vasculature, or the heart (dysrhythmia or anatomic) lead to embolism or intravascular thrombosis.

PATHOLOGY

Edema, neuronal swelling, cellular infiltrate, and cavitation evolving from the first minutes through several months after an ischemic brain injury

GENETICS

Various hereditary and metabolic disorders: neurocutaneous diseases, Down syndrome, collagen disorders, congenital heart disease syndromes, coagulation disorders, hereditary cavernoma or telangiectasia, hyperhomocysteinemia, and others.

EPIDEMIOLOGY

Overall incidence is approximately 2.5 per 100,000, but certain groups are at higher risk (heart disease, sickle cell disease, hereditary thrombophilias).

COMPLICATIONS

- Seizures
- Respiratory insufficiency
- Intracranial hypertension
- Motor, visual, and cognitive deficits
- Autonomic disturbances
- Infection susceptibility

 Differential Diagnosis

- Several disorders may mimic the presentation of stroke:

—Migraine
—Demyelinating disease
—Focal encephalitis
—Postepileptic paralysis (Todd paresis)
—Conversion disorder
—Rarely intracranial neoplasm, abscess, subdural empyema, or mitochondrial disease may present as stroke.

- Underlying causes of stroke include hematologic, circulatory, and cardiac disorders:

—Hematologic: factor V mutation, prothrombin gene mutation, lupus anticoagulant, anticardiolipin/antiphospholipid syndrome, sickle cell, hyperhomocysteinemia, dyslipidemia, proteins S or C, antithrombin III deficiency, asparaginase treatment, hyperviscosity syndromes (including leukemia), thrombocythemia, extreme dehydration, iron deficiency.
—Vascular: carotid or vertebral dissection, intracranial AVM, carotid trauma, moyamoya, cavernous angioma ("occult cerebrovascular malformations"), vasculitis (especially as a result of bacterial meningitis); rarely, aneurysm, Takayasu arteritis, chronic meningitides (tuberculosis, Lyme, or sarcoidosis)
—Cardiac: especially rheumatic heart disease, cyanotic congenital heart disease, or heart failure as a result of acquired or cardiomyopathy, or perioperatively; possible association with mitral prolapse, atrial septal defects; rarely, atrial myxoma, aortic dilatation (Marfan), pulmonary AVM

 Data Gathering

HISTORY

- Occurrence of stroke in specific settings may point to the diagnosis; previous migraines may point to complicated migraine (rare); ask about substance use, prior trauma, infection, excessive bleeding or spontaneous clotting, or history of heart disease.
- Family history of premature thrombosis, hemoglobinopathy, or vascular malformations (e.g., cavernous hemangioma or hereditary hemorrhagic telangiectasia).
- Perinatal stroke may be related to a prepartum, peripartum, or postpartum cerebrovascular event and frequently presents with neonatal seizures. May be associated with multiple gestation.
- Complications of labor or fetal exposure to vasoactive compounds may sometimes be associated.

 Physical Examination

- Note level of alertness and capacity for sustained attention; fluency and appropriateness, and construction of speech; comprehension. Emotional state, subjective or objective pain.
- Vital signs, color, and respiratory pattern may disclose existing or impending respiratory failure as a result of loss of protective airway reflexes.
- General examination should include peripheral pulses and perfusion; palpation and auscultation of the precordium and cervical area may reveal evidence of dysrhythmia or anatomic lesions.
- Other neurologic findings important to note include confrontation visual fields, funduscopy (especially for papilledema), eye movements, facial symmetry, pattern of most severely affected limbs, and extensor response of great toe to plantar stimulation (Babinski sign).
- In the absence of sensory complaints, detailed sensory examination is often fruitless.

Laboratory Aids

TESTS

Laboratory Tests

- Blood chemistry, particularly glucose, should be tested; mild hyperglycemia may reflect stress response; marked elevation (e.g., in diabetics) should be treated, because hyperglycemia may aggravate ischemic brain injury.
- Toxin screen.
- Complete blood count and PT/PTT may prompt important therapeutic decisions.
- Consider lumbar puncture (if neuroradiologic findings show no risk of incipient herniation) to look for evidence of inflammatory/infectious basis.

IMAGING

- Individuals with stable vital signs and suspected stroke should undergo a brain imaging study promptly. Noncontrasted images are important to look for possible hemorrhage and may be followed by contrasted images for possible focal encephalitis, or to identify underlying vascular lesions.
- Many diagnostic questions can be resolved equally well by CT or MRI, although CT may be preferable in suspected subarachnoid hemorrhage; MRI is much more sensitive in the first 24 hours after symptom onset, and may identify venous or sinus thrombosis, or smaller bilateral lesions pointing to systemic embolization.

OTHER TESTS

More extensive testing in undiagnosed cases may include:

- Tests for specific coagulopathies (see Differential Diagnosis, above)
- Varicella serology (may be a common cause of stroke in children)
- Toxin screen (association with cocaine)
- Amino acid screening (for homocysteine)
- Hemoglobin electrophoresis (sickle hemoglobin)
- Lipid profile (hypercholesterolemia)
- Echocardiography (ASD, luminal lesion)
- Carotid Doppler (stenosis/dissection)
- Specialized neuroradiologic studies (MR angiogram, standard angiography)

Emergency Care

- Airway compromise as a result of impaired protective reflexes
- Stroke may present as new onset seizures—follow protocol for emergent treatment of seizures
- Urgent neurosurgical evaluation indicated in cases of large cerebral hemispheric strokes, intracranial hemorrhage, or posterior fossa ischemic stroke (see below)

- Empiric antibiotics indicated in the setting of stroke and fever (abscess, septic emboli, empyema)

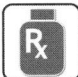

Therapy

- Hospitalization: Patients with radiologically documented or clinically suspected stroke who have stable airway, breathing, and circulation are most often hospitalized for observation and supportive therapy. Those with a diminished or fluctuating level of alertness or with radiographically extensive area(s) of infarction are often monitored in an intensive care unit for changes in respiratory status or signs of increased intracranial pressure.
- Strokes involving the posterior fossa or cerebellum, or affecting a large area of the cerebrum, are of particular concern because of the risk of tentorial or subfalcine herniation; a neurosurgical consult should be obtained for these cases and for those with intracranial hemorrhage above or below the tentorium.
- Consultation with neurology, neurosurgery, cardiology, hematology, or other pediatric subspecialists is often helpful.
- Drugs: In most cases, there is no contraindication to pharmacotherapy appropriate to any identified underlying condition; the decision to use antiplatelet or thrombolytic, therapy or anticoagulation is complex and depends on risk of hemorrhage, experience of the clinician, and potential side effects.
- Rehabilitation and physical therapy may improve outcome and should be instituted as soon as the patient's condition permits.
- Investigational therapies include hypervolemic hemodilution, thrombolytic agents, calcium channel antagonists, and neuroprotective agents such as glutamate receptor antagonists.

Follow-Up

- The usual course in stroke of any cause is for gradual improvement after the acute onset of symptoms. Significant recovery of neurologic function may continue as long as months after the ictus, especially in infants and toddlers.
- Involvement of child developmentalists and/or ophthalmologists in follow-up depends on the etiology and residual deficits of the stroke.
- Remote sequelae that may not be evident for months or years after stroke include epilepsy, hydrocephalus, learning difficulties, short attention span, posture disturbances (especially cerebral palsy), sphincter disturbances, pressure sores, and susceptibility to infection if airway protective reflexes are impaired.

PITFALLS

- Arteriovenous malformations may not be seen on angiography immediately after a primary intracerebral hemorrhage. Some clinicians repeat angiography several weeks or months later.

- CT may be normal in the first 24 hours after nonhemorrhagic stroke. A follow-up study may be necessary.
- Transient ischemic attack (TIA) should prompt a vigorous diagnostic evaluation.

Common Questions and Answers

Q: Will my child have another stroke?
A: The chance of recurrence depends on remediation of the underlying cause. Available evidence suggests that children with no identifiable underlying basis for stroke have a very low recurrence risk.

Q: Aren't there any medicines for acute stroke?
A: Tissue plasminogen activator (TPA) appears to be useful in some cases of adult nonhemorrhagic stroke, but its usefulness in childhood stroke has not been studied.

ICD-9-CM 436

BIBLIOGRAPHY

Ganesan V, Chong WK, Cox TC, Chawda SJ, Prengler M, Kirkham FJ. Posterior circulation stroke in childhood: risk factors and recurrence. *Neurology* 2002;59:1552–1556.

Gunther G, Junker R, Strater R, et al. Symptomatic ischemic stroke in full-term neonates: role of acquired and genetic prothrombotic risk factors. *Stroke* 2000;31:2437–2441.

Hogeveen M, Blom HJ, Van Amerongen M, Boogmans B, Van Beynum IM, Van De Bor M. Hyperhomocysteinemia as risk factor for ischemic and hemorrhagic stroke in newborn infants. *J Pediatr* 2002;141:429–431.

Mercuri E, Barnett A, Rutherford M, Guzzetta A, Haataja L, Cioni G, Cowan F, Dubowitz L. Neonatal cerebral infarction and neuromotor outcome at school age. *Pediatrics* 2004;113:95–100.

Rivkin MJ, Volpe JJ. Strokes in children. *Pediatr Rev* 1996;17(8):265–278.

Yamamoto LG, Yim GK, Bart RD Jr. Emergency department presentations of cerebrovascular disease in children. *Am J Emerg Med* 1999;17:163–171.

Author: Peter M. Bingham

Stuttering

Database

DEFINITION

Stuttering is an involuntary disturbance in the normal fluency and timing of speech that is not appropriate for the age of the speaker. Various patterns are seen:

- Prolongation of sounds or syllables
- Repetition of sounds or syllables or even whole words
- Pauses in the middle of words
- Blocking—either silence or pauses filled with nonsense sounds in middle of words, as if considering what to say next
- Avoidance—word substitutions that are used to skip known problem words; also called circumlocution
- Overemphasis of some syllables or words; also called tension.

Although almost everyone will stutter in a high-tension situation, stuttering is significant when it interferes with the patient's life in academic, occupational, or social arenas. Many children with developmental delays have dysfluencies of speech, but it is not considered stuttering unless it is present more frequently than expected for that level of disability.

ETIOLOGY

- The specific etiology of stuttering is not known, but many factors contribute to stuttering. Stuttering may be more pronounced when a child is fatigued, excited, upset, rushed or exposed to some other stressor (e.g., a move to a new school).
- Environmental factors are thought to have a role in stuttering. Children adopted by a parent who stutters are more likely to stutter than children adopted by a nonstutterer.

PATHOPHYSIOLOGY

Stuttering appears to related to an excessive amount of dopamine in the brain:

- Patients with Parkinson disease often develop adult onset stuttering.
- PET (positron-emission tomography) scans show increased dopamine in the brain of those who stutter.
- Medications that increase brain dopamine (antidepressants), or are dopaminergic (major tranquilizers), can induce stuttering in nonstutterers, although medications that lower dopamine (e.g., clomipramine) may stop stuttering.
- Hundreds of articles have shown many differences between the brains of stutterers and nonstutterers in glucose uptake, dopamine release, and metabolic activity of the basal ganglia, but no one unified physiologic process is well defined to be the cause of stuttering.

GENETICS

Stuttering does cluster in families:

- Monozygotic twins have a higher concordance for stuttering than dizygotic twins
- The more closely related one is to a stutterer, the more likely one is to stutter
- Identical twins have a concordance for stuttering of at least 30%.

EPIDEMIOLOGY

- One percent of all studied populations affected
- Males stutter three times as often as females
- Stuttering is found in every culture and language. The specific language spoken does not increase or decrease the amount of stuttering.
- Stuttering begins between 2 and 7 years of age with 98% of cases presenting by age 10.
- Girls start stuttering several months earlier on average than boys; but they also speak, in general, earlier than boys do.

COMPLICATIONS

- Anxiety and depression, often far out of proportion to the degree of disfluency
- Blocking and hesitation giving an impression of delayed intellectual development
- Voluntary withdrawal from social interaction to avoid embarrassment

ASSOCIATED FINDINGS

- Other language problems: in a recent, large Australian study, 62.8% of 2,628 children who stuttered had other language problems. Boys had these additional problems much more than girls. Of the additional problems, 33% were articulation disorders and 13% phonological disorders. Other frequent problems included learning disabilities, dyslexia and attention-deficit hyperactivity disorder.
- Students with developmental delay or intellectual impairment are found to stutter up to 25% of the time.

PROGNOSIS

- Up to 80% of stutterers spontaneously regress by age 16
- Severity of stuttering does not relate to persistence of stuttering
- The longer stuttering exists, the more likely it will persist

Differential Diagnosis

DEVELOPMENTAL

- Normal development—dysfluencies associated with rapid onset of full speech capabilities that will usually resolve very quickly.
- Cluttering—patients with extremely rapid speech will have dysfluencies that resolve with slowing down of speech.
- Pervasive Developmental Disorder (Autistic Spectrum)—will also have echolalia, tonelessness, and poor eye contact.

NEUROLOGIC

- Tics/Tourettes Syndrome—similar time of onset, initially somewhat similar symptoms. Stuttering is usually not associated with simultaneous physical movement.
- Trauma, tumor, or major central nervous system disease, such as Parkinson Disease, may cause late-onset stuttering.

MEDICATIONS

- Any medication that increases the presence of dopamine may worsen (or cause) stuttering. Examples are SSRI-type antidepressants or major tranquilizers.

Data Gathering

HISTORY

- Is there a family history of stuttering? Stuttering runs in families both by nature and nurture.
- What is age of onset and length of persistence of the problem? Onset is insidious with the child often unaware of the problem. If stuttering starts after the tenth birthday, suspicion of an intracranial mass or brain ischemia should be entertained.
- Does stuttering improve with singing, acting, and in one-to-one situations with family members? Physiologic stuttering is rarely present during oral reading (especially on the second attempt to do the task), singing, acting, and reciting in rhythm. People do not usually stutter while talking to pets or inanimate objects.
- Is the child taking any medications? Especially medications that increase dopamine.
- Has the child had any head trauma? Increased intracranial pressure may lead to stuttering.

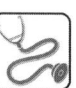
Physical Examination

Although there are no specific physical examination findings of stuttering, some observations of children improve the ability to make this diagnosis.
Stutterers often improve in one-to-one situations with familiar people, so ask the parents to bring in a video recording of the child when talking in public, singing, and talking to a pet or infant.
Observations that may be made in the office that correlate strongly with the diagnosis of stuttering include:

- Multiple repetitions and/or prolongations
- Rising pitch with difficult words
- Grimacing or other physical tension, such as taking deep breaths or jerking the head back when speaking
- Inappropriate emphasis of words not normally emphasized, extremely slow speech, or speech without tone

- Although unwillingness to speak to the examiner is normal, unwillingness to speak to the parent is not

Laboratory Aids

- None currently available, but PET scan may be a useful modality in the future.
- If stuttering begins after the age of 10, or if the patient has additional neurological or developmental problems, a work-up for brain abnormalities should be considered.

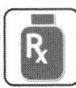

Therapy

Because of the complicated social and psychological sequelae of stuttering, any therapy must work on both improving the child's fluency and on increasing acceptance and tolerance of this problem by the patient and his or her family. In a multicultural learning atmosphere, sensitivity to the learning styles of each social group is paramount in achieving successful results.

SUGGESTIONS FOR PARENTS/FAMILIES

It is important to note that the following suggestions, although very helpful to parents, should be recommended in conjunction with, but not in place of, speech therapy. Parents, lacking the expertise and objectivity of speech therapists, may be too critical of their own children.

- Take time out of each day to speak with the child one-on-one
- Model slow speech.
- Wait for the child to speak. Take turns speaking
- Allow for transition time between activities and tasks.
- Keep a notebook of things that help make speech better and things that elicit stuttering

SPEECH THERAPY

- Stuttering in young children can be resolved with very short courses of therapy, often 3 months or less. Stuttering remains resolved in at least 95% of these early treatment cases. The younger the patient is at the time of referral to speech therapy, the shorter the course of therapy needed, and the more likely that the therapy will be successful.
- Many experts in dysfluency believe that early intervention is more likely to be successful than waiting to start therapy if the stuttering has not spontaneously resolved by the seventh birthday.
- Assessing the success of a program to treat pathology that spontaneously resolves on its own may be problematic, but one of the more successful new programs for young children who stutter is called, the Lidcombe Program of Early Stuttering Intervention. In this intense Australian-developed behavioral therapy program, the belief is that initially stuttering

is physical in nature. Briefly, the program aims to teach the parents and other child caretakers how to praise their children for speaking fluently, and how to correct them occasionally when they do stutter. The parents are trained to measure the frequency of stuttering and carry out the therapy between clinic visits, and they are monitored and supported throughout the whole process by the clinician. Such is the flexibility of the program that the needs and circumstances of each particular family are catered to, and it is unlikely that any two families will carry it out in exactly the same way. The therapy attempts to be fun for the child and ultimately enables the child to speak fluently and to monitor his/her own speech.

OTHER THERAPIES

- A successful new therapy for adolescents and adults is a hearing-aid type device (SpeechEasy) that feeds the individual's speech directly back into an earpiece. Whether this works because patients do not stutter in chorale speech, or it simply reinforces the correct speech, is not known.
- Other devices that make hearing monaural or provide a white noise background in the ear also improve stuttering. The theoretical basis of all these therapies is not clear

ALTERNATIVE THERAPY

- No medications are known to safely reduce stuttering, but acupuncture, hypnosis, and yoga have been used with some success, but not in controlled studies
- Information for families is available through organizations, such as the Stuttering Foundation of America, a nonprofit organization.(www.stutteringhelp.org)

Follow-Up

- If stuttering is reported by the parents in a preschool-aged child, follow up in 1 to 2 months to see if it was only a transitory dysfluency that has resolved. If not, obtain a speech therapy consult for evaluation.

PREVENTION

- There is no known prevention strategy for stuttering

PITFALLS

- Since stuttering waxes and wanes with time, temporary improvement does not equal cure.
- Any behavioral therapy (such as the Lidcombe therapy described above) must be done under the guidance of a well-trained professional because inappropriate criticism may worsen stuttering.
- Waiting to see if stuttering goes away by age 7 is not the best strategy for young children, as was often taught in the past.

Common Questions and Answers

Q. Are some children more prone to stuttering?
A. Yes, "sensitive" children (many different definitions in many different studies) are more likely to stutter, as are the children of highly critical parents.

Q. Should family and friends complete the sentences of children who stutter?
A. No, children who cannot complete a thought should be gently asked to slow down and try again with no time limit set; or, others should simple wait until the child has completed his or her sentence. Children with a stuttering problem should also be praised when they do not stutter.

Q. Do abused children have a high incidence of stuttering?
A. Yes, as previously mentioned, stressful events and environments, such as those experienced by abused children, may elicit and reinforce stuttering.

ICD-9-CM 307.0

BIBLIOGRAPHY

Battle DE. *Communication Disorders in Multicultural Populations.* 3rd Ed. Boston: Butterworth Heinemann, 2002.

Craig A, Hancock K, Tran Y, Craig M, Peters K. Epidemiology of stuttering in the community across the entire life span. *J Speech Lang Hear Res* 2002;45:1097–1105.

Emerick LL, Haynes WO. *Diagnosis and Evaluation in Speech Pathology.* 3rd Ed. Englewood Cliffs, NJ: Prentice-Hall Inc., 1986.

First MB, ed. *Diagnostic and Statistical Manual (DSM-IV-TR).* Washington, DC: American Psychiatric Association, 2000.

Gordon N. Stuttering: incidence and causes. *Dev Med Child Neurol* 2002;44(4):278–281.

Harris V, Onslow M, Packman A, Harrison E, Menzies R. An experimental investigation of the impact of the Lidcombe Program on early stuttering. *J Fluency Disord* 2002;27:203–213; quiz 213–214.

Keating D, Turrell G, Ozanne A. Childhood speech disorders: reported prevalence, comorbidity and socioeconomic profile. *J Paediatr Child Health* 2001;37:431–436.

Rosenfield DB, Viswanath NS. Neuroscience of stuttering. *Science* 2002;295:973.

Stuttering Foundation of America. Videotape: Stuttering and the preschool child. Help for families #70. Memphis, TN: Stuttering Foundation of America, 2000.

Yaruss JS. One size does not fit all: special topics in stuttering therapies. *Semin Speech Lang.* 2003;24:3–6.

Author: Gary A. Emmett

Subdural Hematoma

 Database

DEFINITION

A subdural hematoma (SDH) is a collection of blood between outer pial and inner dural meningeal layers. The bleeding is usually venous in origin, although either cortical arteries or bridging veins may be torn.

PATHOPHYSIOLOGY

- SDHs may be acute or chronic. Arterial SDHs present quickly, whereas venous SDHs may accumulate slowly, remaining undetected for weeks or months. Acute SDHs contain blood, whereas chronic SDHs contain proteinaceous exudate and blood-breakdown products. Rebleeding may be the underlying cause of many chronic SDHs.
- Significant force is usually required for SDH unless there are predisposing circumstances; SDH is only rarely as a result of trivial or minor trauma. However, SDH can occur with relatively minor trauma in individuals with bleeding disorders, children on chronic dialysis, and those with enlarged extracerebral spaces (cortical atrophy).
- Some metabolic disorders, such as glutaric aciduria type I, can be associated with both acute and chronic SDHs.
- SDHs in nonaccidental trauma may be a result of the striking of the infant's head against a surface (like a mattress). The sudden deceleration associated with the impact may tear bridging veins traveling in the subdural space. The term shaking-impact syndrome may be more accurate than shaken-baby syndrome.
- SDHs can also occur after ventricular shunting.

GENETICS

There is no clear genetic predisposition, except when hereditary coagulopathy or metabolic disease is implicated.

EPIDEMIOLOGY

- SDHs occur in all age groups. Neonatal SDHs occur with spontaneous vaginal deliveries, but may be more frequent following deliveries with forceps or vacuum extraction. SDHs related to birth usually resolve.
- SDHs in infants and young children are frequently the result of nonaccidental trauma. Risk factors for nonaccidental trauma include disability or prematurity of the child, unstable family situations, parents of young age, and low socioeconomic status. One study found that fathers were the most frequent perpetrators, followed by boyfriends, female baby-sitters, and mothers, in descending order of frequency.
- SDHs in older children are often the result of motor vehicle accidents, and may be associated with other intracranial injuries, such as diffuse axonal injury.

COMPLICATIONS

- Traumatic SDHs are often associated with cerebral contusions. Other associated injuries include skull fractures, diffuse axonal injury, and penetrating injuries.
- SDHs may result in mass effect, focal neurologic signs, and coma.
- Increased intracranial pressure (ICP) and seizures are other serious complications.

PROGNOSIS

In general, long-term outcome is related to the condition of the child at time of presentation. Prolonged elevation of ICP or significant cerebral edema before treatment is worrisome.

 Differential Diagnosis

- SDHs are almost always traumatic, but separating accidental from nonaccidental trauma may be difficult. Falls in infants may cause linear skull fractures, rarely SDHs.
- Macrocephaly or other signs/symptoms since birth may help to date the origin of the SDH to the perinatal or neonatal period.
- Epidural hematomas, subarachnoid hemorrhages, and acute SDHs cannot be distinguished clinically. The lucid interval sometimes seen with epidural hematomas in adults is not a reliable sign. A head CT should differentiate.

Approach to the Patient

A careful history and detailed physical examination are essential to explore possible causes of the SDH, assess the child's neurologic status, and look for evidence of other injuries. Prompt neuroimaging is critical.

 Data Gathering

HISTORY

- Newborn: SDHs as a result of birth trauma may present with lethargy, pallor, poor feeding, apnea, and seizures.
- Infants and young children: SDHs may also present with a nonspecific history of lethargy, irritability, vomiting, poor feeding, apnea, and seizures.
- Older children present with a history of trauma and alteration of consciousness.
- Chronic SDHs present with nonspecific signs, such as vomiting, irritability, failure to thrive, anemia, and seizures.

 Physical Examination

- Newborns may present with decreased responsiveness, a bulging fontanelle, hypotonia, or hypertonia. Retinal hemorrhages are not specific at this age, because they are seen in up to 40% of newborns following a vaginal delivery.
- Infants and young children may also present with nonspecific physical signs, but focal neurologic signs may be present. Retinal hemorrhages are most often associated with nonaccidental trauma, but they have been reported after accidental trauma leading to SDH. Bilateral retinal hemorrhages with retinal folds or detachments are particularly associated with nonaccidental trauma.
- Other signs of child abuse include burns, lacerations, and bruises in various stages of healing, and belt marks, choke marks, and multiple fractures of different ages.
- Older children present with signs of external head trauma, decreased responsiveness, and focal neurologic signs.

 Laboratory Aids

TESTS

Imaging

- CT scan is the imaging study of choice in acute head trauma with neurologic signs. SDH appears as an extra-axial area of increased density, crescentic in shape, and often associated with cerebral contusion or mass effect. CT also may show evidence of cerebral edema, with loss of gray matter/white matter differentiation and small ventricles.
- Subacute SDHs may be difficult to distinguish from adjacent gray matter on CT scan; loss of gray/white matter differentiation is helpful. Chronic SDHs appear as areas of low density on CT scan, often bilateral.
- MRI is helpful to clarify subacute and chronic SDHs and to identify small SDHs missed by CT.
- Ultrasound is less helpful because it may be difficult to distinguish the subdural space from the subarachnoid space.
- If child abuse is suspected, a skeletal survey or bone scan is useful to look for fractures of different ages.
- Incidental SDH may be found on neuroimaging studies in newborns; frequently no intervention is required other than close follow up.

Emergency Care

Children with SDHs may be critically ill on presentation. The aggressiveness of acute therapy depends on the child's clinical condition. Neuroimaging studies and, if necessary, prompt neurosurgical consultation should be performed.

 Therapy

- The treatment of choice for large, acute SDHs is surgical evacuation. Smaller SDHs may be managed conservatively, with careful monitoring for signs of neurologic deterioration.
- While awaiting surgery, attention to airway, breathing, and circulation (ABCs) is critical. Tracheal intubation should be performed if the child's Glasgow coma score is less than 8 or if airway protective reflexes are impaired.
- Isotonic fluids should be given, because hypotonic fluids may worsen cerebral edema.
- Measures to control ICP include elevating the head of the bed 30 degrees to promote venous drainage and osmotic therapy with mannitol. Intracranial ICP monitoring should be considered. Mild hyperventilation (P_{CO_2} 30 to 35 torr) may be helpful but should not be instituted prophylactically. The efficacy of these measures in improving long-term outcome following large SDHs has not been established. Mild hypothermia and hypertonic saline have been used in some cases of traumatic brain injury in adults, but these are not proven therapies in children.
- Seizures should be treated promptly. Phenytoin is the drug of choice if IV medication is needed, with phenobarbital as a second option. Prophylactic anticonvulsants given for a few weeks are effective in reducing early posttraumatic seizures but do not affect long-term risk of epilepsy.
- Treatment of chronic SDHs is more controversial. If there are no signs of ICP, conservative treatment is reasonable, and most collections will resolve. Subdural taps are indicated if ICP rises. If taps are not successful, a subdural-peritoneal shunt may be placed.
- Treatment of SDHs which develop after ventricular shunting is particularly challenging.

 Follow-Up

- Neurologic sequelae of SDHs are more severe than epidural hematomas because of associated cerebral contusions.
- In general, long-term outcome is related to the condition of the child at the time of surgical evacuation of the hematoma. Prolonged elevation of ICP or significant cerebral edema before surgery indicates a poor prognosis.
- Children generally have a better outcome from head injury than do adults, but children less than 7 years old often do worse than older children, especially if the SDH is the result of nonaccidental trauma.
- Long-term problems include headache, seizures, hydrocephalus, vertigo, difficulty concentrating, poor school performance, fixed neurologic deficits, and neurobehavioral problems.
- Epilepsy eventually develops in approximately 10% to 15% of patients after severe head injury. This risk generally does not warrant the prospective use of prophylactic anticonvulsants.
- Children with neurologic sequelae from head injury may benefit from admission to a rehabilitation hospital.
- Social work services should be consulted in cases of known or suspected child abuse.

PREVENTION

- Parents should be counseled about appropriate methods to channel frustration and anger with infants and children. Shaking an infant when the parent is angry is never appropriate.
- Bicycle helmets, car seats, and seat belts are all valuable in preventing head injuries in children.

PITFALLS

- Be suspicious if the stated history does not fit with the pattern or severity of the injury. Physicians and other health care professionals with experience in child abuse should be consulted early if abuse is suspected.
- Chronic SDHs must be differentiated from benign external hydrocephalus, a self-limited condition characterized by progressive macrocrania and extra-axial fluid collections with the density of spinal fluid. MRI can differentiate benign external hydrocephalus.

 Common Questions and Answers

Q: When did the bleed occur?
A: With chronic SDHs, the time and type of injury may be difficult to establish, because no trauma may be reported and the trauma may have occurred weeks or months before. Neuroimaging can give some indication of the injury's timing.

Q: What limitations should be imposed after an acute SDH?
A: Because SDH may recur with minor trauma, it is prudent to avoid any activities that have significant risk of fall or a blow to the head for weeks to months or until neuroradiologic resolution of the hematoma.

Q: Why are anticonvulsants not used to prevent seizures following SDHs?
A: Seizure medications may be given for a few weeks to prevent early seizures following a SDH. After a few weeks, the risks and side effects of the medications outweigh the risk of developing seizures. If seizures begin at a time remote to the injury, then seizure medications can be restarted.

Q: My baby twisted out of my arms, fell head-first onto a tile floor, and suffered a head injury. Will I be reported for child abuse?
A: Not if the injuries fit with the stated history. In this case, the most likely injury would be a linear skull fracture. If more serious intracranial injuries do occur, they will probably not be associated with retinal hemorrhages or other injuries, such as older fractures in multiple stages of healing.

ICD-9-CM 852.2

BIBLIOGRAPHY

Duhaime AC, Christian CW, Rorke LB, Zimmerman RA. Nonaccidental head injury in infants—the "shaken-baby syndrome." *New Engl J Med* 1998;338:1822–1829.

Haviland J, Russell RI. Outcome after severe nonaccidental head injury. *Arch Dis Child* 1997;77:504–507.

Kochanek PM, Clark RSB, Ruppel RA, Dixon CE. Cerebral resuscitation after traumatic brain injury and cardiopulmonary arrest in infants and children in the new millenium. *Pediatr Clin* 2001;48(3):661–681.

Perrin RG, Rutka JT, Drake JM, et al. Management and outcomes of posterior fossa subdural hematomas in neonates. *Neurosurgery* 1997;40:1190–1199.

Swift DM, McBride L. Chronic subdural hematoma in children. *Neurosurg Clin North Am* 2000;11:439–446.

Authors: Dennis J. Dlugos and Sabrina E. Smith

Sudden Infant Death Syndrome

 ## Database

DEFINITION

Sudden infant death syndrome (SIDS) is sudden and unexpected death of an infant (<1 year old) that remains unexplained after a complete postmortem investigation, including autopsy, death scene evaluation, and review of the case history. SIDS is a diagnosis of exclusion.

By definition, there is no explanation for the death, but investigators have identified the following risk factors:

- History of an apparent life-threatening event (ALTE)
- Poverty
- Lack of prenatal care
- Low birth weight
- Small for gestational age (SGA)
- Prematurity
- Maternal smoking
- Maternal substance abuse
- Prone sleep position
- Soft bedding
- Overheating
- Bed sharing with parents who smoke, drink alcohol, or use other mind-altering drugs

PATHOPHYSIOLOGY

Currently there are three main pathophysiologic mechanisms thought to contribute to SIDS:

- Decreased arousal—theorized to be attributable to the immaturity of the arcuate nucleus of the medulla, an area thought to be important for appropriate physiologic response to carbon dioxide levels
- Asphyxia and rebreathing
- Thermal stress—a condition that is a threat to thermal regulation but may be mild enough to maintain euthermia. Contributors to thermal stress may include infection, increased ambient temperature, soft bedding, prone sleep position, bed sharing, or excess clothing.
- Other potential pathophysiologic contributors include: central apnea associated with brain abnormalities, upper airway obstruction, cardiac arrhythmias, and metabolic diseases such as glycogen storage disease and medium-chain acyl-CoA dehydrogenase deficiency; and environmental factors such as hyperthermia, unsafe bedding, and prone sleeping position.

EPIDEMIOLOGY

- Accounts for 5,000 infant deaths/year in the United States
- Most common cause of death in infants from ages 1 to 6 months
- 1.4 cases per 1,000 live births
- Ninety percent of cases occur before 6 months of age
- Peak incidence: age 2 to 4 months
- SIDS rates decreased by 33% to 50% from the late 1980s and the late 1990s, largely thought to be a result of the Back-to-Sleep campaign
- Black infants have twice the risk of SIDS than Whites.

 ## Differential Diagnosis

INFECTION

- Sepsis (bacterial, viral)
- Pneumonia
- Bronchiolitis
- Myocarditis

ENVIRONMENTAL

- Accidental asphyxiation
- Hyperthermia
- Hypothermia
- Toxins
- Poisonings

TRAUMA

- Child abuse, including nonaccidental suffocation
- Drowning

METABOLIC

- Medium-chain acyl-CoA dehydrogenase (MCAD) deficiency
- Long-chain acyl-CoA dehydrogenase deficiency
- Pyruvate carboxylase deficiency
- Phosphoenolpyruvate carboxykinase deficiency
- Defects in glycogenolysis
- Defects in pyruvate oxidation
- Defects in oxidative phosphorylation
- Biotinidase deficiency
- 3-hydroxy-3-methylglutaric aciduria
- Urea cycle defects
- Lactic acidemias
- Aminoacidopathies

CARDIAC

- Congenital heart disease
- Cardiac arrhythmias

MISCELLANEOUS

- Adrenal insufficiency

 ## Data Gathering

HISTORY

- Previously healthy infant, with or without recent upper respiratory tract infection
- Found unresponsive in the morning or after a nap
- No struggle or crying heard

SPECIAL QUESTIONS

- Have there been previous infant or child deaths in the family? It is unusual to have more than one SIDS death in a family. When multiple SIDS deaths occur in a family, the possibility of sequential homicide needs to be considered.
- When was the last time the baby was seen alive?
- Where was the baby found?
- In what position was the baby found?
- What was the child wearing?
- Were there blankets, stuffed toys, or bumpers at the baby's head?
- Were there any recent illnesses?
- What is the prenatal history?
- Is there a history of previous maternal miscarriages?
- What is the date of the last immunizations?
- Have there been prior medical problems?
- Is there a history of apnea?

 ## Physical Examination

- Postmortem lividity
- Pink, frothy discharge at nose and mouth
- Look for signs of injury.
- Check for dysmorphic features.

 ## Laboratory Aids

- A full autopsy must be done on all infants who die suddenly and unexpectedly.

—A case can be defined as SIDS when:
—There is no gross or microscopic evidence of a significant disease process or trauma
—Other causes are ruled out (infection, cardiac disease, inborn errors of metabolism)
—There is no evidence of alcohol, drug, or toxin exposure

- In infant deaths in which there are nondiagnostic findings on postmortem examination the death is usually termed sudden unexplained infant death (SUIDs) and the cause of death is ruled undetermined.

IMAGING

A postmortem skeletal survey is indicated if there is suspicion of abuse.

Sudden Infant Death Syndrome

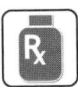 Therapy

Resuscitation is almost always initiated before receiving the baby at the hospital. If rigor mortis or lividity is present, resuscitation efforts should not be initiated.

 Follow-Up

- The medical examiner or coroner's office should be notified of all unexplained infant deaths. Remember an unexplained infant death is not officially SIDS until the autopsy, death scene investigation, and review of the clinical history have been completed.
- All states have multidisciplinary child fatality review teams designed to review child fatalities in an effort to discover unrecognized cases of child abuse and analyze risk factors for child death in an effort to develop strategies to prevent child injury and death.
- Provide support to the family.
- Refer to a SIDS center.

PITFALLS

- Not completing full postmortem examination, including autopsy, death scene review, and careful review of case and family history

PREVENTION

- Use the back sleep position. Avoid the prone sleeping position for young, healthy infants.
- Provide a safe sleeping environment. Use a firm crib mattress. Avoid soft materials, such as pillows, comforters, or sheep skins, in the infant's sleeping environment.
- Encourage use of a crib or bassinet. Avoid use of a chair or couch.
- Avoid overheating.
- Home apnea monitors, although widely used, have not been shown to prevent or decrease mortality related to SIDS.

According to the AAP the following are indications for home apnea monitors:

- Infants who have experienced an ALTE
- Infants with tracheostomies or other airway problems that make them vulnerable to airway compromise
- Infants with metabolic or neurologic problems affecting respiratory control
- Infants with chronic lung disease on home therapies

 Common Questions and Answers

Q: Do all infants who die suddenly and unexpectedly require an autopsy?
A: Yes. It is estimated that autopsy reveals a cause of death in approximately 15% of SIDS deaths. The diagnosis of SIDS cannot be made without an autopsy!

Q: Does SIDS run in families?
A: Recurrence rates in families in which a sibling has died of SIDS vary greatly among studies, but large, controlled studies indicate no increased risk of SIDS in subsequent siblings. In families with recurrent SIDS deaths, especially after the third infant death, the possibility of serial homicide needs to be investigated.

Q: How can you tell the difference between SIDS and intentional suffocation?
A: Because the physical findings of an autopsy cannot distinguish between SIDS and intentional suffocation, other factors related to the death must be considered when attempting to distinguish the two. In comparing the features of suffocated children with the clinical features associated with SIDS, Meadow makes the following comparisons:

- The percent of suffocated children with previous apnea is approximately 90%, compared with less than 10% of SIDS infants.
- Forty-four percent of the suffocated children had a previously unexplained medical problem, whereas greater than 95% of SIDS infants were previously healthy.
- Fifty-five percent of suffocated children were older than 6 months at the time of diagnosis.
- Forty-eight percent of suffocated children had a sibling who had died, compared with 2% of SIDS deaths.

Although these important differences may identify some children who are intentionally suffocated, differentiating fatal abuse by suffocation from SIDS is difficult.

ICD-9-CM 789.0

BIBLIOGRAPHY

American Academy of Pediatrics Task Force on Infant Sleep Position and Sudden Infant Death Syndrome. Changing concepts of sudden infant death syndrome: implications for infant sleeping environment and sleep position. *Pediatrics* 2000;105:650–656.

American Academy of Pediatrics, Committee on Child Abuse and Neglect. Distinguishing sudden infant death syndrome from child abuse fatalities. *Pediatrics* 2001;107:437–441.

American Academy of Pediatrics, Committee on Fetus and Newborn. Apnea, sudden infant death syndrome, and home monitoring. *Pediatrics* 2003;111:914–917.

Cote A, Russo P, Michaud J. Sudden unexpected deaths in infancy: what are the causes? *J Pediatr* 1999;135:437–443.

Kohlendorfer U, Kiechl S, Sperl W. Sudden infant death syndrome: risk factor profiles for distinct subgroups. *Am J Epidemiol* 1998;147:960–968.

Nagler J. Sudden infant death syndrome. *Curr Opin Pediatr* 2002;14:247–250.

Southall DP, Plunkett MC, Banks MW, et al. Covert video recordings of life-threatening child abuse: lessons for child protection. *Pediatrics* 1997;100:735–760.

Authors: Cindy W. Christian and Matthew J. Cox

Suicide

 Database

DEFINITION

- Suicide is an intentional self-harming act that ends life.
- Attempted suicide occurs when the act does not succeed in its goal (also, failed or near suicide).
- Suicidal behavior is any voluntary act that can potentially end one's life.
- Suicidal ideation is defined as thoughts, with or without a specific plan, to end one's own life.

ETIOLOGY

Suicidal behavior in adolescents results from the interaction of long-standing individual and family conditions, social environment, and acute stressors:

- Psychiatric disorders: Suicidal behavior is included in the diagnostic criteria for major depressive episode and borderline personality disorder (DSM-IV). Additionally, psychotic disorders, conduct disturbance, adjustment disorder, and panic disorders have all been found to be associated with suicidal behavior.
- Intense emotional state, in particular shame or humiliation, can be "trigger events" for a suicidal act.
- Personality and social factors can also contribute, such as antisocial behavior, aggressive or impulsive proclivities, and social isolation.
- Suicidal behavior runs in families. There is evidence of a genetic component and of learned or suicidal behavior as a communicative or expressive act.

EPIDEMIOLOGY

- Suicide is the third leading cause of death for the 10 to 14, 15 to 19, and 20 to 24-year-old age groups.
- Approximately 2,000 U.S. adolescents commit suicide, and approximately 2 million attempt suicide annually.
- Adolescent mortality from suicide tripled between the 1950s and the 1990s.
- Overall, suicide accounted for 7.9 deaths per 100,000 persons aged 15 to 19 years in 2001 (12% of all deaths in this age group).
- In 2001, suicide accounted for 1.3 deaths per 100,000 persons aged 10 to 14 years (7% of all deaths in this age group), and for 12.0 deaths per 100,000 persons aged 20 to 24 years (12.6% of all deaths).
- Females attempt suicide at a rate 2 to 4 times that of males. Females are most likely to attempt suicide through ingestion.
- Males complete suicide at a rate 3 to 4 times that of females. Males are most likely to use more lethal methods, such as firearms and hanging, when attempting suicide.
- Completed suicide rates are highest in White and Native American adolescents. Suicide rates for Black males aged 10 to 19 years have increased at a higher rate,

doubling between the years 1980 and 1995. Highest rates of suicide attempts have been reported in Hispanic females.
- Gay, lesbian, bisexual, and questioning youth report higher rates of suicide attempts than their heterosexual peers.
- Risk factors for suicide have been shown to include: previous suicide attempt, mood disorders, substance/alcohol abuse, family history of suicide, family history of mental illness or substance abuse, history of sexual or physical abuse, chronic illness, poor parent-child communication, and the presence of firearms in the home.

PROGNOSIS

- Twenty percent to 50% of those attempting suicide will try again.
- Psychiatric hospitalization has not been shown to decrease risk of attempted suicide in patients with a history of mood disorder or substance abuse.
- Multiple reports show that adolescents who attempt suicide routinely terminate treatment after a few visits.

 Differential Diagnosis

- Central nervous system trauma
—Any insult to the cerebral cortex can result in disinhibitory behaviors.
- Psychiatric disorders, with particular attention to depression, personality disorder, and substance abuse
- Psychosocial trauma or maladjustment
—Emotional or physical abuse, with the suicide attempt being a way to gain attention, obtain help, or to serve as a means of escape
—Feelings of isolation or abandonment, such as following the revelation of pregnancy or homosexuality

 Data Gathering

HISTORY

- Communication should be nonjudgmental and supportive.
- The provider should sensitively ascertain if the patient has a weapon or other method of self-harm.

A comprehensive history should always be obtained or reviewed by a trained mental health worker. Components of a comprehensive history include:

- Method and timing (particularly if method is ingestion)
- Lethality of attempt (e.g., number of pills, seriousness of physical injury)
- Circumstances of attempt (e.g., remote site, public display)
- History of prior attempts
- Level of planning of attempt

- Current affect and psychological status (e.g., feelings and/or level of depression, hopelessness, impulsivity, self-esteem, etc.)
- Family consistency and dynamics
- Pharmaceuticals available at home; what is missing
- History of interpersonal conflict or personal loss
- Family history of suicide
- History of substance use
- History of psychological disorder or disease state
- History of abuse, neglect, or incest
- Social supports and coping strategies
- Feelings of regret or continued desire for self-harm

The following historical information increases the risk for a future, potentially lethal suicide attempt:

- History of potentially lethal attempt
- Family history of suicide or attempted suicide
- Unstable family structure
- Poor social support system, lack of feeling connected

 Physical Examination

- Physical signs or sequelae of prior attempts
- Adolescents do not always have the classic findings of depressed adults.
- Even without a history of ingestion, closely observe vital signs, skin, mucous membranes, and pupils for evidence of toxidrome.
- Examine the skin for signs of physical abuse or self-mutilation.
- If indicated or suspected, examine the genitalia for signs of sexual abuse.
- A complete neurologic examination is essential for the evaluation of intracranial processes, acute mental status changes, and ingestions.

 Laboratory Aids

TESTS

- Serum and urine toxicology screens
- Urine pregnancy test to assess pregnancy as a potential precipitating factor and to recognize potential danger to the fetus
- Acetaminophen level, as it is highly hepatotoxic and used frequently by teenagers
- Other laboratory tests will depend on the history of method of attempt (e.g., trauma labs, metabolic screens).
- Electrocardiograms are indicated for many pharmacologic ingestions, including antidepressants and benzodiazepines.

RADIOGRAPHIC IMAGING

- Abdominal plain film—if history of iron or vitamin ingestion, or severe trauma
- Other imaging studies—may be indicated, depending on method of attempt.

Suicide

 Emergency Care

- ABCs
- Monitoring of behavior and vital signs if history of ingestion
- Decontamination of gastrointestinal (GI) tract and circulation as indicated.
- When available, the Poison Control Center may be very helpful with evaluation and treatment of most drug ingestions.
- Ongoing safety is of primary concern: immediate physical protection (remove all weapons) and enforce around-the-clock observation
- After medical evaluation and stabilization, the need for psychiatric hospitalization or outpatient follow-up should be assessed.

Psychiatric disposition should be determined by, or in conjunction with, a mental health professional. Considerations for admission include:

- Historical factors indicating high risk for repeat attempt
- Ongoing suicidal ideation and/or planning
- Family instability and lack of support
- Altered mental status
- Lack of alternative interventions (e.g., intensive psychiatric follow-up, day treatment program)

When discharge to a caregiver is being considered, the following minimal criteria should be in place at the time of discharge:

- The patient expresses regret and denies ongoing suicidal thoughts.
- The patient is medically stable.
- The patient's family is involved and reports understanding of the seriousness of the attempt.
- The patient and parents agree to contact a health professional or go to the emergency department if suicidal intent recurs. The patient and family must have 24-hour access to mental health or physical health professionals.
- The patient must not have impaired mental status (e.g., severely depressed, psychoses, delirium, intoxication).
- Lethal methods of self-harm are not immediately available to the patient (e.g., guns, dangerous pharmaceuticals).
- Follow-up and treatment of underlying psychological disorders have been arranged. This ideally involves much more than providing a phone number to psychiatric services or asking the family to contact their insurer.
- Acute precipitants and crises have been addressed.
- There is nothing to indicate to the provider that the patient and family will be noncompliant.
- Caregivers and patients are in agreement with the discharge plan.
- Barriers to obtaining follow-up treatment, in particular insurance and fear of stigma, have been addressed and will not preclude the next step toward ongoing treatment.

 Therapy

DRUGS

- For recent ingestions, GI decontamination with activated charcoal may be appropriate, as is the administration of pertinent antidotes (e.g., naloxone for opioids, N-acetylcysteine for acetaminophen).
- While psychotherapy is an essential component to the care of the suicidal adolescent, pharmacotherapy with antidepressants can also play a role, especially given the high association with co-morbid mood disorders.
—Keep in mind when prescribing tricyclic antidepressants (TCAs) their high lethality potential.
—Selective serotonin reuptake inhibitors (SSRIs) have been shown to be effective in treating depressive disorders in adolescents. Use of SSRIs in patients with the potential for suicidal behavior require close monitoring. At least two currently marketed SSRIs that are approved for the treatment of depression in adolescents (venlafaxine, paroxetine) have been shown to be associated with an increase in suicidality.
- Other psychotropic medicines may be used in the acute setting for sedation or psychoses.
- In addition to medication, important psychiatric interventions include acute short-term inpatient psychiatric hospitalization, partial hospitalization (with intensive treatment and support), and outpatient therapy.

 Follow-Up

Long-term psychotherapy (individual and family therapy) is often needed for adolescents who attempt suicide. Improvement may be slow and punctuated by frequent setbacks.

SIGNS TO WATCH FOR

- Acute life stressors
- Failure to comply with therapy or follow-up
- A sudden sense of calm or resolution may occur when a patient has decided to end life.

PREVENTION

Screening of all adolescents for suicidal thoughts and behaviors and associated risk factors should occur at routine office visits and during evaluation of emotional distress or physical symptoms (e.g., chronic headache, abdominal pain). Screening should include:

- Change in level of functioning in school, work, or home
- Changes in mood or affect
- Direct inquiry about suicidal ideation and plans
- Exploration and discussion of coping strategies
- Discussion of social support

If suicidal ideation is reported, the risk of attempt should be assessed. Components of risk assessment include:
- Frequency and timing of suicidal thoughts
- Method of self-injury considered
- Plan to follow through
- History of past suicide attempt
- Consultation with a psychiatrist if there is any question of risk for suicide attempt
- Confidentiality does not extend to potentially suicidal adolescents. Parents, or the appropriate authority, should be made aware of the risk, and a plan, for self-harm on the part of the adolescent.

PITFALLS

- Adolescents often present to medical personnel before attempting suicide. The practitioner should be particularly aware of constitutional or vague complaints, and increased frequency of visits for seemingly diffuse reasons.
- Management must always occur in conjunction with a mental health professional.
- Parents and professionals should avoid minimizing attempts as "not serious" or as "just seeking attention."
- Different laboratories offer different spectra and sensitivities in their toxicology screens. Providers must be familiar with their laboratories and should determine whether additional studies are indicated.

? Common Questions and Answers

Q: Do I keep suicide attempts or plans confidential?
A: No. The limits of confidentiality should be clearly outlined to patients and families at the first visit or early in the patient's adolescence. These limits include anything that will directly place the patient's life in danger, such as suicidal plans, abuse, or homicidal intentions.

Q: If I directly question my patients about suicide, won't that put the idea in their head?
A: No. In most cases, patients will be relieved by having a professional who wants to talk about suicide. There is only risk in asking if nothing is done with the answer. Appropriate referral to mental health services or counseling can save patients' lives.

ICD-9-CM 300.9

BIBLIOGRAPHY

American Academy of Child and Adolescent Psychiatry. Practice parameter for the assessment and treatment of children and adolescents with suicidal behavior. *J Am Acad Child Adolesc Psychiatry* 2001;40(7 Suppl):24S–51S.

Catallozzi M, Pletcher, Schwarz DF. Prevention of suicide in adolescents. *Curr Opin Pediatr* 2001;13:417–422.

Authors: Leonard J. Levine and Jonathan R. Pletcher

Superior Mesenteric Artery Syndrome

 Database

DEFINITION

Superior mesenteric artery (SMA) syndrome is obstruction of the distal duodenum by the superior mesenteric artery or its branches. Also called Wilkie syndrome.

CAUSES

- The mesenteric artery forms an acute downward aortomesenteric angle as it leaves the aorta. The duodenum lies within this angle and in some individuals can be compressed by the SMA anteriorly and the vertebra posteriorly, leading to symptoms of obstruction.
- Some of the conditions that predispose to narrowing of this angle are:

—Increase in lordosis of the back, such as immobilization by body cast, scoliosis surgery, prolonged bed rest in a supine position
—Rapid growth in children
—Weight loss resulting in loss of mesenteric fat, as seen in pediatric AIDS
—In scoliosis surgery weight percentile for height of 5% has been identified as an important risk factor for development of syndrome
—Variations of the ligament of Treitz. A short ligament lifts the third or fourth part of the duodenum into the narrower segment in the aortomesenteric angle.

PROGNOSIS

Most patients improve without need for surgery and are asymptomatic on follow-up.

 Differential Diagnosis

- Anorexia nervosa/bulimia/hysterical
- Luminal obstruction: foreign body
- Intramural obstruction: duplication cyst, web, tumor, bezoar and stricture
- Extramural obstruction: tumor, annular pancreas, bands, adhesions, volvulus, and intussusception
- Dysmotility disorder, which can be a result of an intrinsic neuronal disorder, muscular weakness (holovisceral myopathy), or fibrosis (scleroderma, retroperitoneal fibrosis)

 Data Gathering

HISTORY

- Vomiting (bilious and nonbilious), nausea, postprandial nausea and vomiting, weight loss, early satiety, dehydration, bloating, abdominal pain, and failure to thrive
- The symptoms are chronic and acute, and most patients have vague abdominal pain from 18 months to 10 years in duration.
- None of the symptoms or signs for SMA syndrome are pathognomonic, but a history of weight loss, immobilization, or back surgery followed by symptoms of early satiety, bloating, and vomiting after meals would suggest the diagnosis.

 Physical Examination

- Abdominal pain
- Increased bowel gas
- Dehydration in some cases

 Laboratory Aids

IMAGING

- A plain abdominal radiograph could show gas predominantly in a distended stomach with a dilated proximal duodenum with a sharp cutoff at the level in which the SMA crosses the duodenum.
- An upper contrast radiography would demonstrate passage of contrast when the patient is maneuvered into a prone position, which increases the aortomesenteric angle by gravity.
- A determination of the aortomesenteric angle in severe cases may help in decision making when surgery is contemplated. In normal patients, this angle has a range of 45° to 60°, whereas in patients with SMA syndrome, it is reported to be between 10° and 22°.

Superior Mesenteric Artery Syndrome

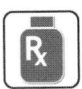 Therapy

- Refeeding to gain weight. Feeding in a prone position may help, but if this fails, a jejunal tube bypassing the obstruction or a period of parenteral feeding can be used.
- Frequent repositioning of patients in body cast
- A decrease in viscosity in feeds has a theoretical advantage.
- Reversal of back surgery may be necessary in some patients.
- Bypass surgery is unnecessary in most cases. Refractory cases in which duodenojejunostomy or derotation surgery has been tried are associated with very good results. The latter surgery consists of dividing the ligament of Treitz, and the whole small intestine is passed beneath the SMA and lies in the right abdomen; the colon is separated from the retroperitoneal attachments and placed in the left abdomen.
- Recently in adults, laparoscopic duodenojejunostomy has been used as a minimally invasive surgical technique for successful management of SMA.

 Common Questions and Answers

Q: When the diagnosis of SMA syndrome is suspected, what sequence do you follow?
A: The logical sequence is to see if the patient improves with refeeding and mobilization first, followed by an imaging study, such as an upper gastrointestinal contrast study. CT does not improve diagnosis, and an aortomesenteric angle study is almost never required.

Q: The following treatment modalities are known to be useful in treatment of SMA syndrome: do nothing, or feed with a jejunal tube, a liquid diet, prone feeding, or TPN. Which program works?
A: All of the above have been used in SMA syndrome. There is a probability that some patients have a functional disorder and do not require any of these feeding modalities. Weight gain has also been accomplished with total parenteral nutrition.

Q: Does radiographic testing or a feeding clinical trial help in confirming the diagnosis?
A: Yes, it may be helpful to confirm the diagnosis if the classic to-and-fro motion of barium is seen on radiographic studies during fluoroscopy. Additionally, a clinical trial of feeding and weight gain often becomes the criteria for confirmation of the diagnosis.

ICD-9-CM 557.1

BIBLIOGRAPHY

Atkin JT, Skandalakis JE, Gray S. The anatomic basis of vascular compression of the duodenum. *Surg Clin North Am* 1974;54:1361–1370.

Gustafsson L. Diagnosis and treatment of superior mesenteric syndrome. *Br J Surg* 1984;71:499–501.

Hoffman RJ, Arpadi SM. A Pediatric AIDS patient with superior mesenteric artery syndrome. *AIDS Patient Care* 2000;14:3–6.

Kim IY, Cho NC, Kim DS, Rhoe BS. Laparoscopic duodenojejunostomy for management of superior mesenteric artery syndrome: two case reports and a review of the literature. *Yonsei Med J* 2003;44:526–529.

Marchant EA, Alvear DT, Fagelman KM. True clinical entity of vascular compression of the duodenum in adolescence. *Surg Gynecol Obstet* 1989;168:381–386.

Shah MA, Albright MB, Vogt MT, Morland MS. Superior mesenteric artery syndrome in scoliosis surgery: weight percentile for height as an indicator of risk. *J Pediatr Orthop* 2003;23:665–668.

Author: Andrew E. Mulberg

Supraventricular Tachycardia

 Database

DEFINITION

Supraventricular tachycardia (SVT) is a tachycardia originating at or above the atrioventricular (AV) node. The heart rates in infants generally range from 220 to 320 beats/minute and in older children range from 150 to 250 beats/minute.

• The majority of infants and children with SVT have structurally normal hearts.
• About 20% of cases of Wolff-Parkinson-White (WPW) syndrome have associated congenital heart disease with Ebstein anomaly, L-looped transposition of the great arteries, and hypertrophic cardiomyopathy being the most common.
• SVT can frequently be precipitated by exercise, infection, fever, or drug exposure (e.g., cold medications).
• SVT is commonly observed in patients who have undergone surgery for congenital heart disease. SVT is frequently observed after the Mustard/Senning procedure, the Fontan operation, and repair of an atrial septal defect.

PATHOPHYSIOLOGY

There are two major mechanisms for SVT:

• Reentry tachycardia: This is the most common mechanism for SVT. It involves a circuit rhythm within the atria (atrial flutter), within the AV node (AV nodal reentry tachycardia), or using an accessory pathway (atrioventricular reentrant tachycardia). Reentrant tachycardias are characterized by sudden onset and termination, regular rate, and responsiveness to pacing maneuvers and direct current cardioversion.
• Automatic tachycardia: This mechanism is responsible for ectopic atrial tachycardia, multifocal atrial tachycardia, and junctional ectopic tachycardia. Automatic tachycardias are characterized by warm-up and cool-down phases, an irregular rate that is sensitive to the body's catecholamine state, and lack of responsiveness to pacing and cardioversion.

GENETICS

WPW syndrome has been noted in several families and an autosomal-dominant mode of inheritance has been demonstrated. About half of the cases of junctional ectopic tachycardia occur in a familial setting with an autosomal dominant mode of inheritance.

EPIDEMIOLOGY

• SVT is the most common arrhythmia in childhood.
• Fifty percent to 60% of pediatric patients present in the first year of life.
• Of patients that present in infancy, 40% to 70% will be asymptomatic by 1 year of age. However, about a third of these patients may experience a reappearance of their tachycardia at an average age of 8 years. The majority of older children who present with SVT will have persistent recurrence of their tachycardia.

COMPLICATIONS

Complications from SVT can arise from one of three causes:

• Persistent tachycardia can lead to congestive heart failure and cardiovascular collapse. This is especially true in the infant who may go unrecognized for 24 to 48 hours.
• A few patients with WPW syndrome (<5%) can have rapid conduction down the accessory pathway. A rapid ventricular response to atrial flutter/fibrillation can potentially cause ventricular fibrillation and sudden death. Patients with WPW syndrome receiving digoxin and/or verapamil are at increased risk.
• Side effects of pharmacologic agents used to treat SVT include bradycardia, other ventricular arrhythmias as a result of the proarrhythmic effects of antiarrhythmic agents (digoxin, procainamide, amiodarone, flecainide), or noncardiac side effects (gastrointestinal, liver, pulmonary, and thyroid dysfunction).

 Differential Diagnosis

• Narrow complex SVT needs to be distinguished from sinus or junctional tachycardia, and sick-sinus syndrome with tachyarrhythmia. Structural heart disease should be excluded in all cases of newly diagnosed SVT.
• Wide complex tachycardia from either aberrantly conducted SVT or SVT with antegrade conduction down an accessory pathway can be seen in a small percentage of patients and may be confused with ventricular tachycardia. As a general rule, unless there are preexisting data that the patient has SVT, wide complex tachycardia should always be interpreted as ventricular tachycardia until proven otherwise.
• Differentiating between types of SVT (reentrant vs. automatic) can be accomplished by evaluating the regularity of the rate, modes of onset and termination, and the tachycardia's responsiveness to pacing and cardioversion.

 Data Gathering

HISTORY

• Infants will manifest signs and symptoms suggestive of low cardiac output if the tachycardia has gone unnoticed for a prolonged period of time. Findings may include tachypnea, retractions, irritability, decreased feedings, excessive sweating, hypotension, poor perfusion, and decreased urine output.
• The toddler and older child may experience palpitations, shortness of breath, chest pain, and dizziness or syncope. It is important to know what the child was doing at the time the arrhythmia started and whether the rhythm had an abrupt onset and termination. Older children often report being able to terminate episodes of tachycardia by performing the Valsalva maneuver (e.g., gagging or standing on their head).

 Physical Examination

The following need to be assessed in all patients presenting with SVT:

• Heart rate
• Respiratory rate
• Blood pressure
• Hydration status
• Peripheral perfusion
• Liver size
• Mental status
• Presence of gallop rhythm on auscultation

 Laboratory Aids

TESTS

• Diagnosis can be made by a 12-lead ECG, 24-hour Holter recording, transtelephonic monitor (TTM), or a transesophageal recording.
• Patients with WPW syndrome have diagnostic ventricular preexcitation (short PR interval and a delta wave) on the surface ECG.
• An exercise stress test and/or electrophysiologic testing may be indicated in older patients with WPW syndrome to help determine the risk of rapid conduction down the accessory pathway.
• Nonpharmacologic maneuvers (ice, vagal) and pharmacologic maneuvers (e.g., IV adenosine, 50 to 300 μg/kg per dose) may distinguish tachycardias that involve the AV node from other types of SVT.

IMAGING

A chest radiograph may reveal cardiomegaly, suggesting congestive heart failure or underlying structural heart disease.

Supraventricular Tachycardia

 Therapy

- Always assess the child's ABCs (airway, breathing, and circulation).
- Initial management of SVT depends on the child's hemodynamic condition.
- Presentation in cardiovascular collapse as a result of SVT warrants treatment with synchronized DC cardioversion (0.5 to 2.0 joules/kg).

REENTRANT SVT

- In a stable child, adenosine (IV bolus 50 to 300 μg/kg) may be used to block the AV node and achieve pharmacologic cardioversion for reentrant SVT that requires the AV node as part of the circuit. The half-life of the drug is less than 10 seconds. Verapamil should be avoided as acute treatment of SVT in children less than 12 months of age because of its vasodilating and negative inotropic effect. Nonpharmacologic vagal maneuvers, including ice to the face, Valsalva, gag, and headstand, may be tried in older children. Pacing via an esophageal catheter may also be used.
- Oral digoxin is the agent of choice in hemodynamically stable SVT needing chronic therapy.
- Digoxin, however, is contraindicated in patients with WPW because it may potentiate faster conduction down the accessory pathway and lead to ventricular fibrillation in some patients.
- β-blockers (propranolol or nadolol) are the treatment of choice in individuals with WPW.
- Procainamide and amiodarone may be used in more resistant cases. β-blockers are usually given to patients with exercise-induced SVT.
- Atrial flutter may be treated with digoxin, procainamide, sotalol, or amiodarone as a single agent or in combination.
- Radiofrequency catheter ablation is an alternative to long-term drug therapy and may be employed for the following reasons: (a) SVT refractory to medical therapy, (b) side effects from the medical regimen, (c) patient choice, (d) life-threatening arrhythmias, (e) rapid conduction properties of an accessory pathway (e.g., WPW), or (f) concomitant congenital or acquired heart disease.

AUTOMATIC SVT

- Automatic tachycardias may be responsive to antiarrhythmics such as procainamide, flecainide (should generally be avoided if the patient has structural heart disease), amiodarone or β-blockers either alone or in different combinations. Ectopic atrial tachycardia and junctional ectopic tachycardia may also be amenable to radiofrequency ablation.

 Follow-Up

- As SVT may recur, neonates and infants generally should receive maintenance therapy for the first year of life and then be observed off medications, assuming that they are not having frequent breakthrough episodes of SVT.
- Individuals with recurrences in the first year of life or those requiring multiple medications should be treated for 1-year to 2-year periods during which they are episode-free, and then closely followed off medications.
- In children presenting beyond infancy, the likelihood for spontaneous resolution of the tachycardia is less likely, and treatment may need to be continued into adulthood. These patients may be considered for a radiofrequency ablation.
- Over-the-counter sympathomimetic cold medications and caffeine products should be avoided, as they may increase the likelihood of SVT.

 Common Questions and Answers

Q: How should infants on chronic therapy be monitored?
A: Parents with infants on chronic therapy for SVT should be educated about counting the heart rate by palpation or auscultation at least one or two times daily. This method of surveillance is just as effective as apnea/bradycardia monitors. Alarm monitors can increase anxiety level by frequent false alarms and are generally not recommended.

Q: What is the concern with verapamil?
A: Verapamil is an L-type calcium channel blocker that blocks conduction in the AV node and is very effective in treating SVT in adults. Since myocardial contractility in infants depends mostly on the transsarcolemmal L-type calcium channels, hypotension and cardiovascular collapse have been reported with its use in children younger than 1 year of age.

Q: What are the indications, success rates, and risks of radiofrequency catheter ablation?
A: Refractory arrhythmias, need for multiple medications, undesirable side effects from the medications, life-threatening events (syncope, cardiac arrest), wide complex tachycardia (cannot determine whether SVT or VT), and elective ablation are some of the indications. The success rate of radiofrequency catheter ablation varies from 80% to 97%, depending on the location of the bypass tract or ectopic focus. The incidence of major complications is less than 2% with the most common being heart block requiring a pacemaker, cardiac perforation, brachial plexus injury, and embolization.

ICD-9-CM 427.89

BIBLIOGRAPHY

Benson DW. Genetic basis of disturbances of cardiac rhythm and conduction. In: Walsh EP, Saul JP, Triedman JK, eds. *Cardiac Arrhythmias in Children and Young Adults with Congenital Heart Disease*. Philadelphia: Lippincott Williams & Wilkins, 2001.

Friedman RA, Walsh EP, Silka MJ, et al. Radiofrequency catheter ablation in children with and without congenital heart disease. *Pacing Clin Electrophysiol* 2002;25:1000–1017.

Kirk CR, Gibbs JL, Thomas R, et al. Cardiovascular collapse after verapamil in supraventricular tachycardia. *Arch Dis Child* 1987;62:1265–1282.

Kugler JD, Danford DA. Management of infants, children, and adolescents with paroxysmal supraventricular tachycardia. *J Pediatrics* 1996;129:324–338.

Paul T, Bertram H, Bokenkamp R, Hausdorf G. Supraventricular tachycardia in infants, children and adolescents: diagnosis, and pharmacological and interventional therapy. *Paediatr Drugs* 2000;2(3):171–181.

Perry JC. Supraventricular tachycardia. In: Garson A, Bricker JT, Fisher DJ, Neish SR, eds. *The Science and Practice of Pediatric Cardiology*. Baltimore: Williams & Wilkins, 1998.

Van Hare, GF. Supraventricular tachycardia. In: Gillete PC, Garson A., eds. *Clinical Pediatric Arrhythmias*. Philadelphia: W.B. Saunders Company, 1999.

Author: Jonathan R. Kaltman

Syncope

 ## Database

DEFINITION

Syncope is loss of consciousness, typically lasting no longer than 1 to 2 minutes, as a result of a transient drop in cerebral perfusion pressure.

PATHOPHYSIOLOGY

Most common mechanism is vasovagal or neurocardiogenic, in which a variety of external stimuli—pain, dehydrated state, emotional upset, carotid pressure—trigger increased vagal tone, leading to slowed heart rate and peripheral vasodilation and decreased cerebral perfusion. Rarer causes include cardiac arrhythmia (heart block or tachyarrhythmia) and intracranial hypertension.

ASSOCIATED CONDITIONS

Syncopal spells in children may be accompanied by a convulsion that usually lasts less than 1 minute (EEG is normal).

 ## Differential Diagnosis

Alternative causes of loss of consciousness not as a result of syncope include:

- Head trauma
- Epilepsy ("temporal lobe syncope")
- Psychogenic
- Stroke, hypoglycemia (rare except in certain metabolic disorders)

Underlying causes of syncope in any age group may include congenital heart malformations, arteriovenous malformation; pulmonary hypertension; intracranial hypertension as a result of hydrocephalus, mass, or pseudotumor; and tachyarrhythmia or heart block (Stokes-Adams).
Other causes of syncope by age group include the following:

- Toddlers

—Pallid or cyanotic breath-holding spells; these occur in response to pain, excitement, or frustration, begin with a deep inspiration or exhalation, although the precipitating "gasp" may not be apparent. (Anemia may be associated.)
—Mastocytosis—syncope preceded by dyspnea

- Older children:

—Prolonged QT syndrome or arrhythmogenic right ventricular dysplasia; may be familial; may occur as unprovoked syncope or as exercise-induced syncope that may resemble an epileptic convulsion
—Adrenal insufficiency
—Dysautonomia—orthostatic hypotension

 ## Data Gathering

HISTORY

- Detailed history of the spell is the most important information used to distinguish syncope from seizure or head trauma.
- Questions addressing a possible family history of sudden death, seizures, or syncope is essential.
- The child or observers may recall "presyncopal" signs—such as warmth, diaphoresis, light-headedness, nausea, palpitations, visual changes—all lasting only a few seconds before loss of consciousness.
- Increasing duration of unconsciousness suggests increasing probability that the event is epileptic, rather than syncopal.
- Generalized tonic-clonic movements may occur with syncope—presyncopal signs point to the nonepileptic nature of the event.
- Details of body position, eye movements, and respiratory pattern

 ## Physical Examination

Key findings to document include:

- Vital signs, peripheral/central pulses
- Orthostatic pulse and blood pressure changes
- Right and left arm blood pressures
- Funduscopy—papilledema?
- Cranial bruits
- Heart sounds (gallop, click, significant murmur?)

Laboratory Aids

Some children may have a clear history of vasovagal syncope and no laboratory testing will be required. If the event is suspected to be symptomatic of a heart condition, ECG and chest radiograph studies may be useful screening tests.

- Children with unexplained syncope may undergo more extensive testing to rule out arrhythmia: echocardiogram, stress test, Holter monitoring, EEG (looking for evidence of epilepsy)
- Other laboratory testing (glucose, CBC, blood gases, echocardiogram, brain imaging, spinal tap) may be appropriate based on clinical suspicion of underlying causes (see Differential Diagnosis, above).

TREATMENT

Clinical intervention is primarily aimed at training the patient in prevention/anticipation:

—Avoiding circumstances predisposing to the most common form of syncope (vasovagal)
—Sitting or lying down when warning signs occur
—Maintaining adequate hydration especially during illness/exertion

- Therapy is otherwise addressed to underlying causes, in the unusual circumstance that one is found.

PITFALLS

- Syncope with exercise always warrants a cardiovascular evaluation, initially with electrocardiogram and echocardiography.
- Recurrent syncope as a result of prolonged QT interval may be missed on routine ECG; QT interval may be prolonged only on treadmill testing or cardiac monitoring.
- Carbon monoxide poisoning may cause syncopal-like spells; ask about potential exposure.
- Epilepsy may rarely mimic a syncopal episode or recurrent presyncopal symptoms; "temporal lobe syncope" seems to occur principally in adults or adolescents.
- A family history of sudden death, syncope, or seizures should trigger further laboratory studies.
- Syncope may trigger a convulsion in an epileptic patient.

Follow-Up

- A record should be kept once a child has had two or more syncopal spells within 6 months.
- Many children outgrow a developmental stage where for unknown reasons they had frequent vasovagal episodes; they may retain a tendency to syncopal spells through adulthood.
- Persistent and frequent spells may prompt more extensive laboratory testing, as described above.

Common Questions and Answers

Q: Do breath-holding spells cause brain damage?
A: Pallid breath-holding spells appear to be uniformly benign; in rare cases, older children with cyanotic breath-holding spells have had neurologic sequelae of recurrent hypoxemia.

Q: What limitations in activity are appropriate for children with recurrent syncope?
A: Precautions should be taken similar to those for children of similar age who have epilepsy—closely monitored water recreation, and restrictions on climbing; however, most children with recurrent syncope do not experience spells in the midst of vigorous activity.

ICD-9-CM 780.2

BIBLIOGRAPHY

Batra AS, Hohn AR. Consultation with the specialist: palpitations, syncope, and sudden cardiac death in children: who's at risk? *Pediatr Rev* 2003;24(8):269–275.

Freed MD. Advances in the diagnosis and therapy of syncope and palpitations in children. *Curr Opin Pediatr* 1994;6(4):368–372.

Friedman MJ, Mull CC, Sharieff GQ, Tsarouhas N. Prolonged QT syndrome in children: an uncommon but potentially fatal entity. *J Emerg Med* 2003;24(2):173–179.

Johnsrude CL. Current approach to pediatric syncope. *Pediatr Cardiol* 2000;21(6):522–531.

Kapoor WN. Syncope. *N Engl J Med* 2000;343:1856–1862.

Rodriguez-Nunez A, Fernandez-Cebrian S, Perez-Munuzuri A, Martinon-Torres F, Eiris-Punal J, Martinon-Sanchez JM. Cerebral syncope in children. *J Pediatr* 2000;136(4):542–544.

Author: Nancy Drucker

Synovitis—Transient

 Database

DEFINITION

A transient inflammatory process resulting in arthralgia and arthritis (especially affecting the hip) and occasionally rash precipitated by an exposure to an infectious agent.

CAUSES

Usually viral (especially upper respiratory but also enteroviruses).

PATHOLOGY

A type III hypersensitivity reaction mediated by immune complex deposition within the skin and joint spaces

EPIDEMIOLOGY

Any age at risk, common in ages 3 to 10, with males affected 1.5 times more commonly

GENETICS

No specific associations

COMPLICATIONS

Questionably associated with subsequent avascular necrosis of femoral head and coxa magna

 Differential Diagnosis

- Infection: Lyme, septic, gonorrhea
- Environment: trauma (fracture, or soft tissue injury), slipped capital femoral epiphysis, avascular necrosis
- Tumors: osteoid osteoma
- Immunologic: juvenile rheumatoid arthritis, spondyloarthropathy.
- Psychological: psychogenic limp, imitative limp
- Miscellaneous: hypothyroidism

 Data Gathering

HISTORY

- Exposure to individuals with viral syndromes
- Day care
- Relatively rapid onset of symptoms, with refusal to bear weight, in a nontoxic appearing child
- Recent nonspecific upper respiratory or gastrointestinal infection

 Physical Examination

Finding: General examination usually benign with occasional low-grade fever.
Significance: Child refuses to bear weight but may tolerate limited ranging of joint. Effusions in peripheral joints are usually small and evanescent.

PROCEDURE

Extreme pain and guarding on passive ranging raises suspicion for septic joint.

 Laboratory Aids

Test: CBC
Significance: Usually mild leukocytosis

Test: ESR
Significance: Usually midrange elevation (35 to 50)

IMAGING

Test: Radiography
Significance: Usually normal or demonstrates small effusion; no evidence of periosteal changes

Test: Ultrasound
Significance: Affected hip joints may have demonstrable effusions

Test: MRI
Significance: Normal signal intensity may help differentiate transient synovitis from septic hip.

Test: Joint aspirate culture
Significance: Be wary of contaminated joint aspiration cultures and that up to 50% of infected joints are culture negative.

PITFALLS

Distinctions between this and a septic joint may be impossible.

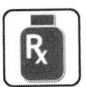 Therapy

DRUGS

• Usually responsive to NSAIDs, such as ibuprofen (up to 10 mg/kg per dose four times a day).
• Very rarely, a short course of oral steroids is necessary.

DURATION

Usually 1 to 3 weeks of a tapering course of NSAIDs is effective.

POSSIBLE CONFLICTS

• Avoid initiation of therapy until septic joint is not in the differential.

 Follow-Up

WHEN TO EXPECT IMPROVEMENT

Usually significant improvement in 24 to 48 hours

SIGNS TO WATCH FOR

Ongoing synovitis despite therapeutic levels of NSAIDs or any bony changes indicates need to change diagnosis.

PROGNOSIS

Excellent, although on occasion patients will experience recurrence of symptoms with subsequent viral syndromes or if there is an underlying spondyloarthropathy.

PITFALLS

Missing a septic hip or, alternatively, overinvestigating transient synovitis with invasive procedures.

 Common Questions and Answers

Q: Are there any chronic sequelae from transient synovitis?
A: Not usually. This is generally a benign disease but there is a questionable association with avascular necrosis of the femoral head.

Q: Is there an association with chronic arthritis?
A: No, there is no known increased risk for chronic arthritis in affected children unless this is the first manifestation of a spondyloarthropathy.

ICD-9-CM 726.90

BIBLIOGRAPHY

Cassidy JT, Petty RE. *Textbook of Pediatric Rheumatology*. 4th Ed. Philadelphia: WB Saunders, 2001.

Del Baccaro MA, Champoux AN, Bockers T, et al. Septic arthritis verus transient synovitis of the hip: the value of screening laboratory tests. *Ann Emerg Med* 1992;21:1418–1422.

Do TT. Transient synovitis as a cause of painful limps in children. *Curr Opin Pediatr* 2000;12:48–51.

Authors: David D. Sherry
Randy Q. Cron, 3rd edition

Syphilis

Database

DEFINITION

Systemic infection caused by the spirochete, *Treponema pallidum*.

Congenital syphilis:
- Transmitted from an infected mother to her unborn or newborn baby.
- Clinical manifestations range from asymptomatic to death or stillbirth.
- Clinical signs include periostitis, osteochondritis, persistent rhinorrhea, maculopapular or
Acquired syphilis:
- Sexually transmitted from an infected to an uninfected individual. Disease becomes a chronic infection via hematogenous spread to ectodermally derived tissues (skin, nervous system, blood vessels).
- Sexual abuse must be considered when syphilis is diagnosed in children.

Stages of Acquired Syphilis

- Primary stage:
—Painless indurated ulcers (chancres), single or multiple, at the site of inoculation about 3 weeks after exposure (range 10 to 90 days); lesions usually resolve without treatment in 3 to 6 weeks.
- Secondary stage:
—Generalized rash, which is often maculopapular and involves the palms and soles
—Condyloma lata, hypertrophic papular lesions
—Fever, malaise, lymphadenopathy
—Signs appear 3 to 6 weeks after initial chancre and may last 2 to 10 weeks
- Relapse:
—Symptoms of secondary syphilis may recur one or more times before the latent period.
- Latent period:
—When left untreated, illness may enter a latent stage; patients are asymptomatic, not contagious; lasts 1 to 40 years or more; patients in this period are seroreactive but there is no other evidence of disease.
—Early latent period: first 4 years of latent period
—Late latent period: subsequent years
- Tertiary stage:
—Up to one-third of those with untreated secondary syphilis may develop tertiary or late disease; this stage can occur many years after the primary infection; may see gummatous changes of the skin, bone, and/or viscera, or cardiovascular syphilis
- Neurosyphilis:
—CNS involvement occurs in 3% to 7% of untreated cases; can develop at any stage of disease; signs include changes in mood/behavior, hyperactive reflexes, impaired memory and/or judgment, and Argyll-Robertson pupils.

COMPLICATIONS

- Stillbirth, spontaneous abortion, perinatal death: 40% of pregnancies in mothers with untreated early syphilis; hydrops fetalis; prematurity; nephrosis; failure to thrive; disseminated intravascular coagulation;

pseudoparalysis of parrot: paralysis of one of the limbs of an infant affected by congenital syphilis and usually unilateral; acute syphilitic leptomeningitis; cranial nerve palsies; hearing loss (e.g., eighth nerve deafness; 10 to 40 years after birth); interstitial keratitis (5 to 20 years after birth); cerebral infarction; seizure disorder; mental retardation; rhagades: cluster of scars radiating around the mouth; mulberry molars: maldevelopment of the cusps in the first molars; clutton joints: painless arthritis of the knees and, rarely, other joints; Hutchinson triad: Hutchinson teeth (notched upper central incisors), interstitial keratitis, eighth nerve deafness; saber shins: anterior bowing of the midportion of the tibia

PROGNOSIS

- The prognosis is better the earlier syphilis is detected and treated. Following appropriate therapy, the disease is usually totally arrested.
- With late findings of syphilis, involving the nervous system and/or cardiovascular system, there may not be clinical improvement.
- Untreated infection in the neonate progresses to neurosyphilis within 1 year.
- Osteochondritis and periostitis in the newborn are usually self-limited and heal in the first 6 months of life.
- Hemolytic anemia seen in congenital syphilis may persist for weeks.

Differential Diagnosis

CONGENITAL SYPHILIS

Infectious

- Herpes simplex virus (HSV); toxoplasmosis; cytomegalovirus; rubella; neonatal hepatitis; osteomyelitis

ACQUIRED SYPHILIS

Infectious

- Chancroid (*Haemophilus ducreyi*); granuloma inguinale (also known as donovanosis; *Calymmatobacterium granulomatis*); Lymphogranuloma venereum (*Chlamydia trachomatis*); scabies; mycotic infections; genital herpes (HSV); venereal warts (human papillomavirus; HPV); scabies; viral exanthem (e.g., enteroviruses may cause a maculopapular rash involving the palms and soles)

Data Gathering

HISTORY

Newborn/Infants

- Always obtain a detailed prenatal history; inquire about all syphilis testing done on the mother; if mother has a history of syphilis, ensure documented treatment; the local department of health should have records on all cases of syphilis.
- Newborns should be evaluated for congenital syphilis if:

—Mother not adequately treated for syphilis
—Mother treated with nonpenicillin regimen, such as erythromycin
—Mother treated adequately but without a fourfold decrease in antibody titers in early or high-titer syphilis
—Maternal syphilis treated less than 1 month (30 days) before delivery
—Maternal syphilis treated prior to pregnancy with insufficient follow-up to assess serologic response to treatment
—Maternal titer has increased fourfold, or if the infant titer is fourfold greater than the mother's titer, or if the infant is symptomatic

Physical Examination

EARLY CONGENITAL SYPHILIS

- Low birth weight; irritability, bulging fontanel, if neurosyphilis is present; alopecia (scalp and eyebrows); fissures in the lips, nares, anus; mucocutaneous lesions; rhinitis ("snuffles") may occur at one to several weeks of age and may be blood-tinged and purulent; lymphadenopathy; pneumonia: check for tachypnea and/or respiratory distress; myocarditis; hepatosplenomegaly with or without jaundice; pseudoparalysis of an extremity; rash: bullous ("syphilitic pemphigus") and/or maculopapular ("blueberry muffin") lesions symmetrically distributed on palms, soles, and other parts of the body; condyloma lata: flat, wart-like, moist lesions around the anus/vagina, chancres

LATE CONGENITAL SYPHILIS

- Bony deformities, such as short maxilla, high-arched palate, saddle nose, mulberry molars, Higoumenakia sign (enlargement of the sternoclavicular portion of the clavicle), protuberance of the mandible, saber shins, scaphoid scapulae
- Rhagades, neurologic involvement

ACQUIRED SYPHILIS

- Primary syphilis: chancre—painless ulcer, single, most commonly located on the genitalia and/or painless; inguinal adenopathy
- Secondary syphilis: may present as flu-like illness—fever, headache, sore throat, nasal discharge, generalized arthralgias and myalgias, malaise, generalized adenopathy (painless and mobile nodes); hepatosplenomegaly; maculopapular rash involving the palms and soles that may involve mucous membranes; condyloma lata (moist, papular lesions); alopecia; signs of meningitis, hepatitis, nephropathy, ocular involvement.

Laboratory Aids

NONTREPONEMAL TESTS

Test: VDRL (Venereal Disease Research Laboratory) or RPR (Rapid Plasma Reagin): measure nonspecific antibodies; RPR more sensitive than VDRL

Significance: used for routine screening; quantitative serum titers generally correlate with disease activity; need to confirm positive results with a treponemal antibody test. Fourfold titer change (e.g., from 1:8 to 1:32) required to document clinically significant change. Titers for different nontreponemal tests are not equivalent; therefore must use same test (and preferably same laboratory) when following serial titers. VDRL/RPR become nonreactive after therapy within 1 year in low-titer (≤1:8) primary syphilis, and within 2 years in secondary and congenital syphilis; tests may remain positive despite therapy ("serofast reaction") in late latent or tertiary syphilis. VDRL (not RPR) used on CSF to rule out neurosyphilis.

TREPONEMAL ANTIBODY TESTS

Tests: FTA-abs (fluorescent treponemal antibody-absorption), TPHA (*T. Pallidum* hemagglutination), MHA-TP (*T. pallidum* antibodies microhemagglutination assay), or EIA (enzyme immunoassay for antitreponemal IgG) Nonquantitative tests which detect antibodies to *T. Pallidum* antigens; used to confirm the diagnosis of syphilis; do not correlate with disease activity; more sensitive and more specific, but more difficult and expensive than nontreponemal tests
Significance: treponemal tests remain positive for life once infected; not useful for measuring treatment effectiveness.

Test: Dark Field Microscopy
Treponemes may be seen on darkfield microscopy of fresh exudate from skin lesions, regional lymph node, placenta, or umbilical cord; or by direct fluorescent antibody staining of acetone-fixed exudate.

Test: Pathology evaluation of the placenta and umbilical cord
Significance: specific fluorescent antitreponemal antibody staining is recommended

Test: CSF analysis
Significance: findings include mononuclear pleocytosis, moderately elevated protein, normal glucose; should be performed in all patients with acquired syphilis of greater than 1 year's duration; in infants, perform when congenital syphilis suspected, if the physical examination is consistent with syphilis, infant titer fourfold greater than that of mother, darkfield or fluorescent antibody test positive on body fluids, and on all children being treated with antibiotics for syphilis. Remember that CSF protein levels in newborns are higher; some are 150 to 200 mg/dL.

RADIOGRAPHIC STUDIES

Test: Long bone plain films
Significance: to rule out metaphyseal osteochondritis and/or diaphyseal periostitis

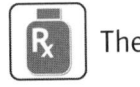 ## Therapy

CONGENITAL SYPHILIS

• Infants <28 days old: Aqueous crystalline penicillin G (50,000 units/kg per dose) IV q

12 hours for first 7 days of life then q 8 hours for a total of 10 days OR Procaine penicillin G (50,000 units/kg per dose) IM q day for 10 days. If more than one day of treatment is missed, must restart 10-day course.
• Infants >28 days old: Aqueous crystalline penicillin G (50,000 units/kg per dose) IV q 6 hours for 10 days

PRIMARY AND SECONDARY SYPHILIS

• Benzathine penicillin G 50,000 U/kg IM (max 2.4 million units) single dose
• Doxycycline 100 mg orally bid OR tetracycline 500 mg orally qid for 14 days for nonpregnant patients allergic to penicillin.
• Less well-studied regimens include ceftriaxone 1gm IM/IV q day for 8 to 10 days OR azithromycin 2 gm PO as a single dose.

EARLY LATENT SYPHILIS (<1 YEAR DURATION)

• Benzathine penicillin G 50,000 U/kg IM (max 2.4 million units) single dose
• Doxycycline 100 mg orally bid OR tetracycline 500 mg orally qid for 14 days for nonpregnant patients allergic to penicillin.

LATE LATENT SYPHILIS OR DISEASE OF UNKNOWN DURATION

• Benzathine penicillin G 50,000 U/kg IM (max 2.4 million units) weekly for 3 consecutive weeks
• Doxycycline 100 mg orally bid OR tetracycline 500 mg orally qid for 4 weeks for nonpregnant patients allergic to penicillin.

TERTIARY SYPHILIS (WITH NO EVIDENCE OF NEUROSYPHILIS)

• Benzathine penicillin G 50,000 U/kg IM (max 2.4 million units) weekly for 3 consecutive weeks

 ## Follow-Up

• Congenital syphilis: Clinical follow-up and serial nontreponemal serologic testing every 2 to 3 months until titer decreases fourfold or test is nonreactive. After adequate treatment, nontreponemal tests should be nonreactive after 6 months; infants with a history of abnormal CSF findings need serial CSF analyses every 6 months until CSF is normal. Infants born to positive mothers, follow-up at 1, 2, 3, 6, and 12 months of age; serologic tests should be performed 3, 6, and 12 months after therapy until they become nonreactive. If titers have not shown a decline by 3 months, retreatment should be considered.
• Primary and secondary syphilis: Clinical follow-up and serial nontreponemal titers at 6 and 12 months posttreatment (more often, if at high risk for reinfection or treatment failure); because it can be difficult to distinguish reinfection from treatment failure, CSF analysis should be considered to rule out neurosyphilis. Nontreponemal titers should drop fourfold within 6 months of treatment of

primary or secondary syphilis, and within 12 to 24 months after treatment of latent or tertiary syphilis.
Latent syphilis: follow the above, but obtain titers at 6, 12 and 24 months posttreatment.

PITFALLS

• All cases should be reported to the local department of (public) health.
• Mothers of infants with congenital syphilis should also be tested for gonorrhea, chlamydia, HIV, and hepatitis B infection.
• In newborns, cord blood testing may result in false-positive nontreponemal tests (from contamination with Wharton jelly) or false-negative results; therefore, serum from the infant is the preferred source of testing.
• False-positive nontreponemal test results may be seen with lab error, autoimmune disease, tuberculosis, lymphoma, viral infections (e.g., EBV, hepatitis, varicella, HIV, and measles), endocarditis, malaria, and intravenous drug abuse .
• False-positive treponemal tests may be seen in other spirochetal diseases (e.g., Lyme disease, leptospirosis), and rarely in autoimmune disease (e.g., SLE) and viral infections.

 ## Common Questions and Answers

Q: Can an infant have congenital syphilis if the mother had a negative VDRL during pregnancy?
A: A mother with a negative VDRL during pregnancy may have acquired syphilis late in pregnancy and transmitted it to her fetus. If the mother was not tested at delivery, then the diagnosis may have been missed

Q: What is the prozone phenomenon?
A: When a nontreponemal test is falsely negative as a result of high concentrations of antibody to *T. pallidum*, diluting the serum will result in positive test results.

Q: What is a Jarisch-Herxheimer reaction?
A: An acute febrile reaction (often accompanied by headache and myalgia) that can occur within the first 24 hours after syphilis treatment, but most often among patients with early syphilis.

ICD-9-CM 079.9

BIBLIOGRAPHY

Centers for Disease Control and Prevention. Congenital syphilis—United States, 2000. *MMWR Morb Mortal Wkly Rep* 2001;50: 573–577.

Centers for Disease Control and Prevention. Primary and secondary syphilis—United States, 2002. *MMWR Morb Mortal Wkly Rep* 2003;52:1117–1120.

Sanchez PJ. Laboratory tests for congenital syphilis. *Pediatr Infect Dis J* 1998;17:70–71.

Authors: Esther K. Chung and Ann B. Bruner

Tapeworm

Database

CAUSES

- *Taenia saginata* (beef tapeworm)
- *Taenia solium* (pork tapeworm)
- *Diphyllobothrium latum* (fish tapeworm)
- *Dipylidium caninum* (dog tapeworm)
- *Echinococcus granulosus*

PATHOLOGY

- Tapeworms cause two major types of zoonotic disease syndromes depending on whether humans are the definitive or intermediate host.
- When humans serve as definitive hosts, adult tapeworms infect the gastrointestinal (GI) tract and interfere with nutrition. These infections are often asymptomatic.
- When humans serve as intermediate hosts for the larval cestode, serious pathology results.

PATHOPHYSIOLOGY

- Beef tapeworm: Cattle (intermediate host) ingest the eggs of *T. saginata* in contaminated feeds. The eggs hatch, releasing embryos. The embryos penetrate the intestinal mucosa, enter the bloodstream, and settle in various tissues where they develop into larvae. Larvae in undercooked meat are consumed by humans and mature into adult tapeworms within the human (definitive host) GI tract. They grow up to 25 m in length.
- Pork tapeworm: Humans are the only definitive host for the adult pork tapeworm, whereas both humans and pigs are intermediate hosts for its embryonic form, cysticercus.

—Pig (intermediate host) ingests *T. solium* eggs. In the intestine, the eggs release embryos that penetrate the mucosa, enter the bloodstream, and settle in various tissues to differentiate into cysticerci (infective larvae). Cysticerci are ingested by humans (definitive host) consuming undercooked pork in which they mature into adult worms in the small intestine. These adult worms can reach a length of 2 to 7 m.
—Humans (intermediate host) ingest food contaminated with human feces containing *T. solium* eggs. The eggs hatch, liberating embryos (oncospheres). Penetration through the intestinal mucosa leads to blood-borne distribution to the brain, subcutaneous tissues, muscle, and eye, in which they develop into cysticerci.

- Fish tapeworm: When sewage containing *D. latum* eggs contaminates freshwater lakes and streams, larvae hatch into the water. These larvae are eaten by crustaceans and fish. Humans are infected when they consume these undercooked fish. The larvae mature into adult tapeworms in the intestines of humans.
- Dog tapeworm: Larvae develop in fleas (intermediate host) after ingestion of the eggs; humans infected through accidental ingestion of infected fleas.

- Echinococcosis (hydatid disease): Humans ingest eggs of *E. granulosus* through contaminated dog feces. After ingestion, the eggs hatch and release embryos (oncospheres) in the small intestine. Penetration through the mucosa leads to blood-borne distribution to the liver, lungs, and other sites, in which development of cysts begins. Within the cysts, new larvae (scolices) develop, accumulate fluid, and encroach on surrounding structures.

EPIDEMIOLOGY

- Beef tapeworm: Widespread in cattle-breeding areas of the world, with a prevalence of >10% in areas of Africa, such as Ethiopia and Kenya, and the former Soviet Union.
- Pork tapeworm: Cysticercosis has a high prevalence in developing areas of Central and South America. In the United States, immigrants account for >90% of cases.
- Fish tapeworm: Infection is most prevalent in populations who consume undercooked fish. In the United States, infected salmon have been implicated in most cases.
- Dog tapeworm: Found in dogs and cats worldwide.
- Echinococcosis: Associated with the practice of feeding sheep viscera to dogs. It is hyperendemic in sheep-raising areas of South America, Australia, and areas of Africa. Also seen in China, central Asia, and the western United States.

COMPLICATIONS

- Cysticercosis: Cysticerci develop in the brain, muscle, eye, or other organs.
- Echinococcosis: Cysts grow slowly, causing symptoms only when they are relatively large. They frequently develop in the liver (50% to 70%) and lung (20% to 30%); 5% to 10% of cysts involve other organs, including the eye, brain, spleen, heart, bone, and kidneys.

—Spontaneous rupture of cysts can cause anaphylaxis.
—Pulmonary lesions cause cough and hemoptysis.
—Bone involvement leads to pathologic fractures.
—Renal involvement can lead to pain and hematuria.

Differential Diagnosis

- Tapeworm infections should be considered in all cases of diarrhea and abdominal pain.
- Larval infection should be considered in individuals with cystic end-organ disease.
- Abdominal pain, anemia, and vitamin B12 deficiency can be seen with fish tapeworm infections, Crohn disease, and intestinal bacterial overgrowth.
- Echinococcal cysts must be differentiated from benign cysts, cavitary tuberculosis, abscesses, and neoplasms.

Data Gathering

HISTORY

Question: Recent travel or immigration?
Significance: Tapeworm infections are more prevalent in other countries.

Question: GI tract complaints?
Significance: Symptoms related to the GI tract include nausea, weight loss, diarrhea, abdominal pain, and intestinal obstruction.

Question: Respiratory tract symptoms?
Significance: Rupture of a pulmonary hydatid cyst as a result of *E. granulosus* causes cough, dyspnea, and hemoptysis.

Question: Partial or generalized seizures?
Significance: New onset seizures are a typical manifestation of neurocysticercosis and some species of Echinococcus. CNS symptoms in neurocysticercosis typically appear 5 to 7 years after initial infection (range, 6 months to 30 years).

Physical Examination

Finding: Pallor
Significance: Signs of anemia secondary to vitamin B12 deficiency can be seen in 2% of fish tapeworm infections. Other signs of pernicious anemia include glossitis, peripheral neuropathy, decreased vibration sense, and ataxia.

Finding: Jaundice
Significance: Hepatic cysts from echinococcosis may be palpable in the right upper quadrant (RUQ); biliary tree extension can lead to obstructive jaundice and cholangitis.

Finding: Cough, wheeze, or signs of respiratory distress
Significance: Rupture of hydatid cysts in echinococcosis can cause an immediate hypersensitivity syndrome or anaphylaxis.

Finding: Abdominal tenderness or dissention
Significance: Fish tapeworm and, rarely, dog tapeworm infections can be complicated by intestinal obstruction.

Finding: Alteration in mental status, signs of elevated intracranial pressure or meningitis
Significance: Neurocysticercosis may present with the above findings. Both neurocysticercosis and vitamin B12 deficiency as a result of fish tapeworm can simulate a psychotic illness with delirium or hallucinations.

Finding: Proglottids in stool
Significance: In dog tapeworm infections, stool examination reveals proglottids that resemble rice or seeds.

Tapeworm

 Laboratory Aids

Test: Beef tapeworm
Significance: Identification of scolex in stool; Ziehl-Neelsen stain of stool or perianal adhesive tape preparations identifies eggs; collection of proglottids in saline with microscopic examination; ELISA test detects *Taenia* antigens in stool.

Test: Pork tapeworm
Significance: ELISA test and immunoblot in combination for parenchymal cysticercosis; stool samples for intestinal worms as for beef tapeworm. Contrast-enhanced CT or MRI of the brain may reveal cysticerci with surrounding edema, granuloma, or calcification.

Test: Fish tapeworm
Significance: Stool samples for eggs and proglottids are diagnostic. Mild eosinophilia (5% to 15%) may be present. Fifty percent of patients have low vitamin B12 levels, 2% have megaloblastic anemia.

Test: Dog tapeworm
Significance: Characteristic egg packets (loose membrane containing up to 20 eggs) may be identified in stool or perianal adhesive tape preparations.

Test: Echinococcosis
Significance: The diagnosis is usually suspected on the basis of clinical or radiologic findings plus a history of residence in an endemic area.

—IgE levels are elevated. Eosinophilia is present in <25% of infected persons. Mild elevation of hepatic enzymes may be present with hepatic hydatid cysts.
—On radiograph, pulmonary cysts demonstrate a sharply demarcated, smooth-bordered cyst; there is a crescent-shaped air level after cyst rupture. Liver and spleen lesions may calcify but only over many years.
—The Casoni skin test (injection of hydatid fluid into the dermis) yields an erythematous papule in <60 minutes in 50% to 80% of infected patients. There is a false-positive result in 30% of uninfected patients.
—Serologic testing is falsely negative in 10% to 50% of cases. False-negative results are more likely in patients with pulmonary hydatid cysts and in children. No current serologic test excludes the diagnosis of hydatid cysts.
—In seronegative persons, a presumptive diagnosis can be confirmed by demonstrating protoscolices or hydatid membranes in the liquid obtained from percutaneous aspiration of the cyst under ultrasound guidance. This procedure is controversial as a result of the risk of anaphylaxis if rupture occurs during aspiration.
—Demonstration of internal septa or daughter cysts (after cyst rupture) by CT, MRI, or ultrasound indicates hydatid cysts. Such findings are present in approximately 50% of patients with unilocular liver cysts.

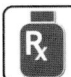 Therapy

• Beef tapeworm:

—Praziquantel: 5 to 10 mg/kg as a single dose; no safety profile exists for children under the age of 4.
—Alternative: Niclosamide: children 11 to 34 kg, 1 g as a single dose; children >34 kg, 1.5 g as a single dose (not available in United States).

• Pork tapeworm:

—Intestinal disease: praziquantel: 5 to 10 mg/kg as a single dose
—Neurocysticercosis: albendazole: 15 mg/kg/day (max. 800 mg/day) in two divided doses for 28 days

Alternative or if albendazole results in only partial response: praziquantel: 50 mg/kg per day in three divided doses for 14 days. Dexamethasone should be given 2 days before cysticidal therapy and continued for a total of 5 to 7 days to decrease the cerebral edema that accompanies release of larval antigens during cysticidal therapy. Anticonvulsant therapy may be required.

• Fish tapeworm: Same as in beef tapeworm. Additionally, supplement with vitamin B12.
• Dog tapeworm: Same as in beef tapeworm.
• Echinococcosis:

—Surgical resection of intact hydatid cysts, especially if >10 cm or secondarily infected.
—Albendazole 15 mg/kg per day (max. 800 mg/day) in two divided doses for 28 days, may require up to three courses of therapy with drug-free intervals of 14 days between courses.

Note: The benzimidazoles, including albendazole, are contraindicated in patients with blood dyscrasias, leukopenia, and liver disease. Prolonged courses require monitoring of liver function and hematopoiesis.
Note: Dexamethasone lowers plasma levels of praziquantel by as much as 50% but raises the level of albendazole by 50%.

PREVENTION

• Adult tapeworms: In general, avoiding contamination of food and drink with human or animal feces. Proper cooking of meat and fish prevents transmission of beef, pork, and fish tapeworms.
• Pork tapeworm: The refrigeration of pork infested with cysticerci at temperatures above 0°C does not affect parasite survival. However, storage of pork for 4 days at −5°C or 1 day at −24°C kills most cysticerci.
• Fish tapeworm: Brief cooking (≥56°C for 5 minutes) or freezing (−18°C for 24 hours) renders the fish safe for consumption.
• Dog tapeworm: Veterinary care of pet with periodic deworming prevents infections.
• Echinococcosis: Control measures can interrupt the life cycle of *E. granulosus* as the cestode moves between sheep and carnivore hosts. Measures include careful disposal of sheep viscera and mass chemotherapy of dogs.

 Follow-Up

• Beef tapeworm: Stool should be checked for eggs and proglottids 1 month after completion of therapy.
• Pork tapeworm: Repeat CNS imaging studies at 2-month intervals (with continued therapy) until successful elimination of parenchymal brain cysticerci.
• Fish tapeworm: Perform stool examination 6 weeks after therapy to test for cure.
• Dog tapeworm: No follow-up stool examination required, but the appearance of proglottids >1 week after therapy indicates treatment failure.
• Echinococcosis: Requires prolonged follow-up with ultrasound or other imaging procedures, depending on the extent and location of the cysts.

 Common Questions and Answers

Q: Can vegetarians develop neurocysticercosis?
A: Yes, because neurocysticercosis results from ingestion of *T. solium* eggs in products contaminated with infected fecal matter. Only gastrointestinal symptoms result from consumption of infected pork.

Q: Is treatment for neurocysticercosis always indicated?
A: The findings are controversial. In many children, the lesion disappears spontaneously within 2 or 3 months. Some studies suggest that a 28-day course of albendazole, even in children whose lesions appear to harbor a dying parasite (edema surrounding the lesion), may lead to a reduction in late seizure recurrences.

ICD-9-CM 123.9

BIBLIOGRAPHY

Anonymous. Drugs for parasitic infections. *Med Lett Drugs Ther* 1998;40:1–12.

Baranwal AK, Singhi PD, Khandelwal N, et al. Albendazone Therapy in children with focal sezures and single small enhancing compalerzed tomographic lesions: a randomized, placebo-controlled double blend trial *Pediatr Infect Dis J* 1998;17:696–700.

Bruckner DA. Helminthic food-borne infections. *Clin Lab Med* 1999;19:639–660.

Garcia HH, Gonzalez AE, Gilman RH. Cysticerosis Working Group in Peru. Diagnosis, treatment and control of Taenia solium cysticercosis. *Curr Opin Infect Dis* 2003;16(5):411–419.

Kalra V, et al. Efficacy of albendazole and short-course dexamethasone treatment in children with 1 or 2 ring-enhancing lesionsof neurocysticercosis: a randomized controlled trial. *J Pediatr* 2003;143:111–114.

Author: Samir S. Shah

831

Tendonitis

 Database

DEFINITION

Inflammation of a tendon or along the tendon sheath

CAUSES

Frequently associated with repetitive motion/overuse activities

PATHOLOGY

Inflammation and microtearing may be present.

EPIDEMIOLOGY

Increases with age and at time of puberty. It may be slightly more common in girls.

GENETICS

Hypermobile individuals may be prone to tendonitis.

COMPLICATIONS

Ongoing pain and predisposition for recurrence

 Differential Diagnosis

- Infection: especially gonococcal disease, septic arthritis, or osteomyelitis
- Environmental: fracture
- Metabolic: homocystinuria
- Congenital: generalized hypermobility, Marfan syndrome, Ehlers-Danlos
- Immunologic: ankylosing spondylitis and the reactive spondyloarthropathies (inflammatory bowel disease, Reiter syndrome), inflammatory arthritides
- Psychological: amplified musculoskeletal pain

 Data Gathering

HISTORY

Question: Trauma or overuse?
Significance: Verify acute nature of injury.

 Physical Examination

Question: Any evidence of hematoma?
Significance: Palpate around and about affected areas, detecting point tenderness especially at tendon insertions and over bony prominences.

Question: Any evidence of bursitis or arthritis?
Significance: Systemic conditions such as spondyloarthropathy can lead to inflammation of tendons, bursa, and joints, and bursitis can mimic the pain of tendonitis.

SPECIAL QUESTIONS

Question: Was a pop or snap felt at the time of the event?
Significance: Sometimes this is felt when tendons and ligaments are torn or avulsed.

 Laboratory Aids

Test: ESR
Significance: Occasionally, an ESR will be helpful to rule out inflammatory conditions if history and/or physical examination are suggestive.

IMAGING

Test: Plain radiograph
Significance: Affected area may be indicated to rule out a fracture, avulsion or identify a bone spur.

FALSE POSITIVES

Patients may have torn ligaments, fractures, or arthritis, not just tendonitis on examination.

Therapy

Rest/reduced use of the affected tendon/muscle group is essential, occasionally requiring splinting

PT/OT

Either self-directed or formal help with resumption of desired activity, through gentle range of motion exercises against low resistance and advanced as tolerated

DRUGS

Nonsteroidal antiinflammatory drugs; rarely do soft tissue steroid injections have a role in children.

DURATION

One to 4 weeks

Follow-Up

WHEN TO EXPECT IMPROVEMENT

Improvement often takes 2 to 6 weeks.

SIGNS TO WATCH FOR

If the provocative activity is resumed too soon, the irritation will recur.

PROGNOSIS

Usually good for children; however, many will suffer recurrences if proper exercises before desired activity are not continued.

PITFALLS

Overdiagnosis in young children, in whom overuse is rare and other diagnoses should be considered; underdiagnosis in older children in whom repetitive activities are likely to occur.

Common Question and Answer

Q: Which activities can result in overuse syndromes and tendonitis?
A: Virtually any repetitive activity in which children engage can cause tendonitis. For example, pain in the tendons of the thumb has occurred in children overusing video games.

ICD-9-CM 726.90

BIBLIOGRAPHY

Almekinders LC, Temple JD. Etiology, diagnosis, and treatment of tendonitis: an analysis of the literature. *Med Sci Sports Exerc* 1998;30:1183–1190.

Athreya BH, Cheh ML, Kingsland LC 3rd. Computer assisted diagnosis of pediatric rheumatic disease. *Pediatrics* 1998;102(4):E48.

Marsh JS, Daigneault JP. Ankle injuries in the pediatric population. *Curr Opin Pediatr* 2000;12(1):52–60.

Micheli LJ, Fehlandt AF. Overuse injuries to tendons and apophyses in children and adolescents. *Clin Sports Med* 1992;11:713–726.

Authors: David D. Sherry, and Randy Q. Cron, 3rd edition

Teratoma

Database

DEFINITION

An embryonal neoplasm that contains tissue derived from all three germ layers (endoderm, mesoderm, and ectoderm). Teratomas are mature or immature and may occur with or without malignant elements. They are a subset of the broader class of germ cell tumors.

PATHOPHYSIOLOGY

- Abnormal migration of germ cells at about the sixth week of embryonal development, causing germ cells to come to rest outside the gonads.
- Mature teratoma: contains well-differentiated, nonmitotic tissues from all three germ layers, such as squamous epithelium, neuronal tissue, muscle, teeth, cartilage, bone, gastrointestinal, and respiratory tract linings.
- Immature teratoma: contains only immature embryonic components of the three germinal layers.
- Divided histologically into four grades, 0 to 3, dependent on immature elements and mitotic activity.
- Teratoma with malignant germ cell elements: foci of malignant tissue that resemble other germ cell tumors such as embryonal carcinoma, endodermal sinus tumor, and choriocarcinoma, in addition to mature or immature tissues.

EPIDEMIOLOGY

- Germ cell tumors account for approximately 3% of childhood malignancies (<15 years) and 15% of malignancies of ages 15 to 19 years.
- Incidence of germ cell tumors as a whole is approximately 2.5 per million in White children and 3.0 per million in Black children under 15 years of age.
- Males and females are equally affected.
- One suggestive epidemiologic association is with high maternal hormone levels during pregnancy.
- More controversial associations include younger gestational age; viral infections including HSV, VZV, CMV, mumps; other congenital anomalies; maternal UTI or tuberculosis; paternal occupation in chemical industries.
- Sacrococcygeal tumors: Most prevalent in infants; females more frequently affected
- Testicular and ovarian tumors: most prevalent in infants and adolescents
- Vaginal tumors: most prevalent in girls under age 3 years
- Mediastinal tumors: average age of the pediatric patient is 3 years, but also found in adolescents; most common extragonadal germ cell tumor in adults

GENETICS

- Most consistent (80% of germ cell tumors) structural chromosomal abnormality is an isochromosome 12p [i(12p)]
- No pattern of inheritance is known.

Differential Diagnosis

- Sacrococcygeal: pilonidal cyst, meningocele, lipomeningocele, hemangioma, abscess, bone tumor, epidermal cyst, chondroma, lymphoma, ependymoma, neuroblastoma, glioma
- Abdominal: Wilms tumor, neuroblastoma, lymphoma, rhabdomyosarcoma, hepatoblastoma, retained twin fetus
- Vaginal: rhabdomyosarcoma (sarcoma botryoides), clear cell carcinoma
- Ovarian: cyst, appendicitis, pregnancy, pelvic infection, hematocolpos, sarcoma, lymphoma, other ovarian tumors
- Testicular: epididymitis, testicular torsion, infarct, orchitis, hernia, hydrocele, hematocele, rhabdomyosarcoma, lymphoma, leukemia, other testicular tumors
- Mediastinal: Hodgkin and non-Hodgkin lymphoma, leukemia, thymoma

Data Gathering

HISTORY

Question: External mass, constipation, urinary abnormalities, lower extremity weakness?
Significance: Sacrococcygeal mass may impinge on nerve structures. Anterior sacrococcygeal mass may have no external component.

Question: Cough, wheeze, dyspnea, hemoptysis, SVC syndrome?
Significance: Suggests anterior mediastinal mass

Question: Blood-tinged vaginal discharge?
Significance: Vaginal teratoma

Question: Abdominal pain, nausea, vomiting, constipation, urinary tract symptoms?
Significance: Ovarian tumors present late with a large mass.

Question: Painless scrotal swelling or painful testicular torsion?
Significance: Testicular mass may be teratoma

Question: Cryptorchidism?
Significance: Associated with germ cell tumors in boys

Physical Examination

Finding: Palpable mass either externally or internally, signs of spinal cord compression?
Significance: Sacrococcygeal tumor

Finding: Vaginoscopy reveals a polyploid lesion arising from the vaginal wall?
Significance: Examination under anesthesia usually necessary

Finding: Palpable abdominal mass, peritoneal symptoms?
Significance: Ovarian mass may be large

Finding: Palpable mass in scrotum?
Significance: Testicular origin

Finding: Decreased breath sounds, consolidation, wheezing, SVC syndrome?
Significance: Mediastinal mass may be an emergency

Laboratory Aids

Test: Serum α-fetoprotein (AFP) and β-human chorionic gonadotropin (β-hCG)
Significance: Pure teratomas are not associated with elevated tumor markers. The elevation of either of these markers indicates the presence of more malignant germ cell elements and requires review of the histologic material.

Test: CBC and chemistry profile, with electrolytes, blood urea nitrogen, creatinine, liver function tests, uric acid, and lactate dehydrogenase
Significance: Workup to rule out other malignancies or associated organ dysfunction

IMAGING

Test: Plain x-ray
Significance: May reveal mature calcified tissues, such as bone or teeth, within the tumor

Test: Chest radiograph
Significance: Shows mediastinal mass

Test: CT scan
Significance: Necessary to evaluate the primary site and regional disease

Test: Chest CT and bone scan
Significance: If malignancy is suspected or proven, these are indicated for evaluation of metastasis.

Test: Ultrasound, if CT is not readily available
Significance: May be helpful, but it will rarely suffice as the sole imaging study of the primary site. May be first evidence of anterior sacrococcygeal mass or to differentiate testicular mass from hydrocele.

Teratoma

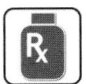

Therapy

- Mature teratoma: full surgical excision, irrespective of the site, is curative.
- Immature teratoma: complete surgical resection is the therapy of choice. In cases of elevated α-fetoprotein, many suggest a short course of postoperative adjuvant chemotherapy.
- Teratoma with malignant components: surgery plus chemotherapy with etoposide, cisplatin or carboplatin, and bleomycin. Patients with residual disease should have additional surgery and additional chemotherapy if total resection not possible. Radiation is reserved for salvage therapy in recurrent disease.

Follow-Up

- Serial physical exams and imaging studies of primary site
- Tumor markers (AFP or β-hCG), if elevated at diagnosis
- If chemotherapy or radiation therapy utilized, need to monitor for secondary malignancies, long term. Short term, need to monitor blood counts, chemistries, renal function, and audiology.

PREVENTION

There is no known prevention for the development of teratomas and other germ cell tumors.

PITFALLS

All that appears to be a teratoma is not. Be prepared for other malignant and nonmalignant histologies on biopsy.

Common Questions and Answers

Q: What is the chance of cure for malignant teratomas?
A: With current chemotherapy as outlined above, disease-free survival is 85%.

Q: Can a benign tumor recur? If so, can it then be malignant?
A: Yes. If there is residual tissue left behind, the tumor can recur. If there were unrecognized areas of malignancy, the recurrence can be a malignant teratoma. The greatest risk for the latter is with the immature teratomas.

ICD-9-CM

Benign 186.9
Sacral 653.7

BIBLIOGRAPHY

Adzick NS, Kitano Y. Fetal surgery for lung lesions, congenital diaphragmatic hernia, and sacrococcygeal teratoma. *Sem Pediatr Surg* 2003;12:154–167.

Allen MS. Presentation and management of benign mediastinal teratomas. *Chest Surg Clin North Am* 2002;12:659–664.

Gobel U, Calaminus G, Engert J, et al. Teratomas in infancy and childhood. *Med Pediatr Oncol* 1998;31:8–15.

Lazar EL, Stolar CJ. Evaluation and management of pediatric solid ovarian tumors. *Semin Pediatr Surg* 1998;7:29–34.

Walsh C, Rushton HG. Diagnosis and management of teratomas and epidermoid cysts. *Urol Clin North Am* 2000;27:509–518.

Weidner N. Germ-cell tumors of the mediastinum. *Semin Diagn Pathol* 1999;16:42–50.

Author: Jane E. Minturn

Tetanus

 Database

DEFINITION

Tetanus is a disease characterized by tonic spasms of the skeletal muscles and occasionally the glottis and larynx as a result of intoxication with an exotoxin tetanospasmin produced by *Clostridium tetani*.

CAUSE

• Tetanus is caused by an anaerobic, spore-forming bacterium, *C. tetani*. In anaerobic conditions, present in wounds with significant tissue damage, inoculated spores become vegetative and produce the disease-causing toxin.
• *C. tetani* is a gram-positive rod found in superficial layers of soil, especially in agricultural areas. Spores may survive in soil for months to years if not exposed to sunlight.
• *C. tetani* spores are found as part of the normal intestinal flora in many domesticated animals, rats, and humans.

PATHOPHYSIOLOGY

• Anaerobic conditions in wounds are promoted by larger amounts of necrosis, the presence of foreign bodies, or other ongoing infections with suppuration.
• *C. tetani* produces two exotoxins, but only tetanospasmin is clinically important.
• Tetanospasmin is one of the most powerful exotoxins known, second in lethality only to botulinum toxin. It seems to travel from the wound site to the central nervous system (CNS) through the neurons.
• The toxin may be absorbed directly into skeletal muscle adjacent to the injury and affects the motor end plates, producing sustained contractions in that area, a condition known as local tetanus.
• Once absorbed into peripheral nerves, the toxin is carried to the CNS
• The toxin has four major effects on the nervous system. At motor end plates in skeletal muscle release of acetylcholine from neurons is inhibited. Toxin also seems to interfere with contraction and relaxation mechanisms directly. In the spinal cord action on interneurons leads to inhibition of antagonist mechanisms and uncontrolled muscle spasms result. In the brain there is also an inhibition of antagonist mechanisms leading to uncontrolled spasms. The toxin also binds to receptors in the medullary center and can lead to direct respiratory depression. Finally, the sympathetic nervous system seems to be affected, leading to profuse sweating, vasoconstriction, labile hypertension, tachycardia, and dysrhythmias, and later hypotension.
• Tetanospasmin does not seem to affect cognitive processes directly. "Tetanic seizures" are actually uncontrolled, generalized tetanic muscle spasms.
• The toxin binds irreversibly to neurons and resolution occurs slowly over 2 to 4 weeks.

• Secondary complications may be associated with findings including pneumonia (often secondary to aspiration), pulmonary hemorrhage, CNS hemorrhage, and fractures, including vertebral body compressions related to the severe tetanic spasms.

EPIDEMIOLOGY

• Tetanus, especially neonatal tetanus, remains a major problem in developing countries but is rare in the developed world because of widespread immunization. In the United States, there are 50 to 200 cases reported annually including occasional cases of neonatal tetanus. About 50% of cases in the United States occur after injuries. Most cases are among the elderly but unimmunized children are also at risk. Rare cases have been reported in patients with seemingly protective levels of antitetanus antibodies.

COMPLICATIONS

• Most complications are related to the severe tetanic muscle contractions experienced by these patients.
• Severe spasm of the paraspinal muscles has led to compression fractures of vertebral bodies.
• Other bones may be broken as well, and muscle hemorrhages are not uncommon. Spasm of the chest wall and laryngospasm may precipitate respiratory failure and arrest. Spasms cause severe pain for patients.
• Spasms also cause dysphagia, hydrophobia, neck stiffness, and urinary retention.
• Repeated or continuous spasms may lead to elevations in body temperature.
• Cerebrovascular hemorrhages may be seen in rare cases, especially in neonatal tetanus.
• Pneumonia, including aspiration, may be a complication.

PROGNOSIS

• With advances in the ability to provide respiratory support in an intensive care setting, the prognosis has improved significantly. Overall mortality rates have decreased from approximately 66% in the 1950s in the United States to 30% in the 1980s.
• Children and young adults have a much better prognosis than older individuals.
• In developing nations, mortality rates remain very high, reflecting an inability to provide technologically advanced tertiary care.
• A more rapid onset of disease and a more rapid progression from trismus to generalized spasms is associated with a more severe course.
• In the absence of complications, recovery is usually complete in survivors without long-term sequelae.
• Signs and symptoms usually progress for about 1 week after presentation before reaching their worst. The patient's condition then plateaus for about 1 week and then gradually improves over 2 to 6 weeks.

 Differential Diagnosis

• Infections: retropharyngeal and peritonsillar abscesses, poliomyelitis, viral encephalitis, and meningoencephalitis may present with trismus or cranial nerve findings that would suggest a diagnosis of tetanus.
• Toxin: dystonic reactions to phenothiazine medications may resemble tetanus in presentation.
• Diphenhydramine will effectively treat these reactions.
• Metabolic: hypocalcemia as a result of rickets or other disorders is usually not as severe as the tetanic contractions seen with tetanus.

 Data Gathering

HISTORY

Question: Incubation period?
Significance: Usually between 3 and 21 days. Cases have been reported with shorter periods, and at times it may be as long as several months. Sites of inoculation farther from the CNS are associated with longer incubation periods.

Question: Pain?
Significance: Local tetanus is associated with painful muscle contractions and stiffness limited to the area near the wound. This may persist for several weeks and resolve, or it may progress to generalized tetanus.

Question: Trismus?
Significance: The classic initial complaint of trismus is seen in about half of cases. Other early complaints include dysphagia, neck pain and stiffness, stiffness and pain in other muscle groups, urinary retention, restlessness, irritability, and headache.

Question: Progression of symptoms?
Significance: Usually occur over the first week but may progress more rapidly.

Question: Neonatal tetanus?
Significance: Usually complicates deliveries in which aseptic conditions were not maintained, and the mother is either unimmunized or not up to date in her immunization status.

 Physical Examination

Finding: Initial presenting sign is usually trismus.
Significance: Persistent trismus gives rise to the classic sardonic smile (wrinkling of the forehead and distortion of the eyebrows and the corners of the mouth).

Finding: Fever?
Significance: Initially, patients are usually afebrile.

Finding: As the disease progresses, other muscle groups develop tetanic contractions. *Significance:* Tonic contractions of the paraspinal muscles lead to a significant opisthotonic posture. Severe spasmodic contractions, "tetanic seizures," also occur. These are extremely painful and can be associated with laryngospasm and tetany of the respiratory musculature with fatal results.

Finding: Tetanus spasms *Significance:* Precipitated by a variety of stimuli including a cold draft, noise, pain, anxiety, and light touch. Because tetanus toxin does not affect the sensorium, the severe anxiety and pain associated with these spasms may precipitate additional spasms.

Finding: Tachycardia, flushing, severe and labile episodes of hypertension and tachycardia *Significance:* Autonomic nervous system involvement. Hypotension may be a late feature of the disease.

Finding: Fever *Significance:* With sustained contractions, fever may develop, although it may also be a result of complications including pneumonia, infected in-dwelling catheters, or infected decubiti.

Finding: Cephalic tetanus *Significance:* Involves only the cranial nerves and occurs after wounds of the face, scalp, or neck. It may also complicate chronic infections of the head and neck including chronic otitis media. Loss of airway control is a frequent and often fatal complication. Cephalic tetanus may progress to generalized tetanus.

 ## Laboratory Aids

Test: Laboratory investigations *Significance:* Yield little useful information in cases of tetanus. Anaerobic wound cultures may rarely yield *C. tetani*. The WBC is usually normal or mildly elevated. CSF studies are unremarkable. EEG and EMG are nonspecific. The diagnosis is made clinically.

 ## Emergency Care

- It is important to recognize the presentation of tetanus so that emergency care may be begun promptly.
- In the emergency department, supportive care including aggressive airway management (including tracheostomy when indicated), ventilatory support, and pharmacologic interventions to promote sedation and muscle relaxation (e.g., diazepam) are the most important therapies.
- Treatment with tetanus immune globulin should be initiated.

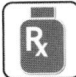 ## Therapy

SPECIFIC

- Specific therapy is aimed at eradication of the vegetative organism and thereby the source of ongoing toxin production and neutralization of any toxin that has not already been irreversibly bound to neurons.
- Human tetanus immune globulin (TIG) should be administered in a dose of 500 to 3,000 units in three divided doses at three separate sites. Repeat doses do not seem to be indicated. Infants with neonatal tetanus should be given a dose of 250 units.
- If TIG is not available, tetanus antitoxin (TAT) may be administered if a skin test for sensitization to this equine-derived product is negative. If the skin test is positive, desensitization must be accomplished before TAT can be administered. The dose of TAT is 50,000 to 100,000 units with half given intramuscularly and half intravenously.
- Penicillin G, 200,000 U/kg per day should be given intravenously in four divided doses for 10 days. Oral tetracycline or intravenous vancomycin may be used in penicillin-sensitive individuals. Cephalosporins are not effective.
- Aggressive surgical débridement and removal of foreign bodies from the infected wound must be undertaken. If a wound is gangrenous, amputation may be considered.
- After resolution of the illness is complete, active immunization is required in individuals who have tetanus.

SUPPORTIVE CARE

- Patients suspected of having tetanus should be rapidly transferred to a tertiary care center capable of providing sophisticated ventilatory and cardiovascular support in an intensive care setting. Transfer should occur early in the disease before these sophisticated techniques are necessary.
- Patients should be kept in a quiet, darkened room with minimum stimulus. Cardiac and respiratory status should be monitored closely.
- Tracheostomy may prevent fatal laryngospasm. It is preferable that this be done on a semiemergent rather than emergent basis.
- Parenteral nutrition is usually required to maintain adequate nutrition and hydration.

DRUGS

- Diazepam should be given to promote sedation and muscle relaxation. A dose of 0.1 to 0.2 mg/kg IV every 4 to 6 hours is an appropriate initial dose. Phenothiazines, especially chlorpromazine, may be helpful if additional sedation is needed. Sedation must be titrated to desired effect and in an attempt to avoid respiratory depression. If spasms cannot be adequately controlled or if laryngospasm or spasm of the respiratory musculature compromises ventilation, then neuromuscular blockade and mechanical ventilation should be instituted.
- Nondepolarizing neuromuscular blocking agents are usually used. Vecuronium in an initial dose of 0.1 to 0.2 mg/kg IV followed by a continuous infusion or hourly dosing intervals seems to have less cardiovascular effects than other agents.
- Beta-blockers are used as needed to manage hypertension, with propranolol in a dose of 0.01 to 0.1 mg/kg every 6 to 8 hours being a popular choice.

PREVENTION

- The mainstays of prevention are good hygiene and aggressive active immunization of all individuals. All wounds should be cleaned thoroughly with soap and water, and foreign bodies should be sought aggressively and removed.
- Tetanus prophylaxis should be initiated at the time of injury in the following manner:

—If the patient has had at least three prior doses of tetanus toxoid, no TIG should be given.
—A dose of tetanus toxoid should be given if it has been longer than 7 years since the last dose or if it has been longer than 5 years and the wound is considered to be dirty or tetanus-prone.
—If the patient has had fewer than three doses of tetanus toxoid, TIG should be given if the wound is considered tetanus-prone. The dose is 250 to 500 U IM. All of these patients should receive tetanus toxoid regardless of the nature of the wound.

 ## Common Question and Answer

Q: What is a tetanus-prone wound?
A: Deep puncture wounds, wounds causing a large amount of tissue necrosis including crushing wounds, large ragged lacerations, and wounds clearly contaminated with soil or feces are generally considered tetanus-prone. All wounds, including minor wounds such as corneal abrasions, insect bites, small lacerations, and burns, may be inoculated with spores and lead to the development of tetanus.

ICD-9-CM 037.0

BIBLIOGRAPHY

Abrahamian FM, Pollack CV Jr, LoVecchio F, et al. Fatal tetanus in a drug abuser with protective antitetanus antibodies. *J Emerg Med* 2000;18(2):189–193.

Brook I. Tetanus in children. *Pediatr Emerg Care* 2004;20:48–51.

Dyce O, Bruno JR, Hong D, et al. Tongue piercing: the new "rusty nail"? *Head Neck* 2000;22(7):728–732.

Loscalzo IL, Ryan J, Loscalzo J, et al. Tetanus: a clinical diagnosis. *Am J Emerg Med* 1995;13:488–490.

Thayaparan B, Nicoll A. Prevention and control of tetanus in childhood. *Curr Opin Pediatr* 1998;10(1):4–8.

Author: James M. Callahan

Tetralogy of Fallot (TOF)

 ## Database

DEFINITION

• Anatomic hallmark is anterior malalignment of infundibular septum:

—A large and unrestrictive ventricular septal defect (VSD)
—Various degrees of right ventricular outflow tract obstruction (RVOTO)
—Overriding aorta
—(Resultant) right ventricular hypertrophy (RVH)

PATHOPHYSIOLOGY

Severity of clinical signs and symptoms are dependent on the degree of RVOTO and related right-to-left shunt.

GENETICS

• Some TOFs are associated with a chromosome 22q11 microdeletion.
• May be associated with other syndromes including Down, Alagille, fetal alcohol, and a variety of limb abnormality syndromes. TOF may also be associated with midline abdominal defects (e.g., omphalocele) as in the pentalogy of Cantrell.

EPIDEMIOLOGY

Three and one-half percent to 8% of all congenital heart disease

COMPLICATIONS

• Paroxysmal hypoxic spells (hypercyanotic spells a.k.a. "tet spell")
• Bacterial endocarditis
• Cerebrovascular accident (CVA) secondary to cyanosis, polycythemia, and microcytic anemia
• Right ventricular dysfunction and ventricular arrhythmia
• Postoperative sudden death (ventricular arrhythmias and/or complete heart block)

PROGNOSIS

• Generally good if treated surgically in a timely manner
• More than 90% of children with TOF are expected to survive to adulthood.

 ## Differential Diagnosis

TOF should be considered in all infants with heart murmur and/or various degrees of cyanosis, and otherwise acyanotic infants or children with history of hypercyanotic spells.

 ## Data Gathering

HISTORY

• Heart murmur in the newborn period
• Various degrees of progressive cyanosis
• History of paroxysmal cyanosis especially when crying or with exercise

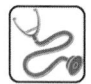 ## Physical Examination

• Various degrees of cyanosis may be present at birth, or may appear later during infancy or childhood as a result of progression of the pulmonary stenosis.
• Normal S1 and single loud S2 secondary to a more anteriorly located aorta
• Systolic ejection murmur at left upper sternal border secondary to RVOTO

 ## Laboratory Aids

Test: ECG
Significance: Right axis deviation ($+90°$ to $180°$), RVH

IMAGING

Test: CXR
Significance: Right aortic arch (30%), decreased pulmonary vascular markings, boot-shaped heart ("coeur en sabot") with concave main pulmonary artery segment

Test: Echocardiogram
Significance: Anterior malalignment type VSD, presence of other VSDs, degree of infundibular stenosis, presence of valvar pulmonary stenosis and/or branch pulmonary artery stenosis, overriding aorta, arch sidedness, coronary artery anatomy

Test: Cardiac catheterization
Significance: Generally not indicated unless there is a concern regarding branch pulmonary artery anatomy, coronary anatomy or multiple additional VSDs that need to be defined prior to surgery.

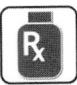 Therapy

MEDICAL

- Hypercyanotic spells:

—Knee-chest position
—Oxygen
—Morphine sulfate (0.1 mg/kg IV or IM)
—Intravenous fluid bolus and/or $NaHCO_3$
—Beta-blocker (esmolol infusion for immediate therapy, propranolol for long term prophylaxis).
—Phenylephrine (0.02 mg/kg IV)

- Polycythemia: oral Fe supplement for iron deficiency to avoid microcytosis
- SBE prophylaxis

SURGICAL

- Palliative surgery: Blalock-Taussig systemic-pulmonary shunt
- Corrective surgery: VSD patch closure and RVOT reconstruction

 Follow-Up

PROGNOSIS

- Surgical mortality is quite low in most centers
- Long-term quality of life in adulthood is comparable to the general population.
- Patients with TOF have a greater risk of requiring additional help in school.
- Residual hemodynamic abnormalities are quite common:

—Pulmonary insufficiency (with transannular patch repair)
—Residual RVOTO
—RV dysfunction in adulthood from volume overload of ventricle
—Left pulmonary artery stenosis
—Residual VSD

- Conduction abnormalities (complete heart block, junctional ectopic tachycardia)
- Supraventricular and ventricular arrhythmias

 Common Questions and Answers

Q: What is the etiology of the "tet spell"?
A: There is an increase in resistance to flow through the RVOT and/or pulmonary vascular bed that leads to a dramatic decrease in pulmonary blood flow and increased right-to-left shunt at the level of the VSD. Therefore, treatment should be aimed at increasing pulmonary blood flow either by decreasing pulmonary vascular resistance (O_2, morphine) or increasing systemic vascular resistance (knee-chest position, phenylephrine) or decreasing dynamic obstruction by decreasing HR and thus increasing RV preload (β-blockers).

Q: When is an optimal time for surgical repair of TOF?
A: At The Children's Hospital of Philadelphia, we recommend elective repair of TOF in early infancy (3 to 6 months). Progressive hypoxemia or recurrent "tet spell" indicates a need for surgical intervention.

ICD-9-CM 745.2

BIBLIOGRAPHY

Cobanoglu A, Schultz JM. Total correction of tetralogy of Fallot in the first year of life: late results. *Ann Thorac Surg* 2002;74(1):133–138.

Hirsch JC, Bove EL. Tetralogy of Fallot. In: Mavroudis C, Backer, eds. *Pediatric Cardiac Surgery,* 3rd Ed. Philadelphia, Mosby, 2003:383–397.

Siwik ES. Moss and Adams: *Heart Diseases in Infants, Children and Adolescents, 5th ed.* Baltimore: Williams & Wilkins, 2001:880–902.

Walker WT, Temple IK, Gnanapragasam JP, Goddard JR, Brown EM. Quality of life after repair of tetralogy of Fallot. *Cardiol Young* 2002;12(6):549–553.

Author: V. Ben Sivarajan

Thalassemia

Database

DEFINITION

- Thalassemia syndromes are hereditary microcytic anemias occurring as a result of mutations that quantitatively reduce globin synthesis.
- Normal hemoglobin is a tetramer of two α and two β chains.

—α-Thalassemia: decrease or lack of α globin synthesis
—β-Thalassemia: decrease or lack of β globin synthesis

PATHOPHYSIOLOGY

- Decrease in either α- or β-globin synthesis leads to fewer completed $\alpha^2\beta^2$ tetramers produced per red cell, which results in a decrease in intracellular hemoglobin and microcytosis.
- Unpaired globin chains precipitate on the red cell membrane causing hemolysis and splenomegaly
- Ineffective erythropoiesis causes hepatosplenomegaly, and bony changes.
- The red cell life span is shortened as a result of hemolysis and splenic sequestration.
- Varying degrees of anemia depending on gene defect.

GENETICS

- α-Thalassemia

—Each cell normally has four α-globin genes, two on each chromosome 16.
—Most mutations in α-thalassemia are large deletions
—The four α-thalassemia syndromes reflect the inheritance of molecular defects affecting the output of one, two, three, or four α genes. See table, α-Thalassemia Syndromes.

- β-Thalassemia

—Each cell normally has two β-globin genes, one on each chromosome 11.
—Most mutation in β-thalassemia are point mutations.
—Many mutations abolish the expression completely ($\beta0$), although others cause variable decrease in quantitative expression ($\beta+$).
—Heterozygous state for β-globin mutation produces β-thalassemia trait.
—Homozygous state produces β-thalassemia major ($\beta0$) or thalassemia intermedia ($\beta+$) or compound heterozygous state.

CLINICAL CLASSIFICATION EPIDEMIOLOGY

- α-Thalassemia

—Predominantly in Chinese subcontinent, Malaysia, Indochina, and Africa, and African-American population.

- β-Thalassemia

—Mediterranean countries, Africa, India, Pakistan, Mideast, and China.

COMPLICATIONS

Most complications occur in patients with homozygous β-thalassemia. They include:

- Skeletal abnormalities secondary to hyperplastic marrow
- Growth retardation
- Congestive heart failure as a result of severe anemia
- Postsplenectomy sepsis
- Gallstones
- Iron overload, which can lead to:

—Cardiac abnormalities: pericarditis, arrhythmias, congestive heart failure (young adults)
—Hepatic abnormalities: cirrhosis and liver failure (onset after second decade usually)
—Endocrine disturbances: delayed puberty, growth retardation, diabetes mellitus, hypothyroidism, hypoparathyroidism

PROGNOSIS

- Life expectancy for β-thalassemia major has improved over the years with regular transfusions and chelation therapy
- Bone marrow transplant from a histocompatible sibling donor may be curative.

Differential Diagnosis

- Differential includes other microcytic anemias

—Iron deficiency anemia—can be distinguished with Fe studies
—Anemia of chronic disease

Data Gathering

HISTORY

Question: Age of onset?
Significance: Severe α-thalassemia or β-thalassemia is symptomatic within first year of life.

Question: Mediterranean, African, or Asian descent?
Significance: Common ethnic background in thalassemia

Question: Familial history of anemia or chronic transfusions?
Significance: Siblings and/or parents may be affected.

Physical Examination

Finding: Pallor
Significance: Indicates anemia

Finding: Heart murmur
Significance: Flow murmurs are often heard in significant anemia. Patients with severe anemia may present with congestive heart failure.

Finding: Variable degrees of icterus
Significance: Hemolysis is part of thalassemia.

Finding: Abnormal facies (frontal bossing)
Significance: Facial bone expansion by hypertrophic marrow in poorly transfused patients with β-thalassemia

Finding: Failure to thrive
Significance: Related to anemia and energy expended in ineffective erythropoiesis

Finding: Variable degrees of hepatosplenomegaly
Significance: Extramedullary hematopoiesis

Laboratory Aids

- CBC with RBC indices

—MCV, MCH, and MCHC are decreased in both α-thalassemia and β-thalassemia

- RDW is usually normal
- Peripheral smear may reveal microcytosis, hypochromia, anisocytosis, poikilocytosis, target cells, nucleated red cells, polychromasia
- Hb 9 to 12 g/dL in α-thalassemia or β-thalassemia trait
- Hb usually 6 to 10 g/dL in HbH disease
- Hb usually 7 to 10 g/dL in β-thalassemia intermedia
- Hb less than 5 g/dL in β-thalassemia major (without transfusions)
- Reticulocyte count

—Usually elevated in HbH and β-thalassemia intermedia and major

- Indirect bilirubin

—May be elevated in severe thalassemia in which there is significant red cell destruction

- Hemoglobin electrophoresis

—α-Thalassemia trait (two defective genes) will have 5% to 10% Hb Bart's (a tetramer of four γ chains) at birth, which should be detected on the newborn screen. This disappears in 1 to 2 months, after which the electrophoresis will be normal in α-thalassemia trait.
—β-thalassemia trait: HbF 1% to 5%, HbA2 3.5% to 8%, remainder HbA. The elevated HbA^2 will distinguish α- from β-thalassemia trait.
—HbH disease (three defective α genes): 5% to 30% HbH (β 4), remainder HbA.
—Hydrops fetalis (four defective α genes): mainly Hb Bart's.
—Thalassemia major (two defective β genes): HbF 20% to 100%, HbA2 2% to 7%, HbA 0% to 80%. In most cases no HbA is detected.

- Iron studies, serum ferritin

—Useful to help distinguish thalassemia from iron deficiency

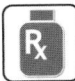 ## Therapy

- Silent carriers and α- and β-thalassemia trait: genetic counseling only
- HbH disease and β-thalassemia intermedia

—Folic acid daily
—Transfusions whenever necessary (aplastic crisis, infection)
—Splenectomy if evidence of hypersplenism
—Cholecystectomy if necessary

- β-thalassemia major

—Regular transfusions of red cells every 3 to 4 weeks to maintain Hb at 9 to 10 g/dL
—Chelation therapy with desferrioxamine to avoid iron overload
—Splenectomy if transfusion requirement more than 200 mL/kg per year
—Folic acid daily
—Penicillin prophylaxis (125 to 250 mg b.i.d.) for all splenectomized patients
—Pneumococcal and *Haemophilus influenzae* vaccine prior to splenectomy
—Cholecystectomy if indicated
—No iron supplements
—Genetic counseling
—Bone marrow transplantation using histocompatible sibling donor can cure the disease and is being increasingly utilized.

 ## Follow-Up

Thalassemia major patients need to be transfused every 3 to 4 weeks. In these patients serum ferritin and liver function tests should be performed every 3 months. Liver biopsy is necessary intermittently to quantitate the status of iron overload accurately.

PREVENTION

Thalassemia can be prevented by identifying and counseling potential parents who can have children with thalassemia. Diagnosis can be made in early pregnancy by chorionic villus sampling.

PITFALLS

Thalassemia trait is often treated presumptively as iron deficiency anemia. Iron studies should be done to confirm the diagnosis if there is no improvement in hemoglobin level after a few weeks of iron therapy.

 ## Common Questions and Answers

Q: Is prenatal testing available?
A: Yes.

Q: In a transfused patient, when does iron overload become a problem and when is chelation started?
A: Usually after the age of 4 years

ICD-9-CM 282.4

BIBLIOGRAPHY

Giardina PJ, Hilgartner MW. Update on thalassemia. *Pediatr Rev* 1992;13(2):55–62.

Giardini C. Treatment of beta-thalassemia. *Curr Opin Hematol* 1997;4(2):79–87.

Gu X, Zeng Y. A review of the molecular diagnosis of thalassemia. *Hematology* 2002;7(4):203–209.

Lo L, Singer ST. Thalassemia: current approach to an old disease. *Pediatr Clin North Am* 2002;49(6):1165–1191.

Piomelli S. Management of thalassemia major (Cooley's anemia). *Semin Hematol* 1995;32(2):262–268.

Piomelli S, Loew T. The management of patients with Cooley's anemia: transfusions and splenectomy. *Hematol Oncol Clin North Am* 1991;5(3):557–569.

Weatherall DJ. The hereditary anaemias. *BMJ* 1997;314:492–496.

Author: Leslie Raffini

α-Thalassemia Syndromes

SYNDROME	CLINICAL FEATURES	α-GLOBIN GENES AFFECTED
Silent carrier	No anemia, normal CBC	1
α-Thalassemia trait	Mild microcytic anemia, usually asymptomatic	2
HbH disease	Moderate microcytic anemia, splenomegaly	3
Hydrops fetalis	Death in utero as a result of severe anemia	4

Tick Fever

 Database

DEFINITION

• Relapsing fever in its endemic form is a vector-borne infection with characteristic recurrent fevers caused by several species of spirochetes of the genus Borrelia. In the United States the vector for endemic relapsing fever are ticks of the genus Ornithodoros. Epidemic relapsing fever is transmitted by the body louse and is no longer found in the United States.
• Colorado tick fever (CTF) is a febrile, usually benign, systemic illness caused by an arbovirus in the family Reoviridae and transmitted by ticks in the genus Dermatocentor.

CAUSES

• Relapsing fever is caused by several spirochetes in the genus *Borrelia* including *B. hermsii*, *B. parkerii*, and *B. turicatae*. Epidemic relapsing fever (louse-borne) is caused by *B. recurrentis*.
• Colorado tick fever is caused by an arbovirus in the family Reoviridae.

PATHOPHYSIOLOGY

• Endemic relapsing fever is characterized by repeated episodes of spirochetemia.
• *Borreliae* are able to undergo plasmid-mediated, antigenic variation. An antibody response against a particular strain leads to immobilization, opsonization, agglutination, and phagocytosis, and symptoms abate. The infecting organism can then again undergo antigenic variation and a recurrent episode of spirochetemia and symptoms occurs. Tick-borne disease may relapse 10 to 12 times before final resolution.
• Transmission of the infecting organism occurs when ticks of the genus *Ornithodoros* take blood meals and then detach themselves. These bites are usually painless, and the tick may remain attached for up to 15 minutes. Ticks are maintained by intermediate hosts including rodents and other small mammals.
• When a tick feeds on an infected individual, spirochetes invade all tissues including the female genital tract. Once infected, ticks remain capable of transmitting disease for many years.
• Additionally, transovarial infection of offspring leads to increased transmission of spirochetes and increased survival.
• In the human host, organisms persist in the central nervous system (CNS), bone marrow, liver, and spleen during remissions. Pathologic findings in humans include petechial hemorrhages on visceral surfaces, hepatosplenomegaly, and a histiocytic myocarditis.
• Pneumonia, CNS hemorrhages, meningitis, disseminated intravascular coagulation (DIC), splenic rupture, hepatic coma, and dysrhythmias may result. Spirochetes may cross the placenta and lead to spontaneous abortion or severe infection in neonates.

• CTF is acquired when infected, adult ticks of the genus *Dermatocentor* (including *D. andersonii*, the wood tick) attach and ingest a blood meal from a human host instead of porcupines, elk, marmot, or deer (usual hosts).
• Ticks are infected while larvae as they feed on viremic, intermediate hosts such as chipmunks and ground squirrels.
• Aseptic meningitis, encephalitis, myocarditis, atypical pneumonia, epididymo-orchitis, and hepatitis have been reported. Generalized hemorrhage and death have been rarely reported in children. Granulocytopenia and thrombocytopenia are often seen.

EPIDEMIOLOGY

• Endemic relapsing fever occurs in the United States among people who are exposed to the habitat of the ticks that serve as vectors. In the United States, most cases are found in the West among people who have spent time in old summer cabins in forested mountain areas. In several series, cabins that were found to be the source of cases contained large rodent nests with infected ticks in them.
• Colorado tick fever is also found among humans who travel to a location where the vector (ticks of the genus *Dermacentor*) is found. The wood tick is found in the Rocky Mountains and western Black Hills at elevations of 4,000 to 10,000 feet. Cases usually occur between April and July when adult ticks are most active. Cases have been reported as early as March and as late as November. Most cases are reported in males, and two-thirds of cases are reported in individuals between the ages of 10 and 49 years.

COMPLICATIONS

• Relapsing fever may be associated with hepatosplenomegaly with necrotic foci. Diffuse histiocytic interstitial myocarditis may be associated with dysrhythmias. Pneumonia, CNS hemorrhages, splenic rupture, meningitis, DIC, hepatitis, and hepatic coma may result. In utero infection may result in fetal loss or severe neonatal infection.
• Treatment may be associated with a marked Jarisch-Herxheimer reaction, which may require intravenous fluids and other supportive measures.
• CTF may lead to aseptic meningitis, encephalitis, myocarditis, atypical pneumonia, hepatitis, and epididymo-orchitis. A prolonged convalescence with persistent lassitude, fatigability, headache, musculoskeletal pain, and fevers may persist for weeks to months in patients who experience persistent viremia.

PROGNOSIS

• Relapsing fever generally responds rapidly to appropriate antibiotic therapy and leaves no significant sequelae. Even when untreated, the vast majority of cases are benign and self-limited.

• Louse-borne, epidemic relapsing fever in developing countries has been associated with mortality rates of up to 40%.
• CTF resolves without sequelae in most patients. Symptoms may persist for at least 3 weeks in a majority of patients. Patients older than 30 years are at a much greater risk of developing prolonged symptoms. Infection usually leads to permanent immunity.

 Differential Diagnosis

• Relapsing fever and CTF resemble each other clinically, but leukopenia is more often seen with CTF. Exposure to ticks or a history of travel to an area where appropriate vectors are found is a helpful clue in diagnosing either disease.
• Relapsing fever and CTF may be misdiagnosed as influenza or enteroviral infections.
• Spirochetes may be seen on peripheral blood smears in cases of relapsing fever.

 Data Gathering

HISTORY

Question: Fever?
Significance: Endemic relapsing fever has a sudden onset of high fever after an incubation period of 5 to 11 days. Patients complain of chills, headache, and myalgias. Symptoms resolve after 3 to 6 days but then recur within several days. Repeated recurrences continue with decreasing severity and lengthening periods of lack of symptoms. CTF has a usual incubation period of 4 days (range, 1 to 14 days). There is a history of tick exposure in 90% of patients. Patients complain of abrupt onset of fever, chills, fatigue, headache, myalgias, photophobia, and stiff neck.

Question: Headache?
Significance: Patients may complain of headache, photophobia, stiff neck, and rash, which usually begins on the trunk. There may be epistaxis.

Question: Other symptoms of CTF?
Significance: Gastrointestinal symptoms, pharyngitis, and rash may be noted by some patients.

Question: How long do symptoms of CTF last?
Significance: In about half of patients symptoms resolve after 2 to 4 days and then recur after 1 to 3 days. Symptoms then last for another 2 to 3 days. Some patients will have a third symptomatic period, whereas others will only have the initial symptomatic period.

Physical Examination

Finding: High fever
Significance: Relapsing patients have high fevers (39°C to 41°C).

Finding: Tender hepatosplenomegaly
Significance: Characteristic of relapsing fever

Finding: A macular rash
Significance: May be seen on the trunk in approximately 10% of cases, but it may fade quickly or become generalized or petechial.

Finding: Meningismus and signs of iridocyclitis
Significance: May be seen

Finding: CTF
Significance: Patients with CTF have mostly nonspecific findings. There are often signs of CNS involvement or meningismus. Myalgias and muscle tenderness are usually seen.

 Laboratory Aids

Test: Peripheral blood smear
Significance: In relapsing fever the diagnosis is often made when spirochetes are noted on a peripheral blood smear. Increased sensitivity can be obtained by examining dehemoglobinized thick smears or buffy coat preparations.

Test: Weil-Felix agglutination tests
Significance: May be positive but are nonspecific. Indirect fluorescent antibody tests are more sensitive but may be falsely positive in cases of Lyme disease.

Test: Specific test for relapsing fever
Significance: Intraperitoneal inoculation of immature laboratory mice with infected blood leads to spirochetemia in the mice and is a specific and sensitive diagnostic tool.

Test: Nonspecific laboratory findings
Significance: Include thrombocytopenia, hyperbilirubinemia, and elevated hepatic transaminases

Test: Electrocardiograms and chest roentgenogram
Significance: Should be performed to exclude the possibility of myocarditis

Test: Diagnostic test for CTF
Significance: May be confirmed by serologic testing, immunofluorescence testing for viral antigens on the surface of red blood cells, or by viral culture

Test: Associated laboratory findings in CTF
Significance: Include leukopenia and thrombocytopenia. Initially, both granulocytopenia and lymphopenia occur. Lymphopenia resolves first, and an atypical lymphocytosis may occur.

Test: CSF studies in CTF
Significance: Pleocytosis may be found, especially in children.

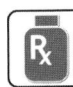 Therapy

DRUGS

- Endemic relapsing fever may be treated with oral tetracycline (in patients older than 8 years of age) or erythromycin at doses of 40 mg/kg per day in four divided doses for 10 days.
- Patients who are symptomatic at the time treatment is begun are at significant risk of developing the Jarisch-Herxheimer reaction (severe fevers, rigors, sweating, hypotension, and prostration) related to rapid clearing of the spirochetemia. In symptomatic patients it is suggested that treatment is initiated with a single dose of oral phenoxymethyl penicillin (7.5 mg/kg) or intravenous penicillin G (10,000 U/kg given over 30 minutes). These therapies should lead to a slower clearing of the organisms and a less severe reaction.
- Close observation, intravenous fluids, and good supportive care are important in treating possible reactions.
- When the patient is afebrile, a course of tetracycline or erythromycin should be completed to prevent relapse, which has been associated with the use of penicillin alone.
- There is no specific therapy for patients with CTF. Ribavirin may be helpful in certain situations. Good supportive care is usually all that is required.

PREVENTION

- Both of these diseases can be prevented by avoidance or elimination of the vector.
- Dwellings should be made of rodent-proof construction. Rodent-nesting materials should be removed from buildings where this is not possible.
- Light-colored, long-sleeved shirts, and long trousers with legs tucked inside of one's socks should be worn when infested areas cannot be avoided. Persons should inspect themselves and each other frequently for adherent ticks.
- Confirmed cases should be reported to health authorities so control measures can be instituted.

ICD-9-CM 066.1

BIBLIOGRAPHY

Boyer KM. Borrelia: relapsing fever. In: Feigin RD, Cherry JD, eds. *Textbook of Pediatric Infectious Disease.* 3rd Ed. Philadelphia: WB Saunders, 1992:1058–1062.

Doan-Wiggins L. Tick-borne diseases. *Emerg Med Clin North Am* 1991;9:303–325.

Klasko R. Colorado tick fever. *Med Clin North Am* 2002;86:435–440.

Tsai TF. Arboviral infections in the United States. *Infect Dis Clin North Am* 1991;5:73–102.

Author: James M. Callahan

Tics

Database

DEFINITION

Tics are rapid, irregular stereotyped movement (motor tics) or vocalizations (vocal tics) that are under partial voluntary control. The movements usually involve the muscles of the face, neck, and shoulder. Tics are often (but not always) brought on by stress or excitement, typically occur in clusters, and they may occur in light sleep. Simple motor tics are blinking; grimacing; neck, arm, or leg jerking; shoulder shrugging; etc. Simple vocal tics include coughing, grunting, barking, yelping, etc. Complex motor tics include jumping, smelling objects, shaking wrists, copropraxia, and echopraxia. Complex vocal tics include coprolalia, echolalia, and neologism.

- Gilles de la Tourette syndrome (GTS) is defined as a condition of chronic vocal and motor tics of more than 1 year's duration.
- Typical onset in childhood with motor tics followed by vocalizations (grunts, snorts, barks); later in adolescence 50% to 60% develop coprolalia and echolalia. Obsessive-compulsive behavior, attention deficits, learning disabilities, and sleep disorders are also frequently seen.
- The natural history of GTS is exacerbation of tics in adolescence, but 80% of children improve as they reach adulthood.
- The lifetime prevalence in GTS has been estimated to be between 0.1 and 1.0 in 1,000.
- The average age of onset is 7 years.

PATHOPHYSIOLOGY

- The pathophysiology of tics or GTS is not known. Rarely, lesions or disease of the caudate nuclei (basal ganglia) may underlie tics.
- Most theories regarding GTS have implicated abnormalities in central dopaminergic transmission, but other neurotransmitters such as serotonin and norepinephrine and sex hormones have been implicated.

GENETICS

No single gene has been associated with tics or GTS. However, tics are frequently seen in families and GTS may be transmitted as an autosomal-dominant trait.

EPIDEMIOLOGY

- Tics can occur in any age group from 2 years up.
- Simple motor tics are considered a part of normal development and occur in 10% to 20% of all school-aged children.
- There is no gender or race preference.

COMPLICATIONS

- Tics are usually harmless. However, patients with complex motor tics that persist for years may develop repetitive motion injuries with arthritic changes of the neck and spine, resulting in increased risk of radiculopathy, disc herniation, and myelopathy.
- Children with tics and particularly GTS are often teased by their peers and have difficulty with social adjustments, isolation, and depression. Comorbid learning difficulties may also contribute to these problems.

PROGNOSIS

Most children outgrow their tics within a year. If the tics last longer than 1 year they may remain as a simple tic disorder or develop into GTS.

Differential Diagnosis

- Movements resembling tics include:

—Hemifacial spasm: a spastic contraction of one-half the muscles of the face. Frequency varies from occasional to constant, but the spasm usually lasts longer than a tic. Spasm results from:
—Abnormal activity in the facial nerve
—Aberrant regeneration after a Bell palsy
—Arteriovenous malformation
—Aneurysms
—Brainstem or posterior fossa tumors
—Idiopathic

Other movements that may be mistaken for tic include

—Chorea
—Myoclonus (also very fast)
—Myokymia (fine repetitive, arrhythmic twitching of muscle bundles around eyes and lips; benign and common; seen in posterior fossa tumors, Guillain-Barré syndrome, and multiple sclerosis)
—Paroxysmal dyskinesia (often familial, movement is more sustained and complex, may be triggered by movement)
—Partial epilepsy: may look like a tic disorder, but there is no voluntary control; EEG may show corresponding abnormalities
—Tremors: simple tics can resemble tremor; tics are more variable and lack the oscillatory appearance of tremor.
—Sleep myoclonus: tics do not occur during sleep; erratic movements during sleep are most commonly benign sleep myoclonus.

Data Gathering

HISTORY

Good record-keeping helps to adjust medication appropriately.

- When did the first tic occur?
- What exacerbates and alleviates the tics?
- History of vocal tics (including throat-clearing, coughing, grunting, sniffing)?
- Is there some degree of voluntary control?
- Have the tics changed in character?
- Evidence of comorbid conditions, especially attention deficit/hyperactivity disorder, obsessive-compulsive disorder, sleep disorders, learning disability.
- Does anyone else in the family have tics?

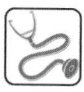

Physical Examination

- General and neurologic examinations are unrevealing. Spontaneous movements or vocalizations may be absent during the visit.
- Often the child can reproduce the tic at will.

Laboratory Aids

Because tics are generally not a symptom of an underlying brain disorder, laboratory testing is usually not indicated.

Test: MRI of the brain
Significance: Not necessarily indicated, but should be normal

Test: EEG
Significance: May be helpful in the rare instance in which there is a concern of partial seizures

Test: Psychological testing
Significance: May be the most useful ancillary assessment (if any testing is to be done) because of high incidence of associated learning disabilities, attention deficit/hyperactivity disorder, obsessive-compulsive disorder

Tics

 ## Therapy

Decision to treat is based on the severity of tics/vocalizations as reported by the child and parent. Medications are not needed in the majority of children with simple tics. Learning and attention difficulties associated with GTS may be the primary focus of attention.

- Haloperidol: started at 0.5 mg q.h.s. and increased each week to effect. A usual maintenance dose is 1 to 3 mg/day divided b.i.d. Side effects include sedation, irritability, decreased appetite, rare neuroleptic malignant syndrome, tardive dyskinesia. Risperdal has similar pharmacodynamic properties to haloperidol and is useful in treatment of GTS but appears to have significantly fewer side effects.
- Pimozide: started at 2 mg/day divided b.i.d., increased 2 mg q week to effect. Maintenance dose is 0.2 mg/kg per day or 10 mg (whichever is less); side effects similar to haloperidol.
- Clonidine: started at 0.05 mg/day, increased 0.05 q week. Maintenance is 0.1 to 0.6 mg/day.
- Sedation is the main side effect; rebound hypertension is a concern if withdrawn rapidly.
- Alternatives include fluphenazine, clonazepam (may cause sedation), and desipramine (primarily used as an antidepressant; potential for arrhythmia).
- Clomipramine may improve associated obsessive-compulsive behavior.
- Fluoxetine may be useful for tics, GTS, particularly when comorbid obsessive-compulsive symptoms are a problem.
- CNS stimulants used for attention deficits, such as Ritalin, may exacerbate tics, or be associated with onset of tics, although they do not appear to cause tic disorder per se, and are not strictly contraindicated for patients with GTS.
- Biofeedback and behavioral modification have been recommended.

 ## Follow-Up

The tics in GTS often become refractory to medication after prolonged use. May help to switch to another drug or to alternate between two drugs.

PREVENTION

Tics cannot be prevented. However, social isolation, adjustment difficulties, and depression can be prevented or minimized by informing teachers, sports coaches, and other caregivers of the child's condition.

PITFALLS

Avoid exclusive focus on the tics in a child: Is he or she adjusting in school? Is there a learning disability? Does he or she have friends? Are there other stressors in the family? GTS is frequently misdiagnosed—there is an approximate 10-year interval between onset of symptoms and treatment.

 ## Common Questions and Answers

Q: My child just started school and now she blinks excessively. When I tell her to stop it just gets worse. What can I do?
A: Mild tics may be considered part of normal development. They can last anywhere from a few weeks to a year, and they usually disappear if you ignore them. If they last longer than a year, they are probably not a simple tic and you should contact your doctor. If there is any concern of eye irritation or a visual disturbance, an ophthalmologic checkup is appropriate.

Q: Our son has been diagnosed with GTS. His tics are increasing in frequency, and now he has developed vocalizations with obscenities. He has already lost his friends in school and was suspended twice last week because of his foul mouth. I tell him to stop but he does not listen. What should I do?
A: Children with GTS cannot control their vocalizations. Swearing is not intentional. Telling a child to control his vocalizations will only increase the level of anxiety and may increase the tics. Once a child has been diagnosed with GTS (particularly if vocalizations are present), it may help to inform teachers, school personnel, and peers about the disease so that misunderstandings can be minimized and the child can feel comfortable at school. A review of medication with the child's physician (child psychiatrist or neurologist) is appropriate.

ICD-9-CM 307.20

BIBLIOGRAPHY

Berardelli A, Curra A, Fabbrini G, Gilio F, Manfredi M. Pathophysiology of tics and Tourette syndrome. *J Neurol* 2003;250(7):781–787.

Coats DK, Paysse EA, Kim DS. Excessive blinking in childhood: a prospective evaluation of 99 children. *Ophthalmology* 2001;108(9):1556–1561.

Deputy SR. Treatment of ADHD in children with tics: a randomized controlled trial. *Clin Pediatr* 2002;41(9):736.

Kurlan R. Tourette syndrome. Treatment of tics. *Neurol Clin* 1997;1592:403–409.

Lumar R, Lang AE. Tourette syndrome. Secondary tic disorders. *Neurol Clin* 1997;15(2):309–331.

McMahon WM, Filloux FM, Ashworth JC, Jensen J. Movement disorders in children and adolescents. *Neurol Clin* 2002;20(4):1101–1124, vii–viii.

Moll GH, Heinrich H, Trott GE, et al. Children with comorbid attention-deficit-hyperactivity disorder and tic disorder: evidence for additive inhibitory deficits within the motor system. *Ann Neurol* 2001;49(3):393–396.

Pappert EJ, Goetz CG, Louis ED, Blasucci L, Leurgans S. Objective assessments of longitudinal outcome in Gilles de la Tourette's syndrome. *Neurology* 2003;61(7):936–940.

Scahill L, Tanner C, Dure L. The epidemiology of tics and Tourette syndrome in children and adolescents. *Adv Neurol* 2001;85:261–271.

Scahill L, Leckman JF, Schultz RT, Katsovich L, Peterson BS. A placebo-controlled trial of risperidone in Tourette syndrome. *Neurology* 2003;60(7):1130–1135.

Author: Peter Bingham and *A. G. Christina Bergqvist 3rd edition*

Toddler's Diarrhea

 ## Database

DEFINITION

Daily painless recurrent passage of three or more large unformed stools, for more than 4 weeks, with onset between 6 and 36 months. The child is normally active and growing and there is no failure to thrive (if caloric intake is adequate) or passage of stools during sleep.
Also known as chronic nonspecific diarrhea and irritable colon of childhood.

CAUSES

• Nutritional factors:

—Excessive consumption of fruit juice (increased sorbitol, fructose) leading to carbohydrate intolerance.
—Diet that is high in fluid but low in fat and fiber.

• Motility disorder, i.e., variant of irritable bowel syndrome of infancy.

PATHOPHYSIOLOGY

• Diarrhea is often preceded by acute gastroenteritis or other viral infection that results in dietary restrictions. Increased oral fluids, including juices are used to compensate for stool losses and prevent dehydration.
• Carbohydrate malabsorption causing osmotic diarrhea
• Capacity of small intestine to absorb fructose is limited. Foods that contain equivalent amounts of fructose and glucose are more readily absorbed because of the additive effect of a glucose-dependent fructose cotransport mechanism. An excess of fructose over glucose will result in fructose malabsorption by the small intestine.
• Sorbitol is nonabsorbable and inhibits fructose absorption and may cause gastrointestinal symptoms.
• Excessive intake of juices high in sorbitol and those with a high fructose to glucose ratio will result in fructose malabsorption and gastrointestinal symptoms.
• Colonic function: possibly, there is a disruption of colonic ability to ferment unabsorbed carbohydrates into short chain fatty acids (SCFA), which maintain colonic function and prevent colon-based diarrhea.
• Motility disorder:

—Persistence of immature bowel motility pattern. Failure of initiation of normal postprandial delayed gastric emptying and rapid transit as a result of persistence of small-bowel fasting motility pattern.
—Meals with high dietary fat delay gastric emptying. This protective mechanism is lost with high-fluid, low-fat meals.

• Low-fiber diet: Dietary fiber (pectin) serves as bulking agent

GENETICS

Family members often report nonspecific gastrointestinal complaints or functional bowel disorders.

EPIDEMIOLOGY

It is the most common cause of prolonged diarrhea without failure to thrive (FTT) in children in the developed world.

PROGNOSIS

Generally good. Carbohydrate-containing fluids contribute to unbalanced nutrition, nonorganic failure to thrive, and also to short stature and obesity.

 ## Differential Diagnosis

All causes of chronic diarrhea should be considered:

• Infection: Intestinal: bacterial, viral, fungal giardiasis, cryptosporidiosis

—Nonintestinal: Urinary tract infection

• Pancreatic: cystic fibrosis, Shwachman-Diamond syndrome, Johannson-Blizzard syndrome, chronic pancreatitis
• Bile acid disorders: chronic cholestasis, terminal ileum disease, bacterial overgrowth
• Carbohydrate malabsorption: Postinfectious-secondary lactose intolerance, sucrase-isomaltase deficiency
• Immunologic: celiac disease, cow's and soy protein intolerance, food allergy, immunodeficiency, AIDS enteropathy
• Miscellaneous: antibiotics, laxatives, fecal retention constipation, abetalipoproteinemia, inflammatory bowel disease, short bowel syndrome, hormone secreting tumors like vasoactive intestinal peptide (VIP)-oma, neuroblastoma, Münchhausen-by-proxy.

—More common conditions to be considered.

Note Most of the diseases listed above cause morbidity and malnutrition. A thorough clinical history, a simple physical examination and limited number of laboratory tests should make an obvious diagnosis of functional diarrhea. It is not a diagnosis of exclusion.

 ## Data Gathering

HISTORY

Question: Nutritional history?
Significance: Essential with attention to the "four Fs": fiber, fluid, fat, and fruit juices

Question: Diarrhea?
Significance: For a toddler it may not be abnormal to have more than three soft and occasionally loose stools a day with visible food remnants.

Question: Stool characteristics?
Significance: Stools foul smelling and contain undigested food particles, with shortened colonic transit time. Presence of blood or mucus suggests another diagnosis.

Question: Timing of diarrhea?
Significance: No stools passed at night and typically the first stool of the day is large and has better consistency than those occurring later on in the day.

Question: Are other children affected?
Significance: Presence of other affected family members or day-care mates makes infectious etiology more likely.

 ## Physical Examination

Normal, children are healthy appearing, eat well, and are growing normally, although weight might be influenced by the dietary measures.

 ## Laboratory Aids

Test: Stool tests and culture
Significance: Negative for white blood cells, blood, and pathogens

Test: Infectious workup
Significance: Negative

Test: Breath hydrogen tests?
Significance: Usually of limited benefit.

Test: Complete blood count (CBC) normal
Significance: No anemia

Test: Serum electrolytes normal
Significance: No dehydration

 ## Therapy

Reassurance on underlying gastrointestinal diseases and normalization of diet.

DIET

- The child's feeding pattern should be normalized according to the "four Fs":

—Overconsumption of fruit juices should be discouraged, especially those that contain sorbitol and a high fructose-to-glucose ratio (apple juice, for example).
—Fiber intake should be normalized by introduction of whole meal bread and fruits.
—Increase dietary fat to at least 35% to 40% of total energy intake. Substitution of low-fat milk with whole milk may be sufficient.
—Restrict fluid intake to less than 150 mL/kg per day, and fruit juices to less than 12 oz/day.
—Improvement occurs within a few days to a couple of weeks after initiating the above therapy.

Parental reassurance is confirmed by good response to dietary therapy.

PREVENTION

Vicious cycle may be initiated after acute gastroenteritis and food restrictions. Parents should be instructed to give an oral rehydration solution (ORS) and resume normal feeding early.

MEDICATIONS

Loperamide is effective in normalizing bowel patterns but only as long as they are given. Medications seem unwarranted for a condition with mostly nutritional etiology that does not hamper growth.

REFERRAL

- Failure of response to the above therapy
- Weight loss despite adequate intake
- Presence of other symptoms like anorexia, irritability, fever, and vomiting
- Blood and mucus in diarrhea

TESTS TO PREPARE FOR CONSULTATION

—Sweat chloride
—Celiac disease panel (antiendomysial antibodies, tissue transglutaminase antibodies, with IgA serum levels)
—Serum albumin
—ESR
—Stool Sudan III stain for fecal fat.

SPECIAL INSIGHTS

- Good history is required because all the illnesses in the differential diagnosis are associated with morbidity, if diagnosis is delayed.
- Consider constipation, if diarrhea alternates with normal or hard stools. KUB will show colonic fecal retention.
- Need to make followup phone call to parents within a few days of instituting diet. If no improvement within a week despite good compliance with dietary recommendations, then rethink diagnosis and consider referral to a specialist.
- Improvement with dietary changes confirms the diagnosis and also reassures the parents.

 ## Common Questions and Answers

Q: Is growth normal in a patient with toddler's diarrhea?
A: Growth is usually normal; weight may be mildly influenced by the prior dietary practices and measures, and failure to thrive has also been reported recently.

Q: What are the components of a successful treatment plan?
A: Attention to the "four Fs": decreased fruit juice intake, increased fat intake, decreased fluid, and increased fiber intake

Q: When should care by a pediatric gastroenterologist be sought?
A: If no response after 2 weeks of compliance with dietary therapy, growth delay or other gastrointestinal or systemic complaints

ICD-9-CM 787.91

564.5 (functional diarrhea)

BIBLIOGRAPHY

Dennison BA. Fruit juice consumption by infants and children: a review. *J Am Coll Nutr* 1996;15(5 suppl):4S–11S.

Ghishan FK. Chronic diarrhea. In: Behrman RE, Kliegman RM, Jenson HB eds. *Nelson Textbook of Pediatrics. Philadelphia:* Saunders, 2004:1276–1283.

Hamdi I, Dodge JA. Toddler diarrhea: observations on the effects of aspirin and loperamide. *J Pediatr Gastroenterol Nutr* 1985;4:362–365.

Hoekstra JH. Toddler diarrhea: more a nutritional disorder than a disease. *Arch Dis Child* 1998;79(1):2–5.

Hoekstra JH, Van den Aker JHL, Kneepkens CMF, et al. Evaluation of 13CO2 breath tests for the detection of fructose malabsorption. *J Lab Clin Med* 1996;127(3):303–309.

Huffman S. Toddler's diarrhea. *J Pediatr Health Care* 1999;13(1):32–33.

Kneepkens CMF, Hoekstra JH. Chronic nonspecific diarrhea of childhood. *Pediatr Clin North Am* 1996;43:375–390.

Lifshitz F, Ament ME, Kleinman RE, et al. Role of juice carbohydrate malabsorption in chronic nonspecific diarrhea in children. *J Pediatr* 1992;120:825–829.

Rasquin-Weber A, Hyman PE, Cucchiara S, et al. Childhood functional gastrointestinal disorders. *Gut* 1999;45(supp II):II60–II68.

Authors: Vered Yehezkely- Schildkraut and Raanan Shamir

Toxic Shock Syndrome (TSS)

 ## Database

DEFINITION

• Toxic shock syndrome (TSS) is an acute febrile illness characterized by myalgia, vomiting, diarrhea, pharyngitis, diffuse desquamating macular erythroderma, mucous membrane and conjunctival erythema, multiorgan system involvement by direct inflammatory damage or ischemia, disseminated intravascular coagulopathy (DIC), and hypotension.
• TSS is most commonly caused by group A β-hemolytic streptococci (GABS or Streptococcus pyogenes) or TSS toxin-1 (TSST-1)-producing strains of *Staphylococcus aureus*. Cases have also been reported in association with group B, C, and G1 streptococci and *Streptococcus mitis*.

Centers for Disease Control and Prevention (CDC) criteria for diagnosis of staphylococcal TSS:

• Fever 38.9°C (102.0°F) or higher
• Diffuse macular erythroderma
• Desquamation 1 to 2 weeks after onset, particularly of palms and soles
• Hypotension below fifth percentile for children, orthostatic changes greater than 15 mm Hg or orthostatic syncope, or dizziness.
• Involvement of three or more organ systems: gastrointestinal, muscular, mucous membrane, renal, hepatic, hematologic or neurologic.

All five of the above criteria with blood culture(s) positive for *S. aureus* only and negative serology for Rocky Mountain spotted fever (RMSF), leptospirosis and measles. Four of five criteria termed probable. Four criteria plus death prior to desquamation yields complete syndrome. CDC criteria for diagnosis of streptococcal TSS:

• Hypotension or shock
• Any two of the following: renal impairment, DIC, thrombocytopenia, hepatic impairment, adult respiratory distress syndrome, erythematous macular rash that may desquamate, soft-tissue necrosis.
• Isolation of group A β-hemolytic streptococci from a normally sterile site constitutes a definite case. Isolation of group A β-hemolytic streptococci from a nonsterile site constitutes a probable case.

Associated risk factors:

• Superabsorbent tampon, diaphragm or contraceptive sponge use
• Local staphylococcal or streptococcal infection
• Surgical wounds
• Childbirth and abortion

EPIDEMIOLOGY

• Early 1980s: over 90% of cases (almost exclusively as a result of *S. aureus*) occurred in menstruating females; associated with "superabsorbent" tampon use. The frequency of cases occurring in menstruating females dropped in the mid-1980s because of changes to less absorbent or different composition tampons. In 1996, fewer than 50% of cases were associated with menstruation.
• Current incidence of menses-related disease: 1 to 5 per 100,000 women of menstrual age per year

—Currently, approximately 60% of cases occur in females.
—Mean age: 22 years
—Incubation period for postoperative *S. aureus*-mediated TSS can be less than 12 hours.
—Streptococcal TSS incidence highest among young children.
—Preceding varicella infection dramatically increases the risk for acquiring invasive disease as a result of GABS including TSS.

COMPLICATIONS

Multisystem organ failure secondary to distributive shock/hypotension including:

• Pulmonary edema
• DIC
• Acute renal failure (oliguric and nonoliguric)
• Hepatic failure
• Myocardial edema and decreased contractility with or without arrhythmias
• "Stunned" myocardium demonstrating severe ventricular contractile dysfunction
• Cerebral edema with toxic or ischemic encephalopathy
• Metabolic disturbances
• Telogen effluvium; temporary hair and nail loss
• Neuropsychologic disturbances including memory loss; abnormal electroencephalogram (EEG) rare

PROGNOSIS

• Recurrences are associated with inadequate treatment (parenteral antibiotics).
• Mortality 5% to 7% for staphylococcal disease. Myocardial and pulmonary failure are the most common causes of death.
• Mortality higher in nonmenstrual TSS (men and women older than 45 years of age) as a result of delayed recognition.
• Death usually occurs within the first few days; may occur as late as 2 weeks following onset.
• Permanent renal damage is extremely rare.

 ## Differential Diagnosis

• Septic shock as a result of *Neisseria meningitidis*
• Streptococcal and staphylococcal Scarletiniform eruptions
• Leptospirosis
• RMSF without characteristic rash
• Fulminant viral infection (e.g., adenovirus)
• Kawasaki disease, although TSS may present simultaneously with Kawasaki

disease. Coronary artery dilatation has been reported in cases presenting as TSS.
• Toxic epidermal necrolysis (TEN)

 ## Data Gathering

HISTORY

Question: Any recent use of tampons, contraceptive sponge, and/or diaphragm? Any surgical including catheters (e.g., intravenous, peritoneal dialysis) or nonsurgical wounds, burns, childbirth, abortion, or puerperal infections?
Significance: These are all known risk factors.

Question: Any other active streptococcal or staphylococcal infections?
Significance: History frequently elicits probable recent infections.

Question: Was there abrupt onset of high fever, rapid-onset hypotension, rapidly accelerated renal failure, and multisystem organ failure?
Significance: These are all historical findings seen in either staphylococcal or streptococcal TSS. Chills, malaise, headache, pharyngitis, fatigue, and dizziness or syncope are also seen frequently.

Question: Was there profuse watery diarrhea (often with fecal incontinence), vomiting, abdominal pain, generalized erythroderma, conjunctival injection, and severe myalgias?
Significance: These are all historical findings seen commonly in staphylococcal TSS but less frequently in streptococcal TSS. The presence of a foreign body is also more common with staphylococcal TSS than streptococcal TSS.

Question: Was there evidence of increasingly painful local soft tissue infection (e.g., abscess, cellulitis, myositis, or necrotizing fasciitis)?
Significance: These are all historical findings seen commonly in streptococcal TSS but less frequently in staphylococcal TSS.

Question: Was the illness associated with the use of superabsorbent tampons?
Significance: Tampons with ingredients such as polyacrylate, polyester foam, cross-linked carboxymethylcellulose; or claims of "superabsorbency" are associated with TSS.

 ## Physical Examination

Finding: Any sign of soft tissue infection such as cellulitis, necrotizing fasciitis, myositis, soft-tissue abscesses, sinusitis
Significance: Often seen prior to TSS

Finding: Overall appearance
Significance: Patients with TSS are always moderately to severely ill.

Finding: Altered vital signs
Significance: Fever, tachycardia, tachypnea, orthostasis or frank hypotension. Tachycardia is the prelude to hypotension.

Toxic Shock Syndrome (TSS)

Finding: Abnormal skin, mucous membranes and soft tissues
Significance: Erythroderma, peripheral cyanosis and edema, bulbar conjunctival hyperemia, subconjunctival hemorrhages, beefy red mucous membranes, and muscle tenderness are seen with TSS.

Finding: Mental status changes
Significance: Altered mental status, including somnolence, agitation, disorientation, obtundation within 24 to 72 hours are seen with TSS.

Finding: Intensity of erythroderma
Significance: May be most intense surrounding the infected focus (e.g., perineum).

Finding: Desquamation
Significance: Begins on trunk and extremities 5 to 7 days after symptom onset. Full thickness desquamation of fingers, toes, palms, and soles begins 10 to 12 days after onset.

Finding: Vesicle or bullae formation, or presence of violaceous hue
Significance: Ominous findings associated with increased fluid loss and potentially hypotensive shock.

 Laboratory Aids

Test: Antibodies to TSST-1 (available for "informational purposes/research only" from Toxin Technology, Inc., www.toxintechnology.com)
Significance: Will be positive several weeks after acute presentation.

Test: Antibodies to antistreptolysin O (ASO), antideoxyribonuclease B, or other streptococcal extracellular products
Significance: May increase 4 to 6 weeks after infection in streptococcal-mediated disease.

Test: Complete Blood Count (CBC)
Significance: usually reveals thrombocytopenia early in the course of disease, thrombocytosis during the recovery phase, anemia early in disease, normal or slightly elevated leukocyte count with left shift and absolute lymphopenia. Neutropenia is more ominous than lymphopenia.

Test: Blood cultures
Significance: Positive in 60% of streptococcal TSS, rarely (<5%) positive in staphylococcal TSS.

Test: Local cultures
Significance: *S. aureus* may be isolated from vagina or cervix in menstrual TSS, or from other infectious focus in nonmenstrual cases. Isolation of group A streptococci from a sterile site is a definite case, although isolation from a nonsterile site constitutes a probable case.

Test: Coagulation studies
Significance: May reveal prolonged prothrombin and partial thromboplastin times (PT/PTT) with or without evidence of DIC; low fibrinogen, elevated fibrin degradation products.

Test: Urinalysis
Significance: May reveal sterile pyuria.

Test: Lumbar puncture
Significance: May reveal CSF pleocytosis.

Test: Creatine phosphokinase (CPK)
Significance: may be elevated reflecting skeletal muscle involvement.

 Emergency Care

- Aggressive fluid resuscitation and often vasopressors in severe cases.
- Correction of coagulopathy and anemia with plasma and blood products.

 Therapy

- Removal of all foreign bodies.
- Surgical debridement with myositis and necrotizing fasciitis; abscess drainage.
- Antibiotics: parenteral administration with antistreptococcal and staphylococcal therapy eradicates source of the toxin, but does not affect the course of the acute illness.
- Use both a bacterial cell wall inhibitor, such as semisynthetic antistaphylococcal penicillins (e.g., nafcillin, oxacillin, dicloxacillin, and cefuroxime or ampicillin/sulbactam) and a protein synthesis inhibitor such as clindamycin to end toxin, enzyme, and cytokine production.
- Continue therapy for 10 to 15 days or until causative bacteria is eradicated on follow-up cultures.
- Clindamycin or erythromycin if patient is penicillin allergic
- Intravenous immunoglobulin (IVIG):
- Placebo-controlled multicenter study did not show a significant benefit in 28-day survival in patients with definite streptococcal TSS.
- Anecdotal reports of efficacy for streptococcal TSS.
- May be considered for infections refractory to aggressive therapy or in patients with infection in an area that cannot be drained.
- Optimal regimen is not known, although single doses of 1 to 2 g/kg, and several days of 150 to 450 mg/kg per day have been studied.
- Corticosteroids: have not been systematically studied.

 Follow-Up

- Poor prognosis is often heralded by development of pulmonary edema, falling cardiac index and rising pulmonary capillary wedge pressure.
- Renal failure and cerebral edema (complication of fluid resuscitation) are other indications of complicated course.
- Temperature usually returns to normal within 2 days.
- Toxin-mediated cardiomyopathy should resolve if fatal arrhythmia does not occur during decompensated stage.
- Gastrointestinal, hepatic, and musculoskeletal changes resolve rapidly with rare permanent sequelae except for muscle weakness.

- Hair and nail loss may occur 4 to 16 weeks after illness onset; should resolve within 5 to 6 months.
- Encephalopathy is common, rarely causes seizures; both usually resolve within 4 to 5 days.

PREVENTION

- Avoidance of tampon use after first episode of TSS.
- Scrupulous wound care.
- Limitation of intravaginal foreign body use (e.g., tampon, sponge) and strict adherence to manufacturer directions.

PITFALLS

- *S. aureus* isolated from nares or vagina may represent a false-positive finding because 10% to 30% of individuals are healthy carriers.
- The production of TSST-1 by isolate is only presumptive evidence unless case meets diagnostic criteria.
- Failure to meet CDC diagnostic criteria.
- Failure to identify soft-tissue or muscular site of local infection.
- Failure to identify or remove foreign body.
- Erythroderma may not be appreciated if patient is already hypotensive.

 Common Questions and Answers

Q: Can TSS recur?
A: Yes. Inadequate eradication of the nidus of infection, as in sinusitis or the case of a foreign body, can lead to recurrent staphylococcal TSS. Also, individuals with some immune system defects may develop recurrent TSS.

Q: Can TSS be diagnosed in persons who have no risk factors?
A: Yes, there have been reports meeting the case definition in which none of the known associated factors were present.

ICD-9-CM: 040.89

BIBLIOGRAPHY

American Academy of Pediatrics. Toxic shock syndrome. In: Pickering LK, ed. *2003 Red Book: Report of the Committee on Infectious Diseases.* 26th Ed. Elk Grove Village, IL: American Academy of Pediatrics; 2003:624–630.

Bisno AL, Stevens DC. Streptococcal infection of skin and soft-tissues. *N Engl J Med* 1996;334:240–245.

Darenberg J, Ihendyane N, Sjolin J, et al. StreptIg-Study-Group. Intravenous immunoglobulin G therapy in streptococcal toxic shock syndrome: a European randomized, double-blind, placebo-controlled trial. *Clin Infect Dis* 2003;37:333–340.

Reich HL, Crawford GH, Pelle MT, James WD. Group B streptococcal toxic shock-like syndrome. *Arch Dermatol* 2004;140(2):163–166.

Author: Mark L. Bagarazzi

Toxoplasmosis

 Database

DEFINITION

Toxoplasma gondii is an intracellular protozoan parasite with a complex life cycle, whose definitive host is the cat. In addition to causing asymptomatic infection and clinical disease in humans, the organism is capable of causing asymptomatic and symptomatic infections in a wide range of mammals and birds.

PATHOPHYSIOLOGY

- Toxoplasmosis is acquired by the ingestion of oocysts or intact viable tissue cysts in inadequately cooked meat.
- After ingestion, the oocysts and cysts are disrupted by the digestive process, and viable infective organisms cross the gastrointestinal lining. Hematologic spread leads to infection of multiple organs, most notably the heart, skeletal muscle, and the brain. There, slowly growing or dormant cysts remain for the patient's lifetime.
- Congenital toxoplasmosis generally occurs during a primary maternal infection. An exception may be when the pregnant woman is severely immunocompromised; congenital infection has occurred in offspring of HIV-infected women with latent toxoplasmosis infection.
- Primary infection in the first trimester is associated with a higher incidence of symptomatic congenital disease, although the majority of congenital infections occur late in pregnancy, and the neonates have subclinical infection at birth. Overall, 30% to 40% of infants born to mothers with primary infection during pregnancy will be congenitally infected.

EPIDEMIOLOGY

- The rate of acquired infection, usually asymptomatic, varies widely through the world and increases with age.
- Seroprevalence rates among pregnant women vary from 4% to 80% worldwide; in the United States a recent serologic survey found 15% of women of childbearing age were seropositive.
- Worldwide, the incidence of congenital infection ranges from 1 to 7/1,000 live births; in the United States incidence is estimated at 0.1 to 1/1,000 live births. It is believed that annually, 400 to 4,000 infants are born in the United States with congenital toxoplasmosis.
- Seventy percent to 90% of children with congenital toxoplasmosis are asymptomatic at birth.
- Late sequelae (chorioretinitis, mental retardation, seizures, sensorineural hearing loss) occur in greater than 50% of untreated infants considered asymptomatic at birth.

COMPLICATIONS

- Congenital infection: retardation, retinitis, hydrocephalus, seizures, microcephaly, sensorineural hearing loss
- Acquired infection (all rare): adenopathy, mononucleosis-like syndrome, myocarditis, pneumonia, meningitis/encephalitis

PROGNOSIS

- Majority of acquired infections are asymptomatic or associated with mild short-lived symptoms.
- Majority of congenital infections are asymptomatic, although late sequelae occur in greater than 50% of untreated infants.
- Symptomatic newborns are at significant risk for sequelae, most frequently neurologic (hydrocephalus, retardation) or ophthalmic (retinitis, blindness).
- Prenatal treatment appears to decrease risk to newborn; therapy of all infected infants appears to improve outcome.

 Differential Diagnosis

- Primary infection: acute disease symptoms of adenopathy, fever, rash: primary EBV, CMV, HIV infection
- For the newborn with microcephaly/ macrocephaly, hepatosplenomegaly, eye disease; other congenital infections: CMV, syphilis, rubella

 Data Gathering

HISTORY

- For acquired infection: history of contact with cats, eating raw or undercooked meat (especially pork)
- For congenital infection: history of maternal exposure or positive titers (IgG and/or IgM)

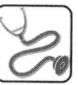 Physical Examination

- Acquired infection: adenopathy, rash, fever, malaise, hepatosplenomegaly
- Congenital infection: microcephaly or macrocephaly, hydrocephalus, chorioretinitis, hepatosplenomegaly, petechiae, sensorineural hearing loss, intracerebral calcifications

 Laboratory Aids

- Screen all pregnant women or their infants in high-incidence areas by use of toxoplasmosis-specific IgM or rise in IgG titer over time.
- Prenatal diagnosis by PCR on amniotic fluid appears promising, with high degree of sensitivity/specificity
- For the at-risk neonate, diagnosis is made by demonstration of specific IgM, IgA, or IgE titers, or rise in IgG titers, and/or clinical symptoms in infant of mother with recent primary infection.
- Head CT or MRI demonstrating calcifications
- Thrombocytopenia
- Early and frequent audiologic and ophthalmic evaluations are a necessity. Many affected infants will have normal neonatal examinations.
- Elevated liver function tests

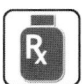 ## Therapy

Pyrimethamine and sulfadiazine for the first year of life for all congenitally infected infants, symptomatic or not. Folic acid is given during the course of therapy to minimize hematologic side effects.

PREVENTION

- Avoidance of undercooked meats
- Seronegative women need to exercise caution in caring for cats.
- Maternal/neonatal antibody screening is important in areas with a significant incidence of toxoplasmosis.
- Treatment of pregnant women with documented seroconversion may prevent congenital infection in many cases.
- If fetal infection is established, aggressive treatment during pregnancy with spiramycin, pyrimethamine, and sulfonamide may ameliorate the severity of the disease in the infant.

 ## Follow-Up

- Continued attention to neurologic development and frequent audiologic and ophthalmic evaluations throughout the first few years of life.
- For children with early symptomatic disease, careful attention to neurologic condition and early intervention services to optimize outcome.

PITFALLS

- Failure to consider diagnosis in at-risk or symptomatic infant.
- Failure to consider the significant risk of late sequelae in asymptomatic exposed/ infected neonate and therefore failure to offer therapy to asymptomatic infected neonate.

 ## Common Questions and Answers

Q: What is the risk of congenital infection in a mother with stable toxoplasmosis?
A: The risk of congenital infection in the offspring of a mother with long-standing toxoplasmosis infection is considered very low; the exception would be for mothers with a significant degree of immunosuppression or deficiency.

Q: What is the risk of congenital infection in offspring of a mother with documented primary infection during pregnancy?
A: Approximately 30% to 40% of infants born to mothers with primary infection during pregnancy will be infected themselves. This rate may be lower if the mother receives therapy (spiramycin or pyrimethamine/ sulfadiazine) prenatally. Of the infected infants, the majority (70% to 90%) are normal at birth; with treatment for 12 months, it appears most will have a favorable outcome.

ICD-9-CM 130.9

BIBLIOGRAPHY

European Multicentre Study on Congenital Toxoplasmosis. Effect of timing and type of treatment on the risk of mother to child transmission of Toxoplasma gondii. *BJOG: an Int J of Obstet Gyn* 2003;110:112–120.

Hill D, Dubey JP. Toxoplasma gondii: transmission, diagnosis and prevention. *Clin Microbiol Infect* 2002;8:634–640.

Jones JL, Lopez A, Wilson M, et al. Congenital toxoplasmosis: a review. *Obstet Gynecol Surv* 2001;56:296–305.

Lynfield R, Guerina NG. Toxoplasmosis. *Pediatr Rev* 1997;18:75–83.

Montoya JG. Laboratory diagnosis of Toxoplasma gondii infection and toxoplasmosis. *J Infect Dis* 2002;185 (Suppl 1):S73–S82.

Roizen N, Swisher CN, Stein MA, et al. Neurological and developmental outcome in treated congenital toxoplasmosis. *Pediatrics* 1995;95:11–20.

Author: Richard M. Rutstein

Tracheitis

Database

DEFINITION

Infection of the trachea associated with airway inflammation and obstruction.

- Acute tracheitis: sudden onset; higher morbidity and mortality.
- Subacute tracheitis: indolent presentation and course; more common among children with prolonged intubation, tracheostomy, and/or underlying respiratory or neurologic conditions.

CAUSES

Bacteria:

- *Staphylococcus aureus* (most common), group A β-hemolytic streptococcus (GABHS), *Moraxella catarrhalis,* and nontypeable *Haemophilus influenzae.*
- *Pseudomonas aeruginosa,* other gram-negative enteric bacteria have been associated with nosocomial infections.
- *Mycobacterium tuberculosis, Mycoplasma pneumoniae, Corynebacterium diphtheria, Haemophilus influenzae* type b (Hib), and respiratory anaerobic bacteria are uncommon pathogens.

Viruses:

- Influenza, parainfluenza, respiratory syncytial, herpes simplex, and measles viruses have been found with bacterial pathogen(s).

Fungi:

- Seen with underlying immunodeficiency disorders or chronic steroid use.

PATHOPHYSIOLOGY

- Epithelial damage from a viral infection or mechanical trauma (endotracheal intubation, surgical procedure) occurs in the trachea at the level of the cricoid cartilage. As a result, the damaged tissue is more susceptible to bacterial superinfection.
- Mucosal damage characterized by marked subglottic edema, copious purulent secretions, and a pseudomembrane (mucosal lining, inflammatory products, and bacteria). These changes lead to marked airway obstruction.
- Toxic shock syndrome may be a consequence if the infection is associated with toxin-producing strains of *Staphylococcus aureus* or *Streptococcus pyogenes.*

EPIDEMIOLOGY

- Affects any age (peak age 2 to 6 years).

—Viral prodrome common.
—Increased incidence during viral respiratory season (fall and winter): up to 75% coinfected with influenza A.
—Gender predisposition unclear (2:1 male to female ratio has been reported).

COMPLICATIONS

- Atelectasis

—Pulmonary edema and pneumonia

- Septicemia

—Staphylococcal toxin syndromes (e.g., toxic shock syndrome)
—Prolonged mechanical ventilation with associated complications (including air leak, infection, pneumothorax, and tracheal stenosis)
—Subglottic stenosis

- Respiratory failure and arrest
- Death (<3.7%)

PROGNOSIS

- Most children recover without any sequelae.

—Younger patients more likely to require intubations and longer hospital stays.
—Children at risk of subacute tracheitis are more likely to have recurrent episodes.

Differential Diagnosis

INFECTIOUS

- Epiglottitis/supraglottitis (presence of supraglottic inflammation)
- Peritonsillar and parapharyngeal abscesses
- Retropharyngeal abscess
- Infectious mononucleosis (Epstein Barr virus)
- Diphtheria (rare)

ENVIRONMENTAL

- Aspiration or inhalation of a caustic substance, including alkali products (e.g., oven cleaner) or smoke
- Foreign body aspiration
- Generalized allergic reaction or anaphylaxis leading to angioedema

TUMORS (rare)

- Papillomas secondary to human papillomavirus (HPV)
- Hamartoma and inflammatory pseudotumor
- Laryngeal tumors

TRAUMA

- Posttraumatic tracheal stenosis
- Blunt trauma to neck

CONGENITAL

- Tracheal stenosis
- Vascular ring and slings
- Laryngotracheal web and clefts
- Laryngotracheomalacia
- Vocal cord paralysis
- Arnold Chiari malformation

Data Gathering

HISTORY

- Hyperpyrexia; nonpainful, brassy cough; noisy respirations; lethargy; dyspnea; rapid progression of airway occlusion (hours to a few days).

—Hoarseness, dysphagia, neck pain, drooling, and croupy cough are less common.
—Presence of upper airway infection.
—Lack of clinical improvement with racemic epinephrine should raise the suspicion for tracheitis.
—An indolent progression of symptoms, including increase of supplemental oxygen requirement and tracheal secretions (thicker and color changes), may be seen in subacute tracheitis.

Physical Examination

Toxic appearance; anxious, agitated, or lethargic; labored breathing with signs of severe respiratory distress (air hunger posture, retractions); pallor or cyanosis; severe stridor; concomitant signs of pneumonia.
Deviated uvula suggests a peritonsillar abscess. Asymmetric lung sounds are often found in patients with foreign bodies in the airway. Generalized lymphadenopathy and splenomegaly are clues for infectious mononucleosis.

Laboratory Aids

Test: Laryngoscopy or bronchoscopy
Significance: Direct visualization and suctioning of obstructed airway is both diagnostic and therapeutic. Findings include a red, edematous and/or eroded trachea and bronchi with purulent secretions and pseudomembrane. Consider in an ill-appearing child with an unclear diagnosis or when the child's condition does not respond to current management.

Test: Tracheal bacterial culture (for aerobic and anaerobic bacteria)
Significance: The gold standard for diagnosis.

Test: Tracheal Gram stain for pathogens and white blood cells (especially polymorphonuclear leukocytes)
Significance: Helps differentiate bacterial infection from colonization.

Test: Blood culture
Significance: Rarely helpful in diagnosis (<50% positive).

Test: Complete blood count (CBC)
Significance: Little diagnostic value, but may show leukocytosis with a left shift.

Test: Erythrocyte sedimentation rate and/or C reactive protein
Significance: May be elevated.

RADIOGRAPHIC STUDIES

Radiographs must be completed in controlled settings by personnel who are trained in airway management.

Test: Lateral and anteroposterior (AP) neck films
Significance: Findings include distention of the hypopharynx, subglottic narrowing, and irregularity of the tracheal wall as a result of mucosal sloughing or the presence of a pseudomembrane.

Test: Chest radiograph
Significance: Obtain if pneumonia, which may be concurrent, is suspected.

 ## Therapy

Rapid assessment of ABCs (airway, breathing, circulation) is essential with emphasis on airway control.

AIRWAY CONTROL

- Supplemental oxygen is usually needed.
- Anticipate and prepare for emergent endotracheal intubation and tracheostomy.
- Endoscopy with suctioning and debridement is often necessary for diagnosis and therapy.
- Subsequent airway suctioning and monitoring prevents adverse outcomes.
- Increased ventilatory support is often required for children with preexisting artificial airways.

DRUGS

- Select antibiotic therapy based on Gram stain and culture results of tracheal secretions.
- One must also consider known prior colonization and institutional pathogens in children with preexisting artificial airway and hospital-acquired infections.

Mild illness: Empiric therapy with amoxicillin-clavulanic acid or a second generation cephalosporin for 10 to 14 days (25 to 45 mg/kg per 24 hr depending on the antibiotic used). Consider a semisynthetic penicillin dicloxacillin (15 to 25 mg/kg per 24 hr) if Hib vaccine completed and clindamycin (10 to 30 mg/kg per 24 hr) if presence of a penicillin allergy.

—Moderate to severe illness: Empiric therapy with a second or third generation cephalosporin or with ampicillin-sulbactam. Consider vancomycin (40 mg/kg per 24 hr) if a hospital-acquired infection is present or if pneumococcal resistance is suspected.
—Anaerobic, pseudomonas, and other gram negative coverage should be considered in children not responding to initial therapy or having preexisting artificial airways.
—Unlike children with croup, nebulized racemic epinephrine does not provide significant relief.
—Duration: Based on clinical response. Usually 10 to 14 days.

 ## Follow-Up

Routine surveillance cultures in children with artificial airways are not recommended. They usually represent colonization in an asymptomatic patient.

SIGNS TO WATCH FOR

- Toxic appearance, excessive secretions, persistent fever, or worsening respiratory distress after introducing antibiotics suggest a resistant organism, an unusual pathogen, or a different diagnosis.

—Recurrent respiratory distress, especially stridor, with subsequent respiratory tract infections suggests underlying tracheal stenosis.
—Sudden deterioration on a ventilator may indicate endotracheal tube obstruction, pneumothorax, or mechanical problems.

PREVENTION

- Routine childhood immunization with Hib and pneumococcal vaccines.
- Influenza vaccination in children identified and targeted by the American Academy of Pediatrics (AAP).

—Avoid overaggressive suctioning of children with artificial airways.

PITFALLS

—Sudden deterioration from tracheal inflammation and secretions. Continuous monitoring necessary.
—Bacterial tracheitis must be considered in all children with sudden upper respiratory distress and hyperpyrexia.

 ## Common Questions and Answers

Q: How can you differentiate a child with severe croup from one with tracheitis?
A: Infectious croup and tracheitis can present with similar features of fever, toxic appearance, respiratory distress, and stridor. Direct endoscopic visualization and culture of the upper airway is the test of choice to distinguish these medical conditions. Croup is commonly associated with parainfluenza virus and a "steeple sign" of the upper trachea on an anteroposterior neck radiograph.

Q: Is influenza A virus a common pathogen of tracheitis?
A: This subject is controversial. Influenza A virus is frequently recovered from tracheal cultures in children who present with tracheitis. It remains unclear, although, if this virus is a pathogen or predisposing factor in tracheitis.

Q: Is the supraglottic area usually involved in tracheitis?
A: No. Unlike epiglottitis, the supraglottic region is usually spared and can help aid in the diagnosis of bacterial tracheitis.

ICD-9-CM 616.0

BIBLIOGRAPHY

Bernstein T, Brilli R, Jacobs B. Is bacterial tracheitis changing? A 14-month experience in a pediatric intensive care unit. *Clin Infect Dis* 1998;27:458–462.

Brook I. Aerobic and anaerobic microbiology of bacterial tracheitis in children. *Pediatr Emerg Care* 1997;13:16–18.

Eckel HE, Widemann B, Damm M, et al. Airway endoscopy in the diagnosis and treatment of bacterial tracheitis in children. *Int J Pediatr Otorhinolaryngol* 1993;27:147–157.

Gallagher PG, Myer CM, III. An approach to the diagnosis and treatment of membranous laryngotracheobronchitis in infants and children. *Pediatr Emerg Care* 1991;7: 337–342.

Jones R, Santos J, Overall J. Bacterial tracheitis. *JAMA* 1979;242:721–726.

Stevenson MD, Gonzalez del Rey JA. Upper airway obstruction: infectious cases. *Clin Pediatr Emerg Care* 2002;3:163–172.

Ward MA. Emergency department management of acute respiratory infections. *Semin Respir Infect* 2002;17(1):65–71.

Author: Charles A. Pohl

Tracheoesophageal Fistula and Esophageal Atresia

 Database

DEFINITION
- Congenital abnormality of the development of the esophagus and trachea.
- In esophageal atresia (EA) the esophagus ends in a blind pouch, generally 10 to 12 cm from the nares. There may also be a distal pouch, with a cord of tissue connecting the two.
- Tracheoesophageal fistula (TEF) is an abnormal communication between trachea and esophagus, often accompanied by other malformations, generally causing respiratory distress in the newborn.
- Five types of lesions, differentiated by anatomy.
—Type C (85%) EA with distal TEF.
—Type A (5% to 10%) isolated EA.
—Type E, also known as "H-type fistula" (3% to 5%): pure TEF without EA—the fistula usually takes an oblique path down from the trachea to the esophagus.
—Type D (1% to 3%) EA with distal and proximal TEF.
—Type B (1%) EA with only proximal TEF.

CAUSES
- Developmental problem occurring before the eighth week of gestation, causing abnormalities in the usual complex process of the separation of the foregut into esophagus and trachea, the mechanism is poorly understood.
- Animal studies suggest that these disorders may be associated with exposure to some teratogens. Adriamycin-exposed rat embryos develop esophageal atresia in a dose dependent frequency.
- In rats, there is evidence that a nonspecific teratogenic insult may lead to ectopic location of the notochord and a deficiency of notochord signaling to foregut mesenchyme, via Shh (Sonic Hedgehog protein), giving rise to esophageal atresia and associated congenital anomalies.

PATHOPHYSIOLOGY
- With TEF, the gastrointestinal (GI) tract can become distended with air as the infant cries or positive pressure ventilation is performed, leading to restriction of diaphragm excursion causing hypoventilation and/or atelectasis.
- With esophageal atresia, the infant is unable to handle oral secretions or feeds and runs the risk of aspiration.
- Distal TEF can cause direct reflux of gastric contents into the airways leading to chemical pneumonitis.
- All of the above can lead to respiratory complications including pneumonia.

GENETICS
Generally sporadic, but there are reports of some familial cases, and there have been reports of autosomal dominant transmission.

- May occur in conjunction with chromosomal abnormalities (~9%) including trisomy 18, trisomy 21, and fragile X syndrome.

EPIDEMIOLOGY
- Incidence: 1 in 2,000 to 4,500 live births.
- Can be isolated, but often associated with other defects: vertebral (50%), cardiac (25% to 30%), GI (10% to 17%)—such as imperforate anus or bowel atresia, renal anomalies (11%), or as part of an association. VATER association includes Vertebral anomalies, imperforate Anus, Tracheoesophageal fistula, Esophageal atresia, Renal anomalies. VACTERL is VATER plus Cardiac and Limb—especially radial—anomalies.

COMPLICATIONS
- Complications are generally pulmonary and depend on the patient's specific anatomy.
- Preoperative complications include pneumonia, sepsis, pneumonitis, respiratory failure.
- Postoperative complications following EA repair occur frequently.
—Anastomotic leak in 10% to 19% requiring re-repair or prolonged chest tube and antibiotic therapy.
—Esophageal strictures in 10% to 40%, especially at the anastomotic site; repeat esophageal dilatation by esophagoscopy is often needed.
—Gastroesophageal reflux disease in these patients (13% to 50%) is likely as a result of intrinsic abnormalities of the esophagus: lower esophageal sphincter tone or esophageal motility anomalies. Therapy generally includes aggressive antireflux medication and possibly fundoplication.
—Fistula recurrence (0% to 10%).
—Injury to recurrent laryngeal nerve.

PROGNOSIS
- Infants with esophageal atresia with proximal TEF have the most severe presentation with life-threatening respiratory compromise presenting in the delivery room.
- H-type TEF may not present with significant disease for months to years, but eventually develop notable chronic cough or recurrent pneumonias.
- Prognosis depends on the type of tracheoesophageal lesion and the presence of comorbid conditions, especially cardiac lesions. Overall survival without cardiac complications is excellent, approaching 100%.
- Surgical complications, especially large esophageal anastomosis leaks cause increased morbidity and/or mortality.
- Adults with these disorders often have problems with swallowing, gastroesophageal reflux, cough, (if tracheomalacia is present), recurrent lung infections.

 Differential Diagnosis

- Gastroesophageal reflux disease. Laryngealtracheoesophageal cleft.
- Accidental perforation of oropharynx by feeding tube can mimic proximal esophageal pouch.
- Esophageal web.
- Esophageal stricture.
- Esophageal duplications.
- Velopharyngeal incompetence.
- Vascular rings, such as double aortic arch.

- Tracheobronchomalacia.
- In older children with recurrent pneumonia—immunodeficiency.

 Data Gathering

HISTORY
Question: Were there any complications during pregnancy?
Significance: With esophageal atresia, mother may have been diagnosed with polyhydramnios as a result of impaired fetal swallowing of amniotic fluid. Prenatal ultrasound can suggest EA by a dilated proximal pouch, reduced intraluminal fluid in the fetal gut, or failure to visualize the fetal stomach.

Question: How does the infant feed?
Significance: With esophageal atresia, from the first hours of life, feeding will result in spitting up, cough, and possible aspiration with resultant cyanosis. The infant may have significant drooling of oropharyngeal secretions—which may be masked by aggressive nursing care with frequent suctioning. The infant with an H-type fistula may have increased choking and cyanosis with feeds and frequent respiratory infections. While symptoms are generally present at birth, diagnosis may be delayed even into adulthood, as these symptoms are nonspecific and often intermittent.

Question: Is the abdomen abnormally flat (scaphoid) or distended?
Significance: A gasless abdomen can indicate esophageal atresia, likely without distal TEF. Abdominal distension can indicate esophageal atresia with distal TEF.

Question: (For an older child) Has there been recurrent respiratory infections?
Significance: While symptoms, retrospectively, are generally present from birth, H-type TEF can be missed in the neonatal period as the presentation is generally nonspecific and intermittent. Older infants and children with TEF generally present with recurrent pneumonia. They may have episodes of choking or cyanosis with feeds, abdominal distention, and have increased sputum production.

 Physical Examination

- Fever or lethargy may be present if there is complicating pneumonia or sepsis.
- Copious drooling with cough as a result of poor clearance of oropharyngeal secretions, if there is esophageal atresia.
- Exam may reveal tachypnea, focal decreased breath sounds with atelectasis; crackles, wheezes, cough with pneumonia or pneumonitis.
- Careful cardiac examination for evidence of associated anomalies. Assess heart tones, murmur, situs, perfusion by pulses, and capillary refill.
- Gasless (flat) or distended abdomen may yield clues to whether esophagus is patent or there is a tracheoesophageal fistula Check for

associated imperforate anus. Kidneys should be palpated for associated renal lesions.
• Cyanosis may be present as a result of cardiac or pulmonary disease or during feeding with aspiration. Limbs should be examined—especially for radial abnormalities.

 ## Laboratory Aids

TESTS

Test: Complete blood count with differential
Significance: Nonspecific test for signs of pneumonia or sepsis. May be part of standard preoperative work-up.

Test: Electrolytes and minerals
Significance: Part of preoperative evaluation; patients can have significant fluid and salt loss through excessive drooling with EA

Test: Creatinine, BUN, urinalysis
Significance: can be helpful to detect concomitant renal anomalies

Test: Other preoperative tests
Significance: Type and screen if blood products are needed. Blood culture, complete blood count, and coagulation studies if sepsis is suspected

RADIOGRAPHIC STUDIES

The goals of radiographic studies are to confirm the diagnosis, locate the site of any tracheo-esophageal fistula (for operative approach), assess the gap size of esophageal atresia (if present), and search for associated anomalies.

Test: Chest radiograph
Significance: A soft 10- to 12-French nasogastric or orogastric feeding tube should be passed into the esophagus; follow-up chest radiograph will either show it terminating or coiling in the blind pouch. A small amount of air can be injected through the feeding tube to distend the blind pouch if it is difficult to visualize.

Test: Fluoroscopic endoscopy
Significance: Occasionally, contrast study of the proximal pouch of an atretic esophagus may be needed to rule out proximal TEF. The standard upper GI series has poor sensitivity for H-type fistulas.

OTHER TESTS

Test: Echocardiography
Significance: Echocardiography can be used to detect associated cardiac anomalies if there are concerning signs such as murmur, hypotension, poor perfusion, or cyanosis.

Test: Bronchoscopy and esophagoscopy
Significance: Bronchoscopy can sometimes directly view dimpling in the trachea at the site of an H-type TEF. Flexible bronchoscopy should be performed with positive distending pressure as fistulae can be hidden by mucosal folds; rigid bronchoscopy may be more sensitive. Simultaneously performed with esophagoscopy, it can also be used to instill small amounts of blue dye into the trachea, with the examiner watching for appearance of the dye in the esophagus.

 ## Therapy

• Surgical referral and intervention is imperative.
• Preoperative management is directed at minimizing respiratory complications. It consists of interventions to reduce aspiration of oral secretions and/or reflux of gastric contents into distal TEF: lateral, semiupright positioning; indwelling suction catheter in blind esophageal pouch (if present); empiric antibiotics; and IV fluids.
• Surgical therapy depends on configuration of the lesion. For EA with distal TEF, gastrostomy may be performed first to facilitate gastric decompression and eventual enteral feeds. Short gap esophageal atresias can undergo primary repair with end-to-end or end-to-side anastomosis.
• The management of long gap EA is more complex. The general approach is delayed repair, after 8 to 12 weeks, as the esophageal pouches exhibit spontaneous growth and hypertrophy. In the meantime, feeds proceed via gastrostomy, and the proximal pouch is evacuated by indwelling suction catheter. Colonic interposition or gastric pull-through procedures are sometimes required to create a neoesophagus, but are more prone to postoperative complications.
• Isolated TEFs are generally ligated by open surgical approach, via incision in the neck (most common) or chest, depending on site of fistula.

 ## Follow-Up

• Postoperative care includes supportive care with pulmonary toilet, prophylactic antibiotics, IV hydration, and slow introduction of feeds by gastrostomy or transpyloric tube. Prior to initiation of oral feeding, contrast esophagram is generally performed to ensure esophageal patency and rule out anastomotic leaks.
• Chest tube should remain in place until drainage stops.
• Long-term follow-up is required to assist with feeding difficulties, to detect late onset complications such as esophageal strictures or reflux with Barrett esophagus. As most of these patients have accompanying tracheomalacia, patients should seek early evaluation and prompt institution of antibiotic therapy for suspected pneumonia.

PITFALLS

• Failure to have a high index of suspicion for a fistula. Clinical presentation of the isolated or recurrent fistula is nonspecific and may be mistaken for gastroesophageal reflux or esophageal dysmotility; 8 of 30 patients required repeat tube-esophagram for detection in one series; and diagnosis by bronchoscopy is difficult. Complicating fistulas can be missed in the context of esophageal atresia repair. The proximal pouch should be dissected to the level of the thoracic inlet and to divide the common wall

between the trachea and esophagus to avoid missing a fistulous connection.
• Postoperative strictures should be suspected if the patient has new episodes of regurgitation, especially in the first few weeks after surgery. The patient should be kept NPO with rapid referral for radiographic diagnosis and possible esophageal dilatation.
• Inadequately treated gastroesophageal reflux disease may encourage esophageal stricture formation. Additionally, severe GERD may encourage Barrett's esophagus and possible esophageal cancer.

 ## Common Questions and Answers

Q: What are the risks and benefits of the surgical repair of esophageal atresia?
A: Without surgical repair, infants are at risk for respiratory complications, including pneumonia and death. Without surgery, it may be difficult to feed the infant. If there are no heart problems, there is an excellent chance that the infant will survive. However, there is likely to be a lifetime risk of relatively minor complications, including the need for frequent medical follow-up.

Q: Will the infant require special care after surgery?
A: Neonates with esophageal atresia generally require daily medication for gastroesophageal reflux disease. Even after repair, they may have significant difficulties with feeding as a result of discoordinated swallowing. Recurrent strictures are fairly common.

ICD-9-CM: 750.3

BIBLIOGRAPHY

Berrocal T, Madrid C, Novo S, Gutierrez J, Arjonilla A, Gomez-Leon N. Congenital anomalies of the tracheobronchial tree, lung, and mediastinum: embryology, radiology, and pathology. *Radiographics* 2004;24:e17.

Little DC, Rescorla FJ, Grosfeld JL, West KW, Scherer LR, Engum SA. Long-term analysis of children with esophageal atresia and tracheoesophageal fistula. *J Pediatr Surg* 2003;38(6):852–956.

Orford J, Manglick P, Cass DT, Tam PP. Mechanisms for the development of esophageal atresia. *J Pediatr Surg* 2001;36(7):985–994.

Tsai JY, Berkery L, Wesson DE, Redo SF, Spigland NA. Esophageal atresia and tracheoesophageal fistula: surgical experience over two decades. *Ann Thorac Surg* 1997;64:778–784.

Upperman JS, Gaines B, Hackman D. H-type congenital tracheoesophageal fistula. *Excerpta Med* 2003;185:599–600.

Zach MS, Eber E. Adult outcomes of congenital lower respiratory tract malformations. *Thorax* 2001;56(1):65–72.

Author: David L. Robinowitz

Tracheomalacia/Laryngomalacia

Database

DEFINITION

- Laryngomalacia (LM)

—Narrowing and collapse of the supraglottic structures of the larynx
—Most common congenital anomaly of the larynx
—Most common noninfectious cause of stridor in children

- Tracheomalacia (TM)

—Narrowing and collapse of the extrathoracic or intrathoracic trachea
—Common cause of chronic wheezing in infants and children
—Classified as primary and secondary:
  —Primary—congenital; results from immature development of the tracheal structures; may occur with other congenital anomalies such as tracheoesophageal fistula, laryngomalacia, and facial anomalies
  —Secondary—acquired in a normally developed trachea after some insult such as prolonged positive-pressure ventilation, recurrent infection or aspiration, or external compression

PATHOPHYSIOLOGY

- Laryngomalacia

—Multiple factors likely involved
—Inward collapse of aryepiglottic folds (cuneiform cartilages) during inspiration
—Elongated, flaccid omega-shaped epiglottis prolapses posteriorly into the pharynx during inspiration
—Immaturity of the laryngeal cartilage results in weakness and collapse during inspiration
—Immaturity of neuromuscular control results in hypotonia of pharyngeal muscles

- Tracheomalacia

—Weakness of the tracheal wall secondary to softening of the anterior cartilaginous rings and to decreased tone of the posterior membranous wall
—During exhalation, increased collapsing pressure across a compliant airway wall causes invagination of the posterior membrane
—With increasing age, the length, area, thickness, and amount of cartilage increases in the anterior rings, and the size and contractility of the membranous wall

Differential Diagnosis

- Laryngomalacia—differential diagnosis of chronic stridor

—Abnormalities of the vocal cords: vocal cord paralysis
—Laryngeal abnormalities: laryngeal cleft, laryngeal web, subglottic hemangioma, papilloma
—Subglottic stenosis (biphasic stridor)

- Tracheomalacia—differential diagnosis of chronic homophonous wheeze

—Structural abnormalities: vascular compression/ring, tracheal stenosis/web, cystic lesion, mass/tumor
—External compression from mediastinal mass, vascular ring
—Nonstructural abnormalities: gastroesophageal reflux disease, retained foreign body, chronic bacterial bronchitis

Data Gathering

HISTORY

Laryngomalacia

- Symptoms may be present at birth or delayed until 1 to 2 months of age.
- Inspiratory stridor
- May be asymptomatic during sleep or quiet breathing
- Worsens with crying, agitation, feeding, upper respiratory infections, supine positioning

TRACHEOMALACIA

- Primary: symptoms may be delayed until 2 to 3 months of age
- Secondary: symptoms delayed until after causative insult occurs
- Expiratory wheeze (or inspiratory stridor if extrathoracic trachea involved)
- Harsh barking cough
- May be asymptomatic during sleep or quiet breathing
- Worsens with crying, agitation, feeding, and upper respiratory infections

Physical Examination

LARYNGOMALACIA

- High-pitched or vibratory, low-pitched inspiratory stridor
- Suprasternal retractions
- Positional changes noted: usually worsens with flexion of neck, supine position
- Stridor transmitted throughout the chest on auscultation

TRACHEOMALACIA

- Homophonous expiratory wheeze (intrathoracic)
- High-pitched inspiratory stridor (extrathoracic)
- Intercostal retractions, worse during acute respiratory infections.

Laboratory Aids

Test: Flexible fiberoptic laryngeoscopy bronchoscopy
Significance:

- Performed during spontaneous breathing
- Most efficient method to evaluate stridor or chronic wheezing
- Visualize the degree and extent of laryngomalacia and/or tracheomalacia
- Evaluate for other airway lesions in the differential diagnosis

Test: Barium swallow
Significance:

- Best noninvasive test to evaluate stridor or chronic wheeze
- Especially of value in evaluation of patients with concomitant swallowing abnormalities
- May see external compression of esophagus from vascular malformation

Test: Chest radiograph
Significance:

- Usually normal in both laryngomalacia and tracheomalacia
- Important to rule out other causes of chronic cough or abnormalities that may cause external airway compression

Test: Airway fluoroscopy
Significance:

- Lateral views are the most useful to visualize the defect
- May be normal; does not rule out diagnosis
- Inspiratory collapsing larynx may be seen in laryngomalacia
- Expiratory narrowing or collapse of the trachea may be seen in tracheomalacia.

Test: MRI
Significance

- Evaluates for thoracic/vascular anomalies that may cause external compression of the airway
- May provide more precise measurements of airway size
- May be performed dynamically to show changes in airway caliber during respiratory cycle

Therapy

- Laryngomalacia

—Usually resolves spontaneously by 15 to 18 months of age
—Observation and reassurance
—Treatment of exacerbating factors, such as upper respiratory infections, asthma or gastroesophageal reflux disease
—Tracheostomy may be needed in severe cases to bypass airway obstruction.
—In rare situations, laryngeal surgery is necessary—epiglottoplasty, resection of arytenoids

- Tracheomalacia

—Usually resolves spontaneously by 18 to 24 months of age
—Observation and reassurance
—Treatment of exacerbating factors, such as upper respiratory infections, asthma or gastroesophageal reflux disease
—Bronchoconstrictor therapy to increase tone of airway wall—bethanecol chloride, ipratropium bromide
—Continuous positive airway pressure (CPAP) may be needed in more severe cases.
—Tracheostomy may be needed in severe cases to bypass lesion or to provide CPAP.
—Humidification of secretions may help some patients, especially during respiratory infections.
—Aortopexy may be needed in severe cases to suspend the anterior trachea and widen the airway.

 ## Follow-Up

Monitor for recurrent respiratory symptoms, poor growth, other exacerbating conditions (asthma, gastroesophageal reflux disease).

PROGNOSIS

- In cases of isolated laryngomalacia and/or tracheomalacia, prognosis is usually excellent.
- In patients with history of tracheoesophageal fistula, vascular ring, or other airway anomalies, tracheal dysfunction may persist after corrective surgery.

PITFALLS

- Missing other causes for presenting symptoms (see Differential Diagnosis)
- Not investigating lower airway in more severe cases of laryngomalacia for other airway anomalies
- Not treating diseases that may exacerbate symptoms and delay spontaneous resolution
- The use of bronchodilators (β^2-agonist) may increase the tracheal wall collapsibility by decreasing muscular tone, thereby making the symptoms worse.
- Bronchoscopy should ideally be done under conscious sedation during spontaneous breathing, to avoid altering vocal cord movement and airway dynamics.
- The use of rigid bronchoscopy may stent open the trachea, making tracheomalacia more difficult to identify.

 ## Common Questions and Answers

Q: When will the symptoms improve?
A: As anatomic structures mature with age, laryngomalacia symptoms may improve by 6 months of age with usual resolution by 18 months of age. Tracheomalacia may last longer, but in both entities symptoms usually resolve completely by age 2 years.

Q: Should all patients have an endoscopic evaluation?
A: No. Diagnosis is usually made based on the appropriate history and physical examination. Infants with mild to moderate typical presentation need only careful monitoring for recurrence or worsening of symptoms and for poor growth. However, airway evaluation should be performed in all cases in which a different pathology is considered or when symptoms worsen or persist past the expected age of resolution.

Q: What should I do when symptoms worsen?
A: Calm the patient, provide humidification of secretions and treatment of intercurrent infection. In cases in which associated bronchospasm is suspected, a trial of steroids or bronchodilators may be considered.

ICD-9-CM 748.3

BIBLIOGRAPHY

Austin J, Ali T. Tracheomalacia and bronchomalacia in children: pathophysiology, assessment, treatment and anaesthesia management. *Paediatric Anaesthesia* 2003;13(1):3–11.

Jacobs I, et al. Tracheobronchomalacia in children. *Arch Otolaryngol Head Neck Surg* 1994;120(2):154–158.

Wright CD. Tracheomalacia. *Chest Surg Clin N Am* 2003;13(2):349–57, viii.

Author: Laura T. Mulreany, MD

Transfusion Reaction

 Database

DEFINITION

Any acute or subacute adverse reaction that develops as a consequence of the administration of blood components. Types include:

- Acute reactions: hemolytic, febrile, allergic, hypervolemia, bacterial sepsis
- Delayed reactions: hemolytic
- Late complications of transfusion: infection, alloimmunization, iron overload, graft-versus-host disease (GVHD)

EPIDEMIOLOGY

Ten percent of blood product recipients develop some type of transfusion reaction.

ACUTE HEMOLYTIC

Cause

Incompatibility of donor RBC antigens and recipient RBC antibodies; usually ABO blood group incompatibility

Pathophysiology

Antigen-antibody interaction leads to complement activation on the surface of the transfused red cells, resulting in acute intravascular hemolysis and vasomotor instability.

 Data Gathering

HISTORY

Fever, chills, abdominal or flank pain, pink or tea-colored urine, tachycardia, hypotension, oliguria

 Laboratory Aids

- Direct Coombs test: positive
- CBC: anemia
- UA: hemoglobinuria
- PT/PTT/fibrinogen/FSP: disseminated intravascular coagulation (DIC)

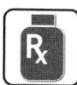 **Therapy**

- As needed to maintain circulation and urine output

—Stop transfusion immediately.
—Hydration
—Pressors
—Diuretics

- Treat DIC with plasma

PREVENTION

Proper labeling of blood specimens and products and correct identification of product and recipient will eliminate most acute hemolytic transfusion reactions.

FEBRILE

Cause

Reaction between recipient antibodies to donor leukocyte or plasma protein antigens

Pathophysiology

Prior exposure to blood products may result in the formation of antibodies to leukocytes or plasma protein antigens; on reexposure the antigen-antibody interaction causes the release of pyrogens; these reactions develop more frequently in individuals with a history of prior transfusion or pregnancy; alternatively, cytokines in the product can cause fever in the recipient.

 Data Gathering

HISTORY

Fever, chills

 Laboratory Aids

- Direct Coombs test
- Blood culture of the patient and product
- Stat gram stain of the product; all should be negative
- This is a diagnosis of exclusion.

 Therapy

Stop transfusion; antipyretics (acetaminophen); may resume transfusion if patient is stable and acute hemolytic transfusion reaction is ruled out.

PREVENTION

Pretransfusion antipyretic or administration of leukodepleted products; the latter is recommended for chronically transfused patients who have a high incidence of febrile transfusion reactions.

ALLERGIC

Cause

Reaction between recipient antibodies and donor plasma proteins; the incidence is sporadic and donor dependent.

Pathophysiology

Unknown

 Data Gathering

HISTORY

Urticaria; sometimes bronchospasm; rarely anaphylaxis

 Laboratory Aids

None

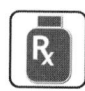 **Therapy**

Stop transfusion; antihistamine (diphenhydramine); steroids or epinephrine in severe reactions

PREVENTION

Pretransfusion antihistamine or administration of washed RBC products (in patients with repeated or severe allergic reactions)

HYPERVOLEMIA

Cause

Administration of an excessive volume of a blood product or infusion at an excessive rate

Pathophysiology

Circulatory overload leading to heart failure

 Data Gathering

HISTORY

Hypertension, dyspnea, rales, cardiac arrhythmia

 Laboratory Aids

CXR: increased pulmonary vascular markings

Therapy

Diuretics (furosemide)

PREVENTION

Administer appropriate volumes (typically 10 mL/kg) at appropriate rate; most RBC transfusions are administered over 3 to 4 hours unless the patient is acutely hypovolemic or actively hemorrhaging; individuals with chronic anemia are frequently euvolemic and should be transfused gradually (smaller volumes over longer time period).

BACTERIAL SEPSIS

Cause

Contaminated blood product; most common in platelet products near the end of their shelf life

Pathophysiology

Intravascular infusion of viable bacteria and endotoxins leads to acute septic shock.

 Data Gathering

HISTORY

Fever, chills, hypotension

 Laboratory Aids

Stat gram stain and blood culture of the transfused product; positive for bacteria

 Therapy

Stop transfusion, fluids if hypotensive, and antibiotics to cover Staphylococcus and Yersinia species

PREVENTION

Sterile technique in blood collection, storage and administration; careful inspection of product prior to transfusion, screening of platelet products by blood banks before they are transfused.

DELAYED HEMOLYTIC

Cause

Incompatibility of donor RBC antigens and recipient RBC antibodies; usually minor blood group antigens

Pathophysiology

Previously transfused individuals who have been sensitized to a minor blood group antigen develop an anamnestic response on reexposure; at the time of the current transfusion, antibody titers are below detectable levels; after the transfusion is complete, titers rise (usually within 3 to 10 days) and extravascular hemolysis occurs.

 Data Gathering

HISTORY

Fever, malaise, dark urine, jaundice; rarely shock, renal failure

 Laboratory Aids

CBC: anemia; bilirubin: elevated; indirect Coombs test (antibody screen): positive; direct Coombs test: positive (mixed field) if done early

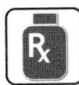 Therapy

Depends on degree of hemolysis; if profound, may need management as described under Acute Hemolytic

PREVENTION

Appropriately performed antibody screen and crossmatch at time of transfusion; check blood bank records for previously identified antibodies.

LATE COMPLICATIONS

Infection

- Posttransfusion hepatitis: caused by hepatitis B or C
- Acquired immunodeficiency syndrome (AIDS): caused by human immunodeficiency virus (HIV)
- Cytomegalovirus (CMV): problematic in individuals with inherited or acquired immunodeficiency states; these individuals should receive CMV-negative products
- Other infection: Epstein-Barr virus, syphilis, malaria, toxoplasmosis, HTLV-I, Chagas disease, babesiosis, filariasis, West Nile virus

Alloimmunization

Formation of antibodies to RBC, platelet, and human leukocyte antigens (HLA) can develop in an individual who has been multiply transfused; this can cause cross-matching problems, febrile transfusion reactions, delayed hemolytic transfusion reactions, and platelet transfusion refractoriness.

Iron Overload

Chronically transfused individuals will accumulate iron as a byproduct of RBC breakdown; an iron-chelating drug (desferrioxamine) will enhance its excretion.

Graft-Versus-Host Disease

Individuals with inherited or acquired T-cell immunodeficiency states can develop GVHD from transfused immunocompetent T cells; can also occur if donor and recipient are related and share HLA types; these individuals should receive irradiated blood products.

 Common Questions and Answers

Q: What is the risk of acquiring certain viral infections?
A: Hepatitis B—1:205,000 units
Hepatitis C—1:1,935,000 units
HIV—1:2,135,000 units

Q: What is the risk of developing bacterial sepsis?
A: 1:50,000 units

Q: Is directed donor blood safer?
A: No, there is no evidence that the infection risk is lower, and some studies suggest that the infection risk actually may be higher.

Q: Is it safe to give a transfusion to a patient with fever?
A: Yes. However, if the temperature rises during the transfusion or if symptoms such as chills or hypotension develop, the transfusion should be stopped and the patient evaluated for a transfusion reaction.

ICD-9-CM 999.8

BIBLIOGRAPHY

AuBuchon JP, Kruskall MS. Transfusion safety: realigning efforts with risks. *Transfusion* 1997;37:1211–1216.

Capon SM, Goldfinger D. Acute hemolytic transfusion reaction, a paradigm of the systemic inflammatory response: new insights into pathophysiology and treatment. *Transfusion* 1995;35(6):513–520.

Dodd RY, Notari EP, Stramer SL. Current prevalence and incidence of infectious disease markers and estimated window-period risk in the American Red Cross blood donor population. *Transfusion* 2002;42:975–979.

Manno CS. What's new in transfusion medicine. *Pediatr Clin North Am* 1996;43:793–808.

Quirolo KC. Transfusion medicine for the pediatrician. *Pediatr Clin North Am* 2002;49:1211–1238.

Schreiber et al. The risk of transfusion transmitted infection. *N Engl J Med* 1996;96:1685–1690.

Author: Cynthia F. Norris

Transient Erythroblastopenia of Childhood

 Database

DEFINITION

An acquired, self-limited suppression of red cell production in an otherwise healthy child.

PATHOPHYSIOLOGY

Unknown. Possible viral etiologies include parvovirus B19 and HHV-6, but this remains hypothetical. A serum inhibitor, such as an IgG directed at the committed erythroid stem cell progenitor, has also been proposed but not yet proven.

GENETICS

There is no simple genetic pattern; familial TEC has been reported (rarely), suggesting a combination of environmental factors and genetic propensity.

EPIDEMIOLOGY

- Mean age at diagnosis is 26 months; less than 10% are older than 3 years of age at diagnosis.
- Slight male predominance (male/female 5.1:3.1)
- There is no seasonal predominance.

COMPLICATIONS

- Cardiovascular compromise secondary to severe anemia is often less than expected given the level of anemia. High-output congestive heart failure is unusual.
- Neurologic symptoms including confusion and transient hemiparesis have been reported but are rare.
- A significant number of patients also have neutropenia (ANC >1,500/μL) during either the acute or recovery phases of the illness.

PROGNOSIS

- All children recover usually within 1 to 2 months from diagnosis (up to 8 months to recovery).
- Prognosis is excellent.
- Recurrence is rare.

 Differential Diagnosis

- Environmental: iron-deficiency anemia
- Metabolic: hypothyroidism
- Congenital: Diamond-Blackfan anemia (this diagnosis usually made within first year of life)
- Neoplasm: leukemia, myelodysplastic syndromes
- Miscellaneous: renal disease, anemia of chronic disease

 Data Gathering

HISTORY

Question: Pallor?
Significance: Typically slow in onset and, therefore, often missed by parents. Often noted by an adult who sees the child less frequently.

Question: Activity level?
Significance: Often preserved because of slow onset of anemia. An extremely anemic child may be irritable, sleepy, and/or lethargic.

SPECIAL QUESTIONS

Question: History of fever, easy bruisability, or frequent/severe infections (especially bacterial)?
Significance: Should alert the clinician to consider other diagnoses such as leukemia and bone marrow failure syndromes.

 Physical Examination

- Child is generally well appearing and not chronically ill.
- Pallor
- Tachycardia secondary to anemia
- Usually no organomegaly, ecchymosis, petechiae, or jaundice

 Laboratory Aids

Test: CBC
Significance: Low Hgb, normal MCV, normal RBC morphology. Total WBC count/morphology and platelet count should be normal; if not, consider leukemias. ANC may be decreased (rarely below 500/μL) but morphology must be normal. RDW may be elevated during recovery.

Test: Reticulocyte count
Significance: Low to zero during anemic phase, should be high during recovery

Test: Chemistry/blood bank
Significance: Bilirubin, LDH, ferritin, iron levels, and Coombs testing should be normal to rule out iron-deficiency anemia and immune hemolysis.

Test: Hemoglobin electrophoresis with quantitative HbF
Significance: Should be normal in TEC, elevated in Diamond-Blackfan anemia

Test: Chest radiograph
Significance: To determine degree of cardiomegaly

Test: Bone marrow aspiration
Significance: May be necessary to rule in TEC and rule out other diagnoses such as Diamond-Blackfan and the leukemias. Presence or absence of early RBC precursors may help predict time to recovery. Maturation of megakaryocytes and the myeloid cell line must be normal, especially if neutropenia is present.

Transient Erythroblastopenia of Childhood

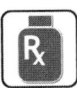 Therapy

- Initial inpatient observation for complications of severe anemia. Daily CBC at least initially to gauge rate of fall of hemoglobin/rise of reticulocyte count and to estimate time to recovery.
- PRBC transfusion only if there is evidence of cardiovascular compromise. If a transfusion is needed, transfuse slowly to prevent fluid overload. A good rule of thumb is to transfuse the same number of mL/kg as the patient's hemoglobin, over 3 to 4 hours. A second transfusion is rarely required.
- Normal activity and diet for age, as tolerated
- Instruct family on signs and symptoms of severe anemia.

DRUGS

No role for prednisone, iron supplements, anabolic steroids, or other immunosuppressive agents. Short-term folic acid may be indicated during reticulocytosis.

 Follow-Up

WHEN TO EXPECT IMPROVEMENT

- Clinic visits weekly to monitor hemoglobin and reticulocytes. (These visits may need to be more frequent in the beginning of the illness and less frequent as recovery becomes evident.)
- Elevation of reticulocyte count is the first sign of recovery.

PREVENTION

There is no known way to prevent TEC.

ISOLATION

Because of possible teratogenicity of parvovirus 19 and contagion within hospital

PITFALLS

- TEC must be an isolated normocytic, normochromic anemia. If the other cell lines are affected or if the anemia is macrocytic, consider bone marrow failure syndromes.
- Iron therapy has no place in the treatment of TEC. Be sure to check RBC indices and reticulocyte count prior to instituting iron therapy for anemia.

 Common Questions and Answers

Q: Can other children in a family get this illness?
A: The cause(s) of this illness in otherwise normal children is unknown. It is very rare for other family members to be affected. It is appropriate to reassure parents regarding this issue.

Q: Are transfusions always necessary?
A: No. Only in cases of heart failure is a transfusion necessary. Most often, children can be managed with watchful waiting.

Q: How can TEC be distinguished from Diamond-Blackfan syndrome?
A: Children with Diamond-Blackfan syndrome are usually less than 1 year old and can have elevated hemoglobin F levels. If a bone marrow aspirate is obtained during the recovery phase of TEC, then the diagnosis will be clear. Often, however, only time will tell. Children with TEC always recover; those with Diamond-Blackfan syndrome do not.

ICD-9-CM 284.8

BIBLIOGRAPHY

Bhambhani K, Inoue S, Sarnaik SA. Seasonal clustering of transient erythroblastopenia of childhood. *Am J Child Dis* 1988;142:175–177.

Cherrick I, Karayalcin G, Lanzkowsky P. Transient erythroblastopenia of childhood: prospective study of fifty patients. *Am J Pediatr Hematol Oncol* 1994;16(4):320–324.

Nathan DG, Oski FA, eds. *Hematology of Infancy and Childhood.* 4th Ed. Philadelphia: WB Saunders, 1993.

Penchansky L, Jordan JA. Transient erythroblastopenia of childhood associated with human herpesvirus type 6, variant B. *Am J Clin Pathol* 1997;108(2):127–132.

Skeppner G, Kreuger A, Elinder G. Transient erythroblastopenia of childhood: prospective study of 10 patients with special reference to viral infections. *J Pediatr Hematol Oncol* 2002;24(4):294–298.

Author: Julie W. Stern

Transient Tachypnea of the Newborn (TTN)

 Database

DEFINITION

Early onset of tachypnea (respiratory rate >60 breaths per minute) following uneventful, normal preterm or term, vaginal or cesarean delivery; sometimes with retractions, expiratory grunting, or cyanosis relieved by minimal oxygenation (<40%).

PATHOPHYSIOLOGY

• Slow or decreased absorption of fetal lung fluid, including fluid accumulation in the interstitial space, resulting in decreased pulmonary compliance, decreased tidal volume and increased dead space
• Mild immaturity of the surfactant system may contribute to decreased pulmonary compliance and result in increased respiratory rate. In some infants with TTN, a decreased amount of phosphatidyl glycerol has been found in their amniotic fluid.

EPIDEMIOLOGY

• Eleven per 1,000 live births (very common)

COMPLICATIONS

• Hypoxia
• Respiratory failure requiring CPAP (continuous positive airway pressure) or mechanical ventilation, rarely

PROGNOSIS

Generally considered a self-limited condition with no recurrence and no residual pulmonary dysfunction. Some studies, however, have demonstrated associations with persistent fetal circulation in the neonatal period and asthma during childhood.

 Differential Diagnosis

RESPIRATORY

• Meconium aspiration
• Respiratory distress syndrome
• Pneumothorax
• Pneumomediastinum

INFECTION

• Pneumonia
• Sepsis

NEUROLOGIC

• Cerebral hypoventilation
• Birth asphyxia

CARDIAC

• Congenital cyanotic heart disease

METABOLIC

• Conditions manifesting as metabolic acidosis

MISCELLANEOUS

• CCAM (congenital cystic adenomatoid malformation)

 Data Gathering

HISTORY

Question: When was the onset of tachypnea? *Significance:* In general, TTN usually presents as early onset of tachypnea (within first few hours of life)

Question: Are there maternal risk factors? *Significance:* Recent research has demonstrated that TTN was twice as likely for infants of mothers with asthma compared to infants of mothers without asthma.

Question: Are there birth-related risk factors? *Significance:* Birth risk factors include maternal sedation, maternal fluid administration, maternal exposure to β-mimetic agents, prolonged labor, cesarean section, preterm birth, fetal asphyxia, and infant male sex. The mechanisms are unknown. The presence of risk factors for other conditions, (e.g., maternal fever) may make a TTN diagnosis less likely and other diagnoses more likely (e.g., pneumonia or sepsis).

 Physical Examination

• Respiratory rate >60 per minute
• Cyanosis, grunting, flaring, intercostal retractions
• Lungs clear on auscultation, without rales or rhonchi
• Absence of signs and symptoms more specific for infection, and neurologic and cardiac conditions (e.g., fever, cyanosis without respiratory distress)

Laboratory Aids

TESTS

Test: Pulse oximetry
Significance: Oxygen saturation should be maintained above 96%

Test: Arterial blood gas
Significance: Metabolic acidosis with base deficit suggests asphyxia

Test: Complete blood count
Significance: Decreased or increased white cell count and increased immature forms (e.g., bands) suggest infection.

Test: Blood culture
Significance: Positive result indicates infection.

RADIOGRAPHIC STUDIES

Test: Chest radiograph
Significance: TTN indicated by prominent central pulmonary vascular markings (central perihilar streaking), fluid lines in the fissures, hyperaeration, flat diaphragm, cardiomegaly, and, occasionally, pleural fluid.

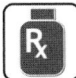 ## Therapy

 ### Emergency Care

- NPO—initially, nothing by mouth until respiratory status stabilized and diagnosis clarified
- Oxygen—may help reduce respiratory distress if patient hypoxic
- CPAP or mechanical ventilation if indicated
- Antibiotics if pneumonia or sepsis suspected
- Furosemide (diuretic) has not been shown to improve TTN

SUPPORTIVE CARE

- Intravenous (IV) fluids if NPO
- Monitoring of respiratory status (e.g., pulse oximetry)

DURATION OF THERAPY

- Typically 2 to 5 days.

 ## Follow-Up

WHEN TO EXPECT IMPROVEMENT

- Rapid respirations slow gradually
- Twelve to 72 hours

SIGNS TO WATCH FOR

- Fever, lethargy, poor feeding, early jaundice
- Persistent or increased need for oxygen

PITFALLS

- Since TTN is a diagnosis of exclusion, it is important to consider and exclude other diagnoses by carefully relying on history, examination, and appropriate laboratory aids.

 ## Common Questions and Answers

Q: Will my baby have breathing problems afterward?
A: No.

Q: Is my baby at risk for breathing problems such as asthma?
A: No. Although, there is a relationship between maternal asthma and TTN, there is no consistent evidence thus far of a relationship between TTN and the development of asthma.

Q: When can my baby go home?
A: When his or her breathing rate is low enough so that she or he feed well, and when she or he no longer requires oxygen.

BIBLIOGRAPHY

Dani C, Reali MF, Bertini G, et al. Risk factors for the development of respiratory distress syndrome and transient tachypnea in newborn infants. *Eur Resp J* 1999;14:155–159.

Demissie K, Marcella SW, Breckenbridge MB, Rhoads GG. Maternal asthma and transient tachypnea of the newborn. *Pediatrics* 1998;102:84–90.

Hook B, Kiwi R, Amini SB, Fanaroff A, Hack M. Neonatal morbidity after elective repeat cesarean section and trial of labor. *Pediatrics* 1997;100:348–353.

Lewis V, Whitelaw A. Furosemide for transient tachypnea of the newborn. *Cochrane Database Syst Rev* 2002;1:CD003064.

Martin RJ, Sosenko I, Bancalari E. Respiratory problems. In: Klaus MH, Fanaroff AA, eds. *Care of the High-Risk Neonate.* 5th Ed. Philadelphia: WB Saunders, 2001:262–263.

Miller MJ, Fanaroff AA, Martin RJ. Respiratory disorders in preterm and term infants. In: Fanaroff AA, Martin RJ, eds. *Neonatal-Perinatal Medicine: Diseases of the Fetus and Infants.* 7th Ed. St. Louis: Mosby Year Books, Inc., 2002:1030–1031.

Whitsett JA, Pryhuber GS, Rice WR, Warner BB, Wert SE. In: Avery G, Fletcher MA, MacDonald MG, eds. *Neonatology, Pathophysiology and Management of the Newborn.* 5th Ed. Philadelphia: Lippincott, Williams & Wilkins, 1999:505–506.

Author: John I. Takayama

Transposition of the Great Arteries

 Database

DEFINITION

• Abnormal anatomic relationship between the great arteries and the ventricles in which the aorta arises from the anatomic right ventricle and the pulmonary artery arises from the anatomic left ventricle.

PATHOLOGY

• In transposition of the great arteries (TGA) the aorta originates anteriorly from the right ventricle and carries desaturated blood to the body, and the pulmonary artery originates posteriorly from the left ventricle and carries oxygenated blood to the lungs. There is fibrous continuity between the pulmonary and mitral valves and subaortic conus (infundibulum) is present. In the normal heart the aorta arises posteriorly from the left ventricle, there is fibrous continuity between the aortic and mitral valves, and subpulmonary conus is present.
• The most common type of TGA, known as D-Transposition or D-TGA is TGA (S,D,D): situs solitus of the atria and viscera (S), dextroventricular segment situs (D), aortic valve annulus to the right of the pulmonary artery (D).
• Other variations include TGA (S,D,L) in which the aortic valve annulus is to the left of the pulmonary artery (L), and TGA (S,L,L) or "corrected transposition," in which there is situs solitus of the atria and viscera (S), levoventricular segment situs (L), and the aortic valve annulus is to the left of the pulmonary artery (L).
• Associated abnormalities: Patent ductus arteriosus (PDA) and patent foramen ovale (PFO) with intact ventricular septum (50%), ventricular septal defect (VSD) (40%), dynamic obstruction of the left ventricular outflow tract (subpulmonary obstruction) (20%), posterior malalignment VSD with left ventricular outflow tract obstruction (subpulmonic stenosis, pulmonary stenosis, pulmonary atresia) (10%), anterior malalignment VSD with right ventricular outflow tract obstruction (subaortic stenosis, aortic stenosis, coarctation of the aorta or interruption of the aortic arch) (10%), coronary branching abnormalities (33%), straddling of the atrioventricular valve, and leftward juxtaposition of the atrial appendages (5%).

PATHOPHYSIOLOGY

• Systemic and pulmonary circulations are separated and function in parallel.
• Desaturated systemic venous blood passes through the right heart to the aorta, although the oxygenated pulmonary venous blood passes through the left heart and returns to the lungs.
• Survival depends on defects that permit mixing between the two circulations (PDA, PFO, VSD).

EPIDEMIOLOGY

• TGA represents 5% to 7% of all congenital heart disease.
• Incidence is 20 to 30 per 100,000 live births, with a 60% to 70% male preponderance.

 Differential Diagnosis

The differential diagnosis for the neonate with transposition of the great arteries is that for the cyanotic neonate.

CARDIAC

• Lesions with ductal-dependent pulmonary blood flow:

—Tricuspid atresia with normally related great arteries
—Tetralogy of Fallot
—Tetralogy of Fallot with pulmonic atresia
—Critical pulmonic stenosis
—Pulmonary atresia with intact ventricular septum
—Ebstein's anomaly
—Heterotaxy (most forms)

• Ductal-independent mixing lesions:

—Total anomalous pulmonary venous connection without obstruction
—Truncus arteriosus

• Lesions with ductal-dependent systemic blood flow:

—Hypoplastic left heart syndrome
—Interrupted aortic arch
—Critical coarctation of the aorta
—Critical aortic stenosis

PULMONARY

Primary Lung Disease

• Airway obstruction

Extrinsic Compression of the Lungs

NEUROLOGIC

• CNS dysfunction

Respiratory Neuromuscular Dysfunction

HEMATOLOGIC

• Methemoglobinemia
• Polycythemia

 Data Gathering

HISTORY

• Infants are of normal birth weight, or sometimes large for gestational age.
• Cyanosis
• Tachypnea often without retractions.
• Poor feeding.

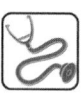 Physical Examination

• General: moderate to severe cyanosis in a large male newborn.
• Cardiovascular: single loud S2, no heart murmur is heard in infants with intact ventricular septum, soft systolic murmur in those infants with a VSD, and a systolic ejection murmur of valvar or subvalvar aortic or pulmonic stenosis may be heard.
• Respiratory: generally there is dyspnea and tachypnea without retractions in the neonate without a VSD; when a large VSD results in congestive heart failure retractions will be present.
• Abdomen: hepatomegaly occurs when there is a large VSD and congestive heart failure.

 Laboratory Aids

TESTS OR STUDIES

• Arterial Blood Gas: hypoxemia (P_{O_2} often in low 30s) unchanged in 100% F_{iO_2}. Infants with marginal mixing have p_{O_2} <20 with metabolic acidosis.
• Chest Radiograph: mild cardiomegaly with an egg-shaped heart with narrow superior mediastinum and increased pulmonary vascular markings (egg on a string)
• Electrocardiogram: initially normal, progressing to right ventricular hypertrophy and right axis deviation
• Echocardiogram: two dimensional echocardiography and color-flow Doppler studies usually provide all of the anatomic and functional information required for management of infants with D-TGA. The study should focus on the alignment of the great arteries and other associated anomalies, specifically defects that promote intercirculatory mixing, the presence of left or right ventricular outflow tract obstruction, and the coronary anatomy.

Therapy

DRUGS

• Correction of metabolic acidosis, hypoglycemia, and hypocalcemia improves myocardial function.
• Prostaglandin E1 (PGE) is used for severe cyanosis to promote mixing at the ductus arteriosus. Instituting PGE1 may increase pulmonary venous congestion if there is an inadequate interatrial communication by increasing the pulmonary blood flow. Side effects of PGE1 include apnea, fever, and hypotension.
• Interventional catheterization
• Balloon atrial septostomy (Rashkind procedure) is used in the severely hypoxemic infant with an intact or restrictive atrial septum to promote intercirculatory mixing at the atrial level and stabilize the neonate prior to definitive or palliative surgery.

SURGERY

Definitive surgery for D-TGA includes procedures that redirect the right- and left-sided pulmonary and systemic venous returns at the atrial, ventricular, and great artery level, and include:

• Atrial inversion: Atrial inversion procedures involve baffling the pulmonary venous blood flow to the tricuspid valve (systemic circulation), and the systemic venous blood flow to the mitral valve (pulmonary circulation). The two atrial inversion operations include, the Mustard procedure, in which prosthetic or pericardial baffles are used to redirect the blood, and the Senning procedure, in which the baffles are made of an atrial septal flap and the right atrial free wall. The Senning or Mustard procedures are used in the following infants:

—Infants with D-TGA with intact ventricular septum who have not been repaired within the first month of life.
—Neonates with D-TGA with intact ventricular septum and moderate to severe pulmonic stenosis.
—Neonates with D-TGA with "unswitchable coronaries"(<1% of cases).

• Ventricular inversion:

—D-TGA with a VSD and severe pulmonic stenosis: The Rastelli operation may be used to redirect blood flow at the ventricular level. In this operation, the left ventricular blood flow is baffled to the aorta by creating an intraventricular tunnel between the VSD and the aortic valve. A conduit is placed from the right ventricle to the pulmonary artery to redirect the right ventricular blood flow.
—D-TGA with a VSD with severe aortic stenosis: The Damus-Kaye-Stansel operation in conjunction with the Rastelli operation may be used to redirect ventricular blood flow.

• Arterial switch: Surgical switching of the great arteries with coronary reimplantation.

PROGNOSIS

• Without treatment, there is a 30% mortality within the first week of life, 50% within the first month, 70% within the first 6 months, and 90% within the first year.
• In most centers, the mortality rate after the arterial switch operation for D-TGA with intact ventricular septum or D-TGA with a VSD is less than 3%. Factors that have been shown to increase the mortality risk include an intramural course of the left coronary artery, retropulmonary course of the left coronary artery, complex arch abnormalities, right ventricular hypoplasia, multiple VSDs, and a straddling atrioventricular valves.

COMPLICATIONS/FOLLOW-UP

• Complications of the intraatrial surgeries include obstruction of pulmonary venous return (<2% of cases), obstruction of systemic venous return (<5% of cases), residual intraatrial baffle shunt (<20% of cases), tricuspid regurgitation (5% to 10%), absence of sinus rhythm (>50% of cases), supraventricular arrhythmias (50%), and moderate to severely depressed right ventricular function (10%). Follow-up is recommended every 6 to 12 months to detect arrhythmias, tricuspid regurgitation, or depressed right ventricular function, which generally occurs years after surgery. Arrhythmias include sinus node dysfunction (marked sinus bradycardia, ectopic atrial rhythm, junctional rhythm or junctional bradycardia) and supraventricular tachycardia, especially atrial flutter.
• Complications after the Rastelli operation include conduit obstruction and complete heart block. Follow-up is recommended every 12 months to monitor for conduit obstruction, left ventricular outflow tract obstruction, and heart block.
• Complications after the arterial switch operation are relatively rare as compared to after the atrial and ventricular inversion operations, and include supravalvar pulmonary stenosis at the anastomotic site (<5% of cases), supravalvar aortic stenosis at the anastomotic site (<5% of cases), neoaortic regurgitation, neoaortic root dilation, and coronary artery obstruction, which may lead to ischemia and infarction. These complications are uncommon and usually hemodynamically insignificant. Mortality results from the following:

—Early mortality is usually related to kinking or obstruction of the coronary arteries during transfer to the neo-aorta, an "unprepared" left ventricle, or hemorrhage from the multiple suture lines.
—Late mortality (1% to 2%) usually occurs from myocardial ischemia, pulmonary vascular obstructive disease, or during reoperation for supravalvular stenosis.
—Follow-up is recommended every 6 to 12 months to monitor for supravalvar aortic or pulmonic stenosis, neoaortic valve insufficiency, and coronary ischemia.

BIBLIOGRAPHY

Bellinger DC, Wypij D, duDuplessis AJ, Rappaport LA, Jonas RA, Wernovsky G, Newburger JW. Neurodevelopmental status at eight years in children with dextro-transposition of the great arteries: the Boston Circulatory Arrest Trial. *J Thorac Cardiovasc Surg* 2003;126(5):1385–1396.

Culbert EL, Ashburn DA, Cullen-Dean G, Joseph JA, Williams WG, Blackstone EH, McCrindle BW. Congenital Heart Surgeons Society. Quality of life of children after repair of transposition of the great arteries. *Circulation* 2003;108(7):857–862.

Formigari R, Toscano A, Giardini A, Gargiulo G, Di Donato R, Picchio FM, Pasquini L. Prevalence and predictors of neoaortic regurgitation after arterial switch operation for transposition of the great arteries. *J Thorac Cardiovasc Surg* 2003;126(6): 1753–1759.

Langley SM, Winlaw DS, Stumper O, et al. Midterm results after restoration of the morphologically left ventricle to the systemic circulation in patients with congenitally corrected transposition of the great arteries. *J Thorac Cardiovasc Surg* 2003;125(6): 1229–1241.

Mavroudis C, Backer CL. Physiologic versus anatomic repair of congenitally corrected transposition of the great arteries. *Sem Thorac Cardiovasc Surg* 2003;6:16–26.

Pasquali SK, Hasselblad V, Li JS, Kong DF, Sanders SP. Coronary artery pattern and outcome of arterial switch operation for transposition of the great arteries: a meta-analysis. *Circulation* 2002;106(20): 2575–2580.

Williams WG, McCrindle BW, Ashburn DA, Jonas RA, Mavroudis C, Blackstone EH. Congenital Heart Surgeon's Society. Outcomes of 829 neonates with complete transposition of the great arteries 12–17 years after repair. *Eur J Cardio-Thoracic Surg* 2003;24(1):1–9.

Author: Bradley S. Marino

Transverse Myelitis

 ## Database

DEFINITION

Inflammation in the spinal cord causing acute/or subacute loss of motor, sensory, and autonomic function, often preceded by midback pain; may be postinfectious, postvaccination, or associated with multiple sclerosis. While acute transverse myelitis (ATM) implies an inflammatory disease of the spinal cord, acute transverse myelopathy is a broader term refers to any process that acutely impairs spinal cord function. Presumed pathophysiology of ATM is autoimmune mediated inflammation and demyelination of the spinal cord. Postinfectious etiology largely predominates in children.

Associated Conditions

• Is most commonly associated with infection.
• May be part of demyelinating disorders.

—May either occur as the first episode of multiple sclerosis (MS) or in the setting of MS.
—Occurs with demyelination of optic nerves (optic neuritis), which is referred to as Devic disease or neuromyelitis optica (NMO).
—Monophasic demyelinating disease acute disseminated encephalomyelitis (ADEM) has multiple demyelinating lesions in the brain and in the spinal cord.

• ATM may be associated with systemic inflammatory diseases (e.g., systemic lupus erythematosus, primary antiphospholipid syndrome, juvenile rheumatoid arthritis, sarcoidosis, connective tissue disease, vasculitis) may present with acute or recurrent transverse myelitis.
• Rarely seen in association with metabolic causes of myelopathy such as vitamin B12 deficiency.
• ATM does not usually occur in association with inherited demyelinating diseases (e.g., adrenomyeloneuropathy/leukodystrophy, Pelizaeus-Merzbacher, globoid cell leukodystrophy, and metachromatic leukodystrophy) which usually present with chronic myelopathy.

EPIDEMIOLOGY

Incidence: 1 to 4/million per year, affecting all ages with bimodal peaks between the ages of 10 and 19 years and 30 and 39 years. Boys and girls are affected equally.

 ## Differential Diagnosis

Presentation of ATM in a toddler may resemble osteomyelitis, arthritis, toxic synovitis, or even an acute abdominal process: extreme irritability, unwillingness to bear weight. In many cases extremity weakness seen in ATM may resemble an acute neuromuscular disorder such as Guillain-Barré syndrome or polymyositis, in which cases the definitive myelopathic signs (spastic tone, hyperreflexia, upgoing toes, sensory level) are not present. GBS is frequently confused with ATM, particularly when the latter does not show typical upper motor neuron findings; normal MRI and the "albuminocytologic dissociation" (high-protein, low cell count) in CSF from patients with GBS helps distinguish the two conditions.
Must exclude other causes of myelopathy which requires different treatment. For example: urgent neurosurgical consultation should be obtained if imaging reveals a surgically remediable cause of myelopathy (e.g., epidural abscess, tumor, AVM); emergent radiation and/or high dose intravenous corticosteroid therapy for neoplastic cord compression.

• Compressive myelopathies:

—Vertebral osteomyelitis/discitis
—Intrinsic or extrinsic tumor
—Spine trauma
—Epidural abscess

• Infectious causes of myelopathy:

—Polio: raises concern of underlying immunodeficiency
—Lyme disease: in children with possible exposure; serology is nonspecific but is sensitive unless antibiotics given early in the course (ablating immune response)
—Syphilis: usually chronic, tertiary form (tabes dorsalis), predominantly involves the posterior column

• Vascular: cord ischemia (postcardiac surgery), cord AVM

 ## Data Gathering

HISTORY

• Most prominent presentation is neurologic dysfunction consistent with a spinal cord injury at a specific level. Bilateral, not necessarily symmetric symptoms are usually present.
• ATM may be suggested by history of back pain, sensory level, urinary, or fecal incontinence/retention. The patient often has lower extremity weakness or inability to bear weight, possibly with decreased spontaneous use of hands.
• Details of the temporal course of the symptoms is important, because sudden onset of weakness raise the possibility of acute structural or vascular causes of myelopathy. In ATM, the onset of spinal cord dysfunction usually progress in 4 hours to 21 days, the patient's signs usually plateau and evolve toward spasticity/hyperreflexia.
• ATM is often preceded by respiratory illness, or vaccination, or systemic illness. One should determine if there is prior history of infection or systemic inflammatory disease
• Other important history includes vascular/ischemia, neoplastica, multiple sclerosis, radiation exposure, trauma, or immunodeficiency, which may suggest other causes of acute myelopathy.

 ## Physical Examination

• Extreme irritability, extent of weakness is assessed by how vigorously the child resists examination.
• Fever, hypertension, tachycardia, meningeal signs may be present, in which cases CNS infection need to be ruled out; point tenderness over the spine may point to trauma or infection.
• Neurologic examination directed to visual acuity and color vision, funduscopic examination for optic nerve head pallor (optic neuritis)
• Increased tone, spastic weakness is usually symmetric, legs more than arms
• Reflexes are usually brisk, with positive Babinski sign.
• Sensory ataxia, a sensory level (a partial level is commonly seen) that may spare joint position and vibration, may be present.
• Sphincter dysfunction can lead to emergent complication of urinary retention or incontinence; check for loss of anal wink, bladder dilatation, and large volume of postvoid residual (>100 mL).

Laboratory Aids

A diagnosis of ATM requires evidence of inflammation of the spinal cord. MRI and CSF analysis are the two most important tests and are mandatory in suspect ATM. Enhancing spinal cord lesion or pleocytosis or increased IgG index is required for the diagnosis. If both tests are negative, repeat tests in 2 to 7 days is recommended.

• The first priority in acute myelopathy is to rule out structural cause—compressive myelopathy.
• Gadolinium-enhanced MRI of spine (above the level that could explain level of weakness or sensory) excludes structural causes of myelopathy and can be diagnostic of transverse myelitis.
• The second priority is to define the presence/absence of spinal cord inflammation and to rule out other CNS infection.

Lumbar puncture is usually done after imaging, often shows normal or slightly increased protein, mild pleocytosis with lymphocyte predominance. Elevation of IgG index and presence of oligo clonal bands are indicative of MS or other systemic inflammatory disease. CSF gram stain, bacterial, viral, and fungal culture, VDRL, lyme antibodies, and PCR of specific viruses should all be negative in ATM.

• Third priority is to define extent of demyelination. Gadolinium-enhanced MRI of the brain and the orbit and evoked potential studies (e.g., visual evoked potential, somatosensory evoked potential) may identify other sites
• Investigation for underlying systemic inflammatory disorder including ESR and ANA; for granulomatous disease or infection including PPD/anergy panel, serum ACE (angiotensin-converting enzyme, elevated in sarcoidosis), RPR, Lyme titer; and for underlying metabolic disorder including VLCFA. Viruses associated with ATM include the herpes viruses (EBV, VZV, HSV), CMV mumps, rubella, influenza, hepatitis A, B, C, HIV. Positive IgM or greater than fourfold increase in IgG levels on two successive tests to a specific infectious agent suggests diagnosis of parainfectious ATM.

 ## Therapy

• Intravenous methylprednisolone may be useful in ATM or other acute demyelinating diseases based on a few observational studies. Intravenous immunoglobulin (IVIG) or plasmapheresis may be a safe and effective therapeutic alternative in patients that do not respond to or intolerant of intravenous methylprednisolone.
• Cyclophosphamide has been reported to be useful in myelitis associated with systemic inflammatory diseases.
• Symptomatic management: anticipate urinary retention to prevent perforated bladder. Bowel/bladder regimen, catheterization, prophylactic antibiotics, stool softeners are often used.
• Unlike acute polyneuropathy (Guillain Barré syndrome), ATM rarely causes respiratory insufficiency unless patients have cervical lesions. In such cases, an intensive care setting to anticipate respiratory distress or autonomic instability, mechanical ventilation, cautious use of antihypertensive agents may be necessary.
• Physical and occupational therapy (PT/OT) may help promote functional recovery and prevent contractures.

 ## Follow-Up

• One-third of individuals with ATM recover completely, with the symptoms mostly resolve (gradually) in 3 to 6 months; one-third are left with moderate disability, and one-third have severe disability. Residual neurologic deficits include fixed weakness, sensory, or autonomic deficits. Sphincter dysfunction improves more slowly than the other deficits. Treatment is largely symptomatic and long term PT/OT may be beneficial.
• Prognostic factors: older age, increased deep tendon reflexes, and presence of Babinski sign may indicate better course. Rapid progression, back pain, and spinal shock predict poor recovery.
• ATM may be the presenting feature of MS, especially in patients with partial ATM and abnormal initial brain MRI, in such cases, follow up MRIs should be considered.

 ## Common Questions and Answers

Q: What makes you think this could be MS instead?
A: History of other neurologic symptoms such as internuclear ophthalmoplegia, optic neuritis, focal weakness and numbness that lasted at least 24 hours to days, have now resolved completely, other lesions on brain/spine MRI at the time of presentation, and subsequent new MRI lesions

Q: What is the usual clinical course?
A: The course of ATM in children proceeds through three stages: (a) initial motor loss precedes sphincter dysfunction in most patients, there is often a sensory loss below certain levels, usually over 2 to 3 days; (b) plateau phase: the mean duration of plateau is 1 week; and (c) a recovery phase.

Q: What causes the pain and irritability commonly seen in children with TM?
A: Pain in TM may be as a result of (a) neuropathic pain from nerve root inflammation, (b) nociceptive pain from dural inflammation, (c) muscle spasm from motor dysfunction, (d) bladder distension from dysautonomia, (e) psychological distress from loss of motor control, or (f) dysesthesia from demyelination of spinothalamic tract.

ICD-9-CM 323.9

BIBLIOGRAPHY

Defresne P, Hollenberg H, Husson B et al. Acute transverse myelitis in children: clinical course and prognostic factors. *J Child Neurol* 2003;18:401–406.

Defresne P, Meyer L, Tardieu M, et al. Efficacy of high dose steroid therapy in children with severe acute transverse myelitis. *J Neurol Neurosurg Psychiatry* 2001;71:272–274.

Meca-Lallana JE, Rodriguez-Hilario H, Martinez-Vidal S et al. Plasmapheresis: its use in multiple sclerosis and other demyelinating processes of the central nervous system. An observation study. *Rev Neurol* 2003; 37:917–926.

Miyazawa R, Ikeuchi Y, Tomomasa T et al. Determinants of prognosis of acute transverse myelitis in children. *Ped Internat* 2003;45:512–516.

Transverse Myelitis Consortium Working Group. Proposed diagnostic criteria and nosology of acute transverse myelitis. *Neurology* 2002;59:499–505.

Weinshenker BG, O'Brien PC, Petterson TM et al. A randomized trial of plasma exchange in acute central nervous system inflammatory demyelinating disease. *Ann Neurol* 1999;46:878–886.

Author: Yang Mao-Draayer

Trichinosis

 Database

DEFINITION

Disease caused by ingestion of inadequately cooked meat containing the nematode (roundworm) Trichinella larvae cysts (parasitic food poisoning).

- Other names: trichinosis, trichinelliasis, trichinellosis

PATHOPHYSIOLOGY

- Trichinella larvae (eggs, cysts, obligate intracellular parasites) in poorly cooked meat (primarily pork) eaten by patient
- Symptoms related to absolute number of ingested larvae
- Organisms released after cyst wall digestion by gastric enzymes, pass to small intestine, invade mucosa with edema, hyperemia, and ulcerations, and then develop into adult worms. Fertilized females release larvae (500 to 5,000) over approximately 2 to 6 weeks. Adult worms then expelled in feces (do not multiply in human host).
- Larvae travel via lymphatic and venules to the bloodstream and into skeletal muscle fibers to grow (10×), coil, and encyst. Muscle fibers enlarge, become edematous; may have granulomatous reactions in nonskeletal muscle, but larvae are only found in skeletal muscle.
- Symptoms occur approximately 7 to 14 days after ingestion, maybe sooner.
- Cysts (hyaline capsules) may calcify over several months to years.

EPIDEMIOLOGY

- Worldwide distribution; virulence varies with location and strain. Reported in Egyptian mummies.
- Seven species (five encapsulated) and three additional phenotypes: most infections from *Trichinella spiralis*
- Infections occur sporadically and in epidemics (families, small communities).
- CDC reported 138 outbreaks from 1973 to 1992 (1,038 cases); 72 U.S. cases from 1997 to 2001 (wild game etiology predominated). Five hundred outbreaks (25,161 cases with 240 deaths) reported from China between 1964 and 2002.
- Approximately 4% of cadavers in 1970 study with evidence of previous infection (other estimates 10% to 20% prevalence; 16% in 1941 study)
- Certain nationalities may be more likely to contract disease as a result of dietary habits.
- Should be considered in patients with recent foreign travel (especially Mexico, Southeast Asia, Africa).
- Most infections involve ingestion of wild game (bear, cougar, hyena, lion, panther, fox), horse, dog (China), seal or walrus meat or poorly cooked pork. Carried by rodents, domesticated animals (dogs, cats), raccoons, opossums, skunks.

- Underlying immune status may effect severity of presentation; disease not transmissible person to person. Infection leads to partial immunity.
- Decreasing number of cases per year in the United States as a result of increased public awareness leading to better-cooked meat, home and commercial freezing, and laws preventing feeding of garbage to swine. Infected pork in the United States reported at 1.4% in 1900; 0% to 0.47% between 1990 and 1996. Consumption of pork per capita in the United States remains relatively constant (~50 lb/person in 1994).

COMPLICATIONS

- Myocarditis (most frequent serious complication), meningoencephalitis, CNS granulomas, pneumonitis, pericardial effusion, pleural effusion, pulmonary embolism or infarction, fatty changes of the liver, glomerulonephritis, severe enteritis, prolonged muscle aches, ocular disturbances (retinal hemorrhages), cardiac complaints, and headaches
- Can be fatal (4 to 8 weeks postinfection)
- Rarely permanent damage

PROGNOSIS

- Usually resolves spontaneously over several months
- Muscle swelling and weakness may persist.
- Poorer prognosis (can be fulminant and fatal) if cardiac, CNS, or pulmonary involvement
- Children may be more symptomatic, but fewer complications and quicker recovery than adults

 Differential Diagnosis

- Infection: viral syndromes, parasitic, spirochetal, gastroenteritis, influenza, sinusitis, typhoid fever, measles, scarlet fever, meningitis, rheumatic fever, encephalitis, encephalomyelitis, poliomyelitis
- Miscellaneous: Fever of unknown origin, dermatomyositis, myocarditis, inflammatory bowel disease, angioneurotic edema, glomerulonephritis, polyneuritis, eosinophilic leukemia, polyarteritis nodosa, nonabsorption syndromes

 Data Gathering

HISTORY

Question: Most ingestions asymptomatic (subclinical)?
Significance: Nonspecific signs and symptoms may mimic other nonspecific illnesses. Lack of specificity of presentation may make diagnosis less obvious in some instances.

Question: Ingestion of poorly cooked or raw meat?

Significance: Infection is transmitted by ingestion of inadequately prepared meat. History of this diet should raise suspicion of potential trichinosis infection.

Question: Ingestion of game animal?
Significance: Game animals have been associated with transmission of trichinosis. This diet may also be associated with less than ideal storage or cooking issues.

Question: Others with same dietary exposure or practice and similar symptoms?
Significance: Because this is a dietary acquired disease, others with similar diet may be at risk of developing trichinosis. Epidemics have been reported in families and communities.

 Physical Examination

- Classic presentation includes myositis, fever, periorbital edema, and eosinophilia
- Symptomatic orderly progression (includes three stages):

—GI stage (first days to week postingestion)
　—Nausea, vomiting, diarrhea (may be prolonged), abdominal pain, cramps, constipation, fever (rare), malaise
—Dissemination ("muscular phase," muscle invasion) stage (weeks 2 to 6)
　—Fever, periorbital edema, myalgias most common symptoms
　—Malaise, fatigue, facial edema and pain, tenderness, swelling, aching, weakness, or fasciculations of muscles (includes extraocular, face, tongue, larynx, neck, shoulder, chest, back, upper extremity muscles, and diaphragm), sweating, cough, rash, retinal hemorrhages, subungual hemorrhage
—Convalescent (encystment) stage (weeks 3 to 6)
　—May have continued, prolonged (months) weakness, myalgias, paralysis, neurologic, circulatory, or metabolic issues

Finding: Other reported signs and symptoms include cough, shortness of breath, hoarseness, headache, dysphagia, conjunctivitis, chemosis, maculopapular, urticarial or petechial rash, trunk or limb edema, conjunctival or splinter (subungual) hemorrhages, facial flushing, photophobia, blurred vision, diplopia, neck mass, cranial nerve abnormalities, meningoencephalitis, seizures, intracranial vessel thrombosis, focal neurologic findings, pericardial effusion

 Laboratory Aids

SPECIFIC TESTS

- Pitfalls

—Serology takes time (3 weeks)
—No stool, body fluid (other than serology), or radiographic aid for routine specific diagnosis
　—Detection of Trichinella-specific DNA by PCR (availability limited)

—Trichinella serology (through CDC or state labs): requires several weeks to become positive; use two tests to increase sensitivity: bentonite flocculation (1:5 or fourfold increase), latex flocculation test, ELISA, immunofluorescence

—Skeletal muscle biopsy (fresh tissue evaluation from patient—can also test suspected meat if available)
—Most direct diagnostic tool, although usually not needed
—Best source swollen muscle, at least 2 weeks postinfection
—Can be negative in infection as a result of sampling error
—Encysted larvae in necrotic muscle fibers surrounded by inflammatory cells
—Granulomatous reaction in nonskeletal muscle, but not encysted larvae

• Skin test: becomes positive in second to third week; does not distinguish between acute or old infection as test remains positive for years after infection

NONSPECIFIC TESTS

• CBC and differential: eosinophilia (to 70%), peaks 10 to 21 days postinfection
• Serum CPK, LDH, SGOT, SGPT often elevated; ESR may be normal or elevated
• ECG: nonspecific ST changes, abnormal with myocarditis
• Imaging studies: small CNS lesions, some with ring calcifications; intravenous enhancement on CT scan
• Electromyography: results resemble polymyositis and inflammatory myopathies

Therapy

• No ideal or totally satisfactory therapy
• Symptomatic: bed rest, salicylates or acetaminophen
• Most recover without specific therapy

MEDICATIONS

Intestinal Phase

• Mebendazole (Vermox)

—Variable dosing recommendations (~10 days)
—200 to 400 mg t.i.d. × 3 days, followed by 400 to 500 mg t.i.d. × 10 days
—May be helpful during the disseminated (muscular) phase
—Successful in animal treatments
—Less toxic than thiabendazole

• Thiabendazole (Mintezol):

—Best if used within 24 hours of ingestion
—25 mg/kg PO for 7 days
—Kills some but not all established larvae
—Does not appear to alter established infection
—Better absorbed than mebendazole, but increased side effects
—Has anti-inflammatory, antipyretic, and analgesic effects

• Albendazole (Albenza)

—Best if used within 24 hours of ingestion
—400 mg PO b.i.d. × 8 to 14 days

• Pyrantel pamoate (Antiminth):

—11 mg/kg per day for 4 days
—Effective against GI worms, not encysted worms

Muscular Phase

—Systemic corticosteroids (high-dose and low-dose):
  —Symptomatic relief
  —Alleviate inflammatory reaction and help if CNS or cardiac involvement
  —May be useful, but unproven
  —Should not be used alone as may prolong or intensify symptomatic disease state

Follow-Up

• Expect improvement over several weeks.
• Cardiac, neurologic, or pulmonary involvement indicates more severe problems.
• Prognosis usually good

PREVENTION

• Isolation
• Standard precautions

Control Measures

—Eat only fully cooked meat, especially pork and ground beef that may have been mixed with pork and game.
—Cook until no trace of pink
—Thermal death at 55°C (for safety, cook to 77°C [170°F] to ensure uniform effect)
—Freeze for 3 weeks at −15°C (5°F).
—Separate (and routinely cleanse) game, pork and other meat grinding equipment.
—Irradiation: May not kill trichinella, but should prevent ability to replicate
—Smoking, salting, and drying meat (including jerky) are not reliable sterilization methods.
—Avoid feeding swine uncooked meat scraps.
—Active rat and rodent control
—Avoid breast-feeding by infected mother.

PITFALLS

• Assuming only pork can transmit disease
• Not considering trichinosis in differential diagnosis

Common Questions and Answers

Q: How can I prevent infection?
A: Be sure meat is fully cooked (internal temperature ≥160°F [71°C], not pink) or has been stored in a freezer at less than −15°C (5°F) for greater than 3 weeks or −29°C (−20°F) for 6 days or −23°C (−10°F) for 10 days). Trichinella larvae in game may be relatively resistant to freezing (frozen bear meat has yielded infective larvae after >2 years of freezing).

Q: Is trichinosis contagious from person to person?
A: No, except through infected breast-milk.

Q: Do special precautions need to be taken when treating a patient with presumed trichinosis?
A: Only good hand washing. No isolation required.

Q: What should we recommend for a patient who has eaten contaminated meat?
A: Treatment with mebendazole or thiabendazole should be considered.

Q: What are the classic hallmarks of trichinosis?
A: Diarrhea, abdominal pain, periorbital edema, myositis, fever, and eosinophilia, especially with history of potentially poorly cooked meat products ingestion.

ICD-9-CM 124

BIBLIOGRAPHY

American Academy of Pediatrics. Trichinosis (Trichinella spiralis). In: Pickering LK, ed. *2000 Red Book: Report of the Committee of Infectious Diseases.* 25th Ed. Elk Grove Village, IL: American Academy of Pediatrics, 2000;587–588, 715, 776–770.

Blancou J. History of trichinellosis surveillance. *Parasite* 2001;8(2 Suppl): S16–S19.

Bolas-Fernandez F. Biological variation in Trichinella species and genotypes. *J Helminthol* 2003;77(2):111–118.

Clausen MR, Meyer CN, Krantz T, et al. Trichinella infection and clinical disease. *QJM* 1996;89(8):631–636.

Grove DI. Tissue nematodes (trichinosis, dracunculiasis, filariasis). In: Mandell GL, Bennett JE, Dolin R, eds. *Principles and Practice of Infectious Diseases.* 5th Ed. Philadelphia: Churchill-Livingstone, 2000;526–528, 1151, 2943–2945.

Liu M, Boireau P. Trichinellosis in China: epidemiology and control. *Trends Parasitol* 2002;18(12):553–556.

McAuley JB, Michelson MK, Schantz PM. Trichinosis infection in travelers. *J Infect Dis* 1991;164:1013–1016.

Moore TA, Nutman TB. Travel medicine: eosinophilia in the returning traveler. *Infect Dis Clin North Am* 1998;12(2):503–521.

Morse JW, Ridenour R, Unterseher P. Trichinosis: infrequent diagnosis or frequent misdiagnosis? *Ann Emerg Med* 1994;24:969–971.

Roy SL, Lopez AS, Schantz PM. Trichinellosis surveillance—United States, 1997–2001. *MMWR Surveill Report Summ Report* 2003; 52(6):1–8.

Author: George Anthony Woodward

Tuberculosis

 Database

DEFINITION

Pediatric tuberculosis (TB) is the disease state caused by *Mycobacterium tuberculosis*, an acid-fast bacillus (AFB). Pediatric TB should be regarded as a spectrum of exposure, from infection to disease, because progression from an infected individual (exposure) to infection and subsequently disease can occur much faster in children under 2 years of age (occurring within the incubation of the disease stated below). Progression through this spectrum is age-dependent, being 40% to 50% for zero up to 2-year-olds, approximately 20% for 2- to 4-year-olds, and 10% to 15% for those 5 years old and over, the 5- to 10-year-olds being the most protected age group. Adolescence is another vulnerable age group.

EPIDEMIOLOGY

• The most common route of infection is via the respiratory tract. TB is spread from a person with disease by droplet nuclei that are inhaled by other individuals. A child becomes infected with TB after close and prolonged contact with an adult or adolescent who has active, untreated infectious disease, usually pulmonary TB, in a poorly ventilated space. The sole risk factor is breathing air containing droplet nuclei that contain the tubercle bacillus. Thus there are individuals who develop TB without knowledge of an infectious contact.
• Congenital infection occurs, rarely, in the setting of an untreated mother in the last trimester of pregnancy.
• Infection with the tubercle bacillus needs to be differentiated from tuberculosis disease.
• The interval between onset of infection and disease is 10 to 12 weeks.
• The greatest chance of disease occurring is within the first 2 years after infection (of developing a positive purified protein derivative [PPD] reaction). However, for infants and children younger than 5 years old, progression through the spectrum of pediatric TB (exposure-infection-disease) is age-dependent (see Definition, above).
• Postpubertal adolescents and immunosuppressed individuals, including persons with diabetes, with chronic renal failure, malnourished individuals, and persons on steroids for whatever reasons (including pulse doses), have higher risks of progression of infection to disease.
• Nationwide, the early 1990s documented an increase in TB in children under 2 years of age in the states where TB is common, this trend has been reversed as a result of adherence to the recommendations for treatment of the American Thoracic Society (ATS)/Centers for Disease Control And Prevention (CDC)/Infectious Disease Society of America (IDSA) Updated 2003—see Bibliography).

PATHOPHYSIOLOGY

• Pathology of disease includes the formation of a primary focus of infection, usually in the lung (Ghon focus), with recruitment of cell-mediated immune responses, which lead to formation of adenopathy of the hilar, cervical, mediastinal, and/or other nodes, depending on the dissemination of infection.
• Development of a PPD reaction is dependent on an adequate cell-mediated immune response, which often is not fully developed in infants younger than 2 years of age and in those infected with overwhelming disease, such as miliary TB or meningitis or large pleural effusions.

COMPLICATIONS

• Missed diagnosis: Failure to consider TB in a child who is failing to thrive and whose PPD is negative
• TB meningitis: Outcome is dependent on the stage at which anti-TB medication is begun.

—If Rx is started at stage I, complete recovery occurs in 94%, with neurologic sequelae in 6%.
—If delayed until stage II, complete recovery occurs in 51%, with neurologic sequelae in 40% and death in 7%.
—If delayed until stage III, complete recovery occurs in 18%, with neurologic sequelae in 61% and death in 20%.

• Miliary TB
• Bony TB: Most commonly spinal
• Renal TB: Presents as a fever of undetermined origin (FUO), with or without urinary symptoms
• Congenital TB manifests with hepatosplenomegaly; may have CSF abnormalities and CXR abnormalities—too young for PPD to be useful.
• Drug toxicity: Pediatric patients are much more tolerant of anti-TB medications than are adults; thus regular monitoring of liver function tests is not routinely required, although clinical monitoring for symptoms such as abdominal pain and loss of appetite on a monthly basis remain the cornerstone for identifying any toxicity.
• Hepatitis with INH, rifampin, and pyrazinamide (PZA); neurologic complications with INH; skin rashes with rifampin; ototoxicity with streptomycin; but ocular toxicity with EMB in the pediatric age group has not been documented, and therefore is a safe drug to use. Management of common side effects and drug interactions may be found in the 2003 ATS/CDC/IDSA: Treatment of Tuberculosis Recommendations (see Bibliography)

PROGNOSIS

• The death rate for untreated TB is 40% over 4 years.
• For miliary TB and meningeal TB, prognosis is dependent on the stage of presentation (see Complications).
• For outbreaks of MDRTB, death rates have ranged from 70% to 90%.

 Differential Diagnosis

TB can do anything malignancy can do.

• Pulmonary infiltrate: other chronic organisms such as Nocardia and histoplasmosis. Infiltrates as a result of bacterial or viral pathogens resolve faster than TB; thus, reevaluation of a suspect in 8 to 12 weeks clarifies this differential.
• Hilar adenopathy: In TB it is usually unilateral, but EBV, adenovirus, pertussis, and malignancy are possible mimickers.
• Miliary disease: pulmonary, hepatosplenomegaly with or without CNS involvement
• Gastrointestinal disease: The most common differential is Crohn disease.
• Meningitis: fungal meningitis, partially treated bacterial meningitis (rarely)

 Data Gathering

HISTORY

Inquire about the factors that are associated with tuberculosis infection:

• Exposure
• Migrant farmers
• Immigration from a high-TB area such as Haiti, Southeast Asia, Africa (any part), South and Central American, or Russia and Eastern Europe
• Higher incidence in Native Americans
• Contact with adults who have active TB
• HIV-positive persons
• Immunosuppressed state
• Incarcerated adolescents and relatives
• Homeless persons
• Poor city dwellers
• Exposure to milk from untested herds
• Malnutrition
• Chronic steroid usage

 Physical Examination

• May reflect underlying disease such as HIV, malnutrition, chronic steroid use
• Pulmonary rales
• Presence of sputum
• May be normal especially in 5- to 10-year-olds

 Laboratory Aids

TESTS
Skin Testing

• The Mantoux test is 5 tuberculin units of PPD administered intradermally.
• The CDC does not recommend routine skin testing in low-risk groups in communities with low prevalence of TB.

- Children at high risk should be tested annually.

—High-risk children include those in contact with adults from regions of the world with high prevalence; children who spend time in homeless shelters, in contact with adults with TB, HIV, and immunosuppressed states; those with Hodgkin disease, lymphoma, diabetes, chronic renal failure, and malnutrition; incarcerated adolescents; and those with exposure to high-risk adults.

- Skin tests become positive 3 to 6 weeks after exposure but may not turn positive for 3 months. Hence the rationale for treating an exposed child with INH and retesting with a PPD in 3 months.

OTHER TESTS

- Culture of sputum, gastric washings, pleural fluid, CSF, urine
- In children, the best source is early-morning gastric washings.
- Culture may take 2 to 3 weeks by the radiometric method.
- Positive cultures are found in fewer than 50% of children.

IMAGING

Chest radiographs may show hilar adenopathy with or without atelectasis. However any infiltrate, pleural effusion in a child with a positive PPD and a risk factor for TB should be considered a TB suspect until proven otherwise. Infiltrates from bacterial or viral pathogens generally clear within 6 to 8 weeks, TB infiltrates tend not to clear as rapidly.

Therapy

HOSPITALIZATION

- Treatment initiated as an outpatient may not be complied with; thus hospitalization reinforces the issue of disease and allows time for education and linkage to TB control programs, which can then supervise direct observed therapy (DOT); however, in the era of managed care, direct linkage of the patient to the local TB control program through the health department and provision of DOT can avert the need to hospitalize for starting therapy, especially because the positivity rate of gastric aspirates for TB is 10% in the best hands.
- In cases of extensive disease, such as miliary or meningitis, and when an adult source case is not known, aggressive attempts should be made to obtain an organism from gastric aspirates, bronchoalveolar lavage, CSF, pleural or joint aspirate, bone aspirate, liver or tissue biopsy, and, in some cases, blood cultures.

ISOLATION POLICIES

- In the past, children under 8 years of age did not require isolation for pulmonary disease, because the disease is usually a primary infection; that is, there is less organism load and more lymphatic enlargement. However, unless one knows that the parent and/or any adult visitors are not contagious, many infection control units require isolation of the child because the family members' state of contagion is unknown at the time of admission.
- Nonpulmonary, such as GI TB, meningitis, bone, joint, also do not require isolation
- Children older than 8 years of age and adolescents should be isolated until they have completed 10 days of four-drug therapy (see Drugs).

DRUGS

- Initial treatment in areas with MDRTB of more than 4%: Until sensitivities are known, a four-drug regimen should be started: INH, 10 mg/kg per day; rifampin, 10 mg/kg per day; PZA, 30 mg/kg per day; and either streptomycin, 20 mg/kg per day (depending on whether it is meningitis or miliary TB, for which a cidal antibacterial agent is desired) or ethambutol, 25 mg/kg per day.
- If the organism is sensitive, treatment with the initial four primary drugs should continue for the first 2 months; at this time point all sputum specimens should be culture negative, followed by 4 months of INH and rifampin. When this regimen is adhered to, prognosis and a complete cure is achieved in 97% to 98% of patients.
- If there is a cavity on CXR or sputum specimens are still culture positive, or the TB is miliary, disseminated or meningeal the duration of treatment needs to be longer—9 to 12 months.

PREVENTION

- Prevention of disease by using INH, 10 mg/kg per day for 9 months orally, or if compliance is an issue, two times a week as DOT at 20 mg/kg, with a maximum dose of 900 mg usually done with the help of a school nurse, child care, or the local TB control program, without breaks in treatment ideally—although one has 12 months to complete the course if a break has been toward the end of treatment one does not need to restart, such treatment is about 90% effective against the development of active TB for 20 years in nonimmunosuppressed children. This recommendation prevents disease in the treated individual and, as a public health measure, interrupts transmission to contacts of the infected person with an efficacy of 90%. Other drugs for latent TB include 4 months of rifampicin if a child is intolerant of INH, 4 months of INH and Rifampin in case of granulomas or fibrosis consistent with Latent TB Infection (LTBI), and finally 6 months of INH by direct observed therapy is the last resort (for a total of 72 doses).
- BCG (bacille of Calmette and Guérin) vaccine is recommended only for infants and children who are PPD-negative, who are continually and intimately exposed to contagious adults or to adults with TB that is resistant to both INH and rifampin, and who cannot take long-term preventative medication or be removed from the contagious adult. These recommendations are currently under review.
- Follow-up and contact tracing are key to making TB a preventable disease.

- Direct observated preventive therapy is preferred for children <5 yrs because of higher risk of progression to disease it treatment of infection not completed.

Common Questions and Answers

Q: If the child has completed a course of INH and is reexposed, what are the risks of infection?
A: One course of preventive therapy is believed to confer immunity to subsequent exposure, even to MDRTB (data are preliminary).

Q: Should all children in close proximity to inner-city areas with a prevalence of TB be screened annually with PPD?
A: No. One needs to consider the risk/benefit. Children under 5 years of age progress to disease more rapidly and are harder to diagnose when ill with TB; therefore, children who are under 5 years of age and live in contact with adults who are at high-risk for TB should be screened.

Q: Because parents return for the PPD reading only 26% to 50% of the time, depending on which clinic they use, are there other ways to ensure that parents receive the PPD reading?
A: This is a tough question. An improved public health surveillance system, use of child care providers, or school programs requiring examination and utility are all shown to be more effective than patient education by the provider. Bottom line ONLY place PPDs on children at risk and explain about TB to the parents—obtain graphic books from CDC to assist you.

ICD-9-CM 011.9

BIBLIOGRAPHY

American Thoracic Society (ATS)/Center for Disease Control And Prevention (CDC)/ Infectious Disease Society of America (IDSA): Treatment of tuberculosis recommendations. *Am J Respir Crit Care Med* 2003;167:603–662.

Diagnostic Standards and Classification of Tuberculosis in Adults and Children. Official statement of the American Thoracic Society and the Centers for Disease Control and Prevention, July 1999. *Am J Respir Crit Care Med* 2000;161(4 pt 1):1376–1395.

Heymann SJ, Brewer TF, Wilson ME, et al. Pediatric tuberculosis: what needs to be done to decrease morbidity and mortality. *Pediatrics* 2000;106(E1).

Neu N, et al. Diagnosis of Pediatric TB in modern era. *Ped Inf Dis J* 1999;18:122–26.

Loeftler AM. Pediatric TB Seminar. *Resp Infection* 2003;18:272–91.

Treatment of TB MMWR Recommends June 2003;52:1–80.

Targeted TB Skin testing and Treatment of Latent TB Infection in Children and Adolescents 2004;114:1175–1201.

Author: Barbara Watson

Tuberous Sclerosis

 Database

DEFINITION

Tuberous sclerosis (TSC) is a neurocutaneous syndrome characterized by hamartomatous growths involving multiple regions of the body, such as the brain, retina, heart, kidney, and skin. First described by Bourneville in 1880, the classic diagnostic triad of adenoma sebaceum, mental retardation, and seizures has been revised to include other manifestations, because many patients with TSC do not exhibit this triad.

CAUSES

TSC either is inherited in an autosomaldominant pattern or results from a spontaneous, sporadic mutation.

PATHOLOGY

Findings reflect the primary tissue in which lesions are identified (*denotes lesions that confirm the diagnosis of TSC).

- Brain

—Three characteristic lesions include *cortical tubers, *subependymal nodules, and giant-cell astrocytomas.
—In tubers, cerebral cortical architecture is disrupted, and these regions may undergo calcification, which can be visible on skull radiographs or brain CT.
—Subependymal nodules consist of large abnormal astrocytes emanating from the lateral ventricular surface.
—Giant-cell astrocytomas are low-grade benign astrocytic neoplasms.

- Skin

—Facial angiofibromas are highly suggestive of TSC and consists of pinkish-yellow plaques on the malar regions and nasolabial folds.
—Ash leaf spots are hypopigmented, hypomelanotic macules occurring anywhere on the body.

- Ungual fibromas are fleshy growths along the lateral borders of the nailbed. Shagreen patches are areas of shaggy, leathery skin typically in the lumbosacral area.

- Retina

—Whitish-yellow angiolipomas or *astrocytic hamartomas occur near the optic nerve head or the retinal periphery, which may calcify.

- Heart
- Rhabdomyomas in the ventricular wall occur in infancy and contain abundant nodules of large eosinophilic cells; this is the most common cardiac tumor of infancy and early childhood.
- Kidney

—Renal cysts, polycystic kidneys, *angiomyolipomas, and, rarely, renal carcinomas

- Other organ systems

—Less commonly affected are the lungs, gastrointestinal tract, spleen, vascular bed, and lymphatics.

GENETICS

Two clearly identified loci for familial and sporadic cases based on linkage analyses are 9q34 and 16p13, corresponding to TSC1 and TSC2 genes, respectively. TSC1 encodes the protein hamartin. The TSC2 gene encodes a protein named tuberin. It is hypothesized that hamartin and tuberin may function as a tumor suppressor. There is a loss of allelic TSC2 heterozygosity in TSC hamartomas, suggesting that an inactivating mutation of the TSC2 occurring in somatic or germ-cell lines reflects a second-hit mutation.

EPIDEMIOLOGY

Current estimates suggest an incidence of 1 in 5,000 to 1 in 15,000 births. Approximately 60% to 70% of cases reflect sporadic mutation; 30% to 40% of cases are familial; it affects males and females equally.

PROGNOSIS

Mental retardation unfortunately will not improve unless cognitive impairment results from uncontrolled seizures. Seizure control is often difficult, and many children require epilepsy surgery to remove cortical tubers or subependymal nodules. Cardiac tumors may require surgical intervention. Renal angiomyolipomas can be embolized angiographically or surgically corrected. Subependymal giant cell astrocytomas that cause hydrocephalus may require resection.

 Differential Diagnosis

Neurocutaneous syndromes in which skin lesions, mental retardation, and seizures are characteristic features should be considered:

- Neurofibromatosis
- Sturge-Weber syndrome
- von Hippel-Lindau disease
- Neurocutaneous melanosis
- Albright syndrome
- Incontinentia pigmenti
- Linear sebaceous nevus

 Data Gathering

HISTORY

- Primary symptoms include seizures, mental defect, and skin lesions.
- Seizures may begin at any time. In infancy, infantile spasms are a common presenting seizure.
- Mental retardation may manifest as developmental delay, but some patients are without cognitive defect.
- Skin lesions may appear in infancy or during early childhood.
- It is important to take a full family history, including consanguinity.
- Inquire about history of TSC, seizures, mental retardation, skin lesions, and cardiac or renal disease/cancers.

Physical Examination

- Need to maintain high level of suspicion for TSC in any patient evaluated with:

—Infantile spasms
—Seizures
—Mental retardation/developmental delay
—Peculiar skin lesions.

- Ash leaf and café-au-lait spots are small (often less than 5 mm) but may be found anywhere on skin and are often present at birth.
- Facial angiofibromas are typically on the face around the nose and cheeks and appears similar to acne, appearing in the later childhood to adolescent years. It does not itch or suppurate.
- Ungual fibromas appear around the nailbed.
- Shagreen patches are brownish, leathery skin patches near the sacrum.
- Funduscopic examination may reveal whitish-yellow areas in epipapillary and peripapillary regions around the optic nerve head. They rarely cause visual impairment.
- Clinical signs of congestive heart failure in infants may be seen with cardiac TSC.
- Flank pain, nausea and vomiting, and hematuria may reflect renal involvement.

PROCEDURE

- In any suspected neurocutaneous syndrome, skin examination with a Wood's lamp may be especially helpful in identifying hypopigmented lesions such as ash leaf spots. Dilated funduscopic examination may also aid in full visualization of optic nerve head.
- One rare sign of TSC is the presence of small dental enamel pits.

Laboratory Aids

TESTS

- Routine blood and CSF laboratory tests are typically normal unless renal function is significantly compromised by renal cysts or renal angiomyolipomas.
- In patients with mental retardation or seizures, EEG is essential to evaluate cerebral activity.
- In infants, an EEG may also help diagnose infantile spasms, which are associated electrographically with a highly disorganized pattern of large-amplitude, asynchronous, sharp waves called hypsarrhythmia.
- Later in childhood, children with TSC may develop the Lennox-Gastaut syndrome, which consists of mental retardation, seizures, and a characteristic EEG pattern of slow (2.5-Hz) spike-wave complexes.

IMAGING

- MRI of the brain with gadolinium administration performed serially every 1 to 2 years will identify tubers, subependymal nodules, and giant-cell tumors. These appear hyperintense on T-weighted images and may enhance with gadolinium. Rarely, a giant-cell astrocytoma may obstruct the foramen of Monro, resulting in hydrocephalus, which can also be detected with MRI.
- Echocardiography can detect cardiac rhabdomyomas in infants with TSC.
- Renal ultrasound (every 1 to 2 years) or CT will demonstrate renal lesions.

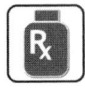

Therapy

DRUGS

Anticonvulsant therapy as needed and ACTH for infantile spasms; medical management of congestive heart failure or cardiac dysrhythmias in TSC patients with cardiac rhabdomyomas

Follow-Up

SIGNS TO WATCH FOR

- A persistent change in mental status may reflect status epilepticus, an expanding mass lesion with obstructive hydrocephalus, or a new CNS neoplasm.
- Worsening renal function may reflect progressive renal involvement.

Common Questions and Answers

Q: Can TSC be transmitted in subsequent pregnancies?
A: An affected individual with the TSC gene mutation has a 50% chance of transmitting the mutation to his or her offspring.

Q: Is genetic testing available?
A: A commercial diagnostic test is under development for TSC1 and TSC2 gene mutations.

Q: Will my child need brain surgery?
A: In the event of refractory seizures, removal of cortical tubers may help seizure control. If a brain tumor is detected by MRI, neurosurgical evaluation is indicated.

ICD-9-CM 759.5

BIBLIOGRAPHY

Crino P, Henske C. New developments in the neurobiology of the tuberous sclerosis complex. *Neurology* 1999;53:1384–1391.

Gomez MR. *Tuberous Sclerosis.* 2nd Ed. New York: Raven Press, 1988.

Jozwiak S, Schwartz RA, Janniger CK, et al. Usefulness of diagnostic criteria of tuberous sclerosis complex in pediatric patients. *J Child Neurol* 2000;15(10):652–659.

Kandt RS. Tuberous sclerosis complex and neurofibromatosis type 1: the two most common neurocutaneous diseases. *Neurol Clin* 2002;20(4):941–964. Erratum in *Neurol Clin* 2003;21(4):983–1004.

Sarnat H. *Cerebral Dysgenesis.* New York: Oxford University Press, 1991.

Webb DW, Osborne JP. Tuberous sclerosis. *Arch Dis Child* 1995;72(6):471–474.

Author: Peter B. Crino

Tularemia

 ## Database

DEFINITION

Tularemia is an infection with *Francisella tularensis*, a small, nonmotile, gram-negative coccobacillus that requires cysteine for growth. Two types have been described:

- Type A (Neartica): found in arthropods; highly virulent to rabbits and humans
- Type B (Palaeartica): found in water and aquatic animals; less virulent
- Tularemia is characterized by six clinical forms, depending on the site of entry:
- Ulceroglandular tularemia constitutes 75% of all cases. A papule, which ruptures and ulcerates, occurs at the site of entry. Lymphadenopathy and hepatosplenomegaly accompany systemic symptoms of fever, chills, and headache.
- Glandular tularemia is identical to the ulceroglandular form, but without a skin lesion.
- Oculoglandular tularemia occurs when the organism gains access via the conjunctival sac, usually from rubbing the eyes with contaminated fingers. The eyelids are inflamed and the conjunctiva is infected. Yellow nodules and ulcers may appear on the palpebral conjunctiva.
- Typhoidal tularemia presents as fever of unknown origin, without localizing lymphadenopathy or skin findings. Shock, pleuropulmonary findings, odynophagia, diarrhea, and bowel necrosis are often associated.
- Oropharyngeal tularemia occurs after the ingestion of infected, improperly cooked meat. An exudative or membranous tonsillitis is seen. Lower gastrointestinal tract involvement with vomiting, diarrhea, and abdominal pain may be associated.
- Pneumonic tularemia occurs after inhalation of the organism. This presentation is seen in laboratory workers and is the most fulminant and lethal form. Tularemia in this form has been produced as a biologic weapon.

PATHOPHYSIOLOGY

- Infection follows contact with rabbits or rodents.
- Ticks or deerflies are the most common vector.
- Entry into the human is via skin or mucous membranes.
- A papule or ulcer may be seen at the inoculation site.
- Bacteremia occurs after a 3- to 5-day incubation period, accompanied by fever and lymphadenopathy.
- The organism produces localized disease in reticuloendothelial organs, with areas of focal necrosis that may form granulomas.

EPIDEMIOLOGY

- *F. tularensis* is found in the northern hemisphere between 30° and 71° latitude.
- Wild mammals (rabbits, hares, squirrels, beavers, and deer) may be infected, and invertebrates (ticks, deerflies, and mosquitoes).
- Humans acquire tularemia after a bite by an infected arthropod or contact with tissues or body fluids of an infected animal.
- Most frequently affected are hunters, trappers, and farmers.

COMPLICATIONS

- Lymph node suppuration occurs in 40% of pediatric patients, regardless of treatment.
- Infection with *F. tularensis* may be complicated by necrotic and granulomatous lesions in the liver and spleen, and parenchymal degeneration.
- A sepsis syndrome with shock, fever, myalgias, and severe headache can be seen.
- Pneumonia and pleural involvement are frequently encountered in adults with typhoidal tularemia.

PROGNOSIS

When recognized and treated with appropriate antibiotics, the course is generally less than 1 month. Mortality is low, except in fulminant disease.

 ## Differential Diagnosis

Tularemia should be considered in the following differentials:

- Fever of unknown origin
- Fever with purulent conjunctivitis
- Fever with hepatosplenomegaly
- Fever with skin ulcer

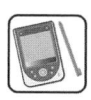 ## Data Gathering

HISTORY

- A history of any of the following contacts with affected animals should be sought: ingestion of wild animal meat, hunting or cleaning wild animals, and playing with dead wild animals.
- History of a recent tick bite is common among affected patients.
- A history of a papule that became ulcerated is classic for the ulceroglandular form.
- Fever greater than 101°F for 2 to 3 weeks is common, with associated weight loss.

Physical Examination

- Skin lesions should be sought.
- Hepatosplenomegaly, purulent conjunctivitis, adenopathy, and exudative tonsillitis are other localized findings.

 Laboratory Aids

TESTS

- Serum agglutination titers to *F. tularensis* are positive if 1:160 or greater.
- A fourfold rise in titers after the second week of illness is characteristic and diagnostic.
- Cultures of blood, skin, ulcers, lymph nodes, gastric washings, and respiratory secretions require special media.
- Laboratory personnel should be made aware of the infection risk from specimens.

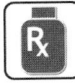 Therapy

- If respiratory compromise is present, oxygen supplementation and/or assisted ventilation must be rapidly addressed.
- Recognition and prompt, aggressive treatment of shock should be a major priority.
- Intravenous antibiotic therapy should be administered. Streptomycin has been used traditionally, but gentamicin (or amikacin) has recently been found to be equally effective. Duration of treatment is usually for 10 days.

 Follow-Up

PREVENTION

Isolation of the Hospitalized Patient

Infection control measures should include protection against secretions and respiratory isolation of the pneumonic form.

Control Measures

- Protective clothing and insect repellent should be used to minimize insect bites.
- Inspection for ticks (and immediate removal) should be routine after outdoor activity in endemic areas.
- Rubber gloves should be worn while cooking or handling wild rabbit meat.
- Laboratory workers should wear rubber gloves and masks when working with potentially infectious specimens.

ICD-9-CM 021.9

BIBLIOGRAPHY

Boyce JM. Francisella tularensis. In: Mandell GL, Douglas GR, Bennett JE, eds. *Principles and Practice of Infectious Diseases*. 3rd Ed. New York: Churchill-Livingstone, 1990: 1742–1746.

Cross JT, Schutze GE, Jacobs RF. Treatment of tularemia with gentamicin in pediatric patients. *Pediatr Infect Dis J* 1995;14(2):152–151.

Dennis DT, Inglesby TV, Henderson DA, et al. Tularemia as a biological weapon: medical and public health management. *JAMA* 2001;285(21):2763–2773.

Ellis J, Oyston PC, Green M, Titball RW. Tularemia. *Clin Microbiol Rev* 2002;15:631–646.

Kaye D. Tularemia. In: Braunwald E, ed. *Harrison's Principles of Internal Medicine*. 14th Ed. New York: McGraw-Hill, 1987:613–615.

Yow MD. Tularemia. In: Oski FA, ed. *Principles and Practice of Pediatrics*. Philadelphia: JB Lippincott, 1990:1132–1133.

Author: Louis M. Bell

Ulcerative Colitis

 ## Database

DEFINITION

Remitting and relapsing inflammation of the large intestine. Hallmark symptoms are abdominal cramping, diarrhea, and bloody stools. There are multiple patterns of presentation in children. Ulcerative colitis (UC) always affects the rectum, with contiguous involvement extending proximally, including up to the entire large intestine.

CAUSES

Multifactorial disease; results from a combination of individual genetic susceptibility and several environmental risk factors that may include:

- Hygiene/exposure to bacteria/parasites/viruses/allergens including endogenous colonic microflora
- Breast-feeding vs. bottle-feeding
- Specific bacteria that colonize the colon
- Dietary influences
- Smoking

PATHOLOGY

- Inflammation and ulceration of colonic mucosa with acute inflammatory cells infiltrating the villi, lamina propria, and crypts, giving rise to crypt abscesses
- Inflammation is mucosal, but can infiltrate all layers of the bowel.
- Site of colon affected:

—Rectum (100%)
—Left side (50% to 60%)
—Pancolitis (10%)

- Small intestine should not be involved, but occasionally the terminal ileum can show some inflammation on radiologic or histologic examination. This is thought to be from refluxed colonic contents through an inflamed ileocecal valve (backwash ileitis).
- Skip lesions are not seen in ulcerative colitis.

GENETICS

- HLA association: Bw52, DR2 (Japan); A2, Bw35, Bw40 (Ashkenazi Jews); A7, A11 (Netherlands)
- Higher concordance in monozygotic than in dizygotic twins

EPIDEMIOLOGY

- Yearly incidence is 2/100,000 in 10- to 19-year-olds
- Twenty percent of patients with UC present before the age of 20
- Incidence peaks between 15 and 30 years of age
- Total prevalence is 50 to 75 per 100,000

COMPLICATIONS

- Bleeding
- Anemia
- Toxic megacolon

—Extraintestinal manifestations:
—Hepatobiliary disease (3% to 5%)
—Uveitis (up to 4%)
—Arthritis affecting large joints (10%)
—Spondylitis (6%)
—Erythema nodosum (>5%)
—Pyoderma gangrenosum (>1%)
—Renal calculi (5%)

- Malignancy risk is 0.51% per year after a decade of onset of disease. The risk for adenocarcinoma of the colon in children who developed disease before 14 years of age is 40% by 40 years of age.
- Colonic stricture

 ## Differential Diagnosis

- Crohn's disease
- Infectious colitis: Salmonella, Shigella, Campylobacter, Yersinia, *Escherichia coli* (enterohemorrhagic), Aeromonas, Amebiasis, *Clostridium difficile*, cytomegalovirus
- Sexually transmitted disease (herpes simplex, lymphogranuloma inguinale, Chlamydia)
- Trauma as a result of anal sex or sexual abuse
- Congenital Hirschsprung enterocolitis
- Bleeding juvenile polyps
- Milk protein allergy
- Eosinophilic colitis
- Autoimmune enteropathy
- Irritable bowel syndrome (IBS)
- Appendicitis
- Hemolytic-uremic syndrome
- Henoch-Schönlein purpura

 ## Data Gathering

HISTORY

A detailed history is important in making the diagnosis:

- Rectal bleeding (90%)
- Abdominal pain (90%)
- Diarrhea (50%)
- Weight loss (10%)
- Growth failure
- Recent travel (enteric infections)
- Antibiotic use (*C. difficile*)
- Family history of IBD
- Appendectomy

 ## Physical Examination

- Fever
- Evidence of weight loss or poor growth
- Signs of anemia
- Uveitis
- Mouth sores
- Arthritis
- Abdominal tenderness and distention

- Perianal/rectal examination (UC should not be associated with perianal disease)
- Evidence of hepatobiliary disease
- Skins lesions, specifically, pyoderma gangrenosum
- Thromboembolic complications

 ## Laboratory Aids

TESTS

- CBC (anemia, iron deficiency)
- Iron studies (iron deficiency)
- ESR (disease activity)
- Electrolytes (hydration)
- Hepatic function panel (hepatobiliary disease)
- pANCA (positive in 80% of UC patients, 20% of Crohn disease patients)
- Stool for blood, white cells (colitis)
- Stool cultures, *C. difficile* toxin A and B (infection)

IMAGING

- Plain abdominal radiograph: perforation, ileus, obstruction, and toxic megacolon. In toxic megacolon, the colon is dilated, and there are multiple air-fluid levels indicative of ileus. Serial x-rays are mandatory.
- Barium enema demonstrates strictures and mucosal disease.
- Upper GI and small-bowel follow-through (UGI/SBFT) can demonstrate the entire gastrointestinal tract to exclude small intestinal disease.
- MRI is gaining efficacy for differentiation between transmural and mucosal inflammation.
- Ultrasound may be useful for evaluating associated hepatobiliary disease.
- Radionuclide imaging (tagged white blood cell scan) can differentiate between Crohn disease (small and large bowel involvement) and UC (only large bowel involvement).

PROCEDURES

- Colonoscopy (with biopsies): to confirm the diagnosis of ulcerative colitis.
- Endoscopic retrograde cholangiopancreatography (ERCP): to detect primary sclerosing cholangitis (3% of UC patients).

PITFALLS

- The combination of positive pANCA and negative ASCA (anti-Saccharomyces cerevisiae antibody) has a reported sensitivity of 60% to 70% and a specificity of 95% to 97% for ulcerative colitis in adults. The sensitivity and specificity is poorer in pediatric patients.
- Inflammation of the small intestine demonstrated by colonoscopy, UGI/SBFT, or radionuclide imaging is indicative of Crohn disease, not UC.
- Perianal disease (perianal skin tags, perianal fistulae, perianal abscess) is indicative of Crohn disease, not UC.

• Infectious colitis (especially *C. difficile*) can mimic the findings of UC. *C. difficile* infection must be evaluated with assays for both toxin A and toxin B, or up to 40% of infections can be missed.

• Toxic megacolon is a surgical emergency. The patient has a dilated colon with breakdown of its barrier to toxins entering the systemic circulation. Signs and symptoms include peritonitis, mental status changes, and fluid and electrolyte imbalance. Plain abdominal radiograph shows a segment or total colonic dilatation. Risk factors include first attack, pancolitis, concurrent use of opiates or anticholinergics, and recent barium enema or colonoscopy.

HOME TESTING

Home testing of stool for occult blood can alert patients and physicians to active disease.

 ## Emergency Care

Emergency care is indicated for fulminant disease. Initial evaluation should include abdominal examination, laboratory evaluation (CBC, ESR, electrolytes), and abdominal obstruction series (supine and upright abdominal films). Surgical consultation should be obtained in cases of suspected toxic megacolon.

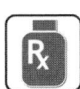 ## Therapy

• Mild disease can be treated with oral mesalamine, topical corticosteroid enema or foam, or mesalamine enema/suppositories.
• Moderate disease: mesalamine, a short course of oral corticosteroid, low-residue diet
• Fulminant disease:

—Hospitalization
—Complete bowel rest with total parenteral nutrition
—Broad-spectrum antibiotics (intravenous ampicillin, gentamicin, and metronidazole)
—Intravenous corticosteroids
—Serial abdominal radiographs
—Frequent examinations
—Stool chart (frequency, amount of blood, and volume of stool output)
—Early surgical consult.

• Traditionally, intravenous cyclosporine had been started in patients with severe disease failing treatment after 2 weeks. Those who responded to cyclosporine were started on oral cyclosporine, which was discontinued after 6 to 8 months. The risk of relapse after discontinuation of cyclosporine is high, and it is useful to start 6-mercaptopurine (6-MP) or azathioprine as maintenance therapy. Infliximab is effective in the treatment of severe UC and may be an alternative to cyclosporine for unresponsive disease.

• Patients who fail therapy with infliximab or cyclosporine or demonstrate chronic unresponsive disease for 6 months should be referred for colectomy.
• Therapy of toxic megacolon is aimed at preventing perforation with decompression of the bowel. Management includes:

—Complete bowel rest
—Discontinuation of anticholinergics and narcotics
—Not performing endoscopy or barium enema
—Broad-spectrum antibiotics; frequent examinations are required.
—Close communication with surgical colleagues is crucial. In the absence of improvement after 24 to 72 hours, the patient requires urgent surgery.

• Maintenance of remission: The corticosteroid dose is tapered and discontinued over weeks to months after initial presentation. Mesalamine is started before discharge.

SURGERY

• Urgently required for perforation, significant and persistent bleeding, toxic megacolon, and failure of medical treatment for fulminant colitis
• Elective consideration for chronic incapacitating disease, growth failure, disease greater than 10 years' duration
• Ileoanal anastomosis and pouch construction is surgery of choice for most pediatric patients

DRUGS

• Methylprednisolone (intravenous): 1 to 2 mg/kg per day (equivalent to prednisone 60 mg maximum)
• Prednisone (oral): 1 to 2 mg/kg per day oral (up to maximum 60 mg/day)
• Mesalamine (oral): 40 to 60 mg/kg per day (maximum 4.8 g/day)
• Mesalamine (enema): 4 g at bedtime
• Mesalamine (suppository): 500 mg b.i.d.
• Hydrocortisone enema: 100 mg qd-b.i.d.
• Hydrocortisone foam: 80 mg qd-b.i.d.
• Cyclosporine (intravenous): 4 mg/kg per day for 2 weeks (therapeutic levels vary depending on the technique used in the laboratory)
• Cyclosporine (oral): 6 to 8 mg/kg per day for 6 to 8 months 6-MP (oral): 1.0 to 1.5 mg/kg to start (keep ANC greater than 500)
• Azathioprine (oral): 2.0 mg/kg (keep ANC greater than 500)
• Infliximab (intravenous): 5 mg/kg infusion 2 weeks apart, then every 6 to 12 weeks as needed.

OTHER

• Severe disease may require nutritional support in the form of nasogastric feedings or total parenteral nutrition
• Annual ophthalmological evaluation for uveitis is recommended
• Psychological resources should be made available for patients and families

• Social work input may be helpful during hospitalizations, particularly during the time of initial diagnosis
• The Crohn and Colitis Foundation of America (www.CCFA.org) and the Crohn's and Colitis Foundation of Canada are nonprofit organizations dedicated to the care and education of people with Crohn's disease and ulcerative colitis.

 ## Follow-Up

Outpatient follow-up with a pediatric gastroenterologist should be arranged. Important parameters to follow as an outpatient include:

• Abdominal symptoms
• Stool frequency/consistency
• Height/weight
• Hemoglobin
• WBC (for patients on immunosuppressives)
• ESR, albumin, bilirubin and liver enzymes
• Fecal occult blood testing
• Colonoscopic cancer screening (patients with long-standing disease)

 ## Common Questions and Answers

Q: Will my child have this disease forever?
A: Some people will have only the initial attack and then be symptom-free, but usually an individual will have episodes of recurrences and remissions. Surgical removal of the colon represents a curative procedure, although some patients may develop inflammation in the pouch created out of the remaining bowel (pouchitis).

Q: What is the cause of ulcerative colitis?
A: Both genetic and environmental factors are important in the development of ulcerative colitis.

Q: What new therapies will be used in the near future?
A: Biologic agents, a type of therapy that uses our recently improved knowledge of the immune system, represent a new type of therapy.

ICD-9-CM 556

BIBLIOGRAPHY

Mamula P, Markowitz JE, Baldassano RN. Inflammatory bowel disease in early childhood and adolescence: special considerations. *Gastroenterol Clin North Am* 2003;32:967–995.

Michetti P, Peppercorn MA. Medical therapy of specific clinical presentations. *Gastroenterol Clin North Am* 1999;28(2):353–370.

Stein RB, Hanauer SB. Medical therapy for inflammatory bowel disease. *Gastroenterol Clin North Am* 1999;28(2):297–321.

Authors: Meena Thayu and Jonathan E. Markowitz

Ureteropelvic Junction Obstruction

 Database

DEFINITION

Ureteropelvic junction (UPJ) obstruction is a partial blockage of the kidney at the point where the renal pelvis transitions into the proximal ureter.

ETIOLOGIES

- Intrinsic: a congenital narrowing of the UPJ, which is most commonly a result of abnormal musculature and fibrosis of this area, resulting in an adynamic segment.
- Extrinsic: kinking at the UPJ, which is most commonly a result of the renal pelvis draping over a lower pole crossing vessel. This type of obstruction can be intermittent.

PATHOPHYSIOLOGY

The obstruction can cause varying degrees of hydronephrosis.

- Mild forms of UPJ obstruction result in dilation of the renal pelvis without loss of function.
- More severe forms result in dilation of the renal pelvis and calyces with loss of renal parenchyma and decreased function.
- In the most severe cases the kidney may have cystic dysplasia and very poor function.
- Congenital hydronephrosis as a result of an intrinsic narrowing is nearly always asymptomatic.
- When the obstruction is intermittent as a result of a crossing vessel, the renal pelvis becomes distended (most commonly a result of transient increase in urine output), which drapes it over the vessel and kinks the ureter, resulting in an acute obstruction. The acute distension of the renal pelvis results in pain (renal colic).

EPIDEMIOLOGY

- Forty-five percent of all cases of prenatal hydronephrosis are a result of UPJ obstruction
- Occurs more commonly in males (M/F 2:1)
- Left-sided lesion more common (66%)
- Bilateral in 10% to 40%
- Fifty percent of patients have an additional genitourinary malformation (most common are vesicoureteral reflux, contralateral UPJ obstruction, multicystic dysplastic kidney, and renal agenesis)
- Of patients with VATER association, 21% have UPJ obstruction and thus should be screened with renal ultrasound

 Differential Diagnosis

- Vesicoureteral reflux: Higher grades of reflux will result in dilation of the upper urinary tract.
- Distal ureteral obstruction: obstruction at the level of the bladder as a result of ureterovesical junction obstruction, ureterocele, or an ectopic ureter.
- Bladder outlet obstruction: dilation of the upper urinary tract secondary to obstruction of the lower urinary tract as a result of posterior urethral valves, urethral atresia, or stricture.
- Megacalycosis: congenital dilation and increased numbers of calyces without significant renal pelvis dilation or obstruction.
- Multicystic-dysplastic kidney: can be difficult to differentiate severe hydronephrosis from cysts by ultrasound. Renal scan will demonstrate no function in multicystic-dysplastic kidneys.
- Triad syndrome: a triad of hypoplastic abdominal wall musculature, bilateral undescended testes, and dilation of the urinary tract (also known as prune-belly syndrome or Eagle-Barrett syndrome).

 Data Gathering

HISTORY

- Antenatal: if unilateral, timing and severity of hydronephrosis, and status of the contralateral kidney. When bilateral or affecting a solitary kidney, renal insufficiency is a concern. The presence of oligohydramnios, increased renal echogenicity, and cystic changes are indicators of poor renal function and dysplasia.
- Postnatal: feeding intolerance/respiratory distress (very rarely caused by massive UPJ obstruction)
- Older children: history of episodic abdominal (may not lateralize well), flank or back pain. Length of episodes (usually 30 minutes to several hours). Associated nausea and vomiting. Relation of episodes to fluid intake. History of urinary tract infections or gross hematuria.

 Physical Examination

Newborn: Palpate kidneys. Affected kidney may feel enlarged but should not be tense. A tense mass can indicate a severe obstruction and should be imaged promptly.
Older child: careful abdominal examination for enlarged kidney and tenderness.
Costal-vertebral angle tenderness.

 Laboratory Aids

TESTS

- Newborn: if bilateral or a solitary kidney need serial assessments of renal function (serum electrolytes and creatinine) starting at 24 to 48 hours of age. With a normal contralateral kidney no immediate laboratory testing is necessary.
- Older children: urinalysis to detect hematuria or pyuria. Culture if infection suspected.

IMAGING

Antenatally detected hydronephrosis: Infants with antenatally detected hydronephrosis typically are evaluated with three imaging studies: a renal/bladder ultrasound, voiding cystourethrogram, and renal scan.

- Renal/bladder ultrasound: In most cases immediate imaging is not necessary. Because of a period of relative oliguria of a newborn in the first 24 to 48 hours of life, an ultrasound may underestimate the degree of hydronephrosis. This should not preclude evaluating an infant during this time as long any normal study is followed up with a repeat study in 4 to 6 weeks. Evaluation should reveal the severity of dilation of the renal pelvis and calyces, changes in the amount and echogenicity of the parenchyma, and presence of cortical cysts. The evaluation of the full bladder is important for excluding dilated distal ureters, thickening of the bladder wall as a result of outlet obstruction, and ureteroceles. In cases of bilateral hydronephrosis, a solitary hydronephrotic kidney, or a tense kidney on physical examination, imaging should be promptly performed.
- Voiding cystourethrogram: This study will detect the presence of vesicoureteral reflux and exclude the presence of posterior urethral valves and other abnormalities of the bladder. The test can be delayed until after discharge from the nursery unless there is concern about posterior urethral valves, in which case it should be performed early.

- Renal scan: This study can quantify the differential renal function or the amount each kidney contributes to overall renal function (the normal differential function is 50% ± 5% for each kidney). The two most commonly used radionuclides are 3-mercaptoacetyl triglycine (MAG-3) and diethylenetriamine pentaacetic acid (DTPA). MAG-3 is the best choice for infants and babies. In addition to the ability to detect diminished function, if there is poor drainage of the affected kidney, furosemide is given to wash out the radiotracer. The time for washing out half of the accumulated radiotracer (T1/2) is often given in the report. A prompt T1/2 (less than 10 minutes) is indicative of a nonobstructed kidney. A slower T1/2 may be indicative of obstruction when it is greater than 20 minutes. An intermediate T1/2 (10 to 20 minutes) is indeterminate for obstruction. Due to effects of hydration, the amount of hydronephrosis, and variables in the timing of the diuretic administration, the T1/2 may be unreliable.
- Intravenous pyelogram (IVP): This study is most useful for evaluating the anatomy of the kidney and the ureters. It can also be used for evaluating an older child with intermittent symptoms if it can be done during a symptomatic episode. A normal study during a symptomatic episode of abdominal or flank pain excludes an intermittent UPJO as the cause of the child's pain. On the other hand, if a normal study is obtained while the child is asymptomatic, an intermittent UPJ obstruction remains a possible cause.
- Magnetic Resonance Imaging (MRI): A new technique being studied that provides both anatomic and functional detail. Dynamic contrast enhanced MRI requires sedation and placement of a bladder catheter. The images are obtained following infusion of Gadolinium-DTPA. Lasix is given 15 minutes before the start of the study. This technique is being studied for use instead of ultrasound and renal scans in the hopes that it will be a more precise tool in deciding whether or not the child requires surgical repair. The studies are currently preliminary but this may be an important technique in the future.

 Therapy

The decision to observe or surgically correct a UPJ obstruction depends on several factors. One must consider the age and overall health of the neonate, the amount of functional impairment of the kidney, whether it is a unilateral or bilateral process, the drainage pattern on renal scan, and whether or not it is symptomatic. There is no strict rule for who should be observed and who should undergo surgery. This decision should be made on an individual basis.

- Antibiotic prophylaxis: Newborns should be started on a once-a-day dose of amoxicillin or cephalexin at one fourth the therapeutic dose. The theory is to suppress the growth of bacteria in the bladder but not give a dose high enough to develop resistant organisms in the intestine. The antibiotic can be switched to trimethoprim/sulfamethoxazole or nitrofurantoin at 3 months of age. The duration that infants should be left on antibiotics is controversial among practicing pediatric urologists. Almost all agree that infants should be started on prophylactic antibiotics at birth. They should be continued at least until the infant undergoes a VCUG to exclude reflux. Several factors including age, sex, and degree of hydronephrosis are taken into account when deciding whether or not to stop the prophylaxis.
- Observation: Infants with hydronephrosis thought to be a result of a narrowing at the UPJ are typically observed when there is preserved function (greater than 40%) in the affected kidney and the contralateral kidney is normal. The pattern of drainage is taken into account, and if there is prompt drainage and normal differential function (50% ± 5%) these patients are followed with less frequent follow-up studies than those with less function or poor drainage. Most patients have follow-up imaging studies done at 3- to 6-month intervals during their first year of life, and they are gradually spaced out as time goes by if the hydronephrosis remains stable or improves.
- Older children with hydronephrosis as a result of a UPJ obstruction are often detected during a symptomatic episode. If the UPJ obstruction is asymptomatic and the function of the kidney is preserved, the child may be observed as well.

- Surgery: The gold standard for the repair of the UPJ obstruction has been a pyeloplasty. During the procedure the narrowed UPJ is most commonly excised and the ureter is reanastomosed to the renal pelvis. This procedure is successful 95% of the time. There are less invasive approaches such as endoscopically incising the narrowing (endopyelotomy) or balloon dilation. These approaches have been used in adults with rates of success in the 50% to 70% range but are considerably less invasive. Endoscopic procedures have not been routinely offered as first-line therapy for the treatment of UPJ obstructions because of their limited experience in children and the lower rates of success. Laparoscopic pyeloplasty is being performed in older children and adolescents and will likely be more common in the next several years. It offers a similar rate of success to a traditional pyeloplasty with decreased perioperative morbidity because of the small incisions for the laparoscopic instruments.

 Common Questions and Answers

Q: My unborn baby has hydronephrosis. My obstetrician told me that it is most likely a UPJ obstruction. Is my baby going to need surgery to correct this?
A: Not necessarily, only about one-third of babies with significant hydronephrosis ultimately require surgical correction.

Q: Will my child's kidney look normal after the surgery to fix it?
A: Often the kidney has less dilation and an improved appearance but not completely normal. Of greater importance is that there is no longer obstruction and the function is preserved or improved.

ICD-9-CM 593.4

BIBLIOGRAPHY

Carr MC. Anomalies and surgery of the ureteropelvic junction in children. In: Walsh PC, Retik AB, Vaughan ED, et al., eds. *Campbell's Urology. 8th Edition. 1995–2006.* Philadelphia: WB Saunders: 2002.

Perez-Brayfield MR, Kirsch AJ, Jones RA, et al. A prospective study comparing ultrasound, nuclear scintigraphy and dynamic contrast enhanced magnetic resonance imaging in the evaluation of hydronephrosis. *J Urol* 2003;170:1330–1334.

Authors: J. Christopher Austin and Michael C. Carr

Urethral Prolapse

Database

DEFINITION

Circular eversion of the distal urethral mucosa through the external urethral meatus.

GENETICS

Predominance in Black females indicates a hereditary pattern.

ETIOLOGY

• Etiology unclear, proposed theories include:

—Poor adherence between smooth muscle layers of the urethra
—Estrogen deficiency

EPIDEMIOLOGY

• Prepubertal girls younger than 10 years of age
• Preponderance among Black females (90% to 100% of patients in reported series)
• Patients above average for height and weight

Differential Diagnosis

• Prolapsing ureterocele (or ectopic ureter, urethral polyp, bladder)
• Sarcoma botryoides
• Condyloma
• Hydrometrocolpos
• Periurethral abscess
• Trauma

Data Gathering

HISTORY

• Ninety-five percent present with bleeding/bloody spotting in underwear.
• Twenty-one percent have dysuria, frequency.
• Occasionally a patient presents with urinary retention.
• Some are asymptomatic and detected only incidentally.

Physical Examination

- Circular (doughnut-shaped) protrusion of urethral meatus with a reddish-purple mass filling the introitus with the urethral meatus at the center.
- Tissue appears inflamed and friable.

IMAGING

- If the appearance is atypical for urethral prolapse, ultrasound may be used to rule out bladder tumor (sarcoma botryoides) or prolapsed ureterocele.
- Urethral prolapse with typical presentation requires no imaging.

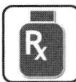 ## Therapy

- Do not try to manually reduce the prolapsed tissue.
- Conservative—Sitz baths followed by topical estrogen cream b.i.d.
- Surgical—Most typical surgical approach is excision of prolapsed segment over a urethral Foley catheter, suturing the proximal urethral margin to the adjacent vestibule.

 ## Follow-Up

Outpatient visit to assess success of estrogen cream or surgical repair

 ## Common Questions and Answers

Q: What is the most common presenting complaint?
A: Bleeding

Q: What is the "first aid" for this problem?
A: Avoid infection and respect the tissue. Keep tissue moist. You may use antibiotic cream. Do not push the tissue back into the urethra.

ICD-9-CM 599.5

BIBLIOGRAPHY

Baldwin D, Landa H. Common problems in pediatric gynecology. *Urol Clin North Am* 1995;22:173.

Kelalis P, King K, Belman A, eds. *Clinical Pediatric Urology*. Philadelphia: WB Saunders, 1992:653–654.

Valerie E, Gilchrists B, Frischer J, et al. Diagnosis and treatment of urethral prolapse in children. *Urology* 1999;54(6):1082.

Authors: Michele Clement and Stephen A. Zderic

Urinary Tract Infection

 Database

DEFINITION

Urinary tract infection (UTI) is growth of bacterial urinary tract pathogen(s) at:

- ≥102 colony-forming units (CFU)/mL for suprapubic aspirate
- ≥104 CFU/mL for urine obtained by catheterization
- ≥105 CFU/mL for urine obtained by clean-catch technique

PATHOLOGY

- Urinary tract pathogens include:

—Common: *Escherichia coli*, *Klebsiella* spp., Enterococcus, *Proteus mirabilis*
—Less common: *Enterobacter cloacae*, group B hemolytic streptococci, Citrobacter, *Staphylococcus aureus*, and *Staphylococcus saprophyticus* (teenage girls)

- A specimen must be obtained sterilely, not by applying a bag to the perineum.
- Ninety percent of patients will also have pyuria (5 WBC/high-power field [HPF] or urine dipstick for leukocyte esterase (LE)] and bacteriuria on examination of the urine.
- Upper tract infection or pyelonephritis: infection of the renal parenchyma; vast majority of febrile babies with a positive culture have upper tract infection.
- Lower tract infection: infection limited to bladder, not involving the kidneys; occurs more in older children and adolescents; no fever.

EPIDEMIOLOGY

- Ascending infection from bladder instrumentation, perineal irritation, bacterial soilage, sexual activity
- Dysfunctional voiding
- Urinary tract abnormalities: vesicoureteral reflux (VUR), neurogenic bladder, urethral obstruction

RISK FACTORS

- Sex/age: boys most at risk for UTI during first year of life; girls until school age and again in adolescence
- Circumcision status: Uncircumcised males have ten times the incidence of UTI compared with circumcised males.
- Race: Beyond the neonatal period, Whites have a higher incidence of UTI; Whites females have the highest rate.
- Abnormal urinary tract: Children with VUR and obstruction are at higher risk for UTI.
- Voiding dysfunction

COMPLICATIONS

- Repeated febrile UTIs in young children may lead to renal scarring.
- Renal scarring in childhood carries a risk of hypertension, preeclampsia, and end-stage renal disease as an adult.

PROGNOSIS

Prompt treatment of febrile UTIs reduces the risk for scarring and its sequelae.

ASSOCIATED ILLNESSES

Approximately 5% to 10% of babies with febrile UTIs (pyelonephritis) are bacteremic.

 Differential Diagnosis

- Lower tract infections

—Urethral irritation for irritants such as bubble baths
—Diabetes
—Excessive drinking
—Masses adjacent to the bladder
—Normal potty training
—Dyes from ingested fluids
—Dehydration with concentrated urine

- Upper tract infections

—Gastroenteritis
—Pelvic inflammatory disease or tubo-ovarian abscess (TOA)
—Appendicitis
—Ovarian torsion

 Data Gathering

HISTORY

- Babies: Symptoms are nonspecific, such as vomiting, irritability, poor feeding, and fever.
- Older children: Classic symptoms of the lower tract include urgency, frequency, dysuria, hesitancy, suprapubic discomfort, hematuria, and malodorous urine. Classic symptoms of the upper tract include chills, nausea, flank pain, and fever.

 Physical Examination

BABIES

- Fever is the most common finding.
- Abdominal pain or distention
- Poor growth or weight gain
- Malodorous urine

OLDER CHILDREN

- Lower tract: suprapubic tenderness
- Upper tract: fever, costovertebral angle tenderness to percussion

SPECIAL QUESTION

Has the young child had a history of UTI, unexplained fevers, or urinary tract anomaly?

PROCEDURE

Suspect UTI in any febrile baby less than 1 year of age , uncircumcised males, or in a preschool girl, even in the absence of signs and symptoms, especially if there is not a definite source of fever, fever has been present ≥2 days, or temperature is ≥39°C.

 Laboratory Aids

TESTS

- Urinalysis: 5 WBC/HPF or bacteria on Gram stain microscopy per HPF.
- Urine dipstick is equivalent to conventional microscopy: trace color changes on the LE test strip indicate 5 WBC/HPF; nitrite indicates the presence of nitrate-splitting bacteria.
- Enhanced urinalysis: 10 WBC/cm³ or higher, or bacteria on Gram stain, may be most sensitive for detecting UTI in the neonate
- Urine culture collected sterilely is the gold standard for diagnosis.

FALSE POSITIVES

Contaminated urine by perineum or stool organisms

PITFALLS

- Ten percent of babies will have a negative urinalysis despite culture or nuclear scan-documented UTI.
- Failure to culture by sterile means: unable to interpret a contaminated urine culture result

HOME TESTING

Urine dipstick for LE or nitrite with first morning void can be used to screen children at risk for repeated infections.

REQUIREMENTS

- Obtain urine sterilely to avoid false-positive results.
- The nitrite test requires urine to be in the bladder for 4 hours; therefore, the first morning specimen is best.

Therapy

UPPER TRACT INFECTION

- Intravenous therapy with ampicillin and gentamicin or third generation cephalosporin, such as ceftriaxone intravenously until clinical improvement (such as defervescence or sterile urine) is the treatment of choice for neonates, infants who may have urinary tract abnormalities, and infants and children who are unable to take oral medications, appear toxic, or may be noncompliant with treatment and follow-up.
- Length of treatment: Complete a 10- to 14-day course orally.
- Outpatient oral treatment for older children and select infants who look well, can take oral fluids, have normal urinary tract anatomy (often by prenatal ultrasound), and have good follow-up.

LOWER TRACT INFECTION

- Oral treatment with amoxicillin (if resistance in community is <20%), trimethoprim-sulfamethoxazole (if older than 2 months of age), cephalexin, cefprozil, amoxicillin and clavulanate orally.
- Length of treatment: 7 to 10 days

PREVENTION

- Teaching correct wiping—front to back—to young children.
- Prophylactic antibiotics for selected children with recurrent infection, VUR, pyelonephritis
- Attention to good voiding habits

 Follow-Up

- Repeat urine culture if persistent fever >3 days, not improving.
- Urinalysis and urine culture for subsequent febrile illnesses
- Renal cortical scan: consider in febrile children if diagnosis is unclear
- Ultrasound: (If prenatal ultrasound beyond 32 weeks gestation was normal, may not be necessary)
- Voiding cystourethrogram (VCUG): all boys, all infants younger than 1 year, history of voiding dysfunction, upper tract infection, or abnormal RCS or ultrasound

PITFALLS

- Not obtaining urine by a sterile method for culturing; unable to interpret contaminated results; not knowing if the child should have a radiographic workup
- Not culturing febrile babies without a documented source of fever; increased risk of long-term sequelae, untreated pyelonephritis

 Common Questions and Answers

Q: Which children require radiologic evaluation after their first UTI?
A: All boys, any girl with an upper tract infection, and all girls younger than 3 years of age (see Follow-Up).

Q: Does a urine culture need to be done if the dipstick or urinalysis is negative?
A: Approximately 10% of febrile infants with pyelonephritis will have a false-negative screening test (dipstick, urinalysis). A sterile urine culture should be done.

ICD-9-CM 599.0

BIBLIOGRAPHY

Al-rifi F, McGillivray D, Tange S, et al. Urine culture from bag specimens in young children: are the risks too high? *J Pediatr* 2000;137:221–226.

American Academy of Pediatrics, Committee on Quality Improvement, Subcommittee on Urinary Tract Infection. Practice parameter: the diagnosis, treatment, and evaluation of the initial urinary tract infection in febrile infants and young children. *Pediatrics* 1999;103:843–852.

Bloomfield P, Hodson EM, Craig JC. Antibiotics for acute pyelonephritis in children (Cochrane Review). In: *The Cochrane Library, Issue 3, 2003.* Oxford Update Software.

Gorelick MH, Shaw KN. Clinical decision rule to identify young febrile children at risk for UTI. *Arch Pediatr Adol Med* 2000;154:386–390.

Gorelick MH, Shaw KN. Screening tests for UTI in children: a meta-analysis. *Pediatrics* 1999;104(5):e1.

Hoberman A, Chao HP, Keller DM, et al. Prevalence of urinary tract infection in febrile infants. *J Pediatr* 1993;23(1):17–23.

Hoberman A, Charron M, Hickey RW, Baskin M, Kearney DH, Wald ER. Imaging studies after a first febrile urinary tract infection in young children. *N Engl J Med* 2003;348:195–202.

Hoberman A, Wald ER, Hickey RW, et al. Oral versus initial intravenous therapy for urinary tract infections in young febrile children. *Pediatrics* 1999;104:79–86.

Michael M, Hodson EM, Craig JC, Martin S, Moyer VA. Short compared with standard duration of antibiotic treatment for urinary tract infection: a systematic review of randomised controlled trials. *Arch Dis Child* 2002;87(2):118–123.

Shaw KN, Gorelick M, McGowan KL, et al. Prevalence of UTI in febrile young children in the emergency department. *Pediatrics* 1998;102(2):1–5.

Wald E. Urinary tract infections in infants and children: a comprehensive overview. *Current Opin Pediatr* 2004;16(1):85–88.

Winberg J. Commentary: progressive renal damage from infection with or without reflux. *J Urol* 1992;148:1733–1734.

Author: Kathy N. Shaw

Urticaria

 Database

DEFINITION

A skin disorder characterized by well-circumscribed and/or coalescent, local or generalized erythematous, raised skin lesions (wheals or welts) of various sizes. Lesions may or may not be pruritic.

- Acute urticaria: lesions lasting less than 6 weeks
- Chronic urticaria: lesions lasting for more than 6 weeks
- Angioedema: subcutaneous swelling with a predilection to areas of loose connective tissue (e.g., face or mucous members involving the lip or tongue).
- Giant urticaria: large wheals and diffuse swelling of the eyelids, hands, genitalia, and mucous membranes (lips and tongue).
- Anaphylaxis: a life-threatening hypersensitivity reaction occurring immediately following exposure to an antigen that involves both local and system reactions including pruritus, urticaria, angioedema, weakness, dyspnea, hypotension, and shock.

ETIOLOGY

The most frequent cause may be viral infections. In 70% to 80% of cases of urticaria, no etiologic agent is identified.
Ingestions—various foods, medications
Direct contact—plants, animals, topical medications
Injections—medications, transfused blood, bee stings, insect, and/or snake bites
Inhalants—pollen, animal dander, molds
Infection—viral (particularly Epstein Barr virus and hepatitis), parasitic, bacterial (particularly Group A Streptococcus)
Systemic—malignancy, autoimmune collagen vascular diseases
Genetic—hereditary angioedema, amyloidosis, C3b inactivator deficiency
Physical—cold-induced, solar-induced, or exercise-induced; pressure, dermographism

PATHOPHYSIOLOGY

- Usually a self-limited allergic (IgE-mediated) reaction occurring secondary to activation of mast cells or basophil-bound IgE antibodies in the skin by an allergen
- Release of histamine from these cells causes vasodilatation and increased vascular permeability, which results in the wheal and flare reaction.

EPIDEMIOLOGY

- Fifteen percent to 20% of the population is affected by urticaria at some time during their life.
- Approximately 1% of those affected by urticaria develop chronic urticaria.
- More common among females than males.

COMPLICATIONS

- Angioedema of the upper respiratory tract can lead to life-threatening obstruction of the laryngeal airway.
- Symptoms can rapidly progress to anaphylaxis.

PROGNOSIS

- Most cases of urticaria in pediatrics are self-limited.
- Etiology of chronic urticaria is identified in less than 20% of cases

 Differential Diagnosis

DERMATOLOGIC

- Insect bites
- Atopic or contact dermatitis
- Erythema multiforme

INFECTIONS

- Bacterial—Group A Streptococcus (with or without scarletiniform rash)

AUTOIMMUNE

- Juvenile rheumatoid arthritis
- Systemic lupus erythematosis
- Celiac disease

TUMORS

- Malignancy

 Data Gathering

HISTORY

Question: Has the child had previous episodes of urticaria?
Significance: Previous episodes of urticaria may provide information about potential allergic triggers.

Question: Has there been ingestion of new foods or medications recently?
Significance: Food and drug allergies are a common cause of urticaria.

Question: Has there been a recent viral illness or symptoms?
Significance: Urticaria is often associated with viral infections in children.

Question: Is there a history of asthma or atopic dermatitis?
Signficance: Asthma and atopic dermatitis are associated with an increased risk of allergic disorders.

Question: Has there been any recent skin contact with plants, topical medications, or animals?
Significance: Contact urticaria occurs at the site of skin contact almost immediately after exposure and may assist in the identification of potential allergens to be avoided in the future.

Question: Are there any known medical problems?
Significance: Systemic illnesses such as connective tissue disorders are associated with urticaria, particularly chronic urticaria.

Question: Are symptoms associated with exercise?
Significance: Exercise-induced anaphylaxis can include presenting with urticaria, and pruritus, angioedema, wheezing, and hypotension.

 Physical Examination

Finding: Wheal and flare lesions or welts
Significance: The classic sign of urticaria and usually serves as the primary clinical sign.

Finding: Facial swelling
Significance: Evidence of angioedema that can lead to life-threatening airway swelling and obstruction.

Finding: Wheezing
Significance: Evidence of life-threatening lower airway edema and bronchial spasm.

Finding: Lymphadenopathy
Significance: May be an indication of underlying malignancy.

Finding: Swollen joints
Significance: May be an indication of an autoimmune disorder.

Laboratory Aids

Test: Skin testing (RAST is an alternative)
Significance: Allergy testing may be useful if food or medications are identified as a potential etiology.

Test: Erythrocyte Sedimentation Rate (ESR), antinuclear antibody (ANA), or rheumatoid factor (RF) (based on clinical symptoms)
Significance: To rule out potential underlying autoimmune disorder.

Therapy

- Emergent treatment of urticaria associated with anaphylaxis:

—Epinephrine 1:1000, 0.01 mL/kg, max 0.03 mL for acute, severe urticaria/angioedema

- Treatment of urticaria not associated with anaphylaxis:

—First generation H1 antihistamines
  —Diphenhydramine (Benadryl) 5 mg/kg per 24 hours divided q 6 hours PO; max 300 mg per 24 hours. Potential side effects: sedation, nausea, vomiting, may cause paradoxical excitement in children.
  —Contraindications: MAO inhibitor use, acute asthma exacerbation, GI, or urinary tract obstruction.
  —Hydroxyzine (Atarax) 2 mg/kg per 24 hours divided q 6 to 8 hours PO, max 600 mg per 24 hours. Potential side effects: may cause dry mouth, drowsiness, tremor, convulsions, blurred vision, hypotension, wheezing, use with caution in asthmatics.
—Second generation H1 antihistamines
  —Cetirizine (Zyrtec)—age 6 to 12 months 2.5 mg PO q day; max 2.5 mg per day ages 12 to 24 months: 2.5 mg PO q day-bid; max 5 mg per day; ages 2 to 6 years 2.5- to 5-mg PO q day; max 5 mg per day ; age >6 years:
  5 to 10 mg PO q day; max 10 mg per day. Potential side effects: headache, pharyngitis, GI symptoms, dry mouth, sedation.
  —Loratidine (Claritin)—ages 2 to 6 years 5 mg PO q day; max 5 mg per day; >6 years 10 mg PO q day; max 10 mg per day; potential side effects: drowsiness, fatigue, dry mouth, headache, palpitations, dizziness.
  —Fexodenadine (Allegra)—ages 6 to 11 years 30 mg PO bid; max dose 60 mg per 24 hours; >12 years 60 mg PO bid; max dose 180 mg per 24 hours. Potential side effects: drowsiness, fatigue, headache, dysmenorrhea, nausea.
—Oral corticosteroids may be considered for cases of severe refractory or chronic urticaria:
  —Prednisone 0.5 to 2 mg/kg per 24 hours PO divided q day or QID for short 2 to 3 day course of acute refractory urticaria; max 80 mg per 24 hours.

—Prednisone 20 mg PO on alternate days with a dosage decrease by 2.5 to 5 mg every 3 weeks depending on patient response for chronic urticaria not resolved by antihistamines.

Follow-Up

- Watch for signs of anaphylaxis (wheezing, angioedema of the face, or oral mucosa that could suggest airway compromise)

PREVENTION

- Avoidance of known triggers (foods, medications, animals, etc.)

PITFALLS

- Identification of all potential causative agents is often not possible

Common Questions and Answers

Q: When should I refer cases of acute urticaria to a specialist?
A: Acute urticaria that may be associated with anaphylactogenic foods, inhalants or medications or that recurs or persists for greater than 6 weeks should be referred to an allergist or immunologist for allergy skin testing, in vitro, or other diagnostic testing as appropriate.

Q: How long should patients with an episode of acute urticaria by observed to prevent missing potentially significant sequelae?
A: Uncomplicated cases that respond to antihistamines may require only a brief observation of 30 minutes to 2 hours. Episodes with associated angioedema or requiring the use of epinephrine should be observed for several hours or overnight.

ICD-9-CM 708.9

BIBLIOGRAPHY

American College of Allergy, Asthma, and Immunology Joint Task Force on Practice Parameters. The diagnosis and management of urticaria: a practice parameter part I: acute urticaria/angioedema part II: chronic urticaria/angioedema. *Ann Allergy Asthma Immunol* 2000;85:521–544.

Dalal I, Levine A, Somekh E, Mizrahi A, Hanukoglu A. Chronic urticaria in children: expanding the "autoimmune kaleidoscope." *Pediatrics* 2000;106:1139–1141.

Greaves MW. Chronic urticaria in childhood. *Allergy* 2000;55:309–320.

Leung DYM. Urticara and Angioedema (Hives). *Behrman: Nelson Textbook of Pediatrics.* 17th Ed. Philadelphia: Saunders, 2004: 778–780.

Zuberbier T, Henz BM. Use of cetirizine in dermatologic disorders. *Ann Allergy Asthma Immunol* 1999;83:476–480.

Author: Ivor Braden Horn

Vaginitis

Database

DEFINITION

- Vaginitis is an inflammatory process of the vagina often caused by infection, but also caused by foreign bodies and other irritants.
- Vulvovaginitis is inflammation of the vulva and vagina, and is more common in prepubertal girls.
- Bacterial vaginosis is an overgrowth of normal vaginal flora, primarily anaerobic, associated with an elevation in vaginal pH, a malodorous discharge and often a sensation of burning. This condition has been referred to as Gardnerella, Hemophilus, and nonspecific vaginitis.
- Vaginal discharge is a vaginal secretion that may or may not be associated with inflammation or infection.

CAUSES

All ages:
- Chemical irritants such as soaps, bubble baths, detergents, and fabric softeners
- Allergic reactions
- Foreign material, such as paper products, sand, and soil
- *Candida albicans*, especially if exposed to antibiotics
- Trauma from repeated rubbing, such as with masturbation
- Sexual abuse

Prepubertal females:
- Diapers and nonbreathable clothing
- Coliform bacteria from the child's toileting practices
- B-hemolytic group A streptococcus
- Infestations, including pinworms and scabies

Postpubertal females:
- Noninflammatory, physiologic leukorrhea
- Bacterial vaginosis
- *Trichomonas*
- *Chlamydia trachomatis*
- Gonorrhea
- Herpes simplex virus, types I and II
- Human papilloma virus (HPV)
- Chancroid
- LGV (lymphogranuloma veneareum)
- Beçhet disease
- Epstein-Barr Virus

PATHOPHYSIOLOGY

- Physiologic leukorrhea is a normally occurring vaginal discharge that is clear or white, nonpruritic, nonirritating, and rarely malodorous. The amount of discharge markedly varies from individual to individual and may be profuse. In menstruating girls, the volume of discharge varies with the menstrual cycle and is especially heavy at ovulation as a result of varying estrogen levels.
- Candidiasis occurs more commonly when the glycogen level in the vaginal mucosa is increased, as in pregnancy and diabetes. Use of antibiotics also increases the occurrence of candidiasis by eliminating competitive organisms.

- For bacterial vaginosis, the inciting cause is not known, but the etiologic cascade involves a decline in levels of lactobacillus leading to an increased pH and increased overgrowth of normal bacterial flora. The change in the vaginal environment decreases the normal defenses against pathogens.
- The normal trauma of sexual intercourse may increase the likelihood of vaginitis by causing microscopic breakdown of the mucosal surface.
- During toileting, wiping from the anus toward the vagina, may introduce bacteria not normal for the vagina and induce a vaginitis.

EPIDEMIOLOGY

- The exact incidence of vaginitis is unknown.
- Candidiasis may present cyclically with menses, possibly as a result of changing estrogen levels.
- Gonorrhea is more likely to be symptomatic at the time of menses as a result of easier access to the upper reproductive tract.
- Body mass index (BMI) at the extremes is associated with increased risk of vulvovaginitis.
- The epidemiology of bacterial vaginosis is not well-known because it is not a reportable disease, and 50% of cases may be asymptomatic.

GENETICS

There is no clear genetic pattern for vaginitis or vulvovaginitis.

COMPLICATIONS

- Pelvic inflammatory disease (PID)
- Scarring in the female reproductive tract
- Pelvic pain syndrome and infertility
- Untreated bacterial vaginosis has been associated with premature labor, premature rupture of membranes, and increased risk of acquiring sexually-transmitted infections (STIs).

PROGNOSIS

When treated, patients with vaginitis, vulvovaginitis, and bacterial vaginosis generally do well.

Differential Diagnosis

- Bacterial vaginosis
- Chlamydia
- Gonorrhea
- Trichomonas
- Candidiasis
- Herpes simplex virus infection
- HPV
- Physiologic leukorrhea
- Psoriasis
- Lichen sclerosis (hypotrophic dystrophy of the vulva)
- Congenital abnormalities, such as ectopic ureter

Data Gathering

HISTORY

Inquiries should include:
- Is discharge present? What is the color, odor and duration? (See chart, Differential Diagnosis of Vaginal Itching in Paramenarchal and Postmenarchal Girls)
- Is the child itchy, or having a burning sensation or dysuria? Itching and burning may be signs of vaginal inflammation. Dysuria raises the suspicion for a urinary tract infection, but burning at the start of micturation (urine touching the vulva) may be seen with vulvovaginal inflammation.
- What conditions make symptoms better or worse? Inflammation may be related to specific clothing, especially tight pants. Nighttime itching/discomfort may signal pinworm infestation.
- Has any treatment been attempted? If so, what? What has worked in the past may work again. The success or failure of over-the-counter products may affect the treatment choices.
- Any other recent health problems? Recent respiratory or gastrointestinal distress increases the risk for group A streptococcal infection.
- Any new medication, especially an antibiotic, introduced around the time of symptom onset? Antibiotics increase the risk for candidal vaginitis.
- Is there a history of sexual activity? STIs should be considered if there is known sexual activity and should be considered even when sexual activity is denied.
- If appropriate, what is the character and time of the last menses? Gonorrhea is associated with increased symptoms at the time of menses. Some girls may have cyclic yeast infections associated with menses.
- Any new chemical exposures such as soaps, spermicides, or feminine hygiene products? Vaginitis often follows vaginal exposure to cleaning and other chemical agents.
- Any chronic illnesses such as diabetes or immunocompromised conditions? Vaginitis is much more common in these situations.
- Any previous similar symptoms? Some people have a tendency toward repeated vaginal inflammation, especially candidiasis.

Physical Examination

- Vital signs including height, weight, and temperature.
- Calculate the BMI.
- Tanner pubertal development scores
- Examine the entire skin for other lesions or dermatoses.
- Abdominal examination to assess for abdominal pain and masses
- Evaluate external genitalia for tenderness, erythema, discharge, ulceration, edema, excoriation, traumatic injuries, warts (HPV), lymphadenopathy, and pigment changes.
- Evaluate vagina for findings above, if possible.

The following table may help with differentiating normal physiologic leukorrhea from three common etiologies:

Laboratory Aids

Common gynecologic tests:

- Odor/whiff test—prepared with 10% KOH.
- Wet mount of the vaginal discharge is mixed with saline for microscopic evaluation (see table).
- pH is measured by nitrazine paper.
- Chlamydial polymerase chain reaction (PCR) assay should be performed on all sexually active patients.
- Culture for gonorrhea may need special media.
- Culture for fungi (yeast).
- Pap test if sexually active.

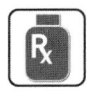

Therapy

NONPHARMACOLOGIC INTERVENTIONS

- Removal of irritant/foreign body: In vaginitis caused by chemical irritants or foreign materials, the practitioner should attempt to identify and remove the cause. On occasion, especially in younger children, intravaginal foreign bodies may have to be removed under anesthesia.
- Promoting good hygiene: Girls should be educated in good toilet hygiene and proper front-to-back wiping.
- Sitz baths: Local treatment should include sitz baths (sitting in plain warm water) followed by air drying of the vulvar area, use of topical emollients (Vaseline or Aquaphor) and topical low-potency steroids (short course) to control inflammation.
- Trauma from repeated rubbing or other causes is treated in the same manner.
- Congenital abnormalities, such as ectopic ureter, will respond to the above regime but will eventually need definitive surgical treatment.

PHARMACOLOGIC INTERVENTIONS

- Topical steroids:
- Lichen sclerosis requires very high potency topical steroids for amelioration. Apply to vulva BID for 2 to 4 weeks. Overuse may lead to thinning of the skin
- In moderate inflammation of the vulva caused by irritants, apply low-potency steroids lightly to vulva BID for 5 to 14 days, until symptoms have subsided for 2 days. Extreme overuse may also lead to skin thinning.
- Antifungal agents including topical butaconazole, miconazole, terconazole applied as directed will relieve vaginal Candidiasis.
- As an alternative, oral fluconazole 6 mg/kg in one dose to maximum dose of 150 mg may be effective.
- Antibiotics are used in many causes of vaginal infection:
- Bacterial vaginosis is treated in older children with metronidazole 500 mg PO BID for 7 days or topically with metronidazole gel or clindamycin cream.
- In infections with coliform bacteria, treat with amoxicillin at 40 mg/kg per day to maximum of 500 mg BID. B-hemolytic group A streptococcus will usually respond to the same dosage of amoxicillin.
- In patients with penicillin allergy, trimethaprim/sulfa, azithromycin, or ciprofloxacin (in older children) is appropriate in either type of bacterial infection.
- Chlamydia is treated with either azithromycin 1,000 mg PO in a single dose or doxycycline 100 mg PO BID for 7 days.
- Gonorrhea is treated with ceftriaxone 125 mg IM or ciprofloxacin 500 mg PO in a single dose. Treat for chlamydia simultaneously unless the child is known not to have chlamydia.
- Trichomonas responds to metronidazole 2 g in a single dose.
- In any infection that raises suspicion of sexual abuse, this suspicion must be reported to the local authorities immediately.
- Other anti-infective agents used in vaginitis include:
- Herpes simplex virus is treated with famciclovir 250 mg TID for 7 to 10 days or with valcyclovir 1 gram PO BID for 7 to 10 days. In recurring herpes simplex virus, prolonged use of these agents may be useful.
- In pinworms, mebendazole 100 mg is taken once by mouth. May be recommended for entire family, but is not used in pregnancy.

Follow-Up

- Follow-up appointment or phone call should be arranged 1 week following the initial diagnosis.
- To prevent recurrence in younger children, avoid irritants such as bubble bath, encourage proper wiping technique and avoid unnecessary antibiotics.

- In sexually active adolescents, consistent use of condoms should be stressed to prevent the spread of STIs.

PITFALLS

- In girls who are Tanner Stage III or greater, antibiotic use may result in the development of candidiasis.
- Telephone therapy of a pruritic vagina as Candidiasis may be incorrect. If a patient using an antifungal is not better in 5 days, she must see the practitioner.

Common Questions and Answers

Q: Is the presence of Gardnerella on vaginal culture sufficient to diagnose bacterial vaginosis?
A: No. The diagnosis of bacterial vaginosis requires three of the following criteria: elevated pH, fishy odor, clue cells on a wet mount, vaginal discharge and/or a positive Gram stain.

Q: Can vaginitis be confused with a urinary tract infection?
A: Yes. Prominent vulvar and vestibular inflammation would strongly suggest a vulvovaginal source.

Q: Can girls be asymptomatic for herpes simplex virus and HPV infections?
A: Yes, sexually active girls may carry these diseases without symptoms.

ICD-9-CM: 616.10

BIBLIOGRAPHY

Brook I. Microbiology and management of polymicrobial female genital tract infections in adolescents. *J Pediatr Adolesc Gynecol* 2002;15(4):217–226.

Jaquiery A, Stylianopoulos A, Hogg G, Grover S. Vulvovaginitis: clinical features, aetiology, and microbiology of the genital tract. *Arch Dis Child* 1999;81:64–67.

Nasraty S. Infections of the female genital tract. *Prim Care* 2003;30(1):193–203, vii.

Nyirjesy P. Vaginitis in the adolescent patient. *Pediatr Clin North Am* 1999;46:733–745.

Quint EH, Smith YR. Vulvar disorders in adolescent patients. *Pediatr Clin North Am* 1999;46:593–606.

Schwebke JR. Gynecologic consequences of bacterial vaginosis *Obstet Gynecol Clin North Am* 2003;30(4):685–694.

Authors: Marianne Ruby and Gary A. Emmett

Differential Diagnosis of Vaginal Infection in Para and Post Menarchal Girls

	NORMAL	BACTERIAL VAGINOSIS	TRICHOMONAS	CANDIDAL VAGINITIS
Inspection	Tanner II or less-pale pink mucosa Tanner III or greater-deeper pink	Possible vulvar erythema	Minimal vulvar changes. Friable cervix	Vulvar erythema, possible Perineal tenderness
Odor	None	Fishy	None	None
Discharge	If present, clear or white	Gray to green	Frothy green to bloody	Cheesy white to yellow
pH	If Tanner III or more <4.5	>4.5	Variable	<4.5
Wet Mount (see Lab. Aids)	Tanner II or less: parabasal epithelial cells Tanner III or greater: lactobacilli may be present None or rare WBCs	Clue cells (epithelial cells with adherent bacteria blurring the cell edge) Rare WBCs	Visible trichomonads. Increased WBCs, possible RBCs	Budding yeast, pseudohyphae Few lactobacilli

Vein of Galen Malformations

Database

DEFINITION

Vein of Galen malformations are congenital arteriovenous malformations (AVMs). The vein of Galen connects the deep cerebral venous system with the intracranial venous sinuses. After draining the internal cerebral veins and basal veins, the vein of Galen flows into the straight sinus.

PATHOPHYSIOLOGY

Vein of Galen malformations may consist of a simple arteriovenous (AV) fistula or a more complicated AVM. Clinical symptoms develop because of high-output congestive heart failure (CHF), cerebral ischemia or hemorrhage, or hydrocephalus. Cerebral ischemia may result from the shunting of blood from the brain parenchyma to the malformation.

GENETICS

- No known genetic predisposition

EPIDEMIOLOGY

Vein of Galen malformations represent about 10% of vascular malformations that present in childhood.

COMPLICATIONS

- High-output CHF, cerebral ischemia or hemorrhage, and hydrocephalus may result from this congenital vascular anomaly.
- Forty percent to 60% of cases present as neonates, almost always with CHF. Occasional infants will present with hydrocephalus, subarachnoid hemorrhage or intraventricular hemorrhage.
- Older infants and children present with hydrocephalus, focal neurologic signs, headache, seizures and subarachnoid hemorrhage.
- In severe cases, 80% of cardiac output may be delivered to the head because of the low vascular resistance within the malformation. Cardiac ischemia may occur because of decreased coronary artery blood flow.
- Some cases are associated with congenital cardiac defects, such as aortic coarctation, atrial septal defect or ventricular septal defect.
- In a recent series, 3 of 34 children had hemorrhagic complications—two children presented with acute intracranial hemorrhage and a third developed acute intracranial hemorrhage following endovascular treatment of the malformation.
- Longer-term complications include mental retardation, seizures, and cerebral palsy.

PROGNOSIS

Prognosis depends on the size of the malformation, the severity of the CHF, and the extent of cerebral injury prior to therapy. Perinatal presentation and choroidal angioarchitecture (multiple arterial feeders from deep vessels that form complex connections) have been associated with worse outcome. Mortality in patients with symptomatic lesions is approximately 50%. Historically, the prognosis has been poor for patients presenting as neonates with CHF, but recent advances in endovascular embolization techniques have improved prognosis.

Differential Diagnosis

- The diagnosis must be considered in any newborn with unexplained CHF (especially high-output failure), hydrocephalus, or intracranial hemorrhage.
- Other causes of high-output CHF in the newborn include anemia, hyperthyroidism, and other AVMs.
- Intracranial hemorrhage may result from other types of AVMs, aneurysms, hemophilic states, hypertension, or trauma in neonates and children. In older children, sickle cell disease, vasculopathies such as moyamoya syndrome and vasculitis can also lead to hemorrhage.
- In older infants and children, presenting symptoms may be nonspecific and raise suspicion of hydrocephalus or a mass lesion.
- Tumors that may obstruct the sylvian aqueduct include common posterior fossa tumors in children, pinealoma, hemangioblastoma, ependymoma, and hamartomas (e.g., in tuberous sclerosis).

Approach to the Patient

First priority is the hemodynamic stability of the patient, because life-threatening CHF may be the presenting symptom. After a history and physical exam, neuroimaging studies must be promptly obtained, so treatment plans can be formulated.

Data Gathering

HISTORY

- Ninety-five percent of newborns with vein of Galen malformations present in CHF. Others present with hydrocephalus, subarachnoid hemorrhage, intraventricular hemorrhage, or failure to thrive.
- Infants and older children usually present with hydrocephalus, headache, seizures, exercise-induced syncope, or subarachnoid hemorrhage. Less common presenting signs include visual loss, syncope, seizures, acute or progressive hemiparesis, developmental regression, epistaxis, and vertigo.

Physical Examination

- In newborns, tachycardia, respiratory distress, hepatomegaly, a continuous cranial bruit heard over the posterior skull, and bounding carotid pulses and peripheral pulses may be present. The resting pulse may increase over time as the volume of blood shunted to the malformation increases. Scalp veins may be dilated.
- As CHF worsens, the peripheral pulses may lose their bounding character, but the prominent carotid pulses persist.
- Older infants and children also may present with CHF but more often demonstrate increased head circumference, focal neurologic signs, and failure to thrive. Proptosis may be noted.

Laboratory Aids

TESTS

As with other AVMs, CBC and blood gases are often normal. Chest radiograph and electrocardiogram may reveal typical changes of high-output CHF, even in patients with resting tachycardia but no overt circulatory symptoms.

Imaging

- Neuroimaging studies are definitive.
- Prenatal diagnosis is now possible with fetal ultrasound. This allows planning for the appropriate location of delivery and postnatal management.
- In newborns, cranial ultrasound shows a large, hypoechoic structure in the region of the vein of Galen. CT shows a high-density mass that enhances with contrast. MRI shows an area of decreased signal intensity or signal void because of high flow within the malformation. CT and MRI will also show areas of cerebral ischemia or hemorrhage.
- MRI can detail the arterial supply and venous drainage of the malformation, but angiography is required before intervention.

Emergency Care

The need for emergency intervention depends on the clinical presentation of the patient. Treatment is usually driven by the severity of the CHF.

Therapy

- Treatment of choice in all ages is endovascular embolization. A venous or arterial approach may be used, depending on the anatomy of the lesion. Direct surgical intervention has unacceptable risks and is no longer recommended.
- Refractory CHF prompts intervention such as embolization of the malformation.
- The initial goal is not total obliteration of the lesion, but a reduction in blood flow to the lesion to improve cardiac function. Embolization can be completed in stages over a few months once CHF is controlled.
- Treatment in older infants and children is indicated to prevent cerebral ischemia from arterial steal or from venous infarction, and to prevent hydrocephalus.
- Therapy for associated conditions may include positive inotropes, diuretics, anticonvulsants, and central nervous system ventricular shunting.
- Radiosurgery (gamma surgery) is a newer treatment option for older children who are clinically stable.

Follow-Up

- Survival depends largely on the severity of the CHF and the age of the patient. In the past, mortality in newborns approached 100%. Today, approximately 50% of newborns with severe CHF will survive. Critically ill infants requiring embolization in the first week of life continue to have the poorest prognosis.
- In one series of 28 children, 45% of those younger than 1 year of age had good outcomes; 61% of those ages 1 to 2 years had good outcomes, and 100% of those older than 2 years had good outcomes. A recent study of neonates and infants reported similar results.
- Resting tachycardia may be an early sign of recurrent CHF in patients previously embolized.
- Ophthalmologic follow-up usually indicated
- A follow-up CT or MRI to evaluate patients with new neurologic signs or symptoms.

PREVENTION

There is no known prevention for this congenital malformation.

PITFALLS

- Overly rapid reduction in blood flow to the malformation can result in overperfusion of normal brain, systemic hypertension, cerebral edema, or hemorrhage.
- Hydrocephalus may occur in patients who have had hemorrhage from the malformation.
- Shunt failure may cause acute hydrocephalus, even if the malformation has not changed.

Common Questions and Answers

Q: Can the malformation recur?
A: AVMs have a propensity to recur. Imaging studies give a good indication of the likelihood of recurrence.

Q: How does the malformation cause seizures?
A: Seizures can result from ischemia, hemorrhage, or acute hydrocephalus associated with the malformation.

ICD-9-CM 747.40

BIBLIOGRAPHY

Borthne A, et al. Vein of Galen malformations in infants: clinical, radiological and therapeutic aspects. *Eur Radiol* 1997;7:1252–1258.

Brunelle F. Arteriovenous malformations of the vein of Galen in children. *Pediatr Radiol* 1997;27:501–513.

Carvalho KS, Garg BP. Cerebral venous thrombosis and venous malformations in children. *Neurol Clin North Am* 2002;20(4):1061–1077.

Fullerton HJ, Aminoff AR, Ferriero DM, Gupta N, Dowd CF. Neurodevelopmental outcome after endovascular treatment of vein of Galen malformations. *Neurology* 2003;61:1386–1390.

Payne BR, Prasad D, Steiner M, Bunge H, Steiner L. Gamma surgery for vein of Galen malformations. *J Neurosurg* 2000;93:229–236.

Authors: Dennis J. Dlugos and Sabrina E. Smith

Ventricular Septal Defect

 Database

DEFINITION

A ventricular septal defect (VSD) is an opening in the ventricular septum.
The ventricular septum can be divided into several portions:

- The canal (a.k.a. inlet) septum
- The membranous septum
- The muscular septum
- The conal (a.k.a. infundibular) septum

There are several corresponding types of VSDs, which have different natural histories and associated problems:

- Inlet VSD: usually part of an AV canal defect (see Atrial Septal Defect); 5% to 7% of all VSDs.
- Conoventricular (a.k.a. perimembranous) VSDs; 80% of all VSDs.
- Muscular VSD: can be single or multiple and of variable size in any given patient; 5% to 20% of all VSDs.
- Conal septal malalignment VSD: the conal septum is not properly aligned with the rest of the ventricular septum, resulting in a defect. Always large and unrestrictive.

—Anterior malalignment is associated with obstruction of the right ventricular (RV) outflow tract (e.g., tetralogy of Fallot)
—Posterior malalignment is associated with obstruction of the left ventricular (LV) outflow tract and aorta (e.g., posterior malalignment VSD with coarctation).

- Conal septal hypoplasia VSD

There also may be multiple VSDs of different types in a single patient.
Many complex forms of congenital heart disease include a VSD.

PATHOPHYSIOLOGY

Direction of shunting (left to right or right to left) depends on the relative pulmonary (PVR) and systemic vascular resistances (SVR). Determinants of the amount of shunting depend on the size of the defect.

- Small VSD: defect imposes high resistance to flow. There is a large LV to RV pressure gradient and a small left to right shunt, directly related to the size of the defect. The work load of the ventricles is normal.
- Moderate sized VSD: defect imposes some resistance to flow, but the amount of shunting can still be large and is affected by the relative PVR and SVR. The RV pressure is normal or only mildly increased.
- Large (unrestrictive) VSD: generally the same size as or larger than the aortic valve orifice. The RV and LV pressures are equal and the amount of shunting is purely determined by the PVR and SVR. The lower the PVR, the greater the degree of left-to-right shunting.

- A large left-to-right shunt leads to increased pulmonary blood flow, left atrial and left ventricular dilation, tachypnea, and congestive heart failure (CHF). Typical onset of CHF is at 2 to 8 weeks of age as the PVR falls postnatally.
- If a large VSD is left untreated, pulmonary vascular disease (irreversible increase in PVR) may develop, leading to reversal of the shunt, cyanosis, and right ventricular failure (Eisenmenger syndrome).

GENETICS

Three percent of children with VSDs have a parent with a VSD. VSD is the most common lesion in trisomy 21, 13, and 18, but >95% of children with VSDs have normal chromosomes. Some lesions that include a conal septal malalignment VSD, such as tetralogy of Fallot or VSD with interrupted aortic arch type B are associated with 22q11 deletions.

EPIDEMIOLOGY

VSD is the most common form of congenital heart disease, occurring in approximately 1.5 to 5.7 per 1,000 live births and 4.5 to 7.0 per 1,000 preterm births; isolated VSD accounts for 20% to 50% of all congenital heart disease; 56% of patients are female.

COMPLICATIONS

- All VSDs

—Endocarditis: overall rate of 15 cases per 10,000 person-years of follow-up

- Moderate to large VSDs

—LV volume overload, left atrial hypertension, CHF, poor growth, Eisenmenger syndrome

- Specific types

—Conoventricular VSDs: development of aortic insufficiency (AI), subaortic membrane, or double-chambered RV
—Conal septal hypoplasia VSDs: development of AI.

PROGNOSIS

- Spontaneous closure: 80% of small muscular VSDs and 8% to 35% of small conoventricular VSDs, usually by age 2 years
- Prognosis with surgical closure is excellent; see Therapy.
- The risk of Eisenmenger syndrome is considered minimal if large VSDs are surgically closed by 2 years of age.

 Data Gathering

HISTORY

- Small VSD: The child is usually asymptomatic, with normal growth and development. Most commonly, a murmur is detected at 1 to 6 weeks of age.
- Moderate VSD: There is poor weight gain, with sparing of longitudinal growth. There may be an increased incidence of respiratory infections. Sweating and fatigue with feeding may be present.
- Large VSD: The symptoms are the same as above but may be more severe.
- Children with Eisenmenger syndrome may have cyanosis, fatigue and symptoms of right heart failure.

 Physical Examination

- Small VSD: The child appears healthy. A systolic thrill along the left sternal border may be palpable. Heart sounds are normal. A harsh, high-pitched, holosystolic or less than holosystolic murmur is best heard at the left lower sternal border. There are no signs of elevated atrial filling pressures, such as hepatomegaly or jugular venous distension.
- Moderate to large defect: Tachycardia and tachypnea are present. The precordial impulse is increased. The S2 is wide, with slight respiratory variation. The P2 component of S2 may be normal or accentuated. A harsh, low-pitched holosystolic murmur is heard at the left lower sternal border. A diastolic rumble at the apex as a result of increased flow across the mitral valve is present if the shunt is ≥ 2:1. Hepatomegaly may be present.
- If AI develops, a high-pitched, early diastolic murmur may be heard along the left sternal border.
- In newborns whose PVR has not yet fallen, S2 is narrowly split or single and the P2 component is loud. The murmur may be unimpressive.
- Likewise, in children with elevated PVR as a result of a long-standing shunt, S2 is narrowly split or single and the P2 component is loud. The murmur may decrease in duration and intensity or disappear.
- Once Eisenmenger syndrome develops (reversal of the shunt as a result of severely elevated PVR) patients manifest cyanosis, clubbing, an increased RV impulse, a single or narrowly split S2 with a loud P2 component and a minimal or absent VSD murmur. There may be a harsh systolic murmur of tricuspid regurgitation, a high-pitched early diastolic murmur of pulmonary insufficiency, or an S3. Jugular venous distension and hepatomegaly indicate high right-sided filling pressures.

Laboratory Aids

TESTS

Electrocardiogram

- Small defect: normal
- Moderate defect: LVH
- Large defect: biventricular hypertrophy and left atrial enlargement
- Eisenmenger syndrome: RVH

Chest Radiograph

- Small defect: normal
- Moderate-large defect: hyperinflation, cardiomegaly, increased pulmonary vascular markings
- Eisenmenger syndrome: normal heart size with prominent central pulmonary arteries and decreased peripheral vascular markings

Echocardiography

- All children with a murmur consistent with a VSD should undergo echocardiography to define the location, size, and number of VSDs and any associated defects. Color Doppler enables visualization of the shunt direction.

Cardiac Catheterization

- Generally reserved for patients with poorly defined anatomy, associated lesions, or for the assessment of pulmonary vascular reactivity in older children with pulmonary hypertension.

 ## Therapy

- Small defect: no intervention; observation and SBE prophylaxis for indicated procedures.
- Moderate-to-large defects: if signs of congestive heart failure develop, digoxin, diuretics, increased caloric intake, and close follow-up are indicated; (See Prophylaxis for indicated procedure)
- Conoventricular and muscular defects may become smaller or close spontaneously. An early surgical repair should be undertaken during infancy if there is evidence of intractable heart failure, failure to thrive, or pulmonary hypertension. Otherwise, the patient can be followed conservatively.
- Conoseptal hypoplasia and malalignment defects do not close spontaneously; surgical closure is indicated in infancy.
- After 1 year of life, a significant left-to-right shunt (Qp:Qs $\geq$ 2:1) is an indication for surgery.
- Children with elevated pulmonary artery pressures (at least half-systemic) should undergo repair before the age of 2 years, even if symptoms of CHF are controlled.
- Development of complications including AI, subaortic membrane, and double-chambered RV are indications for surgical repair.
- Surgical correction may be contraindicated if the PVR is greater than 8 Wood units/m^2.
- Recent series of surgical VSD closure report a mortality of 0.6% to 2.3%.
- Complete heart block occurs in less than 2% of patients.
- Transcatheter device closure may become more widely available for certain anatomic types of VSDs within the next several years.

 ## Follow-Up

A significant residual VSD may need early reoperation.
SBE prophylaxis is recommended for 6 months after complete closure (spontaneous or surgical) of a VSD.

? Common Questions and Answers

Q: Should children with a murmur consistent with a VSD undergo echocardiography?
A: Yes, to define the location, size, and number of VSDs, and any associated lesions.

Q: Should children with VSD have SBE prophylaxis?
A: Yes; also continue SBE prophylaxis for 6 months after complete surgical or spontaneous closure (no residual defect) of a VSD.

Q: Should asymptomatic children with VSD have restricted activity?
A: No, if there are no other problems.

ICD-9-CM 745.4

BIBLIOGRAPHY

Gumbiner CH, Takao A. Ventricular septal defect. In: Garson A, et al., eds. *The Science and Practice of Pediatric Cardiology*. 2nd Ed. Baltimore: Williams & Wilkins, 1998:1119–1140.

Hoffman JI, Kaplan S. The incidence of congenital heart disease. *J Am Coll Cardiol* 2002;39(12):1890–1900.

Kidd L, et al. Second natural history study of congenital heart defects: results of treatment of patients with ventricular septal defects. *Circulation* 1993;87(2 Suppl I):I38–I51.

McDaniel NL. Ventricular and atrial septal defects. *Pediatr Rev* 2001;22(8):265–270.

McDaniel NL, Gutgesell HP. Ventricular septal defects. In: Allen HD, et al., eds. *Moss and Adams' Heart Disease in Infants, Children and Adolescents*. 6th Ed. Philadelphia: Lippincott Williams & Wilkins, 2001:636–651.

Weinberg PM. Anatomy and classification of congenital heart disease. In: Kaiser LR, et al., eds. *Mastery of Cardiothoracic Surgery*. Philadelphia: Lippincott-Raven, 1998:589–602.

Author: Amy H. Schultz

Ventricular Tachycardia

 Database

DEFINITION

Ventricular tachycardia (VT) is a series of three or more repetitive beats originating from the ventricle at a rate faster than 120 bpm. It usually is a wide complex rhythm, but can be narrow in infants. VT may, but not always, have atrioventricular (AV) dissociation.

- Sustained ventricular tachycardia: lasts longer than 30 seconds or causes hemodynamic compromise
- Nonsustained ventricular tachycardia: lasts from 3 beats to 30 seconds without hemodynamic compromise
- May be monomorphic or polymorphic
- Torsades de pointes: associated with congenital long QT syndrome, acquired long QT, and Brugada's syndrome; the QRS complexes gradually change shape throughout the tachycardia.

ETIOLOGY

- Idiopathic
- Myocarditis
- Dilated cardiomyopathy
- Long QT syndrome (LQTS)
- RV dysplasia
- Brugada's syndrome
- Congenital heart disease (CHD) (e.g., tetralogy of Fallot, transposition of the great arteries, aortic stenosis, hypertrophic cardiomyopathy, mitral valve prolapse, Ebstein's anomaly, and pulmonary vascular occlusive disease)
- Ventricular tumors
- Metabolic disturbances (hypoxia, acidosis, hypokalemia/hyperkalemia)
- Drug ingestion (e.g., digitalis toxicity, antiarrhythmic agents)
- Myocardial ischemia (e.g., Kawasaki disease, congenital coronary anomalies)
- Trauma

PATHOPHYSIOLOGY

VT may result from a reentrant mechanism, triggered mechanism, or abnormal automaticity.

GENETICS

Long QT syndrome may be inherited in an autosomal-recessive or autosomal-dominant pattern. It is related to a variety of potential ion channel defects, and may be associated with hearing loss and/or a family history of sudden death. Brugada's syndrome is related to a defect in the cardiac sodium channel and appears to be inherited in an autosomal-dominant pattern.

EPIDEMIOLOGY

VT may present at any age. Premature ventricular contractions (PVCs) have been reported in 0.8% to 2.2% of otherwise healthy children.

COMPLICATIONS

- Cardiovascular compromise (sudden death)
- Acquired cardiomyopathy (from long-standing VT and a lack of AV synchrony)

PROGNOSIS

- Generally very good in patients with idiopathic VT and a structurally normal heart
- Suppression of ventricular ectopy with exercise has a favorable prognosis.
- In patients with heart disease (congenital or acquired) or LQTS, VT may increase the risk of presyncope, syncope, and possibly sudden death.

 Differential Diagnosis

- Supraventricular tachycardia (SVT) with aberrancy
- Antidromic tachycardia (antegrade conduction down an accessory pathway during an AV reciprocating tachycardia, e.g., Wolff-Parkinson-White syndrome)
- Atrial flutter or fibrillation with rapid conduction over an accessory pathway

 Data Gathering

HISTORY

- Mostly asymptomatic
- Palpitations
- Presyncope or syncope
- Exercise intolerance
- Dizziness
- Cardiac arrest

 Physical Examination

- Typically normal; occasional irregularity secondary to frequent PVCs
- Signs of underlying heart disease, if any are present

 Laboratory Aids

TESTS

- Electrocardiogram: three or more consecutive ventricular complexes faster than 120 bpm. The bundle branch morphology (right or left) may point to the site of origin of the VT. Similar morphology to isolated PVCs. May have AV dissociation. Typically, repolarization (T-wave) abnormalities are present. Always measure the QTc in lead II in sinus rhythm. Evaluate for Brugada's syndrome in leads V1 and V2 (right bundle branch block, coved-type ST elevation, and T-wave inversion in the right precordial leads)
- Echocardiogram: Rule out CHD, tumors, and assess ventricular function.
- Ambulatory Holter monitor: Quantitative assessment of ventricular ectopy, frequency of VT, and measurement of QTc interval.
- Exercise stress test (>5 years old): The characteristic response is that benign PVCs are suppressed with exercise and return in the immediate recovery period. Exacerbation or worsening of ventricular arrhythmias is very concerning.
- Cardiac catheterization: Assessment of hemodynamics and possible coronary artery imaging
- Electrophysiologic study indications: (a) diagnosis of a wide complex rhythm; (b) suspected VT in the setting of an abnormal heart, syncope, or cardiac arrest; (c) nonsustained VT in patients with CHD; (d) determination of appropriate medical therapy in a patient with inducible VT; (e) syncope in the setting of palpitations (SVT vs. VT); and (f) characterization of the VT and consideration for radiofrequency ablation. Note: Electrophysiologic studies are generally not helpful in individuals with LQTS.

Therapy

ACUTE

- If the patient is hemodynamically compromised, prompt synchronized direct-current (1 to 2 joules/kg; adult, 100 to 400 joules) cardioversion is indicated. Asynchronous cardioversion for ventricular fibrillation.
- Cardiopulmonary resuscitation as necessary
- Lidocaine (1 mg/kg bolus over 1 minute, followed by an infusion at 20 to 50 mcg/kg per minute, assuming normal kidney function)
- If torsades de pointes, $MgSO_4$ may be given.
- Overdrive ventricular pacing may terminate the tachycardia. However, pacing may accelerate the VT or induce ventricular fibrillation.
- Intravenous amiodarone (side effect: hypotension, responds to volume)

CHRONIC

- Medications

—Class IB (mexiletine and phenytoin); beta-blockers (propranolol, atenolol, nadolol) are used in LQTS and may be effective in exercise-induced VT and postoperative CHD
—Class III (amiodarone and sotalol): avoid in patients with LQTS
—Class IC (flecainide): proarrhythmia, sudden death with proarrhythmia has been reported in patients with structural heart disease while taking class IC agents.

- Atrial pacing at rates slightly faster than VT rates may suppress tachycardia
- Radiofrequency ablation
- Automatic implantable cardioverter defibrillators

 Follow-Up

- Depends on the underlying etiology
- Electrocardiogram, echocardiogram, holter monitor, and exercise stress test

PITFALLS

Misdiagnosis of VT for SVT with aberrancy. A wide complex tachycardia should always be considered to be ventricular tachycardia until proven otherwise.

 Common Questions and Answers

Q: Do frequent single PVCs require treatment?
A: In an otherwise healthy child with a structurally normal heart, normal QT interval, and suppressed PVCs with exercise, no treatment is indicated.

Q: Should siblings of patients with LQTS be evaluated?
A: Yes, siblings and parents (even if asymptomatic) should have an electrocardiogram, Holter monitor, and exercise stress test for definitive evaluation of the QT interval.

ICD-9-CM 427.1

BIBLIOGRAPHY

Antzelevitch C, Brugada P, Brugada B, et al. Brugada syndrome 1992–2002. *J Am Coll Cardiol* 2003;41:1665–1671.

Carboni MP, Garson A Jr. Ventricular arrhythmias. In: Garson A Jr, Bricker JT, Fisher DJ, et al., eds. *The Science and Practice of Pediatric Cardiology*. 2nd Ed. Philadelphia: Williams & Wilkins, 1998:2121–2168.

Garson A Jr, Smith RT, Moak JP, et al. Ventricular arrhythmias and sudden death in children. *J Am Coll Cardiol* 1985;5(6): 134B–137B.

Pfammatter JP, Paul T, et al. Idiopathic ventricular tachycardia in infancy and childhood. *J Am Coll Cardiol* 1999;33: 2067–2072.

Yabek SM. Ventricular arrhythmias in children with an apparently normal heart. *J Pediatr* 1991;119:1–11.

Author: Mitchell I. Cohen

Vesicoureteral Reflux

 ## Database

DEFINITION

Vesicoureteral reflux (VUR) occurs when urine passes backward from the bladder to the ureters or kidneys.

CAUSES

- A combination of abnormal anatomy and abnormal voiding pressure

—Primary VUR results from either a short ureteral tunnel through the bladder wall, or transient high pressure voiding, which occurs normally in the first 18 months of life.
—Patients with primary VUR can expect improvement and even resolution of the VUR with time as the ureteral tunnel grows or when bladder pressures decrease.

- Secondary VUR occurs when there is an associated lesion responsible for the abnormal anatomy or increased intravesical (bladder) pressure.

—Patients with secondary reflux require treatment of their primary problem, and still may require surgery to treat their secondary reflux. Causes of secondary reflux are dysfunctional voiding, neuropathic bladder as a result of spina bifida, ureteroceles, posterior ureteral valves, and prune belly syndrome.
—Although it may seem arbitrary, the distinction between primary and secondary reflux is important because the large prospective trials have been conducted on patients with primary reflux, and it is not appropriate to extend those findings to patients with secondary reflux.
—Another important distinction is whether the diagnosis of VUR was made as a result of a prenatal diagnosis of hydronephrosis, or whether the child presented with urinary tract infection.

PATHOLOGY

VUR in combination with urinary tract infection can lead to pyelonephritis, renal scarring, and possibly end-stage renal disease. Primary VUR is classified into five grades based on the voiding cystourethrogram (VCUG).

- Grade I: reflux into ureter
- Grade II: reflux into renal pelvis without dilation of calyces
- Grade III: blunting of calyces, mild dilation of ureter
- Grade IV: grossly dilated ureter, moderate calyceal dilation with maintained papillary impressions
- Grade V: grossly dilated ureter with loss of papillary impressions

The grading scale is important because spontaneous resolution rates are significantly different between grades I to III and grades IV to V.

GENETICS

Thirty percent of siblings will have low-grade reflux, but the great majority will have been asymptomatic, and renal scarring is rare. Parents with VUR have a 60% chance of having children with reflux. Whether or not to screen siblings is controversial. We elect to screen the patients with a history of recurrent febrile illnesses and girls who have not yet toilet trained.

EPIDEMIOLOGY

VUR occurs in about 1% of children. There are now clearly two different groups of patients:

- Those who were detected prenatally without any history of urinary tract infection (UTI).

—Approximately 30% to 50% of patients with prenatal hydronephrosis have VUR.
—The ratio of males to females in this group is 3:1. This is believed to be caused by a period of high-pressure voiding in boys, which resolves by 18 months.

- Those who were detected after an acute UTI.

—About 30% to 50% of children with UTI will have reflux, and they tend to be 2- to 3-year-old girls.
—Since most children achieve urinary continence by this point, the cause of the UTI tends to be infrequent voiding caused by overlearning the ability to tighten the pelvic floor.

PROGNOSIS

- In primary VUR, 80% of grades I and II reflux, 70% of grade III, 40% of grade IV, and 25% of grade V resolve over a 5-year period.
- The annual rate of spontaneous resolution is between 15% and 20% for grades I to III.
- Bilateral reflux is less likely to resolve than unilateral reflux.
- Patients age 5 or older at presentation are less likely to resolve than those who present at <5 years of age.
- Ultimately the goal is prevention of renal scarring, rather than resolution of the reflux, because low-pressure sterile reflux does not lead to renal scarring.
- The patient's propensity toward UTI must be considered as well as whether the reflux is resolving.

 ## Differential Diagnosis

In the prenatally detected group, hydronephrosis can also be a result of ureteropelvic junction obstruction. The important task is to differentiate primary from secondary VUR so that the parents can be appropriately counseled.

 ## Data Gathering

HISTORY

- Prenatal diagnosis or UTI as presentation
- Family or sibling history of VUR
- Family history of UTI, suggestive of susceptible uroepithelium
- Family history of renal failure
- Voiding history: age at toilet training
- Daytime or nighttime incontinence
- Frequency of urination
- Sensation of emptying the bladder completely
- Signs of dysfunctional voiding:

—Urgency
—Frequency
—Damp underwear
—Associated constipation

- Frequency of bowel movements, suggestive of pelvic floor immaturity
- Evidence of delaying urination:

—Squatting, crossing legs
—Compressing urethra with heel (Vincent's curtsy)

 ## Physical Examination

- Abdominal palpation (mainly to check for hard stool)
- Check for labial adhesions in girls
- Phimosis in boys
- Palpation of spine
- Blood pressure

Vesicoureteral Reflux

 Laboratory Aids

A serum creatinine may be obtained if the renal ultrasound suggests significant renal scarring.

IMAGING

- Renal/bladder ultrasound: This is usually obtained at the time of UTI, or if the patient had a prenatal diagnosis of hydronephrosis, at 1 week of life. The ultrasound is not as sensitive as DMSA scan for renal scarring. The lack of hydronephrosis does not mean that the patient does not have VUR. However, it is a useful tool for following renal growth.
- VCUG: A contrast study is necessary for the first VCUG, to delineate the urethral anatomy in boys, and to accurately grade the reflux in both sexes. Follow-up VCUGs can be performed using radionuclide to decrease the radiation dose to the child.
- DMSA renal scan: The most accurate way to diagnose pyelonephritis and renal scarring. Unfortunately, it is not possible to predict which patients will develop scarring after an acute episode. If the diagnosis of upper tract infection vs. cystitis is important, then the DMSA scan during an acute episode is useful. The DMSA is not usually helpful with nonfebrile UTI in patients older than 6 months of age, because cystitis is rarely associated with high fevers.

 Therapy

- Four prospective randomized controlled trials have concluded that medical management (prophylactic antibiotics) and surgery have essentially equal outcomes in regard to hypertension, growth, and renal scarring. Surgery was more effective at preventing pyelonephritis.
- The rate of renal scarring was equal in the medical and surgical arms of the International Reflux Study. However, the timing of renal scarring was different: in the medically treated arm, new renal scars continued to form during 5 years of follow-up, whereas in the surgical arm, the renal scars stopped within 10 months of surgery. Surgery was 95% successful in correcting reflux with a 4% complication rate. Surgery involves creation of a longer muscular backing for the ureter to create a flap-valve mechanism.
- Patients with low-grade reflux should be maintained on prophylactic antibiotics, because grades I to III have a significant rate of spontaneous resolution. Patients with high-grade reflux should be initially maintained on prophylactic antibiotics, but earlier consideration for surgical correction should be given as a result of the lower rate of spontaneous resolution. Likewise, patients with reflux and renal scarring should be considered for earlier surgery because they have already shown a propensity toward UTI and renal damage.

- Antibiotic prophylaxis does not mean treatment dose antibiotics. The antibiotics chosen are highly concentrated in the urine, and the use of high doses only selects out resistant organisms and leads to complications such as yeast infections. Amoxicillin at 10 to 15 mg/kg qd is used for the first 2 months of life, then trimethoprim/sulfamethoxazole (40 mg/200 mg per 5 mL) at 0.25 mL/kg qd (equivalent to 2 to 3 mg/kg qd of trimethoprim) or nitrofurantoin at 1 to 2 mg/kg qd.
- Patients being managed on antibiotic prophylaxis undergo annual follow-up nuclear VCUG to document improvement or resolution of VUR. Grading is less precise with nuclear VCUG but the radiation dose is lower. Patients who are detected with VUR in infancy should probably have a contrast VCUG at 18 months to 2 years to determine the grade of reflux, because this can improve markedly. A renal ultrasound is also obtained to follow renal growth and check for gross renal scars.
- Indications for crossing over to surgery are:

—Patient or parent wishes
—Noncompliance with medical therapy
—Breakthrough infections while on medical therapy. (This is more of a relative indication. A careful review of voiding habits should be carried out to ensure that dysfunctional voiding is not responsible for the UTI.)
—New renal scarring
—Persistence of reflux after an appropriate period of antibiotic prophylaxis

- The use of injectable bulking agents such as Teflon is popular in Europe. Due to concerns about particle migration, Teflon is not approved for this use in the United States. Many substances have been tried, with at best 80% success rates 1 year after multiple treatments. The minimally invasive nature of these treatments is balanced with a lower success rate. Deflux (dextranomer/hyaluronic acid) is the most commonly used injectable in the United States and may be a more satisfactory form of treatment in the future.
- The management of patients who continue to have VUR after several years of prophylactic antibiotics is controversial. While most feel comfortable taking boys with VUR off antibiotics after age 6 because the risk of renal scarring is decreased and boys are at low risk for UTI, the adolescent girl is at increased risk for complications during pregnancy if she has a past history of UTI. The few studies on this subject seem to indicate that the patients with VUR and recurrent UTI are at risk for pregnancy-related complications whether or not the VUR has been surgically corrected, suggesting that the propensity toward UTI plays a more important factor.

 Follow-Up

Patients with renal scarring should have annual blood pressure checks and urinalysis for proteinuria.
More detailed recommendations can be found in the article by Elder et al. (see Bibliography).

 Common Questions and Answers

Q: How soon after a UTI should the VCUG be performed?
A: Once the patient is clinically stable, afebrile, and sterile urine has been documented, the VCUG can be performed.

Q: Why not operate immediately to repair the reflux when it is diagnosed?
A: Depending on the grade of reflux, many cases will resolve in time. See Therapy.

ICD-9-CM 593.7

BIBLIOGRAPHY

Atala A, Keating MA. Vesicoureteral reflux and megaureter. In: Walsh PC, Retik AB, Vaughn ED, et al., eds. *Campbell's Urology*. 8th Ed. Philadelphia: WB Saunders, 2002.

Decter RM. Vesicoureteral reflux. *Pediatr Rev* 2001;22(6):205–210.

Elder JS, Peters CA, Arant BS, et al. Pediatric vesicoureteral reflux guidelines panel summary report on the management of primary vesicoureteral reflux in children. *J Urol* 1997;157:1846–1851.

Snow BW, Cartwright PC. Vesicoureteral reflux surgery. In: Gillenwater JY, Grayhack JT, Howards SS, et al., eds. *Adult and Pediatric Urology*. 4th Ed. St. Louis: Mosby, 2002.

Walker RD, Atala A. Vesicoureteral reflux and urinary tract infection in children. In: Gillenwater JY, Grayhack JT, Howards SS, et al., eds. *Adult and Pediatric Urology*. 4th Ed. St. Louis: Mosby, 2002.

Yeung CK, Godley ML, Dhillon HK, et al. The characteristics of primary vesico-ureteric reflux in male and female infants with pre-natal hydronephrosis. *Br J Urol* 1997;80:319–327.

Authors: Hsi-Yang Wu and Howard M. Snyder

Viral Hepatitis

 ## Database

DEFINITION

Inflammation of the liver caused by hepatotropic viruses:

- Hepatitis A to E
- Hepatotropic viruses: EBV, CMV, HSV, VZV
- Enterovirus
- Rubella
- Coxsackie B
- Adenovirus
- Parvovirus

In the United States, hepatitis B accounts for 40% of acute viral hepatitis cases, hepatitis A for 30%, and hepatitis C for 20%. Hepatitis C is potentially one of the most devastating diseases in the United States with about 4 million carriers and currently is the single largest cause of liver transplantation in adults. Worldwide HBV is more prevalent but with universal vaccination, will become much less of a burden.

TYPES OF HEPATITIS

Hepatitis A

- Picornavirus with a RNA genome.
- Transmitted by the oral-fecal route.
- Characterized by enteric symptoms associated with right upper quadrant pain, jaundice, diarrhea, pale stools, anorexia, nausea, hepatomegaly, and splenomegaly.
- Incubation period is about 15 to 40 days, and transaminases rise about 1 week after onset of symptoms; recovery is seen in over 95% of patients within 1 to 2 weeks.
- Jaundice is seen in 88% of adults, but is present in only 65% of children with hepatitis A.
- Complications: fulminant hepatitis, cholestatic hepatitis, relapsing hepatitis.
- Mortality: 0.1% to 0.2%
- Chronic sequele: none. Carrier state or chronic hepatitis not reported.

Hepatitis B

- Type 1 Hepadnavirus, DNA genome.
- Transmitted by body fluids.
- Incubation period of 50 to 180 days and has three phases: prodrome, icteric, and convalescence. The prodrome precedes jaundice by 2 to 3 weeks, with vague symptoms of rash and arthralgia resembling serum sickness.
- Jaundice is seen less frequently in children compared with adults, and it may be accompanied by symptoms of fever, fatigue, myalgia, abdominal pain, and pruritus.
- Circulating immune complexes occasionally result in extrahepatic manifestations, which include vasculitis, nephropathy, and acrodermatitis.
- Icteric phase lasts about 4 to 6 weeks, and this is followed by clearance of circulating antigens during the convalescence phase.
- The younger the age of the child with the infection, the higher the likelihood of developing chronic infection. Ninety-five percent of infected neonates, 20% of children, and 10% of adults become carriers after an acute infection.

- Only 5% to 10% lose their carrier status spontaneously.
- Complications: Fulminant hepatitis 1% to 2%.
- Mortality 0.5% to 2% .
- Chronic sequele: Carrier state 10% to 95%, Chronic hepatitis 5% to 10%, Cirrhosis <5%, Hepatocellular carcinoma.

Hepatitis C

- Flavivirus with an RNA genome
- Genotype 1 is prevalent in United States, although genotype 2 and 3 is prevalent in Asia and Africa.
- Causes hepatitis and accounts for a significant number of what was previously called non-A, non-B hepatitis.
- Transmitted by blood and sexual contact.
- Clinical disease is insidious, with a long latency period before levels of ALT start to rise.
- Only about 25% of infected patients have an acute illness that is indistinguishable from other forms of hepatitis.
- May take up to 12 months after exposure for serology to become positive. Detection is by serology or by detection of viral RNA by RT-PCR. Rarely causes fulminant liver failure.
- About 80% will develop viral persistence.
- After chronic hepatitis C virus (HCV) infection, liver functions may remain normal for many years.
- The virus undergoes frequent mutations, which may account for the viral persistence.
- Complications: Fulminant hepatitis 1%,
- Chronic sequele: Carrier state 10% to 20%, Chronic hepatitis 10% to 50%, Cirrhosis 10% to 20%, Hepatocellular carcinoma 5% to 10%.

Hepatitis D

- A viral parasite of the hepatitis B virus. It consists of an HDV antigen and HDV ribonucleic acid surrounded by the hepatitis B viral coat.
- Transmitted by blood or sexual activity
- Causes two types of acute hepatitis:
- Coinfection: Acute hepatitis B and D virus infection occurs simultaneously.
- Coinfection has a mortality rate of 1% to 10%.
- Chronicity in coinfection is less than 5%.
- Superinfection: Acute hepatitis D occurs in a chronic carrier of hepatitis B.
- Superinfection has a mortality rate of 5% to 20%. Fulminant liver failure occurs more frequently in superinfection.
- Chronicity is 75% in superinfection. Chronic HDV causes cirrhosis in 70% to 80% of patients and is a rapidly progressive disease compared with chronic hepatitis B alone.

Hepatitis E

- Causes epidemic hepatitis in areas in which water sanitation is poor
- Transmitted via the oral-fecal route
- Resembles hepatitis A clinically
- Incubation period of 6 weeks and affects young adults mainly
- Higher mortality of 20%, which is higher than hepatitis A, and causes fulminant liver failure in pregnant women. It does not cause chronic hepatitis.

PATHOLOGY

- Acute viral hepatitis tends to affect the liver parenchyma, although chronic viral hepatitis affects portal and periportal areas.
—Features:
  —Spotty necrosis
  —Panlobular disarray
  —Increased cellularity
  —Pleomorphism of hepatocytes
  —Focal parenchymal necrosis
  —Multinucleated hepatocytes, indicating liver regeneration
  —Inflammatory cells line the sinusoids.
—Chronic viral hepatitis is continuing inflammation of the liver for more than 6 months.
—Features:
  —Inflammation in the portal tracts predominantly but also extends into the parenchyma
  —Periportal expansion and fibrosis initially bounded by the limiting plate
  —Extension beyond the limiting plate into the parenchyma (piecemeal necrosis)
  —Portal bridging is the finding of extensive fibrosis that occurs between two portal tracts. When the injury is chronic and severe, attempts by the liver to regenerate lead to nodular changes and, finally, to cirrhosis.

 ## Differential Diagnosis

There are many disorders that give rise to elevated transaminases, and there are clues to a viral origin based on the history, serology, and histologic findings. One often invokes the diagnosis of non-A, non-B, non-C hepatitis when the cause is almost certainly viral but no virus is isolated.

 ## Data Gathering

HISTORY

- In hepatitis transmitted by blood or sexual means, the following risk factors apply:
—Positive family history of hepatitis (B, C)
—Immigrants or travelers from endemic areas, veterinarians, pig farmers (E)
—Institution residents such as day care (A), prisons (B, C)
—IV drug abusers (B, C, D)
—People with multiple sexual partners (B, C, D)
—Health care workers (B, C)
—Patients requiring multiple blood transfusions or hemodialysis (B, C)
—Dietary intake e.g., shellfish (A)
—Many with hepatitis A present with symptoms of gastroenteritis.
—Persistence of elevated transaminases and chronic fatigue syndrome lead to repeat laboratory tests and discovery of viral hepatitis.
—There may be hepatomegaly and splenomegaly with or without jaundice.
—Cholestasis is sometimes seen with tea-colored urine and pale stools.
—Other common symptoms are myalgia, abdominal pain, anorexia, fever, and pale stools.

Laboratory Aids

TESTS

Liver function tests
Prothrombin time
Albumin
Anti-HAV IgM: recent infection
Anti-HAV IgG: past exposure
HBsAg: current infection, either acute or chronic
HBsAb IgM/IgG: resolution of disease
HBeAg: significant infectivity, viral replication
HBeAb: end of severe infectivity (except in precore mutants)
HBcore IgM: early phase of acute infection, not present in chronic hepatitis B
HBV DNA: quantification useful to assess viral load
HBV DNA: qualitative is to screen for presence or absence of viral DNA
HBV mutations: useful to assess resistance to treatment with lamivudine
HDV Ab: exposure to hepatitis D
HCV Ab: exposure
HCV RNA: quantitative—assess viral load, qualitative assess presence/absence virus.
HCV genotype: useful to plan duration of treatment
Liver biopsy to assess the degree of liver damage, assess response to therapy.
Hepatitis B and D
Acute infection: HBsAg+, HBcore IgM+, HBV DNA+, HBe Ag+
Chronic infection high risk: HBsAg+, HBe Ag+, HBsAb−, HBV DNA (high)
Chronic infection low risk: HBsAg+, HBeAg−, HBeAb+, HBV DNA (low/absent)
Chronic active hepatitis: positive serology, elevated ALT/AST, hepatitis on liver biopsy 6 months after first presentation.
HDV coinfection: HBcIgM+, HDV IgM−/−, HDV IgA−
HDV superinfection: HBcIgM−, HDV IgM+, HDV IgA+

Therapy

HEPATITIS A

- No specific therapy is available; patients should avoid going back to the nursery or day-care center for 2 weeks after illness.
- Postexposure prophylaxis with pooled human serum globulin at dose of 0.02 mL/kg for household contacts, intimate exposure contacts, and children and staff in nursery or day-care centers with outbreaks. Preexposure (short-term, 0.02 mL/kg; long-term, 0.06 mL/kg every 4 to 6 months) to travelers to endemic areas.
- Havrix Junior (GSK) vaccine is given by IM injection. Ages 1 to 15 years: two doses of 0.5 mL; the second is given 2 to 4 weeks after the first dose; booster dose 0.5 mL, 6 to 12 months following the initial dose.
- It is sensible for children with liver disease to be vaccinated to prevent its exacerbation.

HEPATITIS B

Postexposure prophylaxis with HBIG is indicated for neonates born to mothers who are hepatitis B carriers, after sexual contact with carriers, and after accidental exposure to infected blood products.

TREATMENT
Hepatitis B

Hepatitis B is treated with interferon, lamivudine, or adefovir. The most successful treatment is still interferon with 33% success rate in meta-analysis of adult studies and this is slightly lower for lamivudine and adefovir.
- Interferon α—5 to 10 MU/m^2 given three times a week for 6 months (not recommended for use in infants and very young childre <2 years).
- Lamivudine (Epivir HBV) (Tablets 100 mg, suspension 5 mg/mL), dose 3 mg/kg per dose for 1 year.
- Adefovir dipivoxil (Hepsera) is approved for the treatment of HBV in adults only at this time. In normal adults with good renal function the dose is 10 mg per day for 48 weeks.
- Pegylated interferon is effective against hepatitis B but is too expensive and not approved yet for use.

HEPATITIS C TREATMENT

- Nonpegylated interferon is not very effective against hepatitis C on its own but in combination with ribavirin (oral, daily) it achieves viral clearance in about 40% of patients.
—Nonpegylated interferon is given subcutaneously three times a week.
- Pegylated interferon (subcutaneous) is given weekly and with ribavirin (oral, daily) achieves viral clearance in 50% to almost 80% depending on the genotype. (In the United States most patients have genotype 1 and this has a success of only about 50%).
—This would make this the treatment of choice once it is approved for use in children.
—Treatment duration depends on genotype: 1 year for genotype 1 and 4, 6 months for genotype 2 and 3.
—Success may be predicted by a two-log fall in viral load after 12 weeks treatment referred to as early viral response (EVR) rate.
—A higher success rate may be achieved by maintaining treatment doses of Pegylated interferon and ribavirin. This may be achieved with the use of erythropoietin, which counters the hemolytic complications of ribavirin and GM-CSF to counter leukopenia caused by Pegylated interferon.
—Psychiatric complications such as depression can be significant and may require addition of antidepressants or discontinuation of medications.
—Doses of Pegylated interferon and ribavirin depend on which product is used. Doses for children are not available.
—Peg-Interferon α-2a (Pegasys, Roche) and Ribavirin (Copegus, Roche)
—Genotype 1 or 4—Pegasys 180 μg weekly, Copegus (>75 kg, 1200 mg, <75 kg, 1,000 mg) for 48 weeks
—Genotype 2 or 3—Pegasys 180 μg weekly, Copegus 800 mg for 24 weeks
—Peg-Interferon α 2b (PEG-Intron, Schering, Rebetol, Schering)
—Dose of PEG-Intron is 1.5 μg/kg per week.
—The recommended dose of REBETOL is 800 mg/day in two divided doses. Duration of treatment is 6 months for genotype 2 and 3, 1 year for genotype 1 and 4.

Common Questions and Answers

Q: Why do patients infected at birth with HBV have a higher incidence of chronicity?
A: This is probably a dose effect, with the infecting dose being higher in vertical transmission than in other forms of transmission. Additionally, early infection increases the time for the virus to integrate into the host genome.

Q: What is the current definition of non-A, non-B (NANB) hepatitis?
A: NANB hepatitis should now be termed non-A to non-E, with all the testing available in modern hospitals. In the past, this probably included patients who are now known to have HCV.

Q: What is the best way of eradicating hepatitis B?
A: Universal vaccination in childhood has been recommended by the U.S. Public Health Service for eradication of HBV. Vaccination is actively pursued in some Asian countries, where the disease affects about a third of the population. However, some babies born to HBsAg+ mothers develop escape mutants of hepatitis B virus.

Q: Should mothers with HCV positivity breast-feed?
A: Based on the fact that viral RNA levels are very low in breast milk, it is felt that transmission of HCV via breast milk is very unlikely.

ICD-9-CM

Hepatitis A 070.1
B 070.30
C 070.51
D 070.52
E 070.53

BIBLIOGRAPHY

American Academy of Pediatrics. Hepatitis B and Hepatitis C. Red Book: 2003 Report of the Committee on Infectious Diseases. 26th Ed. Elk Grove Village, IL: American Academy of Pediatrics, 2003:318–319.

Hochman JA, Balistreri WF. Chronic viral hepatitis: always be current! Pediatr Rev 2003;24(12):399–409.

Koff RS. Hepatitis vaccines. Infect Dis Clin North Am 2001;15(1):83–95.

Laurer GM, Walker BD. Hepatitis C virus infection. N Engl Med 2001;345(1):41–52.

O'Connor JA. Acute and chronic viral hepatitis. Adolesc Med 2000;11(2):279–292.

Popper H, Schaffner F. The vocabulary of chronic hepatitis. N Engl J Med 1997;284:1154–1156.

Yazigi NA, Balistreri W. Acute and chronic viral hepatitis. In: Suchy FJ, eds. Liver disease in children Lippincott Williams & Wilkins, 2001:365–427.

Authors: Vani Gopalareddy and John Tung

Volvulus

Database

DEFINITION

Volvulus is torsion of the gut on itself or on a narrow mesenteric pedicle. It may be acute and complete or chronic and intermittent. Midgut volvulus is the most common form.

CAUSES

Incomplete rotation of the intestine during fetal development is the most common form of malrotation. Incomplete malrotation results in a narrow mesenteric stalk for the midgut loop centered on the superior mesenteric artery and vein, and obstructing bands (Ladd bands) across the duodenum, predisposing to midgut volvulus.

EPIDEMIOLOGY

- Malrotation with midgut volvulus is most common in neonates.
- Fifty percent to 80% of patients with abnormal rotation will be symptomatic in infancy. The majority of patients will present by age 1 year with symptoms of acute bowel obstruction.
- Patients with a rotational anomaly may present with volvulus without any preexisting symptoms.

COMPLICATIONS

- Intermittent or acute obstruction
- Strangulation resulting in ischemia and loss of midgut
- Protein-losing enteropathy can also result from strangulation.

Differential Diagnosis

- Perforated viscus
- Necrotizing enterocolitis
- Meconium ileus or meconium plug syndrome
- Ileal atresia
- Hirschsprung's enterocolitis
- Appendicitis
- Intussusception
- Pyelonephritis

Data Gathering

HISTORY

- Symptoms of acute or recurrent obstruction at birth or in the first year of life
- Recurrent bilious emesis (most important symptom) with acute abdomen
- Feeding intolerance
- Chylous ascites and/or protein-losing enteropathy as a result of lymphatic congestion and bacterial overgrowth. These may present as history of abdominal distension, diarrhea, edema, or generalized/localized extremity swelling
- In older children, recurrent abdominal pain and emesis. Older infants may have symptoms that mimic colic.

Physical Examination

- Abdominal tenderness or fullness with or without distension
- Irritability, lethargy
- Brawny edema of abdominal wall
- Bloody stools or blood-tinged mucus per rectum
- Drawing up of legs
- Tachypnea and tachycardia

Laboratory Aids

TESTS

- May see metabolic acidosis, thrombocytopenia

IMAGING

- Abdominal x-ray may show dilated stomach and duodenum.
- Abdominal ultrasound may show inversion of normal position of superior mesenteric artery (SMA) and vein (SMV; if SMV is located to left of SMA, suggestive of malrotation).
- Upper gastrointestinal tract radiography may show abnormal position of the ligament of Treitz and, in advanced cases, a "corkscrew" appearance of the midgut.
- The radiographic appearance, although, may be confusing because there are at least seven patterns of duodenal malrotation reported. Abdominal x-ray may show "double bubble" sign of duodenal obstruction.
- In the absence of a corkscrew or Z-shaped duodenum, patterns that usually indicate volvulus or obstructing Ladd bands, colon position had greater prognostic implication, especially when the cecum is positioned in the RUQ or LUQ.
- In report by Long et al. (1996), these latter patterns were associated with the highest prevalence of volvulus.
- Barium enema shows an abnormal position of the cecum (but 10% of patients will have normal position of the cecum).
- In cases of colonic volvulus, contrast enema shows beak deformity at site of volvulus.

Therapy

- Emergency surgery is indicated for volvulus.
- Close monitoring of fluids and electrolytes to prevent shock, gastric suction, and intravenous antibiotics (as bowel resection may be required)
- Laparotomy with resection of ischemic portions of the intestine
- Ladd procedure: volvulus is untwisted, transduodenal bands are divided, mesenteric base is broadened, and appendix is removed.
- If the entire midgut is ischemic, the volvulus may be untwisted, with reexploration in 12 to 24 hours.
- Traditional Chinese herbal medicine, dai-kenchu-to (DKT) has been used recently in trial of treatment of obstructive bowel disease in Japan with success.

Follow-Up

- Prognosis depends on extent of involvement and degree of ischemia.
- Monitor closely for feeding intolerance postoperatively.
- Persistent symptoms after surgical repair suggest pseudo-obstructive motility disorder.

PITFALLS

- May take hours to days to become symptomatic
- Symptoms may be mistaken for colic in infants or cyclic emesis in older children.
- Delayed diagnosis may result in strangulation and infarction, leading to short-gut syndrome.

Common Questions and Answers

Q: In what age group is volvulus most common?
A: Midgut volvulus is most common in the neonatal period.

Q: How can the signs and symptoms of volvulus be distinguished from gastroesophageal reflux?
A: Although both intermittent volvulus and gastroesophageal reflux (GER) may present with vomiting, the emesis in GER is not bilious. Bilious emesis, abdominal pain, and lethargy are signs of an abdominal obstruction, requiring further examination.

Q: Should one think of intermittent volvulus in the differential diagnosis of children with presentation of protein-losing enteropathy?
A: In children with unusual presentations of protein-losing enteropathy, especially with emesis as a contributing feature, exclude intermittent volvulus.

Q: Have cases of gastric, small bowel, and colonic volvulus been reported?
A: Yes, but rarely.

- Gastric volvulus patients do not manifest the full spectrum of signs and symptoms such as abdominal distension, vomiting, and abdominal pain. There are two main types of gastric volvulus: organo-axial (longitudinal axis of rotation), mesentericoaxial (transverse avis of rotation through greater and lesser stomach curves). In two-thirds of cases, there is an associated abnormality in which the stomach is affixed to the esophagus.
- Small-bowel volvulus has been reported in association with ascariasis.
- Colonic volvulus (usually sigmoid or cecum) is quite rare in children, and has been associated with Hirschprung's disease. Colonic volvulus also has been seen in mentally handicapped children, many times in association with aerophagia and chronic constipation. Colonic volvulus is a significant cause of death in the mentally handicapped population.

ICD-9-CM

560.2 Volvulus Knotting of intestine, bowel, or colon. Strangulation of intestine, bowel, or colon. Torsion of intestine, bowel, or colon. Twist of intestine, bowel, or colon
560.9, unspecified intestinal obstruction
537.3 Other obstruction of duodenum
Cicatrix of duodenum
Stenosis of duodenum
Stricture of duodenum
Volvulus of duodenum

BIBLIOGRAPHY

Haddock G, Wesson DE. Congenital anomalies. In: Walker WA, Durie PR, Hamilton JR, Walker-Smith JA, Watkins JB, eds. *Pediatric Gastrointestinal Disease*. 3rd Ed. Philadelphia: W.B. Saunders, 2000:378–382, 424–434: 435–444.

Ismail A. Recurrent colonic volvulus in children. *J Pediatr Surg* 1997;32(12): 1739–1742.

Jabra AA, Eng J, Zaleski CG, et al. CT of small-bowel obstruction in children: sensitivity and specificity. *AJR Am J Roentgenol* 2001;177(2):431–436.

Long FR, Kramer SS, Markowitz RI, Taylor GE. Radiographic patterns of intestinal malrotation in children. *Radiographics* 1996;16(3):547–556.

Rodriguez EJ, Gama MA, Ornstein SM, Anderson WD. Ascariasis causing small bowel volvulus. *Radiographics* 2003; 23(5): 1291–1293.

Salas S, Angel CA, Salas N, Murillo C, Swischuk L. Sigmoid volvulus in children and adolescents. *J Am Coll Surg* 2000;190(6): 717–723.

Sarioglu A, Tanyel FC, Buyukpamukco N, Hicsonmez A. Colonic volvulus: a rare presentation of Hirschsprung's disease. *J Pediatr Surg* 1997;32(1):117–118.

Author: Kathleen Graham Lomax

Von Willebrand Disease

 Database

DEFINITION

Von Willebrand disease (vWD) is an inherited bleeding disorder caused by either a quantitative or qualitative abnormality of von Willebrand factor (vWF). It is characterized by mucocutaneous bleeding or bleeding after surgical procedures.

PATHOPHYSIOLOGY

• vWF is a large multimeric protein that allows platelets to adhere to sites of endothelial injury, initiating the primary step in hemostasis-formation of the platelet plug.
• vWF also serves as a carrier for factor VIII in the peripheral circulation, protecting it from degradation. Deficiency of vWF results a shorter factor VIII half-life, causing a lower level of circulating FVIII
• When this protein is either deficient or defective, primary hemostasis is compromised, resulting in a bleeding diathesis characterized by easy bruising, frequent epistaxis, menorrhagia, and prolonged bleeding following surgical procedures.
• vWD is an inherited bleeding disorder; however, acquired forms of vWD have been described in association with hypothyroidism, Wilms tumor, congenital heart disease, EBV infection, and valproate therapy.

CLASSIFICATION

There are three major categories of vWD.

• Type 1: A partial quantitative deficiency of vWF. This is the most common type, accounting for 70% to 80% of patients. This is generally a mild bleeding disorder
• Type 2: A qualitative deficiency of vWF. This is diagnosed in 15% to 20% of patients and there tend to be more significant bleeding symptoms than in type 1. Type 2 vWD is further classified into four subtypes, according to the particular vWF abnormality.
• Type 2A: Loss of the intermediate and high molecular weight multimers. The small multimers are less functional causing the vWF R:Co to be more reduced than the VWF Ag. (see Laboratory Testing)
• Type 2B: An abnormal vWF that spontaneously binds to normal platelets resulting in accelerated clearance of these platelets. This results in mild thrombocytopenia. There is a loss of the high molecular weight multimers in this subtype.
• Type 2N: The mutant vWF does not bind to factor VIII normally. The reduction of Factor VIII activity is greater than in the other types of vWD.
• Type 2M: The vWF fails to bind platelets.
• Type 3: A near complete quantitative deficiency of VWF, which also results in a secondary deficiency of FVIII. This accounts for <5% of patients, and results in a severe bleeding disorder.

GENETICS

• The gene for vWF is found on chromosome 12.
• Type 1 follows an autosomal-dominant inheritance pattern with variable penetrance.
• Type 2 varies, but in general follows an autosomal-dominant inheritance pattern.
• Type 3 follows an autosomal-recessive inheritance pattern. Compound heterozygous patients have been described.

EPIDEMIOLOGY

The prevalence of vWD in the general pediatric population is estimated to be about 1%. Males and females are equally affected.

COMPLICATIONS

• Significant perioperative bleeding can occur, especially with tonsillectomy, but the most common complications are recurrent epistaxis, prolonged bleeding with cuts and abrasions, and menorrhagia.
• Patients with type 3 vWD have a more severe bleeding disorder and can have bleeding complications similar to those seen in hemophilia such as hemarthroses and intracranial hemorrhage.

PROGNOSIS

• VWD type 1 is often a very mild bleeding disorder, and may go undetected.
• Most patients with vWD have a normal life expectancy and, with proper education and treatment, minimal risk for permanent disability.

—Type 3 vWD is a severe bleeding disorder; and life-threatening hemorrhage can occur.

 Differential Diagnosis

• Primary hemostatic disorders

—Platelet function abnormalities, congenital thrombocytopenia
—Mild inherited coagulation factor deficiencies
—Hemophilia (type 3 vWD and type 2N are similar to mild and moderate factor VIII deficiency)

• Acquired and secondary hemostatic disorders

—Mild coagulopathies, resulting in bleeding or a prolongation of the PTT or bleeding time
—Uremia
—Acquired thrombocytopenia
—Drugs that affect platelet function

• Connective tissue disorders

—Ehlers-Danlos syndrome
—Osteogenesis imperfecta
—Scurvy

• Prolonged PTT but no bleeding symptoms

—Inhibitor
—Factor XII deficiency

 Data Gathering

HISTORY

• A family history of vWD or bleeding tendency is an important question in the evaluation for vWD. However, be aware that variation in frequency and severity of bleeding symptoms can occur from person to person, even within an affected family.
• Mucosal bleeding is especially common in vWD; patients who have had tooth extraction without bleeding are unlikely to have vWD.
• Bruising is common, with increased quantity, and quite frequently, increased size (>5 cm), and often in unusual locations with minimal trauma.
• Recurrent and/or prolonged epistaxis
• Menorrhagia occurs in 50% to 75% of women with vWD.
• Excessive posttraumatic or postsurgical bleeding

 Physical Examination

• Bruises: increased number, size, and/or unusual location
• May be entirely normal

Laboratory Aids

TESTS

Screening tests for bleeding disorder:
Prothrombin time (PT)—normal in vWD.
Partial Thromboplastin time (PTT)—may be slightly prolonged as a result of a decrease in FVIII levels.
Platelet count is usually normal (except in the case of type 2B vWD).
Bleeding time is usually prolonged, but may be normal in patients with type 1 vWD (Not recommended as a screening test in young children).
Specific tests used to test for vWD include:

- VWF Antigen: the quantitation of vWF by immunoassay
- VWF Activity or Ristocetin Cofactor: assesses the function of vWF using the antibiotic ristocetin, which induces platelet aggregation in the presence of vWF
- FVIII—Factor VIII clotting activity
- VWF Multimers—the multiple molecular forms of VWF evaluated on agarose gel
- Multimer analysis is important in delineating the type of VWD.

PITFALLS

- The diagnosis of vWD is not always straightforward. Because of normal physiologic variation in plasma levels of vWF and FVIII, repeated measurements over time may be necessary to establish the diagnosis. Thus, a normal laboratory evaluation does not necessarily indicate the absence of disease. The laboratory tests may need to be repeated several times before declaring a patient does not have vWD.
- Normal ranges for vWF are blood type specific, with lower levels in those with blood type O.
- Conditions that may increase vWF levels: the newborn period, surgery, liver disease, hyperthyroidism, high-stress states, pregnancy, inflammatory or infectious disease, steroids, oral contraceptives, and other estrogens.

Therapy

There are several options for the management of bleeding in patients with vWD. Superficial bleeding can usually be stopped by applying local pressure, ice or topical thrombin, particularly in type 1. There are two main approaches to systemic therapy in vWD: increasing the release of endogenous VWF or exogenous replacement of VWF. The appropriate therapy depends on the type of VWD and the clinical scenario.

- DDAVP is a synthetic analog of vasopressin that stimulates endothelial cell release of VWF. It is effective in patients who have functional VWF, as in type 1 VWD. It may be used for some patients with type 2 VWD, but is ineffective in type 3.

—Available in intravenous and intranasal formulations.
—An infusion of 0.3 mg/kg results in approximately threefold to fivefold rise in VWF and FVIII; nasal administration is slightly less effective.
—Side effects include facial flushing, light-headedness, or nausea.
—Prior to use in a surgical setting, patients should have a trial to demonstrate an appropriate response.
—May worsen thrombocytopenia in type 2B and platelet-type vWD
—DDAVP may not be useful when prolonged hemostasis is required. After 24 to 48 hours, there may be depletion of stored VWF, causing it to be ineffective.
—It is important to remember that DDAVP will also cause fluid retention, and in some cases, hyponatremia. This can be avoided with fluid restriction following treatment.

- Humate-P or Alphanate: plasma derived, intermediate purity factor VIII concentrate products with adequate levels (especially large multimers) of vWF

—Therapy of choice for most patients with type 2 vVW and all patients with type 3 vWD
—Useful in type 1 vWD when prolonged hemostasis is necessary

- Aminocaproic acid (Amicar): Stabilizes the fibrin clot. Best for oral mucosal bleeding. The dose is 100 mg/kg given PO every 6 hours.

PREVENTION

- Most patients with mild type 1 vWD do not need activity restrictions.
- Patients with type 3 disease need to avoid contact sports.
- For patients with recurrent epistaxis, measures should be taken to avoid drying of the mucosa by applying petroleum jelly and to reduce trauma to the nasal mucosa by keeping the fingernails short and discouraging nose picking.
- It may be advisable for patients with type 3 vWD to wear an emergency ID bracelet indicating that they have vWD in the event they are involved in an accident that renders them unconscious.

Common Questions and Answers

Q: How can a child have a bleeding disorder if he or she went through surgery without a problem?
A: In vWD, the vWF level can change as a function of stresses in the body. Many conditions will cause the vWF level to rise to a normal level. These conditions include infectious illnesses and pregnancy, and emotional stress. In surgery, the reason for the surgery itself (e.g., appendicitis) may cause enough stress to raise the factor levels to normal and prevent bleeding.

Q: Should the other family members be tested?
A: Yes, even if there is no history of bleeding in family members. Other affected family members may be unaware that they have the disease because vWD can be so mild.

Q: What sports activities can a person with vWD participate in safely?
A: People with type 1 vWD can participate in most activities, although it is usually advised to avoid situations in which significant trauma takes place, such as football, boxing, sky diving, and so forth. Patients with type 3 should try to avoid activities with even moderate trauma. For type 2 patients, the risk of bleeding varies.

Q: Is life expectancy lower in people with vWD?
A: For the majority of patients with vWD, their life expectancy and quality of life will be normal.

ICD-9-CM 286.4

BIBLIOGRAPHY

Batlle J, et al. Advances in the therapy of von Willebrand disease. *Haemophilia* 2002; 8:301–307.

Federici A, Mannuci PM. Advance in the genetics and treatment of von Willebrand disease. *Opin Pediatr* 2002;14:23–33.

Federici A, Mannuci PM. Diagnosis and management of von Willebrand disease. *Haemophilia* 1999;5:S28–S37.

Mannucci PM. Desmopressin (ddavp) in the treatment of bleeding disorders: the first 20 years. *Blood* 1997;90:2515–2521.

Montgomery RR, Gill JC, Scott JP. Hemophilia and von Willebrand disease. In: Nathan DG, Orkin SH, eds. *Hematology of Infancy and Childhood*. 5th Ed. Philadelphia: WB Saunders, 1998:1644–1659.

Schlammadinger A, Boda Z. Laboratory screening and diagnosis of von Willebrand's disease. *Clin Lab* 2002;48(7–8):385–393.

Werner EJ. von Willebrand disease in children and adolescents. *Pediatr Clin North Am* 1996;43(3):683–707.

Authors: Leslie Raffini
Nathan Hanstrom, 3rd edition

Warts

Database

DEFINITION

Warts (verrucae) are benign epithelial tumors on the skin that can occur on any epithelial surface of the body and produce characteristic lesions at various anatomic sites.

TYPES OF WARTS

• Common warts (verruca vulgaris)—rough, minimally scaly papules and nodules on the hands, face, arms, and legs.
• Flat warts (verruca plana)—rough, flat-topped, minimally scaly papules on face and legs.
• Plantar warts (weight-bearing warts)—painful inward-growing papules and plaques on the bottom of the feet.
• Anogenital warts (condyloma acuminata)—subtle skin-colored flat warts or moist, pink to brown, cauliflower-like lesions around the vagina and anal openings.
• Laryngeal warts (laryngeal papillomatosis)—transmitted vertically at delivery and present with stridor and progressive airway obstruction in children.

CAUSES

• Warts are caused by human papillomavirus (HPV), which is a subgroup of papovaviruses, small double-stranded DNA viruses.
• There are over 200 types of HPV.

PATHOPHYSIOLOGY

• The viruses have specific affinity for epidermal cells and cannot replicate in dermal connective tissue cells or other types of nonepithelial tissues.
• After implantation in the epidermis, the viruses enter the nuclei of lower and midepidermal cells. The viruses then take over the machinery of cell production. While replicating themselves, they induce a rapid proliferation of epithelial cells.
• The quantity of the virus, location of the warts, preexisting skin injury and cell-mediated immunity all play a role in the transmission of the disease.

EPIDEMIOGY

• Affects 5% to 10% of children ages 5 and 10 years
• Humans are the only reservoir for HPV.
• HPV can be transmitted by direct skin-to-skin or mucous membrane contact, and by fomites.
• There is an increasing prevalence of anogenital warts in children and young adults. Most children are exposed by nonsexual contact from infected family members and caretakers, but they may also be exposed at the time of birth through an infected birth canal.
• Autoinoculation from common warts at another site should be considered as a possible mode of spread.

COMPLICATIONS

• Irritation and secondary infection of common warts may result in itching and pain.
• Some anogenital warts (HPV types 16, 18, 31, and 45) have neoplastic potential, and may result in cervical carcinoma in women, penile cancer in men, and as anal cancer in men and women.
• Human papilloma viruses have also been associated with melanoma, keratoacanthoma, squamous cell carcinoma, leukoplakia, and oral carcinoma.
• Laryngeal warts can cause stridor and airway obstruction.

PROGNOSIS

• In healthy individuals, 75% of warts will spontaneously resolve without treatment within 3 years.

Differential Diagnosis

• Flat warts: moles, epidermal nevi, tinea vesicolor, milia, mollusum contagiosum, granuloma annulare, folliculitis, lichen nitidus, lichen planus
• Plantar warts: corns, calluses, foreign bodies
• Anogenital warts: irritant contact dermatitis, molluscum contagiosum, skin tags, hemorrhoids

Data Gathering

HISTORY

• Obtain exposure history from family members and caretakers.
• Determine the duration of the warts.
• Elicit any history of immunodeficiency.

Physical Examination

• Common warts: may be solitary or multiple, and range in size from millimeters to centimeters. Linear patterns may be seen from autoinoculation. Filiform or thread-like warts may be seen in the skin creases and on mucous membranes.
• Flat warts: are small, rough, flat-topped and slightly scaly papules. Their size ranges from 1 mm to 3 mm.
• Plantar warts: are painful, inward-growing, hyperkeratotic papules and plaques on the plantar surface of the feet. Due to trauma from weight-bearing, the surface of these lesions may have small black dots from thrombosed blood vessels.
• Anogenital warts: may be skin-colored, flat warts or moist, pink to brown, cauliflower-like lesions in the skin creases and around the vaginal and anal openings. In adolescent and adult males, the warts are localized to the penis. The lesions are brown to slate-blue, pigmented macules and papules.

Laboratory Aids

Tests are rarely needed.

• Biopsy—of flat warts shows koilocytic cells with an eccentric, shrunken nucleus surrounded by a perinuclear halo.
• Electron microscopy—will show the distinctive viral particles.
• Antigen detection and molecular hybridization techniques—have been used in adults to detect HPV in scrapings and biopsies of lesions.
• Pap smears—will show the presence of koilocytic cells in adolescent females with vulvar condyloma

Therapy

Topical irritants and duct tape are inexpensive and easy to use at home.

- Keratolytics—topical irritants such as lactic acid, salicyclic acid, other alpha-hydroxy acids, urea, benzoyl peroxide, and tretinoin cause an inflammatory reaction and are used to remove the excess scale surrounding warts.
- Duct tape (or any durable, occlusive tacky tape)—causes local irritation and stimulates an immune response. Distant warts also resolve, which suggests a systemic immune response. Duct tape has been proven to be more effective than cryotherapy in recent studies.

DESTRUCTIVE TECHNIQUES

- Cryotherapy—involves using liquid nitrogen and deep-freezing the warts. It causes necrosis and blister formation. It is inexpensive, produces a rapid response, and does not require anesthesia. However, the treatment is painful and may lead to infection, scarring, and damage of normal skin.
- Caustic agents—such as topical acids, podophyllum, and podophyllotoxin are applied to pared-down warts. The treatment takes several weeks to months. It may be painful and produce scarring.
- Cantharidin—is a topical applicant that triggers painless intraepidermal blisters. There is a high incidence of wart recurrence and postinflammatory pigment changes.
- Electrocautery and CO_2 laser ablation—require local or general anesthesia. Both treatments can leave scars, and healing of the open wounds may take several months.
- Bleomycin is diluted and injected into the warts under local anesthesia. Edema, crusting and hemorrhage may occur. Healing may take several days.
- Yellow, pulsed, dye laser—generates 585 nm light, which is absorbed by oxyhemoglobin in the skin. The light energy is converted to heat energy. The warts have to be pared down and require repetitive pulsing. There is a small chance of scarring. Treatment may be painful for young children.

IMMUNOTHERAPY AND OTHER TREATMENT MODALITIES

- Contact sensitization—uses an allergen, such as dinitrochlorobenzene or diphenylcyclopropenone. The patient is sensitized to the allergen, and then low concentrations of the same allergen are applied to the warts. This will create a type IV delayed hypersensitivity reaction. The applications are repeated for several months. The treatment can cause severe blistering and systemic reactions.
- Cimetidine—is an H_2 blocker that causes nonspecific stimulation of T lymphocytes; this therapy has not been proven to be effective.
- Intralesional interferon—requires multiple injections given daily for weeks. The treatment is approved for anogenital warts. It is often used in combination with laser therapy.
- Imiquimod—is the first member of a new class of immune response modifiers. It is the first FDA-approved imidazoquinoline. A 5% cream is applied to the warts and results in an increase in the production of cytokines, especially interferon-alpha. The cream is approved for treatment of adults with external anogenital warts for home use. Data have supported efficacy in children with anogenital warts.

Follow-Up

- Patients receiving treatment should be followed-up at 3- to 4-week intervals to check the results and assess for any side effects.

WHEN TO EXPECT IMPROVEMENT

- Spontaneous resolution has been observed in common, flat, genital, and plantar warts. In healthy individuals, 75% of warts regress without treatment within 3 years.
- Any therapy and its side effects must be measured against the high rate of resolution without intervention.
- With the various treatment modalities, a response is generally seen within weeks to several months.

PREVENTION

- Sexual transmission of HPV can be decreased by using condoms. Intercourse should be delayed until all lesions are healed.
- During contact sports, all lesions should be completely covered prior to participation. If the lesions are too extensive to completely cover, the athlete should not be allowed to participate.

PITFALLS

- Underlying immunodeficiency should be considered in any otherwise healthy child with extensive HPV infection. Hereditary severe combined immunodeficiency, acquired immunodeficiency syndrome and selective T-cell immune defects should be considered.
- Treatment of genital warts in children should be carried out in consultation with a dermatologist.

Common Questions and Answers

Q: How can one differentiate corns and/or calluses from warts?
A: Using a #15 blade, pare down the surface of the wart. If the surface is smooth with normal markings without small black dots (thrombosed blood vessels) at the base, then they are not warts.

Q: A child is seen for anogenital warts. What is the role of the physician?
A: The child needs a complete medical examination. The anogenital area should be examined for any signs of sexual abuse. All skin lesions should be documented and possibly photographed. Serologic studies for syphilis and cultures for gonorrhea should be considered. Family members and caretakers should be asked about anogenital and common warts. Parents should be informed that anogenital warts could be caused by sexual abuse, particularly in children over 3 years of age. Consultation with a child abuse expert should be considered.

Q: I am not sure if the lesions are warts. What else can I do in the office to confirm the diagnosis?
A: Apply 3% to 5% acetic acid solution, and the lesions will turn white if they are warts. This, however, is not a sensitive test.

ICD-9-CM

Verruca vulgaris 078.10
Verruca plana 078.19
Verruca plantaris 078.19
Anogenital warts 078.11

BIBLIOGRAPHY

Cohen, B. Warts and children: can they be separated? *Contemp Pediatr* 1997;14:128–149.

Darville, T. Genital warts. *Pediatr Rev* 1999;20:271–272.

Focht, DR, Spicer C, Fairchok MP. The efficacy of duct tape vs cryotherapy in the treatment of verruca vulgaris. *Arch Pediatric Adolesc Med* 2002;156:971–974.

Gibbs, S. Local treatments for cutaneous warts: systemic review. *BMJ* 2002;325:461.

Lynch TJ. Duct tape removes warts. *J Fam Pract* 2003;52:111–112.

Tyring S, Constant M, Marini M, et al. Imiquimod: an international update on therapeutic uses in dermatology. *Int J Dermatol* 2002;41:810–816.

Author: Y. Lily Higgins

West Nile Virus (and Other Arbovirus Encephalitis)

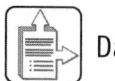 Database

DEFINITION

- West Nile virus (WNV) is an arbovirus (arthropod-borne virus) first recognized in the United States in 1999 during an outbreak of encephalitis in New York City.
- Infection can be asymptomatic; clinical disease is characterized by a simple febrile illness, often associated with myalgias, arthralgias, headaches, conjunctivitis, lymphadenopathy, and a roseolar rash.
- Occasionally (<15% of cases), central nervous system (CNS) manifestations such as encephalitis, aseptic meningitis, or myelitis can be seen.
- Other arboviruses can produce similar syndromes or acute hemorrhagic fevers.

CAUSES

- Arboviruses can be divided into two groups based on the predominant clinical syndrome.
- In the United States, five arboviruses are important causes of encephalitis: WNV, California encephalitis virus (LaCrosse strain), Eastern equine encephalitis (EEE), Western equine encephalitis (WEE), and St. Louis encephalitis.
- Arboviruses such as yellow fever, dengue fever, and Colorado tick fever typically cause acute febrile diseases and hemorrhagic fevers and are not characterized by encephalitis.

PATHOPHYSIOLOGY

- The incubation period for WNV and other arboviral encephalitis agents is 5 to 21 days, usually 1 week.
- The incubation period reflects the time necessary for viral replication, viremia, and subsequent invasion of the CNS.
- Virus replication begins locally at the site of the insect bite, transient viremia leads to spread of virus to liver, spleen, and lymph nodes. With continued viral replication and viremia, seeding of other organs including the CNS occurs.
- Virus can rarely be recovered from blood within the first week of onset of illness but not after neurologic symptoms have developed.

EPIDEMIOLOGY

- Arboviruses are spread by mosquitoes, ticks, and sand flies. The major vector for WNV in the United States is the Culex mosquito. WNV has been spread through blood transfusions and transplanted organs.
- Arboviruses are maintained in nature through cycles of transmission among birds, horses, and small animals. Humans and domestic animals are infected incidentally as "dead-end" hosts.
- Disease among birds has been a hallmark of WNV in the United States, and has served as a sensitive surveillance indicator of WNV activity.

- Each North American arbovirus has specific geographic distributions and is associated with a different ratio of asymptomatic-to-clinical infections. These agents cause disease of variable severity and have distinct age-dependent effects. WNV has now been identified throughout the United States and is also found in Europe, Africa, and Asia.
- The peak incidence of arboviral encephalitis usually occurs during the late summer and early fall. In the South, EEE can be seen throughout the year. Seasonality depends on the breeding and feeding seasons of the arthropod host.
- In 2002, 2,354 cases of meningoencephalitis caused by WNV were reported to the Centers for Disease Control and Prevention (CDC). This made WNV the leading cause of arboviral CNS disease. Encephalitis is most commonly seen in older adults, generally aged >50 years. Cases of WNV in children are unusual.
- A median of three to five cases of WEE and EEE are reported nationally each year. EEE tends to produce a more fulminant illness than LaCrosse or WEE.

COMPLICATIONS

- Optic neuritis
- Seizures
- Coma
- Death
- Guillain-Barré syndrome
- Severe neurologic sequelae
- Myocarditis
- Pancreatitis
- Hepatitis

 Differential Diagnosis

INFECTIOUS

Viral

- Herpes simplex virus (HSV)
- Enteroviruses
- HIV
- HHV-6
- Epstein-Barr virus
- CMV
- Lymphocytic choriomeningitis virus
- Rabies
- Mumps
- Influenza
- Adenovirus

Nonviral

- Cat-scratch disease (*Bartonella henselae*)
- *Mycoplasma pneumoniae*
- Postinfectious encephalomyelitis—generally follows a vague viral syndrome, usually upper respiratory tract, by days to weeks.
- Abscess/subdural empyema
- Meningitis

—Tuberculous
—Cryptococcal or other fungal (histoplasmosis, coccidioidomycoses, blastomycoses)
—Bacterial
—Listeria

- Toxoplasmosis
- *Plasmodium falciparum* infection (malaria)
- Parasites (cysticercosis, echinococcus, amebiasis, trypanosomiasis)

NONINFECTIOUS

- Tumor
- Carcinomatous meningitis
- Systemic lupus erythematosus
- Sarcoidosis
- Vasculitis
- Hemorrhage
- Toxic encephalopathy
- Metabolic disorders

 Data Gathering

HISTORY

- The diagnosis of arboviral infections of the CNS is difficult.

—Characteristic epidemiology that suggests a specific etiology is an important part of the history.
—The season of disease, prevalent diseases within the community, and animal exposures may provide clues to the diagnosis.
—Enteroviral infections are seen in the warmer months (summer and early fall) in temperate climates.
—Mosquito propagation in damp climates during the summer months may increase the likelihood of arthropod-borne viruses.
—History of an animal bite or bat exposure may suggest the possibility of rabies.

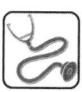 Physical Examination

- Encephalitis caused by arboviruses is characterized by acute onset of fever and headache in almost all patients. Associated symptoms include seizures, altered consciousness, disorientation, and behavioral disturbances. Neurologic signs are more commonly diffuse but may be focal. These clinical findings can help to distinguish patients with meningitis, which is characterized by nuchal rigidity and fever usually without an altered sensorium.
- Other symptoms reported with WNV include arthralgias, myalgias, pharyngitis, conjunctivitis, nausea, vomiting, diarrhea, abdominal pain, and rash. The rash is seen in about 50% of patients and is described as nonpruritic, roseolar, or maculopapular on the chest, back, and arms, which lasts 1 week. Diffuse lymphadenopathy is also common.
- Neurologic examination can reveal motor weakness, increased deep tendon reflexes and extensor plantar responses, tremor, or abnormal movement of extremities.

West Nile Virus (and Other Arbovirus Encephalitis)

 ## Laboratory Aids

The diagnosis of arboviral encephalitis depends on the recognition of epidemiologic risk factors and typical signs and symptoms with the aid of laboratory and radiographic studies.

ROUTINE LABORATORY TESTS

- CBC typically reveals a mild leukocytosis.
- Mild increase in erythrocyte sedimentation rate.
- Mild to moderate CSF pleocytosis predominately mononuclear cells.
- Elevated CSF protein
- Normal CSF glucose

SEROLOGY

- IgM and IgG enzyme-linked immunosorbent assays (ELISAs) for WNV and other arboviruses are performed at state public health laboratories and the CDC.
- The diagnosis of arbovirus encephalitis is made by one of the following:

—Detection of virus-specific IgM antibodies in the CSF is confirmatory.
—A fourfold rise in serum antibody titers is confirmatory. Acute-phase titers should be collected 0 to 8 days after onset of symptoms. Convalescent phase titers should be collected 14 to 21 days after acute specimen. A single negative acute-phase specimen is inadequate for diagnosis, but a positive test can provide evidence of recent infection.
—Isolation of the virus from tissue, blood, or CSF
—PCR to detect viral RNA

RADIOGRAPHIC STUDIES

- Imaging studies such as MRI or CT can assist in ruling out other potential causes of encephalopathy or encephalitis. MRI has proved useful in differentiating postinfectious encephalomyelitis from acute viral encephalitis. The former is characterized by enhancement of multifocal white matter lesions.

EEG

- Diffuse generalized slowing of brain waves. Periodic high-voltage spike waves originating in the temporal lobe region and slow-wave complexes at 2- to 3-second intervals are suggestive of herpes simplex virus infection.

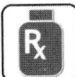 ## Therapy

SPECIFIC

- No specific antiviral therapy is available.
- Supportive therapy including cardiorespiratory function, fluid and electrolyte balance, seizure control, and reduction of intracranial pressure is important.
- Recovery can often be seen after prolonged periods of coma.

PREVENTION

- Public health department efforts focus on surveillance of viral activity to predict and prevent outbreaks.
- Active bird surveillance to detect the presence of WNV activity
- Active mosquito surveillance to detect viral activity in mosquito populations
- Passive surveillance by veterinarians and human health care professionals to detect neurologic illnesses consistent with encephalitis.
- Personal precautions to avoid mosquito bites including use of repellents, protective clothing, screens, and installation of air conditioners
- Vaccines for prevention of most arbovirus infections are not available. A vaccine is available for Japanese encephalitis for travelers to endemic areas who are planning prolonged stays.

INFECTION CONTROL MEASURES

- Standard precautions are recommended for the hospitalized patient.
- Respiratory precautions are recommended when vector mosquitos are present.

 ## Follow-Up

- Prognosis for recovery depends on the specific infecting agent and host factors such as age and underlying illness.
- Neurobehavioral follow-up should be considered in children with severe or complicated disease.

 ## Common Questions and Answers

Q: Should testing for arboviruses, including WNV, be performed on all patients with encephalitis?
A: Diagnostic testing for arboviruses is not recommended for all patients with encephalitis. The prevalence of these diseases is low and the diagnosis of more common causes of childhood encephalitis (e.g., HSV) should be pursued initially. Patients with no other identifiable cause of encephalitis who have epidemiologic risk factors such as geographic location, season, and exposure history suggestive of arbovirus encephalitis should be evaluated. Testing of patients with aseptic meningitis or Guillain-Barré syndrome is low-yield.

ICD-9-CM

Encephalitis arthropod borne 062.0-064
Eastern equine 062.2
Western equine 062.1
Viral 049.8
La Crosse 062.5

BIBLIOGRAPHY

American Academy of Pediatrics. Arboviruses. In: Pickering LK, ed. *2003 Red Book: Report of the Committee on Infectious Diseases.* 26th Ed. Elk Grove Village, IL: American Academy of Pediatrics, 2003:199–206.

Asnis DS, Conetta R, Teixeira AA, et al. The West Nile Virus outbreak of 1999 in New York: the Flushing Hospital experience. *Clin Infect Dis* 2000;30:413–418.

Romero JR, Newland JG. Viral meningitis and encephalitis: traditional and emerging viral agents. *Semin Pediatr Infect Dis* 2003;14(2):72–82.

West Nile Virus Activity U.S. Nov. 20–25 2002 *MMWR Morb Mort Weekly Rep.*

Authors: Jason Newland and Theoklis Zaoutis

Wilms Tumor

 Database

DEFINITION

Wilms tumor is a malignant tumor of the kidney occurring in the pediatric age group. It is also called nephroblastoma.

CAUSES

- Twenty percent of Wilms tumors have a mutation in the WT1 tumor suppressor gene.
- Causes in the remaining 80% of patients is unknown.

PATHOLOGY

- Gross: often cystic with hemorrhages and necrosis; usually no calcification (useful in differentiating from neuroblastoma, which is calcified on plain x-ray); may extend into the inferior vena cava (IVC).
- Histology: triphasic pattern blastemal, epithelial, and stromal cell. Blastemal cells aggregate into nodules like primitive glomeruli; the presence of anaplasia indicates a poor prognosis.

GENETICS

- Fifteen percent to 20% are hereditary in origin.
- Familial cases are more often bilateral and occur at an earlier age.
- A tumor-suppressor gene related to Wilms tumor (WT1) has been localized to chromosome 11p13.
- Mutations of this gene occurs in approximately 20% of Wilms tumors.
- Heterozygous deletions on 11p13 associated with congenital Wilms tumor/aniridia/ genital anomaly/mental retardation syndrome
- Another candidate tumor suppressor gene WT2 has been localized to 11p15.

EPIDEMIOLOGY

- Most common primary malignant renal tumor of childhood
- Five percent to 6% of all childhood cancer
- Incidence: 1 in 10,000 live births
- Higher incidence in Blacks
- More common in girls than boys
- Peak age: 2 to 3 years
- May be associated with aniridia, hemihypertrophy, and cryptorchidism
- Increased incidence in children with neurofibromatosis
- Associated syndromes: WAGR (Wilms tumor, aniridia, GU abnormalities, mental retardation), Beckwith-Wiedemann syndrome (macroglossia, omphalocele, visceromegaly, hemihypertrophy), and Denys-Drash syndrome (ambiguous genitalia, progressive renal failure, and increased risk of Wilms tumor).

COMPLICATIONS

- Extension into IVC
- Metastasis to lungs and liver
- Cardiac toxicity secondary to Adriamycin
- Liver dysfunction secondary to actinomycin D and radiation therapy (XRT)

PROGNOSIS

- Stages I and II: more than 90% cured
- Stage III: 85% cured
- Stage IV: 70% cured

 Differential Diagnosis

- Polycystic kidney
- Renal hematoma
- Renal abscess
- Neuroblastoma
- Other neoplasms of kidney: clear-cell carcinoma, rhabdoid tumor

 Data Gathering

HISTORY

- Abdominal distension
- Abdominal pain (20% to 30% of cases)
- Hematuria (20% to 30% of cases)
- Fever, anorexia, vomiting
- Family history of Wilms tumor
- Rapid increase in abdominal size (suggestive of hemorrhage in the tumor)

 Physical Examination

- Asymptomatic abdominal mass extending from flank toward midline (most common presentation)
- Anemia (secondary to hemorrhage in the tumor)
- Fever
- Hypertension (as a result of increased renin production in 25% of cases)
- Varicocele (indicates obstruction to spermatic vein as a result of tumor thrombus in renal vein or IVC)
- Aniridia, hemihypertrophy, cryptorchidism, hypospadias
- Signs of Beckwith-Wiedemann and neurofibromatosis

 Laboratory Aids

TESTS

- CBC
- Electrolytes
- Urine analysis: for microscopic hematuria
- Liver and kidney function tests

IMAGING

- Ultrasound of abdomen
- Diagnostic of mass of renal origin
- Evaluate for extension of tumor into IVC

—CT scan of abdomen: useful if diagnosis doubtful
—IVP: no longer routinely used
—Chest radiograph: to evaluate for metastatic disease
—Bone scan: only if clear-cell variety on pathology
—CT of head: only for rhabdoid tumors

CLINICOPATHOLOGIC STAGING

- Stage I: Tumor is restricted to one kidney and completely resected. The renal capsule is intact.
- Stage II: Tumor extends beyond the kidney but is completely excised.
- Stage III: Residual nonhematogenous tumor is confined to the abdomen.
- Stage IV: There is hematogenous spread to lungs, liver, bone, or brain.
- Stage V: bilateral disease

FAVORABLE PROGNOSTIC FACTORS

- Tumor weight less than 250 g
- Age at presentation less than 24 months
- Stage I disease
- Favorable histology

POOR PROGNOSTIC FACTORS

- Anaplastic pathology
- Lymph node involvement
- Distant metastasis

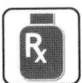 Therapy

SURGERY

• Nephrectomy

—Preoperative chemotherapy in case of very large tumors with IVC extension
—For bilateral disease nephrectomy of more affected side and partial nephrectomy of the other side, followed by chemotherapy and radiation

RADIATION THERAPY

• Not required for stage I and II patients
• Local XRT with 1,000 cGy for stages III and IV
• Whole-lung radiation (1,200 cGy) for pulmonary metastasis

CHEMOTHERAPY

• For stages I and II favorable histology: vincristine (VCR) and actinomycin D (AMD) every 3 weeks for 6 months
• For stages III and IV favorable histology: VCR, AMD, and doxorubicin for 6 to 15 months
• Add cyclophosphamide for higher stage anaplastic tumors

SIDE EFFECTS OF THERAPY

Temporary loss of hair, peripheral neuropathy, impaired function of the remaining kidney over years following radiation, cardiac toxicity with Adriamycin, second malignant neoplasms in few cases

 Follow-Up

• Every 3 months for 18 months, every 6 months for 1 year, and then yearly
• Chest radiograph, urinalysis, and abdominal ultrasound at regular intervals

PITFALLS

Rarely, Wilms tumor may present with polycythemia. It can present as fever of unknown origin without any other signs or symptoms.

 Common Questions and Answers

Q: What should be done to protect the remaining kidney during sports?
A: Children should wear a kidney guard to protect the unaffected kidney during contact sports.

Q: Can a child grow and live normally with one kidney?
A: Yes.

ICD-9-CM 189.0

BIBLIOGRAPHY

Blakely ML, Ritchey ML. Controversies in the management of Wilms' tumor. *Semin Pediatr Surg* 2001;10(3):127–131.

Coppes MJ, Haber DA, Grundy PE. Genetic events in development of Wilms tumor. *N Engl J Med* 1994;331(9):586–590.

Gundy PE, Green DM, et al. Renal Tumors. In: Pizzo PA, Poplack DG, eds. *Principles and Practice of Pediatric Oncology*. 4th Ed. Philadelphia: Lippincott-Raven, 2002.

Kalapurakal JA, Dome JS, et al. Management of Wilm's tumour: current practice and future goals. *Lancet Oncol* 2004;5(1):37–42.

Mrowka C, Schedl A. Wilms' tumor suppressor gene WT1: from structure to renal pathophysiologic features. *J Am Soc Nephrol* 2000;11:S106–S115.

Neville HL, Ritchey ML. Wilms' tumor. Overview of National Wilms' Tumor Study Group results. *Urol Clin North Am* 2000;27(3):435–442.

Petruzzi MJ, Green DM. Wilms tumor. *Pediatr Clin North Am* 1997;44(4):939–952.

Ritchey ML, Haase GM, Shochat SJ. Current management of Wilms' tumor. *Semin Surg Oncol* 1993;9(6):502–509.

Shochat SJ. Wilms' tumor: diagnosis and treatment in the 1990's. *Semin Pediatr Surg* 1993;2(1):59–68.

Authors: Tammy I. Kang and *Sadhna Shankar, 2nd edition*

Wilson Disease

Database

DEFINITION

Wilson disease (WD), also known as hepatolenticular degeneration, is an autosomal-recessive disorder of copper metabolism affecting the liver, brain, kidney, blood, and cornea.

PATHOPHYSIOLOGY

Failure to mobilize copper from liver cells for excretion into bile. An altered copper-transporting protein in hepatocytes results in retention of copper in the liver and impaired incorporation of copper into ceruloplasmin. Pathology related to slow accumulation of copper, first in the liver, leading to cirrhosis, and then in the brain, especially the basal ganglia, leading to impaired motor control and personality changes; kidneys and cornea are also affected.

GENETICS

- Autosomal-recessive inheritance as a result of one of over 200 known defects of the Wilson disease gene (ATP7B) on chromosome 13q14.3, which produces a membrane P-type adenosine triphosphatase (ATPase) protein.
- Heterozygotes generally unaffected.
- Parents of diagnosed individuals can expect a 25% recurrence risk.

EPIDEMIOLOGY

- Incidence in most populations approximately 1:30,000.
- Men and women affected equally; however, fulminant liver failure has 2:1 female to male ratio.
- Age of clinical onset is between 3 years and late middle age, although the majority present between 5 and 35.
- Children usually present with hepatic manifestations; adolescents and young adults tend to present with neurological symptoms.

ASSOCIATED CONDITIONS

- Hepatic: Cirrhosis, acute or chronic hepatitis, fulminant hepatic failure
- Neurologic: Dysarthria, dystonia, tremor, bradykinesia, migraine headaches, insomnia
- Corneal: Kayser-Fleischer rings (granular copper deposits on limbus)
- Renal: Fanconi syndrome, progressive renal failure with alterations in tubular transport of amino acids, glucose, and uric acid, renal tubular acidosis, phosphaturia (rarely with hypophosphatemic rickets), hypercalciuria that may result in stones.
- Hematologic: Hemolytic anemia, thrombocytopenia, leukopenia
- Psychiatric: Depression, mood changes, psychosis, obsessive-compulsive disorder
- Pancreatitis
- Cardiac: Cardiomyopathy, dysrhythmias
- Orthopaedic/rheumatologic: premature osteoporosis, osteomalacia, arthritis
- Endocrinologic: Gynecomastia, delayed puberty; amenorrhea as a result of liver disease; hypoparathyroidism, repeated miscarriages

Differential Diagnosis

- Liver diseases resembling Wilson disease include any cause of hepatitis or fulminant hepatic failure such as viral or autoimmune hepatitis
- Hereditary hypoceruloplasminemia
- Menkes disease
- Neurologic conditions presenting similarly to Wilson disease include Huntington disease (prominent dystonia in children), essential tremor, Hallervorden disease, Sydenham chorea, hereditary dystonia, and other neurodegenerative diseases
- Psychiatric disorders, including clinical depression, psychoses and neuroses

Data Gathering

HISTORY

- In children, symptoms of hepatic disease predominate, ranging in severity from asymptomatic hepatomegaly to chronic hepatitis to fulminant hepatic failure.
- Characteristic neurodevelopmental complications include dysarthria and spastic dystonia, tremor, decreased ability to perform voluntary movements, bradykinesia, personality changes, and poor school performance.
- Nonspecific complaints such as abdominal pain, nausea, anorexia, jaundice, and fatigue.
- A family history of liver disease with or without associated psychiatric symptoms.

Physical Examination

- Vital signs generally normal unless anemia is present
- Ophthalmologic examination: Identification of Kayser-Fleischer rings may require slit lamp
- Heart examination may reveal signs of cardiomyopathy
- Abdominal examination for hepatomegaly with or without splenomegaly; palpate for ascites
- Edema of the extremities
- Full neurologic examination to rule out movement disorders and other neurological deficits; if symptomatic, consultation by a neurologist or movement disorder specialist should be sought
- GU examination may reveal delayed sexual development and/or gynecomastia

Laboratory Aids

TESTS

- Serum ceruloplasmin: Usually low, however 15% to 20% of patients have normal values
- Reduced total serum copper ($<80\ \mu g/dL$) and increased urine copper ($>100\ mg/24$ hours)
- In equivocal cases, marked increase in urinary copper output after initiation of chelation therapy may help in diagnosis
- Liver function tests: Mild to moderate elevations of serum aminotransferase levels; ALT levels may be much lower than AST.
- Screening labs: CBC, PT/PTT, U/A
- Abdominal ultrasound for liver size and pathology
- If neurologic symptoms present, an MRI of the brain with focus on basal ganglia should be obtained prior to initiation of therapy
- Liver biopsy is the definitive procedure for tissue diagnosis and hepatic disease staging, and reveals high parenchymal copper content (usually $>250\ \mu g/g$ dry weight)

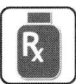 Therapy

- Early diagnosis is essential to limiting morbidity and mortality.
- Copper-chelating agents: Penicillamine or trientine (triethyl tetramine) result in immediate increased excretion of copper; clinical effects may take weeks to months to be seen. In 10% to 50% of cases, a worsening of neurological symptoms follows initiation of Penicillamine therapy. This phenomenon has also been seen with Trientine but is far rarer.
- Low-copper diet for life: restrict copper intake to less than 1 mg/day. Avoid liver and other organ meats, shellfish, nuts, mushrooms and chocolate; drinking water may need to be demineralized.
- Zinc may be and effective treatment for-presymptomatic individuals and is used as maintenance therapy.
- Antioxidants may be a useful adjunct in preventing tissue damage.
- Patients who present in hemolytic crisis may require plasma exchange.
- For severe liver damage, liver transplantation may be indicated.

 Follow-Up

- Patients require life-long dietary copper restriction and chelation therapy.
- Sudden discontinuation of therapy may precipitate fulminant hepatic failure.
- Patients on penicillamine require follow-up examinations, 24-hour urine copper, serum copper, CBC, and U/A before treatment: weekly during the first month, monthly for the first year, and then yearly. They may also need Vitamin B6 supplementation.
- Routine monitoring should include: serum copper and ceruloplasmin, liver biochemistries, and regular physical examination, and yearly 24-hour urinary copper excretion.
- Screen first-degree relatives older than age 3 years with history, physical examination, LFTs, CBC, serum ceruloplasmin, 24-hour urine copper, and ophthalmologic examination for Kayser-Fleischer rings. In addition, genotype or haplotype testing based on the affected relative's genetics should be performed.

PITFALLS

- Wilson disease should be considered in any child, symptomatic or not, with fulminant hepatic failure, hepatomegaly, persistently elevated serum aminotransferase levels, or fatty liver, or in a child with psychosis or neurological changes of unknown etiology. Diagnosis depends on a high index of suspicion and delay in diagnosis increases morbidity and mortality.
- Identification of Kayser-Fleischer rings may require slit-lamp examination by a skilled examiner, especially early in the disease. Absence of Kayser-Fleischer rings does not rule out Wilson disease.

 Common Questions and Answers

Q: Is mutation analysis helpful in screening for Wilson disease?
A: Molecular genetic tests are becoming available for clinical use, however because there are over 200 gene defects known, molecular screening in the general population is not practical. Siblings of patients whose genetic defect is known can be screened using polymerase chain reaction methodology.

Q: Can my patients with Wilson disease have children?
A: Women of reproductive age who are treated can have normal pregnancies. Both penicillamine and trientine appear safe during pregnancy in patients with Wilson disease. Interruption of therapy is not recommended during pregnancy. Offspring have a 1:200 chance of inheriting Wilson disease

ICD-9-CM 275.1

BIBLIOGRAPHY

Feldman. *Sleisenger & Fordtran's Gastrointestinal and Liver Disease*. 7th Ed. Elsevier: 2002,1269–1277.

Jacobs P. Copper. *Dis Mon* 2003;49(10): 589–600.

Roberts E, Schilsky M. A practice guideline on Wilson Disease: AASLD Practice Guidelines. *Hepatology* 2003;37:1475–1492.

Sternlieb I. Wilson's disease. *Clin Liver Dis* 2000;4(1):229–239, viii–ix.

Author: Evan Buxbaum

Wiskott-Aldrich Syndrome

Database

DEFINITION

Wiskott-Aldrich syndrome (WAS) is an X-linked primary immunodeficiency characterized by the classic clinical triad of thrombocytopenia with small platelets, eczema, and recurrent infections with opportunistic and pyogenic infections. It is also associated with IgA nephropathy, autoimmune disorders, and an increased incidence of B cell lymphomas.

CAUSES

- Mutation in gene for Wiskott-Aldrich syndrome protein (WASP)
- WASP is found in hematopoietic cells and is involved in signal transduction from the cell surface to the actin cytoskeleton.
- WASP is activated by Rho GTPase Cdc42, which then initiates polymerization of actin and reorganization of actin cytoskeleton resulting in polarization of cells: Polarized actin mesh in platelets for clotting, polarized actin structures in macrophages for phagocytosis, polarization of T or B cells to form immunologic synapse.

GENETICS

- X-linked recessive disease
- Linkage analyses have localized the defective WASP gene to X p11.22p–11.23.
- Approximately 60% of cases will have a positive family history for WAS.
- X-linked thrombocytopenia (XLT) without the other findings is caused by mutations of the same gene.

EPIDEMIOLOGY

- Incidence is rare.
- Presents in infancy with serious bleeding episodes secondary to thrombocytopenia (e.g., circumcision with increased bleeding, bloody diarrhea, ecchymoses)
- Recurrent infections usually start after 6 months of age. (Bacterial: otitis media, sinusitis, meningitis, sepsis, and pneumonia. Viral infections: HSV, Varicella with systemic complications.)
- Milder phenotypes may lack history of recurrent infections.
- Eczema is usually present by 1 year of age. (May be resistant to therapy, sometimes requiring systemic antibiotics.)

COMPLICATIONS

- Progressive decline in immunologic function with an increase in infections. Humoral and cellular immune systems are affected.
- Increased frequency of autoimmune phenomena such as arthritis and vasculitis. The most common is hemolytic anemia. Vasculitis, Henoch-Schönlein purpura, inflammatory polyarthritis, and inflammatory bowel disease are also observed.
- Approximately 100-fold increased risk of malignancy compared with the general pediatric population. Malignancy is more common in adolescents. Associated with EBV.
- Bleeding episodes can be life-threatening.

Differential Diagnosis

- Other causes of thrombocytopenia such as ITP
- Severe atopic disease with dermatitis and secondary skin infections
- HIV infection
- Hyper-IgE syndrome
- Diagnosis should be considered in any boy who has congenital or early-onset thrombocytopenia with small platelets.
- Definitive diagnosis: male patient, congenital thrombocytopenia ($<70,000/mm^3$), small platelets (mean platelet volume [MPV] <0.5 fL), a mutation in the WASP gene or absent WASP mRNA.

Data Gathering

HISTORY

- Persistent or severe bleeding in infancy as a result of thrombocytopenia
- Recurrent infections, especially by bacteria with capsular polysaccharides (e.g., Pneumococcus)
- Eczema can be of variable severity.
- Older patients may report recurrent viral infections.
- Maternal family history of WAS or XLT

Physical Examination

- Evaluation should focus on presence of infection.
- Dermatologic examination is significant for the extent of eczema and the presence of petechiae or ecchymoses.
- Splenomegaly

Laboratory Aids

TESTS

- CBC with differential
- Platelet count with mean platelet volume and platelet size by Coulter counter; hallmark of WAS is small platelets.
- Immunoglobulin levels typically reveal normal IgG, decreased IgM, and increased IgA and IgE.
- Functional antibody titers and isohemagglutinins; hallmark of WAS is reduced or absent responses to polysaccharide antigens and isohemagglutinins to ABO antigens.
- T- and B-lymphocyte enumeration and mitogen stimulation studies. These may progressively deteriorate with increasing age.

PROCEDURES

- Lymph node biopsy in suspected malignancy
- Bone marrow aspirate to evaluate thrombocytopenia

Therapy

- Antibiotics for acute infections and prophylactically in postsplenectomy patients
- Splenectomy may be helpful for persistent severe thrombocytopenia in select patients. However, this may greatly increase the risk of overwhelming infections with encapsulated organisms.
- Thrombocytopenia precautions: no aspirin and avoidance of situations in which trauma (especially head trauma) is likely to occur, such as contact sports.
- Platelet transfusions may be necessary for severe bleeding. Use irradiated blood products to avoid graft-versus-host disease, and CMV-negative products in case of bone marrow transplantation (BMT).
- IVIG replacement therapy is helpful in managing recurrent infections in some patients.
- BMT should be considered in these patients. If a full match is available, this is the treatment of choice. The overall success rate of HLA-identical BMT is 85%. The use of haploidentical BMT is controversial because of a lower success rate. Cord blood as a source of stem cells is also a curative therapy.
- Consider food allergy as exacerbating factor for eczema.

Follow-Up

- Signs and symptoms of malignancy should be evaluated expeditiously.
- As patients age, a progressive increase in infectious and autoimmune complications may occur.

Common Questions and Answers

Q: What is the life expectancy for WAS patients?
A: Before currently available therapies, most affected patients died in childhood. Currently, many patients live into their third and fourth decades, even without BMT. Major causes of mortality are infections (44%), bleeding (23%), and malignancies (26%). Incidence of malignancy increases in third decade of life. Successfully transplanted patients have a prolonged life expectancy.

Q: Should patients with WAS receive live viral vaccines?
A: These vaccines should be avoided because of the variable cellular immune defects associated with WAS. Any patients receiving IVIG do not require vaccinations.

Q: What is the chance of a sibling having WAS?
A: As with any X-linked disease, there is a 50% chance of another affected male child or asymptomatic carrier female. Genetic counseling should be offered to carrier females.

Q: Can WAS be diagnosed prenatally?
A: In families with affected males, fetal blood sampling can be performed in male fetuses to assess the size of the platelets. Small platelet size and family history of WAS suggests an affected infant.

ICD-9-CM 279.12

BIBLIOGRAPHY

Derry JMD, Ochs HD, Francke U. Isolation of novel gene mutated in Wiskott Aldrich syndrome. *Cell* 1994;78:635–644.

Litzman J, Jones A, Hann I, et al. Intravenous immunoglobulin, splenectomy, and antibiotic prophylaxis in Wiskott-Aldrich syndrome. *Arch Dis Child* 1996;75(5):43–69.

Nonoyama S, Ochs HD. Wiskott-Aldrich syndrome. *Curr Allergy Asthma Rep* 2001;1:430–437.

Ochs HD. The Wiskott-Aldrich syndrome. *Clin Rev Allergy Immunol* 2001;20(1):61–86.

Ochs HD, Skichter SJ, Harker LA, et al. The Wiskott Aldrich syndrome: studies of lymphocytes, granulocytes and platelets. *Blood* 1980;55:243–252.

Schurman SH, Candotti, F. Autoimmunity in Wiskott-Aldrich syndrome. *Curr Opin Rheum* 2003;15(4):446–453.

Shcherbina, A, Candotti, F, Rosen F, O'Donnell ER. High incidence of lymphomas in subgroups of Wiskott Aldrich syndrome patients. *Br J Haematology* 2003;121(3):529.

Snapper, SB., Rosen, FS. A Family of WASPs. *N Engl J Med* 2003;348(4):350–351.

Stites DP, Terr AI. *Basic and Clinical Immunology*. 7th Ed. Norwalk, CT: Appleton-Lange, 1991:346–347.

Sullivan KS, Mullen CA, Blaise RM, et al. A multi-institutional survey of Wiskott Aldrich syndrome. *J Pediatr* 1994;125:876–885.

Thrasher, A. WASp in Immune-System Organization and Function. *Nature Reviews Immunology* 2002;2:635–646.

Winkelstein JA, et al., eds. *Patient and Family Handbook: For the Primary Immune Deficiency Diseases*. 2nd Ed. Immune Deficiency Foundation, 1993.

Author: Elena Perez

Yersinia enterocolitica

 Database

DEFINITION

Yersinia enterocolitica is a facultative, nonlactose-fermenting, urease-positive, gram-negative coccobacillus; 34 serotypes have been recognized with serotypes 0:3, 8, and 9 the most common.

PATHOPHYSIOLOGY

- *Y. enterocolitica* adheres to epithelial cells and mucus, and heat-stable enterotoxins are produced, which play a role in the development of watery diarrhea.
- Another cytotoxin then directly injures the distal small bowel and large bowel, producing the characteristic bloody or mucous diarrhea.
- An enterocolitis develops and usually persists 5 to 14 days and is seen most commonly in the younger age groups.
- A pseudoappendicular syndrome as a result of mesenteric adenitis and/or terminal ileitis is seen more commonly in the older child or young adult.
- Extraintestinal manifestations include pharyngitis, suppurative lymphadenitis, pyomyositis, osteomyelitis, abscess, urinary tract infection, pneumonia, endocarditis, meningitis, peritonitis, panophthalmitis, conjunctivitis, and septic arthritis.
- If septicemia is present, mortality can be as high as 50%.

EPIDEMIOLOGY

- Most infected individuals are young children.
- *Y. enterocolitica* has been isolated from contaminated water, soil, wild and domestic animals, and unpasteurized milk products.
- Epidemics have been noted in the African American population during the winter holidays as a result of exposure to raw chitterlings (pork intestines) prepared for holiday meals.
- Cases as a result of contaminated blood transfusions from asymptomatic carriers of *Y. enterocolitica* 0:3 have been reported.
- Fecal-oral and person-to-person transmission are also possible.
- The incubation period is approximately 1 to 11 days, with symptoms persisting for 5 to 14 days. Symptoms for up to several months have been reported.
- The duration of organism excretion is approximately 6 weeks after diagnosis is made.
- A clinical state of iron overload and deferoxamine therapy are risk factors for developing systemic illness.

COMPLICATIONS

- Postinfectious sequelae of erythema nodosum and reactive arthritis involving weight-bearing joints (occurring 1 to 2 weeks after gastrointestinal symptoms) can occur, although these complications are seen most often in adults.
- Reiter syndrome, myocarditis, glomerulonephritis, erysipelas, chronic diarrhea persisting for months, and hemolytic anemia have also been reported.
- Intestinal perforation and ileocolic intussusception are possible.
- Septicemia is observed in patients with underlying medical conditions.
- Patients with iron overload disorders, e.g., β-thalassemia, hemochromatosis, have an increased susceptibility to *Yersinia* bacteremia.
- Following septicemia, focal abscesses of the liver, kidney, spleen, and lungs have been reported.
- The FDA has reported that contamination of the U.S. blood supply by bacterial infections, although rare, is most frequently a result of *Y. enterocolitica*.

PROGNOSIS

The prognosis is usually quite good, because most infections are gastrointestinal. Systemic disease (septicemia and subsequent secondary spread) has higher morbidity and mortality.

 Differential Diagnosis

Y. enterocolitica should be considered in all patients with a diarrheal illness with bloody or mucous stools with fever and abdominal pain, and in patients with the extraintestinal manifestations described above.

 Data Gathering

HISTORY

- Enterocolitis is the most common manifestation in young children.
- The history taking should include exposure to unpasteurized milk products and raw pork or poultry, especially the preparation of pork chitterlings.
- A history of acute onset of abdominal pain, diarrhea with blood or mucus, and mild fever suggest the diagnosis.
- Abdominal pain can be diffuse or localized to the right lower quadrant, suggestive of pseudoappendicitis as a result of mesenteric adenitis or terminal ileitis.
- Duration of illness is usually 2 to 3 weeks, but may be longer, and 25% of patients will have hematochezia.

 Physical Examination

Because of the wide range of clinical extraintestinal manifestations, the physical examination is nonspecific for this organism.

 Laboratory Aids

TESTS

- Blood, sputum, CSF, urine, and bile cultures do not require selective culture media techniques; stool samples should be plated on selective media such as cefsulodin-triclosan-novobiocin agar. If routine enteric media (MacConkey) are used, a cold enrichment technique will increase recovery of the organism.
- Serologic methods (tube agglutination assay, ELISA) are available with a rise in titers noted 1 week after onset of symptoms and peak titers observed by the second week of illness. These tests identify IgM, IgG, and IgA antibodies against *Y. enterocolitica*.
- Cross-reactivity between *Y. enterocolitica* and *Brucella abortus*, *Rickettsia* species, *Moraxella morganii*, *Salmonella* species, and thyroid tissue antigen make serodiagnosis of limited usefulness.

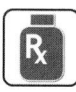 Therapy

- Antimicrobial therapy has been shown to benefit patients with systemic infections, focal extraintestinal infections, and enterocolitis in an immunocompromised host.
- The benefit of treatment of uncomplicated enterocolitis, mesenteric adenitis, or pseudoappendicitis has not been established.
- For most isolates, trimethoprim-sulfamethoxazole, chloramphenicol, aminoglycosides, tetracycline or doxycycline, fluoro quinolones, and third-generation cephalosporins are effective treatment options.
- *Y. enterocolitica* is usually resistant to most penicillins and first-generation cephalosporins.

Follow-Up

• Symptoms of enterocolitis usually abate within 2 weeks of the onset of symptoms, although shedding of the organism in the stool can last at least 6 weeks after diagnosis.
• For extraintestinal manifestations, the expected course is dependent on the specific organ system involved.

PREVENTION

• Infection control: Enteric precautions are indicated for patients with enterocolitis until symptoms resolve.
• General measures: Attempts to eliminate reservoirs and reduce frequency of ingesting contaminated foods and beverages are necessary; uncooked meats, especially pork and unpasteurized milk, and preparation of meats near or during preparation of infant bottles for feeding, are common sources of infection.

PITFALLS

• Not all bacterial colitis presents with bloody or mucus-appearing diarrhea. Therefore, suspicion should exist if the diarrhea is prolonged or environmental exposures pose a risk for developing infection.
• The possibility of *Y. enterocolitica* bacteremia should be considered in blood transfusion–related illnesses, thalassemia, or prior history of liver disease.

 Common Questions and Answers

Q: How long is a child considered infectious with *Y. enterocolitica*?
A: Although the typical course of enterocolitis is approximately 14 days, shedding of the organism in the stool can last at least 6 weeks. Enteric precautions should be discussed with the child's parent or caregiver to ensure infection control.

Q: If there is no history of evidence of bloody or mucous stools, can you exclude *Y. enterocolitica* as the likely infectious agent in a child with diarrhea?
A: No. In fact, early in the course of illness, the diarrhea is more likely to be watery as a result of the enterotoxins produced (see Pathophysiology).

Q: How is the diagnosis of *Y. enterocolitica* determined if you are unable to isolate the organism from a clinical specimen?
A: When a diagnosis cannot be made during acute infection or in the clinical setting of postinfectious complications, a serologic titer of greater than 1:128 is suggestive of previous infection of *Y. enterocolitica*. Keep in mind the possibility of cross-reactivity with *Brucella, Rickettsia, Morganella*, and *Salmonella* species and thyroid antigens.

ICD-9-CM 027.8

(Sepsis) 020.9

BIBLIOGRAPHY

Benavides S, Nicol K, Koranyi K, Nahata MC. Yersinia septic shock following an autologous transfusion in a pediatric patient. *Transfus Apheresis Sci* 2003;28:19–23.

Bottone EJ. *Yersinia enterocolitica*: the charisma continues. *Clin Microbiol Rev* 1997;10:257–276.

Cover TL, Aber RC. *Yersinia enterocolitica*. *N Engl J Med* 1989;321:16–24.

Dennis DT, Chow CC. Plague. *Pediatr Infect Dis J* 2004;23(1):69–71.

Kane DR, Reuman PD. *Yersinia enterocolitica* causing pneumonia and empyema in a child and a review of the literature. *Pediatr Infect Dis J* 1992;11:59–1593.

Krishnan LAG, Brecher ME. Transfusion-transmitted bacterial infection. *Hematol Oncol Clin North Am* 1995;9:167–185.

Lee LA, Taylor J, Carter GP, et al. *Yersinia enterocolitica* 0:3: an emerging cause of pediatric gastroenteritis in the United States. *J Infect Dis* 1991;163:660–663.

Natkin J, Beavis KG. *Yersinia enterocolitica* and *Yersinia pseudotuberculosis*. *Clin Lab Med* 1999;19:523–536.

Peter G, Halsey NA, Marcuse EK, et al. *Yersinia enterocolitica*. *2000 Red Book: Report of the Committee on Infectious Diseases*. 25th Ed. Elk Grove Village, IL: American Academy of Pediatrics, 2000:642–643.

Authors: Louis M. Bell
Philip V. Scribano, 3rd edition

SECTION III
Syndromes Glossary

4p syndrome—characterized by a round face, prominent nasal tip, polydactyly, and scoliosis.

5p syndrome—characterized by macrocephaly; small mandible; long, thin fingers; short, big toes; and anorectal and renal anomalies.

13q syndrome—typically involves malformations of the brain, heart, kidneys, and digits; usually lethal.

Aagene syndrome—hereditary (autosomal-recessive transmission); characterized by recurrent intrahepatic cholestasis, with lymphedema.

Aarskog syndrome—an X-linked recessive disorder characterized by short stature, and musculoskeletal and genital anomalies unknown etiology. Physical features include short stature (90%), hypertelorism, small nose with anteverted nares, broad philtrum and nasal bridge, abnormal auricles and widow's peak, brachyclinodactyly (80%), broad feet with bulbous toes (75%), simian crease (70%), ptosis (50%), syndactyly (60%), "shawl" scrotum (80%), cryptorchidism (75%), inguinal hernia (60%), hyperopic astigmatism, large corneas, ophthalmoplegia, strabismus, delayed puberty, mild pectus excavatum, prominent umbilicus. Radiographs show delayed bone age.

abetalipoproteinemia—recessive transmission; characterized by progressive cerebellar ataxia and pigmentary degeneration of the retina (starts with malabsorption of fat and progresses to ataxia); absent or reduced lipoproteins and low carotene, vitamin A, and cholesterol levels; and acanthocytosis (spiny projections on red blood cells [RBCs]).

acanthosis nigricans (Lawrence-Seip syndrome)—characterized by hyper-pigmented lichenoid plaques in the neck and axilla; may be associated with insulin resistance.

acrodermatitis enteropathica—autosomal-recessive transmission; characterized by zinc deficiency, vesicobullous and eczematous skin lesions in the perioral and perineal areas, cheeks, knees, and elbows; photophobia, conjunctivitis and corneal dystrophy; chronic diarrhea; glossitis; nail dystrophy; growth retardation; and superinfections and *Candida* infections.

Adie syndrome—characterized by a large pupil with little or no reaction to light; pupil may react to accommodation; patients have hyperreflexia.

agenesis of corpus callosum—cause unknown (rarely, X-linked recessive); absence of the major tracts connecting the right and left hemispheres is usually associated with hydrocephalus, seizures, developmental delay, abnormal head size, and hypertelorism.

Alagille syndrome (arteriohepatic dysplasia)—characterized by paucity or absence of intrahepatic bile ducts with progressive destruction of bile ducts; patients have a broad forehead, deep-set eyes that are widely spaced and underdeveloped, a small, pointed mandible, cardiac lesions, vertebral arch defects, and changes in the renal tubules and interstitium.

Albers-Schönberg disease (osteopetrosis tarda, marble bone disease)—most cases are autosomal-dominant, a few are autosomal-recessive; patients are prone to fractures and have mild anemia and craniofacial disproportion; radiologic changes include increased cortical bone density, longitudinal and transverse dense striations at the ends of the long bones, lucent and dense bands in the vertebrae, and thickening at the base of the skull.

Albright syndrome—see **McCune-Albright syndrome.**

Alexander disease—unknown pathogenesis; characterized by megaloencephaly in infants, dementia, spasticity and ataxia; may cause seizures in younger children; patients become mute, immobile, and dependent; hyaline eosinophilic inclusions occur in the footplates of astrocytes in subpial and subependymal regions.

Alport syndrome—several forms are hereditary male-to-male autosomal-dominant, and an X-linked form also exists; characterized by neurosensory deafness and progressive renal failure.

Anderson disease (glycogen storage disease, type IV)—caused by a defect in the glycogen branching enzyme 1, 4-α-glucan branching enzyme; characterized by hepatomegaly and failure to thrive in the first few months, progressing to liver cirrhosis and splenomegaly.

Apert syndrome (acrocephalosyndactyly)—autosomal-dominant; characterized by high and flat frontal bones, underdevelopment of the middle third of the face, hypertelorism and proptosis; a narrow, high, arched palate; a short, beaked nose; and syndactyly of the toes and digits.

arthrogryposis multiplex congenita—characterized by fixed contractures of the middle joints; present at birth.

Asperger syndrome—a developmental disorder on the higher-functioning end of the autism spectrum. These patients, often viewed as brilliant, eccentric, and physically awkward, fail to develop relationships with peers, have repetitive and stereotyped behaviors, usually with hand movements. See *www.aspergersyndrome.org.*

Bart syndrome—autosomal-dominant; congenital aplasia of the skin; characterized by nail defects and recurrent blistering of the skin and mucous membranes.

Bartter syndrome—hypertrophy of the juxtaglomerular apparatus; characterized by hypokalemic alkalosis, hypochloremia, and hyperaldosteronism; patients have normal blood pressure but the renin level is elevated; may lead to mental retardation and small stature.

Beckwith-Wiedemann syndrome—characterized by hypoglycemia, macrosomia, and visceromegaly; patients have umbilical anomalies and renal medullary dysplasia.

Behçet syndrome—unknown cause; involves relapsing iridocyclitis and recurrent oral and genital ulcerations; 50% of patients have arthritis.

blind loop syndrome—stasis of small intestine, usually secondary to incomplete bowel obstruction or a problem of intestinal motility.

Bloch-Sulzberger syndrome (incontinentia pigmenti)—characterized by mental retardation; one-third of patients have seizures and ocular malformations.

Bloom syndrome—autosomal-recessive; characterized by erythema and telangiectasia in a butterfly distribution, photosensitivity, and dwarfism.

Blount disease (tibia vara)—characterized by irregularity of the medial aspect of the tibial metaphysis adjacent to the epiphysis; bowing starts as angulation at the metaphysis.

blue diaper syndrome—defective tryptophan absorption; characterized by bluish stains on the diapers, digestive disturbances, fever, and visual difficulties.

Brill disease (Brill-Zinsser disease)—repeat episode of typhus; caused by a *Rickettsia* infection.

bronchiolitis obliterans—begins with necrotizing pneumonia secondary to viral infection (e.g., adenovirus, influenza, measles); tuberculosis (TB); or inhalation of fumes, talcum powder, or zinc; and involves the obstruction of small bronchi and bronchioles by fibrous tissue.

Byler disease—autosomal-recessive familial cholestasis; characterized by hepatomegaly, pruritus, splenomegaly, elevated bile acids, and gallstones.

Caroli disease—autosomal-recessive; cystic dilatation of the intrahepatic bile ducts; characterized by recurrent bouts of cholangitis and biliary abscesses secondary to bile stasis and gallstones.

cat's eye syndrome—autosomal-dominant; characterized by ocular coloboma, down-slanting eyes, congenital heart disease, and anal atresia.

Charcot-Marie-Tooth disease (peroneal muscular atrophy)—most common cause of chronic peripheral neuropathy; characterized by foot drop, high-arch foot; patients may have stocking-glove sensory loss.

Chèdiak-Higashi syndrome—autosomal-recessive disorder; involves partial oculocutaneous albinism, increased susceptibility to infection, lack of natural killer cells, and large, lysosome-like granules in many tissues; patients have splenomegaly, hypersplenism, hepatomegaly, lymphadenopathy, nystagmus photophobia, and peripheral neuropathy.

Coat disease—telangiectasia of retinal vessels, with subretinal exudate.

Cobb syndrome—intraspinous vascular anomaly and port-wine stains.

Cockayne syndrome—autosomal-recessive; characterized by dwarfism, mental retardation, bird-like facies, premature senility, and photosensitivity.

Cornelia de Lange syndrome—prenatal growth retardation; characterized by microcephaly, hirsutism, anteverted nares, down-turned mouth, mental retardation, and congenital heart defects.

cri du chat syndrome—characterized by growth retardation, mental deficiency, hypotonia, microcephaly, round "moon face," hypertelorism, epicanthal folds, and down-slanting palpebral fissures.

Crigler-Najjar syndrome (congenital nonhemolytic unconjugated hyperbilirubinemia)—type 1 is recessive; a deficiency of uridine diphosphate (UDP) glucuronyl transferase causes a rapid increase in the unconjugated bilirubin level on the first day of life; no hemolysis occurs and patients have no conjugation activity; type 2 is autosomal-dominant and is characterized by variable penetrance and partial activity of UDP glucuronyl transferase.

Cronkhite-Canada syndrome—diffuse intestinal polyps involving large and small intestine; characterized by alopecia, brown skin lesions, and onychatrophia; patients have diarrhea and protein-losing enteropathy (PLE).

Crouzon syndrome (craniofacial dysostosis)—autosomal-dominant with a range of expressivity; characterized by exophthalmos, hypertelorism, and hypoplasia of maxilla; patients have oral cavity anomalies and premature closure of the external auditory meatus.

cyclic neutropenia—syndrome involving lack of granulocyte macrophage colony-stimulating factor (GM-CSF); characterized by fever, mouth lesions, cervical adenitis, and gastroenteritis occurring every 3 to 6 weeks; neutrophil count may be zero.

de Toni-Fanconi-Debré acute syndrome—fatal; infantile myopathy with renal dysfunction; involves abnormal mitochondria and lipid and glycogen accumulation; patient has weak cry, poor muscle tone, poor suck, and lactic acidosis.

De Sanctis-Cacchione syndrome—autosomal-recessive; characterized by xeroderma pigmentosum with mental retardation, dwarfism, and hypogonadism; skin is unable to repair itself after exposure to ultraviolet light; patients may have erythema, scaling bullae, crusting telangiectasia keratoses, photophobia, corneal opacities, and tumors of the eyelids.

Diamond-Blackfan syndrome (congenital hypoplastic anemia)—failure of erythropoiesis; characterized by macrocytic anemia; patients have anemia, pallor, and weakness, no hepatomegaly, elevated fetal hemoglobin, and defect in abduction with retraction of the eye on adduction.

DiGeorge syndrome—thymic hypoplasia with hypocalcemia; patients have tetany, abnormal facies, congenital heart disease, and increased incidence of infection.

Dubin-Johnson syndrome—autosomal-recessive; characterized by elevated conjugated bilirubin, large amounts of coproporphyrin I in urine, and deposits of melanin-like pigment in hepatocellular lysosomes.

Dubowitz syndrome—Children with this syndrome nearly always have a history of intrauterine growth retardation involving both low birth weight and reduced length. Primary microcephaly. Facial characteristics include triangular face; small, receding chin; and broad and sometimes flat nasal bridge. As the child matures, the nasal bridge appears less wide and often becomes prominent, producing a continuous line with the forehead when viewed in profile. Tip of nose is frequently wide, rounded, or prominent, hypertelorism, shortened palpebral fissure that may be slanted, ptosis, sloping and high forehead, scanty hair and eyebrows, ear abnormalities.

Eagle-Barrett syndrome (prune-belly syndrome)—characterized by deficiency of the abdominal musculature, dilatation and dysplasia of the urinary tract, cryptorchidism, dilatation of the posterior urethra, and a hypoplastic or absent prostate.

ectodermal dysplasia—characterized by the poor development, or absence, of teeth, nails, hair, and sweat glands; patients have hyperextensible skin, hypermobile joints, and easy bruisability.

Eisenmenger syndrome—characterized by ventricular septal defect (VSD) with pulmonary hypertension.

Fabry disease—X-linked, lipid storage disease; involves a defect of the ceramide trihexoside α-galactosidase; characterized by tingling and burning in the hands and feet; small, red maculopapular lesions on the buttocks, inguinal area, fingernails, and lips; and an inability to perspire; patients have proteinuria, progressing to renal failure.

Farber syndrome—autosomal-recessive; involves a deficiency of acid ceramidase; characterized by hoarseness; painful, swollen joints; and palpable nodules over affected joints and pressure points.

fetal alcohol syndrome—characterized by a small body, head, and maxillary bone; abnormal palpebral fissures; epicanthal folds; cardiac septal defect; delayed development; and mental deficiency.

fetal hydantoin syndrome—characterized by hypoplasia of the midface, low nasal bridge, ocular hypertelorism, cupid bow upper lip; patients experience slow growth, may have mental retardation, cleft lip, and cardiac malformation.

Friedreich ataxia—mostly autosomal-recessive; appears in late childhood or in adolescence; involves progressive cerebellar and spinal cord dysfunction; patients have high-arched foot, hammer toes, and cardiac failure.

fructose intolerance, hereditary—autosomal-recessive; involves deficiency of fructose-1-phosphate aldolase or fructose 1,6-diphosphatase; characterized by vomiting, diarrhea, hypoglycemic seizures, and jaundice.

Gardner syndrome—characterized by multiple gastrointestinal polyps with malignant transformation, skin cysts, and multiple osteoma.

Gaucher disease—abnormal storage of glucosylceramide in the reticuloendothelial system; three types: (a) adult, or chronic, (b) acute neuropathic, or infantile, (c) subacute neuropathic, or juvenile; characterized by splenomegaly, hepatomegaly, delayed development, strabismus, swallowing difficulties, laryngeal spasm, opisthotonos, and bone pain.

Gianotti-Crosti syndrome—papular acrodermatitis and hepatitis B virus (HBV) infection; usually benign and self-limited.

Gilles de la Tourette syndrome—dominant trait with partial penetrance; characterized by multiple tics (e.g., blinking, twitching, grimacing) and involvement of muscles of swallowing and respiration; patient may exhibit swearing behavior and may have learning disabilities.

Glanzmann disease—autosomal-recessive; involves defective primary platelet aggregation (size and survival of platelets is normal).

Goldenhar syndrome—characterized by oculoauriculovertebral dysplasia and mandibular hypoplasia; patients have a hypoplastic zygomatic arch; malformed, displaced pinnae, and hearing loss.

Goltz syndrome—focal dermal hypoplasia; herniations of fat through thinned dermis produce tan papillomas associated with other skin defects and skeletal anomalies (e.g.,

Gradenigo syndrome

syndactyly, polydactyly, spinal defects); patients also have colobomas, strabismus, and nystagmus.

Gradenigo syndrome—acquired palsy of the abducens nerve and pain in the trigeminal nerve distribution, usually occurs after otitis media; produces diplopia, ocular and facial pain, photophobia, and lacrimation.

Hand-Schüller-Christian disease—see **histiocytosis X.**

Hartnup disease—autosomal-recessive defect in transport of monoamine monocarboxylic amino acids by intestinal mucosa and renal tubules; characterized by photosensitivity and a pellagra-like skin rash; patients may have cerebellar ataxia.

histiocytosis X—(reticuloendotheliosis) formerly called eosinophilic granuloma, Hand-Schüller-Christian disease, or Letterer-Siwe disease; patients may have a few solitary bone lesions or seborrheic dermatitis of scalp, lymphadenopathy, hepatosplenomegaly, tooth loss, exophthalmos, or pulmonary infiltrates.

Hunter syndrome (mucopolysaccharidosis II)—X-linked recessive; characterized by an accumulation of heparan sulfate and dermatan sulfate and enzyme deficiency of l-iduronate sulfatase.

Hurler syndrome (mucopolysaccharidosis IH)—autosomal-recessive; characterized by an accumulation of heparan sulfate and dermatan sulfate, and enzyme deficiency of α-l-iduronidase.

hyper-IgE—characterized by recurrent deep tissue and skin staphylococcal infections; patients have eosinophilia and IgE levels that are 10 times greater than normal.

incontinentia pigmenti—see **Bloch-Sulzberger syndrome.**

Jeune thoracic dystrophy—characterized by respiratory distress, short limbs, and polydactyly; may progress to renal insufficiency.

Job syndrome—characterized by severe staphylococcal infections, chronic skin disease, and cold abscesses; patients may have elevated IgE.

Kallmann syndrome—familial; characterized by isolated gonadotropin deficiency and anosmia.

Kartagener syndrome—characterized by sinusitis, bronchiectasis, and immotile cilia.

Kasabach-Merritt syndrome—characterized by hemangioma and consumption coagulopathy, platelet trapping, and microangiopathic hemolytic anemia.

Kleine-Levin syndrome—characterized by unusual hunger, somnolence, and motor restlessness.

Klinefelter syndrome—XXY karyotype; characterized by seminiferous tubule dysgenesis, testicular atrophy, eunuchoid habitus, and gynecomastia.

Klippel-Feil syndrome—characterized by a short neck, limited neck motion, and low occipital hairline.

Krabbe leukodystrophy—autosomal-recessive; characterized by cerebroside lipidosis and lack of myelin in white matter; usually presents by age 1 year; patients have hyperreflexia, rigidity, swallowing difficulties, lack of development.

Larsen syndrome—usually autosomal-dominant; characterized by hyperlaxity, multiple dislocations, and skin hyperlaxity.

Laurence-Moon-Biedl syndrome—characterized by retinitis pigmentosa, polydactyly, obesity, and hypogonadism.

Lennox-Gastaut syndrome (childhood epileptic encephalopathy)—characterized by severe seizures, mental retardation, and characteristic electroencephalography (EEG) pattern, showing generalized bilaterally synchronous sharp wave and slow wave complexes); patients have seizures starting in infancy; condition is difficult to treat; mental retardation is common.

Lesch-Nyhan syndrome—X-linked recessive disorder; characterized by a defect in purine metabolism; patients have hyperuricemia as a result of diminished or absent hypoxanthine guanine phosphoribosyl transferase (HGPRT) activity, choreoathetosis, compulsive self-mutilation, mental retardation, and growth failure.

Letterer-Siwe disease—component of histiocytosis X; characterized by acute disseminated histiocytosis; patients have seborrheic-looking skin lesions, bone lesions, gingival lesions, and liver and lung infiltrates.

Lowe syndrome (oculocerebral dystrophy)—X-linked recessive; patients have congenital cataracts, glaucoma, hypotonia, hyperreflexia, severe mental retardation, rickets, osteopenia, pathologic fractures, aminoaciduria, and organic aciduria.

Maffucci syndrome—multiple enchondromata and hemangioma of the bone and overlying skin; patients have short stature, skeletal deformities, scoliosis, and limb disproportion.

Marfan syndrome—connective tissue disorder characterized by ectopia lentis; dilatation of the aorta; long, thin extremities; pectus excavatum or carinatum; scoliosis; and pneumothorax.

McCune-Albright syndrome—polyostotic fibrous dysplasia; found more commonly in girls and in patients living on the coast of Maine; characterized by prominent skin discoloration

with ragged edges; patients may have precocious puberty, hyperthyroidism, gigantism headaches, epilepsy, and mental deficiency.

MELAS syndrome—mitochondrial encephalopathy, lactic acidosis, and stroke-like episodes; causes seizures, alternating hemiparesis, hemianopsia, or cortical blindness; patients have lactic acidosis, spongy degeneration of the brain, sensorineural hearing loss, and short stature.

Menkes syndrome—X-linked recessive; patients have short scalp hair, hypopigmentation, hypothermia, growth failure, skeletal defects, arterial aneurysms, seizures, and progressive central nervous system (CNS) failure.

Möbius syndrome—characterized by cranial nerve defects and a hypoplastic tongue or digits.

Morquio syndrome (mucopolysaccharidosis)—characterized by severe skeletal deformities, pectus carinatum, kyphoscoliosis, short neck, hypoplasia of the odontoid processes, C1 and C2 dislocation, neurosensory deafness, and aortic insufficiency.

multiple cartilaginous exostosis—characterized by bony projections near the ends of the tubular bones and ribs, scapula, vertebral bodies, and iliac crest; the exostoses become calcified and cause skeletal deformities; appears after the age of 3 years.

nail-patella syndrome—autosomal-dominant; characterized by dystrophic and hypoplastic nails, hypoplastic patellae and iliac horns, and malformed radial heads; may lead to nephrotic syndrome and renal failure.

Niemann-Pick disease—four types; storage of sphingomyelin and cholesterol causes hepatomegaly; patients are normal at birth but experience delayed development; 50% have a macular cherry red spot.

Noonan syndrome—normal karyotype; syndrome is characterized by cardiac lesions (atrial septal defect [ASD] or pulmonic stenosis); facial changes (palpebral slant, broad flat nose); webbed neck; short stature; a high, arched palate; and malformed ears.

Osler-Weber-Rendu syndrome—hereditary hemorrhagic telangiectasia; patients have telangiectasia in the skin, respiratory tract mucosa, lips, nails, conjunctiva, and nasal and oral mucosae.

Parinaud syndrome—characterized by weakness of upward gaze, poor convergence and accommodation, refractive nystagmus with upward gaze, and pupillary changes.

Patau syndrome—see **trisomy 13.**

Pelizaeus-Merzbacher disease—characterized by dancing eye movements, delayed motor development and spasticity, small head, poor head control, and possible optic atrophy and seizures.

Peutz-Jeghers syndrome—autosomal-dominant; patients have bluish-black macules around the mouth and intestinal polyposis in the small bowel.

Pickwickian syndrome—characterized by obesity and hypoventilation syndrome; patients may have respiratory arrest, restless sleep.

Pierre Robin syndrome—characterized by severe micrognathia, glossoptosis, and cleft palate.

Poland syndrome—characterized by a unilateral hypoplastic pectoral muscle with ipsilateral upper limb deficiency, syndactyly, and a defect of the subclavian artery.

Prader-Willi syndrome—characterized by hypotonia, hypomentia, hypogonadism, obesity, narrow bifrontal diameter, and hypotonia; patients may have a deletion in chromosome 15.

progeria—characterized by premature aging, severe growth failure, atherosclerosis, alopecia, and dystrophic nails.

prune-belly syndrome—see **Eagle-Barrett syndrome.**

Rieger syndrome—sporadic autosomal-dominant; characterized by microcornea with opacity, iris hypoplasia, anterior synechiae, hypodontia, and maxillary hypoplasia.

Riley-Day syndrome—familial dysautonomia; affects sensory and autonomic functions; patients have poor feeding, aspiration, no tears, high threshold to pain, markedly decreased reflexes, smooth tongue and impaired taste, and erratic blood pressure and temperature.

Rotor syndrome—autosomal-recessive; characterized by elevated conjugated bilirubin, elevated coproporphyrin I and coproporphyrin in urine, and normal liver biopsies.

Rubinstein-Taybi syndrome—characterized by broad thumbs and toes, short stature, mental retardation, beaked nose, hypoplastic mandible, and congenital heart defect.

Russell-Silver dwarf syndrome—characterized by intrauterine growth retardation (IUGR), subnormal growth velocity, triangular facies, clinodactyly, simian creases, and genitourinary malformations.

Sandhoff GM2-gangliosidosis type II—characterized by deficient hexosaminidase activity leading to cherry red spot in macula, failure to develop motor skills, blindness, weakness, and seizures.

Sanfilippo type A syndrome (mucopolysaccharidosis IIIA)—autosomal-recessive; characterized by accumulation of heparan sulfate, dermatan sulfate, and sulfatidase.

Sanfilippo type B syndrome (mucopolysaccharidosis IIIA)—autosomal-recessive; characterized by accumulation of heparan sulfate, dermatan sulfate, and α-N-acetylglucosaminidase.

Scheie syndrome (mucopolysaccharidosis IS)—autosomal-recessive; characterized by accumulation of heparan sulfate and dermatan sulfate, and an enzyme defect affecting α-l-iduronidase.

scimitar syndrome—characterized by hypoplasia of the right lung with systemic arterial supply, anomalous right pulmonary vein, and dextroposition of heart.

Seckel syndrome—characterized by intrauterine growth retardation (IUGR), microcephaly, sharp facial features with underdeveloped chin, and mental retardation.

Shwachman syndrome—characterized by pancreatic dysfunction, short stature, bone marrow dysfunction, and skeletal abnormalities.

silo filler disease—acute pneumonitis caused by inhalation of nitrogen dioxide; patients have chills, fever, cough, dyspnea, and cyanosis; associated with a high mortality rate.

Smith-Lemli-Opitz syndrome—characterized by short stature, microcephaly, ptosis, anteverted nares, micrognathia, syndactyly, cryptorchidism, and mental retardation.

Sotos syndrome—characterized by cerebral gigantism, large head and ears, prominent mandible, mental retardation, and poor coordination.

Stickler syndrome—autosomal-dominant; characterized by high myopia, cataract formation, and retinal detachment.

Sturge-Weber syndrome—characterized by a port-wine stain on the face at the first branch of the trigeminal nerve; patients have seizures and mental retardation.

Swyer-James syndrome—characterized by unilateral hyperlucent lung following bronchiolitis obliterans.

Tourette syndrome—see **Gilles de la Tourette syndrome.**

Treacher Collins syndrome—autosomal-dominant with incomplete penetration; characterized by mandibulofacial dysostosis; patients have hypoplastic mandible; hypoplastic zygomatic arches; antimongoloid slant to eyes; deformities of the pinna; and a high, arched palate with or without cleft palate.

trisomy 9—characterized by deep-set eyes, bulbous nasal tip, an anxious facial expression, and cleft lip.

trisomy 13 (Patau syndrome)—characterized by cleft lip, microphthalmia, postaxial polydactyly, and cardiovascular anomalies.

trisomy 18—characterized by a small face, high nasal bridge, short palpebral fissures, micrognathia, small mouth, overriding fingers, and hypoplastic nails; patients have mental retardation and intrauterine growth retardation (IUGR).

tuberous sclerosis—characterized by epiloia; patients have seizures, mental deficiency, adenoma sebaceum foci of intracranial calcification, hypopigmented macules, ash leaf spots, connective tissue nevi (shagreen spots), adenoma sebaceum, and angiofibroma.

Turcot syndrome—characterized by adenomatous colonic polyposis associated with malignant brain tumors, especially glioblastomas.

Turner syndrome—characterized by gonadal dysplasia (streak gonads stem from XO karyotype), short stature, sexual infantilism, atypical facies, low hairline, webbed neck, congenital lymphedema of the extremities, coarctation of the aorta, and increased carrying angle.

Usher syndrome—autosomal-recessive; characterized by retinitis pigmentosa, cataracts, and sensorineural deafness.

vanishing testes syndrome—characterized by bilateral gonadal failure with normal external male genitalia, normal 46, XY karyotype, absent testes, and no male puberty.

VATER syndrome—syndrome involving vertebral defects, analatresia, tracheoesophageal atresia, radial dysplasia, renal dysplasia, and congenital heart defect.

Vogt-Koyanagi-Harada syndrome—characterized by vitiligo, uveitis, dysacousia, and aseptic meningitis.

von Gierke disease (type 1 glycogenosis)—glucose-6-phosphate dehydrogenase (G6PD) is absent in the liver, kidney, and intestinal mucosa; characterized by hypoglycemia under stress (e.g., fasting), hepatomegaly, and seizures.

von Hippel–Landau disease—autosomal-dominant (linked to chromosome 3); characterized by hemangioblastoma of the cerebellum and retina; patients have cystic cerebellar neoplasm with increased intracranial pressure (ICP).

Waardenburg syndrome—autosomal-dominant; characterized by white forelock, heterochromic irides, displacement of the inner canthi, broad nasal root, and confluent eyebrows.

Wegener granulomatosis—necrotizing granulomatous vasculitis of the arteries and veins; involves airways, lungs, and kidneys with resultant rhinorrhea, nasal ulceration, hemoptysis, and cough; patients have hematuria caused by necrotizing vasculitis.

Werner syndrome—autosomal-recessive; characterized by short stature, juvenile cataracts, hypogonadism, gray hair in second decade.

Williams syndrome—characterized by mental retardation, hypoplastic nails, periorbital fullness, supravalvular aortic stenosis, growth delay, and stellate iris.

Wilson-Mikity syndrome—characterized by pulmonary immaturity; occurs in premature infants; patients have slow onset of respiratory distress, retractions, and apnea; may clear in several weeks.

Wiskott-Aldrich syndrome—characterized by thrombocytopenia, severe eczema, and recurrent skin infections.

Wolff-Parkinson-White syndrome—characterized by a short PR interval and slow upstroke of the QRS-delta wave; usually occurs in patients with a normal heart but also may occur in patients with Ebstein anomaly and cardiomyopathy.

Wolman disease—fatal condition characterized by primary xanthomatosis, adrenal insufficiency, vomiting, failure to thrive, steatorrhea, hepatomegaly, and adrenal calcification.

Zellweger syndrome—cerebrohepatorenal syndrome; characterized by hepatic fibrosis and cirrhosis; patients have seizures, mental retardation, hypotonia, glaucoma, congenital stippled epiphyses, and cysts of the renal cortex.

Zollinger-Ellison syndrome—characterized by islet cell tumors that produce duodenal and jejunal ulcers; patients have high gastrin levels and excessive acid secretion.

SECTION IV

Cardiology Laboratory

Ilana Zeltser

Cardiology Laboratory

BLOOD PRESSURE MEASUREMENT

Between 1% and 3% of the pediatric population has hypertension. Most cases of hypertension are early manifestations of essential hypertension. Approximately 10% of children have secondary hypertension, and 80% of these patients have underlying renal parenchymal or renal vascular disease. After renal disease, coarctation or hypoplasia of the aorta is the second most common cause of secondary hypertension.

Accurate determination of the blood pressure is an integral part of the physical examination. The blood pressure cuff must be the correct size; a small cuff will falsely overestimate the blood pressure. The blood pressure cuff should be 50% of the circumference and two-thirds the length of the extremity. Second, the patient should be sitting and calm. Finally, once the cuff is sufficiently inflated, the cuff should then be released slowly at a rate of 3 to 4 mmHg/sec. The first Korotkoff sound corresponds to the systolic pressure, although the fifth Korotkoff sound, the disappearance of sound, represents the diastolic pressure.

The report from the Second Task Force on Blood Pressure Control in Children published standard blood pressure measurements for children from birth to 18 years of age (Figure 1). These reference standards do not distinguish between racial or ethnic groups. In general, blood pressure increases with height, weight, age, and sexual maturation.

Blood pressure is higher in males than in females during the first decade of life and tends to widen around the onset of puberty. Blood pressure follows a circadian rhythm, being highest late in the day and lowest at night while sleeping.

When cardiac disease is suspected, blood pressure measurements should be obtained in all four extremities. A difference of greater than 10 mmHg between upper and lower extremity blood pressures is pathologic and suggests the presence of aortic coarctation, aortic arch hypoplasia or interrupted aortic arch.

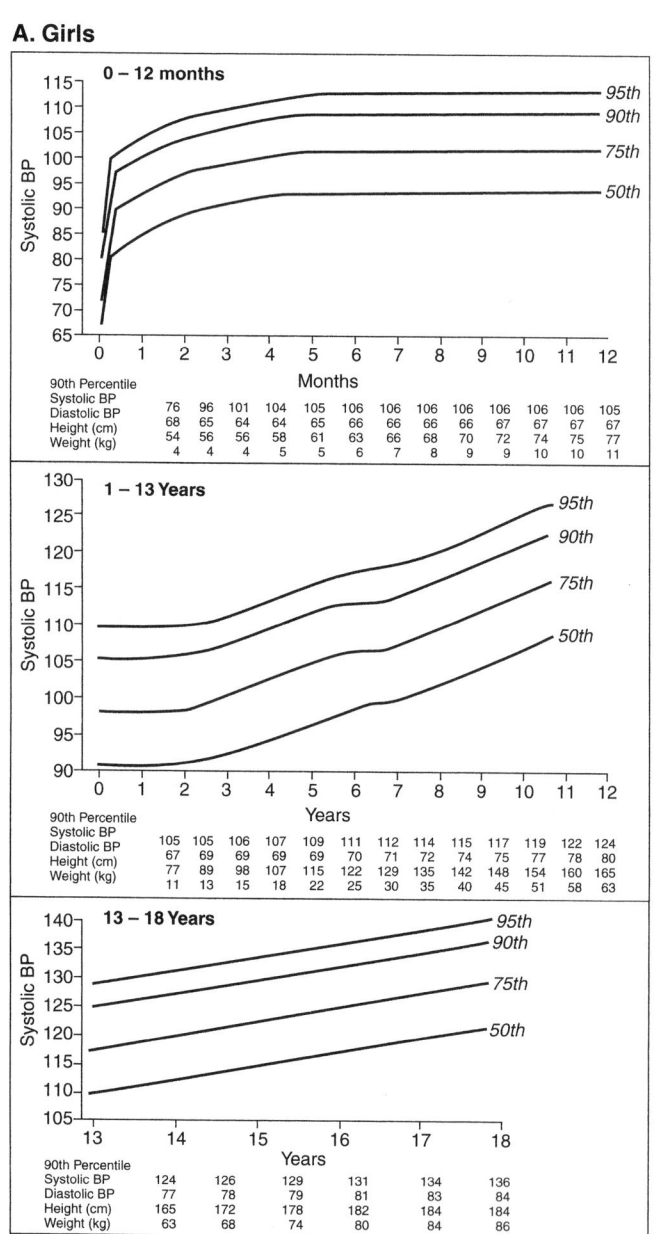

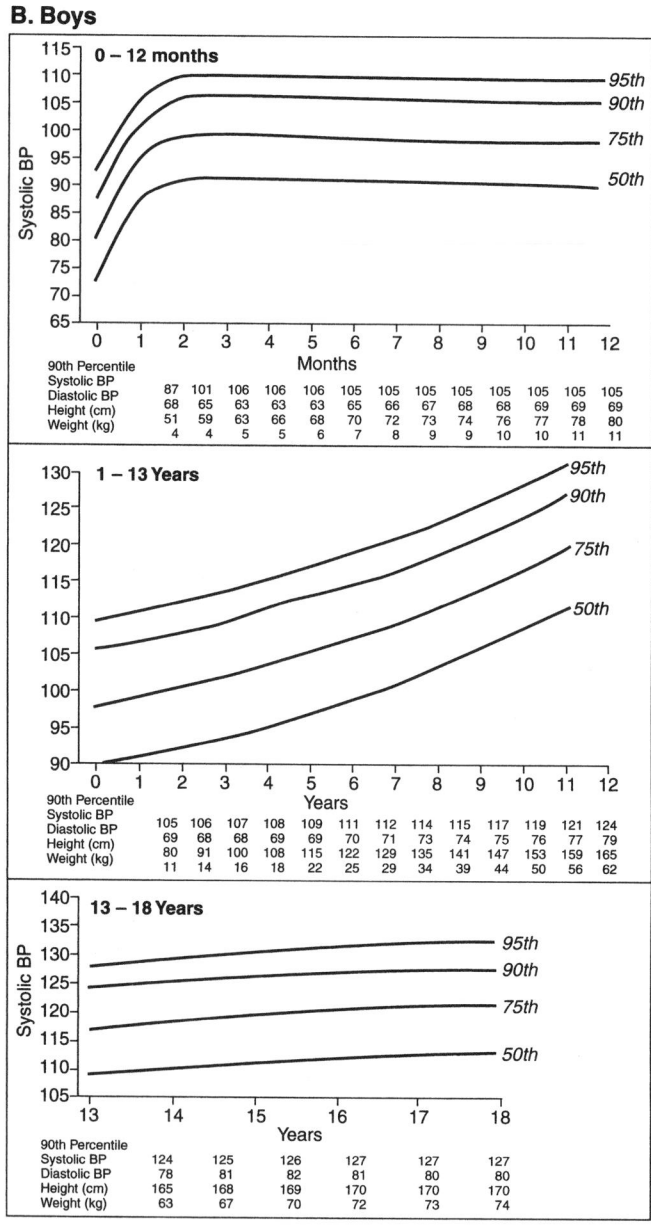

FIGURE 1. Standard blood pressure measurements in accordance with age and gender. A: Girls. B: Boys. BP, blood pressure. (From Horan MJ. Report of the Second Task Force on Blood Pressure Control in Children—1987. Pediatrics 1987;79:1–25, with permission).

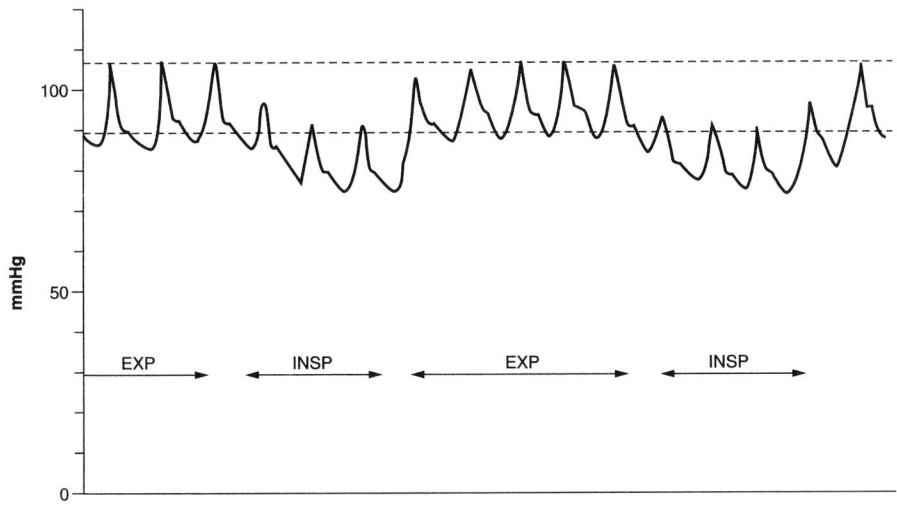

FIGURE 2. Pulsus paradoxus. EXP, expiration; INSP, inspiration. (Modified from Park MK. Pediatric cardiology for practitioners, 3rd ed. St. Louis: Mosby-Year Book 1996:15, with permission).

Pulse Pressure

The pulse pressure is the calculated difference between the systolic and diastolic pressures. A widened pulse pressure is present in: (a) high cardiac output states (anemia, fever, exercise, thyrotoxicosis), (b) diastolic run-off lesions (patent ductus arteriosus, aortic insufficiency, arteriovenous malformations), or (c) complete heart block. Narrow pulse pressure states may reflect: (a) low cardiac output states, (b) mitral or aortic valve stenosis, or (c) pericardial tamponade or constrictive pericarditis.

Hint: Normally, with inspiration, there is a small diminution of the systolic blood pressure compared to the diastolic pressure, resulting in a slight narrowing of the pulse pressure. Pulsus paradoxus exists when this response is exaggerated, and there is a greater than 10 mmHg drop in the systolic blood pressure with inspiration, resulting in narrowing of the pulse pressure. Pulsus paradoxus indicates underlying cardiopulmonary disease and may be associated with cardiac tamponade, constrictive pericarditis, or severe respiratory compromise (e.g., status asthmaticus). See Figure 2 for a schematic illustration of pulsus paradoxus.

CYANOSIS

Central cyanosis can be detected when the absolute concentration of deoxygenated hemoglobin is at least 3 gm/dL in a child with a normal hemoglobin. The best indicator of cyanosis is the tongue, which is free of pigmentation and has a rich vascular supply. Whether or not cyanosis is manifest depends on (a) the hemoglobin and (b) factors that alter the affinity of hemoglobin (temperature, serum pH, level of 2,3-diphosphoglycerate and the percentage of fetal versus adult hemoglobin). For example, a newborn with polycythemia (hemoglobin of 20 g/dL) and an arterial saturation of 80% will have 4 g/dL of deoxygenated hemoglobin and will appear cyanotic. In contrast, an anemic newborn (hemoglobin of 10 g/dL) with an arterial saturation of 80% will have only 2 g/dL of deoxygenated hemoglobin and will not appear cyanotic.

Hint: Central cyanosis should not be confused with acrocyanosis, a common physical finding in newborns as a result of peripheral vasoconstriction.

Hyperoxia Test

In infants with cyanosis and hypoxia, the differential diagnosis includes abnormalities of the cardiovascular, pulmonary, neurologic, and hematologic systems. In all neonates with hypoxemia, the hyperoxia test is a useful diagnostic tool to identify those neonates with a cardiovascular etiology. If a right radial arterial PaO_2 on 100% FiO_2 is less than 150 mmHg, severe congenital heart disease is likely. The infant is presumed to have ductal dependent congenital heart disease and the low PaO_2 is attributed to the obligatory mixing of oxygenated with deoxygenated blood within the circulatory system.

ELECTROCARDIOGRAPHY

The surface electrocardiogram (ECG) reflects the electrical activity in the heart and can provide information regarding the depolarization and repolarization of the heart muscle. The electrical signal represents the propagation of a wavefront through a cardiac chamber. Movement toward a recording electrode results in an upward deflection on the ECG, although movement away produces a negative deflection.

Correct ECG lead placement is of paramount importance in its accurate interpretation. The limb leads create a 360° frontal plane, although the precordial leads view the electrical activity in a horizontal plane (Figure 3). The standard ECG paper speed is 25 mm/sec with an amplitude of 1 mV/mm (Figure 4).

One should establish a systematic approach when interpreting ECGs. After noting the paper speed, standardization, and the patient's age, the signals can be analyzed. One should comment on the following: (a) rhythm, (b) rate, (c) axes of P, QRS, and T waves, (d) PR, QRS, and QT intervals, (e) waveform voltage, and (f) P, QRS, and T wave morphology.

Rhythm

Sinus rhythm occurs when there is a P-wave prior to every QRS complex, and the axis of the P-wave is positive in leads I, II, and aVF.

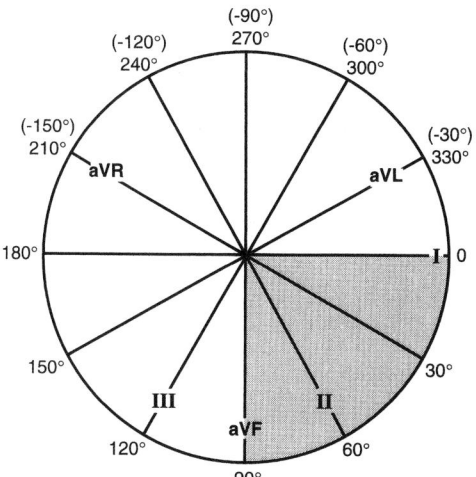

FIGURE 3. Hexaxial reference system (frontal axis). The shaded area represents the normal axis.

Cardiology Laboratory

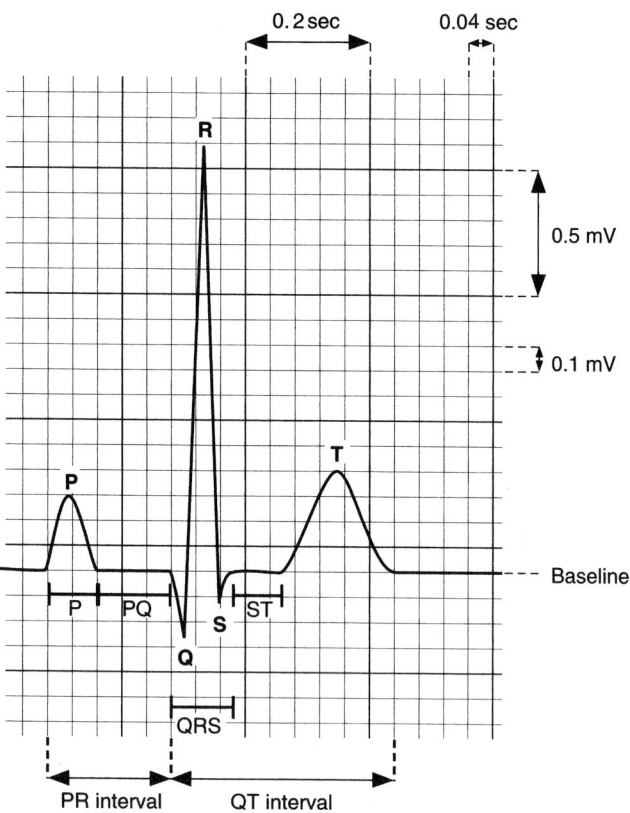

FIGURE 4. A normal electrocardiogram showing waveforms and intervals. The standard paper speed is 25 mm per second; therefore, a single 1-mm box equals 0.04 second, and a large (5-mm) box equals 0.20 second.

Rate

Heart rate norms depend on the patient's age. In general, the heart decreases with increasing age (Table 1). When the ECG is at standard paper speed, 1 mm (one small box) is equal to 0.04 seconds, and 5 mm (one large box) is 0.2 seconds. Thus if there is one QRS complex every 0.2 seconds, then the heart rate is 300 beats/min. If the heart rate is inappropriately fast, then the rhythm may be sinus tachycardia or an arrhythmia. If sinus tachycardia is suspected, an underlying systemic process is usually responsible for stimulating the sinus node. Fever, anxiety, thyrotoxicosis, anemia and myocardial disease are among the more common causes of sinus tachycardia. Alternatively, if the heart rate is inappropriately slow, then the rhythm must be differentiated between sinus bradycardia and an arrhythmia. Sinus bradycardia is common in trained athletes. Other etiologies of sinus bradycardia include increased intracranial pressure, hypothyroidism, malnutrition, anorexia, hypoxia, sinus node dysfunction, electrolyte abnormalities, and pharmaceuticals.

Axes

The limb leads are oriented in a hexaxial reference plane so that the angle between any two leads is 30°. With respect to the P-wave axis, the rhythm should be noted to be originating from the sinus node or an alternative pacemaker. The normal QRS axis changes with age. In the newborn period, the mean vector of depolarization is rightward, reflecting the dominance of the right ventricle in early infancy. As the left ventricular mass increases relative to the right side, the QRS axis shifts more leftward. Table 1 demonstrates expected ranges for the QRS axis with respect to age. When left axis deviation is present, there is frequently left ventricular hypertrophy or a left bundle branch block. Conversely, when right axis deviation is present, there is often right ventricular hypertrophy or a right bundle branch block. When the QRS axis is superior (northwest axis), an endocardial cushion defect or tricuspid atresia are possible. The T-wave represents ventricular repolarization. Within the first 72 hours of life, the T-wave should invert in lead V1. As the left ventricle becomes progressively more dominant, the T-wave axis parallels the QRS axis. Thus, during adolescence, the T-wave becomes upright in lead V1 and the T wave axis becomes leftward. Finally, the QRS-T angle should be ≤90°. When there is an abnormally wide angle, the following are possible: (a) right or left ventricular hypertrophy associated with a strain pattern, (b) a ventricular conduction disturbance, or (c) myocardial dysfunction.

Intervals

Measuring the intervals between deflections on the ECG evaluates the properties of the electrical conduction system. Refer to Table 1 for normal age-corrected values of intervals. The PR interval is measured from the onset of the P-wave to the beginning of the QRS complex and reflects the time for atrial depolarization and delay through the AV node. In general, with age, the heart rate is slower and the PR interval is longer. Abnormal prolongation of the PR interval, or first degree AV block, usually represents a delay in AV node conduction. This delay can be as a result of myocarditis, congenital heart disease, electrolyte abnormalities (hyperkalemia), hypoxia, ischemia, medications, or toxins (e.g., digitalis, quinidine). A short PR interval is present when there is either (a) an abnormal electrical connection between the atrium and ventricle, as seen in Wolff-Parkinson-White syndrome, Lown-Ganong-Levine syndrome, glycogen storage disease, or hypertrophic

Table 1 Heart Rate, PR Interval, and QRS Duration

AGE	HEART RATE (BEATS/MIN) MEAN	HEART RATE (BEATS/MIN) RANGE	PR INTERVAL IN LEAD II (SECONDS) MEAN	PR INTERVAL IN LEAD II (SECONDS) RANGE	QRS DURATION (SECONDS) MEAN	QRS DURATION (SECONDS) RANGE
<1 day	126	95–155	0.106	0.082–0.138	0.05	0.025–0.069
1–7 days	135	100–180	0.107	0.079–0.130	0.05	0.025–0.068
8–30 days	160	120–190	0.100	0.075–0.128	0.053	0.026–0.075
1–3 months	147	95–200	0.098	0.075–0.126	0.052	0.027–0.069
3–6 months	139	114–170	0.105	0.078–0.137	0.053	0.028–0.075
6–12 months	130	95–170	0.105	0.077–0.138	0.055	0.03–0.070
1–3 years	121	95–150	0.113	0.090–0.140	0.056	0.032–0.070
3–5 years	98	70–130	0.119	0.092–0.150	0.058	0.03–0.069
5–8 years	86	65–120	0.124	0.094–0.155	0.059	0.035–0.075
8–12 years	86	65–120	0.129	0.093–0.165	0.062	0.038–0.079
12–16 years	86	65–120	0.135	0.098–0.169	0.065	0.040–0.081

Adapted with permission from Liebman J, Plonsey R, Gillette PC: *Pediatric Electrocardiography*. Baltimore, Williams & Wilkins, 1982, pp 96–97 and Cassels DE, Ziegler RF: *Electrocardiography in Infants and Children*, Philadelphia, WB Saunders, 1966, p 100.

cardiomyopathy. Finally, a variable PR interval suggests either (a) a wandering atrial pacemaker or (b) Wenckebach phenomenon. The QRS interval is measured from the onset of the Q-wave to the completion of the S-wave and represents ventricular depolarization. The QRS duration represents the intraventricular conduction time and is normally less than 0.09 seconds in children younger than 4 years and less than 0.1 seconds in children older than 4 years. When the QRS complex is wide, there is a delay or abnormal propagation of the electrical impulse through the ventricular myocardium. QRS widening is seen with a bundle branch block, preexcitation (e.g., Wolff-Parkinson-White syndrome), intraventricular block, ventricular arrhythmias and ventricular paced rhythms.

Hint: Left bundle branch block is diagnosed when there is a monophasic R wave in lead I and no Q wave in lead V6. Right bundle branch block is diagnosed when there is a wide S wave in leads I and V6, right axis deviation, and an M-shaped (RSR' pattern) QRS complex in lead V1. Left anterior hemiblock can be diagnosed in the setting of left axis deviation associated with right bundle branch block. Finally, the QT interval represents the time it takes for ventricular depolarization and re-polarization. The QT interval is measured from the onset of the Q-wave to the termination of the T-wave. Given that the QT interval should shorten with increasing heart rates, the QT measurement should be adjusted for heart rate using the following formula: QTc = QT measured/square root of the R-R interval. The QTc interval is generally less than 0.45 seconds for infants younger than 6 months, and less than 0.44 seconds for children. The QTc is prolonged in Long QT syndrome wherein there are multi-ple genetic abnormalities of either the cardiac potassium or sodium channels. Other con-ditions that prolong the QTc interval include head injury, myocarditis, medications (such as, procainamide, amiodarone, quinidine) and electrolyte abnormalities (e.g., hypocalcemia, hypomagnesemia, hypokalemia).

Waveforms

Abnormal morphologic characteristics of the waveforms often indicate underlying pathology. When the P-wave amplitude is greater than 3 mm in lead II or lead V1, right atrial enlargement is present. If the P-wave has a duration greater than 0.1 seconds in lead II or is biphasic with a prominent negative component in lead V1, left atrial enlargement is present.
The amplitude of the QRS complex is evaluated in the precordial leads and depends on the child's age. The normal Q-wave represents septal depolarization and is seen in the inferolateral leads. The absence of Q-waves in leads V5 and V6, coupled with the presence of Q-waves in lead V1, is consistent with congenitally corrected transposition of the great arteries (L-TGA). Abnormally tall R-waves in lead V1 or deep S-waves in V5 and V6 represent right ventricular hypertrophy. Similarly, tall R-waves in leads V5 and V6 or deep S-waves in lead V1 represent left

ventricular hypertrophy. Conversely, low-voltage QRS complexes suggest myocarditis, pericarditis, pericardial effusion, or hypothyroidism.
Finally, abnormalities of T-wave morphology can also suggest pathology. For example, tall, peaked T-waves can be seen with ventricular hypertrophy associated with strain, myocardial infarction, or hyperkalemia. Conversely, low-voltage, flat T-waves are associated with electrolyte abnormalities (hypokalemia, hypoglycemia), hypothyroidism, myocarditis, pericarditis, ischemia or medications (i.e., digitalis).

CHEST ROENTGENOGRAM

Despite the increasing use of alternative methods of noninvasive imaging, the plain

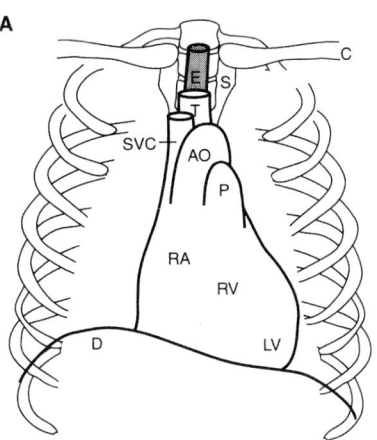

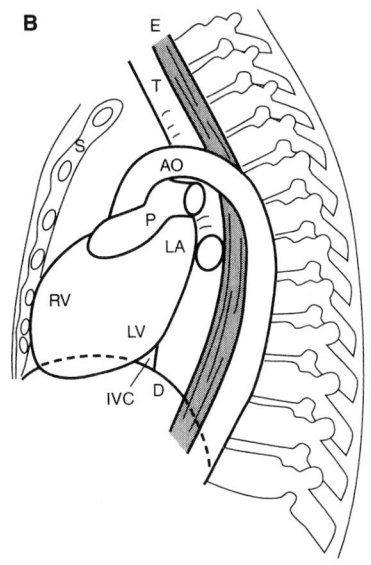

FIGURE 5. Normal cardiac silhouette. A: Anterior-posterior view. B: Lateral view. AO, aorta; C, clavicle; D, diaphragm; E, esophagus; IVC, inferior vena cava; LA, left atrium; LV, left ventricle; P, pulmonary outflow tract; RA, right atrium, RV, right ventricle; S, sternum; T, trachea; SVC, superior vena cava. (Modified from Sapire DW. Understanding and diagnosing pediatric heart disease. East Norwalk, CT: Appleton & Lange, 1991:64, with permission).

chest roentgenogram continues to provide important information to the clinician when cardiac disease is suspected. The study is inexpensive, expedient, readily available, and minimally harmful, and therefore serves as a convenient tool in assessing patients. It can provide important information regarding cardiac size, pulmonary vascularity, and specific cardiac abnormalities. The normal cardiac silhouette in the anterior-posterior and lateral views is shown in Figure 5.

Heart Size

Cardiomegaly, or an enlarged heart, is associated with both congenital and acquired heart disease. Several factors influence the interpretation of cardiac size on a chest radiograph. First, given that the pericardium rests on the diaphragm, the apparent size of the heart will vary with the respiratory cycle and posture. For example, during exhalation or when a patient is in the supine position, the cardiac silhouette is horizontally stretched, and may appear larger. Conversely, during inspiration or in the standing position, the heart is most vertical and appears smaller. Second, the thymic shadow often blends with the cardiac silhouette making an accurate determination of heart size difficult. A quantitative assessment of cardiac size should be made on the inspiratory film, when 9 to 10 ribs are visualized above the level of the diaphragm. The cardiothoracic ratio is then determined by comparing the transverse dimension of the heart relative to the width of the thoracic cavity. The heart is considered enlarged if the cardiothoracic ratio exceeds 0.6 in the anterior-posterior dimension. Individual cardiac chamber sizes can also be assessed on the standard plain film. For example, a large bulge appreciated to the right of the sternum suggests right atrial enlargement. Right ventricular hypertrophy is often demonstrated by an "up-tilting" of the apex of the heart from the diaphragm and an obliteration of the retrosternal space on the lateral projection. Left atrial enlargement is best seen in the lateral view as it displaces or compresses the esophagus. Left ventricular enlargement is best visualized in the anterior-posterior projection and appears as although the apex of the heart is "sagging."

Pulmonary Vascularity

When there is a suspicion of congenital heart disease, the appearance of the pulmonary vascular markings plays an important role in understanding the pathophysiology. In general, when a large left-to-right shunt is present (as in atrial septal defect, ventricular septal defect, patent ductus arteriosus) pulmonary arterial flow is increased and the vessels appear sharp and prominent. In the cyanotic neonate, when there is a paucity of pulmonary vascular markings, one must be suspicious of a right-sided obstructive lesion with a right-to-left shunt. In the case of pulmonary venous congestion, bronchial cuffing, and Kerley B lines, one must suspect pulmonary venous obstructive disease or congestive heart failure.

Cardiology Laboratory

Specific Cardiac Lesions

Distinctive radiographic configurations have been associated with specific cardiac lesions. The "boot-shaped" heart seen in patients with tetralogy of Fallot reflects right ventricular hypertrophy and hypoplasia of the main pulmonary artery segment, causing a concavity of the upper left heart border. In patients with total anomalous pulmonary venous return without obstruction, a "snowman" or "figure-eight" pattern has been described. This radiographic finding represents right atrial and right ventricular enlargement secondary to the large left-to-right shunt and the presence of a large left-sided vertical vein. The chest roentgenogram of a patient with discrete aortic coarctation often shows a prominent indentation of the aorta resembling a "figure 3." The description of

"an egg on a string" is used for the chest x-ray findings in patients with transposition of the great arteries, reflecting the narrowed mediastinum and right heart enlargement.

ECHOCARDIOGRAPHY

In pediatric patients, echocardiography is performed in a systematic manner and obtains subcostal, apical, parasternal, and suprasternal views (Figure 6).

M-Mode Echocardiography

A parasternal short-axis view using M-mode echocardiography reveals a cross section of the left ventricle and can be used to measure dimensions at different points in the cardiac cycle. Most commonly, it is used to obtain a

shortening fraction (SF), calculated in the following manner:

SF = 100 × [(LV end-diastolic dimension − LV end-systolic dimension) / LV end-diastolic dimension]

The normal value for the SF is 28% to 38%, independent of age.

Doppler Echocardiography

Doppler echocardiography detects a frequency shift that reflects the direction and velocity of blood flow. Doppler echocardiography is used to detect valvular insufficiency or stenosis and abnormal flow patterns.

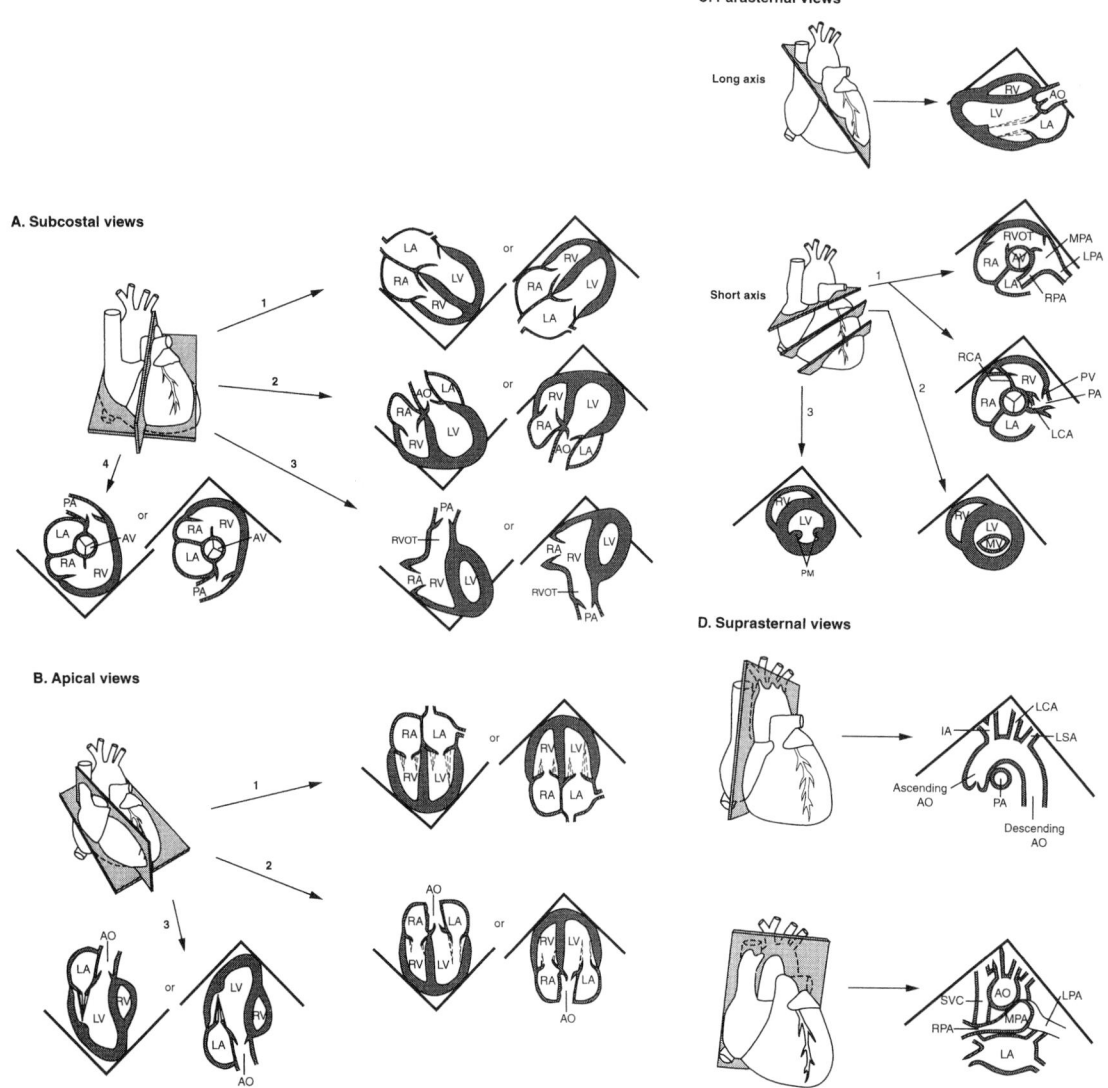

FIGURE 6. Echocardiographic series. The numbers represent different planes along a sweep of the echocardiographic beam. A: Subcostal views. B: Apical views. C: Parasternal views. D: Suprasternal views. AO, aorta; AV, aortic valve; IA, innominate artery; LA, left atrium; LCA, left coronary artery; LPA, left pulmonary artery; LSA, left subclavian artery; MPA, main pulmonary artery; MV, mitral valve; PA, pulmonary artery; PM, papillary muscle; PV, pulmonary valve; RA, right atrium; RCA, right coronary artery; RPA, right pulmonary artery; RV, right ventricle; RVOT, right ventricular outflow tract; SVC, superior vena cava. (Modified from Park MK. Pediatric cardiology for practitioners, 3rd ed. St. Louis: Mosby-Year Book, 1996:70–73, with permission).

Cardiology Laboratory

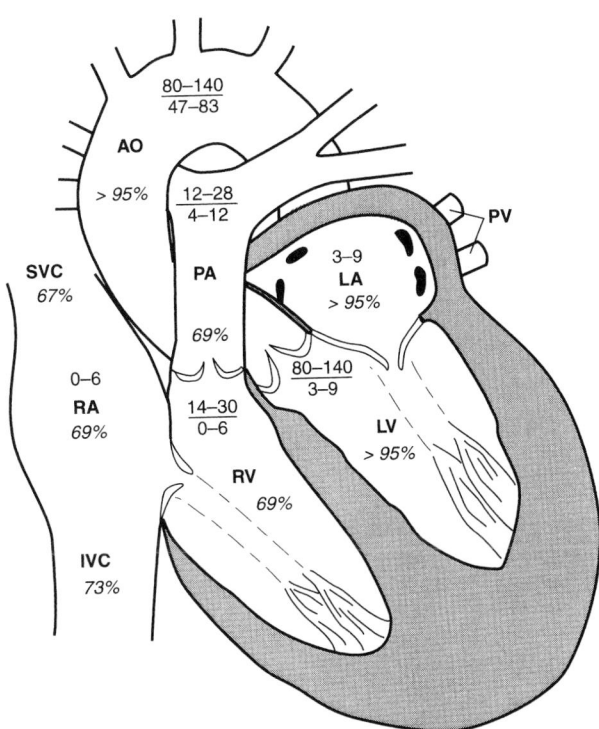

FIGURE 7. Normal pressures (systolic over diastolic, in mmHg), mean pressures, and oxygen saturations for children during cardiac catheterization. The data are based on information compiled from healthy patients between the ages of 2 months and 20 years. AO, aorta; IVC, inferior vena cava; LA, left atrium; LV, left ventricle; PA, pulmonary artery; PV, pulmonary vein; RA, right atrium; RV, right ventricle; SVC, superior vena cava.

CARDIAC CATHETERIZATION

Cardiac catheterization allows sampling of oximetric and hemodynamic data. The normal pressures and oxygen saturations for children are shown in Figure 7. Cardiac catheterization, an invasive procedure, is often used in conjunction with angiography to confirm the diagnosis and physiology of acquired or congenital heart disease. The technique also has therapeutic applications, such as coil embolization of a patent ductus arteriosus, coil embolization of aortopulmonary collaterals, pulmonary artery angioplasty and stent placement, balloon valvuloplasty of semilunar valvular stenosis, and device closure of atrial and some ventricular septal defects.

Shunts

Data obtained from cardiac catheterization can be used to calculate the degree and direction of an intracardiac or extracardiac shunt. The calculation is based on the Fick principle, using oxygen as the indicator. The oxygen content equals the dissolved oxygen (which is usually negligible) plus the oxygen capacity [hemoglobin (g/dL) × 1.36 mL O2/dL × 10] multiplied by the oxygen saturation (as a percentage).

Flow (Q) is equal to the oxygen consumption divided by the arteriovenous oxygen content difference:

$Qp = VO2/PV - PA$
$Qs = VO2/AO - MV$
in which
Qp = pulmonary flow
Qs = systemic flow
VO_2 = oxygen consumption per unit time
PV = pulmonary venous oxygen content
PA = pulmonary arterial oxygen content
MV = mixed venous oxygen content
AO = systemic arterial (aorta) oxygen content
A shunt is calculated with the effective pulmonary blood flow (Qp eff):

$Qp\ eff = VO_2/PV - MV$

A left-to-right shunt is the pulmonary flow less the effective pulmonary flow (Qp – Qp eff), and a right-to-left shunt is the systemic flow less the effective pulmonary flow (Qs – Qp eff).

Resistance

Systemic and pulmonary vascular resistance can also be calculated using the catheterization data. This calculation is based on Ohm's law (resistance equals the pressure change across the vascular bed divided by flow):

$Rs = AO - RA/Qs$
$Rp = PA - LA/Qp$
in which
Rs = systemic resistance
Rp = pulmonary resistance
AO = mean systemic (aorta) pressure
RA = mean right atrial pressure
PA = mean pulmonary artery pressure
LA = mean left atrial pressure
A pulmonary resistance (Rp) of 2.5 Wood units or less is considered within the normal range; however, no vascular bed is static and variations in flow can affect the result obtained.

SECTION V

Surgical Glossary

Aaron E. Carroll and
Nahush A. Mokadam

aortopexy—a procedure in which the aorta is approximated to the anterior thoracic wall; for the treatment of tracheomalacia.

Bishop-Koop procedure—resection of a dilated loop of bowel proximal to meconium obstruction, with end-to-side anastomosis between the proximal bowel and obstructed loop, combined with end ileostomy; for the treatment of meconium ileus.

bladder augmentation—a procedure in which a portion of the intraabdominal gastrointestinal tract is used to increase the volume of the bladder.

Blalock-Taussig shunt—a procedure in which the subclavian artery is anastomosed to the pulmonary artery; for the temporary treatment of tetralogy of Fallot.

Boix-Ochoa procedure—restoration of the intraabdominal esophageal length, repair of the esophageal hiatus, fixation of the esophagus to the hiatus, and restoration of the angle of His; for the treatment of incompetent lower esophageal sphincter.

chordee correction—a procedure in which the corpus spongiosum is moved ventrally and the corpus cavernosa are approximated dorsally; for the treatment of chordee (abnormal penile curvature associated with epispadias or hypospadias).

Clatworthy mesocaval shunt—division of the common iliac veins and side-to-end anastomosis of the inferior mesenteric vein to the left renal vein; for the treatment of portal hypertension.

Cohen procedure—trigonal reimplantation of the ureter; for the treatment of vesicoureteral reflux.

colonic conduit diversion—a procedure involving two stages: (1) a loop diversion using a colonic segment, and (2) an end-to-side anastomosis of the colonic segment to the gastrointestinal tract.

colonic interposition—replacement of the esophagus with a colonic segment; for treatment of esophageal atresia or stricture when gastric mobilization is not feasible.

diaphragmatic plication—surgical shortening of the diaphragm (abdominal, transthoracic, or bilateral); for the treatment of diaphragmatic eventration.

distal splenorenal shunt—see **Warren shunt**.

Drapanas mesocaval shunt—prosthetic graft implantation from the inferior mesenteric vein to the inferior vena cava; for the treatment of portal hypertension.

Duckett transverse preputial island flap—technique in which a flap of foreskin is used to elongate the urethra; for the treatment of hypospadias.

Duhamel procedure—resection of the aganglionic colon above the dentate line with

stable anastomosis to the rectal stump, normally performed in children 6 to 12 months of age for the treatment of Hirschsprung disease (see **Martin modification**).

end-to-side portocaval shunt—procedure in which the portal vein is divided and anastomosed to the inferior vena cava; for the treatment of portal hypertension.

esophagectomy—resection of the esophagus, with gastric pull-up and anastomosis with the cervical esophagus; for the treatment of esophageal atresia or stricture.

Fontan procedure—a procedure in which a graft is created to connect the pulmonary artery to the right atrium; for the treatment of hyperplastic right heart syndrome.

Glenn shunt—a shunt from the superior vena cava to the pulmonary artery; for the treatment of tricuspid atresia or stenosis.

gridiron incision—see **McBurney incision**.

Hegman procedure—surgical release of the tarsal, metatarsal, and intertarsal ligaments; for the treatment of metatarsus adductus.

Heller myotomy—myotomy of the anterior lower esophagus (always accompanied by a Thal fundoplication); for the treatment of achalasia.

ileal loop diversion—resection and implantation of ureters into an isolated ileal segment, with an ileal stoma and primary anastomosis of ileum to cecum.

ileal ureter—ileal interposition between the renal pelvis and bladder when the ureteral length is insufficient for anastomosis; for the treatment of urinary obstruction.

ileocecal conduit diversion—bilateral ureteral diversion and anastomosis to an isolated ileocecal segment and cecostomy with primary anastomosis of ileum to the right colon.

J-pouch—creation of an ileal reservoir in the distal ileum using a J-shaped configuration; used following colectomy.

Jateene procedure—arterial retransposition; for the treatment of transposition of the great vessels.

Kasai procedure—resection of atretic extrahepatic bile ducts and gallbladder with Roux-en-Y anastomosis of the jejunum to the remaining common hepatic duct; for the treatment of biliary atresia or other extrahepatic obstruction.

Kimura procedure (parasitized cecal patch)—a multistep operation in which (1) a side-to-side anastomosis is made with a portion of the distal ileum and the right colon, and (2) an ileoanal pull-through is performed; for the treatment of Hirschsprung disease.

King operation—resection of the knee with placement of a Küntscher rod to fix the femur to the tibia, followed by a Syme amputation

for the treatment of proximal focal femoral deficiency (PFFD).

Koch pouch diversion—a procedure involving bilateral ureteral diversion with anastomosis to a neobladder formed from an isolated ileal segment, combined with an ileal stoma and primary anastomosis of ileum to ileum.

Ladd operation—restoration of intestinal anatomy from a malrotated state; for the treatment of intestinal malrotation.

Lanz incision—an abdominal incision made in the left iliac fossa; for colostomy formation.

left hepatectomy—resection of the left hepatic lobe (medial and lateral segments).

Magpi procedure—distal advancement of the urethral meatus and granuloplasty; for the treatment of hypospadias.

Mainz pouch diversion—a procedure involving bilateral ureteral division with anastomosis to a neobladder formed from isolated cecum and terminal ileum; combined with an ileal stoma and primary anastomosis of the ileum to the right colon.

Martin modification (of Duhamel procedure)—right and transverse colectomy with ileoanal pull-through and side-to-side anastomosis of the remaining left colon to the ileum; procedure preserves some absorptive capacity of the large bowel; for the treatment of total colonic Hirschsprung disease.

McBurney (gridiron) incision—abdominal incision from the anterior superior iliac spine to the umbilicus; used for appendectomy.

Mikulicz procedure—a diverting enterostomy performed proximal to the meconium obstruction without resection; for the treatment of meconium ileus.

mini-Pena procedure—anterior sagittal anorectoplasty; for the treatment of anterior rectoperianal fistula (boys) or rectal-fourchette fistula (girls).

Mitrofanoff technique—a modification of neobladder diversion procedures, in which vascularized appendix is used to create the stoma.

Mustard technique—redirection of blood through an atrial septal defect (ASD) using a pericardial pathway; for the treatment of transposition of the great vessels; because of associated increased turbulence, this technique is not widely used today.

Mustarde procedure—correction, using simple mattress sutures, of a prominent ear with normal or absent antihelical folds.

Nissen fundoplication—a technique involving a 360° wrap of the gastric fundus around the gastroesophageal junction; for the treatment of incompetent lower esophageal sphincter; patient is rendered unable to vomit or belch.

Norwood procedure—a three-stage palliative procedure including (1) atrial septectomy, transection, and ligation of the pulmonary artery, "neoaorta" formation using the proximal pulmonary artery, and creation of a synthetic portoaortal shunt; (2) creation of a Glenn shunt; and (3) performance of a modified Fontan procedure; for the treatment of hypoplastic left heart syndrome.

onlay island flap—a technique in which a flap of foreskin is used to elongate the urethra; for the treatment of hypospadias.

orchidopexy—testicular pull-down and attachment; for the treatment of undescended testis.

orthoplasty—surgical correction of excessive penile curvature.

parasitized cecal patch—see **Kimura procedure**.

Pena procedure—posterior sagittal anorectoplasty performed in children 1 to 6 months of age; for the treatment of imperforate anus.

Pfannenstiel incision—an abdominal incision used to gain access to the lower abdomen and bring pelvic organs within reach without dividing muscular tissue.

pharyngoplasty—elevation of the posterior pharyngeal wall following a primary cleft palate repair (to narrow the pharyngeal space); for the treatment of velopharyngeal incompetence.

Potts shunt—anastomosis of the descending aorta to the pulmonary artery for the permanent treatment of tetralogy of Fallot.

proximal splenorenal shunt—end-to-side anastomosis of the splenic vein to the left renal vein with splenectomy; for the treatment of portal hypertension.

pyeloplasty—resection of an atretic ureter with primary anastomosis to the renal pelvis; for the treatment of ureteropelvic junction obstruction.

Ramstedt operation—relaxation of the pyloric sphincter; for the treatment of pyloric stenosis.

Rashkind procedure—balloon atrial septostomy; for the treatment of palliation of the great vessels.

Rastelli repair—a technique involving the closure of a ventricular septal defect (VSD) with a patch and the creation of a conduit from the distal pulmonary artery to the right ventricle; for the treatment of transposition of the great vessels.

Ravitch procedure—a procedure involving (1) creation of osteotomies between the manubrium and costal cartilages, (2) a greenstick fracture of the manubrium, and (3) the temporary insertion (for 6 to 12 months) of a stabilizing bar; for the treatment of pectus excavatum or pectus carinatum.

right colon pouch—a procedure involving bilateral ureteral division with anastomosis to a neobladder (formed from an isolated segment of the right colon), combined with an ileal stoma and primary anastomosis of the ileum to the transverse colon.

right hepatectomy—resection of the right hepatic lobes (anterior and posterior segments).

rooftop (bilateral subcostal) incision—an abdominal incision used to access the liver and portal structures.

Roux-en-Y anastomosis—division of the jejunum distal to the ligament of Treitz with end-to-side anastomosis of the duodenum to the distal jejunum and anastomosis of the proximal jejunum (typically) to the bile duct.

S-pouch—the creation of an ileal reservoir in the distal ileum using an S-shaped configuration following colectomy.

Santulli-Blanc enterostomy—a modification of the Bishop-Koop procedure that involves the resection of a distal dilated bowel segment with side-to-end anastomosis to the proximal enterostomy; for the treatment of meconium ileus.

Senning procedure (venous switch)—technique involving intraatrial redirection of venous return so that systemic caval return is shunted through the mitral valve to the left ventricle, and pulmonary return is brought through the tricuspid valve to the right ventricle; for the treatment of transposition of the great vessels.

side-to-side portocaval shunt—a procedure in which the portal vein is anastomosed to the inferior vena cava; for the treatment of portal hypertension.

side-to-side splenorenal shunt—side-to-side anastomosis of the splenic vein to the left renal vein; for the treatment of portal hypertension.

Sistrunk operation—complete excision of a thyroglossal duct cyst.

Soave procedure—a technique involving endorectal pull-through; for the correction of rectal resection.

Stamm gastrostomy—placement of an open gastrostomy tube; the opening is designed to close spontaneously on removal of the tube.

Sting procedure—subureteric Teflon injection; for the endoscopic correction of vesicoureteral reflux.

Sugiura procedure—a technique that involves lower esophageal transection and primary anastomosis, devascularization of the lower esophagus and stomach, and splenectomy; for the treatment of esophageal varices.

Swenson procedure—resection of the posterior rectal wall to the dentate line

(aganglionic region); for the treatment of Hirschsprung disease; technically difficult and rarely performed.

Syme amputation—amputation of the foot, calculated to bring the end of the stump above the opposite knee at maturity; for the treatment of proximal focal femoral deficiency (PFFD).

Thal procedure—a procedure involving a 180° anterior wrap of the gastric fundus around the gastroesophageal junction, preserving the patient's ability to vomit and belch; for the treatment of incompetent lower esophageal sphincter.

Thiersch operation—a procedure in which a distal rectal segment that has prolapsed is approximated to the external sphincter muscle; for the treatment of rectal prolapse.

trisegmentectomy—resection of the right hepatic lobe and the quadrate lobe of the liver (right posterior segment, right anterior segment, and medial segment).

ureteropyelostomy—partial resection and side-to-side anastomosis of a partially duplicated ureter.

uretocalycostomy—a technique for the treatment of urinary obstruction involving division of the ureter (distal to the obstruction) and intrarenal anastomosis to the most dependent renal calyx; when the renal pelvis is insufficient for anastomosis, the lower pole of the kidney is resected.

vaginal switch operation—a procedure in which the vagina is separated from the urinary tract; for treatment of duplicated vagina.

Van Ness procedure—rotational 180° osteotomy of the femur in which the foot and ankle are brought to the level of the opposite knee; for prosthetic attachment for the treatment of femoral deficiency.

venous switch—see **Senning procedure**.

ventricular shunt procedure—a procedure in which a Silastic catheter is positioned in a lateral ventricle and tunneled subcutaneously to drain into the central venous system or peritoneal cavity; for the treatment of hydrocephalus

Warren (distal splenorenal) shunt—a procedure in which the splenic vein is anastomosed to the left renal vein; for the treatment of portal hypertension.

Waterston aortopulmonary anastomosis—a procedure involving anastomosis of the ascending aorta and the right pulmonary artery; for the temporary treatment of tetralogy of Fallot.

Whipple procedure—resection of the pancreatic head, duodenum, and gallbladder with gastrojejunostomy, hepatojejunostomy, and pancreaticojejunostomy.

SECTION VI

Laboratory Values

Henry R. Drott

Laboratory Values

Laboratory Values

% Saturation	20%–40%
Absolute B_1 count	76–462/μL
Absolute lymphocytecount (ALC)	1,266–3,022/μL
Absolute T3	919–2,419/μL
Absolute T4	614–1,447/μL
Absolute T8	267–1,133/μL
Absolute T11	1,025–2,587/μL
Acetaminophen	10–20 μg/mL
Acid phosphatase total	2–10 U/L
Alanine aminotransferase (ALT)	5–45 U/L
Albumin	3.7–5.6 g/dL
Aldolase	<6 U/L
Alkaline phosphatase (AP)	130–560 U/L
Alpha$_1$-antitrypsin	210–500 mg/dL
Alpha-fetoprotein (AFP)	0.6–5.6 ng/mL
Amikacin	
Peak	20–30 μg/mL
Trough	0–10 μg/mL
Ammonia	9–33 μmol/L
Amylase	30–100 U/L
Anion gap	7–20 mmol/L
Antithrombin III	91%–128%
Apolipoprotein A-I	102–215 mg/dL
Apolipoprotein B	45–125 mg/dL
Aspartate aminotransferase	
Newborn	35–140 U/L
Child	10–60 U/L
B_1 (TotalBcells)	4%–21%
Bands	0%–4%
Bicarbonate	20–26 mEq/L
Bilirubin	
$\delta\gamma$	0.3–0.6 mg/dL
Neonatal	2.0–12.0 mg/dL
Total	0.6–1.4 mg/dL
Unconjugated	0.2–1.0 mg/dL
Blasts	0%
Caffeine	5–20 μg/mL
Calcium	8.9–10.7 mg/dL
Ionized	1.12–1.30 mmol/L
Stool	0–640 mg/24 h
Carbon dioxide	20–26 mmol/L
Carboxyhemoglobin	0%–2%
CD3+ and CD8+	17.4%–34.2%
CD14+	0%–10%
CD45+ and CD14–	90%–100%
Ceruloplasmin	23–48 mg/dL
CH50	104–356 U/mL
Chloramphenicol	5–20 μg/mL
Chloride	96–106 mmol/L
Sweat	0–40 mmol/L
Cholesterol	111–220 mg/dL
High-density lipoprotein (HDL)	35–82 mg/dL
Low-density lipoprotein (LDL)	59–137 mg/dL
Complement	
C3	
Newborn	67–161 mg/dL
Child	90–187 mg/dL
C4	16–45 mg/dL
Copper	67–147 μg/dL

Laboratory Values (continued)

Cortisol	
AM	10–25 μg/dL
PM	2–10 μg/dL
C-reactive protein (CRP), quantitative	0–1.2 mg/dL
Creatine kinase	
<age 1 year	60–305 U/L
>age 1 year	60–365 U/L
Creatinine	0.6–1.2 mg/dL
Cryoglobulin	
C3	0.0–0.028 mg/dL
IgA	0.0–0.026 mg/dL
IgG	0.0–0.157 mg/dL
IgM	0.0–0.224 mg/dL
Cyclosporin A	150–400 μg/L
Digoxin	0.5–2.0 ng/mL
DNA binding	0–149 IU/mL
D-Xylose, posttest	36–63 mg/dL (25-g dose)
Erythr ocyte sedimentation rate (ESR)	0–20 mm/h
Ethosuximide	25–100 μg/mL
Factor II assay	27%–108%
Factor V assay	50%–200%
Factor VII assay	50%–200%
Factor VIII assay	50%–200%
Factor IX assay	
Newborn	14.5%–58.0%
Child	50%–200%
Factor X assay	50%–200%
Factor XI assay	50%–200%
Ferritin	23–70 ng/mL
Fibrin split products	0–10 μg/mL
Fibrinogen	180–431 mg/dL
G-6-PD assay, quantitative	4.6–13.5 U/gHb
γ-Glutamyltransferase (GGT)	14–26 U/L
Gentamicin	
Peak	4–10 μg/mL
Trough	0–2 μg/mL
Glucose	75–110 mg/dL
CSF	32–82 mg/dL
Whole blood	60–115 mg/dL
Ham test	
Acidified	0%–1%
Unacidified	0%–1%
Haptoglobin	13–163 mg/dL
Hematocrit	36%–46%
Spun	36%–41%
Hemoglobin	13.5–17.0 g/dL
A_1C	3.8%–5.9%
Total	
Newborn	10–18 g/dL
Child	12–16.0 g/dL
HbA$_2$, quantitative	1.8%–3.6%
HbF, quantitative	0%–1.9%
Immunoglobulin A	
Newborn	0–5 mg/dL
Infant	27–169 mg/dL
Child	70–486 mg/dL

Continued

Laboratory Values (continued)

NORMAL LABORATORY VALUES

Immunoglobulin E	
Newborn	0–15 IU/mL
Child	0–200 IU/mL
Immunoglobulin G	
CSF	0.5–6 mg/dL
Child	635–1,775 mg/dL
Immunoglobulin M	
Child	71–237 mg/dL
Iron	50–180 μg/dL
Urine	0–2.0 mg/24h
Iron-binding capacity	250–420 μg/dL
Lactate	
CSF	0–3.3 mmol/L
Plasma	0.6–2.0 mmol/L
Lactate dehydrogenase (LDH)	340–670 U/L
Latex IgE	0–20 U
Lead, blood	0–10.0 μg/dL
Lipase	25–110 U/L
Lyme antibodies (IgG/IgM)	0.00–0.79
Magnesium	1.5–2.5 mg/dL
Mean corpuscular hemoglobin (MCH)	26.0–34.0 pg
Mean corpuscular volume (MCV)	80.0–100.0 μm^3
Mean platelet volume	7.4–10.4 fl
Methemoglobin	0.0%–1.9%
Netilmicin	
Peak	5–10 μg/mL
Trough	0–2 μg/mL
Osmolality	
Urine	
Newborn	50–645 mOsm/kg
Child	50–1,500 mOsm/kg
Whole blood	275–296 mOsm/kg
Partial thromboplastin time	25.0–38.0 seconds
Peroxide hemolysis	0%–20%
Phenobarbital	15–40 μg/mL
Phenytoin	10–20 μg/mL
Phosphorus	2.7–4.7 mg/dL
Platelet aggregation, 10 μm	>60.1%
Platelet count	150–400 10^3/μL
Potassium	3.8–5.4 mmol/L
Prealbumin	22.0–45.0 mg/dL
Primidone	5–12 μg/mL
Procainamide	4–10 μg/mL
Prolactin	2.7–15.2 ng/mL
Protein, 24-hour total	0–150 mg/24h
Protein C	
Immunologic	50%–122%
Functional	59%–116%
Protein S, free	40%–111%

Laboratory Values (continued)

NORMAL LABORATORY VALUES

Protein, total	6.3–8.6 g/dL
Prothrombin time	10–12 seconds
Protoporphyrin, free RBC	30–80 μmol/mol Hb
Pyruvate kinase assay	1.8–2.3 IU/mLRBC
RBC distribution width	11.5%–14.5%
Reptilase	18–22 seconds
Reticulocyte count	0.5%–1.5%
Ristocetin cofactor	48%–220%
Salicylate	<35 mg/dL
Sodium	136–145 mmol/L
Sucrose hemolysis	0%–5%
T3 (total T cells)	69%–86%
T4 (helper T cells)	39%–57%
T4–T8 ratio	0.7–2.5
T8 (suppressor T cells)	18%–45%
T11 (SRBC receptor)	75%–93%
Theophylline	10–20 μg/mL
Thrombin time	11.3–16.3 seconds
Thyroid-stimulating hormone (thyrotropin)	0.5–5.0 μIU/mL
Thyroxine	
Newborn	3.0–14.4 μg/dL
Infant	4.6–13.4 μg/dL
Child	4.5–10.3 μg/dL
Thyroxine-binding globulin	1.8–4.2 mg/dL
Tobramycin	
Peak	4–10 μg/mL
Trough	0–2 μg/mL
Total cell count	100
Total eosinophil count	100–300 mm^3
Total protein	
CSF	
Newborn	40–120 mg/dL
Child	15–40 mg/dL
Urine	0–20 mg/dL
Triglycerides	34–165 mg/dL
Triiodothyronine	0.9–2.25 ng/mL
Trypsin, stool	80–740 μg/g
Urea nitrogen	2–19 mg/dL
Uric acid	2.1–5.0 mg/dL
Urine pH	4.8–7.8
Urine specific gravity; TS meter	1.003–1.1035
Valproic acid	50–100 μg/mL
Vancomycin	
Peak	20–30 μg/mL
Trough	0–12 μg/mL
White blood cell count	
Newborn	9–30 10^3/μL
Child	4.5–11.0 10^3/μL
Zinc	68–94 μg/dL

SECTION VII
Tables

Charles Schwartz

DEVELOPMENT

Table 1   Scoring System: Draw-a-Person Test

ONE POINT ASSIGNED PER FEATURE:

Head present
Neck present
Neck, two dimensions
Eyes present
Eye detail: brows or lashes
Nose present
Nose, two dimensions
  (not round ball)
Mouth present
Lips, two dimensions
Both nose and lips in two
  dimensions
Both chin and forehead shown
Bridge of nose (straight to eyes;
  narrower than base)
Hair I (any scribble)
Hair II (more detail)
Ears present

Fingers present
Correct number of fingers shown
Opposition of thumb shown
  (must include fingers)
Hands present
Arms present
Arms at side or engaged in activity
Feet: any indication
Attachment of arms to legs I
  (to trunk or anywhere)
Attachment of arms and legs II
  (at correct point on trunk)
Trunk present
Trunk in proportion, two dimensions
  (if greater than breadth)
Clothing I (anything)
Clothing II (two articles of clothing)

MENTAL AGE (YR)	POINTS SCORED BY BOYS	POINTS SCORED BY GIRLS
3	4	5
4	7	7
5	11	11
6	13	14
7	16	17
8	18	20

Table 1—*Continued*.   Receptive Language Development

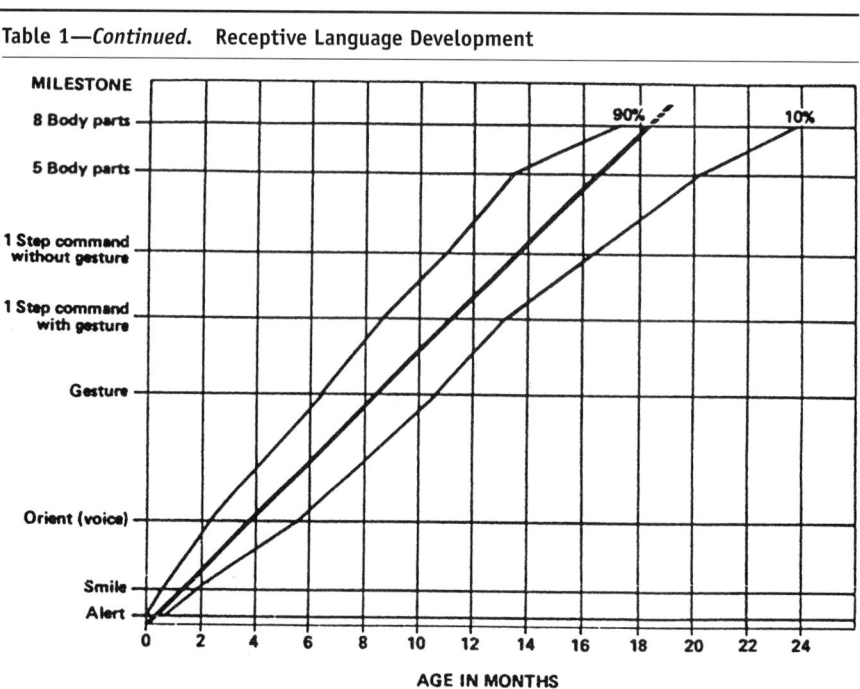

Table 1—*Continued*.   Expressive Language Development

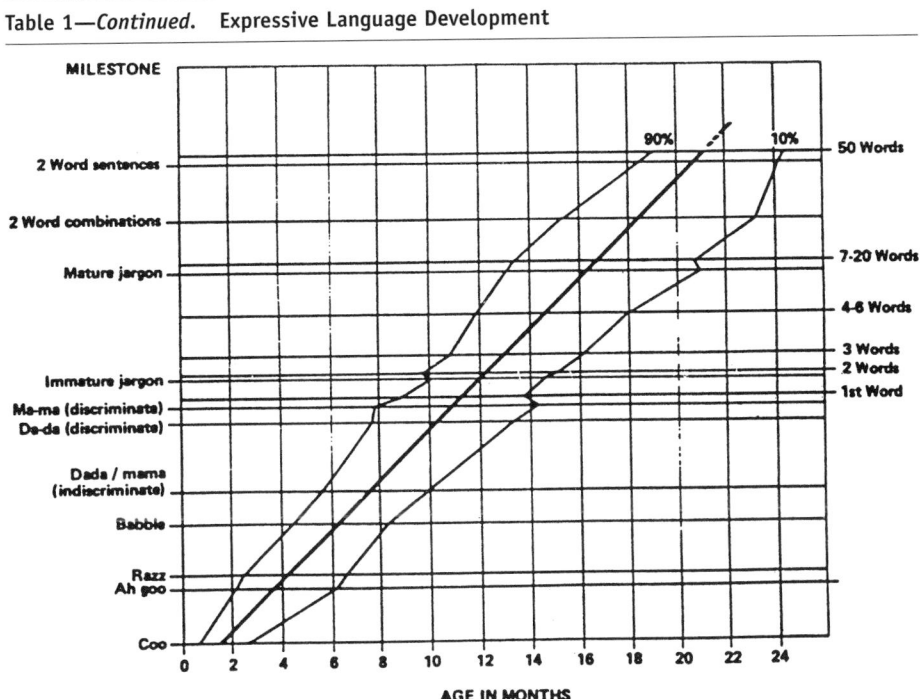

Table 2   Developmental Milestones from Birth to 5 Years

AGE (MONTHS)	ADAPTIVE/FINE MOTOR	LANGUAGE	GROSS MOTOR	PERSONAL–SOCIAL
1	Grasp reflex (hands fisted)	Facial response to sounds	Lifts head in prone position	Stares at face
2	Follows object with eyes past midline	Coos (vowel sounds)	Lifts head in prone position to 45°	Smiles in response to others
4	Hands open	Laughs and squeals	Sits: head steady	Smiles spontaneously
	Brings objects to mouth	Turns toward voice	Rolls to supine	
6	Palmar grasp of objects	Babbles (consonant sounds)	Sits independently	Reaches for toys
			Stands, hands held	Recognizes strangers
			Pulls to stand	
9	Pincer grasp	Says "mama," "dada" nonspecifically, comprehends "no"	Pulls to stand	Feeds self
				Waves bye-bye
				Points to indicate wants
12	Helps turn pages of book	2–4 words	Stands independently	
		Follows command with gesture	Walks, one hand held	
15	Scribbles	4–6 words	Walks independently	Drinks from cup
		Follows command no gesture		Imitates activities
18	Turns pages of book	10–20 words	Walks up steps	Feeds self with spoon
		Points to 4 body parts		
24	Solves single-piece puzzles	Combines 2–3 words	Jumps	Removes coat
		Uses "I" and "you"	Kicks ball	Verbalizes wants
30	Imitates horizontal and vertical lines	Names all body parts	Rides tricycle using pedals	Pulls up pants
				Washes, dries hands
36	Copies circle	Gives full name, age, and sex	Throws ball overhand	Toilet trained
	Draws person with 3 parts	Names 2 colors	Walks up stairs (alternating feet)	Puts on shirt, knows front from back
42	Copies cross	Understands "cold," "tired," "hungry"	Stands on one foot for 2–3 sec	Engages in associative play
48	Counts 4 objects	Understands prepositions (under, on, behind, in front of)	Hops on one foot	Dresses with little assistance
	Identifies some numbers and letters	Asks "how" and "why"		Shoes on correct feet
54	Copies square	Understands opposites	Broad-jumps 24 inches	Bosses and criticizes
	Draws person with 6 parts			Shows off
60	Prints first name	Asks meaning of words	Skips (alternating feet)	Ties shoes
	Counts 10 objects			

Table 2A   Causes of Failure to Thrive

AGE AT ONSET	DIAGNOSTIC CONSIDERATIONS
Before birth (IUGR, prematurity)	Especially in "symmetric" IUGR, consider prenatal infections, congenital syndromes, teratogenic exposures (anticonvulsants, alcohol, etc.)
Neonatal	Incorrect formula preparation; failed breast-feeding; neglect; poor feeding interactions; metabolic, chromosomal, or anatomic abnormality (less common)
3–6 months	Underfeeding (possibly associated with poverty); improper formula preparation; milk protein intolerance; oral-motor dysfunction; celiac disease; HIV infection; cystic fibrosis; congenital heart disease; GE reflux
7–12 months	Autonomy struggles; overly fastidious parent; oral-motor dysfunction; delayed introduction of solids; intolerance of new foods
After 12 months	Coercive feeding; highly distractable child; distracting environment; acquired illness; new psychosocial stressor (divorce, job loss, new sibling, death in the family, etc.)

Reproduced from Frank DA, et al., with permission from the authors.

Table 3   Primitive Reflexes

PRIMITIVE REFLEX	AGE AT DISAPPEARANCE (MONTHS)	DESCRIPTION
Palmar grasp	3–4	Pressing against the palmar surface of the infant's hand results in flexion of all fingers.
Rooting	3–4	Stroking the perioral skin at the corners of the mouth causes the mouth to open and turn to stimulated side.
Galant	2–3	Stroking along the paravertebral area causes lateral flexion of the trunk with the concavity toward the stimulated side.
Moro	4–6	Sudden movement of the head causes symmetric abduction and extension of the arms followed by gradual adduction and flexion of the arms over the body.
Asymmetric tonic neck	4–6	Turning the head to one side leads to extension of extremities on that side and flexion on the contralateral side. This puts the infant in the fencing position.
Tonic labyrinthine	2–3	In supine neck extension leads to shoulder retraction and trunk and lower extremity extension. This is reduced by neck flexion.
Positive support	2–3	Stimulation of the ball of the foot leads to co-contraction of opposing muscle groups, allowing weight to be borne.
Placing/stepping	Variable	When the dorsal surface of one foot touches the underside of a table, the infant places the foot on the table top.

Table 4   Penile and Clitoral Length in the Newborn Infant

GESTATIONAL AGE	LENGTH (MEAN ± SD) (CM)
Male Measure from pubic ramus to the tip of the glans with gentle traction applied.[a]	
30 wk	2.5 ± 0.4
34 wk	3.0 ± 0.4
Term	3.5 ± 0.4
Female Measure with labia majora separated and the prepuce skin retracted.[b]	
Term Infants	4.0 ± 1.24
Preterm infants—The clitoris achieves full size by 24 wk gestation and may appear more prominent relative to the labia in premature infants.	

[a] Feldman KW, Smith DW. Fetal phallic growth and penile standards for newborn male infants. *J Pediatr* 1975;86:395.

[b] Oberfield S, Mondok A, Shanrivar F, et al. Clitoral size in full-term infants. *Am J Perinatol* 1989;6(4):453.

Table 5   Tanner Stages in the Female

STAGE	BREAST	PUBIC HAIR
1	Prepubertal, elevation of papilla only	Prepubertal
2	Enlargement of areola, elevation of breast and papilla ("breast bud")	Sparse, long, straight, slightly pigmented hair along labia
3	Further enlargement of breast and areola with no separation of contour	Hair is darker, curlier, and coarser with increased distribution on pubes
4	Areola and papilla form a second mount above the breast	Adult-type hair limited to pubes with no extension to medial thigh
5	Mature breast	Mature distribution of inverse triangle with spread to medial thighs

Table 6   Tanner Stages in the Male

STAGE	GENITAL DEVELOPMENT	PUBIC HAIR
1	Prepubertal	Prepubertal
2	Enlargement of testes (>4 mL volume) and scrotum with reddening of scrotal skin	Sparse, long, straight, slightly pigmented hair at base of penis
3	Growth of penis, primarily length, with further increase in size of testes and scrotum	Hair is darker and curlier with increased distribution on pubes
4	Further increase in length and breadth of penis with development of glans, increase in testes and scrotum	Adult-type hair limited to pubes with no extension to medial thigh
5	Adult size and shape	Mature distribution with spread to medial thighs and lower abdomen

Table 7   Normal Growth Rates

AGE	EXPECTED GROWTH RATE
First year	25 cm (10 inches)/y
Second year	12.5 cm (5 inches)/y
Childhood	6.25 cm (2.5 inches)/y
Adolescence, boys	15–38 cm (6–15 inches)
Adolescence, girls	15–25 cm (6–12 inches)

Table 8   Head Growth Velocity

FULL-TERM		PRETERM	
2 cm/mo	0–3 months	1 cm/wk	0–2 months
1 cm/mo	3–6 months	0.5 cm/wk	2–4 months
0.5 cm/mo	7–12 months	See full-term	>4 months

Table 9   Illustrations of the Primary and Permanent Dentition. *A* and *B,* The numbers represent the average age of eruption for the teeth, indicated in months for the primary teeth and years for the permanent dentition. *C* and *D,* The names of specific teeth in the primary and permanent dentition are shown.

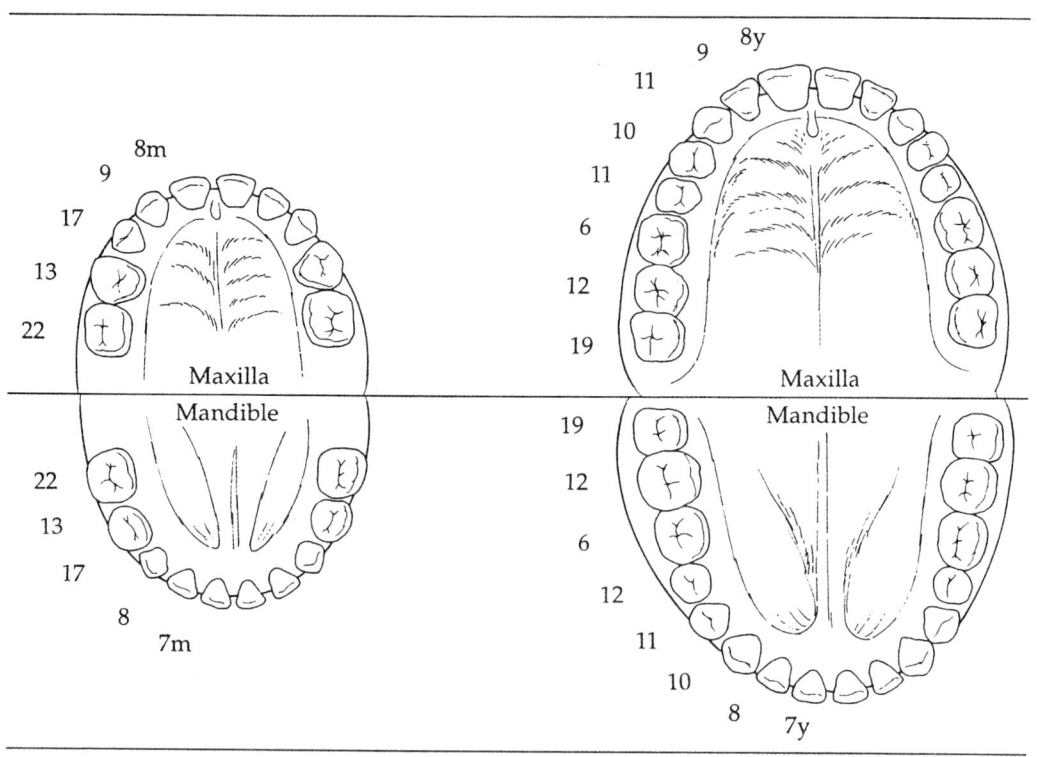

A. Primary Dentition   B. Permanent Dentition

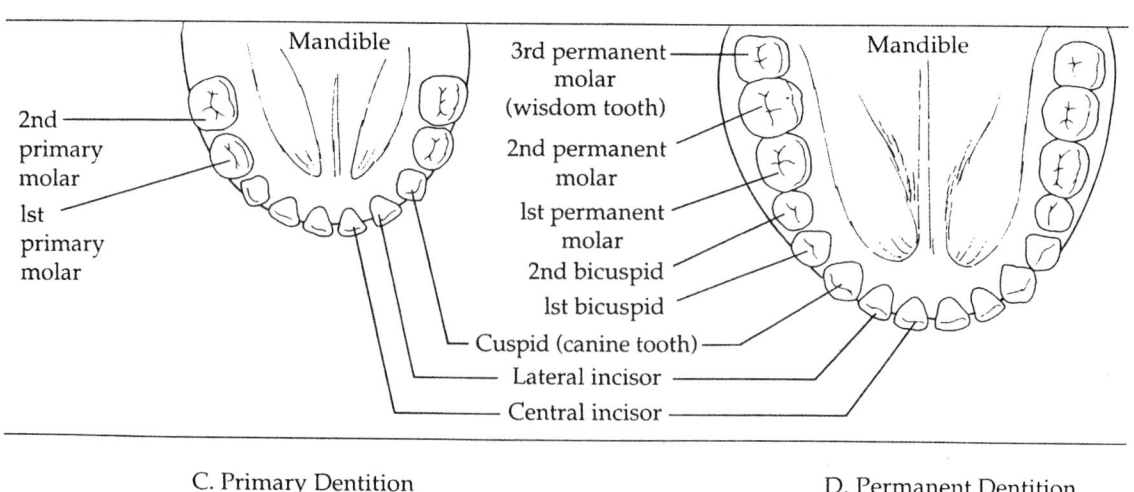

C. Primary Dentition   D. Permanent Dentition

Reproduced with permission from Nazif MM, Davis HW, McKibben DH, Roody MA. Arts of Pediatric Physical Diagnosis-3.

GROWTH CHART

Table 10

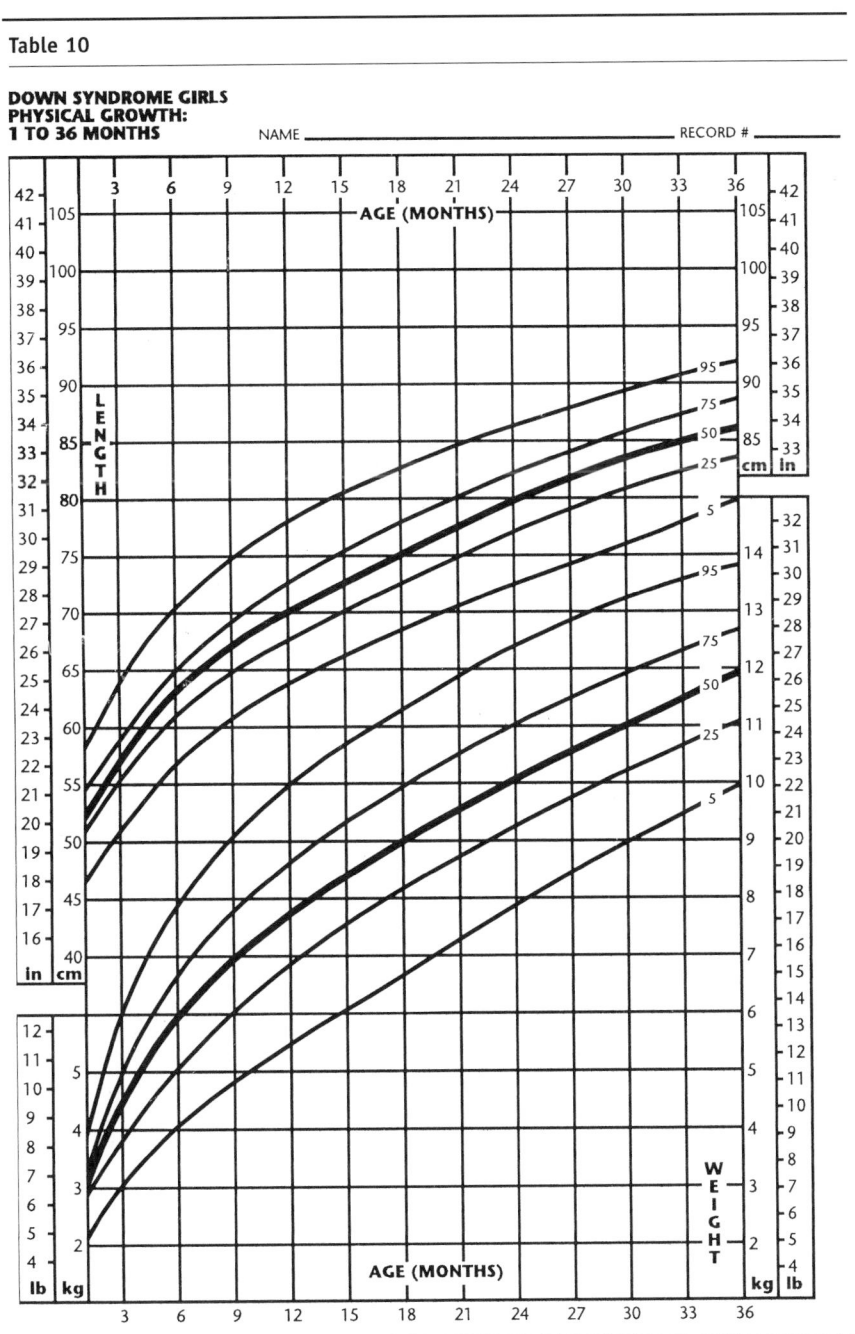

DOWN SYNDROME GIRLS PHYSICAL GROWTH: 1 TO 36 MONTHS

From Cronck C, Crocker AC, Pueschel SM, et al. Growth charts for children with Down syndrome: 1 month to 18 years of age. Pediatrics. 1988;81:102–110, with permission.

Table 10A

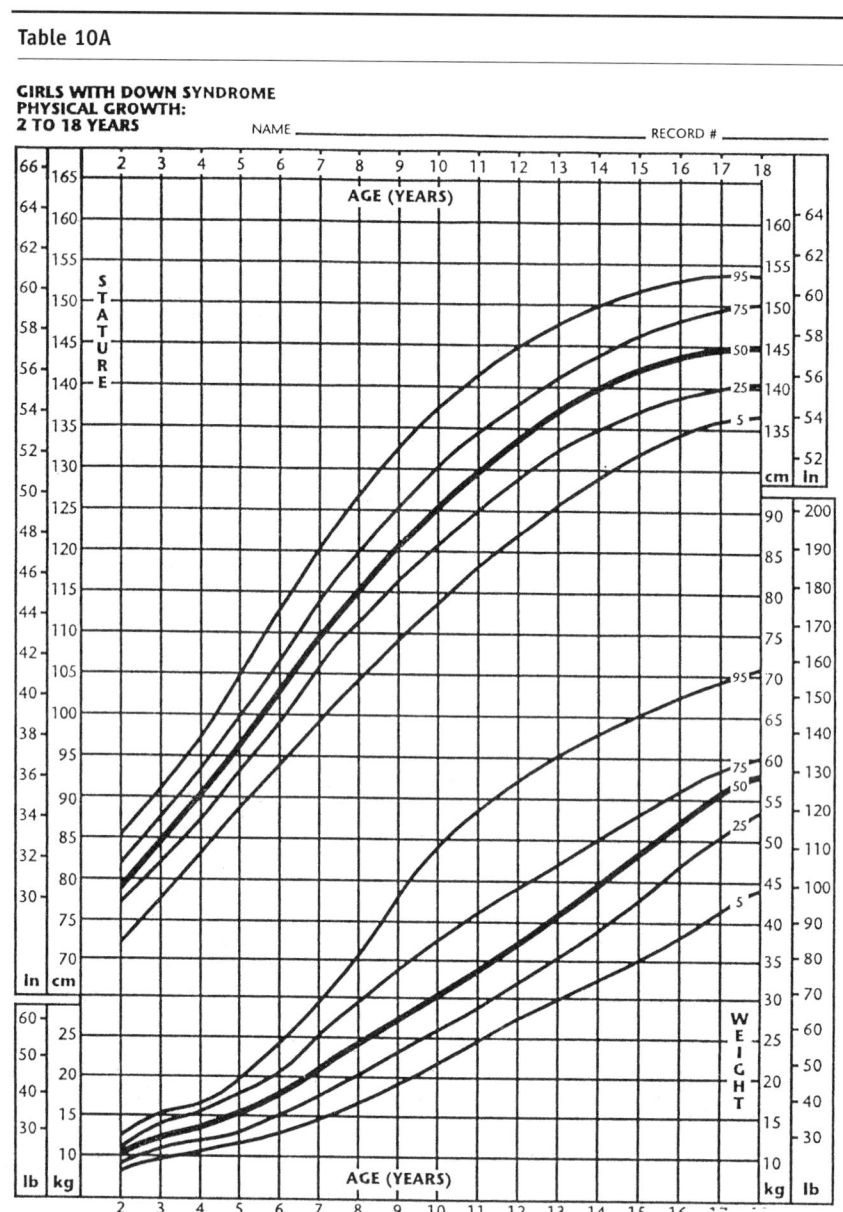

GIRLS WITH DOWN SYNDROME
PHYSICAL GROWTH:
2 TO 18 YEARS

From Cronck C, Crocker AC, Pueschel SM, et al. Growth charts for children with Down syndrome: 1 month to 18 years of age. Pediatrics. 1988;81:102–110, with permission.

Table 11

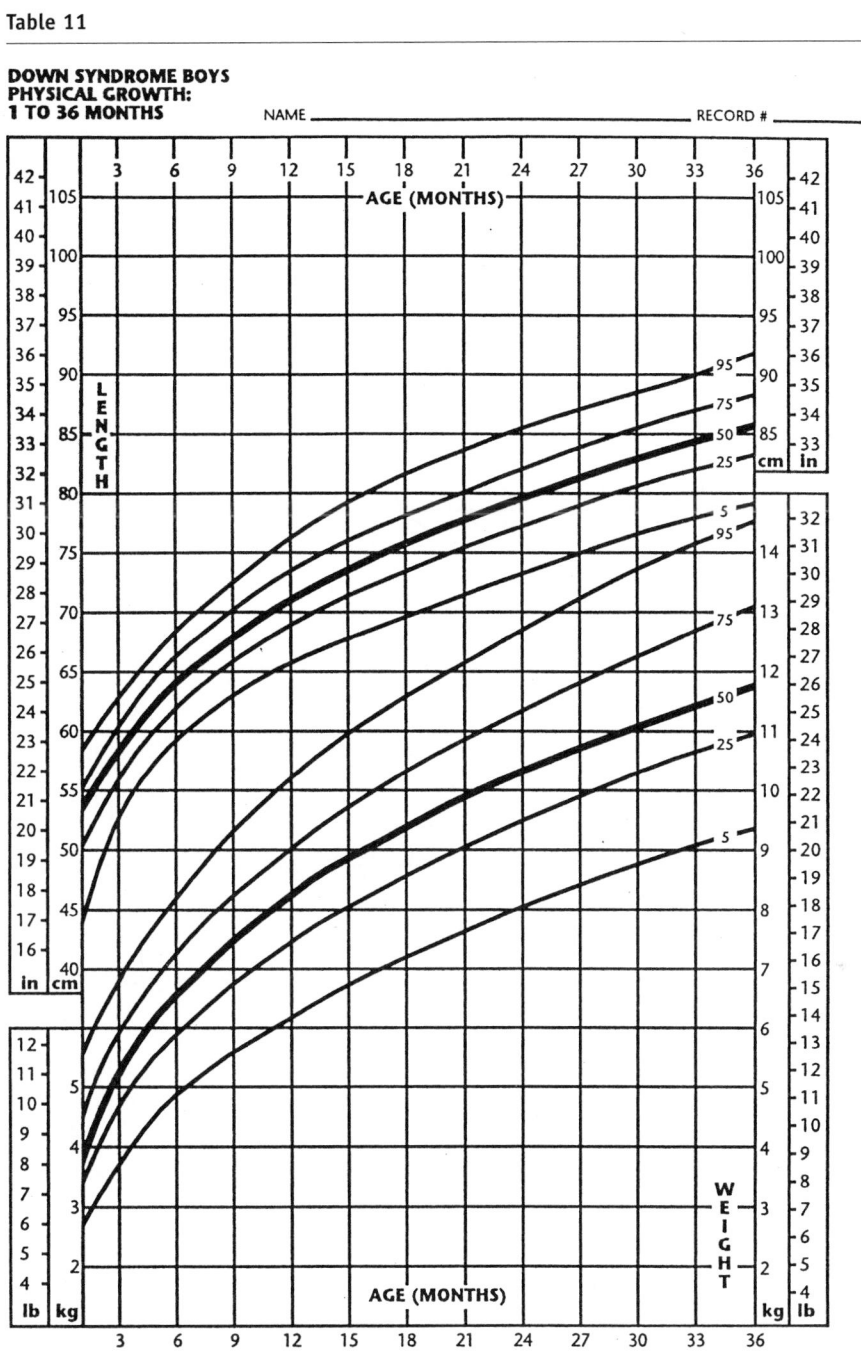

From Cronck C, Crocker AC, Pueschel SM, et al. Growth charts for children with Down syndrome: 1 month to 18 years of age. Pediatrics. 1988;81:102–110, with permission.

Table 11A

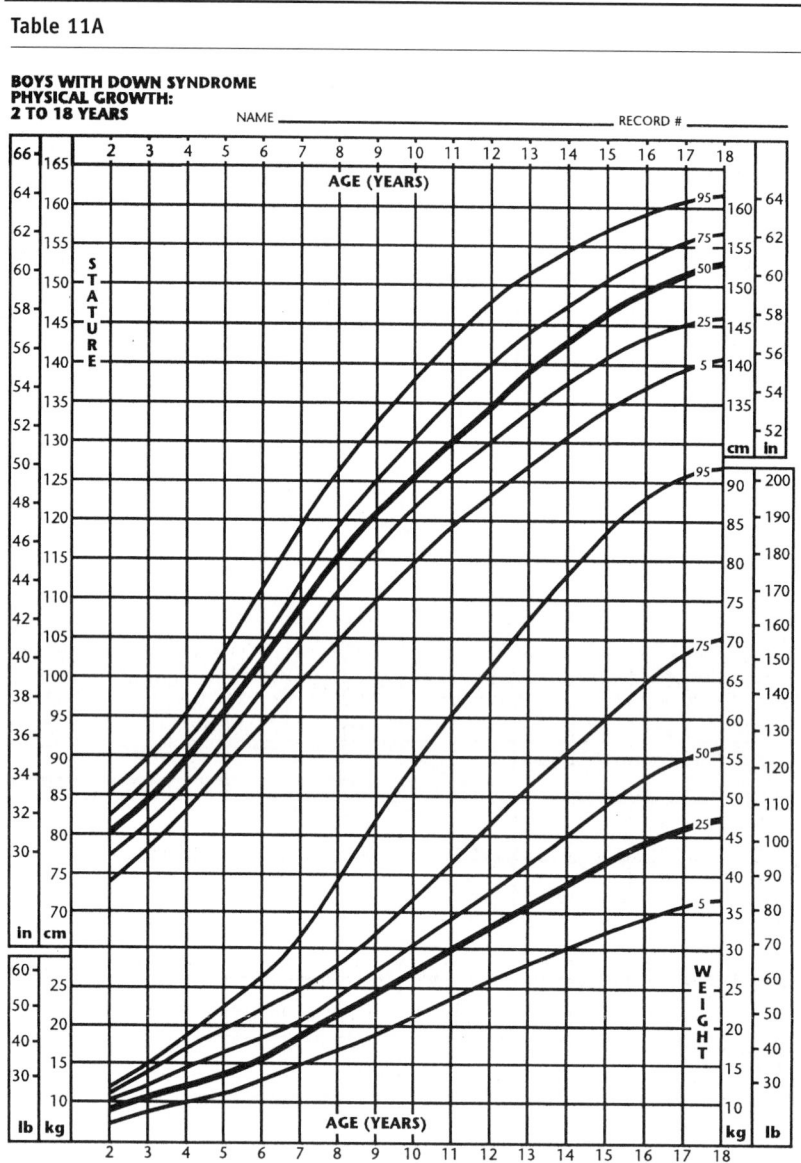

From Cronck C, Crocker AC, Pueschel SM, et al. Growth charts for children with Down syndrome:
1 month to 18 years of age. Pediatrics. 1988;81:102–110, with permission.

Table 12

Recommended Childhood and Adolescent Immunization Schedule
United States · July–December 2004

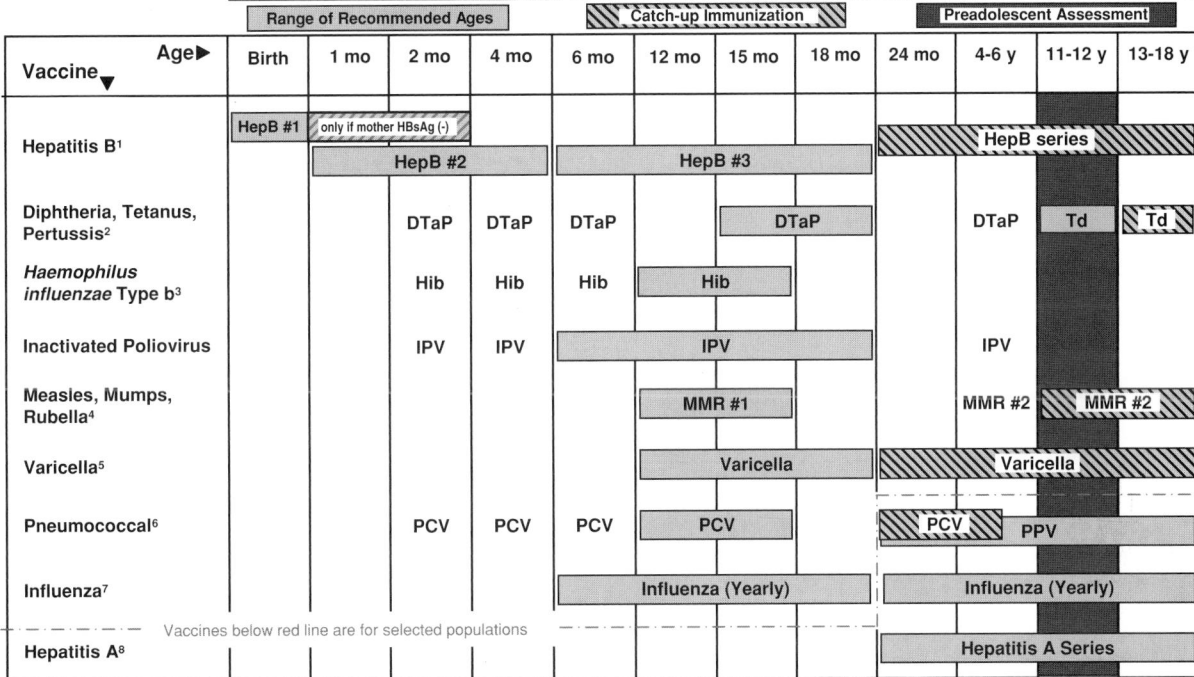

This schedule indicates the recommended ages for routine administration of currently licensed childhood vaccines, as of April 1, 2004, for children through age 18 years. Any dose not given at the recommended age should be given at any subsequent visit when indicated and feasible. ▨▨ Indicates age groups that warrant special effort to administer those vaccines not previously given. Additional vaccines may be licensed and recommended during the year. Licensed combination vaccines may be used whenever any components of the combination are indicated and the vaccine's other components are not contraindicated. Providers should consult the manufacturers' package inserts for detailed recommendations. Clinically significant adverse events that follow immunization should be reported to the Vaccine Adverse Event Reporting System (VAERS). Guidance about how to obtain and complete a VAERS form can be found on the Internet: www.vaers.org or by calling 800-822-7967.

1. Hepatitis B (HepB) vaccine. All infants should receive the first dose of hepatitis B vaccine soon after birth and before hospital discharge; the first dose may also be given by age 2 months if the infant's mother is hepatitis B surface antigen (HBsAg) negative. Only monovalent HepB can be used for the birth dose. Monovalent or combination vaccine containing HepB may be used to complete the series. Four doses of vaccine may be administered when a birth dose is given. The second dose should be given at least 4 weeks after the first dose, except for combination vaccines which cannot be administered before age 6 weeks. The third dose should be given at least 16 weeks after the first dose and at least 8 weeks after the second dose. The last dose in the vaccination series (third or fourth dose) should not be administered before age 24 weeks.

Infants born to HBsAg-positive mothers should receive HepB and 0.5 mL of Hepatitis B Immune Globulin (HBIG) within 12 hours of birth at separate sites. The second dose is recommended at age 1–2 months. The last dose in the immunization series should not be administered before age 24 weeks. These infants should be tested for HBsAg and antibody to HBsAg (anti-HBs) at age 9–15 months.

Infants born to mothers whose HBsAg status is unknown should receive the first dose of the HepB series within 12 hours of birth. Maternal blood should be drawn as soon as possible to determine the mother's HBsAg status; if the HBsAg test is positive, the infant should receive HBIG as soon as possible (no later than age 1 week). The second dose is recommended at age 1–2 months. The last dose in the immunization series should not be administered before age 24 weeks.

2. Diphtheria and tetanus toxoids and acellular pertussis (DTaP) vaccine. The fourth dose of DTaP may be administered as early as age 12 months, provided 6 months have elapsed since the third dose and the child is unlikely to return at age 15–18 months. The final dose in the series should be given at age ≥4 years. **Tetanus and diphtheria toxoids (Td)** is recommended at age 11–12 years if at least 5 years have elapsed since the last dose of tetanus and diphtheria toxoid-containing vaccine. Subsequent routine Td boosters are recommended every 10 years.

3. Haemophilus influenzae type b (Hib) conjugate vaccine. Three Hib conjugate vaccines are licensed for infant use. If PRP-OMP (PedvaxHIB or ComVax [Merck]) is administered at ages 2 and 4 months, a dose at age 6 months is not required. DTaP/Hib combination products should not be used for primary immunization in infants at ages 2, 4 or 6 months but can be used as boosters following any Hib vaccine. The final dose in the series should be given at age ≥12 months.

4. Measles, mumps, and rubella vaccine (MMR). The second dose of MMR is recommended routinely at age 4–6 years but may be administered during any visit, provided at least 4 weeks have elapsed since the first dose and both doses are administered beginning at or after age 12 months. Those who have not previously received the second dose should complete the schedule by the visit at age 11–12 years.

5. Varicella vaccine. Varicella vaccine is recommended at any visit at or after age 12 months for susceptible children (i.e., those who lack a reliable history of chickenpox). Susceptible persons age ≥13 years should receive 2 doses, given at least 4 weeks apart.

6. Pneumococcal vaccine. The heptavalent **pneumococcal conjugate vaccine (PCV)** is recommended for all children age 2–23 months. It is also recommended for certain children age 24–59 months. The final dose in the series should be given at age >12 months. **Pneumococcal polysaccharide vaccine (PPV)** is recommended in addition to PCV for certain high-risk groups. See *MMWR* 2000;49(RR-9):1-35.

7. Influenza vaccine. Influenza vaccine is recommended annually for children aged ≥6 months with certain risk factors (including but not limited to asthma, cardiac disease, sickle cell disease, HIV, and diabetes), healthcare workers, and other persons (including household members) in close contact with persons in groups at high risk (see *MMWR* 2004;53;[RR-6]:1-40) and can be administered to all others wishing to obtain immunity. In addition, healthy children aged 6–23 months and close contacts of healthy children aged 0–23 months are recommended to receive influenza vaccine, because children in this age group are at substantially increased risk for influenza-related hospitalizations. For healthy persons aged 5–49 years, the intranasally administered live, attenuated influenza vaccine (LAIV) is an acceptable alternative to the intramuscular trivalent inactivated influenza vaccine (TIV). See *MMWR* 2004;53;[RR-6]:1-40. Children receiving TIV should be administered a dosage appropriate for their age (0.25 mL if 6–35 months or 0.5 mL if ≥3 years). Children aged ≤8 years who are receiving influenza vaccine for the first time should receive 2 doses (separated by at least 4 weeks for TIV and at least 6 weeks for LAIV).

8. Hepatitis A vaccine. Hepatitis A vaccine is recommended for children and adolescents in selected states and regions and for certain high-risk groups; consult your local public health authority. Children and adolescents in these states, regions, and high-risk groups who have not been immunized against hepatitis A can begin the hepatitis A immunization series during any visit. The 2 doses in the series should be administered at least 6 months apart. See *MMWR* 1999;48(RR-12):1-37.

For additional information about vaccines, including precautions and contraindications for immunization and vaccine shortages, please visit the National Immunization Program Web site at www.cdc.gov/nip/ or call the National Immunization Information Hotline at 800-232-2522 (English) or 800-232-0233 (Spanish).

Approved by the Advisory Committee on Immunization Practices (www.cdc.gov/nip/acip), the American Academy of Pediatrics (www.aap.org), and the American Academy of Family Physicians (www.aafp.org).

Table 13   Recommendations for Routine Immunization of HIV-Infected Children in the United States

VACCINE	KNOWN ASYMPTOMATIC HIV INFECTION	SYMPTOMATIC HIV INFECTION
Hepatitis B	Yes	Yes
DTaP (or DTP)	Yes	Yes
IPV[a]	Yes	Yes
MMR	Yes	Yes[b]
Hib	Yes	Yes
Pneumococcal[c]	Yes	Yes
Influenza[d]	Yes	Yes
Varicella[e]	No	No

Adapted from the American Academy of Pediatrics. In Peter G, ed. *1997 red book: report of the Committee on Infectious Diseases*, 24th ed. Elk Grove Village, IL: American Academy of Pediatrics, 1997.

DTP, diphtheria and tetanus toxoids and pertussis vaccine; DTaP, diphtheria and tetanus toxoids acellular pertussis vaccine; IPV, inactivated poliovirus vaccine; MMR, live-virus measles, mumps, and rubella; Hib, *Haemophilus influenzue* type b conjugate.

[a] Only inactivated polio vaccine (IPV) should be used for HIV-infected children, HIV-exposed infants whose status is indeterminate, and household contacts of HIV-infected patients.

[b] Severely immunocompromised HIV-infected children should not receive MMR vaccine.

[c] Pneumococcal vaccine should be administered at 2 years of age to all HIV-infected children. Children who are older than 2 years of age should receive pneumococcal vaccine at the time of diagnosis. Revaccination after 3 to 5 years is recommended in either circumstance.

[d] Influenza vaccine should be provided each fall and repeated annually for HIV-exposed infants 6 months of age and older, HIV-infected children and adolescents, and for household contacts of HIV-infected patients.

[e] Varicella vaccine is not currently indicated for HIV-exposed or HIV-infected patients, but studies are in progress to determine safety and possible indication.

Table 14   Guide to Tetanus Prophylaxis in Routine Wound Management

HISTORY OF ABSORBED TETANUS TOXOID (DOSES)	CLEAN, MINOR WOUNDS		ALL OTHER WOUNDS[A]	
	TD[B]	TIG[C]	TD[B]	TIG[C]
Unknown or <3	Yes	No	Yes	Yes
≥3[d]	No[e]	No	No[f]	No

Adapted from the American Academy of Pediatrics. In Peter G, ed. *1997 red book: report of the Committee on Infectious Diseases*, 24th ed. Elk Grove Village, IL: American Academy of Pediatrics, 1997.

Td, adult-use tetanus and diphtheria toxoids; TIG, tetanus immune globulin (human).

[a] Such as, but not limited to, wounds contaminated with dirt, feces, soil, or saliva; puncture wounds; avulsions; and wounds resulting from missiles, crushing, burns, or frostbite.

[b] For children <7 years, diphtheria and tetanus toxoids and acellular pertussis (DTaP) or diphtheria-tetanus-pertussis (DTP) is recommended; if pertussis vaccine is contraindicated, diphtheria-tetanus toxoid (DT) is given. For persons ≥7 years of age, Td is recommended.

[c] Equine tetanus antitoxin should be used when TIG is not available.

[d] If only 3 doses of fluid toxoid have been received, a fourth dose of toxoid, preferably an adsorbed toxoid, should be given.

[e] Yes, if more than 10 years since the last dose.

[f] Yes, if more than 5 years since the last dose. (More frequent boosters are not needed and can accentuate side effects.)

Table 15 Suggested Intervals Between Immunoglobulin Administration and Measles Vaccination (MMR or Monovalent Measles Vaccine)

INDICATION FOR IMMUNOGLOBULIN	PREPARATION	ROUTE	DOSE U OR ML	DOSE MG IgG/KG	INTERVAL (MONTHS)[a]
Tetanus	TIG	IM	250 U	10	3
Hepatitis A prophylaxis	IG				
Contact prophylaxis		IM	0.02 mL/kg	3.3	3
International travel		IM	0.06 mL/kg	10	3
Hepatitis B prophylaxis	HBIG	IM	0.06 mL/kg	10	3
Rabies prophylaxis	RIG	IM	20 lU/kg	22	4
Measles prophylaxis	IG				
Standard		IM	0.25 mL/kg	40	5
Immunocompromised host		IM	0.50 mL/kg	80	6
Varicella prophylaxis	VZIG	IM	125 U/10 kg (maximum, 625 U)	20–39	5
Blood transfusion					
Washed RBCs		IV	10 mL/kg	Negligible	0
RBCs, adenine-saline added		IV	10 mL/kg	10	3
Packed RBCs		IV	10 mL/kg	20–60	5
Whole blood		IV	10 mL/kg	80–100	6
Plasma or platelet products		IV	10 mL/kg	160	7
Replacement (or therapy) of immune deficiencies	IGIV	IV	. . .	300–400	8
ITP	IGIV	IV	. . .	400	8
RSV	IGIV	IV	. . .	750	9
ITP		IV	. . .	1000	10
ITP or Kawasaki disease		IV	. . .	1600–2000	11

Adapted from the American Academy of Pediatrics. In: Peter G, ed. *1997 Red Book: Report of the Committee on Infectious Diseases.* 24th ed. Elk Grove Village, IL: American Academy of Pediatrics, 1997.

IG, immune globulin; IGIV, intravenous immune globulin; IM, intramuscular; ITP, immune (idiopathic) thrombocytopenic purpura; IV, intravenous; HBIG, hepatitis B immune globulin; MMR, measles-mumps-rubella vaccine; RBCs, red blood cells; RIG, rabies immune globulin; RSV-IGIV, respiratory syncytial virus intravenous immune globulin; TIG, tetanus immune globulin; VZIG, varicella-zoster immune globulin.

[a] These intervals should provide sufficient time for decreases in passive antibodies in all children to allow for an adequate response to the measles vaccine. Physicians should not assume that children are fully protected against measles during these intervals. Additional doses of IG or measles vaccine may be indicated after exposure to measles.

FEEDING AND NUTRITION

Table 16   Maternal Drug Use During Lactation

AVOID DURING LACTATION		*NO EFFECTS ON INFANT*
Alcohol	Meperidine	Ampicillin
Chloramphenicol	Oral contraceptives	Caffeine
Cimetidine	Paregoric	Cephalosporins
Clindamycin	Phenobarbital	Erythromycin
Codeine	Propoxyphene	Furosemide
Diazepam	Radionuclide material	Haloperidol
Ergot	Sulfonamides	Hydralazine
Iodine	Tetracycline	
Isoniazid		
LSD		
Marijuana		

Adapted from Roberts RJ. *Drug therapy in infants*. Philadelphia: WB Saunders, 1984.

Table 17   Commercially Available Oral Rehydration Fluids (in mEq/L)

	Na$^+$	*K$^+$*	*Cl$^-$*	*BASE*	*GLUCOSE*
Pedialyte	45	20	35	30	2.5
Lytren	50	25	45	30	2.0
Rehydralyte	75	20	65	30	2.5
WHO formula	90	20	80	30	2.0

Table 18   Composition of Infant Formulas (per 100 mL)

NAME (MANUFACTURER)	*Kcal/oz*	*CHO (% of cal/type)*	*Fat (% of cal/type)*	*PRO (% of cal/type)*	*FE (mg)*	*VIT D (IU)*	*mg Ca/mg PO$_4$*
Cow's milk–based standard formulas							
Enfamil (Mead Johnson) with/without iron	20[a]	44%[a] Lactose	48% Palm olein, coconut oil, soy oil, sunflower oil	8% Cow's milk	1.22/0.34	41	52/36
Similac (Ross); with/without iron	20[a]	43% Lactose	48% Soy oil, coconut oil	9% Cow's milk	1.2/0.15	40	49/38
PM 60/75 (Ross)[b]	20	41% Lactose	50% Coconut oil, corn oil	9% Lactalbumin, casein	0.15	40	75/20
Gerber; with/without iron (Gerber)	20[c]	43% Lactose	49% Corn oil, coconut oil	9% Cow's milk	1.21/0.11	40	50/39
Good Start (Carnation)[b]	20[c]	44% Lactose, soy maltodextrin	46% Palm oil, safflower oil, coconut oil	10% Whey and whey protein	1.01	41	43/24
Soy-based standard formulas							
Isomil (Ross)	20	41% Corn syrup, sucrose	49% Coconut oil, soy oil	10% Soy protein isolate	1.2	40	70/50
Prosobee (Mead Johnson)	20	40% Corn syrup solids	48% Coconut oil, soy oil, palm oil	12% Soy protein isolate	1.3	42	63/49

Continued

Table 18 Composition of Infant Formulas (per 50 mL) (continued)

NAME (MANUFACTURER)	Kcal/oz	CHO (% of cal/type)	Fat (% of cal/type)	PRO (% of cal/type)	FE (mg)	VIT D (IU)	mg Ca/mg PO₄
Preterm formulas							
Similac Special Care (Ross)	24[d]	42% Lactose (50%), polycose glucose polymers (50%)	47% MCT oil (50%), soy oil (30%), coconut oil (20%)	11% Nonfat milk whey (60%), casein (75%)	1.5/0.3	122	146/81
Enfamil Premature (Mead Johnson); with/without iron	24[d]	44% Lactose (50%), corn syrup solids	44% MCT oil (75%), soy oil (75%), coconut oil (20%)	12% Lactalbumin (60%), casein (75%)	1.5/0.2	219	134/75
Similac Neocare (Ross)[e]	22	41% Lactose (50%), glucose polymers (50%)	49% MCT oil (25%), LCT oil (75%)	10% Whey (50%), casein (50%)	1.3	59	78/46
Special formulas[f]							
Nutramigen (Mead Johnson)	20	54% Modified corn starch, corn syrup solids	35% Corn oil, soy oil	11% Casein hydrolysate and amino acids	1.25	42	63/42
Pregestimil (Mead Johnson)	20	41% Corn syrup solids, modified corn-starch, dextrose	48% MCT oil (60%), corn oil, soy oil, safflower oil	11% Casein hydrolysate, amino acids	1.25	50	63/42
Portagen (Mead Johnson)	20	46% Corn syrup solids, sucrose	75% MCT oil (85%), corn oil, Lecithin	14% Sodium caseinate	1.25	52	63/47
Alimentum (Ross)[e]	20	41% Sucrose, modified tapioca starch	48% MCT oil (50%), safflower oil (75%), soy oil (10%)	11% Casein hydrolysate, amino acids	1.2	30	70/50
Lactofree (Mead Johnson)	20	42% Corn syrup solids	49% Palm olein, soy oil, coconut oil, sunflower oil	9% Cow's milk protein isolate	1.2	75	55/37
Neocate (Scientific Hospital Supplies, Inc.)	20	47% Corn syrup solids, dextrose, maltose, maltriose, oligosaccharides	41% Hybrid safflower oil, coconut oil, soy oil	12% Synthetic free amino acids	1.2	58	83/62

CHO, carbohydrate; CF, cystic fibrosis; FE, iron; LCT, long-chain triglyceride; MCT, medium-chain triglyceride; PRO, protein.

[a] Also available as 24 kcal/oz and 27 kcal/oz.

[b] Formula with a low renal solute load.

[c] Also available as 24 kcal/oz.

[d] Also available as 20 kcal/oz.

[e] Available only as ready-to-feed.

[f] Indications for Special Formulas

NAME	INDICATIONS
Nutramigen	Cow's milk allergy, severe or multiple food allergies, severe or persistent diarrhea, galactosemia
Pregestimil	Malabsorption, intestinal resection, severe or persistent diarrhea, food allergies
Portagen	Steatorrhea secondary to CF, intestinal resections, pancreatic insufficiency, biliary atresia, lymphatic anomalies, celiac disease
Alimentum	Problems with digestion or absorption, severe or prolonged diarrhea, CF, steatorrhea, food allergies, intestinal resection
Lactofree	Lactose intolerance *without* cow's milk protein intolerance
Neocate	Cow's milk allergy, soy and protein hydrolysate intolerance, multiple food protein intolerance

Table 19   Uncommon Disorders Associated with Obesity

Alström-Hallgren syndrome
Autosomal-recessive trait, obesity, retinal degeneration with blindness in childhood, sensory nerve deafness, diabetes mellitis, small testes in males, and progressive nephropathy in adults.

Carpenter syndrome
Obesity; brachycephaly with craniosynostosis; peculiar facies with lateral displacement of inner canthi and apparent exophthalmos, flat nasal bridge, low-set ears, retrognathism, and high-arched palate; brachydactyly of hands with clinodactyly and partial syndactyly; preaxial polydactyly of feet with partial syndactyly; and mental retardation.

Cohen syndrome
Mild—childhood onset, truncal obesity, persistent hypotonia and muscle weakness, mild mental retardation, characteristic craniofacies with high nasal bridge, maxillary hypoplasia with mild downslant to palpebral fissures, high arched palate, short philtrum, small jaw, open mouth and prominent maxillary central incisors, mottled retina, myopia, strabismus, narrow hands and feet with shortening of metacarpals and metatarsals, simian crease, hyperextensible joints, lumbar lordosis, and mild scoliosis.

Cushing syndrome
Truncal obesity, hypertension, glucose intolerance, hirsutism, oligomenorrhea or amenorrhea, plethora, moon facies, buffalo hump, striae, ecchymoses, increased fatigability and weakness, and personality changes.

Growth hormone deficiency
Short stature, mild-to-moderate obesity.

Hyperinsulinemia (from an insulin-secreting pancreatic tumor, hypersecretion by pancreatic beta cells or a hypothalamic lesion)
Progressive obesity with hyperphagia, normal or excessive growth in stature, and signs and symptoms of hypoglycemia.

Hypothalamic dysfunction (due to tumor, trauma, or inflammation)
Hyperinsulinemia and hyperphagia may be accompanied by headache, papilledema, impaired vision, amenorrhea or impotence, diabetes insipidus, hypothyroidism, adrenal insufficiency, somnolence, temperature dysregulation, seizures, and coma.

Hypothyroidism
Short stature; delayed sexual maturation; delayed union of epiphyses; lethargy; cold intolerance; hoarse voice; menorrhagia; decreased appetite; dry skin; aching muscles and delayed relaxation phase of deep tendon reflexes; progression to dull expressionless face; sparse hair; periorbital puffiness; large tongue; pale, cool, rough-feeling skin; and presence or absence of goiter.

Laurence-Moon-Biedl (Bardet-Biedl) syndrome
Autosomal-recessive trait, truncal obesity, retinal dystrophy/retinitis pigmentosa with progressively decreasing acuity, mental retardation, hypogenitalism, digital anomalies (polydactyly, syndactyly, or both), and nephropathy.

Polycystic ovary (Stein-Leventhal) syndrome
Irregular or absent menses, moderate hirsutism, weight gain shortly after menarche, increased ratio of luteinizing hormone to follicle-stimulating hormone, hyperandrogenemia, and increased levels of estrone with normal levels of estradiol. May occur in association with congenital adrenal hyperplasia, Cushing syndrome, hyperprolactinemia, or insulin resistance.

Prader-Willi syndrome
Obesity, hypotonia, and feeding problems in infancy; hyperphagia in childhood and adolescence; developmental delay; mental retardation; hypogonadism; short stature; small hands and feet; and strabismus.

Pseudohypoparathyroidism (type I)
Short stature, round facies, short metatarsals and metacarpals, subcutaneous calcifications, moderate mental retardation, cataracts, coarse and dry skin, brittle hair and nails, hypocalcemia, and hyperphosphatemia.

Turner syndrome
Short stature, tendency to obesity, ovarian dysgenesis, broad chest with widely spaced nipples, prominent ears, narrow maxilla and small mandible, low posterior hairline, webbed posterior neck, elbow and knee anomalies, nail and skin anomalies, renal anomalies, and hearing impairment.

From Online Mendelian Inheritance in Man.

Table 20 1989 Recommended Daily Dietary Allowance[a]

AGE (YEARS) & SEX GROUP	WEIGHT[b] (KG)	(LB)	HEIGHT[b] (CM)	(IN)	FAT-SOLUBLE VITAMINS VITAMIN A (μg RE)[c]	VITAMIN D (μg)[d]	VITAMIN E (mg TE)[e]	VITAMIN K (μg)	WATER-SOLUBLE VITAMINS VITAMIN C (mg)	THIAMIN (mg)	RIBOFLAVIN (mg)	NIACIN (mg NE)[f]	VITAMIN B6 (mg)	FOLATE (μg)	VITAMIN B12 (μg)
Infants															
0.0–0.5	6	13	60	24	375	7.5	3	5	30	0.3	0.4	5	0.3	25	0.3
0.5–1.0	9	20	71	28	375	10	4	10	35	0.4	0.5	6	0.6	35	0.5
Children															
1–3	13	29	90	35	400	10	6	15	40	0.7	0.8	9	1.0	50	0.7
4–6	20	44	112	44	500	10	7	20	45	0.9	1.1	12	1.1	75	1.0
7–10	28	62	132	52	700	10	7	30	45	1.0	1.2	13	1.4	100	1.4
Males															
11–14	45	99	157	62	1,000	10	10	45	50	1.3	1.5	17	1.7	150	2.0
15–18	66	145	176	69	1,000	10	10	65	60	1.5	1.8	20	2.0	200	2.0
Females															
11–14	46	101	157	62	800	10	8	45	50	1.1	1.3	15	1.4	150	2.0
15–18	55	120	163	64	800	10	8	55	60	1.1	1.3	15	1.5	180	2.0

Adapted from the National Academy of Sciences-National Research Council.

[a] The allowances, expressed as average daily intakes over time, are intended to provide for individual variations among most normal persons as they live in the United States under usual environmental stresses. Diets should be based on a variety of common foods to provide other nutrients for which human requirements have been less well defined.

[b] The median weights and heights of those younger than 19 years were taken from Hammill PVV, et al. Physical growth: National Center for Health Statistics percentiles. *Am J Clin Nutr.* 1979;32:607–629. The use of these figures does not imply that the height-to-weight ratios are ideal.

[c] RE, retinol equivalent. 1 RE = 1 μg retinol or 6 μg beta-carotene.

[d] As cholecalciferol. 10 μg cholecalciferol = 400 IU of vitamin D.

[e] TE, alpha-tocopherol equivalents. 1 TE = 1 mg d-alpha-tocopherol.

[f] NE, niacin equivalent. 1 NE = 1 mg of niacin or 60 mg of dietary tryptophan.

INFECTIOUS DISEASES

Table 21 Risk Factors for Group B Streptococcal Infection

Maternal risk factors
Prolonged rupture of membranes (>18 hours)*
Premature rupture of membranes (<37 weeks' gestation)*
Preterm labor (<37 weeks' gestation)*
Fever >37.9°C (100.2°F)*
History of previous infant with GBS sepsis*
Clinical evidence of chorioamnionitis
GBS bacteriuria*
Multiple gestation
Diabetes

Fetal/neonatal risk factors
Prematurity
Meconium passed in utero
Low 5-minute Apgar score (<6)
Male gender (sepsis four times more common in boys than in girls)

GBS, group B streptococci.

*Risk necessitating intrapartum antibiotic administration per 1996 Centers for Disease Control (CDC) guidelines.

Table 22 Signs and Symptoms of Sepsis in the Newborn

Respiratory distress	Tachypnea (respiratory rate >60/min), grunting, nasal flaring, retractions; sometimes present even without an oxygen requirement or abnormal chest x-ray
Temperature instability	Fever >37.9°C or hypothermia
Poor feeding	Lack of interest, abdominal distention, vomiting, diarrhea
Altered neurologic status	Lethargy, irritability, hypotonia, seizures (especially if meningitis is present)
Apnea	Especially in preterm infants
Poor perfusion	Mottled, grayish, capillary refill >3 s
Tachycardia	Often a late sign
Bulging fontanelle	Meningitis

Table 23 Neutrophil Indices

NEUTROPHIL INDICES	NORMAL VALUES
Absolute neutrophil count (ANC)[a]	$>1,800/mm^3$
Absolute band count (ABC)[b]	$<2,000/mm^3$
I:T ratio[c]	<0.2

[a] ANC = % total neutrophils × WBC count

[b] ABC = % bands × WBC count

[c] I:T = % immature (bands, metamyelocytes, myelocytes): % total (immature + segmented) neutrophils

Table 24   Clinical Features Associated with Congenital Infection

Intrauterine growth retardation
Hydrops
Hepatosplenomegaly
Microcephaly, intracranial calcifications, hydrocephalus
Anemia, thrombocytopenia, petechiae
Jaundice (especially conjugated hyperbilirubinemia)
Pneumonitis
Cardiac malformations, myocarditis
Eye abnormalities (chorioretinitis, cataracts)
Bone abnormalities (osteochondritis, periostitis)

Table 25   Clinical Findings in Congenitally Infected Infants that Suggest a Specific Diagnosis

INFECTION	SUGGESTIVE FINDINGS
Rubella	Cataracts, cloudy cornea, pigmented retina
	"Blueberry muffin" syndrome
	Vertical striation
	Malformation (PDA, pulmonary artery stenosis)
CMV	Microcephaly with periventricular calcifications
	Inguinal hernias in boys
	Petechiae with thrombocytopenia
Toxoplasmosis	Hydrocephalus with generalized calcifications
	Chorioretinitis
Syphilis	Osteochondritis and periostitis
	Eczematoid skin rash
	Mucocutaneous lesions (snuffles)
Herpes	Skin vesicles
	Keratoconjunctivitis
	Acute CNS findings

Modified with permission from Stagno S, Pass RF, Alford CA. Perinatal infections and maldevelopment. In: Bloom AD, James LS, eds. *The fetus and the newborn*, vol 17, Series 1. New York: Wiley-Liss, 1981.

CMV, cytomegalovirus; CNS, central nervous system; PDA, patent ductus arteriosus.

Table 26   Interpretation of Epstein-Barr Virus (EBV) Serology[a]

	IgG-VCA	IgM-VCA	EBV NUCLEAR ANTIGENS	EBV EARLY ANTIGENS
No evidence of infection	<10	<10	<2	<10
Acute infection	>10	≥10	<2	≥ 20
Convalescent infection	>10	Variable	>2	Variable
Remote past infection	≥10	<10	>2	≤ 20

[a] Values are expressed in reciprocal titers as measured by standard immunofluorescence methods.

ABDOMINAL PAIN

Table 27   Classic Clinical Findings in Disorders Characterized by Abdominal Pain

DISORDER	TYPICAL CLINICAL PICTURE	DEFINITIVE DIAGNOSTIC TEST
Peptic ulcer disease	Burning or sharp midepigastric pain that occurs 1–3 hours after meals and is exacerbated by spicy food and relieved by antacids; family history of peptic ulcer disease	Endoscopy
Pancreatitis	Episodic left upper quadrant pain that occurs 5–10 minutes after meals, radiates to the back, and is exacerbated by fatty foods	Pancreatic ultrasound or CT scan Serum amylase level ($\uparrow$)
Urinary tract infection	Suprapubic pain, burning on urination, urinary frequency, urinary urgency	Urine culture Urinalysis
Renal calculi	Severe periodic cramping pain that occurs in the flank and occasionally radiates to the groin; costovertebral angle tenderness; family history of renal calculi	Urinalysis Renal ultrasound
Periappendiceal abscess	Right lower quadrant pain; rebound and direct tenderness; anorexia and vomiting; fever	Barium enema Laparoscopy WBC count ($\uparrow$)
Gallbladder disease	Right upper quadrant pain that occurs 5–10 minutes after meals and is exacerbated by fatty foods; family history of gallstones	Gallbladder ultrasound
Menstrual pain	Cramping suprapubic pain that occurs during the menses	Trial with NSAIDs
Pelvic inflammatory disease (PID)	Suprapubic pain	Cervical culture
Functional abdominal pain (irritable bowel syndrome)	Cramping periumbilical pain that is exacerbated by eating and relieved by defecation	Trial with Metamucil
Lactose intolerance	Cramping periumbilical pain that increases following ingestion of dairy products and is accompanied by flatulence and bloating	Trial with a milk-free diet Breath hydrogen study for lactose deficiency
Inflammatory bowel disease	Right lower quadrant cramping and tenderness; anemia; guaiac-positive stool	Colonoscopy Barium enema Upper gastrointestinal series ESR ($\uparrow$), platelet count ($\uparrow$), WBC count ($\uparrow$)
Esophagitis	Epigastric and substernal pain that is relieved by antacids and exacerbated by lying down; history of iron deficiency; anemia; guaiac-positive stool	Endoscopy
Lead poisoning	Abdominal pain; history of pica; microcytic anemia; basophilic stippling	Serum lead level
Pancreatic pseudocyst	Left upper quadrant pain; recurrent vomiting; history of abdominal pain	Abdominal ultrasound
Sickle cell disease (SCD)	Periumbilical pain that responds to rest and rehydration	Sickle cell preparation Hemoglobin Electrophoresis
Abdominal epilepsy	Periodic severe abdominal pain that is often associated with seizures	Trial with anticonvulsants
Abdominal migraine	Severe abdominal pain; family history of migraine; recurrent headache, fever, and vomiting; unilateral or occipital headache; somatic complaints	Trial with antimigraine medications
Depression	Social withdrawal; decreased activity; irritability; poor attention span; difficulty sleeping	Trial with antidepressant medications
School avoidance	Nonspecific abdominal pain; severe anxiety reaction; pain that is more severe on weekdays and improves on weekends	

Modified with permission from Olson AD. Abdominal pain. In: Stockman JA, ed. *Difficult diagnosis in pediatrics.* Philadelphia: WB Saunders, 1990; p.253.

ESR, erythrocyte sedimentation rate; NSAIDs, nonsteroidal antiinflammatory drugs; WBC, white blood cell; $\uparrow$, increased.

Table 28   Abdominal Masses Commonly Associated with Calcification

Neuroblastoma
Teratoma
    Ovarian
    Sacrococcygeal
Adrenal hematoma
Hepatic hemangioma
Meconium peritonitis

Table 29   Comparison of Functional Constipation and Hirschsprung Disease

	FUNCTIONAL CONSTIPATION	HIRSCHSPRUNG DISEASE
Symptoms as a newborn	Rare	Almost always
Late onset (after 3 years)	Common	Rare
Difficult bowel training	Common	Rare
Stool size	Large	Small, ribbonlike
Urge to defecate	Rare	Common
Obstructive symptoms	Rare	Common
Enterocolitis	Rare	Sometimes
Failure to thrive	Rare	Common
Abdominal distention	Rare	Common
Stool in rectal ampulla	Common	None
Barium enema	Copious stool	Delayed evacuation
	No transition zone	Transition zone
Rectal biopsy	Normal	No ganglion cells
		Increased anticholinesterase staining
Anorectal manometry	Distension of rectum causes relaxation of the internal sphincter	No sphincter relaxation

Table 30   Commonly Used Pediatric Medications that May Cause Cholestasis and Hepatotoxicity

Anticonvulsants
  Phenobarbital
  Diphenylhydantoin
  Carbamazepine
  Valproic acid
Antimicrobials
  Tetracycline
  Erythromycin (estolate preparations)
  Sulfonamides
  Ketoconazole
  Isoniazid
  Rifampin
  Griseofulvin

Immunosuppressants
  Cyclosporine
  Azathioprine
  Methotrexate
Steroids
  Corticosteroids
  Androgens
  Oral contraceptives
Miscellaneous drugs
  Acetaminophen
  Salicylates
  Chlorpromazine
  Cimetidine
  Iron preparations (with overdosage)

A large number of less commonly encountered agents, including antineoplastic agents, antidepressants, antipsychotics, and tranquilizers can also cause cholestasis and hepatotoxicity.

Table 31   Defects in Hepatic Bilirubin Conjugation

DISEASE	DEFECT	GENETICS
Gilbert disease	Underactivity of the transferase, defective uptake of albumin-bound bilirubin from the plasma	Autosomal-recessive
Crigler-Najjar syndrome		
Type I	Complete absence of the transferase enzyme	Autosomal-recessive
Type II	Partial absence of the transferase enzyme (less severe than type I)	Autosomal-dominant

Table 32   Foods and Drugs Mimicking Blood in the Stool

FALSE HEMATOCHEZIA	FALSE MELENA	FALSE HEME-POSITIVE STOOLS
Foods that contain red dye	Spinach	Red meat
Juice	Blueberries	Cherries
Candy	Licorice	Tomato skin
Kool-Aid	Purple grapes	Iron supplements
Jello	Chocolate	
Tomatoes	Grape juice	
Beets	Bismuth subsalicylate	
Cranberries	Iron supplements	

Table 33 Clinical Signs of Dehydration in Children

PARAMETER	MILD	MODERATE	SEVERE
Activity	Normal	Lethargic	Lethargic to comatose
Color	Pale	Gray	Mottled
Urine output	Decreased (<2–3 mL/kg/hr)	Oliguric (<1 mL/kg/hr)	Anuric
Fontanelle	Flat	Depressed	Sunken
Mucous membranes	Dry	Very dry	Cracked
Skin turgor	Slightly decreased	Markedly decreased	Tenting
Pulse	Normal to increased	Increased	Grossly tachycardic
Blood pressure	Normal	Normal	Decreased
Weight Loss	5%	10%	15%

Hypernatremic dehydration may be accompanied by moderate clinical signs. Reprinted with permission from Rogers MC: Shock. In: Rogers MC, Helfaer MA, eds. *Handbook of pediatric intensive care*, 2nd ed. Baltimore: Williams & Wilkins, 1994:140.

Table 34 Therapy for Hyperlipidemia

TYPE	MECHANISM	REDUCTION IN CHOLESTEROL (%)	EFFECT ON VLDL	EFFECT ON HDL	SIDE EFFECT	DOSE
Nonpharmacological therapy American Heart Association diet	Limits exogenous cholesterol	10–15	Decrease	Decrease		N/A
Exercise	Improves insulin resistance	Some decrease	Decrease	Increase		N/A
Weight Loss	Improves insulin resistance	Some decrease	Decrease	Mild increase		N/A
Pharmacological therapy Bile acid resins	Accelerate LDL disposal	20–30	Mild decrease	Mild increase	Epigastric distress, constipation, bloating, interferes with some drug absorption	Up to 24 g/day cholestyramine in divided doses
Nicotinic acid or niacin	Reduces VLDL and LDL synthesis increases HDL	25	50% decrease	30%–40% increase	Flushing, headache, tachycardia, gastrointestinal distress, activation of peptic ulcer disease and inflammatory bowel disease, hepatic dysfunction	Titrate up to 1 g 3 times/day
Probucol	Increases LDL disposal; reduces HDL/LDL	5–15		Decrease	Nausea, diarrhea, flatulence, eosinophelia, hepatic dysfunction, prolongation of QT interval	0.5 g 2 times/day
Gemfibrozil	Enhances VLDL breakdown; decreases VLDL production	Decrease	40%–50% decrease	20%–30% increase	Rarely myositis; should not be used in patients with renal disease, cholelithiasis, or liver dysfunction	600 mg 2 times/day
HMG CoA reductase inhibitor (lovastatin)	Inhibits cholesterol synthesis; increases LDL disposal	30–40			Elevated liver enzymes, myositis, cataracts in animals	20–40 mg 2 times/day

HDL, high-density lipoprotein; HMG CoA, 3-hydroxy-3-methylglutaryl coenzyme A; LDL, low-density lipoprotein; VLDL, very-low-density lipoprotein.

HEPATIC

Table 34A   Expected Liver Span of Infants and Children

	BOYS		GIRLS	
AGE (YR)	MEAN ESTIMATED LIVER SPAN	STANDARD ERROR OF MEAN	MEAN ESTIMATED LIVER SPAN	STANDARD ERROR OF MEAN
6 mo	2.4	2.5	2.8	2.6
1	2.8	2.0	3.1	2.1
2	3.5	1.6	3.6	1.7
3	4.0	1.6	4.0	1.7
4	4.4	1.6	4.3	1.6
5	4.8	1.5	4.5	1.6
6	5.1	1.5	4.8	1.6
8	5.6	1.5	5.1	1.6
10	6.1	1.6	5.4	1.7
12	6.5	1.8	5.6	1.8
14	6.8	2.0	5.8	2.1
16	7.1	2.2	6.0	2.3
18	7.4	2.5	6.1	2.6
20	7.7	2.8	6.3	2.9

From Lawson EE, Grand RJ, Neff RK, et al. *Am J Dis Child* 1978;132:475, with permission.

Table 34B   Review of Liver Function Tests

I. LIVER FUNCTION TESTS

AP	AST	ALT	GGT	5 = NUC
Liver	Hepatocyte	Hepatocyte	Placenta	Biliary
Bone	Muscle	Muscle	Pancreas	
Intestine			Kidney	
Placenta			Bile	
Tumors			Ducts	
			Choroid	

II. "TRUE" LIVER FUNCTION TESTS
Prothrombin time
Albumin
Bile acids and salts
Factor II, V, VII, IX, X
   Vitamin k-dependent factors: II, VII, IX, X

III. LIVER FUNCTION TESTS
Clinical pearls for daily use:

	ALKALINE PHOSPHATASE	γ-GGT
Low	Zinc deficiency	Bile acid deficiency
	Wilson disease	
	Cystic fibrosis	
High	See other List	Cholestasis, ICP

IV. LIVER FUNCTION TESTS
Clinical pearls for daily use: Elevated transaminases and normal bilirubin, GGT, and alkaline phosphatase

Table 34C   Clinical Disease States and Age of Presentation of Hepatomegaly

AGE	CLINICAL DISEASE STATES
Newborn (Birth–2 mo)	Intrauterine and intrapartum acquired infection (TORCH, syphilis, other)
	Erythroblastosis fetalis
	Neonatal hepatitis, α_1-antitrypsin, Alagille syndrome
	Bitiary atresia
	Congestive heart failure
	Congenital paroxysmal atrial tachycardia
	Sepsis
Infant (2–12 mo)	Cystic fibrosis
	Metabolic disease: glycogen storage, α_1-antitrypsin deficiency, galactosemia, tyrosinemia, hereditary fructose intolerance, other
	Neonatal hepatitis, hepatitis B
	HIV infection (AIDS)
	Histiocytosis
	Malnutrition
	Tumors (intrinsic, metastatic)
	Cholelithiasis
	Choledochal cyst
Young child (1–6 yrs)	Viral hepatitis
	Drug-toxic hepatitis
	Parasitic
	Tumor
	Leukemia, lymphoma
Older child, adolescent (7–20 yrs)	Viral hepatitis
	Drug-toxic hepatitis
	Wilson disease
	Chronic active hepatitis
	Congenital hepatic fibrosis
	Focal nodular hyperplasia, adenoma
	α_1-Antitrypsin deficiency
	Reye syndrome
	Sickle cell anemia
	Cholelithiasis
	Juvenile rheumatoid arthritis, lupus erythematosus, sarcoidosis
	Leukemia, lymphoma
	Gonococcal perihepatitis
	Cystic fibrosis
	Diabetes

Adapted from Walker, WA, Mathia RK. *Pediatr Clin North Am* 1975;22:929.

ELECTROLYTES

Table 35   Assessment of Hypernatremia

UNDERLYING CAUSE	ECF VOLUME	URINE OUTPUT	URINE SODIUM	SPECIFIC GRAVITY
Sodium excess	Increased	Normal or increased	Increased	High
Water loss (DI)	Decreased	Increased	Decreased	High
Sodium and water loss (water > sodium)	Normal or decreased	Decreased	Increased	Low

DI, diabetes insipidus; ECF, extracellular fluid.

Table 36   Assessment of Hyponatremia

IF URINE OUTPUT DECREASED AND UNq <20 mEq/L	*IF URINE OUTPUT DECREASED AND UNq >20 mEq/L*	*IF URINE OUTPUT NORMAL OR INCREASED AND UNq >20 mEq/L*	*IF URINE OUTPUT NORMAL OR INCREASED AND UNq >20 mEq/L*
Effective intravascular volume, consider: CHF, nephrotic syndrome, dehydration, liver disease, third spacing conditions	Renal failure or increased ADH	Water intoxication	Renal NaCl wasting 　Nonoliguric renal failure, adrenal 　　insufficiency 　Osmotic diuretic use or osmotic diuresis

Table 37   Conditions Associated with Increased ADH/ADH-Like Effect and Hyponatremia

Pain
Vomiting
CNS disorders: including injuries, infection, tumors
Intrathoracic disorders: including infections, mechanical ventilation
Drugs: narcotics, barbiturates, carbamazepine, NSAIDs, cyclophosphamide, vincristine, others not commonly used in pediatrics

Table 38   Determination of Serum Osmolality

Reliable estimate under most circumstances:
　Serum Osm = 2(Na mEq/L) + 10
Estimate when there is hyperglycemia or azotemia
　Serum Osm = 2(Na) + glucose/18
　　　　　　 + BUN/2.8

Table 39   Drugs Associated with Hyperkalemia

Potassium-sparing diuretics (e.g., spironolactone, triamterene, amiloride)
Potassium supplements (e.g., potassium chloride)
Potassium-containing penicillins
Stored blood
Cyclosporine
Nonsteroidal antiinflammatory drugs (NSAIDs)
Heparin
Angiotensin-converting enzyme (ACE) inhibitors
β-adrenergic blockers
Chemotherapeutic agents

Table 40   Treatment of Hyperkalemia

AGENT	*INDICATION*	*MECHANISM OF ACTION*	*DOSE*	*SIDE EFFECTS/POTENTIAL PROBLEMS*
10% Calcium gluconate	ECG changes	Stabilizes membranes	1 mg/kg IV over 5–10 minutes	Hypercalcemia
Sodium bicarbonate	ECG changes or very high K$^+$ level	Shifts K$^+$ to intracellular compartment	1 mg/kg IV over 5–10 minutes	Sodium load
Glucose plus insulin	ECG changes or very high K$^+$ level	Shifts K$^+$ to intracellular compartment	0.25–0.5 gm/kg glucose plus 0.3 U insulin/gm glucose over 30–60 minutes	Hyper- or hypoglycemia
Kayexalate resin	To remove K$^+$ from body	K$^+$ binds to resin in gut	1 gm/kg PO or PR in 50%–70% sorbitol	Constipation
Furosemide	Symptomatic hyperkalemia	Enhances urinary K$^+$ excretion	1–2 mg/kg IV	May not be enough renal function to be effective
Hemo- or peritoneal dialysis	No renal function	Removes K$^+$ in dialysate	…	Risks associated with dialysis
Exchange transfusion	ECG changes or very high K$^+$ level	Donor blood has had most K$^+$ removed	Double volume	Risks associated with exchange transfusion

ECG, electrocardiogram; IV, intravenous; K$^+$, potassium; PO, orally; PR, parenterally.

Table 41 Drugs Associated with Hypokalemia

Drugs associated with increased renal loss
  Aminoglycoside toxicity
  Amphotericin B
  Cisplatin
  Penicillins in high doses
  Corticosteroids
  Diuretics (except for potassium-sparing ones)
Drugs associated with increased cellular uptake of potassium
  Terbutaline
  Epinephrine
  β-adrenergic agents (e.g., albuterol)
  Theophylline toxicity
  Barium toxicity
  Insulin

Table 42 Oral Potassium Supplements

PREPARATION	FORMULATION	POTASSIUM SUPPLIED
Potassium phosphate	Tablet	1.1, 2.3, or 3.7 mEq
Potassium chloride	Extentabs	10 mEq
	Powder packet	20 mEq
	Effervescent tablets	20 mEq
	Liquid	20 mEq
Potassium citrate	Tablets, crystals, or syrup	1 mEq/mL (Polycitra) or 2 mEq/mL (Polycitra-K)
Potassium gluconate	Liquid	20 mEq/15 mL

Table 43 Commonly Used Calcium Preparations

PREPARATION	ELEMENTAL CALCIUM CONTENT	ROUTE
Calcium gluconate (10%)	1 mL = 9 mg = 0.45 mEq	IV
Calcium chloride (10%)	1 mL = 27 mg = 1.36 mEq	IV
Calcium glubionate (Neocalglucon)	1 mL = 23 mg = 1.12 mEq	PO

Table 44 Calcium Needs

Maintenance calcium (not precisely known)	20–50 mg/kg/d (elemental calcium)
Emergency calcium (for severe symptoms)	10–20 mg/kg (elemental calcium) slow IV with cardiac monitor

RENAL

Table 45 Characteristics of Renal Tubular Acidosis

	TYPE 1	TYPE 2	TYPE 3
Renal function?	Normal	Normal	Normal or decreased
Failure to thrive?	Yes	Yes	Yes
Polyuria or polydipsia?	Yes	Yes	No
Potassium level?	Normal or low	Normal or low	Elevated
Bicarbonate leak?	Usually	Significant	Small
Urine maximally acid?	No (pH > 6)	Yes	Yes
Nephrocalcinosis or nephrolithiasis?	Yes	No	No
Fanconi syndrome?	No	Often	No
Osteomalacia or rickets?	Rarely	If Fanconi syndrome is present	No

Table 46   Toxins Removed by Hemodialysis

TOXIN	MEASURED LEVEL SUGGESTIVE OF NEED FOR HEMODIALYSIS[a]
Acetaminophen	>100 μg/mL in conjunction with antidote
Arsenic	Only with coexistent renal failure
Bromide	>150 mg/dL and severe symptoms
Chloral hydrate	250 mg/dL
Ethanol	600 mg/dL
Ethylene glycol	50 mg/dL
Isopropanol	400 mg/dL
Lithium	4 mEq/L in acute overdose
	As needed for severe symptoms in chronic overdose
Methanol	50 mq/dL
Salicylates	100–120 mg/dL in acute overdose
	60–800 mg/dL in chronic overdose

[a] The decision to perform hemodialysis should be based on physical findings as well as drug levels. A repeat measure should be obtained when the drug level is elevated to ensure that a laboratory error has not occurred. In addition, units of measure should be checked before instituting hemodialysis.

Table 47   Toxins Removed by Charcoal Hemoperfusion[a]

TOXIN	MEASURED LEVEL SUGGESTIVE OF NEED FOR CHARCOAL HEMOPERFUSION
Amitriptyline	Based on signs and symptoms
Chloral hydrate	250 mg/dL
Digitoxin	50 ng/mL with antidotal therapy
Digoxin	15 ng/mL with antidotal therapy
Ethchlorvinyl	150 μg/mL
Glutethimide	40 mg/L
Methaqualone	40 μg/mL
Notriptyline	Based on signs and symptoms
Pentobarbital	50 mg/L
Phenobarbital	100 mg/L
Theophylline	100 μg/mL in acute overdose
	60 μg/mL in chronic overdose

[a] The decision to perform hemoperfusion should be based on physical findings as well as drug levels. A repeat measure should be obtained when the drug level is elevated to ensure that a laboratory error has not occurred. In addition, units of measure should be checked before instituting hemodialysis.

Table 48   Normal Values for Fractional Excretion of Sodium (Fe$_{Na}$)

	PRERENAL ARF	INTRINSIC ARF
Adult or child	<1.0	>2.0
Infant (neonate)	<2.5	>2.5

ARF, acute renal failure.

Table 49   Causes of False-Positive Dipstick Reactions for Urinary Protein

Overlong immersion
Placing reagent strip directly in the urine stream
Alkaline urinary pH (pH >7.0)
Quaternary ammonium compounds and detergents
Pyuria
Bacteriuria
Mucoprotein

Table 50   Drugs that May Cause Hemolytic Anemia in Patients Who Have G6PD Deficiency

Acetanilid	Nitrofurantoin
Doxorubicin	Primaquine
Methylene blue	Pamaquine
Naphthalene	Sulfa drugs

PULMONARY

Table 51   Characteristics of the Three Stages of Parapneumonic Pleural Effusions

	EXUDATIVE STAGE	*FIBRINOLYTIC STAGE*	*ORGANIZING STAGE (EMPYEMA)*
Appearance	Nonpurulent, not turbid	Nonpurulent, not turbid	Purulent, turbid
Fluid consistency	Free flowing	Loculated	Organized
Gram stain and culture results	Negative	Transitional	Positive (before antibiotic treatment)
Glucose	>100 mg/dL	<50 mg/dL	<50 mg/dL
Protein	<3 g/dL	>3 g/dL	>3 g/dL
pH	>7.30	<7.30	<7.30
WBCs	Few	PMNs	PMNs

PMNs, polymorphonuclear neutrophils; WBCs, white blood cells.

Table 52   Pleural Fluid Diagnostic Studies

STUDY	*TRANSUDATE*	*EXUDATE*
Biochemical		
Pleural LDH	<200 IU	≥200 IU
Pleural fluid/serum LDH ratio[a]	<0.6	≥0.6
Pleural fluid/serum protein ratio[a]	<0.5	≥0.5
Specific gravity	<1.016	≥1.016
Protein level	<3.0 g/dL	≥3.0 g/dL
Other studies		
Glucose	*Usually* >40 mg/dL	*Typically* <40 mg/dL
Amylase	May be elevated in some neoplasms, GI trauma, or surgery	
Rheumatoid factor, LE prep, ANA	Are occasionally helpful if collagen vascular disorders are within the differential	
Hematologic		
WBC count	Although high counts (>100/mm^3) are suggestive of an exudate, the results are quite variable	
WBC differential	May actually provide more useful information	
Lymphocyte count	May be elevated in neoplasms, tuberculosis, and some fungal infections	
Segmented neutrophils	May be elevated in bacterial infections, connective tissue disease, pancreatitis, or pulmonary infarction	
Eosinophil count	May be elevated in bacterial infections, neoplasms, and connective tissue diseases	
RBC count	If >100,000/mm^3, is suggestive of trauma, neoplasms, or pulmonary infarction	
Cytology and chromosomal studies	May show evidence of malignant cells or chromosomal abnormalities	
Microbiology		
Gram stain		
Fluid culture for aerobes and anaerobes		
Acid-fast stain (if tuberculosis is in the differential)		
Fungal culture		
Viral culture		
Counterimmune electrophoresis may aid in the detection of a bacterial infection)		

[a] These tests are more reliable in differentiating transudate from exudate than specific gravity or protein level.

Table 53   Normal Blood Gas Values from the Children's Hospital of Philadelphia Blood Gas Laboratory

PARAMETER	AGE OF PATIENT	NORMAL VALUE
pH	1 day	7.29–7.45
	3–24 months	7.34–7.46
	>7 years	7.37–7.41
Pco_2	1 day	27–40 mm Hg
	3–24 months	26–42 mm Hg
	>7 years	34–40 mm Hg
Po_2	1 day	37–97 mm Hg
	3–24 months	88–103 mm Hg
	>7 years	88–103 mm Hg
Base excess	1 day	>8-(−2)
	3–24 months	−7–0
	>7 years	−4-(+2)
HCO_3	1 day	19 mmol/L
	3–24 months	16/24 mmol/L
	>7 years	22–27 mmol/L
α_2 saturation	. . .	94%–99%
Venous pH	. . .	7.32–7.42
Venous CO_2		25–47 mm Hg
Venous O_2		25–47 mm Hg

CO_2, carbon dioxide; HCO_3, bicarbonate; O_2 = oxygen; Pco_2, carbon dioxide tension; Po_2, oxygen tension.

Table 54   Signs of Inhalation Injury

PULMONARY	CNS	SKIN
Tachypnea	Confusion	Facial burns
Stridor	Dizziness	Singed nasal hairs
Hoarseness	Headache	Cyanosis
Rales	Hallucinations	Cherry red color
Wheezing	Restlessness	
Cough	Coma	
Retractions	Seizures	
Nasal flaring		
Carbonaceous sputum		

Table 55   Pulmonary Function Test

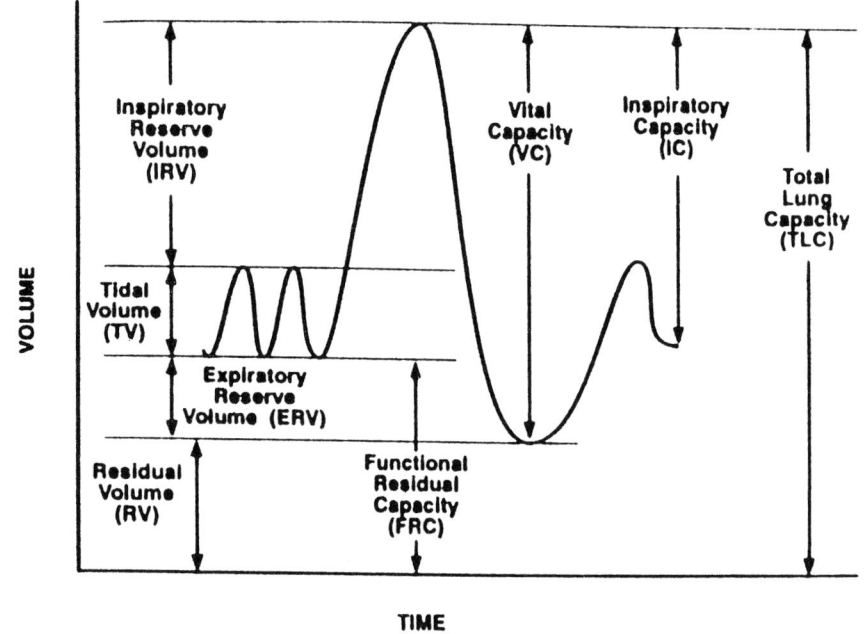

CARDIOVASCULAR

Table 56   Common Causes of Abnormally Wide Splitting of the Second Heart Sound (S_2)

Atrial septal defect (ASD)
Mild pulmonic stenosis
Complete right bundle branch block
Left ventricular paced beats
Massive pulmonary embolus

Table 57   Conditions Causing a Prominent Third Heart Sound (S_3)

Physiologic (infants and children)
Congestive heart failure (CHF)
Ventricular septal defect, with large pulmonary to systemic flow ratio
Mitral insufficiency
Tricuspid insufficiency
Hyperdynamic ventricle with high output (e.g., anemia, thyrotoxicosis, arteriovenous fistula)

Table 58   Conditions Causing a Prominent Fourth Heart Sound (S_4)

Left ventricular outflow tract obstruction (e.g., aortic stenosis)
Right ventricular outflow tract obstruction (e.g., pulmonic stenosis)
Hypertrophic cardiomyopathy
Heart block (atrium contracting against a closed valve)

Table 59   Drugs Associated with Rapid Heart Rates

Prescription drugs
  β-adrenergic agonists (e.g., albuterol)
  Methylxanthines (e.g., theophylline)
  Tricyclic antidepressants (e.g., imipramine)
  Nonsedating histamines (e.g., terfenadine)
Over-the-counter drugs
  Decongestants (e.g., pseudoephedrine)
  Diet aids (phenylpropanolamine)
  Inhaled bronchodilators (e.g., albuterol)
  Caffeine-containing products
Drugs of abuse
  Nicotine
  Cocaine
  Amphetamines
  Alcohol
  Marijuana
  LSD
  Phencyclidine
  Amyl nitrate

Table 60   Causes of Prolonged QT Interval

Congenital
  Hereditary
    Jervell and Lange-Nielsen syndrome: long QT interval, stress-induced syncope, congenital nerve deafness, autosomal-recessive inheritance
    Romano-Ward syndrome: long QT interval, stress-induced syncope, autosomal-dominant inheritance (usually incomplete penetrance)
  Sporadic
Acquired
  Electrolyte abnormalities
    Hypocalcemia
    Hypomagnesemia
  Metabolic disturbances
    Malnutrition
    Liquid protein diets
  Drugs
    Phenothiazines (e.g., haloperidol)
    Tricyclic antidepressants (e.g., imipramine)
    Nonsedating antihistamines (e.g., terfenadine)
    Class Ia antiarrhythmic agents (e.g., quinidine)
    Class III antiarrhythmic agents (e.g., amiodarone)
  CNS trauma
  Cardiac abnormalities
    Ischemia
    Mitral valve prolapse
    Myocarditis
  Intraventricular conduction abnormalities
    Bundle branch blocks

Table 61   Structural Heart Disease Associated with Tachycardia

DEFECT	TYPE OF TACHYCARDIA
Congenital heart disease	
Mitral valve prolapse	SVT, VT
Aortic valve stenosis or regurgitation	VT
Ebstein anomaly of the tricuspid valve	SVT (WPW) commonly, VT less commonly
Tetralogy of Fallot	VT
Mustard/Senning repair of D-TGA	SVT (particularly atrial flutter)
Fontan repair of single ventricle	SVT (particularly atrial flutter)
Cardiomyopathy	
Hypertrophic cardiomyopathy	SVT, VT
Dilated cardiomyopathy	SVT, VT
Arrhythmogenic right ventricular dysplasia	VT (monomorphic, left bundle branch block)
Miscellaneous causes	
Cardiac tumor (atrial myxoma, rhabdomyosarcoma)	VT
Eisenmenger complex (pulmonary vascular disease and pulmonary hypertension)	SVT, VT (depending on tumor site)

D-TGA, D-transposition of the great arteries; SVT, supraventricular tachycardia; VT, ventricular tachycardia; WPW, Wolff-Parkinson-White syndrome.

Table 62   Poisons Causing Tachycardia

Tachycardia and hypertension
   Amphetamines
   Antihistamines
   Cocaine
   LSD/PCP
Tachycardia and hypotension
   β_2-adrenergic agonists
      Albuterol
      Terbutaline
   Carbon monoxide
   Cyclic antidepressants
   Hydralazine
   Iron
   Phenothiazines
   Theophylline
   Any agent causing vomiting, diarrhea, or hemorrhage

LSD, lysergic acid diethylamide; PCP, phencyclidine hydrochloride.

Table 63   Poisons Causing Bradycardia

Bradycardia and hypertension
   α-Adrenergic agonists
      Phenylpropanolamine
      Ephedrine
   Clonidine
   Ergotamine
Bradycardia and hypotension
   α_1-Adrenergic antagonists
      Phentolamine
      Prazosin
   α_1-Adrenergic agonists
      Clonidine
      Tetrahydrozoline
   β-adrenergic antagonists
      Propranolol
      Atenolol
      Metoprolol
   Calcium channel blockers
   Digitalis-containing drugs and plants
   Narcotics
   Organophosphate pesticides
   Sedative/hypnotics

Table 64   Poisons Causing Cardiac Arrhythmias

Atrioventricular block
   Astemizole
   β-Adrenergic antagonists
   Calcium channel blockers
   Clonidine
   Cyclic antidepressants
   Digitalis-containing drugs and plants
Ventricular tachycardia
   Amphetamines
   Carbamazepine
   Chloral hydrate
   Chlorinated hydrocarbons
   Cocaine
   Cyclic antidepressants
   Digitalis-containing drugs or plants
   Phenothiazines (especially thioridazine)
   Theophylline
   Type Ia antiarrhythmic agents
      Quinidine
      Procainamide
   Type Ic antiarrhythmic agents
      Flecainide
      Encainide
Torsades de pointes (multifocal ventricular tachycardia)
   Amantadine
   Cyclic antidepressants
   Lithium
   Nonsedating antihistamines
      Astemizole
      Terfenadine
   Quinidine
   Phenothiazines
   Sotalol

Table 65   Revised Jones Criteria for Diagnosis of Acute Rheumatic Fever

MAJOR CRITERIA	MINOR CRITERIA
Carditis	Fever
Arthritis	Arthralgia
Rash (erythema marginatum)	Elevated ESR, CRP
Chorea (Sydenham)	Prolonged PR interval on ECG
Subcutaneous nodules	History of prior attack of rheumatic fever or rheumatic heart disease

Diagnosis is likely with the presence of two major and one minor criteria, or one major and two minor criteria. Supporting evidence of a preceding streptococcal infection includes a history of recent scarlet fever, a positive throat culture for group A *Streptococcus*, and an increased antistreptolysin 0 (ASO) titer (or titers for other streptococcal antibodies).

Adapted from the Report of the Ad Hoc Committee of the American Heart Association Council on Rheumatic Fever and Congenital Heart Disease. *Circulation* 1984; 69:204A–208A.

CRP, C-reactive protein; ECG, electrocardiogram; ESR, erythrocyte sedimentation rate.

MUSCULOSKELETAL

Table 66   Range of Motion of Major Joints

	FLEXION	EXTENSION	ABDUCTION	ADDUCTION	INTERNAL ROTATION	EXTERNAL ROTATION
Hip	120°	30°	50°	30°	35°	45°
Knee	135°	5°	0°	0°	10°	10°
Ankle	50°	20°	10°	20°	5° (eversion)	5° (inversion)
Shoulder	90°	45°	180°	45°	55°	45°
Elbow	135°	5°	0°	0°	90° (supination)	90° (pronation)
Wrist	80°	70°	20° (radial)	30° (lunar)	0°	0°

Table 67   Characteristics of Synovial Fluid

	APPEARANCE	WBC/MM²	% NEUTROPHILS	% GLUCOSE SYNOVIAL BLOOD
Normal	Clear	<2,000	<40	>50
Infectious	Turbid	>75,000	>75	<50
Inflammatory (JRA, SLE)	Clear/turbid	5,000–75,000	50	≥50
Traumatic	Bloody/Clear	<5,000	<50	>50

Table 68   Relationship Between Short Stature, Bone Age, and Growth Velocity[a]

Bone age delayed—normal growth velocity	Constitutional short stature
Bone age normal—normal growth velocity	Genetic short stature
Bone age delayed—delayed growth velocity	Organic diseases

[a]Velocity = the rate of growth during a year.

ENDOCRINOLOGY

Table 69   Clinical and Biochemical Features of Congenital Adrenal Hyperplasia (CAH)

ENZYME DEFECT	SEXUAL AMBIGUITY FEMALE	SEXUAL AMBIGUITY MALE	ADDITIONAL CLINICAL MANIFESTATIONS	PREDOMINANT STEROIDS
Desmolase	−	+	Salt wasting	...
3β-Hydroxysteroid dehydrogenase	+	+	Salt wasting	17-OH-pregnenolone, DHEA
21-Hydroxylase	+	−	Salt wasting	17-OH-progestone, androstenedione
11-Hydroxylase	+	−	Hypertension	11-Deoxycortisol
17-Hydroxylase	−	+	Hypertension	DOC, corticosterone

DHEA, dehydroepiandrosterone; DOE, deoxycorticosterone.

Table 70   Normal Serum Adrenal Steroid Levels in Newborn Infants

STEROID	PRETERM SICK 24–28 WEEKS	PRETERM SICK 31–35 WEEKS	PRETERM WELL 31–35 WEEKS	FULL TERM
Cortisol (μg/dL)	7.5 ± 4	6 ± 2.7	6.9 ± 3.8	6.2 ± 3.9
17-OH-Preg (ng/dL)	1794 ± 1818	1395 ± 694	942 ± 739	245 ± 291
17-OH-Pro (ng/dL)	651 ± 661	373 ± 317	169 ± 95	36 ± 13[a]
11-deoxycortisol (ng/dL)	662 ± 548	294 ± 239	111 ± 62	87 ± 42
DHEA (ng/dL)	1872 ± 4038	675 ± 502	920 ± 1227	286 ± 238
DHEAS (μg/dL)	467 ± 312	459 ± 209	341 ± 93	162 ± 88
Androstenedione (ng/dL)	479 ± 1032	206 ± 86	215 ± 134	149 ± 67

Data based on information in Lee MM, Rajabopalan L, Berg G, et al. Serum adrenal steroid concentrations in premature infants. *J Clin Endocrinol Metab* 1989;69:1133–1136, and in Wiener D, Smith J, Dahlem S, et al. Serum adrenal steroid levels in healthy term 3-day-old infants. *J Pediatr* 1987;110(1):122–124.

17-OH-Preg, 17-OH-pregnenolone; 17-OH-Pro, 17-OH-progesterone; DHEA, dehydroepiandrosterone; DHEAS, dehydroepiandrosterone sulfate.

[a] 17-OH-Pro values in full-term sick newborns may be double or triple the baseline values. No data are available for other steroid hormones in sick full-term infants.

Table 71   Pharmacokinetics of Common Insulin Preparations

INSULIN PREPARATION	ONSET (HOURS)	PEAK (HOURS)	DURATION OF ACTION (HOURS)
Ultra-rapid-acting (Lispro)	0.25–0.50	1–2	2–3
Short-acting (Regular, Semilente)	0.5–1.0	2–4	4–6
Long-acting (NPH, Lente)	2–4	6–12	18–24
Very long-acting (Ultralente)	6–10	18–24	24–36

NPH, neutral protein Hagedorn insulin.

Table 72   Normal Thyroid Hormone Levels

T_4	Total	7.0–15.0 μg/dL
	Free	0.8–2.3 ng/dL
T_3		100–250 ng/dL
TSH		0.5–5.0 μg/dL

Table 73   Normal Ranges for Gonadotropin and Sex Steroid Levels: Females

	LH (mLU/ml)	FSH (mLU/mL)	ESTRADIOL (ng/dL)	TESTOSTERONE (ng/dL)
0–1 year	0.02–7.0	0.24–14.2	0.5–5.0	<10
Prepubertal	0.02–0.3	1.0–4.2	<1.5	<3–10
Tanner 2	0.02–4.7	1.0–10.8	1.0–2.4	7.0–28
Tanner 3	0.10–12.0	1.5–12.8	0.7–6.0	15–35
Tanner 4	0.4–11.7	1.5–11.7	2.1–8.5	13–32
Tanner 5	0.4–11.7	1.0–9.2	3.4–17.0	20–38
Adult	...	...	...	10–55
Follicular phase	2.0–9.0	1.8–11.2	3.0–10.0	...
Midcycle	18.0–49	6.0–35.0	...	...
Luteal phase	2.0–11.0	1.8–11.2	7.0–30.0	...

FSH, follicle-stimulating hormone; LH, luteinizing hormone.

Table 74   Normal Ranges for Gonadotropin and Sex Steroid Levels: Males

	LH (mLU/mL)	FSH (mLU/mL)	ESTRADIOL (ng/dL)	TESTOSTERONE (ng/dL)
0–1 year	0.02–7.0	0.16–4.1	1.0–3.2	<10
Prepubertal	0.02–0.3	0.26–3.0	<1.5	<3–10
Tanner 2	0.2–4.9	1.8–3.2	0.5–1.6	18–150
Tanner 3	0.2–5.0	1.2–5.8	0.5–2.5	100–320
Tanner 4	0.4–7.0	2.0–9.2	1.0–3.6	200–620
Tanner 5	0.4–7.0	2.6–11.0	1.0–3.6	350–970
Adult	1.5–9.0	2.0–9.2	0.8–3.5	350–1,030

FSH, follicle-stimulating hormone; LH, leuteinizing hormone.

Table 75   Classification of Total and LDL Cholesterol Levels in Children and Adolescents from Families with Hypercholesterolemia or Premature Cardiovascular Disease

CATEGORY	TOTAL CHOLESTEROL, mg/dL	LDL CHOLESTEROL, mg/dL
Acceptable	<170	<110
Borderline	170–199	110–129
High	≥200	≥130

NEUROLOGIC

Table 76   Causes of Ataxia

FORM OF ATAXIA	MAJOR CAUSES	OTHER CAUSES
Acute ataxia	Ingestion	Migraine
	Postinfectious cerebellitis	Neuroblastoma
Acute recurrent ataxia	Migraine	...
	Metabolic disease	
Chronic ataxia	Congenital disorders with mental deficiency	...
Chronic progressive ataxia	Brain tumors	Ataxia-telangiectasia
	Neuroectodermal tumors	Friedreich ataxia

Table 77 Glasgow Coma Scale

Eyes open		Best motor response	
Spontaneously	4	Obey commands	6
To speech	3	Localize pain	5
To pain	2	Withdrawal	4
None	1	Flexion to pain	3
Best verbal response		Extension to pain	2
Oriented	5	None	1
Confused	4		
Inappropriate	3		
Incomprehensible	2		
None	1		

Adapted from Fleisher G, Ludwig S, eds. *Textbook of pediatric emergency medicine,* 3rd ed. Baltimore: Williams & Wilkins, 1993:272.

Table 78 Glasgow Coma Scale (GCS) for Adults and Children and Modified Score for Infants

	GLASGOW COMA SCORE (ADULTS/OLDER CHILDREN)		MODIFIED GLASGOW COMA SCORE (INFANTS)
Eye opening	Spontaneous	4	Spontaneous
	To verbal stimuli	3	To speech
	To pain	2	To pain
	None	1	None
Best verbal response	Oriented	5	Coos and babbles
	Confused speech	4	Irritable, cries
	Inappropriate words	3	Cries to pain
	Nonspecific sounds	2	Moans to pain
	None	1	None
Best motor response	Follows commands	6	Normal spontaneous movements
	Localizes pain	5	Withdraws to touch
	Withdraws to pain	4	Withdraws to pain
	Flexes to pain	3	Abnormal flexion
	Extends to pain	2	Abnormal extension
	None	1	None

Table 79 Drugs that Can Cause Delirium or Coma

DRUG	PHYSICAL FINDINGS
Barbiturates	Small, reactive pupils; hypothermia; flaccidity; doll's eye reflex may be absent
Opiates	Pinpoint, reactive pupils; hypothermia; hypotension; hypoventilation; bradycardia
Psychedelics	Small, reactive pupils; hypertension; hyperventilation; dystonic posturing
Amphetamines	Dilated pupils, hyperthermia, hypertension, tachycardia, arrhythmia
Cocaine	Dilated pupils, hyperthermia, tachycardia
Atropine-scopolamine	Dilated pupils; hyperthermia; flushing; hot, dry skin; supraventricular tachycardia
Glutethimide	Midposition, irregular fixed pupils; hypothermia; flaccidity
Tricyclic antidepressants	Hyperthermia, hypotension, supraventricular tachycardia
Phenothiazines	Hypotension, arrhythmia, dystonia
Methaqualone	Same as with barbiturates; if severe tachycardia, dystonia

From Packer RJ, Berman PH. Coma. In: Fleisher GR, Ludwig S, eds. *Textbook of pediatric emergency medicine,* 3rd ed. Baltimore: Williams & Wilkins, 1993:126, with permission.

Table 80 Prognostic Indicators of Poor Neurologic Outcome in Near-Drowning Victims[a]

At the scene
    Submersion time >4–10 minutes
    Delay in beginning CPR
    Resuscitation >25 minutes
In the emergency department
    Necessity for CPR
    Fixed, dilated pupils
    pH <7.0
    GCS score <5
After initial resuscitation
    Persistent GCS score <5
    Persistent apnea

CPR, cardiopulmonary resuscitation; GCS, Glasgow Coma Scale.

[a] Applies to victims of warm water near-drownings only. Hypothermic victims of cold water near-drownings may have a better prognosis.

Table 81   Relationship of the Lesion to the Physical Findings

LESION	FINDINGS
Upper motor neuron involving corticospinal tract, thalamus, centrum, semiovale, motor cortex	Altered, normal or increased reflexes, bulk normal; strength normal or decreased
Cerebellum	Uncoordinated
Spinal (upper and lower motor)	Local pain, bowel and bladder dysfunction, if anterior horn cells involved, weakness and bulk, decreased absent reflexes, fasciculations
Peripheral	Loss of distal muscles, fasciculations less than spinal lesions; sensation is affected
Muscle	Weakness, muscle atrophy, decreased reflexes, pain, cramping, stiffness
Corticospinal tract	Increased tone, clasp knife character in flexion of arms and extension of legs
Extrapyramidal (basal ganglia)	Rigidity, normal reflexes, absent Babinski, voluntary movement is preserved, may have tremor, chorea, athetosis or dystonia

Table 82   Poisons Causing Coma

Coma with miosis
    Barbiturates and other sedative/hypnotics
    Bromide
    Chloral hydrate
    Clonidine
    Ethanol
    Narcotics
    Organophosphates
    PCP
    Phenothiazines
    Tetrahydrozoline
Coma with mydriasis
    Atropine/diphenoxylate
    Carbon monoxide
    Cyanide
    Cyclic antidepressants
    Glutethimide
    LSD

LSD, lysergic acid diethylamide; PCP, phencyclidine hydrochloride.

Table 83   Poisons Causing Seizures

Amoxapine
Amphetamines
Anticonvulsants
    Phenytoin
    Carbamazepine
Antihistamines and anticholinergic drugs or plants
Camphor
Carbon monoxide
Chlorinated hydrocarbons
Cocaine
Cyanide
Cyclic antidepressants
Isoniazid
Lead
Lidocaine
Meperidine
PCP
Phenothiazines
Phenylpropanolamine
Propoxyphene
Propranolol
Theophylline

PCP, phencyclidine hydrochloride.

Table 84   Differential Diagnosis of Metabolic Neurologic Dysfunction

PROMINENT SYMPTOM	DIAGNOSES TO CONSIDER	DIAGNOSTIC TEST	METABOLIC THERAPY
Myoclonic seizures	Ceroid	DNA, tissue EM	
	Lafora body disease	Muscle biopsy	
	Prion (GSS)	DNA	
	Mitochondrial	DNA, muscle biopsy	CoQ, other vitamins
	Aminoacidopathies	Blood biochemistry	Dietary
	Biotinidase deficiency	Blood biochemistry	Biotin supplement
	Organic acidurias	Blood biochemistry	Dietary, vitamins
Stroke	Homocystinuria	Blood/urine test	B vitamins, betaine
	Mitochondrial	DNA, muscle biopsy	
Coma	Organic aciduria	Blood/urine test	
	MSUD	Blood/urine test	
	Hyperammonemias	Blood test	Dietary
Spasticity	Leukodystrophy	MRI, fibroblast analysis	Dietary
Visual loss	Leukodystrophy	MRI	
	Mitochondrial	DNA, muscle biopsy	
Psychosis	Leukodystrophy	MRI, blood biochemistry, DNA, fibroblast analysis	
	Porphyria	Blood/urine	Avoid precipitants
		Biochemistry	
	Wilson disease	Copper excretion, DNA	Penicillamine
	Homocystinuria	Blood biochemistry	(See above)
	Ceroid	DNA, tissue electron microscopy	
	Huntington disease	DNA	
Microcephaly	Ceroid	DNA, tissue EM	
	Rett syndrome	(Clinical features)	
	Krabbe disease	Blood biochemistry	
Macrocephaly	Storage disorders	DNA, blood biochemistry	
	Canavan disease	Urine biochemistry, DNA	
Neuropathy	Krabbe disease	MRI and blood biochemistry	
	Metachromatic leukodystrophy		
	Porphyria	Blood/urine biochemistry	
	Mitochondrial	DNA, muscle biopsy	
	Friedreich ataxia	(Clinical features)	
	Abetalipoproteinemia		
	Disorders/deficiency of vitamin E	Blood biochemistry	Vitamin E
	Mitochondrial	Vitamin E level	Vitamin E
	Neuroaxonal dystrophy	DNA, muscle biopsy	
		MRI, nerve biopsy	
Myopathy	Fukuyama disease	MRI	
	Mitochondrial	DNA, muscle biopsy	
	Lactic acidoses	Blood biochemistry	
Ataxia	Ataxia telangiectasia	DNA	
	Leukodystrophies	MRI, blood biochemistry	
	Friedreich		
	Mitochondrial	(Clinical features)	
	Hartnup	DNA, muscle biopsy	
	Hyperammonemias	Blood biochemistry	
	Abetalipoproteinemia	Blood biochemistry	
	Sphingolipidoses	Blood biochemistry	
	Machado-Joseph, SCA-1 (hereditary ataxias)	Blood biochemistry, fibroblast analysis, DNA	

Table 85 Acquired Disorders Associated with Progressive Neurologic Dysfunction

STRUCTURAL	HORMONAL	INFECTIOUS	ENVIRONMENTAL	TOXIC	IMMUNOLOGIC
Hydrocephalus	Hypothyroidism	SSPE	Malnutrition/malabsorption syndromes	Lead	Demyelination/multiple sclerosis
Brain tumor	Congenital adrenal hyperplasia (visuospatial deficits)	HIV	Vitamin/trace element deficiency (niacin, thiamine, folic acid, vitamin E, B_{12}, essential fatty acids)	Organic chemicals	Opsoclonus/myoclonus or cerebellar ataxia (neuroblastoma)
Vascular anomalies		Spirochetes	Physical abuse/neglect	Carbon monoxide	Sydenham chorea
				Cocaine, hallucinogens, hypnotics	Rasmussen encephalitis
				Phenytoin (cerebellar degeneration)	

Table 86 Epidural versus Acute Subdural Hematoma

	EPIDURAL HEMATOMA	SUBDURAL HEMATOMA
Common mechanism	Blunt direct trauma, frequently to parietal region	Acceleration-deceleration injury
Etiology	Arterial or venous	Venous (bridging veins below dura)
Incidence	Uncommon	Common
Peak age	Usually >2 years	Usually <1 year
		Peak at 6 months
Location	Unilateral	75% Bilateral
	Commonly parietal	Diffuse, over cerebral hemispheres
Skull fracture	Common	Uncommon
Associated seizures	Uncommon	Common
Retinal hemorrhages	Rare	Common
Decreased level of consciousness	Common	Almost always
Mortality	Rare	Uncommon
Morbidity in survivors	Low	High
Clinical findings	Dilated ipsilateral pupil, contralateral hemiparesis	Decreased level of consciousness
	Period of lucidity prior to acute decompensation and rapid progression to herniation	Irritability, lethargy
Onset	Acute	Acute (within 24 hours), subacute (within 1 day–2 weeks), or chronic (after 2 weeks)
Findings on CT	Convex "lens-shaped" cerebral hemisphere	Concave, diffusely surrounding cerebral hemisphere

CT, computed tomography.

GYNECOLOGICAL

Table 87   Age-Related Prevalence of Principal Laparoscopic Findings in 121 Adolescent Females 11 to 17 Years Old with Acute Pelvic Pain (The Children's Hospital, Boston, 1980–1986)

	NUMBER OF PATIENTS		
DIAGNOSIS	AGE 11–13	AGE 14–15	AGE 16–17
Ovarian cyst	12 (50%)	16 (35%)	19 (37%)
Acute pelvic inflammatory disease	4 (17%)	7 (16%)	10 (19%)
Adnexal torsion	0 (0%)	7 (16%)	2 (4%)
Endometriosis	0 (0%)	2 (4%)	4 (7%)
Ectopic pregnancy	0 (0%)	3 (7%)	1 (2%)
Appendicitis	3 (13%)	4 (9%)	6 (12%)
No pathology	5 (20%)	6 (13%)	10 (19%)
Total	24 (20%)	45 (37%)	52 (43%)

From Goldstein DP. Acute and chronic pelvic pain. *Pediatr Clin North Am* 1989;36(3):576.

Table 88   Key Characteristics of Vaginal Discharges

	PRESENTING SYMPTOMS	DISCHARGE	NONMENSTRUAL pH	AMINE/ WHIFF TEST	VAGINAL SMEAR	TREATMENT
Nonspecific vaginitis	Foul-smelling discharge Itching	Scant to copious Brown to green in color	Variable	Negative	Leukocytes Bacteria and other debris	Improved perineal hygiene
Physiologic leukorrhea	None	Variable Scant to moderate Clear to white	<4.5	Negative	Normal epithelial cells Lactobacilli predominate	None
Bacterial vaginosis	Foul-smelling discharge	Gray-white	>4.7	Positive	Epithelial cells with bacteria ("clue cells") Gram-negative rods	Metronidazole Clindamycin
Candidiasis	Severe itching Vulvar inflammation	White, "curd-like"	<4.5	Negative	Fungal hyphae and buds	Topical or intravaginal imidazoles, triazoles Oral ketoconazole
Trichomonal vaginitis	Copious discharge Itching	Profuse Yellow to green	5.0–6.0	Occasionally present	Motile flagellated organisms	Metronidazole
Foreign body	Foul-smelling discharge	Foul-smelling Purulent Dark brown	Variable (usually >4.7)	Occasionally present	Leukocytes Epithelial cells with bacteria and debris	Remove foreign body Irrigate vagina
Contact vulvovaginitis	Vulvar inflammation Itching Edema	Scant White to yellow	Variable (usually <4.5)	Negative	Leukocytes Epithelial cells	Remove irritant Topical steroids

Table 89   Emergency Contraceptive Pills

INSTRUCTIONS FOR USE

Any of the birth control pills listed below can be used as ECPs. Use only the type of pill your health care provider prescribed for you. Use only one type of pill.

IF YOU ARE TAKING	*NUMBER OF PILLS TO SWALLOW AS SOON AS POSSIBLE (1ST DOSE)*	*NUMBER OF PILLS TO SWALLOW 12 HOURS LATER (2ND DOSE)*
Ovral	2 white pills	2 white pills
Lo/Ovral	4 white pills	4 white pills
Levlen	4 light-orange pills	4 light-orange pills
Nordette	4 light-orange pills	4 light-orange pills
Tri-Levlen	4 yellow pills	4 yellow pills
Triphasil	4 yellow pills	4 yellow pills
Alesse	5 pink pills	5 pink pills

• To reduce the chance of nausea, take an antinausea medicine (like Dramamine II or Benadryl) 1 hour **before** the first ECP dose; repeat according to labeled instructions. This may make you feel tired, so don't drive or drink any alcohol.

• Take the first ECP dose as soon as convenient **WITHIN 3 DAYS (72 HOURS)** after unprotected sex. Try to time the first dose so that the timing of the second dose will be convenient.

• Take the second ECP dose **12 hours after the first dose.**

IMPORTANT: Do not take any extra ECPs. More pills will probably not make the treatment work better. More pills will increase your risk of feeling sick to your stomach.

• Use condoms, spermicides, or a diaphragm if you have sex after taking ECPs until you get your period. Talk to your health care provider about other regular birth control methods you can use in the future.

• Your next period may be a few days early or late.

IMPORTANT: Do a home pregnancy test or see your health care provider if your period has not started **within 3 weeks** after ECP treatment. You may be pregnant.

Source: Program for Applied Technologies (PATH). *Emergency contraception: Resources for providers.* Seattle, 1997. This patient handout may be reproduced without permission of the publisher.

TRAUMA

Table 90   Classification of Burns

TYPE OF BURN	*AFFECTED SKIN LAYER*	*APPEARANCE*
First degree	Epidermis	Erythema, hypersensitivity
Second degree		
Superficial	Upper (papillary) dermis	Erythema, blistering, intact hairs, exquisite pain
Deep	Deep (reticular dermis)	Skin may be white or mottled and nonblanching, or blistered and moist; pain may or may not be present; hairs easily pulled
Third degree	Entire dermis	Dry, white or charred skin; leathery appearance, painless, no hair
Fourth degree	Subcutaneous tissue	Same as third degree; may have exposed muscle and bone

Table 91   "Rule of Nines"

	PERCENT OF BSA		
BODY PART	INFANT	CHILD	ADOLESCENT/ADULT
Head	18%	13%	9%
Anterior trunk	18%	18%	18%
Posterior trunk	18%	18%	18%
Upper extremity (each)	9%	9%	9%
Lower extremity (each)	14%	16%	18%
Genitalia	1%	1%	1%

For small burns, a rough estimate of the affected BSA can be made by comparing the burn with the size of the child's palm (which represents approximately 1% of the BSA).

BSA, body surface area.

TOXICOLOGY

Table 92   Agents with Limited or Uncertain Binding to Activated Charcoal

Iron	Gasoline
Lithium	Mineral seal oil
Heavy metals	Caustics[a]
Arsenic	NaOH
Mercury	KOH
Lead	HCL
Thallium	H_2SO_4
Alcohols	Low-molecular-weight
Methanol	compounds
Ethanol	Cyanide
Isopropanol	Pesticides
Ethylene glycol	Organophosphates
Hydrocarbons	Carbamates
Kerosene	

[a] Administration of activated charcoal may also impede further management.

Table 93   Agents Causing Hypoglycemia in Overdosed Children

Ethanol
Salicylates
Oral hypoglycemic agents
Propranolol
Insulin

Table 94   Poisons Not Detected on the Comprehensive Drug Screen[a]

β-Adrenergic antagonists
Calcium channel blockers
Carbon monoxide
Clonidine
Cyanide
Iron
LSD
Many benzodiazepines (alprazolam, midazolam, lorazepam)
Most plants and mushrooms

[a] Partial listing of some of the most common poisons.

Table 95   Poisons Causing Respiratory Depression or Apnea[a]

Antipsychotic agents	Exotic snake envenomation
Carbamate pesticides	Cobras
Chlorinated hydrocarbons	Sea snakes
Trichloroethylene	Mambas
1,1,1-trichloroethane	Mojave rattlesnake envenomation
Clonidine	Narcotics
Coral snake envenomation	Nicotine
Cyclic antidepressants	Organophosphate pesticides
Ethanol (especially when combined with sedative/hypnotics)	Sedative/hypnotics

[a] Partial list of representative poisons.

Table 96   Poisons Causing an Abnormal Anion Gap[a]

Increased anion gap with metabolic acidosis	Methanol[b]
Carbon monoxide[b]	Salicylates[b]
Cyanide	Theophylline[b]
Ethanol[b]	Decreased anion gap
Ethylene glycol[b]	Bromide
Iron[b]	Lithium[b]
Isoniazid	Hypermagnesemia[b]
	Hypercalcemia[b]

[a] Partial list of representative poisons; anion gap = $Na^+ - (Cl^- + CO_2^-)$.

[b] Specific levels rapidly available.

Table 97 Common Poisons and Antidotes

POISON	ANTIDOTE	ADMINISTRATION
Acetaminophen	N-Acetylcysteine	Loading dose 140 mg/kg, then 17 doses at 70 mg/kg/dose. Dilute 20% solution to 5%–10% with juice or soda to improve palatability.
Anticholinergics	Physostigmine	
Benzodiazepines	Flumazenil	
β-Adrenergic antagonists	Glucagon	
Calcium channel blockers	Glucagon	
	Calcium gluconate 10%	0.3–0.6 mL/kg (8–16 mEq calcium/kg)
Carbon monoxide	Hyperbaric oxygen	
	Sodium thiosulfate 25%[a]	
Cyanide	Sodium nitrate 3%	Dose depends on hemoglobin (see cyanide antidote kit package insert). Do not exceed recommended dosage. Do not give to patients suffering from concomitant carbon monoxide exposure.
	Sodium thiosulfate 25%	Dose depends on hemoglobin (see cyanide antidote kit package insert).
Digitalis	Digitalis Fab fragments	Calculate dose based on level or dose ingested or 10 vials if acute overdose, 5 vials if chronic overdose.
Ethylene glycol	Ethanol	0.6 g/kg load over 1 hour followed by 100 mg/kg/hr infusion
	Pyridoxine	2 mg/kg and thiamine 0.5 mg/kg
Iron	Deferoxamine	5–15 mg/kg/hr IV infusion
Isoniazid	Pyridoxine	
Lead	Lead level 45–69 μg/dL	
	Dimercaptosuccinic acid	10 mg/kg PO three times daily for 5 days, then twice daily for 14 days (may be useful at lower levels)
	or	
	Calcium NaEDTA	50–75 mg/kg/day divided, every 6 hours either IM or by slow IV infusion (IV use not FDA-approved)
	Lead level $\geq$ 70 μg/dL	
	Calcium NaEDTA and	Administer as described above
	British anti-lewisite (BAL)	3–5 mg/kg IM every 4 hours for 5 days
Methanol	Folate	50–100 mg over 6 hours
	4-Methylpyrazole (investigational)	
Methemoglobinemia	Methylene blue 1%	1–2 mg/kg (0.1–0.2 mL/kg)
Narcotics	Naloxone	
Organophosphates	Atropine	0.1–0.5 mg/kg initial dose with additional doses as needed to counteract bronchorrhea
	Pralidoxime	25–50 mg/kg (up to 1 g); for severe cases, consider 10–15 mg/kg/hr infusion
Phenothiazines (dystonia)	Diphenhydramine	1–2 mg/kg IM or IV
	Benztropine	1–2 mg/kg IM or IV

IM, intramuscularly; IV, intravenously; FDA, Food and Drug Administration; NaEDTA, sodium ethylenediaminetetraacetic acid; PO, orally.

[a]Consider for possible cyanide inhalation if the patient suffers from smoke inhalation.

Table 98 Epidemiologic Aspects of Food Poisoning

ORGANISM	PATHOGENESIS	SOURCE	PREVENTION
Salmonella	Infection	Meats, poultry, eggs, dairy products	Proper cooking and food handling, pasteurization
Staphylococcus	Preformed enterotoxin	Meats, poultry, potato salad, cream-filled pastry, cheese, sausage	Careful food handling, rapid refrigeration
Clostridium prefringens	Enterotoxin	Meats, poultry	Avoid delay in serving foods, avoid cooling and rewarming foods
Clostridium botulinum	Preformed neurotoxin	Honey, home-canned foods, uncooked foods	Proper refrigeration (see text)
Vibrio parahaemolyticus	Infection enterotoxin	Sea fish, seawater, shellfish	Proper refrigeration
Bacillus cereus			
Diarrheal type	Sporulation enterotoxin	Many prepared foods	Proper refrigeration
Vomiting type	Preformed toxin	Cooked or fried rice, vegetables, meats, cereal, puddings	Proper refrigeration of cooked rice and other foods
Enterohemorrhagic E. coli 0157-H7	Cytotoxins	Milk, beef	Thorough cooking of beef, consumption of pasteurized milk products
Enterotoxigenic E. coli (traveler's diarrhea)	Enterotoxin	Food or water	Prognosis is not recommended for infants and young children

Table 99   Clinical Aspects of Food Poisoning

ORGANISM	INCUBATION	SYMPTOMS	DURATION	TREATMENT
Bacillus cereus	Vomiting toxin 1–6 hr Diarrhea toxin 6–24 hr	Vomiting ± diarrhea; fever uncommon	8–24 hr	None
Brucella	Several days to months; usually >30 days	Weakness, fever, headache chills, arthralgia, weight loss; splenomegaly		Bactrim, tetracycline
Campylobacter	2–10 days; usually 2–5 days	Diarrhea (often bloody), abdominal pain, fever		Severe infection or immunocompromised; erythromycin, Cipro, or Norfloxacin
Clostridia botulinum	2 hr–8 days; usually 12–48 hr	Poor feeding, weak cry, constipation, diplopia, blurred vision, resp weakness; symmetric descending paralysis		Supportive, trivalent equine antitoxin to prevent further paralysis
Clostridia perfringens	6–24 hr	Diarrhea, abdominal cramps, vomiting and fever uncommon	<24 hr	None
Escherichia coli	→	→		Antibiotics in systemic infections
E. coli 0157:H7	1–10 days; usually 3–4 days	Diarrhea (often bloody), abdominal cramps, little or no fever. Can cause HUS.	5–10 days	Supportive
ETEC	6–48 hr	Diarrhea, abdominal cramps, nausea, fever, and vomiting; Uncommon	5–10 days	Supportive
Listeria monocytogenes	2–6 wk	Meningitis, neonatal sepsis, fever	Variable	Ampicillin and gentamicin
Nontyphoidal Salmonella	6–48 hr	Diarrhea often with fever and abdominal cramps	<7 days	None unless <3 months or immunocompromised
Salmonella typi	3–60 days; usually 7–14 days	Fever, anorexia, malaise, headache, myalgias, ± diarrhea or constipation	3–4 wk	Chloramphenicol, ampicillin, amoxicillin, Bactrim, Cefotaxime, Ceftriaxone
Shigella	12 hr–6 days; usually 2–4 days	Diarrhea (often bloody), frequently fever, abdominal cramps	1 day–1 month	Bactrim, Cipro
Staphylococcus aureus	30 min–8 hr; usually 2–4 hr	Vomiting, diarrhea	<24 hr	None
Vibriosis	4–30 hr	Diarrhea, cramps, nausea, vomiting	Self limited	Usually none. Treatment for patients with liver disease or immunocompromised: Cefotaxime, gentamicin, Chloramphenicol, Tetracycline
Yersinia enterocolitica	1–10 days; usually 4–6 days	Diarrhea, abdominal pain (often severe), mesenteric adenitis, pseudo-appendicular syndrome	1–3 wks	Septicemia or enterocolitis in immunocompromised: cefotaxime, aminoglycosides, tetracycline, Bactrim, chloramphenicol

---

Table 100　Nomogram for Estimating Severity of Acute Poisoning

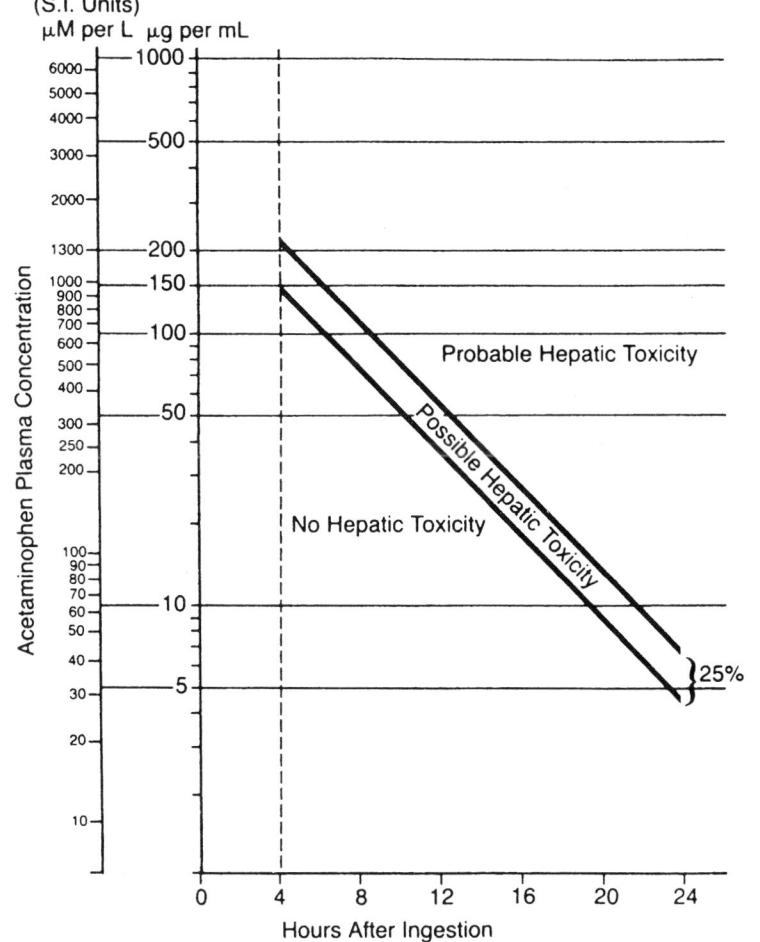

Hours After Ingestion

Table 101　Poisonous Plants

The following are a few common plants that are toxic:

Azalea	Laurel
Buttercup	Lily-of-the-valley
Calla lily	Mistletoe
Creeping Charlie—	Morning glory
ground ivy	Nightshade
Daffodil	Periwinkle
Delphinium	Philodendron
Elderberry	Poison ivy
Holly berries	Poison oak
Hyacinth bulbs	Rhododendron
Hydrangea	Sweet pea
Iris	Tomato vines
Ivy (Boston and	Tulip
English)	Wisteria
Jimson weed	Yew
Larkspur	

Table 102　Helpful Specific Drug Levels

DRUG	TIME TO PEAK BLOOD LEVEL (HOURS POSTINGESTION)	POTENTIAL INTERVENTION
Acetaminophen	4	N-Acetylcysteine administration
Carbamazepine	2–4[a,b]	. . .
Carboxyhemoglobin	Immediate	Hyperbaric oxygen therapy
Digoxin	2–4	Fab (digoxin antibody) fragment
Ethanol	1/2–1[b]	. . .
Ethylene glycol	1/2–1	Ethanol infusion and hemodialysis
Iron	2–4	Deferoxamine administration
Isopropanol	1/2–1[b]	. . .
Lead	5 weeks[a]	Chelation and environmental abatement
Lithium	2–4	Hemodialysis
Methanol	1/2–1	Ethanol infusion and hemodialysis
Methemoglobinemia	Immediate	Methylene blue administration
Phenobarbital	2–4	Alkaline diuresis, multiple-dose activated charcoal
Phenytoin	1–2[a]	Multiple-dose activated charcoal
Salicylates	6–12[a]	Alkaline diuresis, multiple-dose activated charcoal, hemodialysis
Theophylline	1–36[a]	Multiple-dose activated charcoal, whole-bowel irrigation, charcoal hemoperfusion, hemodialysis

[a] Repeated measurement of levels is necessary because of significant variation in time to reach to peak level.

[b] The peak level is predictive of toxicity and clinical course. Adapted from Weisman RS, Howland MA, Verebey K. The toxicology laboratory. In: Goldfrank LR, Flomenbaum NE, Lewin NA, et al., eds. *Goldfrank's toxicologic emergencies,* 5th ed. East Norwalk, CT: Appleton & Lange, 1994:105.

GONOCOCCAL INFECTIONS

Table 103 Regimens for the Treatment of Pelvic Inflammatory Disease (PID) in Adolescents

---

Outpatient regimens
  Regimen A
    Ofloxacin, 400 mg PO twice daily for 14 days
PLUS

    Metronidazole, 500 mg PO twice daily for 14 days
  Regimen B
    Ceftriaxone, 250 mg IM once
OR

    Cefoxitin (2 mg IM) plus probenecid (1 g PO) in a single dose
      concurrently once
OR

    Another parenteral third-generation cephalosporin (e.g., ceftizoxime
      or cefotaxime)
PLUS

    Doxycycline, 100 mg orally twice daily for 14 days
Inpatient regimens
  Parenteral regimen A
    Cefotetan, 2 g IV every 12 hours
OR

    Cefoxitin, 2 g IV every 6 hours
PLUS

    Doxycycline, 100 mg IV or PO every 12 hours
  Parenteral regimen B
    Clindamycin, 900 mg IV every 8 hours
PLUS

    Gentamicin loading dose IV or IM (2 mg/kg of body weight),
      followed by a maintenance dose (1.5 mg/kg) every 8 hours; single
      daily dosing may be substituted

The safety and effectiveness of fluoroquinolones (e.g., ciprofloxacin, ofloxacin, nurfloxacin, enoxacin) in patients younger than 18 years, pregnant women, and lactating women has not been established; therefore, fluoroquinolones are presently not recommended in these patients.

IM, intramuscularly; IV, intravenously; PO, orally.

Table 104   Uncomplicated Gonococcal Infection: Treatment in Children Beyond the Newborn Period and in Adolescents. Recommended Antimicrobial Regimens Include Therapy for Presumed Concomitant Infection with *Chlamydia trachomatis*[a]

DISEASE	PREPUBERTAL CHILDREN WHO WEIGH <100 LB (45 KG)	DISEASE	PATIENTS WHO WEIGH >100 LB (45 KG) AND ARE 9 YEARS OR OLDER
Uncomplicated vulvovaginitis, urethritis, proctitis, or pharyngitis	Ceftriaxone, 125 mg IM,[b] in a single dose **OR** Spectinomycin[c] (max 2 g), IM, in a single dose **PLUS** Erythromycin,[e] 40 mg/kg/d in divided doses for 7 d	Uncomplicated endocervicitis, or urethritis	Ceftriaxone, 125 mg IM,[b] in a single dose **OR** Ciprofloxacin,[d] 500 mg orally, in a single dose **OR** Cefixime, 400 mg orally, in a single dose **OR** Ofloxacin,[d] 400 mg orally, in a single dose **OR** Spectinomycin,[c] 2 g IM, in a single dose **PLUS** Doxycycline, 100 mg orally, twice daily for 7 d[f] **OR** Azithromycin, 1 g orally, in a single dose

[a] Hospitalization should be considered, especially for patients who have been treated as outpatients and have failed to respond, and for those who are unlikely to adhere to treatment regimens.

[b] Some clinicians believe the discomfort of an IM injection can be reduced by using 1% lidocaine as a diluent.

[c] Spectinomycin is not recommended for treatment of pharyngeal infections; in persons who cannot take a cephalosporin, a quinolone, or spectinomycin, a 5-d oral regimen of trimethoprim-sulfamethoxazole may be given.

[d] Quinolones are contraindicated for persons younger than 18 years, pregnant women, and nursing women.

[e] Doxycycline can be given instead of erythromycin if the child is 9 years or older.

[f] Tetracycline, 500 mg, four times daily, can be substituted for doxycycline.

From American Academy of Pediatrics. In: Peter G, ed. *1994 Red book: report of the Commitee on Infectious Diseases,* 23rd ed. Elk Grove Village, IL: American Academy of Pediatrics, 1994:199, with permission.

Table 105   Complicated Gonococcal Infection: Treatment for Children Beyond the Newborn Period and for Adolescents[a]

DISEASE	PREPUBERTAL CHILDREN WHO WEIGH <100 LB (45 KG)	DISEASE	PATIENTS WHO WEIGH >100 LB (45 KG) AND ARE 9 YEARS OR OLDER
Ophthalmia, peritonitis, bacteremia, or arthritis	Ceftriaxone, 50 mg/kg/d (max 1 g/d) IV or IM,[c] once daily for 7 d	Gonococcal pharyngitis Pelvic inflammatory disease	Ceftriaxone, 125 mg IM,[c] in a single dose See Table 86

[a] In all cases, in addition to the recommended treatment for gonococcal infection, doxycycline (100 mg orally, twice daily for 7 d), tetracycline (500 mg, 4 times daily for 7 d), or azithromycin (1 g orally, in a single dose) is recommended on the presumption that the patient has concomitant infection with *Chlamydia trachomatis,* for children younger than 9 y and pregnant women, erythromycin is recommended.

[b] Hospitalization is required; follow-up cultures are necessary to ensure that treatment has been effective.

[c] Some clinicians believe the discomfort of IM injection can be reduced by using 1% lidocaine as a diluent.

[d] Such as the arthritis-dermatitis syndrome.

[e] Spectinomycin is not recommended for treatment of pharyngeal gonococcal infection. For patients who cannot take a cephalosporin, spectinomycin, or a quinolone, a 5-d oral regimen of trimethoprim-sulfamethoxazole may be given.

[f] Alternatively, parenteral therapy can be discontinued 24–48 h after improvement begins and a 7-d course is completed with an appropriate oral antimicrobial. Some experts advise a 10- to 14-d course of therapy.

From American Academy of Pediatrics. In: Peter G, ed. *1994 Red book: report of the Commitee on Infectious Diseases,* 23rd ed. Elk Grove Village, IL: American Academy of Pediatrics, 1994:200, with permission.

MISCELLANEOUS

Table 106   Late Effects of Chemotherapy and Radiation

CHEMOTHERAPY AGENT	POSSIBLE LATE EFFECTS
Cyclophosphamide	Azoospermia, amenorrhea, hemorrhagic cystitis, secondary malignancies
Doxorubicin, daunomycin	Cardiomyopathy/pericarditis, secondary leukemia
Methotrexate, actinomycin	Avascular necrosis, hepatitis or cirrhosis, learning disabilities with intrathecal use
Vincristine	Neuropathies
Steroids	Obesity, avascular necrosis, osteoporosis, cataracts
Cisplatin	Gynecomastia, nephritis, thrombotic thrombocytopenic purpura
Etoposide	Secondary leukemia

RADIATION	
Cranium/brain	Short stature or short trunk, obesity, learning disabilities, leukoencephalopathy, cranial neuropathies, alopecia, cataracts, hypothyroidism, second malignancies (brain, thyroid)
Head and neck	Nasolacrimal duct obstruction, chronic conjunctivitis, chronic otitis media, alopecia, cataracts, dental abnormalities, voice changes, facial deformities, neuropathies, esophagitis, second malignancies (thyroid, soft tissue sarcomas, bone tumors)
Mediastinum	Cardiomyopathy, hypothyroidism, second malignancies (thyroid, acute myeloid leukemia, breast cancer), pneumonitis/fibrosis, reduced cell-mediated immunity
Lungs	Pneumonitis or fibrosis
Spine	Short stature or short trunk, scoliosis, hypothyroidism, second malignancies (thyroid), delayed puberty
Bones	Atrophy or hypoplasia, avascular necrosis, osteoporosis, second malignancies (bone and soft-tissue sarcomas), osteochondromas
Total nodes	Reduced cell-mediated immunity, bone marrow dysfunction

Table 107   Red Eye: Common Causes by Location

CONJUNCTIVA	ADNEXA	GLOBE
Infectious conjunctivitis	Chalazion/hordeolum	Corneal abrasion
Neonatal conjunctivitis	Dacryocystitis	Foreign body
Allergic conjunctivitis	Orbital cellulitis	
Periorbital cellulitis		

Table 108   Human Papilloma Viruses: Preferred Sites of Infectivity

CLINICAL TYPE	HPV TYPE
Verruca vulgaris (common warts)	1, 2, 4, 7, 26, 27, 29
Verruca plana (flat warts)	3, 10, 28, 41
Verruca plantaris (plantar warts)	1, 2, 4
Anogenital warts	1–6, 10, 11, 13, 16, 18, 31, 33, 35, 39, 41, 42
Laryngeal warts	6, 11, 13, 30, 40
Anogenital carcinoma	11, 16, 18, 31, 33, 42, 47
Bowenoid papulosis	16, 18, 30
Epidermodysplasia verruciformis	5, 8–10, 12, 14, 15, 17, 19–25, 16–38, 40

Table 109   Proper Child Safety Seat Use Chart: Buckle Everyone; Children Age 12 and Under Sit in Back!

	INFANTS	TODDLER	YOUNG CHILDREN
Weight	Birth to 1 year up to 20–22 lbs	Over 1 year and >20–40 lbs	>40–80 lbs
Type of seat	Infant only or rear-facing convertible	Convertible/forward-facing	Belt positioning booster seat
Seat position	Rear-facing only	Forward facing	Forward facing
Guidelines	Children to 1 year and at least 20 lbs in rear-facing seats. Harness straps at or below shoulder level	Harness straps should be at or above shoulders. Most seats require top slot for forward-facing	Belt positioning booster seats must be used with both lap and shoulder belts. Make sure the lap belt fits low and tight across the lap/upper thigh area and the shoulder belt fits snug crossing the chest and shoulder to avoid abdominal injuries
Warning	All children age 12 and under should ride in the back seat	All children age 12 and under should ride in the back seat	All children age 12 and under should ride in the back seat

From National Highway Traffic Safety Administration, *www.nhtsa.dot.gov.*

Medications

Monica Darby

MEDICATIONS

Table 1   Medications

DRUG	DOSE	DOSAGE FORMS
Acetaminophen (Feverall, Tylenol)	*Orally or rectally:* Infants under age 3 months: 15 mg/kg repeated every 8 hours. Children: 10–15 mg/kg repeated every 4–6 hours, up to 5 doses daily. Adults: 325–650 mg every 4–6 hours or 1 g t.i.d. or q.i.d. Do not exceed 4 g/day.	Drops: 100 mg/mL Suspension: 160 mg/5 mL Suppositories: 120 mg, 325 mg, 650 mg Tablets: 160 mg, 325 mg, 500 mg Tablets, chewable: 80 mg Also available in combination with codeine; see codeine monograph.
Acetazolamide (Diamox)	*Orally or IV:* Children and adults: 8–30 mg/kg per day in 4 divided doses. Do not exceed 1 g/day. *Altitude sickness (adults):* 250 mg every 8–12 hours beginning 24–48 hours before ascent and continuing for at least 48 hours after arrival.	Injection: 500 mg Tablets: 250 mg
Acetylcysteine (Mucomyst, Mucosil)	*Acetaminophen poisoning:* 140 mg/kg PO followed by 70 mg/kg for 17 doses administered every 4 hours until acetaminophen levels are nontoxic. Usually administered as a 5% solution diluted in juice or soda. *Inhalation* (administer 10% solution undiluted): Infants: 2–4 mL repeated t.i.d. or q.i.d. Children and adolescents: 6–10 mL repeated t.i.d. or q.i.d.	Solution for inhalation: 10% or 20% in 10-mL and 30-mL vials
Acyclovir (Zovirax)	*Oral doses for children and adults:* *Varicella zoster (chickenpox):* 80 mg/kg per day in 4 divided doses for 5 days. Do not exceed 800 mg/dose (3,200 mg/day). *Herpes simplex virus:* Children: 1,200 mg/m^2/day in 4–5 divided doses. Adults: 200 mg every 4 hours while awake (5 doses daily). Chronic suppressive therapy at a dose of 400 mg b.i.d. may be used for up to 1 year or longer. *IV doses for children and adults:* *Neonatal HSV encephalitis:* *Full term infants:* 30–60 mg/kg per day in 3 divided doses for 10–14 days. *Premature infants* ≤1,200 g: 20 mg/kg per day in 2 divided doses. *HSV encephalitis:* 1,500 mg/m^2 per day in 3 divided doses for at least 10 days and up to 21 days. *Other HSV infections:* 750 mg/m^2 per day in 3 divided doses for 7 days. *Varicella zoster infections:* 1,500 mg/m^2 per day in 3 divided doses for 7 days. *Topically:* apply ointment every 3 hours up to 6 times daily for 7 days. Use a disposable finger cot or glove when applying the ointment to avoid transmission of the virus. Dosage may need to be adjusted in patients with renal dysfunction.	Capsules: 200 mg Injection: 500-mg, 1-g vials Ointment: 5%, 15 g Suspension: 200 mg/5 mL
Adenosine (Adenocard)	IV (given via rapid push followed by a saline flush): Children: 0.1 mg/kg initially, followed by doses increasing in 0.05 mg/kg increments every 2 minutes to a maximum dose of 0.35 mg/kg or 12 mg/dose. Adults: 6 mg followed by 12 mg with a repeat dose of 12 mg, if needed.	Injection: 3 mg/mL 2-mL vial)

Continued

Table 1   Medications   (continued)

DRUG	DOSE	DOSAGE FORMS
Albumin, human (Albuminar, Albutein, Plasbumin)	*IV* (as a 5% solution for hypovolemic patients or 25% for fluid- or sodium-restricted patients): Children: 0.5–1 g/kg infused over 2–4 hours. May repeat to a maximum of 6 g/kg/day. Adults: 25 g infused over 2–4 hours. Usually not to exceed 125 g/day.	Injection: 5% (50 mL, 250 mL, 500 mL); 25% (20 mL, 50 mL, 100 mL)
Albuterol (Proventil, Ventolin)	*Oral:* Age 2–<6: 0.3–0.6 mg/kg per day in 3 divided doses to a maximum of 12 mg/day. Age ≥6–≤12: 6–8 mg/day in 3–4 divided doses to a maximum of 24 mg/day. Over age 12: 6–16 mg/day in 3–4 divided doses to a maximum of 32 mg/day. *Inhalation:* *Metered-dose inhaler:* Under age 12: 1–2 inhalations q.i.d. Over age 12: 1–2 inhalations up to 6 times a day. *Nebulization:* 0.01–0.05 mL/kg usually repeated every 4–6 hours, but may be administered more frequently in severely ill patients under controlled conditions.	Aerosol: 90 μg/actuation Solution for inhalation: 0.5% Syrup: 10 mg/5 mL Tablets: 2 mg, 4 mg Tablets, extended release: 4 mg, 8 mg
Allopurinol (Zyloprim)	*Orally:* Under age 6: 150 mg/day in 3 divided doses. Age 6–10: 300 mg/day in 2 or 3 divided doses. Over age 10: 600–800 mg/day in 2 or 3 divided doses. Note: The metabolism of mercaptopurine and azathioprine is decreased by allopurinol. Decrease dose of mercaptopurine or azathioprine by 75%.	Tablets: 100 mg, 300 mg
Alprostadil (Prostin VR Pediatric)	A continuous infusion beginning at a dose of 0.05–0.1 μg/kg per min. Dosage may be adjusted downward or gradually upward based on the patient's response. Usual dosage range is 0.01–0.4 μg/kg per min.	Injection: 500 μg/mL (1-mL vial)
Aluminum acetate (Domeboro, Burow's Solution)	*Topically:* as a wet dressing or soak 2–4 times daily for 30 minutes at a time. Usual concentrations are 1:10, 1:20, or 1:40. *Ear:* 4–6 drops in the ear at first every 2–3 hours, then every 4–6 hours until itching or burning subsides.	Powder (packets): 1 packet/pint of water = 1:40 dilution Solution otic, 1:10 dilution with 2% acetic acid
Aluminum and magnesium hydroxides (Maalox, Maalox Plus, Mylanta)	Children: 5–10 mL 4–6 times daily or more frequently. Adults: 15–30 mL 4–6 times daily or more frequently.	Suspension: aluminum hydroxide 225 mg and magnesium hydroxide 200 mg/5 mL Suspension with simethicone: as above with simethicone 25 mg/5 mL
Amantadine (Symmetrel)	*Orally* for prophylaxis or treatment of influenza A: Children 1–9 years of age: 5–9 mg/kg/day in 2 divided doses Children 10 years of age and adults: 200 mg daily in 1 or 2 divided doses	Solution: 50 mg/5 mL Capsules: 100 mg
Amikacin (Amikin)	*IV* (dose should be based on ideal body weight): Neonates: 0–4 weeks, <1,200 g: 7.5 mg/kg per dose every 18–24 hours. ≤7 days of age: 1,200–2,000 g: 7.5 mg/kg per dose every 12–18 hours. >2,000 g: 10 mg/kg per dose every 12 hours. Over 7 days of age: 1,200–2,000 g: 7.5 mg/kg per dose every 8–12 hours. >2,000 g: 10 mg/kg per dose every 8 hours. Infants and children: 15–22.5 mg/kg per day in 3 divided doses daily. The dose for the treatment of nontuberculous mycobacterial infections is 15–30 mg/kg per day in 2 divided doses, to a maximum of 1.5 g/day as part of a multiple-drug regimen.	Injection: 50 mg/mL, 250 mg/mL

Continued

Table 1　Medications　(continued)

DRUG	DOSE	DOSAGE FORMS
Amikacin (Amikin) (*continued*)	Adults: 15 mg/kg/day in 2–3 divided doses. Dosage adjustment is required in patients with renal dysfunction.	
Aminocaproic acid (Amicar)	*IV:* Children: 100 mg/kg over the first hour followed by an infusion of 33.3 mg/kg per hr to a maximum daily dose of 30 g. Older children and adults: 4–5 g over the first hour followed by an infusion of 1 g/hr for 8 hours or until control is achieved. Orally: doses are the same or alternatively, 100 mg/ kg may be administered every 4–6 hours to a maximum of 5 g/dose.	Injection: 250 mg/mL (20-mL vial) Solution: 1.25 g/5 mL (16-oz bottle) Tablets: 500 mg
Amiodarone (Cordarone)	*Orally:* Children (use body surface area for children age 1 year or under): loading dose of 10–15 mg/kg per day or 600–800 mg/1.73 m^2/day in 1–2 divided doses for 4–14 days or until adequate control of arrhythmia is achieved or prominent adverse effects occur. Then reduce dosage to 5 mg/kg per day or 200–400 mg/1.73 m^2/day as a single dose for several weeks. A further dose reduction to 2.5 mg/kg per day should be attempted if the arrhythmia does not recur. Adults: loading dose of 800–1,600 mg/day in 1–2 divided doses for 1–3 weeks, followed by dose of 600–800 mg/day in 1–2 divided doses for 1 month. Maintenance dose usually 400 mg/day, but may be lower for supraventricular arrhythmias. *IV:* Children (only limited information is available): initial loading dose of 5 mg/kg over 1 hour followed by a continuous infusion of 5 μg/kg per min has been used. The continuous infusion dosage may be increased to 10 μg/kg per min and then to 15 μg/kg per min until the desired effect is achieved. Adults: loading dose of 150 mg administered over 10 minutes (15 mg/min) followed by 360 mg over 6 hours at a rate of 1 mg/min, followed by the maintenance dose of 540 mg over 18 hours at a rate of 0.5 mg/min. If necessary, maintenance infusion of 0.5 mg/min may be continued past the initial 24 hours. Additional bolus doses of 150 mg may be administered over 10 minutes for breakthrough arrhythmias.	Injection: 50 mg/mL Tablets: 200 mg
Amitriptyline (Elavil, Endep)	*Orally:* *Chronic pain:* 0.1 mg/kg per day at bedtime initially, advancing to 0.5–2 mg/kg per day over a 2–3 week period. *Depression:* 1 mg/kg per day to start, advancing to a maximum of 5 mg/kg or 100 mg, whichever is less. Adolescents and adults: 25–50 mg at bedtime or in divided doses, increasing daily doses by 25 mg to a maximum of 100 mg/day for adolescents and 300 mg for adults. Dosage should be decreased to the lowest effective dose after symptom control has been reached.	Tablets: 10 mg, 25 mg, 50 mg, 75 mg, 100 mg, 150 mg

Continued

Table 1   Medications   (continued)

DRUG	DOSE	DOSAGE FORMS
Amoxicillin (Amoxil, Polymox, Trimox, Wymox)	*Orally:* Children ≤20 kg: 20 mg/kg per day in 3 divided doses for urinary tract infections. 40 mg/kg per day in 3 divided doses for otitis media, upper respiratory infection, or skin infections. Acute otitis media due to highly resistant strains of *S. pneumoniae* may require doses of 80–90 mg/kg per day in 3 divided doses. Children >20 kg and adults: 750 mg/day in 3 divided doses for urinary tract infections or 1,500 mg/day in 3 divided doses for otitis media, upper respiratory infections, or skin infections. Maximum daily dose is 3 g. *Endocarditis prophylaxis:* 50 mg/kg (up to 2 g) 1 hour before procedure	Capsules: 250 mg, 500 mg Drops: 50 mg/mL Suspension: 125 mg/5 mL, 250 mg/5 mL Tablets, chewable: 125 mg, 250 mg
Amoxicillin and clavulanic acid (Augmentin, Augmentin ES-600)	*Orally* (based on the amoxicillin component): 20–40 mg/kg per day in 3 divided doses to a maximum of 1.5 g/day, or 25–45 mg/kg per day in 2 divided doses to a maximum of 1.75 g/day using the b.i.d. formulation of the drug. Use the higher doses for respiratory tract infections and otitis media. Otitis media infections caused by multidrug-resistant pneumococcus: 80–90 mg/kg per day in 2 divided doses using the Augmentin ES-600 suspension to avoid higher than recommended doses of clavulanic acid.	Suspension: amoxicillin 125 mg and clavulanic acid 31.25 mg/5 mL; b.i.d. formulation—amoxicillin 200 mg and clavulanic acid 28.5 mg/5 mL; amoxicillin 250 mg and clavulanic acid 62.5 mg/5 mL; b.i.d. formulation—amoxicillin 400 mg and clavulanic acid 57 mg/5 mL; b.i.d. formulation—amoxicillin 600 mg and clavulanic acid 42.9 mg/5 mL Tablets: amoxicillin 250 mg and clavulanic acid 125 mg; amoxicillin 500 mg and clavulanic acid 125 mg; b.i.d. formulation—amoxicillin 875 mg and clavulanic acid 125 mg Tablets, chewable: amoxicillin 125 mg and clavulanic acid 31.25 mg; b.i.d. formulation—amoxicillin 200 mg and clavulanic acid 28.5 mg; amoxicillin 250 mg and clavulanic acid 62.5 mg; b.i.d. formulation—amoxicillin 400 mg and clavulanic acid 57 mg
Amphotericin B (Fungizone)	*IV* (infusion over 2–8 hours): *Test dose* (infusion over 30 minutes) <10 kg: 0.1 mg in 1 mL D_5W. ≥10 kg: 1 mg in 10 mL D_5W. *Therapeutic dose:* begin with 0.25–0.5 mg/kg immediately following test dose. Doses may be doubled on each subsequent day to a maximum of 1 mg/kg as the patient tolerates. Once therapy is established, alternate day doses at a maximum of 1.5 mg/kg per day may be used. Bladder irrigations of 15–50 mg daily in 1 L of sterile water instilled over 24 hours have been used to treat bladder infections.	Injection: 50-mg vial
Amphotericin B, cholesteryl (Amphotec)	*IV* (infusion at a rate of 1 mg/kg per hr): Children and adults: 3–4 mg/kg per day as a single infusion. Doses of 6 mg/kg per day have been used to treat invasive Candida or Cryptococcus infections. Admix with 5% dextrose injection to a final concentration of about 0.6 mg/mL for administration over 3–4 hours. In patients who tolerate the longer infusion time well, the time can be shortened to 2 hours.	Injection: 50-mg vial

Continued

Table 1 Medications (continued)

DRUG	DOSE	DOSAGE FORMS
Amphotericin B, liposomal complex (Abelcet)	*IV* (infusion over 2 hours): Children and adults: 5 mg/kg/day in a single infusion. Admix with 5% dextrose to a final concentration of 1 mg/mL. A final concentration of 2 mg/mL may be used for pediatric patients or patients requiring fluid restriction.	Suspension for injection: 5 mg/mL

Ampicillin (Omnipen, Polycillin, Principen, Totacillin)	*IV:*
	Meningitis:
	  Neonates under age 7 days:
	    <2,000 g: 100 mg/kg per day in 2 divided doses.
	    ≥2,000 g: 150 mg/kg per day in 3 divided doses.
	  Neonates over age 7 days:
	    <1,200 g: 100 mg/kg per day in 2 divided doses.
	    1,200–2,000 g: 150 mg/kg per day in 3 divided doses.
	    >2,000 g: 200 mg/kg per day in 4 divided doses.
	  Infants and children: 150–300 mg/kg per day in 4–6 divided doses to a maximum of 12 g/d.
	  Adults: 150–200 mg/kg per day in 6–8 divided doses to a maximum total daily dose of 14 g.
	Moderate infections:
	  Neonates under age 7 days:
	    <2,000 g: 50 mg/kg per day in 2 divided doses.
	    >2,000 g: 75 mg/kg per day in 3 divided doses.
	  Neonates under age 7 days:
	    <1,200 g: 50 mg/kg per day in 2 divided doses.
	    1,200–2,000 g: 75 mg/kg per day in 3 divided doses.
	    >2,000 g: 100 mg/kg per day in 4 divided doses.
	  Infants, children, and adults: 50–100 mg/kg per day in 4–6 divided doses to a maximum total dose of 12 g/day.
	Orally (mild to moderate infections):
	  Children <20 kg: 50–75 mg/kg per day in 4 divided doses. Do not exceed adult doses for the same degree of infection.
	  Children >20 kg and adults: 1–2 daily (250–500 mg/dose) in 4 divided doses.
		Capsules: 250 mg, 500 mg
		Injection: 125-mg, 250-mg, 500-mg, 1-g, 2-g vials
		Suspension: 125 mg/5 mL, 250 mg/5 mL, 500 mg/ 5 mL

Ampicillin and sulbactam sodium (Unasyn)	*IV:*
	  Infants and children: 150 mg/kg per day (100 mg ampicillin + 50 mg sulbactam) in 3–4 divided doses.
	  Adults: 1.5–3 g (1–2 g ampicillin + 0.5–1 g sulbactam) given every 6 hours.
		Injection: 1.5 g (1 g ampicillin + 0.5 g sulbactam), 3 g (2 g ampicillin + 1 g sulbactam)

Amrinone (Inocor)	*IV:* a bolus dose of 0.75 mg/kg administered over 2–3 minutes is followed by a maintenance infusion of 3–5 μg/kg per min for neonates or 5–10 μg/kg per min for infants, children, or adults. The bolus doses may be repeated at 30-minute intervals to a total of 3 mg/kg. Total daily dose should not exceed 10 mg/kg.	Injection: 5 mg/mL

Aspirin (Anacin, Ascriptin, Bufferin, Easprin, Ecotrin)	*Orally or rectally:*
	Analgesic, antipyretic:
	  Children: 10–15 mg/kg every 4–6 hours.
	  Adults: 325–1,000 mg every 4–6 hours, up to 4 g/day.
		Suppositories: 300 mg, 325 mg, 600 mg, 650 mg
		Tablets: 325 mg, 500 mg, 650 mg
		Tablets, chewable: 81 mg
		Tablets, extended release: 165 mg, 325 mg, 500 mg, 650 mg, 975 mg

Continued

Table 1   Medications   (continued)

DRUG	DOSE	DOSAGE FORMS
Aspirin (Anacin, Ascriptin, Bufferin, Easprin, Ecotrin) (*continued*)	*Antiinflammatory:* Children ≥25 kg: 60–90 mg/kg per day in 3–4 divided doses initially, with a usual range of 80–100 mg/kg per day. Monitor serum levels. Children >25 kg and adults: 2.4–3.6 g/day in 4 divided doses. Maximum total daily dose usually should not exceed 5.4 g. *Kawasaki syndrome:* 100 mg/kg per day in 4 divided doses until fever resolves; then 3–8 mg/kg once daily for 6–10 weeks after onset of the disease, or longer.	Also available in buffered formulation, enteric-coated tablets, and chewing gum.
Atenolol (Tenormin)	*Orally:* Children: initially 0.8–1 mg/kg per day in a single dose. Dosage may be increased to 1.5 mg/kg/day or a maximum of 2 mg/kg per day if necessary. Adults: initially 25–50 mg/day, increasing to 50–100 mg/day as needed. The maximum dose for hypertension is 100 mg; for angina, 200 mg.	Tablets: 25 mg, 50 mg, 100 mg
Atomoxetine (Strattera)	*Orally:* Children ≤70 kg: 0.5 mg/kg per day initially to a maximum of 1.2 mg/kg per day. Doses may be given as a single daily dose or as two divided doses. Adolescents and adults >70 kg: 40 mg daily initially, increasing to a maximum daily dose of 100 mg.	Capsules: 10 mg, 18 mg, 25 mg, 40 mg, 60 mg
Atropine sulfate	*Preoperative orally or IM:* 0.02 mg/kg to a maximum dose of about 1 mg. *Bradycardia:* 0.02 mg/kg with a minimum dose of 0.1 mg and a maximum dose of 0.5 mg in children, 1 mg in adolescents, and 2 mg in adults. *Ophthalmic:* 1–2 drops of 0.5–1% solution in the eye.	Injection: 0.3 mg/mL, 0.4 mg/mL, 0.5 mg/mL, 0.8 mg/mL, 1 mg/mL Ointment, ophthalmic: 0.5%, 1% Solution, ophthalmic: 0.5%, 1%, 2%
Attapulgite (Kaopectate)	*Orally* (dose after each loose bowel movement, up to 7 times a day): Age 3–5: 7.5 mL or 1 tablet. Age 6–12: 15 mL or 2 tablets. Over age 12: 30 mL or 4 tablets.	Suspension: 600 mg/15 mL Tablets, chewable: 300 mg
Azathioprine (Imuran)	*IV or orally:* Children and adults: initially 3–5 mg/kg per day as a single dose. Maintenance doses are usually 1–3 mg/kg per day. Note: Metabolism of azathioprine is decreased by allopurinol; decrease dose of azathioprine by 75%.	Injection: 100-mg vial Tablets: 50 mg
Azelastine (Astelin)	*Intranasal metered dose spray:* 12 years of age and adults: 2 sprays in each nostril twice daily	Solution, nasal: 137 μg/metered spray
Azithromycin (Zithromax)	*Orally:* *Otitis media* (6 months of age and older): 10 mg/kg (to a maximum of 500 mg) on the first day followed by 5 mg/kg per day (to a maximum of 250 mg) for 4 days. *Pharyngitis/tonsillitis:* 2 years of age and older: 12 mg/kg per day (to a maximum of 500 mg) for 5 days. Adults: 500 mg on the first day followed by 250 mg/day for 4 days. *Uncomplicated chlamydia infection:* 1 g as a single dose for patients >8 years of age weighing at least 45 kg. *Gonorrhea:* 2 g for patients weighing at least 45 kg *Chancroid:* 20 mg/kg to a maximum dose of 1 g	Capsules: 250 mg Suspension: 100 mg/5 mL, 200 mg/5 mL, 1-g packet

Continued

Table 1   Medications   (continued)

DRUG	DOSE	DOSAGE FORMS
Aztreonam (Azactam)	*IV or IM:* Children over age 1 month: 60–100 mg/kg per day in 3–4 divided doses. Doses of up to 200 mg/kg per day have been used in severe infections. Maximum total daily dose is 8 g. Adults: 1–2 g every 6–8 hours, depending on the severity of the infection. Dose adjustment is necessary in renal impairment.	Injection: 500-mg, 1-g, 2-g vials
Bacitracin; bacitracin and polymyxin B (Polysporin); bacitracin, neomycin, and polymyxin B (Neosporin)	*Topically:* apply to affected area 1–3 times daily. *Ophthalmic:* apply to eyes every 3–4 hours.	Ointment, ophthalmic (all three): 3.5-g tube Ointment, topical (all three): 15-g, 30-g tubes
Beclomethasone dipropionate (Beclovent, Beconase, Vancenase, Vanceril)	*Intranasal:* Age 6–12: 1 inhalation in each nostril t.i.d. Over age 12 and adults 1 inhalation in each nostril b.i.d. or q.i.d. or 2 inhalations in each nostril b.i.d. *Intranasal aqueous formulation:* Children ≥6 years of age and adults: 1–2 sprays in each nostril b.i.d. Vancenase AQ 84 μg: 1–2 sprays in each nostril daily. *Oral inhalation:* Age 6–12: 1–2 inhalations t.i.d. or q.i.d. or 2–4 inhalations b.i.d. Do not exceed 10 inhalations/day. Over age 12 and adults: 2 inhalations t.i.d. or q.i.d. not to exceed 20 inhalations/day. Vanceril 84 μg Double Strength: use 1/2 the doses recommended above.	Intranasal aerosol spray: 42 μg/spray Intranasal nasal suspension spray pump: 42 μg/spray Intranasal nasal suspension spray pump double strength: 84 μg/spray Oral inhalation aerosol: 42 μg/spray Oral inhalation aerosol double strength: 84 μg/spray
Betamethasone (Diprolene, Diprosone, Maxivate, Uticort, Valisone)	Apply a thin film to the skin 1–3 times daily. Avoid application to the face, groin, or axillae.	Benzoate (Uticort): 0.025% cream, lotion, gel Dipropionate, augmented (Diprolene): 0.05% cream, lotion, gel, ointment Dipropionate (Diprosone): 0.05% cream, lotion, ointment, 0.1% aerosol Dipropionate with clotrimazole (antifungal) [Lotrisone] Valerate (Valisone): 0.01% cream, lotion, ointment
Bethanechol (Urecholine)	*Orally:* *Gastroesophageal reflux:* Children: 0.1–0.2 mg/kg given at least 30 minutes before a meal. Up to 4 doses/day may be given. Adults: 10–50 mg up to q.i.d. *Urinary retention:* Children: 0.6 mg/kg/day in 3–4 divided doses. Adults: 10–50 mg/dose up to q.i.d.	Tablets: 25 mg
Bisacodyl (Dulcolax)	*Orally* (higher doses for evacuation, lower for laxation): Age 3–12: 5–10 mg as a single dose. Over age 12: 5–15 mg as a single dose. Tablets are enteric coated and must not be chewed or crushed. *Rectally:* Under age 2: 5 mg/day as a single dose. Age 2–11: 5–10 mg/day as a single dose. Age 12 or over: 10 mg/day as a single dose.	Suppositories: 5 mg, 10 mg Tablets, enteric coated: 5 mg
Brompheniramine (Dimetane)	*Orally:* <6 years of age: 0.125 mg/kg per dose 4 times a day to a maximum of 8 mg/day. 6–12 years of age: 2–4 mg given 3–4 times a day to a maximum of 16 mg/day. Over age 12: 4–8 mg every 4–6 hours to a maximum of 24 mg/day. Extended-release tablets may be given in as 8 mg b.i.d. or t.i.d. or 12 mg b.i.d.	Elixir: 2 mg/5 mL Tablet: 4 mg, 8 mg, 12 mg Tablets, extended release: 8 mg, 12 mg

Continued

Table 1   Medications   (continued)

DRUG	DOSE	DOSAGE FORMS
Budesonide (Pulmicort, Rhinocort)	*Intranasal metered dose spray:* Children ≥6 years of age and adults: 8 sprays (4 sprays in each nostril) as a single dose in the morning or as 2 divided doses. Dosage may be decreased to the lowest number of sprays that controls symptoms. *Oral inhalation powder:* Children 6–12: 1 to 2 puffs b.i.d. Over age 12 and adults: 2 to 4 puffs b.i.d. *Oral inhalation suspension for nebulization:* All patients: 0.5 mg to 2 mg daily as a single daily dose or in 2 divided doses.	Aerosol, nasal: 50 μg/actuation Oral inhalation powder: 200 mcg/actuation Oral inhalation suspension: 0.25 mg/2 ml, 0.5 mg/2 ml
Bumetanide (Bumex)	*Orally or IV:* Neonates: 0.01–0.05 mg/kg per dose every 24–48 hours. Infants and children: 0.015–0.1 mg/kg per dose every 6–24 hours to a maximum of 10 mg/day. Adults: 0.5–1 mg/dose IV or 0.5–2 mg/dose orally once or twice daily to a maximum of 10 mg/day.	Injection: 0.25 mg/mL Tablets: 0.5 mg, 1 mg, 2 mg
Caffeine	*Orally or IV:* *Loading dose:* 10 mg/kg caffeine base. If theophylline has been administered within the previous 3 days, a modified dose (50%–75% of loading dose) may be given. *Maintenance:* 2.5 mg/kg caffeine base 24 hours after the loading dose. Dosage may be adjusted based on the patient's response and the results of serum level monitoring. Do not use caffeine and sodium benzoate injection in neonates.	Injection: 10 mg/mL Solution: 10 mg/mL
Calcitriol (Calcijex, Rocaltrol)	Individualize to maintain normal serum calcium levels. *Orally:* *Hypocalcemia in premature infants:* 1 μg/day for 5 days. *Renal failure:* Children 0.25–2 μg/day (hemodialysis) or 0.014–0.041 μg/kg per day (no hemodialysis). Adults: 0.25–1 μg/day. *IV:* *Hypocalcemia in premature infants:* 0.05 μg/kg per day for 4 days. *Renal failure:* Children: 0.01–0.05 μg/kg 3 times weekly (hemodialysis). Adults: 0.5–3 μg 3 times weekly (hemodialysis).	Capsules: 0.25 μg, 0.5 μg Injection: 1 μg/mL, 2 μg/mL (1-mL ampules) Solution: 1 μg/mL
Calcium salts	See dosage forms for calcium content of various salts. Dosage should be adjusted based on the desired response and serum calcium levels. *IV (gluconate or chloride salts):* *Cardiac resuscitation:* Calcium gluconate: Children: 60–100 mg/kg per dose to a maximum of 3 g. Adults: 500 mg–1 g/dose. Calcium chloride: Children: 20 mg/kg per dose to a maximum of 1 g. Adults: 2–4 mg/kg per dose to a maximum of 1 g.	Calcium acetate = 25% Ca = 250 mg Ca per 1 g Ca acetate Calcium carbonate = 40% Ca = 400 mg Ca per 1 g Ca carbonate Calcium chloride = 27% Ca = 270 mg Ca per 1 g Ca chloride Calcium citrate = 21% Ca = 210 mg Ca per 1 g Ca citrate Calcium glubionate = 6.5% Ca = 65 mg Ca per 1 g Ca glubionate Calcium gluconate = 9% Ca = 90 mg Ca per 1 g Ca gluconate

Continued

Table 1   Medications   (continued)

DRUG	DOSE	DOSAGE FORMS
Calcium salts (continued)	*Hypocalcemia* (usually the gluconate salt): Neonates: 200–800 mg/kg per day, usually as a continuous infusion. Infants and children: 200–500 mg/kg per day as a continuous infusion or in 4 divided doses. Adults: 2–15 g/day as a continuous infusion or in divided doses. *Orally (carbonate, glubionate, or lactate salts):* Neonates: 20–80 mg calcium/kg per day in 4–6 divided doses. Infants and children: 20–40 mg calcium/kg per day in 4–6 divided doses. Adults: 400 mg-1.2 g calcium/day or more.	Calcium lactate = 13% Ca = 130 mg Ca per 1 g Ca lactate Injection: Chloride salt: 1 g (100 mg/mL) = 27 mg Ca/mL Gluconate salt: 1 g (100 mg/mL) = 9 mg Ca/mL Suspension: carbonate salt: 1.25 g/5 mL = 500 mg Ca/5 mL Syrup: glubionate salt: 1.8 g/5 mL = 115 mg Ca/5 mL Tablets: Acetate salt: 667 mg = 169 mg Ca (PhosLo) Carbonate salt: 650 mg = 260 mg Ca; 1.25 g = 500 mg Ca; 1.5 g = 600 mg Ca Citrate salt: 950 mg = 200 mg Ca (Citracal); 2376 mg = 500 mg Ca (Citracal Liquitab) Gluconate salt: 500 mg = 45 mg Ca; 650 mg = 58.5 mg Ca; 975 mg = 87.75 mg Ca; 1 g = 90 mg Ca Lactate salt: 325 mg = 42.25 mg Ca; 650 mg = 84.5 mg Ca
Calfactant (Infasurf)	*Intratracheally:* 3 mL/kg divided into 2–4 aliquots. Patients should be ventilated and repositioned between aliquots.	Suspension, intratracheal: 8 mL
Captopril (Capoten)	*Orally:* Neonates: 0.01–0.05 mg/kg up to t.i.d., initially. Dose may be increased incrementally to a maximum of 0.5 mg/kg administered as frequently as every 6 hours (2 mg/kg per day). Infants and children: 0.15–0.3 mg/kg up to t.i.d., initially. Dose may be increased incrementally to a maximum of 6 mg/kg per day in divided doses. Adolescents and adults: 12.5–25 mg every 8–12 hours, initially. May be titrated upward to a maximum of 6 mg/kg per day or 450 mg.	Tablets: 12.5 mg, 25 mg, 50 mg, 100 mg
Carbamazepine (Carbatrol, Tegretol, Tegretol-XR)	*Orally:* initially 5–10 mg/kg per day in 2–4 divided doses, increasing slowly to a maximum of 30 mg/kg per day (1.6–2.4 g in adults). Suspension formulation should be administered in 3–4 daily doses; regular tablet formulations may be administered in 2–3 divided doses, extended release formulations may be administered in 2 divided doses.	Capsules, extended release: 200 mg, 300 mg. Suspension: 100 mg/5 mL Tablets, chewable: 100 mg Tablets: 200 mg Tablets, extended release: 100 mg, 200 mg, 400 mg
Carbamide peroxide (Debrox, Gly-Oxide)	*Ear:* instill up to 5–10 drops in the ear and allow to remain there for several minutes or longer. *Orally:* apply several drops to the affected area up to q.i.d.	Drops, oral: 10% (Cank-aid, Gly-Oxide, Orajel Brace-aid Rinse) Drops, otic: 6.5% (Auro Ear Drops, Debrox, Murine Ear Drops)
Cefaclor (Ceclor)	*Orally:* 20–40 mg/kg per 24 hr in 2–3 divided doses to a maximum of 2 g/24 hr.	Capsules: 250 mg Suspension: 125 mg/5 mL, 250 mg/5 mL
Cefadroxil (Duricef, Ultracef)	*Orally:* Children: 30 mg/kg per day in 2 divided doses to a maximum of 2 g/day. Adults: 1–2 g/day in a single or 2 divided doses.	Capsules: 500 mg Suspension: 125 mg/5 mL, 250 mg/5 mL, 500 mg/5 mL Tablets: 1 g
Cefazolin (Ancef, Kefzol)	*IV or IM:* 50–100 mg/kg per day in 3 divided doses to a maximum of 6 g/day. Usual adult doses are 500 mg-2 g/dose every 8 hours Dosing adjustment is necessary in renal impairment.	Injection: 250-mg, 500-mg, 1-g vials
Cefdinir (Omnicef)	*Orally:* Age 6 months to 12 years: 14 mg/kg per day in 1 or 2 divided doses. >12 years or 43 kg: 600 mg daily in 1 or 2 divided doses.	Capsules: 300 mg Suspension: 125 mg/5 mL

Continued

Table 1 Medications (continued)

DRUG	DOSE	DOSAGE FORMS

Cefixime (Suprax)	*Orally:*
	  Children: 8 mg/kg per day in 1 or 2 divided doses to a maximum of 400 mg.
	  Adults: 400 mg/day in 1 or 2 divided doses.
	Otitis media: use suspension formula because higher serum levels are reached at the same dose when the suspension is administered.
		Suspension: 100 mg/5 mL
		Tablets: 200 mg, 400 mg

Cefotaxime (Claforan)	*IV:*
	Sepsis:
	  Infants and children: 100–120 mg/kg per day in 3–4 divided doses.
	  Adults: 1–2 g every 6–8 hours.
	Meningitis:
	  Neonates under age 1 week: 50 mg/kg every 12 hours.
	  Neonates age 1 week or over: 50 mg/kg every 8 hours.
	  Infants over 4 weeks and children: 200 mg/kg per day in 4 divided doses. A dose of 300 mg/kg per day in 4 divided doses has been used for the treatment of pneumococcal meningitis. Maximum total daily dose is 12 g.
	  Adults: 2 g every 4–6 hours.
	  Dosing adjustment is necessary in renal impairment.
		Injection: 1-g, 2-g vials

Cefoxitin (Mefoxin)	*IV:*
	  Neonates: 90–100 mg/kg per day in 3 divided doses.
	  Children: 80–160 mg/kg per day depending on the severity of the infection in 4 divided doses.
	  Adults: 1–2 g every 6–8 hours to a maximum total daily dose of 12 g.
		Injection: 1-g, 2-g vials

Cefpodoxime (Vantin)	*Orally* (with food to enhance absorption):
	  Children: 10 mg/kg per day in 2 divided doses to a maximum of 400 mg/day (otitis media) or 200 mg/day (pharyngitis/tonsillitis).
	  Adults: 200 mg/day in 2 divided doses for upper respiratory or uncomplicated urinary tract infection, 400 mg/day in 2 divided doses for lower respiratory tract infection (community-acquired pneumonia), 800 mg/day in 2 divided doses (skin, skin structure infection).
	  Dosage adjustment is necessary in severe renal impairment.
		Suspension: 50 mg/5 mL, 100 mg/5 mL
		Tablets: 100 mg, 200 mg

Cefprozil (Cefzil)	*Orally:*
	  Children:
	    Otitis media: 30 mg/kg per day in 2 divided doses to a maximum total daily dose of 1 g.
	    Pharyngitis, tonsillitis: 15 mg/kg per day in 2 divided doses to a maximum total daily dose of 500 mg.
	  Adults:
	    Lower respiratory tract: 500 mg every 12 hours.
	    Upper respiratory tract and skin: 500 mg every 24 hours.
	  Dosage adjustment is necessary in renal impairment.
		Suspension: 125 mg/5 mL, 250 mg/5 mL
		Tablets: 250 mg, 500 mg

Continued

Table 1   Medications   (continued)

DRUG	DOSE	DOSAGE FORMS
Ceftazidime (Fortaz, Tazicef, Tazidime)	*IV:* *Neonates:* <2,000 g: 60 mg/kg per day in 2 divided doses. ≥2,000 g: 90 mg/kg per day in 3 divided doses. Infants and children: 90–150 mg/kg per day in 3 divided doses to a maximum total daily dose of 6 g. Adults: 3–6 g/day in 3 divided doses. Dosage adjustment is necessary in renal impairment.	Injection: 500 mg, 1 g, 2 g
Ceftriaxone (Rocephin)	*IV or IM:* *PPNG (uncomplicated pharyngeal, urethral, endocervical, rectal):* <45 kg: 125 mg IM as a single dose. ≥45 kg: 250 mg IM as a single dose. *PPNG (ophthalmia):* >20 kg: 1 g IM as a single dose. *Infants born to a mother infected with PPNG:* 50 mg/kg IM to a maximum of 125 mg as a single dose. *Other serious infections (not including meningitis):* Children: 50–75 mg/kg per day in 2 divided doses. Do not exceed 2 g/day. Adults: usually 1–2 g as a single daily dose or in 2 divided doses. *Otitis media, chancroid:* 50 mg/kg as a single dose given IM. *Meningitis:* Children: 100 mg/kg per day in 1–2 divided doses to a maximum total daily dose of 4 g.	Injection: 250-mg, 500-mg, 1-g, 2-g vials
Cefuroxime (Ceftin, Kefurox, Zinacef)	*Orally* (administer with food to enhance absorption): *Otitis media* (all ages): 30 mg/kg per day in 2 divided doses to a maximum total daily dose of 1 g. *Other infections* (all ages): 20 mg/kg per day in 2 divided doses to a maximum total daily dose of 500 mg. *IV:* Children: 50–100 mg/kg per day in 3–4 divided doses. A dose of 150 mg/kg per day in 3 divided doses is recommended for bone and joint infections. Do not exceed adult doses below. Adults: 2.25–4.5 g/day in 3 divided doses. Higher dose is necessary for severe infections and bone and joint infections. Dosage adjustment is necessary in renal impairment.	Injection: 750-mg, 1.5-g vials Suspension (axetil): 125 mg/5 mL Tablets: 125 mg, 250 mg, 500 mg
Cephalexin (Keflet, Keflex)	*Orally:* Children: 50–100 mg/kg per day in 4 divided doses for otitis media and serious infections. Doses of 25–50 mg/kg per day in 2–4 divided doses may be used for less serious infections. Do not exceed adult doses. Adults: 1–4 g/day in 4 divided doses.	Capsules: 250 mg, 500 mg Drops: 100 mg/mL Suspension: 125 mg/5 mL, 250 mg/5 mL Tablets: 250 mg, 500 mg, 1 g
Cetirizine (Zyrtec)	*Orally:* Age 2–5 years: 2.5 mg/day. Dose may be increased to 5 mg/day as a single or 2 divided doses. Age 6 years–adults: 5–10 mg/day as a single dose.	Syrup: 1 mg/mL Tablets: 5 mg, 10 mg
Charcoal (Actidose-Aqua, Actidose with Sorbitol, CharcoAid, Liqui-Char)	*Orally:* usually available as premixed solutions. Solutions containing sorbitol should not be used for multiple doses because diarrhea will occur. Do not administer concomitantly with ipecac because charcoal will adsorb and inactivate the ipecac. Do not administer with milk, ice cream, or sherbet because adsorptive capacity of the charcoal will be decreased.	Liquid: 25 g/120 mL, 30 g/240 mL, 50 g/240 mL Liquid, with sorbitol: 25 g/120 mL, 50 g/240 mL

Continued

Table 1 Medications (continued)

DRUG	DOSE	DOSAGE FORMS

Charcoal (Actidose-Aqua, Actidose with Sorbitol, CharcoAid, Liqui-Char) (*continued*)	Single dose:
	   Children: 1–2 g/kg up to 15–30 g as soon as possible after the ingestion, preferably after emesis.
	   Adults: 30–100 g.
	   Dose should be 5 to 10 times the amount of the ingested poison.
	Multiple dose (products without sorbitol):
	   Infants: 1 g/kg every 4–6 hours.
	   Children and adults: 1–2 g/kg (up to 60 g) every 2–6 hours.	

Chloral hydrate (Aquachloral, Noctec)	*Orally or rectally:* *Sedation before procedures:* 60–75 mg/kg 30 minutes to 1 hour before the procedure. May repeat with a half-dose (30–37.5 mg/kg) if the first dose is ineffective. Do not exceed 120 mg/kg or 2 g total. *Sedation for anxiety:* 25 mg/kg per day in divided doses every 6–8 hours to a maximum of the usual adult dose of 750 mg/day. Continuous therapy, especially in infants, is not recommended.	Capsules: 250 mg, 500 mg Suppositories: 324 mg, 500 mg, 648 mg Syrup: 500 mg/5 mL

Chloramphenicol (Chloromycetin)	*IV or orally:*
	   Neonates under age 7 days: 25 mg/kg per day in a single daily dose.
	   Neonates age 7–21 days: 50 mg/kg per day in 2 divided doses daily.
	   Infants and children: 50–75 mg/kg per day in 4 divided doses to a maximum total daily dose of 4 g.
	   Adults: 50 mg/kg per day in 4 divided doses to a maximum total daily dose of 4 g.
	   Serum levels must be monitored closely, especially in neonates and infants, and patients with renal or hepatic impairment.
		Capsules: 250 mg
		Injection: 1-g vial

Chlorothiazide (Diuril)	*Orally:*
	   Infants under age 6 months: 20–40 mg/kg per day in 2 divided doses.
	   Children: 20 mg/kg per day in 2 divided doses.
	   Adults: 0.5–1 g/day in 1 or 2 divided doses.
	IV:
	   Infants under age 6 months: 20–40 mg/kg per day in 2 divided doses, but doses of 2–8 mg/kg per day may be sufficient in some patients.
	   Children: 4–20 mg/kg per day in 2 divided doses.
	   Adults: 0.5–1 g/day.
		Injection: 500 mg
		Suspension: 250 mg/5 mL
		Tablets: 250 mg, 500 mg

Chlorpromazine (Thorazine)	*Nausea and vomiting or psychosis:*
	   Over age 6 months: 0.3–0.5 mg/kg IV every 6–8 hours or 0.5–1 mg/kg PO every 4–6 hours or 1 mg/kg rectally every 6–8 hours as needed. Do not exceed adult doses.
	   Adults: 25–50 mg IV every 6–8 hours or 10–25 mg PO every 4–6 hours or 50–100 mg rectally every 6–8 hours. Doses may be increased in the treatment of psychoses; some adults may require as much as 800 mg/day until control is achieved. Dose should then be decreased to the usual maintenance levels of 200 mg/day for adults.
		Injection: 25 mg/mL
		Oral concentrate: 30 mg/mL, 100 mg/mL
		Suppositories: 25 mg, 100 mg
		Syrup: 10 mg/5 mL
		Tablets: 10 mg, 25 mg, 50 mg, 100 mg, 200 mg

Cholestyramine resin (Cholybar, Questran, Questran Light)	*Orally:*
	   Children: 240 mg/kg per day of the resin administered in 3 divided doses.
	   Adults: 3–4 g t.i.d. or q.i.d.
	   Doses should be administered mixed in liquids (4 g in 2–6 oz) or with pulpy fruits (applesauce or pineapple).
	   Many drugs bind with cholestyramine in the GI tract. Drugs should be administered 1 hour before or 4 hours after cholestyramine. Patients should also be cautioned to ingest plenty of fluids to avoid constipation and fecal impaction.
		Bar: 4 g resin/bar (Cholybar)
		Powder: 4 g resin/9 g powder (Questran); 4 g resin/5 g powder (Questran Light, contains aspartame)

Continued

Table 1 Medications (continued)

DRUG	DOSE	DOSAGE FORMS

Cimetidine (Tagamet)	*Orally, IV:*
	 Initial dose:
	    Neonates: 5–10 mg/kg per day in 2–3 divided doses daily.
	    Infants: 10–20 mg/kg per day in 2–4 divided doses daily.
	    Children: 20–40 mg/kg per day in 4 divided doses daily.
	    Adults: 300 mg every 6 hours. Orally, doses of 800 mg at bedtime or 400 mg b.i.d. may be used.
	    Doses may be adjusted upward, especially in hypersecretory states, as necessary to maintain the gastric pH of 5 or greater. A maximum total daily dose of 2.4 g should not be exceeded.
	 Dosage must be adjusted in renal impairment.
		Injection: 150 mg/mL
		 Liquid: 300 mg/5 mL
		 Tablets: 200 mg, 300 mg, 400 mg, 800 mg

Ciprofloxacin (Ciloxan, Cipro)	The drug is not approved for use in patients under age 18 due to possible adverse effects; consider risk vs. benefit if for use in patients under age 18.
	 Orally (on an empty stomach):
	    Children: 20–30 mg/kg per day in 2 divided doses; up to 40 mg/kg per day may be used for patients with cystic fibrosis. Do not exceed 1.5 g/day.
	    Adults: 500–1,500 mg/day in 2 divided doses.
	 IV (administer over 1 hour at a concentration of 1–2 mg/mL):
	    Children: 15–20 mg/kg per day in 2 divided doses; up to 30 mg/kg per day may be used in patients with cystic fibrosis. Do not exceed 800 mg/day.
	    Adults: 400–800 mg/day in 2 divided doses.
	    Dosage must be adjusted in patients with renal dysfunction.
	 Ophthalmic: administer 1–2 drops every 2 hours while awake for 2 days and then every 4 hours while awake for 5 days.
		Injection: 10 mg/mL
		 Solution, ophthalmic: 3.5%
		 Tablets: 250 mg, 500 mg, 750 mg

Citrate and citric acid (Bicitra, Polycitra, Shohl's Solution)	*Orally (dilute in water or juice):*
	    Infants and children: 2–3 mEq/kg per day in 3–4 divided doses.
	    Adults: 15–30 mL given q.i.d.
	    Giving doses with meals decreases the saline laxative effect.
		Content per 1 mL*

Clarithromycin (Biaxin)	*Orally:*
	    Children: 15 mg/kg per day in 2 divided doses, not to exceed 1 g/day.
	    Adults: 500 mg-1 g/day in 2 divided doses.
		Suspension: 125 mg/5 mL, 250 mg/5 mL
		 Tablets: 250 mg, 500 mg

Clindamycin (Cleocin)	*IV:*
	    Neonates under age 7 days:
	       ≤2,000 g: 10 mg/kg per day in 2 divided doses.
	       >2,000 g: 15 mg/kg per day in 3 divided doses.
	    Neonates over age 7 days:
	       <1,200 g: 10 mg/kg per day in 2 divided doses.
	       1,200–2,000 g: 15 mg/kg per day in 3 divided doses.
	       >2,000 g: 20 mg/kg per day in 3–4 divided doses.
	    Infants and children: 25–40 mg/kg per day in 3–4 divided doses.
	    Adults: 1.2–2.7 g/day in 2–4 divided doses.
	       Maximum total daily dose should not exceed 4.8 g and should be used for life-threatening infections only.
		Capsules: 150 mg
		 Injection: 150 mg/mL
		 Solution, oral: 75 mg/5 mL
		 Solution, topical: 1%

Continued

Table 1 Medications (continued)

DRUG	DOSE	DOSAGE FORMS
Clindamycin (Cleocin) (*continued*)	*Orally:* Infants and children: 15–25 mg/kg per day in 3–4 divided doses for moderate to severe infections. Adults: 150–450 mg every 6–8 hours to a maximum total daily dose of 1.8 g. *Topically:* apply to the affected area b.i.d. Avoid the eyes, abraded skin, and mucous membranes.	
Clonazepam (Klonopin)	*Orally:* Under age 10 or <30 kg: initially 0.01–0.03 mg/kg/day in 2–3 divided doses. Dose may be increased gradually (every third day) until seizures are controlled or adverse effects are seen. The usual maintenance dose range is 0.1–0.2 mg/kg per day. Adults >30 kg: initially 1.5 mg/day in 3 divided doses. Dose may be increased by 0.5–1 mg every third day to a maximum total daily dose of 20 mg. Usual maintenance dose is 0.05–0.2 mg/kg per day.	Tablets: 0.5 mg, 1 mg, 2 mg
Clonidine (Catapres)	*Orally:* *Hypertension:* 5 to 10 μg/kg per day in 2 to 3 divided doses. In patients who experience sedation, the doses may be divided such that the patient receives a larger dose at bedtime and a smaller dose in the morning. Dose may be incrementally increased if necessary to 25 μg/kg/day to a maximum dose of 0.9 mg/day. *Attention deficit/hyperactivity disorder:* 5 μg/kg per day in 4 divided doses has been used in some patients who have failed conventional therapy.	Tablet: 0.1 mg, 0.2 mg, 0.3 mg
Clorazepate dipotassium (Tranxene)	*Orally:* Age 9–12: initially 3.75–7.5 mg b.i.d. Dose may be increased by 3.75 mg at weekly intervals to a maximum total daily dose of 60 mg. Over age 12 and adults: up to 7.5 mg up to t.i.d. May be increased by 7.5 mg at weekly intervals to a maximum total daily dose of 90 mg.	Capsules or tablets: 3.75 mg, 7.5 mg, 15 mg Tablets: 11.25 mg, 22.5 mg
Clotrimazole (Lotrimin, Mycelex)	*Vaginal cream:* 1 full applicator at bedtime for 7–14 days. *Vaginal suppository:* 1 suppository intravaginally at bedtime for 7 days or 2 at bedtime for 3 days or 500 mg as a single dose. *Topically:* apply to affected areas b.i.d.	Cream, topical: 1% (30-g tube) Cream, vaginal: 1% (45-g tube) Solution, topical: 1% (30-mL squeeze bottle) Suppositories, vaginal: 100 mg, 500 mg
Codeine	*Orally:* *Analgesic:* 0.5–1 mg/kg every 4–6 hours as needed, to a maximum of 60 mg. Usual adult dose is 30 mg. *Antitussive:* 0.2–0.25 mg/kg every 4–6 hours as needed, to a maximum of 30 kg. *SC:* same doses as above may be used, although the oral route is only two thirds as effective as the SC route. It should not be used IV. (For IV route, use morphine)	Injection (phosphate): 30 mg/mL, 60 mg/mL Solution, oral (phosphate): 15 mg/5 mL Tablets (sulfate): 15 mg, 30 mg, 60 mg Also available in various combinations with acetaminophen: Elixir, oral: 12 mg codeine with 120 mg acetaminophen Tablets: 7.5 mg codeine with acetaminophen 300 mg (Tylenol w/Codeine No. 1), 15 mg codeine with acetaminophen 300 mg (Tylenol w/Codeine No. 2), 300 mg codeine with acetaminophen 300 mg (Tylenol w/Codeine No. 3), 60 mg codeine with acetaminophen 300 mg (Tylenol w/Codeine No. 4)
Colfosceril palmitate (Exosurf Neonatal)	*Intratracheally:* should be used only by physicians familiar with its administration. The usual dose is 5 mL/kg divided equally between the two lungs. Second and third doses may be administered at 12-hour intervals. The infant should be suctioned before administration of colfosceril and ventilator settings should be decreased, depending on the patient's response.	Powder, lyophilized: 108 mg/10 mL

Continued

Table 1   Medications   (continued)

DRUG	DOSE	DOSAGE FORMS
Colistin, neomycin, and hydro-cortisone (Coly-Mycin S Otic)	*Otic* (shake bottle well before administering): Children: 3 drops in the affected ear t.i.d. or q.i.d. Adults: 4 drops in the affected ear t.i.d. or q.i.d.	Suspension, otic: 5 mL
Cortisone acetate (Cortone Acetate)	Depends on the use of the drug and patient response. *Orally:* *Physiologic replacement:* 0.5–0.75 mg/kg per day in 3 divided doses. *Antiinflammatory:* 2.5–10 mg/kg per day in 3–4 divided doses. *IM:* *Physiologic replacement:* 0.25–0.35 mg/kg per day as a single dose. *Antiinflammatory:* 1–5 mg/kg per day in 1 or 2 divided doses. In patients requiring physiologic replacement, dosage may need to be increased during periods of stress, including perioperatively and during illness.	Injection: 50 mg/mL Tablets: 5 mg, 10 mg, 25 mg
Cosyntropin (Cortrosyn)	*IV:* Under age 2: 0.125 mg. Over age 2 and adults: 0.25 mg.	Injection: 0.25 mg
Co-trimoxazole (trimethoprim and sulfamethoxazole; Bactrim, Septra)	*Orally or IV (based on trimethoprim):* Over age 2 months and adults: *Treatment doses:* 　*Mild to moderate infections (urinary tract or otitis media):* 8 mg trimethoprim/kg per day in 2 divided doses. Maximum dose is 320 mg trimethoprim/day. 　*Pneumocystis carinii pneumonitis:* 20 mg trimethoprim/kg per day in 4 divided doses. *Prophylaxis doses:* 　Urinary tract infection: 2 mg trimethoprim/kg per day as a single dose. 　*Pneumocystis carinii:* 150 mg/m2 per day in 1 or 2 divided doses daily on 3 consecutive or alternating days per week. 　Dosage adjustment is necessary in patients with renal impairment. 　IV doses must be administered over 60–90 minutes and should be well diluted (1 mL injection in 25 mL infusate).	Injection: 16 mg trimethoprim and 80 mg sulfamethoxazole per 1 mL Suspension: 8 mg trimethoprim and 40 mg sulfamethoxazole per 1 mL Tablets: 80 mg trimethoprim and 400 mg sulfamethoxazole Tablets, double strength: 160 mg trimethoprim and 800 mg sulfamethoxazole
Cromolyn sodium (Crolom, Intal, Nasalcrom, Opticrom)	Children: *Metered-dose inhaler:* 2 inhalations q.i.d. *Spinhaler dry inhalation:* contents of 1 capsule q.i.d. *Nebulizer solution:* 20 mg nebulized q.i.d. *Intranasal spray:* 1 spray in each nostril 3–6 times daily. *Ophthalmic:* 1–2 drops in each eye 4–6 times daily.	Capsules, powder for inhalation: 20 mg Inhalation, metered dose: 800 μg/spray Solution, nasal: 5.2 mg/spray Solution, nebulizer: 20 mg/2 mL Solution, ophthalmic: 4%
Crotamiton (Eurax)	*Topically:* apply a thin layer to all skin surfaces from the neck to the toes and soles of the feet. Be sure to apply to all surfaces, including skin folds. Avoid the face and mucous membranes, including the urethral meatus. A second coat is applied 24 hours later. A cleansing bath should follow 48 hours after the second application. Treatment may be repeated after 7–10 days if the mites reappear. It is safe for use in infants and young children. If signs of irritation or hypersensitivity appear, remove the product immediately by bathing. Contaminated clothing and bed linens should be washed to avoid reinfestations.	Cream: 10% Lotion: 10%

Continued

Table 1   Medications   (continued)

DRUG	DOSE	DOSAGE FORMS
Cyclosporine (Neoral, Sandimmune)	NOTE: The two are not bioequivalent. Clinical condition and serum levels must be monitored carefully when a patient's therapy is changed from one to the other, especially in patients receiving large doses (>10 mg/kg per day) of Sandimmune who are changed to Neoral therapy because significant drug toxicity may result. *Orally:* *Sandimmune:* initially 10–18 mg/kg per day (dose dependent on organ being transplanted) in 2 divided doses, tapering over several weeks with frequent monitoring to a maintenance dose usually in the range of 5–10 mg/kg per day. *Neoral:* initially about 10 mg/kg per day in 2 divided doses, tapering over several weeks based on clinical condition and serum levels. *Conversion from Sandimmune to Neoral:* Consult with pharmacist *IV (Sandimmune only):* 5–6 mg/kg per day in 1 or 2 divided doses. Each dose should be administered over at least 2 hours.	Capsules (Neoral): 25 mg, 100 mg Capsules (Sandimmune): 25 mg, 50 mg, 100 mg Injection (Sandimmune): 50 mg/mL Solution, oral (Neoral and Sandimmune): 100 mg/mL
Dantrolene sodium (Dantrium)	*Orally:* *Spasticity:* Children >5 years of age: 0.5 mg/kg given b.i.d. initially, but frequency may be increased gradually to t.i.d. or q.i.d. The maximum dose is 100 mg q.i.d. Adults: 25 mg daily initially, with increases in frequency and dose to a maximum of 400 mg/day in 4 divided doses. *Malignant hyperthermia prophylaxis:* 4–8 mg/kg per day in 3–4 divided doses daily for 1–2 days prior to surgery. *Intravenously:* *Malignant hyperthermia prophylaxis:* 2.5 mg/kg administered over 1 hour about 1.25 hours before surgery. Repeat doses may be necessary. *Malignant hyperthermia crisis:* 1 mg/kg given rapidly. Repeat doses may be necessary, but it is usually not necessary to exceed 2.5 mg/kg. Maximum dose should not exceed 10 mg/kg.	Capsules: 25 mg, 50 mg, 100 mg Injection: 20 mg
Deferoxamine (Desferal)	*Children:* *Acute iron intoxication:* 15 mg/kg per hr IV continuous infusion; maximum 6 g/24 hr. *Chronic iron overload:* 20–25 mg/kg per day IM or 500 mg-2 g IV with each unit of blood transfused, or 20–40 mg/kg per day SC over 8–12 hours up to 1–2 g/day.	Injection: 500-mg vial
Desmopressin acetate (DDAVP)	*Intranasally:* *Nocturnal enuresis in patients over age 6:* 20 μg at bedtime with half of dose in each nostril. Dose may be increased or decreased depending on the patient's response. Usual range is 10–40 μg/day. *Diabetes insipidus in patients age 7 years-adults:* initially 5 μg/day as a single dose or in 2 divided doses. Dosage should be titrated to the patient's response. The usual range is 5–40 μg/day.	Injection: 4 μg/mL Solution, nasal: 100 μg/mL/2.4 mL bottle with calibrated intranasal tube Spray, intranasal: 10 μg/actuation metered dose Tablets: 0.1 mg, 0.2 mg

Continued

Table 1   Medications   (continued)

DRUG	DOSE	DOSAGE FORMS

Desmopressin acetate (DDAVP) (*continued*)	*Orally:*
	Diabetes insipidus:
	  Children: initially, 0.05 mg/dose with careful monitoring to prevent hyponatremia or water intoxication.
	  Over age 12 and adults: initially, 0.05 mg b.i.d. Dosage may then be adjusted to maintain normal diurnal water turnover. The usual total daily dosage is in the range of 0.1–1.2 mg and may be administered in 2–3 divided doses.
	Nocturnal enuresis in children over age 12:
	  0.2–0.4 mg/day at bedtime.
	IV:
	To increase factor VIII levels: 0.3 μg/kg over 30 minutes.
	Diabetes insipidus: adult doses are 2–4 μg/day in 2 divided doses or approximately one tenth of the intranasal dose necessary to control the patient's symptoms, if that is known.	

Dexamethasone (Decadron, Hexadrol, Maxidex)	*IV or orally:* *Bacteria meningitis:* 0.6 mg/kg per day in 4 divided doses for the first 4 days of antibiotic therapy. It must be started at the same time or before the first dose of antibiotic. *Cerebral edema:* 1–1.5 mg/kg per day in 4 divided doses to a maximum total daily dose of 16 mg. *Antiemetic therapy (chemotherapy-induced emesis):* 20 mg/m^2 per day in 4 divided doses. *Airway edema or extubation:* 0.5–2 mg/kg per day in 4 divided doses beginning 24 hours before and continuing for at least 24 hours after extubation. Doses should be tapered when discontinuing long-term therapy. *Ophthalmic:* instill drops or apply ointment t.i.d. or q.i.d.	Elixir: 0.5 mg/5 mL Injection: 4 mg/mL, 10 mg/mL, 20 mg/mL, 24 mg/mL Ointment, ophthalmic: 0.05% Solution, ophthalmic: 0.05% Solution, oral: 1 mg/mL Tablets: 0.25 mg, 0.5 mg, 0.75 mg, 1 mg, 1.5 mg, 2 mg, 4 mg, 6 mg

Dextroamphetamine sulfate (Dexedrine)	*Orally:*
	  Age 3–5: 2.5 mg/day given in the morning. Dosage may be increased 2.5 mg/day until a response is realized or side effects appear. Usual range is 0.1–0.5 mg/kg per day to a maximum of 40 mg.
	  Age 6 or older: 5 mg/day in the morning or at noon. Dosage may be increased in 5-mg increments at weekly intervals. Usual range is 0.1–0.5 mg/kg per day to a maximum of 40 mg.
		Capsules, sustained release: 5 mg, 10 mg, 15 mg
		Tablets: 5 mg, 10 mg

Diazepam (Diastat Rectal, Valium)	*IV:* *Status epilepticus:* 0.05–0.3 mg/kg administered over 2–3 minutes and repeated every 15–30 minutes to a total maximum dose of 0.75 mg/kg or 30 mg, whichever is less. May be repeated in 2–4 hours, if necessary. *Sedation:* 0.04–0.2 mg/kg every 2–4 hours to a maximum of 0.6 mg/kg within an 8-hour period. *Orally for sedation or muscle relaxant:* 0.12–0.8 mg/kg per day in 3–4 divided doses to an adult dose of 6–40 mg/day. *Rectally (round dose off to closest dose available from manufacturer):* Children 2–5 years of age: 0.5 mg/kg. Children 6–11 years of age: 0.3 mg/kg Children $\geq$12 years of age and adults: 0.2 mg/kg. Dose may be repeated every 4–12 hours as necessary.	Gel, rectal (in rectal delivery system): 2.5 mg, 5 mg, 10 mg, 15 mg, 20 mg Injection: 5 mg/mL Solution, oral: 5 mg/5 mL Solution, concentrated oral: 5 mg/mL Tablets: 2 mg, 5 mg, 10 mg

Continued

Table 1   Medications   (continued)

DRUG	*DOSE*	*DOSAGE FORMS*
Diazoxide (Hyperstat IV, Proglycem)	*IV* (hypertensive emergency): 1–3 mg/kg to a maximum of 150 mg. Dose may be repeated in 5–15 minutes. *Orally* (hypoglycemia due to hyperinsulinism): Newborns and infants: initially 8 mg/kg per day in 2 or 3 divided doses. May be increased incrementally if response is inadequate to a maximum of 15 mg/kg per day. Children and adults: 3 mg/kg per day in 2 or 3 divided doses initially. May be increased to a maximum of 8 mg/kg per day.	Capsules: 50 mg Injection: 15 mg/mL Suspension, oral: 50 mg/mL
Dicloxacillin (Dycill, Dynapen, Pathocil)	*Orally:* Children <40 kg: 25–50 mg/kg per day in 4 divided doses. Doses of 50–100 mg/kg per day in 4 divided doses are necessary for follow-up oral therapy of osteomyelitis. Children ≥40 kg and adults: 125–500 mg/dose every 6 hours.	Capsules: 250 mg, 500 mg Suspension, oral: 62.5 mg/5 mL
Didanosine (ddI [dideoxyinisine]; Videx)	*Orally:* doses must be given at 12-hour intervals on an empty stomach, but because the drug is degraded by gastric acids, each formulation contains buffers. *Infants and children:* 180–300 mg/m^2 per day in 2 divided doses. If the tablet formulation is used, children over age 1 should receive 2 tablets per dose to assure sufficient buffering. Children under age 1 may receive doses in a single tablet. *Adults:* <60 kg: 125 mg (tablets) or 167 mg (buffered powder) per dose twice daily. ≥60 kg: 200 mg (tablets) or 250 mg (buffered powder) per dose twice daily.	Powder for oral solution, buffered (single-dose packets): 100 mg, 167 mg, 250 mg, 375 mg Powder for oral solution, pediatric (mixed with an antacid at the time it is dispensed by the pharmacist): 10 mg/mL tablets, buffered, chewable/dispersible: 25 mg, 50 mg, 100 mg, 150 mg
Digoxin (Lanoxicaps, Lanoxin)	Should be based on lean body weight. Dosage adjustment is required in patients with impaired renal function. Total digitalizing dose (TDD) is administered as follows: half TDD initially, then one fourth TDD 8–12 hours later, then one fourth TDD 8–12 hours after that. Maintenance doses are administered in 2 divided doses beginning 12 hours after the last digitalizing dose. Patients should be under continuous cardiographic monitoring during digitalization. IM doses are the same as oral doses, but that route of administration should be avoided.[†]	Capsules, liquid filled (Lanoxicaps): 0.05 mg, 0.1 mg, 0.2 mg (90%–100% bioavailable) Elixir: 0.05 mg/mL (75%–87% bioavailable) Injection: 0.1 mg/mL, 0.25 mg/mL (100% bioavailable IV) Tablets: 0.125 mg, 0.25 mg, 0.5 mg (60%–80% bioavailable)
Dihydroergotamine (D.H.E.)	*Intravenously:* Children 6 to 9 years of age: 100–150 mcg/dose repeated every 6 hours to a maximum of 8 doses. Children 10–12 years of age: 200 mcg/dose repeated every 6 hours to a maximum of 8 doses. Adolescents up to 16 years of age: 250-500 mcg/dose repeated every 6 hours to a maximum of 8 doses. Adults: 500 mcg repeated hourly to a maximum of 2 mg (6 mg/week)	Injection: 1 mg/mL

Dimercaprol (BAL [British antilewisite])	*Deep IM:*
	Lead toxicity:
	Severe poisoning: 4 mg/kg 6 times a day for 3–5 days.
	Arsenic, mercury, or gold toxicity:
	Mild:
	  Days 1 and 2: 3 mg/kg q.i.d.
	  Day 3: 3 mg/kg b.i.d.
	  Days 4–14: 3 mg/kg every day.
		Injection: 100 mg/mL (3-mL ampule)

Continued

Table 1   Medications   (continued)

DRUG	DOSE	DOSAGE FORMS
Dimercaprol (BAL [British antilewisite]) (continued)	*Severe:* Days 1 and 2: 3 mg/kg 6 times a day. Day 3: 3 mg/kg q.i.d. Days 4–14: 3 mg/kg b.i.d.	
Diphenhydramine (Benadryl, Benylin, Nytol, Sleep-Eze 3, Sominex Formula 2)	*IV, orally, IM:* Children: 5 mg/kg per day in 3 or 4 divided doses to a maximum of 300 mg/day. Adults: 10–50 mg repeated as often as every 4 hours, not to exceed 400 mg/day. The drug may cause paradoxical excitement in children.	Capsules: 25 mg, 50 mg Elixir (14% alcohol): 12.5 mg/5 mL Injection: 10 mg/mL, 50 mg/mL Syrup (5% alcohol): 12.5 mg/5 mL Tablets: 25 mg, 50 mg
Dobutamine hydrochloride (Dobutrex)	*IV infusion:* 2–15 μg/kg per min to a maximum of 40 μg/kg per min. Start at the lower end of the range and titrate upward based on the patient's response.	Injection: 12.5 mg/mL
Docusate sodium (dioctyl sodium sulfosuccinate; Colace, D-S-S, Doxinate)	*Orally* (in 1–4 divided doses with a glass of water): Infants and children under age 3: 10–40 mg/day. Age 3–6: 20–60 mg/day. Age >6–12: 40–150 mg/day. Over age 12 and adults: 50–500 mg. Do not administer with mineral oil because absorption of the mineral oil may be increased.	Capsules: 50 mg, 100 mg, 240 mg, 250 mg Liquid: 150 mg/15 mL Solution: 50 mg/mL Syrup: 50 mg/15 mL, 60 mg/15 mL Also available in combination with stimulant laxatives, including senna, phenolphthalein, and casanthranol.
Dopamine hydrochloride (Dopastat, Intropin)	*Continuous IV infusion:* initially 1 μg/kg per min titrated upward based on patient's response to a maximum of 20 μg/kg per min in neonates or 50 μg/kg per min in all other patients. The hemodynamic effects of dopamine occur only at doses >15 μg/kg per min.	Injection in 5% dextrose: 0.8 mg/mL, 1.6 mg/mL, 3.2 mg/mL (premixed infusions) Injection: 40 mg/mL, 80 mg/mL, 160 mg/mL
Dornase alfa (Pulmozyme)	*Inhalation via approved compressor:* Children >5 years of age and adults: 2.5 mg/day.	Solution, inhalation: 2.5 mg/2.5 mL
Doxycycline (Doryx, Doxy-100, Vibramycin)	*Orally or IV:* Children under age 8: should not be used unless there is no alternative. $\geq$age 8: 2–5 mg/kg per day to a maximum of 200 mg/day in 1 or 2 divided doses. Adults: 100–200 mg/day in 1 or 2 divided doses. Inpatient treatment of PID 100 mg IV b.i.d. with cefoxitin 2 g IV every 6 hours for at least 4 days or 2 days after patient improves, whichever is longer. Doxycycline should be continued orally to complete 10–14 days of therapy.	Capsules or tablets: 50 mg, 100 mg Injection: 100 mg, 200 mg
d-Xylose (wood sugar; Xylo-Pfan)	*Orally* (prepared as a 5%–10% aqueous solution): 14.5 g/m^2 to a maximum dose of 25 g. Alternatively, a dose of 500 mg/kg may be used. Infants should fast for 4–5 hours before the dose and children should fast overnight. Blood xylose levels are then measured to determine extent of intestinal absorption.	Powder for preparing oral solutions: 25 g
Edetate calcium disodium (Calcium Disodium Versenate, Calcium EDTA)	*Mild to moderate lead poisoning:* 25–50 mg/kg. *Severe lead poisoning:* up to 75 mg/kg per 24 hr not to exceed 1.5 g/day. *Usual dosage* (children): *Asymptomatic lead toxicity:* *Initial:* up to 1 g/m^2 per 24 hr in a continuous IV drip if possible or in 2–4 divided doses for 5 days. Subsequent courses: up to 50 mg/kg per 24 hr in a continuous IV drip if possible or in 2–4 divided doses for 3–5 days.	Injection: 200 mg/mL For intravenous infusion, dilute to a maximum concentration of 5 mg/mL with D$_5$W or normal saline. Infusions should be administered either continuously or over 1–2 hours if intermittent doses are used. Rapid infusion may increase intracranial pressure.

Continued

Table 1   Medications   (continued)

DRUG	DOSE	DOSAGE FORMS
Edetate calcium disodium (Calcium Disodium Versenate, Calcium EDTA) (continued)	*Symptomatic lead toxicity or lead encephalopathy:* Initial: up to 1.5 g/m² per 24 hr in a continuous IV drip if possible or in 6 divided doses for 5–7 days; give with dimercaprol (BAL). Subsequent courses: as for asymptomatic toxicity above.	
Edrophonium (Enlon, Reversol, Tensilon)	*Myasthenia gravis diagnosis:* Infants: Initially 0.1 mg; if no response, follow with an additional 0.4 mg for a maximum total dose of 0.5 mg. Children: Initial: 0.04 mg/kg followed by 0.16 mg/kg if no response; maximum total dose is 10 mg. Adults: 0.2 mg/kg up to 10 mg. Administer 2 mg initially, then titrate dose. *Titration of therapy:* 0.04 mg/kg one time; if strength improves, an increase in neostigmine or pyridostigmine dose is indicated.	Injection: 10 mg/mL May precipitate cholinergic crisis.
Enalapril, enalaprilat (Vasotec)	*Orally:* initially 0.1 mg/kg per day in 1 or 2 divided doses to the usual adult dose of 2.5–5 mg/kg per day. Dosage may be increased as required to a maximum of 0.5 mg/kg per day or 40 mg. *IV:* 5–10 μg/kg (up to 0.625–1.25 mg) may be administered every 8–24 hours as necessary for control of hypertension. Dosage must be decreased in patients with compromised renal function and also should be decreased in patients who are hyponatremic or volume depleted, in severe congestive heart failure, or in those who are receiving diuretics. The oral dosage form (enalapril) is a product that is not stable in aqueous media. The injectable dosage form (enalaprilat) is the active form, but is not absorbed from the GI tract.	Injection: 1.25 mg/mL Tablets: 2.5 mg, 5 mg, 10 mg, 20 mg
Enoxaparin (Lovenox)	*SC:* *Prophylaxis:* Infants <2 months of age: 0.75 mg/kg per dose every 12 hours Infants ≥2 months of age and children: 0.5 mg/kg per dose every 12 hours. Adults >45 kg: 30 mg every 12 hours. *Treatment of DVT or PE:* Infants <2 months of age: 1.5 mg/kg per dose every 12 hours Infants ≥2 months of age and children: 1 mg/kg per dose every 12 hours Adults >45 kg: 1 mg/kg per dose every 12 hours. Doses should be adjusted based on anti-factor Xa levels.	Injection: 100 mg/mL
Epinephrine (Adrenalin, Vaponefrin)	*IV for asystole, or pulseless arrest:* Neonates: 0.01–0.03 mg/kg (0.1–0.3 mL/kg of a 1:10,000 solution) every 3–5 minutes as necessary. Infants to adults: 0.1 mg/kg to a maximum of 1 mg; may be repeated every 3–5 minutes as necessary. A continuous infusion may be started at a dose of 0.1–1 μg/kg per min and titrated to effect. *Nebulization:* 0.25–0.5 mL of a 2.25% racemic epinephrine solution diluted in 2.5–3 mL of normal saline for inhalation.	Aerosol: 0.2–0.3 mg/spray, depending on brand (Bronkaid Mist, Primatene Mist, AsthmaHaler Mist) Injection: 1:10,000 (0.1 mg/mL), 1:1,000 (1 mg/mL) Injection prefilled automatic syringe: 1:200 (EpiPen delivers 0.3 mg IM, EpiPen Jr. delivers 0.15 mg IM) Solution, racemic for inhalation: 2.25% (AsthmaNefrin, S-2, Vaponefrin)

Continued

Table 1   Medications   (continued)

DRUG	DOSE	DOSAGE FORMS
Epoetin alfa (erythropoietin; Epogen, EPO, r-HuEPO)	*IV or SC:* initially 50–100 U/kg administered 1–3 times weekly until the hematocrit reaches 30%–33%. Dosage should be lowered if the hematocrit exceeds that range or increases by more than 4 points in a 2-week period. It may be increased if the hematocrit does not reach the target range or fails to increase by 5–6 points in an 8-week period. The usual maintenance dose is 25 U/kg 3 times weekly. Hematocrit and serum iron levels should be monitored frequently. Blood pressure should also be monitored frequently.	Injection: 2,000 U/mL, 4000 U/mL, 10,000 U/mL

Ergocalciferol (vitamin D$_2$, acti-vated ergosterol; Calciferol, Drisdol)	1 μg = 40 U.
	Orally:
	  Healthy infants and children: 400 U/day.
	  Infants and children with malabsorption syndromes: 1,000 U/day.
	  Children with liver disease: 4,000–8,000 U/day.
	  Children with vitamin D-dependent rickets: 3,000–5,000 U/day.
	  Nutritional rickets with normal absorption: 1,000–5,000 U/day; with malabsorption: 10,000–25,000 U/day.
	IM: should be retained for patients with rickets due to severe vitamin D-deficiency. The dose for vitamin D-resistant rickets ranges from 50,000–500,000 U/day, for hypoparathyroidism from 50,000–200,000 U/day, and for familial hypophosphatemia from 10,000–80,000 U/day. The range between therapeutic and toxic doses is narrow. Patients must be closely monitored.
		Capsules: 50,000 U (1.25 mg)
		Injection (in sesame oil): 500,000 U/mL (12.5 mg/mL)
		Solution, oral: 8,000 U/mL (200 μg/mL)

Erythromycin (E-Mycin, Ery-Tab, Eryc, Erythrocin, E.E.S., Ilosone, Pediamycin)	*Orally* (do not exceed 2 g/day):
	  Neonates: 20–30 mg/kg per day in 2 or 3 divided doses.
	  Infants and children:
	    Base or ethylsuccinate: 30–50 mg/kg per day in 3 or 4 divided doses.
	    Estolate: 20–50 mg/kg per day in 3 or 4 divided doses.
	  Adults:
	    Base, estolate, or stearate: 250–500 mg every 6–12 hours.
	  Ethylsuccinate: 400–800 mg every 6–12 hours.
	Endocarditis prophylaxis (penicillin-allergic patients): 20 mg/kg to a maximum of 1 g 2 hours before the procedure and 10 mg/kg to a maximum of 500 mg 6 hours later.
	Bowel preparation (erythromycin base, only): 20 mg/kg to a maximum of 1 g administered at 1:00, 2:00, and 11:00 p.m. on the day before surgery, usually combined with neomycin and mechanical cleansing of the bowel.
	IV: 15–20 mg/kg per day to a maximum of 4 g/day administered in 4 divided doses.
	Ophthalmic ointment for prophylaxis of neonates: apply a 0.5–1 cm ribbon of the ointment to each conjunctival sac.
	Topically for acne: apply to the affected areas b.i.d. The skin should be washed, rinsed well, and dried before applying the erythromycin. Keep away from the eyes, nose, and mouth.
		Base:
		Capsules, enteric-coated pellets; 250 mg
		Ointment, ophthalmic: 0.5%
		Solution, topical: 1.5%, 2%
		Tablets, enteric-coated: 250 mg, 333 mg, 500 mg
		Tablets, film-coated: 250 mg, 500 mg
		Estolate:
		Capsules: 250 mg
		Suspension: 125 mg/5 mL, 250 mg/5 mL
		Tablets: 500 mg
		Ethylsuccinate:
		Suspension: 200 mg/5 mL, 400 mg/5 mL
		Tablets, chewable: 200 mg
		Tablets: 400 mg
		Stearate: Tablets: 250 mg, 500 mg

Continued

Table 1   Medications   (continued)

DRUG	*DOSE*	*DOSAGE FORMS*
Erythromycin and sulfisoxazole (Eryzole, Pediazole)	*Orally* (based on the erythromycin content): Up to age 2 months: 40–50 mg/kg per day in 3 or 4 divided doses to a maximum of 2 g/day. Alternatively, the following patient weights may be used: 8–15 kg: 2.5 mL every 6 hours. 16–23 kg: 5 mL every 6 hours. 24–44 kg: 7.5 mL every 6 hours. ≥45 kg: 10 mL every 6 hours.	Suspension: 200 mg erythromycin and 600 mg sulfisoxazole per 5 mL
Etanercept (Enbrel)	Subcutaneously for the treament of rheumatoid arthritis: 0.4 mg/kg to a maximum dose of 25 mg given twice weekly 72 to 96 hours apart. Injection sites should be rotated.	Injection, powder for reconstitution: 25 mg
Ethacrynic acid (Edecrin)	*Orally:* 1 mg/kg administered 1–2 times daily. Do not exceed the usual adult dose of 50–100 mg/day. *IV:* 0.4–1 mg/kg up to 50 mg administered 1 or 2 times daily. Serum electrolytes must be closely monitored during ethacrynic acid therapy.	*Injection:* 50 mg Tablets: 25 mg, 50 mg
Ethambutol (Myambutol)	*Orally* (patient should be old enough to cooperate with an eye exam; optic neuritis is an adverse effect): Children: 15 mg/kg/day in a single dose. Adolescents and adults: 15–25 mg/kg per day in a single dose. Do not exceed 2.5 g/day.	Tablets: 100 mg, 400 mg
Ethosuximide (Zarontin)	*Orally:* Under age 6: 15 mg/kg per day in 2 divided doses to a maximum of 250 mg/dose. ≥age 6: 250 mg b.i.d. Dose may be increased by 250 mg/day every 4–7 days to a maximum of 1.5 g/day or 40 mg/kg per day.	Capsules: 250 mg Syrup: 250 mg/5 mL
Famotidine (Pepcid)	*Orally, IV:* Infants >3 months of age to 1 year of age: 1 mg/kg/day in 2 divided doses may be used for GERD. Children and adults: 1 mg/kg/day in 2 divided doses up to 80 mg/day may be used for GERD. A dose of 0.5 mg/kg up to 40 mg may be used for peptic ulcer or esophagitis.	Injection: 5 mg/mL Powder for oral suspension: 40 mg/5 mL Tablets: 10 mg, 20 mg, 40 mg
Fentanyl citrate (Sublimaze)	*IV* (slowly over a period of 3–5 minutes to avoid chest wall rigidity and to titrate to effect): Children: 1–2 μg/kg may be repeated at 30- to 60-minute intervals. For continuous therapy, after a bolus dose, a dose of 1 μg/kg per hr initially may be increased or decreased as necessary to response. Older children and adults: 0.5–1 μg/kg (25–50 μg) may be repeated at 30- to 60-minute intervals. The doses listed are analgesic/sedation doses. Doses used for general anesthesia may be higher. *Orally (Oralet):* Children ≥2 years of age who weigh 15–40 kg: 5–15 μg/kg to a maximum of 400 μg. Children ≥40 kg and adults: 5 μg/kg to a maximum of 400 μg.	Injection: 50 μg/mL Lozenge, oral transmucosal (Oralet): 100 μg, 200 μg, 300 μg, 400 μg
Ferrous sulfate (Feosol, Fer-In-Sol)	*Orally* (doses are expressed as elemental iron; ferrous sulfate contains 20% iron): *Iron deficiency anemia:* Children: 3–6 mg/kg per day depending on the severity of the deficiency. Higher doses should be administered in 3 divided doses; moderate doses may be administered in 2 divided doses to avoid GI upset. For prophylaxis, 1–2 mg/kg per day in a single dose may be used. Adults: 120–240 mg iron daily in 2–4 divided doses. For prophylaxis, 60 mg iron daily as a single dose.	Capsules: 50 mg Fe Drops: 15 mg Fe/0.6 mL Elixir: 44 mg Fe/5 mL Syrup: 18 mg Fe/5 mL Tablets: 60 mg Fe, 65 mg Fe

Continued

Table 1   Medications   (continued)

DRUG	DOSE	DOSAGE FORMS
Ferrous sulfate (Feosol, Fer-In-Sol) (continued)	Administration between meals increases absorption, but may result in more GI upset. Do not administer with antacids, eggs, or milk because they may decrease absorption of the iron.	
Fexofenadine (Allegra)	*Orally:* Children 6–11 years: 30 mg twice a day Over age 12: 60 mg twice a day or 180 mg daily.	Tablet: 30 mg, 60 mg, 180 mg
Fluconazole (Diflucan)	*Orally or IV:* *Oropharyngeal or esophageal candidiasis:* 6 mg/kg (up to 200 mg) on the first day; then 3 mg/kg per day (up to 100 mg). *Systemic candidiasis or cryptococcal meningitis:* 12 mg/kg (up to 400 mg) on the first day; then 6 mg/kg/day (up to 200 mg). *Prevention of candidiasis in bone marrow transplant:* 12 mg/kg per day (up to 400 mg) beginning several days before anticipated onset of neutropenia and continued until 7 days after neutrophil count is >1,000/mm^3. *Vaginal candidiasis:* 150 mg as a single dose. Dosage should be adjusted in patients with renal dysfunction.	Injection: 2 mg/mL (ready to administer) Suspension: 10 mg/mL, 40 mg/mL Tablets: 50 mg, 100 mg, 150 mg, 200 mg
Flucytosine (Ancobon)	*Orally:* Neonates: 50–100 mg/kg per day in 1–2 divided doses. Children and adults: 50–150 mg/kg per day in 4 divided doses. Dosage must be adjusted in renal impairment.	Capsules: 250 mg, 500 mg
Fludrocortisone (Florinef)	*Orally:* Infants and children: 0.05–0.1 mg/day. Adults: 0.05–0.2 mg/day.	Tablets: 0.1 mg
Flumazenil (Mazicon, Romazicon)	*IV:* Children (little information is available on dosing in children) The following are guidelines only: 0.01 mg/kg (to a maximum of 0.2 mg) initially, followed by 0.005 mg/kg (to a maximum of 0.2 mg) every minute until a total cumulative dose of 1 mg has been reached. Adults: *Reversal of sedation:* 0.2 mg over 15 seconds; may repeat 0.2-mg dose every 60 seconds to a maximum of 1 mg. May repeat doses every 20 minutes to a maximum of 3 mg in 1 hour. *Benzodiazepine overdose:* 0.2 mg over 30 seconds, then 0.3 mg over 30 seconds if desired level of consciousness is not reached. Additional 0.5-mg doses may be given every minute until a cumulative dose of 3 mg has been reached. If a partial response is noted, further 0.5-mg doses may be given until a cumulative dose of 5 mg is reached. Resedation may occur in patients who received long-acting benzodiazepines.	Injection: 0.1 mg/mL
Flunisolide (AeroBid, Nasalide)	*Intranasal spray:* Age 6–14: 1 spray in each nostril t.i.d. or 2 sprays in each nostril b.i.d. initially. Maintenance dose is usually 1 spray in each nostril daily. Over age 14 and adults: 2 sprays in each nostril b.i.d. or t.i.d. initially. After symptoms are controlled, dosage should be decreased to the lowest dose that will prevent symptoms from recurring. That may be as little as 1 spray in each nostril once daily for perennial rhinitis. The maximum dose is 4 sprays to each nostril daily.	Oral inhalation: 250 μg/spray Spray, intranasal: 25 μg/metered spray

Continued

Table 1   Medications   (continued)

DRUG	DOSE	DOSAGE FORMS

Flunisolide (AeroBid, Nasalide) (*continued*)	*Oral inhalation:*
	    Children 6–15 years of age: 2 inhalations twice a day.
	    Adults: 2 inhalations twice a day initially, increasing to a maximum of 8 inhalations daily.
	    Improvement in symptoms may take from several days to several weeks to occur, but therapy should not be continued for more than 3 weeks in the absence of efficacy. Dosage should be decreased to the lowest effective dose when symptoms abate.	

Fluocinolone acetonide (Fluonid, Flurosyn, Synalar, Synemol)	*Topically:* apply a thin layer to the affected area b.i.d. to q.i.d. Use the lowest effective potency product. Absorption is greater if the product is covered by anything that is occlusive (plastic pants, tight diapers).	Cream: 0.01%, 0.025%, 0.2% Ointment: 0.025% Shampoo: 0.01% Solution: 0.01%

Fluoride (Fluoritab, Karidium, Luride, Pediaflor)	*Orally:* dosage should be based on the fluoride content of the water supply. Long-term supplementation in areas with fluoridated water may result in dental fluorosis and osseous changes.*
	    Fluoride content of drinking water <0.3 ppm:
	        Birth-6 months: do not supplement.
	        >6 months–3 years: 0.25 mg/day.
	        >3–6 years: 0.5 mg/day.
	        >6–16 years: 1 mg/day.
	    Fluoride content of drinking water 0.3–0.6 ppm:
	        Birth-3 years: do not supplement.
	        3–6 years: 0.25 mg/day.
	        >6–16 years: 0.5 mg/day.
	    Fluoride content of drinking water >0.6 ppm: do not supplement.
	Dental gel: usually applied by a dentist.
	Rinses: over-the-counter rinses may be used for patients over age 6 on a daily basis and contain 0.01%–0.02% fluoride.
		Most multivitamin combinations are available in formulations containing appropriate amounts of fluoride (Poly-Vi-Flor drops or chewable tablets, Tri-Vi-Flo drops, Vi-Daylin/F drops and chewable tablets).
		Products containing only fluoride:
		Drops: 0.125 mg/drop, 0.25 mg/drop, 0.5 mg/mL
		Solution: 0.2 mg/mL (may be used orally or as a rinse)
		Tablets, chewable: 0.5 mg, 1 mg

Fluticasone (Flonase, Flovent)	*Intranasal metered dose spray*
	    Children ≥4 years of age: 1 spray in each nostril daily. Dosage may be increased to 2 sprays in each nostril daily if necessary.
	    Adults: 2 sprays in each nostril daily.
	Oral aerosol inhalation:
	    Children ≥12 years of age and adults: 88 μg twice daily for patients not previously treated with corticosteroids to a maximum of 440 μg twice daily in patients who were previously treated with inhaled corticosteroids.
	Oral powder inhalation:
	    Children 4–12 years of age: 50 μg twice daily to a maximum of 100 μg twice daily.
	    Children >12 years of age and adults: 100 μg twice a day up to 500 μg twice a day based on the patient's previous corticosteroid needs. Patients who previously required oral corticosteroids may require up to 1,000 μg twice a day.
		Powder, oral inhalation: 50 μg (delivers 44 μg), 100 μg (delivers 88 μg), 250 μg (delivers 220 μg)
		Spray oral inhalation: 44 μg/actuation, 110 μg/actuation, 220 μg/actuation
		Suspension, nasal: 50 μg/actuation

Fluticasone and Salmeterol (Advair)	*Oral powder inhalation:* Children >12 years of age and adults: 1 inhalation twice daily using the product that most closely matches the patient's previous steroid dosage. Use the lowest dose product for steroid naïve patients.	Powder for oral inhalation: 100 mcg fluticasone/50 mcg salmeterol/puff, 250 mcg fluticasone/50 mcg salmeterol/puff, 500 mcg fluticasone/50 mcg salmeterol/puff.

Continued

Table 1   Medications   (continued)

DRUG	DOSE	DOSAGE FORMS

Folic acid (Folvite)	*Orally, parenterally:*
	    Infants: 50 μg/day.
	    Age 1–10: 1 mg/day initially, then 0.1–0.4 mg/day.
	    Age 11 and over, and adults: 1 mg/day initially, then
	        0.5 mg/day.
		Injection: 5 mg/mL, 10 mg/mL
		Tablets: 0.1 mg, 0.4 mg, 0.8 mg, 1 mg

Fomepizole (Antizol, 4-MP,
    4-methylpyrazole)
	IV (diluted to <25 mg/mL):
	    Children: not well studied
	    Adults: 15 mg/kg loading dose, then 10 mg/kg/dose
	        every 12 hours for 4 doses, then 15 mg/kg/dose
	        every 12 hours until level is <20 mg/dL. Doses
	        should be given every 4 hours during hemodialysis
	        since the drug and its metabolites are
	        hemodialyzable.
		Injection: 1 gm/mL

Fosphenytoin-See phenytoin		

Furosemide (Lasix)	*Orally, IV, or IM:*
	    Premature neonates (oral absorption may be poor):
	        1–2 mg/kg every 12–24 hours. Oral doses up to
	        4 mg/kg may be used.
	    Children: 1–2 mg/kg every 6–12 hours but not to
	        exceed 6 mg/kg/day.
	    Adults: 20–80 mg/day in divided doses to a maximum
	        of 600 mg/day.
	Serum electrolyte levels should be monitored closely.
		Injection: 10 mg/mL
		Solution: 10 mg/mL, 40 mg/5 mL
		Tablets: 20 mg, 40 mg, 80 mg

Gabapentin (Neurontin)	*Orally* (as add-on therapy):
	    Patients 3–12 years of age: 10–15 mg/kg per day in
	        3 divided doses. The maintenance dose for patients
	        3–4 years of age is usually about 40 mg/kg per day
	        and for patients 5 years and older is 25–35 mg/kg
	        per day.
	    Age >12 years–adults: initially, 300 mg on day 1,
	        followed by rapid titration to 300 mg t.i.d. The usual
	        maintenance dosage range is 900–1,800 mg/day in 3
	        divided doses to a maximum daily dose of 3,600 mg.
	It is not necessary to monitor gabapentin levels or the
	    levels of other antiepileptic drugs the patient may be
	    taking because there are no significant drug
	    interactions. Withdrawal of gabapentin therapy should
	    be accomplished over a period of at least 1 week.
		Capsules: 100 mg, 300 mg, 400 mg
		Solution: 250 mg/5 mL

Ganciclovir (Cytovene, DHPG)	*IV* (as an infusion over 1 hour):
	    Induction: 10 mg/kg per day in 2 divided doses for
	        2–3 weeks.
	    Maintenance: 5 mg/kg per day as a single dose for
	        7 days a week to 6 mg/kg per day for 5 days a
	        week.
	Orally:
	Maintenance therapy only: in adults, a dose of 1,000 mg
	    t.i.d. with food is used. There are no guidelines for oral
	    use in children.
	Dosage must be adjusted in patients with renal
	    dysfunction.
		Capsules: 250 mg, 500 mg
		Injection: 500-mg vial

Gentamicin (Garamycin)	*IV or IM* (in obese patients it should be based on ideal,
	    rather than actual, body weight):
	    Neonates under age 7 days:
	        <1,000 g: 2.5 mg/kg every 24 hours.
	        1,000–1,500 g: 2.5 mg/kg every 18 hours.
	        >1,500 g: 2.5 mg/kg every 12 hours.
	    Neonates over age 7 days:
	        1,200–2,000 g: 2.5 mg/kg every 8–12 hours.
	        >2,000 g: 2.5 mg/kg every 8 hours.
		Injection: 10 mg/mL, 40 mg/mL
		Ointment, ophthalmic: 0.3%
		Solution, ophthalmic: 0.3%

Continued

Table 1   Medications   (continued)

DRUG	*DOSE*	*DOSAGE FORMS*
Gentamicin (Garamycin) (*continued*)	ECMO patients: 2.5 mg/kg every 18 hours. Infants and children under age 5: 2.5 mg/kg every 8 hours. Age 5–10: 2 mg/kg every 8 hours. Over age 10 and adults: 5 mg/kg per day administered in 3 divided doses. *Ophthalmic solution:* 1–2 drops in the affected eye every 2–4 hours. More frequent application (up to every hour) may be used initially in severe infections. *Ophthalmic ointment:* apply a ribbon of ointment to the eye b.i.d. or t.i.d. *Intrathecal/intraventricular* (use only a preservative-free product): Neonates: 1 mg/day as a single dose. Children over age 3 months: 1–2 mg/day. Older children and adults: 4–8 mg/day. Dosage must be adjusted in renal dysfunction. Serum levels should be monitored during therapy in all patients.	
Glucagon	*IV, IM, or SC:* *Hypoglycemia* (dose may be repeated in 20 minutes if necessary): Neonates: 0.025 mg/kg per dose. Children: 0.025–0.1 mg/kg/dose to a maximum of 1 mg. Adults: 0.5–1 mg/dose. *Infusion for the treatment of neonatal hyperinsulinemia:* 1–5 ng/kg per min to start and titrate to response. The infusion must be delivered by a pump to maintain a steady rate. Glucose levels must be monitored hourly until they are stable in an acceptable range. Rebound hypoglycemia may occur if the infusion is suddenly discontinued. *Diagnostic aid during radiography:* 0.25–2 mg 10 minutes before the procedure.	Injection: 1 mg-vial, 10 mg-vial (1 mg = 1 U)
Glycopyrrolate (Robinul)	*IM:* *Preoperatively:* Under age 2: 4.4–8.8 μg/kg 30–60 minutes before the procedure. $\geq$ age 2-adults: 4.4 μg/kg 30–60 minutes before the procedure. *Orally:* *To control respiratory secretions* (glycopyrrolate is poorly absorbed from the GI tract): 50 μg/kg administered t.i.d. or q.i.d. *Reversal of neuromuscular blockade:* 0.2 mg for each 1 mg neostigmine or 5 mg pyridostigmine administered.	Injection: 0.2 mg/mL Tablets: 1 mg, 2 mg
Gonadorelin HCl (Factrel, LHRH [luteinizing hormone-release hormone], GnRH [gonadotropin-releasing hormone])	*IV:* 2–5 μg/kg to a maximum of 100 μg.	Injection: 100 μg
Griseofulvin (Microsize products: Fulvicin U/F, Grifulvin V, Grisactin; Ultramicrosize products: Fulvicin P/G, Grisactin Ultra, Gris-PEG)	Absorption of griseofulvin from the GI tract is somewhat dependent on the size of the particles of griseofulvin. The ultramicrosize is absorbed about 1.5 times as well as the microsize. Absorption is also increased by administering the dose with a fatty meal. Duration of therapy is dependent on the site of infection and ranges from 2–4 weeks for tinea corporis, to 4–8 weeks for tinea capitis and tinea pedis, to 3–6 months for tinea unguium.	Microsize: Capsules: 125 mg, 250 mg Suspension: 125 mg/5 mL Tablets: 250 mg, 500 mg Ultramicrosize: Tablets: 125 mg, 165 mg, 250 mg, 330 mg

Continued

Table 1   Medications   (continued)

DRUG	DOSE	DOSAGE FORMS

Griseofulvin (Microsize products: Fulvicin U/F, Grifulvin V, Grisactin; Ultramicrosize products: Fulvicin P/G, Grisactin Ultra, Gris-PEG) (continued)	Children:
	  Microsize: 15–20 mg/kg per day in 1 or 2 divided doses.
	  Ultramicrosize: 10–13 mg/kg per day in 1 or 2 divided doses.
	Older children and adults:
	  Microsize: 500 mg–1 g/day in a single or 2 divided doses. Use higher dose for tinea pedis or tinea unguium.
	  Ultramicrosize: 660–750 mg/day in a single or 2 divided doses.
	During long-term therapy, renal, hepatic, and hematopoietic function should be monitored.
	Patients should also be cautioned to avoid sunlight because photosensitivity reactions have occurred.	

Haloperidol (Haldol)	*Orally:*
	Age 3–12:
	  Agitation or hyperkinesia: 0.01–0.03 mg/kg per day once daily.
	  Tourette disorder: 0.05–0.075 mg/kg per day in 2 or 3 divided doses.
	  Psychotic disorders: 0.05–0.15 mg/kg per day in 2 or 3 divided doses.
	  IM: 1–3 mg every 4–8 hours; maximum, 0.1 mg/kg per day.
	  Dose should be individually adjusted to patient. Not recommended for children under age 3. Oral dosage range is 2–100 mg/24 hr.
		Injection: 5 mg/mL
		Solution, concentrated oral: 2 mg/mL
		Tablets: 1 mg, 2 mg, 5 mg, 10 mg

Heparin sodium	*IV:*
	  Anticoagulation:
	    Children and adults:
	      Continuous infusion: 50 U/kg then 15–25 U/kg per hr. Dose may be increased by 2–4 U/kg per r every 6–8 hours based on the results of the APTT.
	      Intermittent infusion: 50–100 U/kg every 4 hours. This method is less desirable than continuous infusion.
	  Line flushing:
	    Central catheters: may be flushed as infrequently as once daily with 2–3 mL of solution containing 10 U/mL for patients under age 1 or 100 U/mL for patients age 1 or older.
	  Peripheral catheters, locks: usually flushed every 6–8 hours with 10 U/mL concentration with a volume determined by the length of the catheter, but usually about 1 mL.
	Lines should be flushed before and after medication or blood administration or if blood is seen in the catheter.
	Preservative-free heparin solutions should be used for all line flushes in children under age 2 months.
		Injection: 1,000 U, 5,000 U, 10,000 U, 20,000 U, 40,000 U/mL
		Injection, preservative-free: 1,000 U, 5,000 U, 10,000 U/mL
		Solution, lock flush: 10 U/mL, 100 U/mL (available preserved and preservative-free)

Hydralazine (Apresoline)	*Orally:*
	  Children: 0.75–1 mg/kg per day in 2–4 divided doses, but not to exceed 25 mg/dose initially. May be increased slowly over 3 or 4 weeks to a maximum of 7.5 mg/kg per day (or 200 mg).
	  Adults: initially 10 mg q.i.d. May be increased by 10–25 mg/dose every 2–5 days to a maximum of 300 mg/day.
		Injection: 20 mg/mL
		Tablets: 10 mg, 25 mg, 50 mg, 100 mg

Continued

Table 1   Medications   (continued)

DRUG	DOSE	DOSAGE FORMS
Hydralazine (Apresoline) (*continued*)	*IV* (ratio of oral to IV dosing is about 4:1): Children: initially 0.1–0.2 mg/kg (to a maximum of 20 mg) every 4–6 hours. May be increased to a maximum of 1.7–3.5 mg/kg per day. Adults: initially 10–20 mg every 4–6 hours. May be increased to 40 mg/dose. Dose must be adjusted in renal impairment.	
Hydrochlorothiazide (Esidrix, HydroDIURIL, Oretic)	*Orally* (chlorothiazide, which is available as a suspension, is usually a better choice for children requiring low doses): Children over age 6 months: 2 mg/kg per day in 2 divided doses. Adults: 25–100 mg/day in 1 or 2 doses.	Tablets: 25 mg, 50 mg, 100 mg
Hydrocortisone (Cortef, Cortenema, Cortifoam, Cortril, Hydrocortone, Solu-Cortef)	*Orally:* *Congenital adrenal hyperplasia:* initially 30–36 mg/m^2 per day divided as one third in the morning and two thirds in the evening or one fourth in the morning, one fourth midday, and half in the evening. *Physiologic replacement:* 0.5–0.75 mg/kg per day. *Antiinflammatory:* 2.5–10 mg/kg per day in 3 or 4 divided doses. *IV:* *Adrenal insufficiency:* Infants and young children: 1–2 mg/kg bolus, then 25–150 mg/day in 3 or 4 divided doses. Older children: 1–2 mg/kg bolus, then 150–250 mg/day in 3 or 4 divided doses. Adults: 15–240 mg/day in 1 or 2 divided doses. *Antiinflammatory:* Infants and children: 1–5 mg/kg per day in 2–4 divided doses. Adults: 15–240 mg every 12 hours. *Shock* (succinate salt): Children: 50 mg/kg then in 4 hours or every 24 hours as needed. Adults: 500 mg-2 g every 2–6 hours. *Rectal retention enemas:* 1 enema nightly for 21 days. May be continued for a longer period if effective or discontinued if no effect is seen. *Intrarectal foam:* 1 full applicator rectally nightly or b.i.d. for 2 or 3 weeks. Absorption of hydrocortisone may be greater from the foam formulation than the enema. Discontinue if not effective after 3 weeks. *Topically* (low-potency corticosteroid in most formulations): apply a thin layer to the affected area t.i.d. or q.i.d.	Cream, topical: 0.5%, 1%, 2.5% Enema: 100 mg/60 mL (Cortenema) Foam, intrarectal: 90 mg/full applicator (Cortifoam), rectal/anal 1% (Proctofoam-HC) Injection (sodium phosphate): 50 mg/mL Injection (sodium succinate): 100-mg, 250-mg, 500-mg, 1-g vials Ointment, topical: 0.5%, 1%, 2.5% Suspension (cypionate): 10 mg/5 mL Tablets: 5 mg, 10 mg, 20 mg
Hydromorphone (Dilaudid)	*IV:* Young children: 0.015–0.03 mg/kg every 3–4 hours. Older children and adults: 1–4 mg every 3–4 hours. *Orally:* Young children: 0.04–0.07 mg/kg every 3–4 hours. Older children and adults: 1–6 mg every 3–4 hours depending on size and pain severity. *To convert a patient from oral to IV therapy:* start with a ratio of 5:1. Ratios of up to 2:1 may be required in some patients on long-term chronic therapy. *To convert a patient from IV to oral therapy:* in a patient who is receiving a stable dose, use an IV to oral ratio of 1:3.	Injection: 1 mg/mL, 2 mg/mL, 4 mg/mL, 10 mg/mL Solution, oral: 1 mg/mL Suppositories, rectal: 3 mg Tablets: 2 mg, 4 mg, 8 mg

Continued

Table 1   Medications   (continued)

DRUG	DOSE	DOSAGE FORMS

Hydromorphone (Dilaudid) (*continued*)	Equianalgesic doses:
	  Oral: 7.5 mg hydromorphone = 30 mg morphine.
	  Parenteral: 1.5 mg hydromorphone = 10 mg morphine.	

Hydroxyzine (Atarax, Vistaril)	*Orally:*
	  Children: 2 mg/kg per day in 3 or 4 doses.
	  Adults: 100–400 mg/day in 3 or 4 doses. Use lower doses for pruritus and higher doses for sedation.
	Parenterally: the use of hydroxyzine parenterally (IM, IV, SC) has been associated with severe adverse effects at the site of the injection. The reactions are characterized by local discomfort, sterile abscess, erythema, and tissue necrosis. Phlebitis and hemolysis have been reported after IV administration. The manufacturers recommend administration by deep IM injection into a well-developed large muscle. SC infiltration of the drug from an IM injection or extravasation of an IV injection must be avoided.
		Capsule (pamoate): 25 mg, 50 mg, 100 mg
		Injection for IM use: 25 mg/mL, 50 mg/mL
		Solution, oral: 10 mg/5 mL
		Suspension, oral (pamoate): 25 mg/5 mL
		Tablets: 10 mg, 25 mg, 50 mg, 100 mg

Ibuprofen (Advil, Motrin, Nuprin)	*Orally:*
	Antipyretic:
	  Age 6 months–12 years (repeat doses up to every 6 hours):
	    Temperature <39°C (102.2°F): 5 mg/kg per dose.
	    Temperature ≥39°C (102.2°F): 10 mg/kg per dose.
	  Over age 12 and adults: 200–400 mg/dose to a maximum of 1,200 mg/day.
	Juvenile rheumatoid arthritis: 30–70 mg/kg per day in 4 divided doses to a maximum of 2,400 mg/day.
	Adult antiinflammatory dose: 400–800 mg every 6–8 hours to a maximum of 3,200 mg/day.
		Suspension, oral: 100 mg/5 mL
		Tablets: 200 mg, 300 mg, 400 mg, 600 mg, 800 mg

Imipenem and cilastatin (Primaxin)	*IV infusion over 1 hour* (expressed as mg of imipenem):
	  Children: 50–100 mg/kg per day in 4 divided doses to a maximum of 4 g/day.
	  Adults: 2–4 g/day in 3 or 4 divided doses.
	Dosage adjustment is required in renal impairment.
		Injection: imipenem 250 mg and cilastatin 50 mg, imipenem 500 mg and cilastatin 500 mg

Imipramine (Tofranil)	*Orally:*
	Enuresis in children under age 6: initially 25 mg 1 hour before bedtime nightly. Dose may be increased to 50 mg in children age 6–12 or 75 mg in children over age 12 if the initial dose is ineffective.
	Depression:
	  Children: 1.5 mg kg/day in 1–4 divided doses initially. May be increased in increments of about 1 mg/kg per day to a maximum of 5 mg/kg per day.
	  Adolescents: 25–50 mg/day increased gradually to a maximum of 100 mg/day in a single or divided doses.
	  Adults: 75–100 mg/day increased gradually to a maximum of 300 mg/day in a single or divided doses.
	  Dosage should be decreased to the minimum effective dose after symptom control has been achieved.
		Tablets: 10 mg, 25 mg, 50 mg

Continued

Table 1   Medications   (continued)

DRUG	*DOSE*	*DOSAGE FORMS*
Imipramine (Tofranil) (*continued*)	*Doses used to treat pain:* generally lower than those used in the treatment of depression. A starting dose of 0.2–0.4 mg/kg per day administered at bedtime may be used initially. A gradual increase to 1–3 mg/kg per day may be necessary for some patients. Administration of the total daily dose at bedtime may decrease the daytime sedative effects.	
Immune globulin, intramuscular	*IM:* *Measles prophylaxis:* 0.25 mL/kg within 6 days of exposure. In immunocompromised patients, use 0.5 mL/kg (15 mL maximum). *Hepatitis A preexposure prophylaxis:* Risk of exposure within 3 months: 0.02 mL/kg. Risk of exposure greater than 3 months: 0.06 mL/kg. *Hepatitis A postexposure:* 0.02 mL/kg given within 2 weeks of exposure. *Immunodeficiency:* IV has largely replaced use of the IM form. An initial dose of 1.2 mL/kg is followed with doses of 0.6 mL/kg at 2–4-week intervals. The usual maximum volumes are 20–30 mL in infants and small children and 30–50 mL in adults.	Injection, IM: 165 $\pm$ 15 mg (of protein) per mL (2 mL and 10 mL)
Immune globulin, intravenous (Gamimune N, Gammagard S/D, Gammar-P IV, Iveegam, Polygam S/D, Sandoglobulin, Venoglobulin-I, Venoglobulin-S)	*IV as a slow infusion:* The rate of infusion varies from product to product but should always be initiated at a very slow rate and may be increased every 30 minutes to the manufacturer's maximum recommended rate or less as the patient tolerates. Infusion-related reactions usually abate if the rate of infusion is decreased. Anaphylactic hypersensitivity reactions may occur and are more likely in patients with IgA deficiency. *Immunodeficiency syndromes:* 100–400 mg/kg every 2–4 weeks. *Idiopathic thrombocytopenic purpura:* either 400 mg/kg per day for 2–5 consecutive days or 1 g/kg per day for 1 or 2 consecutive days may be used for induction. Maintenance doses are usually 400 mg/kg per dose every 4–6 weeks but may be increased to 800–1,000 mg/kg if the lower dose is insufficient and are based on platelet counts and clinical response. *Kawasaki disease:* usually 2 g/kg as a single dose. Alternatively, 400 mg/kg per day for 4 days may be used.	Gamimune N: 5% or 10% solution in vials Gammagard S/D: powder with diluent to make 5% solution Gammar-P IV: powder with diluent to make 5% solution Iveegam: powder with diluent to make 5% solution Polygam S/D: powder with diluent to make 5% solution Sandoglobulin: powder with diluent to make 3%, 6%, or 12% solution Venoglobulin-I: powder with diluent to make 5% solution Venoglobulin-S: solution 5%, 10%
Indomethacin IV (Indocin IV)	*IV push:* Further dilution of the reconstituted injection may result in precipitation of insoluble indomethacin. An initial 0.2 mg/kg per dose is followed by 2 doses based on the patient's postnatal age (PNA) *at the time of the first dose:* PNA <48 hours: 0.1 mg/kg at 12- to 24-hour intervals. PNA 2–7 days: 0.2 mg/kg at 12- to 24-hour intervals. PNA >7 days: 0.25 mg/kg at 12- to 24-hour intervals. The patient's renal and hepatic function should be monitored. Oral use in children is generally not recommended.	Injection (sodium trihydrate): 1 mg

Continued

Table 1   Medications   (continued)

DRUG	*DOSE*	*DOSAGE FORMS*
Insulin	*IV:* *Treatment of diabetic ketoacidosis:* loading dose of 0.1 U/kg followed by a continuous infusion of 0.1 U/kg/hr (usual range 0.05–0.2 U/kg per hr) to maintain steady, but slow, decrease of serum glucose levels of 80–100 mg/dL per hr. Only regular insulin should be used by this route. *SC:* *Maintenance:* most patients require 0.5–1 U/kg per day in 2–4 divided doses depending on how well controlled the patient's glucose levels have been. Patients should be warned not to change insulins without prior approval of their physicians. If regular insulin is to be mixed with other types of insulin, the regular insulin should always be measured first. Extemporaneously prepared doses of mixed insulins should be used as soon as possible after mixing to minimize the amount of the regular insulin that will be bound by excess protamine or zinc in the other insulin. The activity of regular insulin has a time to onset of 1/2 to 1 hour, peaks at 2–3 hours, and has a duration of 5–7 hours. The activity of isophane (NPH) insulin has a time to onset of about 1–2 hours, peaks at 4–12 hours, and has a duration of 18–24 hours.	All insulins below are 100 U/mL. Aspart (NovoLog): human Extended zinc (Ultralente) insulin: human, Glargine (Lantus) insulin: human Isophane (NPH) insulin: available in pork or human Lispro (Humalog) insulin: human Regular insulin: available in pork or human, Fixed combinations: regular insulin 30 U/mL with isophane insulin 70 U/mL; available as pork or human; regular insulin 50 U/mL with isophane insulin 50 U/mL available as human; aspart insulin 30 U/mL with aspart protamine insuilin 70 U/mL, human; lispro 25 U/mL with lispro protamine 75 U/mL
Ipecac	*Orally* (followed by 10–20 mL/kg (up to 300 mL) of water. May be repeated after 20 minutes if vomiting does not occur): Age 6–12 months: 5–10 mL. Age >1–12 years: 15 mL. Over age 12 years: 30 mL. Do not administer at the same time as activated charcoal, or with milk or carbonated beverages.	Syrup
Ipratropium bromide (Atrovent)	*Oral metered dose inhalation:* Children 3–14 years of age: 1–2 inhalations t.i.d. Children >14 years of age and adults: 2 inhalations q.i.d. Maximum dose should not exceed 12 inhalations in 24 hours. *Nebulization* Children 3–14 years of age: 125–250 μg t.i.d. Children >14 years of age and adults: 500 μg 3 to 4 times daily.	Aerosol, metered dose: 18 μg/actuation Solution for nebulization: 0.02%, 2.5 mL
Isoniazid (isonicotinic acid hydrazide, isonicotinyl hydrazide; INH, Nydrazid)	*Orally or IM:* *Treatment:* Children: 20 mg/kg per day in 1 or 2 divided doses (up to 300 mg/day). Adults: 5 mg/kg per day up to 300 mg; 10 mg/kg should be used for disseminated disease. *Prophylaxis:* Children: 10 mg/kg per day in a single dose up to 300 mg/day. Adults: 300 mg/day. Liver function should be monitored during therapy because hepatitis may occur at any time. Patients whose diets are low in milk or meat should receive pyridoxine supplements at a dose of about 10–50 mg/day.	Injection: 100 mg/mL Solution, oral: 50 mg/5 mL (with sorbitol 70%) Tablets: 100 mg, 300 mg

Continued

Table 1   Medications   (continued)

DRUG	DOSE	DOSAGE FORMS

Isoproterenol (Isuprel)	*IV* (by continuous infusion): 0.05–3 μg/kg per min up to 2–20 μg/min.
	Oral inhalation: 1–2 metered doses up to 6 times daily.
	Nebulization:
	   Age 2–9: 0.25 mL (1:200) in 2.5 mL normal saline solution up to every 4 hours.
	   Over age 9: 0.5 mL (1:200) in 2.5 mL normal saline solution up to every 4 hours.
		Aerosol, metered dose inhaler: 1:400 (0.25%)
		Injection: 1:5,000 (0.2 mg/mL, 1 mg/5 mL)
		Solution for inhalation: 1:200 (0.5%)

Ketoconazole (Nizoral)	*Orally* (acid must be present in the GI tract for the dissolution and absorption of ketoconazole):
	   Children: 3.3–6.6 mg/kg per day in 1 or 2 divided doses to a maximum dose of 400 mg/day.
	   Adults: 200–400 mg/day in a single dose.
	Do not administer antacids or H_2 antagonists at the same time as ketoconazole.
	Monitor liver function during therapy.
	Topically: apply to the affected area once or twice daily.
	Shampoo for dandruff: apply shampoo and lather, allow to remain on the scalp for at least 1 minute before rinsing. Reapply shampoo and lather again, allow to remain on the scalp for 3 minutes, and then rinse. Treatments should be done twice weekly with at least 3 days between treatments, for 4 weeks. The frequency of subsequent treatments should be determined individually.
		Cream: 2%
		Shampoo: 2%
		Tablets: 200 mg

Lamivudine (Epivir)	*Orally:*
	   Age 3 months–12 years: 4 mg/kg b.i.d., to a maximum of 150 mg b.i.d.
	   Adolescents and adults: 150 mg b.i.d.
	   Dosage adjustment may be necessary in patients with renal dysfunction.
		Solution: 10 mg/mL
		Tablets: 150 mg

Leuprolide acetate (Lupron, Lupron Depot)	*SC:*
	   Anterior pituitary gonadotropic testing: 10 μg/kg per dose.
	   Precocious puberty: 50 μg/kg per day. Dosage may be titrated upward in 10-μg/kg increments if suppression of ovarian or testicular function is incomplete.
	   IM for precocious puberty (higher doses may be necessary for younger children. Doses should be based on the patient's weight and age): Girls over age 8 and boys over age 9: 0.3 mg/kg (minimum 7.5 mg) repeated every 4 weeks using the depot product. Dosage may be increased in 3.75 mg increments every 4 weeks until an effective dose is achieved. Therapy should generally be discontinued at age 11 for girls or age 12 for boys.
		Injection for SC use (Lupron): 5 mg/mL
		Injection, suspension for IM use (Lupron Depot): 3.75 mg, 7.5 mg

Levalbuterol (Xopenex)	*Ihalation:*
	   Age 6–11 years: 0.31 mg/dose 3 times a day to a maximum dose of 0.63 mg 3 times a day.
	   Over age 11 years and adults: 0.63 mg 3 to 4 times a day to a maximum of 1.25 mg 3 times a day with close monitoring for adverse effects.
		Solution for inhalation 0.63 mg/3 mL and 1.25 mg/3 mL

Levothyroxine sodium (Levothroid, Synthroid)	*Orally:*
	   Age 0–6 months: 8–10 μg/kg or 25–50 μg/day.
	   Age >6–<12 months: 6–8 μg/kg or 50–75 μg/day.
	   Age 1–5: 5–6 μg/kg or 75–100 μg/day.
	   Age 6–12: 4–5 μg/kg or 100–150 μg/day.
	   Over age 12 and adults: 2–3 μg/kg or >150 μg/day.
	IV: one half to three fourths of the oral dose for children or about half the oral dose for adults. The parenteral form of the drug is very unstable and should be used immediately after reconstitution without admixing with other solutions.
		Injection: 200 μg, 500 μg
		Tablets: 25 μg, 50 μg, 75 μg, 88 μg, 100 μg, 112 μg, 125 μg, 150 μg, 175 μg, 200 μg, 300 μg

Continued

Table 1   Medications   (continued)

DRUG	DOSE	DOSAGE FORMS
Lidocaine hydrochloride (Xylocaine)	*IV for cardiac arrhythmias:* 1 mg/kg loading dose followed by a continuous infusion of 20–50 μg/kg per minute. The loading dose may be repeated twice at 10- to 15-minute intervals, if necessary. *Infiltration for local anesthesia:* dose depends on procedure, degree, and duration of anesthesia required and the vascularity of the site. Maximum recommended dose is 4.5 mg/kg. Doses should not be repeated sooner than 2 hours. *Topical:* apply to affected area as needed. Maximum dose should not exceed 3 mg/kg or be repeated within 2 hours. Patients treated with oral lidocaine viscous should be cautioned about the hazards of biting the numbed areas and swallowing difficulties.	Aerosol, metered dose: 10% (for use before endotracheal intubation) Injection: 0.5%, 1%, 1.5%, 2%, 4%; 0.5% with epinephrine 1:200,000; 1% with epinephrine 1:100,000 or 1:200,000; 1.5% with epinephrine 1:200,000; 2% with epinephrine 1:100,000 or 1:200,000 Jelly: 2% Liquid, viscous: 2% Ointment: 2.5%, 5% Solution, topical: 2%, 4%
Lindane (gamma benzene hexachloride; Kwell)	*Topically:* *Pediculosis:* apply 15–30 mL of shampoo to the scalp and lather for 4–5 minutes, then rinse. The hair should be combed with a fine-toothed comb to remove nits. Treatment may be repeated after 1 week, if necessary. *Scabies:* apply a thin layer of the lotion to the skin from the neck to the toes (include the head in infants). The lotion should be removed by bathing after 6 hours for infants, 6–8 hours for children or 8–12 hours for adults. Treatment may be repeated after 1 week, if necessary. Percutaneous absorption may occur and cause toxicity. Do not apply to inflamed or raw skin.	Lotion: 1% Shampoo: 1%
Loperamide (Imodium)	*Orally:* *Acute diarrhea* (dosage is for the initial 24 hours): Age 2–age 6 (13–20 kg): 1 mg t.i.d. Age >6–8 (20–30 kg): 2 mg b.i.d. Age >8–12 (>30 kg): 2 mg t.i.d. Adults: 4 mg initially followed by 2 mg after each unformed stool to a maximum of 8 mg in 24 hours (16 mg/24 hr under a physician's care). For subsequent days, use a dose of 0.1 mg/kg for children after each loose stool, but do not exceed dosage guidelines for the first day *Chronic diarrhea:* Children: 0.08–0.24 mg/kg per day in 2 or 3 doses daily to a maximum of 2 mg/dose. Adults: 4 mg followed by 2 mg after each unformed stool until symptoms are controlled, then decreased to the lowest dose that will control symptoms. Usual maintenance dose is 4–8 mg/day.	Capsules: 2 mg Solution, oral: 1 mg/5 mL Tablets: 2 mg
Loracarbef (Lorabid)	*Orally* (administer doses on an empty stomach): Age 6 months-12 years: *Otitis media:* 30 mg/kg per day in 2 divided doses. Administer only the suspension for otitis because it is absorbed more quickly and results in higher blood levels. *Other infections:* 15 mg/kg per day in 2 divided doses. Older children and adults: 200–400 mg/day in 2 divided doses.	Capsules: 200 mg Suspension, oral: 100 mg/5 mL, 200 mg/5 mL
Loratadine (Claritin)	*Orally:* Age 2–12: 5 mg/day in a single dose. Adults >30 kg: 10 mg/day in a single dose.	Tablets: 10 mg

Continued

Table 1   Medications   (continued)

DRUG	DOSE	DOSAGE FORMS
Lorazepam (Ativan)	*IV:* *Status epilepticus:* 　Neonates: 0.05 mg/kg over 2–5 minutes. Dose may be repeated in 10–15 minutes. 　Infants and children: 0.1 mg/kg over 2–5 minutes to a maximum of 4 mg/dose. A second dose of 0.05 mg/kg may be given. 　Adolescents: 0.07 mg/kg over 2–5 minutes to a maximum of 4 mg. Dose may be repeated in 10–15 minutes. 　Adults: 4 mg over 2–5 minutes. Dose may be repeated in 10–15 minutes. *Adjunct to antiemetic therapy:* 0.02–0.04 mg/kg up to every 6 hours. 　Do not exceed a maximum of 2 mg/ dose. *Orally or IV:* *Anxiety and sedation:* 　Infants and children: 0.03–0.04 mg/kg per day, in 3–4 divided doses. 　Adults: 2–6 mg/day, usually orally, in 2 or 3 divided doses.	Injection: 2 mg/mL, 4 mg/mL Solution, oral: 2 mg/mL Tablets: 0.5 mg, 1 mg, 2 mg
Magnesium citrate (Citrate of Magnesia, Evac-Q-Mag)	*Orally* (chill for better palatability): 　Under age 6: 2–4 mL/kg. 　Age 6–12: 100–150 mL. 　Over age 12: 150–300 mL.	Solution: 300 mL (carbonated; contains 3.85–4.71 mEq Mg/5 mL)
Magnesium gluconate (Almora, Magonate, Magtrate)	*Orally* (expressed in terms of mEq of magnesium): 　Children: 0.5–0.75 mEq/kg per day in 3 or 4 divided doses. 　Adults: 2.2–4.4 mEq administered b.i.d. or t.i.d.	Liquid: 1,000 mg/5 mL (54 mg Mg = 4.4 mEq Mg) Tablets: 500 mg (27 mg Mg = 2.2 mEq Mg)
Magnesium hydroxide (Milk of Magnesia)	*Orally:* 　Under age 2: 0.5 mL/kg per dose. 　Age 2–5: 5–15 mL/day. 　Age 6–12: 15–30 mL/day. 　Over age 12: 30–60 mL/day.	Suspension: contains about 13.7 mEq Mg/5 mL
Magnesium sulfate (Epsom Salts)	*IV* (expressed in terms of magnesium sulfate [and mEq Mg]): *Hypomagnesemia* (monitor serum magnesium levels closely): 　Neonates: 25–50 mg/kg (0.2–0.4 mEq/kg) every 8–12 hours for 2–3 doses. 　Infants and children: 25–50 mg/kg (0.2–0.4 mEq/kg) every 4–6 hours for 3 or 4 doses with a maximum single dose of 2,000 mg (16 mEq). Doses up to 100 mg/kg have been used in severe hypomagnesemia. 　Adults: 1 g (8 mEq) every 6 hours for 4 doses. Doses of 2–3 g (16–24 mEq) have been used for severe hypomagnesemia. *Maintenance dose:* 30–60 mg/kg per day (0.25–0.5 mEq/kg per day) in 3 or 4 divided doses. *Management of seizures or hypertension in children:* 25–100 mg/kg (0.2–0.8 mEq/kg) every 4–6 hours as needed. Administer the drug slowly (over 1–2 hours) in a concentration not greater than 10 mg/mL. Blood pressure should be monitored frequently during infusions because hypotension has been reported with too-fast administration.	Injection: 500 mg/mL (4 mEq magnesium = 49 mg Mg)

Continued

Table 1   Medications   (continued)

DRUG	DOSE	DOSAGE FORMS
Mannitol (Osmitrol)	*IV:* initial dose of 2 g/kg followed by doses of 0.25–0.5 g/kg every 4–6 hours. A test dose of 0.2 g/kg (to a maximum of 12.5 g) over 3–5 minutes should produce a urine flow of about 1 mL/kg per hr for 2 or 3 hours. It should be used for patients with marked oliguria or inadequate renal function.	Injection: 5%, 10%, 15%, 20%, 25%

Mebendazole (Vermox)	*Orally:*
	Over age 2 and adults:
	  Enterobiasis (pinworm): 100 mg as a single dose. May be repeated at 2 weeks.
	  Ascariasis (roundworm), trichuriasis (whipworm), hookworm, or mixed infections: 200 mg/day in 2 divided doses for 3 days. A second course may be administered 3–4 weeks later.
		Tablets, chewable: 100 mg

Meperidine hydrochloride (Demerol)	Oral doses are about half as effective as IV doses but are generally used for less severe pain; therefore, the doses listed are for all routes of administration, but that should be kept in mind if a patient is being switched from parenteral to oral therapy. Children: 1–1.5 mg/kg every 3–4 hours. A single dose of 3 mg/kg (to a maximum of 100 mg) may be used preoperatively. Adults: 50–150 mg every 3–4 hours. Dosage adjustment is necessary in renal impairment. Long-term or high-dose therapy may result in accumulation of normeperidine, an active metabolite that is a CNS stimulant, especially in patients with renal failure.	Injection: 25 mg/mL, 50 mg/mL, 75 mg/mL, 100 mg/mL Solution, oral: 50 mg/5 mL Tablets: 50 mg, 100 mg

Meropenem (Merrem IV)	*IV:*
	Mild to moderate infections:
	  Age 3 months–adults: 60 mg/kg per day in 3 divided doses to a maximum total daily dose of 3 g.
	Meningitis:
	  Age 3 months–adults: 120 mg/kg per day in 3 divided doses to a maximum total daily dose of 6 g.
		Injection: 500 mg, 1 g

Mesalamine (Asacol, Pentasa, Rowasa)	*Orally:* Adults: 1 g (capsules) q.i.d. or 800 mg (tablets) t.i.d. *Rectally:* 4 g enema administered at bedtime daily. The enema should be retained overnight (8 hours) for best results. The oral forms of the drug are formulated with an enteric coating to slowly release the drug.	Capsules (Pentasa): 250 mg Suspension, rectal: 4 g/60 mL Tablets (Asacol): 400 mg

Metaproterenol (Alupent, Metaprel)	*Orally:*
	  Under age 6: 1.3–2.6 mg/kg per day in 3 or 4 divided doses.
	  Age 6–9 (<27 kg): 10 mg/dose t.i.d. or q.i.d.
	  Over age 9 (>27 kg) and adults: 20 mg/dose t.i.d. or q.i.d.
	Oral inhalation:
	  Over age 12 and adults: 2–3 inhalations every 3–4 hours, up to 12 inhalations daily.
	Nebulizer:
	  Age 6–12: 0.1 mL of a 5% solution diluted in 0.9% sodium chloride solution to 3 mL, repeated up to every 4 hours.
	  Over age 12 and adults: 0.2–0.3 mL of 5% solution (or 2.5 mL of 0.4% or 0.6% commercially available diluted solution) administered t.i.d. or q.i.d.
		Inhalation: Aerosol: 0.65 mg/inhalation spray
		Solution: 5%, 0.4% in normal saline solution, 0.6% in normal saline solution
		Solution, oral: 10 mg/5 mL
		Tablets: 10 mg, 20 mg

Continued

Table 1   Medications   (continued)

DRUG	DOSE	DOSAGE FORMS
Methylene blue (Urolene Blue)	*IV for methemoglobinemia:* 1–2 mg/kg injected slowly over a period of several minutes. The dose may be repeated in 1 hour, if necessary. *Orally for adults with chronic methemoglobinemia:* 100–300 mg/day.	Injection: 10 mg/mL Tablets: 65 mg
Methylphenidate (Concerta, Metadate, Ritalin)	*Orally:* Over age 6: initially 0.3 mg/kg per day (2.5–5 mg/dose) before breakfast and lunch. That may be increased to the usual dosage range of 0.5–1 mg/kg per day or a maximum of 2 mg/kg per day or 60 mg. The sustained-release form may be given as a single dose at breakfast.	Capsules, extended release: (Metadate CD) 10 mg, 20 mg, 30 mg; (Ritalin LA) 20 mg, 30 mg, 40 mg Tablets: 5 mg, 10 mg, 20 mg Tablets, extended release: 20 mg Tablets, osmotic extended release (Concerta): 18 mg, 27 mg, 36 mg, 54 mg
Methylprednisolone (A-methaPred, Depo-Medrol, Medrol, Solu-Medrol)	*IV:* *Status asthmaticus:* 1 mg/kg every 6 hours. *Acute spinal cord injury:* 30 mg/kg over 15 minutes followed in 45 minutes by an infusion of 5.4 mg/kg per hr for 23 hours. *Shock:* 30 mg/kg and may be repeated every 4–12 hours, but not to continue for longer than 48–72 hours. *"Pulse" therapy for lupus nephritis in older children and adults:* 1 g/day for 3 days. A dose of 30 mg/kg every other day for 6 doses has been used for children. *Orally:* Children: 0.117–1.6 mg/kg per day in 4 divided doses. Adults: 2–60 mg/day in 4 divided doses. *Intraarticular, intralesional doses (acetate):* 4–40 mg or up to 80 mg for large joints every 1–5 weeks.	Injection (acetate; Depo-Medrol): 20 mg/mL, 40 mg/mL, 80 mg/mL Injection (sodium succinate): 40-mg, 125-mg, 500-mg, 1-g, 2-g vials Tablets: 2 mg, 4 mg, 8 mg, 16 mg, 24 mg, 32 mg
Metoclopramide (Maxolon, Octamide, Reglan)	*Orally or IV:* *Gastroesophageal reflux:* Children: initially 0.1–0.5 mg/kg per day in 4 divided doses before meals. Dosage may be increased to a maximum of 0.8 mg/kg per day. Adults: 10–15 mg 30 minutes before meals and at bedtime. *IV:* *Intubation of GI tract or radiographic exam:* Under age 6: 0.1 mg/kg. Age 6–14: 2.5–5 mg. Adults: 10 mg. *Antiemetic in chemotherapy-induced nausea:* 1–2 mg/kg administered 30 minutes before the chemotherapy and every 2–4 hours as necessary thereafter to a maximum of 3 doses. Extrapyramidal reactions are common at this dose and may be treated with diphenhydramine IV (1 mg/kg up to 50 mg) every 6 hours.	Injection: 5 mg/mL Solution, oral: 5 mg/5 mL, 10 mg/5 mL Tablets: 5 mg, 10 mg
Metolazone (Zaroxolyn)	*Orally:* Infants and children: 0.2–0.4 mg/kg per day in 1–2 divided doses. Adults: 2.5–5 mg/day for the treatment of hypertension. Edema due to cardiac or renal disease may require doses of 5–20 mg/day.	Tablets: 2.5 mg, 5 mg, 10 mg
Metronidazole (Flagyl, Protostat)	*Orally or IV:* *Anaerobic bacterial infections* (IV initially, then orally): Infants other than neonates to adults: 30 mg/kg per day in 4 divided doses, not to exceed 4 g/day. *Amebiasis* (usually orally): Infants and children: 35–50 mg/kg per day in 3 divided doses. Adults: 500–750 mg every 8 hours.	Injection: available 5 mg/mL ready to infuse solution or 500-mg vial Tablets: 250 mg, 500 mg

Continued

Table 1   Medications   (continued)

DRUG	DOSE	DOSAGE FORMS

Metronidazole (Flagyl, Protostat) (*continued*)	*Other parasitic infections* (usually orally):
	    Infants and children: 15–30 mg/kg per day in
	        3 divided doses.
	    Adults: 250 mg every 8 hours or a single 2-g dose.
	Pelvic inflammatory disease:
	    Adults: 500 mg every 12 hours.
	Antibiotic-associated pseudomembranous colitis:
	    Infants and children: 20 mg/kg per day in 4 divided
	        doses.
	    Adults: 250–500 mg t.i.d. or q.i.d.
	Oral doses may be taken with food to minimize stomach
	    upset.	

Midazolam (Versed)	*IV* (titrate dose slowly to avoid excessive dosing):
	Conscious sedation:
	    Children: 0.05 mg/kg just before the procedure to a
	        maximum dose of 2 mg. Dose may be repeated
	        every 3 or 4 minutes up to 4 times.
	    Adults: 0.5–2 mg over 2 minutes. Titrate to effect
	        by repeating doses every 2–3 minutes to a usual
	        dose of 2.5–5 mg.
	Infusion for sedation during mechanical ventilation:
	    administer a loading dose of 0.05–0.2 mg/kg followed
	    by a continuous infusion of 1–2 μg/kg per min and
	    titrate to effect.
	Orally: 0.5 mg/kg to a maximum dose of 15 mg.
	Intranasally: 0.2–0.3 mg/kg per dose.
	The intranasal route of administration is not FDA
	    approved.
		Injection: 1 mg/mL, 5 mg/mL
		Solution: 2 mg/mL

Mineral oil	*Orally* (do not administer concomitantly with docusate):
	    Children: 5–20 mL/day.
	    Adults: 15–45 mL/day.
	Rectally (as a retention enema):
	    Children: 30–60 mL.
	    Adults: 60–150 mL.
		Enema: 133 mL
		Liquid

Mometasone Elocon	*Topically:*
	    Apply a thin film to the affected area once daily. The
	        cream and ointment have been used twice daily.
		Cream: 0.1%
		Lotion: 0.1%
		Ointment: 0.1%

Montelukast (Singulair)	*Orally:*
	    Children 2–6 years of age: 4 mg once daily.
	    Children >6–14 years of age: 5 mg once daily.
	    Children >14 years of age and adults: 10 mg once
	        daily.
		Tablets, chewable: 4 mg, 5 mg
		Tablets: 10 mg

Morphine sulfate (Astramorph PF, Duramorph, MSIR, MS Contin, Roxanol)	*IV or IM:*
	    Neonates and infants under age 6 months: these
	        patients are particularly sensitive to the respiratory
	        depressant effects of opiates; therefore, the doses
	        recommended are lower:
	        0.03 mg/kg every 3 or 4 hours. Infusions have been
	        used in neonatal patients at a dose of
	        0.01 mg/kg per hour. The dose may be increased if
	        necessary but should not exceed 0.015–0.02 mg/
	        kg per hour.
	    Infants over 6 months and children: 0.025–0.1 mg/kg
	        every 3 to 6 hours. Doses of up to 2.5 mg/kg have
	        been used in severe pain such as sickle cell or cancer
	        pain. The usual maximum dose is 10 mg.
	    Adults: 2.5–10 mg every 2–6 hours.
	Epidurally: 0.5–5 mg in the lumbar region. Dose may be
	    repeated every 24 hours. Maximum dose is
	    10 mg/24 hr.
	Intrathecally: one tenth of epidural dose or about
	    0.2–1 mg/dose. Repeat doses are not recommended.
		Injection: 0.5 mg/mL, 1 mg/mL, 2 mg/mL,
		    3 mg/mL, 4 mg/mL, 5 mg/mL, 8 mg/mL,
		    10 mg/mL, 15 mg/mL
		Solution: 10 mg/5 mL, 20 mg/5 mL, 20 mg/mL
		Suppositories: 5 mg, 10 mg, 20 mg, 30 mg
		Tablets: 15 mg, 30 mg
		Tablets, controlled release: 15 mg, 30 mg, 60 mg,
		    100 mg

Continued

Table 1 Medications (continued)

DRUG	DOSE	DOSAGE FORMS
Morphine sulfate (Astramorph PF, Duramorph, MSIR, MS Contin, Roxanol) (continued)	*Orally:* prompt-release preparations are administered every 3 or 4 hours; controlled-release preparations are administered every 8–12 hours. Oral doses are about one third as effective as IV doses. Infants over 6 months and children: 0.3 mg/kg every 3 or 4 hours (prompt release) or 0.3–0.6 mg/kg every 8–12 hours (extended release). Adults: 10–30 mg every 3–4 hours (prompt release) or 15–30 mg every 8–12 hours (extended release).	
Mumps virus vaccine (Mumpsvax)	*SC into the outer aspect of the upper arm:* 0.5 mL at age 15 months or older. Trivalent MMR vaccine is preferred for most vaccinations. Federal law requires that the date of administration, manufacturer, lot number, and expiration date of the vaccine, and the name, title, and address of the person administering the dose be entered into the patient's permanent medical record. It also requires providers to distribute information on vaccines before each vaccination.	Injection: $\geq$20,000 $TCID_{50}$/0.5 mL
Mupirocin (pseudomonic acid A; Bactroban)	*Topically:* *Impetigo:* apply ointment to affected area t.i.d. for 3–5 days. *Lacerations, minor suture infections or abrasions:* apply cream to the affected area t.i.d. for 10 days. *Intranasal Staphylococcus aureus infection:* apply half of the contents of a unit-dose tube of intranasal cream into each nostril 2–4 times daily for 5–14 days.	Cream (as mupirocin calcium): 2% mupirocin Cream, intranasal (as mupirocin calcium): 2% Ointment: 2%
Nafcillin (See oxacillin)	Neonates: 60 mg/kg per 24 hr in 4–6 divided doses. Children: 100–200 mg/kg per 24 hr in 4–6 divided doses.	Injection: 500 mg, 1 g, 2 g
Nalbuphine (Nubain)	*Parenterally:* *Reversal of morphine infusion side effects:* 0.025–0.05 mg/kg repeated every 6 hours as necessary. *Analgesia:* Children over age 10 months: 0.1–0.14 mg/kg every 3–6 hours as necessary to a maximum dose of 10 mg. Adults: 10–20 mg every 3–6 hours. Its use in narcotic-dependent patients may cause symptoms of withdrawal.	Injection: 10 mg/mL, 20 mg/mL
Naloxone (Narcan)	*IV (preferred), IM, or SC:* *Neonatal opiate depression:* 0.01 mg/kg every 2 or 3 minutes until the desired response is obtained. Additional doses may be necessary at 1–2-hour intervals. *Opiate overdosage:* 0.1 mg/kg to a dose of 2 mg administered every 2 or 3 minutes until 5 doses (up to 10 mg) have been given. If the depressive condition is not reversed, causes other than opiate ingestion should be considered. Additional doses may be necessary because the duration of effect of the opiate is generally longer than that of naloxone. The drug may also be administered via continuous infusion, especially if higher doses are necessary. *Postoperative narcotic reversal (partial reversal):* 0.005–0.01 mg/kg every 2–3 minutes until the desired degree of reversal is achieved. Care should be taken to avoid excessive dosage because that might result in a decrease in analgesia and an increase in blood pressure.	Injection (neonatal): 0.02 mg/mL Injection: 0.4 mg/mL, 1 mg/mL

Continued

Table 1   Medications   (continued)

DRUG	DOSE	DOSAGE FORMS
Naproxen (Aleve, Naprosyn)	*Orally:* 5–10 mg/kg every 8–12 hours to a maximum daily dose of 1 g.	Suspension: 125 mg/5 mL Tablets: 250 mg, 375 mg, 500 mg
Nelfinavir (Viracept)	*Orally* (to be used in combination with nucleoside analogs): Age 2–13: 60–90 mg/kg per day in 3 divided doses with food. Adolescents and adults: 750 mg/dose t.i.d.	Powder: 50 mg/g (1 g scoop provided to measure doses) Tablets: 250 mg
Neomycin, polymyxin B, and hydrocortisone (Cortisporin)	*Ophthalmic:* Solution: 1–2 drops to the affected eye every 4–6 hours; apply finger pressure to the lacrimal sac for 1 minute after instillation. Ointment: apply about half-inch ribbon of ointment to the eye t.i.d. or q.i.d. *Otic* (both a suspension and a solution formulation are available. The solution form may sting when instilled, but allows the ear canal to be examined easily): instill 3–4 drops into the affected ear t.i.d. or q.i.d.	Ointment, ophthalmic: neomycin 0.35%, bacitracin 400 U, polymyxin B 10,000 U, and hydrocortisone 1% Solution or suspension, otic: neomycin 5 mg/mL, polymyxin B 10,000 U/mL, and hydrocortisone 1% Suspension, ophthalmic: neomycin 0.35%, polymyxin B 10,000 U, and hydrocortisone 1%
Neomycin sulfate (Mycifradin)	*Orally:* *Bowel preparation:* 15 mg/kg (up to 1 g) at 1 PM, 2 PM, and 11 PM on the day before surgery (with erythromycin, cleansing enemas). *Hepatic coma:* 50–100 mg/kg per day in 3 or 4 divided doses up to 12 g/day.	Solution, oral: 125 mg/5 mL Tablets: 500 mg
Neostigmine (Prostigmin)	IM: *Myasthenia gravis test:* 0.04 mg/kg single dose IV: *Reversal of nondepolarizing neuromuscular blockade after surgery in conjunction with atropine or glycopyrrolate:* Infants: 0.025–0.1 mg/kg per dose. Children: 0.025–0.08 mg/kg per dose. Adults: 0.5–2.5 mg, total dose not to exceed 5 mg.	Injection: 0.25 mg/mL, 0.5 mg/mL, 1 mg/mL
Nitrofurantoin (Furadantin, Macrodantin)	*Orally:* *Active infection:* Children: 5–7 mg/kg per day in 4 divided doses to a maximum of 400 mg/day. Adults: 200–400 mg/day in 4 divided doses. *Chronic suppression therapy:* Children: 1–2 mg/kg per day in 1 or 2 divided doses. Adults: 50–100 mg at bedtime daily. Administer with food or milk to decrease rate of absorption because high peak levels are associated with increased GI upset.	Capsules (macrocrystals): 25 mg, 50 mg, 100 mg Suspension: 25 mg/5 mL
Nitroprusside sodium (Nipride, Nitropress)	*IV as a continuous infusion:* 0.3–0.5 μg/kg per min initially, then titrate to effect. Usual dose is 3 μg/kg per min. The maximum dose is 10 μg/kg per min. Cyanide toxicity may occur during prolonged therapy or in patients with hepatic dysfunction. Administration of sodium thiosulfate may decrease blood cyanide levels. Thiocyanate may accumulate in patients with renal impairment.	Injection: 50 mg Protect solutions from light. Do not use if highly colored (blue, green, or red).
Norepinephrine (Levarterenol, Levophed, Noradrenalin)	*IV as a continuous infusion:* initially 0.05–0.1 μg/kg per min, titrated to response. Maximum dose: 1–2 μg/kg per min.	Injection: 1 mg/mL
Nystatin (Mycostatin, Nilstat)	*Orally:* Neonates: 100,000 U administered q.i.d. Infants: 200,000 U administered q.i.d. Children and adults: 400,000–1 million U administered q.i.d. *Topically:* apply ointment or cream to the affected area t.i.d. or q.i.d.	Cream: 100,000 U/g (also available with triamcinolone, a topical steroid [Mycolog]) Ointment: 100,000 U/g (also available with triamcinolone, a topical steroid [Mycolog]) Suspension: 100,000 U/mL Tablets: 500,000 U (intestinal infections only) Troches: 200,000 U

Continued

Table 1   Medications   (continued)

DRUG	DOSE	DOSAGE FORMS
Octreotide (somatostatin analog; Sandostatin)	*IV or SC:* the subcutaneous route is generally preferred because absorption is not immediate and the activity is somewhat prolonged. The drug may also be administered as a continuous infusion. Pediatric experience is limited, but initial doses of 1–10 μg/kg with total daily doses of 2–50 μg/kg in 2–4 divided doses. Usual adult doses are 50 μg 1 or 2 times daily initially, then titrate dose to the patient's response. The long-term effects of octreotide on growth hormone release have not been determined.	Injection: 50 μg/mL, 100 μg/mL, 200 μg/mL, 500 μg/mL, 1,000 μg/mL

Ofloxacin (Floxin Otic, Ocuflox)	*Ophthalmic infections:*
	Bacterial conjunctivitis: 1–2 drops in the affected eye every 2–4 hours while awake for 2 days, then 4 times a day for up to 5 more days.
	Bacterial keratitis: 1–2 drops in the affected eye every 30 minutes while awake and 4–6 hours after retiring for 2 days, then every hour while awake for up to 4–6 more days, then 4 times a day until cure is affected.
	Otic infections:
	Otitis externa:
	    Children 1–12 years of age: 5 drops in the affected ear canal twice a day for 10 days.
	    Children >12 years of age and adults: 10 drops in the affected ear canal twice a day for 10 days.
	Suppurative otitis media in patients with perforated tympanic membranes: 10 drops in the affected ear twice a day for 14 days. The tragus of the ear should be pumped several times to make sure the solution is in the ear canal and the patient should remain in a position with the ear up for 5 minutes.
	Otitis media in patients with tympanostomy tubes:
	    5 drops in the affected ear twice a day for 10 days. The tragus of the ear should be pumped as above and the patient should remain in a position with the ear up for 5 minutes.
		Solution, ophthalmic: 0.3%
		Solution, otic: 0.3%

Olopatadine (Patanol)	*Ophthalmic:* Children ≥3 years of age to adults: 1–2 drops in each eye twice daily at 6–8 hours intervals.	Solution, ophthalmic: 0.1%

Omeprazole (Prilosec)	*Orally with food or a meal:*
	    Children: while safety and efficacy in children has not been established, a dose of 0.6–0.7 mg/kg per day as a single dose in the morning has been used. If necessary, a second dose may be given 12 hours later. The usual range of doses used is 0.3–3.3 mg/kg per day.
	    Adults: 20 mg daily. Higher doses may be used for pathologic hypersecretory conditions. The usual starting dose is 60 mg daily, but doses of up to 360 mg daily have been used. Doses >80 mg/day should be given in 2–3 divided doses.
	    Capsules: 10 mg, 20 mg, 40 mg. The capsules contain enteric coated spheres. If the patient is unable to swallow capsules, the spheres may be put into an acidic juice, such as apple juice, for administration. Do not crush the spheres. The spheres may be crushed for administration through a jejunostomy tube if a 650-mg tablet of sodium bicarbonate is added.
		Capsules: 10 mg, 20 mg, 40 mg. The capsules contain enteric coated spheres. If the patient is unable to swallow capsules, the spheres may be put into an acidic juice, such as apple juice, for administration. Do not crush the spheres. The spheres may be crushed for administration through a tube if a 650 mg tablet of sodium bicarbonate is added to the diluent.

Oseltamivir (Tamiflu)	*Orally (within 2 days of onset of symptoms):* ≥13 years of age: 75 mg twice a day for 5 days.	Capsules: 75 mg. Powder for suspension: 12 mg/mL

Continued

Table 1   Medications   (continued)

DRUG	DOSE	DOSAGE FORMS

Oxacillin (Bactocill)	*IV:*
	Neonates under age 7 days:
	  <2,000 g: 50 mg/kg per day in 2 divided doses.
	  ≥2,000 g: 100 mg/kg per day in 2 divided doses.
	Neonates over age 7 days:
	  <1,200 g: 50 mg/kg per day in 2 divided doses.
	  1,200–2,000 g: 75 mg/kg per day in 3 divided doses.
	  >2,000 g: 100 mg/kg per day in 4 divided doses.
	Infants and children (depends on severity and site of infection)
	  Mild to moderate infections: 50 mg/kg per day in 4 divided doses.
	  Severe infections, including osteomyelitis: 100–200 mg/kg per day in 4–6 divided doses.
	Total maximum dose is 12 g/day.
	Adults:
	  Mild to moderate infections: 250–500 mg every 6 hours.
	  Severe infections: 1–2 g every 4–6 hours.
	Orally:
	  Infants and children: 50–100 mg/kg per day in 4 divided doses.
	  Adults: 500 mg–1 g every 4–6 hours.
		Capsules: 250 mg, 500 mg
		Injection: 250 mg, 500 mg, 1 g, 2 g, 4 g, 10 g
		Solution, oral: 250 mg/5 mL

Oxybutynin (Ditropan)	*Orally:*
	  Children ≥age 5: 0.2 mg/kg per dose given 2–3 times daily.
	  Children over age 5: 5 mg administered b.i.d. or t.i.d.
	  Adults: 5 mg b.i.d. or t.i.d., to a maximum of q.i.d.
		Solution, oral: 5 mg/5 mL
		Tablets: 5 mg

Oxcarbazepine (Trileptal)	*Orally:*
	  Children 4 to 16 years of age: 8 to 10 mg/kg/day (to a maximum of 600 mg daily) initially, with increases over a 2 week period to a maximum dose of 900 mg daily for patients weighing 20 to 29 kg, 1,200 mg daily for patients weighing >29 kg to 39 kg and 1,800 mg daily for patients weighing >39 kg.
	  Adults: 600 mg daily in 2 divided doses initially, increasing over 1 week to the usual maintenance dos of 1,200 mg daily. Maximum daily dose is 2,400 mg.
		Suspension: 60 mg/mL
		Tablets: 150 mg, 300 mg, 600 mg

Oxycodone	*Orally (oxycodone component for combination products):*
	  Children: 0.05–0.15 mg/kg per dose every 4 to 6 hours.
	  Adults: 5 mg every 6 hours initially; may be increased to 10 mg every 4 hours if necessary. Higher doses may be necessary for severe pain, using a plain oxycodone product.
		Capsule: 5 mg
		Solution: 1 mg/mL
		Solution (concentrate): 20 mg/mL
		Tablets: 5 mg, 15 mg, 30 mg
		Also available in fixed combinations with acetaminophen or aspirin in capsule, liquid and tablet dosage forms.

Palivizumab (Synagis)	*Intramuscularly:* Infants and children up to 2 years of age: 15 mg/kg/dose given every month during RSV season, usually October through April.	Injection, lyophilized powder: 50 mg and 100 mg

Continued

Table 1   Medications   (continued)

DRUG	DOSE	DOSAGE FORMS
Pancrelipase (Cotazym, Cotazym-S, Creon, Pancrease MT, Ultrase, Zymase)	*Orally:* depends on the condition being treated and the dietary content of the patient. Dosage is usually determined by the fat content of the diet. The usual starting dose is 4,000–8,000 U of lipase activity before or with each meal or snack for children age 1–7, 4,000–12,000 U for children age >7–12, or 4,000–33,000 U for adults. Further dosage adjustments may be made based on the patient's symptoms. The newer, enteric-coated products are designed to release the enzymes at pH >6 and are therefore more resistant to destruction by gastric acids.	Capsules, delayed release, containing enteric-coated spheres, microspheres, or microtablets‡

Penicillamine (Cuprimine, Depen)	Do not exceed a dose of 30 mg/kg per day.
	Rheumatoid arthritis:
	Children:
	   Initial: 3 mg/kg per day (≤250 mg/day) for 3 months, then 6 mg/kg per day (500 mg/day) in divided doses b.i.d. for 3 months. Maximum: 10 mg/kg per day in 3 or 4 divided doses.
	Wilson disease:
	   Children: 20 mg/kg per day in 4 divided doses.
		Capsules: 125 mg, 250 mg
		Tablets: 250 mg

Penicillin G, aqueous (potassium and sodium salts)	*IV:*
	Neonates under age 7 days:
	   <2,000 g: 25,000 U/kg every 12 hours. For meningitis, use 50,000 U/kg every 12 hours.
	   >2,000 g: 20,000 U/kg every 8 hours. For meningitis, 50,000 U/kg every 8 hours.
	Neonates over age 7 days:
	   <2,000 g: 25,000 U/kg every 8 hours. For meningitis, 50,000 U/kg every 8 hours.
	>2,000 g: 25,000 U/kg every 6 hours. For meningitis, 50,000 U/kg every 6 hours.
	   Infants and children: 100,000–250,000 U/kg/day in 6 divided doses. Up to 500,000 U/kg/day may be used for severe infections to a maximum of 20 million U/day.
	   Adults: 2–20 million U/day in 6 divided doses.
	The potassium salt contains 1.7 mEq of potassium and 0.3 mEq of sodium per 1 million U.
	The sodium salt contains 2 mEq of sodium per 1 million U.
	The potassium salt must be administered slowly at high doses due to the effect of the potassium.
		Injection, potassium salt: 1 million U, 5 million U, 10 million U
		Injection, sodium salt: 5 million U

Penicillin G procaine, benzathine	*Deep IM:* results in low but prolonged serum levels. May be given as a single daily dose. A dose of penicillin G benzathine will result in low serum levels for up to 4 weeks.
	   Newborns: avoid use in these patients because sterile abscess and procaine toxicity are of greater concern.
	Infants: 50,000 U/kg up to 600,000 U.
	Children and adults: 600,000–1.2 million U/day.
	   Maximum dose is 4.8 million U.
		Injection, benzathine: 600,000 U/mL
		Injection, benzathine and procaine: combined equal parts of each in 300,000 U, 600,000 U, 1.2 million U, 2.4 million U; 900/300 (900,000 U benzathine, 300,000 U procaine)
		Injection, procaine: 600,000 U/mL

Penicillin V potassium (phenoxymethylpenicillin; Pen Vee K, V-Cillin K, Veetids)	*Orally:*
	   Children: 25–50 mg/kg per day in 4 divided doses.
	   Adults: 125–500 mg/dose every 6 hours.
	Prophylaxis:
	   Under age 5: 125 mg b.i.d.
	   Over age 5 and adults: 250 mg b.i.d.
		Liquid, oral: 250 mg/5 mL
		Tablets: 125 mg, 250 mg, 500 mg

Continued

Table 1   Medications   (continued)

DRUG	DOSE	DOSAGE FORMS
Pentobarbital (Nembutal)	*Orally, IM:* *Sedation before surgery:* 　Children: 2–6 mg/kg per day to a maximum of 　　100 mg *IV:* *For sedation before procedures:* dose should be 　administered slowly and incrementally to avoid 　oversedation. Patients must be closely observed. 　Dosing is very patient-specific. The rate of 　injection should not exceed 1 mg/kg per min 　(50 mg/min in adults). Allow at least 1 minute 　to reach full effect. 　Children: initially 2 mg/kg to a maximum of 100 mg. 　　Incremental doses of 1–2 mg/kg may be used to a 　　maximum total dose of 200 mg. 　Adults: initially 100 mg. Incremental doses of 　　100–200 mg may be given to a maximum dose of 　　500 mg for healthy adults. *Barbiturate coma:* 10–15 mg/kg administered over 　1–2 hours, followed by a maintenance infusion of 　1 mg/kg per hr. Dosage may be increased to 　2–3 mg/kg per hr to maintain burst suppression on 　EEG. Hypothermia may necessitate a decrease in 　dosage. *Rectally* (do not divide suppositories): 　4.5–9 kg: 30 mg. 　>9–18 kg: 30–60 mg. 　19–36 kg: 60 mg. 　>36–50 kg: 60–120 mg. 　>50 kg: 120–200 mg.	Capsules: 50 mg, 100 mg Elixir: 20 mg/5 mL Injection: 50 mg/mL Suppositories: 30 mg, 60 mg, 120 mg, 200 mg
Permethrin (Elimite Cream, Nix Cream Rinse)	*Scabies:* 　Children >2 months of age and adults: apply cream 　　from head to toe. Wash cream off after 8–14 hours. 　　May be reapplied after 1 week if live mites appear. *Head lice:* apply cream rinse to hair that has been 　thoroughly washed, rinsed and towel dried. Saturate 　hair and scalp with cream rinse. Also apply to the 　ears and hairline at the nape of the neck. Rinse off 　after 10 minutes and remove remaining nits with the 　comb provided. May be repeated after 1 week if 　necessary.	Cream, topical 5% Cream rinse: 1%
Phenobarbital	*IV or orally:* *Loading doses (usually IV for status epilepticus):* 　Neonates: 20 mg/kg in a single or 2 divided doses. 　Infants, children and adults: 15–18 mg/kg a single or 　　2 divided doses. 　Allow 15–30 minutes for the drug to distribute into 　　the CNS and for the seizures to stop. *Maintenance doses:* 　Neonates: 5 mg/kg per day in 2 divided doses. 　Infants: 5–6 mg/kg per day in 2 divided doses. 　Age 1–5: 6 mg/kg per day in 2 divided doses. 　Age >5–12: 4 mg/kg per day in 1 or 2 divided doses. 　Over age 12 and adults: 1–2 mg/kg per day in 1 or 　　2 divided doses.	Elixir: 15 mg/5 mL, 20 mg/5 mL Injection (sodium): 30 mg/mL, 60 mg/mL, 65 mg/mL, 　130 mg/mL Tablets: 15 mg, 30 mg, 60 mg, 100 mg
Phentolamine mesylate	*Test dose (pheochromocytoma):* 1 mg IM or IV.	Injection: 5-mg ampul
Phenylephrine (Neo-Synephrine, Mydfrin ophthalmic)	*Intranasally* (do not use for longer than 3–5 days): 　Under age 6: 0.125% solution 2–3 drops every 　　4 hours as needed. 　Age 6–12: 0.25% solution 2–3 drops or 1–2 sprays 　　every 4 hours as needed.	Drops only: 0.125% Injection: 10 mg/mL Solution, nasal drops or spray: 0.25%, 0.5%, 1% Solution, ophthalmic: 2.5%, 10%

Continued

Table 1   Medications   (continued)

DRUG	*DOSE*	*DOSAGE FORMS*

Phenylephrine (Neo-Synephrine, Mydfrin ophthalmic) (*continued*)	Over age 12 and adults: 0.5% solution 2–3 drops or 1–2 sprays every 4 hours as needed. 1% solution may be used in adults with extreme congestion.
	Ophthalmic:
	  Infants: 1 drop of 2.5% solution 15–30 minutes before procedure.
	  Children and adults: 1 drop of 2.5% or 10% solution; may repeat in 15–30 minutes.
	IV for severe hypotension or shock: a bolus dose of 5–20 μg/kg (2–5 mg in adults) may be repeated every 10–15 minutes. For infusion, initial doses of 0.1–0.5 μg/kg per min are titrated to effect.	

Phenytoin (Dilantin) and fosphenytoin (Cerebyx)	Care must be taken when changing from one dosage form of the drug to another because some contain phenytoin sodium and some contain the free acid form of the drug. The free acid form is used for the Infatabs and the suspension. Phenytoin sodium is used for the injection and capsules. Phenytoin sodium contains 92% phenytoin. Injection labeled as 50 mg/mL phenytoin sodium contains 46 mg of phenytoin and capsules labeled 100 mg contain 92 mg phenytoin.
	Fosphenytoin should be ordered in terms of phenytoin equivalents.
	The patient's serum levels should be monitored whenever the dosage form is changed. In addition, the different brands of phenytoin capsules have different dissolution characteristics. Dilantin capsules are considered extended and may be dosed in adults as a single daily dose. The serum level range usually associated with clinical effectiveness is 10–20 μg/mL; that associated with mild to moderate toxicity may be as low as 25–30 μg/mL.
	Loading dose (IV or PO): 15–20 mg/kg in a single or divided doses.
	Maintenance dose (IV or PO): 5 mg/kg per day in 2 or 3 divided doses initially and then adjusted to response and serum levels. Usual ranges based on age (divided into 2 or 3 doses daily):
	  Neonates: 5–8 mg/kg per day.
	  Age 6 months-3 years: 8–10 mg/kg per day.
	  Age 4–6: 7.5–9 mg/kg per day.
	  Age 7–9: 7–8 mg/kg per day.
	  Age 10–16: 6–7 mg/kg per day.
	  Adults: 5–6 mg/kg per day may be given as a single dose if extended-capsule preparation is used.
	Higher doses are required in infants and young children due to lower absorption of the drug from the GI tract.
	IV doses of phenytoin should be administered at a maximum rate of about 1 mg/kg per min (50 mg/min in adults) to avoid cardiovascular side effects. The injection is not compatible with many solutions or medications. The line must be flushed well with saline before administration to avoid precipitation of phenytoin in the line. Extravasation of the drug must also be avoided because it is very alkaline and may cause severe tissue necrosis. Thorough flushing of the vessel after phenytoin administration will also decrease the incidence of local tissue inflammation that may occur even in the absence of extravasation.
		Capsule, phenytoin sodium, extended: 30 mg, 100 mg
		Injection, for phenytoin: 75 mg/1 mL (equivalent to 50 mg phenytoin sodium)
		Injection, phenytoin sodium: 50 mg/mL
		Suspension, phenytoin: 125 mg/5 mL
		Tablet, chewable, phenytoin: 50 mg

Continued

Table 1   Medications   (continued)

DRUG	DOSE	DOSAGE FORMS
Phenytoin (Dilantin) and fosphenytoin (Cerebyx) (*continued*)	Fosphenytoin injection should be diluted with either 5% dextrose or normal saline to a concentration of 1.5–25 mg of phenytoin equivalents (2.3–37.5 mg fosphenytoin) per mL of diluent and may be administered at a rate of 2–3 mg phenytoin equivalents/kg per min (100–150 mg phenytoin equivalents/min in adults).	
Phosphate (potassium and/or sodium)	Should be guided by the patient's serum phosphorus and potassium levels. Severe deficits should be replaced by the IV route because the oral route may result in diarrhea and oral absorption is unreliable. In general, the deficit should be made up by incorporating it into the patient's maintenance fluids. Intermittent infusions should follow the guidelines outlined below for potassium infusions because the IV form is potassium phosphate and each 3 mmol of phosphate will also deliver 4.4 mEq of potassium. The guidelines below are meant for use in patients with severe hypophosphatemia (<1 mg/dL in adults): Neonates: 0.5 mmol/kg up to 1–2 mmol/kg per day. Children: 0.15–0.3 mmol/kg with subsequent doses only after serum levels are checked and if the patient is symptomatic. Adults: 0.08 mmol/kg (uncomplicated hypophosphatemia) or 0.16 mmol/kg for prolonged deficits. Do not exceed 0.24 mmol/kg per day (serum phosphorus ≥0.5 mg/dL) or 0.5 mmol/kg per day (serum phosphorus <0.5 mg/dL). IV doses should be administered over a 6-hour period. *Maintenance doses:* Children: 0.5–1.5 mmol/kg per day. Adults: 15–30 mmol/day. *Orally:* should be taken with food to increase GI tolerance. Each packet or capsule should be mixed in 75 mL of water. Tablets should be taken with a full glass of water. *Maintenance doses:* Children: 2–3 mmol/kg per day in 4 divided doses. Adults: 32–64 mmol/day (4–8 packets) in 4 divided doses. Do not administer at the same time as aluminum- and/or magnesium-containing antacids, sucralfate, or calcium because they may act to bind phosphorus.	Injection (potassium phosphate): 3 mmol (94 mg) phosphorus and 4.4 mEq potassium per milliliter Packets or capsules (Neutra-Phos): 250 mg (8 mmol) phosphorus, 7 mEq potassium, and 7 mEq sodium Packets or capsules (Neutra-Phos K): 250 mg (8 mmol) phosphorus, 14.25 mEq potassium Tablets (K-Phos Neutral): 250 mg (8 mmol) phosphorus, 1.1 mEq potassium, and 13 mEq sodium Tablets (Uro-KP-Neutral): 250 mg (8 mmol) phosphorus, 1.27 mEq potassium, and 10.9 mEq sodium
Phytonadione (vitamin K; AquaMEPHYTON, Konakion, Mephyton)	*IM or SC:* *Hemorrhagic disease of the newborn, prophylaxis:* 0.5–1 mg within 1 hour of birth and again 6–8 hours later, if needed. *Treatment:* 1–2 mg/day. *Treatment of deficiency caused by malabsorption or decreased synthesis or due to drugs (administer IV cautiously and slowly):* Children: 1–2 mg/day. Adults: 10 mg/day *Treatment of oral anticoagulant overdose:* Infants: 1–2 mg repeated every 4–8 hours. Children and adults: 2.5–10 mg repeated in 6–8 hours. *Orally:* *Prevention of deficiency in malabsorption:* Children: 2.5–5 mg every other day or daily. Adults: 5–25 mg/day.	Injection: 2 mg/mL, 10 mg/mL Tablets: 5 mg

Continued

Table 1   Medications   (continued)

DRUG	DOSE	DOSAGE FORMS

Piroxicam (Feldene)	*Orally:*
	  Children: 0.2–0.3 mg/kg per day in a single daily dose to a maximum of 15 mg/day.
	  Adults: 10–20 mg/day in a single dose.
		Capsules: 10 mg, 20 mg

Polyethylene glycol electrolyte solution (Colyte, GoLYTELY, Miralax, NuLytely)	*Orally after a 3–4-hour fast for bowel cleansing:*
	  Children: 25–40 mL/kg per hr.
	  Adults: 240 mL every 10 minutes.
	The patient should continue to drink the solution until the rectal effluent is clear. Rapid drinking of each portion is more effective than slow consumption. The first bowel movement should occur about an hour after starting. The solution is more palatable if chilled, but must not be poured over ice. Nothing, including other flavorings, should be added to the solution.
	Nasogastric tube administration:
	  Adults: 240 mL every 10 minutes.
	Constipation (Miralax):
	  Adults: 1 capful (17 g) mixed in 8 oz of water or juice daily
		Powder for oral solution to make 4 L (GoLytely): PEG3350 236 g, sodium sulfate 22.74 g, sodium bicarbonate 6.74 g, sodium chloride 5.86 g, and potassium chloride 2.97 g
		Powder for oral solution to make 4L (Colyte): PEG3350 227.1 g, sodium sulfate 21.5 g, sodium bicarbonate 6.36 g, sodium chloride 5.53 g, and potassium chloride 2.82 g.
		Powder for oral solution to make 4L (Nulytely): PEG3350 420 g, sodium bicarbonate 5.72 g, sodium chloride 11.2 g, potassium chloride 1.48 g
		Powder (Miralax): PEG3350: 255 g, 527 g

Potassium chloride	*Orally:* liquid doses must be well diluted before administration to avoid GI adverse effects. Capsules or tablets should be taken with a full glass of water. Capsules may be opened and emptied onto a soft food, but the beads should not be crushed or chewed. Total daily dose may be given in 1 or 2 divided doses if tolerated, or may be given in 3 or 4 divided doses to decrease GI upset. Dose is usually based on each patient's requirements and may depend on concurrent medications or medical conditions that result in potassium losses. The following may be used as general guidelines:
	Normal daily requirement for either PO or IV replacement:
	  Newborn: 2–6 mEq/kg per day.
	  Children: 2–3 mEq/kg per day.
	  Adults: 40–80 mEq/day.
	During diuretic therapy:
	  Children: 1–2 mEq/kg per day.
	  Adults: 20–40 mEq/day.
	For treatment of hypokalemia:
	  Children: 2–5 mEq/kg per day.
	  Adults: 40–100 mEq/day.
	IV: doses should be well diluted. Usually they are incorporated into the patient's daily fluid requirement. The maximum desirable concentration is 80 mEq/L. Greater concentrations should be used cautiously and only in patients with documented hypokalemia with a serum potassium level <2.5 mEq/L.
		Capsules, controlled release: 8 mEq (600 mg), 10 mEq (750 mg)
		Injection, concentrated: 2 mEq/mL, 3 mEq/mL
		Liquids: 20 mEq/15 mL (10%), 30 mEq/15 mL (15%), 40 mEq/15 mL (20%)
		Powders, effervescent packets: 15 mEq, 20 mEq, 25 mEq
		Tablets, effervescent: 20 mEq, 25 mEq, 50 mEq
		Tablets, extended release: 6.7 mEq (500 mg), 8 mEq (600 mg), 10 mEq (750 mg)
		Other potassium salts are also available and may be desirable in patients who are acidotic. They include bicarbonate, citrate, acetate, and gluconate salts.

Continued

Table 1   Medications   (continued)

DRUG	DOSE	DOSAGE FORMS
Potassium chloride (*continued*)	In the case of a patient in whom a shorter infusion of potassium is necessary, the following guidelines may be used: Maximum concentration of the solution must not exceed 30 mEq/100 mL (1 mEq/3 mL) and rate of infusion should not exceed 1 mEq/kg per hour in children or 40 mEq/hour in adults. The solutions should be infused using a pump to control the infusion rate. Infusion over 2–3 hours (0.3–0.5 mEq/kg per hour) is more desirable. Administration of doses greater than 0.3 mEq/kg per hour should be done only if the patient has an ECG monitor in place. Solutions should be mixed well to prevent layering of the potassium chloride, which may result in inadvertent rapid administration.	

Prednisolone and prednisone	*Orally:* depends on the condition being treated and the patient's response. The lowest dose possible should be used. Withdrawal of long-term therapy must be accomplished slowly by gradually tapering the dose. The guidelines below may be used for initial dosing.
	Children:
	  Antiinflammatory or immunosuppressive: 0.1–2 mg/kg per day in 1–4 divided doses.
	  Acute asthma: 1–2 mg/kg per day in 1 or 2 divided doses for up to 5 days.
	  Inflammatory bowel disease: 1–3 mg/kg per day in 1–2 divided doses.
	Nephrotic syndrome: 2 mg/kg per day in 3 or 4 divided doses.
	Organ transplants: 1 mg/kg per day in 2 divided doses, tapering gradually to 0.15 mg/kg per day or lowest effective dose.
		Prednisolone:
		  Liquid, as sodium phosphate: 5 mg/5 mL (Pediapred), 15 mg/5 mL (OraPred)
		  Syrup (Prelone): 15 mg/5 mL
		  Tablets: 5 mg
		Prednisone:
		  Solution: 5 mg/5 mL
		  Syrup (Liquid Pred): 5 mg/5 mL
		  Tablets: 1 mg, 2.5 mg, 5 mg, 10 mg, 20 mg, 50 mg

Primidone (Mysoline)	*Orally:*
	  Under age 8: initially 50–125 mg/day at bedtime or in 2 divided doses. Increase dose by 50–125 mg/day at weekly intervals to the normal range of 125–250 mg t.i.d. or 10–25 mg/kg per day.
	  Over age 8 and adults: initially 125–250 mg/day at bedtime or in 2 divided doses. Increase dose by 125–250 mg/day at weekly intervals to the usual maintenance dose of 250 mg t.i.d. or q.i.d. Do not exceed 500 mg q.i.d. (2 g).
	Primidone is metabolized to phenobarbital and phenyl-ethylmalonamide (PEMA).
	Phenobarbital levels should be monitored in addition to primidone levels.
		Suspension: 250 mg/5 mL
		Tablets: 50 mg, 250 mg

Probenecid (Benemid)	*Uricosuric:*
	  Children under age 2: not recommended.
	  Age 2–14:
	    Initial: 25 mg/kg for 1 dose.
	    Maintenance: 40 mg/kg per 24 hr in 4 divided doses.
		Tablets: 500 mg

Procainamide (Procanbid, Pronestyl)	*IV:*
	  Children: loading dose of 3–6 mg/kg to a maximum of 100 mg over 5 minutes. This may be repeated every 5–10 minutes to a maximum of 15 mg/kg. Follow with a maintenance infusion at a dose of 20–80 μg/kg per minute.
	  Adults: loading dose of 50–100 mg, repeated every 5–10 minutes to a maximum of 15–18 mg/kg or 1–1.5 g. Follow with a maintenance infusion at a usual dose of 3–4 mg/min (range 1–6 mg/min).
		Capsules, immediate release: 250 mg, 375 mg, 500 mg
		Injection: 100 mg/mL, 500 mg/mL
		Tablets, immediate release: 250 mg, 375 mg, 500 mg
		Tablets, sustained release: 250 mg, 500 mg, 750 mg, 1,000 mg
		Tablets, sustained release, 12-hour duration (Procanbid): 500 mg, 1,000 mg

Continued

Table 1   Medications   (continued)

DRUG	DOSE	DOSAGE FORMS
Procainamide (Procanbid, Pronestyl) (continued)	*Orally* (immediate-release products must be administered every 3 hours; controlled-release products must be administered every 6 hours or every 12 hours depending on the formulation used): Children: 15–50 mg/kg per day to a maximum dose of 4 g/day. Adults: usual range is 1–4 g/day in divided doses as above.	
Prochlorperazine (Compazine)	*Orally or rectally as an antiemetic:* 0.4 mg/kg per day in 3 or 4 divided doses or alternatively by the patient's weight: 9–14 kg: 2.5 mg every 12–24 hours as needed, to a maximum of 7.5 mg/day. >14–18 kg: 2.5 mg every 8–12 hours as needed, to a maximum of 10 mg/day. >18–39 kg: 2.5 mg every 8 hours or 5 mg every 12 hours as needed, to a maximum of 15 mg/day. >40 kg: Rectally: 25 mg every 12 hours. Orally: 5–10 mg t.i.d. or q.i.d. *IM* (IV is not recommended in children): 0.13 mg/kg; may be repeated if necessary up to t.i.d. or q.i.d. Usual adult dose is 5–10 mg every 4 hours to a maximum of 40 mg/day.	Capsules, sustained release: 10 mg, 15 mg, 30 mg Injection: 5 mg/mL Suppositories: 2.5 mg, 5 mg, 25 mg Syrup: 5 mg/5 mL Tablets: 5 mg, 10 mg, 25 mg
Promethazine (Phenergan)	*Antihistamine* (usually orally): Children: 0.1 mg/kg every 6 hours during the day. A dose of 0.5 mg/kg may be used at bedtime. Adults: 12.5 mg every 6 hours during the day with a 25-mg dose at bedtime. *Antiemetic* (orally, IV, IM, or rectally): Children: 0.5 mg/kg up to every 4 hours. Adults: 12.5–25 mg every 4 hours as needed. *Motion sickness* (orally): Children: 0.5 mg/kg 30 minutes to 1 hour before traveling; then every 12 hours as needed. Adults: 25 mg 30 minutes to 1 hour before traveling; then every 12 hours as needed. *Sedation* (all routes): Children: 0.5–1 mg/kg every 6 hours as needed. Adults: 25–50 mg every 6 hours as needed.	Injection: 25 mg/mL, 50 mg/mL Suppositories: 12.5 mg, 25 mg, 50 mg Syrup: 6.25 mg/5 mL, 25 mg/5 mL Tablets: 12.5 mg, 25 mg, 50 mg
Propranolol (Inderal)	*Orally:* *Arrhythmias:* Children: 0.5–1 mg/kg per day in 3 or 4 divided doses. Dosage may be titrated upward at 3- to 7-day intervals to the usual range of 2–4 mg/kg per day. If higher doses are necessary, up to 16 mg/kg per day (up to 640 mg) may be used. Adults: usually 10–30 mg every 6–8 hours. *Hypertension:* Children: 0.5–1 mg/kg per day in 2–4 divided doses, increasing at 3- to 7-day intervals to the usual range of 1–5 mg/kg per day. Adults: 40 mg b.i.d., increasing at 3- to 7-day intervals to a maximum dose of 640 mg/day. *Migraine prophylaxis:* Children: 0.6–1.5 mg/kg per day in 3 divided doses. Adults: 80 mg/day in 3 or 4 divided doses. Dose may be increased to a maximum of 240 mg/day in divided doses.	Capsules, sustained release: 60 mg, 80 mg, 120 mg, 160 mg Injection: 1 mg/mL Solution: 4 mg/mL, 8 mg/mL Tablets: 10 mg, 20 mg, 40 mg, 60 mg, 80 mg, 90 mg

Continued

Table 1 Medications (continued)

DRUG	DOSE	DOSAGE FORMS

Propranolol (Inderal) (continued)	*Tetralogy spells:*
	  Children: 1–2 mg/kg every 6 hours.
	Thyrotoxicosis:
	  Neonates: 2 mg/kg per day in 2–4 divided doses.
	  Children: 1 mg/kg per day q.i.d.
	  Adolescents and adults: 10–40 mg every 6 hours.
	IV: reserve for life-threatening arrhythmias. To be administered as an IV bolus *slowly* under ECG monitoring. The IV dose is much smaller than the oral dose.
	  Children: 0.01–0.1 mg/kg to a maximum of 1 mg for arrhythmias. For tetralogy spells, 0.15–0.25 mg/kg, which may be repeated once after 15 minutes.
	  Adults: 1–3 mg. A second dose may be given, if necessary, after 2 minutes.	

Propylthiouracil	*Orally:* Initially:
	  Neonates: 5–10 mg/kg per day in 3 divided doses.
	  Under age 10: 5–7 mg/kg per day in 3 divided doses.
	  ≥age 10: 150–300 mg/day in 3 divided doses.
	  Adults: 300 mg/day in 3 divided doses.
	After control of symptoms has been achieved, the dose may be decreased to the lowest dose possible, usually one-third to two-thirds of the initial dose, administered in 3 doses daily.
		Tablets: 50 mg

Protamine sulfate	*IV:* 1 mg of protamine sulfate neutralizes 90 mg of lung-derived heparin or 115 U of intestinal mucosa-derived heparin. Because heparin disappears rapidly from the circulation, the dose of protamine decreases rapidly with time elapsed since the heparin infusion. The dose of protamine necessary after 30 minutes is half the dose above and that necessary after 2 hours is one fourth the dose above. Because protamine itself is an anticoagulant, avoid overdosing. Protamine should be administered slowly, over a 1-minute period, and the dose should not exceed 50 mg.	Injection: 10 mg/mL

Protirelin (Thyrel TRH)	*IV* (as a bolus over 15–30 seconds with the patient remaining supine for an additional 15 minutes):
	  Children: 7 μg/kg to a maximum of 500 μg.
	  Adults: 500 μg.
		Injection: 500 μg/mL

Psyllium (Fiberall, Hydrocil, Konsyl, Metamucil, Perdiem Fiber, Serutan).	*Orally* (each dose should be accompanied by a full glass of water or other liquid):
	  Children: half the adult dose (1/2 to 1 packet or 1.7–3.4 g of psyllium) once daily to t.i.d.
	  Adults: 1–2 packets or 3.4–6.8 g of psyllium once daily to t.i.d.
		Powder: ~3.4 g/dose
		Powder, effervescent

Pyrantel pamoate (Antiminth)	*Orally* (may be taken with juice or milk and without regard to the ingestion of food): 11 mg/kg to a maximum of 1 g.	Suspension: 50 mg/mL

Ranitidine (Zantac)	*Orally:*
	  Children: 2–4 mg/kg per day in 2 divided doses initially. Dose may be higher, up to 8 mg/kg per day in GERD and hypersecretory conditions.
	  Adults: 150 mg b.i.d. or 300 mg at bedtime. Dose may be higher or more frequently administered. Up to 6 g/day has been used in hypersecretory conditions.
		Injection: 25 mg/mL
		Syrup: 15 mg/mL
		Tablets: 75 mg, 150 mg, 300 mg

Continued

Table 1   Medications   (continued)

DRUG	DOSE	DOSAGE FORMS
Ranitidine (Zantac) (continued)	*IV:* Children: 1–2 mg/kg per day in 3 or 4 divided doses. Do not exceed 6 mg/kg per day or 300 mg/day Adults: 50 mg every 6–8 hours. Do not exceed 400 mg/day. Dosage should be adjusted for renal dysfunction.	
Ribavirin (Virazole)	Aerosol administered via the manufacturer's small particle aerosol generator (SPAG). 6 g of the drug are solubilized in sterile water and aerosolized over 12–18 hours daily for 3–7 days. Therapy must be started within the first 3 days of lower respiratory tract infection due to RSV. The manufacturer recommends against using the drug for patients who require assisted ventilation. Precipitation of the drug in respiratory equipment has occurred, as has accumulation of fluid in tubing. Either condition may compromise the patient.	Powder for reconstitution for aerosol: 6 g
Rifampin (Rifadin, Rimactane)	*Orally* (on an empty stomach): *Tuberculosis:* Children: 10–20 mg/kg per day as a single daily dose to a maximum of 600 mg. Adults: 600 mg/day. *Meningococcal carriers:* Under age 1 month: 10 mg/kg per day in 2 divided doses for 2 days. Infants and children: 20 mg/kg per day in 2 divided doses for 2 days, to a maximum dose of 1,200 mg/day. Adults: 600 mg/dose b.i.d. for 2 days. *Haemophilus influenzae type b prophylaxis:* Under age 1 month: 10 mg/kg per day as a single dose for 4 days. Over age 1 month and children: 20 mg/kg per day as a single dose for 4 days. Adults: 600 mg/day for 4 days. *IV* (over 30 minutes to 3 hours): same doses as for the oral route. Rifampin may cause a red-orange discoloration of the sweat, urine, tears, and other body fluids; soft contact lenses may be permanently stained.	Capsules 150 mg, 300 mg Injection: 600 mg Suspension: not commercially available, but may be made by mixing the powder from the capsules with simple syrup to form a 10 mg/mL suspension. Such suspensions are stable for 4 weeks at room temperature or refrigerated.
Rimantadine (Flumadine)	*Orally:* Under age 10: 5 mg/kg once daily to a maximum dose of 150 mg. Over age 10 and adults: 100 mg b.i.d. Therapy may be continued for up to 6 weeks. Rimantadine does not completely prevent an immune response to influenza vaccine; therefore, vaccination is not contraindicated. Rimantadine should be continued for 2–4 weeks after vaccination to allow for antibody production.	Syrup: 50 mg/5 mL Tablets: 100 mg
Ritonavir (Norvir)	*Orally with food to increase absorption:* Children 2–12 years of age: 250 mg/m^2 per dose given twice a day initially to decrease the nausea that usually occurs. The dose is gradually increased by 50 mg/m^2 per dose every 2–3 days as tolerated to a maximum of 400 mg/m^2 per dose (or 600 mg/dose). Children >12 years of age and adults: 300 mg/dose twice daily initially, increasing by 100 mg/dose over 3–5 days to a maximum dose of 600 mg twice a day.	Capsule, liquid filled: 100 mg Solution, oral: 80 mg/mL

Continued

Table 1   Medications   (continued)

DRUG	DOSE	DOSAGE FORMS
Salmeterol (Serevent, Serevent Diskus)	*Salmeterol is a long-acting drug and must not be used for acute exacerbations of asthma, is not a substitute for the use of steroids and should not be used without steroids for the treatment of chronic asthma.* *Powder (Diskus) for oral inhalation:* 　Children ≥4 years of age to adults: 1 inhalation (50 μg) twice daily about 12 hours apart is used for chronic asthma. *Metered dose inhalation:* 　Children ≥12 years of age and adults: 2 inhalations (42 μg) twice daily about 12 hours apart. For exercise-induced asthma, 1 puff should be inhaled 30–60 minutes prior to exercise and may be repeated 12 hours later. Patients on regular twice a day doses should not add a third dose prior to exercise.	Inhalation, metered dose: 21 μg/actuation Inhalation, powder: 50 μg/foil blister
Scopolamine (hyoscine; Isopto Hyoscine)	*IM, SC, or IV:* 　Children: 0.006 mg/kg to a maximum dose of 0.3 mg. 　Adults: 0.3–0.65 mg. *Ophthalmic:* 　Children: 1 drop (up to q.i.d. for uveitis). 　Adults: 1–2 drops (up to q.i.d. for uveitis).	Injection: 0.3 mg/mL, 0.4 mg/mL, 0.86 mg/mL, 1 mg/mL Solution, ophthalmic: 0.25%
Sermorelin acetate (growth hormone-releasing hormone; Geref)	*IV (in the morning after an overnight fast):* 　1 μg/kg IV push followed by a 3-mL saline flush.	Injection: 50-μg vials
Silver sulfadiazine (Silvadene, SSD, Thermazene)	*Topically:* applied to a thickness of 1/16-inch under sterile conditions (using a sterile glove) once or b.i.d. to a clean, debrided wound. Wound should always be covered with cream; reapply if it rubs off.	Cream: 10 mg/g
Sodium bicarbonate (baking soda, NaHCO$_3$)	*IV:* *Cardiac arrest* (only after adequate ventilation has been established): 1 mEq/kg IV push initially; may repeat with a dose of 0.5 mEq/kg. Further doses should not be given until the patient's acid-base status has been determined. In infants, the concentration should not exceed 4.2% (0.5 mEq/mL). *Metabolic acidosis* (after measurement of blood gases and pH): 　Children: mEq HCO$_3$ = 0.3 × weight (kg) × base deficit (mEq/L) *OR* mEq HCO$_3$ = 0.5 × weight (kg) × (24-serum HCO$_3$ [mEq/L]). 　Adults: mEq HCO$_3$ = 0.2 × weight (kg) × base deficit (mEq/L) *OR* mEq HCO$_3$ = 0.5 × weight (kg) × (24-serum HCO$_3$ [mEq/L]). Doses should be administered slowly with frequent monitoring of acid-base balance. *Orally:* *Urine alkalinization* (titrate dose to desired pH): 　Children: 1–10 mEq/kg per day in divided doses. 　Adults: 48 mEq initially followed by 12–24 mEq every 4 hours. Doses up to 192 mEq/day have been used.	Injection: 4.2% (0.5 mEq/mL), 7.5% (0.9 mEq/mL), 8.4% (1 mEq/mL) Tablets: 325 mg, 650 mg
Sodium polystyrene sulfonate (Kayexalate)	*Orally:* 　Children: base the dose on the exchange rate of 1 mEq K$^+$/g of resin in smaller children. 　Alternatively, a dose of 1 g/kg every 6 hours may be used. 　Adults: 15 g administered once daily to q.i.d. *Rectally as a retention enema:* 　Children: 1 g/kg every 2–6 hours. 　Adults: 30–50 g every 6 hours.	Powder Suspension: 15 g/60 mL (with sorbitol)

Continued

Table 1   Medications   (continued)

DRUG	DOSE	DOSAGE FORMS
Sodium polystyrene sulfonate (Kayexalate) (continued)	Enemas should be retained for as long as possible to increase ion exchange. Evacuation of the enema should be followed by a nonsodium-containing cleansing enema. Sorbitol is frequently used for making solutions because it helps to prevent constipation. Administer cautiously to patients who may be at risk of serum sodium level increases. It is not totally selective for potassium; small amounts of calcium and magnesium may also be lost.	
Sodium sulfacetamide (Ak-Sulf, Bleph-10, Cetamide, Sodium Sulamyd)	*Topically to the eye:* Solutions: apply 1–2 drops in the affected eye up to every 2 or 3 hours while awake. Ointment: apply to the eye once daily to q.i.d. Drops will cause burning or stinging sensation. Ointment will cause blurred vision.	Ointment, ophthalmic: 10% Ointment, ophthalmic: 10% with prednisolone 0.2%, 0.25%, or 0.5% Suspension, ophthalmic: 10%, 15%, 30% Suspension, ophthalmic: 15% with phenylephrine 0.125% (Vasosulf) Suspension, ophthalmic: 10% with prednisolone 0.2%, 0.25%, or 0.5%
Spironolactone (Aldactone)	*Orally:* *Edema* (response may not be evident for up to 5 days): Children: 1–3 mg/kg per day in 1 or 2 divided doses. Adults: 100 mg/day with a range of 25–200 mg/day. Primary aldosteronism: Children: 125–375 mg/m^2 per day in divided doses. Adults: 400 mg/day in 1 or 2 divided doses.	Tablets: 25 mg, 50 mg, 100 mg (a stable suspension may be made by crushing tablets and suspending the powder in simple syrup or cherry syrup.)
Stavudine (Zerit)	*Orally:* Age 6 months-15 years: dose has not been established, but doses of 1–2 mg/kg per day have been well tolerated. Adults: <60 kg: 30 mg b.i.d. ≥60 kg: 40 mg b.i.d. Dosage must be adjusted in patients with renal dysfunction.	Capsules: 15 mg, 20 mg, 30 mg, 40 mg
Streptomycin	*IM:* Newborn: 20–30 mg/kg per 24 hr in 2 divided doses for 10 days. Children: 20–40 mg/kg per 24 hr in 2 divided doses for 10 days. Adults: 1–2 g in 1 or 2 doses daily. Maximum dose 2 g/24 hr.	Injection: 400 mg/mL
Sucralfate (Carafate)	Sucralfate is not absorbed from the GI tract. It may bind with other drugs administered at the same time, lowering their effectiveness; therefore, it should be administered at least 2 hours before or after other drugs. *Orally:* Children: dosage has not been established, but 40–80 mg/kg per day in 4 divided doses has been used. Adults: 1 g q.i.d. The dose for stomatitis or mucositis is about 500 mg–1 g of suspension swished around the mouth and then spit out or swallowed, repeated q.i.d.	Suspension: 1 g/10 mL Tablets: 1 g
Sulfasalazine (Azulfidine)	*Orally:* Over age 2: initially 40–60 mg/kg per day in 3–6 divided doses (not to exceed 6 g/day) then decreasing to a maintenance dose of 20–40 mg/kg per day in 4 divided doses to a maximum dose of 2 g/day.	Tablets: 500 mg Tablets, enteric coated: 500 mg

Continued

Table 1   Medications   (continued)

DRUG	*DOSE*	*DOSAGE FORMS*
Sulfasalazine (Azulfidine) (*continued*)	Adults: initially 3–4 g/day in equally divided doses. Although doses as high as 12 g/day have been used, they are generally accompanied by an increased incidence of adverse effects. Maintenance doses are usually 2 g/day in 4 divided doses. The drug may cause a yellow discoloration of urine and skin.	
Sulfisoxazole (Gantrisin)	*Orally:* Over age 2 months: 150 mg/kg per day in 4 or 6 divided doses to a maximum daily dose of 6 g. An initial dose of 75 mg/kg may be given. Adults: 2–4 g initially followed by 4–8 g/day in 4–6 divided doses.	Solution or suspension: 500 mg/5 mL Tablets: 500 mg
Sumatriptan (Imitrex)	*SC:* Children ≥6 years of age and ≤30 kg: 0.06 mg/kg or 3 mg. Children >30 kg and adults: 6 mg. A second dose may be given at least 1 hour after the first dose if necessary. Do not exceed 2 doses in 24 hours.	Injection: 12 mg/ml
Tacrolimus (FK-506, Prograf)	Patients are usually treated concurrently with an adrenal corticosteroid. *Orally:* Children: 0.1–0.5 mg/kg per day in 2 divided doses. Adults: 0.15–0.3 mg/kg per day in 2 divided doses. Doses may be decreased to a lower maintenance dose. *IV* (as a continuous infusion): Children: 0.1 mg/kg per day. Adults: 0.05–0.1 mg/kg per day. Conversion to oral therapy should take place as soon as the patient is able to tolerate oral medication.	Capsules: 1 mg, 5 mg Injection: 5 mg/mL
Terbinafine (Lamisil AF)	*Topically:* ≥12 years of age: apply to affected area and surrounding skin for at least 1 week, but not more than 4 weeks.	Cream: 1%
Terbutaline (Brethine, Bricanyl)	*Orally:* Under age 12: initially 0.05 mg/kg t.i.d., increased gradually as required to a maximum of 0.15 mg/kg t.i.d. or total of 5 mg/24 hr. Over age 12: initially 2.5 mg t.i.d. Maintenance: usually 5 mg or 0.075 mg/kg t.i.d. *Parenteral, SC:* Under age 12: 0.01 mg/kg to a maximum of 0.3 mg every 15–20 minutes for 3 doses. Over age 12: 0.25 mg, repeated in 15–30 minutes if needed once only; a total dose of 0.5 mg should not be exceeded within a 4-hour period. *Inhalation:* 2 puffs every 4–6 hours.	Aerosol, oral: 0.2 mg/activation Injection: 1 mg/mL (1-mL ampul) Tablets: 2.5 mg, 5 mg
Tetracycline (Achromycin V, Panmycin, Robitet, Sumycin)	*Orally* (should be given on an empty stomach): Over age 8: 25–50 mg/kg per day in 4 divided doses. Adults: 1–2 g/day in 2–4 divided doses.	Capsules: 250 mg, 500 mg Suspension: 125 mg/5 mL Tablets: 250 mg, 500 mg
Theophylline	*IV or orally for apnea in infants:* Premature neonates (postconceptional age under 40 weeks): 2 mg/kg per day in 2 divided doses. Term neonates under age 4 weeks: 5 mg/kg loading dose followed by 2–4 mg/kg per day in 2 or 3 divided doses. Term neonates over age 4 weeks: 5–7.5 mg/kg loading dose followed by 3–6 mg/kg per day in 3 divided doses.	*Immediate release:* Capsules: 100 mg, 200 mg Injection in D_5W: 0.4 mg/mL, 0.8 mg/mL, 1.6 mg/mL, 2 mg/mL, 3.2 mg/mL, 4 mg/mL Solution: 27 mg/5 mL, 50 mg/5 mL, 90 mg/5 mL (provided by 105 mg/5 mL of aminophylline) Tablets: 100 mg, 125 mg, 200 mg, 250 mg, 300 mg

Continued

Table 1   Medications   (continued)

DRUG	DOSE	DOSAGE FORMS
Theophylline (*continued*)	*Acute bronchospasm* (all dosing should be based on lean body weight): Loading dose: 1 mg/kg will increase serum theophylline concentration by 2 μg/mL. Patients who have received no theophylline in the previous 24 hours may be given 6 mg/kg. Patients who have received theophylline within the previous 24 hours may receive 3 mg/kg. Serum theophylline level should be monitored 30 minutes after the end of a bolus infusion. Loading dose should be administered IV over 30 minutes or PO using an immediate-release product. For patients requiring a continuous IV infusion of theophylline, it should be started at the completion of the bolus dose at the following rate for children: Age 6 months-1 year: 0.5 mg/kg per hr. Age >1–9: 0.9 mg/kg per hr. Age >9–12 and adolescent smokers: 0.8 mg/kg/hr. Age >12–16 (nonsmokers): 0.7 mg/kg per hr. Theophylline levels should be monitored 12–24 hours after beginning the infusion and daily while therapy continues. *Oral therapy for chronic bronchospasm:* Age 6 months-1 year: 12–18 mg/kg per day. Age >1–9: 20–24 mg/kg per day. Age >9–12 and adolescent smokers: 20 mg/kg per day. Age >12–16 (nonsmokers): 18 mg/kg per day. Over age 16 (nonsmokers): 13 mg/kg per day (not to exceed 900 mg/day).	*Controlled release:* Capsules and tablets of various strengths and release properties: Frequency of dosing must be based on the characteristics of the product chosen. Immediate-release products must be administered every 6 hours. Extended-release products may be administered every 8–12 hours or even every 24 hours in adolescents using products designed for daily administration. Serum levels should be monitored frequently during early therapy to maintain serum levels between 10–20 μg/mL. After a stable dose is achieved, monitoring should be done at least every 6–12 months.

Ticarcillin (Ticar)	*IV (for the treatment of severe infections):*
	Neonates under age 1 week:
	    <2 kg: 75 mg/kg every 12 hours.
	    ≥2 kg: 75 mg/kg every 8 hours.
	Neonates from age 1–4 weeks:
	    <2 kg: 75 mg/kg every 8 hours.
	    ≥2 kg: 100 mg/kg every 8 hours.
	Infants over age 4 weeks and children:
	    200–300 mg/kg per day in 4–6 divided doses.
	Children weighing over 40 kg and adults:
	    200–300 mg/kg per day in 4–6 divided doses to a maximum daily dose of 24 g.
	Dosage must be adjusted in patients with renal or hepatic dysfunction.
		Injection: 1 g, 3 g, 6 g (20-g and 30-g pharmacy bulk packages)

Ticarcillin and clavulanate potassium (Timentin)	*IV (may be expressed in terms of ticarcillin content alone or in terms of the fixed ratio [30:1] of the commercially available combination product):* Children: <60 kg: 200–300 mg/kg per day of ticarcillin (207–310 mg of ticarcillin/clavulanic acid) in 4–6 divided doses. ≥60 kg: 3 g ticarcillin + 0.1 g clavulanic acid (3.1 g of combination) every 4–6 hours to a maximum of 24 g of ticarcillin daily. Dosage must be adjusted in patients with renal or hepatic dysfunction.	Injection: 3 g ticarcillin + 0.1 g clavulanic acid labeled as a combined total potency of 3.1 g (pharmacy bulk package containing 30 g ticarcillin + 1 g clavulanic acid)
Tobramycin (Nebcin, TobraDex, Tobrex)	*IV:* Infants and children: 7.5 mg/kg per day in 3 divided doses. Older children and adults: 5 mg/kg per day in 3 divided doses.	Injection: 10 mg/mL, 40 mg/mL Ointment, ophthalmic: 0.3% Ointment, ophthalmic: 0.3% with dexamethasone 0.1% Solution, ophthalmic: 0.3% Solution, ophthalmic: 0.3% with dexamethasone 0.1%

Continued

Table 1　Medications　(continued)

DRUG	DOSE	DOSAGE FORMS
Tobramycin (Nebcin, TobraDex, Tobrex) (continued)	Patients with cystic fibrosis usually require higher doses (10 mg/kg per day in 3 divided doses). Dosage may be increased based on the results of serum level monitoring. Dosage must be adjusted in patients with renal dysfunction. *Ophthalmic:* 　Ointment: apply a 1-cm ribbon of ointment to the eye b.i.d. or t.i.d. 　Solution: apply 1–2 drops into the eye up to every 30–60 minutes in severe infections or every 3–4 hours for moderate infections.	
Tolmetin (Tolectin)	*Orally for rheumatoid arthritis:* 　Over age 2: initially 20 mg/kg per day in 3 or 4 divided doses, adjusted to the patient's response. Usual maintenance dosage range is 15–30 mg/kg per day. 　Adults: 600 mg-1.8 g/day in 3 divided doses.	Capsules: 400 mg Tablets: 200 mg, 600 mg
Topiramate (Topomax)	*Orally* 　Children 2–16 years of age: initially, 1–3 mg/kg per day (or 25 mg) given daily at bedtime for 1 week. Gradually increase dose by 1–3 mg/kg per day and increase frequency to twice daily to the usual maintenance dosage range of 5–9 mg/kg per day. 　Children >16 years of age and adults: initially, 50 mg daily in two divided doses, then increase at weekly intervals by 50 mg/day to a usual adult dose range of 200–400 mg daily in 2 divided doses.	Capsule, sprinkle: 15 mg, 25 mg Tablet: 25 mg, 100 mg, 200 mg. Tablets should not be crushed since the drug has a very bitter taste. Broken tablets should be used immediately as the drug is not stable.
Trazodone (Desyrel)	*Orally:* 　Children 6–18 years of age: 1.5-2 mg/kg per day in 2 divided doses, increasing gradually to a maximum dose of 6 mg/kg per day in 3 divided doses. 　Adolescents: 25-50 mg/day, increased gradually to a maximum of 150 mg/day in divided doses. 　Adults: 150 mg/day in 3 divided doses increased gradually to a maximum of 600 mg/day.	Tablets: 50 mg, 100 mg, 150 mg, 300 mg
Tretinoin (retinoic acid; Retin-A)	*Topically:* apply to the affected area once daily after cleaning, generally at bedtime. Avoid application to areas not being treated. Use should be discontinued if severe reddening, swelling, or peeling occurs. After healing, therapy may be restarted with the same or a different formulation administered less frequently.	Cream: 0.025%, 0.05%, 0.1% Gel: 0.01%, 0.025% Solution: 0.05%
Trifluridine (Viroptic)	*Topically to the eye:* apply 1 drop every 2 hours while awake until re-epithelialization has occurred. Maximum daily dose of 9 drops should not be exceeded. After re-epithelialization has occurred, dosage should be reduced to 1 drop every 4 hours for an additional 7 days to prevent recurrence, but the total length of therapy should not exceed 21 days.	Solution, ophthalmic: 1%
Trimethobenzamide (Tigan)	*IM* (not for infants or young children): 200 mg t.i.d. or q.i.d. *Rectally* (not for neonates or infants): 　<13.6 kg: 100 mg t.i.d. or q.i.d. 　13.6–45 kg: 100–200 mg t.i.d. or q.i.d. 　>45 kg: 200 mg t.i.d. or q.i.d. *Orally:* 　13.6–45 kg: 100–200 mg t.i.d. or q.i.d. 　>45 kg: 250 mg t.i.d. or q.i.d. Alternatively, a dose of 5 mg/kg administered t.i.d. or q.i.d. rectally or orally may be used.	Capsules: 100 mg, 250 mg Injection: 100 mg/mL Suppositories: 100 mg, 200 mg

Continued

Table 1   Medications   (continued)

DRUG	DOSE	DOSAGE FORMS
Trimethoprim (Primsol, Proloprim, Trimpex)	*Orally:* *UTI:* Infants and children <12 years of age: 4–6 mg/kg/day in 2 divided doses for 10 days. Children ≥12 years of age and adults: 100 mg twice daily or 200 mg once daily for 10 days *Pneumocystis carinii* pneumonia treatment (given with dapsone): 15–20 mg/kg per day in 4 divided doses.	Solution: 50 mg/5 mL Tablet: 100 mg, 200 mg
Tropicamide (Mydriacyl, Ocu-Tropic, Tropicacyl)	*Topically to the eye:* 1 to 2 drops into the eye(s) 15–20 minutes before exam. 0.5% solution is usually sufficient for exam. If cycloplegia for refraction is necessary, 1% solution must be used and repeated in 5 minutes. Exam must take place within 30 minutes because its effect is short.	Solution, ophthalmic: 0.5%, 1%
Valproic acid, valproate sodium, and divalproex sodium (Depacon, Depakene, Depakote)	*Orally* (expressed in terms of valproic acid): initially 15 mg/kg per day increasing by 5–10 mg/kg per day at weekly intervals until seizures are controlled or side effects occur. Usual maximum total daily dose is 60 mg/kg. Frequency of administration in part depends on dosage form, but dosage is usually divided. To prevent adverse GI effects, capsules (valproic acid) and solution are usually administered in 2 or 3 divided doses. Divalproex usually may be administered in 2 divided doses. The usual therapeutic serum concentration range is 50–100 μg/mL. The oral solution has been administered rectally in patients who are NPO by diluting it 1:1 with tap water and administering it as a retention enema. *IV* (over 1 hour): for patients who are not on valproic acid therapy, use the dosing and frequency of administration guidelines outlined above for oral dosing. For patients already on valproic acid therapy, use the patient's total oral daily dose and frequency of dosing for the IV route. The use of the injectable form for periods of more than 14 days has not been studied.	Capsules (divalproex sodium): 125 mg valproic acid Capsules (valproic acid): 250 mg Injection: 100 mg/mL Solution (valproate sodium): 250 mg valproic acid/5 mL Tablets (divalproex sodium): 125 mg, 250 mg, 500 mg valproic acid
Vancomycin (Lyphocin, Vancocin, Vancoled)	*IV* (over at least 1 hour): Neonates under age 7 days: <1,000 g: 10 mg/kg every 24 hours. 1,000–2,000 g: 10 mg/kg every 18 hours. >2,000 g: 10 mg/kg every 12 hours. Neonates age 7–30 days: <1,000 g: 10 mg/kg every 18 hours. 1,000–2,000 g: 10 mg/kg every 12 hours. >2,000 g: 10 mg/kg every 8 hours. Infants age 31–60 days: 10 mg/kg every 8 hours. Infants over age 2 months and children: 40 mg/kg/day in 4 divided doses to a maximum dose of 2 g/day. Adults: 0.5 g every 6 hours or 1 g every 12 hours. Dosage adjustment is necessary in renal impairment. Higher doses, up to 60 mg/kg per day, may be required in children with staphylococcal central nervous system infections. *Intrathecal:* Neonates: 5–10 mg/day. Children: 5–20 mg/day. Adults: 20 mg/day.	Capsules: 125 mg, 250 mg Injection: 500 mg, 1 g, (5-g, 10-g pharmacy bulk packages) Solution, oral: 1 g, 10 g

Continued

Table 1   Medications   (continued)

DRUG	DOSE	DOSAGE FORMS
Vancomycin (Lyphocin, Vancocin, Vancoled) (*continued*)	*Orally* (not absorbed; do not use for systemic infections): Children: 40 mg/kg per day in 4 divided doses to a maximum daily dose of 2 g. Adults: 0.5–2 g/day in 3 or 4 divided doses.	
Verapamil (Calan, Isoptin, Verelan)	*IV* (push over 2 to 3 minutes): Under age 1: 0.1–0.2 mg/kg (usually 0.75–2 mg). Age 1–16: 0.1–0.3 mg/kg to a maximum of 10 mg. May be repeated once in 30 minutes if not effective. Over age 16: 0.075–0.15 mg/kg (5–10 mg) with a repeat dose in 30 minutes if necessary. *Orally* (not well established in children): Age 1–5: 4–8 mg/kg per day in 3 divided doses or about 40–80 mg every 8 hours. Over age 5: 80 mg every 6–8 hours. Adults: 240–480 mg/day in 3 or 4 divided doses (1–2 doses daily using extended-release products for the treatment of hypertension).	Capsules, extended release: 120 mg, 180 mg, 240 mg Injection: 2.5 mg/mL Tablets: 40 mg, 80 mg, 120 mg Tablets, extended release: 120 mg, 180 mg, 240 mg
Vitamin A (Aquasol A)	*Orally:* *For malabsorption syndromes* (water miscible product): Under age 8: 5,000–15,000 U/day. Over age 8 and adults: 10,000–50,000 U/day. *For severe deficiency with xerophthalmia:* Age 1–8: 5,000 U/kg per day for 5 days or until recovery. Over age 8 and adults: 500,000 U/day for 3 days, then 50,000 U/day for 14 days, then 10,000–20,000 U/day for 2 months. *Deficiency* (without corneal change): Under age 1: 10,000 U/kg per day for 5 days, then 7,500–15,000 U/day for 10 days. Age 1–8: 5,000–10,000 U/kg per day for 5 days, then 17,000–35,000 U/day for 10 days. Over age 8 and adults: 100,000 U/day for 3 days, then 50,000 U/day for 14 days. *Dietary supplementation:* Infants up to age 6 months: 1,500 U/day. Age >6 months–3 years: 1,500–2,000 U/day. Age 4–6: 2,500 U/day. Age 7–10: 3,300–3,500 U/day. Over age 10 and adults: 4,000–5,000 U/day.	Capsules: 10,000 U, 25,000 U, 50,000 U
Vitamin E (alpha tocopherol, alpha tocopheryl acetate, tocopherol polyethylene glycol succinate [TPGS], Aquasol E)	*Orally* (water miscible or water soluble TPGS products are recommended, especially for patients with malabsorption): *Deficiency:* Infants: 25–50 U/day. *Children with malabsorption:* 15–25 U/kg per day to raise and maintain plasma tocopherol levels. Patients with cystic fibrosis, thalassemia, or sickle-cell disease may require larger daily doses (400–800 U/day). Adults: 60–75 U/day.	Capsules: 100 U, 200 U, 400 U, 600 U, 1,000 U Capsules, water miscible: 100 U, 200 U, 400 U Solution, water miscible: 50 U/mL Solution (TPGS): 400 U/15 mL
Warfarin sodium (Coumadin)	*Orally:* Infants and children: 0.1 mg/kg per day with a range of 0.05–0.34 mg/kg per day adjusted to achieve the desired PT. Adults: 5–15 mg/day initially for 2–5 days until desired PT is reached. Usual maintenance dosage range is 2–10 mg/day.	Tablets: 1 mg, 2 mg, 2.5 mg, 4 mg, 5 mg, 7.5 mg, 10 mg

Continued

Table 1   Medications   (continued)

DRUG	*DOSE*	*DOSAGE FORMS*
Zafirlukast (Accolate)	*Orally on an empty stomach:* Children 7–12 years of age: 10 mg twice daily. Children >12 years of age and adults: 20 mg twice daily.	Tablet: 10 mg, 20 mg
Zalcitabine (ddC, Hivid)	*Orally:* Under age 13: 0.01 mg/kg per dose given every 8 hours. Adolescents age 13-adults: 0.75 mg every 8 hours on an empty stomach. Adjust dose in patients with renal dysfunction.	Tablets: 0.375 mg, 0.75 mg
Zanamivir (Relenza)	*Oral inhalation:* Children ≥12 years of age and adults: 2 inhalations twice a day for 5 days beginning within 2 days of the onset of symptoms.	Powder for inhalation with device: 5 mg/actuation
Zidovudine (Retrovir)	*Orally:* Age 3 months-12 years: 180 mg/m^2 every 6 hours to a maximum of 200 mg every 6 hours. Dosage may be decreased in patients who develop anemia and/or granulocytopenia. Adults: *Asymptomatic:* 100 mg every 4 hours while awake (500 mg/day). *Symptomatic:* 100 mg every 4 hours (600 mg/day). *IV:* Age 3 months-13 years: 0.5–1.8 mg/kg/hr as a continuous infusion or 100 mg/m^2 by infusion over 1 hour every 6 hours. Adults: 1–2 mg/kg every 4 hours 6 times daily. *Maternal-fetal HIV transmission prevention:* Maternal (>14 weeks of pregnancy): 100 mg every 4 hours while awake (500 mg/day) until the onset of labor. During labor and delivery, 2 mg/kg over 1 hour followed by a continuous IV infusion of 1 mg/kg per hour until the umbilical cord is clamped. Infant: 2 mg/kg orally every 6 hours starting within 12 hours of birth and continuing for 6 weeks. For infants unable to tolerate oral drugs, 6 mg/kg per day IV in 4 evenly divided doses may be used. Dosage adjustment is necessary in severe renal impairment.	Capsules: 100 mg Injection: 10 mg/mL Solution: 50 mg/5 mL
Zinc	Response may not occur for 6–8 weeks. *Orally:* Infants and children: 0.5–1 mg/kg per day of elemental zinc in 1–3 divided doses. Adults: 25–50 mg elemental zinc t.i.d. *Acrodermatitis enteropathica:* 10–45 mg/day elemental zinc. Zinc sulfate 4.4 mg = 1 mg elemental zinc (220 mg = 50 mg).	Zinc sulfate (23% zinc): Capsules: 220 mg (50 mg zinc) Injection: 1 mg/mL, 5 mg/mL (zinc) Tablets: 66 mg (15 mg zinc), 110 mg (25 mg zinc), 220 mg (45 mg zinc) Zinc gluconate (14.3% zinc): Tablets: 10 mg (1.4 mg zinc), 15 mg (2 mg zinc), 50 mg (7 mg zinc), 78 mg (11 mg zinc)

*See Table 83.2 for a discussion of the content of each milliliter of these products.

†See Table 83.3 for dosage recommendations.

‡See Table 83.4 for the lipase, amylase, and protease content of each form of pancrelipase.

Table 2 Citric Acid and Citrate Dosage Forms (Content per 1 mL)

PRODUCT	SODIUM CITRATE	POTASSIUM CITRATE	CITRIC ACID	BICARBONATE EQUIVALENT
Bicitra solution	100 mg (1 mEq Na)	...	66.8 mg	1 mEq
Oracit solution	98 mg (1 mEq Na)	...	128 mg	1 mEq
Polycitra K solution	...	220 mg (2 mEq K)	66.8 mg	2 mEq
Polycitra-LC solution	100 mg (1 mEq Na)	110 mg (1 mEq K)	66.8 mg	2 mEq

Table 3 Digoxin Dosing

| | TOTAL DIGITALIZING DOSE (μG/KG) | | DAILY MAINTENANCE DOSE (μG/KG DIVIDED IN 2 DOSES) | |
AGE	PO	IV	PO	IV
Preterm infant	20–30	15–25	5–7.5	4–6
Full-term infant	25–40	20–30	6–10	5–8
1 month to 2 years	35–60	30–50	10–15	7.5–12
2 years to adult	30–40	25–35	7.5–15	6–9
Maximum dose	0.75–1.5 mg	0.5–1 mg	0.125–0.5 mg	0.1–0.4 mg

PO, orally; IV, intravenously.

Table 4 Pancrelipase Dosage Forms

	LIPASE (USP UNITS)	AMYLASE (USP UNITS)	PROTEASE (USP UNITS)
Capsules (enteric-coated or delayed-release microspheres)			
Creon-5, Lipram-CR5	5,000	16,000	18,750
Creon-10, Lipram-CR10	10,000	33,200	37,500
Creon-20, Lipram-CR20	20,000	66,400	75,000
Lipram 4500, Pancrease, Ultrase	4500	20,000	25,000
Lipram-PN10, Pancrease MT-10	10,000	30,000	30,000
Lipram-PN 16, Pancrease MT-16	16,000	48,000	48,000
Lipram-PN 20, Pancrease MT-20	20,000	56,000	44,000
Lipram-UL 12, Ultrase MT 12	12,000	39,000	39,000
Lipram-UL 18, Ultrase MT 18	18,000	58,500	58,500
Lipram-UL 20, Ultrase MT 20	20,000	65,000	65,000
Pancrease MT-4	4,500	12,000	12,000
Pancrecarb MS-4	4000	25,000	25,000
Pancrecarb MS-8	8000	40,000	45,000
Powder (not enteric-coated)			
Viokase (per 0.7 g)	16,800	70,000	70,000
Tablets/capsules (not enteric-coated)			
Ku-Zyme HP, Panokase, Plaretase 8000, Viokase 8	8,000	30,000	30,000
Viokase-16	16,000	60,000	60,000

Index

Page numbers in boldface indicate major discussion; page numbers in italics denote figures; those followed by "t" denote tables.

Index

Index

Index

Index

Index

Index

Index

Index

Index

Index

Index

Index

Index

Index

Index

Index

Index

Index